# HANDBOOK OF ATTACHMENT

# Also Available

Attachment in Adulthood:
Structure, Dynamics, and Change, Second Edition
*Mario Mikulincer and Phillip R. Shaver*

# HANDBOOK OF
# ATTACHMENT

*Theory, Research,
and Clinical Applications*

THIRD EDITION

Edited by
JUDE CASSIDY
PHILLIP R. SHAVER

THE GUILFORD PRESS
New York London

**Library of Congress Cataloging-in-Publication Data**

Handbook of attachment : theory, research, and clinical applications / edited by Jude Cassidy,
Phillip R. Shaver. — Third edition.
    pages cm
 Includes bibliographical references and index.
 ISBN 978-1-4625-2529-4 (hardcover)
 1. Attachment behavior.  2. Attachment behavior in children.  I. Cassidy, Jude.  II. Shaver, Phillip R.
 BF575.A86H36 2016
 155.9′2—dc23

                                                                2015030511

*With respect and gratitude for*
*the pioneering work of*
*John Bowlby and Mary Ainsworth*

# About the Editors

**Jude Cassidy, PhD,** is Distinguished Scholar-Teacher and Professor of Psychology at the University of Maryland, College Park, and Director of the Maryland Child and Family Development Laboratory. Her research interests include socioemotional development from infancy through adolescence, with an emphasis on attachment and family relationships; social, cognitive, and regulatory mechanisms through which children's early family experiences come to influence later well-being and relationships; and early intervention designed to reduce the risk of insecure attachment and mental disorders. Her research has been funded by the National Institute of Mental Health, the National Institute of Child Health and Human Development, the National Institute on Drug Abuse, the Substance Abuse and Mental Health Services Administration, and the Zanvyl and Isabelle Krieger Fund. Dr. Cassidy serves as coeditor of the journal *Attachment and Human Development* and is on the editorial boards of *Journal of Clinical Child and Adolescent Psychology* and *Infant Mental Health Journal*. She is a Fellow of the Association for Psychological Science (APS) and the American Psychological Association (APA), and is a recipient of the Boyd R. McCandless Young Scientist Award from APA Division 7 (Developmental Psychology).

**Phillip R. Shaver, PhD,** is Distinguished Professor Emeritus of Psychology at the University of California, Davis. He has published several books and over 250 journal articles and book chapters. Dr. Shaver's research focuses on attachment, human motivation and emotion, close relationships, personality development, and the effects of meditation on behavior and the brain. He is a Fellow of both the APA and the APS, and has served as executive officer of the Society of Experimental Social Psychology (SESP) and as president of the International Association for Relationship Research (IARR). Dr. Shaver is a recipient of Distinguished Career Awards from the SESP, the IARR, and the Society for Personality and Social Psychology, and an honorary doctorate from the Faculty of Social Sciences at the University of Stockholm, Sweden.

# Contributors

**Joseph P. Allen, PhD,** Department of Psychology, University of Virginia, Charlottesville, Virginia

**Elizabeth Allison, DPhil,** Research Department of Clinical, Educational and Health Psychology, University College London, London, United Kingdom

**Camilla Azis-Clauson, BSc,** Social, Genetic and Developmental Psychiatry Centre, Institute of Psychiatry, Psychology, and Neuroscience, King's College London, London, United Kingdom

**Marian J. Bakermans-Kranenburg, PhD,** Centre for Child and Family Studies, Leiden University, Leiden, The Netherlands

**Jay Belsky, PhD,** Department of Human Ecology, University of California, Davis, Davis, California

**Lisa J. Berlin, PhD,** School of Social Work, University of Maryland, Baltimore, Baltimore, Maryland

**Gurit E. Birnbaum, PhD,** Baruch Ivcher School of Psychology, Interdisciplinary Center Herzliya, Herzliya, Israel

**Kelly K. Bost, PhD,** Department of Human and Community Development Family Resiliency Center, University of Illinois at Urbana–Champaign, Urbana, Illinois

**Audrey Brassard, PhD,** Department of Psychology, Université de Sherbrooke, Sherbrooke, Quebec, Canada

**Inge Bretherton, PhD,** Department of Human Development and Family Studies, University of Wisconsin–Madison, Madison, Wisconsin

**Preston A. Britner, PhD,** Department of Human Development and Family Studies, University of Connecticut, Storrs, Connecticut

**Laura E. Brumariu, PhD,** Derner Institute of Psychology, Adelphi University, Garden City, New York

**Chloe Campbell, PhD,** Research Department of Clinical, Educational and Health Psychology, University College London, London, United Kingdom

**Lauren M. Carter, BA,** Curry School of Education, University of Virginia, Charlottesville, Virginia

**Jude Cassidy, PhD,** Department of Psychology, University of Maryland, College Park, College Park, Maryland

**James A. Coan, PhD,** Department of Psychology, University of Virginia, Charlottesville, Virginia

**Judith A. Crowell, MD,** Division of Child and Adolescent Psychiatry, Department of Psychiatry and Behavioral Sciences, Stony Brook University Medical Center, Stony Brook, New York

**Michelle DeKlyen, PhD,** Center for Research on Child Well-Being, Princeton University, Princeton, New Jersey

**Mary Dozier, PhD,** Department of Psychology, University of Delaware, Newark, Delaware

**Katherine B. Ehrlich, PhD,** Institute for Policy Research and Department of Psychology, Northwestern University, Evanston, Illinois

**R. M. Pasco Fearon, PhD,** Research Department of Clinical, Educational and Health Psychology, University College London, London, United Kingdom

**Brooke C. Feeney, PhD,** Department of Psychology, Carnegie Mellon University, Pittsburgh, Pennsylvania

**Judith A. Feeney, PhD,** School of Psychology, University of Queensland, Queensland, Australia

**Peter Fonagy, PhD,** Research Department of Clinical, Educational and Health Psychology, University College London, and The Anna Freud Centre, London, United Kingdom

**Nathan A. Fox, PhD,** Child Development Lab, Department of Human Development, University of Maryland, College Park, College Park, Maryland

**R. Chris Fraley, PhD,** Department of Psychology, University of Illinois at Urbana–Champaign, Champaign, Illinois

**María Teresa Frías, PhD,** Department of Psychology, University of California, Davis, Davis, California

**Carol George, PhD,** Department of Psychology, Mills College, Oakland, California

**Pehr Granqvist, PhD,** Department of Psychology, Stockholm University, Stockholm, Sweden

**Mark T. Greenberg, PhD,** Prevention Research Center, Pennsylvania State University, University Park, Pennsylvania

**Jacquelyn T. Gross, MS,** Department of Psychology, University of Maryland, College Park, College Park, Maryland

**Amie A. Hane, PhD,** Department of Psychology, Williams College, Williamstown, Massachusetts

**Cindy Hazan, PhD,** Department of Human Development, Cornell University, Ithaca, New York

**Erik Hesse, PhD,** Department of Psychology, University of California, Berkeley, Berkeley, California

**Myron A. Hofer, MD,** Department of Psychiatry and Sackler Institute for Developmental Psychobiology, Columbia University, New York, New York

**Carollee Howes, PhD,** Psychological Studies in Education Program, Graduate School of Education and Information Studies, University of California, Los Angeles, Los Angeles, California

**Skyler D. Jackson, BA,** Department of Psychology, University of Maryland, College Park, College Park, Maryland

**Deborah Jacobvitz, PhD,** Department of Human Ecology, College of Natural Sciences, University of Texas at Austin, Austin, Texas

**Susan M. Johnson, PhD,** Department of Psychology, University of Ottawa, and Ottawa Couple and Family Institute, Ottawa, Ontario, Canada

**Jason D. Jones, PhD,** Department of Psychology, University of Maryland, College Park, College Park, Maryland

**Kathryn A. Kerns, PhD,** Department of Psychology, Kent State University, Kent, Ohio

**Lee A. Kirkpatrick, PhD,** Department of Psychology, College of William and Mary, Williamsburg, Virginia

**Roger Kobak, PhD,** Department of Psychology, University of Delaware, Newark, Delaware

**Alicia F. Lieberman, PhD,** Child Trauma Research Program, University of California, San Francisco, and San Francisco General Hospital, San Francisco, California

**Patrick Luyten, PhD,** Faculty of Psychology and Educational Sciences, University of Leuven, Leuven, Belgium; Research Department of Clinical, Educational and Health Psychology, University College London, London, United Kingdom

**Karlen Lyons-Ruth, PhD,** Department of Psychiatry, Cambridge Hospital, Harvard Medical School, Cambridge, Massachusetts

**Stephanie D. Madsen, PhD,** Department of Psychology, McDaniel College, Westminster, Maryland

**Carol Magai, PhD,** Department of Psychology, Long Island University, Brooklyn, New York

**Robert S. Marvin, PhD,** Department of Psychiatric Medicine, Child and Family Psychiatry, University of Virginia, Charlottesville, Virginia

**Judi Mesman, PhD,** Centre for Child and Family Studies, Leiden University, Leiden, The Netherlands

**Mario Mikulincer, PhD,** Baruch Ivcher School of Psychology, Interdisciplinary Center Herzliya, Herzliya, Israel

**Gregory E. Miller, PhD,** Institute for Policy Research and Department of Psychology, Northwestern University, Evanston, Illinois

**Jonathan J. Mohr, PhD,** Department of Psychology, University of Maryland, College Park, College Park, Maryland

**Joan K. Monin, PhD,** Department of Chronic Disease Epidemiology, Social and Behavioral Science Division, Yale School of Public Health, New Haven, Connecticut

**Kristine A. Munholland, MSW, PhD,** Department of Human Development, Washington State University Vancouver, Vancouver, Washington

**Robert C. Pianta, PhD,** Curry School of Education, University of Virginia, Charlottesville, Virginia

**H. Jonathan Polan, MD,** Department of Psychiatry, Weill Cornell Medical College and New York Presbyterian Hospital, New York, New York

**Glenn I. Roisman, PhD,** Institute of Child Development, University of Minnesota, Minneapolis, Minnesota

**Beth S. Russell, PhD,** Department of Human Development and Family Studies, University of Connecticut, Storrs, Connecticut

**Michael Rutter, MD,** Social, Genetic and Developmental Psychiatry Centre, Institute of Psychiatry, Psychology and Neuroscience, King's College London, London, United Kingdom

**Abraham Sagi-Schwartz, PhD,** Center for the Study of Child Development, University of Haifa, Haifa, Israel

**Phillip R. Shaver, PhD,** Department of Psychology, University of California, Davis, Davis, California

**Jeffry A. Simpson, PhD,** Department of Psychology, University of Minnesota, Minneapolis, Minnesota

**Arietta Slade, PhD,** Yale Child Study Center, Yale University, New Haven, Connecticut

**Judith Solomon, PhD,** Child FIRST Program, Department of Pediatrics, Bridgeport Hospital, Bridgeport, Connecticut

**Susan Spieker, PhD,** Department of Family and Child Nursing, Center on Human Development and Disability, University of Washington, Seattle, Washington

**L. Alan Sroufe, PhD,** Institute of Child Development, University of Minnesota, Minneapolis, Minnesota

**Jessica A. Stern, BA,** Department of Psychology, University of Maryland, College Park, College Park, Maryland

**K. Chase Stovall-McClough, PhD,** Child Study Center, Institute for Trauma and Stress, New York University School of Medicine, New York, New York

**Stephen J. Suomi, PhD,** Laboratory of Comparative Ethology, Eunice Kennedy Shriver National Institute of Child Health and Human Development, National Institutes of Health, Bethesda, Maryland

**Joseph S. Tan, MA,** Department of Psychology, University of Virginia, Charlottesville, Virginia

**Ross A. Thompson, PhD,** Department of Psychology, University of California, Davis, Davis, California

**Marinus H. van IJzendoorn, PhD,** Center for Child and Family Studies, Leiden University, Leiden, The Netherlands

**Brian E. Vaughn, PhD,** Department of Family and Child Development, Auburn University, Auburn, Alabama

**Amanda P. Williford, PhD,** Center for Advanced Study of Teaching and Learning, Curry School of Education, University of Virginia, Charlottesville, Virginia

**Susan S. Woodhouse, PhD,** Department of Education and Human Services, Lehigh University, Bethlehem, Pennsylvania

**Kristyn Zajac, PhD,** Department of Psychiatry and Behavioral Sciences, Medical University of South Carolina, Charleston, South Carolina

**Charles H. Zeanah, MD,** Department of Psychiatry and Behavioral Sciences, Tulane University, New Orleans, Louisiana

**Debra M. Zeifman, PhD,** Department of Psychology, Vassar College, Poughkeepsie, New York

# Preface

It seems unlikely that either John Bowlby, when he first wondered about the relation between maternal deprivation and juvenile delinquency, or Mary Ainsworth, when she answered an advertisement in a London newspaper to work as a postdoctoral researcher with Bowlby, dreamed for a moment that their theoretical efforts would spawn one of the broadest, most profound, and most creative lines of research in 20th- and 21st-century psychology. Yet that is exactly what happened. Anyone who conducts a literature search on the topic of "attachment" will turn up more than 30,000 entries that have appeared since the beginning of 1975 (three times the number we discovered when preparing the 2008 second edition of this volume). And the entries are spread across scores of physiological, clinical, developmental, and social psychology journals; medical and social work journals; and authored books and edited anthologies. The literature spans everything from the prenatal period to old age and considers all kinds of relationships: parent–child, sibling, friendship, teen romance, and adult sexual.

In the study of social and emotional development, attachment theory is the most visible and empirically grounded conceptual framework guiding today's research. In the growing clinical literature on the effects of early parent–child relationships, including troubled and abusive relationships, attachment theory is prominent. In the rapidly expanding field of research on close relationships in adolescence and adulthood—including the study of romantic, marital, or "pair-bond" relationships, and their formation, maintenance, and dissolution—attachment theory is one of the most influential theoretical approaches, as it also is in the field of couples counseling. Among researchers who study bereavement, Bowlby's volume on loss is a continuing source of insight and intellectual inspiration.

Attachment theory is one of the best examples of the value of deep, coherent theorizing in contemporary psychology. It is a model of the process by which scientists move back and forth between clear conceptualizations and penetrating empirical research, with each pole of the dialectic influencing the other over an extended period of time. Attachment theory today is in many respects similar to attachment theory 40 years ago, but it has become much more specific, more multifaceted, and more deeply anchored in a wide variety of powerful research methods, including new ones such as behavioral genetics and functional magnetic resonance imaging. Because the theory was remarkably insightful and accurate from the beginning, and because Ainsworth was such an effective researcher, the initial studies inspired by the theory were largely supportive of the theory's basic ideas, but they were also surprising and provocative in certain respects. The theory encountered considerable criticism at first, as any new scientific theory should. Yet the many honors accorded to Bowlby and Ainsworth toward the ends of their careers symbolize the considerable respect their work now engenders. The present volume is further testimony to the lasting nature of their impressive contributions to psychological science.

One problem created by the enormous literature on attachment, and by attachment theory's continual evolution in the light of new research, is that few scholars, researchers, and clinicians are familiar with the entire body of work. In order to make optimal use of the theory as a researcher, clinician, or teacher, one has to know what Bowlby and Ainsworth originally said; what subsequent research has revealed; what measures of attachment have been developed and what they measure; and what recent theoretical and empirical developments contribute to our overall understanding of attachment relationships and personality development. The purpose of this third edition of the *Handbook of Attachment* is to satisfy these important professional needs. The book will prove useful to anyone who studies attachment processes, uses attachment theory in clinical work, or teaches courses and seminars that touch on, or focus on, attachment. It will be an excellent single resource for courses devoted to attachment theory and research. It will also be of great interest to anyone in the general public who wishes to think more effectively about close relationships of all kinds.

The first edition of the *Handbook*, published in 1999, was extensively read, frequently cited, and influential in affecting research and clinical applications of attachment theory and research. We were deeply gratified by the field's response to the volume, which inspired everything from graduate seminars and clinical discussion groups to theoretical debates, major new research programs, and systematic tests of clinical interventions. It helped spawn a much more diverse and deeply probing research field. The second edition of the *Handbook*, published in 2008, had the same effect, and its influence grew as attachment research and its clinical applications became better known internationally. The theory's influence is now evident all over the world, and its literature includes publications in many different languages. Because psychology and psychiatry have moved energetically in the directions of neuroscience, psychophysiology, and behavioral genetics, there are many new findings to incorporate into an expanded attachment theory. And because federal granting agencies have become increasingly interested in "translational" research—research that moves basic research findings more quickly into the realm of clinical and community applications—there is a great deal of new information about intervention procedures and outcomes.

As volume editors, we have dealt with the many new developments in two ways. First, we have added new chapters to reflect the changing nature of the field. In 2008, new additions to the second edition included chapters on social neuroscience, affect regulation, attachment in the middle childhood years, foster care, divorce, and attachment in an aging population. In this third edition, we have retained and updated those chapters while commissioning additional new ones on attachment, genetics, and epigenetics; attachment and psychoneuroimmunology; attachment and sexual mating; attachment and empathy, altruism, and prosocial behavior; and attachment and school readiness. The volume ends with a brilliant overview and evaluation of the field, "The Place of Attachment in Development," by a distinguished attachment-research pioneer, L. Alan Sroufe.

Second, we charged the authors of previously included chapters, as well as new authors who have taken over territories covered by previous chapters, with a specific task. We asked authors to specifically describe the current state of theory and research *in comparison to that outlined in the earlier chapter.* We asked: Have new conceptualizations emerged? Have former conceptualizations dropped by the wayside? Why? Have connections with other areas of research provided new insights? What empirical progress has been attempted and made? If little progress has been made, why? In short, in the earlier editions, we portrayed "the state of the field." Now that we are on our third edition, an important goal is to present, in addition to the current state of the field, an overview of how the field has changed, stagnated, shifted, provided insights, opened up new questions, borrowed, fallen short, or failed—along with providing some guidance concerning how best to help the field move even further forward.

Part I, "Overview of Attachment Theory," provides an updated primer on the theory. The first two chapters correspond roughly to the first and second volumes of Bowlby's seminal trilogy, *Attachment and Loss.* In Chapter 1, "The Nature of the Child's Ties," Jude Cassidy explains the central construct of attachment theory, first expounded by Bowlby in the first volume of *Attachment and Loss.* In Chapter 2, "Attachment Disruptions, Reparative Processes, and Psychopathology," Roger Kobak, Kristyn Zajac, and Stephanie D. Madsen explain topics that Bowlby addressed in *Separation: Anxiety and Anger,* the second volume of his trilogy. In Chapter 3, "Attachment, Loss, and Grief: Bowlby's Views, New Developments, and Current Controversies," R. Chris Fraley and Phillip R. Shaver discuss theory and research related to topics addressed by Bowlby in the third volume of *Attachment and Loss.* Chapter 4, by Inge Bretherton and Kristine A. Munholland, deals with a core construct in attachment theory: internal working models. In this new version of their chapter, "The Internal Working Model Construct in Light of Contemporary Neuroimaging Research," the authors focus on contributions from cognitive and affective neuroscience, scientific fields that have grown enormously in prominence during the past decade.

Part II, "Biological Perspectives," begins with Chapter 5, by Jeffry A. Simpson and Jay Belsky, "Attachment Theory within a Modern Evolutionary Framework." Bowlby valued evolutionary theory and the associated ethological approach to animal research, from which he borrowed extensively—to the chagrin of some of his British psychoanalytic colleagues. This is one of several ways in which he was ahead of his time (the emphasis on cognitive "internal working models" being another). Chapter 6, by H. Jonathan Polan and Myron A. Hofer, is titled "Psychobiological Origins of Infant Attachment and Its Role in Development." The pioneering rodent research that Hofer and his colleagues conducted over a period of decades shows that regulation of basic bodily processes in infants is multidimensional, meaning that the "attachment system" initially conceptualized by Bowlby as a single, unified system can be characterized in much greater detail.

Adding to these insights from animal research is Chapter 7, by Stephen J. Suomi, "Attachment in Rhesus Monkeys." Bowlby and Ainsworth's theorizing about human attachment processes was strongly influenced by primate researchers, and their perspective continues to bear fruit. In recent years, Suomi and other researchers have included in their work research on epigenetic changes related to care received from parents, offering new ways to understand the long-range effects of early social experiences on later physical and psychological health (addressed throughout this volume).

Chapters 8 and 9 are new to the *Handbook.* Chapter 8, "Attachment, Parenting, and Genetics," by Marian J. Bakersman-Kranenburg and Marinus H. van IJzendoorn, delves further into the ideas raised by Suomi, with special emphasis on human genetics, epigenetics, and effects of early experiences with caregivers. In Chapter 9, "Attachment and Psychoneuroimmunology," Katherine B. Ehrlich, Gregory E. Miller, Jason D. Jones, and Jude Cassidy explore connections between the quality of care one receives in at-

tachment relationships and subsequent immune functioning.

In Chapter 10, "Attachment and Temperament as Intersecting Developmental Products and Interacting Developmental Contexts Throughout Infancy and Childhood," Brian E. Vaughn and Kelly K. Bost discuss the complex relations between attachment, viewed primarily as affected by social experiences, and temperament, viewed primarily as a product of genes and psychobiology. In Chapter 11, "Studying the Biology of Human Attachment," Amie A. Hane and Nathan A. Fox describe both well-established and recently developed methods for studying attachment-related psychobiological processes. One of the recent methods, functional magnetic resonance imaging, is then described in much more detail in Chapter 12, by James A. Coan, "Toward a Neuroscience of Attachment." Coan explains social baseline theory, a companion for attachment theory that focuses on the human brain's tendency to treat social connectedness, rather than independence, as a default state.

Part III of the volume, "Attachment in Infancy and Childhood," addresses the age periods that were the original focus of Bowlby's theorizing and Ainsworth's seminal research methods and findings. In Chapter 13, "Normative Development: The Ontogeny of Attachment in Childhood," Robert S. Marvin, Preston A. Britner, and Beth S. Russell explain the species-typical development of human attachments over the first few years of life. As attachment theory has become popular worldwide and inspired scores of new measures and research streams, an increasingly small proportion of researchers know the details of the developmental processes at the heart of the theory. Marvin and colleagues provide an excellent starting point for anyone wishing to understand the early development of attachment. Chapter 14, "Precursors of Attachment Security," by R. M. Pasco Fearon and Jay Belsky, reviews the extensive body of research on the early determinants of security and insecurity. In Chapter 15, "Attachment Relationships in the Context of Multiple Caregivers," Carollee Howes and Susan Spieker explain what is known about the attachment-related effects of having multiple caregivers, an issue that became increasingly controversial as more women in developed societies entered the workforce. Howes and Spieker show that there is no simple answer to the question of whether early day care is "good" or "bad" for children. The answer depends on the quality of care and its temporal extent.

Among Bowlby's main concerns were the

long-term effects of early attachment-related experiences on later personality development and long-term life outcomes. In Chapter 16, "Early Attachment and Later Development: Reframing the Questions," Ross A. Thompson explains what is known about early attachment and subsequent development. The "reframing" referred to in the chapter subtitle includes different ways of characterizing internal working models, taking continuity of sensitive or insensitive care into account, considering biological/health effects of attachment, and exploring the connections among attachment, emotions, emotion understanding, and emotion regulation.

Because Bowlby and Ainsworth focused mainly on attachment in infancy, it took some time for researchers to redirect attention to the nature and fate of attachment processes in middle childhood. That is the subject of Chapter 17, "Attachment in Middle Childhood," by Kathryn A. Kerns and Laura E. Brumariu. They show that although relations with peers become increasingly important, parents remain the principal attachment figures, even though children become more active participants in the parent–child relationship. The authors also discuss the continuing lack of resolution concerning how to measure attachment during middle childhood. The last chapter in Part III, Chapter 18, "The Measurement of Attachment Security and Related Constructs in Infancy and Early Childhood," by Judith Solomon and Carol George, deals with the extremely important issue of measurement. When Bowlby was beginning his theoretical journey as a young psychoanalyst, he was part of a psychoanalytic milieu in which several key theorists, such as Anna Freud and Donald Winnicott, were concerned with social aspects of mental development in infancy. Although they, like Bowlby, had interesting ideas based on clinical observations of children, they did not have anyone to operationalize and test those ideas empirically. By collaborating with Ainsworth, a creative and well-trained researcher, Bowlby benefited from the huge volume of scientific information being built upon Ainsworth's early work. In 1982, he revised the 1969 first volume of his attachment trilogy in light of new data. Today, attachment theory is much more firmly anchored in psychological science than the observations and insights of Bowlby's psychoanalytic peers, thanks largely to the measures described in this chapter.

Part IV, "Attachment in Adolescence and Adulthood," deals with age periods in which there has been a huge explosion of research in recent years. This growth is indicated by the large number of chapters in this part, including a new one on attachment and sexuality. Chapter 19, "The Multiple Facets of Attachment in Adolescence," by Joseph P. Allen and Joseph Tan, covers the rise of research on adolescent attachment to parents and peers. As adolescents strive to attain greater autonomy from parents while continuing to rely on parents as a safe haven and secure base, many interesting issues come to the surface, and these have been the focus of fascinating new research. Adolescents have increasingly complex and important relationships with peers, including in many cases romantic/sexual relationships. The notion that romantic or marital relationships involve attachment was somewhat controversial when it first began to attract attention in the late 1980s. In Chapter 20, Debra M. Zeifman and Cindy Hazan consider "Pair Bonds as Attachments: Mounting Evidence in Support of Bowlby's Hypothesis," concluding that romantic relationships definitely qualify as attachment relationships. Their chapter leads smoothly into Chapter 21, "Adult Romantic Attachment: Developments in the Study of Couple Relationships," by Judith A. Feeney. She explains how the concepts of attachment and attachment relationships have inspired a monumental growth of attachment research in social and personality psychology over the past 30 years. Chapter 22, "Attachment and Sexual Mating: The Joint Operation of Separate Motivational Systems," by Gurit E. Birnbaum, summarizes this growing topic area. Because psychological scientists, like society more generally, have become aware of and interested in same-sex relationships, the study of attachment has been extended into that domain. In Chapter 23, "Same-Sex Romantic Attachment," Jonathan J. Mohr and Skyler D. Jackson summarize and comment on this research area.

Social/personality researchers who study adult attachment have been concerned with one of the key issues in attachment theory more generally: emotion regulation. Delving into this topic area allows attachment researchers to use a wide variety of methods developed by scholars who study social cognition and emotions, as well as the methods of cognitive and affective neuroscience. Mario Mikulincer and Phillip R. Shaver review the extensive recent research in Chapter 24, "Adult Attachment and Affect Regulation." Just as attachment research was gradually extended from infancy to middle childhood, adolescence, and early adulthood, it is now being pursued in studies discussed in Chapter 25, "Attachment in

Middle and Later Life," by Carol Magai, María Teresa Frías, and Phillip R. Shaver. This topic area is likely to become much more active as large proportions of the adult populations of industrialized countries move into old age.

As already mentioned, the early science of infant–parent attachment depended heavily on Ainsworth's creation of new measuring instruments. As research was extended into adolescence and adulthood, new measures were needed and created. One of the most influential approaches is discussed in Chapter 26, "The Adult Attachment Interview: Protocol, Method of Analysis, and Empirical Studies: 1985–2015," by Erik Hesse. The AAI and a host of alternative measures, including many that use self-report questionnaires, are further examined by Judith A. Crowell, R. Chris Fraley, and Glenn I. Roisman in Chapter 27, "Measurement of Individual Differences in Adult Attachment." These two chapters are must-reads for anyone wishing to conduct studies of adult attachment and related issues.

Although attachment theory is not a theory of psychopathology per se, and does not characterize insecure attachment as a form of psychopathology, many connections exist between attachment insecurity and vulnerability to psychopathology, whether mild or severe. Thus, Part V of this volume is titled "Psychopathology and Clinical Applications." Chapter 28, by Michelle DeKlyen and Mark T. Greenberg, deals with "Attachment and Psychopathology in Childhood." When Ainsworth created her Strange Situation procedure for coding various forms of infant–parent attachment, she designated three main patterns. Later, Main and Solomon added a fourth category, labeled "disorganized/disoriented," now usually abbreviated as "disorganized." Karlen Lyons-Ruth and Deborah Jacobvitz summarize the fascinating literature in Chapter 29, "Attachment Disorganization from Infancy to Adulthood: Neurobiological Correlates, Parenting Contexts, and Pathways to Disorder." For anyone interested in links between attachment and psychopathology, or the treatment of psychopathology, this chapter is crucial.

Not every infant or young child is raised by a biological mother, as was the case in the sample that Ainsworth and her colleagues studied in the early days of attachment research. Some children are raised by someone other than a biological parent. In Chapter 30, Mary Dozier and Michael Rutter discuss "Challenges to the Development of Attachment Relationships Faced by Young Children in Foster and Adoptive Care." Chapter 31,

in parallel with Chapter 28 on attachment and psychopathology in childhood, focuses on "Attachment States of Mind and Psychopathology in Adulthood" and was written by K. Chase Stovall-McClough and Mary Dozier. Because so much is now known about parenting influences on early attachment, there are a number of well-designed and carefully evaluated programs, discussed in Chapter 32, "Prevention and Intervention Programs to Support Early Attachment Security: A Move to the Level of the Community," by Lisa J. Berlin, Charles H. Zeanah, and Alicia F. Lieberman. In Chapter 33, "Attachment and Adult Psychotherapy: Theory, Research, and Practice," Arietta Slade explains how knowledge of attachment theory and research can guide psychotherapy. In Chapter 34, "Reconciling Psychoanalytic Ideas with Attachment Theory," Peter Fonagy, Patrick Luyten, Elizabeth Allison, and Chloe Campbell explain the historical and contemporary relations between psychoanalytic approaches and attachment theory, including current integrations in which attachment theory is viewed much more favorably by psychoanalysts than it was during Bowlby's lifetime. In Chapter 35, "Couple and Family Therapy: An Attachment Perspective," Audrey Brassard and Susan M. Johnson explain how attachment theory has been incorporated into influential contemporary approaches to couple counseling.

Part VI, "Systems, Culture, and Context," provides a sampling of the many other topic areas into which attachment theory and research have been extended. In a new chapter for this edition, Chapter 36, "Caregiving," Brooke C. Feeney and Susan S. Woodhouse explain how attachment theory's construct of the "caregiving behavioral system" is proving useful in the study of relationships of many kinds. Chapter 37, "Cross-Cultural Patterns of Attachment: Universal and Contextual Dimensions," by Judi Mesman, Marinus H. van IJzendoorn, and Abraham Sagi-Schwartz, explores the important issue of cross-cultural similarities and differences in attachment relationships and dynamics. In Chapter 38, another new chapter created for this edition, "A Lifespan Perspective on Attachment and Care for Others: Empathy, Altruism, and Prosocial Behavior," Phillip R. Shaver, Mario Mikulincer, Jacquelyn T. Gross, Jessie A. Stern, and Jude Cassidy review the large and growing literature linking attachment security with caring feelings and behavior across the lifespan. In Chapter 39, "Attachment and Religious Representations and Behavior," Pehr Granqvist and Lee A. Kirkpatrick show how the concept of attachment fits with religious notions of reliance on a personal god, and how individual differences in attachment, assessed with both interviews and questionnaires, relate to differences in religious conceptions and experiences.

Divorce, an important form of separation and loss, was not explored in detail by Bowlby and Ainsworth, but has become increasingly important as it has become more common. This kind of separation and loss is examined in Chapter 40, "Divorce through the Lens of Attachment Theory," by Brooke C. Feeney and Joan K. Monin. In Chapter 41, "Attachment and School Readiness," new to this edition, Amanda P. Williford, Lauren M. Carter, and Robert C. Pianta show that school readiness is not simply a matter of cognitive or academic preparation, but instead depends heavily on skills linked to the kind of security that attachment researchers study. Finally, Michael Rutter and Camilla Azis-Clauson discuss, in Chapter 42, "Implications of Attachment Theory and Research for Child Care Policies," the ways in which attachment theory and research could and should affect social policy.

Part VII, "Perspectives on Attachment," contains a single conceptual analysis by L. Alan Sroufe, "The Place of Attachment in Development." This chapter summarizes the many accomplishments of attachment theorists and researchers, evident in the previous chapters, but also raises some concerns. Says Sroufe, "Like any major theory in the social sciences, with success come certain hazards. These include overextensions of the theory (thinking it can explain everything, including things for which it was not designed), misunderstanding and misapplication, and even complacency" (p. 997). We are grateful to have this senior and highly awarded researcher cap the volume with important ideas for future consideration, research, and applications. As the research extends in new directions and raises new issues for consideration, we assume that the theory will continue to evolve in complexity and usefulness.

## Acknowledgments

As can be discerned from its heft, this handbook is huge in scope, with thousands of references, including hundreds that are new to this edition. It has taken many talented people's time and dedication to bring it to fruition. Our first thanks go to the international cast of chapter authors—busy

people all—who agreed not only to write for the volume, but also to tailor their chapters to our specific needs. As you will see, the chapters are not like ones in the usual anthologies, in which authors simply spell out their own ideas and research programs without much regard for what other authors in the same volume are saying. Here, each author or set of authors looks seriously at the history of the area under discussion and explains how work in that area is progressing, what new conclusions are being drawn, and how the work might be applied. In many places, the authors refer to other chapters in the volume, making it easier to see how different topics are connected. Many of the chapters were vetted by colleagues, and all were carefully commented upon and edited by both of us. Several of the chapters went through multiple drafts. The chapter authors, all people with considerable experience and very high standards, were remarkably cooperative with our editorial plans and interventions. The book is unusually approachable, readable, and understandable as a result.

We had wonderful assistance from the professionals at The Guilford Press. Seymour Weingarten, Editor-in-Chief, helped conceptualize the first edition and get us involved with it; he then remained incredibly supportive, patient, and enthusiastic throughout the process of creating the second and third editions. C. Deborah Laughton, Judith Grauman, and Carolyn Graham were enormously helpful on a daily basis, responding quickly and helpfully to our many queries. We were fortunate in having Marie Sprayberry serve as our copyeditor for the previous two editions, and thank Jacquelyn Coggin this time around. Laura Specht Patchkofsky was our multitalented production editor. Paul Gordon designed a lovely cover. Deanna Butler composed a very detailed subject index. Behind the scenes of any large and long effort such as this one, there are scores of other professionals who quietly do excellent work without ever personally meeting the beneficiaries of their labor. We thank them, sincerely, as a group.

We are also extremely grateful to our families. In the preface to the first edition of the *Handbook*, we noted that we had both become first-time parents while editing that initial volume; we now note that we have both become first-time parents of college students while editing this current edition. It's not easy to study and write about attachment day after day while telling your own family members that you'll be with them in a while, when urgent editorial tasks are finished. The contradiction between sensitivity and responsiveness to chapter authors and sensitivity and responsiveness to loved ones at home is palpable. Certainly it is enlightening and personally gratifying for people who study attachment to experience its ramifications in everyday life.

Finally, we wish to thank each other. Collaborating on a large project like this is somewhat like running a family business. It requires open, honest communication about both shared and divergent opinions. Over the years of working on three editions of this book, we have been guests in each other's homes; eaten some great conference meals together; discussed every chapter in great detail; and begun to collaborate on research, not just on book editing. It's rare for two professors at universities thousands of miles apart to sustain such a good and deep working relationship, especially when we come from different parts of psychology and conduct different kinds of research. Sharing conceptual and editing problems, thoughts about attachment theory and research, computer screens in different cities, and reactions to the book as it developed has been extremely rewarding. We heartily congratulate and thank each other.

As we did with the first edition, we dedicate this volume to the memories of John Bowlby and Mary Ainsworth. They not only had great ideas, which they were able to transform into excellent research; they provided a model of how people can work together to create a large intellectual edifice that has many beneficial consequences for other professionals and for the people whose lives they work to improve.

JUDE CASSIDY
PHILLIP R. SHAVER

# Contents

# III. ATTACHMENT IN INFANCY AND CHILDHOOD

# IV. ATTACHMENT IN ADOLESCENCE AND ADULTHOOD

## V. PSYCHOPATHOLOGY AND CLINICAL APPLICATIONS

# PART I

## OVERVIEW OF ATTACHMENT THEORY

# Chapter 1

# The Nature of the Child's Ties

## Jude Cassidy

John Bowlby's work on attachment theory can be viewed as starting shortly after his graduation from Cambridge University, with the observations he made when working in a home for maladjusted boys. Two boys, both of whom had suffered disruptions in their relationships with their mothers, made important impressions on him. Bowlby's more systematic retrospective examination, published over a decade later as "Forty-Four Juvenile Thieves: Their Characters and Home Life" (Bowlby, 1944), as well as the observations of others (Bender & Yarnell, 1941; Goldfarb, 1943), convinced him that major disruptions in the mother–child relationship are precursors of later psychopathology. Bowlby's observations led not only to his belief that the child's relationship with the mother is important for later functioning, but also to a belief that this relationship is of critical immediate importance to the child. Bowlby, along with his colleague James Robertson, observed that children experienced intense distress when separated from their mothers, even if they were fed and cared for by others. A predictable pattern emerged—one of angry protest followed by despair (Robertson & Bowlby, 1952). Bowlby came to wonder why the mother is so important to the child.

At the time, the two widely accepted theories that offered explanations for the child's tie to the mother were both secondary drive theories. Psychoanalytic and social learning theorists alike proposed that an infant's relationship with the mother emerges because she feeds the infant (e.g., Freud, 1910/1957; Sears, Maccoby, & Levin, 1957), and that the pleasure experienced upon having hunger drives satisfied comes to be associated with the mother's presence. When Bowlby was first developing attachment theory, he became aware of evidence from animal studies that seriously called this perspective into question. Lorenz (1935) noted that infant geese became attached to parents—even to objects—that did not feed them. Harlow (1958) observed that infant rhesus monkeys, in times of stress, preferred not the wire mesh "mother" that provided food, but the cloth-covered "mother" that afforded contact comfort. Soon systematic observations of human infants were made, and it became evident that babies too became attached to people who did not feed them (Ainsworth, 1967; Schaffer & Emerson, 1964). Years later, Bowlby recalled that

> this [secondary drive] theory did not seem to me to fit the facts. For example, were it true, an infant of a year or two should take readily to whomever feeds him, and this clearly is not the case. But, if the secondary drive dependency theory was inadequate, what was the alternative? (1980b, p. 650)

Because he found himself dissatisfied with traditional theories, Bowlby (1969/1982) sought a new explanation through discussion with colleagues from fields such as evolutionary biology, ethology, developmental psychology, cognitive science, and control systems theory. He drew on all of these fields to formulate the innovative proposition that the mechanisms underlying the infant's tie to the mother originally emerged as a result of evolutionary pressures. For Bowlby, this strikingly strong tie, evident particularly when disrupted, results not from an associational learning process (a secondary drive), but rather from a biologically based desire for proximity that arose through the process of natural selection. Bowlby (1958, 1960a, 1960b) introduced attachment theory in a series of papers, the first of which was "The Nature of the Child's Tie to His Mother." All of the major points of attachment theory were presented there in at least rudimentary form, providing, as Bretherton (1992) noted, "the first basic blueprint of attachment theory" (p. 762). These ideas were later elaborated in Bowlby's trilogy, *Attachment and Loss* (1969/1982, 1973, 1980a).

A member of Bowlby's research team during this period of initial formulation of attachment theory was a developmental psychologist visiting from Canada, Mary Salter Ainsworth. Her serendipitous connection with Bowlby—a friend had shown her a newspaper advertisement for a developmental research position—proved fortunate for the development of attachment theory. Ainsworth conducted two pioneering naturalistic observation studies of mothers and infants in which she applied the ethological principles of attachment theory as a framework. One of these investigations was conducted in the early 1950s in Uganda; the other was carried out in the early 1960s in Baltimore. These inquiries provided the most extensive home observation data to date and laid the foundation for Ainsworth's contributions to attachment theory, as well as for Bowlby's continued formulations. Ainsworth later created an assessment tool, the "Strange Situation," that triggered the productive flowering of the empirical study of individual differences in attachment quality—the research that is largely responsible for the place of attachment theory in contemporary psychology and psychiatry.

This chapter summarizes Bowlby's initial ethological approach to understanding the child's tie to the mother, along with elaborations based on more recent research and theorizing. First, I discuss the biological bases of attachment, describing the evolutionary roots of attachment behavior, the attachment behavioral system and its organization, the role of context in the system's operation, the role of emotion, the role of cognition, and individual differences in attachment. Second, I examine

the attachment system in relation to other behavioral systems: the exploratory, fear, sociable, and caregiving systems. Third, I consider the nature of the child's attachment bond to the people to whom he or she is attached (Bowlby called these people "attachment figures"), and describe how attachments differ from other affectional bonds. Finally, I discuss multiple attachments. Although Bowlby's idea that attachment is a lifespan phenomenon was present in his earliest writings (e.g., 1956), as was the idea that people other than the mother often serve as attachment figures (1958), his principal focus was the tie to the mother during childhood, and I maintain that focus in this chapter (but see my discussion of multiple attachments later in this chapter).

## Biological Bases of Attachment Behavior

The most fundamental aspect of attachment theory is its focus on the biological bases of attachment behavior (Bowlby, 1958, 1969/1982). *Attachment behavior* has the predictable outcome of increasing proximity of the child to the attachment figure (usually the mother). Some attachment behaviors (smiling, vocalizing) are signaling behaviors that alert the mother to the child's interest in interaction, and thus serve to bring her to the child. Other behaviors (crying) are aversive and bring the mother to the child to terminate them. Some (approaching and following) are active behaviors that move the child to the mother.

### An Evolutionary Perspective

Bowlby proposed that during the time in which humans were evolving substantially (he called this "the environment of evolutionary adaptedness"), genetic selection favored attachment behaviors because they increased the likelihood of child–mother proximity, which in turn increased the likelihood of protection and provided survival advantage. In keeping with the evolutionary thinking of his time, Bowlby emphasized survival of the species in his earliest theoretical formulations. By the time he revised *Attachment* (Volume 1 of his trilogy, *Attachment and Loss*; Bowlby, 1969/1982), he noted that advances in evolutionary theory included the understanding that for all behavioral systems, including attachment, "the ultimate outcome to be attained is always the survival of the genes an individual is carrying" (p. 56). (For a more extensive discussion of attachment and this notion of "reproductive fitness," see Simpson & Belsky, Chapter 5, this volume.)

In the environment of evolutionary adaptedness, infants who were biologically predisposed to stay close to their mothers were less likely to be killed by predators, and it was for this reason that Bowlby referred to protection from predators as the "biological function" of attachment behavior. Because of this biological function of protection, Bowlby considered infants to be predisposed particularly to seek their attachment figures in times of threat or distress. In a basic Darwinian sense, then, the proclivity to seek proximity is a behavioral adaptation in the same way that a fox's white coat on the tundra is an adaptation. As Bowlby (1988) noted in his final collection of lectures, later revisions of evolutionary theory make the notion of a "principal" biological function (i.e., Bowlby's initial selection of protection) unnecessary; the multiple benefits of attachment (e.g., feeding, learning about the environment, self-regulation, social interaction) all contribute to its conveying an evolutionary advantage. Within this framework, attachment is considered a normal and healthy characteristic of humans throughout the lifespan, rather than a sign of immaturity that needs to be outgrown.

### The Attachment Behavioral System

Attachment behaviors are thought to be organized within an "attachment behavioral system." Bowlby (1969/1982) borrowed the behavioral system concept from ethology to describe a species-specific system of behaviors that leads to certain predictable outcomes, at least one of which contributes to survival and reproductive fitness. The concept of behavioral systems involves inherent motivation. There is no need to view attachment as the by-product of any more fundamental processes or "drive," and children are thought to become attached to individuals irrespective of whether their physiological needs are met. This idea, as already mentioned, is supported by evidence indicating that in contrast to what secondary drive theories lead one to expect (e.g., Freud, 1910/1957; Sears et al., 1957), attachment is not a result of associations with feeding (Ainsworth, 1967; Harlow, 1962; Schaffer & Emerson, 1964). Furthermore,

findings that infants become attached even to abusive mothers (Bowlby, 1956) suggest that the system is not driven simply by pleasurable associations. Bowlby's notion of the inherent motivation of the attachment system is compatible with Piaget's (1954) formulation of the inherent motivation of the child's interest in exploration.

Central to the concept of the attachment behavioral system is the notion that several attachment behaviors are organized within the individual in response to a particular history of internal and external cues. Sroufe and Waters (1977) emphasized that the attachment behavioral system is "not a set of behaviors that are constantly and uniformly operative" (p. 1185). Rather, the "functional equivalence" of behaviors is noted, with a variety of behaviors having similar meanings and serving similar functions. As Bowlby (1969/1982) noted, "whether a child moves toward a mother by running, walking, crawling, shuffling or, in the case of a thalidomide child, by rolling, is thus of very little consequence compared to the set-goal of his locomotion, namely proximity to mother" (p. 373). The behaviors chosen in a particular context are the ones the infant finds most useful at that moment and with that caregiver. With development, the child gains access to a greater variety of ways of achieving proximity and learns which ones are most effective in which circumstances. Indeed, as Sroufe and Waters pointed out, this organizational perspective helps to explain stability within the context of both developmental and contextual changes. Thus, an infant may maintain a stable internal organization of the attachment behavioral system in relation to the mother over time and across contexts, yet the specific behaviors used in the service of this organization may vary greatly. For example, whereas a nonmobile infant may be expected to cry and reach out to the mother for contact, a mobile child may achieve the same goal of establishing contact by crawling or toddling after her.

This emphasis on the organization of the attachment behavioral system also helps to explain its operation in a "goal-corrected" manner. Unlike certain reflexes that, once activated, maintain a fixed course (e.g., sneezing, rooting), the attachment behavioral system enables the individual to respond flexibly to environmental changes while attempting to attain a goal. Bowlby used the analogy of a heat-seeking missile: Once launched, the missile does not remain on a preset course; rather, it incorporates information about changes in the target's location and adjusts its trajectory accordingly. Similarly, the infant is capable of considering changes in the mother's location and behavior (as well as other environmental changes) when attempting to maintain proximity to her. And the flexible use of a variety of attachment behaviors, depending on the circumstances, affords the infant greater efficiency in goal-corrected responses. For instance, an infant may see the mother starting to leave in an unfamiliar environment and may desire to increase proximity to her. The infant may begin by reaching for her and then following her (changing course as she moves); if this fails, the infant may try calling or crying.

Bowlby's approach to the organization of attachment behavior involves a control systems perspective. Drawing on observations of ethologists who described instinctive behavior in animals as serving to maintain them in a certain relation with the environment for long periods of time, Bowlby proposed that a control systems approach could also be applied to attachment behavior. He described the workings of a thermostat as an example of a control system. When a room gets too cold, the thermostat activates the heater; when the desired temperature is reached, the thermostat turns the heater off. Bowlby described children as wanting to maintain a certain proximity to their mothers. When a separation becomes too great in distance or time, the attachment system becomes activated, and when sufficient proximity has been achieved, it is terminated. Bowlby (following Bretherton, 1980; see Bowlby, 1969/1982) later described the attachment system as working slightly differently from a thermostat—as being continually activated (with variations of relatively more or less activation), rather than being completely turned off at times. According to Bowlby, the child's goal is not an object (e.g., the mother), but rather a state—a maintenance of the desired distance from the mother, depending on the circumstances. Bowlby described this idea of behavioral homeostasis as similar to the process of physiological homeostasis, whereby physiological systems (e.g., blood pressure and body temperature) are maintained within set limits. Like physiological control systems, a behavioral control system is thought to be organized within the central nervous system. According to Bowlby (1969/1982), the distinction between the two is that the latter is "one in which the set-limits concern the organism's relation to features of the environment and in which the limits are maintained by behavioral rather than physiological means" (p. 372).

## The Role of Context

The child's desired degree of proximity to the attachment figure is thought to vary under differing circumstances, and Bowlby (1969/1982) was interested in understanding how these different circumstances contribute to relative increases and decreases in activation of the attachment system. Thus, he described two classes of conditions that contribute to activation of the attachment system, both of which indicate danger or stress. One relates to conditions of the child (e.g., illness, fatigue, hunger, or pain). The other relates to conditions of the environment (e.g., the presence of threatening stimuli); particularly important are the location and behavior of the mother (e.g., her absence, withdrawal, or rejection of the child). Interactions among these causal factors can be quite complex: Sometimes only one needs to be present, and at other times several are necessary. In regard to relative deactivation of the attachment system, Bowlby made it clear that his approach had nothing in common with a model in which a behavior stops when its energy supply is depleted (e.g., Freud, 1940/1964). In Bowlby's ethological view, attachment behavior stops in the presence of a terminating stimulus. For most distressed infants, contact with mother is an effective terminating stimulus. Yet the nature of the stimulus that serves to terminate attachment behavior differs according to the degree of activation of the attachment system. If the attachment system is intensely activated, contact with the mother may be necessary to terminate it. If it is moderately activated, the presence or soothing voice of the mother (or even of a familiar substitute caregiver) may suffice. In either case, the infant is viewed as using the mother as a "safe haven" to return to in times of trouble. In summary, proximity seeking is activated when the infant receives information (from both internal and external sources) that a goal (the desired distance from the mother) is not met. It remains activated until the goal is achieved, and then it stops.

## The Role of Emotion

According to Bowlby (1979), emotions are strongly associated with attachment:

> Many of the most intense emotions arise during the formation, the maintenance, the disruption, and the renewal of attachment relationships. The formation of a bond is described as falling in love, maintaining

a bond as loving someone, and losing a partner as grieving over someone. Similarly, threat of loss arouses anxiety and actual loss gives rise to sorrow; whilst each of these situations is likely to arouse anger. The unchallenged maintenance of a bond is experienced as a source of joy. (p. 130)

It is likely that these affective responses originally resulted from evolutionary pressures. An infant predisposed to experience positive emotions in relation to an attachment and sadness with its loss may actively work to maintain attachments that in turn contribute to the infant's enhanced chances of survival and reproductive fitness.

Bowlby also viewed emotions as important regulatory mechanisms within attachment relationships, noting, for instance, that anger and protest, as long as they do not become excessive and destructive, can serve to alert the attachment figure to the child's interest in maintaining the relationship (Bowlby, 1973; see Kobak, Zajac, & Madsen, Chapter 2, this volume). More recently, attachment theorists have noted the ways in which the regulation of emotions is used in the service of maintaining the relationship with the attachment figure, and they have noted that individual differences in attachment security have much to do with the ways in which emotions are responded to, shared, communicated about, and regulated within the attachment relationship (Cassidy, 1994; Cassidy & Berlin, 1994; Cassidy & Kobak, 1988; Kobak & Duemmler, 1994; Thompson, 2013; see also Thompson, Chapter 16, this volume).

### The Role of Cognition

Drawing on cognitive information theory, Bowlby (1969/1982) proposed that the organization of the attachment behavioral system involves cognitive components—specifically, mental representations of the attachment figure, the self, and the environment—all of which are largely based on experiences. Bretherton (1991) suggested that repeated attachment-related experiences become organized as scripts, which in turn become the building blocks of broader representations (see also Vaughn et al., 2006). (This emphasis on the importance of an individual's actual experiences was another way in which Bowlby's theory differed from that of Freud, which emphasized instead the role of internally generated fantasies.) Bowlby referred to these representations as "representational models" and as "internal working models." According to him, these models allow individuals to anticipate

the future and to make plans, thereby operating most efficiently. (There is in fact evidence that even young children are capable of using representations to make predictions about the future; see Heller & Berndt, 1981.) The child is thought to rely on these models, for instance, when making decisions about which attachment behavior(s) to use in a specific situation with a specific person. Representational models are considered to work best when they are relatively accurate reflections of reality, and conscious processing is required to check and revise models in order to keep them up to date. Extensive discussion of these cognitive models is provided by Bretherton (1990; Bretherton & Munholland, Chapter 4, this volume) and by Main, Kaplan, and Cassidy (1985); see also Baldwin (1992) for a review of similarities between these models and a variety of constructs within the literatures on developmental, social, clinical, and cognitive psychology. Bowlby (1969/1982, 1973, 1979, 1980a) also discussed the role within the attachment system of other cognitive processes, such as object permanence, discrimination learning, generalization, nonconscious processing, selective attention and memory, and interpretative biases (see also Dykas & Cassidy, 2011; Sherman, Rice, & Cassidy, 2015).

### Individual Differences

In extending the biological emphasis of Bowlby's initial theorizing, Main (1990) proposed that the biologically based human tendency to become attached is paralleled by a biologically based ability to be flexible to the range of likely caregiving environments. This flexibility is thought to contribute to variations associated with quality of attachment. Whereas nearly all children become attached (even to mothers who abuse them; Bowlby, 1956), not all are securely attached. Striking individual differences exist. Secure attachment occurs when a child has confident expectations of the attachment figure as available and responsive when needed. Infants are considered to be insecurely attached when they lack such confidence. Bowlby's early clinical observations led him to predict that just as feeding does not cause attachment in infants, so individual differences in feeding (e.g., breast vs. bottle feeding) do not contribute to individual differences in attachment quality. In one of his earliest writings, Bowlby (1958) predicted that the important factor is "the extent to which the mother has permitted clinging and following, and all the behavior associated with them, or has refused them" (p. 370). This prediction has since gained empirical support (e.g., Ainsworth, Blehar, Waters, & Wall, 1978; see also De Wolff & Van IJzendoorn, 1997). (Precursors and outcomes associated with individual differences in attachment security are discussed in detail in this volume by Fearon & Belsky, Chapter 14, and Thompson, Chapter 16; see also Kobak et al., Chapter 2, and Fraley & Shaver, Chapter 3, for discussions of theory related to major separations and losses as linked to individual differences in attachment.)

## Attachment in Relation to Other Behavioral Systems

The attachment behavioral system can be fully understood only in terms of its complex interplay with other biologically based behavioral systems. Bowlby highlighted two of these as being particularly related to the attachment system in young children: the exploratory behavioral system and the fear behavioral system. The activation of these other systems is related to activation of the attachment system. Activation of the fear system generally heightens activation of the attachment system. In contrast, activation of the exploratory system can, under certain circumstances, reduce activation of the attachment system. As any parent knows, providing a novel set of car keys can at least temporarily distract a baby who wants to be picked up, as long as the infant's attachment system is not intensely activated. These two behavioral systems are discussed in this section, as are the sociable and caregiving behavioral systems.

### The Exploratory System

The links between the exploratory behavioral system and the attachment behavioral system are thought to be particularly intricate. According to Bowlby, the exploratory system gives survival advantages to the child by providing important information about the workings of the environment: how to use tools, build structures, obtain food, and negotiate physical obstacles. Yet unbridled exploration with no attention to potential hazards can be dangerous. The complementary yet mutually inhibiting nature of the exploratory and attachment systems is thought to have evolved to ensure that while the child is protected by maintaining proximity to attachment figures, he or she nonetheless gradually learns about the environment through exploration. According to Ainsworth (1972), "the dynamic equilibrium between these two behavioral systems is even more significant for development (and for survival) than either in isolation" (p. 118).

The framework that best captures the links between the attachment and exploratory systems is that of an infant's use of an attachment figure as a "secure base from which to explore"—a concept first described by Ainsworth (1963) and central to attachment theory (Ainsworth et al., 1978; Bowlby, 1969/1982, 1988). On the basis of her observations during the infant's first year of life, Ainsworth referred to an "attachment–exploration balance" (Ainsworth, Bell, & Stayton, 1971). Most infants balance these two behavioral systems, responding flexibly to a specific situation after assessing both the environment's characteristics and the caregiver's availability and likely behavior. For instance, when the infant experiences the environment as dangerous, exploration is unlikely. Furthermore, when the attachment system is activated (perhaps by separation from the attachment figure, illness, fatigue, or unfamiliar people and surroundings), infant exploration and play decline. Conversely, when the attachment system is not activated (e.g., when a healthy, well-rested infant is in a comfortable setting with an attachment figure nearby), exploration is enhanced. Thus attachment, far from interfering with exploration, is viewed as fostering exploration. Bowlby (1973) described as important not only the physical presence of an attachment figure but also the infant's belief that the attachment figure will be available if needed. A converging body of empirical work, in which maternal physical or psychological presence was experimentally manipulated, has provided compelling evidence of the theoretically predicted associations between maternal availability and infant exploration (Ainsworth & Wittig, 1969; Carr, Dabbs, & Carr, 1975; Rheingold, 1969; Sorce & Emde, 1981).

### The Fear System

The fear behavioral system is also thought to be closely linked to the attachment system. For Bowlby, the biological function of the fear system, like that of the attachment system, is protection. It is biologically adaptive for children to be frightened of certain stimuli. Without such fear, survival and reproduction would be reduced.

Bowlby (1973) described "natural clues to danger"—stimuli that are not inherently dangerous, but that increase the likelihood of danger. These include darkness, loud noises, aloneness, and looming. Because the attachment and fear systems are intertwined, so that frightened infants increase their attachment behavior, infants who find these stimuli frightening are considered more likely to seek protection and thus to survive to pass on their genes for this tendency. Although Bowlby acknowledged the role of factors such as genetics, his focus was on environmental influences. The presence or absence of the attachment figure is thought to play an important role in the activation and regulation of an infant's fear system, such that an available and accessible attachment figure makes the infant much less susceptible to fear, and there is evidence that this is so (Morgan & Ricciuti, 1969; Sorce & Emde, 1981). In fact, even photographs of the mother can calm a fearful infant, as can "security blankets" for children who are attached to such objects (Passman & Erck, 1977; Passman & Weisberg, 1975).

### The Sociable System

A complete understanding of the attachment behavioral system rests on an understanding of its distinction from the sociable (or "affiliative") behavioral system.[1] Although Bowlby did not discuss this behavioral system as extensively as he did some others, he did point out, as have other theorists, that the sociable system is distinct from the attachment behavioral system. Bowlby (1969/1982, p. 229) wrote:

> "Affiliation" was introduced by Murray (1938): "Under this heading are classed all manifestations of friendliness and goodwill, of the desire to do things in company with others." As such it is a much broader concept than attachment and is not intended to cover behavior that is directed towards one or a few particular figures, which is the hallmark of attachment behavior.

According to Ainsworth (1989), it is "reasonable to believe that there is some basic behavioral system that has evolved in social species that leads individuals to seek to maintain proximity to conspecifics, even to those to whom they are not attached or otherwise bonded, and despite the fact that wariness is likely to be evoked by those who are unfamiliar" (p. 713). Harlow and Harlow (1965) described the "peer affectional system

through which infants and children interrelate . . . and develop persisting affection for each other" as an "affectional system" distinct from those involving infant and parents (p. 288). Bronson (1972) referred to affiliation as an "adaptive system" present in infancy and separate from attachment. Bretherton and Ainsworth (1974) examined the interplay among several behavioral systems in infants, including the sociable and the attachment systems, and Greenberg and Marvin (1982) examined this interplay in preschool children. Hinde (1974) described nonhuman primates' play with peers, which he identified as different from mother–child interaction, as "consum[ing] so much time and energy that it must be of crucial adaptive importance" (p. 227).

The *sociable system* is thus defined as the organization of the biologically based, survival-promoting tendency to be sociable with others. An important predictable outcome of activation of this system is that individuals are likely to spend at least part of their time in the company of others. Given evidence from the primate literature that individuals in the company of others are much less likely to be killed by predators (Eisenberg, 1966), it seems reasonable to assume that humans too would derive the important survival advantage of protection from associating with others. The sociable system is likely to contribute to an individual's survival and reproductive fitness in other important ways: Primates biologically predisposed to be sociable with others increase their ability to gather food, build shelter, and create warmth; they learn about the environment more efficiently; and they gain access to a group of others with whom they may eventually mate (see Huntingford, 1984, for a review). Strong evidence of the importance of the sociable system for the development of young nonhuman primates comes from several studies, most notably those of Harlow (1969) and his associates, in which monkeys reared with their mothers but without peers were seriously hindered in their social development and could not mate or parent effectively (see also Miller, Caul, & Mirsky, 1967).

Observations of both humans and other primates clearly show differences between the attachment and sociable systems in what activates behavior, in what terminates behavior, and in the way behaviors are organized (Bretherton & Ainsworth, 1974; Harlow, 1969; Vandell, 1980). The sociable system is most likely to be activated when the attachment system is not activated. According to Bowlby,

A child seeks his attachment-figure when he is tired, hungry, ill, or alarmed and also when he is uncertain of that figure's whereabouts; when the attachment-figure is found he wants to remain in proximity to him or her and may want also to be held or cuddled. By contrast, a child seeks a playmate when he is in good spirits and confident of the whereabouts of his attachment-figure; when the playmate is found, moreover, the child wants to engage in playful interaction with him or her. If this analysis is right, the roles of attachment-figure and playmate are distinct. (1969/1982, p. 307)

Lewis, Young, Brooks, and Michalson (1975) interpreted their observations of pairs of 1-year-olds and their mothers similarly: "Mothers are good for protection, peers for watching and playing with" (p. 56).

### The Caregiving System

In one of his earliest writings, Bowlby (1956) pointed out that further understanding of attachment could be gained from examination of the mother's tie to her infant. Bowlby later (1984) wrote briefly about "parenting behavior" from a biological perspective as "like attachment behavior, . . . in some degree preprogrammed" (p. 271). He described the biologically based urge to care for and protect children, yet he simultaneously viewed individual differences in the nature of parenting as emerging largely through learning (yet see Bakermans-Kranenburg & Van IJzendoorn, Chapter 8, this volume, for recent evidence of genetic influences on parenting in humans; see also Mileva-Seitz, Bakermans-Kranenburg, & Van IJzendoorn, in press). Although Bowlby wrote little about this topic, his ethological perspective, his ideas about interrelated behavioral systems, and his interest in attachment-related processes across the lifespan lend themselves readily to an elaboration of the parental side of what he (Bowlby, 1969/1982) called the "attachment–caregiving social bond." Solomon and George (1996; George & Solomon, 1996, 2008) have filled this void, writing in detail about the "caregiving system"; see also Feeney & Woodhouse, Chapter 36, this volume).

It can be difficult to delineate precisely which aspects of parenting behavior should be considered part of the caregiving system. I propose that the term "caregiving system" be used to describe a subset of parental behaviors—only those behaviors designed to promote proximity and comfort when the parent perceives that the child is in real or potential danger or distress. The chief behavior within this system is retrieval of the infant from a potentially dangerous situation (Bowlby, 1969/1982); others include calling, reaching, grasping, restraining, following, soothing, and rocking.[2]

Just as the child's interactions with the parent involve more than the attachment system (e.g., a child may approach the father not for comfort but for play), so other parental systems may be activated during interactions with the child (Bowlby, 1969/1982). These various behavioral systems can all be viewed as enhancing the child's survival and reproductive fitness (e.g., teaching, feeding, playing). A parent may be differentially responsive to a child when each of these different parental behavioral systems is activated (e.g., sensitive when teaching or feeding, yet insensitive when the caregiving system is activated). The predominance of each of these parental behavioral systems varies considerably both across and within cultures. For instance, as Bretherton (1985) pointed out, among Mayan Indians in Mexico, mothers rarely serve as playmates for their infants but are quite available and responsive as caregivers (Brazelton, 1977). Similarly, Ainsworth (1990) noted that "the mothers of Ganda babies who were securely attached to them almost never played with them, even though they were highly sensitive caregivers" (p. 482; see also Mesman, Van IJzendoorn, & Sagi-Schwartz, Chapter 37, this volume). Within-culture variation exists as well: Within a particular culture, one mother may be a readily available attachment figure, yet stodgy and inept in the role of playmate; another mother may be comfortable in interaction with her children only in her roles as teacher or coach when attention is focused on a task or skill, and may be uncomfortable with attachment-related interactions. Main, Hesse, and Kaplan (2005, p. 292) have proposed that such parental discomfort (anxiety) may emerge when infant behavior interferes with parents' ability to preserve "the state of mind that had seemed optimal for maintenance of the relationship to their own parents during childhood." (For additional discussion of the ways in which particular parents experience discomfort when faced with particular child behavior, see Cassidy et al., 2005; Jones, Cassidy, & Shaver, 2015.)

As is the case with the child's attachment system, the predictable outcome of activation of the caregiving system is parent–child proximity, and a central biological function is protection of the child. In most cases, both parent and child work together to maintain a comfortable degree of proximity. If the child moves away, the parent will retrieve him or her; if the parent moves away, the child will follow or signal for the parent to return. Following Bowlby's (1969/1982) thinking, it seems likely that when the caregiving system is relatively activated, the child's attachment system can be relatively deactivated; attachment behaviors are not needed because the parent has assumed responsibility for maintaining proximity. If the caregiving system is not relatively activated, then the child's attachment system becomes activated, should the context call for it. This is one reason why the mother's leaving is particularly disturbing to a child and particularly likely to activate attachment behavior. This "dynamic equilibrium" (Bowlby, 1969/1982, p. 236) contributes to understanding the notion of the mother's providing "a secure base from which to explore." The mother's monitoring of infant–mother proximity frees the infant from such monitoring and permits greater attention to exploring. For instance, if, when visiting a new park, a mother actively follows the infant in his or her explorations, the infant is much more likely to cover a wide area than if the mother sits on a bench talking with friends. Empirical support for this proposition comes from a study in which the simple act of a mother diverting her attention away from the infant to a magazine in a brief laboratory procedure reduced the quality of infant exploration (Sorce & Emde, 1981). (As usual, the role of context is key; there are times when parental caregiving behaviors do not free the child to explore, but instead cue the child to potential danger, thereby activating the child's fear system and thus the attachment system.)

Yet parent and child do not always agree on what distance between them is desirable. For example, a mother's caregiving system may be activated (with or without her fear system) and prompt her to retrieve an infant whose activated exploratory system leads him or her to prefer to move away. Parents and their children may also differ in terms of how their priorities guide activation of their behavioral systems. For instance, when an infant's attachment system is activated in the presence of the mother, the infant's sole wish is for her to respond. Although such infant behavior is usually a powerful activating stimulus for the mother's caregiving system, the mother may choose among several competing needs and may or may not provide care (Trivers, 1974). The child's concern is immediate and focused; the mother's concerns may be more diffuse and long-range. The mother may have to leave the infant

to work to support the family (in which case activation of her food-getting behavioral system has taken precedence over her caregiving system). Or she may have several children (or a romantic partner) to whose needs she must attend. Main (1990) has proposed that from an evolutionary perspective, maternal insensitivity to a particular child may be useful to the mother if it maximizes the total number of surviving offspring (see also Simpson & Belsky, Chapter 5, this volume).

As is true for many behavioral systems, activation of the caregiving system results from both internal and external cues. Internal cues include presence of hormones, cultural beliefs, parental state (e.g., whether the parent is tired or sick), and activation of other parental behavioral systems (e.g., exploratory, food-getting, fear, attachment). External cues include state of the environment (e.g., whether it is familiar, whether there is danger, whether others are present and who these others are), state of the infant (e.g., whether the infant is sick or tired), and behavior of the infant (e.g., whether he or she is exhibiting attachment behavior). Activation of the caregiving system has crucial implications for the infant, who cannot otherwise survive. Ethologists have suggested that infants therefore have evolved characteristics that serve to activate the caregiving system: their endearing "babyish" features (the large rounded head with the high forehead, the small nose) and their thrashing arm movements. Attachment behaviors, of course, motivate parents to respond; even aversive behaviors, such as crying, typically motivate parents to provide care in order to terminate them. Given that an infant's attachment system is activated by stimuli that indicate an increased risk of danger (e.g., loud noise, looming objects), a parent who increases proximity when a child's attachment behavior is activated increases the likelihood of being able to protect the child, should the danger prove real. Similarly, when the parent perceives or expects danger that the child does not, parental proximity also increases the likelihood of survival. Thus, it is likely that the close link between the child's attachment and fear systems is paralleled by a close link between the parent's caregiving and fear systems, such that when a parent's fear system is activated, so too is his or her caregiving system.

Fear is only one of the powerful emotions likely to be linked to the caregiving system. Just as attachment is associated with powerful emotions (Bowlby, 1979), so is the caregiving system. These emotions may in fact be as strong as any an individual experiences in his or her lifetime. The birth of a first child (which establishes the adult as a parent) is often accompanied by feelings of great joy; threats to the child are accompanied by anxiety; the death of a child brings profound grief. This intertwining of the caregiving system with intense emotions may result from selective pressures during evolution: Enhanced reproductive fitness may result when, for instance, a parent's anxiety about threats to a child prompts the parent to seek effective interventions.

The role of parental soothing as a component of the caregiving system merits consideration. Why would a parent who safely holds a crying child out of reach of a large barking dog continue to comfort the child? Why would a parent pick up a distressed child whom the parent perceives to be in no danger? What could be the role of such soothing behaviors? I propose that soothing behaviors serve indirectly to facilitate the parent's monitoring of potential or real dangers to the child. Parental provision of contact usually comforts a distressed child. If the child continues to be distressed for a substantial time following contact, there may be another threat of which the parent is unaware. Through continuing attempts to soothe the child, the parent gains information about threat to the child. The parent may not realize, for instance, that the child has a painful splinter in his or her foot. Furthermore, there are many ways in which inconsolable crying beyond early infancy can signal (or contribute to) serious health problems. And a parent will not know whether crying is inconsolable unless the parent attempts to console. Moreover, the evolution of a parental tendency to soothe is understandable to the extent that soothing returns an overwrought child to a state of equilibrium in which he or she can engage in other activities more likely to enhance reproductive fitness, such as exploration or sociability. See also Shaver, Mikulincer, Gross, Stern, and Cassidy, Chapter 38, this volume, for discussion of the evolutionary basis of parental soothing of child distress.

Important questions about the caregiving system remain, including links between the parental caregiving and child attachment systems. First, given that there are times when the child's distress does not stem from activation of his or her attachment system, research could examine whether it is best to consider parental behavior in response to such distress as part of the caregiving system. For instance, it seems plausible that a child may get upset because his or her exploratory system is

frustrated, and that the child's distress prompts the mother to pick the child up and comfort him or her. It may be that the mother's behavior then contributes to the child's attachment-related expectations about the mother's likely responses to his or her distress, and thus to the formation of the child's representational model of the mother. Second, research is needed to determine how separate the caregiving system is from other parental systems, and whether it is only the parent's behaviors within the caregiving system that affect the child's attachment system. Third, it is unclear whether it is best to think of a single parental caregiving system in humans or of separate maternal and paternal caregiving systems. Harlow has proposed separate maternal and paternal systems in primates (Harlow, Harlow, & Hansen, 1963). If two separate systems exist in humans, there must be considerable overlap, even though genetic, hormonal, and cultural factors may contribute to differences in the specific characteristics of these systems.[3]

## The Attachment Bond

Whereas *attachment behavior* is behavior that promotes proximity to the attachment figure, and the *attachment behavioral system* is the organization of attachment behaviors within the individual, an *attachment bond* refers to an affectional tie. Ainsworth (1989) described an attachment bond *not* as dyadic, but rather as characteristic of the individual, "entailing representation in the internal organization of the individual" (p. 711). Thus, this bond is not one between two people; it is instead a bond that one individual has to another individual who is perceived as stronger and wiser (e.g., the bond of an infant to the mother). A person can be attached to a person who is not in turn attached to him or her; as described below, this is usually the case with infants and their parents.[4]

The attachment bond is a specific type of a larger class of bonds that Bowlby and Ainsworth referred to as *affectional bonds*. Throughout the lifespan, individuals form a variety of important affectional bonds that are not attachments. To make it completely clear what an attachment bond is, one needs to delineate what it is not. Ainsworth (1989) described the criteria for affectional bonds, and then the additional criterion for attachment bonds. First, an affectional bond is persistent across time, not transitory. Second, an affectional bond involves a specific person—a figure who is not interchangeable with anyone else. This bond reflects "the attraction that one individual has for another *individual*" (Bowlby, 1979, p. 67, original emphasis). For instance, the sadness associated with the loss of a close friend is not lessened by the fact that one has other close friends. Bowlby emphasized specificity when he stated: "To complain because a child does not welcome being comforted by a kind but strange woman is as foolish as to complain that a young man deeply in love is not enthusiastic about some other good-looking girl" (1956, p. 589). Third, the relationship is emotionally significant. Fourth, the individual wishes to maintain proximity to or contact with the person. The nature and extent of the proximity/contact desired vary as a function of a variety of factors (e.g., age and state of the individual, environmental conditions). Fifth, the individual feels distress at involuntary separation from the person. Even though the individual may choose separation from the figure, the individual experiences distress when proximity is desired but prevented. In addition to these five criteria, an additional criterion exists for an attachment bond: In times of distress, the individual seeks security and comfort in the relationship with the person (Ainsworth, 1989). (The attachment is considered "secure" if one achieves security and "insecure" if one does not; it is the seeking of security that is the defining feature. See also Hinde, 1982; Weiss, 1982.) It is this final criterion that leads attachment researchers to refer to "parental bonds" to children and "child attachments" to parents: When the roles are reversed and a parent attempts to seek security from a young child, it is "almost always not only a sign of pathology in the parent but also a cause of it in the child" (Bowlby, 1969/1982, p. 377). (The situation is viewed differently later in life, when a middle-aged offspring takes care of an increasingly infirm and dependent parent; see Magai, Frías, & Shaver, Chapter 25, this volume.)

The existence of an attachment bond cannot be inferred from the presence or absence of attachment behavior. To begin with, it is important to remember that most behaviors can serve more than one behavioral system (Bretherton & Ainsworth, 1974; Sroufe & Waters, 1977). Thus, for instance, every approach does not serve the attachment system; even though approach can be an attachment behavior, it can also be an exploratory or sociable behavior. Yet it is also the case that distressed infants separated from their mothers may seek comfort from strangers (Ainsworth et al., 1978; Bretherton, 1978; Rheingold, 1969).

Nonetheless, an enduring attachment bond of an infant to a stranger cannot be assumed to exist, and it is thus possible for an infant to direct attachment behavior to an individual to whom he or she is not attached. Some babies will stop crying when comforted by a stranger, but observations in the Strange Situation reveal that this comfort is generally not as satisfying as that provided by the mother (Ainsworth et al., 1978).

Similarly, even during a period when the child is directing no attachment behavior to the parent, the child is still attached. When, for instance, a contented child is in comfortable surroundings with the mother present, the attachment system is not likely to be activated to a level that triggers attachment behavior. Thus, activation of attachment behavior is largely situational; it may or may not be present at any given time. The attachment bond, however, is considered to exist consistently over time, whether or not attachment behavior is present. Bowlby (1969/1982) pointed out that even the cessation of behavior during a long separation cannot be considered an indication that the attachment bond no longer exists.

The strength of attachment behaviors is sometimes mistakenly regarded as reflecting the "strength" of the attachment bond. There are striking variations in strength of activation of attachment behaviors across contexts and across children. Yet no evidence exists that these variations in themselves map onto variations in child–mother attachment in any meaningful way. According to Ainsworth (1972, p. 119),

> to equate strength of attachment with strength of attachment behavior under ordinary nonstressful circumstances would lead to the conclusion that an infant who explores when his mother is present is necessarily less attached than one who constantly seeks proximity to his mother, whereas, in fact, his freedom to explore away from her may well reflect the healthy security provided by a harmonious attachment relationship.

Ainsworth characterized individual differences in relationships with an attachment figure as variations in quality rather than in strength. Similarly, it is a mistake to label as "very attached" a young child who clings fearfully to the mother; such attachment behavior may reflect insecure attachment or secure use of the mother as a safe haven, depending on the context.

Given that the strength of attachment behaviors should not be confused with the strength of an attachment bond, is strength nonetheless a useful dimension on which to consider an attachment bond? One might assume that Bowlby's proposition that children develop "attachment hierarchies" (discussed in the following section) implies that some attachments are stronger than others. Although Bowlby himself did occasionally use this terminology—for example, "How do we understand the origin and nature of this extraordinarily strong tie between child and mother?" (Bowlby, 1988, p. 161)—such usage was relatively rare, particularly when he was comparing one attachment with another (when doing so, he referred instead to "secure" and "insecure" attachments). Ainsworth (1982a) suggested that Hinde's (1979) notion of "penetration," as opposed to notions of either strength or intensity, provides a more useful framework for characterizing an attachment bond. According to Hinde, penetration is a dimension of relationships that describes the centrality of one person to another's life—the extent to which a person penetrates a variety of aspects of the other person's life. Ainsworth pointed out that the concept of penetration is particularly useful when considering the changing nature of a child's attachment to the parent as the child grows older. She proposed that it may be more appropriate not to talk of the bond as becoming "weaker," but rather as characterizing a relationship that penetrates fewer aspects of the growing child's life as he or she comes to spend more time away from the parents and to develop new relationships.

For Bowlby (1969/1982), there are two important propositions about the nature of the attachment bond within the larger context of a relationship. First, the attachment bond reflects only one feature of the child's relationship with the mother: the component that deals with behavior related to the child's protection and security in time of stress. The mother may serve not only as an attachment figure but also as playmate, teacher, or disciplinarian. These various roles are not incompatible, and it is possible that two or more roles may be filled by the same person. Thus, for example, a child may direct attachment behavior to the mother when he or she is frightened, yet at other times interact with her in ways relatively unrelated to attachment (e.g., play). Consequently, it would be a mistake to label as an attachment behavior a child's approach to the mother in order to engage in peekaboo. As Bretherton (1980) noted, a behavior may serve different behavioral systems at different times, even when it is directed to the same individual. Yet it is important to note that

even though a mother may be a frequent playmate for her 5-year-old, it does not negate the fact that this relationship is essentially characterized as an attachment relationship. Bowlby (1969/1982, p. 378) summarized his position on this issue: "A parent–child relationship is by no means exclusively that of attachment–caregiving. The only justification, therefore, for referring to the bond between a child and his mother in this way is that the shared dyadic programme given top priority is one of attachment–caregiver."

Second, an attachment bond cannot be presumed to exist even though a relationship may contain an attachment component. As noted earlier, the fact that a 1-year-old distressed about separation from the mother will direct his or her attachment behaviors to a friendly stranger does not mean that the relationship with the stranger involves an attachment bond. This is true even in more ongoing relationships, such as relationships with peers. A young child may routinely direct attachment behavior to a close friend and feel comfort in the friend's presence (particularly in a context such as school, when a parent is not present), without that relationship's involving an attachment bond. This is evident from the fact that the loss of such a friend usually does not have the devastating effects on the child that loss of a true attachment figure (e.g., a parent) has. Thus, even though children may at times turn to friends for comfort (Hazan & Zeifman, 1994), these friendships need not be attachment relationships.

## Multiple Attachments

Bowlby stated three principal propositions about multiple attachments in infancy. First, most young infants are thought to form more than one attachment. According to Bowlby (1969/1982), "almost from the first, many children have more than one figure to whom they direct attachment behavior" (p. 304).[5] Indeed, empirical observations have revealed that the majority of children become attached to more than one familiar person during their first year (Ainsworth, 1967; Schaffer & Emerson, 1964). According to Bowlby (1969/1982), "responsiveness to crying and readiness to interact socially are amongst the most relevant variables" (p. 315) in determining who will serve as an attachment figure. In most cultures, this means that the biological parents, older siblings, grandparents, aunts, and uncles are most likely to serve as attachment figures. Generally, the mother's role as an attachment figure is clear. The father is also particularly likely to become an additional attachment figure early in the infant's life. Observational studies have revealed that fathers are competent caregivers (Belsky, Gilstrap, & Rovine, 1984), and that children use their fathers as attachment figures (Ainsworth, 1967). Ainsworth noted the special infant–father relationship that sometimes emerged in Uganda:

> It seemed to be especially to the father that these other attachments were formed, even in the cases of babies who saw their fathers relatively infrequently. One can only assume that there was some special quality in the father's interaction with his child—whether of tenderness or intense delight—which evoked in turn a strength of attachment disproportionate to the frequency of his interaction with the baby. (p. 352)

Furthermore, there is evidence that individual differences in quality of infant–father attachment are related to paternal behavior: Infants are more likely to be securely attached to fathers who have been sensitively responsive to them (see Van IJzendoorn & De Wolff, 1997, for meta-analytic findings). Evidence has also emerged that siblings (Stewart & Marvin, 1984; Teti & Ablard, 1989) and day care providers (Ahnert, Pinquart, & Lamb, 2006) can serve as attachment figures. In unusual and stressful situations, infants can even become attached to other infants (see A. Freud & Dann's [1951] observations of child survivors of a concentration camp). Howes and Spieker (Chapter 15, this volume) provide an extensive discussion of multiple attachment figures.

Second, although there is usually more than one attachment figure, the potential number of attachment figures is not limitless. Bretherton (1980, p. 195) has described the infant as having a "small hierarchy of major caregivers," which is in contrast to the larger group of individuals with whom the infant has other sorts of relationships (Weinraub, Brooks, & Lewis, 1977). Marvin, VanDevender, Iwanaga, LeVine, and LeVine (1977) reported that most Hausa infants observed in Nigeria were attached to no more than three or four attachment figures; Grossmann and Grossmann (1991) reported similar observations for a sample of German infants.

Third, although most infants have multiple attachment figures, it is important not to assume that an infant treats all attachment figures as equivalent, or that they are interchangeable; rather, as mentioned earlier, an "attachment hierarchy" is thought to exist. According to Bowlby (1969/1982), "it is a mistake to suppose that a young child diffuses his attachment over many figures in such a way that he gets along with no strong attachment to anyone, and consequently without missing any particular person when that person is away" (p. 308). Bowlby proposed that this strong tendency for infants to prefer a principal attachment figure for comfort and security be termed "monotropy" (see also Ainsworth, 1964, 1982b).[6] Bowlby cited as evidence of this phenomenon the tendency of children in institutions to select, if given the opportunity, one "special" caregiver as their own (see Burlingham & Freud, 1944). Ainsworth (1982b, p. 19) described responses to major separations from and losses of attachment figures as further support for the idea that a hierarchy exists: "The child would tolerate major separations from subsidiary figures with less distress than comparable separations from the principal attachment figure. Nor could the presence of several attachment figures altogether compensate for the loss of the principal attachment figure."[7] (For similar findings, see Heinicke & Westheimer, 1966.)

Also consistent with this hierarchy notion are data from observational studies of both mothers and fathers, which show that most infants prefer to seek comfort from their mothers when distressed; in the mother's absence, however, an infant is likely to seek and derive comfort and security from other attachment figures as well (Kagan, Kearsley, & Zelazo, 1978; Lamb, 1976a, 1976b, 1978; Rutter, 1981; see also Ainsworth, 1967; Schaffer & Emerson, 1964). For a review of the relatively few experimental studies examining attachment hierarchies, and a discussion of the relevant methodological issues, see Colin (1996; for data and discussions of attachment hierarchies beyond infancy, see also Kobak, Rosenthal, & Serwik, 2005; Kobak, Rosenthal, Zajac, & Madsen, 2007; Rosenthal & Kobak, 2010).

What determines the structure of an infant's attachment hierarchy? Colin (1996) listed a likely set of contributing factors: "(1) how much time the infant spends in each figure's care; (2) the quality of care each provides, (3) each adult's emotional investment in the child, and (4) social cues" (p. 194).

Why would monotropy have evolved as a tendency of human infants? Neither Bowlby nor Ainsworth addressed this question. I propose three possibilities, all of which may operate simultaneously. The fact that there may be multiple ways in which the tendency toward monotropy contributes to infant survival and reproductive fitness increases the likelihood of its emerging through genetic selection. First, the infant's tendency to prefer a principal attachment figure may contribute to the establishment of a relationship in which that one attachment figure assumes principal responsibility for the child. Such a relationship should increase the child's likelihood of survival by helping to ensure that care of the child is not overlooked. This system seems more practical than the alternative, wherein a large number of caregivers have equal responsibility for a large number of offspring; this latter system might leave any individual child "falling between the cracks."

Second, monotropy may be most efficient for the child. When faced with danger, the child does not have to make a series of assessments and judgments about who may be most readily available, most responsive, and best suited to help. Rather, the child has a quick, automatic response to seek his or her principal attachment figure.

Third, monotropy may be the child's contribution to a process I term *reciprocal hierarchical bonding*, in which the child matches an attachment hierarchy to the hierarchy of the caregiving in his or her environment. Evolutionary biologists writing on parental investment (e.g., Trivers, 1972) have suggested that adults vary in their investment in offspring largely as a function of the extent to which this investment contributes to the transmission of the adults' genes (i.e., their reproductive fitness). Following this reasoning, it should be most adaptive for the child to use as a principal attachment figure the person who, correspondingly, is most strongly bonded to him or her (i.e., the person who provides the most parental investment and has the most to gain—in terms of reproductive fitness—from the baby's healthy development). In most cases, it is the biological mother who has the greatest biological investment in the child. With the exception of an identical twin, there is no one with whom the child shares more genes than the mother (50%). Although the biological father and siblings also share 50% of their genes with a child, their investments are nonetheless considered to be less because (1) only the mother can be certain of a true biological connection; (2) the mother devotes her body and bodily resources to the infant for 9 months of pregnancy and often nurses the child for a considerable period thereafter; and (3) the mother has fewer opportunities to produce additional offspring than fathers and siblings do.

If this process of reciprocal hierarchical bonding exists, it may help to explain not only monotropy, but also, in part, why the biological mother is generally the principal attachment figure.

The infant's selection of the principal attachment figure occurs over time, and it is important to consider why it takes a period of time for this centrally important attachment to crystalize rather than happening immediately, as it does in some other mammals. Jay Belsky (personal communication, October 15, 2007) has proposed two possible explanations, in addition to the obvious fact that human newborns do not possess the skills needed to form attachments because of their immature status at birth. First, the mother may not survive childbirth; many surely did not do so during our ancestral past. Second, the infant needs to be able to discern which individual is making the intensive investment upon which he or she is so dependent—a judgment that is likely to take some time.

Given the existence of multiple attachments, what is the course of their development across the lifespan? As noted earlier, two or three attachments usually develop during the infant's first year. These are usually with other family members or other people closely involved in the child's care. By middle childhood, when the child is spending more time with people outside the family, opportunities for new attachments may arise. In adolescence and young adulthood, individuals usually begin to develop attachments to sexual partners. Although attachments to parents typically remain throughout life, the later attachments may become the most central ones in the individual's adult life.

When considering multiple attachments, theorists are faced with several sets of questions. One of these has to do with similarities versus differences in quality across different attachments (i.e., concordance rate). To what extent are a child's attachments to different caregivers similar? Studies examining concordance rate yield inconsistent results. Some studies reveal independence of attachment across caregivers (Belsky & Rovine, 1987; Grossmann, Grossmann, Huber, & Wartner, 1981; Main & Weston, 1981); other studies reveal similarity of attachment across caregivers (Goossens & Van IJzendoorn, 1990; Steele, Steele, & Fonagy, 1996); and two meta-analytic studies have revealed significant but weak concordance between attachment to mother and attachment to father (Fox, Kimmerly, & Schafer, 1991; Van IJzendoorn & De Wolff, 1997; for additional discussion, see Berlin, Cassidy, & Appleyard, 2008).

Another question relates to the integration of multiple attachments. If a child's attachments are similar, he or she may develop a consistent set of internal working models of attachment figures, him- or herself, and relationships. Yet what if the child is faced with attachments that contribute to conflicting models? What if the child's experiences with one parent contribute to a model of the attachment figure as sensitively responsive and of the self as worthy of such care, but negative experiences with the other parent contribute to very different models? If differing models of attachment figures eventually become integrated, how does this happen? In relation to models of the self, Bretherton (1985) asked over two decades ago: "Is an integrated internal working model of the self built from participation in a number of nonconcordant relationships? If so, how and when? Or are self models, developed in different relationships, only partially integrated or sometimes not at all?" (p. 30). Researchers have made little progress in answering these questions.

Still another question about multiple attachments relates to the issue of how these different attachments influence children's functioning. It could be that the attachment to the principal attachment figure, usually the mother, is most influential. On the other hand, it could be that one attachment is most influential in some areas and another is most influential in other areas. Or perhaps having at least one secure attachment, no matter who the attachment figure is, serves as a protective factor to facilitate the child's functioning across areas. Relatively little empirical work has addressed these possibilities, given that most research examining the sequelae of attachment focuses only on infant–mother attachment. The research that is available suggests that when a child is securely attached to one individual and insecurely attached to another, the child behaves more competently when the secure relationship is with the mother than when it is with the other attachment figure (Easterbrooks & Goldberg, 1987; Howes, Rodning, Galluzzo, & Myers, 1988; Main et al., 1985; Main & Weston, 1981; Sagi-Schwartz & Aviezer, 2005). These same studies indicate, however, that the best-functioning individuals have two secure relationships, whereas the least competent children have none. Mesman and colleagues (Chapter 37, this volume) review the cross-cultural data and report similar evidence that multiple secure attachments enhance children's functioning; more extensive discussion of models of the influence of multiple attachments can be found in that chapter.

## Summary and Theoretical Extensions

This chapter has addressed the issues that Bowlby presented in his initial ethological approach to understanding the nature of a child's tie to the mother. Bowlby's observations led him to be dissatisfied with the explanations provided by existing theories and prompted him to consider alternative explanations. Drawing on the thinking of evolutionary biologists, cognitive scientists, control systems theorists, and developmental psychologists, he initiated what proved to be one of the earliest and most influential of the neo-Darwinian theories of evolutionary psychology, tackling the problem of the ways humans evolved to master the primary task of genetic transmission: survival through infancy and childhood to reproductive age (see Simpson & Belsky, Chapter 5, this volume).

For this third edition of the *Handbook of Attachment*, authors were asked to consider changes, or the lack thereof, that have occurred since earlier *Handbook* editions. Given the historical nature of this chapter, I approach this task in terms of considering current perceptions of the original theory. Perhaps one day I will write: "We now know that Bowlby's initial theory was incorrect in the following ways." This is not yet the case. Although it is likely I am plagued by the restricted vision that characterizes "insiders" in most fields, my view is that Bowlby and Ainsworth's original ideas have held up well, while providing a remarkably fruitful foundation for related ideas and studies.

Bowlby's original focus was on the then radical ideas about the evolutionary underpinnings of human attachments and the importance of individual variation in the quality of these attachments for subsequent development. Because Bowlby understandably devoted his attention to setting the foundations of his revolutionary ideas, he left considerable room for deeper examination of the underpinnings and connections of components of his theory, and extensions into new territory.

Although nothing that has emerged from the thousands of studies produced over the past 40 years has led to a serious challenge to the core theory, what has changed since the time of Bowlby's initial writings, and indeed during the 15 years since the initial edition of this handbook, is that subsequent theorists and researchers have extended and enriched Bowlby's thinking. I mention only a few of these extensions here.

Some of the most important theoretical advances relate to greater specificity of the *mecha-*

*nisms* through which early attachment experiences influence so many aspects of later child and adult functioning (see Thompson, Chapter 16, for discussion of these influences). As described earlier, the central mechanism on which Bowlby focused was the experience-based internal working model (IWM; see Bretherton & Munholland, Chapter 4, this volume). Yet despite his claim of the causal importance of IWMs, Bowlby never wrote a sole definitive work about this purported mechanism of influence. Rather, his formulation of the building, revising, and maintenance of IWMs is distributed across multiple works (Bowlby, 1969/1982, 1973, 1979, 1980a, 1988). Bretherton and Muholland (2008) noted that Bowlby's thinking about IWMs "was not a fully worked-out theory, but a promising conceptual framework to be filled in by others" (p. 103). Thus, subsequent theorists have offered varied conceptualizations of IWMs (Bretherton, 1990; Main et al., 1985; Thompson, 2006; Weinfield, Sroufe, Egeland, & Carlson, 2008; see Sherman et al., 2015, for theory and a review of research about infant capacities during the first year of life necessary to support the development of the IWM). Moreover, Bretherton's elegant analysis of how the capacities involved in the IWM are associated with neural processes is a substantial new contribution to the theoretical understanding of IWMs (Bretherton & Munholland, Chapter 4, this volume; see also Coan, Chapter 12, this volume).

Two other important theoretical extensions also relate to potential mechanisms linking early attachment experiences with later psychological functioning, one of which involves physiological processes. At the same time that experiences with caregivers are contributing to the formation of IWMs, they are also likely to set into motion a variety of nonrepresentational, physiological regulatory processes that play important roles in children's developing attachment systems. These physiological processes in turn can explain how early attachments come to influence child functioning, including greater understanding of the link between the attachment and fear behavioral systems. For instance, there is now evidence that experiences within the attachment relationship can influence the functioning of the hypothalamic–pituitary–adrenal (HPA) axis and child stress reactivity (Bernard & Dozier, 2010; Luijk et al., 2010; Nachmias, Gunnar, Mangelsdorf, Parritz, & Buss, 1996; Spangler & Grossmann, 1993; see Hane & Fox, Chapter 11, this volume). The fact that Bowlby paid relatively little attention to these infant physiological processes is surprising given that he studied medicine as an undergraduate stu-

dent at Cambridge, and given that the education about ethology that he received largely from Robert Hinde was so central to his early theorizing about why humans become attached to their caregivers. Yet Bowlby's focus on mental representations is understandable considering that much of his writing took place during a time when many branches of science were focused on the "cognitive revolution," and most of the research related to physiology in the mother–infant relationship in humans was not yet available. Attention to the role of noncognitive processes in explaining the link between early experience and later functioning, as well as the interconnections between cognitive and noncognitive processes, has grown in recent years; this focus extends Bowlby's theory to a new level of specificity without contradicting his initial perspective (Polan & Hofer, Chapter 6, this volume; see also Cassidy, Ehrlich, & Sherman, 2013).

A third mechanism through which early attachment experiences influence later functioning is emotion regulation. Although Bowlby talked extensively about emotions (and indeed the concept of IWM is thought to contain both cognitive and affective components), the concept of emotion regulation was not as well developed when Bowlby was writing as it is currently. The notion that children's emotion regulation capacities develop within the context of attachment relationships, and then mediate the link between attachment and social functioning, for both children and parents, is now widely accepted across developmental, clinical, neuroscience, and social psychological perspectives (Calkins & Leerkes, 2011; Cassidy, 1994; Thompson, 2013; see Shaver et al., Chapter 38, and Thompson, Chapter 16, both this volume).

The continued rigor of attachment theory requires that it be able to incorporate theoretical and empirical advances from other areas of science. I mention three of these, with a focus on infancy and childhood. First, because attachment theory is so firmly based in evolutionary theory, continuing revision of evolutionary theory brings with it a need to rethink some components of attachment theory. Simpson and Belsky (Chapter 5, this volume) focus on these considerations, and I do not review them here. Second, the recent conceptualization of genetically based differential susceptibility to environmental influence has implications for attachment theory. It is reasonable to expect that Bowlby, like most developmentalists of his time, assumed that environmental factors affect most children in similar ways; more recent theory and research suggest that this is not the case (Van

IJzendoorn, Belsky, & Bakermans-Kranenburg, 2012). Attachment theory can readily incorporate ideas of differential susceptibility (in this volume, see Bakermans-Kranenburg & Van IJzendoorn, Chapter 8, and Vaughn & Bost, Chapter 10, for discussions of attachment and the notion of differential susceptibility).

    Third, the empirical work most likely to have an important impact on the understanding of attachment is that concerning epigenetic processes. Just as Darwin speculated about genes while not understanding how they actually work, so Bowlby, while focusing on the environment, recognized the existence of a role for genes without understanding what this role might be. Certainly he did not realize that the environment could bring about changes in gene expression. It was not until Meaney's research (e.g., Caldji et al., 1998; Francis, Diorio, Liu, & Meaney, 1999) on maternal licking and grooming, and arched-back nursing, which affects the demethylation of genes related to receptor sites in the hippocampus, that scientists began to focus on environmental, including social, influences on genetic processes. The work of Meaney and his colleagues opened the door for research into what experiences contribute to the expression of particular genes in humans, and whether attachment experiences can moderate gene expression. Again, however, this exciting new development does not alter the main tenets of attachment theory.

    In summary, Bowlby and Ainsworth's initial ideas and the newer extensions of them, some of which I have mentioned here, have inspired the creation of the huge research literature discussed throughout this volume. The torrent of new ideas, studies, and research methods shows no sign of letting up, and it is likely to continue enriching rather than overturning attachment theory.

## Acknowledgments

The writing of this chapter was supported by Grant Nos. RO1-MH50773 from the National Institute of Mental Health and RO1-HD36635 from the National Institute of Child Health and Human Development.

## Notes

1. See Greenberg and Marvin (1982; also Ainsworth, 1989) for discussion of the advantages of the term *sociable system* rather than *affiliative system*. For data and more extensive discussion related to the interplay of the sociable system with other behavior sys-

tems, see Ainsworth and colleagues (1978), Bretherton (1978), Bretherton and Ainsworth (1974), Cassidy and Berlin (1999), and Greenberg and Marvin (1982).

2. This perspective differs somewhat from that of Bowlby (1969/1982, p. 240), who described "maternal retrieval behavior" as distinct from other parenting behavior, with the former having the predictable outcome of proximity and the biological function of protection. It is unclear, however, what for Bowlby would constitute a behavioral system. The position taken here is that retrieval is the parental equivalent to child proximity seeking; it is a behavior, not a behavioral system. The relevant behavioral system would be what here is called the "caregiving system," which includes a variety of behaviors, one of which is parental retrieval of the child. This perspective, along with that of Solomon and George (1996), also differs from the one proposed by Bretherton, Biringen, and Ridgeway (1991). Their view incorporates the notion of a "parental side of attachment," in which the parent's bond to the child is considered part of the attachment system, in part because of its great emotional power.

3. Within the modern evolutionary perspective, the existence of separate maternal and paternal caregiving systems is readily understood. Both mothers and fathers are concerned with their own reproductive fitness. Yet because mothers and fathers may differ substantially in the extent to which the survival of any one child enhances this fitness, their parenting behavior may differ. Compared to fathers, mothers have more to gain in terms of reproductive fitness from each child, for several reasons (e.g., mothers' certainty about parental status, shorter reproductive lifespan, longer interchild intervals, and greater energy expenditure per child during pregnancy and lactation; see Trivers, 1972).

4. Consensus is lacking about terminology related to the attachment bond. The description provided here is Ainsworth's (1989) and reflects Bowlby's most common usage. Yet in the second edition of the first volume of his trilogy, *Attachment and Loss*, Bowlby (1969/1982) described a bond as "a property of two parties," and labeled the child–parent bond as the "attachment–caregiving" bond (p. 377). In contrast to the implied notion of an "attachment relationship," Ainsworth (1982b) stated:

> That there is a "relationship" between mother and child, in Hinde's (1979) sense, from the time of the infant's birth onward, and that the nature of this relationship stems from the interaction between them, is not to be gainsaid, but neither the mother-to-infant bond nor the emergent infant-to-mother attachment seems to me to comprehend all the important aspects of this relationship. (p. 24)

Bretherton (1985) also pointed out the limits of considering an attachment to be a "property of two parties": "A representational view of relationships . . . underscores that the two partners have, in another sense, two relationships: the relationship as mentally represented by the attached person and by the attachment figure" (p. 34). Ainsworth (personal communication, June 15, 1986) suggested that the most appropriate way to consider an "attachment relationship" is as a "shorthand" designation for "a relationship in which the attachment component is central" (see also Ainsworth, 1990).

5. There has been some confusion over Bowlby's position on this issue. Lamb, Thompson, Gardner, and Charnov (1985), for instance, mistakenly stated, "Bowlby was firmly convinced that infants were initially capable of forming only one attachment bond" (p. 21). In fact, from his earliest writings on (1958, 1969/1982), Bowlby described the role of multiple attachment figures. Bowlby (1969/1982) noted that "it has sometimes been alleged that I have expressed the view . . . that mothering 'cannot be safely distributed among several figures' (Mead, 1962). No such views have been expressed by me" (p. 303).

6. Starting with his earliest writings, Bowlby (e.g., 1958) used the term *principal attachment-figure* or *mother-figure* rather than the term *mother*. This usage underscored Bowlby's belief that although this figure is usually the biological mother, it is by no means necessarily so. From the beginning, Bowlby recognized that the figure's status (father, adoptive parent, grandmother, aunt, nanny) is less important than the nature of the figure's interactions with the infant.

7. One of the most moving passages of Bowlby's writing illustrates how one attachment figure can be more centrally important to a child's well-being than others:

> About four weeks after mother had died, [4-year-old] Wendy complained that no one loved her. In an attempt to reassure her, father named a long list of people who did (naming those who cared for her). On this Wendy commented aptly, "But when my mommy wasn't dead I didn't need so many people—I needed just one." (Bowlby, 1980a, p. 280).

# References

Ahnert, L., Pinquart, M., & Lamb, M. E. (2006). Security of children's relationships with nonparental care providers: A meta-analysis. *Child Development, 74,* 664–679.

Ainsworth, M. D. S. (1963). The development of infant–mother interaction among the Ganda. In B. M. Foss (Ed.), *Determinants of infant behavior* (Vol. 2, pp. 67–112). New York: Wiley.

Ainsworth, M. D. S. (1964). Patterns of attachment behavior shown by the infant in interaction with his mother. *Merrill–Palmer Quarterly, 10,* 51–58.

Ainsworth, M. D. S. (1967). *Infancy in Uganda: Infant care and the growth of attachment.* Baltimore: Johns Hopkins University Press.

Ainsworth, M. D. S. (1972). Attachment and dependency: A comparison. In J. L. Gewirtz (Ed.), *Attachment and dependency* (pp. 97–137). Washington, DC: Winston.

Ainsworth, M. D. S. (1982a). *Attachment across the lifespan.* Unpublished lecture notes, University of Virginia, Charlottesville, VA.

Ainsworth, M. D. S. (1982b). Attachment: Retrospect and prospect. In C. M. Parkes & J. Stevenson-Hinde (Eds.), *The place of attachment in human behavior* (pp. 3–30). New York: Basic Books.

Ainsworth, M. D. S. (1989). Attachments beyond infancy. *American Psychologist, 44,* 709–716.

Ainsworth, M. D. S. (1990). Some considerations regarding theory and assessment relevant to attachments beyond infancy. In M. T. Greenberg, D. Cicchetti, & E. M. Cummings (Eds.), *Attachment in the preschool years: Theory, research, and intervention* (pp. 463–488). Chicago: University of Chicago Press.

Ainsworth, M. D. S., Bell, S. M., & Stayton, D. J. (1971). Individual differences in Strange-Situation behavior of one-year-olds. In H. R. Schaffer (Ed.), *The origins of human social relations* (pp. 17–52). New York: Academic Press.

Ainsworth, M. D. S., Blehar, M., Waters, E., & Wall, S. (1978). *Patterns of attachment: A psychological study of the Strange Situation.* Hillsdale: Erlbaum.

Ainsworth, M. D. S., & Wittig, B. A. (1969). Attachment and exploratory behaviour of one-year-olds in a strange situation. In B. M. Foss (Ed.), *Determinants of infant behaviour* (Vol. 4, pp. 111–136). London: Methuen.

Baldwin, M. W. (1992). Relational schemas and the processing of social information. *Psychological Bulletin, 112,* 461–484.

Belsky, J., Gilstrap, B., & Rovine, M. (1984). The Pennsylvania Infant and Family Development Project: I. Stability and change in mother–infant and father–infant interaction in a family setting at one, three, and nine months. *Child Development, 55,* 692–705.

Belsky, J., & Rovine, M. (1987). Temperament and attachment security within the Strange Situation: An empirical rapprochement. *Child Development, 58,* 787–795.

Bender, L., & Yarnell, H. (1941). An observation nursery. *American Journal of Psychiatry, 97,* 1158–1174.

Berlin, L. J., Cassidy, J., & Appleyard, K. (2008). The influence of early attachments on other relationships. In J. Cassidy & P. R. Shaver (Eds.), *Handbook of attachment: Theory, research, and clinical applications* (2nd ed., pp. 333–347). New York: Guilford Press.

Bernard, K., & Dozier, M. (2010). Examining infants' cortisol responses to laboratory tasks among children varying in attachment disorganization: Stress reactivity or return to baseline? *Developmental Psychology, 46,* 1771–1778.

Bowlby, J. (1944). Forty-four juvenile thieves: Their characters and home life. *International Journal of Psycho-Analysis, 25,* 19–52, 107–127.

Bowlby, J. (1956). The growth of independence in the young child. *Royal Society of Health Journal, 76,* 587–591.

Bowlby, J. (1958). The nature of the child's tie to his

mother. *International Journal of Psycho-Analysis, 39,* 350–373.

Bowlby, J. (1960a). Grief and mourning in infancy. *Psychoanalytic Study of the Child, 15,* 3–39.

Bowlby, J. (1960b). Separation anxiety. *International Journal of Psycho-Analysis, 41,* 1–25.

Bowlby, J. (1973). *Attachment and loss: Vol. 2. Separation: Anxiety and anger.* New York: Basic Books.

Bowlby, J. (1979). *The making and breaking of affectional bonds.* London: Tavistock.

Bowlby, J. (1980a). *Attachment and loss: Vol. 3. Loss: Sadness and depression.* New York: Basic Books.

Bowlby, J. (1980b). By ethology out of psycho-analysis: An experiment in interbreeding. *Animal Behavior, 28,* 649–656.

Bowlby, J. (1982). *Attachment and loss: Vol. 1. Attachment.* New York: Basic Books. (Original work published 1969)

Bowlby, J. (1984). Caring for the young: Influences on development. In R. S. Cohen, B. J. Cohler, & S. H. Weissman (Eds.), *Parenthood: A psychodynamic perspective* (pp. 269–284). New York: Guilford Press.

Bowlby, J. (1988). *A secure base.* New York: Basic Books.

Brazelton, T. B. (1977). Implications of infant development among the Mayan Indians of Mexico. In P. H. Leiderman, S. R. Tulkin, & A. Rosenfeld (Eds.), *Culture and infancy* (pp. 151–187). New York: Academic Press.

Bretherton, I. (1978). Making friends with one-year-olds: An experimental study of infant–stranger interaction. *Merrill–Palmer Quarterly, 24,* 29–52.

Bretherton, I. (1980). Young children in stressful situations: The supporting role of attachment figures and unfamiliar caregivers. In G. V. Coelho & P. I. Ahmed (Eds.), *Uprooting and development* (pp. 179–210). New York: Plenum Press.

Bretherton, I. (1985). Attachment theory: Retrospect and prospect. In I. Bretherton & E. Waters (Eds.), Growing points of attachment theory and research. *Monographs of the Society for Research in Child Development, 50*(1–2, Serial No. 209), 3–38.

Bretherton, I. (1990). Open communication and internal working models: Their role in the development of attachment relationships. In R. A. Thompson (Ed.), *Nebraska Symposium on Motivation: Vol. 36. Socioemotional development* (pp. 59–113). Lincoln: University of Nebraska Press.

Bretherton, I. (1991). Pouring new wine into old bottles: The social self as internal working model. In M. Gunnar & L. A. Sroufe (Eds.), *Minnesota Symposium on Child Psychology: Vol. 23. Self processes in development* (pp. 1–41). Hillsdale, NJ: Erlbaum.

Bretherton, I. (1992). The origins of attachment theory: John Bowlby and Mary Ainsworth. *Developmental Psychology, 28,* 759–775.

Bretherton, I., & Ainsworth, M. D. S. (1974). Responses of one-year-olds to a stranger in a strange situation. In M. Lewis & L. A. Rosenblum (Eds.), *The origins of fear* (pp. 131–164). New York: Wiley.

Bretherton, I., Biringen, Z., & Ridgeway, D. (1991). The parental side of attachment. In K. Pillemer & K. McCartney (Eds.), *Parent–child relations through life* (pp. 1–22). Hillsdale: Erlbaum.

Bretherton, I., & Munholland, K. A. (2008). Internal working models in attachment relationships: A construct revisited. In J. Cassidy & P. R. Shaver (Eds.), *Handbook of attachment: Theory, research, and clinical applications* (pp. 102–127). New York: Guilford Press.

Bronson, G. (1972). Infants' reactions to unfamiliar persons and novel objects. *Monographs of the Society for Research in Child Development, 37*(3, Serial No. 148), 1–46.

Burlingham, D., & Freud, A. (1944). *Infants without families.* London: Allen & Unwin.

Caldji, C., Tannenbaum, B., Sharma, S., Francis, D., Plotsky, P. M., & Meaney, M. J. (1998). Maternal care during infancy regulates the development of neural systems mediating the expression of fearfulness in the rat. *Proceedings of the National Academy of Sciences USA, 95,* 5335–5340.

Calkins, S. D., & Leerkes, E. M. (2011). Early attachment processes and the development of emotional self-regulation. In K. D. Vohs & R. F. Baumeister (Eds.), *Handbook of self-regulation: Research, theory, and applications* (2nd ed., pp. 355–373). New York: Guilford Press.

Carr, S. J., Dabbs, J., & Carr, T. S. (1975). Mother–infant attachment: The importance of the mother's visual field. *Child Development, 46,* 331–338.

Cassidy, J. (1994). Emotion regulation: Influences of attachment relationships. In N. Fox (Ed.), The development of emotion regulation. *Monographs of the Society for Research in Child Development, 59*(2–3, Serial No. 240), 228–249.

Cassidy, J., & Berlin, L. J. (1994). The insecure/ambivalent pattern of attachment: Theory and research. *Child Development, 65,* 971–991.

Cassidy, J., & Berlin, L. J. (1999). Understanding the origins of childhood loneliness: Contributions of attachment theory. In K. J. Rotenberg & S. Hymel (Eds.), *Loneliness in childhood and adolescence* (pp. 34–55). New York: Cambridge University Press.

Cassidy, J., Ehrlich, K. B., & Sherman, L. J. (2013). Child–parent attachment and response to threat: A move from the level of representation. In M. Mikulincer & P. R Shaver (Eds.), *Nature and development of social connections: From brain to group* (pp. 125–144). Washington, DC: American Psychological Association.

Cassidy, J., & Kobak, R. (1988). Avoidance and its relation to other defensive processes. In J. Belsky & T. Nezworski (Eds.), *Clinical implications of attachment* (pp. 300–323). Hillsdale, NJ: Erlbaum.

Cassidy, J., Woodhouse, S., Cooper, G., Hoffman, K., Powell, B., & Rodenberg, M. S. (2005). Examination of the precursors of infant attachment security: Implications for early intervention and intervention research. In L. J. Berlin, Y. Ziv, L. M. Amaya-

Jackson, & M. T. Greenberg (Eds.), *Enhancing early attachments: Theory, research, intervention, and policy* (pp. 34–60). New York: Guilford Press.

Colin, V. L. (1996). *Human attachment*. New York: McGraw-Hill.

De Wolff, M. S., & Van IJzendoorn, M. H. (1997). Sensitivity and attachment: A meta-analysis on parental antecedents of infant attachment. *Child Development, 68*, 571–591.

Dykas, M. J., & Cassidy, J. (2011). Attachment and the processing of social information across the lifespan: Theory and evidence. *Psychological Bulletin, 137*, 19–46.

Easterbrooks, A., & Goldberg, W. (1987, April). *Consequences of early family attachment patterns for later social–personality development*. Paper presented at the biennial meeting of the Society for Research in Child Development, Baltimore, MD.

Eisenberg, J. F. (1966). The social organization of mammals. *Handbuch Zoologie, 8*, 1–92.

Fox, N. A., Kimmerly, N. L., & Schafer, W. D. (1991). Attachment to mother/attachment to father: A meta-analysis. *Child Development, 62*, 210–225.

Francis, D. D., Diorio, J., Liu, D., & Meaney, M. J. (1999). Nongenomic transmission across generations of maternal behavior and stress response in the rat. *Science, 286*, 1155–1158.

Freud, A., & Dann, S. (1951). An experiment in group upbringing. *Psychoanalytic Study of the Child, 6*, 127–168.

Freud, S. (1957). Five lectures on psycho-analysis. In J. Strachey (Ed., & Trans.), *The standard edition of the complete psychological works of Sigmund Freud* (Vol. 11, pp. 3–56). London: Hogarth Press. (Original work published 1910)

Freud, S. (1964). An outline of psycho-analysis. In J. Strachey (Ed., & Trans.), *The standard edition of the complete psychological works of Sigmund Freud* (Vol. 23, pp. 139–207). London: Hogarth Press. (Original work published 1940)

George, C., & Solomon, J. (1996). Representational models of relationships: Links between caregiving and attachment. *Infant Mental Health Journal, 17*, 198–216.

George, C., & Solomon, J. (2008). The caregiving system: A behavioral systems approach to caregiving. In J. Cassidy & P. R. Shaver (Eds.), *Handbook of attachment: Theory, research, and clinical applications* (2nd ed., pp. 833–856). New York: Guilford Press.

Goldfarb, W. (1943). The effects of early institutional care on adolescent personality. *Journal of Experimental Education, 12*, 106–129.

Goossens, F. A., & Van IJzendoorn, M. (1990). Quality of infants' attachments to professional caregivers: Relations to infant–parent attachment and daycare characteristics. *Child Development, 61*, 832–837.

Greenberg, M., & Marvin, R. S. (1982). Reactions of preschool children to an adult stranger: A behavioral systems approach. *Child Development, 53*, 481–490.

Grossmann, K., & Grossmann, K. E. (1991). Newborn behavior, early parenting quality, and later toddler–parent relationships in a group of German infants. In J. K. Nugent, B. M. Lester, & T. B. Brazelton (Eds.), *The cultural context of infancy* (Vol. 2, pp. 3–38). Norwood, NJ: Ablex.

Grossmann, K. E., Grossmann, K., Huber, F., & Wartner, U. (1981). German children's behavior towards their mothers at 12 months and their fathers at 18 months in Ainsworth's Strange Situation. *International Journal of Behavioral Development, 4*, 157–181.

Harlow, H. F. (1958). The nature of love. *American Psychologist, 13*, 673–685.

Harlow, H. F. (1962). The development of affectional patterns in infant monkeys. In B. M. Foss (Ed.), *Determinants of infant behavior* (Vol. 1, pp. 75–88). New York: Wiley.

Harlow, H. F. (1969). Age-mate or affectional system. In D. S. Lehrman, R. A. Hinde, & E. Shaw (Eds.), *Advances in the study of behavior* (Vol. 2, pp. 334–383). New York: Academic Press.

Harlow, H. F., & Harlow, M. K. (1965). The affectional systems. In A. M. Schrier, H. F. Harlow, & F. Stollnitz (Eds.), *Behavior of non-human primates* (Vol. 2, pp. 287–334). New York: Academic Press.

Harlow, H. F., Harlow, M. K., & Hansen, E. W. (1963). The maternal affectional system of rhesus monkeys. In H. R. Rheingold (Ed.), *Maternal behavior in mammals* (pp. 254–281). New York: Wiley.

Hazan, C., & Zeifman, D. (1994). Sex and the psychological tether. In K. Bartholomew & D. Perlman (Eds.), *Advances in personal relationships: Vol. 5. Attachment processes in adulthood* (pp. 151–177). London: Jessica Kingsley.

Heinicke, C., & Westheimer, I. (1966). *Brief separations*. New York: International Universities Press.

Heller, K. A., & Berndt, T. J. (1981). Developmental changes in the formation and organization of personality attributions. *Child Development, 52*, 683–691.

Hinde, R. A. (1974). *Biological bases of human social behavior*. New York: McGraw-Hill.

Hinde, R. A. (1979). *Towards understanding relationships*. London: Academic Press.

Hinde, R. A. (1982). Attachment: Some conceptual and biological issues. In C. M. Parkes & J. Stevenson-Hinde (Eds.), *The place of attachment in human behavior* (pp. 60–70). New York: Basic Books.

Howes, C., Rodning, C., Galluzzo, D. C., & Myers, L. (1988). Attachment and child care: Relationships with mother and caregiver. *Early Childhood Research Quarterly, 3*, 703–715.

Huntingford, F. (1984). *The study of animal behavior*. London: Chapman & Hall.

Jones, J. D., Cassidy, J., & Shaver, P. R. (2015). Parents' self-reported attachment styles: A review of links with parenting behaviors, emotions, and cognitions. *Personality and Social Psychology Review, 19*, 14–76.

Kagan, J., Kearsley, R., & Zelazo, P. (1978). *Infancy: Its place in human development*. Cambridge, MA: Harvard University Press.

Kobak, R., Rosenthal, N., & Serwik, A. (2005). The

attachment hierarchy in middle childhood: Conceptual and methodological issues. In K. A. Kerns & R. A. Richardson (Eds.), *Attachment in middle childhood* (pp. 71–88). New York: Guilford Press.

Kobak, R., Rosenthal, N., Zajac, K., & Madsen, S. (2007). Adolescent attachment hierarchies and the search for an adult pair bond. *New Directions in Child and Adolescent Development, 117,* 57–72.

Kobak, R. R., & Duemmler, S. (1994). Attachment and conversation: Toward a discourse analysis of adolescent and adult security. In K. Bartholomew & D. Perlman (Eds.), *Advances in personal relationships: Vol. 5. Attachment processes in adulthood* (pp. 121–149). London: Jessica Kingsley.

Lamb, M. (1976a). Effects of stress and cohort on mother–infant and father–infant interaction. *Developmental Psychology, 12,* 435–443.

Lamb, M. (1976b). Interactions between two-year-olds and their mothers and fathers. *Psychological Reports, 38,* 447–450.

Lamb, M. (1978). Qualitative aspects of mother– and father–infant attachments. *Infant Behavior and Development, 1,* 265–275.

Lamb, M., Thompson, R. A., Gardner, W. P., & Charnov, E. L. (1985). *Infant–mother attachment.* Hillsdale, NJ: Erlbaum.

Lewis, M., Young, G., Brooks, J., & Michalson, L. (1975). The beginning of friendship. In M. Lewis & R. A. Rosenblum (Eds.), *Friendship and peer relations* (pp. 27–60). New York: Wiley.

Lorenz, K. E. (1935). Der Kumpan in der Umwelt des Vogels: Der Artgenosse als auslösendes Moment sozialer Verhaltungsweisen [The companion in the bird's world: The fellow-member of the species as releasing factor of social behavior]. *Journal of Ornithology, 83,* 137–213, 289–413.

Luijk, M. P. C. M., Saridjan, N., Tharner, A., Van IJzendoorn, M. H., Bakermans-Kranenburg, M. J., Jaddoe, et al. (2010). Attachment, depression, and cortisol: Deviant patterns in insecure-resistant and disorganized infants. *Developmental Psychobiology, 52*(5), 441–452.

Main, M. (1990). Cross-cultural studies of attachment organization: Recent studies, changing methodologies, and the concept of conditional strategies. *Human Development, 33,* 48–61.

Main, M., Hesse, E., & Kaplan, N. (2005). Predictability of attachment behavior and representational processes at 1, 6, and 19 years of age. In K. E. Grossmann, K. Grossmann, & E. Waters (Eds.), *Attachment from infancy to adulthood: The major longitudinal studies* (pp. 245–304). New York: Guilford Press.

Main, M., Kaplan, N., & Cassidy, J. (1985). Security in infancy, childhood, and adulthood: A move to the level of representation. In I. Bretherton & E. Waters (Eds.), Growing points of attachment theory and research. *Monographs of the Society for Research in Child Development, 50*(1–2, Serial No. 209), 66–104.

Main, M., & Weston, D. (1981). The quality of the toddler's relationship to mother and to father: Related to conflict behavior and the readiness to establish new relationships. *Child Development, 52,* 932–940.

Marvin, R. S., VanDevender, T. L., Iwanaga, M. I., LeVine, S., & LeVine, R. A. (1977). Infant–caregiver attachment among the Hausa of Nigeria. In H. McGurk (Ed.), *Ecological factors in human development* (pp. 247–259). Amsterdam: North Holland.

Mead, M. (1962). A cultural anthropologist's approach to maternal deprivation. In *Deprivation of maternal care: A reassessment of its effects* (Public Health Papers No. 14). Geneva, Switzerland: World Health Organization.

Mileva-Seitz, V. R., Bakermans-Kranenburg, M., & Van IJzendoorn, M. H. (in press). Genetic mechanisms of parenting. *Hormones and Behavior.*

Miller, R., Caul, W., & Mirsky, I. (1967). Communication of affect between feral and socially isolated monkeys. *Journal of Personality and Social Psychology, 7,* 231–239.

Morgan, G. A., & Ricciuti, H. N. (1969). Infants' responses to strangers during the first year. In B. M. Foss (Ed.), *Determinants of infant behaviour* (Vol. 4, pp. 253–272). London: Methuen.

Murray, H. A. (1938). *Explorations in personality.* New York: Oxford University Press.

Nachmias, M., Gunnar, M., Mangelsdorf, S., Parritz, R., & Buss, K. (1996). Behavioral inhibition and stress reactivity: The moderating role of attachment security. *Child Development, 67,* 508–522.

Passman, R. H., & Erck, T. W. (1977, March). *Visual presentation of mothers for facilitating play in childhood: The effects of silent films of mothers.* Paper presented at the biennial meeting of the Society for Research in Child Development, New Orleans, LA.

Passman, R. H., & Weisberg, P. (1975). Mothers and blankets as agents for promoting play and exploration by young children in a novel environment: The effects of social and nonsocial attachment objects. *Developmental Psychology, 11,* 170–177.

Piaget, J. (1954). *The construction of reality in the child.* New York: Basic Books.

Rheingold, H. (1969). The effect of a strange environment on the behaviour of infants. In B. M. Foss (Ed.), *Determinants of infant behaviour* (Vol. 4, pp. 137–166). London: Methuen.

Robertson, J., & Bowlby, J. (1952). Responses of young children to separation from their mothers. *Courrier du Centre International de l'Enfance, 2,* 131–142.

Rosenthal, N., & Kobak, R. R. (2010). Assessing adolescents' attachment hierarchies: Differences across developmental periods and associations with individual adaptation. *Journal of Research on Adolescence: 20,* 678–706.

Rutter, M. (1981). *Maternal deprivation reassessed* (2nd ed.). New York: Penguin.

Sagi-Schwartz, A., & Aviezer, O. (2005). Correlates of attachment to multiple caregivers in kibbutz children from birth to emerging adulthood: The Haifa longitudinal study. In K. E. Grossmann, K. Grossmann, & E. Waters (Eds.), *Attachment from infancy to adulthood: The major longitudinal studies* (pp. 165–197). New York: Guilford Press.

Schaffer, H. R., & Emerson, P. E. (1964). The development of social attachments in infancy. *Monographs of the Society for Research in Child Development, 29*(3, Serial No. 94), 1–77.

Sears, R. R., Maccoby, E. E., & Levin, H. (1957). *Patterns of child rearing.* Evanston, IL: Row, Peterson.

Sherman, L. J., Rice, K., & Cassidy, J. (2015). Infant capacities related to building internal working models of attachment figures: A theoretical and empirical review. *Developmental Review, 37,* 109–141.

Solomon, J., & George, C. (1996). Defining the caregiving system: Toward a theory of caregiving. *Infant Mental Health Journal, 17,* 183–197.

Sorce, J., & Emde, R. (1981). Mother's presence is not enough: Effect of emotional availability on infant explorations. *Developmental Psychology, 17,* 737–745.

Spangler, G., & Grossmann, K. E. (1993). Biobehavioral organization in securely and insecurely attached infants. *Child Development, 64,* 1439–1450.

Sroufe, L. A., & Waters, E. (1977). Attachment as an organizational construct. *Child Development, 48,* 1184–1199.

Steele, H., Steele, M., & Fonagy, P. (1996). Associations among attachment classifications of mothers, fathers, and their infants. *Child Development, 67,* 541–555.

Stewart, R., & Marvin, R. S. (1984). Sibling relations: The role of conceptual perspective-taking in the ontogeny of sibling caregiving. *Child Development, 55,* 1322–1332.

Teti, D., & Ablard, K. E. (1989). Security of attachment and infant–sibling relationships. *Child Development, 60,* 1519–1528.

Thompson, R. A. (2006). The development of the person: Social understanding, relationships, self, conscience. In W. Damon & R. M. Lerner (Series Eds.) & N. Eisenberg (Vol. Ed.), *Handbook of child psychology: Vol. 3. Social, emotional, and personality development* (6th ed., pp. 24–98). Hoboken, NJ: Wiley.

Thompson, R. A. (2013). The socialization of emotion and emotion regulation in the family. In J. J. Gross (Ed.), *Handbook of emotion regulation* (2nd ed., pp. 237–250). New York: Guilford Press.

Trivers, R. L. (1972). Parental investment and sexual selection. In B. Campbell (Ed.), *Sexual selection and the descent of man, 1871–1971* (pp. 136–179). Chicago: Aldine-Atherton.

Trivers, R. L. (1974). Parent–offspring conflict. *American Zoologist, 14,* 249–264.

Vandell, D. L. (1980). Sociability with peer and mother during the first year. *Developmental Psychology, 16,* 355–361.

Van IJzendoorn, M. H., Belsky, J., & Bakermans-Kranenburg, M. J. (2012). Serotonin transporter genotype 5HTTLPR as a marker of differential susceptibility?: A meta-analysis of child and adolescent gene-by-environment studies. *Translational Psychiatry, 2,* e147.

Van IJzendoorn, M. H., & De Wolff, M. S. (1997). In search of the absent father—meta-analyses of infant–father attachment: A rejoinder to our discussants. *Child Development, 68,* 604–609.

Vaughn, B. E., Waters, H. S., Coppola, G., Cassidy, J., Bost, K. K., & Verissimo, M. (2006). Script-like attachment representations and behavior in families and across cultures: Studies of parental secure base narratives. *Attachment and Human Development, 8,* 179–184.

Weinfield, N. S., Sroufe, L. A., Egeland, B., & Carlson, E. (2008). Individual differences in infant-caregiver attachment: Conceptual and empirical aspects of security. In J. Cassidy & P. R. Shaver (Eds.), *Handbook of attachment: Theory, research, and clinical applications* (2nd ed., pp. 78–101). New York: Guilford Press.

Weinraub, M., Brooks, J., & Lewis, M. (1977). The social network: A reconsideration of the concept of attachment. *Human Development, 20,* 31–47.

Weiss, R. S. (1982). Attachment in adult life. In C. M. Parkes & J. Stevenson-Hinde (Eds.), *The place of attachment in human behavior* (pp. 171–184). New York: Basic Books.

# Chapter 2

# Attachment Disruptions, Reparative Processes, and Psychopathology

## Theoretical and Clinical Implications

Roger Kobak
Kristyn Zajac
Stephanie D. Madsen

In the *Separation* volume of his attachment trilogy, Bowlby (1973) dramatically expanded his theory to account for the contribution of attachment processes to personality development, defensive processes, and psychopathology. In the first section, "Security, Anxiety, and Distress," he used young children's responses to separations to illustrate how a child's perception of a threat to a caregiver's availability elicits feelings of anxiety, anger, and sadness. The second section, "An Ethological Approach to Human Fear," highlighted how lack of access to an available caregiver amplifies the normal fear response to dangerous situations and contributes to pathological levels of fear and anxiety. The final section, "Individual Differences in Susceptibility to Fear: Anxious Attachment," considered how severe or prolonged threats to caregiver availability could contribute to anxious attachment. Bowlby posited that these attachment disruptions become internalized as working models, shape negative interpersonal expectancies, and increase risk for adult psychopathology. In many respects, the theoretical advances in the *Separation* volume established the framework for the next four decades of research on attachment and psychopathology.

We review in this chapter the three major theoretical advances in the *Separation* volume and their implications for the role of attachment in the development and maintenance of psychopathology. We begin with Bowlby's (1973) and Ainsworth's (1990) views that the attachment behavioral system monitors a caregiver's *availability and responsiveness*. This perspective dramatically shifted the focus of attachment research from the study of young children's separations from caregivers to investigations of the quality of *emotional communication* in maintaining attachment bonds. We stress that momentary threats to caregiver availability or responsiveness typically activate *reparative processes* that serve to restore confidence in the attachment bond. Second, Bowlby used young children's reactions to prolonged physical separations from caregivers as a prototype for explaining how more prolonged or severe threats to caregiver availability contribute to anxiety, defenses, and symptomatic expressions of attachment needs. We suggest that these more severe threats to caregiver availability or responsiveness represent a broader class of *attachment injuries or disruptions*. Furthermore, when these injuries remain unrepaired or unresolved, they increase an individual's vulnerability for psychopathology. Finally, Bowlby used working models or internalized expectancies for caregiver availability and responsiveness to explain both continuity and change in an individual's developmental pathway. We conclude with suggestions for how further investigation of emotional communication, attachment injuries, reparative processes and internalized expectancies for caregivers can guide clinical assessment and treatment of attachment problems experienced by young children, adolescents, and adults.

We note that in order to focus on these three theoretical advances of Bowlby's *Separation* volume, we omit major portions of our previous chapter in the second edition of the *Handbook of Attachment*. That earlier chapter (Kobak & Madsen, 2008) provided an account of the historical context that shaped the evolution of Bowlby's thinking and led up to his clarification of the attachment system's set-goal. Our account in that chapter also highlights Ainsworth's contributions to attachment theory. By translating theory into empirical observations and research methodology, Ainsworth tested and refined Bowlby's ideas and succeeded in communicating the core premises of attachment theory to a much wider audience. Readers interested in Bowlby and Ainsworth's contributions to the evolution of attachment theory may want to return to our earlier chapter.

## Emotionally Attuned Communication and Reparative Processes Maintain Secure Attachment Bonds

The *Separation* volume marked a critical shift in defining the set-goal of the attachment system. The early studies of young children's reactions to prolonged physical separations from their caregivers implied that the set-goal of the child's attachment system was monitoring simple physical proximity to a caregiver (Sroufe & Waters, 1977). However, by 3 or 4 years of age, physical separations no longer elicited the same reactions nor presented as serious a threat to the child's bond with a parent. Even in the case of infants, naturalistic observations provided compelling evidence that children monitored not only their caregivers' physical proximity but also their *responsiveness* or ability to provide protection and support during moments of danger, distress, or high need (Ainsworth, 1962). As a result, throughout the *Separation* volume,

Bowlby (1973) stressed a new and broader view of the attachment system. In addition to monitoring the caregivers' whereabouts and physical proximity, Bowlby referred to the attachment system as designed to continuously monitor the caregiver's *availability and responsiveness* (Bowlby, 1969/1982).

The expanded view of the child's attachment system shifted attention from observing reactions to separations to observing patterns of *emotional communication* in caregiver–child dyads. In Bowlby's (1969/1982) view, the child's emotions served essential motivational and communicative functions in maintaining the child's attachment setgoal within a comfortable range. For Ainsworth and the researchers who followed, the child's emotional signals and behaviors became a window to the attachment system and provided a context for observing caregiver sensitivity to those signals and behaviors (Ainsworth, Blehar, Waters, & Wall, 1978). When access to a sensitive caregiver was assured, infants could comfortably attend to other matters, such as exploring, affiliating, or resting. However, if the child became distressed, he or she would initiate behaviors to gain assurance and comfort from the caregiver. If efforts to reestablish contact failed or resulted in an insensitive response from the caregiver, infants would protest and direct *anger* toward the caregiver or, alternatively, develop avoidant strategies.

Careful consideration of the motivational and communicative functions of emotions allowed Ainsworth to make inferences about other behavioral systems, such as fear, exploration, and affiliation. As a result, a caregiver's interpretations of a child's displays of fear, anger, or sadness had to be understood as reflecting the child's goals in a particular context. In addition to monitoring a caregiver's availability and responsiveness, young children use emotions to signal how they monitor danger in the environment, explore new learning opportunities, and enjoy social exchanges. Fear signals the child's appraisal of danger, anger signals frustration at the interruption of an enjoyable or goal-directed activity, and sadness signals the child's despair at losing a desired toy or object. Ainsworth's sensitivity ratings focused on how caregivers attended to, interpreted, and responded to their infants' signals in a variety of contexts that took into account children's changing signals and motivational goals. Sensitivity to infant signals required caregivers continually to adapt their inferences about the child's emotional cues to account for the degree to which the child's attachment, exploration, and fear behavioral systems were activated (Ainsworth & Wittig, 1969). The interplay between the attachment and exploration systems was described as the infant's use of the mother as a "secure base" from which to explore. This balance between the attachment system, whose function is protection, and the exploration system, whose function is learning, provided a mechanism that allowed the child to learn and develop without straying too far away from the caregiver or remaining away for too long (Ainsworth et al., 1978).

Subsequent researchers have struggled with capturing the full complexity of Ainsworth's sensitivity construct and its ratings of acceptance–rejection, accessibility–ignoring, cooperation–interference, and sensitivity (Bretherton, 2013). For example, a caregiver might correctly interpret and respond to the child's signals of distress, yet fail to recognize the child's exploratory behaviors, resulting in an intrusive response. Another caregiver might be quite responsive to the child's exploratory activity but be averse to close bodily contact that would provide the child with a sense of comfort and protection when distressed. At the heart of Ainsworth's sensitivity construct was the notion that the caregiver could make accurate inferences about the child's emotional state and respond appropriately. To read an infant's signals accurately, make inferences about the infant's motivational states, and respond appropriately, caregivers need to adopt the child's perspective. This capacity for *empathic reading and responding* to an infant's changing needs and motivations has been described as *mentalizing* or accurately drawing inferences about the child's wishes, desires, and intentions (Sharp & Fonagy, 2008). This mentalizing capacity has been studied in terms of "mind-mindedness" or the caregiver's ability to understand accurately and comment on the child's mind (Meins, 2013). Research assessing individual differences in mentalizing capacities relies on what caregivers say when interacting with or discussing their child after watching brief replays of video clips featuring their child (Oppenheim & Koren-Karie, 2013).

## Emotionally Attuned Communication and Reparative Processes in Childhood and Adolescence

Efforts to study emotionally attuned communication with older children and adults require observ-ing interactions that test caregiver sensitivity and the child or adult's appraisals of the caregiver's availability and responsiveness. Because the attachment system is less frequently activated in older children and adults (Ainsworth, 1990), assessments of emotionally attuned communication can benefit from more structured laboratory or home observations. These paradigms can be designed to elicit interactions that allow observers to rate caregiver sensitivity and the child or adult's expectancies for caregiver availability and responsiveness. In many respects, these structured paradigms draw on particular aspects of daily interactions that Ainsworth observed in the home or village settings. *Safe haven episodes* provide a prototype for activating the attachment systems with cues to danger or threats to a caregiver's availability posed by brief physical separations. These episodes are defined by interactions in which the individual becomes distressed, injured, frightened, or endangered, and actively seeks comfort and protection from the caregiver. Some investigators have used intimidating laboratory equipment or discussions of distressing events to evaluate emotional communication (Simpson, Collins, Tran, & Haydon, 2007). From a behavioral systems perspective, these interactions represent the synchronous operation of the fear and attachment systems. Emotionally attuned interactions can be evaluated by attending to how the individual signals a need for contact and comfort, and the caregiver's response to those signals.

In contrast to safe haven episodes, *secure base episodes* are subtler and occur when the individual faces uncertainty in new or challenging situations. In these situations, an available and responsive caregiver typically responds with encouragement and support. From a behavioral systems perspective, these episodes require the individual to balance exploratory, fear, and attachment motivations in ways that use the caregiver as a resource to support new learning and master new challenges. These situations may become more salient at later phases of development as the individual becomes more self-reliant and less exposed to emergency situations that call for protective responses from the caregiver (Waters & Cummings, 2000). As a result, these types of interactions may play an increasingly important role in shaping the individual's expectancies or forecasts regarding his or her caregiver's availability and responsiveness beyond infancy.

Beginning in early childhood, interactions that require cooperative *negotiation of goal conflicts* play an increasingly important role in maintaining attachment bonds (Kobak & Duemmler, 1994). The nature of these goal conflicts changes with development. In early childhood, conflicts often involve coordinating the child's need for autonomy and self-assertion with the parent's goal of providing rules to ensure safety and encouraging the internalization of those rules to foster self-regulation (Kochanska & Murray, 2000). In adolescence, the child's need for autonomy must be coordinated with the caregiver's need to monitor, reduce risky behaviors, and ensure safety (Smetana, 2010). In adult attachment relationships, conflicts often center on managing finances, child-rearing differences, or communication. To maintain a "goal-corrected partnership," these goal conflicts require that both individuals engage in cooperative conversations (Bowlby, 1969/1982) that test each individual's capacity to communicate his or her own perspective while empathizing and reflecting on the partner's goals, needs, wishes, and desires. Observational coding of these conversations has consistently linked cooperative negotiation of differences to secure expectancies for caregiver availability and responsiveness (Allen, Moore, Kuperminc, & Bell, 1998; Kobak, Cole, Ferenz-Gillies, Fleming, & Gamble, 1993; Obsuth, Henninghausen, Brumariu, & Lyons-Ruth, 2014).

Momentary threats to caregiver availability or responsiveness present frequent challenges to maintaining emotionally attuned communication in attachment dyads. These momentary threats, including brief separations, goal conflicts, or competing demands on the caregiver's time and attention, are common in all attachment relationships. Furthermore, such threats typically initiate *reparative processes* that are motivated by a desire to reestablish contact and restore confidence in the relationship. To restore confidence in the caregiver effectively, the individual must directly signal distress and initiate contact; subsequently, the caregiver must accurately read these signals and empathically respond to the individual's need for contact and comfort. An attuned and timely caregiver response typically completes the reparative episode and restores confidence in the caregiver's availability and responsiveness. These *reparative episodes* have been well documented among infants and their caregivers. For instance, laboratory paradigms have used the "still face procedure" to test the infant's reaction to a nonresponsive caregiver (Tronick, 2007). In this procedure, after a period in which the infant becomes distressed and dysregulated, the caregiver and the infants quickly reestablish synchronous interaction, thus restoring

the child's confidence in the caregiver's availability. Ainsworth's Strange Situation also illustrates how the infant's confidence in the caregiver can be restored following the distress induced by being left alone in a strange environment (Ainsworth et al., 1978). Following this perceived threat to the caregiver's availability, secure children actively seek contact with the caregiver, effectively gain comfort, and restore their confidence in the caregiver's availability and responsiveness.

## Severe or Prolonged Disruptions, Defensive Process, and Psychopathology

States of anxiety and depression that occur during the adult years, and also psychopathic conditions, can, it is held, be linked in a systematic way to the states of anxiety, despair, and detachment described by Burlingham and Freud.

—JOHN BOWLBY (1973, pp. 4–5)

In contrast to the relatively brief threats to caregiver availability that typically activate repair processes, *attachment disruptions* are defined as prolonged or severe threats to a caregiver's availability or responsiveness that create fundamental fear and uncertainty about the caregiver's availability or capacity to respond in moments of danger. When disruptions remain unrepaired, the individual becomes vulnerable to persistent feelings of fear, anger, or sadness, and to defensive strategies that reduce the individual's ability to engage in emotionally attuned communication with caregivers. At moments of high stress, the defenses are likely to break down and result in symptomatic expressions of attachment needs and feelings. In contrast to common forms of insensitive care and insecure attachment, attachment disruptions represent severe threats to the attachment bond and constitute a significant risk for the development and maintenance of psychopathology.

### Dysfunctional Emotional and Defensive Responses to Attachment Disruptions

The mechanisms linking attachment disruptions to psychopathology can be found in Bowlby and Robertson's close observations of 2- to 4-year-old children's reactions to prolonged separations from their caregivers (e.g., Bowlby, Robertson, &

Rosenbluth, 1952; Robertson, 1953, 1962). Their descriptions provide a prototype for how disruptions elicit emotional reactions and defensive processes that impair relationship functioning and distort expressions of attachment needs. The observations documented how children's emotional reactions may become dysfunctional when they no longer serve a reparative function of signaling and eliciting a comforting response from a caregiver. These phases, labeled "protest," "despair," and "detachment," echoed many of the descriptions of children's responses to separation provided by other observers (e.g., Burlingham & Freud, 1944; Heinicke & Westheimer, 1966).

Protest is the initial phase, typically lasting from a few hours to a week or more. For example, in one of Bowlby's and Robertson's observations, protest began at the moment a parent prepared to leave a child at the nursery or hospital. The child signaled separation distress in a variety of ways, such as crying loudly, showing anger, following the mother, pounding the door, or shaking his or her cot. Any sight or sound might produce a temporary respite, as the child eagerly checked to see whether it was a sign of the mother's return. The dominant attitude during this phase was hope that the mother would return, and the child actively attempted to regain contact with her. During this phase, efforts by alternative adults to comfort or soothe the child typically were met with little success, and some children actively spurned potential caregivers. Although crying gradually subsided over time, it commonly recurred, especially at bedtime or during the night. Searching for the missing parent often continued on a sporadic basis over a number of days. During the protest phase, the dominant emotions were fear, anger, and distress. Fear and distress signaled a child's appraisal of danger at being separated from a primary attachment figure, while anger served to mobilize and sustain the child's efforts to reestablish contact with the mother.

The despair phase, which succeeded protest, was marked by behaviors suggesting increased hopelessness about the mother's return. Although a child might continue to cry intermittently, active physical movements diminished, and the child withdrew or disengaged from people in the environment. Bowlby (1973) compared this phase to deep mourning, in that the child interpreted the separation as a loss of the attachment figure. He suggested that adults often misinterpreted the reduced activity and withdrawal as signs of the child's recovery from the distress of separation. Sadness accompanied this withdrawn state. Heinicke and Westheimer (1966) also noted that hostile behavior, directed toward another child or toward a favorite object brought from home, tended to increase over time.

A child's active turning of attention to the environment marked the final phase, detachment. In this phase, the child no longer rejected alternative caregivers, and some children even displayed sociability toward other adults or peers. The nature of this phase became most evident during reunion with the mother. A child who reached the phase of detachment showed a striking absence of joy at the mother's return; instead of enthusiastically greeting her, the detached child was likely to appear apathetic. In the Heinicke and Westheimer (1966) study, varying degrees of detachment were reported among 10 children following separations that lasted from 12 days to 21 weeks. On their initial reunion, two of the children seemed not to recognize their mothers, and the other eight children either turned or walked away from their mothers. Children often alternated between crying and showing blank, expressionless faces. Some degree of detachment persisted following the reunions, with five of the mothers complaining that their children treated them like strangers. For many children, detachment and neutrality alternated with clinging and showing fear that the mother might leave again. Following the reunions, children appeared to feel frightened by home visits from observers they knew from the nursery.

## Attachment Disruptions among Older Children, Adolescents, and Adults

The phases of protest (anger), despair (sadness), and defensive detachment observed in young children's reactions to prolonged separations from their caregivers provided a prototype for understanding older children's and adults' emotional responses to other types of attachment disruptions. The dysregulated emotions, interpersonal difficulties, and symptomatic expressions that accompany severe threats to caregiver availability often contribute to psychopathology (e.g., Adam & Chase-Lansdale, 2002; Carlson, Egeland, & Sroufe, 2009; Kobak, Little, Race, & Acosta, 2001). Unfortunately, in many cases, the problematic reactions, feelings, and behaviors that result from attachment disruptions are often more evident than the threats to caregiver availability that contributed to those problems. As a result, the role that attachment disruptions play in the emergence of psychopathology may remain undetected by standard psychiatric assessments and procedures.

In reviewing the literature on older children, adolescents, and adults, it is useful to distinguish between two types of pathogenic attachment disruptions. One type is analogous to the threat to caregiver availability encountered by young children who experience prolonged separations. Although older children and adults are much less likely to perceive prolonged physical separation as a threat to the attachment bond, these individuals remain vulnerable to fears of abandonment or loss of a caregiver. Examples of these disruptions include unexplained separations, perceived loss of the caregiver through desertion or death, and lack of access to a caregiver in a moment of high need. The second type of attachment disruption results from a breakdown in the caregiving system that leads to nearly complete failure of the caregiver to provide protection and guidance. These disruptions represent severe threats to the caregiver's responsiveness and include abdication of the caregiving role, betrayal, and threatening or frightening behavior. Such threats allow the individual to develop strategies for maintaining the relationship with a caregiver who is physically available but unable to serve as a source of safety and protection.

### Severe or Prolonged Threats to Caregiver Availability

The perception of physical accessibility remains the most fundamental appraisal of an attachment figure's availability. With age, there are dramatic advances in the cognitive mapping of the attachment figure's whereabouts, the resources for seeking proximity, and the types of distal communication with the attachment figure. Although these advances make distance less of an obstacle to maintaining an attachment bond, the notion that the individual can reunite with the attachment figure if necessary remains a crucial aspect of the caregiver's availability. Furthermore, when lines of communication are closed or cut off, older children and adults can perceive physical separations as a major threat to maintaining an attachment bond. For instance, separations in which a caregiver leaves in an angry or unexplained manner may disrupt a child's ability to plan for reunion and leave the child uncertain about the parent's whereabouts. Bowlby (1973) cited a research study

by Newson and Newson (1968) describing how a 4-year-old had become anxious and clingy following her father's desertion of the family 3 months earlier. The child's mother speculated that her child's difficulty with staying at day care resulted from her fear that the mother would also not come back—a speculation supported by the child's repeatedly saying to the mother, "Do you love me? You won't leave me, Mummy, will you?" (Bowlby, 1973, p. 214).

Witnessing violence between parents may also threaten a child's confidence in the parents' availability (Davies & Cummings, 1995, 1998). The child's appraisal of marital violence is likely to include fear that harm may come to one or both parents. In addition, parents living with constant conflict and fear are likely to have reduced capacities to attend to the child. Thus, in addition to fear of harm to the parents, attachment anxiety is increased by uncertainty about the parents' ability to respond to the child's distress and the lack of open communication with both parents. Even in situations with less extreme conflict, parents who become emotionally disengaged from one other and decide to separate or divorce may create fears in the child that the parents will also decide to leave the child. The notion that a parent may leave and not return creates a fundamental threat to physical accessibility. Most parents who divorce make efforts to communicate with the child and reassure the child of their continued availability, which substantially reduces the perceived threat (Bretherton, 1995; see also B. C. Feeney & Monin, Chapter 40, this volume).

Hostile verbal communication creates additional possibilities for attachment disruptions. For instance, without actually leaving, a parent can threaten to leave or to send the child away. Such behavior may occur in disciplinary contexts when the parent has become angry and exasperated with the child. As an example, Bowlby quoted a mother from the Newson and Newson (1968; emphasis added) study:

"I used to threaten him with the Hartley Road Boys' Home, which isn't a Home anymore; and since then, I haven't been able to do it; but I can always say I shall go down town and see about it you know. And Ian says, "Well, if I'm going with Stuart (7) it won't matter"; so I say, "Well, you'll go to different ones— you'll go to one Home, and *you'll* go to another." But it really got him worried, you know, and I really got him ready one day and I thought I'll take him a walk round, *as if* I was going, you know, and he really *was* worried. In fact, I had to bring him home, he started to cry. He saw I was in earnest about it—he *thought* I was, anyway. And now I've only got to threaten him. I say "It won't take me long to get you ready.'"

It is difficult to document the frequency of such statements because many parents are ashamed to admit them to researchers. However, in his review of parenting studies, Bowlby reported that the incidence of such statements was as high as 27% in the Newson and Newson (1968) study of families in England and 20% in a study of parents in the United States (Sears, Maccoby, & Levin, 1957).

Threats of suicide by a desperate parent may elicit even greater anxiety about the parent's availability. In addition to the obvious threat to the parent's physical accessibility, the child is faced with the fear of violence and the prospect of loss. These threats often occur in the context of hostile and conflict-filled relations, which may create the impression that the child's angry feelings toward the parent are responsible for the parent's desperation and despair. Bowlby noted that many children are not only exposed to threats of suicide, but may also actually witness suicide attempts. A parent may also make statements that attribute responsibility for future abandonment to the child. Statements to the child, such as "You will be the death of me," or threats of abandonment that follow a child's misbehavior are likely to confound attachment-related fears with feelings of guilt. This kind of attribution not only shakes the child's confidence in the parent's availability but also leads to negative perceptions of the self.

Over 400,000 children in the United States currently experience prolonged physical separations from biological parents (Zeanah, Shauffer, & Dozier, 2011). Because foster care families have replaced residential nurseries for children removed from the care of their biological parents, new questions about the effects of attachment disruptions with biological parents and the potential formation of bonds to foster parents have been investigated (Stovall-McClough & Dozier, 2004; see Dozier & Rutter, Chapter 30, this volume). These studies suggest that infants and young children in foster care will display attachment behaviors toward their new caregivers within the first few weeks of placement; however, it is uncertain whether such behaviors necessarily indicate the formation of an attachment bond because they do not predict the long-term stability of the placement. In contrast, the foster parent's "commitment" to the foster child measured early in the relationship is a strong predictor of the long-term stability of the placement and of adoption (Dozier & Lindhiem, 2006). These findings illustrate that assessment of foster parents' feelings of commitment to the child yield a better prediction of bond formation than either home or laboratory assessments of the foster child's attachment behavior. The importance of maintaining an enduring attachment bond is further highlighted by a prospective study of foster and maltreated children. Higher rates of behavior problems were found in children who had been placed in foster care compared with children who remained placed with maltreating caregivers, with whom they presumably had maintained an attachment bond (Lawrence, Carlson, & Egeland, 2006). Children who enter the child welfare system not only experience prolonged separation from their biological parents but also face the challenge of repairing the bonds with biological parents or developing an attachment with an alternative caregiver.

## Severe or Chronic Threats to Caregiver Responsiveness

The complete absence of an appropriate caregiving response in situations that normally call for nurturance or guidance constitutes a severe threat to confidence in the caregiver's responsiveness to the child's attachment needs. Main and Solomon (1986) first called attention to this type of disruption when they observed a relatively small group of infants who showed unusual behaviors in the Strange Situation, marked by fear, freezing, and disorientation. They assigned these infants to a new classification: "disorganized/disoriented" (D).

The infant D classification has been consistently linked to a variety of adjustment difficulties and to psychopathology (Groh, Roisman, Van IJzendoorn, Bakermans-Kranenburg, & Fearon, 2012; Lyons-Ruth & Jacobvitz, Chapter 29, this volume). In a 6-year longitudinal study, children who were classified as D in infancy developed aggressive behavior problems in preschool and elementary school at much higher rates than other children (Lyons-Ruth, 1996; Lyons-Ruth, Alpern, & Repacholi, 1993; Moss, Cyr, & Dubois-Comtois, 2004; Moss et al., 2006). Longitudinal data from the Minnesota Longitudinal Project indicate that the infant D classification predicts adjustment problems consistently from childhood through adolescence, and that it specifically predicts dissociative symptoms (Carlson, 1998; Sroufe, 2005).

Main and Hesse (1990) traced infants' disorganized behavior to children's perceptions of their caregivers as "frightened or frightening," signaling severe threats to caregiver responsiveness. A potential explanation for caregivers' difficulty in responding to their children's attachment needs was uncovered in interviews about their own childhoods. Parents of D infants showed unusual difficulties discussing loss and trauma during the Adult Attachment Interview (AAI; Hesse & Main, 2006; see Hesse, Chapter 26, this volume). These difficulties were evident from momentary lapses in "monitoring discourse or reason" that included disorientation, loss of monitoring of discourse, and reports of extreme behavioral reactions. The internal focus of these parents, resulting from their own preoccupation with unresolved loss and traumatic experience, was thought to interfere drastically with their capacity to respond to their infants (Main & Hesse, 1990).

Subsequent researchers have further investigated the links among caregiver behavior, severe threats to a caregiver's responsiveness, and disorganized attachment among older children and adolescents (Solomon & George, 2011). Prolonged failure to respond appropriately to the child's needs has been described by George and Solomon (2008) as *caregiver abdication*. This term describes a general breakdown in the caregiving system that includes frightening, maltreating, neglecting, or failing to protect children. These caregiving failures are thought to result from caregivers being flooded and overwhelmed by their own fears, resulting in feelings of helplessness in caring for their children. As children mature, they develop new capacities to manage the feelings of confusion, fear, anger, and sadness that accompany perceptions of the caregiver as frightened or frightening. As a result, older children who perceive severe threats to caregiver responsiveness may develop "controlling strategies" for managing their relationship with the caregiver. These strategies may reduce the child's feelings of confusion and helplessness and provide more predictable interactions with the caregiver that ensure maintenance of the attachment bond. Two types of controlling/disorganized strategies have been observed in caregiver–child interactions: a controlling–hostile pattern and a controlling–caregiving pattern (Lecompte & Moss, 2014; Main & Cassidy, 1988; Obsuth et al., 2014; Solomon & George, 2011; Zanetti, Powell, Cooper, & Hoffman, 2011; see also Solomon & George, Chapter 18, this volume). These patterns have been consistently associated with increased risk for child and adolescent psychopathology.

In addition to the disorganized patterns observed in caregiver–child dyads, severe threats to caregiver responsiveness may also undermine trust and communication in adult attachment relationships. For instance, disruptions in adult relationships are often marked by intense negative affect and by the adults' feelings of helplessness and anger in attempting to respond to their partners' needs. A common dysfunctional pattern of interaction occurs when one partner rigidly pursues the other in a manner that is perceived as critical or nagging, and the partner responds by emotionally disengaging. Such disengagement can take a variety of forms, including contemptuous or aloof responses, silent stonewalling, or actual physical withdrawal from the partner (Gottman, 1994). Although this disengagement may be an effort to escape from a painful interaction, it paradoxically heightens anxious and angry feelings associated with a perceived threat to the partner's availability or responsiveness (Johnson & Greenman, 2006; see Brassard & Johnson, Chapter 35, this volume). Unfortunately, fear of losing the partner or of being hurt is often mixed with defensive anger. As a result, events that have been perceived as threats to the partner's availability or responsiveness are often hidden behind cycles of blame and defensive responses that dominate much of a distressed couple's interactions.

## Internal Working Models: Continuity and Change in Developmental Pathways

Bowlby (1973) viewed the transaction between the individual's internal working models and the caregiving environment as the central dynamic that shapes an individual's developmental pathway from infancy through adulthood (Kobak, Cassidy, Lyons-Ruth, & Ziv, 2006). His developmental pathways model accounted for both continuity and change in adaptation. Continuity in a developmental pathway was maintained by internalized expectations for caregiver availability and responsiveness that in turn shaped the individual's interpretation of behavior with caregivers and partners in close relationships. Confident expectancies in a caregiver's availability tended to promote adaptive functioning, while negative or insecure expectancies tended to leave an individual vulnerable to subsequent difficulties. The model also allowed for changes in a pathway. For instance, changes in the caregiving environment could alter an individual pathway in both positive and negative directions, leading to subsequent revisions in an individual's internal model. Attachment disruptions in childhood, adolescence, or adulthood could have profound effects in shifting an individual's trajectory regarding relationship difficulties and psychopathology.

## Internal Working Models and Attachment Disruptions

Bowlby posited internal working models as a mechanism through which interactions with caregivers are internalized. These "working models" or expectancies forecast the caregiver's availability and responsiveness, and allow individuals to adapt their communications with caregivers to assure maintenance of the attachment bond. Expectancies form the core of internal working models and anticipate how the caregiver will respond in variety of contexts given the individual's changing needs and goals. A child who experiences consistent responses that are attuned to his or her changing motivational states will develop confident expectancies in the caregiver's availability and responsiveness. These expectancies conform to a "secure base script" that anticipates how attachment-related events with a particular caregiver typically unfold (e.g., "If I am distressed, I can go to my mother and she will comfort me"; Bretherton & Munholland, 2008; Cassidy, Jones, & Shaver, 2013; Mikulincer, Shaver, Sapir-Lavid, & Avihou-Kanza, 2009; Waters & Rodrigues-Doolabh, 2001; Waters & Waters, 2006).

Internal working models that are organized by secure base scripts provide individuals with valuable resources for coping with attachment disruptions. Secure expectancies predispose individuals toward openly signaling their needs and assuming that these signals will elicit a timely and effective caregiver response. As a result, emotions are more likely to serve their adaptive functions of motivating effective behavior and signaling needs to others. This sense of emotional efficacy in turn allows individuals to develop confidence to explore new situations and master new skills. Thus, nonattachment motivational systems such as exploration and affiliation can take precedence over attachment concerns to facilitate new learning and social interaction (Waters & Cummings, 2000). Older adolescents and adults who have developed the internal resources associated with secure internal working models are likely to show more resilience when they encounter a threat to caregiver availability, as well as a reduced risk for developing psy-

chopathology (Carlson et al., 2009). In contrast, those with insecure internal models may be particularly vulnerable to attachment disruptions and at greater risk for emotional and defensive reactions that undermine relational functioning and increase symptomatic expressions of attachment needs.

Ainsworth's patterns of attachment in the Strange Situation provided initial evidence for the development and assessment of internal working models. Her laboratory observations demonstrated that, by 1 year of age, infants had begun to internalize expectancies for caregiver availability and responsiveness, subsequently organizing how they communicated and behaved toward the caregiver when they were distressed. Later researchers (e.g., Bretherton, 1985; Main, Kaplan, & Cassidy, 1985) extended the assessment of internal models to older children and adults (see Bretherton & Munholland, Chapter 4, this volume). Many of the assessments designed to infer expectancies for caregiver availability and responsiveness share a common strategy of eliciting narratives of events that would typically activate the attachment system and lead an individual to seek protection or comfort from the caregiver. The AAI uses structured prompts designed to elicit memories of times when an individual would normally need comfort or support from the caregiver. Other assessments rely on projective methods or word prompts to generate narratives that can be coded for their degree of adherence to or deviation from the secure base script. Expectancies for caregiver responsiveness can be inferred at the level of behavior or by observing how individuals communicate when they are distressed or in need of support (Kobak & Duemmler, 1994).

Much of the research that followed Ainsworth's work assumed considerable continuity in internal working models from infancy through adulthood (Kobak & Zajac, 2011). Although longitudinal research generally yielded some support for the continuity hypothesis, these effects tend to be quite modest and suggest that internal working models are open to considerable change and revision between early childhood and late adolescence (Booth-LaForce et al., 2014; Haydon, Roisman, Owen, Booth-LaForce, & Cox, 2014; Sroufe, Egeland, Carlson, & Collins, 2005). This substantial instability highlights the need to consider how ongoing experiences in attachment relationships, as well as an individual's exposure to attachment disruptions, may create "lawful discontinuities" in internal working models. In Bowlby's view, internal working models become not only more complex over the course of childhood and adolescence but also more resistant to change. However, even in adulthood, these models may be amenable to change resulting from new experiences in relationships with partners.

The internal working model concept is essential to understanding the resources an individual brings to coping with attachment disruptions. Expectancies that organize the internal working model that predate the disruption can amplify or reduce the response to the disruption and its impact on relationship functioning and psychopathology. Individuals with secure internal models (organized by confident expectancies for caregiver availability) are likely to bring more resources to interpreting and coping with the relationship disturbance. Not only does a secure internal model enable the individual to cope more effectively, but it is also likely to facilitate more direct emotionally attuned communication with caregivers. The capacity for communicating vulnerable emotions and attachment needs may be very useful in gaining comfort and protection from alternative caregivers or in signaling the individual's need to restore confidence in the disrupted relationship. In situations where alternative caregivers are not available, the confident expectancies and emotional self-efficacy that characterize a secure model may be useful in helping the individual understand the source of the disruption and to maintain resilience in managing attachment-related distress. Unfortunately, the effects of attachment disruptions such as loss or trauma often co-occur with insecure models and expectancies for insensitive care (Zajac & Kobak, 2009). As a result, the insecure models will amplify problematic reactions to attachment disruptions. These models are more likely to activate defensive processes resulting in distorted and symptomatic expression of the anger, fear, and sadness that accompany severe threats to caregiver availability or responsiveness.

## The Caregiver's Capacity for Repairing Attachment Disruptions

The caregiver's capacity to empathize and respond sensitively to feelings of hurt, anger, and sadness is the other major factor that moderates the impact of attachment disruptions on relationship functioning and psychopathology. Efforts to assess the contributions of the caregiving environment to continuity and change in developmental pathways have lagged behind efforts to measure internal working models. The degree to which a caregiver's ability or inability to provide sensitive care remains stable across development requires further

study, as does the chronic versus transitory nature of factors that overwhelm caregivers and lead to abdication of the caregiving role. The caregiver's capacity to restore trust following an attachment disruption is premised on the notion that the caregiver can recover from (or effectively manage) the factors that produced the disruption. Examples of events that are more amenable to recovery include a caregiver's serious illness or hospitalization, psychological or substance abuse disorders that lead to treatment or remission, and major transitions in adult relationships (e.g., separation and divorce) that allow the caregiver to reestablish a stable support network. Factors that are more chronic and less amenable to recovery include economic adversity, personality disorders that undermine stable relationship functioning, and repeated exposure to loss and/or trauma (Kobak, Cassidy, & Ziv, 2004).

When a caregiver can overcome or manage the adversity that contributed to separation from the child or caregiving abdication, repair is possible. For instance, if an available and responsive caregiver were able to attend to the relationship following a disruption, the disruption could be repaired and confidence in a caregiver's availability and responsiveness restored. The caregiver's central challenges in repairing a disrupted attachment are understanding and empathizing with the child's injured feelings, even when those feelings may be hidden by defensive detachment or expressed in angry and distorted ways that initially distance the caregiver. Responding to these challenges tests the caregiver's ability to be the stronger and wiser person in a damaged relationship (Zanetti et al., 2011). Whereas reestablishing contact and effectively gaining comfort from the primary caregiver might repair some disruptions, other disruptions may be resolved by establishing or strengthening an attachment relationship with an alternative caregiver. These efforts are likely to be most successful when supported by other adults in the caregiver's life or possibly by help from a professional therapist or coach.

## Therapeutic Change: Repairing or Resolving Attachment Disruptions

Attachment-based therapies share the common goal of increasing security in attachment relationships, so that those relationships can serve as a resource for helping the individual to manage major sources of stress more effectively. These treatments may target the caregiver and the caregiver's capacity to empathize with the child, emotionally attuned communication in the attachment dyad, and the child or adult's internal working model of the caregiver (Kobak, Zajac, Herres, & Krauthamer-Ewing, 2015). The extent to which attachment disruptions are implicated in attachment-based treatments vary along a continuum (Kobak et al., 2006). On one end are individuals with secure or mildly insecure relationships who encounter severe stress or adversity and require support in managing these problems. These individuals have not likely been exposed to a major disruption, and treatments can focus on improving communication. On the other end of the continuum are individuals who have experienced prolonged or severe threats to caregiver availability and responsiveness, and have developed rigid defenses that distort expressions of attachment needs and feelings. These individuals may require more supportive exploration of attachment disruptions and internal working models in order to repair negative expectancies and defensive reactions that accompany the disruption.

Bowlby (1988) wrote most extensively about individual therapy with adults. The goal of his approach was (1) to provide a secure base from which to access painful expectancies regarding caregiver availability that had been shut away from conscious processing and (2) to allow the client to test the validity of those expectancies in light of current experience. This type of treatment often begins by linking symptomatic expressions of fear and anger to disturbances in attachment relationships. In doing so, a clinician can help the client experience and integrate painful experiences to gain control over symptoms. Accessing previously avoided experiences makes it possible for the individual to update working models and reduce defensively distorted emotions that contribute to miscued communication. Although this description of adult therapy focuses on intrapersonal working models, intrapersonal change is premised on the notion that the interpersonal relationship with the therapist provides a model of open communication about attachment-related experiences (see Slade, Chapter 33, this volume).

## Treatments for Caregivers of Young Children

Two of the major attachment-based therapies for young children provide support for caregivers on both ends of the continuum of attachment disturbances and child psychopathology. The Attachment and Biobehavioral Catch-Up (ABC) program focuses on identifying, commenting on,

and reinforcing caregiver sensitivity at moments when the child needs comfort; in this way, parents are encouraged to take initiative in the interaction (Bernard et al., 2012; Bernard, Meade, & Dozier, 2013). This intervention has proven effective at increasing caregivers' ability to respond sensitively to children's signals for nurturance and reciprocal interaction in ways that produce enhanced biological regulation for the child. Similarly, the Circle of Security project encourages caregivers to explore how their internal worlds shape their perceptions and reactions to their child (Marvin, Cooper, Hoffman, & Powell, 2002; Powell, Cooper, Hoffman, & Marvin, 2013). In doing so, the intervention is intended to enhance caregivers' capacities for self-regulation, self-awareness of filters that interfere with accurately reading the child's signals, and empathic attunement and response to the child's attachment and exploratory signals. Research has demonstrated the effectiveness of the Circle of Security in changing children's attachment classifications from disorganized to organized (Hoffman, Marvin, Cooper, & Powell, 2006). Other attachment interventions such as toddler–parent psychotherapy focus more on the impact of parents' working models derived from childhood experience on current parent–child interactions (Lieberman, 1992). This approach has produced increased attachment security in a randomized trial with mothers diagnosed with major depressive disorder (Toth, Gravener-Davis, Guild, & Cicchetti, 2013; see Berlin, Zeanah, & Lieberman, Chapter 32, this volume, for a review of early intervention programs designed to enhance attachment security).

## Attachment-Based Treatment for Adolescents and Adults

Adolescents and adults have established internal working models that have become more resistant to change over the course of development, thus complicating attachment-based therapy. Furthermore, the negative expectancies that organize internal models are often distorted by well-established defensive strategies that make attachment needs and feelings less apparent to caregivers or therapists. The challenge for attachment-based therapists is to support caregivers in seeing beyond these defensive processes to underlying attachment needs. Connect, a group program for the caregivers of antisocial adolescents, approaches this problem with an extensive 10-session program designed to direct caregivers' attention to adolescents' hidden attachment needs (Moretti & Obsuth, 2009). In doing so, the curriculum encourages an empathic shift in caregivers that recognizes adolescents' vulnerability and allows for more attuned responding to adolescents' attachment and autonomy needs.

Attachment-based family therapy (ABFT) is designed to uncover adolescents' attachment disruptions or threats to caregiver availability or responsiveness in order to structure a reparative conversation with the caregiver (Diamond et al., 2010). ABFT was designed to treat depressed and suicidal adolescents, using the adolescent's suicidal despair to understand why the he or she could not rely on the caregiver at a moment of distress. After eliciting attachment narratives that support negative expectancies for caregiver availability or responsiveness, the therapist prepares the adolescent to discuss these episodes directly with the caregiver. Caregivers are given advance preparation to support a validating and empathic stance toward the adolescent's vulnerability and attachment needs. The goals of the reparative conversation are to allow the adolescent to signal attachment needs directly and to encourage the caregiver to shift from seeing a depressed and suicidal adolescent to seeing a child in need of understanding, protection, and comfort. Once the therapist establishes a reparative conversation, treatment centers on conversations about the adolescent's challenges and difficulties outside the family, allowing the caregiver to provide a secure base for understanding and support.

Attachment-based marital therapists face similar challenges in treating distressed couples. Marital distress is presumed to be motivated by fears about a partner's availability and responsiveness. As a result, the therapist is faced with the challenge of uncovering "attachment injuries" or perceived threats to a partner's availability and responsiveness (Kobak, Hazan, & Ruckdeschel, 1994; see also Brassard & Johnson, Chapter 35, this volume). Shifting from an externally focused attentional set, in which a partner is viewed as primarily a source of danger, to a more internally focused awareness of the fear and distress caused by the threat to the attachment relationship can be a critical step in marital therapy. When the fears that accompany perceived threats to a partner's availability are openly communicated, the high level of conflict and disengagement found in distressed marriages can be deescalated (Johnson, 1996, 2003). Johnson's approach uses emotion-focused techniques to help distressed partners access attachment fears and vulnerabilities that are

hidden behind angry and defensive interaction sequences. This approach has produced increased levels of marital satisfaction in the majority of couples completing treatment (Makinen & Johnson, 2006; see also Brassard & Johnson, Chapter 35, this volume).

## Summary

Bowlby's *Separation* volume established the framework for understanding how disturbances in attachment relationships are implicated in the development and maintenance of psychopathology. Although insensitive care and insecure attachment have provided much of the focus for attachment research in nonclinical populations, Bowlby was concerned with more extreme breakdowns in caregiving that we have termed "attachment disruptions." These severe or prolonged threats to a caregiver's availability or responsiveness activate defensive process and symptomatic expressions of attachment-related anger, fear, and sadness that severely compromise an individual's ability to cope with normal stressful and developmental challenges. Caregivers and therapists who work with individuals who have experienced attachment disruptions can use Bowlby's framework to assess the nature of the disruption, determine the degree to which disturbance is implicated in presenting problems, and, most importantly, to develop treatment designed to repair or resolve injuries resulting from attachment disruptions.

## References

Adam, E. K., & Chase-Lansdale, P. L. (2002). Home sweet home(s): Parental separations, residential moves, and adjustment problems in low-income adolescent girls. *Developmental Psychology, 38,* 792–805.

Ainsworth, M. D. S. (1962). The effects of maternal deprivation: A review of findings and controversy in the context of research strategy. In *Deprivation of maternal care: A reassessment of its effects* (p. 97). Geneva, Switzerland: World Health Organization.

Ainsworth, M. D. S. (1990). Some considerations regarding theory and assessment relevant to attachments beyond infancy. In M. T. Greenberg, D. Cicchetti, & E. M. Cummings (Eds.), *Attachment in the preschool years* (pp. 463–488). Chicago: University of Chicago Press.

Ainsworth, M. D. S., Blehar, M. C., Waters, E., & Wall, S. (1978). *Patterns of attachment: A psychological study of the Strange Situation.* Hillsdale, NJ: Erlbaum.

Ainsworth, M. D. S., & Wittig, B. A. (1969). Attachment and exploratory behavior of one-year-olds in a strange situation. In B. M. Foss (Ed.), *Determinants of infant behaviour* (Vol. 4, pp. 129–173). London: Methuen.

Allen, J. P., Moore, C., Kuperminc, G., & Bell, K. (1998). Attachment and adolescent psychosocial functioning. *Child Development, 69*(5), 1406–1419.

Bernard, K., Dozier, M., Bick, J., Morrarty, E. L., Lindhiem, O., & Carlson, E. (2012). Enhancing attachment organization among maltreated children: Results of a randomized clinical trial. *Child Development, 83*(2), 623–636.

Bernard, K., Meade, E. B., & Dozier, M. (2013). Parental synchrony and nurturance as targets in an attachment based intervention: Building upon Mary Ainsworth's insights about mother–infant interaction. *Attachment and Human Development, 15*(5–6), 507–523.

Booth-LaForce, C., Groh, A. M., Burchinal, M. R., Roisman, G. I., Owen, M. T., & Cox, M. J. (2014). Caregiving and contextual sources of continuity and change in attachment security from infancy to late adolescence. *Monographs of the Society for Research in Child Development, 79*(3), 67–84.

Bowlby, J. (1973). *Attachment and loss: Vol. 2. Separation: Anxiety and anger.* New York: Basic Books.

Bowlby, J. (1982). *Attachment and loss: Vol. 1. Attachment.* New York: Basic Books. (Original work published 1969)

Bowlby, J. (1988). *A secure base: Parent–child attachment and healthy human development.* New York: Basic Books.

Bowlby, J., Robertson, J., & Rosenbluth, D. (1952). A two-year-old goes to hospital. *Psychoanalytic Study of the Child, 7*, 82–94.

Bretherton, I. (1985). Attachment theory: Retrospect and prospect. In I. Bretherton & E. Waters (Eds.), Growing points of attachment theory and research. *Monographs of the Society for Research in Child Development, 50*(1–2, Serial No. 209), 3–35.

Bretherton, I. (1995). A communication perspective on attachment relationships and internal working models. *Monographs of the Society for Research in Child Development, 60*(2–3), 310–329.

Bretherton, I. (2013). Revisiting Mary Ainsworth's conceptualization and assessments of maternal sensitivity–insensitivity. *Attachment and Human Development, 15*(5–6), 460–484.

Bretherton, I., & Munholland, K. A. (2008). Internal working models in attachment relationships: Elaborating a central construct in attachment theory. In J. Cassidy & P. R. Shaver (Eds.), *Handbook of attachment: Theory, research, and clinical applications* (pp. 102–127). New York: Guilford Press.

Burlingham, D., & Freud, A. (1944). *Infants without families.* London: Allen & Unwin.

Carlson, E. A. (1998). A prospective longitudinal study of disorganized/disoriented attachment. *Child Development, 69*, 1107–1128.

Carlson, E. A., Egeland, B., & Sroufe, L. A. (2009). A prospective investigation of the development of borderline personality symptoms. *Development and Psychopathology, 21*(4), 1311–1334.

Cassidy, J., Jones, J. D., & Shaver, P. R. (2013). Contributions of attachment theory and research: A framework for future research, translation, and policy. *Development and Psychopathology, 25*(4, Pt. 2), 1415–1434.

Davies, P. T., & Cummings, E. M. (1995). Children's emotions as organizers of their reactions to interadult anger: A functionalist perspective. *Developmental Psychology, 31*(4), 677–684.

Davies, P. T., & Cummings, E. M. (1998). Exploring children's emotional security as a mediator of the link between marital relations and child adjustment. *Child Development, 69*(1), 124–139.

Diamond, G. S., Wintersteen, M. B., Brown, G. K., Diamond, G. M., Gallop, R., Shelef, K., et al. (2010). Attachment-based family therapy for adolescents with suicidal ideation: A randomized controlled trial. *Journal of the American Academy of Child and Adolescent Psychiatry, 49*(2), 122–131.

Dozier, M., & Lindhiem, O. (2006). This is my child: Differences among foster parents in commitment to their young children. *Child Maltreatment, 11*, 338–345.

George, C., & Solomon, J. (2008). The caregiving system: A behavioral systems approach to parenting. In J. Cassidy & P. R. Shaver (Eds.), *Handbook of attachment: Theory, research, and clinical applications* (pp. 833–856). New York: Guilford Press.

Gottman, J. (1994). *What predicts divorce?* Hillsdale, NJ: Erlbaum.

Groh, A. M., Roisman, G. I., Van IJzendoorn, M. H., Bakermans-Kranenburg, M. J., & Fearon, R. P. (2012). The significance of insecure and disorganized attachment for children's internalizing symptoms: A meta-analytic study. *Child Development, 83*(2), 591–610.

Haydon, K. C., Roisman, G. I., Owen, M. T., Booth-LaForce, C., & Cox, M. J. (2014). VII. Shared and distinctive antecedents of Adult Attachment Interview state-of-mind and inferred-experience dimensions. *Monographs of the Society for Research in Child Development, 79*(3), 108–125.

Heinicke, C., & Westheimer, I. (1966). *Brief separations.* New York: International Universities Press.

Hesse, E., & Main, M. (2006). Frightened, threatening, and dissociative parental behavior in low-risk samples: Description, discussion, and interpretations. *Development and Psychopathology, 18*, 309–343.

Hoffman, K. T., Marvin, R. S., Cooper, G., & Powell, B. (2006). Changing toddlers' and preschoolers' attachment classifications: The Circle of Security intervention. *Journal of Consulting and Clinical Psychology, 74*, 1017–1026.

Johnson, S. M. (1996). *Creating connection: The practice of emotionally focused marital therapy.* New York: Brunner/Mazel.

Johnson, S. M. (2003). Attachment theory: A guide for couple therapy. In S. M. Johnson & V. E. Whiffen (Eds.), *Attachment processes in couple and family therapy* (pp. 103–123). New York: Guilford Press.

Johnson, S. M., & Greenman, P. S. (2006). The path to a secure bond: Emotionally focused couple therapy. *Journal of Clinical Psychology, 62,* 597–609.

Kobak, R., Cassidy, J., Lyons-Ruth, K., & Ziv, Y. (2006). Attachment, stress and psychopathology: A developmental pathways model. In D. Cicchetti & D. Cohen (Eds.), *Handbook of developmental psychopathology* (pp. 333–369). New York: Cambridge University Press.

Kobak, R., Cassidy, J., & Ziv, Y. (2004). Attachment-related trauma and posttraumatic stress disorder: Implications for adult adaptation. In J. A. Simpson & W. S. Rholes (Ed.), *Adult attachment: Theory, research, and clinical implications* (pp. 388–407). New York: Guilford Press.

Kobak, R., Cole, H. E., Ferenz-Gillies, R., Fleming, W. S., & Gamble, W. (1993). Attachment and emotion regulation during mother–teen problem solving: A control theory analysis. *Child Development, 64*(1), 231–245.

Kobak, R., Hazan, C., & Ruckdeschel, K. (1994). From symptom to signal: An attachment view of emotion in marital therapy. In S. M. Johnson & L. Greenberg (Eds.), *Emotions in marital therapy* (pp. 46–71). New York: Brunner/Mazel.

Kobak, R., Little, M., Race, E., & Acosta, M. C. (2001). Attachment disruptions in seriously emotionally disturbed children: Implications for treatment [Special issue]. *Attachment and Human Development, 3,* 243–258.

Kobak, R., & Madsen, S. (2008). Disruptions in attachment bonds: Implications for theory, research and clinical intervention. In J. Cassidy & P. R. Shaver (Eds.), *Handbook of attachment: Theory, research, and clinical applications* (2nd ed., pp. 88–105). New York: Guilford Press.

Kobak, R., & Zajac, K. (2011). Rethinking adolescent states of mind: A relationship/lifespan view of attachment and psychopathology. In D. Cicchetti & G. I. Roisman (Eds.), *Minnesota Symposium on Child Psychology: The origins and organization of adaptation and maladaptation* (pp. 185–229). Hoboken, NJ: Wiley.

Kobak, R., Zajac, K., Herres, J., & Krauthamer-Ewing, S. (2015). Attachment based treatments for adolescents: The secure cycle as a framework for assessment, treatment and evaluation. *Attachment and Human Development, 17*(2), 220–239.

Kobak, R. R., & Duemmler, S. (1994). Attachment and conversation: A discourse analysis of goal-corrected partnerships. In K. Bartholomew & D. Perlman (Eds.), *Advances in personal relationships: Vol. 5. Attachment processes in adulthood* (pp. 121–149). London: Jessica Kingsley.

Kochanska, G., & Murray, K. T. (2000). Mother–child mutually responsive orientation and conscience development: From toddler to early school age. *Child Development, 71,* 417–431.

Lawrence, C. R., Carlson, E. A., & Egeland, B. (2006). The impact of foster care on development. *Development and Psychopathology, 18,* 57–76.

Lecompte, V., & Moss, E. (2014). Disorganized and controlling patterns of attachment, role reversal, and caregiving helplessness: Links to adolescents' externalizing problems. *American Journal of Orthopsychiatry, 84*(5), 581–589.

Lieberman, A. (1992). Infant–parent psychotherapy with toddlers. *Development and Psychopathology, 4,* 559–574.

Lyons-Ruth, K. (1996). Attachment relationships among children with aggressive behavior problems: The role of disorganized early attachment patterns. *Journal of Consulting and Clinical Psychology, 64,* 64–73.

Lyons-Ruth, K., Alpern, L., & Repacholi, B. (1993). Disorganized infant attachment classification and maternal psychosocial problems as predictors for hostile–aggressive behavior in the preschool classroom. *Child Development, 64,* 572–585.

Main, M., & Cassidy, J. (1988). Categories of response to reunion with the parent at age six: Predictable from infant attachment classifications and stable over a 1-month period. *Developmental Psychology, 24,* 415–426.

Main, M., & Hesse, E. (1990). Parents' unresolved traumatic experiences are related to infant disorganized attachment status: Is frightening and/or frightened parental behavior the linking mechanism? In M. T. Greenberg, D. Cicchetti, & E. M. Cummings (Eds.), *Attachment in the preschool years* (pp. 121–160). Chicago: University of Chicago Press.

Main, M., Kaplan, N., & Cassidy, J. (1985). Security in infancy, childhood and adulthood: A move to the level of representation. In I. Bretherton & E. Waters (Eds.), Growing points of attachment theory and research. *Monographs of the Society for Research in Child Development, 50*(1–2, Serial No. 209), 66–104.

Main, M., & Solomon, J. (1986). Discovery of a new, insecure disorganized/disoriented attachment pattern. In T. B. Brazelton & M. Yogman (Eds.), *Affective development in infancy* (pp. 95–124). Norwood, NJ: Ablex.

Makinen, J. A., & Johnson, S. M. (2006). Resolving attachment injuries in couples using emotionally focused therapy: Steps toward forgiveness and reconciliation. *Journal of Consulting and Clinical Psychology, 74,* 1055–1064.

Marvin, R., Cooper, G., Hoffman, K., & Powell, B. (2002). The Circle of Security project: Attachment-based intervention with caregiver-pre-school child dyads. *Attachment and Human Development, 4*(1), 107–124.

Meins, E. (2013). Sensitive attunement to infants' internal states: Operationalizing the construct of mind-mindedness. *Attachment and Human Development, 15*(5–6), 524–544.

Mikulincer, M., Shaver, P. R., Sapir-Lavid, Y., & Avihou-Kanza, N. (2009). What's inside the minds of securely and insecurely attached people?: The secure-base script and its associations with attachment-style dimensions. *Journal of Personality and Social Psychology*, 97(4), 615–633.

Moretti, M., & Obsuth, I. (2009). Effectiveness of an attachment-focused manualized intervention for parents of teens at risk for aggressive behaviour: The Connect Program. *Journal of Adolescence, 32*, 1347–1357.

Moss, E., Cyr, C., & Dubois-Comtois, K. (2004). Attachment at early school age and developmental risk: Examining family contexts and behavior problems of controlling-caregiving, controlling-punitive, and behaviorally disorganized children. *Developmental Psychology, 40*, 519–532.

Moss, E., Smolla, N., Cyr, C., Dubois-Comtois, K., Mazzarello, T., & Berthiaume, C. (2006). Attachment and behavior problems in middle childhood as reported by adult and child informants. *Development and Psychopathology, 18*, 425–444.

Newson, J., & Newson, E. (1968). *Four years old in an urban community*. Chicago: Aldine.

Obsuth, I., Hennighausen, K., Brumariu, L. E., & Lyons-Ruth, K. (2014). Disorganized behavior in adolescent–parent interaction: Relations to attachment state of mind, partner abuse, and psychopathology. *Child Development*, 85(1), 370–387.

Oppenheim, D., & Koren Karie, N. (2013). The insightfulness assessment: Measuring the internal processes underlying maternal sensitivity. *Attachment and Human Development*, 15(5-6), 545–561.

Powell, B., Cooper, G., Hoffman, K., & Marvin, B. (2013). *The Circle of Security Intervention: Enhancing attachment in early parent–child relationships*. New York: Guilford Press.

Robertson, J. (1953). *A two-year-old goes to hospital: A scientific film record* (film). Nacton, UK: Concord Film Council.

Robertson, J. (1962). *Hospitals and children: A parent's eye view*. New York: Gollancz.

Sears, R. R., Maccoby, E., & Levin, H. (1957). *Patterns of child rearing*. Evanston, IL: Row, Peterson.

Sharp, C., & Fonagy, P. (2008). The parent's capacity to treat the child as a psychological agent: Constructs, measures and implications for developmental psychopathology. *Social Development*, 17(3), 737–754.

Simpson, J. A., Collins, W. A., Tran, S., & Haydon, K. C. (2007). Attachment and the experience and expression of emotions in romantic relationships: A developmental perspective. *Journal of Personality and Social Psychology, 92*, 355–367.

Smetana, J. G. (2010). *Adolescents, families, and social development*. Hoboken, NJ: Wiley.

Solomon, J., & George, C. (2011). *Disorganized attachment and caregiving*. New York: Guilford Press.

Sroufe, L. A. (2005). Attachment and development: A prospective, longitudinal study from birth to adulthood. *Attachment and Human Development, 7*, 349–367.

Sroufe, L. A., Egeland, B., Carlson, E. A., & Collins, W. A. (2005). Placing early attachment experiences in developmental context. In K. Grossmann, K. E. Grossmann, & E. Waters (Eds.), *Attachment from infancy to adulthood: The major longitudinal studies* (pp. 48–97). New York: Guilford Press.

Sroufe, L. A., & Waters, E. (1977). Attachment as an organizational construct. *Child Development, 48*, 1184–1199.

Stovall-McClough, K. C., & Dozier, M. (2004). Forming attachments in foster care: Infant attachment behaviors during the first 2 months of placement. *Development and Psychopathology, 16*, 253–271.

Toth, S. L., Gravener-Davis, J. A., Guild, D. J., & Cicchetti, D. (2013). Relational interventions for child maltreatment: Past, present, and future perspectives. *Development and Psychopathology, 25*(4, Pt. 2), 1601–1617.

Tronick, E. (2007). *The neurobehavioral and social–emotional development of infants and children*. New York: Norton.

Waters, E., & Cummings, E. M. (2000). A secure base from which to explore close relationships. *Child Development, 71*(1), 164–172.

Waters, H. S., & Rodrigues-Doolabh, L. (2001, March). *Are attachment scripts the building blocks of attachment representations*. Paper presented at the biennial meeting of the Society for Research in Child Development, Washington, DC.

Waters, H. S., & Waters, E. (2006). The attachment working models concept: Among other things, we build script-like representations of secure base experiences. *Attachment and Human Development, 8*(3), 185–197.

Zajac, K., & Kobak, R. (2009). Caregiver unresolved loss and abuse and child behavior problems: Intergenerational effects in a high-risk sample. *Development and Psychopathology, 21*(1), 173–187.

Zanetti, C. A., Powell, B., Cooper, G., & Hoffman, K. (2011). The Circle of Security intervention: Using the therapeutic relationship to ameliorate attachment security in disorganized dyads. In J. Solomon & C. George (Eds.), *Disorganized attachment and caregiving* (pp. 318–342). New York: Guilford Press.

Zeanah, C. H., Shauffer, C., & Dozier, M. (2011). Foster care for young children: Why it must be developmentally informed. *Journal of the American Academy of Child and Adolescent Psychiatry, 50*(12), 1199–1201.

# Chapter 3

# Attachment, Loss, and Grief
## Bowlby's Views, New Developments, and Current Controversies

R. Chris Fraley
Phillip R. Shaver

For most of his life, evolutionary theorist Charles Darwin—one of John Bowlby's intellectual heroes—suffered from a perplexing set of symptoms, including recurrent and persistent gastric pains, nausea, and heart palpitations. These are common symptoms of hyperventilation syndrome, a condition that can be triggered by trauma, stress, or bereavement. In Bowlby's (1990) final book, *Charles Darwin: A New Life*, he attributed Darwin's symptoms to suppressed and unresolved grief following the death of his mother when he was 8 years old. Bowlby emphasized that Darwin's father did not allow his children to speak about their deceased mother following her death, and that Darwin suffered fainting spells and other signs of hyperventilation from then on.

Bowlby believed that the suppression of grief inhibits a sequence of painful emotional reactions that, unless allowed to run their natural course, can lead to psychological and physical ill health. Although his final book was primarily concerned with understanding Darwin's loss in particular, Bowlby had been deeply concerned with the psychological consequences of loss more generally throughout his own career. In his first empirical study, Bowlby (1946) argued that loss of a primary attachment figure is a predisposing factor in juve-

nile delinquency. Decades later, in his landmark trilogy, *Attachment and Loss*, bereavement and grief were the focus of the entire third volume, *Loss: Sadness and Depression* (Bowlby, 1980).

Although Bowlby's ideas about grief changed over the course of his career, he continued to view loss of an attachment figure as an important influence on personality development. He considered suppressed and unresolved grief to be pathogenic forces, and portrayed grief itself as a natural feature of what he called the "attachment behavioral system"—a system "designed" by natural selection to discourage prolonged separation of an individual from his or her primary attachment figures (see Cassidy, Chapter 1, this volume).

Our main aim in this chapter is to summarize Bowlby's contributions to the study of bereavement. In addition, we review research, theoretical developments, and controversies that have emerged recently in the study of bereavement, and we discuss the implications of these developments for attachment theory. We begin with a brief overview of the volume *Loss: Sadness and Depression*. We discuss Bowlby's thoughts about the function and course of mourning, patterns of "disordered" mourning, and how these patterns may be products of the way the attachment system is orga-

40

nized. We then discuss recent themes in the study of bereavement that are inspired by or relevant to Bowlby's theory. Specifically, we discuss recent criticisms that the phases of grief that Bowlby discussed were too rigid. Next, we discuss current controversies concerning complicated grief and whether it is distinct from other psychological disorders. We also review how these controversies are playing out in diagnostic reform efforts. Next, we review debates about the absence of grief and how recent research on patterns of bereavement can be integrated with Bowlby's ideas to provide a more nuanced view of what the relative absence of grief does and does not reveal about psychological adaptation. We also review empirical research on how individual differences in attachment organization are related to grief reactions and highlight what we consider to be some of the advances in this area, as well as the gaps that require further research. We also return to the issue of continuing bonds—a theme that was discussed in depth in the 1999 and 2008 editions of this chapter. Finally, we review a recent theoretical model of bereavement that integrates many of Bowlby's ideas concerning bereavement with emerging themes in the study of autobiographical memory, identity, and complicated grief reactions.

## An Attachment Perspective on Separation and Bereavement

Bowlby's thoughts on loss and grief were developed over several decades, but they were expressed most completely in his 1980 volume, in which he addressed a wide range of issues (e.g., whether children are capable of grieving, and whether they can harbor multiple conflicting representations of loss events). Two of Bowlby's aims are particularly relevant to this chapter. First, he wished to show that seemingly irrational or "immature" reactions to loss, such as disbelief, anger, searching, and sensing the continued presence of a lost attachment figure, are understandable when viewed from an ethological or evolutionary perspective. Second, he wished to show that how an individual responds to loss stems partly from the way his or her attachment system has become organized over time. He thought that people whose attachment systems are organized in such a way that they chronically anticipate rejection and loss (i.e., those who are anxious with respect to attachment concerns) or defensively suppress attachment-related feelings

(i.e., avoidant or compulsively self-reliant individuals) are likely to suffer from psychological and physical distress following bereavement.

## The Function and Course of Mourning in Infancy and Adulthood

One of Bowlby's most important contributions to the literature on bereavement was his ethological perspective on attachment and loss. He observed that in order to survive, infants of many species require protection and care from older individuals. To obtain this protection, evolution has resulted in infants having several physical adaptations (e.g., large eyes and facial expressions of emotion) and behavioral adaptations (e.g., crying and reaching) that attract and hold the attention of potential caregivers. In addition to these more basic adaptations, infants possess a motivational system (the attachment system) designed by natural selection to regulate and maintain proximity between infants and their caregivers (see Cassidy, Chapter 1, this volume). When an attachment figure is judged to be sufficiently available and responsive, an infant is thought to experience what Sroufe and Waters (1977) called *felt security*, allowing the infant to explore the environment and engage in playful social interactions. In contrast, when the attachment figure is judged to be inaccessible or unresponsive, the infant experiences anxiety and vigorously attempts to reestablish contact by protesting, searching, approaching, and clinging.

The following passage illustrates the protest of a 16-month-old girl after learning that her father would be leaving her in the nursery for an extended time.

> When Dawn sensed that her father was leaving, she again whined "Mm, mm, mm," and as he got up she broke into a loud cry and clutched him around the neck. Father became upset, put her down and tried to console her. . . . As he was departing through the door, she almost knocked her head on the floor. When the nurse picked her up, she continued to scream but later comforted herself by sucking her finger and some candy. (Heinicke & Westheimer, 1965, pp. 94–95)

According to Bowlby (1969/1982), these "protest" reactions are biologically functional because in the environment of evolutionary adaptedness they would have kept infants close to their protective attachment figures (see also Archer, 1999). This natural anxiety and yearning for an attachment figure motivate continued searching and calling until either success is attained or all efforts are exhausted. Viewed in this light, many of the seemingly perplexing reactions to separation and loss (e.g., continuing to yearn and search even when a lost caregiver is objectively irretrievable) appear more reasonable and, in many situations, adaptive. By doing everything possible to prevent the loss of attachment figures or by successfully reuniting with temporarily absent or distracted attachment figures, infants would have substantially increased their chances of survival, and ultimately their reproductive fitness.

During the protest phase of separation and loss, infants generally react very forcefully. However, the intensity of these reactions eventually wanes if the separation is extended, as is the case following a caregiver's death. Anxiety, anger, and denial give way to sadness and hopelessness. This second phase, which Bowlby (1980) called "despair," is thought to be a natural result of failure to bring about the attachment figure's return. A third phase, which Bowlby at first called "detachment," marks an apparent recovery and gradual renewal of interest in other activities and social relationships. The term *detachment* is misleading, however, because Bowlby (e.g., 1973) and his coworkers provided evidence that reunion with a lost attachment figure, who may at first be treated coolly or warily, can suddenly cause a powerful upsurge in attachment behavior (e.g., crying, persistent following and clinging). The apparent "detachment," therefore, is not a simple wearing away or diminishing of the attachment bond; it is a sign of defensive suppression of attachment responses that have repeatedly failed to bring about the attachment figure's return.

Although Bowlby was primarily concerned with understanding infant–caregiver attachment, he considered adult romantic or pair-bond relationships within the same theoretical framework he used to explain infant attachment. Bowlby (1969/1982, 1980) and his colleagues (e.g., Parkes, 2006; Parkes & Weiss, 1983; Weiss, 1975) observed that adults who lose or are separated from their romantic attachment figures (e.g., a spouse) undergo a series of reactions similar to those observed in infants. As an illustration, consider the following passage from *Death's Door* (Gilbert, 2006), a book about grief and the autobiographical literature it has spawned:

In an account of his 34-year-old wife's death from breast cancer, the memoirist David Collins summarizes with poignant precision the rationale underlying his feeling that "I wanted to die too—so I could be with her." Explaining "so freshly present she seemed [that] I had this thought: *I could follow her*," he adds, "I just wanted to go after her, not let her get away. I wanted to find her again. Hadn't I found her once [before]?" (p. 3, original emphasis)

When a separation turns into a permanent loss, the protest phase may be marked by enduring preoccupation with the missing person. It is not uncommon for people—even adults—to experience intense yearning for a lost mate, and to continue for some time to find it surprising or disquieting when aspects of the normal routine are interrupted by the attachment figure's conspicuous but still shocking absence.

The hardest thing for me, I think, is at night. We have a neighbor [who] works the second shift and we hear his pickup truck every night. And my husband would always say something like, "When's he going to get his brakes fixed?" And every night I'm sitting here when he comes along, and that's when I really think about my husband, because he would always say something. (Parkes & Weiss, 1983, p. 87)

Once the bereaved individual realizes that the partner will not be returning (which can sometimes occur even before the partner dies, if he or she has suffered a long and irrevocable decline because of a terminal illness; e.g., Bonanno, Moskowitz, Papa, & Folkman, 2005), some degree of sadness and of mental or physiological disorganization is likely. For both adults and children, this phase is characterized by sleeping and eating disturbances, social withdrawal, loneliness, and dysphoria. (In some cases, the stress may hasten the bereaved individual's own death; Hart, Hole, Lawlor, Smith, & Lever, 2007; see M. Stroebe, Schut, & Stroebe, 2007, for a review.) As Weiss (1973) noted, the feelings of loneliness stem specifically from the absence of the attachment figure and cannot be fully alleviated by the presence of others (see W. Stroebe, Stroebe, Abakoumkin, & Schut, 1996, for empirical evidence on this point). Although many bereaved individuals definitely derive comfort from the presence of close, supportive friends or family members, who can be viewed as parts of a hierarchy of attachment figures (Bowlby, 1969/1982), a support network does not necessarily fill the emotional gap left by a specific missing attachment figure. According to Bowlby, attachment bonds are person-specific and involve many memories and feelings unique to a history of interactions with that particular person.

Bowlby's (1980) writings about loss in adult-hood were based on the phases of mourning observed in young children (protest, despair, and detachment). But he supplemented these phases with a new initial phase, "numbing." This phase was added because research and clinical observations indicated that mourners often fail to register the loss of the attachment figure at first, presumably because the event is too painful to accept or it seems cognitively incomprehensible. The following example describes the initial numbing reaction of a woman whose husband died suddenly and unexpectedly. At the morgue, she found it difficult to acknowledge that her husband was dead.

> I didn't believe it. I stayed there for twenty minutes. I rubbed him, I rubbed his face, I patted him, I rubbed his head. I called him, but he didn't answer. And I knew if I called him he'd answer me because he's used to my voice. But he didn't answer me. They said he was dead, but his skin was just as warm as mine. (Parkes & Weiss, 1983, p. 84)

Importantly, on the basis of adults' ability to talk about their troubling experiences and to deal cognitively and emotionally with loss, Bowlby used the term *reorganization* rather than *detachment* to characterize the way people come to terms with loss. As we explain in detail later, this change is important because it reflects Bowlby's belief that many mourners do not, and do not wish to, "detach" defensively from their lost attachment figure; instead, they rearrange their representations of self and the lost figure so that a continuing bond *and* adjustment to post-loss circumstances are possible.

As might be expected, given Bowlby's ethological perspective on separation and loss, there is considerable evidence that grief responses are characteristic of many species, not just humans (Archer, 1999). For animals born without the capacity to care for themselves, the loss of a primary attachment figure evokes intense protest, and leads eventually to what seems to human observers to be sorrow and despair (see Bowlby, 1969/1982). For example, in one of the earliest studies on attachment in rhesus macaques, Seay, Hansen, and Harlow (1962) separated 5-month-old rhesus infants from their mothers for a 3-week period. The infants reacted at first with extreme signs of protest and agitation, including screeching and attempting to break the barriers separating them from their mothers. When these attempts failed to es-

tablish contact, the infants became lethargic and withdrawn. Such responses are also characteristic of some nonprimate species that exhibit attachment behavior (including elephants; e.g., Poole, 1996). Konrad Lorenz (1963), one of the ethologists whose work influenced Bowlby's ideas, provided an illustration of these emotional reactions in the greylag goose:

> The first response to the disappearance of the partner consists in the anxious attempt to find him again. The goose moves about restlessly by day and night, flying great distances and visiting all places where the partner might be found, uttering all the time the penetrating trisyllabic long-distance call. . . . The searching expeditions are extended farther and farther, and quite often the searcher himself gets lost, or succumbs to an accident. . . . All the objectively observable characteristics of the goose's behaviour on losing its mate are roughly identical with those accompanying human grief. (pp. 200–201)

Cross-cultural research on humans also attests to the prevalence of these emotional and behavioral responses to loss (Rosenblatt, 2008; Rosenblatt, Walsh, & Jackson, 1976). As W. Stroebe and Stroebe (1987) observed, however, the specific ways in which grief is manifested vary substantially across cultures. Some societies are structured in ways that accentuate, and perhaps romanticize, the anxiety, anger, and yearning experienced after a loss. For example, Mathison (1970) described the rituals of certain Trobriand Islanders. As part of mourning, a widow is expected to cry for several days. In contrast, the display of emotion is restricted to a brief period among the Navajo. After this time, a widow is expected to return to her normal everyday activities and not to speak of the deceased (Miller & Schoenfeld, 1973). Nevertheless, despite the variability in mourning rituals observed by cultural anthropologists, the loss of a loved one appears to be very distressing in every part of the world and throughout recorded history (Rosenblatt et al., 1976).

## Bowlby's Conceptualization of Disordered Mourning

Bowlby expected the majority of people who lose someone they love to experience and express negative feelings, revise and reorganize relevant internal working models, and eventually establish a satisfactory way of moving on with life. But given his clinical interests, Bowlby was also concerned with understanding disordered forms of mourning. His analysis of these disordered forms suggested that they can be arrayed along a single conceptual dimension running from "chronic mourning" to "prolonged absence of conscious grieving" (Bowlby, 1980, p. 138).[1] Chronic mourning is characterized by protracted grief and prolonged difficulty in normal functioning. Individuals who suffer in this way may find themselves overly preoccupied with thoughts of their missing partner and unable to return to normal functioning for months or even years after the loss. In contrast, an absence of grief is characterized by a conspicuous lack of conscious sorrow, anger, or distress. According to Bowlby, individuals exhibiting this pattern may express relatively little distress following the loss, continue in their jobs or activities without any noticeable disruption, and seek little support or solace from friends and family. It was Bowlby's belief that this manner of reacting to loss can lead to difficulties in long-term adjustment if a person has lost someone to whom he or she is deeply attached.

For a while, modern clinicians agreed with Bowlby's description of these patterns of grief (e.g., Middleton, Raphael, Martinek, & Misso, 1993; W. Stroebe & Stroebe, 1987). According to Middleton and colleagues (1993), most clinicians distinguished between two forms of disordered mourning: chronic and delayed. *Chronic mourning* is characterized by prolonged symptoms of depression and anxiety, possibly also with aspects of posttraumatic stress disorder (PTSD). Chronic mourning might also include what some clinicians and attachment researchers call *unresolved grief* (e.g., Ainsworth & Eichberg, 1991; Main & Hesse, 1990; Zisook & DeVaul, 1985), although the precise meaning of this term varies across theorists. As we discuss later, the form of chronic mourning that Bowlby emphasized is currently generating a great deal of attention among clinicians and bereavement researchers because, in the extreme, it represents a debilitating condition.

Similar to Bowlby's description of a prolonged absence of conscious grieving, *delayed mourning* is characterized by denial of distress and a continuation of normal affairs without substantial disruption. This category of disordered mourning is similar to what Parkes (1965) referred to as "inhibited" mourning and what Deutsch (1937) called "absent" mourning. As we discuss later, there is disagreement among contemporary bereavement scholars as to whether delayed or absent grieving is a "disordered" form of grief (e.g., Bonanno, 2009).

It is noteworthy that variants of the two major endpoints of Bowlby's (1980) continuum of grief patterns have been identified in multiple ways throughout the history of attachment research. In the literatures on both infant and adult attachment relationships, researchers have focused on individuals who experience intense distress after losing attachment figures and on those who apparently experience little distress following loss or separation. Although this research has not focused exclusively on irretrievable losses (e.g., death of a spouse), it provides important insights into the nature of bereavement because, according to Bowlby, the same psychological mechanisms underlie reactions to both brief and permanent separations.

One of the earliest researchers to study reactions to separation from an attachment figure was Mary Ainsworth. As Solomon and George describe (Chapter 18, this volume), Ainsworth developed the Strange Situation assessment procedure (Ainsworth, Blehar, Waters, & Wall, 1978) to investigate the interplay of attachment and exploration in a controlled laboratory setting. She and her colleagues identified three major patterns of infant–mother attachment: secure, resistant, and avoidant. Of special interest here is the fact that these patterns can be arrayed along a dimension ranging from intense and chronic distress to an absence or avoidance of distress.

Resistant infants in the Strange Situation exhibit a tendency to remain focused on their attachment figure (rather than playing wholeheartedly with attractive toys provided by the experimenter), to cry profusely during separations, and to refuse to calm down once their attachment figure returns. In other words, they exhibit a miniature version of grief, becoming extremely distressed by separation, then finding it impossible to "resolve" this distress when conditions seem to call for resolution. Avoidant infants in the Strange Situation are marked by what might be called a cool, if somewhat tense, nonchalance regarding their attachment figure's whereabouts, and—at least in some cases—an active ignoring of her or him when the figure returns following a separation. This can be viewed as a small, short-term version of failure to become anxious, angry, or bereft in the face of loss. Secure infants fall somewhere in between the two major insecure groups, often reacting with distress to separations but also being quick to achieve resolution once their attachment figure returns.

Research on adults' reactions to separation from or loss of attachment figures also indicates that responses can be arrayed along a conceptual dimension running from absent to chronic distress. As noted earlier, research by Parkes and his colleagues (Parkes, 1965, 2006; Parkes & Weiss, 1983) suggested that some individuals experience chronic anxiety, whereas others report little impact of the loss on their well-being. In our own research on relationship breakups (Fraley, Davis, & Shaver, 1998) and marital separations (Fraley & Shaver, 1998), we have also identified reactions falling along this dimension. Specifically, after separation from a romantic partner or spouse, some individuals report experiencing intense anxiety and depression. Moreover, naturalistic observations indicate that these individuals are likely to cling to their partners and actively resist separation (Fraley & Shaver, 1998). In contrast, some individuals appear less distressed when separated from their romantic or marital partner. They are unlikely to protest separation and appear to be relatively unaffected by it. (See Sbarra & Emery, 2005, for an intensive longitudinal investigation of the emotional sequelae of relationship dissolution; also, see Sbarra & Hazan, 2008, for an integrative overview of research on the experience of and recovery from relationship breakups and losses.)

## Chronic Grief and the Organization of Attachment

One of Bowlby's key ideas was that whether an individual exhibits a healthy or problematic pattern of grief following separation depends on the way his or her attachment system has become organized over the course of development. Individuals who experience chronic grief are thought to have organized their attachment behavior around the implicit belief that attachment figures will not be consistently accessible or dependable. As Bowlby argued, these expectations have their roots in an individual's history of attachment experiences.

By persistently searching for an attachment figure and doing everything possible to prevent separation, the anxious-ambivalent individual increases the chance that he or she will be able to retain the attachment figure's attention and care. Thus, the individual's mind is organized in a way that keeps him or her chronically "searching" for cues regarding the attachment figure's availability and presence. When the attachment figure's availability is questionable, this hypervigilance manifests itself in clinginess, jealousy, and inability to focus or concentrate on other activities. In the absence of the attachment figure, however, this vigilance manifests itself in persistent searching behavior, yearning, anxiety, and depression. Because the mind has become organized to detect cues of unavailability or unresponsiveness, a real loss continues to prime the attachment system, making extreme anxiety and sorrow difficult to avoid.

Following bereavement, adults characterized as insecure, dependent, anxious, or fearful are often those who suffer from chronic mourning (Parkes & Weiss, 1983). Parkes (1965; Parkes & Weiss, 1983) described the "grief-prone personality," a construct modeled after Bowlby's description of anxiously attached individuals and empirically associated with poor outcomes in Parke's studies. These individuals were intensely anxious, yearned deeply for their lost spouses, and had extreme difficulty in adjusting to prior losses.

## The Absence of Grief and the Organization of Attachment

Bowlby (1980) believed that the prolonged absence of conscious grieving was a defensive reaction to loss, one that has the potential to break down and give rise to intense feelings of grief and sorrow. He also entertained the possibility that the suppression of grief can have adverse effects on physical health, as illustrated by the example of Charles Darwin that opens this chapter.

According to Bowlby, the relative absence of grief exhibited by some individuals following loss is a facet of a more general pattern of personality organization, which he called "compulsive self-reliance." He believed that that compulsive self-reliance stems from early attachment experiences in which the expression of emotion was discouraged: "Not infrequently, it seems, a person who grows up to assert his independence of affectional ties has [grown up in a context where] affectional bonds are little valued, attachment behavior is regarded as childish and weak and is rebuffed, all expression of feeling is frowned upon and contempt expressed for those who cry" (1980, pp. 224–225). Bowlby believed that, over time, such experiences can lead an individual to assert his or her independence and self-sufficiency, even in situations involving permanent losses.

In Chapter 4 of *Loss*, Bowlby (1980) offered a sophisticated account of the defense mechanisms that may regulate an individual's experience of grief and sorrow, and explained why these mechanisms may pose problems for psychological well-being. He believed that the process of *defensive exclusion*—a deliberate or automatic redirection of attention away from painful thoughts and feelings about the loss—can eventually lead to the development of dissociated memory systems for the loss experience. Because these memories still exist, albeit in an unintegrated form, they can continue to influence emotion and behavior without the person understanding how or why.

Bowlby believed that people who fail to acknowledge the implications of a loss have the potential to be vulnerable to subsequent physical and psychological distress for two reasons. First, if representations of the experience become relatively dissociated from other representations in memory, people may have a difficult time sensitizing themselves to the events and thoughts surrounding the loss; they tend not to work through the walled-off memories and expectations. Because the dissociated representations are infrequently activated, it is difficult to habituate naturally to the emotions associated with them. When this is the case, it may take no more than subtle, but personally meaningful, stimuli to reactivate representations of the attachment or the loss and to bring about feelings of anxiety and distress. As an example, Bowlby noted that individuals who fail to express grief in the early months of bereavement may break down when an anniversary takes place or when some other reminder of the attachment figure summons to mind fragmented memories and feelings for the deceased. For a less defensive individual, these events may not elicit heightened distress because the meaning of the events and their connections to other aspects of the individual's life have been integrated into current representations of the world. For the defensive person, in contrast, these unintended reactions have the potential to be disarming or disorienting.

Bowlby also believed that dissociated or segregated memory systems can lead to long-term physical or psychological distress because their partial activation continues to prime the attachment system—a theme that is reemerging in recent models of bereavement (see Maccallum & Bryant, 2013). For example, seemingly mundane events, such as making dinner, can elicit stressful reactions and tax a person's physical resources if those activities were previously organized around the now-deceased attachment figure. A bereaved individual, however, may not recognize the source of these reactions if he or she has not fully acknowledged the loss or come to recognize the loss-related meaning implicit in these activities. Repeated activation of inexplicable and partially suppressed negative emotions may eventually have a negative impact on psychological or physical well-being.

## Current Research Issues and Perspectives

### Stages of Grief

One controversy that continues to hold a visible place in the bereavement literature concerns the extent to which people move through discrete phases or stages of grief. Critics of stage models have often identified Bowlby as an advocate for these models due to the fact that he called attention to the phases of numbing, protest, despair, and reorganization (e.g., Klass, Silverman, & Nickman, 1996; Wortman & Boerner, 2007). As several researchers have observed, however, the stage model does not seem to characterize the mourning process adequately (Wortman & Boerner, 2007). Some people, for example, seem to move in and out of various phases over the course of bereavement. Moreover, there appears to be considerable variation in how people respond to loss, both cross-culturally and at the level of individual differences. These kinds of observations have led several scholars (e.g., Wortman & Boerner, 2007) to reject the stage model and to seek alternative ways of understanding the bereavement process (e.g., Neimeyer, 2012).

Although we agree that overly rigid interpretations of stage models have been influential in popular culture (see Konigsberg, 2011, for a discussion), it is a mischaracterization of Bowlby's views to associate him with a rigid stage perspective. It is clear from Bowlby's writings that he believed that there are different phases of mourning, and that some phases (e.g., numbing) are more likely to peak shortly after a loss rather than later. But Bowlby clearly did not believe that people needed to pass through one phase before entering another. Nor did he believe that these phases were mutually exclusive, such that a person experiencing a yearning for his or her partner could not also be experiencing despair, loneliness, and depression. For example, in his 1980 volume he wrote, "Admittedly these phases [of numbing, protest, despair, and reorganization] are not clear cut, and any one individual may oscillate for a time back and forth between any two of them" (p. 85). The reason Bowlby called attention to these phases is that he viewed them as reflecting different functions within his ethological framework. Protest responses, for example, represent attempts to reunite with a missing attachment figure. And reorganization reflects the challenging process of trying to make sense of the world and one's place in it without the lost attachment figure. When viewed from this perspective, the adaptive function of the phases discussed by Bowlby can be better appreciated.

In short, the phases Bowlby (1980) described were attempts to characterize the way in which people tend to experience separation and loss. Most of the data he drew upon came from samples of relatively young people from North America, Australia, and Great Britain, and he acknowledged the limitation of such data for generalizing beyond those samples (pp. 84–85). Although some scholars find it convenient to associate Bowlby with a rigid stage perspective (e.g., Holland & Neimeyer, 2010), we believe that doing so undermines his emphasis on the function of these responses and ties him to a particular perspective that was foreign to him.

## Complicated Grief and The DSM

Recent research suggests that the majority of bereaved individuals experience negative emotions, physiological disorganization, and health problems to only a modest or moderate degree, and that they react with considerable acceptance and resilience (Bonanno, 2004; Bonanno et al., 2002, 2005). Nevertheless, about 10–15% of individuals suffer more extreme grief reactions (Bonanno & Kaltman, 2001; Lichtenthal, Cruess, & Prigerson, 2004). In recent years, one of the most active areas of research in the study of bereavement has been concerned with understanding these extreme grief reactions and identifying ways to define, measure, and treat complicated or prolonged grief. This work is especially pertinent to Bowlby's theory because of his emphasis on chronic grief and his attempts to understand its origins.

The fourth, text revised edition of the *Diagnostic and Statistical Manual of Mental Disorders* (DSM-IV-TR; American Psychiatric Association, 2000) classified negative reactions to bereavement under such rubrics as depression, PTSD, or adjustment disorders. To the extent that normal grieving does not involve reactions extreme enough to warrant a clinical label or clinical intervention (Bonanno, 2004), it seems important to distinguish normal grieving from more extreme reactions. As such, there has been a substantial amount of discussion and debate about how to define and measure such reactions and whether complicated grief reactions warrant their own DSM diagnostic classification (Prigerson et al., 2009; Shear et al., 2011; M. Stroebe et al., 2000).

Debates about the boundaries of complicated grief and its status as a psychological disorder became especially pronounced in the years leading up to the publication of DSM-5 in 2013. Two issues, in particular, captivated much scholarly attention among bereavement researchers. The first was the controversial removal of the "bereavement exclusion" (BE) that was present in the previous two DSM editions. The BE holds that an individual should not be diagnosed as having a depressive disorder if he or she has recently lost a loved one. The rationale for this exclusion is that depressive symptoms are common following loss and may not be indicative of a psychological disorder that requires intervention. As Shear and colleagues (2011) note, the BE was designed to limit overdiagnosis of depression. But the proposed (and eventual) removal of the BE from the DSM-5 generated considerable controversy. Some writers—especially those in the popular media—perceived it as an attempt to pathologize bereavement (Adler, 2012). But others defended the revision, noting that the removal of the BE does not compel clinicians to diagnose a bereaved person as having major depressive disorder (MDD); instead, the removal of the BE provides an opportunity to ensure that someone who might need additional treatment has the opportunity to obtain it. Removal of the BE has the potential to be useful because loss is a significant life stressor and can potentially be a trigger for MDD among those with an existing vulnerability (Bowlby, 1980). Moreover, removal of the BE seems appropriate from an attachment–theoretical perspective on loss because although grief itself is a natural response to the loss of an attachment figure, it has the potential to become crippling and to interfere with adaptation. In such cases, it would be useful for those experiencing complicated grief to get treatment.

The second major issue concerns whether complicated grief itself merits its own diagnostic category. Although some scholars have been making a case for the new category for decades (e.g., Horowitz et al., 1997), there was an especially large amount of work on this topic in anticipation of DSM-5. Shear and colleagues (2011) observed that complicated grief meets many of the criteria that are commonly used to identify psychological disorders. For example, one of the consequences of complicated grief is clinically significant distress or disability. Moreover, complicated grief appears to be distinct from other psychological disorders, such as MDD and PTSD. People experiencing MDD, for example, often have profound feelings of self-doubt and low efficacy. In contrast, self-esteem is not typically impaired among those suffering from prolonged grief.

Researchers who advocate a separate diagnostic category for complicated grief have developed inventories, such as the commonly used Inventory of Complicated Grief (ICG; Prigerson et al., 2009), which can be used for both research purposes and diagnostic purposes. Moreover, several recommendations exist on how to classify a person as suffering from complicated grief (Forstmeier & Maercker, 2007; Horowitz et al., 1997; Prigerson, Vanderwerker, & Maciejewski, 2008; Shear et al., 2011). Prigerson and colleagues (2009), for example, proposed that people be classified as experiencing complicated grief if they have the following symptom set: severe yearning at least 6 months following the loss of a loved one, as well as five of nine other symptoms: emotional numbing, being stunned, feeling life is meaningless, mistrust of others, bitterness, difficulty accepting the loss, identity confusion, avoidance of the reality of the loss, and difficulty moving on with life.

Factor-analytic studies support the claim that complicated, prolonged grief is separable from depression and anxiety (e.g., Boelen, van den Bout, & de Keijser, 2003; Ogrodniczuk et al., 2003; Prigerson et al., 1996). A few studies have shown that various indicators of adjustment—psychological, behavioral (e.g., friend or observer reports), and physiological—are predicted by measures of complicated or prolonged grief, even after researchers statistically control for scores on measures of other clinical conditions, such as depression and PTSD (e.g., Bonanno et al., 2007; Simon et al., 2007). In short, much of the empirical research on these issues seems consistent with the notion that complicated grief (1) can be debilitating, (2) is not isomorphic with depression and anxiety, and (3) may be treatable using interventions that target the lost relationship and the feelings people have regarding the loss (e.g., Sandler et al., 2008).

Despite the advocacy for complicated grief as a DSM diagnostic category, complicated grief was not, in fact, included in the 2013 revision of the DSM. (It was discussed in the Appendix but not formally recognized as a diagnostic category.) We suspect that many researchers will continue to fight for its inclusion in future revisions. The World Health Organization is currently developing the *International Classification of Diseases*, version 11. One of the proposed additions is prolonged grief disorder (Maercker et al., 2013), defined in ways that are highly similar to other characterizations of complicated grief.

## The Absence of Grief

Another theme that we highlighted in the 1999 and 2008 editions of this chapter, absence of grief, continues to be salient in bereavement research. When Bowlby was originally formulating his thoughts on attachment and loss, there were relatively few large-scale empirical studies available on the topic, and much of his inspiration regarding absent grief came from clinical case studies on loss, such as those by Deutsch (1937).

This is important because contemporary bereavement researchers have highlighted the numerous limitations of trying to understand various forms of grieving, such as relative absence of grief, using clinical case studies and nonprospective designs. One such limitation is that cases often come to the attention of clinicians and health care workers because a bereaved client is struggling emotionally or interpersonally; that is, the outcome (e.g., difficulties with depression or anxiety) is already known. It is tempting in such circumstances to conclude that the relative lack of grief symptoms at a prior point in time may have been a predictor of pathology on the client's part. But the counterfactual is missing. Without an estimate of the proportion of people expressing a relative lack of grief symptoms that do not come to the attention of clinicians or health care workers, there is no basis for assuming that the absence of grief is a prospective indicator of adjustment difficulties post-loss. Another limitation is that much of the early research that inspired Bowlby was not based on prospective designs. It often drew on retrospective accounts (which may be of questionable accuracy) and did not allow individuals' long-term outcomes to be tracked.

One of the important features of recent bereavement research is the use of prospective designs and nonclinical populations (e.g., Carnelley, Wortman, Bolger, & Burke, 2007). This is crucial for our purposes because it enables researchers to examine the long-term outcomes of people who express relatively few symptoms of grief, depression, and anxiety shortly after the loss of a loved one. Bonanno and his colleagues have done some of the most important work in this area (for reviews, see Bonanno, 2009; Wortman & Boemer, 2007). One of the key contributions of this work is the documentation of heterogeneity in the ways people respond and adapt to loss. To appreciate the richness of the various patterns, it is useful to consider grief symptoms at two points in time: shortly after a loss and again months later. When the severity of grief symptoms is crossed with time, four potential bereavement trajectories emerge (see Figure 3.1).

The first, what Bonanno and his colleagues (e.g., Bonanno, 2009) call *common grief*, is characterized by high levels of grief shortly after the loss, followed by a gradual decline in grief-related symptoms over time. In many respects, this is the prototypical form of grief observed in Western cultures. Another potential pattern, *chronic grief*, is characterized by elevated grief symptoms across time. Individuals exhibiting this pattern are highly likely to meet the diagnostic criteria for complicated grief (see Prigerson et al., 2009). Another theoretical pattern is characterized by low levels of symptoms at both time points, a pattern that Bonanno and his colleagues call *resilience*. A final pattern characterizes people who exhibit few

symptoms early on, but show elevated symptoms at a subsequent assessment. Bonanno and his colleagues call this pattern *delayed grief*, which is expected if the relative lack of grief in the early phases of loss is a risk factor for the development of symptoms later on (Bonanno & Field, 2001).

One of Bonanno's important findings is that individuals who express relatively few symptoms of grief shortly after a loss are also likely to express relatively few, rather than more, symptoms later on. That is, the resilient pattern is relatively common in empirical studies, whereas the delayed pattern rarely occurs (e.g., Bonanno et al., 2002). People who show a relative absence of grief 3 months post-loss, for example, are much more likely to continue to show few grief symptoms months down the road.

What are the implications of these findings for Bowlby's ideas on the absence of grief? We believe that these studies convincingly demonstrate that people who are not suffering from extreme symptoms of grief shortly after a loss are unlikely to be suffering from those symptoms at a later point in time. Moreover, we believe that Bonanno's work does a service to the field by demonstrating that when people appear not to be "suffering enough,"

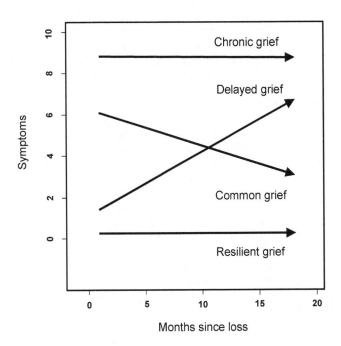

**FIGURE 3.1.** Prototypical patterns fo bereavement. From Fraley and Bonanno (2004). Copyright 2004 by Sage Publications, Inc. Adapted by permission.

according to friends and family, it does not mean that they are grieving "incorrectly." In fact, one of the key contributions of Bonanno's work is its demonstration that it is quite common to exhibit resilience following a loss. Yet the norms in Western culture can lead bereaved individuals to wonder whether they are doing something wrong if they are not grieving enough.

Having said this, we should add that some writers have been too quick to dismiss Bowlby's ideas in light of the finding that the relative absence of grief is a predictor of long-term adaptation. There are two important ideas in Bowlby's writings that suggest that these dismissals may be premature. First, in Bowlby's discussion of the absence of grief, he was largely concerned with what we refer to as *off-diagonal* cases. To better explain this idea, consider Figure 3.2, which presents a 2 × 2 table that classifies people with respect to two factors: (1) the expression of grief shortly after a loss (low vs. high) and (2) long-term psychological outcome (negative vs. positive). Based on Bonanno's research, it seems that there is a moderate negative association between these factors. That is, people who are most visibly distressed by loss are less likely than those who are not to exhibit signs of psychological adjustment later in time (Cell A). Similarly, those who are less visibly distressed by loss are more likely than those who are more visibly distressed to exhibit better psychological adjustment later in time (Cell D).

In his discussion of the absence of grieving, Bowlby was not claiming that there is a positive association between these variables, such that people who fail to express grief shortly after loss will be at greater risk for psychological maladjustment than those who express extreme distress shortly after loss. Indeed, he was aware of the evidence that one of the best predictors of poor outcomes later in time is poor outcomes shortly after loss (Bowlby, 1980, p. 148). Bowlby was calling attention to the fact that there are people on the off-diagonal of Figure 3.2—people who do not report symptoms of grief shortly after a loss but who nonetheless exhibit poor adjustment in the long run (e.g., Cell C). The important message for Bowlby and other clinicians was this: Just because someone is expressing relatively few symptoms of grief shortly after the loss of an attachment figure does not mean they will adapt smoothly to the loss. Some of these individuals may be suppressing the expression of their grief and, if so, there is a chance that those defenses will break down at

some point and reveal more clearly the impact of the loss on the individual's emotional functioning.

The second point is that Bowlby was concerned primarily with the *absolute* absence of grief rather than with the fact that some people grieve less than others. Bonanno's focus, in contrast, is individual differences in, or *relative ranks*, with respect to grieving. The individuals who are classified as resilient in Bonanno's taxonomy are not showing an initial "absence" of grief, absolutely speaking. Instead, relative to others, their grief is less intense and less debilitating. Indeed, Bonanno is careful to note that people who are not grieving strongly are not simply unaffected by the loss; they are simply managing the loss in a way that enables them to move forward in adaptive ways. That is, they seem relatively secure from an attachment–theoretical perspective (Fraley & Bonanno, 2004).

One question that remains is whether people who exhibit Bonanno's resilient profile are homogenous in their psychological functioning. In the case of young Darwin, for example, it seemed clear to Bowlby that Darwin harbored great pain following the loss of his mother. But Darwin did not feel that he could express those feelings to others, at least not without being reprimanded. This strikes us as a form of absence of grief that is quite different from what might be observed if, in fact, someone was relatively resilient and able to move forward with life tasks without becoming overwhelmed. Similarly, both of these forms of grief seem different from what might result if a person was not deeply attached to the person who was lost.

Thus, our intuition is that people who exhibit a resilient pattern following a loss may represent a mixture of subpopulations. The majority, in fact, may be managing the loss relatively well. They may be deeply affected by it, but are finding meaning in their lives, continuing forward with life goals, and not getting submerged in the painful feelings that can result from loss. But some may not have been given the opportunity to grieve in the way they felt necessary (see Doka, 2008, for an interesting discussion of "disenfranchised" grief). And some who exhibit this pattern may have lost someone who was not a central figure in their lives or in their identities.

Although Bowlby thought that the absence of grief was sometimes a defensive reaction to covert distress, he also noticed that there are exceptions to this pattern. Consider the following quotations from *Loss* (Bowlby, 1980):

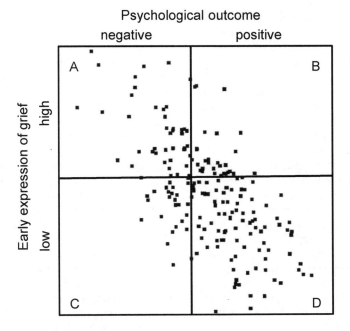

**FIGURE 3.2.** The consideration of "off-diagonal" cases in discussions of the absence of grief.

Some of those who proclaim their self-sufficiency are in fact relatively immune to loss. (p. 213)

Not everyone [characterized by an assertion of independence of affectional ties] develops a highly organized personality, however. In many the hardness and self-reliance are more brittle and it is from amongst these persons, it seems likely, that a substantial proportion of all those who at some time in their life develop a pathological response to loss are recruited. (p. 225)

Some individuals having this disposition [of compulsive self-reliance] have made such tenuous ties with parents, or a spouse or a child that, when they suffer loss, they are truly little affected by it. (p. 211)

Individuals disposed strongly to assert their self-sufficiency fall on a continuum ranging from those whose proclaimed self-sufficiency rests on a precarious basis to those in whom it is firmly organized. (p. 211)

The more frequently a child is rejected or experiences a separation, moreover, and the more anxious and distressed he becomes the more frequent and painful are the rebuffs he is likely to receive and the thicker therefore will grow his protective shell. In some persons, indeed, the shell becomes so thick that affectional relationships are attenuated to a point at which loss ceases almost to have significance. Immune to mourning they may be; but at what a price! (p. 240)

These quotations reveal two trends in Bowlby's thinking. They suggest that he thought some people who exhibit an absence of grief are truly unperturbed by loss, or are at least less perturbed than others, because (1) they have never established a close, emotional attachment to their partners in the first place; and/or (2) their defenses have become so "thick," or highly organized, that it is possible to defensively regulate their emotions fairly effectively.

Research and theory concerning infant–caregiver attachment has generally adhered to the idea that almost all infants become emotionally attached to their primary caregivers. Therefore, following separation or loss, avoidant behavior on the part of infants involves the suppression of *true* feelings of rejection and distress. In adult romantic relationships, however, we may encounter a kind of defensive process that does not normally unfold in the context of infant–caregiver relationships. Specifically, an adult can avoid becoming attached to his or her romantic partner, even in the course of an extended relationship. When the relationship ends, such a person may not experience intense anxiety and sorrow; moreover, few long-term difficulties should be encountered in such a case because the loss is not deeply traumatic.

Recall that Bowlby believed that part of the recovery process entails rearranging one's representations of the world in a way that integrates the reality of the loss with one's implicit assumptions about the world. People vary, however, in the extent to which their assumptions about the world are organized around their relationship partners. When a person is relatively unattached to his or her partner, the relationship will be less important to his or her sense of well-being and security. The partner or the partnership will not be a valued aspect of the self, and the person's memories and goals will not be extensively organized around the partner. The absence of distress in these cases may reflect a true absence of grief and not just a defensive disguise of painful feelings.

We expand on these issues in the next section, where we review some of the recent empirical research on responses to loss and on individual differences in attachment organization. Here, however, we note that Bowlby suggested that the kinds of defensive strategies people use to regulate attachment-related experiences and behavior have not only the potential to be dysfunctional but may also reflect, in some people, a chronic pattern of nonengagement, one that has the potential to blunt their interpersonal experiences and cause pain to their relationship partners and families. This important "side effect" should be added to what Bowlby had in mind when he exclaimed, "At what a price!" In other words, although these individuals may not experience debilitating symptoms of grief at any point following a loss; that is, because of their defensive strategies, such individuals are of clinical interest because their defenses may be preventing them from building relationships that are emotionally and personally meaningful and rewarding for their relationship partners.

## Research on Attachment Styles and Reactions to Loss

A key component of Bowlby's theoretical analysis was that the ways in which people mourn, and the degree to which these patterns are adaptive in the long run, can be understood partly in terms of their attachment histories. Specifically, Bowlby (1980) thought that adults with anxious attachment histories (i.e., histories of insecurity, inconsistent care, and persistent frustration of attachment-related needs) would be more likely to exhibit prolonged or chronic grief, whereas individuals for whom attachment-related needs had

been consistently rebuffed or rejected would be more likely to express few overt signs of grief.

In the late 1980s, a number of researchers began to develop taxonomies of individual differences in attachment organization for adults (e.g., Hazan & Shaver, 1987; Main, Kaplan, & Cassidy, 1985). Hazan and Shaver (1987), for example, proposed a three-group taxonomy involving security, avoidance, and anxious-ambivalence, based on the patterns of attachment that had been documented by Ainsworth and her colleagues using the strange situation paradigm (Ainsworth et al., 1978; for a review, see Fraley & Shaver, 2000). When Bowlby's ideas are considered in the context of Hazan and Shaver's three-category model, the theoretical links between attachment organization and grief are clear: Secure individuals should be distressed by the loss of a loved one but find it easier than others to adapt to the loss. Anxious-ambivalent or preoccupied individuals should exhibit a pattern characterized by chronic grief, whereas avoidant individuals should show an apparent absence of overt grief symptoms (see Field & Sundin, 2001; Shaver & Tancredy, 2001; Wayment & Vierthaler, 2002).

Contemporary research on bereavement in adults has begun to examine Bowlby's ideas concerning individual differences (e.g., Mikulincer & Shaver, 2008). There is growing evidence that individuals who are high in attachment-related anxiety are more likely than those who are low in anxiety to have complicated grief reactions (Field & Sundin, 2001; Fraley & Bonanno, 2004; Wayment & Vierthaler, 2002). For example, Field and Sundin (2001) found that anxious attachment, assessed 10 months after the death of a spouse, predicted higher levels of psychological distress 14, 25, and 60 months after the loss. More recently, Meier, Carr, Currier, and Neimeyer (2013) examined prolonged grief symptomology in a sample of 656 bereaved young adults. They found that attachment-related anxiety was associated with grief symptoms, even after they controlled for loss-related circumstances (e.g., relationship to the deceased, violent vs. nonviolent loss). Conceptually similar findings were reported by Waskowic and Chartier (2003), Wayment and Vierthaler (2002), and Wijngaards-de Meij and colleagues (2007).

How do avoidant people fare in response to loss? This particular issue is more challenging to address because theoretical models of avoidance have evolved over time. In the early 1990s, Bartholomew introduced an alternative model of individual differences that makes a critical distinction between different kinds of avoidant strategies (see Bartholomew & Horowitz, 1991). Specifically, Bartholomew distinguished between fearful-avoidant and dismissing-avoidant attachment patterns. According to Bartholomew, fearfully avoidant adults, while organizing their behavior in a defensive manner, tend to do so as an attempt to quell their insecurities. Because they are explicitly afraid of being hurt or rejected, they avoid opening up to others and try to avoid becoming emotionally invested in them. The avoidant strategies of dismissing individuals, in contrast, appear to be organized around the goal of self-reliance or independence. Although dismissing individuals may avoid opening up to and depending on others, it is because they consciously see little need to forge close emotional bonds with others, not because they consciously fear being hurt. Theoretically, this strategy is motivated by a history of rejection, but consciously it is rooted in a desire to be autonomous and self-reliant.

Importantly, Griffin and Bartholomew (1994) argued that these theoretical "prototypes" can be arrayed along two conceptual dimensions that researchers have come to call *attachment-related anxiety* and *attachment-related avoidance* (see Fraley & Shaver, 2000; Mikulincer & Shaver, 2007). This first dimension captures variation in the degree to which people are vigilantly attuned to attachment-related concerns (Fraley & Shaver, 2000). A highly anxious person, for example, may worry that his or her attachment figure is unresponsive, whereas a less anxious person may feel relatively secure about attachment-related matters. The second dimension captures variation in people's tendencies to use avoidant versus proximity-seeking strategies to regulate attachment-related behavior, thought, and feeling. People on the high end of this dimension tend to withdraw from intimacy in close relationships, whereas people on the low end of this dimension are more comfortable opening up to others and relying on others as a safe haven and secure base (Fraley & Shaver, 2000).

The classic Hazan and Shaver categories, as well as Bartholomew's four theoretical prototypes, can be viewed as linear combinations of these two dimensions (see Griffin & Bartholomew, 1994). For example, a prototypical fearful individual is relatively attentive to attachment-related concerns (i.e., is high on the anxiety dimension) and typically employs avoidant strategies to regulate his or her feelings and behavior (i.e., is high on the avoidance dimension). By contrast, a proto-

typically dismissive individual also employs avoidant strategies but is less attentive to or downplays attachment-related concerns (i.e., is low on the anxiety dimension). A prototypically secure individual is low on both of these dimensions.

One of the valuable features of this two-dimensional model is that it distinguishes different kinds of defensive patterns. The classic Hazan and Shaver conception of avoidance implied that avoidance stems from conscious insecurities, thereby conflating dismissing-avoidance with fearful-avoidance (see Fraley & Shaver, 2000). However, once the distinction between different forms of avoidance is recognized, it can be seen that the association between these forms of avoidance and grief reactions may be more nuanced.

Theoretically, the two-dimensional model implies that attachment-related anxiety is the primary driver of complicated and severe grief. This hypothesis is based on the assumption that the control systems underlying attachment-related vigilance, which are tapped by measures of the anxiety dimension, may produce maladaptive grief responses (see Fraley & Shaver, 2000). Theoretically, highly anxious people are more vigilant and insecure regarding the psychological accessibility and availability of their loved ones. Thus, when their loved one is missing, they should not only experience distress but that distress should also be triggered more easily by day-to-day reminders (both physical and psychological) of the loved one's absence. Over a period of time, the repeated activation of these stressful emotions, coupled with the failure of attachment behavior to reunite the person with his or her loved one, may heighten feelings of distress, hopelessness, and despair.

This two-dimensional model suggests that avoidance, by itself, may not lead to difficulties adjusting to a loss. Fraley and colleagues (1998), for example, argued that avoidant strategies of emotion regulation (e.g., withdrawing from situations that make one feel vulnerable) can be just as effective as proximity-seeking strategies (e.g., turning to others for support or comfort) in regulating attachment-related distress. According to Fraley and colleagues, avoidant individuals sometimes appear vulnerable because researchers do not always distinguish between fearful-avoidance and dismissing-avoidance, thereby conflating attachment-related anxiety and avoidance. Once the distinction is made between different patterns of avoidance, it is reasonable to expect some avoidant individuals (i.e., those who are fearfully avoidant) to have difficulty adjusting to loss because they are highly anxious with respect to attachment concerns, but we might expect other avoidant individuals (i.e., those who are dismissingly avoidant) to have less difficulty adjusting to loss because they are not as anxious with respect to attachment concerns.

What does the empirical research indicate? Relatively few bereavement studies have attempted to assess attachment-related anxiety and avoidance independently. Among those that have, however, the evidence is mixed. Fraley and Bonanno (2004) studied a sample of 59 bereaved individuals, assessing attachment style shortly after the loss and examining symptoms of grief, depression, and PTSD at 4 and 18 months postloss. Replicating previous findings (e.g., Field & Sundin, 2001; Wayment & Vierthaler, 2002), they found that attachment-related anxiety predicted elevated levels of depression, grief, and PTSD across time. But they also found that individual differences in attachment-related avoidance were not related to negative outcomes. In the context of Bartholomew's model, then, this implies that adjustment was most challenging for avoidant people who were fearfully avoidant. But those who were dismissingly avoidant showed patterns of adaption that were comparable to those who were secure. This implies that defensive strategies were not effective among fearfully avoidant individuals, but may have been effective among dismissingly avoidant individuals.

In a more recent study, Jerga, Shaver, and Wilkinson (2011) examined self-report data from 368 adults who completed an online survey measuring their attachment style, relationship characteristics, loss circumstances, and grief symptoms. Consistent with other findings regarding anxiety, they found that attachment-related anxiety was associated with prolonged grief symptoms. They also found, however, that people who were generally more avoidant were more likely to report long-term difficulties in adjusting to loss. When considered in the context of Bartholomew's model, this implies that the avoidant people who experienced the most severe distress were fearfully avoidant. Dismissing-avoidant individuals, by comparison, experienced fewer disruptions in functioning (but were not as resilient as those who were secure). Similar findings were reported by Boelen and Klugist (2011), who found that both anxiety and avoidance were correlated concurrently with complicated grief symptoms in a sample of 438 bereaved individuals.

Mancini, Robinaugh Shear, and Bonanno (2009) found that marital adjustment may moderate the association between avoidance and complicated grief in a sample of individuals who had lost their spouses. They found a three-way interaction among attachment-related anxiety, avoidance, and marital adjustment, indicating that dismissing individuals had low levels of grief symptoms if they reported high marital functioning. However, among dismissing individuals who reported low marital functioning, grief symptoms were as high as those of fearful and preoccupied (anxious but not avoidant) individuals.

In their important study, Meier and colleagues (2013) compared a subgroup of individuals who had experienced a violent loss with a control group that was not bereaved. They found that the general health of the nonbereaved individuals was better than that of the bereaved ones, but more importantly, that avoidance was negatively correlated with health in the bereaved group. This suggests that especially stressful or traumatic events might undermine the utility of avoidant strategies that in other circumstances might function relatively effectively (see Mikulincer & Shaver, 2008, for an in-depth discussion of this point). Similar findings were reported by Fraley, Fazzari, Bonanno, and Dekel (2006), who studied stress and coping in a sample of individuals who survived the World Trade Center attacks in 2001. Fraley and colleagues found that highly avoidant individuals had elevated levels of PTSD and depressive symptoms compared to secure individuals. Again, this context was an extremely traumatic one and may have revealed some vulnerabilities that may not be evident under less threatening circumstances. (For further evidence that cognitive and emotional loads can render avoidant defenses unsuccessful, see Berant, Mikulincer, & Shaver, 2008; Mikulincer, Dolev, & Shaver, 2004.)

What are the implications of these findings for Bowlby's ideas about attachment organization and reactions to loss? First, these findings suggest that people who are relatively secure adapt to loss with the fewest complications. They exhibit symptom patterns that overlap with both the common grief and resilient patterns reviewed previously (e.g., Bonanno, 2009). Second, the data consistently indicate that people who are relatively high in attachment-related anxiety are at greater risk of experiencing severe symptoms of grief, depression, and anxiety—the kinds of indicators that are found in complicated grief in recent diagnostic systems. Third, these data, combined with contemporary models of individual differences in attachment organization, lead to some important nuances in the way we understand avoidance and loss. On the one hand, some forms of avoidance are linked to difficulties in adjustment because of their overlap with anxiety. That is, fearfully avoidant individuals, despite their avoidant tendencies, are likely to experience high levels of dysfunction following loss. But those who are relatively dismissing are not necessarily likely to experience severe emotional disruptions. The evidence concerning whether dismissing individuals function at levels comparable to secure individuals is not yet entirely clear, but, in either case, it seems safe to suggest that avoidance, in and of itself, is not an unambiguous predictor of disruption following loss.

## Continuing Bonds: A Controversy Concerning Detachment and Resolution

A dramatic challenge to Bowlby's account of loss appeared in *Continuing Bonds: New Understandings of Grief* (Klass et al., 1996). The authors of that anthology claimed that the modernist emphasis on extreme individualism and mechanistic science mistakenly led Freud and Bowlby to view mourning as a biological, rigidly sequenced process with a fixed healthy endpoint: *decathexis* or *detachment*, defined by Klass and colleagues as complete severance of the emotional bond to a lost attachment figure. In the first edition of this chapter (Fraley & Shaver, 1999), we examined the evidence and rationale for this "postmodern" position and found it wanting—partly because it unfairly caricatured Bowlby's views, and partly because it ignored the possibility of unresolved grief associated with fearful or disorganized attachment. Nevertheless, we credited some of the book's insights and showed how they might be incorporated into attachment theory. We carried this discussion forward in our chapter in the 2008 second edition of this volume.

Since that last edition, the discussion of *Continuing Bonds* in the bereavement literature has waned to some extent. Thus, our goals here are to bring the issue to the attention of new readers and briefly highlight some recent research that speaks to the conditions under which continuing bonds with the deceased can be beneficial.

### What Did Bowlby Say about Continuing Bonds?

Some writers have claimed that Bowlby advocated an abrupt and complete detachment from a lost at-

tachment figure. Bowlby (1980), however, reacted against that recommendation. Instead, he argued that the grief reactions that many clinicians apparently viewed as immature or pathological—searching, yearning, and sometimes expressing anger or ambivalence toward the lost attachment figure—are normal aspects of the functioning of the attachment system. It was part of Bowlby's general approach to attachment phenomena to be sympathetic to people of any age, and in any circumstances, whose attachment behavioral system was activated by distress or by unavailability or loss of an attachment figure.

Even Freud, at least in his personal correspondence, did not agree with the position that subsequent writers attributed to him. In our view, the notion of decathexis from mental representations of a lost attachment figure, when stripped of its outdated theoretical language (concerning the investment and disinvestment of psychic energy), refers to a commonly experienced emotional reaction when one suddenly remembers a deceased attachment figure and realizes once again that he or she is gone. This often happens when one has a glancing thought or memory of the deceased person and is jolted by the realization that the thought or related expectation is no longer appropriate. This can occur scores or hundreds of times over many weeks or months and is a normal part of coming to terms with a loss that is not yet fully represented in all of one's unconscious and preconscious memories. As elements of "internal working models" of the lost attachment figure are called up unexpectedly (by situations or associations), altered to acknowledge the loved one's death, and forgotten again as one returns to current activities and concerns, the emotional charge associated with them typically decreases—partly by virtue of habituation and desensitization, partly by virtue of being reorganized into more realistic, updated working models (Shaver & Tancredy, 2001). But this does not mean that the bereaved person's attachment to the lost figure is erased from memory; far from it.

Some of the misunderstandings concerning Bowlby's position might be due to his use of the term *detachment*, which was originally coined to describe a defensive reaction to the return of a temporarily absent attachment figure. When infants are separated from their attachment figures, they protest before eventually exhibiting sadness. Eventually they seem to recover and begin to explore their environments with renewed interest; they seem once again to be interested in other people. However, if an absent attachment figure returns, Bowlby (1969/1982) noted that many children respond with coolness and an absence of attachment behavior, as if they are punishing the attachment figures for abandoning them or are unsure how to organize their conflicting desires to seek comfort and express anger. Bowlby emphasized that this defensive response is best described as "apparent" detachment because once the children reaccept their attachment figure's care, they are particularly clingy and hypervigilant, not wanting to let the figure out of sight.

In contrast, when discussing bereavement, Bowlby used the term *reorganization* rather than *detachment*. It was not his belief that, as part of the process of adapting to loss, a person needs to detach from his or her loved one. Indeed, for Bowlby, part of the process of reorganization involved finding ways to integrate the loved one—his or her legacy, memory, and continued psychological presence—into one's identity, plans, and life. The following quotations from Bowlby (1980) are illuminating in this respect:

> There is no reason to regard any of these experiences as either unusual or unfavourable, rather the contrary. For example, in regard to the Boston widows Glick, [Weiss, and Parkes] (1974) report: "Often the widow's progress toward recovery was facilitated by inner conversations with her husband's presence. . . . This continued sense of attachment was not incompatible with increasing capacity for independent action" (p. 154). . . . [I]t seems likely that for many widows and widowers it is precisely because they are willing for their feelings of attachment to the dead spouse to persist that their sense of identity is preserved and they become able to reorganize their lives along lines they find meaningful. (p. 98; emphasis added)

> [A secure] person . . . is likely to possess a representational model of attachment figure(s) as being available, responsive and helpful and a complementary model of himself as at least a potentially lovable and valuable person. . . . On being confronted with the loss of someone close to him such a person will not be spared grief; on the contrary he may grieve deeply. . . . [But] he is likely to be spared those experiences which lead mourning to become unbearable or unproductive or both. . . . Since he will not be afraid of intense and unmet desires for love from the person lost, he will let himself be swept by pangs of grief; and tearful expression of yearning and distress will come naturally. During the months and years that follow he will probably be able to organize life afresh, *fortified perhaps by an abiding sense of the lost person's continuing and benevolent presence.* (pp. 242–243; emphasis added)

## Subsequent Writings on the Construct of Continuing Bonds

The continuing bonds book, which was based more on qualitative than quantitative data, stimulated a flurry of more quantitative studies, many of which were reviewed by Boerner and Heckhausen (2003). They concluded, in line with our analysis (Fraley & Shaver, 1999), that "Different types of connections [with the deceased] may be more or less adaptive" (p. 211). They also emphasized that when such connections were obtained in correlational studies, it was unclear which variable—grief severity or continuing bonds—was cause and which was effect, or what third factor might have caused the two variables to be related.

Subsequent studies (e.g., Field & Friedrichs, 2004; Field, Gal-Oz, & Bonanno, 2003) obtained results inconsistent with some of the earlier ones and also failed to discern causal relationships among key variables. In a review of this literature, M. Stroebe and Schut (2005) concluded that it was impossible to tell whether continuing bonds were generally beneficial or detrimental when coping with bereavement. In most studies, continuing bonds (at least as measured) were associated with grief severity, not with resolution. But this fact seemed partially attributable to content overlap in measures of grief severity and continuing bonds (Schut, Stroebe, Boelen, & Zijerveld, 2006). In fact, most operationalizations of the continuing bonds construct seemed inadvertently to make continuing bonds a part of grieving. To make matters more confusing, Lalande and Bonanno (2007) found that the relation between continuing bonds and grief severity, assessed over time, differs between persons in the United States and China.

Our earlier suggestion (Fraley & Shaver, 1999) that continuing bonds can take either secure or insecure forms, and in particular can be part of "unresolved" or "disorganized" attachment, has been most fully developed by Field (2006), who points out that there is a difference between, on the one hand, thinking positively about a deceased attachment figure's admirable and loving qualities and incorporating some of this figure's positive qualities and goals into oneself, and, on the other hand, being haunted by the person's sudden (imagined) appearance or being confused about whether the person is or is not still available in the physical world. Viewed from this perspective, which is based on Main's (1991) conception of unresolved grief, the empirical studies conducted so far do not seem adequate to resolve arguments about such bonds. A coded interview, based on insights from research with the AAI, might be more productive. The goal would be to determine how a person represents, relates to, and talks about (coherently or incoherently) a particular deceased attachment figure (see Hesse, Chapter 26, this volume, for details).

Our conclusions are similar regarding therapeutic interventions based on the continuing bonds construct. Whereas many psychotherapists were apparently taught in the past to help bereaved clients decathect and detach from mental representations of deceased attachment figures, many are now being taught to help bereaved clients continue their bonds with lost loved ones (e.g., Neimeyer, 2012). In light of attachment theory and research, it would make more sense to help each person articulate his or her experiences and ideas about the loss, and move toward models of the lost attachment figure and the relationship that are maximally compatible with maintaining a secure stance toward the future. In cases in which a person's memories and continuing bonds are positive, there is no reason to alter them (and perhaps no reason for them to be a focus of psychotherapy; Bonanno, 2004). In cases in which a person's emotions and mental representations seem deeply conflicted, painful, disorganized, and incoherent, therapeutic interventions should be focused on more than continuing bonds per se (some examples can be found in an article by Malkinson, Rubin, & Witztum, 2006).

## The Cognitive Attachment Model of Bereavement

Maccallum and Bryant (2013) have recently proposed a cognitive attachment model (CAM) of prolonged grief. The model is explicitly designed to account for why some individuals experience symptoms of prolonged grief following the loss of a loved one. The model is partially rooted in attachment theory, but it also integrates contemporary models emphasizing self-identity and autobiographical memory: for example, Shear and Shair's (2005) biobehavioral model; Boelen, van den Hout, and van den Bout's (2006) cognitive-behavioral model; and Stroebe and Schut's (1999) dual process model.

According to Maccallum and Bryant (2013), the primary task in bereavement is "the revision of self-identity to incorporate the reality of the loss and enable the development of new goals, life roles, and attachments that are independent of the deceased" (p. 719). This process is facili-

tated, according to the CAM, when people are able to activate, pursue, and develop goals that are not dependent on a sense of self or identity that is rooted in the deceased. Maccallum and Bryant (2013, p. 720) write that "recalling memories of the deceased, even positive memories, would make salient the discrepancy between desired goals (e.g., reunion with the deceased) and reality, triggering loss-related memories and yearning."

In this framework, a person's identity is conceptualized as varying along a continuum ranging from merged to independent. A *merged identity* is one in which the bereaved person's identity is constructed around or entwined with the deceased. The person's sense of self, his or her goals, and his or her roles are interwoven with those of the deceased. An *independent identity*, in contrast, is one in which core aspects of the self are not based exclusively on the deceased. This is not to imply that the person construes him- or herself as being fully autonomous or distinct from the deceased individual, but that he or she possesses self-elements that are not exclusively grounded in the deceased.

According to this framework, individuals with a merged self-identity are at greater risk for developing complicated grief symptoms because the discrepancy between personal goals and the post-loss situation is frequently made salient. This in turn has the potential to influence the way in which autobiographical memory processes play out, leading to the preferential retrieval of memories involving the lost individual, appraisals that generate stress, and emotion regulation strategies that reinforce those maladaptive appraisals and perpetuate grief. Indeed, research suggests that individuals experiencing complicated grief are more likely to provide self-defining memories that involve the deceased (e.g., Maccallum & Bryant, 2008). Moreover, Boelen, Keijsers, and van den Hout (2012) found that self-concept clarity was dramatically reduced following loss and that symptoms of grief were more pronounced among those who experienced larger changes in self-concept clarity.

Maccallum and Bryant (2008) propose that anxious attachment may predispose people to develop merged self-identities, which in turn can affect autobiographical memory processes in ways that make the loss more salient and make adaptation more challenging. They also suggest that anxious attachment functions as a moderator of some of these pathways, although those ideas are not fully fleshed out.

One valuable feature of the CAM is that it brings together many core ideas that have been discussed throughout this chapter. For example, it highlights the role that continuing bonds may play in coping with loss, and it helps to clarify that the extent to which a person's identity is organized around the deceased may be one of the key predictors of both the intensity of the grief and the kind of challenges that must be faced as part of the recovery process. One way in which we think the CAM could be usefully expanded in the future is by disaggregating the merged versus independent identity dimension. In the CAM framework, a merged identity is one in which the person's sense of self is tightly connected to the lost individual. In our reading of Maccallum and Bryant's work, it is not always clear whether this dimension combines (1) the extent to which the lost person is a valued element of one's identity and (2) the extent to which the person's identity is rooted in other domains. To appreciate the distinction, it might be helpful to consider an economic metaphor. A person can invest all of his or her money in one company. Alternatively, a person can diversify his or her investments, placing some in real estate, some in tech stocks, and so on. Even within a diverse portfolio, however, a person can choose whether to invest a large or small portion of assets in one particular area. There is potential variation, then, in how (1) diverse the portfolio is and (2) what proportion of a person's assets are invested in any one domain.

In the case of loss, there can be variability in the extent to which a person is emotionally invested in the lost individual. Some people's identities are firmly grounded in their relationship, whereas other people's identities are more independent. But with this difference held constant, some people have a more diverse portfolio of goals, responsibilities, and competencies. In other words, if we take the two extremes of Maccallum and Bryant's (2008) self-identity dimension (i.e., merged and independent) and split those, it is possible to form a 2 × 2 table in which people vary in (1) the extent to which their identity is merged with that of the lost individual (e.g., high vs. low) and (2) the extent to which their identity is diversified and contains elements that are distinct from their relationship with the lost individual (e.g., high vs. low). It seems to us that the amount of distress that a person experiences following loss might vary largely as a function of the emotional investment the person has in the lost relationship, but that the ease or difficulty with which the person adapts to the loss will vary more as a function of whether his or her identity is also organized

around goals and tasks that are not integral to the lost relationship.

We find this distinction helpful in considering an attachment perspective because one of the hallmarks of having a secure attachment is that the bond enables the individual to explore the world in a more confident and autonomous manner. As a result, a person with a secure base is likely to develop a number of relationships and competencies that, while facilitated by the secure attachment bond, are not entwined with or dependent on that particular attachment relationship. Importantly, this conceptualization may help reconcile some of the apparent discrepancies between attachment theory on one hand, and Bonanno's research on resilience on the other. When oscillating between a loss-focused mindset and a restoration-focused mind-set (Stroebe & Schut, 1999), it might be most beneficial for a bereaved person to have in place a set of relationships, responsibilities, and plans that have meaning and significance that are independent of the lost person.

## Summary and Conclusion

The first time the full significance of [my father, John Bowlby's] work struck me was during a family walk ... just after his paper on "The nature of the child's tie to his mother" was first published [in 1958]. He said to me, "You know how distressed small children get if they're lost and can't find their mother and how they keep searching? Well, I suspect it's the same feeling that adults have when a loved one dies, they keep on searching too. I think it's the same instinct that starts in infancy and evolves throughout life as people grow up, and becomes part of adult love." I remember thinking, well, if you're right, you're on to something really big!
—RICHARD BOWLBY (2005, pp. vi–vii)

From a combination of attachment theory and numerous clinical case studies, Bowlby (1980) developed a conception of loss, grief, and mourning that remains the deepest and most comprehensive available. His theory is recognized as one of the major explanations of bereavement, and it has generated an enormous amount of research on reactions to loss and individual differences in the way people respond to and adapt to loss. Not surprisingly, Bowlby's theory has also generated criticism and controversy. In this chapter, we have considered some of the main criticisms of the theory. In each case, we considered the possibility that critics have mischaracterized Bowlby's views in an effort to supersede them. But we have also acknowledged that data collected and reported long after Bowlby's death make it clearer that many people weather losses without becoming disorganized, depressed, or vulnerable to later breakdown; that positive emotion plays a role in resilience following loss; and that the stages Bowlby inferred from studies of young children's separations from and reunions with their parents may not apply directly or without modification to the course of normal grieving.

The field of bereavement studies has made several advances over what existed in Bowlby's era. There are beginning to be prospective longitudinal studies, which allow us to see how prebereavement experiences and mental health affect postbereavement reactions. A clearer distinction is emerging between normal grief and complicated or prolonged grief (the latter is likely to be a consequence, in part, of preexisting anxious attachment). There is a more explicit recognition of continuing bonds, and that those bonds can be either adaptive or maladaptive. The clinical application of the new and old insights will require considerable judgment and training because there is no one-size-fits-all form of therapy that will work or be helpful for every bereaved individual.

Bowlby was not able to answer every important question about grief and mourning. Nevertheless, having reconsidered his work in light of what came before and what has come since, we are humbled by his ability to incorporate so much of the available evidence while keeping an eye on a coherent, comprehensive, and deep theory of human attachment and loss. His work will continue to inform researchers and clinicians interested in bereavement.

## Note

1. Bowlby (1980) also discussed "compulsive caregiving" as a disordered form of mourning. Because of space limitations and the relative lack of research examining this pattern, we do not discuss it further in this chapter.

## References

Adler, J. (2012). Crazy sad: The madness of pathologizing grief. *New York Magazine*. Retrieved from *http://nymag.com/news/intelligencer/grief-2012-5*.

Ainsworth, M. D. S., Blehar, M. C., Waters, E., & Wall, S. (1978). *Patterns of attachment: A psychological study of the Strange Situation*. Hillsdale, NJ: Erlbaum.

Ainsworth, M. D. S., & Eichberg, C. (1991). Effects on infant–mother attachment of mother's unresolved loss of an attachment figure, or other traumatic experience. In C. M. Parkes, J. Stevenson-Hinde, & P. Marris (Eds.), *Attachment across the life cycle* (pp. 160–183). London: Routledge.

American Psychiatric Association. (2000). *Diagnostic and statistical manual of mental disorders* (4th ed., text rev.). Washington, DC: Author.

Archer, J. (1999). *The nature of grief: The evolution and psychology of reactions to loss*. New York: Routledge.

Bartholomew, K., & Horowitz, L. M. (1991). Attachment styles among young adults: A test of a four-category model. *Journal of Personality and Social Psychology, 61*, 226–244.

Berant, E., Mikulincer, M., & Shaver, P. R. (2008). Mothers' attachment style, their mental health, and their children's emotional vulnerabilities: A 7-year study of mothers of children with congenital heart disease. *Journal of Personality, 76*, 31–65.

Boelen, P. A., Keijsers, L., & van den Hout, M. A. (2012). The role of self-concept clarity in prolonged grief disorder. *Journal of Nervous and Mental Disease, 200*, 56–62.

Boelen, P. A., & Klugkist, I. (2011). Cognitive behavioral variables mediate the associations of neuroticism and attachment insecurity with prolonged grief disorder severity. *Anxiety, Stress, and Coping, 24*, 291–307.

Boelen, P. A., van den Bout, J., & de Keijser, J. (2003). Traumatic grief as a disorder distinct from bereavement-related depression and anxiety: A replication study with bereaved mental health care patients. *American Journal of Psychiatry, 160*, 1339–1341.

Boelen, P. A., van den Hout, M. A., & van den Bout, J. (2006). A cognitive-behavioral conceptualization of complicated grief. *Clinical Psychology: Science and Practice, 13*, 109–128.

Boerner, K., & Heckhausen, J. (2003). To have and have not: Adaptive bereavement by transforming mental ties to the deceased. *Death Studies, 27*, 199–226.

Bonanno, G. (2004). Loss, trauma, and human resilience: Have we underestimated the human capacity to thrive after extremely aversive events? *American Psychologist, 59*, 20–28.

Bonanno, G. (2009). *The other side of sadness: What the new science of bereavement tells us about life after loss*. New York: Basic Books.

Bonanno, G. A., & Field, N. P. (2001). Evaluating the delayed grief hypothesis across 5 years of bereavement. *American Behavioral Scientist, 44*, 798–816.

Bonanno, G. A., & Kaltman, S. (2001). The varieties of grief experience. *Clinical Psychology Review, 21*, 705–734.

Bonanno, G. A., Moskowitz, J. T., Papa, A., & Folkman, S. (2005). Resilience to loss in bereaved spouses, bereaved parents, and bereaved gay men. *Journal of Personality and Social Psychology, 88*, 827–843.

Bonanno, G. A., Neria, Y., Mancini, A., Coifman, K.

G., Litz, B., & Insel, B. (2007). Is there more to complicated grief than depression and posttraumatic stress disorder?: A test of incremental validity. *Journal of Abnormal Psychology, 116,* 342–351.

Bonanno, G. A., Wortman, C. B., Lehman, D., Tweed, R., Sonnega, J., Carr, D., et al. (2002). Resilience to loss, chronic grief, and their pre-bereavement predictors. *Journal of Personality and Social Psychology, 83,* 1150–1164.

Bowlby, J. (1946). *Forty-four juvenile thieves: Their characters and home-life.* London: Bailliere, Tindall, & Cox.

Bowlby, J. (1973). *Attachment and loss: Vol. 2. Separation: Anxiety and anger.* New York: Basic Books.

Bowlby, J. (1980). *Attachment and loss: Vol. 3. Loss: Sadness and depression.* New York: Basic Books.

Bowlby, J. (1982). *Attachment and loss: Vol. 1. Attachment.* New York: Basic Books. (Original work published 1969)

Bowlby, J. (1990). *Charles Darwin: A new life.* New York: Norton.

Bowlby, R. (2005). Introduction. In J. Bowlby, *The making and breaking of affectional bonds* (Routledge Classics ed.). New York: Routledge.

Carnelley, K. B., Wortman, C. B., Bolger, N., & Burke, C. T. (2007). The time course of grief reactions to spousal loss: Evidence from a national probability sample. *Journal of Personality and Social Psychology, 91,* 476–492.

Deutsch, H. (1937). Absence of grief. *Psychoanalytic Quarterly, 6,* 12–22.

Doka, K. J. (2008). Disenfranchised grief in historical and cultural perspective. In M. S. Stroebe, R. O. Hansson, W. Stroebe, & H. A. W. Schut (Eds.), *Handbook of bereavement research and practice: 21st century perspectives* (pp. 223–240). Washington, DC: American Psychological Association.

Field, N. P. (2006). Continuing bonds in adaptation to bereavement: Introduction. *Death Studies, 30,* 709–714.

Field, N. P., & Friedrichs, M. (2004). Continuing bonds in coping with the death of a husband. *Death Studies, 28,* 597–620.

Field, N. P., Gal-Oz, E., & Bonanno, G. A. (2003). Continuing bonds and adjustment at 5 years after the death of a spouse. *Journal of Consulting and Clinical Psychology, 71,* 110–117.

Field, N. P., & Sundin, E. C. (2001). Attachment style in adjustment to conjugal bereavement. *Journal of Social and Personal Relationships, 18,* 347–361.

Forstmeier, S., & Maercker, A. (2007). Comparison of two diagnostic systems for complicated grief. *Journal of Affective Disorders, 99,* 203–211.

Fraley, R. C., & Bonanno, G. A. (2004). Attachment and loss: A test of three competing models on the association between attachment-related avoidance and adaptation to bereavement. *Personality and Social Psychology Bulletin, 30,* 878–890.

Fraley, R. C., Davis, K. E., & Shaver, P. R. (1998). Dismissing-avoidance and the defensive organization of emotion, cognition, and behavior. In J. A. Simpson & W. S. Rholes (Eds.), *Attachment theory and close relationships* (pp. 249–279). New York: Guilford Press.

Fraley, R. C., Fazzari, D. A., Bonanno, G. A., & Dekel, S. (2006). Attachment and psychological adaptation in high exposure survivors of the September 11th attack on the World Trade Center. *Personality and Social Psychology Bulletin, 32,* 538–551.

Fraley, R. C., & Shaver, P. R. (1998). Airport separations: A naturalistic study of adult attachment dynamics in separating couples. *Journal of Personality and Social Psychology, 75,* 1198–1212.

Fraley, R. C., & Shaver, P. R. (1999). Loss and bereavement: Attachment theory and recent controversies concerning "grief work" and the nature of detachment. In J. Cassidy & P. R. Shaver (Eds.), *Handbook of attachment: Theory, research, and clinical applications* (pp. 735–759). New York: Guilford Press.

Fraley, R. C., & Shaver, P. R. (2000). Adult romantic attachment: Theoretical developments, emerging controversies, and unanswered questions. *Review of General Psychology, 4,* 132–154.

Gilbert, S. M. (2006). *Death's door: Modern dying and the ways we grieve.* New York: Norton.

Griffin, D. W., & Bartholomew, K. (1994). Models of the self and other: Fundamental dimensions underlying measures of adult attachment. *Journal of Personality and Social Psychology, 67,* 430–445.

Hart, C. L., Hole, D. J., Lawlor, D. A., Smith, G. D., & Lever, T. F. (2007). Effect of conjugal bereavement on mortality of the bereaved spouse in participants of the Renfrew/Paisley Study. *Journal of Epidemiology and Community Health, 61,* 455–460.

Hazan, C., & Shaver, P. (1987). Romantic love conceptualized as an attachment process. *Journal of Personality and Social Psychology, 52*(3), 511–524.

Heinicke, C. M., & Westheimer, I. J. (1965). *Brief separations.* New York: International Universities Press.

Holland, J. M., & Neimeyer, R. A. (2010). An examination of stage theory of grief among individuals bereaved by natural and violent causes: A meaning-oriented contribution. *OMEGA: Journal of Death and Dying, 61*(2), 103–120.

Horowitz, M. J., Siegel, B., Holen, A., Bonanno, G. A., Milbrath, C., & Stinson, C. H. (1997). Diagnostic criteria for complicated grief disorder. *American Journal of Psychiatry, 154,* 904–910.

Jerga, A. M., Shaver, P. R., & Wilkinson, R. B. (2011). Attachment insecurities and identification of at-risk individuals following the death of a loved one. *Journal of Social and Personal Relationships, 28,* 891–914.

Klass, D., Silverman, P. R., & Nickman, S. L. (Eds.). (1996). *Continuing bonds: New understandings of grief.* Washington, DC: Taylor & Francis.

Konigsberg, R. D. (2011). *The truth about grief: The myth*

*of its five stages and the new science of loss*. New York: Simon & Schuster.

Lalande, K. M., & Bonanno, G. A. (2007). Culture and continuing bonds: A prospective comparison of bereavement in the United States and the People's Republic of China. *Death Studies, 30*, 303–324.

Lichtenthal, W. G., Cruess, D. G., & Prigerson, H. G. (2004). A case for establishing complicated grief as a distinct mental disorder in DSM-V. *Clinical Psychology Review, 24*, 637–662.

Lorenz, K. (1963). *On aggression*. New York: Bantam.

Maccallum, F., & Bryant, R. A. (2008). Self-defining memories in complicated grief. *Behaviour Research and Therapy, 46*, 1311–1315.

Maccallum, F., & Bryant, R. A. (2013). A Cognitive Attachment Model of prolonged grief: Integrating attachments, memory, and identity. *Clinical Psychology Review, 33*(6), 713–727.

Maercker, A., Brewin, C. R., Bryant, R. A., Cloitre, M., Reed, G. M., van Ommeren, M., et al. (2013). Proposals for mental disorders specifically associated with stress in the International Classification of Diseases–11. *Lancet, 381*, 1683–1685.

Main, M. (1991). Metacognitive knowledge, metacognitive monitoring, and singular (coherent) vs. multiple (incoherent) model of attachment: Findings and directions for future research. In C. M. Parkes, J. Stevenson-Hinde, & P. Marris (Eds.), *Attachment across the life cycle* (pp. 127–159). London: Tavistock/Routledge.

Main, M., & Hesse, E. (1990). Parents' unresolved traumatic experiences are related to infant disorganized attachment status: Is frightened and/or frightening parental behavior the linking mechanism? In M. T. Greenberg, D. Cicchetti, & E. M. Cummings (Eds.), *Attachment in the preschool years: Theory, research, and intervention* (pp. 161–182). Chicago: University of Chicago Press.

Main, M., Kaplan, N., & Cassidy, J. (1985). Security in infancy, childhood, and adulthood: A move to the level of representation. *Monographs of the Society for Research in Child Development, 50*(1–2, Serial No. 209), 66–104.

Malkinson, R., Rubin, S. S., & Witztum, E. (2006). Therapeutic issues and the relationship to the deceased: Working clinically with the two-track model of bereavement. *Death Studies, 30*, 797–815.

Mancini, A. D., Robinaugh, D., Shear, K., & Bonanno, G. A. (2009). Does attachment avoidance help people cope with loss?: The moderating effects of relationship quality. *Journal of Clinical Psychology, 65*, 1127–1136.

Mathison, J. (1970). A cross-cultural view of widowhood. *Omega: Journal of Death and Dying, 1*, 201–218.

Meier, A. M., Carr, D. R., Currier, J. M., & Neimeyer, R. A. (2013). Attachment anxiety and avoidance in coping with bereavement: Two studies. *Journal of Social and Clinical Psychology, 32*(3), 315–334.

Middleton, W., Raphael, B., Martinek, N., & Misso, V. (1993). Pathological grief reactions. In M. S. Stroebe, W. Stroebe, & R. O. Hansson (Eds.), *Handbook of bereavement: Theory, research, and intervention* (pp. 44–61). New York: Cambridge University Press.

Mikulincer, M., Dolev, T., & Shaver, P. R. (2004). Attachment-related strategies during thought-suppression: Ironic rebounds and vulnerable self-representations. *Journal of Personality and Social Psychology, 87*, 940–956.

Mikulincer, M., & Shaver, P. R. (2007). *Attachment in adulthood: Structure, dynamics, and change*. New York: Guilford Press.

Mikulincer, M., & Shaver, P. R. (2008). An attachment perspective on bereavement. In M. Stroebe, R. O. Hansson, H. A. W. Schut, & W. Stroebe (Eds.), *Handbook of bereavement research and practice: 21st century perspectives* (pp. 87–112). Washington, DC: American Psychological Association.

Miller, S. I., & Schoenfeld, L. (1973). Grief in the Navajo: Psychodynamics and culture. *International Journal of Social Psychiatry, 19*, 187–191.

Neimeyer, R. A. (Ed.). (2012). *Techniques of grief therapy: Creative practices for counseling the bereaved*. New York: Routledge.

Ogrodniczuk, J. S., Piper, W. E., Joyce, A. S., Weideman, R., McCallum, M., Azim, H. F., et al. (2003). Differentiating symptoms of complicated grief and depression among psychiatric outpatients. *Canadian Journal of Psychiatry, 48*, 87–93.

Parkes, C. M. (1965). Bereavement and mental illness. *British Journal of Medical Psychology, 38*, 388–397.

Parkes, C. M. (2006). *Love and loss: The roots of grief and its complications*. New York: Taylor & Francis.

Parkes, C. M., & Weiss, R. S. (1983). *Recovery from bereavement*. New York: Basic Books.

Poole, J. H. (1996). *Coming of age with elephants*. New York: Hyperion.

Prigerson, H. G., Bierhals, A. J., Kasl, S. V., Reynolds, C. F., III, Shear, M. K., Newsom, J. T., et al. (1996). Complicated grief as a disorder distinct from bereavement-related depression and anxiety: A replication study. *American Journal of Psychiatry, 153*, 1484–1486.

Prigerson, H. G., Horowitz, M. J., Jacobs, S. C., Parkes, C. M., Aslan, M., Goodkin, K., et al. (2009). Prolonged grief disorder: Psychometric validation of criteria proposed for DSM-V and ICD-11. *PLoS Medicine, 6*, e1000121.

Prigerson, H. G., Vanderwerker, L. C., & Maciejewski, P. K. (2008). A case for inclusion of prolonged grief disorder in DSM-V. In M. S. Stroebe, R. O. Hansson, H. A. W. Schut, & W. Stroebe (Eds.), *Handbook of bereavement research and practice: Advances in theory and intervention* (pp. 165–186). Washington, DC: American Psychological Association.

Rosenblatt, P. C. (2008). Grief across cultures: A review and research agenda. In M. S. Stroebe, R. O. Hansson, W. Stroebe, & H. A. W. Schut (Eds.), *Handbook*

of bereavement research and practice: 21st century perspectives (pp. 207–222). Washington, DC: American
Psychological Association.

Rosenblatt, P. C., Walsh, R. P., & Jackson, D. A. (1976).
*Grief and mourning in cross-cultural perspective*. New
Haven, CT: Human Relations Area Files.

Sandler, I. N., Wolchik, S. A., Ayers, T. S., Tein, J. Y.,
Coxe, S., & Chow, W. (2008). Linking theory and
intervention to promote resilience in parentally bereaved children. In M. S. Stroebe, R. O. Hansson,
W. Stroebe, & H. A. W. Schut (Eds.), *Handbook of
bereavement research and practice: 21st century perspectives*. Washington, DC: American Psychological Association.

Sbarra, D. A., & Emery, R. E. (2005). The emotional sequelae of nonmarital relationship dissolution: Analysis of change and intraindividual variability over
time. *Personal Relationships, 12,* 213–232.

Sbarra, D. A., & Hazan, C. (2008). Coregulation, dysregulation, self-regulation: An integrative analysis
and empirical agenda for understanding adult attachment, separation, loss, and recovery. *Personality and
Social Psychology Review, 12,* 141–167.

Schut, H. A. W., Stroebe, M. S., Boelen, P. A., & Zijerveld, A. M. (2006). Continuing relationships with
the deceased: Disentangling bonds and grief. *Death
Studies, 30,* 757–766.

Seay, B., Hansen, E., & Harlow, H. F. (1962). Mother–
infant separation in monkeys. *Journal of Child Psychology and Psychiatry, 3,* 123–132.

Shaver, P. R., & Tancredy, C. M. (2001). Emotion,
attachment, and bereavement: A conceptual commentary. In M. S. Stroebe, W. Stroebe, R. O. Hansson, & H. Schut (Eds.), *Handbook of bereavement
research: Consequences, coping, and care* (pp. 63–88).
Washington, DC: American Psychological Association.

Shear, M. K., & Shair, H. (2005). Attachment, loss, and
complicated grief. *Developmental Psychobiology, 47,*
253–267.

Shear, M. K., Simon, N., Wall, M., Zisook, S., Neimeyer,
R., Duan, N., et al. (2011). Complicated grief and re-
lated bereavement issues for DSM-5. *Depression and
Anxiety, 28*(2), 103–117.

Simon, N. M., Shear, K. M., Thompson, E. H., Zalta, A.
K., Perlman, C., Reynolds, C. F., et al. (2007). The
prevalence and correlates of psychiatric comorbidity

in individuals with complicated grief. *Comprehensive
Psychiatry, 48,* 395–399.

Sroufe, L. A., & Waters, E. (1977). Attachment as an
organizational construct. *Child Development, 48,*
1184–1199.

Stroebe, M., & Schut, H. (1999). The dual process
model of coping with bereavement: Rationale and
description. *Death Studies, 23,* 197–224.

Stroebe, M., & Schut, H. (2005). To continue or relinquish bonds: A review of consequences for the bereaved. *Death Studies, 29,* 477–494.

Stroebe, M., Schut, H., & Stroebe, W. (2007). Health
outcomes in bereavement. *Lancet, 370,* 1960–1973.

Stroebe, M., van Son, M., Stroebe, W., Kleber, R.,
Schut, H., & van den Bout, J. (2000). On the clas-
sification and diagnosis of pathological grief. *Clinical
Psychology Review, 20,* 57–75.

Stroebe, W., & Stroebe, M. (1987). *Bereavement and
health: The psychological and physical consequences of
partner loss.* New York: Cambridge University Press.

Stroebe, W., Stroebe, M., Abakoumkin, G., & Schut, H.
(1996). The role of loneliness and social support in
adjustment to loss: A test of attachment versus stress
theory. *Journal of Personality and Social Psychology, 70,*
1241–1249.

Waskowic, T. D., & Chartier, B. M. (2003). Attachment
and the experience of grief following the loss of a
spouse. *Omega: Journal of Death and Dying, 47,* 77–91.

Wayment, H. A., & Vierthaler, J. (2002). Attachment
style and bereavement reactions. *Journal of Loss and
Trauma, 7,* 129–149.

Weiss, R. S. (1973). *Loneliness: The experience of social
and emotional isolation.* Cambridge, MA: MIT Press.

Weiss, R. S. (1975). *Marital separation.* New York: Basic
Books.

Wijngaards-de Meij, L., Stroebe, M., Schut, H., Stroebe,
W., van den Bout, J., van der Heijden, P. G. M., et al.
(2007). Patterns of attachment and parents' adjustment to the death of their child. *Personality and Social
Psychology Bulletin, 33,* 537–548.

Wortman, C. B., & Boerner, K. (2007). Beyond the
myths of coping with loss: Prevailing assumptions
versus scientific evidence. In H. S. Friedman & R.
C. Silver (Eds.), *Foundations of health psychology*
(pp. 285–324). New York: Oxford University Press.

Zisook, S., & DeVaul, R. A. (1985). Unresolved grief.
*American Journal of Psychoanalysis, 45,* 370–379.

# Chapter 4

# The Internal Working Model Construct in Light of Contemporary Neuroimaging Research

Inge Bretherton
Kristine A. Munholland

The notion that brains do in fact provide more or less elaborate models that can be made to conduct, as it were, small-scale experiments within the head is one that appeals to anyone concerned to understand the complexities of behavior and especially human behavior. . . . In order to understand human behavior it is difficult to do without such a hypothesis—which squares, of course, with such introspective knowledge of our own mental processes as we have.

—JOHN BOWLBY (1969, pp. 80–81)

In formulating attachment theory (1969/1982, 1973, 1980, 1988) Bowlby maintained that an individual's mental health from the cradle to the grave is intimately tied to relationships with attachment figures who afford emotional support and physical protection. He addtionally claimed that the security-enhancing quality of these relationships turns not only on attachment partners' momentary behavior toward one another but also on the translation of their habitual interaction patterns into relationship representations—or, as he called them, *internal working models* (IWMs), a term he did not regard as purely metaphorical (M. D. S. Ainsworth, personal communication, n.d.). IWMs, in Bowlby's view, help both members of an attachment dyad, whether parent and child, or adult couple, to anticipate, interpret, and guide reciprocal interactions.

Bowlby discovered the IWM construct in the writings of an eminent scientist interested in the neural basis of animal memory, J. Z. Young (1964), while rethinking what he considered to be scientifically outdated explanations of the psychoanalytic "internal world." The originator of the IWM construct, however, was the innovative cognitive psychologist, Kenneth Craik (1943). Unfortunately, Craik's work was cut short by his early death.

Although Bowlby (1969/1982, p. 80) occasionally used other, more static descriptions for mental representation such as "cognitive map" or "image," he favored IWM because that term connotes a dynamic representational system that allows humans to imagine (or internally simulate) habitually experienced sequential patterns of social interaction. More explicitly than Craik (1943), Bowlby maintained that in order to make plans for achieving desired goals, humans must acquire not only an IWM of their environment, but also a working knowledge of their own behavioral skills and potentialities in that environment (which he initially called an "organismic model"). Note that whereas Bowlby (1973, 1980, 1988) emphasized the role of IWMs in attachment relationships, his initial notion of representation as IWM-building included interactions with the physical, as well as the social, environment and was limited neither to attachment relationships nor to other social relationships (Bowlby, 1969/1982). He considered emotional appraisals to be an integral aspect of working models.

Despite the centrality of the IWM construct in Bowlby's thinking about representation, he never developed a systematic overall account of the formation, development, function, and intergenerational transmission of IWMs. His views on these topics are hence scattered across the three volumes of his seminal trilogy *Attachment and Loss* (1969/1982, 1973, 1980) and his final book on attachment, *A Secure Base* (1988). In an attempt to capture the essence of Bowlby's IWM-related proposals, we included a large selection of verbatim quotes from his works in our 2008 chapter of this handbook. In this revised chapter, we begin with a much briefer summary of Bowlby's IWM tenets (keeping close to his own wording and providing page numbers for easy reference), and then discuss their fit with related developmental research on event memory. Our primary focus, however, is on IWM-relevant neuroimaging research that has proliferated in the last 20 years. We believe that Bowlby would have incorporated findings from these studies into his writings had they been available to him. We conclude with reflections on ways in which neuroimaging research can affirm, expand, and clarify our thinking about working models in attachment relationships.

## Bowlby's Major Postulates Regarding IWMs

1. Whereas IWMs play an important role in human attachment relationships, Bowlby's IWM construct is restricted neither to humans nor to relationship representations. As Bowlby (1969/1982, p. 48) stressed: "Members of all but the most primitive phyla are possessed of equipment that enables them to organize such information as they have about the world into schemata or maps." IWMs, in his view, derive from an organism's selective processing of interactions with the physical and so-

cial environment, but the complexity and type of IWMs that an organism can build depends on and is limited by the particular organism's perceptual and effector equipment.

2. Organisms with more adequate working models can make more accurate predictions and organisms whose models are more comprehensive can make predictions in a greater number of situations (Bowlby, 1969/1982, p. 81). Making accurate predictions improves the likelihood of the organisms' survival and eventual reproduction.

3. In humans, the function of working models is to transmit, store, and manipulate information regarding behavioral choices for achieving the set-goals of behavioral systems (Bowlby, 1969/1982, p. 80), including but not limited to the attachment system, and to aid in the evaluation of alternative courses of action by means of *internal simulation* (Bowlby, 1988, pp. 130, 165).

4. In humans, IWMs include selective appraisals that are often, but not necessarily, experienced as conscious feelings or, as Bowlby preferred, "felt." Thus, input representing features of the environment and the self is appraised in terms of value (good, bad) and categorized in terms of potential actions based on behavioral choices made previously (1969/1982, p. 112). Individuals who are aware of these prior appraisals can use them to monitor their own current states, urges, and situations. Their facial expressions or postures, moreover, can transmit valuable information regarding these appraisals to companions.

5. By allowing an individual to profit from past experiences, rather than having to react de novo to momentary influences and perturbations, IWMs ensure a certain degree of continuity in an individual's interpretation of and interaction with the social and physical world.

6. However, to be of use in novel situations, it must be possible to extend IWMs imaginatively to potential realities, not merely to apply them to similar recurrent events (1969/1982, p. 81).

7. A key feature *within* a person's working model of the world is who his or her attachment figures are, where they may be found, and how they are likely to respond. Likewise, a key feature in a person's working models of the self is whether he or she feels accepted by attachment figures and is confident that they will respond to bids for support. "On these complementary IWMs of self with attachment figures depends an individual's confi-

dence that attachment figures, in general, will be readily available—most of the time, occasionally, or almost never" and whether he will approach the world with confidence when faced with alarming situations, either by tackling them effectively or seeking support (see Bowlby, 1973, p. 203). Said differently, IWMs of self with attachment figures "increasingly become a property of the child himself" (Bowlby, 1988, p. 129).

8. To function adequately, infants' embryonic working models of self and attachment figure(s) must be updated in step with their developing communicative, social, and cognitive abilities. The same holds for a parent's working models of the developing child and self as attachment figure. Despite the time lag that is inevitably associated with IWM updating, under normal circumstances the "currently operative models continue to be reasonably good *simulations* of himself and his parents in interaction" (Bowlby, 1988, p. 130, emphasis added). More radical updating may, however, be called for as a consequence of family transitions, accidents, chronic illness, or loss (Bowlby, 1969/1982, pp. 82, 348).

8. Although IWM-building begins *before* the onset of speech, language acquisition allows children to draw on and learn from the working models of others (Bowlby, 1969/1982, p. 83). Parents transmit to the child the images they have of the child "not only by how each treats him, but by what each says to him" (Bowlby, 1988, p. 130). There are circumstances, however, under which parents may exert pressure on the child to "adopt and confirm a parent's false models—of self, of child and of their relationships" (1973, p. 322).

9. Young children's growing competence in perspective taking enables them to develop a degree of insight into their parents' feelings and motives, hence allowing them to influence their parents' independent goals. This transforms the child–parent relationship into a partnership (Bowlby, 1969/1982, p. 268).

10. Infant–caregiver relationship patterns worked out in the first 12 months tend to persist at least for the next few years because the IWMs of two people are in play. Given that each member of the pair expects the other to behave in a certain way and tends to try to evoke from the other the behavior he or she expects, reciprocal expectations tend to be confirmed, thus increasing the

stability of their relationship patterns and IWMs (Bowlby, 1969/1982, p. 347).

11. According to Bowlby, "many of the mental processes of which we are most keenly conscious are processes concerned with the building of models, with revising and extending them, checking them for internal consistency or drawing on them for making a novel plan to reach a set-goal. Although it is certainly not necessary for all such processes always to be conscious, it is probably necessary for some of them to be so sometimes" (Bowlby, 1969/1982, pp. 82–83).

12. When—in analogy to a physical skill—cognitive and action components of IWMs become highly ingrained or overlearned, they are applied automatically and without conscious awareness. When IWMs are well adapted, this is an advantage, but when automated IWMs are not well adapted, and parental or internal (superego) rules forbid their reappraisal, revising IWMs becomes an arduous task that may be undertaken only slowly or not at all (Bowlby, 1980, pp. 54–56).

13. Much psychopathology can be attributed to fully or partially out-of-date IWMs that are fraught with inconsistencies and confusions because defensive processes (e.g., denial, self-deception, distortion, and misattribution) obstruct adaptive IWM revisions (Bowlby, 1969/1982, p. 80). Under some circumstances, such defensive processes lead individuals to invert the attachment relationship and construct an IWM of self as caregiver of a helpless or rejecting attachment figure, or else individuals may become morbidly preoccupied with relationship-related emotional pain (Bowlby, 1980, p. 68).

14. Although Bowlby (1973, p. 208) saw adult personality "as a product of an individual's interaction with key figures, especially of his interactions with attachment figures, during his years of immaturity, nowhere in his attachment trilogy (1969/1982, 1973, 1980) did he envisage that a child might construct qualitatively different IWMs in relation to different attachment figures. After Main and Weston (1981), among others, reported such differences in many families, Bowlby (1988, pp. 128–129) acknowledged that little is known about the relative influence on personality development of the child's relationship with father and mother, that different facets of personality might be differentially influenced by mother and father,

and that male and female children might be differentially affected. He then speculated that, during the early years, the model of self-interacting-with-mother may be most influential because, in most cultures, the mother is likely to be the child's principal caregiver.

15. The term *internalization* as applied by Bowlby (1988, p. 129) did not refer to the process of forming relationship-specific attachment IWMs, but to the process whereby relationship-specific IWM patterns increasingly become a "property of the child himself." He proposed that these internalized patterns or some derivative thereof were likely to be imposed on new relationships, sometimes "despite the absence of fit" (Bowlby, 1988, pp. 127, 170).

## IWMs in Light of Developmental Research on Event Representation

When Bowlby (1969/1982) incorporated the IWM construct into attachment theory, the notion of representation as working model building and revision was unheard of in the academic literature on infant and adult memory, cognition, emotion, and language. Aside from Piaget's (1951, 1952) theory of assimilation and accommodation in the context of sensorimotor schemas and emergent representations, there was little empirical evidence with which Bowlby could support his IWM hypotheses.

Only in the late 1970s did new insights and empirical work on scripts in story understanding, conducted by Schank and Abelson (1977), and research on young children's developing event representations, by Nelson and Gruende (1981), offer empirical evidence in line with Bowlby's notion that humans can mentally simulate interpersonal transaction patterns with attachment figures (Bretherton, 1985, pp. 31–32). Nelson's (1996) revised conceptualization of experiential event memory made the fit with Bowlby even clearer.

For Nelson (1996) as well as Bowlby (1969/1982, 1980), the everyday function of representation is to guide actions in the present and anticipate future events/interactions in light of what has generally happened in the past. Events, in this context, are defined as "whole scenes unfolding over time that involve people and/or other animates acting over time and in particular places" (Nelson, 2005, p. 360). Whereas Nelson had initially assumed that infants' and toddlers' recall ability was limited to generic events or scripts, she retracted that view when research showed that even 16-month-olds can demonstrate their memory for unique events they had experienced in a laboratory by *reenacting them* in the same context weeks to months later (see Bauer & Wewerka, 1995). Following Donald's (1993) terminology, Nelson called this reenactive type of early remembering "mimetic," but nevertheless maintained that young children's world models are derived from their generalized event representations (GERs). GERs, in her view, develop when each new instance of a recurring event overwrites memories of the previous one.

Nelson (1996) treated generic event memory as distinct from the episodic and semantic memory systems, as proposed by the eminent memory theorist Tulving (1972), whose ideas subsequently influenced Bowlby (1980). Tulving defined episodic memories as temporally dated, autobiographical episodes or events ("I remember that . . ."), but regarded semantic memories as undated and unlocalized *factual* knowledge ("I know that . . ."). Although GERs are not by necessity undated or unlocalized (i.e., "I remember" can also apply to them), Tulving subsumed generic events into his definition of the semantic system. Nelson argued, more plausibly in our view, that GERs are the *source* from which general knowledge categories are created. Thus, children might learn to group an item into a general "food" category because it can fill the same "slot" in a generic event or script, such as "lunch at the day care center." Nelson further suggested that GERs can provide a framework for organizing autobiographical memories of unique events, a view close to that subsequently adopted by Tulving (2002). Finally, Nelson explained that GERs are not to be confused with procedural (skill) memory which, as defined by Sherry and Schacter (1987), operates outside awareness. Event memory, she noted, "is a form of representation that involves a degree of conscious awareness" (Nelson, 1996, p. 62).

Around age 2, many toddlers take tentative steps toward translating unique and generic nonverbal/mimetic memories into verbal narratives to be shared with others, particularly if their efforts are encouraged by supportive and sensitive caregivers who expand on their children's contributions through affirmations, questions, and evaluative language (e.g., Fivush & Vasudeva, 2002; Laible & Thompson, 2000; Newcombe & Reese,

2004). Concurrently, they acquire a rudimentary ability to translate *others'* verbal narratives back into their own meaningful event representations, although fuller mastery of these communicative/representational processes extends over the preschool years and beyond (Nelson, 1996). A fascinating account of a young child's solitary verbal rehearsal of daily routines and unique happenings before falling asleep was published by Nelson in 1989.

### Relationship Scripts

Because young children's capacity for generating verbal event representations was initially examined in the context of emotionally neutral scripts, some attachment researchers objected to the use of this term in relation to IWMs. They maintained that the script notion could not apply to attachment relationships, which are never affectively neutral. However, Nelson's GER construct can easily be extended to include affects and intentions (Bretherton, 1990). Moreover, whereas event schemas as defined by Nelson would allow classes of people (e.g., caregivers in general) to fill the agent and recipient "slots" in a GER, there is no reason why a child should not construct generic relationship-specific representations of, say, "self with father" that are restricted to this particular relationship.

However, if conceptualized as a mere collection of GERs, an IWM of self with a specific other would be unworkable. A better approach would be to regard working models as an organized, multilayered, partially hierarchical network or web of interrelated GERs with different levels of generality (Bretherton, 1985, 1990; Bretherton & Munholland, 2008). In such a network, habitual, experience-near, relationship-specific scenarios would serve as inputs to higher-order general categories. At an experience-near level, relationship-specific attachment memories in infancy would be nonverbal, based on experiential GERs of the way a particular mother cuddled, comforted, and interacted with her child. These GERs could then serve, along with other mother–infant scenarios, as the basis of a more general but still relationship-specific IWM (e.g., expressed verbally as "When I feel bad/sad, Mom helps me feel better"). Such a mother-specific "secure base script" (a term coined by Waters & Waters, 2006) represents basic trust in not only the specific parent's ability to provide emotional support and protection, but also her perceived willingness and availability to

do so. Bowlby (1980, p. 62) sometimes conceptualized working models at this general scriptlike level, that is, as "generalizations of mother, father, and self." However, at other times, he (Bowlby, 1988, p. 128) used a more experience-near description, referring to a child's model "of mother and her ways of communicating and behaving towards him, and a comparable model of his father, together with the complementary models of himself." In our view, these levels work together. Without access to underlying experience-near GERs (as in Bowlby, 1988), trust in attachment figures could neither come into being or be sustained—whether in infancy or later. Trait adjectives such as *trustworthy* or *loving* are but stand-ins for highly general event categories that are meaningful only because of underlying experience-near GERs (see also Waters, Crowell, Elliott, Corcoran, & Treboux, 2002).

The question whether general expectations about others, especially close others, derive from experiences with several attachment and other key figures (as Bowlby suggested in 1973), or primarily from a child's IWMs of self with his or her *principal* attachment figure (as Bowlby surmised in 1988) has not been definitively answered. In partial support of combined influences, Main and Weston (1981) showed that toddlers deemed secure both with mother and father in separate Strange Situations showed greater readiness to engage with a friendly stranger than infants deemed insecure with one parent and not the other. Lowest scores were given to infants with two insecure attachments. Likewise, Van IJzendoorn, Sagi, and Lambermon (1992) showed that children with secure relationships to father, mother, and child care provider in infancy had greater ego resilience as kindergartners. At variance with these findings, Main, Kaplan, and Cassidy (1985) and Grossmann, Grossmann, and Kindler (2005), as well as others, reported that infant attachment classifications to mother, but not father, predicted the quality of representational attachment measures in early childhood and at school entry (assessed with separation pictures). There is as yet no firm consensus on when and how children develop and apply generalized expectations in new relationships and whether these expectations are more predictable from primary or aggregated attachment classifications. We still await an exhaustive meta-analysis of results from longitudinal studies that include relationships with multiple attachment figures (see Howes & Spieker, Chapter 15, this volume, for discussion of multiple attachment figures).

## The IWM Construct in Light of Neuroimaging Studies

Not only can children as young as 3 years of age provide rudimentary verbal descriptions of sequentially ordered generic events, as shown by Nelson and Gruendel (1981), even more complex interpersonal event representations are possible at this age if children are permitted to combine verbal with enactive or mimetic narration by using family figures and small props to create attachment- and other family-related stories (Bretherton, Ridgeway, & Cassidy, 1990; Oppenheim, Emde, & Warren, 1997). But what are the brain processes that underlie these developing abilities? Do they justify Bowlby's claim that the human brain constructs mental models in a more than metaphoric sense, and do emerging neuroimaging discoveries line up with Bowlby's views and the event memory literature?

Partial answers to these questions from neuroimaging research have revealed that Bowlby's notions about "a working model in the brain" were remarkably prescient. A rapidly growing number of studies, only a small selection of which can be reviewed and discussed here, have consistently demonstrated links between perception/representation and brain structure/functioning that are congruent with Bowlby's IWM notion. Moreover, as memory theorist Barsalou (2009) has repeatedly explained, these findings also accord with contemporary approaches to cognition, emotion, and event memory according to which representations are contextually situated, grounded in experience, and embodied (see also Damasio, 1999; Decety & Grèzes, 2006; Glenberg, 1997). Instead of assuming that representations consist of amodal symbols (e.g., logical propositions, data structures, and procedures as advocated by Pylyshyn, 1973), neuroimaging studies reveal that mental models rely on the same brain sites that subserve perception (e.g., vision, audition, touch), action (e.g., movement), proprioception (balance), and interoception (e.g., visceral, emotional, and cognitive states).

Admittedly, the most commonly used neuroimaging methods are not yet as precise as one might wish. For example, the two methods for assessing increases of local blood flow in specific brain regions (positron emission tomography [PET] and functional magnetic resonance imaging [fMRI]) have less than ideal temporal and spatial resolution. Transcranial magnetic stimulation (TMS), although useful for temporarily and reversibly inactivating or hyperactivating specific cortical sites, cannot reach cortical areas buried in cerebral fissures or sulci; and event-related potentials (ERPs), capable of assessing the precise timing of cortical responses, are less exact than desirable regarding the location of these responses. New methods for revealing neural interconnections (magnetic resonance diffusion tractography) are promising, although researchers cannot always discern the functions of these connections, and case studies of single-cell recordings performed before or during brain surgery can test only a limited number of neurons. In addition, deficits following so-called focal brain injuries often involve more than the region of interest (for additional discussion of technical and measurement issues related to this topic, see Sarter, Berntson, & Cacioppo, 1996). Finally, developmental neuroimaging studies are as yet few and far between. Nevertheless, many insights obtained with these brain imaging methods are giving new meaning to and expanding upon Bowlby's (1969/1982, 1973, 1980) IWM notions.

## IWMs Enabled by the Organization of Modal and Multimodal Cortical Sites

To be capable of simulating future events based on past experiences with people and objects, IWMs must retain configural aspects of these events in their physical and social context. An ever-increasing number of neuroimaging studies suggests that this is achieved, in the first instance, by the orderly conveyance of signals from the peripheral body and sensory organs to specialized primary motor, extero-, and interoceptive cortical sites, after preprocessing in various subcortical way stations. These cortical sites hence reflect the layout of the body (musculoskeletal, somatosensory, and visceral) and the structure of its exteroceptive organs (e.g., retinotopic for vision, audiotopic for hearing).[1]

Note that cortical body maps include not only the well-known primary sensory and motor "homunculi" familiar from textbook illustrations, but a considerable number of auxiliary, somatotopically or topographically organized, secondary and tertiary sites that analyze, sharpen, and integrate signals from the primary maps into meaningful perceptions and motor commands for goal-directed actions. At least three body-reflective motor maps in each frontal lobe (primary, premotor, and supplementary motor) harbor increasingly complex neural prescriptions or schemas for coordinated actions (Fernandino & Iacoboni, 2010). More than two somatosensory body maps are aligned alongside each other in the parietal lobes just behind the central fissure, specializing in skin, deep muscle, and joint sensations. Finally, hidden behind the Sylvan fissure that delimits the frontal from the temporal lobes, the insulae process interoceptive (evaluative) information about the current physiological/visceral condition of the body.

Before the advent of PET and fMRI methods, neural activity in cortical fissures and sulci could not be adequately probed, and the insula was hence largely inaccessible to study. It is now known that the *posterior* part of the insula receives input from all parts of the autonomic nervous system and engenders interoceptive sensations of pain, temperature, itch, sensual/libidinal touch; muscular, visceral, and vestibular sensations; and vasomotor activity, hunger, thirst, and "air hunger." In the insula's *anterior* portion, these sensory-discriminative visceral signals are rerepresented together with their positive and negative affective qualities, indicating the current state of the physical "me" (Craig, 2009; see also Damasio, 1999), findings that are consistent with Bowlby's contention that emotional appraisal processes are a vital aspect of IWMs. The insula has somatotopic organization, at least with respect to painful temperature sensations (Brooks, Zambreanu, Godinez, Craig, & Tracey, 2005) as well as muscle and cutaneous pain (Henderson, Gandevia, & Macefield, 2007). Electrical stimulation in the insula can elicit pain experiences in specific body locations (Mazzola, Isnard, Peyron, & Maugière, 2012).

In the occipital lobes, five or more retinotopically organized sites process different aspects of vision (e.g., visual area 4 processes color and visual area 5 processes motion). Beyond these general purpose sites, the more specialized fusiform face area (FFA; in the inferior occipitotemporal lobes) responds selectively to familiar faces, particularly their unique featural configurations (see reviews by Kanwisher & Yovel, 2006). Patients with focused lesions in the FFA can recognize neither the faces of familiar persons nor their own reflections in a mirror (prosopagnosia; Damasio, 1999).

Adjacent to the FFA is the extrastriate body area (EBA; *extrastriate* means outside the striate or striped primary visual cortex). The EBA captures static and moving images of human—and to a lesser extent animal—body forms, but not faces. Subregions within the EBA respond to viewing specific body parts, such as hands (Downing, Jiang, Shuman, & Kanwisher, 2001). According to Astafiev, Stanley, Shulman, and Corbetta (2004), EBA neurons are also somatotopically activated during an individual's own body movements. TMS of this area disrupts the meaningful perception of nonfacial body parts (Urgesi, Berlucci, & Aglioti, 2004).

The primary auditory cortices in the superior temporal gyrus are tonotopically organized, in line with the pitch-sensitive organization of the cochlea and are supplemented by surrounding secondary (belt) and tertiary (parabelt) sites, with many subdivisions whose distinct functions are not yet well understood but that are believed to specialize in rhythm and melody recognition in speech and music (Kaas & Hackett, 2000).

In sum, peripheral neurons transmit signals indicating the where and what of actions, skin and joint sensations, vision, audition, proprioception, and autonomic functioning to corresponding primary somatotopic and topographic cortical sites, where they are further processed. They are thence transmitted to secondary and tertiary areas before they can be experienced as meaningful. Damage to these auxiliary cortical processing sites results in various *agnosias* (or inability to comprehend the meaning of what is seen, touched, or heard) even when the primary motor and perceptual sites are intact. That there are specialized areas underpinning the perception of faces and bodies points to their importance in relating to and understanding others.

## Multimodal Integration

Experience and IWMs are multimodal and hence require the integration of unimodal activation patterns. One somatotopically organized area subserving such integration is the superior temporal sulcus (STS). The STS is recruited when study participants view motions of head, body, and limbs, including eye gaze direction, facial expressions, purposeful movement of lips and mouth during speech, and walking (see review by Haxby, Hoffman, & Gobbini, 2000). A developing ability to detect and understand aspects of biological motion has been empirically documented in infants as young as 4 to 6 months of age (Fox & McDaniel, 1982). In adults, TMS of the STS temporarily disrupts the ability to perceive biological movements in terms of meaningful actions.

Another important multimodal site is located near the temporoparietal junction (TPJ; where the temporal and parietal lobes join). It integrates multisensory (visual, auditory, skin, vestibular, and insular) input. Lesions at this location, especially in the right TPJ, can disrupt the sense that one's body is one's own (self-location) and can engender out-of-body experiences, such as seeing oneself floating above one's body, as well as other illusions regarding agency or perspective (Blanke & Arzy, 2005).

Multimodal integration of limb, head, and body movements in visual (retinotopic) space, spatial navigation, spatial imagery, mental rearrangement/rotation of objects, and a host of other integrative functions, including perspective taking, appear to be supported by the medial and lateral parietal cortices, but their organization in humans is still not well understood.

### Affordance-Related Multimodal Integration

The notion that perception serves action was already implied in Lewin's (1933) proposal that humans from infancy onward construe their psychological environment or "life space" in terms of the actions it invites, repels, permits, or prohibits in relation to current goals and competencies (known as *Aufforderungscharakter*, sometimes inappropriately translated as "valence"). Gibson (1977), using the English term *affordance*, subsequently showed that humans interpret aspects of the perceptual world in terms of the specific actions they afford.

Consistent with the notion of affordance, fMRI studies have shown that people who view manipulable objects register these objects' potential uses at the neural level. For example, when participants look at tools that require the use of hands, neurons fire not only in visual areas but also in the "hand" location of the supplementary motor area and in somatotopic cerebellar sites (Grèzes & Decety, 2001; see also Martin, Wiggs, Ungerleider, & Haxby, 1996). Likewise, mere pictures of appetizing food engage sites involved in evaluation of the actual taste and reward value of food (Simmons, Martin, & Barsalou, 2005), a reason why admiring still-life paintings in an art museum can lead to feelings of hunger.

### Social Observation–Action Matching

An effect with enormous social implications for IWM construction was serendipitously discovered in a study of monkeys by Rizzolatti, Fadiga, Gallese, and Fogassi (1996). Using microelectrodes to record the activity of single neurons in the premotor cortices of awake monkeys, these authors noticed that a subset of cells in a monkey's premotor cortex, dubbed *mirror neurons*, displayed the very same discharge pattern (1) when the monkey spontaneously performed a specific goal-directed hand action (e.g., picking up a peanut or tearing paper) and (2) when it merely observed another monkey doing so, even if part of the observed action had to be inferred from sound alone.

Probing the possible mirroring activity of single neurons in living human brains is possible only under extraordinary circumstances (e.g., exploration of cortical layout prior to epilepsy- or tumor-related surgery). However, the much earlier finding that human newborns are already able to imitate mouth opening, tongue protrusion, lip pursing, finger movements, and even some facial expressions (e.g., Meltzoff & Moore, 1977) suggested that mirror systems might be found in humans, too.

In one of the many subsequent fMRI studies confirming this hypothesis in adults, video clips of *other* individuals performing specific mouth, hand, and foot movements activated the mouth, hand, and foot areas in participants' *own* premotor map, while simultaneously triggering corresponding parietal neurons that capture the spatial aspects of body movements (Buccino et al., 2001). In a review of the now voluminous mirror neuron literature, Rizzolatti and Sinigaglia (2010) concluded that mirror neurons are activated when people observe others' goal-directed (intentional) actions but not when they view mere body displacements. They contend that mirror neurons hence allow individuals to understand others experientially or "from the inside." Note, however, that this propensity is affected by learning. For example, expert piano players, but not novices, exhibit strong cortical premotor responses while watching a soundless videotape of another expert player at the keyboard. This effect would presumably also apply to social interactions, and hence to social IWM construction (Bangert et al., 2006).

At least in humans, neural mirror systems extend beyond action to emotion. In an fMRI study by Carr, Iacoboni, Dubeau, Mazziotta, and Lenzi (2003), participants' imitation of happy, sad, angry, surprised, disgusted, and fearful emotional facial expressions registered in the same neural sites as when they viewed another person perform these expressions (the face area of participants' premotor and presupplementary motor maps, a subdivision in Broca's area, and the mouth area of the STS). Interoceptive appraisal sites (the anterior insula and amygdala) were also engaged. Results for each separate emotion were not assessed in this study.

Regarding specific emotions, Wicker and colleagues (2003) found that participants' anterior insula responded not only when they sniffed a foul-smelling substance themselves but when they looked at video clips of others' disgust expressions. The authors' interpretation of this finding is captured in the pithy title of their article: "Both of Us Disgusted in My Insula." In another fMRI study, participants' anterior insulae were activated by experiencing pain and witnessing others' facial pain expressions (Botvinick et al., 2005).

### Distinguishing Self from Other

If one's own actions and emotions recruit the same modal and multimodal cortical sites as observation of others' corresponding actions and emotion expressions, neural processes must exist that enable individuals to *distinguish* self from other. Ruby and Decety (2004) addressed this issue in a PET study by asking participants to imagine how *they* would feel and how their *mothers* would feel in three neutral and three emotional situations. In addition to the expected activations common to both conditions, the authors noted responses in the right somatosensory cortex that occurred exclusively when participants considered their own feelings. In contrast, the multimodal TPJ lit up only when participants imagined their mothers' feelings and thoughts. This suggested that, in addition to locating the self within the body, as noted earlier, the TPJ also plays a role in distinguishing feelings of self from feelings of others.

With respect to pain and self–other differentiation, the anterior insula responds to pain when it is directly administered to participants and when they observe other individuals in pain, whereas the posterior insula and somatosensory (SII) cortices are activated only when painful stimuli are administered to the self (Mazzola, Faillenot, Barral, Maugière, & Peyron, 2012).

### Remembering and Imagining

So far we have discussed neural responses to ongoing actions/emotions in self and others. However, of crucial importance for an understanding of working models "in the brain," it turns out that these very same modal and multimodal cortical sites also subserve *remembering* or *imagining* one's own or others' actions, feelings, or situations. For example, neurons in the STS respond not only when individuals perceive the meaning of others' biological motion but also when they imagine *themselves* as protagonists in a story (Vogeley et al., 2001), solve false-belief tasks, and consider moral dilemmas (see comprehensive review of social cognitive neuroscience studies by Frith & Frith, 2006). Other studies revealed strong TPJ activations when participants responded to stories involving others' mental states and beliefs (Saxe & Kanwisher, 2003). In short, direct experiences and mental simulations appear to rely on the same modal and multimodal brain sites, a topic to which we return in the section on memory.

### Summary

Mental model building, we propose, begins with the transduction of peripheral body signals into neural motor, exteroceptive, and interoceptive neural firing patterns. That is, incoming signals from the periphery are conveyed in orderly fashion to specialized cortical areas via subcortical way stations. These somatotopically and topographically organized brain regions extract modal meanings in stages. Processed modal signals are then combined and coordinated into multimodal activation patterns that generate conscious unified motor and sensory images imbued with positive and negative emotional feelings of self, other, and self-with-other, relying on processes that are imitative/replicative (although not in the strict literal sense) and at the same time analytic/constructive.

These processes are imitative/replicative because the spatial and temporal structure of somatotopically and topographically organized modal and multimodal neural activation patterns are preserved and can be neurally reinstated when events are remembered and can even be generated de novo when imagining novel events. Put forth as a hypothesis by Damasio (1999) and others, the reinstatement notions have since been multiply confirmed (e.g., Naselaris, Olman, Stansbury, Ugurbil, & Gallant, 2015; Nyberg, Habib, McIntosh, & Tulving, 2000; Wheeler, Petersen, & Buckner, 2000). To be clear, we are not making the naive proposal that the brain contains pictures, but that neural patterns that give rise to ongoing experience can be partially reinstated in the service of planning, appraising, and thinking (Nadel & Peterson, 2013).

Brain processes are also analytic and integrative. As already noted, sensory and motor signals are not just relayed from the periphery to the cortex, but undergo considerable pre-processing in subcortical way-stations before they arrive at their primary cortical destinations. They are then further analyzed in secondary and tertiary modal cortices that extract and sharpen increasingly specialized meanings, including features promoting social interaction (e.g., facial configurations) before being integrated in multimodal regions such as the STS or TPJ.

Regarding the phenomenon of *social* action–observation matching, it appears that in the course of evolution, a capacity for shared subjectivity or experiential understanding of others' behavior and feelings became possible via dual use of various modal and multimodal somatotopic and topographic cortical sites. That this capacity has its beginnings in early infancy is consistent with the previously cited evidence for neonatal imitation and early perception of biological motion, as well as research on early intersubjectivity (Trevarthen & Hubley, 1978), the emergence around 9–12 months of a capacity for joint attention (Bruner, 1975), and mastery of intersubjective gestural communication (Bates, Camaioni, & Volterra, 1974; Bretherton & Bates, 1979).

We do not yet understand the processes whereby activation patterns, separately generated in various modal and multimodal cortical sites, are amalgamated into one unified experience or translated into IWMs of multimodal experience and interactions. Time-locked neural activation has been suggested (e.g., Damasio, 1989) as one possibility, but the unity of experience might also be supported by the many documented interconnections among modal areas (such bidirectional links between motor, auditory, and somatosentory cortices; see Mazzola, Faillenot, et al., 2012). In addition, neuroimagining studies offer emerging insights into how the motor, exteroceptive, and interoceptive/evaluative sites we have described contribute to further processing in cortical regions responsible for the appraisal and selection of alternative courses of action, the topic we consider next.

## IWMs and Behavioral Choice

A major function of IWMs, according to Bowlby (1969/1982), is to generate plans for attaining desired goals (including but not limited to attachment system set-goals), and to evaluate their potential effectiveness for attaining adaptive outcomes. In this section we review neuroimaging studies that shed light on the proposed involvement of IWMs, particularly their evaluative aspects, in influencing behavioral choice. Relevant research relates mostly to adults and only rarely to attachment–caregiving processes; it nevertheless demonstrates important phenomena regarding IWM-guided goal-directed behavior.

In the developmental literature, executive functions such as planning, goal-directed problem solving, and working memory are generally attributed to the prefrontal cortex (PFC) as a whole. The PFC region comprises that portion of the frontal lobes not occupied by primary and supplementary motor sites and the attention-regulating (oculomotor) frontal eye fields. It is slow to develop, reaching full maturity only in adolescence (Fuster, 2001) and early adulthood (Sowell, Thompson, Holmes, Jernigan, & Toga, 1999).

In contrast to developmental psychologists, neuroimaging researchers have focused on three or four identified major subdivisions of the PFC: the orbitofrontal cortex (OFC; situated behind the orbits for the eyes); the ventromedial prefrontal cortex (VMPFC; between the two hemispheres); and the dorsolateral prefrontal cortex (DLPFC; on the upper and outer side of the prefrontal lobes). For good reasons that will become apparent, some investigators (e.g., Amodio & Frith, 2006; Fuster, 2001) include the anterior cingulate cortex (ACC) in the VMPFC. The cingulate cortex with anterior and posterior portions is a medial structure that encircles the corpus callosum like a cingulum, or collar.

Research has shown that dense connections within each PFC subdivision are complemented by systematic links of the subdivisions to each other, suggesting that they have both differentiated and collaborative functions. In addition, each subdivision has distinct reciprocal connections to various somatosensory, interoceptive, and multimodal cortical sites, as well as to subcortical reward nuclei (see reviews by Botvinick, 2008; Fuster, 2001; Miller & Cohen, 2001). Given these complex arrangements, Fuster (2001) cautioned that the workings of the PFC as an executive region cannot be fully understood without considering each of the subdivisions, their interactions, and their communication with modal sites and neural processing hubs across the whole fronto-temporal–parietal network. Further advances in research are required to implement these recommendations, but useful insights with bearings on IWMs and their uses can nevertheless be gleaned from studies that reveal the OFC (and to some extent, the anterior insula) as priority-setting regions whose signals are processed in the anterior cingulate cortex (ACC) for regulating emotional appraisal-guided behavioral choices.

## The Orbitofrontal Cortex

Early researchers held that the OFC's sole function was cognitive, to inhibit highly practiced, automated responses that conflicted with the effective execution of a task. However, both neuroimaging and lesion studies have revealed that the human OFC plays a much more complex role than was once assumed. Patients with OFC-focused injuries tend to undergo extensive personality changes; exhibit impulsive, instinctually disinhibited behavior and coarse humor; and show disregard for social and moral principles. They make counterproductive, highly risky decisions in their day-to-day social and attachment relationships, and employ maladaptive strategies in neuroimaging studies involving experimental gambling tasks (Damasio, 1999). Whereas such patients do well on IQ tests and can verbally explain beneficial choices that they *could* or *should* make, they find themselves unable to act on these constructive alternatives while executing the task in the MRI scanner. In addition, there is limited evidence that infants with this kind of prefrontal damage are even more severely afflicted. Not only do they fail to express (and seemingly fail to experience) social emotions of sympathy, embarrassment, or guilt, they are also unable to develop an understanding of social rules and to recognize rule violations. It appears that in such cases, the brain is not developmentally adaptable enough to make up for the damage (Anderson, Bechara, Damasio, Tranel, & Damasio, 1999).

Given the empirically confirmed contribution of an intact OFC to constructive decision making and social relationships, and given its location in the prefrontal (supposedly executive) region of the brain, it is somewhat surprising that the OFC has no direct links to motor cortices. Rather, OFC functions appear to be *sensory–evaluative*, by linking diverse inputs from several primary and auxiliary *sensory* cortices with positive and negative affective qualities (Rolls, 1996). Examples are the pleasant or unpleasant flavor of food (Rolls & Grabenhorst, 2008), the size of expected monetary rewards and losses, and—especially important for

interpersonal relationships and as shown in several fMRI studies reviewed below—differential OFC activations to the faces of loved ones and to faces of fair versus unfair companions. The OFC also generates flexible responses to sudden changes in others' positive or negative emotional expressions.

Nitschke and colleagues (2004) showed, for example, that mothers exhibited much stronger OFC activations to never-before-seen facial photos of their own infants as contrasted with faces of unfamiliar infants. Viewing their own infants, moreover, was associated with significantly more positive self-reported maternal mood. Strong, preferential maternal OFC activations, interpreted by the authors as evidence of maternal love, were also seen in a study in which mothers were confronted with a much more stringent comparison of their own versus *liked, familiar* children (Bartels & Zeki, 2004). Strathearn, Li, Fonagy, and Montague (2008, p. 49) commented that preferential engagement of maternal cortical (OFC) and subcortical reward-processing areas when viewing their own infants' *smiling* faces attested to "the reward value or salience of the infant's face to the mother, which may in turn relate to maternal sensitivity or conversely, child neglect." We suspect that if it were easier to conduct neuroimaging studies with infants, preferential activations to maternal faces, indicative of attachment, could also be demonstrated.

Differential OFC responses are evident as well after participants experience positive or negative social interactions with previously unfamiliar companions, as revealed in a two-phase experiment by Singer, Kiebel, Winson, Dolan, and Frith (2004). In Phase I, participants played an Internet game with fair and unfair coplayers (actually, computer programs simulating such coplayers whose purported facial photos were taped to the monitor). In the subsequent, neuroimaging phase, said to be unrelated, participants were asked to identify the gender of a collection of facial photos, including the purported coplayers. Faces of the *prosocial* coplayers evoked significantly stronger positive OFC responses than other faces in the collection and were subsequently rated as better liked than their unfair counterparts, suggesting that differential OFC responses were prompted by conscious evaluations of the coplayers' behavior in Phase I.

The OFC also responds during so-called reversal-learning experiments when a rapid evaluative switch is required because a previously rewarded choice is suddenly no longer effective or is punished (e.g., when a chosen face no longer smiles, but frowns; see Kringelbach & Rolls, 2003). Patients with OFC lesions lack the capacity to respond flexibly to rapidly changing reward contingencies.

OFC appraisals of reward and punishment (Rolls, 1996), and with respect to pain, affective pain signals from the insula (Medford & Critchley, 2010) influence ACC functions of monitoring and guiding behavioral choices that we discuss next after briefly considering related proposals by Bowlby.

### The Anterior Cingulate Cortex

In a largely ignored chapter on appraising and feeling, Bowlby (1969/1982, p. 105) emphasized the importance of emotional appraisals in making choices among alternative means for reaching a goal (attachment related or otherwise). The processes he described are uncannily relevant to current accounts of the ACC's function and include monitoring progress toward a goal, registering its successful attainment, and taking account of outcomes and consequences for learning. Whereas Bowlby (1980, pp. 53–54) saw routine IWM-guided behavior as being based on ingrained habits that may no longer be consciously accessible, he believed that conscious evaluation was required for "juxtaposing information of varying kinds," "preparing an array of alternative plans and sub-plans, then evaluating them, thus making possible high-level decisions." These ideas square quite well with current neuroimaging studies according to which the guidance of *habitual* choices is relegated to subcortical control, whereas ACC involvement is called on for reward-related behavioral guidance in the not infrequent instances when several possible behavioral choices conflict.

Until quite recently, the ACC was regarded as a paleomammalian limbic–emotional structure (as proposed by MacLean, 1973). However, consistent with an executive role, anatomical evidence has revealed that the anterior midsegment of the human cingulate cortex (henceforth the aMCC, also known as the dorsal ACC) is best regarded as a motor specialization of neocortex, containing spindle neurons for corticocortical communication found only in apes and humans (Allman, Hakeem, Erwin, Nimchinsky, & Hof, 2001). Relatedly, monkey and human studies have shown that the aMCC contains two somatotopically organized motor sites with efferent and afferent links to all primary and subsidiary motor

cortices, as well as the spinal cord (Paus, 2001). Moreover, suggesting a social-communicative role, "facial" neurons within the head region of these aMCC motor maps send signals to the subcortical facial nucleus that controls muscles of the upper face involved in expressing negative emotions and cognitive confusion (Shackman et al., 2011).

In line with the anatomical findings, an executive decision-making or -fostering function of the aMCC has been demonstrated in surprisingly diverse situations that, at first glance, seem to have little in common (e.g., resolving cognitive conflict, as in Stroop tasks; selecting optimal strategies in games involving gains and losses; solving moral dilemmas; and responses to pain). In a comprehensive meta-analysis Shackman and colleagues (2011, p. 161) confirmed closely overlapping aMCC activations during diverse tasks calling for cognitive problem solving, or effective avoidance of pain and negative emotions/outcomes. They concluded that what these tasks shared was the "need to determine optimal courses of action in the face of uncertainty, that is, to exert control." Their analyses showed that aMCC activation is heightened by action–outcome uncertainty, and by having to select adaptive responses appropriate to the type of problem or threat encountered (we suggest that this *could* include protective and attachment behaviors, but relevant studies do not yet exist).

Single-neuron studies of monkeys and humans provide some insight into various steps of appraisal-based behavioral decisions. Some aMCC cells are triggered in anticipation of increases or reductions in expected rewards, whereas others warn of or signal erroneous choices for future error correction (Bush et al., 2002). With respect to pain, while probing cells in awake patients before partial ACC ablation, Hutchison, Davis, Lozano, Tasker, and Dostrovsky (1999) detected neurons that fired *prospectively* as a hot or sharp implement approached the patients' hand, while others were triggered *vicariously* or *empathically* as a syringe touched the experimenter's hand. The authors suggest that nociceptive-specific neurons in the ACC may mediate diverse responses, such as alerting and orienting to the potentially threatening stimulus, evaluating and anticipating the threat and executing an appropriate escape response, as well as learning and memory to avoid future unpleasant encounters. Undercutting the notion that this region is *primary* for the "suffering aspects" of pain, research has shown that whereas electrical stimulation of the insula elicits pain experiences (Mazzola, Isnard, Peyron, & Maugière, 2012), direct stimulation of the aMCC does not. Rather, it evokes nonspecific urges "to act," "to overcome a challenge," or "to figure your way out of something" consistent with an appraisal-guided executive role (Parvizi, Rangarajan, Shirer, Desai, & Greicius, 2013).

Few human aMCC studies have been directly informed by attachment theory and research, and in some that *were*, overt behavioral choices were not asked for because the primary aim was to compare experienced pain with vicarious/empathic pain or distress. However, in a neuroimaging study of maternal responses to infant crying, Lorberbaum and colleagues (2002) found not only the expected vicarious/empathic neural activations in mothers' aMCC, but also reported that some mothers mentioned urges to help the crying infant. In a study of romantic couples, self-described as truly, deeply, and madly in love, Bartels and Zeki (2000) noted preferential insula and aMCC activations when participants viewed a loved partner's versus a best friend's facial photo. They also found that these responses covaried with stronger self-reported feelings of love and sexual arousal vis-à-vis the partner. During this task, Bartels and Zeki detected hippocampal activations (traditionally linked to memory) that may have been related to recalling interactions with the partner while viewing his or her image. However, the authors did not further discuss the possible significance of their hippocampus findings.

With respect to fMRI studies in which participants observe pain suffered by unfamiliar others, the default response was vicarious activation of the same aMCC locations that are triggered by self-experienced pain (see review and meta-analysis by Lamm, Decety, & Singer, 2011). However, participants' empathic aMCC pain responses were much reduced when the same experiment was performed after they were treated unfairly during a game with previously unfamiliar coplayers. During a subsequent purportedly unrelated task, participants rated unfair coplayers as substantially less liked than fair coplayers while viewing a collection of photos that included these players (Singer et al., 2006). We suspect that participants experienced a lesser behavioral urge to intervene on behalf of the unfair individuals (male participants admitted to a desire for exacting revenge). What is of interest here is not the expectable effects of another's unfairness, but that the participants' appraisal-related decision processes could, to some extent, be tracked by aMCC modulation.

Additional fMRI and ERP studies reviewed by Lavin and colleagues (2013) documented that hostile prior social interaction with an individual not only lowered the normal intensity of participants' empathic aMCC activations when that individual suffered pain but made task errors or lost expected rewards. Other studies reported that group membership (favoring ingroup members) affected the intensity with which pain and error empathy registered in participants' aMCC. Hence, a simple dichotomy between relationship-specific and general IWMs is likely to be too simplistic. Lavin and colleagues concluded that the aMCC is an integrative executive site for human social decision making, social outcome monitoring, and empathy.

## Summary

Strong preferential OFC activations when participants view faces of significant others (infant, child, or adult) lead us to infer that their relationship-specific IWMs have invested these individuals with strong positive value (i.e., feelings of affection and love). Even experimentally induced liking and disliking of previously unfamiliar individuals registers differentially in the OFC.

Evaluative signals from the OFC and insula influence emotion-guided aMCC behavioral monitoring and choice processes. These are manifest when an infant's distress elicits a mother's urge to intervene and when expected empathic aMCC activations vis-à-vis unfair companions are downregulated. This and other aMCC research underscores the alerting and informative role that positive and negative emotions play in monitoring and guiding behavioral choices in social relationships (Damasio, 2010). Such processes are also likely to be involved in the construction of relationship-specific and general IWMs, their revision, and their consolidation.

Given that the aMCC communicates not only with the OFC and anterior insula but also with other prefrontal, motor, parietal, and medial temporal sites, as well as with subcortical regions, much remains to be understood about its role of emotional guidance in behavioral choice within this larger network. It is particularly puzzling that the influence of memory (let alone IWMs) is almost never mentioned in aMCC neuroimaging studies, not only because remembered emotional experiences inform behavioral decisions but also because the aMCC and OFC are known to receive input from the hippocampus, which is known to be involved in memory processing (Aggleton, 2012). In the next section we focus on neuroimaging research that suggests new approaches to memory processes relevant to IWM construction and use.

## Memory Research and the Prospective–Imagining Brain

As noted earlier, Bowlby's (1980) IWM-related theorizing was strongly influenced by Tulving's (1972) proposition that humans possess two distinct declarative (awareness–accessible) memory systems, one termed "episodic" and the other "semantic." Bowlby described *episodic memory* as personally experienced information, stored sequentially in terms of temporally dated episodes and temporospatial relations that retain their perceptual properties. *Semantic memory*, in his view, consisted of generalized propositions about the world, derived either from personal experience or knowledge learned from others. The storage of "images of parents and self" would therefore also be "of at least two distinct types." Memories of specific interactions and conversations would be stored episodically, whereas "generalizations about mother, father, and self, enshrined in what I am terming working models or representational models" would be "stored semantically (in either analogical, propositional, or some combined format)" (for all quotations in this paragraph, see Bowlby, 1980, p. 62).

Bowlby stressed that having two distinct types of memory storage could be problematic if a child's episodic memory of a troubling experience such as sexual abuse was disavowed or denied by a parent who did not wish the child to understand its meaning. Incorporating this idea into his theory of defensive processes, Bowlby proposed that to allay anxiety caused by seeing attachment figures in a bad light, a child in such situations was likely to defensively exclude or repress his or her own episodic memories and retain conscious access only to semantically stored knowledge acquired from parents.

In 2002, 30 years after his initial propositions about two forms of declarative memory, Tulving made it known that his earlier conception of episodic memory (which Bowlby adopted) was now outdated. He redefined episodic memory as a neurocognitive mind/brain system underpin-

ning the *capacity to reexperience or mentally relive* personal events that had occurred in the past at a particular time and place, or to *pre-experience or pre-live* events that might occur in the future. This required a special kind of past and future awareness, dubbed "autonoësis," in contrast to noësis, or the retrieval of factual information from semantic memory. In 2009, Tulving and Szpunar further elaborated (1) that reliving the past or pre-experiencing the future required the stored information to be isomorphic with what is or could be in the world, reminiscent of Bowlby's working model notion; (2) that episodic memory depended on semantic memory with which it shared many, but not all, neural underpinnings; (3) that both episodic and semantic remembering required consciousness and a sense of self; (4) that neither episodic nor semantic remembering depended on language, although language greatly facilitated them; and (5), that autonoëtic consciousness had evolved because humans with this capacity were better able to predict what might happen in the future and could thus avoid or at least anticipate potentially threatening or otherwise detrimental events. This statement is at partial variance with Bowlby because of Tulving and Szpunar's exclusive focus on episodic (and not semantic) memory in generating predictions.

## Retrospective and Prospective Memory

Several years after Tulving put forth the notion of autonoësis, or past and future episodic time travel, several neuroscience teams almost simultaneously discovered that *envisioning future episodes* activates the very same cortical network as *recalling past personal* episodes (reviewed by Schacter & Addis, 2007). What came to be called the "core network" comprises the medial and prefrontal PFC, the medial temporal lobe (MTL), including the hippocampus, the posterior cingulate cortex, and the medial parietal cortex (also known as "precuneus")—all major integrative hubs (often termed *association areas*). This core network substantially overlaps what Raichle, MacLeod, Snyder, Powers, Gusnard, and Shulman (2001) identified as the "default network." Contrary to expectations, the default network was particularly active between fMRI task-related episodes, when individuals were supposedly resting but were actually daydreaming or mulling over past events (see review by Buckner, Andrews-Hanna, & Schacter, 2008). It is beyond the scope of this chapter to discuss the core network in detail, or to compare it with the default network, whose functioning is currently undergoing considerable rethinking. We focus instead on componential and combinatorial aspects of memory construction and imagination that emerged from this research and that have considerable implications for elaborating our ideas on IWM construction.

The core network findings led Schacter and Addis (2007) to advance the *constructive episodic simulation hypothesis*, according to which humans can envision plausible future episodes by extracting and then flexibly recombining event components derived from remembered episodes. Schacter and Addis maintained that these components (sometimes called "bits and pieces") were widely distributed across different brain sites rather than being stored as a "literal copy" in a single location.

In the same year, Hassabis and MacGuire (2007) reported that participants also recruited the core network while imagining a *fictitious* event not obviously linked to remembered or predicted personal situations. Focusing particularly on the function of the hippocampus and adjoining sites in the MTL, Hassabis and MaGuire hypothesized that *scene construction* was the common underlying process, which they defined as

> mentally generating, maintaining and visualizing a complex, coherent scene or event. This is achieved by the retrieval and integration of relevant informational components, stored in their modality-specific areas, the product of which has a coherent spatial context and can then later be manipulated and visualized. (p. 299)

Additional support for this hypothesis came from Hassabis, Kumaran, Vann, and Maguire's (2007) discovery that people with bilateral hippocampal injuries, long known for their inability to form new episodic memories, also struggled when asked to imagine personal futures. These patients' descriptions lacked spatial coherence and consisted of isolated fragments rather than connected scenes, again highlighting the role of the hippocampus in retrieving and integrating various event components into a coherent spatial and temporal whole. Related to more complex aspects of IWM construction than discussed so far, these findings and those reviewed below support and broaden Bowlby's notion that IWMs need to be extendable to novel situations. We also believe these findings to be important for conceptions of IWM-related future planning and defensive processes.

## New Views of MTL and Hippocampal Functions

Inklings that the hippocampus is indispensable for forming *new* episodic and semantic memories first emerged from Scoville and Milner's (1957) case study of the famous patient H. M., whose hippocampus was removed because of uncontrollable epilepsy. This study gave rise to the assumption that the hippocampus played a merely temporary role in consolidating short-term into long-term memories that would then be stored in other (nonspecified) cortical sites and be recallable without hippocampal intervention. However, current evidence that the hippocampus also participates in episodic memory retrieval and the construction of future, as well as fictive, episodes calls for a revised conceptions of MTL and hippocampal functions.

Complicating the issue still further were findings that the hippocampal formation is needed for successfully distinguishing among simultaneously displayed, highly similar but not identical complex visual scenes, and that an adjoining MTL site (the perirhinal cortex) enables discrimination among complex objects that share most but not all features (see review by Lee, Yeung, & Barense, 2012). Additionally, Zeidman, Mullally, and Maguire (2014) confirmed that the anterior hippocampus is active during scene perception (assessed with photos of locations, many including people and suggesting action), as well as during imagined scene construction (assessed with two-word cues for locations). In summary, perceiving/understanding, recalling, and imagining scenarios in context appear to rely on multiple uses of the same MTL and hippocampal substrates, although how these processes are differentiated from each other is not yet understood.

Zeidman and colleagues (2014) noted that scene construction, in comparison to scene perception, evoked significantly stronger (temporary) connectivity between the anterior hippocampus and primary visual sites, the dorsolateral PFC, inferior parietal lobe, and the STS. They hence concluded that the anterior hippocampus is involved in building an *internal model* of both perceived and imagined scenes, whereas the posterior hippocampus is activated only by scene perception and analyzes visual–spatial scene features. Relatedly, Bosch, Jehee, Fernández, and Doeller (2014) demonstrated that stimulus-specific, recognizable activation patterns that were evident during scene perception were reinstated in visual areas (V1 to V3) during recall, with tentative confirmation that reinstatement was mediated by the hippocampus.

## SUMMARY

Neuroimaging research affirms that the hippocampal formation and surrounding MTL are recruited when humans perceive and simulate (remember and imagine) complex scenarios that, in our view, are important in IWM construction. They offer contextual and spatial frames for the modal, multimodal, and evaluative processes described earlier and provide neural underpinnings for the event representation research discussed earlier. Via hippocampal and MTL signals, neural activations initially evoked by perceiving whole episodes in spatiotemporal context can apparently be reinstated in modal and multimodal areas. This makes it possible to relive/refeel them in memory and even to prelive/pre-feel or vividly imagine fictive events. However, the mental "editing" involved in *assembling* event components in the service of remembering or producing coherent spatiotemporal scenarios, let alone a life story, can at present only be guessed at (see detailed speculations by Damasio, 2010). Nor is there consistent evidence or explicit discussion of how the experience of reconstructing remembered scenes from "bits and pieces" is neurally different from doing so when constructing imagined future or fictitious scenes. This gap may be filled when we gain a more complete understanding of the function played by the now known, enormously complicated interconnections among MTL and hippocampal subdivisions and by the organization of distinct inputs to and outputs from hippocampal subfields to other cortical sites (Aggleton, 2012).

## Semantic Memory/Knowledge, Categorizing, and Summarizing

If semantic memory is synonymous with world knowledge, then its purview is considerably vaster than that of episodic memory (see an up-to-date assessment of current debates in this field by Yee, Chrysikou, & Thompson-Schill, 2013). In this section, we restrict our focus to three IWM-related semantic memory topics: a simulation approach to category formation, various levels of summarizing temporal events, and the grounding of language in simulations.

### Simulation and Concepts

Barsalou (2009) regards mental simulation (in contrast to amodal representation) as a basic brain strategy supporting a broad range of memory and cognitive processes. In one of several studies that take a simulation approach to concept formation, Barsalou and Wiemer-Hastings (2005) asked students to generate thoughts about concrete concepts (*bird, sofa*) and abstract concepts (*truth, freedom*). Rather than coming up with feature lists or dictionary definitions, the students' responses included considerable contextual information, not only for concrete but also for abstract concepts (e.g., freedom: "people on TV saying whatever they want to be saying"; truth: "when what you are saying is not a lie"). In addition to parts and properties of objects, participants mentioned related behavior, evaluations, goals, and introspections, including beliefs. Introspections were more frequent in descriptions of abstract concepts (*truth*). Participants did not simulate exemplars of concrete and abstract concepts in isolation, but in the context of a variety of summarized and unique situations (how something feels, what can be done with it, in what settings various exemplars of it would be used or experienced, whether or not one likes it/them). Different aspects of the concept were called upon in different simulated contexts (e.g., a chair in a kitchen vs. a dentist's office), and descriptions drew on both unique and generic/semantic memories.

This is as far as we can take this discussion here. Note, however, that the above mentioned category findings call for a consideration of language in relation to simulation (and hence verbally expressed IWMs), a topic we address after considering summarized events.

### Summarized Events

To examine Tulving's (2002) claim that episodic memories (usually prefaced with "I remember that . . .") are distinct from memories for generic events (usually prefaced with "I know that . . ."), Barsalou (1988) asked random individuals at his university to participate in a survey at the beginning of the fall semester. The tape-recorded task was to spend 5 minutes recalling summer activities in any order that came to mind. The authors primarily expected recounts of specific events.

Most participants, however, responded with a chronological sequence of several extended events (e.g., a challenging job for 2 months, followed by a trip to Europe and several weeks at home. They then filled in more details with summarized events ("On my days off we always went to the beach") and specific events ("We went to see a play at the outdoor theater"), although the latter were mentioned less frequently. Given the 5-minute time limit, participants' use of longer time frames is not surprising per se. What is noteworthy is the lack of a strict distinction between episodic and semantic remembering, made possible by language labels that permit various levels of temporal summarization.

An even more extended time frame (lifetime periods or "My time in college was stressful") was reported in a study of autobiographical interviews by Conway, Singer, and Tagini (2004), suggesting that IWMs could be organized within such temporal frames.

## The Grounding of Verbal Event Descriptions in Simulations

The category and event summary studies by Barsalou and colleagues raise questions regarding the nature of links between mental simulation and verbally reported IWM-related memories in interviews and clinical contexts. These led Barsalou (2012) to make the following provocative points: (1) Verbal accounts must ultimately be grounded in multimodal mental simulations, and situated categories (as described earlier) are central to processing language structure as expressive of meaning; (2) lexical meanings and simulated, nonverbal concepts are not identical, but have much in common; (3) verbal accounts are too incomplete to be understood without at least some shared situated knowledge; and (4) people construct situation models in the course of attempting to understand texts; hence, reasoning is often difficult if a concrete situation cannot be imagined (Yeh & Barsalou, 2006).

## Simulation in Clinical Perspective

Clinically oriented studies relevant to the IWM construct adopted notions of simulation akin to Barsalou's before neuroimaging studies began to proliferate. We review some of them here because they discuss both advantages and drawbacks rather than focusing primarily on the adaptiveness of past and future episodic thinking. They are helpful because they can shed light on individual differences in IWM construction that are related to mental health and psychopathology.

We begin by discussing the effectiveness of prospective simulations, then consider the phenomenon of overgeneral memory, and lastly present findings about defensive processes as related to self-defining autobiographical memories.

## Effective Prospective Simulations

Elaborating on propositions by Bowlby (1980), Taylor, Pham, Rivkin, and Armor (1998) posited that simulations have constructive purposes beyond the predictable turns of events. Thus, people may revisit a troubling scenario to pinpoint when and why an interaction went awry, then imaginatively substitute what they might or should have said for use during a future, similar occasion. Or they may relive an accident or near accident in order to reflect on how to exercise greater vigilance when encountering similar situations. Likewise, simulating possible emotional repercussions of an upcoming situation may be helpful in facing a related situation in reality. However, when such simulations take the form of obsessive ruminations without resolution, they are likely to be detrimental to mental health.

Empirical evidence that some types of prospective simulation are more constructive than others emerged from a study by Taylor and colleagues (1998) that distinguished *process* from *outcome* simulations. Engaging in process simulation implies plans that detail the successive steps necessary for reaching a goal (and include seeking instrumental help and engaging in cognitive reappraisal). Such plans also reduce anxiety. Outcome simulations, in contrast, focus on the pleasure or relief on having reached the goal, but they proved less effective because participants failed to reckon with the effort and steps required to actually attain the goal.

## Overgeneral Memory and Psychopathology

Relevant to linguistic markers for "state of mind" used in Adult Attachment Interview (AAI) classifications (Hesse, Chapter 26, this volume), clinical research has revealed associations between psychopathology and *overgeneral memory*, defined as retrieving only generic events even when detailed autobiographical memories were specifically requested. The effect held for clinically and subclinically depressed groups, as well as for individuals with unresolved trauma (e.g., sexual and physical abuse in childhood). Overgeneral memory has also been linked to experiencing accidents, war, cancer, and PTSD, and pervades interviews even when clients are not recalling traumatic memories. Overgeneral memory has been explained as truncated memory search for aversive episodes and is associated with dysfunction in executive control and with rumination involving global, undifferentiated self-representations (see studies cited by Williams, 2006).

## Self-Defining Memories and Defense

What is remembered long-term and reasons why, are topics that have been relatively neglected by neuroimaging researchers who often employ shorter delays (minutes, hours, or days, but not years) between a new experience and related episodic remembering. Focusing on long-term remembering, Conway and colleagues (2004) stressed that many autobiographical memories and even much semantic knowledge will be semiforgotten or irretrievably lost if not periodically retrieved. They pointed out that the comparatively few episodic memories that *are* retained in the very long term tend to be appraised as self-defining and for this reason become integrated with a person's autobiographical knowledge base (including IMWs of self-in-relationships). Such memories tend to be affectively intense and vivid, associated with long-term goals and identity concerns, and are easily accessed because of frequent rehearsal.

Relating self-defining memories to defensive processes, Conway and colleagues (2004) drew on a wealth of past research and theorizing too voluminous to cite. They proposed that the content of autobiographical memory is affected by tensions between two potentially conflicting goals, termed adaptive correspondence and self-coherence. They claim that adaptive correspondence may suffer when discrepancies between an individual's goal-structure and current behavior or experience pose a threat to self-coherence. In such situations, episodic memories may be distorted in the service of unrealistic self-enhancement and even self-deprecation, or they may be repressed altogether to leave the individual's goal structure (or life story) unchallenged. We suggest that such effects could explain defensive processes in IWM-guided perception, IWM construction, and related behavioral choice.

Noting obvious overlaps between their conception of autobiographical memory and secure-autonomous, dismissing, preoccupied, and unresolved "states of mind with respect to attachment" reflected in the AAI (Main, 1995), Conway and colleagues (2004) described three cases in which AAI status was meaningfully related to performance during a self-defining memory task. However, whether their conclusions hold in the overall study has not yet been reported.

## Discussion and Reflections

Let us first acknowledge that in order to place boundaries around the task we set for ourselves in this chapter, we have left aside important domains that are potentially involved in working model construction. These include subcortical appraisal processes that feed into cortically supported simulations; the action of hidden regulators involved in direct limbic-to-limbic mother–infant communication that are described with greater emphasis with respect to animals by Polan and Hofer (Chapter 6, this volume) and with greater emphasis on human infants by Trevarthen and Aitken (2003) and Schore (1994); the potentiation of specific brain systems, including the OFC, by neurohormones such as oxytocin; the effects of stress on the developing hypothalamic–pituitary–adrenal system (e.g., Gunnar, 2003; see also Hane & Fox, Chapter 11, this volume); and emerging insights about genetic and epigenetic influences on social functioning (reviewed in Hofer, 2014; see also Bakermanns-Kranenburg & Van IJzendoorn, Chapter 8, this volume).

Recognizing these limitations, we reflect on potential contributions that the simulation approach can make to an expanded understanding of human IWM construction and use. Whereas not all neuroscientists subscribe to the simulation view, support for it has grown so substantially since the last edition of this handbook that only a small selection of findings could be included in this chapter.

### Embodiment and Simulation

Mental models that can be made to "work" or conduct simulations must preserve the temporal, spatial, and psychological relation–structure of the experiences they represent, as Craik (1943) proposed and Bowlby (1969/1982) reiterated. Neuroimaging studies have revealed how the human brain conserves configural and relational information as it is transmitted from the body and perceptual organs to cortical regions via subcortical processing stations. These cortical regions are the very ones that also allow us to vividly *reexperience* the past and imagine future and fictive events by reinstating or evoking the appropriate modal and multimodal cortical activations. What is more, many of these sites also enable us to experientially apprehend others' meaningful behavior, sensations, and feelings, not only while interacting with them, but also while thinking about them.

Mental simulation, moreover, can spill over into bodily activations beyond the brain, so that we experience others through our physical and autonomic responses as well. For example, facial or bodily muscles can be covertly yet measurably active when individuals consciously or unconsciously resonate to or mirror the behaviors and emotions of others (Glenberg, 1997). Such effects are usually not assessed in neuroimaging studies because relative immobility (including head restraints) is required to prevent motor interference during scanning. Together with neuroimaging studies, such findings imply that experiences in close relationships are likely to leave their imprint on not only our brains/minds but also our physical being.

The embodiment findings also suggest that questions about detailed memories of childhood loss and abuse experiences, such as those evoked during the AAI, are likely to awaken psychological conflict and negative mood in individuals who have not been able to resolve such experiences (Conway et al., 2004). Steele and Steele (2005) confirmed, for example, that interviewees' negative emotions before responding to the AAI were not predictive of secure–insecure AAI classifications, whereas negative emotions after the interview were. Those with autonomous-secure status felt positive about the opportunity to reflect openly and coherently on important childhood and current relationships, whereas those classified as dismissing and preoccupied felt worse. Unfortunately the requirement to remain as immobile as possible in the scanner makes it exceedingly difficult to conduct AAIs and related interview assessments in conjunction with neuroimaging (for a lone, ingenious clinical study related to this topic, see Buchheim et al., 2012).

## Analytic and Constructive Processes: Experience, Memory, and Imagination

IWM building involves a number of depictive/imitative and constructive processes that have hitherto been mostly taken for granted. The somatotopic and topographic layout of cortical modal and multimodal sites enables site-to-site coordination of signals (i.e., coordinated information as to where a specific bodily injury is seen and felt), but this does not fully explain how our brains construct a unified experience. Moreover, multimodally integrated information must be further integrated with value judgments (OFC, insula) and linked to context. The latter seems to require MTL processing and signals to modal cortices that manage to reinstate a semblance of past modal and multimodal cortical activations, and can seemingly also evoke them de novo when individuals imagine or listen to accounts of future and fictive events (hence stories can induce laughter or tears). How such reinstatements are accomplished in detail is still a mystery, but there is ever-increasing evidence that they occur.

Additional isuues are raised by findings that the same motor, sensory, and interoceptive appraisal sites are used for experiencing self and others. This means that the seemingly self-evident knowledge that an individual owns his or her own body and feelings, and that these are separate from those of others, cannot be taken for granted, but must be based on neural processes of self–other differentiation that are only beginning to be understood. Another, usually taken-for-granted ability whose brain underpinnings are not fully understood is engaging in mental time travel while remaining aware of the present. Greater knowledge of how these differentiating processes are performed might lead to better insights into how they can go awry during development, and how they can interfere with adequate IWM construction.

Observational and clinical infant research (e.g., Ainsworth, Bell, & Stayton, 1974; Stern, 1985; Trevarthen & Hubley, 1978) revealed decades ago that infants and children develop relationships and relationship-specific IWMs optimally in the context of responsive early communication and care by attachment figures (see also the special issue of *Attachment & Human Development* on maternal sensitivity, edited by Grossmann, Bretherton, Waters, & Grossmann, 2013). Neuroscience findings that link quality of parental care to brain development in infancy have "tangibly" affirmed these long-known observational results, but to date neuroscience research is mostly limited to general evidence for brain growth, appropriate synaptic pruning, and the developmental schedule of myelination. Because neuroimaging research with infants and young children is challenging, we still lack details about the involvement of relationship and other experiences in the early patterning of cortical motor, exteroceptive, and interoceptive sites. Such knowledge would give us some much-needed insight into how infants' and young children's capacities for mental simulations develop at the neural level.

### IWMs, Imagination, and Defense

Bowlby's (1988) proposal that attachment IWMs consist of semantically stored summary representations needs rethinking, especially with respect to his account of defensive processes (Bowlby, 1980). We urge that Bowlby's rather tentatively stated ideas on memory and defense not be elevated to the status of dogma (see related statements by Fonagy & Target, 2007). It would be a mistake to neglect potentially useful insights for updating and revising theoretical ideas regarding IWM construction and defensive processes offered by discoveries in the field of neuroscience, as well as by discoveries in the study of emotion, representation, narratives, and language.

Neuroimaging studies suggest that our capacity to imagine plausible futures and fictive events draws on "bits and pieces" of remembered events (although deliberate transformations of whole events could also play a role). We know that the ability to invent a different past from the one we experienced or remember, and to simulate plausible desired and undesired futures (whether plausible or not) begins early with the emergence of simple story enactment in pretend play, continues in daydreaming, and makes art and literature possible, but detailed developmental studies of these abilities and their meaning with respect to attachment IWMs are still lacking given that current efforts in attachment research tend to dwell on measurement improvement and reliability.

The componential aspects of remembering and imagining that have been suggested by neuroimaging studies could shed light on the occurrence of memory errors, misattributions, intrusions, and event fragmentation caused by partial forgetting of event components, whether defensively motivated or not (Schacter et al., 2012). That imagined emotional episodes become more believable with repetition is empirical confirmation of the persuasive power of wishful thinking (Szpunar & Schacter, 2013).

Autobiographical studies show that defensive memory distortions are common when an individual's experiences or conduct pose threats to self-coherence and thus challenge existing goal structures. Such processes could be explored in AAI and other attachment interview texts, although with the proviso that *self-coherence* as defined by Conway and colleagues (2004) refers to individuals' attempts to create a *superficially* consistent life story by distorting construals of the past or present. This definition of coherence differs greatly from

Main's (1995) proposal that coherent AAI accounts are supported by a secure-autonomous state of mind, associated with the ability to acknowledge and *integrate* positive and negative aspects of relationships into a vivid, detailed, believable, and *coherent* narrative (see also Cassidy, 2001).

Finally, although the dictum that an unexamined life is not worth living suggests that reflection on experience is always worthwhile, clinicians caution that prospective simulation can be used both productively and counterproductively.

### Simulation and Language

We have presented a view of remembering as simulation that involves neural reinstatement of vivid experiences, without paying much attention to the role of language. As MacWhinney (2005) cogently pointed out, simulation and language work together because they evolved together for many millennia, but language does not seem suited as an ungrounded symbol system on its own.

Whereas words are largely based on arbitrary (amodal) sounds rather than simulations, it is important to acknowledge that this may not always have been so, given the many words that imitate sounds (onomatopoeia) and that iconic gestures frequently accompany oral conversations, with or without the speakers' awareness (McNeill, 2005). We have noticed, for example, that spontaneous depictive or enactive gestures are common during the Parent Attachment Interview. One mother (taking the perspective of her child) tapped herself gently on the cheek while describing the child's affectionate behavior toward her, and another hugged herself in the same context (Bretherton, unpublished research). It might be of interest to examine videotaped AAIs for such embodied meanings, which, if concordant with narration, could be related to a secure-autonomous AAI state of mind.

Concerning the componential and constructive nature of event perception and event memory at the neural level, we suspect that this may have made language as a componential representational and communicative system possible. However, word sequences have to make explicit what simulations can do with mental mimesis. In contrast to mental or physical enactments, language must use explicit devices for expressing temporal, spatial, causal, and personal relations, including tenses to mark past and future, spatial words, and implicitly code perspective taking with deictic expressions such as this (near me) and that (near you).

Language, on the other hand, has useful properties that mimesis does not. These allow us to convey "facts" and evaluative attitudes in the same expression (e.g., a father dismissing his mother's affectionate behavior as "lovey-dovey"). Such meanings would be difficult to impart via enactment alone, although tone of voice, or a throwaway gesture could perhaps express such double meanings. Language also contributes uniquely to category creation by providing "handles" for complex situated categories as described by Barsalou (1988); for summarized experiences within longer and shorter time frames (e.g., infancy, wedding); and for multifaceted, abstract concepts, such as love and truth, that a single simulation can only partially express (Barsalou & Wiemer Hastings, 2005). Language can also provide handles for typologies that are grounded in vast amounts of patterned situated information, as exemplified by AAI and Strange Situation classifications)

## Consciousness

Although it is often claimed that IWMs operate mostly at the unconscious level or are exclusively unconscious, this is not quite what Bowlby (1980) stated. In line with the literature on controlled and automatic processing, he pointed out that as interaction patterns become increasingly habitual and ingrained, they also become more automatic and hence less open to conscious control and revision. As previously noted, there is supporting evidence for this distinction at the neural level. The aMCC is no longer recruited when choices become highly habitual.

Attachment researchers often characterize the unconscious or implicit operation of IWMs as *procedural*. We should recognize, however, that this usage differs from implicit motor skill memory for which the term was originally coined. Furthermore, skill memory in people with an intact hippocampus is unconscious/implicit only in some respects. They may not be able to describe precisely how they move their limbs during swimming or dancing, how they produce grammatical sentences, and how they interact with another person, but they can imagine performing these skills, are aware of their skill level, and know that a skill can be improved by observational analysis and deliberate practice.

As Barsalou (2009) and others have pointed out, implicit or unconscious top-down use of mental models during ongoing perception does not imply that explicit aspects of such models thereof cannot be called to mind while reflecting on past or future. Furthermore, while acknowledging the general consensus that an enormous amount of the brain's processing occurs outside awareness and at subcortical levels, let us not forget that persons who are bereft of a cortex, because of prenatal injury, are also bereft of much human experience (Damasio, 2010). We suggest that the notion of unconscious/unconscious IWMs functioning requires rethinking.

## Attachment IWMs: Feelings of Love and Affection

Our analyses here cannot speak to how the brain creates the preferential evaluations that make some figures, whether child, parent, or mate, more important than others, whether in interaction or thought. We know that infant preferences for parental figures begin very early, but how this preference is implemented in the brain and built into IWMs is not fully understood (for suggestions, see Swain et al., 2014). We can point out, however, that with respect to research with adults (parents or partners), the effect of such preferences, once established, is strikingly evident in differential OFC activations by the faces of loved ones, even when compared with familiar, liked others.

In a much-cited statement, Bowlby (1980, p. 40) described preferential valuations inherent in intense feelings of love and affection toward children by parents, toward parents by children, and by romantic partners toward each other:

> Many of the most intense emotions arise during the formation, the maintenance, the disruptions, and the renewal of attachment relationships. The formation of a bond is described as falling in love, maintaining a bond as loving someone, and losing a partner as grieving over someone. Similarly threat of loss arouses anxiety and actual loss gives rise to sorrow; while each of these situations is likely to arouse anger. The unchallenged maintenance of a bond is experienced as a source of security and the renewal of a bond as a source of joy.

In the current literature on attachment, however, much emphasis has been given to monadic aspects of attachment, such as describing individuals with a secure-autonomous AAI status as feeling "secure within themselves" (Main, Hesse, & Kaplan, 2005) or explaining a secure stance in the Adult Attachment Projective as reliance on an "internalized secure base" (George & West, 2004). Valuing of attachment relationships has been associated with these monadic aspects, but feelings of love and longing in attachment relationships and inherent in IWMs have been largely neglected. The capacity to experience these feelings and evoke them in memory may have evolved because they fostered familial care seeking and caregiving, and hence survival (also see, in this volume, Zeifman & Hazan, Chapter 20, and Simpson & Belsky, Chapter 5). We suggest that their importance and role in attachment relationships and relationship IWMs deserves much greater attention.

## Acknowledgments

We wish to express our gratitude to Rose Addis, Lawrence Barsalou, Martin Conway, Peter Fonagy, Myron Hofer, Claus Lamm, Eleanor McGuire, Laure Mazzola; Katherine Nelson, Lyn Nadel, Tania Singer, Colwyn Trevarthen, and Brian MacWinney for kindly and promptly responding to questions and sharing materials. Any interpretive errors of their or others' work are, of course, ours. We also thank the editors for their patience and helpful supportive critiques.

## Note

1. To avoid confusion we interject here that Damasio (1999, p. 23) used the terms *model of the body in the brain* and *body map* to refer to the moment-to-moment, coordinated, multimodal flow of activation pattern in the various neural sites that (jointly) represent the current state of the body rather than, as we do, referring to the somatotopic layout of various modal and multimodal cortical sites.

## References

Aggleton, J. P. (2012). Multiple anatomical systems embedded within the primate medial temporal lobe: Implications for hippocampal function. *Neuroscience and Biobehavioral Reviews, 36,* 1579–1596.

Ainsworth, M. D. S., Bell, S. M., & Stayton, D. (1974). Infant–mother attachment and social development: "Socialization" as a product of reciprocal responsiveness to signals. In P. M. Richards (Ed.), *The integration of a child into a social world* (pp. 99–135). Cambridge, UK: Cambridge University Press.

Allman, J. M., Hakeem, A., Erwin, J. M., Nimchinsky, E., & Hof, P. (2001). The anterior cingulate cortex: The evolution of an interface between emotion and cognition. *Annals of the New York Academy of Sciences, 935,* 107–117.

Amodio, D. M., & Frith, C. D. (2006). Meeting of minds: The medial frontal cortex and social cognition. *Nature Reviews Neuroscience, 7,* 268–277.

Anderson, S., Bechara, A., Damasio, H., Tranel, D., & Damasio, A. (1999). Impairment of social and moral behavior related to early damage in the prefrontal cortex. *Nature Neuroscience, 2,* 1032–1037.

Astafiev, S. V., Stanley, C. M., Shulman, G. L., & Corbetta, M. (2004). Extrastriate body area in human occipital cortex responds to the performance of motor actions. *Nature Neuroscience, 7,* 548–548.

Bangert, M., Peschel, T., Schlaug, G., Rotte, M., Drescher, D., Hinrichs, et al. (2006). Shared networks for auditory and motor processing in professional pianists: Evidence from fMRI conjunction. *NeuroImage, 30,* 917–926.

Barsalou, L. W. (1988). The content and organization of autobiographical memories. In U. Neisser & E. Winograd (Eds.), *Remembering reconsidered: Ecological and traditional approaches to the study of memory* (pp. 193–243). Cambridge, UK: Cambridge University Press.

Barsalou, L. W. (2009). Simulation, situated conceptualization, and prediction. *Philosophical Transactions of the Royal Society B, 364,* 1281–1289.

Barsalou, L. W. (2012). The human conceptual system. In M. J. Spivey, K. McRae, & M. Joanisse (Eds.), *The Cambridge handbook of psycholinguistics* (pp. 239–258). Cambridge, UK: Cambridge University Press.

Barsalou, L. W., & Wiemer-Hastings, K. (2005). Situating abstract concepts. In D. Pecher & R. A. Zwaan (Eds.), *Grounding cognition* (pp. 129–163). Cambridge, UK: Cambridge University Press.

Bartels, A., & Zeki, S. (2000). The neural basis of romantic love. *NeuroReport, 11,* 3829–3834.

Bartels, A., & Zeki, S. (2004). The neural correlates of maternal and romantic love. *NeuroImage, 21,* 1155–1166.

Bates, E., Camaioni, L., & Volterra, V. (1975). The acquisition of performatives prior to speech. *Merrill–Palmer Quarterly, 21,* 205–226.

Bauer, P. J., & Wewerka, S. S. (1995). One- to two-year-olds' recall of events: The more impressed, the more expressed. *Journal of Experimental Child Psychology, 59,* 475–496.

Blanke, O., & Arzy, S. (2005). The out-of-body experience: Disturbed self-processing at the temporo-parietal junction. *Neuroscientist, 11,* 16–24.

Bosch, S. E., Jehee, J. F. M., Fernandez, G., & Doeller, C. F. (2014). Reinstatement of associative memories in early visual cortex is signaled by the hippocampus. *Journal of Neuroscience, 34,* 7493–7500.

Botvinick, J., Iha, P., Bylsma, L. M., Fabian, S. A., Solomon, P. E., & Prkachin, K. M. (2005). Viewing facial expressions of pain engages cortical areas involved in the direct experience of pain. *NeuroImage, 25,* 312–319.

Botvinick, M. (2008). Hierarchical models of behavior and prefrontal function. *Trends in Cognitive Sciences, 12,* 201–206.

Bowlby, J. (1973). *Attachment and loss: Vol. 2. Separation: Anxiety and anger.* New York: Basic Books.

Bowlby, J. (1980). *Attachment and loss: Vol. 3. Loss: Sadness and depression.* New York: Basic Books.

Bowlby, J. (1982). *Attachment and loss: Vol. 1. Attachment.* New York: Basic Books. (Original work published 1969)

Bowlby, J. (1988). *A secure base.* New York: Basic Books.

Bretherton, I. (1985). Attachment theory: Retrospect and prospect. In I. Bretherton & E. Waters (Eds.), Growing points of attachment theory and research. *Monographs of the Society for Research in Child Development, 50*(1–2, Serial No. 209), 3–35.

Bretherton, I. (1990). Open communication and internal working models: Their role in the development of attachment relationships. In R. A. Thompson (Ed.), *Nebraska Symposium on Motivation: Vol. 36. Socioemotional development* (pp. 59–113). Lincoln: University of Nebraska Press.

Bretherton, I., & Bates, E. (1979). The emergence of intentional communication. In I. C. Užgiris (Ed.), *Social interaction and communication during infancy* (pp. 81–100). San Francisco: Jossey-Bass.

Bretherton, I., & Munholland, K. A. (2008). Internal working models in attachment relationships: A construct revisited. In J. Cassidy & P. R. Shaver (Eds.), *Handbook of attachment: Theory, research, and clinical applications* (pp. 102–127). New York: Guilford Press.

Bretherton, I., Ridgeway, D., & Cassidy, J. (1990). Assessing internal working models of the attachment relationship: An Attachment Story Completion Task for 3-year-olds. In D. Cicchetti, M. Greenberg, & E. M. Cummings (Eds.), *Attachment in the preschool years: Theory, research, and intervention* (pp. 272–308). Chicago: University of Chicago Press.

Brooks, J. C., Zambreanu, L., Godinez, A., Craig, A. D., & Tracey, I. (2005). Somatotopic organization of the human insula to painful heat studied with high resolution functional imaging. *NeuroImage, 27,* 201–209.

Bruner, J. S. (1975). The ontogenesis of speech acts. *Journal of Child Language, 2,* 1–19.

Buccino, G., Binkofski, F., Fink, G. R., Fadiga, L., Fogassi, L., Gallese, V., et al. (2001). Action observation activates premotor and parietal areas in a somatotopic manner: An fMRI study. *European Journal of Neuroscience, 13,* 400–404.

Buchheim, A., Viviani, R., Kessler, H., Kächele, H., Cierpka, M., et al. (2012). Changes in prefrontal-limbic function in major depression after 15 months of long-term psychotherapy. *PLoS ONE, 7,* e33745.

Buckner, R. L., Andrews-Hanna, J. R., & Schacter, D. L. (2008). The brain's default network: Anatomy, function, and relevance to disease. *Annals of the New York Academy of Sciences, 1124,* 1–38.

Bush, G., Vogt, B. A., Holmes, J., Dale, A. M., Greve, D., Jenike, M. A., et al. (2002). Dorsal anterior cingulate cortex: A role in reward-based decision making. *Proceedings of the National Academy of Sciences, 99,* 523–528.

Carr, L., Iacoboni, M., Dubeau, M.-C., Mazziotta, J. C., & Lenzi, G. L. (2003). Neural mechanisms of empathy in humans: A relay from neural systems for imitation to limbic areas. *Proceedings of the National Academy of Sciences, 100,* 5497–5502.

Cassidy, J. (2001). Truth, lies, and intimacy: An attachment perspective. *Attachment and Human Development, 3,* 121–155.

Conway, M. A., Singer, J. A., & Tagini, A. (2004). The self and autobiographical memory: Correspondence and coherence. *Social Cognition, 22,* 491–529.

Craig, A. D. (2009). How do you feel—now?: The anterior insula and human awareness. *Nature Reviews Neuroscience, 10,* 59–70.

Craik, K. (1943). *The nature of explanation.* Cambridge, UK: Cambridge University Press.

Damasio, A. (1989). Time-locked multiregional retroactivation: A systems level proposal for the neural substrates of recall and recognition. *Cognition, 33,* 25–62.

Damasio, A. (2010). *The self comes to mind: Constructing the conscious brain.* New York: Pantheon.

Damasio, A. R. (1999). *The feeling of what happens.* New York: Harcourt Brace.

Decety, J., & Grèzes, J. (2006). The power of simulation: Imagining one's own and other's behavior. *Brain Research, 1079,* 4–14.

Donald, M. (1993). Précis of origins of the modern mind: Three stages in the evolution of culture and cognition. *Behavioral and Brain Sciences, 16,* 737–791.

Downing, P. E., Jiang, Y., Shuman, M., & Kanwisher, N. (2001). A cortical area selective for visual processing of the human body. *Science, 293,* 2470–2473.

Fernandino, L., & Iacoboni, M. (2010). Are cortical motor maps based on body parts or coordinated actions?: Implications for embodied semantics. *Brain and Language, 112,* 44–53.

Fivush, R., & Vasudeva, A. (2002). Remembering to relate: Socioemotional correlates of mother–child reminiscing. *Journal of Cognition and Development, 3,* 73–90.

Fonagy, P., & Target, M. (2007). The rooting of the mind in the body: New links between attachment theory and psychoanalytic thought. *Journal of the American Psychoanalytic Association, 55,* 411–456.

Fox, R., & McDaniel, C. (1982). The perception of biological motion by human infants. *Science, 218,* 486–487.

Frith, C. D., & Frith, U. (2006). How we predict what other people are going to do. *Brain Research, 1079,* 36–46.

Fuster, J. M. (2001). The prefrontal cortex—an update: Time is of the essence. *Neuron, 30,* 319–333.

George, C., & West, M. (2004). The Adult Attachment Projective: Measuring individual differences in attachment security using projective methodology. In M. Hersen (Series Ed.) & M. Hilsenroth & D. Segal (Vol. Eds.), *Comprehensive handbook of psychological assessment: Vol. 2. Personality assessment* (pp. 431–447). Hoboken, NJ: Wiley.

Gibson, J. J. (1977). The theory of affordances. In R. Shaw & J. Bransford (Eds.), *Perceiving, acting, and knowing: Toward and ecological psychology* (pp. 127–143). Hoboken, NJ: Wiley.

Glenberg, A. M. (1997). What memory is for. *Behavioral and Brain Sciences, 20,* 1–55.

Grèzes, J., & Decety, J. (2001). Functional anatomy of execution, mental simulation, observation, and verb generation of actions: A meta-analysis. *Human Brain Mapping, 12,* 1–19.

Grossmann, K., Grossmann, K. E., & Kindler, H. (2005). Early care and the roots of attachment and partnership representations. In K. E. Grossmann, K. Grossmann, & E. Waters (Eds.), *Attachment from infancy to adulthood: The major longitudinal studies* (pp. 98–136). New York: Guilford Press.

Grossmann, K. E., Bretherton, I., Waters, E., & Grossmann, K. (2013). Maternal sensitivity: Observational studies honoring Mary Ainsworth in her 100th year [Special issue)]. *Attachment and Human Development, 15,* 443–681.

Gunnar, M. (2003). Integrating neuroscience and psychological approaches in the study of early experiences. *Annals of the New York Academy of Sciences, 1008,* 238–247.

Hassabis, D., Kumaran, D., Vann, S. D., & Maguire, E. A. (2007). Patients with hippocampal amnesia cannot imagine new experiences. *Proceedings of the National Academy of Sciences, 104,* 1726–1731.

Hassabis, D., & Maguire, E. (2007). Deconstructing episodic memory with construction. *Trends in Cognitive Sciences, 11,* 299–306.

Haxby, J. V., Hoffman, E. A., & Gobbini, M. I. (2000). The distributed human neural system for face perception. *Trends in Cognitive Sciences, 4,* 223–233.

Henderson, L. A., Gandevia, S. C., & Macefield, V. G. (2007). Somatotopic organization of the processing of muscle and cutaneous pain in the left and right insula cortex: A single-trial fMRI study. *Pain, 128,* 20–30.

Hofer, M. (2014). The emerging synthesis of development and evolution: A new biology for psychoanalysis. *Neuropsychoanalysis: An Interdisciplinary Journal for Psychoanalysis and the Neurosciences, 16,* 3–22.

Hutchison, W. D., Davis, K. D., Lozano, A. M., Tasker, R. R., & Dostrovsky, J. O. (1999). Pain-related neurons in the human cingulate cortex. *Nature Neuroscience, 2,* 403–405.

Kaas, J. H., & Hackett, T. A. (2000). Subdivisions of auditory cortex and processing streams in primates. *Proceedings of the National Academy of Sciences, 97,* 11793–11799.

Kanwisher, N., & Yovel, G. (2006). The fusiform face area: A cortical region specialized for the perception of faces. *Philosophical Transactions of the Royal Society of London B, 361,* 2109–2128.

Kringelbach, M. L., & Rolls, E. T. (2003).Neural correlates of rapid reversal learning in a simple model of human social interaction. *NeuroImage, 20,* 1371–1383.

Laible, D. J., & Thompson, R. (2000). Mother–child discourse, attachment security, shared positive affect and early conscience development. *Child Development, 71,* 1424–1440.

Lamm, C., Decety, J., & Singer, T. (2011). Meta-analytic evidence for common and distinct neural networks associated with directly experienced pain and empathy for pain. *NeuroImage, 54,* 2492–2502.

Lavin, C., Melis, C., Mikulan, E., Gelormini, C., Huepe, D., & Ibañez, A. (2013). The anterior cingulate cortex: An integrative hub for human socially driven interactions. *Frontiers in Neuroscience, 7,* 1–4.

Lee, A. C. H., Yeung, L.-K., & Barense, M. D. (2012). The hippocampus and visual perception. *Frontiers of Human Neuroscience, 6,* 1–17.

Lewin, K. (1933). Environmental forces. In C. Murchison (Ed.), *A handbook of child psychology* (2nd ed., pp. 590–625). Worcester, MA: Clark University Press.

Lorberbaum, J. P., Newman, J. D., Horwitz, A. R., Dubno, J. R., Lydiard, R. B., Hamner, M. B., et al. (2002). A Potential role for thalamocingulate circuitry in human maternal behavior. *Biological Psychiatry, 51,* 431–445.

MacLean, P. (1973). A triune concept of the brain and behavior. In T. J. Boag & D. Campbell (Eds.), *The Hincks Memorial Lectures* (pp. 6–66), Toronto: University of Toronto Press.

MacWhinney, B. (2005). Language evolution and human development. In B. J. Ellis & D. J. Bjorklund (Eds.), *Origins of the social mind: Evolutionary psychology and child development* (pp. 383–410). New York: Guilford Press.

Maguire, E. A., & Mullally, S. L. (2014). Memory, imagination, and predicting the future: A common brain mechanism? *The Neuroscientist, 20,* 220–234.

Main, M. (1995). Recent studies in attachment. In S. Goldberg, R. Muir, & J. Kerr (Eds.), *Attachment theory: Social, developmental, and clinical perspectives* (pp. 407–474). Hillsdale, NJ: Analytic Press.

Main, M., Hesse, E., & Kaplan, N. (2005). Predictability of attachment behavior and representational processes at 1, 6 and 19 years of age. In K. E. Grossmann, K. Grossmann, & E. Waters (Eds.), *Attachment from infancy to adulthood: The major longitudinal studies* (pp. 245–304). New York: Guilford Press.

Main, M., Kaplan, K., & Cassidy, J. (1985). Security in infancy, childhood, and adulthood: A move to the level of representation. In I. Bretherton & E. Waters (Eds.), Growing points of attachment theory and research. *Monographs of the Society for Research in Child Development, 50*(1–2, Serial No. 209), 66–104.

Main, M., & Weston, D. R. (1981). The quality of the toddler's relationship to mother and to father: Related to conflict behavior and the readiness to establish new relationships. *Child Development, 52,* 932–940.

Martin, A., Wiggs, C. L., Ungerleider, L. G., & Haxby, J. V. (1996). Neural correlates of category-specific knowledge. *Nature, 379,* 649–652.

Mazzola, L., Faillenot, I., Barral, F. G., Maugière, F., & Peyron, R. (2012). Spatial segregation of somatosensory and pain activations in the human operculo-insular cortex. *NeuroImage, 60,* 409–418.

Mazzola, L., Isnard, J., Peyron, R., & Maugière, F. (2012). Stimulation of the human cortex and the experience of pain, *Brain, 135,* 631–640.

McNeill, D. (2005). *Gesture and thought.* Chicago: University of Chicago Press.

Medford, N., & Critchley, H. D. (2010). Conjoint activity of anterior insular and anterior cingulate cortex: Awareness and response. *Brain Structure and Function, 214,* 535–549.

Meltzoff, A. N., & Moore, M. K. (1977). Imitation of facial and manual gestures by human neonates. *Science, 198,* 75–98.

Miller, E. K., & Cohen, J. D. (2001). An integrative theory of prefrontal cortex function. *Annual Review of Neuroscience, 24,* 167–202.

Nadel, L., & Peterson, M. A. (2013). The hippocampus: Part of an interactive posterior representational system spanning perceptual and memorial systems. *Journal of Experimental Psychology: General, 142,* 1242–1254.

Naselaris, T., Olman, C. A., Stansbury, D. E., Ugurbil, K., & Gallant, J. L. (2015). A voxel-wise encoding model for early visual areas decodes mental images of remembered scenes. *NeuroImage, 105,* 215–228.

Nelson, K. (1989). *Narratives from the crib.* Cambridge, MA: Harvard University Press.

Nelson, K. (1996). *Language in cognitive development: Emergence of the mediated mind.* New York: Cambridge University Press.

Nelson, K. (2005). Evolution and development of human memory systems. In B. J. Ellis & D. J. Bjorklund (Eds.), *Origins of the social mind: Evolutionary psychology and child development* (pp. 354–382). New York: Guilford Press.

Nelson, K., & Gruendel, J. (1981). Generalized event representations: Basic building blocks of cognitive development. In M. E. Lamb & A. Brown (Eds.), *Advances in developmental psychology* (Vol. 1, pp. 131–158). Hillsdale, NJ: Erlbaum.

Newcombe, R., & Reese, E. (2004). Evaluations and orientations in mother–child narratives as a function of attachment security: A longitudinal investigation. *International Journal of Behavioral Development, 28,* 230–245.

Nitschke, J. B., Nelson, E. E., Rusch, B. D., Fox, A. S., Oakes, T. R., & Davidson, D. J. (2004). Orbitofrontal cortex tracks positive mood in mothers viewing pictures of their newborn infants. *NeuroImage, 21,* 583–592.

Nyberg, L., Habib, R., McIntosh, A. R., & Tulving, E.

(2000). Reactivation of encoding-related brain activity during memory retrieval. *Proceedings of the National Academy of Sciences, 97,* 11120–11124.

Oppenheim, D., Emde, R. N., & Warren, S. (1997). Children's narrative representations of mothers: their development and associations with child and mother adaptation. *Child Development, 68,* 127–139.

Parvizi, J., Rangarajan, V., Shirer, W. R., Desai, N., & Greicius, M. D. (2013). The will to persevere induced by electrical stimulation of the human cingulate gyrus, *Neuron, 80,* 1359–1367.

Paus, T. (2001). Primate anterior cingulate cortex: Where motor control, drive and cognition interface. *Nature Reviews Neuroscience, 2,* 417–424.

Piaget, J. (1951). *Play, dreams, and imitation.* New York: Norton.

Piaget, J. (1952). *The origins of intelligence in children.* New York: Norton.

Pylyshyn, Z. W. (1973). What the mind's eye tells the mind's brain: A critique of mental imagery. *Psychological Bulletin, 80,* 1–24.

Raichle, M. E., MacLeod, A. M., Snyder, A. Z., Powers, W. J., Gusnard, D. A., & Shulman, G. L. (2001). A default mode of brain function. *Proceedings of the National Academy of Sciences, 98,* 676–682.

Rizzolatti, G., Fadiga, L., Gallese, V., & Fogassi, L. (1996). Premotor cortex and the recognition of motor actions. *Brain Research: Cognitive Brain Research, 3,* 131–141.

Rizzolatti, G., & Sinigaglia, C. (2010). The functional role of the parieto-frontal mirror circuit: Interpretations and misinterpretations. *Nature Reviews Neuroscience, 11,* 264–274.

Rolls, E. T. (1996). The orbitofrontal cortex. *Philosophic Transactions of the Royal Society of London B, 351,* 1433–1444.

Rolls, E. T., & Grabenhorst, F. (2008). The orbitofrontal cortex and beyond: From affect to decision-making, *Progress in Neurobiology, 86,* 216–244.

Ruby, P., & Decety, J. (2004). How would *you* feel versus how do you think *she* would feel?: A neuroimaging study of perspective-taking with social emotions. *Journal of Cognitive Neuroscience, 16,* 988–999.

Sarter, M., Berntson, G. G., & Cacioppo, J. T. (1996). Brain imaging and cognitive neuroscience: Toward strong inference in attributing function to structure. *American Psychologist, 51,* 13–21.

Saxe, T., & Kanwisher, N. (2003). People thinking about people: The role of the temporo-parietal junction in "theory of mind." *NeuroImage, 19,* 1835–1842.

Schacter, D. L., & Addis, D. R. (2007). The cognitive neuroscience of constructive memory: Remembering the past and imagining the future. *Philosophical Transactions of the Royal Society of London B, 362,* 773–786.

Schacter, D. L., Addis, D. R., Hassabis, D., Martin, V. C., Spreng, R. N., & Szpunar, K. K. (2012). The future of memory: Remembering, imagining, and the brain. *Neuron, 76,* 677–694.

Schank, R. C., & Abelson, R. P. (1977). *Scripts, plans, goals, and understanding.* Hillsdale, NJ: Erlbaum.

Schore, A. N. (1994). *Affect regulation and the origin of the self.* Hilldale, NJ: Erlbaum.

Scoville, W. B., & Milner, B. (1957). Loss of recent memory after bilateral hippocampal lesions. *Journal of Neurology, Neurosurgery, and Psychiatry, 20,* 11–21.

Shackman, A., Salomons, T. V., Slagter, H. A., Fox, A. S., Winter, J. J., & Davidson, R. J. (2011). The integration of negative affect, pain and cognitive control in the cingulate cortex. *Nature Reviews Neuroscience, 12,* 153–167.

Sherry, D. F., & Schacter, D. L. (1987). The evolution of multiple memory systems. *Psychological Review, 94,* 439–454.

Simmons, W. K., Martin, A., & Barsalou, L. W. (2005). Pictures of appetizing foods activate gustatory cortices for taste and reward. *Cerebral Cortex, 15,* 1602–1608.

Singer, T., Kiebel, S. J., Winston, J. S., Dolan, R. J., & Frith, C. D. (2004). Brain responses to the acquired moral status of faces. *Neuron, 41,* 653–662.

Singer, T., Seymour, B., O'Doherty, J., Stephan, K. E., Dolan, R. J., & Frith, C. D. (2006). Empathic neural responses are modulated by the perceived fairness of others. *Nature, 439,* 466–469.

Sowell, E. R., Thompson, P. M., Holmes, C. J., Jernigan, T. L., & Toga, A. W. (1999). *In vivo* evidence for post-adolescent brain maturation in frontal and striatal region. *Nature Neuroscience, 2,* 859–861.

Steele, H., & Steele, M. (2005). Understanding and resolving emotional conflict: The London parent–child project. In K. E. Grossmann, K. Grossmann, & E. Waters (Eds.), *Attachment from infancy to adulthood: The major longitudinal studies* (pp. 137–164). New York: Guilford Press.

Stern, D. N. (1985). *The interpersonal world of the infant.* New York: Basic Books.

Strathearn, L., Li, J., Fonagy, P., & Montague, P. R. (2008). What's in a smile?: Maternal brain responses to infant facial cues. *Pediatrics, 122,* 40–51.

Swain, J. E., Kim, P., Spicer, J., Ho, S. S., Dayton, C. J., Elmadih, A., et al. (2014). Approaching the biology of human parental attachment: Brain imaging, oxytocin and coordinated assessments of mothers and fathers. *Brain Research, 1580,* 78–101.

Szpunar, K. K., & Schacter, D. L. (2013). Get real: Effects of repeated simulation and emotion on the perceived plausibility of future experiences. *Journal of Experimental Psychology: General, 142,* 323–327.

Taylor, S. E., Pham, L. B., Rivkin, I. D., & Armor, D. A. (1998). Harnessing the imagination: Mental simulation, self-regulation, and coping. *American Psychologist, 53,* 429–439.

Trevarthen, C., & Aitken, K. J. (2003). Regulation of brain development and age-related changes in infants' motives: The developmental function of "regressive" periods. In M. Heimann (Ed.), *Regression periods in human infancy.* (pp. 107–184). Mahwah, NJ: Erlbaum.

Trevarthen, C., & Hubley, P. (1978). Secondary intersubjectivity: Confidence, confiding, and acts of meaning in the first year. In A. Lock (Ed.), *Action, gesture, and symbol* (pp. 183–229). London: Academic Press.

Tulving, E. (1972). Episodic and semantic memory. In E. Tulving & W. Donaldson (Eds.), *Organization of memory* (pp. 381–403). New York: Academic Press.

Tulving, E. (2002). Episodic memory: From mind to brain. *Annual Review of Psychology, 53,* 1–25.

Tulving, E., & Szpunar, K. K. (2009). Episodic memory. *Scholarpedia, 4,* 3332.

Urgesi, C., Berlucci, G., & Aglioti, S. M. (2004). Magnetic stimulation of extrastriate body area impairs visual processing of nonfacial body parts. *Current Biology, 14,* 2130–2134.

Van IJzendoorn, M. H., Sagi, A., & Lambermon, M. W. (1992). The multiple caregiver paradox: Some data from Holland and Israel. *New Directions in Child Development, 57,* 5–24.

Vogeley, K., Bussfeld, P., Newen, A., Herrmann, S., Happe, F., Falkai, P., et al. (2001). Mind reading: Neural mechanisms of theory of mind and self-perspective. *NeuroImage, 14,* 170–181.

Waters, E., Crowell, J., Elliott, M., Corcoran, D., & Treboux, D. (2002). Bowlby's secure base theory and the social/personality psychology of attachment styles: Work(s) in progress. *Attachment and Human Development, 4,* 230–242.

Waters, H. S., & Waters, E. (2006). The attachment working models concept: Among other things, we build script-like representations of secure base experiences. *Attachment and Human Development, 8,* 185–197.

Wheeler, M. E., Petersen, S. E., & Buckner, R. L. (2000). Memory's echo: Vivid remembering reactivates sensory-specific cortex. *Proceedings of the National Academy of Sciences, 101,* 11125–11129.

Wicker, B., Keysers, C., Plailly, J., Royet, J.-P., Gallese, V., & Rizzolatti, G. (2003). Both of us disgusted in my insula: The common neural basis of seeing and feeling disgust, *Neuron, 3,* 655–664.

Williams, J. M. G. (2006). Capture and rumination, functional avoidance and executive control (CaRFAX): Three processes that underly overgeneral memory. *Cognition and Emotion, 20,* 548–568.

Yee, E., Chrysikou, E. G., & Thompson-Schill, S. L. (2013). Semantic memory. In K. Ochsner & S. Kosslyn (Eds.), *Oxford handbook of cognitive neuroscience: Vol. 1. Core topics* (pp. 353–374). Oxford, UK: Oxford University Press.

Yeh, W., & Barsalou, L. W. (2006). The situated nature of concepts. *American Journal of Psychology, 119,* 349–384.

Young, J. Z. (1964). *A model for the brain.* London: Oxford University Press.

Zeidman, P., Mullally, S. L., & Maguire, E. A. (2014). Constructing, perceiving, and maintaining scenes: Hippocampal activity and connectivity. *Cerebral Cortex, 10,* 3836–3855.

# PART II

# BIOLOGICAL PERSPECTIVES

# Chapter 5

# Attachment Theory within a Modern Evolutionary Framework

Jeffry A. Simpson
Jay Belsky

> It has often been assumed that animals were in the first place rendered social, and that they feel as a consequence uncomfortable when separated from each other, and comfortable whilst together, but it is a more probable view that these sensations were first developed in order that those animals which would profit by living in society, should be induced to live together, . . . for with those animals which were benefited by living in close association, the individuals which took the greatest pleasure in society would best escape various dangers; whilst those that cared least for their comrades and lived solitary would perish in greater numbers.
> —CHARLES DARWIN (1871, Vol. 1, p. 80)

As this quotation indicates, Charles Darwin was an attachment theorist. Although he focused on "society" (instead of significant others) and "comrades" (instead of attachment figures), Darwin was the first scientist to appreciate the full extent to which human social nature is a product of selection pressures. John Bowlby, who not only admired Darwin's theoretical vision but was one of his biographers (see Bowlby, 1991), spent most of his brilliant career treading the intellectual path that Darwin started paving. Integrating ideas from Darwin's theory of evolution by natural selection, object relations theory, control systems theory, evolutionary biology, and the fields of ethology and cognitive psychology, Bowlby (1969/1982, 1973, 1980) developed a grand synthesis of social and personality development across the lifespan, which is now known as attachment theory. One

reason why attachment theory is so generative and prominent today is its deep intellectual ties to fundamental principles of evolution.

In many respects, however, attachment theory and its adherents have not kept up with developments in evolutionary biology. In fact, beyond acknowledging that attachment behavior evolved via natural selection to facilitate the survival of infants in the environment of evolutionary adaptedness (EEA), surprisingly little attachment-related research and writing addresses the importance of either reproduction and reproductive fitness as the target of natural selection or the role of environmental conditions, including parenting, in regulating the development of reproductive strategies. These are critical issues that we address in this chapter.

As we shall see, attachment theory is one of a handful of major middle-level evolutionary theories. Bowlby's interest in the cognitive, emotional, and behavioral ties that bind humans to one another began with an astute observation. Across all human cultures and most primate species, young and vulnerable infants display a specific sequence of reactions following separation from their stronger, older, and wiser caregivers. Immediately following separation, most infants *protest*, typically crying, screaming, and throwing temper tantrums as they search for their caregivers. Bowlby surmised that vigorous protest during the early phases of caregiver absence is a good initial strategy to promote survival. Intense protests usually draw the attention of caregivers to their infants, who, during evolutionary history, would have been susceptible to injury or predation if left unattended.

If loud and persistent protests fail to retrieve the caregiver, infants enter a second stage, *despair*, during which their movement declines and they fall silent. From an evolutionary standpoint, Bowlby realized that despondency is a good "second" strategy to promote survival. Excessive movement could result in accident or injury, and loud protests combined with movement may draw predators. Thus, if protests fail to retrieve the caregiver, the next best survival strategy would be to avoid actions that might increase the risks of self-inflicted harm or predation.

Bowlby also observed that, after a period of despair, infants who are not reunited with their caregivers enter a third stage: *detachment*. During this phase, the infant begins to resume normal activity without the caregiver, learning to behave in an independent and self-reliant manner. Bowlby (1969/1982) conjectured that the function of detachment is to permit the formation of emotional bonds with new caregivers. He reasoned that emotional ties with previous caregivers must be relinquished before new bonds can be formed. From the standpoint of evolution, detachment allows infants to cast off old emotional ties and begin the process of forming new ones with caregivers who may be willing to provide the attention and resources necessary for survival.

Bowlby believed that the cognitive, emotional, and behavioral reactions that characterize each stage reveal the operation of an innate attachment system. The main reason why the attachment system evolved and remains so deeply ingrained in human nature is that it provided a good solution to one of the most difficult adaptive problems our ancestors faced—how to increase the probability of survival through the most perilous years of social and physical development. Inspired

by Darwin, Bowlby believed that the attachment system was genetically "wired" into many species through directional selection during evolutionary history.

There were, of course, limitations to Bowlby's and other early attachment theorists' understanding and application of evolutionary thinking, many of which Bowlby sought to correct as he developed attachment theory (see Belsky, 1999; Simpson, 1999). One shortcoming was his initial focus on the differential survival of species rather than individuals. Another shortcoming was his focus on the survival function of attachment rather than the implications it has for differential reproduction. To enhance reproductive fitness, individuals must not only survive to reproductive age, but they also must successfully mate and raise children, who then must mate and raise their own children, and so on. Fortunately, as we shall see, some contemporary attachment theorists have shifted attention to how attachment phenomena and processes in childhood are systematically linked to the enactment of different reproductive strategies in adulthood (Belsky, in press; Belsky, Steinberg, & Draper, 1991; Chisholm, 1996, 1999). However, because individuals cannot reproduce without first surviving to reproductive age, Bowlby wisely built the foundation of attachment theory on this vital precursor to ultimate reproductive fitness.

Early attachment theorists also held the erroneous view that most rearing environments in the EEA were benign, resulting in the secure attachment pattern being "species-typical" (e.g., Ainsworth, 1979; Main, 1981). The EEA, however, was not nearly as uniform, resource-rich, or benign as many early attachment theorists envisioned (e.g., Edgarton, 1992), which means that no single attachment pattern should have been primary or species-typical. In fact, as we shall see, the adoption of different attachment patterns (in children) or orientations (in adults) most likely reflect evolved, often unconsciously enacted tactics that probably improved *reproductive fitness* in response to the specific environments in which individuals grew and developed in ancestral times and perhaps still today. Reproductive fitness reflects the extent to which an individual's genes are present in his or her descendants. The concept of inclusive fitness (described below) highlights the important distinction between genes present in direct descendants (i.e., children) and those present in indirect descendants (e.g., grandchildren, nieces, nephews). From an evolutionary standpoint, the maximization of reproductive or inclusive fitness is the goal of all living organisms, including humans, and thus is the target of natural selection.

Perhaps the biggest impediment to Bowlby's understanding of evolution, however, was the undeveloped state of evolutionary thinking when he began formulating attachment theory in the 1950s and 1960s. The foundation of attachment theory was well established long before several significant "middle-level" theories of evolution—theories that address the major adaptive problems with which humans were confronted during our evolutionary history—were introduced in the 1970s. As a consequence, Bowlby was not privy to much of what is now known as the "modern" evolutionary perspective when he started erecting the tenets of attachment theory. Until recently, few of the modern middle-level evolutionary theories were systematically linked with mainstream attachment theory and research. We hope to facilitate this process.

The overarching goal of this chapter is to place attachment theory in a modern (neo-Darwinian) evolutionary perspective. The chapter had seven sections. The first briefly reviews theoretical developments that have transformed Darwin's (1859, 1871) original theory of natural selection into the modern evolutionary perspective. We also discuss where attachment theory fits within the hierarchy of evolutionary principles and middle-level theories. The second section describes the major adaptive problems that our ancestors had to overcome given the probable nature of the environments they inhabited in the course of the past 100,000 years, focusing on the most stable features of the social EEAs that humans probably inhabited.

The third section addresses how the two major components of attachment theory—the normative component and the individual-difference component—fit within a modern evolutionary view of human behavior. In discussing normative attachment, we briefly review the species-typical course through which attachment bonds develop across the lifespan. Different patterns or styles of attachment are construed as adaptive, ecologically contingent behavioral strategies that should have facilitated reproduction in adulthood given the probable environments that individuals would inhabit as adults.

Section four reveals how another major middle-level theory of evolution—Trivers's (1974) theory of parent–offspring conflict—sheds new light on several attachment-related phenomena, including how and why parents and children negotiate issues of weaning, parental investment, and the child's eventual independence. In the fifth section, we review and evaluate several attachment/life history models, most of which articulate how and why different attachment patterns in childhood might affect the trajectory of social and personality development, culminating in divergent reproductive strategies in adulthood. In the final two sections, we discuss some unresolved issues and promising new directions for research, and offer concluding comments.

## The Place of Attachment Theory in Modern Evolutionary Thinking

Though it remains one of the greatest intellectual accomplishments in the history of science, Darwin's (1859) original theory of evolution was incomplete and imprecise. Darwin's thinking was constrained by several factors. First, his theory predated our understanding of genes and patterns of inheritance. Second, because Darwin did not focus on genes as the principal units on which natural selection operates, he could not explain why some organisms engage in self-sacrificial or nonreproductive behavior. This enigma was not solved until Hamilton (1964) introduced the concept of *inclusive fitness* (i.e., the notion that differential gene replication is what truly drives evolution). Third, Darwin had only a faint understanding of how sexual recombination and genetic mutations provide the variation from which better adaptations and new species are selected. Fourth, he did not fully appreciate the degree to which specific adaptations have both benefits and costs. Similar to many theorists of his time, Darwin focused more on the benefits bestowed by certain adaptations, without fully factoring in their associated costs (Cronin, 1991). Darwin's brilliance, however, allowed him to envision how natural selection might operate *without* the benefits of all this later knowledge.

### The Rise of Modern Evolutionary Theories

Few theoretical advances occurred in the evolutionary sciences for more than a century after Darwin published his second landmark book, *The Descent of Man, and Selection in Relation to Sex*, in 1871. This state of affairs changed in the mid-

1960s. With the development of inclusive fitness theory, Hamilton (1964) introduced kin selection. By focusing on the gene rather than the individual organism as the primary unit on which selection operates, Hamilton solved the biggest paradox that Darwin never unraveled, namely, that during the evolutionary struggle for reproductive fitness, some organisms forgo reproduction to assist the reproductive efforts of their biological relatives.

Hamilton solved this riddle by realizing that an individual's total (inclusive) fitness depends on his or her own reproductive output plus the total reproductive output of all kin who share some portion of the individual's genes. If genes are the units on which selection operates, and if individuals can facilitate the reproductive output of their biological relatives, there would be situations in which it would pay to sacrifice one's own reproductive output, including one's life, to facilitate the reproduction of close relatives. Unlike Darwin, Hamilton could calculate the degree to which pairs of individuals are likely to share novel genes. On average, parents share half of their genes with their children, full siblings share half of their genes with each other, grandparents share one-fourth of their genes with their grandchildren, aunts and uncles share one-fourth of their genes with their nieces and nephews, and first cousins share one-eighth of their genes.

Armed with this knowledge, Hamilton confirmed that self-sacrificial behavior could have been selected in situations where the costs of engaging in an act were less than the benefits to be gained times the degree to which individuals were biologically related (i.e., altruistic behavior should occur when $C < Br$, where $C$ = costs, $B$ = benefits, and $r$ = the degree of relatedness; see Simpson, 1999). For example, while it would make sense to sacrifice one's own life to save at least two biological children (each of whom shares 50% of the parent's genes), one would have to save many more nieces or nephews (who carry fewer genes) to achieve the same fitness benefits. Hamilton's intellectual breakthrough marked the dawn of the modern evolutionary perspective. Indeed, inclusive fitness theory is the overarching theory of natural selection from which virtually all middle-level evolutionary theories are derived. Although Hamilton's research was not cited by Bowlby (1969/1982), Bowlby's first major statement on attachment proved to be one of the first middle-level evolutionary theories. In developing attachment theory, Bowlby sought to understand and explain how our ancestors successfully solved the first major barrier to inclusive fitness—how to survive the perils and dangers of infancy.

Several important theoretical advances followed in the 1970s, many of which were spearheaded by Robert Trivers. In 1971, he introduced the theory of reciprocal altruism, which explains why organisms with inherently "selfish" genes should, at times, behave cooperatively with non-kin. The development of this theory was important for attachment theory given the presumed links between early attachment security–insecurity and the development of empathy and prosocial behavior. Trivers identified some of the specific conditions under which selective reciprocal altruism ought to enhance an individual's inclusive fitness. Axelrod (1984) then demonstrated mathematically how a quid pro quo strategy of helping others (i.e., a tit-for-tat strategy) can evolve and become stable amid other competing strategies.

In 1972, Trivers unveiled the theory of parental investment and sexual selection. According to this theory, different amounts of parental investment in children govern sexual selection, which explains why females and males in many species differ on certain physical attributes (e.g., relative body size) and behavioral characteristics (e.g., aggressiveness). Trivers argued that, in species in which one sex *initially* invests more time, effort, resources, and energy in producing and raising offspring (usually women, in the case of humans), the other sex (usually men) should compete to mate with the higher-investing sex. The intense *intra*sexual competition that results should have produced some of the modal physical, behavioral, and emotional differences witnessed between the sexes. This leads one to wonder whether we should expect similarities or differences in attachments to mothers versus fathers.

In 1974, Trivers introduced the theory of parent–offspring conflict, which explains why parents and their children—individuals who share half their genes and, thus, should be jointly invested in passing them on to future generations—experience conflict: Their individual self-interests are not identical. Because this theory has several fascinating implications for how attachment patterns between children and their caregivers can be understood, it is discussed in greater detail below. For now, though, it is important to recognize that this theoretical precept challenges the common assumption that parents are motivated to be unconditionally devoted to their offspring rather than "strategic allocators" of time, attention, and other resources.

In recent years, life history theory (Charnov, 1993; Kaplan & Gangestad, 2005) has become a unifying perspective within the evolutionary sciences. To leave descendants, individuals must solve multiple problems associated with survival, growth, development, and reproduction across the lifespan. Depending on life circumstances, an individual's time, effort, and energy can be allotted to *somatic effort* (i.e., investing in growth and development of one's own body to facilitate survival enroute to later reproduction) or *reproductive effort* (i.e., funneling effort toward progeny). Reproductive effort has two components: *mating effort* (i.e., locating, courting, and retaining suitable mates) and *parenting effort* (i.e., gestating, giving birth, postnatal child care, and teaching/socialization). Life history theory explains how individuals should best allocate somatic versus reproductive effort given their past, current, and anticipated (future) life circumstances, as well as their health and well-being.

## Attachment Theory in the Hierarchy of Evolutionary Theories

Inclusive fitness theory, which encompasses both Darwin's concept of fitness due to one's own reproduction (i.e., direct descendants: children) and Hamilton's notion of fitness due to the reproduction of one's biological relatives (i.e., indirect descendants: grandchildren, nieces, etc.), is the superordinate theory of evolution from which all middle-level evolutionary theories flow. The middle-level theories, which include reciprocal altruism (Trivers, 1971), sexual selection and parental investment (Trivers, 1972), parent–offspring conflict (Trivers, 1974), and attachment (Bowlby 1969/1982), address the specific adaptive problems that humans faced and had to resolve during evolutionary history. Thus, they reside one level below inclusive fitness theory. Because life history theory addresses how individuals should allocate their finite resources across the entire lifespan, it interconnects and integrates the middle-level theories. Each middle-level theory in turn has a small set of basic principles that reside at the next level down (see Simpson, 1999). Most evolutionary hypotheses and predictions are derived from these basic principles.

Sexual selection and parental investment theory, for instance, contains two major principles relevant to mate selection. The theory suggests that the search for mates is governed by the degree to which prospective mates (1) are likely to be good investors in and providers for future offspring, and (2) have desirable attributes (e.g., physical attractiveness or other mate-attracting features) that could be passed on genetically to offspring (Gangestad & Simpson, 2000). Specific predictions and hypotheses are then derived from each of these principles.

Attachment theory also has two primary theoretical components. The *normative component* of attachment theory makes predictions about relatively universal, stable patterns of behavior, particularly in response to situations in which individuals feel ill, fatigued, afraid, or upset (Bowlby, 1969/1982). The *individual-difference component* offers predictions about the ontogenic origins and developmental sequelae of different patterns or orientations (styles) of attachment, including why each pattern or style should be "adaptive" in certain environments.

Even though each middle-level evolutionary theory addresses a specific set of adaptive problems, many of them have overlapping implications for social behavior. Kin selection theory, for example, also stipulates when conflict should arise between parents and their children; parent–offspring conflict theory specifies when reciprocal altruism should emerge between different sets of pair-bonded parents; and reciprocal altruism theory addresses when men and women might strive to attain status and ascend social hierarchies in groups (Simpson, 1999). In some cases, middle-level theories generate different hypotheses and predictions regarding a given outcome. For some phenomena, therefore, there is no single evolutionary prediction, particularly if competing middle-level theories are involved (Buss, 1995). What is most important to appreciate is that predictions derived from evolutionary theorizing *are* empirically testable.

## Stable Features of the Social EEA

In order to understand the context in which the attachment system evolved and the problems it was designed to "solve," one must consider the physical and social environments that humans most likely inhabited during evolutionary history. Although attachment theorists have speculated about what the EEA may have been like (especially the physical EEA; see Bowlby, 1969/1982), less consideration has been given to the *social* EEA (Simpson & Belsky, 2008).

For most of our evolutionary history, humans were hunters and gatherers (Cronk, 1999; Kelly, 1995) who lived in small, cooperative groups (Brewer & Caporael, 2006; Eibl-Eibesfeldt, 1989). Most people within a tribe were biologically related to one another, and strangers were encountered rather infrequently, mainly during intertribal trading, social contact, or war (Wright, 1994). Though people occasionally migrated in and out of their natal groups, most remained in the same tribe their entire lives. Men and women formed long-term pair bonds (Cronk, 1999), but serial monogamy was probably most common (Fisher, 1992). Children were born approximately 4 years apart and were raised with considerable help from extended family and perhaps even non-kin (Wright, 1994); few children were raised exclusively by their biological parents. Humans, in fact, were probably "cooperative breeders" who shared childrearing with their kin (Hrdy, 1999, 2005). Younger children most likely spent considerable time being socialized by older children (Eibl-Eibesfeldt, 1989) if they survived premature death, especially during the first 5 years of life. Both men and women were involved in securing food, with men doing most of the hunting and women doing most of the gathering (Wood & Eagly, 2002). Participation in the daily functioning of small, cooperative groups may in fact have been the predominant survival strategy of early humans (Brewer & Caporael, 2006). These likely features of the social EEA must be considered when conceptualizing attachment theory within an evolutionary framework.

## Normative and Individual-Difference Components of Attachment

As mentioned earlier, attachment theory has two primary components: (1) a normative component that explains modal or species-typical patterns and stages of attachment in humans (e.g., "How and why are attachment bonds formed?"), and (2) an individual-difference component that explains deviations from modal or normative patterns and stages (e.g., "How and why do different patterns of attachment exist?"). The attempt to account for both species-typical patterns of behavior and predictable individual differences is a hallmark of nearly all major middle-level evolutionary theories.

## Normative Features of Attachment

There are three normative features of attachment that have especially important ties to evolutionary principles (Simpson & Belsky, 2008): the "synchronization" of infant–parent responses/behaviors during the first few months of life, young children's need to maintain contact with and seek proximity to their caregivers, and the basic stages through which attachment propensities develop.

### Synchronized Capabilities

Compared to most other species, human infants are born in an underdeveloped and premature state (Kaplan, Lancaster, & Hurtado, 2000). From the moment of birth, however, human infants are "prepared" to bond with their caregivers (Simpson, 1999), and several ways in which mothers behave—at birth and early in development—seem to operate in *synchrony* with the capabilities and limitations of their infants, facilitating infant–caregiver bonds (Simpson & Belsky, 2008). For example, mothers typically exaggerate their facial expressions, change them more slowly, and maintain visual contact for longer periods of time when interacting with infants than with others (Eibl-Eibesfeldt, 1989). When talking to infants, mothers engage in "motherese" (Fernald, 1985), slowing their speech, accentuating certain syllables, and speaking one octave above normal speech (Grieser & Kuhl, 1988). These patterns of behaving are preferred by most young infants and are well suited to their developing visual and auditory capacities. Systems that operate in a synchronous, lock-and-key fashion between codependent individuals, as those just highlighted do, are often a telltale sign of evolved adaptations.

### Contact Maintenance and Proximity Seeking

According to Bowlby (1980), attachment behaviors include actions that promote proximity between children and their attachment figures. Young children engage in three classes of behavior to establish or maintain proximity to their caregivers (Bowlby, 1969/1982). *Signaling behaviors* (e.g., vocalizing, smiling) tend to draw caregivers toward the child, usually for positive interactions. *Aversive behaviors* (e.g., crying, screaming) bring caregivers to children, typically to terminate the aversive reactions. *Active behaviors* (e.g., approaching, following) move the child toward the caregiver. Though different phenotypically, these behaviors all serve the same evolutionary function—to keep vulnerable infants in close physical proximity to their caregivers, thereby increasing their chances of survival. Since death prior to reproduction was the first major threat to inclusive fitness, Bowlby reasoned that directional selection shaped the attachment system in humans, establishing the foundation of our social nature.

### Phases of Development

According to Bowlby (1969/1982), attachment propensities develop through four phases in humans (see also Marvin, Britner, & Russell, Chapter 13, this volume). In the first phase, which takes place between birth and age 2–3 months, infants respond to a wide variety of social stimuli and people without exhibiting strong preferences for one attachment figure. Although Bowlby may have overestimated how open young infants are to contact comfort from multiple caregivers, he was correct in believing that infants are malleable in terms of whom they can and do bond with during the opening months of life. The early openness of the system may have facilitated survival—and may, therefore, have been selected—in a world where the risk of maternal death resulting from delivery and/or its complications was far more common than it is today.

During the second phase, which occurs between age 2–3 months and about 7 months, infants display greater discrimination in social responsiveness. They begin, for instance, to distinguish caregivers and family members from strangers, selectively prefer certain persons, and direct their attachment behaviors toward specific attachment figures. Such discrimination should have helped the infant "reel-in" the caregiver, further facilitating survival (in the service of eventual reproduction), and thus resulting in its selection.

In the third phase, which extends from age 7 months to roughly 3 years, children play a more active role in seeking proximity and initiating social contact. During this phase, they also start developing internal working models (i.e., beliefs, expectancies, and attitudes about relationships based on experiences with attachment figures) of themselves and significant others (Bowlby, 1973). This is also when the three primary "functions" of attachment are first seen in the child's behavior: *proximity maintenance* (staying near to, and resist-

ing separations from, the attachment figure), *safe haven* (turning to the attachment figure for comfort and support), and *secure base* (using the attachment figure as a base from which to engage in nonattachment behaviors). If children in this phase have prolonged separations from their attachment figures, they experience the three stages of response to separation: protest, despair, and detachment. For reasons outlined earlier, these responses should also have aided and abetted survival and reproduction, thereby leading to their selection.

The fourth phase, which begins around age 3, marks the beginning of behaviors that signal goal-corrected partnerships with attachment figures. Given the further development of their language skills and theory-of-mind capabilities, children start to see the world from the perspective of their interaction partners. This allows them to incorporate the goals, plans, and desires of their partners into their own decision making, which results in the negotiation of joint plans and activities. These unique abilities should also have facilitated the formation and maintenance of pair bonds and, thus, may have been selected by evolutionary processes.

As children move through the toddler years, their desire for physical proximity is gradually replaced by a desire to maintain psychological proximity (i.e., felt security; Sroufe & Waters, 1977). Early in adolescence, overt manifestations of attachment bonds with parents subside, and the three functions of attachment—proximity maintenance, safe haven, and secure base—are gradually transferred from parents to peers and romantic partners as adolescents enter adulthood (Furman & Simon, 1999). During this final stage, the centrality of reproduction as an evolutionary process becomes more obvious and direct instead of indirect (i.e., through enhancing survival).

### Individual Differences in Attachment

Although infants are biologically predisposed to form attachment bonds to their caregivers, the type of bonds they form ought to depend on the conditions in which they are raised, as Bowlby (1969/1982) and Ainsworth (1979) proposed. Perceptions of environmental conditions, in turn, should be filtered through evolved psychological mechanisms, including sensation (e.g., physical warmth), perception (e.g., caregiver responsivity), and representations (e.g., internal working models). Such psychological mechanisms are typically activated by specific environmental cues, resulting in "optimal" ecologically contingent strategies that evolved to solve specific adaptive problems posed by certain kinds of environments (Buss, 1995; Tooby & Cosmides, 1992).[1]

Infants, of course, do not have the cognitive ability to appraise the quality of local environmental conditions, such as whether the environment is safe, plentiful, and rich in resources versus threatening, harsh, and impoverished. However, they *do* have the ability, which is well appreciated by attachment theory, to determine whether caregivers are sensitive, responsive, and attentive to their biological needs. Such information ought to provide clues about the nature and quality of current—and perhaps future—environmental conditions (Belsky, 1997; Chisholm, 1996; Frankenhuis, Gergely, & Watson, 2013). If caregivers in evolutionary history were able to devote the time, effort, and energy necessary to be sensitive, responsive, and attentive to the needs of their children, the local environment was probably safe and sufficiently rich in resources, broadly defined. In contrast, if caregivers were insensitive, nonresponsive, and devoted less attention to their children, the local environment was probably less resource-rich and perhaps even dangerous.

Ainsworth's Strange Situation is well suited to detect different patterns of attachment because it presents infants with two common cues to danger in the EEA: being left alone, and being left with a stranger. Examining reunions between mothers and their 12- to 18-month-old infants, Ainsworth, Blehar, Waters, and Wall (1978) identified three primary attachment patterns in young children: secure, anxious-ambivalent, and anxious-avoidant. Upon reunion, securely attached children use their caregivers to regulate and attenuate their distress, resuming other activities (e.g., exploration, play) rather quickly after calming down. Anxious-avoidant children retract from their caregivers upon reunion, opting to control and dissipate their negative affect in an independent, self-reliant manner. Anxious-ambivalent children make inconsistent and conflicted attempts to derive comfort and support from their caregivers, intermingling clinginess with outbursts of anger (see Fearon & Belsky, Chapter 14, and Solomon & George, Chapter 18, this volume).

Each attachment pattern reflects a different "strategy" that would have solved adaptive problems posed by different kinds of rearing environments (Belsky, 1997; Chisholm, 1996; Main,

1981). Mothers of securely attached infants tend to be available and responsive to the needs and signals of their infants (Ainsworth et al., 1978; De Wolff & Van IJzendoorn, 1997). Largely because of this, secure children do not have to worry about the availability and responsiveness of their caregivers, which allows them to concentrate on other life tasks.

Anxious-ambivalent children have caregivers who tend to behave inconsistently toward them (Ainsworth et al., 1978), sometimes because of poor or deficient parenting skills (Isabella, Belsky, & von Eye, 1989; Lewis & Feiring, 1989). Among children who are maltreated, anxious-ambivalent children are more likely to have been victims of parental neglect (Youngblade & Belsky, 1989). Thus, the demanding nature of anxious-ambivalent children may reflect an ecologically contingent strategy designed to obtain, retain, or improve greater parental attention and care (Cassidy & Berlin, 1994; Main & Solomon, 1990). For children with such parents, this behavioral strategy would have increased proximity to caregivers, solicited better care, and improved the child's chances of survival (and eventually reproduction).

Avoidant children usually have caregivers who are cold and rejecting (Ainsworth et al., 1978). Among maltreated children, avoidant children are more likely to have suffered physical or emotional abuse from their parents (Youngblade & Belsky, 1989). The evolutionary origins of avoidance, however, may be more complex and multifaceted than those of anxious-ambivalence. Bowlby (1980) conjectured that avoidance allows infants to disregard cues that might activate the attachment system. If such cues were fully processed, avoidant infants might recognize the true inaccessibility and rejecting demeanor of their primary caregivers, which could be incapacitating.

Two additional evolutionary explanations for avoidance in childhood have been proposed. According to Main (1981), the distant, self-reliant behavior that characterizes avoidant infants enables them to maintain reasonably close proximity to belligerent or overwhelmed caregivers without driving them away. Avoidance, in other words, may have evolved to overcome deficiencies in caregiving provided by highly distressed, hostile, or unmotivated parents. During evolutionary history, this behavioral strategy would have increased the survival of infants who, if they put too many demands on their parents, might have been abandoned. Alternatively, earlier reproduction may facilitate inclusive fitness in some circumstances, especially in harsh environments with few resources (Trivers, 1985). If maternal rejection was a valid proximal cue of the severity of future environments, avoidant tendencies might motivate children not only to move away from their parents earlier but also to become more opportunistic and risk taking, thereby facilitating survival and early reproduction in arduous environments (Belsky, 1997; Belsky et al., 1991). Moreover, if the stress experienced by insecure children undermined their health, internal bodily signals indicating declining health and increased morbidity or mortality may also have played a role in strategically regulating development (Belsky, 2014; Rickard, Frankenhuis, & Nettle, 2014).

As children enter adolescence, cumulative experiences in relationships are further assimilated into internal working models, which are continuously being updated and revised. These models reflect the degree to which individuals (1) believe they are worthy of love and affection, and (2) view significant others as loving and affectionate (Mikulincer & Shaver, 2007). Unlike in childhood, however, the attachment system in adulthood becomes integrated with the mating and caregiving systems (Shaver, Hazan, & Bradshaw, 1988), making adult attachment orientations (styles) more challenging to interpret than attachment patterns in children.

## Attachment Theory and Parent–Offspring Conflict Theory

One middle-level evolutionary theory that has considerable relevance to attachment theory is parent–offspring conflict theory (Trivers, 1974). According to this theory, children (who share 50% of their genes with parents and full siblings) should want greater investment from their parents than their parents have been selected to provide. As a result, parents and offspring have slightly divergent reproductive interests, which result in conflict that peaks during the final stages of weaning. Stated another way, the evolutionary interests of parents and their infants are not perfectly aligned, which means that what is good for the child is not necessarily good for the parent, and vice versa. Unlike many current applications of attachment theory, the modern evolutionary perspective does not romanticize or idealize parent–child relationships.

## Parent–Offspring Conflict Theory and Parental Investment

According to Trivers (1972), parental investment involves any actions performed by a parent for his or her offspring that increase the offspring's chances of survival, while reducing the parent's ability to invest in other current or future offspring. The level of investment depends on the costs and benefits associated with a given parental act or behavior. *Costs* are defined as units of forgone reproductive success by other current or future offspring, and *benefits* are defined as units of reproductive success of the current offspring (Trivers, 1974). In humans, acts of investment include allocating time, effort, energy, or resources to children through activities such as feeding, protecting, sheltering, and teaching. The amount of investment that children seek and parents offer should hinge on how both parties view the costs and benefits of different forms of parental investment.

When infants are young and highly dependent on their parents for care and resources, the costs of investment to parents are low and the benefits to infants are high from the reproductive standpoint of each party. During the early stages of childrearing, therefore, the reproductive interests of parents and their offspring coincide reasonably well, but not perfectly. However, as infants grow, consume more resources, and become more self-sufficient, the reproductive interests of parents and offspring diverge. From the parents' perspective, the costs of investment continue to rise over time while the benefits the infant derives from additional investment asymptotes. During this phase, directing investment to new offspring could enhance parents' reproductive success more than continuing to invest in an increasingly autonomous, self-sufficient child. This is the point at which weaning takes place in most cultures.

Given that children share only half of their genes with their parents and full siblings, two of their siblings must survive and successfully reproduce to propagate the infant's genes fully to future generations. Thus, infants should "devalue" the costs of investment incurred by their parents by 50%, expecting twice as many benefits as their parents have been selected to provide. Children and parents, therefore, should experience conflict until, from the perspective of the parent, the cost of parental investment is more than twice the benefit to the infant (or, from the perspective of the child, the cost of parental investment exceeds self-benefit). When this point is reached, the child's inclusive fitness would be reduced if he or she continued to demand additional investment. Conflict should then subside as the child accepts the diversion of parental investment to other siblings.

Attachment theory does not fully recognize and account for the somewhat different reproductive interests of infants and their caregivers. Instead, scholars often assume that the evolutionary interests of parents and their children are largely equivalent and that, barring significant abnormalities, each child should be of equal "reproductive value" to its parents. Both of these assumptions are questionable. The reproductive value of a child should depend on several factors (Daly & Wilson, 1981; Trivers, 1974), including attributes of (1) the infant (e.g., his or her health, normality), (2) the mother (e.g., her health, age, ability to provide for the infant), (3) the father (e.g., the certainty of his paternity, his resources, his willingness to invest in the infant), (4) the nuclear family (e.g., the number of existing children, their birth spacing, the presence of stepsiblings), and (5) the local environment (e.g., whether or not resources are available to minimize the costs and maximize the benefits of further parental investment). When the costs of investing in a given child are disproportionately high relative to the benefits, parents should display preferential investment in certain children (Daly & Wilson, 1981). In some instances, attachment insecurity might arise from conditions that lower parental investment. Lower levels of investment should be evident in inadequate or poor caregiving behaviors, such as parental inattentiveness, neglect, rejection, abuse, and infanticide in extreme cases.

Cross-cultural research reveals that parental investment is, in fact, lower in families that have at least one biologically unrelated parent; when fathers question their paternity; when infants are ill, weak, or deformed; during periods of famine; when families are poor or lack social support; when mothers are very young; when families have too many children; and when birth spacing is too short (Daly & Wilson, 1988; Hrdy, 1999).

## Parental Investment and Attachment

Relatively little is known about whether the conditions that reduce parental investment actually *cause* insecure attachment in children, primarily because it is unethical to employ such experimental interventions. However, strong links have been chronicled between certain contextual factors and

the quality of parental care, which *is* causally related to attachment security (Fearon & Belsky, Chapter 14, this volume). These factors include parental psychological health and well-being (e.g., Belsky & Jaffee, 2006), quality of marital/romantic partner relations (e.g., Krishnakumar & Buehler, 2000), and social support/connectedness (e.g., Andresen & Telleen, 1992). This research indicates that the greater the well-being, marital quality, and social support, the more sensitive, responsive, stimulating, and less detached (or hostile) the parenting tends to be. These "determinants of parenting" (Belsky, 1984) are also related to attachment security in the expected direction, such that better conditions instill greater security, which fosters better parental well-being (e.g., Atkinson et al., 2000; Jacobson & Frye, 1991). There is even evidence that parenting is the proximate mediator linking these more distal contextual factors with attachment security (e.g., Crittenden, 1985).

## Evolutionary Models of Social Development across the Lifespan

Attachment theory addresses social and personality development "from the cradle to the grave" (Bowlby, 1979, p. 129). Most early attachment research, however, investigated certain barriers to inclusive fitness (e.g., problems associated with infant survival) to the relative exclusion of other barriers (e.g., problems associated with mating and reproduction). Even though some early attachment theorists (e.g., Main, 1981) conjectured that different attachment patterns in children might reflect different evolved strategies for promoting survival under certain rearing conditions, childhood attachment patterns were not theoretically tied to the development of different adult romantic attachment styles and mating orientations until the early 1990s, when Belsky and his colleagues (1991) published an influential paper on human social development from an evolutionary/attachment perspective.

## Life History Theory

More recent theoretical developments have been guided by life history theory (LHT) (Charnov, 1993). LHT addresses how and why individuals allocate time, energy, and resources to different traits, behaviors, and life tasks when they are faced with tradeoff decisions that could influence their reproductive fitness (Kaplan & Gangestad, 2005). In particular, LHT models the selection pressures in our ancestral past that should have determined when, and the conditions under which, individuals allocated time, energy, and resources to physical development, growth, reproduction, body repair, or aging.

According to most life history models, individuals can increase their reproductive fitness in two general ways (Parker & Maynard Smith, 1991). First, they can "invest" in traits or attributes that affect the timing of their mortality (i.e., the age at which they die). Second, they can "invest" in traits or attributes that influence the timing of their fertility (i.e., the age and rate at which they reproduce). Many life history traits/attributes, however, have countervailing effects on mortality and fertility (Kaplan & Gangestad, 2005). Traits or attributes that improve fertility through more frequent or more intense mating effort, for example, usually shorten survival, because many of the traits that make people (particularly men) more attractive to the opposite sex compromise the immune system (Grafen, 1990). Moreover, the allocation of energy and resources to growth during development tends to retard fertility when individuals are young, but enhance it once individuals mature sexually (Charnov, 1993). And the allocation of time, energy, and resources needed to ensure that one's children grow to be strong and healthy typically undermines one's own future fertility and survival.

Because one "can't have it all," individuals must negotiate three fundamental tradeoffs during their lives: (1) whether to invest in present (immediate) reproduction or future (delayed) reproduction; (2) whether to invest in higher quantity or higher quality offspring; and (3) whether to invest in mating effort or parenting effort. The way in which each tradeoff is resolved ought to depend on several factors, including the demands of the local environment (e.g., how taxing it is, the number of pathogens it contains, whether biparental care is required); the health, skills, abilities, and resources available to an individual at that time; the health, skills, abilities, and resources of others (e.g., kin, potential mates, competitors); and so forth.

### The Belsky, Steinberg, and Draper Model

Inspired by LHT and earlier research on father absence during childhood (Draper & Harpending, 1982), Belsky and colleagues (1991) developed the first evolution-based and attachment-oriented

lifespan model of human social development. According to this model, the main evolutionary function of early social experience is to "prepare" children for the social and physical environments they are likely to encounter during their lifetime. The model focuses primarily on rate of development (i.e., faster vs. slower) and therefore offspring quantity versus quality tradeoffs. Ellis (2004) has labeled it "psychosocial acceleration theory" even though the theory addresses both slower and faster development. Certain information gleaned from the early environment should allow individuals to adopt an appropriate reproductive strategy—one that, on average, best increases inclusive fitness—in future environments. Hinde (1986), for example, proposed that if maternal rejection is induced by harsh environments in which competition for limited resources is intense, offspring who are aggressive and noncooperative should have higher reproductive fitness as adults than those who do not display these attributes. Conversely, offspring raised in environments with abundant resources could increase their fitness by adopting a more cooperative and communal orientation in adulthood.

The five-stage Belsky and colleagues (1991) model proposes that (1) early contextual factors in and around the family of origin (e.g., level of stress, spousal harmony, financial resources) affect (2) early childrearing experiences (e.g., level of sensitive, supportive, and responsive caregiving). These experiences then affect (3) psychological and behavioral development (e.g., attachment patterns, internal working models) that in turn influence (4) somatic development (i.e., how quickly sexual maturation is reached) and eventually (5) the adoption of specific ways of mating and parenting. These stages are linked sequentially, but earlier stages may statistically interact to predict later outcomes. Early contextual factors in the family of origin, for instance, can interact with early childrearing experiences to forecast the rate of somatic development.

Belsky and colleagues (1991) hypothesized that two developmental trajectories culminate in two reproductive strategies in adulthood (although they could also be opposite ends of a single continuum rather than discrete vs. continuous phenotypes). One strategy entails a short-term, opportunistic orientation toward close relationships, especially with regard to mating and parenting, in which sexual intercourse occurs earlier in life, romantic pair bonds are short-lived and less stable, and parental investment is lower. This orientation is geared to increase the *quantity* of offspring. The second strategy entails a long-term, investing orientation toward mating relationships in which sexual intercourse occurs later in life, romantic pair bonds are stronger and more enduring, and parental investment is greater. This orientation maximizes offspring *quality*. A critical and novel prediction derived from this model involving rate of development is that early rearing experiences should influence the timing of puberty. Specifically, sexual maturation should occur earlier for individuals who develop along the "quantity trajectory" than for those who develop along the "quality trajectory."

A large body of evidence supports the Belsky and colleagues model (for reviews, see Belsky, 2012; Ellis, 2004; Simpson & Belsky, 2008). For example, consistent with nonevolutionary perspectives, greater socioemotional stress in families is associated with more insensitive, harsh, rejecting, inconsistent, and unpredictable parenting practices. Economic hardship (McLoyd, 1990), occupational stress (Bronfenbrenner & Crouter, 1982), marital discord (Belsky, 1981; Emery, 1988), and psychological distress (McLoyd, 1990) are all precursors of more hostile and/or detached parenting styles. Conversely, greater social support and more economic resources facilitate warmer and more sensitive childrearing practices (Lempers, Clark-Lempers, & Simons, 1989), perhaps because less taxed parents are more patient with or tolerant of their young children (Belsky, 1984).

The link between parental sensitivity and the psychological and behavioral development of children is also well established, consistent with both attachment theory and many other theories (e.g., social learning, emotion socialization, life course). During the first year of life, insensitive and unresponsive caregiving predicts the development of insecure attachments (De Wolff & Van IJzendoorn, 1997), which in turn forecasts behavior problems later in development. Insecurely attached 2-year-olds, for instance, are less tolerant of frustration (Matas, Arend, & Sroufe, 1978). Insecurely attached preschoolers are more socially withdrawn (Waters, Wippman, & Sroufe, 1979), less likely to display sympathy to distressed peers (Waters et al., 1979), less willing to interact with friendly adults (Lutkenhaus, Grossmann, & Grossman, 1985), and less well liked by their classmates (LaFreniere & Sroufe, 1985). During elementary school, insecure children have more severe behavior problems, especially aggression and disobedience (Lewis, Fiering, McGuffog, & Jaskir, 1984). According to Belsky and colleagues (1991), these

behaviors are governed by insecure working models, which prepare the child for opportunistic advantage taking and, therefore, noncommunal relationships later in life.

The most novel part of the model concerns what predicts the rate of somatic development. Belsky and colleagues (1991) hypothesized that children exposed to greater socioemotional stress develop insecure attachments, exhibit behavior disorders, and should reach puberty—and thus reproductive capacity—earlier than children without these attributes. According to life history logic (Chisholm, 1993, 1999; Kaplan & Gangestad, 2005), environments in which resources are scarce, relationship ties are tenuous, and mortality risks are elevated should cause more energy and effort to be allocated to rapid physical development, early mating, and short-term romantic pair bonds. This developmental strategy should increase the chances of reproducing before dying (or should have done so in our ancestral past). On the other hand, environments in which resources are plentiful and relationship ties are reciprocal and enduring should lead to effort being channeled to further somatic development, later sexual maturity, delayed mating, and longer-term romantic pair bonds that contribute to greater parental investment. In more benign environments, reproductive fitness could be enhanced by deferring reproduction until (1) individuals have acquired the skills and resources needed to maximize the quality of each offspring, and (2) offspring can benefit from all of the embodied capital that humans need to reproduce successfully.

Several strands of evidence support these predictions (Belsky, 2012). First, greater parent–child warmth, cohesion, and positivity predict delayed pubertal development in both prospective longitudinal studies (Ellis, McFadyen-Ketchum, Dodge, Pettit, & Bates, 1999; Graber, Brooks-Gunn, & Warren, 1995) and retrospective or concurrent ones (Kim, Smith, & Palermiti, 1997; Miller & Pasta, 2000). Second, greater parent–child conflict and coercion predict earlier pubertal timing in both prospective longitudinal studies (Ellis & Essex, 2007; Moffitt, Caspi, Belsky, & Silva, 1992) and retrospective or concurrent ones (Kim et al., 1997). Third, the happier and/or less conflict-ridden the parental relationship, the later pubertal maturation occurs in girls, both in prospective longitudinal studies (Ellis et al., 1999; Ellis & Garber, 2000) and in nonprospective ones (Kim et al., 1997). Indeed, early insecure attachment—measured at age 15 months—forecasts earlier age of menarche and both onset and completion of pubertal development (Belsky, Houts, & Fearon, 2010). These results cannot be easily explained by traditional attachment theory, but they are central to psychosocial acceleration theory. Not all studies have found puberty-related links like those just highlighted. Steinberg (1988), for instance, did not find associations between the amount of family conflict/coercion and pubertal timing in girls. However, family experience–pubertal developmental links consistent with psychosocial acceleration theory have recently emerged in studies that take into account genetic confounding, either via sibling designs (Tithers & Ellis, 2008) or natural experiments (Pesonen et al., 2008).

Almost all of these findings are based on studies involving girls. Although it was once thought that this gender disparity could be attributable to the greater difficulty of measuring puberty in males, this fact does not seem to explain these sex differences. New theorizing by James, Ellis, Schlomer, and Garber (2012) has noted that the early versus later reproduction tradeoff central to Belsky and colleagues' (1991) original theorizing is more pressing for females, whereas that between somatic development and reproduction is more pressing for males, who must engage in considerable intrasexual competition for mates. Recent empirical work by this team provides evidence consistent with this important insight (James et al., 2012).

Evidence relevant to the final stages of the Belsky and colleagues (1991) model (i.e., the mating strategies individuals adopt in adulthood) comes from two sources: (1) research linking adult attachment styles to mating and romantic relationship functioning, and (2) research bridging adult attachment and parenting practices. Individuals who report being more securely attached to romantic partners are less likely to have promiscuous sexual attitudes or engage in extrapair sex (Brennan & Shaver, 1995); are more likely to desire only one sexual partner over a 30-year period (Miller & Fishkin, 1997); and, if female, have sexual intercourse at a later age than their insecure counterparts (Bogaert & Sadava, 2002). Securely attached adults also have more satisfying romantic relationships (J. A. Feeney, Chapter 21, this volume), display less negative affect and more constructive conflict resolution tactics when interacting with romantic partners (Simpson, Rholes, & Phillips, 1996), and engage in more self-disclosure and are more responsive to self-disclosures by partners (Mikulincer & Nachshon, 1991). Consequently, secure adults are also less likely to divorce or separate (J. A. Feeney, Chapter 21, this volume), have longer lasting romantic relationships (Hazan & Shaver, 1987), and report greater commitment to and trust in their dating partners (Simpson, 1990) and spouses (Fuller & Fincham, 1995).

These findings, although consistent with Belsky and colleagues' (1991) original model, are limited due to their cross-sectional nature and their focus on romantic (rather than childhood) attachment assessments. Recent longitudinal research using data from the Minnesota Longitudinal Study of Risk and Adaptation has provided even more direct support for the model (see Simpson, Collins, & Salvatore, 2011). Simpson, Collins, Tran, and Haydon (2007), for example, have documented links between attachment security (assessed in the Strange Situation at 12 months) and how individuals experience and express conflict with their romantic partners 20 years later. Specifically, individuals classified as insecure at age 1 tend to experience and express relatively more negative emotions in their romantic relationships in their early 20s, and this effect appears to be mediated through their lower social competence in grade school and their less secure same-sex friendships at age 16.

Supporting the Belsky and colleagues (1991) model, adult attachment is also associated with differential expectations about children and parenting even before individuals have children. Rholes, Simpson, Blakely, Lanigan, and Allen (1997), for instance, found that insecurely attached college students anticipate being more easily aggravated by their young children if/when they become parents, expect to be more strict disciplinarians, believe they will express less warmth toward their children, and are less confident about their ability to relate well to them. In addition, avoidant college students believe they will derive less satisfaction from caring for their young children and express less interest in having them. Once they have children, avoidant parents report feeling less emotionally close to their first newborn child as soon as 2 weeks after birth (Wilson, Rholes, Simpson, & Tran, 2007), and avoidant mothers are less emotionally supportive of their preschooler children, adopting a detached, controlling, or instrumentally focused mode of relating to them (Crowell & Feldman, 1991; Rholes, Simpson, & Blakely, 1995). (For a review of studies of self-reported adult attachment patterns and parenting characteristics, see Jones, Cassidy, & Shaver, 2015.)

Furthermore, mothers classified as secure on the Adult Attachment Interview (AAI) (who in many cases received greater warmth and contingent care from their own parents) are more sensitive to and supportive of the needs of their children (Hesse, 2008, Chapter 26, this volume; Van IJzendoorn, 1995). For example, attachment security is linked with greater warmth and more appropriate structuring of learning tasks by fathers and mothers (Adam, Gunnar, & Tanaka, 2004), greater emotional support in various situations (Crowell & Feldman, 1991), less negativity (Slade, Belsky, Aber, & Phelps, 1999), and greater awareness of the child's needs (Das Eiden, Teti, & Corns, 1995).

### The Chisholm Model

Chisholm (1993, 1996) extended Belsky and colleagues' (1991) thinking by proposing a slightly revised and expanded model of alternative reproductive strategies, one that focuses on the immediate versus delayed reproduction life history tradeoff. This work advanced our thinking in three significant ways. First, it drew attention to local mortality rates as being the critical cues that humans monitor to regulate their rate of development and, ultimately, their reproductive strategies. After all, high mortality rates ought to have been a direct barometer of the difficulty of local environments, and they should have been associated with poorer caregiving in the EEA. According to Chisholm (1993, 1996), parental indifference or insensitivity—being a valid cue of local mortality rates—would have motivated children to develop avoidant working models and behaviors that should have increased fitness in such arduous environments. Low mortality rates, which should have signaled more hospitable environments, should have been associated with better and more attentive caregiving. Sensitive parenting, in other words, should have conveyed to children that premature death was less likely, resulting in secure working models and behaviors that enhanced fitness in benign environments.

Consistent with Chisholm's theorizing is evidence connecting adverse life conditions with expectations regarding longevity and the timing of reproduction later in life (Nettle, 2010; Nettle & Cockerill, 2010). For example, as life expectancy declines in a local area, the probability of women reproducing by age 30 increases (Wilson & Daly, 1997), and teen mothers who expect to die at a younger age are more likely to become mothers at an earlier age (Johns, 2003). Such findings are consistent with Geronimus's (1996) "weathering hypothesis," which states that early birth is a strategic response to the rapid decline in health among women, especially poor women, in their 30s and 40s. This underscores the value of treating local mortality rates as a powerful cue in the development of alternative reproductive strategies.

Besides highlighting the importance of local mortality rates, Chisholm (1999) also called attention to *time preference*—the tendency to discount the future by favoring smaller, immediate rewards over larger, delayed ones—as the psychological mechanism linking early rearing experiences with the timing of future mating and parenting behavior. Individuals raised in harsh or unpredictable (i.e., insecurity-inducing) environments, in which waiting for rewards could result in leaving no descendants, ought to prefer immediate payoffs, even if delayed ones might be significantly better (Wilson & Daly, 2005).

Chisholm's (1996) third major contribution was his identification of two parent-based threats to the survival and growth of children in the EEA—parents' *inability* and *unwillingness* to invest in offspring—to which children should have evolved to detect and respond. Thus, the secure attachment pattern is a facultative adaptation to parents' ability *and* willingness to provide high investment, as reflected in their warm/sensitive caregiving. The avoidant attachment pattern, in contrast, is an adaptation to parents' unwillingness to invest (regardless of their ability), reflected in their cold/rejecting caregiving. Finally, the anxious-ambivalent pattern is an adaptation to parents' inability to invest, reflected in their inconsistent/unpredictable caregiving.

The Belsky and colleagues and Chisholm models have both played important roles in getting scholars to think more deeply about how and especially *why* early experiences shape subsequent development, something that many developmental psychologists have simply taken for granted. Both models, however, have been expanded and further refined by the infusion of additional evolutionary considerations. First, neither model addresses all of the factors that, from an evolutionary standpoint, should govern the adoption of specific reproductive strategies in adulthood. Mate selection is contingent on a multitude of factors, ranging from a potential mate's genetic quality to his or her ability to accrue and share resources, to his or her capacity to impart knowledge and information to offspring (Gangestad & Simpson, 2000).

In addition, psychosocial acceleration theory, as originally conceptualized, was not sufficiently sensitive to the different roles that men and women assume in reproduction (Buss & Schmitt, 1993; Geary, 2005). This inspired James and colleagues (2012) and Del Giudice (2009) to develop sex-differentiated models that accentuate the different life history tradeoffs that females and males must negotiate. For females, the critical tradeoff is between early and later reproduction; for males, it is between growth and reproduction. Despite these limitations, the Belsky and colleagues and Chisholm models represent important advances in our understanding of attachment and social development across the lifespan.

## The Del Giudice Model

Del Giudice (2009) has developed a model that incorporates sex differences within an explicitly attachment/evolutionary framework and, in so doing, extends psychosocial acceleration theory in some novel ways. Recent cross-cultural research indicates that boys are more likely to be avoidantly attached in middle childhood, whereas girls tend to be anxious (reviewed in Del Giudice, 2009; for an alternative view, see Van IJzendoorn & Bakermans-Kranenburg, 2010). Del Giudice argues that sex differences in attachment patterns in middle childhood might have adaptive significance for both children and adults because they reflect the enactment of sex-specific life history strategies. Consistent with Belsky and colleagues (1991), early psychosocial stress and insecure attachment patterns are viewed as cues of heightened environmental risk, which shift development toward reproductive strategies that facilitate current reproduction over later reproduction and emphasize mating effort over parenting effort. In line with well-established sex differences between mating and parenting effort (Geary, 2005), insecure males typically enact avoidant strategies, whereas insecure females enact anxious ones, both of which increase subsequent investment from kin and mates. (Females ought to become avoidant, however, when environmental risks become high.)

The most novel part of the model is the proposal that sex differences in attachment should emerge in middle childhood—for reproductive-fitness-related reasons—rather than occurring earlier in development, which is the focus of psychosocial acceleration theory. Indeed, adrenarche (the early stages of sexual maturation) is theorized

to be a "developmental switch-point," reorganizing attachment during middle childhood, which then has several important implications for ties between attachment patterns and sexual development across the lifespan. Specifically, at the start of middle childhood, insecure children's attachment patterns become sex-biased, shunting reproductive strategies down sex-optimal developmental pathways. Because attachment security versus insecurity early in childhood is a good barometer of local ecological risk, it has been retained by evolution as a stable, prototype-like behavioral trait (Fraley, 2002). These early strategies, however, are disposable phenotypes that can be modified later in development if they no longer match the environmental demands to which the developing child is exposed. This is important, Del Giudice (2009) claims, because avoidant and anxious attachment patterns have different adaptive value for boys and girls with regard to competition in same-sex peer groups in middle childhood.

According to Del Giudice (2009), the strongest selection pressure on attachment patterns in middle childhood should come from intrasexual competition within peer groups when children start competing with others for status, attention, and resources. Negotiations within these groups should be particularly challenging for insecurely attached children, who can no longer count on their nuclear family members to buffer them from all the inherent stress and failures. The avoidant behavioral pattern, which is characterized by heightened aggression, excessive self-reliance, and inflated self-esteem, is used more effectively by males to attain higher status and popularity in middle childhood peer groups (Benenson, 2014). Girls, in contrast, shift to anxious patterns that help them utilize "tend-and-befriend" tactics (Taylor et al., 2000), which are more effective at promoting ascension and success within their social groups.

Successful social strategies, of course, do not always involve competitive status seeking. If environmental conditions are safe/predictable, and monogamy and high paternal investment define the local mating system, low-risk, cooperative strategies ought to maximize males' long-term fitness better, with less male avoidance (i.e., greater security) resulting in less male–male competition and lower conflicts of interest between mothers and fathers.

Maternal and paternal attachment might also differentially affect the behavioral strategies that children adopt in middle childhood. Maternal and paternal investments are differentially responsive to extrinsic risk (Quinlan, 2007), which could alter children's life history strategies in novel ways. The level of paternal investment, for instance, often contains more diagnostic information about the amount of male–male competition, polygyny, and paternal involvement within the local environment, which could shape children's levels of competitiveness and risk taking (especially in boys), as well as the adoption of avoidant versus anxious attachment patterns (particularly in girls). Future research needs to test these hypotheses and determine whether genotypic variability also affects the regulation of these life history-related traits.

## The Ellis Model

Whereas psychosocial acceleration theory called attention to family dynamics, including marital and parent–child relational experiences in regulating the development of reproductive strategies (Belsky et al., 1991), Ellis and colleagues (1999; Ellis & Garber, 2000) drew upon Draper and Harpending's (1982) focus on father absence and Trivers's (1972) parental investment theory to hypothesize that fathers have a special role in the development of girls' reproductive strategies. Belsky and colleagues (1991) viewed early father absence as a marker of stress in the family of origin and appreciated the influence of the quality of both mothering and fathering. Ellis (2004), on the other hand, suggests that father absence or stepfather presence is a particularly salient, evolutionarily privileged cue of paternal investment that signals low, unpredictable, or changing levels of paternal investment in families.

Father absence does, in fact, predict accelerated pubertal development among girls, both in prospective studies in which girls are followed from childhood into adolescence (e.g., Campbell & Udry, 1995; Ellis & Garber, 2000; Ellis et al., 1999) and in retrospective studies of adults (e.g., Doughty & Rodgers, 2000; Hoier, 2003; Quinlan, 2003). Similar effects, however, have not been found in African American samples (e.g., Campbell & Udry, 1995; Rowe, 2000). In addition, research does not always find greater predictive power of fathering or the father–child relationship over mothering and the mother–child relationship (e.g., Ellis, Shirtcliff, Boyce, Deardorff, & Essex, 2011). All too often, evidence of father effects on pubertal development comes from studies that

do not include measures of mothers (see Belsky, 2012).

Nevertheless, research does indicate that the earlier father absence occurs in a child's life (especially within the first 5 years), the more strongly it predicts the speed of female pubertal development (e.g., Ellis & Garber, 2000; Quinlan, 2003). Stepfather presence may also affect pubertal timing, perhaps accounting for some of the father absence effects (Ellis, 2004). Supporting this view, greater conflict between the mother and stepfather combined with earlier stepfather presence in the home is especially influential in accelerating pubertal development in girls (Ellis & Garber, 2000). Consistent with Belsky and colleagues' (1991) emphasis on the quality of parent–child relationships, Ellis and colleagues (1999) also found that girls' pubertal development is delayed the more time fathers spend caring for their daughters during the first 5 years of life and the more fathers have positive/affectionate interactions with their daughters at age 5.

Thus, there are good theoretical and even empirical grounds for *not* treating mothers and fathers as interchangeable agents of influence in understanding how childhood experiences shape reproductive strategies. Greater attention should be paid to the presence of biologically unrelated male figures in the home during development and to the differential influence of maternal and paternal investment (i.e., quality of parenting).

## The Hazan–Zeifman and Kirkpatrick Models

Scholars have also attempted to explain the nature and strength of adult romantic pair bonds from a life history/attachment perspective. Hazan and Zeifman (1999; Zeifman & Hazan, 2008), for example, propose that adult romantic relationships are an instantiation of attachment relationships formed earlier in life. They point out many similarities between childhood attachment to caregivers and adult attachment to close peers and romantic partners (also see Shaver et al., 1988). Both infants and adults, for example, display similar reactions to separation from or loss of their attachment figures. In addition, people value qualities in prospective mates that parallel those they valued in their caregivers, and children and adults behave similarly when seeking close contact, physical intimacy, and affection from their attachment figures. Parent–child and adult–adult attachment relationships also pass through a similar set of developmental stages.

Hazan and Zeifman (1999) suggest that the primary evolutionary function of secure attachment in adult relationships is to increase the likelihood of stable and enduring pair bonds so mates can provide better mutual support (see also Zeifman & Hazan, Chapter 20, this volume). Pair bonding, therefore, is conjectured to enhance the reproductive fitness of both parents and their offspring. Adult mating strategies are, in fact, related to the pair-bond status of one's parents, with father absence and greater marital discord in the family of origin predicting earlier sexual maturation, short-term mating strategies in adulthood, and less stable marriages (Belsky, 1999). Children who have more pair-bonded parents, by comparison, should adopt long-term mating strategies and emphasize quality rather than quantity of investment when they have their own children (Hazan & Zeifman, 1999). (See the earlier evidence linking positive marital and partner relationships with more supportive parenting and greater likelihood of having secure offspring.) More strongly pair-bonded partners should also contribute to their own reproductive success by providing each other with greater support, which is associated with better long-term physical and mental health and more regular ovulation patterns (Zeifman & Hazan, 1997).

Partially in response to this model, Kirkpatrick (1998) claims that adult attachment styles evolved to enhance reproductive fitness based on early childhood experiences, but he questions whether security and protection are the *primary* functions of adult attachment. Instead, Kirkpatrick suggests that components of the caregiving system (e.g., love) may have been co-opted during evolutionary history to cement romantic pair bonds in adulthood, and that—similar to the views of Belsky and colleagues and Chisholm—adult attachment styles primarily reflect evolved reproductive strategies.

One of the principal life history tradeoffs involves allocating time and energy to mating effort versus parenting effort. Kirkpatrick (1998) argues that it was not always adaptive or advantageous for women and men to enact long-term, monogamous mating strategies (see also Gangestad & Simpson, 2000). Consequently, adult attachment styles may be a "mechanism" for choosing the best mating strategy given the nature of one's early childhood experiences and the quality of early parental investment. Individuals who receive consistently sensitive and responsive parenting should develop

secure working models, resulting in the adoption of long-term, committed mating strategies. These individuals should also develop greater trust and intimacy in their relationships (Simpson, 1990) and should fall in love with partners who have higher mate value (Hazan & Shaver, 1987), which they do. Avoidant individuals, in contrast, should have less committed relationships, pursue short-term mating strategies, and have more unrestricted sociosexual orientations, which they do (Simpson, Wilson, & Winterheld, 2004). And anxious persons should desire and want to pursue long-term mating strategies, yet their strong desire to be attractive to and merge with their romantic partners ought to result in short-term sexual relationships that are unstable (Kirkpatrick, 1998). Given these findings, Kirkpatrick (1998) believes that features of the caregiving system—especially love operating as a "commitment device" (Fletcher, Simpson, Campbell, & Overall, 2015; Frank, 1988)—could have been co-opted to bind and stabilize long-term romantic pair bonds.

## Conceptualizing the Early Developmental Environment

According to life history thinking, the quality of the environment early in life can exert long-lasting effects on psychosocial development, including the development of specific mating and parenting strategies in both males and females, and different rates of pubertal timing in females. In conceptualizing the early rearing environment, Ainsworth and her colleagues (1978) have identified sensitive responsiveness as a key factor regulating the development of secure versus insecure attachment patterns. Moreover, Chisholm (1996, 1999) has suggested that because parenting quality is a good barometer of local mortality rates, it serves as a powerful, evolved cue that shapes the development of secure versus insecure attachment patterns and, therefore, the development of slow versus fast reproductive strategies in adulthood.

These observations become especially interesting in light of a recent cross-species analysis by Ellis, Figueredo, Brumbach, and Schlomer (2009), who examined the environmental factors that regulate the development of different reproductive strategies in assorted species and made a critical distinction between exposure to harsh versus exposure to unpredictable environments early in life. Security, of course, emanates from warm, sensitive, and consistently responsive caregiving, whereas insecurity stems from cold, insensitive, and inconsistent (or unpredictable) caregiving.

From a cross-species perspective, *harshness* refers to age-specific rates of morbidity–mortality in the local environment. In Western societies, harshness is indexed by socioeconomic status (SES), given that lower levels of SES are linearly related to nearly all forms of morbidity and mortality (Ellis et al., 2009). And, of course, such distal contextual conditions are associated with harsher, less supportive, and less responsive parenting (McLoyd, 1998). The harsher and poorer the environment, the higher the rate of morbidity (e.g., illness, injury) and mortality (death) at every age in a society. *Unpredictability* refers to stochastic changes (fluctuations) in the harshness of environmental conditions across time and may therefore incorporate inconsistent or unpredictable parenting. Unpredictability is signaled by important changes in the ecology of the family that directly affect parents and/or their children, such as frequent changes in the job status of parents, residential changes, and parental transitions such as divorce and remarriage (see Belsky, Schlomer, & Ellis, 2012; Simpson, Griskevicius, Kuo, Sung, & Collins, 2012). Although a great deal of research by developmentalists studying attachment has unwittingly blended the two dimensions—especially at the proximate level when operationalizing sensitive parenting—Ellis and colleagues' (2009) model suggests that harshness and unpredictability might have independent effects on life history-relevant behaviors in young adulthood. However, this model does not delineate when each form of stress ought to forecast specific life history traits in adolescence or adulthood, and it does not speak to the origins of attachment security.

To date, only a few prospective longitudinal studies have tested the effects of environmental unpredictability and harshness in childhood on later behavior in direct response to Ellis and colleagues' (2009) theorizing. Brumbach, Figueredo, and Ellis (2009) found that exposure to both greater environmental unpredictability and harshness measured in adolescence independently predicted faster life history strategies in adolescence, such as engaging in more deviant social behavior. Belsky and colleagues (2012) observed that being raised in more unpredictable environments during the first 5 years of life forecasted having more sexual partners by age 15, both directly and as mediated by maternal depressive symptoms and maternal sensitivity (which were also assessed during childhood). Simpson and colleagues (2012)

reported that individuals exposed to less predictable environments between ages 0 and 5 displayed a faster life history strategy at age 23, having more sexual partners, engaging in more aggressive and delinquent behaviors, and being associated with criminal activities. Exposure to either harsh environments or experiencing unpredictability in later childhood (ages 6–16), however, did not predict these outcomes. Viewed together, these findings indicate that unpredictable childhood environments exert unique effects on risky behavior later in life, consistent with adopting a faster life history strategy, and there may be a developmentally sensitive window for assessing unpredictability. They also raise intriguing questions about whether one can distinguish harsh versus warm parenting from consistent/predictable versus inconsistent/unpredictable parenting when examining the interactional origins of attachment patterns.

A recent longitudinal study has investigated the effects of early unpredictability on parenting 30 years later. Using data from the Minnesota Longitudinal Study of Risk and Adaptation, Szepsenwol, Simpson, Griskevicius, and Raby (2015) found that for males, exposure to greater unpredictability during the first 5 years of life forecasts less parental involvement/investment and less supportive parenting behavior in men who have children. These effects, however, were mediated through the quality of care that mothers gave their male children and the attachment representations of childhood that these males harbored in adulthood. Specifically, males (but not females) exposed to greater unpredictability during the first 5 years of life had mothers who were rated by observers as providing less sensitive care/support (i.e., less predictable warmth) between years 0 and 5, which in turn predicted them having more insecure attachment representations at age 26 (assessed by the AAI). Age 26 AAI insecurity, in turn, forecasted less observer-rated parental involvement/investment as well as less supportive behavior in adulthood. This evidence is important because it links unpredictability to actual parenting behavior, which is a critical component of Belsky and colleagues' (1991) original model.

## Unresolved Issues, Promising Directions, and Conclusions

We have covered only a few of the several unresolved issues and promising directions for future research. Two of the most perplexing questions center on why maternal sensitivity accounts for only a portion of the variance in children's attachment status and why the intergenerational transmission of attachment patterns is not stronger than it is (Van IJzendoorn & Bakermans-Kranenburg, 1997). LHT might be able to provide solutions to these puzzles.

Applying evolutionary bet-hedging logic, Belsky (1997; Belsky & Pluess, 2009) and Boyce and Ellis (2005; Ellis, Boyce, Belsky, Bakermans-Kranenburg, & Van IJzendoorn, 2011) have theorized that children should differ in their susceptibility to parental influence. Belsky and his colleagues suggest that differential susceptibility could be adaptive for parents, children, and their siblings if a parent's attempt to "prepare" his or her children for the future environment is mistaken due to the inherent unpredictability of future conditions. This would explain why, from an evolutionary standpoint, differential susceptibility to parental influence is witnessed within families. It would also explain why intergenerational transmission effects are weaker than expected. There is even more evidence, both observational and experimental, that children vary in their susceptibility to parenting and other influences (Belsky & Pluess, 2009, 2013). Most notable is discovery of a recent gene × environment interaction by Manuck, Craig, Flory, Halder, and Ferrell (2011), which indicates that the theory-distinguishing prediction of psychosocial acceleration theory— that exposure to an adverse rearing environment predicts earlier sexual maturation—holds for girls who carry one version of estrogen receptor genes but not another. Given that most attachment-related research is still not informed by a differential-susceptibility perspective, past research may have both under- and overestimated certain effects of rearing experiences on attachment outcomes— underestimated for those individuals who are more susceptible, and overestimated for those who are less susceptible.

If the early rearing environment regulates the development of reproductive strategies, which now seems likely, we need to determine exactly *how* certain environmental cues actually shape attachment patterns and reproductive strategies. Frankenhuis and Panchanathan (2011) have proposed that among those who are more susceptible to environmental regulation, the timing of "commitment" to a particular course of development (e.g., secure attachment, slower physical development) may depend on the clarity of the contextual cues. When cues are clear and consistent, a "reading" of them may lead to earlier commitment, but when they are less clear or when more time is required to decipher the environmental "tea leaves," individuals may defer commitment to one developmental pathway versus another. Attachment and developmental theorists should contemplate the implications of this possibility. Might some children who appear insecure early in life but then develop secure representations have experienced less consistent sensitive caregiving cues and, therefore, required more time before "committing" to such a developmental pathway? If so, could this explain why the presumed developmental antecedents of early attachment patterns are neither as strong nor as reliable as attachment theorists initially expected?

Time also comes into play when one considers the intergenerational transmission of attachment. To date, transmission has been assumed to be a single-generation process (e.g., a mother's attachment status shapes her child's attachment status via her parenting), with little consideration of the possible impact of grandparents, great-grandparents, and so forth. The evolutionary concept of intergenerational phenotypic inertia (Kuzawa, 2005), however, suggests that some forms of influence may endure across multiple generations, even when the most proximate generational experiences are at odds with the modal family trajectory. In particular, this model proposes that individuals should place greater diagnostic weight on conditions that have endured over multiple generations (e.g., repeated insecurity) rather than just the preceding one (e.g., one case of security), especially when the latter is inconsistent with the former. One might wonder whether an exclusive focus on the immediately preceding generation accounts in part for the intergenerational "transmission gap" that Van IJzendoorn (1995) identified.

This raises another set of issues. Although evolutionary forces should have shaped developmental trajectories, organisms also evolved to respond adaptively to rapid changes in local environments. The field of behavioral ecology, in fact, models such adaptive behaviors (see Gangestad & Simpson, 2007). In addition, the strategic pluralism model (Gangestad & Simpson, 2000) proposes that human females evolved to base mating decisions (including decisions about parenting qualities in mates) on two dimensions—the extent to which prospective mates display evidence of (1) viability (i.e., good health or other desirable mate-attracting attributes that could be passed on genetically to offspring) and (2) investment potential (in both the romantic relationship and any resulting offspring). In pathogen-prevalent environments, women should place more weight on men's viability attributes, so the "good genes" of such mates might be passed on to their children. In environments that demand heavy investment in children or biparental care, women should place greater importance on men's investment potential to enhance the likelihood of offspring survival. Given their different life experiences, adults who have different attachment histories and styles may evaluate, calibrate, or apply each mate dimension somewhat differently. This returns us to the mate value of relationship partners. Avoidant women, for instance, may expect and require less paternal investment in light of their independence and self-reliance and, given their mistrust of others, they may want less. Anxious women, in contrast, may expect and demand greater investment given their chronic concerns about relationship loss and abandonment.

Epigenetics research may also advance our understanding of intergenerational attachment issues. Animal research has shown that maternal grooming of newborn female rat pups does not just calibrate pups' stress–response system when they are adults and raise their own offspring; through nongenetic mechanisms, such care also influences the development of the *grand-offspring* of the original grooming mother (Cameron et al., 2005). These findings are important because they partially explain the attachment–mothering intergenerational cycle, in that rearing experiences stimulate gene action, which launches a cascade of developmental processes and outcomes leading to different reproductive strategies in adulthood, which are then transmitted intergenerationally by nongenetic means. This evidence raises further intriguing questions about possible gene × environment interactions; indeed, work by Caspi and colleagues (2002) supports differential susceptibility to parental influence by showing that the impact of rearing effects (e.g., child maltreatment) on the development of opportunistic, antisocial behavior varies depending on genotype. What remains unclear, however, is whether individuals who possess genetic "vulnerabilities" succumb to environmental risks, or whether early rearing experiences activate certain genes that then facilitate opportunistic, antisocial behavior.

Finally, like all too many developmental scientists who lack foundational knowledge about evolutionary theory, virtually all thinking and writing to date about attachment (and even the development of reproductive strategies) has presumed that malleable children have their development regulated primarily by their rearing experiences. Yet as Trivers (1974) pointed out more than four decades ago, the fact that parents and children share on average only 50% of their genes means that their biological interests are not isomorphic, and they are therefore bound to experience conflicts of interest (see also Schlomer, Del Giudice, & Ellis, 2011). Del Giudice (2012) has noted that this may explain why children—even highly malleable ones—do not simply "take instructions" from their parents. What are the implications of this observation for understanding the development of attachment patterns specifically and for developmental plasticity more generally?

In conclusion, attachment theory is an evolutionary theory of human social behavior "from the cradle to the grave" (Bowlby, 1979, p. 129). Although the theory's initial ties to evolution focused on how the normative and individual-difference components of attachment should have promoted infant survival, recent work has revealed how attachment patterns across the lifespan—including adult romantic attachment styles—may have evolved to increase reproductive fitness. These theoretical advances are important for several reasons. Until recently, attachment theorists have not addressed *why* early developmental experiences should be systematically related to later life outcomes, *why* intergenerational transmission of attachment should exist, or *why* maternal sensitivity should shape attachment security in children. Traditionally, attachment theorists and researchers have focused on *how* these processes work. Recent applications of LHT *within* attachment theory have rectified this deficiency, directing attention to questions of both ultimate *and* proximate causation. These theoretical advances are also important because they suggest that adult attachment styles might *not* be inconsequential evolutionary "artifacts" of the attachment system in children. According to life history accounts, the attachment system in young children should have facilitated survival and development through the perilous years of early childhood, not just psychological health and well-being. In adulthood, the attachment system may further enhance inclusive fitness via the adoption of environmentally contingent, alternative reproductive strategies, not just satisfaction and happiness in close relationships.

In the future, attachment scholars need to anchor more of their thinking and research within a modern evolutionary framework. As Dobzhansky (1973) once exclaimed, "Nothing in biology makes sense except in the light of evolution" (p. 125). The same claim applies to much of psychology in general, and to much of developmental and social psychology in particular. We strongly advocate treading the intellectual path first paved by Darwin and extended by Bowlby and other modern evolutionary theorists. Various middle-level evolutionary theories—especially parent–offspring conflict theory, parental investment and sexual selection theory, and a life-history framework—have a tremendous amount to offer scholars interested in attachment phenomena across the lifespan. Significant future advances in attachment theory and research are likely to rest on the successful and complete integration of attachment theory into a modern evolutionary perspective.

## Note

1. The term *strategy* refers to a set of coevolved anatomical, physiological, psychological, and/or behavioral traits designed by natural selection to increase inclusive fitness. It does *not* imply foresight, conscious awareness, or premeditation. The term *optimal* does *not* imply that natural selection produces a single, perfect phenotype. *Optimal strategies* are sets of coevolved traits that tend to increase inclusive fitness in specific environments given various tradeoffs.

## References

Adam, E., Gunnar, M., & Tanaka, A. (2004). Adult attachment, parent emotion, and observed parenting behavior. *Child Development, 75,* 110–122.

Ainsworth, M. D. S. (1979). Infant–mother attachment. *American Psychologist, 34,* 932–937.

Ainsworth, M. D. S., Blehar, M. C., Waters, E., & Wall, S. (1978). *Patterns of attachment: A psychological study of the Strange Situation.* Hillsdale, NJ: Erlbaum.

Andresen, P., & Telleen, S. (1992). The relationship between social support and maternal behavior and attitudes: A meta-analytic review. *American Journal of Community Psychology, 20,* 753–774.

Atkinson, L., Paglia, A., Coolbear, J., Niccols, A., Parker, K. C. H., & Guger, S. (2000). Attachment security: A meta-analysis of maternal mental health correlates. *Clinical Psychology Review, 20,* 1019–1040.

Axelrod, R. (1984). *The evolution of cooperation.* New York: Basic Books.

Belsky, J. (1981). Early human experience: A family perspective. *Developmental Psychology, 17,* 3–23.

Belsky, J. (1984). The determinants of parenting: A process model. *Child Development, 55,* 83–96.

Belsky, J. (1997). Attachment, mating, and parenting: An evolutionary interpretation. *Human Nature, 8,* 361–381.

Belsky, J. (1999). Modern evolutionary theory and patterns of attachment. In J. Cassidy & P. R. Shaver (Eds.), *Handbook of attachment: Theory, research and clinical applications* (pp. 141–161). New York: Guilford Press.

Belsky, J. (2012). The development of human reproductive strategies: Progress and prospects. *Current Directions in Psychological Science, 21,* 310–316.

Belsky, J. (2014). Toward an evo-devo theory of reproductive strategy, health and longevity. *Perspectives in Psychological Science, 9,* 16–18.

Belsky, J. (in press). Childhood experiences and reproductive strategies. In R. Dunbar & L. Barrett (Eds.), *Oxford handbook of evolutionary psychology.* Oxford, UK: Oxford University Press.

Belsky, J., Houts, R. M., & Fearon, R. (2010). Infant attachment security and the timing of puberty: Testing an evolutionary hypothesis. *Psychological Science, 21,* 1195–1201.

Belsky, J., & Jaffee, S. (2006). The multiple determinants of parenting. In D. Cicchetti & D. Cohen (Eds.), *Developmental psychopathology: Vol. 3. Risk, disorder and adaptation* (2nd ed., pp. 38–85). New York: Wiley.

Belsky, J., & Pluess, M. (2009). Beyond diathesis stress: Differential susceptibility to environmental influences. *Psychological Bulletin, 135,* 885–908.

Belsky, J., & Pluess, M. (2013). Beyond risk, resilience and dysregulation: Phenotypic plasticity and human development. *Development and Psychopathology, 25,* 1243–1261

Belsky, J., Schlomer, G. L., & Ellis, B. J. (2012). Beyond cumulative risk: Distinguishing harshness and unpredictability as determinants of parenting and early life history strategy. *Developmental Psychology, 48,* 662–673.

Belsky, J., Steinberg, L., & Draper, P. (1991). Childhood experience, interpersonal development, and reproductive strategy: An evolutionary theory of socialization. *Child Development, 62,* 647–670.

Benenson, J. (2014). *Warriors and worriers.* New York: Oxford University Press.

Bogaert, A. F., & Sadava, S. (2002). Adult attachment and sexual behavior. *Personal Relationships, 9,* 191–204.

Bowlby, J. (1973). *Attachment and loss: Vol. 2. Separation: Anxiety and anger.* New York: Basic Books.

Bowlby, J. (1979). *The making and breaking of affectional bonds.* London: Tavistock.

Bowlby, J. (1980). *Attachment and loss: Vol. 3. Loss.* New York: Basic Books.

Bowlby, J. (1982). *Attachment and loss: Vol. 1. Attachment.* New York: Basic Books. (Original work published 1969)

Bowlby, J. (1991). *Charles Darwin: A new life.* New York: Norton.

Boyce, W. T., & Ellis, B. J. (2005). Biological sensitivity to context. *Development and Psychopathology, 17,* 271–301.

Brennan, K. A., & Shaver, P. R. (1995). Dimensions of adult attachment, affect regulation, and romantic relationship functioning. *Personality and Social Psychology Bulletin, 21,* 267–283.

Brewer, M. B., & Caporael, L. R. (2006). An evolutionary perspective of social identity: Revisiting groups. In M. Schaller, J. A. Simpson, & D. T. Kenrick (Eds.), *Evolution and social psychology* (pp. 143–161). New York: Psychology Press.

Bronfenbrenner, U., & Crouter, A. (1982). Work and family through time and space. In S. Kamerman & C. Hayes (Eds.), *Families that work* (pp. 39–83). Washington, DC: National Academy Press.

Brumbach, B. H., Figueredo, A. J., & Ellis, B. J. (2009). Effects of harsh and unpredictable environments in adolescence on development of life history strategies: A longitudinal test of an evolutionary model. *Human Nature, 20,* 25–51.

Buss, D. M. (1995). Evolutionary psychology: A new paradigm for psychological science. *Psychological Inquiry, 6,* 1–30.

Buss, D. M., & Schmitt, D. P. (1993). Sexual strategies theory: A contextual evolutionary analysis of human mating. *Psychological Review, 100,* 204–232.

Cameron, N. M., Champagne, F. A., Parent, C., Fish, E. W., Ozaki-Kuroda, K., & Meaney, M. (2005). The programming of individual differences in defensive responses and reproductive strategies in the rat through variations in maternal care. *Neuroscience and Biobehavioral Reviews, 29,* 843–865.

Campbell, B. C., & Udry, J. R. (1995). Stress and age at menarche of mothers and daughters. *Journal of Biosocial Science, 27,* 127–134.

Caspi, A., McClay, J., Moffitt, T. E., Mill, J., Martin, J., Craig, I. W., et al. (2002). Role of genotype in the cycle of violence in maltreated children. *Science, 297,* 851–854.

Cassidy, J., & Berlin, L. J. (1994). The insecure/ambivalent pattern of attachment: Theory and research. *Child Development, 65,* 971–991.

Charnov, E. L. (1993). *Life history invariants.* Oxford, UK: Oxford University Press.

Chisholm, J. S. (1993). Death, hope, and sex: Life-history theory and the development of reproductive strategies. *Current Anthropology, 34,* 1–24.

Chisholm, J. S. (1996). The evolutionary ecology of attachment organization. *Human Nature, 7,* 1–38.

Chisholm, J. S. (1999). *Death, hope, and sex.* New York: Cambridge University Press.

Crittenden, P. M. (1985). Social networks, quality of child rearing, and child development. *Child Development, 56,* 1299–1313.

Cronin, H. (1991). *The ant and the peacock.* Cambridge, UK: Cambridge University Press.

Cronk, L. (1999). *That complex whole: Culture and the evolution of human behavior.* New York: Westview.

Crowell, J., & Feldman, S. (1991). Mothers' working models of attachment relationships and mother and child behavior during separation and reunion. *Developmental Psychology, 27,* 597–605.

Daly, M., & Wilson, M. I. (1981). Abuse and neglect of children in evolutionary perspective. In R. D. Alexander & D. W. Tinkle (Eds.), *Natural selection and social behavior: Recent research and new theory* (pp. 405–416). Oxford, UK: Blackwell.

Daly, M., & Wilson, M. [I.] (1988). *Homicide.* New York: Aldine de Gruyter.

Darwin, C. (1859). *On the origins of species.* London: John Murray.

Darwin, C. (1871). *The descent of man, and selection in relation to sex.* London: John Murray.

Das Eiden, R., Teti, D. M., & Corns, K. M. (1995). Maternal working models of attachment, marital adjustment, and the parent–child relationship. *Child Development, 66,* 1504–1518.

De Wolff, M., & Van IJzendoorn, M. (1997). Sensitivity and attachment: A meta-analysis on parental antecedents of infant attachment. *Child Development, 68,* 571–591.

Del Giudice, M. (2009). Sex, attachment, and the development of reproductive strategies. *Behavioral and Brain Sciences, 32,* 1–21.

Del Giudice, M. (2012). Fetal programming by maternal stress: Insights from a conflict perspective. *Psychoneuroendocrinology, 37*(10), 1614–1629.

Dobzhansky, T. (1973). Nothing in biology makes sense except in the light of evolution. *American Biological Teacher, 35,* 125–129.

Doughty, D., & Rodgers, J. L. (2000). Behavior genetic modeling of menarche in US females. In J. L. Rodgers, D. C. Rowe, & W. B. Miller (Eds.), *Genetic influences on human fertility and sexuality* (pp. 169–181). Boston: Kluwer.

Draper, P., & Harpending, H. (1982). Father absence and reproductive strategy: An evolutionary perspective. *Journal of Anthropological Research, 38,* 255–273.

Edgarton. R. (1992). *Sick societies: Challenging the myth of primitive harmony.* New York: Free Press.

Eibl-Eibesfeldt, I. (1989). *Human ethology.* New York: Aldine de Gruyter.

Ellis, B. J. (2004). Timing of pubertal maturation in girls. *Psychological Bulletin, 130,* 920–958.

Ellis, B. J., Boyce, W. T., Belsky, J., Bakermans-Kranenburg, M. J., & Van IJzendoorn, M. H. (2011). Differential susceptibility to the environment: an evolutionary-neurodevelopmental theory. *Development and Psychopathology, 23,* 7–28.

Ellis, B. J., & Essex, M. J. (2007). Family environments, adrenarche, and sexual maturation: A longitudinal test of a life history model. *Child Development, 78,* 1799–1817.

Ellis, B. J., Figueredo, A. J., Brumbach, B. H., & Schlomer, G. L. (2009). Fundamental dimensions of environmental risk: The impact of harsh versus unpredictable environments on the evolution and development of life history strategies. *Human Nature*, *20*, 204–268.

Ellis, B. J., & Garber, J. (2000). Psychosocial antecedents of variation in girls' pubertal timing. *Child Development*, *71*, 485–501.

Ellis, B. J., McFadyen-Ketchum, S., Dodge, K. A., Pettit, G. S., & Bates, J. E. (1999). Quality of early family relationships and individual differences in the timing of pubertal maturation in girls. *Journal of Personality and Social Psychology*, *77*, 387–401.

Ellis, B. J., Shirtcliff, E. A., Boyce, W. T., Deardorff, J., & Essex, M. J. (2011). Quality of early family relationships and the timing and tempo of puberty: Effects depend on biological sensitivity to context. *Development and Psychopathology*, *23*, 85–99.

Emery, R. (1988). *Marriage, divorce, and children's adjustment*. Beverly Hills, CA: Sage.

Feeney, J. A. (2008). Adult romantic attachment: Developments in the study of couple relationships . In J. Cassidy & P. R. Shaver (Eds.), *Handbook of attachment: Theory, research and clinical applications* (2nd ed., pp. 456–502). New York: Guilford Press.

Fernald, A. (1985). Four-month-old infants prefer to listen to motherese. *Infant Behavior Development*, *8*, 181–195.

Fisher, H. E. (1992). *Anatomy of love: The natural history of monogamy, adultery, and divorce*. New York: Norton.

Fletcher, G. J. O., Simpson, J. A., Campbell, L., & Overall, N. C. (2015). Pair-bonding, romantic love, and evolution: The curious case of Homo sapiens. *Perspectives on Psychological Science*, *10*, 20–36.

Fraley, R. C. (2002) Attachment stability from infancy to adulthood: Meta-analysis and dynamic modeling of developmental mechanisms. *Personality and Social Psychology Review*, *6*, 123–151.

Frank, R. H. (1988). *Passions within reason: The strategic role of the emotions*. New York: Norton.

Frankenhuis, W. E., Gergely, G., & Watson, J. S. (2013). Infants may use contingency analysis to estimate environmental states: An evolutionary, life-history perspective. *Child Development Perspectives*, *7*, 115–120.

Frankenhuis, W. E., & Panchanathan, K. (2011). Individual differences in developmental plasticity may result from stochastic sampling. *Perspectives on Psychological Science*, *6*, 336–347.

Fuller, T. L., & Fincham, F. D. (1995). Attachment style in married couples: Relation to current marital functioning, stability over time, and method of assessment. *Personal Relationships*, *2*, 17–34.

Furman, W., & Simon, V. A. (1999). Cognitive representations of adolescent relationships. In W. Furman, B. B. Brown, & C. Feiring (Eds.), *The development of romantic relationships in adolescence* (pp. 75–98). New York: Cambridge University Press.

Gangestad, S. W., & Simpson, J. A. (2000). The evolution of human mating: Trade-offs and strategic pluralism. *Behavioral and Brain Sciences*, *23*, 573–587.

Gangestad, S. W., & Simpson, J. A. (Eds.). (2007). *The evolution of mind: Fundamental questions and controversies*. New York: Guilford Press.

Geary, D. C. (2005). Evolution of paternal investment. In D. M. Buss (Ed.), *The handbook of evolutionary psychology* (pp. 483–505). New York: Wiley.

Geronimus, A. T. (1996). What teen mothers know. *Human Nature*, *7*, 323–352.

Graber, J., Brooks-Gunn, J., & Warren, M. (1995). The antecedents of menarcheal age. *Child Development*, *66*, 346–359.

Grafen, A. (1990). Biological signals as handicaps. *Journal of Theoretical Biology*, *144*, 517–546.

Grieser, D. L., & Kuhl, P. K. (1988). Maternal speech to infants in a tonal language: Support for universal prosodic features in motherese. *Developmental Psychology*, *24*, 14–20.

Hamilton, W. D. (1964). The genetical evolution of social behaviour. *Journal of Theoretical Biology*, *7*, 1–52.

Hazan, C., & Shaver, P. R. (1987). Romantic love conceptualized as an attachment process. *Journal of Personality and Social Psychology*, *52*, 511–524.

Hazan, C., & Zeifman, D. (1999). Pair bonds as attachments: Evaluating the evidence. In J. Cassidy & P. R. Shaver (Eds.), *Handbook of attachment: Theory, research, and clinical applications* (pp. 336–354). New York: Guilford Press.

Hesse, E. (2008). The Adult Attachment Interview: Protocol, method of analysis, and empirical studies. In J. Cassidy & P. R. Shaver (Eds.), *Handbook of attachment: Theory, research and clinical applications* (2nd ed., pp. 552–598). New York: Guilford Press.

Hinde, R. A. (1986). Some implications of evolutionary theory and comparative data for the study of human prosocial and aggressive behaviour. In D. Olweus, J. Block, & M. Radke-Yarrow (Eds.), *Development of anti-social and prosocial behaviour* (pp. 13–32). Orlando, FL: Academic Press.

Hoier, S. (2003). Father absence and age at menarche. *Human Nature*, *14*, 209–233.

Hrdy, S. B. (1999). *Mother nature*. New York: Ballantine.

Hrdy, S. B. (2005). Evolutionary context of human development: The cooperative breeding model. In C. S. Carter, L. Ahnert, K. E. Grossmann, S. B. Hrdy, M. E. Lamb, S. W. Porges, et al. (Eds.), *Attachment and bonding: A new synthesis* (pp. 9–32). Cambridge, MA: MIT Press.

Isabella, R., Belsky, J., & von Eye, A. (1989). Origins of infant–mother attachment: An examination of interactional synchrony during the infant's first year. *Developmental Psychology*, *25*, 12–21.

Jacobson, S. W., & Frye, K. F. (1991). Effect of maternal social support on attachment: Experimental evidence. *Child Development*, *62*, 572–582.

James, J., Ellis, B. J., Schlomer, G. L., & Garber, J. (2012). Sex-specific pathways to early puberty, sexual debut, and sexual risk taking: Tests of an integrated evolutionary-developmental model. *Developmental Psychology*, *48*, 687–702.

Johns, S. E. (2003). *Environmental risk and the evolution-*

*ary psychology of teenage motherhood*. Unpublished doctoral thesis, University of Bristol, Bristol, UK.

Jones, J. D., Cassidy, J., & Shaver, P. R. (2015). Parents' self-reported attachment styles: A review of links with parenting behaviors, emotions, and cognitions. *Personality and Social Psychology Review, 19*(1), 44–76.

Kaplan, H. S., & Gangestad, S. W. (2005). Life history theory and evolutionary psychology. In D. M. Buss (Ed.), *The handbook of evolutionary psychology* (pp. 68–95). New York: Wiley.

Kaplan, H. S., Lancaster, J., & Hurtado, A. M. (2000). A theory of human life history evolution. *Evolutionary Anthropology, 9*, 156–185.

Kelly, R. L. (1995). *The foraging spectrum: Diversity in hunter-gatherer lifeways*. Washington, DC: Smithsonian Institution Press.

Kim, K., Smith, P. K., & Palermiti, A. L. (1997). Conflict in childhood and reproductive development. *Evolution and Human Behavior, 18*, 109–142.

Kirkpatrick, L. A. (1998). Evolution, pair-bonding, and reproductive strategies. In J. A. Simpson & W. S. Rholes (Eds.), *Attachment theory and close relationships* (pp. 353–393). New York: Guilford Press.

Krishnakumar, A., & Buehler, C. (2000). Interparental conflict and parenting behaviors: A meta-analytic review. *Family Relations, 49*, 25–44.

Kuzawa, C. W. (2005). Fetal origins of developmental plasticity: Are fetal cues reliable predictors of future nutritional environments? *American Journal of Human Biology, 17*, 5–21.

LaFreniere, P. J., & Sroufe, L. A. (1985). Profiles of peer competence in the preschool: Interrelations between measures, influence of social ecology, and relation to attachment history. *Developmental Psychology, 21*, 56–69.

Lempers, J., Clark-Lempers, D., & Simons, R. (1989). Economic hardship, parenting, and distress in adolescence. *Child Development, 60*, 25–49.

Lewis, M., & Feiring, C. (1989). Infant, mother, and mother–infant interaction behavior and subsequent attachment. *Child Development, 60*, 831–837.

Lewis, M., Feiring, C., McGuffog, C., & Jaskir, J. (1984). Predicting psychopathology in six-year-olds from early social relations. *Child Development, 55*, 123–136.

Lutkenhaus, P., Grossmann, K. E., & Grossmann, K. (1985). Infant–mother attachment at twelve months and style of interaction with a stranger at the age of three years. *Child Development, 56*, 1538–1542.

Main, M. (1981). Avoidance in the service of attachment: A working paper. In K. Immelmann, G. Barlow, M. Main, & L. Petrinovich (Eds.), *Behavioral development: The Bielefeld Interdisciplinary Project* (pp. 651–693). New York: Cambridge University Press.

Main, M., & Solomon, J. (1990). Procedures for identifying disorganized/disoriented infants in the Ainsworth Strange Situation. In M. T. Greenberg, D. Cicchetti, & E. M. Cummings (Eds.), *Attachment in the preschool years: Theory, research, and intervention* (pp. 121–160). Chicago: University of Chicago Press.

Manuck, S. B., Craig, A. E., Flory, J. D., Halder, I., & Ferrell, R. E. (2011). Reported early family environment covaries with menarcheal age as a function of polymorphic variation in estrogen receptor-$\alpha$ gene. *Development and Psychopathology, 23*, 69–83.

Matas, L., Arend, R., & Sroufe, L. A. (1978). Continuity in adaptation in the second year: The relationship between quality of attachment and later competence. *Child Development, 49*, 547–556.

McLoyd, V. C. (1990). The declining fortunes of black children: Psychological distress, parenting, and socioemotional development in the context of economic hardship. *Child Development, 61*, 311–346.

McLoyd, V. C. (1998). Social disadvantage and child development. *American Psychologist, 53*, 185–204.

Mikulincer, M., & Nachshon, O. (1991). Attachment styles and patterns of self-disclosure. *Journal of Personality and Social Psychology, 61*, 321–331.

Mikulincer, M., & Shaver, P. R. (2007). *Attachment in adulthood: Structure, dynamics, and change*. New York: Guilford Press.

Miller, C., & Fishkin, S. A. (1997). On the dynamics of human bonding and reproductive success. In J. A. Simpson & D. T. Kenrick (Eds.), *Evolutionary social psychology* (pp. 197–235). Mahwah, NJ: Erlbaum.

Miller, W. B., & Pasta, D. J. (2000). Early family environment, reproductive strategy and contraceptive behavior. In J. L. Rodgers, D. C. Rowe, & W. B. Miller (Eds.), *Genetic influences on human fertility and sexuality* (pp. 183–230). Boston: Kluwer.

Moffitt, T. E., Caspi, A., Belsky, J., & Silva, P. A. (1992). Childhood experience and the onset of menarche: A test of a sociobiological model. *Child Development, 63*, 47–58.

Nettle, D. (2010). Dying young and living fast: Variation in life history across English neighborhoods. *Behavioral Ecology, 21*, 387–395.

Nettle, D., & Cockerill, M. (2010). Development of social variation in reproductive schedules: A study of an English urban area. *PLoS ONE, 5*, e12690.

Parker, G. A., & Maynard Smith, J. (1991). Optimality theory in evolutionary biology. *Nature, 348*, 27–33.

Pesonen, A., Raikkonen, K., Heinonen, K., Kajantie, E., Forsen, T., & Eriksson, J. G. (2008). Reproductive traits following a parent–child separation trauma during childhood: A natural experiment during World War II. *American Journal of Human Biology, 20*, 345–351.

Quinlan, R. J. (2003). Father absence, parental care, and female reproductive development. *Evolution and Human Behavior, 24*, 376–390.

Quinlan, R. J. (2007). Human parental effort and environmental risk. *Proceedings of the Royal Society of London B, 274*, 121–125.

Rholes, W. S., Simpson, J. A., & Blakely, B. S. (1995). Adult attachment styles and mothers' relationships with their young children. *Personal Relationships, 2*, 35–54.

Rholes, W. S., Simpson, J. A., Blakely, B. S., Lanigan,

L., & Allen, E. A. (1997). Adult attachment styles, the desire to have children, and working models of parenthood. *Journal of Personality, 65*, 357–385.

Rickard, I. J., Frankenhuis, W. E., & Nettle, D. (2014). Why are childhood family factors associated with timing of maturation?: A role for internal prediction. *Perspectives on Psychological Science, 9*, 3–15.

Rowe, D. C. (2000). Environmental and genetic influences on pubertal development. In J. L. Rodgers, D. C. Rowe, & W. B. Miller (Eds.), *Genetic influences on human fertility and sexuality* (pp. 147–168). Boston: Kluwer.

Schlomer, G. L., Del Giudice, M., & Ellis, B. J. (2011). Parent–offspring conflict theory: An evolutionary framework for understanding conflict within human families. *Psychological Review, 118*, 496–521.

Shaver, P. R., Hazan, C., & Bradshaw, D. (1988). Love as attachment: The integration of three behavioral systems. In R. J. Sternberg & M. L. Barnes (Eds.), *The psychology of love* (pp. 68–99). New Haven, CT: Yale University Press.

Simpson, J. A. (1990). Influence of attachment styles on romantic relationships. *Journal of Personality and Social Psychology, 59*, 971–980.

Simpson, J. A. (1999). Attachment theory in modern evolutionary perspective. In J. Cassidy & P. R. Shaver (Eds.), *Handbook of attachment: Theory, research, and clinical applications* (pp. 115–140). New York: Guilford Press.

Simpson, J. A., & Belsky, J. (2008). Attachment theory within a modern evolutionary framework. In J. Cassidy & P. R. Shaver (Eds.), *Handbook of attachment: Theory, research, and clinical applications* (2nd ed., pp. 131–157). New York: Guilford Press.

Simpson, J. A., Collins, W. A., & Salvatore, J. E. (2011). The impact of early interpersonal experience on adult romantic relationship functioning: Recent findings from the Minnesota Longitudinal Study of Risk and Adaptation. *Current Directions in Psychological Science, 20*, 355–359.

Simpson, J. A., Collins, W. A., Tran, S., & Haydon, K. C. (2007). Attachment and the experience and expression of emotions in adult romantic relationships: A developmental perspective. *Journal of Personality and Social Psychology, 92*, 355–367.

Simpson, J. A., Griskevicius, V., Kuo, S. I., Sung, S., & Collins, W. A. (2012). Evolution, stress, and sensitive periods: The influence of unpredictability in early versus late childhood on sex and risky behavior. *Developmental Psychology, 48*, 674–686.

Simpson, J. A., Rholes, W. S., & Phillips, D. (1996). Conflict in close relationships: An attachment perspective. *Journal of Personality and Social Psychology, 71*, 899–914.

Simpson, J. A., Wilson, C. L., & Winterheld, H. A. (2004). Sociosexuality and romantic relationships. In J. H. Harvey, A. Wenzel, & S. Sprecher (Eds.), *Handbook of sexuality in close relationships* (pp. 87–112). Mahwah, NJ: Erlbaum.

Slade, A., Belsky, J., Aber, J. L., & Phelps, J. L. (1999). Maternal representations of their relationship with their toddlers. *Developmental Psychology, 35*, 611–619.

Sroufe, L. A., & Waters, E. (1977). Attachment as an organizational construct. *Child Development, 48*, 1184–1199.

Steinberg, L. (1988). Reciprocal relation between parent–child distance and pubertal maturation. *Developmental Psychology, 24*, 122–128.

Szepsenwol, O., Simpson, J. A., Griskevicius, V., & Raby, K. L. (2015). The effect of unpredictable early childhood environments on parenting in adulthood. *Journal of Personality and Social Psychology, 109*, 1045–1067.

Taylor, S. E., Klein, L. C., Lewis, B. P., Gruenewald, T. L., Gurung, R. A. R., & Updegraff, J. A. (2000). Biobehavioral responses to stress in females: Tend-and-befriend, not fight-or-flight. *Psychological Review, 107*, 411–429.

Tithers, J. M., & Ellis, B. J. (2008). Impact of fathers on daughters' age of menarche: A genetically and environmentally controlled sibling study. *Developmental Psychology, 44*, 1409–1420.

Tooby, J., & Cosmides, L. (1992). Psychological foundations of culture. In J. Barkow, L. Cosmides, & J. Tooby (Eds.), *The adapted mind* (pp. 19–136). New York: Oxford University Press.

Trivers, R. L. (1971). The evolution of reciprocal altruism. *Quarterly Review of Biology, 46*, 35–57.

Trivers, R. L. (1972). Parental investment and sexual selection. In B. Campbell (Ed.), *Sexual selection and the descent of man, 1871–1971* (pp. 136–179). Chicago: Aldine-Atherton.

Trivers, R. L. (1974). Parent–offspring conflict. *American Zoologist, 14*, 249–264.

Trivers, R. L. (1985). *Social evolution.* Menlo Park, CA: Benjamin/Cummings.

Van IJzendoorn, M. H. (1995). Adult attachment representations, parental responsiveness, and infant attachment: A meta-analysis on the predictive validity of the Adult Attachment Interview. *Psychological Bulletin, 117*, 387–403.

Van IJzendoorn, M. H., & Bakermans-Kranenburg, M. J. (1997). Intergenerational transmission of attachment: A move to the contextual level. In L. Atkinson & K. J. Zucker (Eds.), *Attachment and psychopathology* (pp. 135–170). New York: Guilford Press.

Van IJzendoorn, M. H., & Bakermans-Kranenburg, M. J. (2010). Stretched until it snaps: Attachment and close relationships. *Child Development Perspectives, 4*, 109–111.

Waters, E., Wippman, J., & Sroufe, L. A. (1979). Attachment, positive affect, and competence in the peer group: Two studies in construct validation. *Child Development, 50*, 821–829.

Wilson, C. L., Rholes, W. S., Simpson, J. A., & Tran, S. (2007). Labor, delivery, and early parenthood: An attachment theory perspective. *Personality and Social Psychology Bulletin, 33*, 505–518.

Wilson, M., & Daly, M. (1997). Life expectancy, economic inequality, homicide and reproductive timing in Chicago neighbourhoods. *British Medical Journal, 314,* 1271–1274.

Wilson, M., & Daly, M. (2005). *Carpe diem:* Adaptation and devaluing the future. *Quarterly Review of Biology, 80,* 55–60.

Wood, W., & Eagly, A. H. (2002). A cross-cultural analysis of the behavior of men and women: Implications for the origins of sex differences. *Psychological Bulletin, 128,* 699–727.

Wright, R. (1994). *The moral animal.* New York: Vintage.

Youngblade, L. M., & Belsky, J. (1989). Child maltreatment, infant–parent attachment security, and dysfunctional peer relationships in toddlerhood. *Topics in Early Childhood Special Education, 9,* 1–15.

Zeifman, D., & Hazan, C. (1997). Attachment: The bond in pair-bonds. In J. A. Simpson & D. T. Kenrick (Eds.), *Evolutionary social psychology* (pp. 237–263). Mahwah, NJ: Erlbaum.

Zeifman, D., & Hazan, C. (2008). Pair bonds as attachments: Reevaluating the evidence. In J. Cassidy & P. R. Shaver (Eds.), *Handbook of attachment: Theory, research, and clinical applications* (2nd ed., pp. 436–455). New York: Guilford Press.

## Chapter 6

# Psychobiological Origins of Infant Attachment and Its Role in Development

H. Jonathan Polan
Myron A. Hofer

John Bowlby (1969/1982) was the first to give the psychological concept of human attachment a strong base in evolutionary theory. He was convinced that early attachment is evidence of a previously unrecognized motivational system present in both mammals and birds, which had been selected during evolution for the survival value of the protection it afforded offspring through the emotional bond that develops between infant and mother. The strong tendency for young to stay close to their mothers, and their apparent emotional distress upon separation, was the core behavioral indicator of what Bowlby viewed as a basic instinct organized according to the principle of goal-corrected feedback—a concept borrowed from engineering, which had proved useful in understanding physiological adaptation and homeostasis.

With the discovery of qualitatively different patterns of attachment in children and of mental representations in mothers (Bowlby's "internal working models"), attachment research moved quickly in these new directions, as if the nature of the "bond" and the separation response were well understood. But for many behavioral scientists studying early development experimentally, evidence from their research did not fit Bowlby's concept of a *unitary* attachment system at work within the mother–infant interaction. Instead, they found a number of relatively independent systems organized to carry out functions such as searching, following, orienting, early learning and memory, thermoregulation, vocalizing, and other early expressions of affect, each with its own organizing principles. In addition, Bowlby's concepts did not lend themselves easily to laboratory research with animals, and, occasionally, seemed to lead to a frustrating form of circular reasoning. For example, an infant's attachment bond was inferred from the infant's response to separation (Bowlby, 1973), which itself was explained as a consequence of disruption of the attachment bond.

Evolutionary principles give us a conceptual common ground that can be shared by neuroscience, psychology, and psychoanalysis, providing answers to questions about how the human mind and brain have come into being and why they have their present form. The historical nature of both development and evolution bridges the gap between the "reductionist" emphasis of the molecular/cellular neurosciences and the "holistic" emphasis on the meaning of events that is the central focus of psychoanalytically oriented clinicians. Early human development traverses a series of levels of scale and organization—from the multicellular interactions of the embryo to the inte-

117

grated systems and behavior of the fetus, to the emerging cognitive and affective capacities of the child. The biological, behavioral, and psychological processes at work at those levels of organization seem very different. But the new properties that emerge at each level arise from the combined operation of simpler processes taking place at the previous level. Understanding those transitions, and the emergence of new properties at higher levels, is one of the central issues for research in early human development, as well as for attempts to integrate neuroscience, psychology, and psychoanalysis.

In the second edition of this handbook, Simpson and Belsky (2008) extended the evolutionary theoretical approach, begun by Bowlby, to the possible long-term developmental effects of early attachment patterns and the transmission of these patterns across generations. They described the contribution of different developmental attachment patterns for enhancing reproductive fitness, as well as simple survival in the next generation. For example, a secure attachment pattern may prepare offspring best in a predictable, secure environment in which prolonged parental investment in offspring is possible; however, the insecure patterns may be more adaptive in chaotic, dangerous, and depriving environments in which fearful responses maximize short-term survival and early sexual maturation maximizes the number of offspring produced.

New discoveries regarding the genetic mechanisms of early development over the past decade have provided the basis for an integration of the fields of evolutionary and developmental biology (for a review, see Carroll, 2005). Development can now be viewed as a major source of potentially adaptive variation for selection to act upon in the course of evolution. We have learned that genes are not only instruments of inheritance in evolution but also targets of molecular signals originating both within the organism and in the environment outside it. These signals regulate development. Rapid progress in understanding these molecular genetic mechanisms has revealed an unexpected potential for plasticity, which can enable a relatively few evolutionarily conserved cellular processes to be linked together by differential gene expression into a variety of adaptive patterns that respond to environmental changes, as well as to genetic mutations. The resulting plasticity allows a variety of developmental pathways, evident in both behavior and physiology, to be generated from the same genome. This discovery of the cen-

tral role for the regulation of gene expression in development and novel epigenetic mechanisms mediating this regulation have at last provided a specific locus and mechanism for the frustratingly vague and much-debated concept of gene–environment interaction (see Bakermans-Kranenberg & Van IJzendoorn, Chapter 8, this volume).

These advances in our understanding of both development and evolution have given us a new way to understand the psychological constructs and life history consequences of early attachment. In this chapter, we outline how the strategy of uncovering the component processes underlying the psychological constructs that have been proposed in the study of early human attachment, and the perspective of evolutionary developmental biology, offer new and potentially useful ways of thinking about attachment and, from this, creating new ways to help patients.

The term *early attachment* has a number of different meanings in the psychological literature. In its most general sense, it refers to a set of behaviors we observe in infants, and to the feelings and thought processes (conscious and/or unconscious) we suppose infants to have, based on our own experiences and the psychological concepts we ourselves have formed as individual human beings or learned from others. Within this range of usage of the word *attachment*, several different schools of thought have emerged—some within psychoanalysis and others within different schools of psychodynamic psychotherapy. Common to all, however, are three themes: (1) some sort of emotional tie or bond that is inferred to develop in an infant for its caretaker, which allows the infant to identify its own mother and keeps the infant physically close; (2) a series of physiological and behavioral responses to separation that constitute the infant's emotional reaction to interruption of that bond; and (3) the existence of different patterns and qualities of interaction between infants and mothers that have important long-term effects on the infant's subsequent development, and that lead to a repetition of particular patterns of mothering by daughters in the next generation. These three central concepts of attachment theory have been extremely useful clinically, but they leave a number of observations unexplained and questions unanswered, as we explain below.

We use recent psychobiological research to provide answers to questions left open by attachment theory, and we organize the answers by the three concepts just outlined. The answers emerging from our laboratory research with animals, and from research by others, have tended to support clinical observations, but they have also extended them in unexpected ways. We cannot settle questions of human nature by studying other animals, but we can generate new hypotheses, concepts, and ways of thinking that ultimately may apply to our clinical work with patients.

## Development of the Bond

Exclusive, or preferential, orienting toward and proximity seeking by offspring toward their mothers are defining behaviors of filial attachment, requiring offspring to recognize their mothers and distinguish between maternal and nonmaternal stimuli. Although rat pups cannot see or hear until at least postnatal day (PND) 11, their sense of smell is competent at birth. Rat pups begin discriminating familiar from unfamiliar odors immediately after birth based on learning *in utero* (Hepper, 1987) and postnatally (Gregory & Pfaff, 1971; Johanson, Turkewitz, & Hamburgh, 1980; Nyakas & Endroczi, 1970). We asked whether pups could also discriminate *among the familiar odors* in their environment—specifically, their mothers and their home shavings. That ability would be evidence of *filial* attraction, not simply a nonspecific orientation toward *any* familiar cues, and its onset would mark an important developmental milestone for the infant.

In a two-choice test chamber, pups as young as 4–5 days old crawled closer to their mothers' odor than to that of their home nest shavings. Furthermore, pups increased maternal preference after overnight isolation, demonstrating early development of a motivational component. As little as 0.5°C of additional warmth on the mothers' side of the test chamber caused even 2-day-olds to express a preference for maternal odor over that of equally familiar home nest shavings (Polan & Hofer, 1998). Thus, preference for the odor of mothers over home shavings is acquired between PNDs 1 and 2.

We and others found some rather surprising reinforcers of the early olfactory learning that support the emergence of maternal preference behavior. Classical olfactory conditioning during the first 9 PNDs involves reinforcers that neither satisfy an obvious physiological need state nor are themselves attractive (Sullivan, Hofer, & Brake, 1986). Examples include pinching the tail, vigorous repetitive stroking with a soft brush (Sullivan & Hall, 1988), and mild foot shock (Camp & Rudy, 1988). Each of these artificial reinforcers appears to imitate something that a mother typically does to her pups. When she returns to the nest after foraging, she often steps on the pups, picks them up with her teeth, carries them, and licks them vigorously before replacing them in the litter pile. Tail pinching may mimic being stepped on, and stroking may mimic being licked; perhaps mild shock mimics the sensation of teeth gripping the skin when the mother transports her pups. What these and the other primary reinforcers in neonates (even milk ingestion) have in common is that they are vigorously behaviorally arousing to pups.

Thus, a wide variety of stimuli that mimic specific maternal behaviors toward the pups, and all that vigorously activate pups, support the learning of a preference for a novel odor with which they are paired (reviewed in Sullivan & Hall, 1988; Wilson & Sullivan, 1994). Norepinephrine plays a key role in mediating this activation-dependent associative preference learning during a sensitive period extending through the first postnatal week and a half (see next section).

What advantage might there be in newborn rats' predisposition to learn approach responses to a wide range of unconditioned stimuli—some of which are noxious? This ability was likely selected in evolution precisely because it enables pups to learn from the widest range of maternal interactions and cues, learning about their mother each time she reenters the nest up to 20 times a day. By stepping on, retrieving, licking, crouching over, and providing milk to them, the mother powerfully conditions an attraction in her pups to her own odor and tactile cues. This approach conditioning substantiates Bowlby's (1969/1982) positing of an imprinting-like basis for the formation of mammalian attachment. By activating stimuli during the 9-day sensitive period, and beyond that for cues originally conditioned during the sensitive period (Sullivan, 1996), it is the *functional equivalent* of imprinting in an altricial mammalian species.

Preference behavior, essentially a choice of the direction of movement on a horizontal surface, though profoundly revealing as a model of filial attachment, greatly oversimplifies the full repertoire of maternally directed orienting behaviors (MDOBs) we observed in the nest. A rat pup is born into a three-dimensional "sandwich" world, consisting of the substrate of its nest materials beneath it and the canopy of its mother's belly looming above as she hovers over the litter.

In this environment, the newborn pup must (1) burrow under the mother's abdominal surface and (2) orient and maintain itself in relation to her ventrum, so that (3) contact with her body will permit heat transfer, protection, nipple grasp, and access to ongoing maternal cues that regulate the pup's endocrinological, physiological, and behavioral processes. In this world, the mother's body is both the *source* of stimuli to which the pups are responding and the *superstructure* upon which the pups organize their responses in three dimensions.

To determine precisely what maternal stimuli guided these complex pup behaviors, we modeled the mother's ventral body surface with overhead "roof" surfaces featuring increasingly dam-like tactile and olfactory cues. Under even the least mother-like roof, a wire mesh, pups became aroused, crawled, turned supine onto their backs, and audibly barked. Once supine, some pups planted their feet against the overlying mesh and crawled on their backs. Thus, an overhead mesh roof evokes behaviors that appear identical in form to those we observed in the nest, by which pups orient toward and seek proximity to the maternal ventrum. Under roof surfaces that featured increasingly mother-like cues, 2- to 3-day-olds engaged in correspondingly higher frequencies of the behaviors (Polan & Hofer, 1999a), showing that early maternally directed proximity-seeking behaviors are not simple reflexes stimulated by nonspecific inputs, but are graded responses to specific maternal features.

We next asked whether these behaviors might respond to changes in the pups' motivational state. Operationally, we asked how a period of acute overnight deprivation might affect the expression of the maternally directed orienting and proximity-seeking behaviors. We found that maternal deprivation significantly *enhanced* responding to sufficiently mother-like surfaces but did not affect behavior in the absence of maternal stimuli. Therefore, motivation specifically modulates maternally directed orienting behaviors, but not undirected behaviors performed in isolation.

Finally, to understand how early in development the entire repertoire of behaviors is present and when they come under the sensory guidance of maternal features, we tested newborn pups that were deprived just before and after their very first nursing bout. After the first nursing experience, the behaviors were already subject to sensory guidance by maternal features, whereas before any nursing occurred, pups performed the behaviors vigorously but independently of the type of stimulus encountered (Polan, Milano, Eljuga, & Hofer, 2002). Thus, the first experience of nursing organizes an important transition in the control of these orienting behaviors from reflex-like action patterns to responsiveness to specific maternal features.

## New Views of Sensitive Periods

Since the original descriptions of avian imprinting by Lorenz and Tinbergen, the concept of sensitive periods has occupied attachment researchers with a view toward pinpointing the sources and mechanisms of psychopathology and devising preventions. Mammalian sensitive periods were thought to be confined to *precocial* species such as sheep, whose grazing in open terrain requires the infant's attachment bond to be literally "up and running" within hours after birth. The identification of maternal licking and grooming in rats as the stimulus that promotes long-term programming of the hypothalamic–pituitary–adrenocortical (HPA) axis led to discovery of an apparent sensitive period in the development of attachment in an *altricial* mammal. *Handling*, or brief daily maternal separation during infancy, which promotes extra maternal licking and grooming upon reunion, causes permanent down-regulation of the HPA axis and a high tolerance for stress in adulthood. To be effective, handling has to be initiated within the first postnatal week (Meaney & Aitken, 1985).

This sensitive period for HPA axis programming by maternal behavior coincides with a sensitive period for early olfactory learning, which also depends on maternal behavior, as described earlier. Olfactory preference learning is our best current model for how learned preferences for maternal cues begin to establish mother-seeking attachment behaviors in the infant. The sensitive period for this kind of learning extends through PND 9. Learning of maternal odor cues depends on behavioral stimulation, which serves as the unconditioned stimulus (US) that is paired with the odor. Up through PND 9, all sufficiently arousing stimuli—whether presumed pleasant ones, such as stroking with a soft brush (mimicking the mother's licking), or aversive ones, such as a tail pinch or foot shock that mimic maternal rough handling—cause pups to seek proximity with and prefer the odor with which they are paired (Camp & Rudy, 1988; Sullivan et al., 1986). During this sensitive period, it is difficult to condition *avoidance* behavior to an odor paired with any exteroceptive US. This strong predominance of preference learning over avoidance learning can be seen as an evolutionarily determined developmental adaptation that serves an infant's need to form a bond to its mother.

Abruptly at PND 10, however, the behavior learned from odor–shock pairings reverses direction to become the more adult-like response, avoidance, and stroking no longer conditions proximity seeking or preference for a new odor. Sullivan, Landers, Yeaman, and Wilson (2000) determined a special brain mechanism for preference learning during this pre-PND 10 sensitive period: an overactive locus ceruleus, a midbrain nucleus that mediates arousal, releasing large amounts of the neuromodulator norepinephrine at its synapses in the olfactory bulb. When stroking is paired with a new odor, the olfactory signals reaching the bulb converging with the norepinephrinergic signals from the midbrain are transduced into a new response pattern—approach behavior—when the odor is next encountered. This simple learning circuit omits brain regions involved in adult learning, in particular the amygdala, which later is crucial in fear conditioning. During the sensitive period for olfactory preference learning, the amygdala is kept "offline" even during aversive stimulation (Moriceau & Sullivan, 2005). This special early learning process, which strongly favors preference learning and inhibits avoidance learning, may well be the basis by which infant mammals, from puppies to humans, form strong attachments to even abusive caregivers (Scott, 1963).

Although the amygdala is kept "offline" from the olfactory learning circuit, it is hardly inactive during the sensitive period. Rather, it initiates the long-term processes of HPA axis programming by maternal licking and grooming. Adult animals that, as infants, experienced high levels of licking and grooming have a "toned-down" stress axis, which has an attenuated "on" switch in the form of decreased secretion of corticotropin-releasing hormone by the hypothalamus, and an augmented "off" switch in the form of extra corticosterone receptors in the hippocampus. The amygdala is the first brain locus to register added daily maternal care. By PND 6, after just 4 days of augmented maternal care, the amygdala's central nucleus increases production of corticotropin-releasing factor, which induces the production of the stress hormone corticosterone, and, by PND 9, decreases the expression of glucocorticoid receptors (GRs) (Fenoglio, Brunson, Avishai-Eliner,

Chen, & Baram, 2004), which detect corticosterone in the brain and provide feedback to reduce its production. These changes occur long before the permanent increase in GR expression in the hippocampus, and, although transient, may be part of the cascade of events that establishes the permanent changes in HPA axis regulation in the hypothalamus and hippocampus. These early changes in elements of the corticosterone response system in the amygdala also have a surprising immediate influence on the circuits for olfactory learning. An early boost in corticosterone levels hastens the end of the sensitive period, turning off preference learning and ushering in precocious avoidance learning (Moriceau, Wilson, Levine, & Sullivan, 2006).

Thus, the period from birth through PND 9 harbors at least two sensitive periods: one for the emergence of the attachment relationship itself, which equips the pup to survive the immediately demanding transition to postnatal life; and another that, in a sense, is banked for the pup's later benefit, the emotional tuning of its adult life, as a legacy of its rearing, but that under emergency conditions even alters the duration of the first sensitive period, as we describe below. Through evolution's conservative economy of form and function, the pup's nervous system is equipped to generate both kinds of behavioral plasticity from the same maternal care behaviors, licking and grooming.

Sullivan's group recently found a "transitional sensitive period," immediately following the sensitive period, lasting from PND 10 to PND 15 (Sevelinges et al., 2011), during which odor–shock conditioning can produce either a more adult-like fear/avoidance response or a preference/approach response typical of the sensitive period. Remarkably, the mother's presence acts as a "switch" between these two forms of learning during this transitional sensitive period. When the mother (or just her odor) is present, the amygdala disengages, resulting in preference/approach learning, just as in the sensitive period, but when the mother is absent, the amygdala is engaged by the odor–shock conditioning, resulting in a more adult-like fear/avoidance response. Thus, during the transitional sensitive period, the mother provides the pup with a "social buffer," blocking the new amygdala-dependent stress-induced fear/avoidance learning when the pups are with her (Bisaz & Sullivan, 2012).

The mechanism of action of this maternal switch is the mother's regulation of the pups' own production of the stress hormone corticosterone.

Her presence suppresses the pups' stress-induced corticosterone secretion, which limits the amount of corticosterone reaching, and activating, the amygdala (Moriceau & Sullivan, 2006). A quiescent amygdala permits odor–shock conditioning to continue to produce the approach/preference learning typical of younger pups. In essence, the transitional sensitive period is a window prior to weaning and the pups' emergence from the nest, during which maternal presence and stress interact to pivot the direction of pups' new learning from approach to avoidance, or vice versa. Thus, this interval can be seen as an adaptive shaper of how pups will face weaning and emergence from the nest: If a stressful environment pressures the mother to be absent from the nest for long stretches, perhaps due to poor foraging conditions, pups will acquire more fear/avoidance responses to novel experiences, equipping them for harsh conditions outside the postweaning nest.

Taking these insights a step further, Sullivan's group is using the odor–shock conditioning paradigm to model the formation of attachment despite maternal abuse. As discussed earlier, the conditioned odor cue (conditioned stimulus [CS]) that has been paired with shock functions as a maternal odor; that is, pups prefer it to the odor of familiar clean bedding and are stimulated by it to attach to the mother's nipples even after her natural odor has been removed. And, this odor's potency as an attachment cue is retained even after the sensitive period ends (Sullivan et al., 2000). For comparison, to model attachment to nonabusive maternal care, other pups were conditioned by pairing an odor with soft brush strokes, mimicking typical maternal licking and grooming behaviors. Both conditioning treatments were performed on PND 8, and the results were tested by exposure to the CS, or to the natural maternal odor, the next day (Raineki, Moriceau, & Sullivan, 2010).

When tested under *nonstressful* conditions, both groups of pups showed equally strong attachment behaviors and brain activity patterns. Specifically, brain activity was the expected sensitive period response to conditioned odors: robust olfactory bulb engagement in response to either the CS or the natural maternal odor, and no activation of the amygdala to either odor (Raineki et al., 2010). But when tested under physiological stress induced by administering exogenous corticosterone, the two groups' responses diverged dramatically. The odor–shock (abuse model) pups' attachment behaviors toward the conditioned odor were nearly erased, while the odor–stroke (typical care model) pups' attachment behaviors toward the odor were

fully intact. Moreover, the odor–shock pups had altered brain responses to the conditioned odor (i.e., strong activation of the amygdala), while odor–stroke pups did not (Raineki et al., 2010).

A more naturalistic model of maternal abuse validated these findings: From PND 3 to PND 8, litters were reared with a dam that was stressed by being given insufficient bedding material to make an adequate nest. Such a dam gives less maternal care and more rough handling; possibly as a result, her pups have high circulating levels of corticosterone, show reduced attachment behaviors toward her, and react to her odor with amygdala activation (Raineki et al., 2010). Both models show that an attachment that forms despite abusive maternal behavior functions normally under benign environmental conditions, but, under stress, undergoes behavioral breakdown and altered neural function, even during the sensitive period. These events may mark the earliest psychobiological manifestations of the vulnerability to later psychopathology that emerge from maternal maltreatment as development proceeds, as we now discuss.

## Sensitive Period Seeds of Psychopathology

Since maltreatment in nature is unlikely to be confined to a sensitive period, Sullivan's group exposed pups to odor–shock conditioning beginning in the sensitive period (at PND 8) and continuing into the transitional sensitive period (through PND 12). They found that the fear/avoidance learning that would be expected at PND 13 is blocked, even in the mother's absence. Instead, the odor preference response learned in the sensitive period persists into the transitional sensitive period (Moriceau, Raineki, Holman, Holman, & Sullivan, 2009). Under these conditions, corticosterone secretion and amygdala activity during the transitional sensitive period are suppressed to the low levels of sensitive period pups (Moriceau et al., 2009). The conditioned odor, having acquired a mother-like valence during the sensitive period, continues to mimic the mother's influence as a social buffer in the transitional sensitive period.

Such pups develop later behavioral abnormalities that resemble psychiatric symptoms that often affect abused children later in life. Pups reared with either kind of maternal maltreatment—daily odor–shock or insufficient bedding—showed deficits in social behavior with another pup as early as the preweaning period (PND 20), and a depression-like behavior, increased immobility on the Porsolt forced swim test, occurred in adolescence (Raineki, Cortés, Beinoue, & Sullivan, 2012). Elegant immunohistochemical and pharmacological assessments demonstrated that excess activation of the amygdala during the forced swim test was the cause of this depression-like behavior in these maltreated adolescents (Raineki et al., 2012).

This depressive predisposition of maltreated pups persists into adulthood when another symptom appears, lack of preference for a sweet drink versus water, which can be interpreted as anhedonia (Sevelinges et al., 2011). Amygdala dysfunction is again implicated as the neural basis of these behaviors. Strikingly, however, there is an apparent paradox embedded in the adult outcome. When the odor that was associated with shock in infancy was supplied during the adult behavioral and neural tests, all results normalized (Sevelinges et al., 2011). Moreover, this odor continued to elicit a preference response in the adults (Sevelinges et al., 2011), and when the adults were reconditioned by pairing this odor with shock, the resulting fear response and amygdala activation were attenuated (Sevelinges et al., 2007). Moreover, these adults had infant-like olfactory bulb activation when compared to adults that had never experienced the odor–shock pairing in infancy (Moriceau et al., 2009). Thus, early maternal maltreatment is a double-edged sword: One edge induces adult depression, whereas the other provides a safety signal in the adult that blunts new fear learning and relieves the depressive behaviors (Sevelinges et al., 2011). It is as if the adult offspring holds the abusive mother in its long-term memory as an ambivalent object, mirroring how she was originally experienced in infancy. And in blunting the fear associated with dangers encountered in adulthood, the remembered maternal odor could predispose the adult to repeat the abuse of the early attachment. This parallels the phenomenon of revictimization—the higher probability that adults who have been abused as children will be abused in adulthood (Messman-Moore & Long, 2003)—and suggests that the rat or mouse models could reveal mechanisms underlying this important clinical phenomenon.

## Responses to Separation

Behavioral systems that maintain an infant in close proximity to the mother and promote physical attachment to the nipple do not fulfill our criteria for a fully developed attachment system. Another essential component is a particular set of responses to maternal separation. In fact, Bowlby's attachment theory was developed to explain the separation responses that became all too evident during the societal devastations of World War II (Bowlby, 1969/1982). It was maternal separation that revealed the existence of a deeper layer of processes beneath the apparently simple interactions of mother and infant. The behavioral and physiological responses of the infant to separation, in Bowlby's conception, were consequences of the danger inherent in the "disruption" of an "affectional bond" that had been formed as part of an integrated psychophysiological organization that Bowlby called "the attachment behavioural system." More recent research, however, has revealed a network of simple behavioral and biological processes underlying these psychological constructs that we use to define and understand early human social relationships.

Experiments in our laboratory have shown that infant rats have complex and lasting responses to maternal separation, similar to those of primates, and that these responses occur in a number of different physiological and behavioral systems. We found that the slower developing components (Bowlby's "despair" phase) were *not* an integrated psychophysiological response, as had been supposed, but were the results of a novel mechanism (reviewed in Hofer, 1994). As separation continued, each individual system of the infant rat responded to the loss of one or another of the components of the infant's previous interactions with its mother. Providing one of these components to a separated pup (e.g., maternal warmth) maintained the level of brain biogenic amine function underlying the pup's general activity level, but it had no effect on other systems. For example, the pup's cardiac rate continued to fall, regardless of whether supplemental heat was provided. The heart rate, normally maintained by sympathetic autonomic tone, was found to be regulated by provision of milk to neural receptors in the lining of the pup's stomach. With loss of the maternal milk supply, sympathetic tone fell and cardiac rate was reduced by 40% in 12–18 hours.

By studying a number of additional systems, such as those controlling sleep–wake states, activity level, sucking patterns, exploratory behavior and isolation calling, we found different components of the mother–infant interaction (e.g., olfaction, taste, touch, warmth, and texture) that either up-regulated or down-regulated each of these functions. We therefore concluded that in maternal separation, all of these regulatory components of the mother–infant interaction are withdrawn at once. This widespread loss creates a pattern of increases, as well as decreases, in the levels of function of the infant's systems depending on whether the particular system had been up- or down-regulated previously by specific components of mother–infant interactions. We called these *hidden regulators* because they were not evident from simply observing the ongoing mother–infant relationship.

One of the best-known responses to maternal separation is the infant's separation cry, a behavior that occurs in a wide variety of species, including humans. In the rat, this call is in the ultrasonic range. Pharmacological studies by Susan Carden in our laboratory and by a number of others showed that the ultrasonic vocalization (USV) response to isolation is attenuated or blocked in a dose-dependent manner by clinically effective anxiolytic drugs that act at benzodiazepine and serotonin receptors (reviewed in Hofer, 1996). Conversely, USV rates are increased by compounds known to be anxiogenic in humans.

This evidence strongly suggests that separation produces an early affective state in rat pups that is expressed by the rate of infant calling. This calling behavior (and its inferred underlying affective state) develops as a communication system between mother and pup. Infant rat USVs are a powerful stimulus for the lactating rat, capable of causing her to interrupt an ongoing nursing bout, initiate searching outside the nest, and direct her search toward the source of the calls. The mother's retrieval response to the pup's vocal signals then results in renewed contact between pup and mother. This contact in turn quiets or comforts the pup.

The separation and comfort responses in "classical" attachment theory are described in terms of a single affective system, as expressions of interruption and reestablishment of a social bond. Instead, we found multiple regulators of infant ultrasonic calling "hidden" within the physical contact and behavioral interactions between mother and pup, including warmth, touch, texture, shape, and milk, as well as the mother's own scent (Hofer, 1996). The full "comfort" quieting response was elicited only when all sensory modalities were presented together, and maximum calling rates occurred when all were withdrawn at once. In essence, we found parallel regulatory systems involving different sensory systems, with the rate of infant calling reflecting both the composition and the sum total of effective maternal regulatory stimuli present at any given time.

In the case of the most complex behaviors we studied, sleep–wake state organization, a *temporal patterning* of the intragastric delivery of milk and of tactile stimulation to the pups was necessary to maintain the pups normal sleep–wake state patterns through their 24-hour separation from their mothers. These rhythmic patterns of central brain states are evidently organized by the timing of the mother's periodic nursing bouts, as well as nutrient and sensorimotor exchanges with her under normal conditions.

For human infants, still more complex interactions such as attunement, imitation, and play are likely to have regulatory effects on developing infants' cognitive and affective systems. In this way, all these different interactions would appear to participate in the early formation of human infants' mental representations of their first relationship.

## Hidden Regulators of Early Development

As we began to understand the infant's separation response as one of loss—loss of a number of individual regulatory processes that were hidden within the interactions of the previous relationship—an important implication of this finding emerged: These ongoing regulatory interactions can shape the course of development of an infant's brain and behavior throughout the preweaning period when mother and infant remain in close proximity. We could now think of mother–infant interactions as regulators of normal infant development, with variations in the intensity and patterning of these interactions gradually shaping infant behavior and physiology. Supporting this idea, Kuhn and Schanberg (1998) published a series of studies in which they found that removal of the mother from rat pups produced a rapid (30-minute) fall in the pups' growth hormone (GH) levels, and that vigorous tactile stroking of maternally separated pups (mimicking maternal licking) prevented this fall in GH. There are several biological similarities between this maternal deprivation effect in rats and the growth retardation that occurs in some variants of human reactive attachment disorders of infancy (Chatoor, Ganiban, Colin, Plummer, & Harmon, 1998). Applying this new knowledge about the regulation of GH to low-birthweight, prematurely born babies, Field and coworkers (1986) joined the Schanberg group and used a combination of stroking and limb movement, administered three times a day for 15 minutes each time, and continued through the infants' 2 weeks of hospitalization. This intervention increased weight gain, head circumference, and behavioral development test scores in relation to those of a randomly chosen control group, with enhanced maturational effects discernible many months later. Clearly, early regulators are effective in humans, and over time periods as long as several weeks to months.

These processes go beyond the adaptive evolutionary role of the attachment "bond" as a protection against predators, as proposed by Bowlby (1969/1982). The rapid onset and prolonged duration of processes keeping infants close to their mothers, described earlier, provide the necessary conditions for long-term regulatory effects of early mother–infant interactions on infants' development. The processes underlying infants' proximity maintenance are likely to have evolved together with the hidden regulatory interactions because the two, acting together, created a developmental mechanism capable of shaping the offsprings' adaptive capabilities, as well as maternal behavior in the next generation, through selection over evolutionary time.

## Lasting Effects of Early Relationships

One of the major tenets of attachment theory is the idea that an infant's early attachment pattern can have long-term developmental effects—in particular on the infant's early mental representations (which Bowlby sometimes called "internal working models" or "representational models"), on his or her later relationships with his or her own children, and on broader aspects of behavior, such as levels of anxiety and aggression, and the quality of social interactions. As described early in this chapter, such a transgenerational developmental system could evolve as a result of the competitive advantages to be gained by young who are shaped by their parents, in advance, to deal most effectively with the kind of environment they are likely to face as adolescents and adults.

What basis do we have for this evolutionary interpretation, or even for the existence of such very long-term developmental effects of variations in maternal behavior? In the 1980s, we began to

test the possible long-term developmental effects of the "hidden maternal regulators" we had uncovered within the mother-infant interactions in our separation studies. By observing naturally occurring variations in mother–infant interactions of an inbred strain of genetically identical rats that had been selectively bred as an animal model for hypertension, we were able to identify three maternal behaviors, observed in the first 2 postnatal weeks, that were correlated with the severity of hypertension in their offspring as adults (Myers, Brunelli, Shair, Squire, & Hofer, 1989). The use of genetically identical strains ensured that any differences between the adult offspring of different mothers could not be attributed to different genes being passed on to these offspring, but instead to differences in each mother's behavior toward them as infants. The behaviors we found most closely correlated with offspring blood pressure included the amount of maternal licking and grooming, the time mothers spent in a highly stimulating high-arched resting position, and their level of contact time. Thus, we were able to conclude that differences in specifiable patterns of mothers' interactions with their pups could produce developmental effects on autonomic/endocrine systems regulating blood pressure that lasted into adulthood. But we had no clue as to how these differences in maternal behavior were translated into changes in their pups' blood pressure regulation as adults.

The work of Michael Meaney, Frances Champagne, and their colleagues over the past decade and a half has greatly enlarged our understanding of the cell/molecular processes underlying the lasting effects of early mother-infant interactions on adult offspring behavior and physiology (reviewed in Chapter 8 by Bakermans-Kranenberg and Van IJzendoorn). In summary, they found that normally occurring differences between rat mothers involving the maternal behaviors we had described in our studies systematically modified the long-term development of the adrenocortical stress response and behavioral fear response of their adult offspring, with lower levels of these interactions leading to greater adrenocortical and fear responses. Then, in a remarkable series of cell biological experiments, Meaney and his colleagues (1996) were able, first, to trace the effects of these maternal behaviors to changes in offsprings' hippocampal glucocorticoid receptors. These receptors sense the level of endogenous adrenocortical hormone and inhibit this hormonal response to stress—a form of inhibitory feedback, as in a thermostat. Next, they traced these effects to differences in the expression levels of genes regulating the number of active receptors, differences produced by newly discovered epigenetic processes acting outside the genes themselves but regulating their activity. Importantly, identical effects were found in cross-fostered pups born to other mothers, ruling out direct genetic inheritance of the traits. These findings linked differences in normally occurring levels of mother–infant interactions to molecular processes regulating gene expression in the brains of the developing young. Meaney and colleagues found similar epigenetic effects involving not only a variety of stress responses but also learning processes, aggression, and sexual and maternal behavior, as described below.

In more general terms, what these studies have done is uncover some of the component processes through which different patterns of early mother–infant interactions can regulate the long-term development of physiological and behavioral systems of offspring, extending into their adult lives. Given that the number of genes now known to be involved in this kind of long-term regulation number in the hundreds, it seems likely that the effects of different early mother–infant interaction patterns are more extensive and may well involve even more systems than those already identified.

As discussed earlier, we know that attachment patterns tend to be repeated by daughters in the next generation—an effect thought to be mediated by processes of psychological representation (Bowlby's "internal working models"). Now we have good evidence for biological processes that underlie and contribute to this transgenerational process as well. Frances Champagne, when she was in Meaney's laboratory (Champagne, Diorio, Sharma, & Meaney, 2001), found that mothers with high or low levels of licking/grooming and high-arched nursing position pass these maternal behavior patterns on to their daughters, along with the different levels of adult adrenocortical and fear responses just described. They could link this transgenerational effect on maternal behaviors to increases, or decreases, in the activity of genes regulating oxytocin receptors in the 1-week-old pups' developing brain systems that later become central to their maternal behavior as adults, the medial preoptic area and lateral septum.

How do these widespread biological effects fit into the evolutionary perspective on attachment described at the beginning of this section? The changes in offspring physiology and behavior generated by the two different mother–infant interaction types showed widespread, recognizable

"preadaptations" to two different kinds of environments. Low levels of maternal interaction resulted in more fearful adult offspring with heightened startle responses and intense adrenocortical responses to stress (Claessens et al., 2011; Zhang, Chretien, Meaney, & Gratton, 2005). In other studies (e.g., Liu, Diorio, Day, Francis, & Meaney, 2000), researchers found that the offsprings' capacity for avoidance learning was enhanced, whereas their spatial learning and memory were relatively impaired, as reflected in slower hippocampal synapse growth. In addition to transmitting their own low-level maternal behavior pattern to their offspring, young adults in this group showed more rapid sexual maturation (vaginal opening), greater sexual receptivity, more rapidly repeated sexual encounters, and a higher rate of pregnancy following mating than offspring of high-interaction-level mothers. These differences appear to be suited to a harsh, unpredictable, and threatening environment with few resources—an environment in which intense defensive responses, fearful avoidance of threats, and early increased sexual activity would be likely to result in both enhanced individual survival and more offspring born in the next generation.

In experimental support of this theoretical prediction, Champagne and Meaney (2006) went on to demonstrate that the experience of stress during rat mothers' pregnancies reduced their subsequent licking and grooming of their pups, leading to the pups later developing the very behavioral characteristics just described.

High levels of mother–infant interaction in turn were found to lead to a pattern of slower sexual development, more exploration than fear of novelty, a predisposition to learn spatial maps rather than avoidance responses, and lower levels of adrenocortical responses—traits that would be liabilities in very harsh environments, but that allow optimal adaptation to a stable, supportive environment with abundant new opportunities and resources.

This remarkable research is revealing a network of biological processes—extending down to the regulatory mechanisms within the genome—that appear to be developmental and evolutionary precursors of the psychological processes, such as enduring mental representations, that are fundamental to concepts of human attachment. From an evolutionary perspective, maternal behavior not only prepares an infant for its likely adult environment but also can exert a transgenerational propagation of maternal behavior, extending effects into a third generation and beyond. They provide not only a more generationally limited but also a more flexible way of passing biological information forward into the future, from one generation to the next, resembling the cultural inheritance of ideas, beliefs, and psychological predispositions. They fit remarkably well with previous human studies of transgenerational continuity in attachment patterns (e.g., Main, Kaplan, & Cassidy, 1985). Most recently, transgenerational effects of early experience acting through male or female germline genes in rodents have been reported (Curley & Mashoodh, 2010; Dias & Ressler, 2014), opening a new chapter in this story, one that awaits scientific assessment of its extent and importance in nature.

## Applying the New Tools of Molecular Biology

One of the major insights of molecular biology is that genes—once viewed as static repositories of the information contained in the organism's basic plan, akin to a house's blueprint that is rolled up and stored away after construction—are active participants in all cellular processes throughout life, and their ongoing contributions are regulated from moment to moment. Now it is possible to manipulate the genes that are thought to regulate the biology and behavioral processes of attachment and separation. Genetic engineering can delete a gene (i.e., "knock it out"), add extra copies of it (a "transgene"), or add copies that make a dysfunctional product, which dominates the endogenous gene's normal product (a "transdominant negative"). One can then infer the gene's function from the consequences of these manipulations. To avoid "false-negative" results due to developmental compensation mechanisms, or "false-positive" results due to the mutation occurring in brain regions responsible for nonspecific behavioral disruptions, we can make "conditional" genetic manipulations that target specific parts of the brain, or that can be activated or deactivated at specific times in development.

Now, with the sequencing of the mouse genome, and the technology to introduce very precise mutations into the mouse oocyte's DNA, the mouse is beginning to take center stage in the study of filial attachment. To exploit the genetic techniques requires a mouse model of infant–mother attachment with enough behavioral and physiological detail to allow the investiga-

tion of important questions in depth. Behavioral researchers have now established that murine infant–mother attachment has all the essential elements that have made the rat model so productive, specifically, MDOBs, separation USVs, olfactory preference learning during a sensitive period, and a transport response to maternal retrieval.

We showed that the earliest manifestations of attachment, neonatal MDOBs, emerge in mice from PND 0 to 3, with the same motor action patterns in response to nearness of the mother's ventral body surface seen in same age rats (Masson et al., 2006). Mouse pups call in the ultrasonic range when separated from their mother and potentiate the rate of calling after brief reunion and reseparation (Moles, Kieffer, & D'Amato, 2004), just as do rats.

Sullivan's group has recently demonstrated a sensitive period for olfactory preference learning in infant mice that appears identical to that of same-age rats in all behavioral and neurophysiological aspects so far studied (Roth et al., 2013), including the support of a behavioral attachment to the mother, even in the face of treatment that is aversive or abusive.

The transport (or carry) response has also been shown to be present in both mice and rats, but unlike MDOBs, USVs, and olfactory preference learning, it has been explored more fully in mice than in rats. Elegant studies by the Kikusui, Kato, and Kuroda group (Esposito et al., 2013; Yoshida et al., 2013) revealed its developmental course, motor patterns, and sensory elicitors, and the accompanying physiological "calming" (reduced heart rate and ultrasonic calling). They also showed remarkably close parallels to the human infant's motor and physiological calming responses to being picked up and carried by his or her mother (Esposito et al., 2013).

Only a few models of the impact of genes on the filial behavior of infants and juvenile mice have so far been studied. In one, our collaborators knocked out the gene for glutaminase type 1 (GLS1), the enzyme responsible for most of the brain's main excitatory neurotransmitter, glutamate (Masson et al., 2006). Newborns that lack both copies of the gene (also called "null" or "knockout" mice) die within 1 or 2 days after birth, lacking milk in the stomach, whereas their siblings that have one copy of the gene (i.e., the heterozygotes) survive and develop, on gross inspection, normally.

We found that the nulls' failure to obtain milk was not due simply to behavioral debilitation. They were as active as their heterozygote and wild-type littermates, but the nulls' MDOBs were disorganized. Under the mother's ventrum, the nulls attained, but failed to maintain, the supine orientation and emitted far too little audible calling (barking) when encountering the mother, whereas they engaged in undirected and inappropriately high frequencies of mouthing and licking, even when not in the mother's presence. These behavioral anomalies suggest that the nulls failed either to recognize the mother or to organize an appropriate response to her.

The heterozygotes had a behavioral phenotype intermediate between the nulls and wild types on all measures, demonstrating that they were not in fact "normal." Their mild deficit of glutamate neurotransmission caused them to hold the supine orientation under the mother's ventrum for less than half the time typical of the wild types. Supination is critical for the pup to be able to locate a nipple and nurse, and its absence is devastating for the null pups. But if supination is performed competently, even low amounts of it are evidently enough for the heterozygotes to survive and grow. As adults, the heterozygotes showed deficits of hippocampus-dependent contextual fear learning (Gaisler-Salomon et al., 2012). Whether they have deficits in the affective or social behavior domain has not yet been determined.

Another study examined the effects of the gene for the mu opioid receptor on the infant mouse's isolation-induced USV. As described earlier, USV is analogous to the human infant's separation cry and is regarded as a necessary indicator of the establishment of a "filial attachment bond" (Hofer, 1996). The mu receptor mediates the behavioral and physiological effects of many natural rewards. It has also been hypothesized to mediate the infant's response to social isolation, but the pharmacological evidence is controversial. Isolation-induced USV was recorded (1) for infant mice null for the mu receptor gene and (2) for wild-type controls (Moles et al., 2004). The knockouts exhibited significantly less USV during the first 2 postnatal weeks, and failed to "potentiate" their calling rates after being reexposed briefly to their mothers and then reisolated. However, the knockouts' sensitivity to physical (cold) or social (strange male) threats was not impaired; nor were the knockouts grossly deficient in olfactory competence. This study of the mu receptor knockout mouse lends support to the hypothesis that the infant's mu opioid receptor plays a specific role in mediating the reinforcing properties of maternal

stimuli. Neither of these knockout studies is definitive, but they represent the leading edge of emerging work on the effects of candidate genes on the formation and competence of filial behaviors.

A third study illustrates two other approaches taken in molecular studies to shed light on attachment (Gross et al., 2002). The investigators used a genetic model to examine the development of an emotion, anxiety, that figures critically in attachment. They knocked out the gene for the 1A type of receptor for serotonin—a neurotransmitter that is central to the maintenance of normal mood and affect and, when dysfunctional, permits pathological anxiety and depression. Since stimulation of the serotonin 1A receptor is anxiolytic, the knockout mouse was more anxious than the wild type on behavioral tests including exploration and food-sampling in a novel open (i.e., anxiety-provoking) field. When the researchers used the molecular method of turning the knocked-out gene's expression back on in the mouse's forebrain, they found that when this rescue occurred, in just the first 2 postnatal weeks, normal emotional responsiveness in adulthood was restored.

As shown by this study, we can now determine, at the molecular level, the quality, quantity, and timing of developmental provisions that support the emergence of normal emotional capacities. We know that experiences of maternal separation or variations in maternal care reprogram the stress axis, leading to altered levels of anxiety and stress responsiveness in adulthood (Cameron et al., 2005; Meaney et al., 1996). Meaney and others have hypothesized that maternal separation, and the altered maternal behaviors that occur with reunion, are transduced in part by the pups' serotonin systems. The serotonin 1A receptor knockout provides evidence that serotonin is indeed part of the mechanism by which altered infant separation and attachment experiences can reprogram the stress axis and its affective manifestation, anxiety.

## Perspectives for Future Research

We concluded our chapter in the second edition of this handbook (Polan & Hofer, 2008) with a set of questions for future investigation. Some of these have been partially answered and explained in the main body of this chapter. We summarize these here, address others below, and now add some new questions arising in part from the answers to the old ones and in part from the new perspectives that molecular methods have opened up.

We asked a set of related questions: Are early attachment experiences or their biological substrates responsible for the quality of adult attachment or the development of psychiatric disorders in adulthood? Are the processes of preference learning and stress axis programming during the sensitive period reversible, and, if so, what implications might this have for the treatment of abuse, neglect, or early abandonment?

The new information covered in this chapter allows us to summarize the answers as follows. We now understand that maternal maltreatment creates both vulnerability to psychopathology across development and a safety signal in adulthood. The discovery of symptoms in multiple realms of emotional behavior—social interaction deficits, signs of depression, and abnormal fear processing—and the brain substrates of these reveal the outlines of the developmetal psychopathology of abusive attachment. Many details remain to be filled in. Nevertheless, we have sufficient behavioral, neurohumoral, and neural-circuit-level correlates of abusive attachment to suggest that the rodent models can be used for preclinical tests of primary preventions and early interventions for the later complicating psychopathologies. And we have learned that, paradoxically, the maternal cue that was associated with abuse in infancy still attracts the adult offspring, diminishes adult fear learning, and relieves depression. This suggests a new animal model of the role of ambivalent early object representations in the important clinical phenomenon of revictimization (Messman-Moore & Long, 2003).

We also asked: What is the precise relation between the development of proximity seeking (MDOBs) and separation or loss responses? Is the achievement of one necessary for the emergence of the other?

In the previous edition, we interpreted the increase in MDOBs in 2- to 3-day-old pups after an overnight separation from their mothers as evidence for the development of a "motivational" component in this behavioral system (Polan & Hofer, 2008). But the increase could also be viewed as an affect-driven intensification of these behaviors that evolved in response to the dangers posed by separation, or may be shaped by the loss of regulatory processes that had been "hidden" within the ongoing mother–infant interactions that normally inhibit or down-regulate MDOBs. Future research exploring the underlying neurobiological and behavioral mechanisms of MDOBs will help us to integrate these possible interpretations.

Finally, we asked whether there are genetically based differences in the neural and endocrine substrates for attachment and separation processes and, if so, how these might interact with the environmental and genetic mechanisms described earlier. Study of associations of human gene polymorphisms and attachment security has been limited by the same difficulty of replication that has slowed the entire field of genetic association and complex behavior (Roisman, Booth-LaForce, Belsky, Burtf, & Groh, 2013). As statistical power and methods improve, candidate genes found in humans can be tested for phenotypes and biological mechanisms in mice.

We now offer for this edition the following three questions for future investigations:

1. It has become clear that neonatal intensive care units (NICUs) are not only a source of (necessary) physical trauma for premature infants, but also of unavoidable, prolonged periods of mother–infant separation. Yet this situation has not become a major area for research on early attachment processes. The effects of the prolonged separations are almost as important for the mother as for the premature infant, so the development of infant attachment (as well as of maternal caregiving) under these circumstances will be an exceptionally interesting and growing area for future attachment research.

2. The limits and overall significance of epigenetic processes for development and evolution are not yet fully established. Although developmental processes are now established as a major source of variation for natural selection to act upon (the subject of the new academic field of study: evolutionary developmental biology), there are a number of well-established processes for such effects. Thus, the discovery of novel *epi*genetic mechanisms for transgenerational change (many in the area of attachment research) has generated skepticism among molecular geneticists who ask: How frequent and widespread such epigenetic effects actually are in nature? We should have some answers by the time the fourth edition of this handbook is undertaken.

3. What are the intervening links between particular behaviors of rat mothers toward their infants and the establishment of epigenetic "marks" on specific genes in her pups' brains? A complex paper by the Meaney group (Hellstrom,

Dhir, Diorio, & Meaney, 2012) has worked out the cascade of cell and molecular events that bridges the gap between the dam's licking behavior on the one hand and the epigenetic events regulating the exon-1$_7$ promoter of the glucocorticoid receptor gene in her offsprings' brains. But since many (literally hundreds) of the pups' brain genes are regulated by (presumably many different) dam–pup interactions, there is much more that we have yet to learn about these complex behavioral–genomic events.

## References

Bisaz, R. & Sullivan, R. M. (2012). Developmental neurobiology of the rat attachment system and its modulation by stress. *Behavioral Sciences, 2,* 79–102.

Bowlby, J. (1973). *Attachment and loss: Vol. 2. Separation: Anxiety and anger.* New York: Basic Books.

Bowlby, J. (1982). *Attachment and loss: Vol. 1. Attachment* (2nd ed.). New York: Basic Books. (Original work published 1969)

Cameron, N. M., Champagne, F. A., Carine, P., Fish, E. W., Ozaki-Kuroda, K., & Meaney, M. J. (2005). The programming of individual differences in defensive responses and reproductive strategies in the rat through variations in maternal care. *Neuroscience and Biobehavioral Reviews, 29,* 843–865.

Camp, L. L., & Rudy, J. W. (1988). Changes in the categorization of appetitive and aversive events during postnatal development of the rat. *Developmental Psychobiology, 21,* 25–42.

Carroll, S. B. (2005). *Endless forms most beautiful: The new science of evo devo and the making of the animal kingdom.* New York: Norton.

Champagne, F., Diorio, J., Sharma, S., & Meaney, M. J. (2001). Naturally occurring variations in maternal care in the rat are associated with differences in estrogen-inducible central oxytocin receptors. *Proceedings of the National Academy of Sciences USA, 98,* 12736–12741.

Champagne, F. A., & Meaney, M. J. (2006). Stress during gestation alters postpartum care and the development of offspring in a rodent model. *Biological Psychiatry, 59,* 1227–1235.

Chatoor, I., Ganiban, J., Colin, V., Plummer, N., & Harmon, R. J. (1998). Attachment and feeding problems: A reexamination of nonorganic failure to thrive and attachment insecurity. *Journal of the American Academy of Child and Adolescent Psychiatry, 37*(11), 1217–1224.

Claessens, S. E. F., Daskalakis, N. P., van der Veen, R., Oitzl, M. S., de Kloet, E. R., & Champagne, D. L. (2011). Development of individual differences in stress responsiveness: An overview of factors mediating the outcome of early life experiences. *Psychopharmacology, 214,* 141–154.

Curley, J., & Mashoodh, R. (2010). Parent-of-origin and trans-generational germline influences on behavioral development: The interacting roles of mothers, fathers and grandparents. *Developmental Psychobiology, 52,* 312–330.

Dias, B. G., & Ressler, K. J. (2014). Parental olfactory experience influences behavior and neural structure in subsequent generations. *Nature Neuroscience, 17,* 89–96.

Esposito, G., Yoshia, S., Ohnishi, R., Tsuneoka, Y., del Carmen Rostagno, M., Yokota, S., et al. (2013). Infant calming responses during maternal carrying in humans and mice. *Current Biology, 23,* 739–745.

Fenoglio, K. A., Brunson, K. L., Avishai-Eliner, S., Chen, Y., & Baram, T. Z. (2004). Region-specific onset of handling-induced changes in corticotropin-releasing factor and glucocorticoid receptor expression. *Endocrinology, 145,* 2702–2706.

Field, T. M., Schanberg, S. M., Scafidi, F., Bauer, C. R., Vega-Lahr, N., Garcia, R., et al. (1986). Tactile/kinesthetic stimulation effects on preterm neonates. *Pediatrics, 77,* 654–658.

Gaisler-Salomon, I., Wang, Y., Chuhma, N., Zhang, H., Golumbic, Y. N., Mihali, A., et al. (2012). Synaptic underpinnings of altered hippocampal function in glutaminase-deficient mice during maturation. *Hippocampus, 22,* 1027–1039.

Gregory, E. H., & Pfaff, D. W. (1971). Development of olfactory guided behavior in infant rats. *Physiology and Behavior, 6,* 573–576.

Gross, C., Zhuang, X., Stark, K., Ramboz, S., Oosting, R., Kirby, K., et al. (2002). Serotonin 1A receptor acts during development to establish normal anxiety-like behaviour in the adult. *Nature, 416,* 396–400.

Hellstrom, I. C., Dhir, S. K., Diorio, J. C., & Meaney, M. J. (2012). Maternal licking regulates hippocampal glucocorticoid receptor transcription through a thyroid hormone–serotonin–NGFI-A signaling cascade. *Philosophical Transactions of the Royal Society B, 367,* 2495–2510.

Hepper, P. G. (1987). The amniotic fluid: An important priming role in kin recognition. *Animal Behaviour, 35,* 1343–1346.

Hofer, M. A. (1994). Early relationships as regulators of infant physiology and behavior. *Acta Paediatrica Supplement, 397,* 9–18.

Hofer, M. A. (1996). Multiple regulators of ultrasonic vocalization in the infant rat. *Psychoneuroendocrinology, 21,* 203–217.

Johanson, I. B., Turkewitz, G., & Hamburgh, M. (1980). Development of home orientation in hypothyroid and hyperthyroid rat pups. *Developmental Psychobiology, 13,* 331–342.

Kuhn, C. M., & Schanberg, S. M. (1998). Responses to maternal separation: Mechanisms and mediators. *In-*

ternational Journal of Developmental Neuroscience, 16, 261–270.

Liu, D., Diorio, J., Day, J. C., Francis, D. D., & Meaney, M. J. (2000). Maternal care, hippocampal synaptogenesis and cognitive development in rats. Nature Neuroscience, 3, 799–806.

Main, M., Kaplan, N., & Cassidy, J. (1985). Security in infancy, childhood, and adulthood: A move to the level of representation. In I. Bretherton & E. Waters (Eds.), Growing points of attachment theory and research. Monographs of the Society for Research in Child Development, 50(1–2, Serial No. 209), 66–104.

Masson, J., Darmon, M., Conjard, A., Chuhma, N., Ropert, N., Thoby-Brisson, M., et al. (2006). Mice lacking brain/kidney phosphate-activated glutaminase have impaired glutamatergic synaptic transmission, altered breathing, disorganized goal-directed behavior and die shortly after birth. Journal of Neuroscience, 26, 4660–4671.

Meaney, M. J., & Aitken, D. H. (1985). The effects of early postnatal handling on hippocampal glucocorticoid receptor concentrations: Temporal parameters. Brain Research, 354, 301–304.

Meaney, M. J., Diorio, J., Francis, D., Widdowson, J., LaPlante, P., Caldji, C., et al. (1996). Early environmental regulation of forebrain glucocorticoid receptor gene expression: Implications for adrenocortical responses to stress. Developmental Neuroscience, 18, 49–72.

Messman-Moore, T. L., & Long, P. J. (2003). The role of childhood sexual abuse sequelae in the sexual revictimization of women: An empirical review and theoretical reformulation. Clinical Psychology Review, 23, 537–571.

Moles, A., Kieffer, B. L., & D'Amato, F. R. (2004). Deficit in attachment behavior in mice lacking the mu-opioid receptor gene. Science, 304, 1983–1986.

Moriceau, S., Raineki, C., Holman, J. D., Holman, J. G., & Sullivan, R. M. (2009). Enduring neurobehavioral effects of early life trauma mediated through learning and corticosterone suppression. Behavioral Neuroscience, 3(Article 22), 1–13.

Moriceau, S., & Sullivan, R. M. (2005). Neurobiology of infant attachment. Developmental Psychobiology, 47, 230–242.

Moriceau, S., & Sullivan, R. M. (2006). Maternal presence serves as a switch between learning fear and attraction in infancy. Nature Neuroscience, 9, 1004–1006.

Moriceau, S., Wilson, D. A., Levine, S., & Sullivan, R. M. (2006). Dual circuitry for odor–shock conditioning during infancy: Corticosterone switches between fear and attraction via amygdala. Journal of Neuroscience, 26, 6737–6748.

Myers, M. M., Brunelli, S. A., Shair, H. N., Squire, J. M., & Hofer, M. A. (1989). Relationships between maternal behavior of SHR and WKY dams and adult blood pressures of cross-fostered F1 pups. Developmental Psychobiology, 22, 55–67.

Nyakas, C., & Endroczi, E. (1970). Olfaction guided approaching behaviour of infantile rats to the mother in maze box. Acta Physiologica Academiae Scientiarum Hungaricae, 38, 59–65.

Polan, H. J., & Hofer, M. A. (1998). Olfactory preference for mother over home nest shavings by newborn rats. Developmental Psychobiology, 33, 5–20.

Polan, H. J., & Hofer, M. A. (1999). Maternally-directed orienting behaviors of newborn rats. Developmental Psychobiology, 34, 269–279.

Polan, H. J., & Hofer, M. A. (2008). Psychobiological origins of infant attachment and separation responses. In J. Cassidy & P. R. Shaver (Eds.), Handbook of attachment: Theory, research, and clinical applications (2nd ed., pp. 158–172). New York: Guilford Press.

Polan, H. J., Milano, D., Eljuga, L., & Hofer, M. A. (2002). Development of rats' maternally directed orienting from birth to day 2. Developmental Psychobiology, 40, 81–103.

Raineki, C., Cortés, M. R., Beinoue, L., & Sullivan, R. M. (2012). Effects of early life abuse differ across development: Infant social behavior deficits are followed by adolescent depressive-like behaviors mediated by the amygdala. Journal of Neuroscience, 32, 7758–7765.

Raineki, C., Moriceau, S., & Sullivan, R. M. (2010). Developing a neurobehavioral animal model of infant attachment to an abusive caregiver. Biological Psychiatriy, 67, 1137–1145.

Roisman, G. I., Booth-LaForce, C., Belsky, J., Burtf, K. B., & Groh, A. M. (2013). Molecular-genetic correlates of infant attachment: A cautionary tale. Attachment and Human Development, 15, 384–406.

Roth, T. L., Raineki, C., Salstein, L., Perry, R., Sullivan-Wilson, T. A., Sloan, A., et al. (2013). Neurobiology of secure infant attachment and attachment despite adversity: A mouse model. Genes, Brain and Behavior, 12, 673–680.

Scott, J. P. (1963). Process of primary socialization in canine and human infants. Monographs of the Society for Research in Child Development, 28(1, Serial No. 85), 1–47.

Sevelinges, Y., Moriceau, S., Holman, P., Miner, C., Muzny, K., Gervais, R., et al. (2007). Enduring effects of infant memories: Infant odor–shock conditioning attenuates amygdala activity and adult fear conditioning. Biological Psychiatry, 62, 1070–1079.

Sevelinges, Y., Mouly, A.-M., Raineki, C., Moriceau, S., Forest, C., & Sullivan, R. M. (2011). Adult depression-like behavior, amygdala and olfactory cortex functions are restored by odor previously paired with shock during infant's sensitive period attachment learning. Developmental Cognitive Neuroscience, 1, 77–87.

Simpson, J. A. & Belsky, J. (2008). Attachment theory within a modern evolutionary framework. In J. Cassidy & P. R. Shaver (Eds.), Handbook of attachment: Theory, research, and clinical applications (2nd ed., pp. 131–157). New York: Guilford Press.

Sullivan, R. M. (1996, November). *Neural correlates of neonatal olfactory learning*. Paper presented at the meeting of the International Society for Developmental Psychobiology, Washington, DC.

Sullivan, R. M., & Hall, W. G. (1988). Reinforcers in infancy: Classical conditioning using stroking or intra-oral infusions of milk as UCS. *Developmental Psychobiology, 21,* 215–223.

Sullivan, R. M., Hofer, M. A., & Brake, S. (1986). Olfactory-guided orientation in neonatal rats is enhanced by a conditioned change in behavioral state. *Developmental Psychobiology, 19,* 615–623.

Sullivan, R. M., Landers, M., Yeaman, B., & Wilson, D. A. (2000). Good memories of bad events in infancy. *Nature, 407,* 38–39.

Wilson, D. A., & Sullivan, R. M. (1994). Neurobiology of associative learning in the neonate: Early olfactory learning. *Behavioral and Neural Biology, 61,* 1–18.

Yoshida, S., Esposito, G., Ohnishi, R., Tsuneoka, Y., Okabe, S., Kikusui, T., Kato, T., et al. (2013). Transport response is a filial-specific behavioral response to maternal carrying in C57Bl/6 mice. *Frontiers in Zoology, 10,* 50.

Zhang, T. Y., Chretien, P., Meaney, M. J., & Gratton, A. (2005). Influence of naturally occurring variations in maternal care on prepulse inhibition of acoustic startle and the medial prefrontal cortical dopamine response to stress in adult rats. *Journal of Neuroscience, 25,* 1493–502.

# Chapter 7

# Attachment In Rhesus Monkeys

Stephen J. Suomi

Attachment is not an exclusively human phenomenon. Although the theory that John Bowlby developed during the 1950s and 1960s, and refined during the 1970s, reflected his clinical observations of infants and young children, it also had a strong biological foundation stemming in large part from his long-standing interest in ethological studies of developmental phenomena in animals, especially nonhuman primates (van der Horst, Van der Veer, & Van IJzendoorn, 2007). Indeed, it can be argued that Bowlby (1969/1982) specifically tailored the basic biological features of his attachment theory to account for clear-cut commonalities in the strong behavioral and emotional ties that infants typically develop with their mother, not only across virtually all of humanity but also among our closest evolutionary relatives.

Around the time that Bowlby published, with James Roberston, his seminal studies of mother-infant separation due to hospitalization (Robertson & Bowlby, 1952), he was also becoming familiar with the classic ethological studies of filial imprinting in precocial birds. During this period he developed a close friendship with the Cambridge University ethologist Robert Hinde, who at the time was in the process of shifting his own basic research interests from song learning in birds to mother–infant interactions in rhesus monkeys. Hinde soon had rhesus monkey mothers raising babies in small, captive social groups (e.g., Hinde, Rowell, & Spencer-Booth, 1964), and Bowlby came to recognize patterns of behavior

of the infant monkeys toward their mothers—but not toward other adult females in the group—that strikingly resembled recurrent response patterns of human infants and young children he had observed over years of clinical practice (van der Horst et al., 2007). During the same period, Bowlby became intrigued by the research of Harry Harlow, documenting the attachments that rhesus monkey infants developed with artificial ("surrogate") mothers, differing systematically with respect to certain physical features (Harlow, 1958; Harlow & Suomi, 1970).

Indeed, virtually all of the classic features of human infant behavior that Bowlby's attachment theory specifically ascribed to our evolutionary history could be clearly observed in the patterns of mother-directed activity exhibited by rhesus monkey infants, as described by Hinde, Harlow, and other primate researchers. For Bowlby (1958, 1969/1982), the fact that rhesus monkey infants and human babies share unique physical features, behavioral propensities, and emotional liabilities linked to highly specific social situations was consistent with the view that they also share significant parts of their respective evolutionary histories. He argued that these features, present in newborns of each species but often largely absent (or at least largely obscured) in older individuals, reflect successful adaptions to selective pressures over millions of years. To Bowlby, those characteristics common to both human and monkey infants represented evolutionary success stories that should be viewed as beneficial, if not essential, for promoting the survival of both the individual infant and the species.

What are those common characteristics, and what is their relevance for attachment theory? This chapter begins with a description of how attachment relationships between rhesus monkey infants and their mothers are typically established and maintained throughout development. Next, those features that are unique to attachment relationships are examined. Attachment relationships in rhesus monkeys and other primates are subject to influence from a variety of sources, and some of these influences are reviewed next. Some long-term behavioral and biological consequence of different early attachment experiences are then examined in detail. Finally, the implications for attachment theory of recent findings regarding cross-generational transmission of specific attachment patterns in rhesus monkey families are discussed.

## Normative Patterns of Infant–Mother Attachment in Rhesus Monkeys

The first detailed longitudinal studies of species-normative attachment relationships in rhesus monkeys were carried out a half-century ago (e.g., Hansen, 1966; Harlow, Harlow, & Hansen, 1963; Hinde & Spencer-Booth, 1967). These seminal investigations provided descriptions of infant behavioral development and emerging social relationships that not only appear remarkably accurate today but also have repeatedly been shown to generalize to other rhesus monkey infants growing up across a variety of natural and captive settings, as well as to infants of many other Old World monkey and ape species (see Higley & Suomi, 1986, for one of many comprehensive reviews). Virtually all infants in these species spend their initial days, weeks, and (for infant apes) months of life in near-continuous physical contract with their biological mothers, typically clinging to their mothers' ventral surface for most of their waking (and virtually all of their sleeping) hours each day.

Newborn rhesus monkeys clearly and consistently display four of the five "component instinctual responses" that Bowlby (1958) listed as universal human attachment behaviors in his initial monograph on attachment: sucking, clinging,

crying, and following (the fifth, smiling, is seen in chimpanzee but not in monkey infants). On their first postnatal day they can discriminate pictures and videos of faces from nonfacial stimuli, by the end of their first week of life they come to prefer female faces over male faces, and by 3 weeks of age they prefer faces of conspecifics to those of other species, including closely related primate species (Simpson, Paukner, Suomi, & Ferrari, 2015).

Some rhesus monkey infants, like some human infants, are also able to imitate specific facial expressions of their mother shortly after birth (Ferrari et al., 2006; Paukner, Ferrari, & Suomi, 2013), although this form of "mirroring" behavior largely disappears after the first 10–14 days of life (Paukner et al., 2013). Electroencephalographic (EEG) recordings from scalp electrodes have revealed a distinctive EEG "signature" (suppression of mu rhythms at low frequencies) that can be detected during bouts of imitative behavior on the first postnatal day, gets stronger and more distinctive over the first week, and appears to be modifiable by particular experiences with facial stimuli (Vanderwert et al., 2012, 2015). All of these response patterns involving face-to-face interactions arguably serve to facilitate efforts on the part of the infant to obtain and maintain physical contact with or proximity to its mother (Paukner et al., 2013).

Rhesus monkey mothers, in turn, provide their newborns with essential nourishment, physical and psychological warmth (e.g., Harlow, 1958), and protection from the elements, potential predators, and even other members of the infant's immediate family (e.g., jealous older siblings). During this time, a strong and enduring social bond inevitably develops between mother and infant, a bond that is unique in terms of its exclusivity, constituent behavioral features, and ultimate duration. The attachment bond that a rhesus monkey infant typically develops with its mother is like no other social relationship it will ever experience during the rest of its life, except (in reciprocal form) when a female grows up to have infants of her own. For a male infant, this bond will last at least until puberty, whereas for a female, it will be maintained as long as mother and daughter are both alive (Suomi, 1995).

In their second month of life, most rhesus monkey infants start using their mother as a "secure base" from which to begin exploring their immediate physical and social environment. At this age, monkey infants are inherently curious (Harlow, 1953), and most attempt to leave their mother for brief periods as soon as they become physically capable of doing so. Mothers typically monitor these attempts quite closely, and they often physically restrain their infant's efforts—or retrieve them if they have wandered beyond arm's length—at the slightest sign of potential danger. Several studies (e.g., Hinde & White, 1974) have demonstrated that at this stage of infant development the mother is primarily responsible for maintaining mutual contact and/or proximity. With the emergence of social fear in the infant's emotional repertoire between 2 and 3 months of age—seemingly analogous to the appearance of "stranger anxiety" in 9- to 12-month-old human infants (Sackett, 1966; Suomi & Harlow, 1976)—this pattern reverses, and thereafter the infant is primarily responsible for inititating and maintaining proximity and physical contact with its mother. Once an infant monkey has become securely attached to its mother and begins to use her as an established base from which to make exploratory ventures toward stimuli that have caught its interest, it soon learns that if it becomes frightened or is otherwise threatened by the stimuli it has sought out, it can always run back to its mother, who usually is able to provide immediate safety and comfort via mutual ventral contract. Initiation of ventral contract with the mother has been shown to promote rapid decreases in the infant's hypothalamic–pituitary–adrenal (HPA) activity (as indexed by lowered plasma cortisol concentrations) and in sympathetic nervous system arousal (as indexed by reductions in heart rate), along with other physiological changes commonly associated with soothing (e.g., Gunnar, Gonzalez, Goodlin, & Levine, 1981; Mendoza, Smotherman, Miner, Kaplan, & Levine, 1978; Reite, Short, Seiler, & Pauley, 1981).

As they grow older, most monkey infants voluntarily spend increasing amounts of time at increasing distances from their mothers, apparently confident that they can return to their mother's protective care without interruption or delay should circumstances so warrant. The presence of their mother as a secure base clearly promotes exploration of their ever-expanding physical and social world (Dienske & Metz, 1977; Harlow et al., 1963; Simpson, 1979). On the other hand, some rhesus monkey infants develop less secure attachment relationships with their mothers, and their subsequent exploratory behavior becomes compromised (e.g., Arling & Harlow, 1967; McCormack, Sanchez, Bardi, & Maestripieri, 2006), consistent with Bowlby's observations regarding

human attachment relationships (e.g., Bowlby, 1969/1982, 1988), which I discuss later.

At approximately 3 months of age, monkey infants typically start developing distinctive social relationships with other members of their social group. Increasingly, these come to involve their peers—other infants of similar age and comparable physical, cognitive, and socioemotional capabilities. Following weaning (usually in the fourth and fifth months) and essentially until puberty (during the third or fourth year), play with peers represents the predominant social activity of young monkeys (Ruppenthal, Harlow, Eisele, Harlow, & Suomi, 1974; Suomi, 1979a). During this time social play becomes increasingly gender-specific and sex-segregated (i.e., males tend to play more with males, and females with females; Harlow & Lauersdorf, 1974). Play interactions with peers also become more and more behaviorally and socially complex, such that by the third year, the play bouts typically involve patterns of behavior that appear to simulate almost the entire range of adult social activity (e.g., Suomi & Harlow, 1976). By the time they reach puberty, most rhesus monkey juveniles have had ample opportunity to develop, practice, and perfect behavioral routines that will become crucial for normal functioning in adult life, especially patterns involved in reproduction and in dominance/aggressive interactions (Suomi, 1979b). Virtually all of these juveniles will also have maintained close ties with their mothers throughout their juvenile years (e.g., Berman, 1982).

The onset of puberty is associated with dramatic life transitions for both male and female rhesus monkeys, involving not only major hormonal alterations, pronounced growth spurts, and other obvious physical changes, but also major social changes for both sexes (Suomi, Rasmussen, & Higley, 1992). Males experience the most dramatic and serious social disruption: They typically leave their natal troop, severing all social ties not only with their mothers and other kin but also with all others in that troop. Most adolescent males soon join all-male "gangs," and after several months to a year, typically attempt to enter a different troop, usually composed entirely of individuals largely unfamiliar to them. Field studies have revealed substantial individual differences among these males in the timing of their emigration, in the basic strategies they follow in attempting to join other established social groups, and in their ultimate success or failure in these efforts (Howell et al., 2007; Mehlman et al., 1995). It is clearly a time of great risk for most of them. Adolescent females, by contrast, almost never leave their maternal family or natal social group (Lindburg, 1971). Puberty for them is instead associated with increases in social activities directed toward maternal kin, typically at the expense of interaction with unrelated peers. Rhesus monkey females continue to be involved in family social affairs for the rest of their lives, even after they cease having infants of their own. Thus, their experiences with specific attachment relationships tend to be lifelong (Suomi, 1998).

## Unique Aspects of Primate Infant–Mother Attachment Relationships

Is infant–mother attachment fundamentally different from the other social relationships a young rhesus monkey (or, for that matter, a human infant) will establish during its lifetime? Clearly, some aspects of the attachment relationship are exclusive to the mother–infant dyad because the mother is the exclusive source of not only for all that passes through the placenta but also a prenatal environment uniquely attuned to her own circadian and other biological rhythms. In addition, there is increasing evidence of predictable fetal reactions that can be traced to specific activities (including vocalizations) of the mother, perhaps providing the basis for exclusive multimodal protocommunication between mother and fetus (e,g., Busnell & Granier-Deferre, 1981; DeCasper & Fifier, 1980; Fifer, 1987; Novak & Stuart, 2007; Schneider, 1992). Such types of prenatal stimulation are, of course, routinely (and exclusively) provided by pregnant females in all placental mammalian species.

Some of these unique aspects of maternal support and stimulation are basically continued into an infant's initial postnatal weeks and months, including, obviously, the mother's status as the primary (if not sole) source of its nutrition. Mothers also keep sharing their own specific antibodies with their infants postnatally via the nursing process. Moreover, the essentially continuous contact or proximity between a mother and her newborn provides the infant with extended exposure to its mother's odor, taste (of milk, at least; see Dettmer, Woodward, & Suomi, 2015), relative warmth, sound, and sight, representing a range and intensity of social stimulation seldom, if ever, provided by any other family or group members. In addition, rhesus monkey mothers continue to communi-

cate their internal circadian and other biological rhythms to their offspring via extended ventral–ventral contact, and there is some evidence that their offspring typically develop synchronous parallel rhythms during their initial weeks of life (Boyce, Champoux, Suomi, & Gunnar, 1995). As before, these maternally specific postnatal aspects of infant support and stimulation are not limited to primates but instead are characteristic of mothers in many other mammalian species, at least until the time of weaning (e.g., Hofer, 1995). But other aspects of a rhesus monkey mother's relationship with her infant are not shared by all mammalian mothers, not even by mothers of some other primate species.

What are these unique features of a rhesus monkey (and human) mother's relationship with her infant? It turns out that they are the very characteristics that Bowlby made the defining features of maternal attachment: (a) the mother's ability to reduce fear in her infant via direct social contact and other soothing behavior, and (b) the mother's capacity to provide a secure base to support her infant's exploration of the environment. Numerous longitudinal studies of rhesus monkey social ontogeny, carried out in both laboratory and field environments, have consistently found that mothers have a virtual monopoly on these capabilities—or at least the opportunity to express them with their infants (e.g., Berman, 1982; Ferrari, Paukner, Ionica, & Suomi, 2009; Harlow & Harlow, 1965). Thus, rhesus monkey infants rarely, if ever, use other group members (even close relatives) as secure bases, or even as reliable sources of ventral contact (Suomi, 1979a). Moreover, on those occasions when they "mistakenly" seek the company of someone other than their own mother, they are unlikely to experience decreases in physiological arousal comparable to those resulting from contact with their mother; instead, they are likely to experience *increases* in arousal.

The attachment relationship a rhesus monkey infant establishes with its mother differs in additional fundamental ways from all other social relationships it will ever develop during its lifetime. Although, as previously noted, rhesus monkeys routinely establish a host of distinctive relationships with different siblings, peers, and adults of both sexes throughout development, each of these relationships is strikingly different from the initial attachment they establish to their mother in terms of primacy, constituent behaviors, reciprocity, and course of developmental change (Suomi, 1979a, 2002). Given these findings, perhaps Bowlby was not entirely correct when he argued that the infant's attachment to the mother provides the *prototype* for all of its subsequent social relationships (Bowlby, 1969/1982) because, at least for rhesus monkeys, the relationship an infant establishes with its mother is like no other. On the other hand, Bowlby was absolutely correct (at least for rhesus monkeys) when he argued that the nature of the specific attachment relationship an infant develops with its mother can profoundly affect both concurrent and future relationships the infant may develop with others in its social sphere, as I discuss in detail later.

A somewhat different issue concerns the question of whether attachment phenomena as Bowlby originally defined them generalize to other species, including other primates. As outlined earlier, Bowlby clearly believed that basic features of attachment phenomena are essentially homologous in rhesus monkey infants and human babies, but are these characteristic features of attachment seen in other mammalian species as well? It all depends on how one defines *attachment,* or related terms such as *partner preference* or *imprinting.*

Without question, infant preference for the mother (and vice versa) represents an exceedingly ubiquitous phenomenon across most mammalian and avian species, as well as in numerous other taxa (Wilson, 1975). One specific (and, for Bowlby, a particularly relevant) form of partner preference involves *imprinting.* According to Lorenz's (1937) classical definition, imprinting is restricted to those partner preferences that are (1) acquired during a critical period, (2) irreversible, (3) generally species-specific, and (4) typically established prior to any behavioral manifestation of the preference. According to a slightly broadened version of this definition, imprinting-like phenomena can be observed in numerous insect, fish, avian, and mammalian species, including most, if not all, primates (Immelmann & Suomi, 1981).

On the other hand, it can be argued that infant–mother attachment as Bowlby (1958, 1969/1982) originally defined it represents a special case of imprinting that may itself be limited largely to Old World monkeys, apes, and humans (Suomi, 1995). To be sure, infants of all the other primate species (i.e., prosimians and New World monkeys) are initially at least as dependent on their mothers for survival, and spend at least as much time in physical contact with them, as do rhesus monkey (and human) infants (Higley & Suomi, 1986). In these other primate species, however, the predominant form of mother–infant physical contact is usually different (dorsal–ventral vs. ventral–ventral); the frequency and diversity of mother–infant interactions are generally reduced; the patterns of developmental change are also different (often dramatically so); and, most importantly, the specific defining features of attachment are largely absent.

Consider the case of capuchin monkeys (*Cebus apella,* a.k.a. *Sapajus libidinosus*), a highly successful New World species whose natural habitat covers much of South America, including both Amazonian and Andean regions. These primates are remarkable in many respects, not the least of which is an amazing capability for manufacturing and using tools to manipulate their physical environment both in captivity and in their natural habitats (Darwin, 1794; Visalberghi, 1990; Visalberghi et al., 2007). In this respect they are probably superior to rhesus monkeys and, for that matter, all other primates except humans and perhaps chimpanzees. On the other hand, capuchin mother–infant relationships seem somewhat primitive by rhesus monkey standards.

A capuchin monkey infant spends virtually all of its first 3 months of life clinging to its mother's back, moving ventrally only during nursing bouts (Welker, Becker, Hohman, & Schafer-Witt, 1987). During this time there is very little visual, vocal, or grooming interaction between mother and infant, in marked contrast to rhesus monkey infants, who by 1 month of age are already actively interacting with their mother in extensive one-on-one bouts involving a wealth of visual, auditory, olfactory, tactile, and vestibular stimulation, and who typically are already beginning to use their mother as a secure base. When capuchin monkeys finally get off their mother's backs in their fourth month, they seem to be surprisingly independent and can spend long periods away from their mother without getting visibly upset. If frightened, they are almost as likely to seek protective contact from other group members as from their mothers (Byrne & Suomi, 1995). At this age and thereafter, capuchin monkey youngsters spend only about one third as much time grooming their mother as do rhesus, and their other activities with her are not markedly different from their activities with siblings, peers, or unrelated adults (Byrne & Suomi, 1995; Welker, Becker, & Schafer-Witt, 1990), which is in sharp contrast to rhesus monkeys of comparable age. All in all, capuchin monkey infants, compared to rhesus monkeys, seem far less attached to their biological mothers in terms of the prominence of the relationship, the relative uniqueness of constituent behaviors, and the nature and degree of secure-base-mediated exploration. One wonders how Bowlby's attachment theory might have looked if Hinde and Harlow had been studying capuchin rather than rhesus monkeys!

Comparative studies of infant–mother relationships in other New World monkey and prosimian species indicate that in most cases the relationships more closely resemble those of capuchin monkeys than those of rhesus monkeys (e.g., Fragaszy, Baer, & Adams-Curtis, 1991); in a few species (e.g., some marmosets and tamarins), the mother is not even an infant's primary caregiver (Higley & Suomi, 1986). To be sure, infants in all these primate species appear to be *imprinted* on their mothers, according to Lorenz's (1937) definition. However, attachment involves considerably more developmental complexity and reciprocity, especially with respect to secure-base phenomena, than do classical notions of imprinting. It can therefore be argued that, strictly speaking, attachment represents a special, *restricted* case of imprinting. Moreover, because infant–mother attachment is most apparent in humans and their closest phylogenetic kin, it may also represent a relatively recent evolutionary adaptation among primates (Suomi, 1995).

## Conflict in Rhesus Monkey Infant–Mother Relationships

The relationships that rhesus monkeys develop with their mothers over time involve many behavioral patterns that go beyond attachment phenomena per se (Hinde, 1976). Indeed, a rhesus monkey female is extensively involved in a wide variety of interactions with her mother virtually every day that both are alive (and a male is thus involved every day until adolescence). However, this does not mean that all of these interactions are uniformly positive and pleasant. To the contrary, conflicts between mothers and offspring are frequent and often predictable, if not inevitable, occurrences in everyday rhesus monkey social life.

Sociobiological theorists have long argued that although mothers and infants share many genes and (therefore) many long-term goals, their short-term interests are not always mutual; hence, periodic conflict is inevitable (Trivers, 1974). Regardless of the validity of this view, an obvious instance of parent–offspring conflict occurs for virtually every rhesus monkey infant at approximately 20 weeks of age, when its mother begins to wean it from her own milk to solid food. Whether this process begins because the mother "wants" her infant to cease nursing (so she can stop lactating, begin cycling, and be able to produce another offspring, as sociobiologists have proposed); because she "knows" that she cannot continue to produce enough milk to sustain her infant's rapidly growing energy requirements; or because her infant's erupting teeth make nursing increasingly uncomfortable is certainly open to question. What *is* clear is that weaning is almost always associated with significant changes in the basic nature of the infant's relationship with its mother, and those changes are seldom placid (e.g., Hinde & White, 1974).

Mothers, for their part, make increasingly frequent efforts to deny their infants access to their nipples, albeit with considerable variation in the precise form, timing, and intensity of their weaning behavior, ranging from the exquisitely subtle to what borders on abuse. Infants, on the other hand, dramatically increase their efforts to obtain and maintain physical contact with their mothers, even when nipple contact is not attainable. As with mothers, there is substantial variation in the nature, intensity, and persistence of the infants' efforts to prevent or at least delay the weaning process (Berman, Rasmussen, & Suomi, 1993). In virtually all cases, an infant's newfound preoccupation with maintaining maternal contact clearly inhibits its exploratory behavior, and noticeably alters and diminishes its interactions with peers (and often other kin) as well. Indeed, it usually takes a month or more (if at all) before those interaction patterns return to some semblance of normality (Hinde & White, 1974; Ruppenthal et al., 1974). Weaning therefore appears to undermine basic attachment security for the infant, perhaps permanently in some cases.

Postweaning "normality" for a young rhesus monkey seldom lasts for more than a few additional weeks before a second form of conflict with its mother typically arises. Most mothers return to reproductive receptivity at about the time their infants are 6–7 months old, at which point the mothers begin actively soliciting selected adult males for the next 2 or 3 months (rhesus monkeys are seasonal breeders in nature). Throughout this period, they may enter into consort relationships with several different males, typically lasting 1–3 days each. During this time, a female and her chosen partner usually leave the main body of the monkey troop for most (if not all) of the time they are together, often seeking relative seclusion to avoid harassment or other interruptions from other troop members (Manson & Perry, 1993). At the same time, a mother's offspring from the previous year's consort tends to be ignored, actively avoided, or even physically rejected by both the mother and her current mate (Berman, Rasmussen, & Suomi, 1994).

Not surprisingly, most rhesus monkey yearlings become quite upset in the face of such functional maternal separations; indeed, a few actually develop dramatic behavioral and physiological symptoms that parallel Bowlby's (1960, 1973) descriptions of separation-induced depression in human infants and young children (Suomi, 1995). Most of their cohorts likewise exhibit an initial period of intense protest following loss of access to their mothers but soon begin directing their attention elsewhere. Interestingly, female offspring "left behind" by their mothers during consorts tend to seek out other family members during their mothers' absence, whereas young males are more likely to increase interactions with peers while their mothers are away (Berman et al., 1994). These gender differences in the prototypical response to maternal separation at 6–7 months of age thus appear to presage the much more dramatic gender differences in life course that emerge during adolescence and continue throughout adulthood.

It would seem that a rhesus monkey mother would always have the upper hand in conflicts with her offspring during both weaning and breeding periods, given her great size and strength advantage over even the most persistent 5- to 7-month-old infant. A number of research findings, however, suggest that infants bring resources of their own into these conflicts. For example, Simpson, Simpson, Hooley, and Zunz (1981) reported that infants who remained in physical contact with their mothers more and explored less during the preweaning months were more likely to delay the onset of weaning by several weeks, and in some cases even to preempt their mothers' cycling during the normal breeding season; this pattern was especially clear for male infants. Berman and colleagues (1993) found that, in a semi-field environment, infants who achieved the most frequent nipple contacts with their mothers during the breeding season had mothers who were least likely to conceive, even if they entered into relationships with multiple consorts during that period. The end result in both cases was that these

infants could, by their own actions, "postpone" their mothers' next pregnancy for another year, thus gaining additional opportunities for unfettered access to her not shared by agemates whose mothers had become pregnant during the same period. In the process, such an infant was also able to postpone by at least a year the appearance of a new source of conflict—that of "rivalry" with the mother's next infant.

The birth of a new sibling has major consequences for a yearling rhesus monkey. From that moment on, the yearling's relationship with the mother is altered dramatically, especially with respect to attachment-related activities. No longer is a yearling the primary focus of its mother's attention. Instead, many of its attempts to use her as a source of security and comfort are often ignored or rebuffed, especially when its newborn sibling is nursing or merely clinging to the mother's ventrum (Suomi, 1982). Moreover, whenever the yearling tries to push its younger sibling off the mother, to obstruct its access to her, or to disrupt its activity when it moves away from her, the mother's most likely response is to physically punish the yearling quickly, without warning, and often with considerable severity. In contrast, the mother seldom, if ever, punishes the younger sibling when it interrupts the yearling's attempts to interact with her or otherwise disrupts the yearling's activities (Berman, 1992).

Thus, the arrival of a younger sibling inevitably alters the yearling's attachment relationship with its mother. This relationship generally continues to wane (i.e., proximity-seeking and secure-base exploratory behavior both diminish) throughout the rest of the childhood years, especially after the birth of each succeeding sibling. For males, the waning process continues into puberty, eventually culminating with their natal troop emigration, which effectively terminates any remnant of their relationship with their mothers. Although attachment-related activities likewise decline throughout childhood for females, the daughters tend to increase other forms of affiliative interaction with their mothers (e.g., mutual grooming bouts), most notably after they start having offspring of their own. Coincidentally, episodes involving obvious conflict with their mothers become increasingly frequent for both male and female offspring as they approach puberty; thereafter, any semblance of attachment-like behavior directed toward mothers is infrequent at best among daughters and, of course, impossible for sons once they have left their natal troop (Suomi, 1998).

## Factors Influencing Attachment Relationships in Rhesus Monkeys

Although Bowlby (1969/1982) believed that attachment has a strong biological basis and represents the product of evolutionary processes, he also observed that there is substantial variation among mother–infant dyads in fundamental aspects of their attachment relationships, and he recognized the potential developmental significance of such variation. Indeed, he lived to see his collaborator Mary Ainsworth's Strange Situation assessment paradigm become almost reified in its identification and characterization of different "patterns" (groups A, B, C, and, more recently, D) and even "subgroups" of human infant–mother attachment relationships (e.g., Ainsworth, Blehar, Waters, & Wall, 1978; Main & Solomon, 1986). Perhaps not surprisingly, there appears to be comparable variation in the attachment relationships formed by different rhesus monkey mother–infant dyads. Indeed, there exist compelling parallel examples in rhesus monkey attachment relationships to each of the major human attachment types, if not at least some of the subtypes (Higley & Suomi, 1989). Moreover, a substantial body of research has identified numerous factors that can significantly influence the nature and ultimate developmental trajectory of these different attachment relationships. Some of these influences derive from factors external to the mother-infant dyad, and others appear to be derived from specific behavioral and biological features of the mother and the infant themselves.

With respect to external factors, numerous studies carried out over the past half century have demonstrated that most rhesus monkey mothers are usually highly sensitive to those aspects of their immediate physical and social environment that pose a potential threat to their infants' well-being, and they appear to adjust their maternal behavior accordingly. Both laboratory and field studies have consistently shown that mothers from low-ranking families typically are much more restrictive of their infant's exploratory efforts than are mothers from high-ranking matrilines, whose maternal style tends to be more "laissez-faire" (e.g., Fairbanks, 1996). The standard interpretation of these findings has been that low-ranking mothers risk reprisal from others if they try to intervene whenever their infants are threatened, so they minimize such risk by restricting their infants' exploration. High-ranking mothers usually

have no such problem and hence can afford to let their infants explore as they please (Suomi, 1998). Other studies have found that mothers generally become more restrictive and increase their levels of infant monitoring when their immediate social environment becomes less stable, such as when major changes in dominance hierarchies take place or when a new male joins the social group (Fairbanks, 1989). They also tend to monitor their infant's social activities with peers more closely and become more restrictive with respect to the range of social partners with whom they allow their infants to interact as the size of their troop increases (Berman, Rasmussen, & Suomi, 1997). For those infants whose opportunities to explore and to interact with peers are chronically limited during their first few months of life, their ability to develop species-normative relationships with others in their social group (especially peers) can be compromised, often with long-term consequences for both the infants and the troop itself (Suomi, 1999).

Changes in various aspects of the physical environment, such as the food supply becoming less predictable, have also been associated with alterations in the day-to-day relationships between monkey mothers and their infants, with significant short-term and surprising long-term consequences for the infants as they mature. In a series of landmark studies with bonnet macaques (*Macaca radiata*), Rosenblum and his colleagues (e.g., Rosenblum & Paully, 1984) developed a laboratory procedure that provided for experimental manipulation of the amount of time and effort a mother must spend to obtain the nutrition needed to satisfy her own and her infant's daily needs, specifically, a low-foraging demand (LFD) condition in which food is available *ab lib* and a high-foraging demand (HFD) condition in which the mother must spend several hours each day to obtain equivalent nutrition for both her infant and herself, but for which there is no food deprivation per se). These researchers found that although there were no major differences among bonnet macaque infants reared under either condition, there were profound consequences for infants whose mothers experienced a *shift* in foraging conditions (e.g., from LFD to HFD and back) every 2 weeks, a condition termed variable foraging demand (VFD) condition, even if this condition was in place for only a period of 12 weeks. They observed major changes in the amount of time and the manner in which the mothers interacted with their infants during VFD periods, largely due to changes in the way the mothers were interacting with each other within their social group (Andrews & Rosenblum, 1991). The end result was that the attachment relationships of VFD mothers and infants became less secure (Andrews & Rosenblum, 1993).

Offspring raised by VDF mothers exhibited persistent effects of this experience when compared with those raised either in the LDF or HDF conditions only. As juveniles they showed less social affiliation, greater affective withdrawal, and more subordinate behavior toward others in their social group (Andrews & Rosenblum, 1994; Rosenblum, Forger, Noland, Trost, & Coplan, 2001). They also exhibited a different profile of HPA activity, with higher cerebrospinal fluid (CSF) concentrations of corticotropin-releasing factor (CRF) but, interestingly, lower CRF concentrations of cortisol than did non-VFD subjects, not only as infants immediately following the VFD manipulation (as did their mothers) but actually continuing well into adulthood (Coplan et al., 1996; Matthew et al., 2002). Interestingly, these VDF effects on offspring HPA activity patterns were significantly less pronounced for offspring of socially dominant mothers. Moreover, these effects were not limited to the HPA system: Infants whose mothers experienced VFD also had significantly higher CSF levels of 5-hydroxyindoleacetic acid (5-HIAA; the primary central serotonin metabolite), somatostatin, and homovanillic acid (HVA; the primary central dopamine metabolite) than did those whose mothers experienced only the LFD condition (Coplan et al., 1998). Significant VDF–LDV differences were also found in growth hormone levels and in several measures of immune response that also persisted into adulthood (Coplan et al., 2000). In summary, these findings clearly indicate that environmental factors that fall short of what might be characterized as truly traumatic in nature but are sufficient to alter attachment relationships between a mother monkey and her infant can have profound and long-lasting consequences not only for the infant's subsequent behavioral and emotional development but also for the functioning of a variety of biological systems throughout its ontogeny and beyond.

## Individual Differences in Infant-Mother Relationships

Numerous other studies have shown that differences among monkey mothers' characteristic maternal "style" can also affect the type of attachment relationships they develop with their offspring, even when they are living in the same physical and social–environmental settings. Although a comprehensive review of the relevant literature is beyond the scope of this chapter, it is worth noting that most primate females tend to be remarkably consistent in the specific manner in which they rear their infants, at least after their initial pregnancy (Higley & Suomi, 1986; Suomi, 1987). It is also worth noting that some of the differences one can observe among monkey mothers' respective maternal styles can be related to specific temperamental characteristics they displayed as infants, as well as the nature of the attachment relationship they formed with their own mothers (e.g., Champoux, Byrne, Delizio, & Suomi, 1992; Suomi, 1995, 1999; Suomi & Ripp, 1983).

It is now apparent that differences in maternal style can have major and lasting consequences for not only for the attachments their offspring develop to them but also, as in the case of external environmental influences described earlier, their offspring's behavioral and biological functioning throughout life. One of the most dramatic examples of the effects of differential maternal style comes from the work of Maestripieri and his colleagues at the Yerkes National Primate Center field facility near Atlanta, where large breeding groups of rhesus monkeys are maintained in outdoor corrals. These investigators observed that successive generations of females in several long-standing matrilines maintained in this setting physically abuse most of their offspring to a degree not seen in other families. Most of the abuse occurs during their infant's first month of life and is rarely seen after the third month (Maestripieri, McCormack, Higley, Lindell, & Sanchez, 2006). In addition, these abusive mothers also tend to exhibit unusually high levels of infant rejection (i.e., preventing their infant from obtaining ventral or nipple contact, or pushing it away if such contact has been already established) and these high rates of rejection continue long after all incidents of abuse have ceased (McCormack et al., 2006). Thus, for females living in these families, high levels of infant neglect and abuse appear to be the norm rather than the exception across successive generations of mothers.

Such extreme styles of maternal care are not without behavioral and biological consequences for infants growing up in these matrilines. The maternally abused and neglected infants exhibit much higher rates of screams, tantrums, and other behavioral indices of obvious distress throughout their first 6 months of life, long after they are no longer being physically abused, than do offspring of nonabusive mothers. They also appear to become much more emotionally reactive than their nonabused agemates, including delayed independence from their mothers, less environmental exploration, and much lower levels of social play during this same developmental period (McCormack et al., 2006). In addition, as was the case for monkey infants whose mothers were exposed to VFD conditions during their initial 6 months, physically abused infants exhibit deviations from the normative pattern of HPA activity and central serotonin metabolism shown by nonabused infants, and these aberrant patterns continue well into the juvenile years, if not beyond. However, it appears that the nature of these deviations is quite different from that seen in VFD infants: Maltreated infants exhibit unusually high levels of HPA reactivity in their first month, but thereafter, HPA reactivity appears to be blunted relative to that of nonabused infants, and abused infants have significantly *lower* CSF concentrations of 5-HIAA, exactly the opposite of infants growing up under VFD conditions (Maestripieri et al., 2006; Sanchez, 2006). Moreover, it has now been well documented that a high proportion of females who experienced such abuse and rejection by their mothers early in life grow up to be maltreating mothers themselves (Maestripieri & Carroll, 1998). These and other findings clearly support the proposition that individual differences in maternal style, including attachment-related activities, among rhesus monkey mothers can have profound consequences for the behavioral and biological functioning of their offspring throughout development, especially when the differences are extreme. (For discussion of precursors of individual differences of attachment in humans, see Fearon & Belsky, Chapter 14, this volume.)

## The Role of Infant Temperament

Finally, variance in rhesus monkey attachment relationships may come in part from differences among infant monkeys' temperamental characteristics and the physiological processes that underlie their behavioral expression early in life. Researchers studying rhesus and other monkey species in both laboratory and field settings have long recognized developmentally stable individual differences along certain temperamental dimensions.

One dimension involves relative *fearfulness*, as reflected by individual differences in prototypical behavioral and biological responses to environmental novelty and/or challenge. Some monkey infants consistently respond to such mildly stressful situations with obvious behavioral expressions of fear and anxiety, as well as significant (and often prolonged) cortisol elevations, unusually high and stable heart rates, and dramatic increases in norepinephrine metabolism (e.g., Capitanio, Rasmussen, Snyder, Laudenslager, & Reite, 1986; Clarke & Boinski, 1995; Kalin & Shelton, 1989; Suomi, 1981, 1991; Suomi, Kraemer, Baysinger, & Delizio, 1981). These distinctive behavioral and physiological features appear early in infancy; they show remarkable interindividual stability throughout development; and there is increasing evidence that they are highly heritable (Dettmer & Suomi, 2014; Higley et al., 1993; Williamson et al., 2003).

One consequence of these behavioral and biological proclivities is that such "high-reactive" infants tend to spend more time with their mothers and less time with peers during their initial weeks and months of life. High-reactive young monkeys are also more likely to exhibit depressive-like reactions to functional maternal separations during the breeding season, as described earlier, than the rest of their birth cohort (Berman et al., 1994; Suomi, 1995). On the other hand, a high-reactive infant may ultimately be more "successful" than others in its peer group in postponing its mother's next pregnancy and, eventually, a new sibling rival for her attention (Berman et al., 1993; Simpson et al., 1981; Suomi, 1998). These and other findings provide impressive evidence that temperamental reactivity on the part of the infant can influence, if not substantially alter, fundamental aspects of its relationship with its mother throughout development.

Another temperamental dimension for which there are obvious individual differences among rhesus monkey infants is relative impulsivity, especially in social settings in which inappropriately impulsive behavior often leads to aggressive exchanges. This temperamental pattern is most readily apparent in peer play interactions. Impulsive males in particular seem unable to moderate their behavioral responses to rough-and-tumble play initiations from peers, instead escalating initially benign play bouts into full-blown, tissue-damaging aggressive exchanges, disproportionately at their own expense (Higley, Chaffin, & Suomi, 2011; Higley, Suomi, & Linnoila, 1996). Prospective longitudinal studies have shown that individuals that develop such response patterns typically exhibit poor state control and significant deficits in visual orienting capabilities during their first month of life (Champoux, Suomi, & Schneider, 1994). They also tend to exhibit chronically low rates of central serotonin metabolism, a prominent inhibitory neurotransmitter implicated in ubiquitous aspects of metabolic, regulatory, and emotional functioning (Coccaro & Murphy, 1990). In particular, impulsive and aggressive monkeys consistently have lower CSF 5-HIAA than their peers throughout development (e.g., Champoux, Higley, & Suomi, 1997; Higley, King, et al., 1996; Higley & Suomi, 1996; Mehlman et al., 1994; Shannon et al., 2005). As is the case for high reactivity, these behavioral and biological characteristics of impulsive aggression are remarkably stable throughout development, and they appear to be highly heritable (Higley et al., 1993; Higley & Suomi, 1996).

Highly impulsive rhesus monkeys typically develop difficult attachment relationships with their mothers. They seem to be unusually fussy in their initial weeks (reflecting their generally poor state control; see Champoux et al., 1994), and their conflicts with their mother intensify substantially during and shortly after the time of weaning (Suomi, 1998). As they grow older, highly impulsive youngsters usually continue to exhibit difficulties in their social interactions with their mothers, with peers, and with others in their social group, and these social problems generally carry over into adolescence and adulthood—and sometimes into the next generation (Higley & Suomi, 1996; Higley et al., 2011; Suomi, 2006). (For discussion of attachment and temperament in humans, see Vaughn & Bost, Chapter 10, this volume.)

## Effects of Differential Attachment Relationships on Long-term Developmental Trajectories for Rhesus Monkeys

Although considerable evidence from both field and laboratory studies has shown that individual differences among rhesus monkeys in certain temperamental characteristics tend to be quite stable from infancy to adulthood and are at least in part heritable, this does not mean that these behavioral and physiological features are necessarily fixed at birth or are immune to subsequent environmen-

tal influence. On the contrary, an increasing body of evidence from laboratory studies has demonstrated that prototypical behavioral and biological response patterns can be modified substantially by certain early experiences, especially those involving attachment relationships. This is perhaps most clearly illustrated by the results of experimental studies in which monkey infants have been separated from their biological mother at or shortly after birth and reared in the presence of other monkeys, species, or a variety of animate or inanimate objects. In most of these circumstances, rhesus monkey infants readily develop Bowlby-like attachments with whomever or whatever might be available, although some potential attachment objects are clearly preferred to others. The classic case is Harlow's (1958) seminal studies involving cloth- and wire-covered surrogates that Bowlby found so compelling (e.g., Bowlby, 1969/1982), but there have been many others. Over the years rhesus monkey infants have been reported to become attached to unrelated adult female conspecifics, adult male conspecifics, adult females from other primate species, dogs, cats, hobby horses, and a range of variations on the original Harlow cloth surrogate (e.g., Dettmer & Suomi, 2014; Mason & Gerson, 1975). Mason & Kenney, 1978; Redican & Mitchell, 1973). It is clearly in their nature to become attached, but attachments with these different classes of individuals and objects often have vastly different consequences, especially for different infants.

One extensive set of studies has focused on rhesus monkey infants raised with peers instead of their biological mothers. Infants in these studies were permanently separated from their biological mothers at birth; hand-reared in a neonatal nursery for their first weeks of life; housed with same-age, like-reared peers for the rest of their first 6–7 months; then moved into larger social groups containing both peer-reared and mother-reared agemates. During their initial months, these infants readily developed strong social attachment bonds to each other, much as mother-reared infants develop attachments to their own mothers (Harlow, 1969). However, perhaps because peers are not nearly as effective as typical monkey mothers in reducing fear in the face of novelty, or in providing a secure base for exploration, the attachment relationships that these peer-reared infants developed were almost always dysfunctional in nature (Suomi, 1995). As a result, although peer-reared monkeys showed completely normal physical and motor development, their early exploratory behavior was somewhat limited. They seemed reluctant to approach novel objects, and they tended to be shy in initial encounters with unfamiliar peers (Suomi, 2006, 2011).

Even when peer-reared youngsters interacted with their same-age cagemates in familiar settings, their emerging social play repertoires were usually retarded in frequency, intensity, and complexity. One explanation for their relatively poor play performance is that their cagemates had to serve as both attachment figures and playmates, a dual role that neither mothers nor mother-reared peers have to fulfill. Another explanation is that they faced difficulties in developing sophisticated play repertoires with basically incompetent play partners. Perhaps as a result of either or both of these factors, peer-reared youngsters typically dropped to the bottom of their respective dominance hierarchies when they were grouped with mother-reared monkeys their own age (Higley, King, et al., 1996).

Several prospective longitudinal studies have found that peer-reared monkeys consistently exhibit more extreme behavioral, HPA axis, and other neurochemical reactions to social separations than do their mother-reared cohorts, even after they have been living in the same social groups for extended periods (Higley & Suomi, 1989; Shannon, Champoux, & Suomi, 1998). Such differences in prototypical behavioral reactions to separation persist from infancy to adolescence, if not beyond. Interestingly, the separation reactions of peer-reared monkeys seem to mirror those that occur naturally in high-reactive mother-reared subjects. In this sense, early rearing by peers appears to have the effect of making rhesus monkey infants generally more high-reactive than they might have been if reared by their biological mothers (Suomi, 1997).

Early peer-rearing has another long-term developmental consequence for rhesus monkeys: It tends to make them more impulsive, especially if they are males. Peer-reared males initially exhibit aggressive tendencies in the context of juvenile play; as they approach puberty, the frequency and severity of their aggressive episodes typically exceeds those of mother-reared group members of similar age. Peer-reared females tend to groom (and be groomed by) others in their social group less frequently and for shorter durations than their mother-reared counterparts, and, as noted earlier, they usually stay at the bottom of their respective dominance hierarchies (Higley, King, et al., 1996; Higley et al., 2011). These differences between peer-reared and mother-reared

agemates in aggression, grooming, and dominance remain relatively robust throughout the preadolescent and adolescent years (Higley, Suomi, et al., 1996). Peer-reared monkeys also consistently show lower CSF concentrations of 5-HIAA than their mother-reared counterparts. These group differences in 5-HIAA concentrations appear well before 6 months of age, and they remain stable at least throughout adolescence and into early adulthood (Higley & Suomi, 1996; Shannon et al., 2005). Thus, peer-reared monkeys as a group resemble the impulsive subgroup of wild-living (and mother-reared) monkeys not only behaviorally but also in terms of decreased serotonergic functioning (Suomi, 1997).

Other laboratory studies of peer-reared monkeys have disclosed additional differences with their mother-reared counterparts, differences that are not readily apparent in free-ranging populations of rhesus monkeys. Peer-reared adolescent monkeys consistently consume larger amounts of alcohol under comparable ad lib conditions than their mother-reared agemates (Higley, Hasert, Suomi, & Linnoila, 1991; Higley et al., 2011). Recent follow-up studies have demonstrated that the peer-reared subjects quickly develop a greater tolerance for alcohol; this can be predicted by their central nervous system serotonin turnover rates, which in turn appear to be associated with differential serotonin transporter availability (Heinz et al., 1998). Peer-reared adolescent and adult males require larger doses of the anesthetic ketamine to reach a comparable state of sedation. They also exhibit significantly higher rates of whole-brain glucose metabolism under mild isoflurane anesthesia, as determined by positron emission tomography (PET) imaging, than mother-reared controls (Doudet et al., 1995). Additional studies involving PET imaging have reported that peer-reared juveniles have significantly lower levels of serotonin binding potential and cerebral blood flow in multiple brain regions than do their mother-reared counterparts (Ichise et al., 2006) and that there are rearing condition differences in serotonin I-A receptors in various brain regions as well (Spinelli et al., 2010). Structural magnetic resonance imaging (sMFI) studies comparing mother- versus peer-reared juveniles have revealed significant structural differences. For example, peer-reared subjects have an enlarged vermis, as well as larger dorsomedial prefrontal cortical and dorsal anterior cingulated cortical regions, which can be attributed to similar differences in early rearing conditions early in life (Spinelli, Chefer, Suomi, Barr,

& Stein, 2009). Thus, the development of early attachments to peers in the absence of the mother can have significant long-term consequences for monkeys at levels of not only behavioral expression and emotional regulation but also neuroendocrine function, neurotransmitter metabolism, drug sensitivity, and even brain structure and function. Long-term follow-up studies have revealed that some of these consequences persist well into adulthood (Corcoran et al., 2012). (For discussion of the developmental trajectories associated with individual differences in attachment in humans, see Thompson, Chapter 16, and Ehrlich, Miller, Jones, & Cassidy, Chapter 9, both in this volume.)

## Gene–Environment Interactions Involving Different Forums of Early Attachment Relationships

Clearly, a range of adverse early experiences, be they exposure to a mother dealing with the demands of a VFD environment, experience with an abusive and rejecting mother, or peer rearing in the absence of attachment opportunities with any adult, can have significant developmental consequences for individuals at multiple levels of analysis. It also seems apparent that heritable factors might influence individual developmental trajectories at one or more levels of analysis as well. But do these genetic and environmental factors operate separately, or do they interact in some fashion? Research over the past several years has demonstrated several significant *interactions* between specific genetic and experiential factors in shaping developmental trajectories for rhesus monkeys.

For example, the serotonin transporter gene (*5-HTT*), a candidate gene for impaired serotonergic function (Heils et al., 1996), has length variation in its promoter region that results in allelic variation in *5-HTT* expression. A heterozygous short allele (LS) confers low transcriptional efficiency to the *5-HTT* promoter relative to the homozygous long allele (LL), raising the possibility that low *5-HTT* expression may result in decreased serotonergic function (Lesch et al., 1996). Comparative studies have shown that rhesus monkeys possess a homologous serotonin transporter gene, as well as essentially the same allelic variation structurally and functionally (Lesch et al., 1997).

Several studies have now demonstrated that the consequences of having the LS allele differ dramatically for peer-reared monkeys and their mother-reared counterparts. For example, Champoux and colleagues (2002) examined the relation between early rearing history and *5-HTT* polymorphic status on measures of neonatal neurobehavioral development during the first month of life and found evidence of some sort of *maternal buffering*. Specifically, infants possessing the LS allele who were being reared in the laboratory neonatal nursery showed significant deficits in measures of attention, activity, and motor maturity relative to nursery-reared infants possessing the LL allele, whereas both LS and LL infants who were being reared by competent mothers exhibited normal values for each of these measures. One interpretation of this interaction is that effective mother-rearing, including the development of secure attachment relationships, appeared to *buffer* any potentially deleterious effects of the LS allele on these measures. Similarly, Bennett and colleagues (2002) found that CSF *5-HIAA* concentrations did not differ as a function of *5-HTT* status for securely attached mother-reared juvenile subjects, whereas among peer-reared juveniles, individuals with the LS allele had significantly lower CSF *5-HIAA* concentrations than those with the LL allele. Once again, mother rearing appeared to buffer any potentially deleterious effects of the LS allele on serotonin metabolism. A similar pattern appeared with respect to aggression: High levels of aggression were shown by peer-reared juveniles with the LS allele, whereas mother-reared LS monkeys exhibited low levels that were comparable to those of both mother-reared and peer-reared LL subjects, again suggesting a buffering effect of maternal rearing (Barr et al., 2003).

An even more dramatic pattern of gene–environment (G × E) interaction was revealed by an analysis of alcohol consumption data: Whereas peer-reared monkeys with the LS allele consumed more alcohol than peer-reared monkeys with the LL allele, the reverse was true for mother-reared subjects, with individuals possessing the LS allele actually showing relatively low levels of alcohol consumption (Barr et al., 2004). Similar evidence of maternal buffering with respect to differing patterns of alcohol response and consumption were reported by Schwandt and colleagues (2010). Here, the LS allele appeared to represent a significant *risk* factor for excessive alcohol consumption among monkeys with adverse early attachment experiences but a significant *protective* factor for mother-reared subjects, most of whom had experienced positive attachment experiences with their mother.

In summary, peer-reared monkeys with the LS allele displayed deficits in measures of neurobehavioral development during their initial weeks of life and reduced serotonin metabolism and excessive alcohol consumption as adolescents compared with those possessing the LL allele. In contrast, mother-reared subjects with the LS allele were characterized by normal early neurobehavioral development and serotonin metabolism, as well as reduced risk for excessive alcohol consumption later in life compared with their mother-reared counterparts with the LL allele. It could be argued on the basis of these findings that having the LS allele of the *5-HTT* gene may well lead to psychopathology among monkeys with adverse early rearing histories but actually be adaptive for monkeys who develop a secure early attachment to their mothers.

A parallel "maternal buffering" pattern of G × E interaction involving a polymorphism in the monoamine oxidase A (MAOA) gene was found for levels of aggressive behavior exhibited by mother-reared and peer-reared rhesus monkey juveniles; here, peer-reared subjects with the less functionally efficient MAOA allele had significantly higher levels of aggression than mother-reared subjects carrying the same allele and both mother- and peer-reared subjects carrying the more functionally efficient allele (Newman et al., 2005), essentially replicating findings reported for humans (e.g., Caspi et al., 2002). In addition, similar patterns of G × E interactions have been reported regarding functional polymorphisms in other rhesus monkey genes, including the corticotropin-releasing hormone (*CRH2A*) receptor gene (Barr et al., 2008), the neuropeptide Y (*NPY*) gene (Lindell et al., 2010), the *mu* opioid receptor (*OMRM1*) gene (Barr et al., 2008), the dopamine receptor *DRD1 5′UTR* gene (Newman et al., 2009), and the brain-derived neurotrophic factor (*BDNF*) receptor gene (Cirulli et al., 2009), among others, and a variety of behavioral and biological outcomes (e.g., Schwandt et al., 2011). For each of these "candidate" genes the significant G × E findings basically followed the same "maternal buffering" pattern (i.e., peer-reared monkeys carrying the functionally less efficient allele exhibited significant deficits relative to peer-reared subjects carrying the same allele), whereas peer-reared monkeys carrying the more efficient allele showed levels that were equivalent to, in a few cases, or

even better than those of mother-reared monkeys for most of the behavioral or biological measures that were the focus of each study.

The implications of these recent findings may be considerable with respect to the cross-generational transmission of these behavioral and biological characteristics in that, as previously mentioned, the particular attachment style of a monkey mother tends to be mirrored by her daughters when they grow up and become mothers themselves (Fairbanks, 1989; Maestripieri, 2005). If similar buffering is indeed experienced by the next generation of infants carrying, for example, the LS *5-HTT* polymorphism, then having had their own mothers develop a secure attachment relationship with them when they were infants may well provide the basis for a nongenetic means of transmitting its apparently adaptive consequences to that new generation. On the other hand, if contextual factors such as changes in dominance rank, instability within the troop, or changes in the availability of food were to alter a young mother's care of her infants in ways that compromised such buffering (e.g., Dettmer, Novak, Meyer, & Suomi, 2014; Dettmer et al., 2015), one might expect any offspring carrying the LS polymorphism to develop some, if not all, of the problems described earlier.

(For discussion of G × E interactions in humans in this volume, see Bakermans-Kranenburg & Van IJzendoorn, Chapter 8; Simpson & Belsky, Chapter 5; and Vaughn & Bost, Chapter 10.)

## Cross-Generational Consequences of Early Attachment Relationships: Implications for Human Attachment Theory

One of the most intriguing aspects of the long-term consequences of different early attachment experiences, especially in light of the speculation outlined earlier, is the apparent transfer of specific features of maternal behavior across successive generations. Several studies of rhesus monkeys and other Old World monkey species have demonstrated strong continuities between the type of attachment relationship a female infant develops with her mother and the type of attachment relationship she develops with her own infant(s) when she becomes a mother herself. In particular, the pattern of ventral contact a female infant has with her mother (or mother substitute) during her initial months of life is a powerful predictor of the pattern of ventral contact she will have with her own infants during their first 6 months of life (Champoux et al., 1992; Fairbanks, 1989, 1996). This predictive cross-generational relationship appears to be as strong in females who were foster-reared from birth by unrelated multiparous females as it is for females reared by their biological mothers. An even more impressive demonstration of cross-generational transmission of maternal characteristics comes from Maestripieri (2005), who cross-fostered female infants of abusive mothers to nonabusive multiparous females and also cross-fostered offspring of nonabusive mothers to unrelated females with a prior history of abuse. Maestripieri found that whereas approximately half of the female offspring of nonabusive mothers who were reared by abusive foster mothers grew up to be abusive toward their own offspring, *none* of the female offspring of abusive mothers who had nonabusive foster mothers subsequently abused their own infants! These findings clearly demonstrate that cross-generational transmission of at least some aspects of mother–infant attachment necessarily involves nongenetic mechanisms (cf. Suomi & Levine, 1998). What those nongenetic mechanisms might be, and through what developmental processes they might they act, are questions at the heart of extensive ongoing investigations, in particular those examining genomewide *epigenetic* changes contingent on different early social experiences (see Provencal et al., in press).

Two published studies investigated the effects of differences in early social rearing (mother rearing vs. a form of peer rearing) on genomewide patters of messenger RNA (mRNA) expression in leukocytes, and on methylation patterns in prefrontal cortex (PFC) and in T-cell lymphocytes, respectively. The research involving mRNA expression examined expression patterns in differentially reared 4-month-old infants. In all, 521 genes were significantly more expressed in mother-reared infants than in peer-reared infants, whereas the reverse was the case for another 717 genes. In general, peer-reared infants showed enhanced expression in genes involved in inflammation, T-lymphocyte activation and cell proliferation, and suppression of antiviral and antibacterial responses (Cole et al., 2012). Since that initial study, the same investigators have embarked on a prospective longitudinal study in which differentially reared subject were sampled at 14 days, 30 days, 6–7 months, and every 4 months thereafter, until they reached puberty. Data from that prospective longitudinal study are currently being analyzed.

The other study involved genomewide analyses of methylation patterns in differentially reared monkeys when they were adults. This study compared such patterns in PFC tissue and T-cell lymphocytes obtained from 8-year-old monkeys differentially reared for their initial 6–7 months of life and thereafter maintained under identical conditions until adulthood (Provencal et al., 2012). These analyses revealed that (1) more than 4,400 genes were differentially methylated in both PFC and lymphocytes; (2) although there was considerable tissue specificity, approximately 25% of the affected genes were identical in both PFC and lymphocytes; and (3) in both PFC and lymphocytes, methylated promoters tended to cluster both by chromosomal region and gene function. The same research team has since completed the data collection in a prospective longitudinal study of genomewide methylation patterns in lymphocytes, obtaining samples at exactly the same ages and from exactly the same monkeys as in the aforementioned longitudinal study of genomewide mRNA expression. Data from this second longitudinal study are also currently under analysis, although preliminary results have revealed that at least some of the massive rearing condition differences already present after the first month appear to be *reversible* during the second year after the original rearing conditions have been experimentally altered (Provencal et al., in press).

Proponents of human attachment theory have long focused on possible cross-generational continuities in attachment styles. Some authors have posited the likely existence of strong cross-generational continuities, such that mothers who experienced secure attachments when they were infants might tend to raise infants who are securely attached to them, whereas those who experienced avoidant or ambivalent attachments with their own mothers might tend to promote avoidant or ambivalent attachments as mothers themselves (e.g., Main, 1995). Moreover, current attachment theorists attribute these postulated infancy-to-parenthood continuities in attachment type to "internal working models" initially based on early memories and periodically transformed by more recent experience. Most of the empirical findings that have led to these hypotheses have come from comprehensive interviews of adults (e.g., with the Adult Attachment Interview) retrospectively probing memories of events and experiences. On the other hand, some of the most powerful empirical support for apparently parallel long-term continuities in attachment behavior from the nonhuman primate literature comes from prospective longitudinal observations and physiological recordings, both in controlled experimental settings and in naturalistic habitats, as reviewed earlier.

One insight that the nonhuman primate data bring to discussions about long-term consequences of early experiences is that strong developmental continuities can unfold *in the absence of language or complex imagery.* It is difficult to argue that rhesus monkeys, for example, possess sufficient cognitive capabilities to develop anything remotely analogous to human internal working models requiring considerable self-reflection, given that they are clearly not fully capable of human-like self-awareness or self-recognition (e.g., Gallup, 1977; Povinelli, Parks, & Novak, 1992). Given those restricted capabilities, what cognitive, emotional, and mnemonic processes might underlie these empirically documented behavioral continuities, and do they have any parallels in human nonverbal mental processes? (See Cassidy, Ehrlich, and Sherman [2013] for discussion of noncognitive mechanisms of links between early experience and later functioning in humans.)

Alternatively, one might argue that working models are *exclusively* human constructions that are built upon a basic foundation that is essentially biological in nature and universal among the more advanced primate species. According to this view, cognitive constructions per se may not be necessary for long-term developmental or cross-generational continuities in attachment phenomena to transpire. That is, such continuities are essentially "programmed" to occur in the absence of major environmental disruption and are in fact the product of strictly biological processes that reflect the natural evolutionary history of advanced primate species, human and nonhuman alike. If this is the case, then working models (or other comparable cognitive processes) scaffolded on existing basic biological foundations perhaps actually represent a "luxury" for humans that might enable individuals to reinforce cognitively those postulated underlying biological foundation, in which case the predicted developmental continuity might actually be strengthened.

On the other hand, the existence of a working model that has the potential to be *altered* by specific experiences (and/or insights) in late childhood, adolescence, or adulthood might provide a basis for breaking an otherwise likely continuity between one's early attachment experiences and subsequent performance as a parent (i.e., make it possible to break an otherwise likely cross-generational cycle), especially when one is confronted with a recurrent cycle of early adversity. These important issues deserve not only further theoretical consideration but also empirical investigation. As Bowlby (1988) himself said, "All of us, from cradle to the grave, are happiest when life is organized as a series of excursions, long or short, from the secure base provided by our attachment figure(s)" (p. 62). Research with nonhuman primates has clearly provided compelling evidence in support of a strong biological foundation for attachment-like phenomena. Indeed, such a foundation may well serve as a secure base for future excursions in the realm of attachment research.

## References

Ainsworth, M. D. S., Blehar, M., Waters, E., & Wall, S. (1978). *Patterns of attachment.* Hillsdale, NJ: Erlbaum.

Andrews, M. W., & Rosenblum, L. A. (1991). Security of attachment in infants raised in variable- or low-demand environments. *Child Development, 62,* 686–693.

Andrews, M. W., & Rosenblum, L. A. (1993). Assessment of attachment in differentially reared infant monkeys (*Macaca radiata*). *Journal of Comparative Psychology, 107,* 84–90.

Andrews M. W., & Rosenblum, L. A. (1994). The development of affiliative and agonistic patterns in differentially reared monkeys. *Child Development, 65,* 1398–1404.

Arling, G. L., & Harlow, H. F. (1967). Effects of social deprivation on maternal behavior of rhesus monkeys. *Journal of Comparative and Physiological Psychology, 64,* 371–377.

Barr, C. S., Dvoskin, R. L., Gupte, M., Sommer, W., Sun, H., Schwandt, M. L., et al. (2009). Functional CRH variation increases stress-induced alcohol consumption in primates. *Proceedings of the National Academy of Sciences, 106,* 14593–14598.

Barr, C. S., Newman, T. K., Becker, M. L., Parker, C. C., Champoux, M., Lesch, K. P., et al. (2003). The utility of the non-human primate model for studying gene by environment interactions in behavioral research. *Genes, Brain and Behavior, 2,* 336–340.

Barr, C. S., Newman, T. K., Lindell, S., Champoux, M., Lesch, K. P., Suomi, S. J., et al. (2004). Interaction between serotonin transporter gene variation and rearing condition in alcohol preference and consumption in female primates. *Archives of General Psychiatry, 61,* 1146–1152.

Barr, C. S., Schwandt, M. L., Lindell, S. G., Higley, J. D., Maestripieri, D., Goldman, D., et al. (2008). Variation at the mu-opioid receptor gene (OPRM1) influences attachment behavior in primates. *Pro-*

*ceedings of the National Academy of Sciences*, *105*, 5277–5281.

Bennett, A. J., Lesch, K. P., Heils, A., Long, J. C., Lorenz, J. G., Shoaf, S. E., et al. (2002). Early experience and serotonin transporter gene variation interact to influence primate CNS function. *Molecular Psychiatry*, *7*, 118–122.

Berman, C. M. (1982). The ontogeny of social relationships with group companions among free-ranging rhesus monkeys: I. Social networks and differentiation. *Animal Behavior*, *30*, 149–162.

Berman, C. M. (1992). Immature siblings and mother–infant relationships among free-ranging rhesus monkeys on Cayo Santiago. *Animal Behavior*, *44*, 247–258.

Berman, C. M., Rasmussen, K. L. R., & Suomi, S. J. (1993). Reproductive consequences of maternal care patterns during estrus among free-ranging rhesus monkeys. *Behavioral Ecology and Sociobiology*, *32*, 391–399.

Berman, C. M., Rasmussen, K. L. R., & Suomi, S. J. (1994). Responses of free-ranging rhesus monkeys to a natural form of maternal separation: I. Parallels with mother–infant separation in captivity. *Child Development*, *65*, 1028–1041.

Berman, C. M., Rasmussen, K. L. R., & Suomi, S. J. (1997). Group size, infant development, and social networks: A natural experiment with free-ranging rhesus monkeys. *Animal Behavior*, *53*, 405–421.

Bowlby, J. (1958). The nature of the child's tie to his mother. *International Journal of Psychoanalysis*, *39*(9), 350–373.

Bowlby, J. (1960). Separation anxiety. *International Journal of Psychoanalysis*, *41*, 89–113

Bowlby, J. (1973). *Attachment and loss*: Vol. 2. *Separation*. New York: Basic Books.

Bowlby, J. (1982). *Attachment and loss*: Vol. 1. *Attachment* (rev. ed.). New York: Basic Books. (Original work published 1969)

Bowlby, J. (1988). *A secure base*. New York: Basic Books.

Boyce, W. T., Champoux, M., Suomi, S. J., & Gunnar, M. R. (1995). Salivary cortisol in nursery-reared rhesus monkeys: Interindividual stability, reactions to peer interactions, and altered circadian rhythmicity. *Developmental Psychobiology*, *28*, 257–267.

Busnell, M.-C., & Granier-Deferre, C. (1983). And what of fetal audition? In A. Oliverio & M. Zappella (Eds.), *The behavior of human infants* (pp. 93–126). New York: Plenum.

Byrne, G. D., & Suomi, S. J. (1995). Activity patterns, social interaction, and exploratory behavior in *Cebus apella* infants from birth to 1 year of age. *American Journal of Primatology*, *35*, 255–270.

Capitanio, J. P., Rasmussen, K. L. R., Snyder, D. S., Laudenslager, M. L., & Reite, M. (1986). Long-term follow-up of previously separated pigtail macaques: Group and individual differences in response to unfamiliar situations. *Journal of Child Psychology and Psychiatry*, *27*, 531–538.

Caspi, A., McClay, J., Moffitt, T. E., Mill, J., Martin, J., Craig, I. W., et al. (2002). Role of genotype in the cycle of violence in maltreated children. *Science*, *297*, 851–854.

Cassidy, J., Ehrlich, K. B., & Sherman, L. J. (2013). Child–parent attachment and response to threat: A move from the level of representation. In M. Mikulincer & P. R Shaver (Eds.), *Nature and development of social connections: From brain to group* (pp. 125–144). Washington, DC: American Psychological Association.

Champoux, M., Bennett, A. J., Shannon, C., Higley, J. D., Lesch, K. P., & Suomi, S. J. (2002). Serotonin transporter gene polymorphism, differential early rearing, and behavior in rhesus monkey neonates. *Molecular Psychiatry*, *7*, 1058–1063.

Champoux, M., Byrne, E., Delizio, R. D., & Suomi, S. J. (1992). Motherless mothers revisited: Rhesus maternal behavior and rearing history. *Primates*, *33*, 251–255.

Champoux, M., Higley, J. D., & Suomi, S. J. (1997). Behavioral and physiological characteristics of Indian and Chinese-Indian hybrid rhesus macaque infants. *Developmental Psychobiology*, *31*, 49–63.

Champoux, M., Suomi, S. J., & Schneider, M. L. (1994). Temperamental differences between captive Indian and Chinese-Indian hybrid rhesus macaque infants. *Laboratory Animal Science*, *44*, 351–357.

Cirulli, F., Francia, N., Brachi, I., Antonucci, M., Aloe, L., Suomi, S. J., et al. (2009). Changes in plasma levels of BDNF and NGF reveal a gender-selective vulnerability to early adversity in rhesus macaques. *Psychoneuroendocrinology*, *34*, 172–180.

Clarke, A. S., & Boinski, S. (1995). Temperament in nonhuman primates. *American Journal of Primatology*, *37*, 103–125.

Coccaro, E. F., & Murphy, D. L. (1990). *Serotonin in major psychiatric disorders*. Washington, DC: American Psychiatric Press.

Cole, S. W., Conti, G., Arevalo, J. M., Ruggiero, A. M., Heckman, J. J., & Suomi, S. J. (2012). Transcriptional modulation of the developing immune system by early life social adversity. *Proceedings of the National Academy of Sciences USA*, *109*, 20578–20583.

Coplan, J. D., Andrews, M. W., Rosenblum, L. A., Owens, M. J., Friedman, S., Gorman, J. M., et al. (1996). Persistent elevations of cerebrospinal fluid concentrations of corticotropin-releasing factor in adult nonhuman primates exposed to early-life stressors: Implications for the pathophysiology of mood and anxiety disorders. *Proceedings of the National Academy of Sciences*, *93*, 1619–1623.

Coplan, J. D., Trost, R. C., Owens, M. J., Cooper, T. B., Gorman J. M., Nemeroff, C. B., et al. (1998). Cerebrospinal fluid concentrations of somatostatin and biogenic amines in grown primates reared by mothers exposed to manipulated foraging conditions. *Archives of General Psychiatry*, *55*, 473–477.

Coplan, J. D., Smith, E. L., Trost, R. E., Scharf, B. A., Altemus, M., Bjornson, J., et al. (2000). Growth hormone response to clonidine in adversely reared young adult primates: Relationship to serial cerebrospinal fluid corticotropin-relaeasing factor concentrations. *Psychiatric Research, 95*, 93–102.

Corcoran, C. A., Pierre, P. J., Haddad, T., Bice, C., Suomi, S. J., Grant, K. A., et al. (2012). Long-term effects of differential early rearing in rhesus macaques: Behavioral reactivity in adulthood. *Developmental Psychobiology, 55*, 546–555.

Darwin, E. (1794). *Zoonomia, or the laws of organic life.* London: Johnson.

DeCasper, A. J., & Fifer, W. P. (1980). Of human bonding: Newborns prefer their mother's voices. *Science, 208*, 1174–1176.

Dettmer, A. M., Murphy, A. M., Guitarra, D., Slonnacker, E., Rosenberg, K. L., Novak, M. A., et al. (in press). Cortisol in mother's milk predicts later infant social behavior and later cognitive functioning in rhesus monkeys. *Child Development.*

Dettmer, A. M., Novak, M. A., Meyer, J. S., & Suomi, S. J. (2014). Population density-dependent hair cortisol concentrations in rhesus monkeys (*Macaca mulatta*). *Psychoneuroendocrinology, 42*, 59–67.

Dettmer, A. M., & Suomi, S. J. (2014). Nonhuman primate models of neuro-psychiatric disorders: Influence of early experiences, genetics, and epigenetics. *ILAR Journal, 55*(2), 361–370.

Dettmer, A. M., Woodward, R. A., & Suomi, S. J. (2015). Reproductive consequences of a matrilineal overthrow in rhesus monkeys. *American Journal of Primatology, 77*, 347–352.

Dienske, H., & Metz, J. A. J. (1977). Mother–infant body contact in macaques: A time interval analysis. *Biology of Behaviour, 2*, 3–21.

Doudet, D., Hommer, D., Higley, J. D., Andreason, P. J., Moneman, R., Suomi, S. J., et al. (1995). Cerebral glucose metabolism, CSF 5-HIAA, and aggressive behavior in rhesus monkeys. *American Journal of Psychiatry, 152*, 1782–1787.

Fairbanks, L. A. (1989). Early experience and cross-generational continuity of mother–infant contact in vervet monkeys. *Developmental Psychobiology, 22*, 669–681.

Fairbanks, L. A. (1996). Individual differences in maternal style: Causes and consequences for mothers and offspring. *Advances in the Study of Behavior, 25*, 59–611.

Ferrari, P. F., Paukner, A., Ionica, C. S., & Suomi, S. J. (2009). Reciprocal face-to-face communication between rhesus macaque mothers and their newborn infants. *Current Biology, 19*, 1768–1772.

Ferrari, P. F., Visalberghi, E., Paukner, A., Fogassi, L., Ruggiero, A., & Suomi, S. J. (2006). Neonatal imitation in infant macaques. *PLoS Biology, 4*, 1501–1508.

Fifer, W. P. (1987). Neonatal preference for mother's voice. In N. A. Krasnagor, E. M. Blass, M. A. Hofer, & W. P. Smotherman (Eds.), *Perinatal development: A psychobiological perspective* (pp. 39–60). New York: Academic Press.

Fragaszy, D. M., Baer, J., & Adams-Curtis, L. (1991). Behavioral development and maternal care in tufted

capuchins (*Cebus apella*) and squirrel monkeys (*Saimiri sciureus*) from birth through seven months. *Developmental Psychobiology, 24*, 375–393.

Gallup, G. G. (1977). Self-recognition in primates: A comparative approach to the bidirectional properties of consciousness. *American Psychologist, 32*, 329–338.

Gunnar, M. R., Gonzalez, C. A., Goodlin, B. L., & Levine, S. (1981). Behavioral and pituitary–adrenal responses during a prolonged separation period in rhesus monkeys. *Psychoneuroendocrinology, 6*, 65–75.

Hansen, E. W. (1966). The development of maternal and infant behavior in the rhesus monkey. *Behaviour, 27*, 109–149.

Harlow, H. F. (1953). Mice, monkeys, men, and motives. *Psychological Review, 60*, 23–35.

Harlow, H. F. (1958). The nature of love. *American Psychologist, 13*, 673–685.

Harlow, H. F. (1969). Age-mate or peer affectional system. In D. S. Lehrman, R. A. Hinde, & E. Shaw (Eds.), *Advances in the study of behavior* (Vol. 2, pp. 333–383). New York: Academic Press.

Harlow, H. F., & Harlow, M. K. (1965). The affectional systems. In A. M Schrier, H. F. Harlow, & F. Stollnitz (Eds.), *Behavior of nonhuman primates* (Vol. 2, pp. 287–334). New York: Academic Press.

Harlow, H. F., Harlow, M. K., & Hansen, E. W. (1963). The maternal affectional system of rhesus monkeys. In H. L. Rheingold (Ed.), *Maternal behavior in mammals* (pp. 254–281). New York: Wiley.

Harlow, H. F., & Lauersdorf, H. E. (1974). Sex differences in passions and play. *Perspectives in Biology and Medicine, 17*, 348–360.

Harlow, H. F., & Suomi, S. J. (1970). The nature of love—simplified. *American Psychologist, 25*, 161–168.

Heils, A., Teufel, A., Petri, S., Stober, G., Riederer, P., Bengel, B., et al. (1996). Allelic variation of human serotonin transporter gene expression. *Journal of Neurochemistry, 6*, 2621–2624.

Heinz, A., Higley, J. D., Gorey, J. G., Saunders, R. C., Jones, D. W., Hommer, D., et al. (1998). *In vivo* association between alcohol intoxication, aggression, and serotonin transporter availability in nonhuman primates. *American Journal of Psychiatry, 155*, 1023–1028.

Higley, J. D., Chaffin, A. C., & Suomi, S. J. (2011). Impulsivity and aggression as personality traits in nonhuman primates. In A. Weiss & J. King (Eds.), *Primate personality and temperament* (pp. 257–284). New York: Springer.

Higley, J. D., Hasert, M. L., Suomi, S. J., & Linnoila, M. (1991). A new nonhuman primate model of alcohol abuse: Effects of early experience, personality, and stress on alcohol consumption. *Proceedings of the National Academy of Sciences, 88*, 7261–7265.

Higley, J. D., King, S. T., Hasert, M. F., Champoux, M., Suomi, S. J., & Linnoila, M. (1996). Stability of individual differences in serotonin function and its relationship to severe aggression and competent social behavior in rhesus macaque females. *Neuropsychopharmacology, 14*, 67–76.

Higley, J. D., & Suomi, S. J. (1986). Parental behaviour in primates. In W. Sluckin & M. Herbert (Eds.), *Parental behaviour in mammals* (pp. 152–207). Oxford, UK: Blackwell.

Higley, J. D., & Suomi, S. J. (1989). Temperamental reactivity in nonhuman primates. In G. A. Kohnstamm, J. E. Bates, & M. K. Rothbard (Eds.), *Handbook of temperament in children* (pp. 153–167). New York: Wiley.

Higley, J. D., & Suomi, S. J. (1996). Reactivity and social competence affect individual differences in reaction to severe stress in children: Investigations using nonhuman primates. In C. R. Pfeffer (Ed.), *Intense stress and mental disturbance in children* (pp. 3–58). Washington, DC: American Psychiatric Press.

Higley, J. D., Suomi, S. J., & Linnoila, M. (1996). A nonhuman primate model of Type II alcoholism?: Part 2. Diminished social competence and excessive aggression correlates with low CSF 5-HIAA concentrations. *Alcoholism: Clinical and Experimental Research, 20*, 643–650.

Higley, J. D., Thompson, W. T., Champoux, M., Goldman, D., Hasert, M. F., Kraemer, G. W., et al. (1993). Paternal and maternal genetic and environmental contributions to CSF monoamine metabolites in rhesus monkeys (*Macaca mulatta*). *Archives of General Psychiatry, 50*, 615–623.

Hinde, R. A. (1976). On describing relationships. *Journal of Child Psychology and Psychiatry, 17*, 1–19.

Hinde, R. A., Rowell, T. E., & Spencer-Booth, Y. (1964). Behavior of socially living monkeys in their first six months. *Proceedings of the Zoological Society of London, 143*, 609–649.

Hinde, R. A., & Spencer-Booth, Y. (1967). The behaviour of socially living rhesus monkeys in their first two and a half years. *Animal Behaviour, 15*, 169–176.

Hinde, R. A., & White, L. E. (1974). Dynamics of a relationship: Rhesus mother–infant ventro–ventro contact. *Journal of Comparative and Physiological Psychology, 86*, 8–23.

Hofer, M. A. (1995). Hidden regulators: Implications for a new understanding of attachment, separation, and loss. In S. Goldberg, R. Muir, & J. Kerr (Eds.), *Attachment theory: Social, developmental, and clinical perspectives* (pp. 203–230). Hillsdale, NJ: Analytic Press.

Howell, S., Westergaard, G. C., Hoos, B., Chavanne, T. J., Shoaf, S. E., Cleveland, A., et al. (2007). Serotonergic influences on life-history outcomes in free-ranging male rhesus macaques. *American Journal of Primatology, 69*, 851–865.

Ichise, M., Vines, D. C., Gura, T., Anderson, G. M., Suomi, S. J., Higley, J. D., et al. (2006). Effects of early life stress on [¹¹C] DABS PET imaging of serotonin transporters in adolescent peer- and mother-reared rhesus monkeys. *Journal of Neuroscience, 26*, 4638–4643.

Immelmann, K., & Suomi, S. J. (1981). Sensitive phases in development. In K. Immelmann, G. W. Barlow, L.

Petrinovich, & M. Main (Eds.), *Behavioral development: The Bielefeld Project* (pp. 395–431). New York: Cambridge University Press.

Kalin, N. H., & Shelton, S. E. (1989). Defensive behaviors in infant rhesus monkeys: Environmental cues and neurochemical regulation. *Science, 243*, 11718–11721.

Lesch, K. P., Bengel, D., Heils, A., Sabol, S. Z., Greenberg, B. D., Petri, S., et al. (1996). Association of anxiety-related traits with a polymorphism in the serotonin transporter gene regulatory region. *Science, 274*, 1527–1531.

Lesch, K. P., Meyer, J., Glatz, K., Flugge, G., Hinney, A., Hebebrand, J., et al. (1997). The 5-HT transporter gene-linked polymorphic region (*5-HTTLPR*) in evolutionary perspective: Alternative biallelic variation in rhesus monkeys. *Journal of Neural Transmission, 104*, 1259–1266.

Lindburg, D. G. (1971). The rhesus monkey in north India: An ecological and behavioral study. In L. A. Rosenblum (Ed.), *Primate behavior: Developments in field and laboratory research* (Vol. 2, pp. 1–106). New York: Academic Press.

Lindell, S. G., Schwandt, M. L., Sun, H., Sparenborg, J., Bjoerk, K., Kasckow, J. W., et al. (2010). Functional *NPY* variation as a factor in stress resilience and alcohol consumption in rhesus macaques. *Archives of General Psychiatry, 67*, 423–431.

Lorenz, K. (1937). Der Kumpan in der Ümwelt des Vogels [The sidekick in the environment of the bird]. *Journal für Ornithologie, 83*, 137–213, 289–413.

Main, M. (1995). Recent studies in attachment: Overview, with selected implications for clinical work. In S. Goldberg, R. Muir, & J. Kerr (Eds.), *Attachment theory: Social, developmental, and clinical perspectives* (pp. 407–474). Hillsdale, NJ: Analytic Press.

Main, M., & Solomon, J. (1986). Discovery of a new, insecure disorganized/disoriented attachment pattern. In T. B. Brazelton & M. Yogman (Eds.), *Affective development in infancy* (pp. 95–124). Norwood, NJ: Ablex.

Maestripieri, D. (2005). Early experience affects the intergenerational transmission of infant abuse in rhesus monkeys. *Proceedings of the National Academy of Sciences, 102*, 9726-9729.

Maestripieri, D., & Carroll, K. A. (1998). Risk factors for infant neglect and abuse in group-living rhesus monkeys. *Psychological Science, 9*, 143–145.

Maestripieri, D., McCormack, K. M., Higley, J. D., Lindell, S. G., & Sanchez, M. M. (2006). Influence of parenting style and offspring behavior and CSF monoamine metabolites in cross-fostered and noncrossfostered rhesus macaques. *Brain and Behavioral Research, 175*, 90–95.

Manson, J. H., & Perry, S. E. (1993). Inbreeding avoidance in rhesus macaques: Whose choice? *American Journal of Physical Anthropology, 90*, 335–344.

Mason, W. A., & Gerson, G. (1975). Effects of surrogate mobility of the development of rocking and other behaviors in rhesus monkeys: A study with artificial mothers. *Developmental Psychobiology, 8,* 197–211.

Mason, W. A., & Kenney, M. D. (1974). Re-direction of filial attachments in rhesus monkeys: Dogs as mother surrogates. *Science, 183,* 201–211.

Matthew, S. J., Coplan, J. H., Smith, E. L., Scharf, B. A., Owens, M. J., Nemeroff, C. B., et al. (2002). Cerebrospinal fluid concentrations of biogenic amines and corticotropin-releasing factor in adolescent non-human primates as a function of the timing of adverse early rearing experiences. *Stress, 5,* 185–193.

McCormack, K. M., Sanchez, M. M., Bardi, M., & Maestripieri, D. (2006). Maternal care patterns and behavioral development of rhesus macaque abused infants in the first 6 months of life. *Developmental Psychobiology, 48,* 537–550.

Mehlman, P. T., Higley, J. D., Faucher, I., Lilly, A. A., Taub, D. M., Vickers, J., et al. (1994). Low cerebrospinal fluid 5-hydroxyindoleacetic acid concentrations are correlated with severe aggression and reduced impulse control in free-ranging nonhuman primates (*Macaca mulatta*). *American Journal of Psychiatry, 151,* 1485–1491.

Mehlman, P. T., Higley, J. D., Faucher, I., Lilly, A. A., Taub, D. M., Vickers, J. M., et al. (1995). CSF 5-HIAA concentrations are correlated with sociality and the timing of emigration in free-ranging primates. *American Journal of Psychiatry, 152,* 907–913.

Mendoza, S. P., Smotherman, W. P., Miner, M., Kaplan, J., & Levine, S. (1978). Pituitary–adrenal response to separation in mother and infant squirrel monkeys. *Developmental Psychobiology, 11,* 169–175.

Newman, T. K., Parker, C. C., Suomi, S. J., Goldman, D., Barr, C. S., & Higley, J. D. (2009). DRD1 5′UTR variation, sex, and early stress influence alcohol consumption in rhesus macaques. *Genes, Brain, and Behavior, 8,* 626–630.

Newman, T. K., Syagailo, Y, Barr, C. S., Wendland, J., Champoux, M., Graessle, M., et al. (2005). Monoamine oxidase A gene promoter polymorphism and infant rearing experience interact to influence aggression and injuries in rhesus monkeys. *Biological Psychiatry, 57,* 167–172.

Novak, X., & Stuart, M. F. (2007). Tethering with maternal and fetal catheterization as a model for studying pre- and post-natal continuities. In G. P. Sackett, G. C. Ruppenthal, & E. Elias (Eds.), *Nursery rearing of nonhuman primates in the 21st century* (pp. 513–536). New York: Springer.

Paukner, A., Ferrari, P. F., & Suomi, S. J. (2013). A comparison of neonatal imitation abilities in human and macaque infant. In M. Banaji & S. Gelman (Eds.), *Navigating the social world: What infants, children, and other species can teach us* (pp. 133–138). New York: Oxford University Press.

Povinelli, D. J., Parks, K. A., & Novak, M. A. (1992). Role reversal by rhesus monkeys, but no evidence of empathy. *Animal Behavior, 43,* 269–281.

Provencal, N., Massert, R., Nemoda, Z., & Suomi, S. J. (in press). Alterations in DNA methylation and hydroxymethylation due to parental care in rhesus macaques. In D. Spengler & E. Binder (Eds.), *Epigenetics and neuroendocrinology: Clinical focus on psychiatry.* New York: Springer.

Provencal, N., Suderman, M., Guillemin, C., Massart, R., Ruggiero, A., Wang, D., et al. (2012). Signature of maternal rearing in the methylome in rhesus monkey prefrontal cortex and T cells. *Journal of Neuroscience, 32,* 15626–15642.

Redican, W., & Mitchell, G. D. (1973). A longitudinal study of paternal behavior in adult male rhesus monkeys: I. Observations on the first dyad. *Developmental Psychology, 8,* 135–136.

Reite, M., Short, R., Seiler, C., & Pauley, J. D. (1981). Attachment, loss, and depression. *Journal of Child Psychology and Psychiatry, 22,* 141–169.

Robertson, J., & Bowlby, J. (1952). Responses of young children to separation from their mothers. *Cours du Centre International de l'Enfance, 2,* 131–142.

Rosenblum, L. A., Forger, C., Noland, S., Trost, R. C., & Coplan, J. D. (2001). Response of adolescent bonnet macaques to an acute fear stimulus as a function of early rearing conditions. *Developmental Psychobiology, 39,* 40–45.

Rosenblum, L. A. & Paully, G. S. (1984). The effects of varying demands on maternal and infant behavior. *Child Development, 55,* 305–314.

Ruppenthal, G. C., Harlow, M. K., Eisele, C. D., Harlow, H. F., & Suomi, S. J. (1974). Development of peer interactions of monkeys reared in a nuclear family environment. *Child Development, 45,* 670–682.

Sackett, G. P. (1966). Monkeys reared in isolation with pictures as visual input: Evidence for an innate releasing mechanism. *Science, 154,* 1468–1472.

Sanchez, M. M. (2006). The impact of early adverse care on HPA development: Nonhuman primate models. *Hormones and Behavior, 50,* 623–631.

Schneider, M. L. (1992). Delayed object permanence in prenatally stressed rhesus monkey infants. *Occupational Therapy Journal of Research, 12,* 96–110.

Schwandt, M. L., Lindell, S. G., Chen, S. C., Higley, J. D., Suomi, S. J., Heilig, M., et al. (2010). Alcohol response and consumption in adolescent rhesus macaques: Life history and genetic influences. *Alcohol – An International Biomedical Journal, 44,* 67–80.

Schwandt, M. L., Lindell, S. G., Higley, J. D., Suomi, S. J., Heilig, M., & Barr, C. S. (2011). OPMR1 gene variation influences hypothalamic-pituitary-adrenal axis function in response to a variety of stressors in rhesus macaques. *Psychoneuroendocrinology, 36,* 1303–1311.

Shannon, C., Champoux, M., & Suomi, S. J. (1998). Rearing condition and plasma cortisol in rhesus monkey infants. *American Journal of Primatology, 46,* 311–321.

Shannon, C., Schwandt, M. L., Champoux, M., Shoaf, S. E., Suomi, S. J., Linnoila, M., et al. (2005). Maternal absence and stability of individual differences in CSF 5-HIAA concentrations in rhesus monkey infants. *American Journal of Psychiatry, 162*, 1658–1664.

Simpson, E. A., Paukner, A., Suomi, S. J., & Ferrari, P. F. (2015). Neonatal imitation and its sensory-motor mechanism. In P. F. Ferrari & G. Rizzolatti (Eds.), *New frontiers in mirror neuron research* (pp. 296–314). Oxford, UK: Oxford University Press.

Simpson, M. J. A. (1979). Daytime rest and activity in socially living rhesus monkey infants. *Animal Behaviour, 27*, 602–612.

Simpson, M. J. A., Simpson, A. E., Hooley, J., & Zunz, M. (1981). Infant-related influences on birth intervals in rhesus monkeys, *Nature, 290*, 49–51.

Spinelli, S., Chefer, S., Carson, R., Jagoda, E., Lang, L., Heilig, M., et al. (2010). Effects of early life stress on serotonin 1A receptors in juvenile rhesus monkeys as measured by positron emission tomography. *Biological Psychiatry, 67*, 1145–1153.

Spinelli, S., Chefer, S., Suomi, S. J., Barr, C. S., & Stein, E. (2009). Early-life stress induces long-term morphological changes in primate brain. *Archives of General Psychiatry, 66*, 658–665.

Suomi, S. J. (1979a). Differential development of various social relationships by rhesus monkey infants. In M. Lewis & L. A. Rosenblum (Eds.), *Genesis of behavior: The child and its family* (Vol. 2, pp. 219–244). New York: Plenum Press.

Suomi, S. J. (1979b). Peers, play, and primary prevention in primates. In M. Kent & J. Rolf (Eds.), *Primary prevention in psychopathology: Vol. 3. Social competence in children* (pp. 127–149). Hanover, NH: University Press of New England.

Suomi, S. J. (1981). Genetic, maternal, and environmental influences on social development in rhesus monkeys. In A. B. Chiarelli & R. S. Corruccini (Eds.), *Primate behavior and sociobiology: Selected papers (Part B) of the VIII Congress of the International Primatological Society, 1980* (pp. 81–87). New York: Springer-Verlag.

Suomi, S. J. (1982). Sibling relationships in nonhuman primates. In M. E. Lamb & B. Sutton-Smith (Eds.), *Sibling relationships: Their development and significance* (pp. 284–309). Hillsdale, NJ: Erlbaum.

Suomi, S. J. (1987). Genetic and maternal contributions to individual differences in rhesus monkey biobehavioral development. In N. A. Krasnagor, E. M. Blass, M. A. Hofer, & W. P. Smotherman (Eds.), *Perinatal development: A psychobiological perspective* (pp. 397–420). New York: Academic Press.

Suomi, S. J. (1991). Up-tight and laid-back monkeys: Individual differences in the response to social challenges. In S. Brauth, W. Hall, & R. Dooling (Eds.), *Plasticity of development* (pp. 27–56). Cambridge, MA: MIT Press.

Suomi, S. J. (1995). Influence of Bowlby's attachment theory on research on nonhuman primate biobehavioral development. In S. Goldberg, R. Muir, & J. Kerr (Eds.), *Attachment theory: Social, developmental, and clinical perspectives* (pp. 185–201). Hillsdale, NJ: Analytic Press.

Suomi, S. J. (1997). Early determinants of behaviour: Evidence from primate studies. *British Medical Bulletin, 53*, 170–184.

Suomi, S. J. (1998). Conflict and cohesion in rhesus monkey family life. In M. Cox & J. Brooks-Gunn (Eds.), *Conflict and cohesion in families* (pp. 283–296). Mahwah, NJ: Erlbaum.

Suomi, S. J. (1999). Developmental trajectories, early experiences, and community consequences: Lessons from studies with rhesus monkeys. In D. P. Keating & C. Hertzman (Eds.), *Developmental health and the wealth of nations: Social, biological, and educational dynamics* (pp. 185–200). New York: Guilford Press.

Suomi, S. J. (2002). Parents, peers, and the process of socialization in primates. In J. G. Borkowski, S. L. Ramey, & M. Bristol-Power (Eds.), *Parenting and the child's world: Influences on academic, intellectual, and social-emotional development* (pp. 265–279). Mahwah, NJ: Erlbaum.

Suomi, S. J. (2006). Risk, resilience, and gene × environment interactions in rhesus monkeys. *Annals of the New York Academy of Sciences, 1094*, 52–62.

Suomi, S. J. (2011). Risk, resilience, and gene–environment interplay in primates. *Journal of the Canadian Academy of Child and Adolescent Psychiatry, 20*, 289–297.

Suomi, S. J., & Harlow, H. F. (1975). The role and reason of peer friendships. In M. Lewis & L. A. Rosenblum (Eds.) *Friendships and peer relations* (pp. 310–334). New York: Basic Books.

Suomi, S. J., & Harlow, H. F. (1976). The facts and functions of fear. In M. Zuckerman & C. D. Spielberger (Eds.), *Emotions and anxiety: New concepts, methods, and applications* (pp. 3–34). Hillsdale, NJ: Erlbaum.

Suomi, S. J., Kraemer, G. W., Baysinger, C. M., & Delizio, R. D. (1981). Inherited and experiential factors associated with individual differences in anxious behavior displayed by rhesus monkeys. In D. G. Klein & J. Rabkin (Eds.), *Anxiety: New research and changing concepts* (pp. 179–200). New York: Raven Press.

Suomi, S. J., & Levine, S. (1998). Psychobiology of intergenerational effects of trauma: Evidence from animal studies. In Y. Danieli (Ed.), *International handbook of multigenerational legacies of trauma* (pp. 623–637). New York: Plenum Press.

Suomi, S. J., Rasmussen, K. L. R., & Higley, J. D. (1992). Primate models of behavioral and physiological change in adolescence. In E. R. McAnarney, R. E. Kriepe, D. P. Orr, & G. D. Comerci (Eds.), *Textbook of adolescent medicine* (pp. 135–139). Philadelphia: Saunders.

Suomi, S. J., & Ripp, C. (1983). A history of motherless mother monkey mothering at the University of Wisconsin Primate Laboratory. In M. Reite & N Caine (Eds.), *Child abuse: The nonhuman primate data* (pp. 49–77). New York: Alan R. Liss.

Trivers, R. L. (1974). Parent–offspring conflicts. *American Zoologist, 14,* 249–264.

Van der Horst, F. C. P., Van der Veer, R., & Van IJzendoorn, M. H. (2007). John Bowlby and ethology: An annotated interview with Robert Hinde. *Attachment and Human Development, 9,* 1–15.

Vanderwert, R. E., Ferrari, P. F., Paukner, A., Bower, S. B., Fox, N. A., & Suomi, S. J. (2012). Spectral characteristics of the newborn rhesus macaque EEG reflects fundamental cortical activity. *Physiology and Behavior, 107,* 787–791.

Vanderwert, R. E., Simpson, E. A., Paukner, A., Suomi, S. J., Fox, N. A., & Ferrari, P. F. (2015). Early social experience affects neural activity to affiliative gestures in newborn nonhuman primates. *Developmental Neuroscience, 47,* 243–252.

Visalberghi, E. (1990). Tool use in Cebus. *Folia Primatologica, 54,* 146–154.

Visalberghi, E., Frazasgy, D., Ottoni, E., Izar, P., de Oliveria, M. G., & Andrade, F. R. D. (2007). Characteristics of hammer stones and anvils used by wild bearded capuchin monkeys (*Cebus libidinosus*) to crack open palm nuts. *American Journal of Physical Anthropology, 132,* 426–444.

Welker, C., Becker, P., Hohman, H., & Schafer-Witt, C. (1987). Social relations in groups of the black-capped capuchin *Cebus apella* in captivity: Interactions of group-born infants during their first 6 months of life. *Folia Primatologica, 49,* 33–47.

Welker, C., Becker, P., & Schafer-Witt, C. (1990). Social relations in groups of the black-capped capuchin (*Cebus apella*) in captivity: Interactions of group-born infants during their second half-year of life. *Folia Primatologica, 54,* 16–33.

Williamson, D. E., Coleman, K., Bacanu, S. A., Devlin, B., Rogers, J., Ryan, N. E., et al. (2003). Heritability in fearful–anxious endophenotypes in infant rhesus macaques: A preliminary study. *Biological Psychiatry, 53,* 284–291.

Wilson, E. O. (1975). *Sociobiology.* New York: Cambridge University Press.

# Chapter 8

# Attachment, Parenting, and Genetics

Marian J. Bakermans-Kranenburg
Marinus H. van IJzendoorn

## Attachment

Without doubt, forming attachments, as defined by Bowlby (1969/1982), is a genetic characteristic of human beings. The most general definition of attachment is one that considers it to be an inborn bias of human infants to seek proximity to a protective caregiver in times of stress, distress, illness, and other physical or psychological discomfort. Human offspring would not be able to survive without the care of a stronger or more experienced conspecific who is able to regulate body temperature, food intake, and stress levels because young infants cannot take care of these basic physiological and psychological needs by themselves. The early environment of evolutionary adaptedness among humans required the basic ability to become emotionally attached in order to survive and enhance inclusive fitness (Bowlby, 1969/1982).

Attachment, however, is also strongly dependent on the environment. Although all infants are born with the ability to become attached to a protective caregiver, they differ in the way in which this competence is expressed. Infants differ rather drastically in the quality of their attachment relationships, and attachment theory hypothesizes that this "attachment performance" is largely, albeit not exclusively, environmentally determined. Differences in attachment behaviors and relationships emerge in the course of the first few years of life as a consequence of childrearing experiences with parents and other caregivers. Infants may develop secure or insecure attachments in response to a more or less sensitive or predictable social environment. The parallel to language development is useful here. Every child is born with the capacity to learn a language, but the specific language environment determines the kind of language to be learnt.

Paradoxically, the search for the genetic foundation of attachment seems to be inspired by two contrasting goals. On the one hand, cross-cultural researchers who study attachment wish to document the balance between universal and culture-specific influences on attachment *competence*, in order to test the core hypothesis that every human infant is born with a bias to become attached (see Mesman, Van IJzendoorn, & Sagi-Schwartz, Chapter 37, this volume). On the other hand, the behavioral and molecular genetics studies of attachment are aimed at elucidating the genetic versus environmental determination of attachment *performance*, with the assumption (on the part of attachment researchers) that attachment differences are mainly rooted in variations in the environment in which an infant grows up. Here we focus on the genetics of individual differences in attachment behavior and relationship quality.

## Behavioral Genetics of Attachment

Twins have been a great source of information about human development. The comparison of monozygotic (MZ, or identical) twins, whose structural DNA is exactly the same, with dizygotic (DZ, or fraternal) twins, who share on average half of their DNA, is an experiment by nature. If children within an MZ twin pair are more similar to each other in terms of attachment (or any other trait) than children within a DZ twin pair, one might conclude that genetic similarity matters. In the case of strong similarity of attachment between MZ twins and much smaller similarity between DZ twins, attachment would be considered highly heritable. This conclusion is warranted, of course, only when we assume that parents do not treat MZ and DZ twins differently. The equal environments assumption has been examined and found to be valid for a variety of phenotypes (Cronk et al., 2002), but for parenting relevant to attachment development this information is not available.

Only a few, rather small twin studies of infants' and preschoolers' attachments have been reported (Bakermans-Kranenburg, Van IJzendoorn, Bokhorst, & Schuengel, 2004; Bokhorst et al., 2003; Finkel, Wille, & Matheny, 1998; O'Connor & Croft, 2001; Ricciuti, 1992; Roisman & Fraley, 2008), and the majority of these studies did not find differences in attachment similarity between MZ and DZ twin pairs. In general about 50% of the variance in attachment security could be attributed to the shared environment (parenting influences that make children within the same family similar), and about 50% of the variation could be explained by unique influences (that make children within a family more dissimilar) and measurement error. There seemed to be no room for genetic influences. Interestingly, the shared environmental variance in attachment security showed substantial overlap with the shared environmental variance in observed maternal sensitivity, suggesting that parental sensitivity is indeed an important part of the (shared) environment shaping children's attachment patterns (Fearon et al., 2006).

The only exception to the rule that young children's attachment security is not heritable was the study in which Finkel and colleagues (1998) found considerable heritability for attachment, but unfortunately used an attachment measure that was originally meant to assess temperament. In the study by Bokhorst and colleagues (2003), temperamental reactivity was estimated to be highly heritable, whereas attachment security was mainly environmentally based. In a study of infant–father attachment using the Attachment Q-Sort (AQS; Vaughn & Waters, 1990), high heritability of temperament went with low heritability of attachment security to the father, using the same measure and the same sample as Bakermans-Kranenburg and colleagues (2004). It is important to note that the developmental roots of attachment and temperament seem to be different, which underlines their conceptual and functional differences (Groh et al., in press; Van IJzendoorn & Bakermans-Kranenburg, 2012; see Vaughn & Bost, Chapter 10, this volume).

Disorganized attachment has rarely been studied with a twin design. Disorganized attachment is observed in children who are maltreated or otherwise frightened by parental behavior, for example because their parents struggle with unresolved loss or other potentially traumatic experiences (Cyr, Euser, Bakermans-Kranenburg, & Van IJzendoorn, 2010; Schuengel, Bakermans-Kranenburg, & Van IJzendoorn, 1999; see Lyons-Ruth & Jacobvitz, Chapter 29, this volume). Disorganized attachment behaviors include, among others, frightened facial expressions; freezing or stilling of behavior; or avoidance in distress, when a parent returns following a brief separation in the Strange Situation (Main & Solomon, 1990). Heritability estimates of disorganized attachment approach zero, and in remarkable contrast to attachment security, no trace of shared environmental influence can be found (Bokhorst et al., 2003). Variance in disorganized attachment seems to be explained almost exclusively by a unique environment. This suggests that unique experiences with the parents trigger children's disorganized attachment. It may also imply a large error component in the assessment of disorganized attachment, which, indeed, is by far the most difficult part of the attachment coding system to master. Of course, low statistical power should be taken into account when considering the absence of heritability: The modest sample size and skewed distribution of disorganized attachment result in large confidence intervals around the estimates.

In several cases the influence of genetics on traits or characteristics such as cognitive development has been shown to increase with age. The influence of the environment seems to decrease as children grow older, undergo a variety of influences outside the family, and are more able to shape their own environments. Indeed, genetic studies of individual differences in mental development and temperament confirm this view (e.g., Plomin, 1994; but see Haworth, Dale, & Plomin, 2009, for contrasting effects). In the largest twin study on attachment to date, Fearon, Shmueli-Goetz, Viding, Fonagy, and Plomin (2014) used the semistructured Child Attachment Interview (CAI; Shmueli-Goetz, Target, Fonagy, & Datta, 2008) in a sample of 551 twin pairs age 15 years. The CAI is modeled after the Adult Attachment Interview (see Hesse, Chapter 26, this volume), assessing attachment security in terms of coherence of discourse when discussing childhood attachment experiences. Surprisingly, the authors found correlations between attachment security in MZ twins that were about twice as strong as correlations in DZ twins, and they concluded that attachment in this sample of young adolescents was about 40% heritable, whereas the influence of the shared environment was negligible (Fearon et al., 2014).

Of course, this finding might point at a genuine developmental phenomenon of increasing genetic influence with growing age. It should be noted, however, that adolescence is a somewhat difficult age period for the measurement of attachment because many adolescents are in the middle of a potentially confusing struggle for independence from their parents. This might be the reason that in this and other studies, dismissing attachments seem to be temporarily overrepresented (Bakermans-Kranenburg & Van IJzendoorn, 2009). Fearon and colleagues (2014) found insecure-preoccupied attachments in only 5% of the cases, and unresolved attachments in only 3% of their subjects, so any conclusion about heritability of adolescent attachment is limited to the specific security-dismissing dimension (see also Van IJzendoorn & Bakermans-Kranenburg, 2014). Clearly, more longitudinal studies going beyond adolescence are needed to test whether heritability of attachment indeed increases with age, and well into adulthood. One relevant study included adopted sibling pairs from the Iowa Adoption Studies who, on average, were 39 years old when the AAI was administered (Caspers, Yucuis, Troutman, Arndt, & Langbehn, 2007). Concordance rates showed substantial similarity of attachment representations between the siblings, although they were genetically unrelated; they only grew up in the same family. These findings do not support the idea of increased heritability with age, but they do point to an important role for shared environmental influences. Thus, the findings reported by Fearon and colleagues may be specific to adolescence.

## Molecular Genetics of Attachment

Behavioral genetics studies of the kinds discussed so far involve inferring heritability from phenotypic (dis-)similarities between MZ and DZ twins, but participants' genetic makeup itself is not assessed. This indirect method of inferring heritability has several drawbacks, including dependence on the specific population distribution of relevant environmental and genetic features. In an environment with sufficient food for everyone, physical growth would appear to be much more heritable than in an environment with large variation in food supply. In contrast, in molecular genetics studies, structural DNA patterns are assessed directly, often with great precision, and variation in the environment does not play a critical role in estimating heritability except when the environment influences the expression of genes. (We discuss this issue—the study of epigenetics—later in this chapter.)

The first molecular genetics study of attachment, published by Gervai's Hungarian team (Lakatos et al., 2000), was conducted on a rather small, low-risk Hungarian sample ($N = 95$ infants) and is an example of the candidate gene approach (i.e., focusing on a particular gene of interest). It revealed a strong association between the dopamine receptor D4 gene (*DRD4*) and infant disorganized attachment. Child carriers of the *DRD4* 7-repeat allele appeared to run a fourfold elevated risk of disorganized attachment. The T-variant of the -521 (C/T) single-nucleotide polymorphism (SNP) in the regulatory region of the *DRD4* gene increased the risk for disorganization even further (Lakatos et al., 2002). *DRD4* had already acquired a bad reputation as a "risk" genotype for impulsivity, addiction, and attentional problems, and the neurotransmitter dopamine had been found to be involved in motivational and reward mechanisms (Robbins & Everitt, 1999). But did this *DRD4* genotype also deserve a bad reputation in relation to attachment?

Although the link between *DRD4* and attentional and motivational issues seemed to make the association with disorganization somewhat plausible, the findings were surprising against the background of the behavior genetics study of disorganization by the Leiden team (Bokhorst et al., 2003), which did not find any evidence for genetic influences on disorganized attachment. DNA was therefore collected in the Leiden twin sample to replicate the Hungarian findings, but without success (Bakermans-Kranenburg & Van IJzendoorn,

2004). Several other replication attempts followed, but the picture did not change: Across a series of studies (total $N$ = 542) the combined effect size of the association between *DRD4* and disorganization was close to zero (Bakermans-Kranenburg & Van IJzendoorn, 2007). Compared to the combined effect size across studies of the association between parental frightening or anomalous behavior and disorganized attachment (Cohen's $d$ = 0.72, total $N$ = 644; Madigan et al., 2006), this was a disappointing outcome for advocates of genetic influences on attachment.

More molecular genetics studies involving candidate genes have been conducted in recent years. Some of the studies indicated a potential role for candidate genes. For example, Spangler, Johann, Ronai, and Zimmermann (2009) reported an association between attachment disorganization and the short variant of the serotonin transporter-linked polymorphic region (*5-HTTLPR*), qualified by an interaction with maternal responsiveness (see below). This genotype, one of the usual suspects in the study of psychiatric genetics, is considered to be a "risk" factor for depression and anxiety. Fearon and colleagues (Frigerio et al., 2009) studied the associations between several gene polymorphisms implicated in the serotonin and dopamine systems (*5-HTTLPR, COMT, GABRA6, DRD4, DRD4/-521*) and attachment security as well as attachment disorganization in an Italian sample of 100 infants, but no association survived stringent statistical tests.

To date, the largest candidate gene study on attachment is the combination of the Generation R study, a large cohort study in Rotterdam, the Netherlands, and the National Institute of Child Health and Human Development (NICHD) Study of Early Child Care and Youth Development (SECCYD), which includes more than 1,000 infants in all (Luijk, Roisman, et al., 2011). It was the first study to replicate key findings across two relatively large samples. Associations of candidate genes involved in the dopamine, serotonin, and oxytocin systems (*DRD4, DRD2, COMT, 5-HTTLPR, OXTR*) with attachment security and disorganization were examined. The only replicable significant finding was the association between *COMT* and attachment disorganization. Children with the Val/Met genotype had higher disorganization scores (combined effect size $d$ = 0.22). This codominant risk model for *COMT* Val158Met was consistent across both samples but it is difficult to explain. Perhaps the broader range of plasticity in heterozygotes (the Val/Met carriers) increased sus-

ceptibility to environmental influences or, in case of a frightening environment, to dysregulation of emotional arousal (Luijk, Roisman, et al., 2011).

With increasing age, the heritability of traits might become more pronounced, as discussed earlier. In a German sample of 167 adults, the associations of adult attachment representations (using the AAI) and two candidate genes, *5-HTTLPR* and *DRD4*, were examined (Reiner & Spangler, 2010). Carriers of *DRD4* 7-repeat alleles were significantly more often securely attached and received higher coherence scores compared to carriers of the other alleles. The authors suggested that this main effect was qualified by an interaction with recollections of a loving caregiver, but because this "loving" scale was part of the AAI coding system for attachment representations, the variable cannot be considered an independent assessment of past childrearing environments. *5-HTTLPR* was not significantly associated with adult attachment, with or without taking reported experiences into account. The absence of molecular genetic evidence for heritability diverges from the Fearon and colleagues (2014) behavior genetics finding, but converges with the Caspers and colleagues (2007) results in adoptive families.

Failure to find replicable main effects of candidate genes is not unique for attachment security or disorganization. Publication bias may account for the lack of replicable genetic findings because initially positive results may be selectively published, whereas numerous negative results may remain unpublished. This is the so-called "winner's curse" (for an example involving the oxytocin receptor gene, see Bakermans-Kranenburg & Van IJzendoorn, 2013). Candidate genes are the proverbial needle in a haystack and cannot be solely or largely responsible for complex behaviors or traits such as attachment security. Candidate genes might serve as important and valid indices for broader underlying genetic pathways that modulate the production, transport, and reuptake of neurotransmitters involved in attachment–related behaviors and emotions. When isolated from the environment, however, it seems overly optimistic to expect them to explain more than a small amount of variance in the attachment phenotype.

### Genomewide Association Studies and Genomewide Complex Trait Analysis

At least two ways to try to solve the complex puzzle of genetic determination of variance in attachment security and disorganization remain to be explored. The first is to expand the number of genes involved in the hunt for attachment genes using the method of genomewide association studies (GWAS; Plomin, 2013) and related approaches such as genetic pathway analysis (Plomin & Simpson, 2013) and genomewide complex trait analysis (GCTA; Benjamin et al., 2012). The second approach is broadening the focus to include the interaction between genes and environment (G × E) instead of limiting the search to main effects. Here we briefly discuss the GWAS, genetic pathways, and GCTA approaches; in the next section we discuss G × E studies of attachment.

GWAS differ from the candidate gene approach in associating a large part of the genome with a complex phenotype, such as attachment, in a hypothesis-free manner. Instead of including the usual genetic suspects with known biological functions, the GWAS approach covers the 1 million or so independent SNPs that are markers of the most common genotypic variation in humans. Using linkage disequilibrium to prune the number of markers, 1 million SNPs may efficiently represent the 16 million SNPs of the human genome. In the GWAS approach, associations of these SNPs with the targeted phenotype are tested with, of course, massive correction for multiple testing by an increase of the significance threshold to $p <$ .00000005 to avoid chance results.

Although the GWAS approach was successfully used in the detection of the genetic basis of some diseases (e.g., macular degeneration) and led to new treatments, application to behavioral phenotypes and complex psychological traits has so far been disappointing. Plomin (2013) summarized GWAS results on reading, mathematics, and general cognitive ability, and showed that less than 0.5% of the variance could be explained by a small number of GWAS hits. The amazingly large gap between GWAS-based estimates of heritability and heritability found in twin studies is called the *missing heritability problem* (Manolio et al., 2009; Plomin & Simpson, 2013; Van IJzendoorn et al., 2011). The gap made Plomin (2013) sigh: "Gene hunters are still recovering from the shock of finding that the largest associations account for so little variance in the population" (p. 109).

In an exploratory effort to apply GWAS to attachment security and disorganization in the Generation R sample ($N = 641$), no significant hit was found, and the suggestive hits ($p < .00005$) did not replicate in an independent sample of similar size. Of course, the sample size was way too small

for the small effects to be expected on the basis of previous GWAS (Plomin & Simpson, 2013). But it is difficult to imagine how samples 100 times larger might ever be assembled given the time-consuming "gold-standard" attachment assessments at our disposal, let alone the usefulness of finding genes accounting for less than 1% of the variance in attachment.

Alternative approaches that may require fewer subjects are genetic pathways and GCTA, which might be more powerful in discovering the genetic basis of complex traits (Plomin, DeFries, Knopik, & Neiderhiser, 2013). Genetic pathways are functionally related genotypes potentially consisting of hundreds of SNPs that are associated with the phenotype as one block (Ramanan, Shen, Moore, & Saykin, 2012; Wang, Li, & Hakonarson, 2010), thus requiring less correction for multiple testing. GCTA pairs every individual in a sample with every other genetically unrelated individual and correlates any similarity in genotype with the phenotypic similarity within each pair (Yang, Lee, Goddard, & Visscher, 2011). When genotypic similarities go together with stronger similarity in a trait, the genetic component of the trait can be estimated (see Pappa, Fedko, et al., 2015, for an example). Both approaches have been used in Generation R (Jaddoe et al., 2012), the largest ethnically homogeneous (Caucasian) attachment sample to date, but these efforts have again failed to yield significant effects (Pappa, Szekely, et al., 2015).

## G × E Effects

Overall, main-effects studies of the genetics of attachment have not yielded impressive effects. Given Bronfenbrenner's (1979) idea that *main effects are in the interactions* (see also Rutter, 2006), it seemed sensible to examine gene-by-environment (G × E) effects on attachment. Certain genotypes may act as a "risk factor" that makes it more likely that insensitive or frightening and anomalous parenting will result in insecure or disorganized infant attachment. Alternatively, genes may act as "susceptibility factors" that increase the effects of both sensitive and insensitive parenting on children's positive or negative outcomes (Bakermans-Kranenburg, & Van IJzendoorn, 2010; Belsky, Bakermans-Kranenburg, & Van IJzendoorn, 2007; Ellis, Boyce, Belsky, Bakermans-Kranenburg, & Van IJzendoorn, 2011).

Although some have argued that the search for G × E effects is warranted only when genetic main effects have been established (Munafò, Durrant, Lewis, & Flint, 2009; Risch et al., 2009), this point of view is not correct, as is evident from the following example: Imagine that for a specific gene, environmental effects are absent for one gene variant but present for the other gene variant. Imagine further that for this second gene variant, good outcomes are observed under favorable conditions and bad outcomes under unfavorable conditions. This pattern of effects, *for better and for worse*, in a specific subgroup, as proposed by the differential susceptibility model, has been documented in many studies (for reviews and meta-analytic evidence see Bakermans-Kranenburg, & Van IJzendoorn, 2011; Belsky & Pluess, 2009; Van IJzendoorn, Belsky, & Bakermans-Kranenburg, 2012). In that case G × E effects are found in the absence of a genetic main effect (the two directions *within* one genotype cancel each other out; Bakermans-Kranenburg & Van IJzendoorn, 2015).

Two types of G × E studies of attachment can be distinguished, depending on the role of attachment quality as an environmental factor or as an outcome. In both types of studies, the genetic factor is the moderator. In the first scenario, attachment security is used as an index of a supportive environment, for example, with emotion regulation or cortisol reactivity to a stressor as outcomes. The pertinent question in these studies is whether genotypes moderate the association between attachment quality (predictor) and these outcomes. In the second scenario, the moderating role of genotype in the association between caregiving quality (predictor) and attachment quality (outcome) is examined. We first review studies with attachment quality as the observed environmental predictor, then studies with attachment as outcome.

## Attachment as Environment

Attachment security was used as an indirect index of a supportive caregiving environment in a G × E study of child self-regulation (Kochanska, Philibert, & Barry, 2009). Infant–mother attachment was assessed at 15 months, and children's ability to self-regulate was assessed at 25, 38, and 52 months. Among children who carried a short 5-HTTLPR allele, those who were insecurely attached developed poor regulatory capacities, whereas those who were securely attached developed as good regulatory capacities as children without the short allele. For children with two long alleles, attachment security did not predict self-regulation.

In a study of 7-year-old Dutch children, emotion regulation was observed during a stressful public speaking task, the Trier Social Stress Test for Children (TSST-C). 5-HTTLPR moderated the association between attachment security as assessed with the Attachment Story Completion Task (Bretherton, Ridgeway, & Cassidy, 1990; Cassidy, 1988) and electrodermal reactivity during the TSST-C. There was a fan-shaped interaction pattern: Children with a secure attachment representation, as well as two long (LL) alleles, were less stressed during the TSST-C than all other children (Gilissen, Bakermans-Kranenburg, Van IJzendoorn, & Linting, 2008). Children who had the "double protection" of both the LL genotype and secure attachment were the only ones who experienced low levels of stress, perhaps indicating how much support is needed for being unconcerned about giving a public speech.

In a study with 4- to 6-year-old Norwegian children, the COMT gene polymorphism moderated the effect of disorganized attachment (assessed at age 4 with the doll play story completion task) on social development. Children homozygous for the COMT*val* allele who were highly disorganized at age 4 became more aggressive over time and showed reduced social competence compared to highly disorganized children with one or two *met* alleles (Hygen, Guzey, Belsky, Berg-Nielsen, & Wichstrom, 2014).

Finally, Luijk and colleagues (2010) related attachment security to cortisol reactivity levels during the Strange Situation procedure and tested the moderating role of HPA-axis-related SNPs (*BclI*, *rs41423247*; *TthIIII*, *rs10052957*; *GR-9b*, *rs6198*; *N363S*, *rs6195*; *ER22/23EK*, *rs6189*, and *6190*; and *FKBP5 rs1360780*) in more than 300 14-month-old infants. *FKBP5 rs1360780* was related to cortisol reactivity and a double-risk for heightened cortisol reactivity was found in infants with one or two T-alleles of the *FKBP5* SNP and an insecure-resistant attachment relationship with their mother.

## Attachment as Outcome

Based on data from the Minnesota Longitudinal Study, Raby and colleagues (2012) found no moderating effect of the 5-HTTLPR genotype on the association between maternal sensitivity and attachment security. This study thus failed to replicate the G × E findings of Barry, Kochanska, and Philibert (2008), who observed mothers' sensitivity at

7 months during lengthy naturalistic interactions combining Ainsworth, Blehar, Waters, and Wall's (1978) scales with time-sampled, event-triggered ratings of mothers' responses to each child signal. Infant attachment was assessed at 15 months. Infants with the short 5-HTTLPR allele and insensitive mothers were more likely to be insecure than were infants with the same genotype whose mothers were sensitive, but infants with the LL genotype scored high on attachment security independent of the variation in maternal responsiveness.

Surprisingly, similar results emerged in conditions of severe deprivation. It is no wonder that institutional care has been shown to lead to insecure and disorganized attachment (Van IJzendoorn et al., 2011), since institutional care has so many characteristics of structural neglect (minimal physical resources, unfavorable staffing patterns, and socioemotionally inadequate caregiver–child interactions) that it fails to respond to children's basic need for stable and positive personal relationships, as well as adequate care and stimulation. In these conditions, environmental effects may be expected to overrule any genetic or G × E effect. However, some children appear to be surprisingly resilient to the adverse environment, and in a small hypothesis-generating study, the potentially moderating role of 5-HTTLPR was explored (Bakermans-Kranenburg, Dobrova-Krol, & Van IJzendoorn, 2011). The study involved Ukrainian preschoolers reared in institutional settings or with their biological families. 5-HTTLPR moderated the association between caregiving environment and attachment disorganization. Children with a short allele showed more attachment disorganization and less attachment security when they grew up in an institution than when they lived in a family, but when children had the LL genotype, they were not more disorganized when they grew up in an institution than children growing up in their biological families.

This seems to suggest that the protective role of the 5-HTTLPR LL genotype is not limited to moderately adverse environments (as shown by, e.g., Barry et al., 2008; Gilissen et al., 2008) but also exists in extremely untoward circumstances. Notably, the findings are in line with the outcomes of adoptees in the English and Romanian Adoptee Study (Kumsta et al., 2010), in which adoptees with the LL genotype showed the lowest levels of emotional problems during adolescence even when they experienced severe early institutional deprivation, and with results of the Bucharest Early Intervention Project, in which children with

the LL genotype showed low levels of indiscriminate social behavior irrespective of their living arrangement (institutionalized care or high-quality foster care; Drury et al., 2012).

For disorganized attachment, Spangler and colleagues (2009) found an interaction between maternal responsiveness and child 5-HTTLPR: Children with the short allele were more often disorganized when maternal responsiveness was low. Maternal responsiveness was observed during a 30-minute session, in which the mother was asked to complete a questionnaire but to respond to the infant as she usually would. Responsiveness was indexed with an aggregated score that combined the number and promptness of maternal responses to infant signals, irrespective of the (emotional) quality of the response. The proportion of disorganized infants increased with the number of short alleles, but only in the low responsiveness group (Spangler et al., 2009).

Van IJzendoorn and Bakermans-Kranenburg (2006) examined whether infants with the DRD4 7-repeat allele were more susceptible to parental unresolved loss and anomalous parenting behavior than infants without this allele. This turned out to be the case: Maternal unresolved loss or trauma was associated with infant disorganization in children with the DRD4 7-repeat allele, whereas children without this allele did not have higher scores for disorganized attachment when their mothers were unresolved. However, children with the DRD4 7-repeat allele who had mothers without unresolved loss showed the lowest levels of attachment disorganization. These findings support the notion that the DRD4 7-repeat allele constitutes not a genetic risk but a genetic marker of differential susceptibility (Ellis et al., 2011). The differential susceptibility model is described more extensively in the section on intervention (see below).

Gervai and colleagues (2007), combining a low-risk Hungarian and a high-risk U.S. sample, found that maternal affective communication was related to disorganized attachment in children without the DRD4 7-repeat allele and not in carriers of the DRD4 7-repeat allele. In light of the meta-analytic results (Bakermans-Kranenburg & Van IJzendoorn, 2011, 2015), the latter outcome is not convergent with the general finding of higher susceptibility of carriers of the 7-repeat allele, and this may have to do with the ethnically heterogeneous U.S. sample in the Gervai and colleagues (2007) study.

The moderating role of DRD4 was also found for the adult equivalent of disorganized attachment, unresolved loss or trauma, as assessed with the AAI. Participants were adopted adults from the Iowa Adoption Studies, interviewed with the AAI when they were on average 39 years old (Bakermans-Kranenburg, Van IJzendoorn, Caspers, & Philibert, 2011). Participants with the *DRD4* 7-repeat allele with independently reported parental problems in their adoptive families had the highest scores for unresolved loss or trauma, whereas participants with the *DRD4* 7-repeat allele who did not experience parental problems had the lowest ratings. Among participants without the *DRD4* 7-repeat allele, parental problems during childhood did not make a difference for unresolved loss or trauma, again pointing to heightened susceptibility to environmental influences for carriers of the *DRD4* 7-repeat allele.

In the Generation R study, two genes involved in the regulation of stress responses were examined: those for the glucocorticoid receptor (GR) and mineralocorticoid receptor (MR) (Luijk, Tharner, et al., 2011). In more than 500 infant–parent dyads, maternal sensitivity was observed during a psychophysiological assessment using Ainsworth's rating scales for sensitivity (Ainsworth et al., 1978). Moreover, maternal extreme insensitivity was observed, including withdrawal and neglect, and intrusive, negative, aggressive, or otherwise harsh parental behaviors (Out, Bakermans-Kranenburg, & Van IJzendoorn, 2009). There were no main effects of MR or GR on infant attachment. However, infants with the minor MR allele (G) were more securely attached if their mothers were more sensitive, and less securely attached if their mothers showed more extremely insensitive behaviors, whereas these associations were not present in children without the G allele. No main or interaction effects were found for attachment disorganization.

Based on the combination of two large cohorts, the Generation R study and the NICHD SECCYD, the interactions between candidate genes involved in the dopamine, serotonin, and oxytocin systems (*DRD4, DRD2, COMT, 5-HTTLPR, OXTR*) and maternal sensitivity were examined in more than 1,000 Caucasian infants in total. G × E interaction effects were not replicable across the two samples (Luijk, Roisman, et al., 2011).

Even though the combined sample size in this latter study was substantial, and indeed the largest available to examine the interplay between genetics and parenting, predicting attachment with state-of-the-art observational measures, the power to detect G × E effects may have been in-

sufficient. The power of correlational G × E studies is inherently limited by several factors (see Bakermans-Kranenburg & Van IJzendoorn, 2015; Van IJzendoorn & Bakermans-Kranenburg, 2015): The distributions of genotypes and parenting quality tend to be skewed, and genetic and environmental factors may not be independent because through passive or evocative gene–environment correlation (rGE), parenting may be related to either the parent's or the child's genotype. Unmeasured genotypes that elicit specific parental behaviors may play a role and, last but not least, power is reduced by measurement errors. Selective recruitment and attrition, processes that are unavoidable in cohort studies, result in low numbers of participants in the eccentric parts of the distribution, with consequences for the distribution of the interaction term. Duncan and Keller (2011) argued that the primary reason for reduced power to detect interactions in nonexperimental studies is that the variance of the product term tends to be low. Thus, replication and meta-analysis to document the replicability of any finding is essential (Cumming, 2014). At the same time, experimental designs constitute a powerful alternative to examine G × E effects (see the section "Interventions from a G × E Perspective").

## Epigenetics

In the past, behavioral and molecular genetics researchers assumed that the genetic makeup of every individual is invariable, originating from conception and remaining basically the same across the lifespan, except in rare cases of mutations through radiation or other toxic influences. This assumption is valid as far as it pertains to the structural properties of the double helix of DNA. But even MZ twins with identical DNA structures may grow apart in gene expression. They may develop radically different disease patterns because of changes in the epigenome that influences and regulates the expression of genes. Fraga and colleagues (2005) found, for example, that a 3-year-old MZ twin pair had about 1,000 genes with differential gene expression, whereas a 50-year-old MZ twin pair had more than 5,000 differently expressed genes. Differences in the epigenome increase with age and with nonshared environmental influences, implying that they are larger when twins have spent more time in separate environments.

One of the most widely studied epigenetic mechanisms is *methylation,* which is, simply put, the blocking of gene expression through the linking of a methyl (CH$_3$) molecule to one of the bases, cytosine, at a CpG site (cytosine–phosphate–guanine) located in a gene promoter region. Methylation might be loosely compared to a cork on a bottle of champagne, down-regulating the escape of bubbles (the messenger RNA [mRNA]) and thus modulating the level of protein and enzyme production encoded for by the specific gene (Van IJzendoorn, Bakermans-Kranenburg, & Ebstein, 2011). Epigenetic studies of rodents (e.g., Meaney, 2010; Szyf, Weaver, Champagne, Diorio, & Meaney, 2005) have made clear that the caregiving environment (e.g., the amount of licking and grooming and arched-back nursing that parents provide) may radically alter methylation patterns and, consequently, gene expression in the pups, and not just in the pups exposed to sensitive parenting (or deprived thereof) but even in these pups' offspring (Meaney, 2010). In particular, altered methylation of the GR gene induces long-term changes in response to stress, affecting the next generation (Weaver et al., 2004; Zhang & Meaney, 2010).

One of the first epigenetic studies on human development that is relevant for attachment theory was conducted by Meaney's team (McGowan et al., 2009). They examined the brains of deceased young males stored in the Quebec Suicide Brain Bank, matching suicide victims with and without a history of abuse, and comparing these two groups with age- and gender-matched victims of fatal accidents. They found that through methylation, GR gene expression in the hippocampus of the suicide victims was decreased, but only when they had experienced child abuse. Hippocampal GRs play a crucial role in down-regulating the HPA axis, which is responsible for the level of the stress hormone cortisol. In other studies, similar epigenetic alterations have been found as a result of child maltreatment (Beach et al., 2010; Perroud et al., 2013) or structural neglect in orphanages (Naumova et al., 2012), and in adolescent children whose mothers were exposed to intimate partner violence during pregnancy (Radtke et al., 2011).

The first epigenetic study of adult attachment was conducted with participants in the Iowa Adoption Studies (Van IJzendoorn et al., 2010). The AAI was administered, and participants ($N = 143$) reported on any loss or other potentially traumatic event during their childhood years in the adoptive family. The AAI scale for Unresolved Loss or Trauma was not associated with 5-HTTLPR. When the level of methylation was taken into account, genotype predicted Unresolved Loss or Trauma. Carriers of the long variant of 5-HTTLPR showed more Unresolved Loss or Trauma but only when more methylation was observed. Thus, the potentially protective effect of the long variant seemed to be mitigated by the effects of methylation suppressing the activity of this variant. The short variant of 5-HTTLPR appeared to be associated with more Unresolved Loss or Trauma but only with low levels of methylation. Unexpectedly, high levels of methylation of the short variant led to lower Unresolved Loss or Trauma, a finding that still needs an explanation (Van IJzendoorn et al., 2010). What this study shows, however, is that genetic effects on attachment might be hidden behind interactions with epigenetic changes, which in turn might be critically dependent on environmental input, such as abusive or neglectful parenting. This first study on methylation and attachment is relatively small and should be considered exploratory.

Jones-Mason (2011) administered the AAI to 101 participants of various ethnic backgrounds (half of them Asian American, one-third European American). DNA was genotyped for 5-HTTLPR as well as GR, and methylation analyses were conducted in the upstream regions of these genotypes. GR methylation was not associated with any of the variables. The author suggested that in the Asian American group, more methylation in the 5-HTTLPR short allele carriers was associated with less Unresolved Loss or Trauma, and that methylation seemed to have protected them from the potentially traumatizing effects of low socioeconomic status (SES). Similarly, in the Iowa Adoption Study, high methylation in carriers of the short alleles might have blunted their susceptibility to the environment, resulting in low Unresolved Loss or Trauma scores. Because of ethnic heterogeneity and the lack of power for multivariate analyses, the Jones-Mason (2011) study can only be used as a takeoff point to generate hypotheses to be tested in larger and more homogeneous samples.

At present, the study of the epigenetics of attachment is in an embryonic stage and much more work needs to be done to find out whether epigenetics mediates the influence of insensitive and abusive parenting on the development of attachment relationships and representations.

## Parenting

The study of intergenerational transmission of attachment involves the assessment of adult attachment representations in the parent and relating these representations to infant–parent attachment quality (see Hesse, Chapter 26, this volume; Van IJzendoorn, 1995). For the study of intergenerational transmission of *parenting*, it would be ideal if we could observe parents interacting with their offspring, then come back two or three decades later and observe the toddlers of the first wave now interacting with their own offspring. This is exactly what has been done by Kovan, Chung, and Sroufe (2009). They videotaped interactions of parents and their 2-year-old offspring, and did so again several decades later, when the offspring had children of their own who were approximately 2 years of age. Comparing the interactions across the two generations, they found substantial similarity in parenting behaviors ($r = .43$), even when various confounds were taken into account.

Can genetic factors play a role in the explanation of intergenerational transmission of parenting? Unfortunately, traditional studies of parents and their biological children cannot disentangle the effects of shared genes from those of the environment. As with attachment, genetically informative twin or adoption studies are needed to examine the etiology of parenting.

## Behavioral Genetics of Parenting

Two types of behavioral genetic studies of parenting can be found. The first is that of *parent-based twin designs*. Such studies involve adult twin siblings parenting their offspring, and heritability estimates are computed based on a comparison of the similarity between MZ twins' and DZ twins' parenting. In terms of estimations of variance explained by genetic factors, shared environmental factors, and nonshared environment, parent-based twin designs are directly comparable to twin studies on infant attachment. Such studies, however, are scarce. One of the obvious reasons is that twin siblings—notwithstanding the anecdotal and proverbial similarity of their life courses—usually do not have children at the same point in time. The comparability of parenting behaviors in case of divergent timing, numbers, gender, and ages of children is thus hampered.

The second type of study involves parents of twins and is called a *child-based twin design*. These studies compare the similarity between parents of MZ twins and DZ twins. The extent to which parenting behavior toward MZ twin siblings is more similar than parenting behavior toward DZ twin

siblings indicates genetic influence on parenting because genetically influenced characteristics of the children (e.g., temperament) apparently elicit these parenting behaviors. Child-based genetic effects on parenting are thus indicative of evocative rGE: The child's genetic makeup evokes certain parenting behaviors, and these are child-driven genetic influences on parenting.

Shared environmental influences on parenting are due to parents' own characteristics (personality or parenting attitudes), or due to similar behaviors of siblings that result from siblings' shared experiences, regardless of their degree of genetic relatedness. These shared environmental influences include factors such as family SES and cultural environment because they increase similarity in the parenting that children receive. Somewhat counterintuitively, this implies that in child-based twin studies, effects of parents' genes are included in estimates of the shared environment. Last, parents may treat siblings differently for reasons unrelated to the children's genetically influenced characteristics, such as the specific experiences they have with each of their children, with nonshared environmental effects as a result. As always, measurement errors are included in the nonshared environmental effect estimates. It is important to note that child-based twin designs cannot be informative regarding the impact of the parents' own genes or early experiences on their parenting. Only parent-based twin designs can be used to estimate these genetic and (shared and nonshared) environmental effects.

## Parent-Based Twin Designs

A recent meta-analysis of behavioral genetics studies of parenting identified a modest number of six unique parent-based studies (Klahr & Burt, 2014). Most studies were based on questionnaires; in only one study (Neiderhiser et al., 2004) were these combined with observations. Heritability estimates in individual studies varied greatly, ranging from 0% for maternal overprotection to 48% for parental authoritarianism. Distinguishing three dimensions of parenting (i.e., warmth, control, and negativity), combined genetic estimates were moderate for parental warmth and negativity (28–37%), but zero for parental control. Nonshared environmental influences accounted for the largest proportion of variance (63–90%). Heritability estimates were similar for father and mothers. The substantial role for nonshared environmental influences points to parents' unique experiences and the specific conditions in which they find themselves, including the relationship with their spouses and characteristics of their children.

## Child-Based Twin Designs

The same meta-analysis identified 27 studies with child-based twin designs, presenting combined estimates for genetic, shared environmental, and nonshared environmental influences on parental warmth, control, and negativity (Klahr & Burt, 2014). Estimates were largely similar across these three parenting dimensions, with genetic influences ranging from 23 to 40%, shared environmental influences, from 27 to 39%, and nonshared environmental influences, from 32 to 44%. Remember that the genetic influences represent child evocative rGE effects on parenting. Evocative genetic influences on parenting were larger for negativity than for warmth and control, whereas shared environmental influences were largest for warmth, and nonshared environmental influences were largest for control.

Shared environmental influences in child-based twin studies may, among other things, reflect genetic influences in parent-based studies; the results for parental warmth may point in that direction, since moderate genetic estimates for warmth were found in parent-based studies. In child-based twin studies maternal control and negativity were explained to a greater extent by genetic influences than paternal control and negativity. Fathering was more influenced by shared environmental factors than was mothering. Unfortunately, and similar to parent-based twin studies, most child-based twin studies used questionnaire measures of parenting. Notably, observer-rated parenting yielded lower estimates of heritability than child-report or parent-report; for observed parenting, genetic influences on warmth and negativity were not significant.

## Evocative Gene–Environment Correlation

In the meta-analysis of parent-based and child-based twin studies, genetic influences on negativity were found in both types of studies. This may indicate a process in which, in addition to potential passive rGE (parents give their genes, as well as the environment, to their children), children inherit the genetic tendency toward negative behavior from their parents, then through evocative rGE elicit negative parental behavior in their parents (Klahr & Burt, 2014).

Indeed, in a recent child-based twin study in the United Kingdom, Oliver, Trzaskowski, and Plomin (2014) found that the negative side of parenting showed significantly more genetic influence than the positive side. Again, a weakness of the design was that self-reports were used, and that the same parent completed the questionnaire twice, once for each twin sibling, creating nonindependent scores with similar response biases. Importantly, a different U.K. child-based twin study (Jaffee et al., 2004) showed a genetic effect for harsh parenting but not for physical maltreatment; in other words, the child's behavior may evoke harsh discipline, but risk factors for physical maltreatment are more likely to reside in characteristics of the parent and the environment.

The disadvantages of self-reports were overcome in a multivariate child-based twin study of observed parental sensitivity as related to attachment, a study that was somehow left out of Klahr and Burt's (2014) meta-analyses. Fearon and colleagues (2006) examined the extent to which genetic and environmental aspects of maternal sensitivity accounted for the pattern of similarity and dissimilarity of twins' attachments to their mothers (see the section "Behavioral Genetics of Attachment"). Bivariate behavioral genetics modeling is based on the pattern of within-twin and cross-twin correlations to estimate genetic, shared environmental, and nonshared environmental correlations between two measures (Plomin, DeFries, McClearn, & McGuffin, 2001). No genetic factor (residing in the infants) explained differences in maternal sensitivity. The variance in maternal sensitivity was explained by shared environmental (66%) and nonshared environmental (34%) factors. Thus, in line with attachment theory, shared environmental effects were found to underlie the association between maternal sensitivity and attachment security. The shared environmental component of maternal sensitivity accounted for approximately one-third of the twins' similarity in attachment security. Note that this shared environmental component may reflect genetic influences on the level of the parent, perhaps in line with the findings for parental warmth. Exploring the nonshared environmental effect, it appeared that sensitivity toward Twin 2 (that was *not* shown to Twin 1) affected Twin 1's attachment security *positively*. The attachment security of one child thus depends on the relationship the parent has with the other child, and not just on his or her parenting behavior. These findings underscore the importance of effects of relationships within a family system (Hinde & Stevenson-Hinde, 1988) and point to the need for studies including more than one child per family.

## Molecular Genetics of Parenting

The gene systems that have been examined in relation to parenting behavior converge with the gene systems that have been central to studies of attachment. These are genes related to the neurotransmitters dopamine and serotonin, and to the neuropeptide oxytocin. Here we first review studies on potential main effects of these genes on human parenting, then review G × E studies. Our focus is on human parenting. A review that also includes nonhuman mammals can be found elsewhere (Mileva-Seitz, Bakermans-Kranenburg, & Van IJzendoorn, in press).

### Dopamine

What makes dopamine-related gene polymorphisms candidate genes for associations with parenting? Part of the answer lies in the demonstrated implication of dopamine for maternal behavior in rats (Miller & Lonstein, 2005; Stolzenberg et al., 2007). Individual differences in their licking and grooming behavior have been found to be related to variations in dopamine levels in the nucleus accumbens (Champagne et al., 2004). Another part of the answer can be found in studies of humans. Dopamine is related to motivational and reward mechanisms (Robbins & Everitt, 1999), and infants are expected to be rewarding to parents, motivating parents to respond to them and initiate and maintain interaction with them. Variation in dopaminergic system genes may therefore be related to variation in parenting.

In a sample of more than 200 mother–child dyads, Lee and colleagues (2010) tested the association between the dopamine transporter (DAT1) gene and three dimensions of observed maternal parenting behavior (positive parenting, negative parenting, and total maternal commands). The sample consisted of a group of children with attention-deficit/hyperactivity disorder (ADHD) and demographically matched comparison children without ADHD. The observed interaction included free play, as well as tasks that were frustrating for the child (e.g., cleanup, sit and count geometric shapes, play while the mother reads a

magazine and takes a telephone call). Maternal DAT1 was significantly associated with negative parenting and commands, also when child disruptive behavior and various other confounds were taken into account. Mothers with the 9/9 genotype showed the least negative parenting: Mothers with the 9/9 and 10/10 genotypes showed less negative parenting than mothers with the 9/10 genotype, and mothers with the 9/9 genotype used fewer commands than mothers with the 9/10 and 10/10 genotypes. DAT1 genotype was not related to positive parenting.

In the Maternal Adversity, Vulnerability, and Neurodevelopment (MAVAN) study, Mileva-Seitz and colleagues (2012) found an association between genetic variation in several SNPs in the DRD1 and DRD2 genes, and maternal orienting away and infant-directed vocalizing during 20 minutes of free play at 6 months. In three out of five DRD1 SNPs (rs 265981, rs4532, and rs686) the heterozygote group oriented away from the infant less frequently than the two homozygous genotypes, which may be associated with dopamine-related distractibility. Two of the three DRD2 SNPs were associated with infant-directed vocalizing: rs6277 and rs1799732. Although the observations were also rated with Ainsworth's sensitivity rating scales (Ainsworth et al., 1978), the associations with DRD1 and DRD2 polymorphisms were not found with these more global sensitivity ratings, but only with the frequencies of the discrete maternal behaviors. The absence of an association with global ratings for maternal sensitivity replicated findings of Mills-Koonce and colleagues (2007), who in a mixed sample of African American and European American families found no relation between DRD2 and maternal sensitivity or negativity during free play. The authors suggest that discrete behavioral tendencies may show stronger molecular genetic associations than complex phenotypes such as overall sensitivity (Mileva-Seitz et al., 2012).

### Serotonin

The serotonin transporter gene 5-HTTLPR has been studied extensively in relation to depression (e.g., Caspi et al., 2003; Lesch et al., 1996), biased attention for emotional information (Pergamin-Hight, Bakermans-Kranenburg, Van IJzendoorn, & Bar-Haim, 2012), and increased amygdala activation in response to emotional stimuli (Hariri et al., 2002). Usually short and long alleles are distinguished, but strictly speaking, taking into account an adjacent upstream polymorphism, three allelic variants exist: S, LG (functionally similar to S), and LA. Short alleles (including LG) are associated with lower transcription of *5-HTT* mRNA, which encodes for a protein involved in serotonin reuptake. Some, but not all, studies on *5-HTTLPR* and parenting take this additional allelic variant into account. Given the increased attention to emotional stimuli found in carriers of the short allele, the expected direction of the association between *5-HTTLPR* and parenting quality is not unequivocal: Carriers of the short allele may be more attentive to children's emotional signals and respond more promptly and sensitively than carriers of the long alleles, but they may also be more easily overwhelmed by negative child signals and more prone to depression, with compromised parenting as a result.

In the previously mentioned MAVAN study, Mileva-Seitz and colleagues (2011) found support for the former hypothesis: At 6 months postpartum, mothers with the short allele were more sensitive during their interactions with their infants, and they less often oriented away from their infants.

Pener-Tessler and colleagues (2013) found that in families with twins, maternal positive parenting was related to *5-HTTLPR* in different ways for mothers of boys and mothers of girls: In mothers of boys, positive parenting significantly decreased with the number of maternal short alleles, whereas in mothers of girls, positive parenting nonsignificantly increased with the number of short alleles. Three-way interactions, however, are notoriously difficult to replicate.

In a Dutch study, maternal sensitivity was observed in a community sample of 159 white, middle-class mothers with their 2-year-old toddlers at risk for externalizing behavior problems. The dyads were asked to solve puzzles that were too difficult for the child, and mothers were instructed to help their child in the way they usually did. Mothers' supportive presence, intrusiveness, and clarity of instruction were rated on 7-point scales drawn from Egeland and colleagues (1990). These observation scales extend Ainsworth and colleagues' (1978) original scales with an age-appropriate concept of sensitivity that includes the developmental domain of coping with cognitive challenges. The short allele was related to lower levels of maternal sensitive responsiveness (Van IJzendoorn, Bakermans-Kranenburg, & Mesman, 2008).

## Oxytocin

Given the important role of oxytocin in parturition, breastfeeding, and parenting (for a review, see Galbally, Lewis, Van IJzendoorn, & Permezel, 2011), it is only natural that research on parenting has examined associations between various aspects of maternal behavior and oxytocin-related genes. Moreover, oxytocin receptor levels were found to be related to maternal behavior in various types of mammals (Carter, 2014; Dwyer, 2008; Insel & Shapiro, 1992). With regard to studies of human mothers, a few have focused on single-nucleotide polymorphisms (SNPs) in the *OXT* peptide gene, and somewhat more studies have included SNPs in the *OXTR* receptor gene.

Although the functionality of these polymorphisms has not yet been demonstrated, two SNPs in the third intron of *OXTR* have been suggested as particularly promising candidates to explain differences in oxytocinergic functioning: *rs53576* and *rs2254298* (Meyer-Lindenberg, Domes, Kirsch, & Heinrichs, 2011). For both SNPs, the A alleles are hypothesized to confer risk in comparison to the G alleles. It should be noted, however, that a meta-analysis covering 82 studies, 48 ($N = 17,559$) for *OXTR rs53576* and 34 ($N = 13,547$) for *OXTR rs2254298*, with five domains of outcomes (biology, personality, social behavior, psychopathology, and autism), did not yield significant combined effect sizes for any of the domains, or for all domains combined (Bakermans-Kranenburg & Van IJzendoorn, 2013).

Notably, only one study on parenting was included in the meta-analysis (Bakermans-Kranenburg & Van IJzendoorn, 2008). That specific study tested the association between *OXTR rs53576* and sensitive parenting of mothers in interaction with their 2-year-old toddlers at risk for externalizing behavior problems. Controlling for differences in maternal education, depression, and marital discord, parents with the A allele showed lower levels of sensitive responsiveness to their toddlers.

Since then, a number of additional studies on oxytocin-related genes and parenting have been conducted. Replication of the effect found in the first study was provided by the Twin Study of Behavioral and Emotional Development in Children (TBED-C), including 500 families with twins ages 6–10 years old (Klahr, Klump, & Burt, 2015). Three dimensions of parenting were observed—warmth, negativity, and control—for both fathers and mothers. Parents as well as children were genotyped for *OXTR rs53576*. Child *OXTR* genotype did not predict the type of parenting received, and the father's genotype was also not associated with his parenting behavior. But the mother's genotype was related to maternal warmth; mothers with the AA genotype showed less warmth in interaction with their children than mothers with the GG or AG genotypes. Importantly, the association between maternal *OXTR* genotype and warmth was unchanged when controlling for child *OXTR* genotype, age, and gender (i.e., controlling for child-driven evocative effects).

In a longitudinal study of children with ADHD and matched controls, selection of 40 mothers was based on their extreme scores on positive or negative parenting of their 4- to 6-year-old children to maximize variation in parenting (Michalska et al., 2014). Parenting was observed during free play and a series of tasks, for a total of about 20 minutes, and 15 years later, mothers were exposed to pictures of their own and other children in a functional magnetic resonance imaging (fMRI) session. *OXTR rs53576* and *rs1042778* were both associated with quality of parenting, although only *rs53576* survived correction for multiple testing. In contrast with studies reviewed earlier, not the G allele but the A allele was associated with higher levels of positive parenting. Note, however, that an interaction with ethnicity suggested that the association with parenting might be different for African American mothers (almost half of the sample) and European American mothers. Looking at pictures of their own child rather than an unknown child, A-allele carriers showed greater activation in the orbitofrontal cortex (OFC, involved in orienting toward, monitoring, and evaluating infant cues and emotional stimuli in general) and the anterior cingulate cortex (ACC, involved in regulating emotional responses). Finally, when exposed to pictures of their own child's inappropriate versus appropriate behavior, A-allele carriers showed more right hippocampus activation. As the activation of oxytocin receptors in the hippocampus is related to inhibited behavioral reaction to stress in rats (Cohen et al., 2010), this may suggest that increased hippocampal activation helps to inhibit a strong negative behavioral reaction to child transgressing behavior.

In another small study, adult females without children of their own were exposed to bouts of infant crying. Cries produce autonomic arousal in adults, which in turn facilitates a quick response to the infant in order to terminate the cry (Del Vecchio, Walter, & O'Leary, 2009). Almost half of the variance in adults' cardiac reactivity to an experimental paradigm with bouts of infant crying of varying pitch (Crowe & Zeskind, 1992) was shown to be explained by genetic factors in a behavioral genetic study with adult twins (Out, Pieper, Bakermans-Kranenburg, & Van IJzendoorn, 2010), and this cry paradigm was thus used to test whether *OXTR rs53576* would be related to variation in reactivity to cry sounds. Women with the GG genotype had greater heart rate responses to infant cries, but only when they had low depression scores (Riem, Pieper, Out, Bakermans-Kranenburg, & Van IJzendoorn, 2011). The participants were female twins, and the results were replicated in their twin sisters.

In an Israeli study, three SNPs were investigated: *OXTR rs2254298* and *rs1042778*, and *CD38 rs3796863* (Feldman et al., 2012). CD38 is a regulator of oxytocin release and has been found related to autism spectrum disorders (Munesue et al., 2010). In mice without *CD38*, reduced oxytocin levels and marked deficits in social and maternal behavior were observed (Jin et al., 2007). During the observation, infants sat on an infant seat, parents sat next to them, and parents were asked to play with their infants as they would typically do. Gaze synchrony and parental touch were coded. Parents with the *CD38* CC genotype touched their infants less frequently than those carrying the A allele, and parents with the *OXTR rs1042778* TT genotype touched their infant less than parents carrying the G allele. For gaze synchrony, no genetic effects were found.

In the MAVAN study mentioned earlier, two polymorphisms in the oxytocin peptide gene (*OXT rs2740210, rs4813627*) and one polymorphism in the oxytocin receptor gene (*OXTR rs237885*) were genotyped and related to mother–infant interaction (Mileva-Seitz et al., 2013). At 6 months, the two *OXT* SNPs were related to infant-directed vocalizing, though not to maternal sensitivity, as assessed with Ainsworth's maternal sensitivity scales (Ainsworth et al., 1978). A allele carriers showed less infant-directed vocalizing. Because the two SNPs were in high linkage disequilibrium (i.e., specific allelic combinations were found more often than would be expected based on the allele frequencies in the sample), they cannot be considered independent effects, and the effect may also be due to some other SNP in linkage disequilibrium with these two SNPs. *OXT rs2740210* was also related to breast-feeding duration, with replication in an independent sample (Jonas et al., 2013). The *OXTR* (*rs237885*) genotype was not related to vocalizing, maternal sensitivity, or breastfeeding.

Although the role of oxytocin in parenting is undisputed, variations in the *OXT* peptide gene and in the *OXTR* receptor gene have not yet produced a convincing picture of associations between particular polymorphisms and sensitive parenting. The link between particular *OXTR* genotypes and parenting has been suggested as an important direction for research into parenting (Taylor, 2008), but so far the results are at best promising and not as consistent as might be expected on the basis of animal research. The possibility to have much more control over environmental variation in animal studies may allow for stronger genetic effects in studies of parenting in rats compared to studies on human parenting.

In a similar vein, findings regarding associations between maternal dopamine- and serotonin-related genotypes and observed parenting are inconclusive. All studies published so far have been based on relatively small samples. The lack of convergence in the results points to the risk of chance results, and replication in larger samples is badly needed. Unfortunately, in the two large studies with child genotype and attachment data reviewed earlier (Generation R and NICHD SEC-CYD), measures of parenting quality are available, but maternal DNA has not (yet) been genotyped.

Of course, genes may play additive or interactive roles that so far have not been taken into account. Dopamine and oxytocin work together to regulate behavioral responses to social stimuli. In rats, there is a direct effect of oxytocin on dopamine release within the mesocorticolimbic dopamine system (Shahrokh, Zhang, Diorio, Gratton, & Meaney, 2010). In a similar way, genetic variants in dopamine- and oxytocin-related genes may interact to affect parenting in humans. This may be an important future step for studies on parenting, along with the examination of genetic pathways and genomewide association studies (see earlier sections on GWAS and GCTA).

## G × E Interactions

G × E interactions may explain why some parents are more affected and others are less affected by disadvantageous childhoods or concurrent daily stresses in responding sensitively to their offspring's signals (Rutter, 2006). For example, in the MAVAN study, *OXT rs2740210* moderated the effect of early life experiences on breastfeeding through depression. In women with the CC genotype, childhood abuse experiences were related to lower maternal mood at 6 months postpartum, which in turn was associated with reduced breastfeeding duration across the first year (Jonas et al., 2013). Parents may also be differentially susceptible to environmental influences *for better and for worse*. In an Israeli study with mothers of twins, mothers with the *DRD4* 7-repeat allele who experienced more stress around childbirth (e.g., their twin children had low gestational age, low birthweight, and prolonged stay at the neonatal intensive care unit) were less sensitive when interacting with their children at age 3.5 than other mothers, whereas mothers with the *DRD4* 7-repeat allele whose children had few complications around birth showed the highest levels of sensitivity (Fortuna et al., 2011).

Including not only *DRD4* but also *COMT* gene polymorphisms, mothers and toddlers were observed in a series of problem-solving tasks, and parents reported on their daily hassles (Van IJzendoorn et al., 2008). The two dopamine-related genes moderated the negative influence of daily hassles on sensitive parenting behavior to their offspring. In parents with the combination of genes leading to the least efficient dopaminergic system functioning (COMT*val* allele, *DRD4* 7-repeat allele), more daily hassles were associated with less sensitive parenting, but in this group, lower levels of daily hassles were associated with more sensitive parenting. The other combinations of *COMT* and *DRD4* polymorphisms did not show significant associations between daily hassles and maternal sensitivity.

The latter two studies (Fortuna et al., 2011; Van IJzendoorn et al., 2008) yielded interaction effects that are reminiscent of the G × E effect found for infant disorganization (Van IJzendoorn & Bakermans-Kranenburg, 2006). Remember that in this study, infants with the *DRD4* 7-repeat allele were more susceptible to parental unresolved loss than infants without this allele. Infants with the *DRD4* 7-repeat allele and mothers with unresolved loss had relatively high levels of infant disorganization, but infants with the *DRD4* 7-repeat allele and mothers without unresolved loss showed the lowest levels of attachment disorganization. In children without this allele, maternal unresolved loss was not related to disorganized attachment.

Here similar patterns of results emerge: Parents with the *DRD4* 7-repeat allele (and, in one study, an additional COMT*val* allele) were more affected by stress than parents without this specific genotype. Under conditions of stress, they were among the least sensitive parents, but lower levels of stress were accompanied by an increase in caregiving sensitivity, much stronger so than in parents without this genotype. The role of *DRD4* as a susceptibility marker may therefore not be limited to children but may extend to adults as well. Support for this idea is also provided by the Iowa Adoption Studies, showing that adults with the *DRD4* 7-repeat allele were most susceptible to the absence or presence of parental problems in their adoptive families (Bakermans-Kranenburg, Van IJzendoorn, et al., 2011). Differential susceptibility has important implications for interventions. Susceptible individuals, whether parents or children, may profit more from interventions that systematically improve the environment.

## Genetically Moderated Intervention Efficacy

Interventions with the aim of enhancing parental sensitivity or reducing attachment insecurity are manifold (see Berlin, Zeanah, & Lieberman, Chapter 32, this volume). They vary in scope and intensity, from brief and focused to covering a broad range of topics and approaches over a period of several years. What the vast majority of these interventions have in common is that their impact is only modest, with intervention effects that are disappointing in relation to the large investments in terms of time and money. In this section we delineate the role of genetics in explaining differences in susceptibility to intervention that may mask the efficacy of interventions in specific groups (Bakermans-Kranenburg & Van IJzendoorn, 2015).

### Differential Susceptibility

The differential susceptibility model is of particular importance to intervention research. If environmental effects are more pronounced for specific groups compared to others, the effect of interventions will also be stronger for some than for others. As a consequence, the average intervention effect would underestimate the effectiveness/efficacy in the most susceptible groups. This is a completely different perspective on intervention, and for that reason, we dig somewhat deeper into differential susceptibility in general and into genetic differential susceptibility in particular.

The first three decades of G × E research were characterized by approaches such as the transac-

tional/dual-risk (Sameroff, 1983), cumulative risk (Rutter, 2010), and diathesis–stress models (Monroe & Simons, 1991). These approaches share a focus on psychopathology: Children with a vulnerable constitution ("risk" genes) and poor developmental experiences (e.g., insensitive parenting, low-quality child care, stressful life experiences) are expected to be at increased risk for bad outcomes. A typical example would be that children with the *5-HTTLPR* short allele were more often disorganized when maternal responsiveness was low (Spangler et al., 2009), or that infants with the minor MR allele (G) were less securely attached if their mothers showed extremely insensitive behaviors, whereas these associations were not present in children without the G allele (Luijk, Tharner, et al., 2011). The G allele might easily be indicated as the "risk allele." In the latter study, however, infants with the G allele were more securely attached if their mothers were more sensitive. Genetic variation in MR thus modulated infants' sensitivity to care, for better (increased susceptibility to maternal sensitive behavior) and for worse (increased vulnerability to maternal extreme insensitivity), and it would be a mistake to consider the G allele a risk allele when it also enhances the chance of developing secure attachments with sensitive caregivers.

In short, the same genotype that makes individuals vulnerable to adversity may also make them disproportionately likely to benefit from contextual support (Belsky et al., 2007). The differential susceptibility hypothesis proposes that in positive environments, "vulnerable" children may flourish even more than their peers who are less susceptible to both supportive and unsupportive environments (Bakermans-Kranenburg & Van IJzendoorn, 2007; Belsky et al., 2007; Ellis et al., 2011). The differential susceptibility model is not so much complementary to the diathesis–stress model; it is fundamentally different from it. Its evolutionary foundation implies that certain genotypes must be called "susceptibility" genes instead of "risk" genes (Bakermans-Kranenburg & Van IJzendoorn, 2015).

Evidence for genetic moderation of environmental effects according to the differential susceptibility model has been specifically tested for serotonin- and dopamine-related gene polymorphisms, although other genotypes have been identified as potential markers of susceptibility as well (e.g., monoamine oxidase A [*MAOA*], brain-derived neurotrophic factor [*BDNF*], MR). The first G × E differential susceptibility study showed that children with the *DRD4* 7-repeat allele displayed the most externalizing behavior at 39 months, when their mothers were observed to be insensitive during home observations at 10 months of age, but the least externalizing behavior when their mothers were highly sensitive (Bakermans-Kranenburg & Van IJzendoorn, 2006). The findings of this pioneering small study were confirmed in a meta-analysis on dopamine-system-related genotypes (15 studies, $N = 1,232$). The combined effect sizes for the association between adverse rearing influences and behavioral disturbance amounted to $r = .37$ for carriers of the "risk alleles" and only $r = .10$ for the comparisons without the risk alleles. But the combined effect sizes for association between support and better adaptation were $r = .31$ for carriers of the putatively risk alleles, and $r = -.03$ for those without the risk alleles (Bakermans-Kranenburg & Van IJzendoorn, 2011). Thus, genotypes that in adverse contexts put children at risk for behavior problems allowed them to benefit more from support.

For *5-HTTLPR* as a genetic susceptibility marker, quite similar meta-analytic results were found, but with a difference depending on the inclusion of samples with mostly non-Caucasian and mixed ethnicities (Van IJzendoorn et al., 2012). In the total set of studies (77 studies, $N = 9,361$) children with short alleles were more negatively affected by adverse contexts than carriers of two long alleles with regard to negative outcomes, but they did not benefit significantly more from positive environments. The pattern of results was thus convergent with the diathesis–stress model; with short alleles as "risk alleles" rendering individuals more vulnerable to environmental adversity but not more open to supportive contexts. In studies with predominantly ( >80%) Caucasian participants (52 studies, $N = 6,626$), carriers of short alleles were more sensitive to negative ($r = .18$) as well as positive ($r = .17$) environmental influences than individuals with two long alleles ($r = .04$ for negative environments, $r = .05$ for positive environments), in accordance with the differential susceptibility model. These differences point to ethnicity as an important moderator in G × E studies, including genetic differential susceptibility studies.

Most of these first studies that formed the basis for the two meta-analyses were correlational. More often than not, the studies did not specifically aim at testing the "bright side" of better outcomes in carriers of "risk alleles" in positive environments. In a way, this is an advantage because

it implies that those results that were derived as part of the meta-analytical process were not the focus of the specific study, which counters the risk of publication bias. The crucial test of the differential susceptibility model is, however, whether in randomized controlled trials (RCT) individuals with the susceptible genotypes profit more from interventions, that is, from experimental improvement of the environment.

## Interventions from a G × E Perspective

G × E experiments (or G × eE [*experimental* E) are RCTs with random assignment of participants to intervention and control groups. G × E experiments have at least three advantages compared to correlational G × E studies (see Van IJzendoorn & Bakermans-Kranenburg, 2015).

First, G and E are uncorrelated. Correlational G × E studies may test for gene–environment correlation (rGE) and set it aside when the genetic marker is not correlated with the environmental factor, but this provides no definite proof of the absence of rGE, because unmeasured genes may be related to the environmental factor under study. In RCTs, the environment is manipulated in standard ways, and randomization breaks any possible rGE. Only random assignment to experimental and control conditions can disentangle genetic and environmental factors (Van IJzendoorn, Bakermans-Kranenburg, Belsky, et al., 2011).

Second, G × E experiments decrease the risk of unequal measurement errors in the G × E equation. If genetic assessments are done in a careful way but broad or "quick-and-dirty" measures are used for the environment (e.g., self-reported retrospective childhood experiences), the error components are smaller for G than for E, creating risks for type I and type II errors. Experiments with well-defined, standardized manipulations of specific dimensions of the environment reduce measurement error in E. Of course, ineffective interventions do not contribute to a reduction of measurement error in E. Assessing the change in the environment is important to check the impact of the manipulation and to examine dose–response relations between environmental change and outcome in the experimental condition. As an example, in a study on the efficacy of the Video-feedback Intervention to promote Positive Parenting and Sensitive Discipline (VIPP-SD) in the reduction of child externalizing behavior, the way in which parental discipline strategies were affected by the intervention was measured, and the change in parental strategies was related to decreased externalizing behavior in children with the *DRD4* 7-repeat allele (Bakermans-Kranenburg et al., 2008).

Third, G × E experiments have more statistical power compared to rGE studies. Experimental studies make participants in the experimental condition maximally different from participants in the control condition, and this creates more variance in the product term. Correlational studies tend to contain few observations at the extremes of the distribution and many observations close to the center of the distribution. Selective recruitment and attrition, especially in the tails of the distribution, are responsible for this effect, and they can hardly be avoided. Experimental G × E studies lead to better distributed variables, and as a result, the power can be more than 10 times larger compared to correlational studies (McClelland & Judd, 1993). This is not a trivial issue because lack of power has been identified as one of the major problems in G × E research.

Randomized controlled intervention studies thus offer great opportunities to examine G × E interaction effects. Randomized controlled intervention studies can also provide insight in variation in intervention effectiveness among different groups. This is an important step in uncovering which intervention works best for whom, and provides hints relating to the mechanisms involved. Finally, they enable testing of whether the dopamine-related and serotonin-related genotypes that emerge as "susceptibility" factors from correlational G × E studies are indeed related to larger intervention effects.

## Meta-Analysis of Genetic Differential Susceptibility Experiments

In the past decades, a number of genetic differential susceptibility experiments have been conducted. These RCTs address the question of whether intervention effects are moderated by a genetic susceptibility marker. In a meta-analysis of these experiments, we tested whether genotypes that were once considered risk factors and that were later suggested to be susceptibility (or "plasticity") factors were related to larger intervention effects.

Twenty-two RCTs could be identified (Van IJzendoorn & Bakermans-Kranenburg, 2015), some of which had attachment as the outcome— for example, the intervention study of maltreat-

ing families conducted by Cicchetti, Rogosch, and Toth (2011), and the Bucharest Early Intervention Project (Brett et al., 2015; Nelson, Fox, & Zeanah, 2014). The 22 RCTs included 3,257 participants in total, 38% of whom were carriers of susceptibility genes. The combined effect size of the interventions for carriers of the susceptible genotypes amounted to $r = .33$, which is a large effect even in terms of Cohen's (1988) conventional criteria. In contrast, the hypothesized nonsusceptible group was less affected by the interventions; the combined size of the intervention effects in this group was not significant, $r = .08$. Intervention effects were thus much stronger in the a priori hypothesized susceptible group.

In the 14 studies with predominantly ( >80%) Caucasian participants ($N = 2,060$), the findings were replicated, with significantly larger intervention effects for the susceptible genotypes ($r = .26$) than for the nonsusceptible genotypes ($r = .12$). Considering the genetic marker of susceptibility, dopamine-related genes were indeed markers of susceptibility. The 11 studies with dopamine-related genotypes as moderators showed larger intervention effects in susceptible genotype groups ($r = .35$) than in nonsusceptible genotypes ($r = -.00$). Seven studies with *5-HTTLPR* as moderator showed significant combined effects in the susceptible genotype group ($r = .30$) but also in the nonsusceptible genotype group ($r = .16$); the difference between these two effect sizes was in the expected direction but not statistically significant ($p = .15$).

As an important final step, the difference between the effect sizes for the susceptible and nonsusceptible groups within each study was computed. The combined effect size for the difference between susceptible and nonsusceptible genotypes within studies was significant, with a medium effect size. We tested this combined effect size for publication bias and did not find any, which indicates that the combined effect size was not based on selective publication of studies that reported significant moderation of intervention effects by genotype at the expense of studies that did not find such moderation.

## Conclusion

The study of the role of genetics in explaining differences in attachment security began only around the year 2000, so it is a relatively young branch of the growing attachment tree. On the one hand, this is remarkable because attachment theory might be considered the first application of evolutionary theory to human development—after Charles Darwin but before so-called "evolutionary psychology" emerged. From evolutionary theory, John Bowlby (1969/1982) derived one of the core hypotheses of current attachment theory, the idea that every human infant is born with an innate bias to become attached to a protective conspecific. The genetic basis of this specieswide bias and related behavior in the various stages of attachment development has not yet received any attention.

On the other hand, attachment theory has always emphasized environmental influences, more specifically, effects of parenting, on the development of individual differences in attachment relationships and representations. Central to attachment theory is the idea that attachment starts as a dyadic construct, shaped mostly by parents, to be gradually internalized by the child and to become a defining feature of the growing individual. Behavior genetics studies seem to confirm this idea because most twin and adoption studies document the large role of the environment in explaining variance of attachment security and disorganization at a young age.

For three reasons, one should be careful deriving strong conclusions from behavior genetics. First, twin studies partition variation in attachment within a specific population and environment, and results are therefore sample-specific and dependent on variation in the environment. In more homogeneous environments, higher estimations for heritability are found. Second, results pertain to the group level, and should not be taken to indicate individual genetics. Third, the influence of genetics might grow with age, and twin studies on attachment beyond adolescence are lacking. As a relatively new development, GCTA extends behavior genetics in that it is not dependent on twin studies. Similar to behavioral genetics, GCTA leads to estimates of heritability without pointing at specific genes or gene pathways that play a role in the phenotype.

Molecular genetics has been used as a tool in search for specific genotypes related to parenting and to attachment security and disorganization. However, few, if any, clues for finding "attachment genes" have emerged. Considering the complex phenotypic signature of attachment and the necessarily limited sample sizes involved in studies of infant or adult attachment, this should not come as

a surprise. In fact, the search for main effects in genetics of human behaviors and disorders has been generally disappointing even to the most influential and optimistic gene hunters (Plomin, 2013). Ever larger samples account for ever smaller variance in traits on the level of singular genotypes. Gene pathways, mirroring more closely complex neurobiological endophenotypes of attachment, such as the dopamine system, may characterize the next generation of molecular genetics studies.

It seems safe to conclude that the intergenerational transmission gap between parental and child attachments (Van IJzendoorn, 1995) cannot be bridged by genes alone or by separate accounts of genetic and environmental input. G × E interactions may be better suited for this challenge. Correlational studies have documented the important role of G × E interactions in explaining human development, and experimental studies have provided even more compelling evidence of the importance of the interplay between genes and environments. In particular, the concept of genetic differential susceptibility generates support for the hypothesis derived from Belsky's (1997) notion that children might differ in their openness to parenting influences in a *for better and for worse* manner. Although conclusive evidence is still missing, particularly in the area of attachment, genetic makeup might make some children vulnerable to the development of insecure attachments in less supportive environments, whereas the same genetic endowment enables children to profit more from supportive environments (i.e., sensitive parenting). This is a new perspective on the old issue of the transmission gap, to be explored more carefully in the next decade of attachment studies. In a clinical and practical sense, the implication is that the efficacy of attachment-based interventions may have been over- and underestimated depending on the proportions of susceptible parents or children.

In his revised edition of the trilogy *Attachment*, Bowlby (1969/1982) has already argued that the antithesis of innate versus acquired behavioral traits is unreal and unproductive: "Just as area is a product of length multiplied by width so every biological character ... is a product of the interaction of genetic endowment with environment" (p. 38). Meaney (2001) attributes this wonderful rectangle metaphor to Donald Hebb and dates it back to the 1960s of the previous century. Meaney adds that it is impossible to explain to the general public that one ever could make sense of a rectangle by studying only length isolated from width, or the other way around. Nevertheless, this is exactly what has happened in the study of human development, including attachment. Genetic differential susceptibility, incorporating epigenetics, may offer a viable window to study the interplay between genes and environment in attachment.

## References

Ainsworth, M. D. S., Blehar, M. C., Waters, E., & Wall, S. (1978). *Patterns of attachment: A physiological study of the Strange Situation.* Hillsdale, NJ: Erlbaum.

Bakermans-Kranenburg, M. J., Dobrova-Krol, N. A., & Van IJzendoorn, M. H. (2011). Impact of institutional care on attachment disorganization and insecurity of Ukrainian preschoolers: Protective effect of the long variant of the serotonin transporter gene (5HTT). *International Journal of Behavioral Development, 36,* 11–18.

Bakermans-Kranenburg, M. J., & Van IJzendoorn, M. H. (2004). No association of the dopamine D4 receptor (*DRD4*) and *-521 C/T* promoter polymorphisms with infant attachment disorganization. *Attachment and Human Development, 6,* 211–218.

Bakermans-Kranenburg, M. J., & Van IJzendoorn, M. H. (2007). Research review: Genetic vulnerability or differential susceptibility in child development: The case of attachment. *Journal of Child Psychology and Psychiatry, 48,* 1160–1173.

Bakermans-Kranenburg, M. J., & Van IJzendoorn, M. H. (2008). Oxytocin receptor (*OXTR*) and serotonin transporter (*5-HTT*) genes associated with observed parenting. *Social Cognitive and Affective Neuroscience, 3,* 128–134.

Bakermans-Kranenburg, M. J., & Van IJzendoorn, M. H. (2009). The first 10,000 Adult Attachment Interviews: Distributions of adult attachment representations in non-clinical and clinical groups. *Attachment and Human Development, 11,* 223–263.

Bakermans-Kranenburg, M. J., & Van IJzendoorn, M. H. (2010). Parenting matters: Family science in the genomic era. *Family Science, 1,* 25–35.

Bakermans-Kranenburg, M. J., & Van IJzendoorn, M. H. (2011). Differential susceptibility to rearing environment depending on dopamine-related genes: New evidence and a meta-analysis. *Development and Psychopathology, 23,* 39–52.

Bakermans-Kranenburg, M. J., & Van IJzendoorn, M. H. (2013). A sociability gene?: Meta-analysis of oxytocin receptor (*OXTR*) genotype effects in humans. *Psychiatric Genetics, 24,* 45–51.

Bakermans-Kranenburg, M. J., & Van IJzendoorn, M. H. (2015). The hidden efficacy of interventions: Gene × environment experiments from a differential susceptibility perspective. *Annual Review of Psychology, 66,* 381–409.

Bakermans-Kranenburg, M. J., Van IJzendoorn, M. H.,

Bokhorst, C. L., & Schuengel, C. (2004). The importance of shared environment in infant–father attachment: A behavioral genetic study of the Attachment Q-Sort. *Journal of Family Psychology, 18,* 545–549.

Bakermans-Kranenburg, M. J., Van IJzendoorn, M. H., Caspers, K., & Philibert, R. (2011). *DRD4* genotype moderates the impact of parental problems on unresolved loss or trauma. *Attachment and Human Development, 13,* 253–270.

Barry, R. A., Kochanska, G., & Philibert, R. A. (2008). G × E interaction in the organization of attachment: Mothers' responsiveness as a moderator of children's genotypes. *Journal of Child Psychology and Psychiatry, 49,* 1313–1320.

Beach, S. R. H., Brody, G. H., Todorov, A. A., Gunter, T. D., & Philibert, R. A. (2010). Methylation at *SLC6A4* is linked to family history of child abuse: An examination of the Iowa adoptee sample. *American Journal of Medical Genetics B: Neuropsychiatric Genetics, 153,* 710–713.

Belsky, J. (1997). Theory testing, effect-size evaluation, and differential susceptibility to rearing influence: The case of mothering and attachment. *Child Development, 68,* 598–600.

Belsky, J., Bakermans-Kranenburg, M. J., & Van IJzendoorn, M. H. (2007). For better and for worse: Differential susceptibility to environmental influences. *Current Directions in Psychological Sciences, 16,* 300–304.

Belsky, J., & Pluess, M. (2013). Genetic moderation of early child-care effects on social functioning across childhood: a developmental analysis. *Child Development, 84,* 1209–1225.

Benjamin, D. J., Cesarini, D., van der Loos, M. J. H. M., Dawes, C. T., Koelinger, P. D., & Magnusson, P. K. E. (2012). The genetic architecture of economic and political preferences. *Proceedings of the National Academy of Sciences USA, 109,* 8026–8031.

Bernstein, D. P., Stein, J. A., Newcomb, M. D., Walker, E., Pogge, D., Ahluvalia, T., et al. (2003). Development and validation of a brief screening version of the Childhood Trauma Questionnaire. *Child Abuse and Neglect, 27,* 169–190.

Bokhorst, C. L., Bakermans-Kranenburg, M. J., Fearon, R. M., Van IJzendoorn, M. H., Fonagy, P., & Schuengel, C. (2003). The importance of shared environment in mother–infant attachment security: A behavioral genetic study. *Child Development, 74,* 1769–1782.

Bowlby, J. (1982). *Attachment and loss: Vol. 1. Attachment* (2nd ed.). New York: Basic Books. (Original work published 1969)

Bretherton, I., Ridgeway, D., & Cassidy, J. (1990). Assessing internal working models of attachment relationships: An attachment story completion task for 3-year-olds. In M. T. Greenberg, D. Cicchetti, & E. M. Cummings (Eds.), *Attachment in the preschool years: Theory, research and intervention* (pp. 87–119). Chicago: University of Chicago Press.

Brett, Z. H., Humphreys, K. L., Smyke, A. T., Gleason, M. M., Nelson, C. A., Zeanah, C. H., et al. (2015). Serotonin transporter linked polymorphic region (5-HTTLPR) genotype moderates the longitudinal impact of early caregiving and attachment on externalizing behavior. *Development and Psychopathology*, 27(1), 7–18.

Bronfenbrenner, U. (1979). *The ecology of human development*. Cambridge, MA: Harvard University Press.

Carter, C. S. (2014). Oxytocin pathways and the evolution of human behavior. *Annual Review of Psychology*, 65, 10.1–10.23.

Caspers, K., Yucuis, R., Troutman, B., Arndt, S., & Langbehn, D. (2007). A sibling adoption study of adult attachment: The influence of shared environment on attachment states of mind. *Attachment and Human Development*, 9, 375–391.

Caspi, A., Sugden, K., Moffitt, T. E., Taylor, A., Craig, I. W., Harrington, H., et al. (2003). Influence of life stress on depression: Moderation by a polymorphism in the 5-HTT gene. *Science*, 301, 386–389.

Cassidy, J. (1988). Child–mother attachment and the self in six-year-olds. *Child Development*, 59, 121–134.

Champagne, F., Chretien, P., Stevenson, C. W., Zhang, T. Y., Gratton, A., & Meaney, M. J. (2004). Variations in nucleus accumbens dopamine associated with individual differences in maternal behavior in the rat. *Journal of Neuroscience*, 24, 4113–4123.

Cicchetti, D., Rogosch, F. A., & Toth, S. L. (2011). The effects of child maltreatment and polymorphisms of the serotonin transporter and dopamine D4 receptor genes on infant attachment and intervention efficacy. *Development and Psychopathology*, 23, 357–372.

Cohen, H., Kaplan, Z., Kozlovsky, N., Gidron, Y., Matar, M. A., & Zohar, J. (2010). Hippocampal microinfusion of oxytocin attenuates the behavioural response to stress by means of dynamic interplay with the glucocorticoid–catecholamine responses. *Journal of Neuroendocrinology*, 22, 889–904.

Cohen, J. (1988). *Statistical power analysis for the behavioral sciences* (2nd ed.). London: Routledge.

Cronk, N. J., Slutske, W. S., Madden, P. A. F., Bucholz, K. K., Reich, W., & Heath, A. C. (2002). Emotional and behavioral problems among female twins: An evaluation of the equal environments assumption. *Journal of the American Academy of Child and Adolescent Psychiatry*, 41, 829–837.

Crowe, H. P., & Zeskind, P. S. (1992). Psychophysiological and perceptual responses to infant cries varying in pitch: Comparison of adults with low and high scores on the Child Abuse Potential Inventory. *Child Abuse and Neglect*, 16, 19–29.

Cumming, G. (2014). The new statistics: Why and how. *Psychological Science*, 25, 7–29.

Cyr, C., Euser, E. M., Bakermans-Kranenburg, M. J., & Van IJzendoorn, M. H. (2010). Attachment security and disorganization in maltreating and high-risk families: A series of meta-analyses. *Development and Psychopathology*, 22, 87–108.

Del Vecchio, T., Walter, A., & O'Leary, S. G. (2009). Affective and physiological factors predicting maternal response to infant crying. *Infant Behavior and Development*, 32, 117–122.

Drury, S. S., Gleason, M. M., Theall, K. P., Smyke, A. T., Nelson, C. A., Fox, N. A., et al. (2012). Genetic sensitivity to the caregiving context: The influence of 5HTTLPR and BDNF val66met on indiscriminate social behavior. *Physiology and Behavior*, 106, 728–735.

Duncan, L. E., & Keller, M. C. (2011). A critical review of the first 10 years of candidate gene-by-environment interaction research in psychiatry. *American Journal of Psychiatry*, 168, 1041–1049.

Dwyer, C. M. (2008). Individual variation in the expression of maternal behaviour: A review of the neuroendocrine mechanisms in the sheep. *Journal of Neuroendocrinology*, 20, 526–534.

Egeland, B., Erickson, M. F., Clemenhagen-Moon, J. C., Hiester, M. K., & Korfmacher, J. (1990). *24 Months Tools Coding Manual* (Project STEEP revised 1990 from mother–child project scales). Unpublished manuscript, University of Minnesota.

Ellis, B. J., Boyce, W. T., Belsky, J., Bakermans-Kranenburg, M. J., & Van IJzendoorn, M. H. (2011). Differential susceptibility to the environment: A neurodevelopmental theory. *Development and Psychopathology*, 23, 7–28.

Fearon, P., Shmueli-Goetz, Y., Viding, E., Fonagy, P., & Plomin, R. (2014). Genetic and environmental influences on adolescent attachment. *Journal of Child Psychology and Psychiatry*, 55(9), 1033–1041.

Fearon, R. M. P., Van IJzendoorn, M. H., Fonagy, P., Bakermans-Kranenburg, M. J., Schuengel, C., & Bokhorst, C. L. (2006). In search of shared and nonshared environmental factors in security of attachment: A behavior-genetic study of the association between sensitivity and attachment security. *Developmental Psychology*, 42, 1026–1040.

Feldman, R., Zagoory-Sharon, O., Weisman, O., Schneiderman, I., Gordon, I., Maoz, R., et al. (2012). Sensitive parenting is associated with plasma oxytocin and polymorphisms in the OXTR and CD38 genes. *Biological Psychiatry*, 72, 175–181.

Finkel, D., Wille, D. E., & Matheny, A. P., Jr. (1998). Preliminary results from a twin study of infant–caregiver attachment. *Behavior Genetics*, 28, 1–8.

Fortuna, K., Van IJzendoorn, M. H., Mankuta, D., Kaitz, M., Avinun, R., Ebstein, R. P., et al. (2011). Differential genetic susceptibility to child risk at birth in predicting observed maternal behavior. *PLoS ONE*, 6, e19765.

Fraga, M. F., Ballestar, E., Paz, M. F., Ropero, S., Setien, F., Ballestar, M. L., et al. (2005). Epigenetic differences arise during the lifetime of monozygotic twins. *Proceedings of the National Academy of Sciences USA*, 102, 10604–10609.

Frigerio, A., Ceppi, E., Rusconi, M., Giorda, R., Raggi, M. E., & Fearon, P. (2009). The role played by the interaction between genetic factors and attachment in the stress response in infancy. *Journal of Child Psychology and Psychiatry, 50,* 1513–1522.

Galbally, M., Lewis, A., Van IJzendoorn, M. H., & Permezel, M. (2011). The role of oxytocin in maternal–infant relationships: A systematic review of human studies. *Harvard Review Psychiatry, 19,* 1–14.

Gervai, J., Novak, A., Lakatos, K., Toth, I., Danis, I., Ronai, Z., et al. (2007). Infant genotype may moderate sensitivity to maternal affective communications: Attachment disorganization, quality of care, and the *DRD4* polymorphism. *Social Neuroscience, 2,* 307–319.

Gilissen, R., Bakermans-Kranenburg, M. J., Van IJzendoorn, M. H., & Linting, M. (2008). Electrodermal reactivity during the Trier social stress test for children: Interaction between the serotonin transporter polymorphism and children's attachment representation. *Developmental Psychobiology, 50,* 615–625.

Groh, A., Narayan, A. J., Bakermans-Kranenburg, M. J., Roisman, G. I., Vaughn, B. E., Fearon R. M. P., et al. (in press). Attachment and temperament in the early life course: A meta-analytic review. *Child Development.*

Hariri, A. R., Mattay, V. S., Tessitore, A., Kolachana, B., Fera, F., Goldman, D., et al. (2002). Serotonin transporter genetic variation and the response of the human amygdala. *Science, 297,* 400–403.

Haworth, C. M. A., Dale, P. S., & Plomin, R. (2009). The etiology of science performance: Decreasing heritability and increasing importance of the shared environment from 9 to 12 years of age. *Child Development, 80,* 662–673.

Hinde, R. A., & Stevenson-Hinde, J. (Eds.). (1988). *Relationships within families: Mutual influences.* Oxford, UK: Clarendon Press.

Hygen, B. W., Guzey, I. C., Belsky, J., Berg-Nielsen, T. S., & Wichstrom, L. (2014). Catechol-O-methyltransferase Val158Met genotype moderates the effect of disorganized attachment on social development in young children. *Development and Psychopathology, 26,* 947–961.

Insel, T. R., & Shapiro, L. E. (1992). Oxytocin receptors and maternal behavior. *Annals of the New York Academy of Sciences, 652,* 122–141.

Jaddoe, V. W., van Duijn, C. M., Franco, O. H., van der Heijden A. J., Van IJzendoorn M. H., de Jongste, et al. (2012). The Generation R Study: Design and cohort update 2012. *European Journal of Epidemiology, 27,* 739–756.

Jaffee, S. R., Caspi, A., Moffitt, T. E., Polo-Tomas, M., Price, T. S., & Taylor, A. (2004). The limits of child effects: Evidence for genetically mediated child effects on corporal punishment but not on physical maltreatment. *Developmental Psychology, 40,* 1047–1058.

Jin, D., Liu, H. X., Hirai, H., Torashima, T., Nagai, T., Lopatina, O., et al. (2007). CD38 is critical for social behaviour by regulating oxytocin secretion. *Nature, 446,* 41–45.

Jonas, W., Mileva-Seitz, V., Girard, A. W., Bisceglia, R., Kennedy, J. L., Sokolowski, M., et al. (2013).

Genetic variation in oxytocin rs2740210 and early adversity associated with postpartum depression and breastfeeding duration. *Genes, Brain and Behavior, 12,* 681–694.

Jones-Mason, K. M. (2011). Attachment processes and gene–environment interactions: Testing two initial hypotheses regarding the relationship between attachment, and methylation of the glucocorticoid receptor gene (*NR3C1*) and the serotonin transporter gene (*SLC6A4*). Doctoral dissertation, University of California, Berkeley. Retrieved from *http://escholarship.org/uc/item/86d940pw.*

Klahr, A. M., & Burt, S. A. (2014). Elucidating the etiology of individual differences in parenting: A meta-analysis of behavioral genetic research. *Psychological Bulletin, 140,* 544–586.

Klahr, A. M., Klump, K., & Burt, S. A. (2015). A constructive replication of the association between the oxytocin receptor gene and parenting. *Journal of Family Psychology, 29*(1), 91–99.

Kochanska, G., Philibert, R. A., & Barry, R. A. (2009). Interplay of genes and early mother–child relationship in the development of self-regulation from toddler to preschool age. *Journal of Child Psychology and Psychiatry, 50,* 1331–1338.

Kovan, N. M., Chung, A. L., & Sroufe, L. A. (2009). The intergenerational continuity of observed early parenting: A prospective, longitudinal study. *Developmental Psychology, 45,* 1205–1213.

Kumsta, R., Stevens, S., Brookes, K., Schlotz, W., Castle, J., Beckett, C., et al. (2010). 5HTT genotype moderates the influence of early institutional deprivation on emotional problems in adolescence: Evidence from the English and Romanian Adoptee (ERA) study. *Journal of Child Psychology and Psychiatry, 51,* 755–762.

Lakatos, K., Nemoda, Z., Toth, I., Ronai, Z., Ney, K., Sasvari-Szekely, M., et al. (2002). Further evidence for the role of the dopamine D4 receptor (*DRD4*) gene in attachment disorganization: Interaction of the exon III 48-bp repeat and the -521 C/T promoter polymorphisms. *Molecular Psychiatry, 7,* 27–31.

Lakatos, K., Toth, I., Nemoda, Z., Ney, K., Sasvari-Szekely, M., & Gervai, J. (2000). Dopamine D4 receptor (*DRD4*) gene polymorphism is associated with attachment disorganization in infants. *Molecular Psychiatry, 5,* 633–637.

Lee, S. S., Chronis-Tuscano, A., Keenan, K., Pelham, W. E., Loney, J., van Hulle, C. A., et al. (2010). Association of maternal dopamine transporter genotype with negative parenting: Evidence for gene × environment interaction with child disruptive behavior. *Molecular Psychiatry, 15,* 548–558.

Lesch, K. P., Bengel, D., Heils, A., Sabol, S. Z., Greenberg, B. D., Petri, S., et al. (1996). Association of anxiety-related traits with a polymorphism in the serotonin transporter gene regulatory region. *Science, 274,* 1527–1531.

Luijk, M. P. C. M., Roisman, G. I., Haltigan, J. D., Tiemeier, H., Booth-LaForce, C., Van IJzendoorn, M. H., et al. (2011). Dopaminergic, serotonergic, and oxytonergic candidate genes associated with infant attachment security and disorganization?: In search of main effects and G × E interactions. *Journal of Child Psychology and Psychiatry, 52,* 1295–1307.

Luijk, M. P. C. M., Tharner, A., Van IJzendoorn, M. H., Bakermans-Kranenburg, M. J., Jaddoe, V. W. V., Hofman, A., et al. (2011). The association between parenting and attachment security is moderated by a polymorphism in the mineralocorticoid receptor gene: Evidence for differential susceptibility. *Biological Psychology, 88,* 37–40.

Luijk, M. P. C. M., Velders, F., Tharner, A., Bakermans-Kranenburg, M. J., Van IJzendoorn, M. H., Jaddoe, V. W. V., et al. (2010). FKBP5 and resistant attachment predict cortisol reactivity in infants: Gene–environment interaction. *Psychoneuroendocrinology, 35,* 1454–1461.

Madigan, S., Bakermans-Kranenburg, M. J., Van IJzendoorn, M. H., Moran, G., Pederson, D. R., & Benoit, D. (2006). Unresolved states of mind, anomalous parental behavior, and disorganized attachment: A review and meta-analysis of a transmission gap. *Attachment and Human Development, 8,* 89–111.

Main, M., & Solomon, J. (1990). Procedures for identifying infants as disorganized/disoriented during the Ainsworth Strange Situation. In M. T. Greenberg, D. Cicchetti & E. M. Cummings (Eds.), *Attachment in the preschool years: Theory, research, and intervention* (pp. 121–160). Chicago: University of Chicago Press.

Manolio, T. A., Collins, F. S., Cox, N. J., Goldstein, D. B., Hindorff, L. A., Hunter, D. J., et al. (2009). Finding the missing heritability of complex diseases. *Nature, 461,* 747–753.

McClelland, G. H., & Judd, C. M. (1993). Statistical difficulties of detecting interactions and moderator effects. *Psychological Bulletin, 114,* 376–390.

McGowan, P. O., Sasaki, A., D'Alessio, A. C., Dymov, S., Labonte, B., Szyf, M., et al. (2009). Epigenetic regulation of the glucocorticoid receptor in human brain associates with childhood abuse. *Nature Neuroscience, 12,* 342–348.

Meaney, M. J. (2001). Nature, nurture, and the disunity of knowledge. *Annals of the New York Academy of Sciences, 935,* 50–61.

Meaney, M. J. (2010). Epigenetics and the biological definition of gene × environment interactions. *Child Development, 81,* 41–79.

Meyer-Lindenberg, A., Domes, G., Kirsch, P., & Heinrichs, M. (2011). Oxytocin and vasopressin in the human brain: Social neuropeptides for translational medicine. *Nature Reviews Neuroscience, 12,* 524–538.

Michalska, K. J., Decety, J., Liu, C., Chen, Q., Martz, M. E., Jacob, S., et al. (2014). Genetic imaging of the association of oxytocin receptor gene (*OXTR*) polymorphisms with positive maternal parenting. *Frontiers in Behavioral Neuroscience, 8,* 1–10.

Mileva-Seitz, V., Fleming, A. S., Meaney, M. J., Mastroi-

anni, A., Sinnwell, J. P., Steiner, M., et al. (2012). Dopamine receptors D1 and D2 are related to observed maternal behavior. *Genes, Brain and Behavior, 11,* 684–694.

Mileva-Seitz, V., Kennedy, J., Atkinson, L., Steiner, M., Levitan, R., Matthews, S. G., et al. (2011). Serotonin transporter allelic variation in mothers predicts maternal sensitivity, behavior and attitudes toward 6-month-old infants. *Genes, Brain and Behavior, 10,* 325–333.

Mileva-Seitz, V., Steiner, M., Atkinson, L., Meaney, M. J., Levitan, R., Kennedy, J. L., et al. (2013). Interaction between oxytocin genotypes and early experience predicts quality of mothering and postpartum mood. *PLoS ONE, 8,* e61443.

Mileva-Seitz, V. R., Bakermans-Kranenburg, M. J., & Van IJzendoorn, M. H. (in press). Genetic mechanisms of parenting. *Hormones and Behavior.*

Miller, S. M., & Lonstein, J. S. (2005). Dopamine D1 and D2 receptor antagonism in the preoptic area produces different effects on maternal behavior in lactating rats. *Behavioral Neuroscience, 119,* 1072–1083.

Mills-Koonce, W. R., Propper, C. B., Gariepy, J.-L., Blair, C., Garrett-Peters, P., & Cox, M. J. (2007). Bidirectional genetic and environmental influences on mother and child behavior: The family system as the unit of analyses. *Development and Psychopathology, 19,* 1073–1087.

Monroe, S. M., & Simons, A. D. (1991). Diathesis–stress theories in the context of life stress research: Implications for the depressive disorders. *Psychological Bulletin, 110,* 406–425.

Munafò, M. R., Durrant, C., Lewis, G., & Flint, J. (2009). Gene–environment interactions at the serotonin transporter locus. *Biological Psychiatry, 65,* 211–219.

Munesue, T., Yokoyama, S., Nakamura, K., Anitha, A., Yamada, K., Hayashi, K., et al. (2010). Two genetic variants of CD38 in subjects with autism spectrum disorder and controls. *Neuroscience Research, 67,* 181–191.

Naumova, O. Y., Lee, M., Koposov, R., Szyf, M., Dozier, M., & Grigorenko, E. L. (2012). Differential patterns of whole-genome DNA methylation in institutionalized children and children raised by their biological parents. *Development and Psychopathology, 24,* 143–155.

Neiderhiser, J. M., Reiss, D., Pedersen, N. L., Lichtenstein, P., Spotts, E. L., Hansson, K., et al. (2004). Genetic and environmental influences on mothering of adolescents: A comparison of two samples. *Developmental Psychology, 40,* 335–351.

Nelson, C. A., Fox, N. A., & Zeanah, C. H. (2014). *Romania's abandoned children: Deprivation, brain development, and the struggle for recovery.* Cambridge, MA: Harvard University Press.

O'Connor, T. G., & Croft, C. M. (2001). A twin study of attachment in preschool children. *Child Development, 72,* 1501–1511.

Oliver, B. R., Trzaskowski, M., & Plomin, R. (2014).

Genetics of parenting: The power of the dark side. *Developmental Psychology, 50*, 1233–1240.

Out, D., Bakermans-Kranenburg, M. J., & Van IJzendoorn, M. H. (2009). The role of disconnected and extremely insensitive parenting in the development of disorganized attachment: Validation of a new measure. *Attachment and Human Development, 11*, 419–443.

Out, D., Pieper, S., Bakermans-Kranenburg, M. J., & Van IJzendoorn, M. H. (2010). Physiological reactivity to infant crying: A behavioral genetic study. *Genes, Brain and Behavior, 9*, 868–876.

Pappa, I., Fedko, I. O., Mileva-Seitz, V. R., Hottenga, J. J., Bakermans-Kranenburg, M. J., Bartels, M., et al. (2015). SNP heritability of behavior problems in childhood: Genome-wide complex trait analysis. *Journal of the American Academy of Child and Adolescent Psychiatry, 54*, 737–744.

Pappa, I., Szekely, E., Mileva-Seitz, V. R., Luijk, P. C. M., Bakermans-Kranenburg, M. J., Van IJzendoorn, M. H., et al. (2015). Beyond the usual suspects: A multidimensional genetic exploration of infant attachment disorganization and security. *Attachment and Human Development 17*, 288–301

Pener-Tessler, R., Avinun, R., Uzefovsky, F., Edelman, S., Ebstein, R. P., & Knafo, A. (2013). Boys' serotonin transporter genotype affects maternal behavior through self-control: A case of evocative gene–environment correlation. *Development and Psychopathology, 25*, 151–162.

Pergamin-Hight, L., Bakermans-Kranenburg, M. J., Van IJzendoorn, M. H., & Bar-Haim, Y. (2012). Variations in the promoter region of the serotonin-transporter gene (*5HTTLPR*) and biased attention for emotional information: A meta-analysis. *Biological Psychiatry, 71*, 373–379.

Perroud, N., Salzmann, A., Prada, P., Nicastro, R., Hoeppli, M.-E., Furrer, S., et al. (2013). Response to psychotherapy in borderline personality disorder and methylation status of the BDNF gene. *Translational Psychiatry, 3*, e207.

Plomin, R. (1994). Interface of nature and nurture in the family.of children. In W. B. Carey & S. C. McDevitt (Eds.), *Prevention and early intervention: Individual differences as risk factors for the mental health of children: A festschrift for Stella Chess and Alexander Thomas* (pp. 179–189). New York: Brunner/Mazel.

Plomin, R. (2013). Child development and molecular genetics: 14 years later. *Child Development, 84*, 104–120.

Plomin, R., DeFries, J. C., Knopik, V. S., & Neiderhiser, J. M. (2013). *Behavioral genetics* (6th ed.). New York: Worth.

Plomin, R., DeFries, J. C., McClearn, G. E., & McGuffin, P. (2001). *Behavior genetics* (4th ed.). New York: Worth.

Plomin, R., & Simpson, M. A. (2013). The future of genomics for developmentalists. *Development and Psychopathology, 25*, 1263–1278.

Raby, K. L., Cicchetti, D., Carlson, E. A., Cutuli, J. J., Englund, M. M., & Egeland, B. (2012). Genetic and caregiving-based contributions to infant attachment: Unique associations with distress reactivity and attachment security. *Psychological Science, 23*, 1016–1023.

Radtke, K..M., Rufl, M., Gunter, H. M., Dohrmann, K., Schauer, M., Meyer, A., et al. (2011). Transgenerational impact of intimate partner violence on methylation in the promoter of the glucocorticoid receptor. *Translational Psychiatry, 1*, e21.

Ramanan, V. K., Shen, L., Moore, J. H., & Saykin, A. J. (2012). Pathway analysis of genomic data: Concepts, methods, and prospects for future development. *Trends in Genetics, 28*, 323–332.

Reiner, I., & Spangler, G. (2010). Adult attachment and gene polymorphisms of the dopamine D4 receptor and serotonin transporter (5-HTT). *Attachment and Human Development, 12*, 209–229.

Ricciuti, A. E. (1992). Child–mother attachment: A twin study. *Dissertation Abstracts International, 54*, 3364–3364.

Riem, M. M. E., Pieper, S., Out, D., Bakermans-Kranenburg, M. J., & Van IJzendoorn, M. H. (2011). Oxytocin receptor gene and depressive symptoms associated with physiological reactivity to infant crying. *Social Cognitive and Affective Neuroscience, 6*, 294–300.

Risch, N., Herrell, R., Lehner, T., Liang, K. Y., Eaves, L., Hoh, J., et al. (2009). Interaction between the serotonin transporter gene (*5-HTTLPR*), stressful life events, and risk of depression: A meta-analysis. *Journal of the American Medical Association, 301*, 2462–2471.

Robbins, T. W., & Everitt, B. J. (1999). Motivation and reward. In F. E. Bloom, S. C. Landis, J. L. Robert, L. R. Squire, & M. J. Zigmond (Eds.), *Fundamental neuroscience* (pp. 1246–1260). San Diego, CA: Academic Press.

Roisman, G. I., & Fraley, R. C. (2008). A behavior-genetic study of parenting quality, infant attachment security, and their covariation in a nationally representative sample. *Developmental Psychology, 44*, 831–839.

Rutter, M. (2006). *Genes and Behavior: Nature–nurture interplay explained.* Oxford, UK: Blackwell.

Rutter, M. (2010). Gene–environment interplay. *Depression and Anxiety, 27*, 1–4.

Sameroff, A. J. (1983). Developmental systems: Contexts and evolution. In P. Mussen (Ed.), *Handbook of child psychology* (pp. 237–294). New York: Wiley

Schuengel, C., Bakermans-Kranenburg, M. J., & Van IJzendoorn, M. H. (1999). Frightening maternal behavior linking unresolved loss and disorganized infant attachment. *Journal of Consulting and Clinical Psychology, 67*, 54–63.

Shahrokh, D. K., Zhang, T.-Y., Diorio, J., Gratton, A., & Meaney, M. J. (2010). Oxytocin–dopamine interactions mediate variations in maternal behavior in the rat. *Endocrinology, 151*, 2276–2286.

Shmueli-Goetz, Y., Target, M., Fonagy, P., & Datta, A.

(2008). The Child Attachment Interview: A psychometric study of reliability and discriminant validity. *Developmental Psychology, 44*, 939–956.

Spangler, G., Johann, M., Ronai, Z., & Zimmermann, P. (2009). Genetic and environmental influence on attachment disorganization. *Journal of Child Psychology and Psychiatry, 50*, 952–961.

Stolzenberg, D. S., McKenna, J. B., Keough, S., Hancock, R., Numan, M. J., & Numan, M. (2007). Dopamine D1 receptor stimulation of the nucleus accumbens or the medial preoptic area promotes the onset of maternal behavior in pregnancy-terminated rats. *Behavioral Neuroscience, 121*, 907–919.

Szyf, M., Weaver, I. C. G., Champagne, F. A., Diorio, J., & Meaney, M. J. (2005). Maternal programming of steroid receptor expression and phenotype through DNA methylation in the rat. *Frontiers in Neuroendocrinology, 26*, 139–162.

Taylor, S. E. (2008). Genetic contributions to sensitive parenting. *Social Cognitive and Affective Neuroscience, 3*, 89–90.

Van IJzendoorn, M. H. (1995). Adult attachment representations, parental responsiveness, and infant attachment: A meta-analysis on the predictive validity of the Adult Attachment Interview. *Psychological Bulletin, 117*, 387–403.

Van IJzendoorn, M. H., & Bakermans-Kranenburg, M. J. (2006). DRD4 7-repeat polymorphism moderates the association between maternal unresolved loss or trauma and infant disorganization. *Attachment and Human Development, 8*, 291–307.

Van IJzendoorn, M. H., & Bakermans-Kranenburg, M. J. (2012). Integrating temperament and attachment: The differential susceptibility paradigm. In M. Zentner & R. L. Shiner (Eds.), *Handbook of temperament* (pp. 403–424). New York: Guilford Press.

Van IJzendoorn, M. H., & Bakermans-Kranenburg, M. J. (2014). Confined quest for continuity: The categorical versus continuous nature of attachment. *Monographs of the Society for Research in Child Development, 79*, 157–167.

Van IJzendoorn, M. H., & Bakermans-Kranenburg, M. J. (2015). Genetic differential susceptibility on trial: Meta-analytic support from randomized controlled experiments. *Development and Psychopathology, 27*(1), 151–162.

Van IJzendoorn, M. H., Bakermans-Kranenburg, M. J.,

Belsky, J., Beach, S., Brody, G., Dodge, K. A., et al. (2011). Gene-by-environment experiments: A new approach to finding the missing heritability. *Nature Reviews Genetics, 12*, 881–881.

Van IJzendoorn, M. H., Bakermans-Kranenburg, M. J., & Ebstein, R. P. (2011). Methylation matters in child development: Toward developmental behavioral epigenetics. *Child Development Perspectives, 4*, 305–310.

Van IJzendoorn, M. H., Bakermans-Kranenburg, M. J., & Mesman, J. (2008). Dopamine system genes associated with parenting in the context of daily hassles. *Genes, Brain and Behavior, 7*, 403–410.

Van IJzendoorn, M. H., Belsky, J., & Bakermans-Kranenburg, M. J. (2012). Serotonin transporter genotype 5HTTLPR as a marker of differential susceptibility?: A meta-analysis of child and adolescent gene-by-environment studies. *Translational Psychiatry, 2*, e147.

Van IJzendoorn, M. H., Caspers, K., Bakermans-Kranenburg, M. J., Beach, S. R. H., & Philibert, R. (2010). Methylation matters: Interaction between methylation density and 5HTT genotype predicts unresolved loss or trauma. *Biological Psychiatry, 68*, 405–407.

Van IJzendoorn, M. H., Palacios, J., Sonuga-Barke, E. J. S., Gunnar, M. R., Vorria, Y., McCall, R., et al. (2011). Children in institutional care: Delayed development and resilience. *Monographs of the Society for Research in Child Development, 76*, 8–30.

Vaughn, B. E., & Waters, E. (1990). Attachment behavior at home and in the laboratory: Q-Sort observations and strange situation classifications of one-year-olds. *Child Development, 61*, 1965–1973.

Wang, K., Li, M., & Hakonarson, H. (2010). Analysing biological pathways in genome-wide association studies. *Nature Reviews Genetics, 11*, 843–854.

Weaver, I. C., Cervoni, N., Champagne, F. A., D'Alessio, A. C., Sharma, S., Seckl, J. R., et al. (2004). Epigenetic programming by maternal behavior. *Nature Neuroscience, 7*, 847–854.

Yang, J. A., Lee, S. H., Goddard, M. E., & Visscher, P. M. (2011). GCTA: A tool for genome-wide complex trait analysis. *American Journal of Human Genetics, 88*, 76–82.

Zhang, T. Y., & Meaney, M. J. (2010). Epigenetics and the environmental regulation of the genome and its function. *Annual Review Psychology, 61*, 439–466.

# Chapter 9

# Attachment and Psychoneuroimmunology

Katherine B. Ehrlich
Gregory E. Miller
Jason D. Jones
Jude Cassidy

At the core of attachment theory is the notion that the availability of a responsive and dependable caregiver is critical to healthy development across the lifespan (Bowlby, 1973, 1980, 1982). During the first several decades of the scientific study of attachment, developmental, clinical, and social researchers focused primarily on how attachment shapes individuals' social and emotional functioning. More recently, researchers have undertaken investigations of the links between attachment and physiological systems, shedding light on the ways in which attachment security may influence various systems in the body. For example, some studies have identified individual differences in infants' autonomic nervous system activity during the Strange Situation procedure (e.g., Sroufe & Waters, 1977), and other work has demonstrated individual differences in neuroendocrine stress reactivity to novel stimuli as a function of infant attachment classification and temperament (e.g., Nachmias, Gunnar, Mangelsdorf, Parritz, & Buss, 1996). Furthermore, recent evidence suggests that attachment figures can attenuate adults' threat-responsive neural activity following a stressor (e.g., Coan, Schaefer, & Davidson, 2006). These studies provide some of the first evidence for connections between attachment and psychophysiology

(see also Dozier & Kobak, 1992; Eisenberger et al., 2011), and this area of research continues to generate new insights into the dynamic connections between attachment and physiological systems.

During the years that Bowlby was developing his theory of attachment, other researchers were focused on the connections among psychological processes, neural and endocrine activity, and immune functioning, a field that became known as *psychoneuroimmunology* (PNI) (Ader, 1980, 2001; Ader & Cohen, 1975; Solomon & Moos, 1964; for a review, see Kiecolt-Glaser, McGuire, Robles, & Glaser, 2002). This interdisciplinary area of research has revealed the ways in which emotions, social support, and stressful life experiences—in addition to many other psychosocial and behavioral factors—are connected to immune and endocrine function, and to physical health. These studies show how the social world can "get under the skin" to affect immune and neuroendocrine systems in ways that might have consequences for later health.

With the exception of a few studies, these two areas of research—attachment and psychoneuroimmunology—have proceeded independently of each other. Yet it is becoming increasingly clear that many of the same guiding principles of attachment theory, which explain why early experiences with caregivers have long-lasting connections to social and emotional health, may also explain how attachment-based experiences can shape individuals' immune processes and physical health across development. At the same time, conceptual models guiding research on connections between social experiences and immune functioning (e.g., Fagundes, Glaser, & Kiecolt-Glaser, 2013; Miller, Chen, & Parker, 2011) are instrumental in providing a foundation for how attachment experiences might be associated with the immune system. Furthermore, evidence suggests that attachment is associated with physical health outcomes in childhood and adulthood (Anderson, Gooze, Lemeshow, & Whitaker, 2012; Anderson & Whitaker, 2011; McWilliams & Bailey, 2010; Puig, Englund, Simpson, & Collins, 2013).

Our goal in this chapter is to provide an introduction for attachment researchers who may be unfamiliar with the field of PNI. We begin with a theoretical framework for the study of attachment and the immune system, drawing on existing theoretical models that outline how social experiences can become embedded in the body (e.g., Miller et al., 2011; Uchino, Cacioppo, & Kiecolt-Glaser, 1996). Consistent with the notion that attachment experiences are important for social and emotional health from "the cradle to the grave" (Bowlby, 1979, p. 129), we propose that connections between attachment and the immune system can be observed across the lifespan. We then provide a general overview of common indicators of immune system function, with a specific focus on inflammation, which is the predominant focus of contemporary human PNI research. We present some preliminary evidence for a connection between attachment experiences and inflammatory processes, followed by a review of relevant research that has examined links between attachment-related social factors (e.g., maternal warmth) and various biological mechanisms. To date, studies of attachment and inflammation have focused on adult samples, but when available, we include studies that have examined relevant caregiving experiences and immune function in children. We conclude with a discussion of future directions for this emerging area, as well as some words of caution for researchers who are interested in embarking on this ambitious interdisciplinary work. Because other chapters in this handbook cover research on the neuroscience of attachment (see Coan, Chapter 12) and links between attachment and the endocrine system (see Hane & Fox, Chap-

ter 11), our review focuses on attachment and its potential links to the immune system.

## Attachment, Stress Regulation, and Inflammation: A Theoretical Framework

In this section, we describe our thinking about how attachment-related experiences may be associated with inflammation. A large body of research supports the notion that stressful experiences are associated with inflammation, and we begin this section with a review of an existing model that explains how stressors shape inflammatory processes over time. We then describe how attachment-related stress regulatory capabilities and the presence (or absence) of a secure base may contribute to inflammatory processes. After that, we describe two models that may explain how attachment orientations are associated with inflammatory processes.

### Stress and Inflammation

Stressful experiences are thought to alter inflammatory processes via the autonomic nervous system. Fibers from the sympathetic nervous system directly connect brain regions involved in emotion processing and regulation to the lymphoid organs, where immune responses take place. Evidence from animal studies suggests that stressful experiences can increase the density of these fibers (e.g., Sloan et al., 2007), which release epinephrine, norepinephrine, and other neurotransmitters. These neurotransmitters in turn bind to receptors on white blood cells, resulting in changes to their patterns of trafficking, cytokine release, proliferation, and differentiation. Hormonal pathways also influence immune processes. Immune cells respond to cortisol, oxytocin, and other molecules whose expression can be affected by stress (e.g., Fries, Ziegler, Kurian, Jacoris, & Pollak, 2005; Miller et al., 2009).

Miller and colleagues (2011) outlined how stressful experiences in childhood are associated with inflammatory processes. In this model, exposure to chronic stressors incites a *proinflammatory phenotype*, which becomes embedded within key cells of the immune system: monocytes and macrophages. According to this model, these cells (which play a critical role in the initial immune response to injury and infection) become programmed to launch exaggerated responses to stimuli and become desensitized to inhibitory signals (e.g., from cortisol; described in more detail in the next section). Across development, this proinflammatory phenotype can result in chronic, low-grade inflammation, which is increasingly recognized in the biomedical literature as a fundamental contributor to many of the chronic diseases of aging, including cardiovascular disease, diabetes, stroke, some cancers, and various autoimmune conditions (Danesh, Collins, Appleby, & Peto, 1998; Libby, Ridker, & Hansson, 2009; Ridker, 2007; Yeh & Willerson, 2003). Inflammation is especially likely to occur when individuals face severe and chronic stressors, in part because these stressful experiences take a toll on individuals' self-regulation resources. As a result, individuals are more likely to develop unhealthy lifestyle practices (e.g., poor diet, smoking, substance use, sedentary behavior) and form poor social relationships. These factors in turn have been associated with inflammation (Miller et al., 2011).

### Attachment and Stress Regulation

Attachment theory suggests that individuals develop capacities for regulating stress as a result of experiences with caregivers in times of distress. Bowlby (1982) proposed that children develop experience-based mental representations of their caregivers' availability and responsiveness during times of need. These representations, or *internal working models*, develop as early as the first year of life and reflect the extent to which the child perceives the parent as a "secure base" from which to explore and as a "safe haven" to which to return in times of threat or distress. Over time, as children become more autonomous, they learn regulatory strategies for managing their own emotions but continue to seek comfort from attachment figures when distressed. Even in adulthood, individuals use attachment figures (e.g., parents, romantic partners) for support and comfort when upset (Ainsworth, 1989; Mikulincer & Shaver, 2007).

According to attachment theory, access to a secure base is critical because it provides a sense of security that enables individuals to explore the world and seek help or comfort when confronted with threat (Bowlby, 1973). In other words, individuals who have a secure base feel assured that, when faced with difficulties, someone will be available to come to their aid; this assurance allows them to confront stressors without becoming overwhelmed. Furthermore, within close relationships, secure individuals are able to engage in open, flexible expression of emotions, thus allowing expression and mitigation of negative feelings. In contrast, individuals without a secure base have not had the experience of being able to rely on a consistent caregiver to meet their emotional needs, and as a result, they struggle to manage their negative emotions.

Of course, not everyone has a history of experiences with caregivers in which negative feelings were acknowledged, comforted, and alleviated. Some individuals may have experienced minimizing or punitive responses from their attachment figures, and others may have experienced inconsistently available attachment figures who were only sometimes responsive to their needs. These individuals, who are likely to be classified as insecurely attached, are unable to use their attachment figures effectively as a secure base and safe haven (Ainsworth, Blehar, Waters, & Wall, 1978). As a result, these individuals develop strategies for managing their negative emotions (Main, 1990), either by minimizing, suppressing, and denying their negative feelings (labeled *attachment-related avoidance*), or by maximizing and heightening their distress in order to capture the attention of attachment figures (labeled *attachment anxiety*). Although these strategies may be adaptive for bringing coherence to an inconsistent or unsupportive caregiving environment, they are ineffective for long-term stress regulation (see Mikulincer & Shaver, Chapter 24, this volume). Indeed, individuals who are high in avoidant and/or anxious attachment have more depressive symptoms, anxiety, and substance use problems than do secure individuals (see DeKlyen & Greenberg, Chapter 28, and Stovall-McClough & Dozier, Chapter 31, both in this volume).

### Models Linking Attachment and Inflammation

We propose that associations between attachment orientations and inflammatory processes are likely to occur in one of two principal forms. First, we expect there to be direct links between insecure attachment and inflammation. Insecurely attached individuals have difficulty regulating stress, and exposure to chronic stressors may foster the proinflammatory phenotype described earlier (e.g., Miller et al., 2011). Second, we argue that attachment orientation may serve as an important moderator of the already documented connections between psychosocial stressors and inflammation (e.g., Glaser & Kiecolt-Glaser, 2005; Segerstrom

& Miller, 2004). For example, attachment security may buffer against the heightened inflammatory consequences associated with low socioeconomic status (SES) (e.g., Miller et al., 2011). Conversely, insecurely attached individuals who are also facing chronic or acute stressors may have greater inflammatory responses than securely attached individuals who are experiencing similar levels of stress. We discuss these models in more detail in "Future Directions."

In the next section, we provide an overview of some of the most common biological measures that indicate inflammation in the body. After that, we describe research that has used these measures to examine connections between attachment-related indices and inflammatory processes.

## Biological Measures of Interest

In the last several decades, significant progress has been made in understanding biological correlates of social experiences, such as social isolation, maltreatment, and poverty, and it is plausible that attachment-related experiences are among these important influences on underlying biologic processes. In this section, we describe some of the most common measures of the immune system, with a specific emphasis on indicators of inflammation because of their influence on many of the chronic diseases of aging.

This section is divided into four parts. In the first part, we review systemic measures of inflammation, which provide an index of circulating inflammation in the body. After that, we discuss functional measures of inflammatory processes, which provide information about the extent to which an individual's immune system is aggressive in its response to pathogens and sensitive to signals to reduce the inflammatory response. We then review several indicators of gene regulation, including epigenetic modifications and gene expression. In the final part of this section, we review a number of laboratory-based measures of the immune system; these laboratory measures require a deliberate (though minor) injury to an individual, oftentimes to the skin, with systematic follow-up measures regarding repair and recovery.

### Systemic Inflammation

Inflammation occurs when cells of the innate immune system, including neutrophils, dendritic cells, monocytes, and macrophages, gather at the site of an infection or injury. These cells attempt to eliminate the pathogen, rid the body of infected tissue, repair any damage the pathogen caused, and begin the process of healing. The inflammatory response is essential for survival: Without it, minor injuries or infections would be lethal. The inflammatory response must be carefully regulated, however; otherwise, inflammation can become persistent and disseminated, thereby contributing to multiple chronic diseases.

Inflammation is orchestrated by signaling molecules known as cytokines, which are released by immune cells and the damaged tissue. The major cytokines involved with inflammation are interleukins 1 and 6 (IL-1, IL-6), and tumor necrosis factor alpha (TNF-$\alpha$). Researchers sometimes use concentrations of these molecules in circulation as a rough estimate of ongoing inflammatory activity. However, these cytokines are fairly unstable in blood, so a more common approach is to measure C-reactive protein (CRP), a molecule produced by the liver during inflammation. CRP provides a reliable index of low-grade chronic inflammation over the preceding month or so, and is prognostic of morbidity and mortality from a number of chronic diseases of aging. CRP's role is particularly well established in the progression of cardiovascular disease, where, in apparently healthy individuals, it presages disease risk in a roughly dose–response manner.

To be most effective in research studies, researchers should attempt to measure inflammation at multiple time points, which allows for a better understanding of both *stability* and *change* in inflammation over time. Longitudinal studies, with multiple assessments of inflammation, will help to clarify the extent to which attachment-related experiences predict chronic disparities in inflammation. These types of studies will also help to clarify whether such experiences can precipitate changes in inflammation, whether favorable or unfavorable. For inflammation to be involved in accelerating some diseases, such as atherosclerosis, the inflammation would need to be long-standing. Only with multi-wave studies can researchers ascertain whether inflammation is transitory or chronic. On the other hand, short bursts of inflammation could initiate a cascade of biological processes, ultimately leading to a heart attack (Maseri & Fuster, 2003). One important caveat is that most studies of inflammation capture ongoing inflammatory activity in peripheral blood rather than inflammation in tissues or organs where disease processes are happening (e.g., the coronary arteries for heart disease, the joints for rheumatoid arthritis). The assumption is that blood provides a window to inflammatory activity at these sites. The available research generally supports this assumption, and suggests that, if anything, blood-based measures underestimate the association between stressors and inflammation in tissue (Glaser et al., 1999).

To date, the majority of PNI studies have focused on proinflammatory processes, which is not surprising given the role of inflammation in the progression of chronic disease. But anti-inflammatory signals play an important role in regulating the balance of inflammatory activity. Some cytokines, such as IL-10, are involved in terminating the inflammatory response. These cytokines act as "brakes" and help prevent inflammatory responses from proceeding in an unchecked manner. Thus, researchers should include measures of both pro- and anti-inflammatory signals to capture a more comprehensive picture of how the immune system responds to social experiences.

Measures of systemic inflammation are arguably the best starting point for attachment researchers who are interested in expanding their research to include inflammation. These measures are relatively easy to obtain, with only a peripheral blood draw or finger prick needed to obtain samples. Many hospitals process samples at an affordable rate, allowing researchers to minimize costs associated with necessary laboratory facilities. Moreover, the clinical implications of chronic inflammation are clear. Studies have shown that elevated CRP predicts adults' cardiovascular events in a roughly dose–response manner, even within the normal range of values (Ridker, 2003). Notably, CRP is often viewed as a marker rather than as a causal actor in the progression toward disease. Other cytokines (e.g., IL-1, TNF-α) play a more direct role in the generation of inflammation that contributes to plaque formation that may trigger later coronary events. Despite these advantages, measures of some indices, such as CRP, may be less appropriate for samples with children and adolescents. At younger ages, children often have levels of CRP that are below the detection threshold for standard assays, which may contribute to a "floor effect" when trying to link attachment experiences to inflammation. Although this issue is less of a concern for other measures of inflammation, such as TNF-α, IL-6, and IL-8, these measures often lack variability in scores, and the clinical implications of low scores are unclear. Given these developmental considerations, researchers working with children and adolescents may want to explore the possibility of using functional measures of inflammation, which are described in more detail in the next section.

## Functional Measures of Inflammatory Processes

As described earlier, systemic measures reflect the amount of ongoing inflammation circulating in peripheral blood. Functional measures, in contrast, provide insight into how cells respond when confronted with pathogens (e.g., bacteria) or signaling molecules (e.g., cortisol). It is unclear whether functional measures are diagnostic or predictive of chronic disease, but they are useful for capturing individual differences in proinflammatory response patterns that, if sustained, could put individuals on an accelerated trajectory toward chronic disease.

When macrophages encounter signs of injury or infection, one of their initial responses is to secrete cytokines, including IL-1-β, IL-6, and TNF-α. These molecules attract cells to the site, activate their killing functions, call in other more specialized cells, and initiate systemic processes (e.g., fever) that decapacitate the invading microorganisms. As mentioned earlier, this inflammatory response is critical for survival from acute infections and injuries. However, it must be carefully regulated because, if sustained in an unchecked manner, inflammation can bring about tissue damage and contribute to chronic diseases (Hotamisligil, 2006; Libby & Theroux, 2005).

Cortisol plays an important role in helping the body regulate immune responses, particularly inflammation. Cortisol binds to glucocorticoid receptors located in immune cells and, under normal circumstances, this complex regulates the magnitude and duration of inflammation, helping to ensure that the response does not overshoot in a manner that causes tissue damage (Sapolsky, Romero, & Munck, 2000; Sternberg, 2006). Over time, however, long-term exposure to stress can result in the desensitization of glucocorticoid receptors to cortisol, particularly in the cells (monocytes and macrophages) that initiate and sustain most inflammatory responses (e.g., Marques, Silverman, & Sternberg, 2009; Miller et al., 2008; Raison & Miller, 2003; Rohleder, Marin, Ma, & Miller, 2009). One result of this desensitization is that cortisol has a reduced ability to regulate these cells' responses to infections and injuries, which gives rise to chronic low-grade inflammation even in the absence of acute events (Miller, Cohen, &

Ritchey, 2002; Raison & Miller, 2003). Thus, reduced sensitivity to the anti-inflammatory effects of cortisol may contribute to a poorly regulated inflammatory response to injuries, infections, and other stimuli.

Of course, researchers cannot easily expose participants (particularly children) to infection or injuries (but see Eisenberger, Inagaki, Mashal, & Irwin, 2010, for an example of exposing adults to endotoxins, and Cohen, Doyle, Turner, Alper, & Skoner, 2004, for an example of exposing participants to viral challenge). Instead, researchers collect white blood cells and then expose these cells to bacteria *in vitro*, a process known as *microbial challenge*. Cells are then cultured with a bacterial stimulus, such as lipopolysaccharide (LPS), which is a molecule found in the outer membrane of gram-negative bacteria. Following a predetermined incubation period (e.g., 24 hours), *supernatants* (i.e., the remaining fluids minus the white blood cells) are harvested, and researchers can determine the amount of cytokines produced following exposure to LPS. Greater levels of inflammatory cytokine production (e.g., IL-6) are indicative of a more aggressive inflammatory response. Again, as described earlier, an acute aggressive response may be advantageous when combating a pathogen or responding to an injury because it can accelerate repair and recovery; on the other hand, if this aggressive inflammatory response persists over an extended period of time, individuals may be susceptible to tissue damage and accelerated aging. As such, interpretation of stimulated cytokine production responses will depend on the context in which the inflammatory response occurs.

In addition to measuring how aggressively an individual's cells respond to bacterial challenges, researchers can measure the extent to which cells are sensitive to the anti-inflammatory signals from cortisol, which is a measure known as *glucocorticoid sensitivity*. This procedure is often conducted in unison with the microbial challenge procedure described earlier. To perform this assessment, cells are incubated with bacteria (e.g., LPS), as well as doses of hydrocortisone in varying concentrations. Following the incubation period, cytokine levels are measured across the different doses of hydrocortisone, which can then be used to create a dose–response curve. The area under the curve reflects the participant's glucocorticoid sensitivity; larger values indicate that the immune cells are *less sensitive* to cortisol's anti-inflammatory signals. In other words, glucocorticoid sensitivity reflects the extent to which the cytokine response

is tightly controlled and responsive to signals to attenuate it.

These measures often provide more variability in inflammatory processes, compared to systemic measures of inflammation, and this variability can be helpful for detecting links between inflammatory processes and social experiences. Nevertheless, these assessments are considerably more complicated to perform than systemic measures of inflammation. One complication is that cell cultures need to be prepared with fresh (i.e., not frozen) blood under sterile conditions, and by a technician experienced with this methodology. Thus, close proximity to a laboratory equipped to process blood samples and greater technical expertise is needed. These measures are also significantly more expensive than most systemic measures, which can be a limiting factor for most research laboratories with tight budgets. As such, studies of connections between attachment and functional measures of inflammatory processes might be best conducted in collaboration with laboratories that already incorporate these research techniques.

### Epigenetic Modifications and Gene Expression

All cells within an individual carry an identical DNA sequence that is established at conception and fixed for life. (Lymphocytes and cells that have acquired mutations are exceptions to this rule.) The DNA sequence serves as a blueprint for *transcription*, the process whereby cells synthesize RNA molecules—a process known as *gene expression*. RNA molecules are later translated into proteins that cells use for structural and functional purposes. Not all genes are active at all times, however, and some genes are thought to be "socially sensitive," altering their expression patterns as a function of social experiences (Cole, 2013).

The term *epigenetics* refers to stable changes in gene expression activity that arise without changes in the DNA sequence (Jaenisch & Bird, 2003; Jirtle & Skinner, 2007). A principal function of epigenetic alterations is to allow cells to develop and maintain specialized functions. For example, epigenetic alterations can modify a cell's ability to transcribe a particular gene into RNA. Because RNA serves as a template for the translation of proteins, these epigenetic alterations often (although not always) have downstream influences on how much of the gene's protein is ultimately synthesized. When this process takes place across many different genes, it can give rise to significant phenotypic diversity among cells of the body. This variability is thought to play a role in the long-term development of physical disease (e.g., Rakyan, Down, Balding, & Beck, 2011), although the nature of these pathways remains largely unknown.

Epigenetic modifications to DNA typically occur in one of two ways (Whitelaw & Garrick, 2006). The first modification is DNA methylation, which involves the attachment or removal of a methyl group to cytosine residues in a gene's promoter. The methyl groups prevent transcription factors from interacting with DNA to modulate gene expression, which makes the gene inactive. The second form of epigenetic modification involves changes to the chromatin structure that packages the DNA. This process occurs by attaching or removing chemicals from the histone proteins that hold DNA within the cell's nucleus. These proteins cause the DNA near the gene to become more or less tightly coiled, which makes it more or less difficult for RNA polymerase and transcription factors to access their promoters (Whitelaw & Garrick, 2006).

Assessments of epigenetic modifications and gene expression can take a variety of forms. Measurement of epigenetic modifications typically relies on microarray analysis of DNA methylation patterns. This process assesses the presence of methylation at multiple sites in each of many thousands of different genes (e.g., these analyses can quantify the proportion of sites that are methylated). Quantification of messenger RNA (mRNA) can be done by focusing on candidate genes or thousands of genes using DNA microarrays. Although the cost of this technology has dropped substantially, costs remain high, making this assessment prohibitively expensive for some researchers. Nevertheless, these assessments provide unique insight into early mechanisms that go on to shape systemic inflammation, and greater utilization of these methods will be an important direction for future research.

It may be that attachment experiences bring about changes in methylation patterns, which in turn affect expression of mRNA and then synthesis of cytokines and other proteins that are involved with inflammation. The notion that caregiving experiences could bring about epigenetic changes has already been demonstrated in animal models (Weaver et al., 2004), wherein maternal caregiving experiences triggered changes in methylation and acetylation patterns for the glucocorticoid receptor gene in the offspring hippocampus.

These epigenetic modifications affected regulation of the hypothalamic–pituitary–adrenal (HPA) axis—the hormonal system that controls the release of cortisol in response to stress. Some preliminary evidence suggests that similar processes occur in early human social experiences (e.g., Bick et al., 2012; McGowan et al., 2009). But to date, most of these investigations with human samples have focused on childhood maltreatment rather than attachment security, and have relied mostly on white blood cells and buccal cells rather than cells in the brain, where these epigenetic effects would be most relevant to individual differences in emotion regulation and stress responsivity. Thus, future epigenetic research would be most helpful if methylation data were supplemented with studies of functional consequences for gene expression (e.g., by quantifying mRNA expression).

## Laboratory Measures of the Immune System

For studies using the measures described in the previous sections of this chapter, participant burden is quite minimal. Researchers collect peripheral blood samples, and all subsequent processing and analysis steps are done without direct interaction with participants. We now describe several techniques that require more direct involvement with participants. These measures require the administration of a minor injury, typically to the skin, with follow-up assessments to examine repair and recovery. Although considerably more invasive than standard venipuncture, these procedures provide an opportunity to observe how the immune system repairs damaged tissue. The skin is the largest organ in the body and is often viewed as the first layer of defense of the immune system (Salmon, Armstrong, & Ansel, 1994). Cytokines play an important role in maintaining skin barrier function and are recruited to repair damaged tissue. Stress is thought to slow cytokine production at the site of damaged skin tissue (e.g., Glaser et al., 1999; Kiecolt-Glaser, Marucha, Malarkey, Mercado, & Glaser, 1995). By temporarily disrupting the skin's surface, researchers can examine the length of time needed for recovery, as well as clinical indicators of wound healing (e.g., cytokine production).

Of the two skin disruption measures, the less invasive measure utilizes a tape stripping procedure to disrupt the skin barrier and is followed by examination of skin barrier recovery (Fluhr, Feingold, & Elias, 2006). Prior to the procedure, researchers measure the vapor pressure gradient in the layers close to the skin surface, which reflects the skin's ability to prevent water loss. Then, researchers repeatedly apply tape to the surface of the skin (anywhere from five to 60 times, on average), which disrupts the site and removes the superficial layer of dead skin on the surface. Following this treatment, researchers take periodic assessments of the vapor pressure gradient to quantify the skin's recovery from the tape-stripping procedure. Delayed skin barrier recovery is indexed by slower return to baseline pressure gradient.

The second procedure involves the administration of skin blisters to the forearm of participants (Kuhns, DeCarlo, Hawk, & Gallin, 1992). Researchers create small, standardized blisters using a suction blister device. Following generation of the blisters, trained assistants remove the top of the blister and attach a collection device to the site to collect fluid from each wound over a predetermined period of time. This procedure is often accompanied by a behavioral task, such as a conflict or support-seeking discussion with a spouse, to examine links between observed behaviors and wound healing (e.g., Kiecolt-Glaser et al., 2005). Blister healing can be assessed using measures of the vapor pressure gradient.

Participants generally report minimal discomfort from these procedures, and there is little risk for long-term injury. Not surprisingly, however, this procedure requires significant participant compliance, often involving overnight stays in the hospital/laboratory setting in order to collect blister fluid over the course of a day. Researchers frequently control for diet by standardizing food intake over the course of the study to minimize variation due to individual differences in health behaviors. The administration of blister wounds is not appropriate for studies with children, but it has yielded important insights into connections between stress and immune functioning in adults (e.g., Kiecolt-Glaser et al., 2005).

## Attachment and Inflammation: Empirical Evidence

In the previous section, we highlighted the various immune measures at the disposal of researchers who are interested in exploring associations between attachment and immune functioning. In this section, we review the empirical evidence for links between attachment (and attachment-related constructs) and inflammation. We have focused

our review on measures of inflammation given increasing evidence that inflammation plays an important role in the progression of many chronic diseases. We note, however, that other studies have examined links between attachment and other measures of immune functioning, including measures of the adaptive immune system (e.g., Picardi et al., 2007, 2013); review of these studies is beyond the scope of this chapter, however.

Below, we first review the sparse literature on the associations between attachment and inflammation. Then, we review studies that have demonstrated links between attachment-relevant constructs (e.g., maltreatment in childhood, marital quality in adulthood) and inflammatory processes.

Almost all of the research in this area has focused on adults, with examination of links between individual differences in self-reported adult attachment style and laboratory measures of inflammatory responses to some type of stressor. Self-report measures of adult attachment style yield scores on two dimensions: attachment-related avoidance and anxiety. Avoidance reflects the extent to which individuals are uncomfortable with intimacy and emotional disclosure in close relationships. Anxiety reflects the extent to which individuals fear rejection and abandonment, and desire high intimacy and closeness in relationships (Shaver & Mikulincer, 2002).

Two studies examined how attachment-related avoidance and anxiety relate to individuals' inflammatory responses following interactions with their romantic partners that were designed to be mildly stressful (Gouin et al., 2009; Robles, Brooks, Kane, & Dunkel Schetter, 2013). In these studies, couples participated in two consecutive laboratory visits. During one visit, each partner discussed a personal concern (i.e., something the individual would like to change about him- or herself). During the other visit, the partners were instructed to discuss and try to resolve sources of conflict in their relationship. Gouin and colleagues (2009) measured serum levels of IL-6 at each visit, whereas Robles and colleagues (2013) measured skin barrier recovery following a tape-stripping procedure (described in detail earlier) at each visit. The results of the Gouin and colleagues study revealed that individuals higher in attachment-related avoidance produced more IL-6 following the relationship conflict discussion than did individuals lower in avoidance, after researchers adjusted for various inflammation-related covariates. No significant attachment-related differences in IL-6 production emerged during the personal concern discussion visit, and attachment anxiety was unrelated to inflammatory responses to either discussion task. No gender differences emerged in the link between attachment style and IL-6 production. The finding that attachment style was associated with inflammatory responses only after the conflict discussion is consistent with theory suggesting that attachment-related individual differences are likely to be most evident under conditions of threat or stress (Bowlby, 1982). The authors proposed a potential behavioral mechanism underlying the link between attachment and IL-6 production, which may also account for the fact that significant findings emerged for avoidance only. Greater avoidance, but not anxiety, was associated with more negative behaviors and fewer positive behaviors during the conflict discussion. Prior research with the same sample revealed that a higher frequency of negative behavior during both discussions was associated with larger IL-6 responses (Kiecolt-Glaser et al., 2005, discussed further in the next section).

Although Gouin and colleagues (2009) found that links between attachment style and IL-6 emerged for both men and women, Robles and colleagues (2013) identified gender differences in the association between attachment style and skin barrier recovery during the two visits. Specifically, among females, greater attachment-related avoidance was related to slower skin barrier recovery across both discussion tasks, indicating a delay in tissue repair following the procedure. In contrast, among males, greater attachment anxiety was related to slower skin barrier recovery during the discussion about a personal concern only. These results provide additional support for a link between attachment style and inflammatory responses. Contrary to the authors' expectations, however, greater attachment anxiety among females was associated with *faster* skin barrier recovery across both discussion tasks. Drawing from the animal literature pertaining to physiological responses to repeated social threats or injuries, the authors speculated that the faster skin barrier recovery among anxious women may reflect a "preparative" response to anticipated social injury (i.e., lack of support from or rejection by a romantic partner) that facilitates a rapid inflammatory response to injury. Additional research is needed to replicate these findings and clarify the reasons for the unexpected positive association between attachment anxiety and skin healing in women.

A third study examined the association between adult attachment style and inflammatory response to a different type of acute stressor: coronary artery bypass graft surgery (CABG; Kidd et al., 2014). Cardiac patients completed a self-report measure of attachment style prior to surgery. Serum levels of IL-6, CRP, and TNF-$\alpha$ were measured before and after surgery. Attachment style was unrelated to postsurgery levels of CRP and TNF-$\alpha$. However, greater attachment anxiety (but not avoidance) was related to higher levels of IL-6 following surgery, after adjusting for presurgery IL-6 levels. These results provide additional evidence for a link between attachment style and inflammatory responses to a stressor; however, the pattern of findings differed from the pattern observed in the study by Gouin and colleagues (2009) that examined IL-6 responses to a laboratory-based conflict discussion. Whereas Gouin and colleagues found that avoidance, but not anxiety, predicted greater IL-6 production following a stressor, Kidd and colleagues (2014) found that anxiety, but not avoidance, predicted greater IL-6 production. Although speculative, the inconsistent findings across these two studies could be due to differences in the type of stressor (i.e., laboratory-based discussion vs. surgical procedure), poststressor consequences (i.e., momentary discomfort in relationship following conflict vs. extensive recovery following the surgery), and sample characteristics (i.e., healthy adults vs. adults suffering from heart disease). It is also important to note that Kidd and colleagues found that attachment style was only related to one out of three measured inflammatory markers. Future research will help determine whether attachment style is associated with other measures of inflammatory responses to a stressor.

To our knowledge, only one study has examined the association between self-reported attachment style and systemic inflammation (i.e., inflammation that is not in response to a specific stressor). In a sample of mostly white, healthy married couples, Uchino and colleagues (2013) did not find any significant links between attachment style and levels of IL-6, CRP, or fibrinogen. Because this is only study to test the association between adult attachment style and systemic inflammation, and the participants did not complete the full attachment style measure (10 selected items from a 36-item scale), it is hard to reach any firm conclusions from these null findings. Additional research will shed light on whether attachment style plays a role in systemic inflammation or is more reliably related to inflammatory responses to acute stressors.

Only one study has examined how attachment prior to adulthood prospectively predicts systemic inflammation in adulthood. Using longitudinal data from the Maryland Adolescent Development in Context Study (MADICS; principal investigators: Jacquelynne S. Eccles & Arnold J. Sameroff), we (Jones et al., 2015) examined the prospective association between perceptions of parents as a secure base and adult CRP levels in an African American sample. The secure base construct reflects the degree to which adolescents feel they can depend on their parents in time of need or distress. Although perception of parents as a secure base is not a measure of attachment per se, the secure base construct is central to attachment theory, and the ability to rely on one's parent(s) as a secure base is the defining feature of attachment security (Ainsworth et al., 1978; Bowlby, 1988).

In early adolescence (~12 years) and early adulthood (~20 years), participants rated the extent to which they felt they could depend on their parents in times of need—the core feature of a secure base. When participants were 32 years old, we conducted home interviews and collected serum to measure CRP. We hypothesized that perceptions of parents as a secure base in early adolescence would predict lower CRP levels in adulthood. We advanced no specific hypotheses about perceptions of parents as a secure base in early adulthood. To test our prediction that the perceived ability to depend on parents for support in times of need specifically would predict adult CRP (as opposed to other forms of support), we also included measures of more general parental support not specific to the secure base function (e.g., providing praise for successful accomplishments) and peer support in the analyses. As expected, after adjusting for inflammation-related confounds (e.g., tobacco and alcohol use, body mass index), perceptions of parental secure base support in early adolescence, but not peer support or other forms of parental support, predicted lower CRP values at age 32. None of the support variables in early adulthood predicted CRP at 32 years.

As discussed at the beginning of this chapter, one possible mechanism by which having a secure base may influence systemic inflammation is stress regulation. Given that stress is associated with elevated levels of inflammatory markers (Glaser & Kiecolt-Glaser, 2005), the enhanced emotion regulation and coping skills that having a secure base promotes may result in lower levels of inflammation in adulthood. Mounting evidence suggests that caregiving experiences influence the calibration and ongoing regulation of the child's HPA axis (Gunnar & Quevedo, 2007), and it may be that HPA axis functioning acts as a mechanism linking early secure base experiences with adult inflammatory activity. It is noteworthy that only parental

secure base support in early adolescence, but not early adulthood, predicted adult CRP. This finding is consistent with recent conceptualizations of adolescence as a sensitive period during which experiences may have long-lasting influences on development (Steinberg, 2005). Additional longitudinal research will help to shed light on how the timing of parental secure base experiences relates to later inflammation.

In summary, the studies reviewed here provide initial evidence for links between individual differences in attachment and inflammatory functioning, particularly inflammatory responses to an acute stressor. However, it is important to note that in one study, attachment style was significantly related to only one of three inflammatory markers (Kidd et al., 2014) and in another, attachment style was unrelated to three markers of systemic inflammation (Uchino et al., 2013). In addition, the available evidence is inconsistent with regard to which dimension of adult attachment is related to inflammatory responses, and the findings of Robles and colleagues (2013) indicate the possibility of gender differences. Clearly, the links between attachment and inflammation are complicated, and much more work needs to be done. Nonetheless, the few studies reviewed in the section provide an important foundation upon which future studies can build.

## Attachment-Related Constructs and Inflammation

Although few studies have examined links between attachment specifically and inflammatory activity, several studies have reported associations between constructs that are related to attachment and inflammatory outcomes. In this section, we first review studies within the domain of parent–child relationships, followed by studies within the domain of romantic relationships.

### Parent–Child Relationships and Inflammation

#### Childhood Maltreatment and Harsh Family Climate

A parent who is abusive or neglectful is the antithesis of a secure base for a child. Although nonmaltreated children are likely to turn to their attachment figure in times of threat, maltreated children are faced with a difficult paradox in which their attachment figure is both the source of the threat and the source of protection (Main & Hesse, 1990). This paradox may result in a lack of an organized strategy for dealing with threats or stressors, which in turn may have negative consequences for immune functioning. Not surprisingly, low rates of secure attachment and high rates of disorganized attachment have been observed in samples of children of maltreating parents (e.g., Cicchetti, Rogosch, & Toth, 2006). In addition, one meta-analysis suggests that the effect of maltreatment on attachment security is large (Cyr, Euser, Bakermans-Kranenburg, & Van IJzendoorn, 2010). Thus, although maltreatment is not a measure of attachment, it has important implications for child attachment security.

Mounting evidence suggests that childhood maltreatment is associated with elevated levels of inflammatory markers in adulthood (see Coelho, Viola, Walss-Bass, Brietzke, & Grassi-Oliveira, 2013, for a review of 20 studies). For example, in the Dunedin Longitudinal Study, childhood maltreatment (a composite of observed maternal rejection at age 3, parent-reported harsh discipline at ages 7 and 9, repeated caregiver changes through age 11, and physical abuse retrospectively reported at age 26) predicted higher CRP at age 32 (Danese et al., 2009; Danese, Pariante, Caspi, Taylor, & Poulton, 2007). Similarly, older adults who reported abuse during childhood had significantly higher circulating IL-6 levels and marginally higher TNF-α levels than adults who did not report being abused as children (Kiecolt-Glaser et al., 2011). Interestingly, one study of women found that retrospectively reported sexual abuse, but not physical abuse, during adolescence was associated with heightened CRP and IL-6 in adulthood (Bertone-Johnson, Whitcomb, Missmer, Karlson, & Rich-Edwards, 2012). Studies utilizing retrospective reports of a harsh, chaotic, and unsupportive family environment also revealed associations between such an environment and heightened inflammatory activity in adolescence and adulthood (Miller & Chen, 2010; Slopen et al., 2010).

In addition to examining systemic inflammation, several studies have tested the association between childhood maltreatment and inflammatory responses to acute stressors in adulthood. For example, Carpenter and colleagues (2010) found that adults who reported maltreatment during childhood showed elevated levels of IL-6 following the Trier Social Stress Test (an acute laboratory stressor) relative to adults who did not report maltreatment during childhood. Similar results

have emerged in relation to naturally occurring daily stressors. Gouin, Glaser, Malarkey, Beversdorf, and Kiecolt-Glaser (2012) found that adults who reported childhood abuse showed greater IL-6 responses to daily stressors than did adults who did not report childhood abuse.

## Warm and Supportive Parenting

The studies reviewed here provide compelling evidence for a link between negative parenting practices (i.e., maltreatment) and later inflammation. A related question is whether positive experiences with caregivers are also associated with inflammation in adulthood. Although research in this area is limited, the tentative answer to this question appears to be yes.

In a sample of adults who grew up in low-SES homes, a risk factor for heightened inflammation in adulthood (e.g., Pollitt et al., 2007), those who retrospectively reported high maternal warmth during childhood exhibited reduced proinflammatory signaling in adulthood relative to those who reported low maternal warmth (Chen, Miller, Kobor, & Cole, 2011). In addition, evidence suggests that psychosocial interventions with at-risk children may protect individuals from later heightened inflammation. In a study by Miller, Brody, Yu, and Chen (2014), low-SES African American children and their mothers were randomly assigned to either the Strong African American Families (SAAF) program—a program designed to improve family relationships, parenting behaviors, and children's self-esteem—or a control condition when children were 11 years old. Children who participated in the SAAF intervention had lower levels of six markers of inflammation (IL-1-β, IL-6, IL-8, IL-10, TNF-α, and interferon gamma [IFN-γ]) at age 19 compared to children in the control condition. Mediation analyses suggested that the effects of the SAAF program on later inflammation were partly attributable to improved parenting quality. These studies provide preliminary evidence suggesting that positive parenting practices may be a protective factor that buffers at-risk children from subsequent elevated levels of inflammatory markers. An interesting direction for future research is examination of whether links emerge between positive parenting practices and inflammatory outcomes in low-risk samples.

In summary, the studies in this section indicate links between aspects of the parent–child relationship relevant to attachment and inflammatory activity. Much of this work is based on retrospective self-reports of childhood experiences with parents. Prospective studies and the inclusion of observational measures of parenting that are not susceptible to self-report biases would help advance research in this area. In addition, future research should include other measures of parenting and the parent–child relationship. For example, parental sensitivity holds a privileged position within the attachment framework. An interesting question for future research is how early parental sensitivity relates to later inflammation and whether global sensitivity or sensitivity in response to child distress specifically is more strongly predictive of inflammatory functioning.

## Romantic Relationships and Inflammation

Nearly three decades of research indicate that adult attachment has major implications for how individuals think, feel, and behave in the context of romantic relationships (see J. A. Feeney, Chapter 21, for a review). Furthermore, the majority of adults consider a spouse or romantic partner to be their principal attachment figure (Zeifman & Hazan, Chapter 20). Thus, although romantic relationship functioning is not a measure of attachment, attachment plays an important role in couple relationships, with secure individuals typically reporting more positive romantic relationships than do insecure individuals. Several studies have examined associations between various aspects of romantic relationship functioning and markers of inflammation. We review these studies below.

### Relationship Quality

Two studies using data from the National Survey of Midlife Development in the United States (MIDUS) examined how self-reported marital strain and marital support relate to inflammatory markers in married adults (Donoho, Crimmins, & Seeman, 2013; Whisman & Sbarra, 2012). Whisman and Sbarra included all married participants who participated in the biomarker component of the MIDUS study, whereas Donoho and colleagues (2013) focused specifically on MIDUS participants who had been married for 10 years or longer. Interestingly, both studies found that marital support was associated with lower levels of inflammation in women only. Furthermore, Whis-

man and Sbarra (2012) found that age moderated the association between marital support and IL-6 levels in women: Marital support was related to lower IL-6 levels only among women 53 years old or younger. The link between marital strain and inflammation was inconsistent across the two studies. Donoho and colleagues found that marital strain was associated with higher levels of IL-6 among both men and women, but this association disappeared after adjusting for biobehavioral factors associated with inflammation. Whisman and Sbarra found that marital strain was associated with heightened IL-6, but only among women 53 years old or younger. Given prior evidence that being married (vs. unmarried) is associated with lower levels of inflammation for men only (Sbarra, 2009), one possible interpretation of the gender differences observed in these two studies is that just being married has beneficial health effects for men but, for women, the salutary effects of marriage are much more dependent on marital quality. This interpretation is also consistent with evidence that the effects of marital interactions on physiology are stronger for women than for men (see Kiecolt-Glaser & Newton, 2001, for a review). It is unclear why links between relationship quality and inflammation emerged for younger women only. Given that the mean age of menopause in the United States is 51 years (National Institute on Aging, 2010), 2 years prior to the age cutoff reported by Whisman and Sbarra, it is possible that hormonal changes are involved in observed age differences, although more research is needed to explore whether changes in hormones can explain the age effects observed by Whisman and Sbarra.

Two other aspects of romantic relationship quality that have been examined in relation to inflammatory activity include self-reported couple mutuality and ambivalence about one's spouse. In a study of women with rheumatoid arthritis (RA), perceptions of more couple mutuality—conceptualized as one's own and one's partner's levels of empathy, engagement, authenticity, zest, diversity, and empowerment in the relationship (Genero, Milller, Surrey, & Baldwin, 1992) —were associated with lower levels of inflammation (indicated by erythrocyte sedimentation rate [ESR] 6 months later; Kasle, Wilhelm, McKnight, Sheikh, & Zautra, 2010). The link between mutuality and ESR remained significant after researchers controlled for disease-modifying antirheumatic and anti-inflammatory drugs, suggesting that positive couple relationships may have benefits for RA patients beyond the benefits associated with traditional pharmacological treatments.

In a study of middle-aged and older adult married couples, Uchino and colleagues (2013) examined how perceived spousal ambivalence (i.e., rating a spouse as a source of both positivity and negativity) in three different contexts relates to serum levels of IL-6, fibrinogen, and CRP. Participants reported how positively and negatively they perceived their spouses during support-seeking, capitalization (i.e., when happy or excited), and routine daily interactions. Participants who simultaneously reported both positive and negative perceptions of their spouse in a support-seeking context had higher levels of IL-6 and fibrinogen, and marginally higher levels of CRP, compared to participants who held completely positive perceptions of their spouse. Perceived spousal ambivalence during capitalization was associated with higher fibrinogen only. No links emerged between perceived spousal ambivalence during routine daily interactions and the markers of inflammation. These findings highlight the importance of taking into account relational context (i.e., support-seeking vs. capitalization) when examining links between romantic relationships and inflammation. Although this study suggests that ambivalent perceptions of one's spouse are worse than completely positive perceptions in terms of inflammatory outcomes, it does not shed light on how ambivalent perceptions compare to completely negative perceptions of one's spouse. However, as the authors note, there are likely few individuals in long-term marriages who have completely negative perceptions of their spouse. Future research involving couples who have been married for shorter periods of time or who have relationship difficulties could provide insight into how ambivalent perceptions of one's spouse compare to completely negative perceptions.

### Observed Behavior during Marital Interaction

Kiecolt-Glaser and colleagues (2005) instructed married couples to engage in personal concerns and marital conflict discussions across two consecutive laboratory visits. Using the Rapid Marital Interaction Coding System (Heyman, 2004), the researchers rated each couple's level of hostility during the two discussions. Partners' hostility scores were combined, and couples were classified as high conflict or low conflict using a median split. The researchers then examined how hostility during the interactions related to blister wound healing and circulating levels of inflammatory markers following the interactions. Couples high in observed hostility had blister wounds that healed more slowly compared to those of couples low in observed hostility. In addition, highly hostile couples showed larger increases in IL-6 and TNF-$\alpha$ levels the morning after the conflict discussion compared to the personal concern discussion, whereas hostile couples low in hostility showed similar increases in IL-6 across both discussions and smaller increases in TNF-$\alpha$ levels after the conflict discussion compared to the personal concern discussion. These findings suggest that hostility in the marital relationship has a deleterious effect on inflammatory regulation, with implications for the speed of wound healing.

### Loss of Spouse

The loss of a spouse is, in most cases, the loss of a principal attachment figure. In the third volume of his trilogy, Bowlby (1980) devoted considerable space to discussing the psychological consequences of the loss of an attachment figure. In addition to psychological difficulties, substantial research has documented the negative health consequences associated with the loss of a spouse (e.g., Martikainen & Valkonen, 1996). Schultze-Florey and colleagues (2012) compared circulating levels of inflammatory cytokines in bereaved versus married/partnered individuals. The results revealed that bereaved individuals had higher levels of IL-6 compared to nonbereaved individuals. These results suggest that heightened systemic inflammation may be one mechanism by which the loss of a spouse results in negative health outcomes.

In summary, the studies reviewed in this section demonstrate links between aspects of romantic relationships relevant to attachment and inflammatory activity. As is the case with the studies of the parent–child relationship, much of this work is based on self-reports of marital functioning (the study by Kiecolt-Glaser et al. [2005] is a notable exception). Additional studies utilizing observational measures of couple interactions will help to advance knowledge in this area. An interesting question for future research is whether adult attachment style has an indirect effect on inflammatory activity through romantic relationship functioning. An abundance of research has shown that attachment style predicts many different aspects of romantic relationship functioning (see J. A. Feeney, Chapter 21, this volume, for a review), and the studies reviewed here indicate that couple relationships are associated with inflammatory markers. Thus, an indirect effects model seems tenable, and such a model could advance our understanding of the processes by which attachment influences inflammatory outcomes.

Research on the role of attachment in inflammation is only just beginning, and much work remains. The studies reviewed in this section offer initial support for how an attachment theory perspective can provide a useful framework for gaining insight into inflammatory processes in adolescence and adulthood. In addition to the evidence for direct links between attachment and inflammation, there is growing evidence that both predictors (e.g., maltreatment) and outcomes (e.g., marital quality) of attachment security and insecurity are associated with inflammation. Taken together, these findings suggest that attachment is a useful and potentially important construct to consider (as a predictor, mediator, or moderator) when examining associations between relationships and inflammation.

## Future Directions

As we mentioned earlier, sufficient evidence exists to warrant further study of the ways in which attachment may be associated with immune functioning in general, and inflammatory processes in particular. We are excited about the many opportunities for advancing the scientific study of attachment and immune processes, and we are confident that researchers who choose to bridge these two areas of study will find that this research adds to the field's understanding of the role of attachment across the lifespan. As others have argued (e.g., Kiecolt-Glaser, 2009), it will be important for researchers to acquire training across disciplines in order to develop sound research studies. As a note of caution, we advise attachment researchers to form collaborations with researchers who already have an established program of PNI research. These partnerships will ensure that research questions are grounded in appropriate theory, that study designs take into account the practical realities of conducting biomedical research, and that proper analytical techniques are used. Below, we have identified several opportunities for future research.

### Establishing Basic Links

As we reviewed earlier, although a large body of research has examined links between inflammation and measures that are correlated with attachment (e.g., warmth, marital quality), only a handful of studies have tested links between measures of attachment and inflammatory processes. As such, a critical first step is to build a foundation of studies that examine these associations in a diverse set of samples, with children and adults, and with different measures of attachment (e.g., self-reports, observations, interviews). These studies will help refine our understanding of how attachment is associated with inflammation and other immune processes, and whether this pattern should be expected to emerge across development, at key developmental transition periods, or only within specific age groups (e.g., later in life, when inflammation becomes increasingly prevalent). We have no reason to suspect that these hypothesized links will be limited to particular racial or ethnic groups; nevertheless, examination of these proposed links across diverse sample populations will be important for determining whether these proposed connections are robust across populations.

Two questions are important to keep in mind as researchers continue with studies of attachment and immune functioning. First, what are the limits of attachment as a predictor of immune function and physical health? We cannot expect attachment to predict *all* indicators of immune functioning. In this chapter, our focus has been on inflammation, which is part of the innate immune response that begins within hours of exposure to infection. Although we have deliberately excluded studies of *adaptive immunity* (the branch of the immune system involved in acquired or "learned" immunity), there is some evidence that attachment may play a role in adaptive immune responses as well (see Picardi et al., 2007, 2013). Some models of stress–immune system links, however, propose that stress may differentially affect innate and adaptive immune responses (Fagundes et al., 2013; Segerstrom & Miller, 2004). Thus, an important direction for future research will be to chart the contours of attachment's relation to various dimensions of immune functioning. The second question that researchers need to keep in mind is: In what ways can attachment add to the existing body of research on links between inflammatory processes and other relationship factors, such as warmth, hostility, and support? Some researchers will understandably be concerned that attempts to study links between attachment and inflammation simply constitute a rebranding of existing research that has examined relationship characteristics and inflammatory processes. One way to tackle this concern is to include measures of additional nonattachment components of relationships in analytical models in order to compare the unique role of attachment in shaping inflammatory processes (e.g., Jones et al., 2015). Our hypothesis is that attachment—and the presence of a secure base in particular—represents a unique characteristic that should help people when confronted with stressful experiences. As we move forward with this research, it will be important to consider how attachment can add to our growing understanding of how the social environment contributes to health and disease.

### Special Populations

Much of the work on psychosocial processes associated with inflammation has been done with healthy samples of children and adults, under the premise that if the risk exposure is sustained over time (e.g., if individuals experience poverty for long periods), then people will experience chronic inflammation and therefore be at risk for disease later in life. Another option is to do research with people who are already sick in order to examine how psychosocial influences shape disease-relevant inflammatory processes, and whether these changes in inflammation result in changes in disease symptoms.

Some examples of the value of a disease-centered approach can be found in studies of children with asthma (e.g., Chen & Schreier, 2008; Kaugars, Klinnert, & Bender, 2004; Marshall, 2004; Wright, 2008). Asthma, a chronic respiratory disorder and one of the most common chronic diseases in childhood, affecting over 7 million children in the United States (Bloom, Cohen, & Freeman, 2012), is a complex multifactorial disease, characterized by reversible airway hyperactivity and obstruction that develops in response to allergens, pollutants, irritants, and other stimuli (Busse & Lemanske, 2001). The immune system plays a key role in many cases of asthma, launching exaggerated responses to stimuli that cause mucus production, airway constriction, and difficulties breathing. In recent years, researchers have documented associations between psychosocial factors and the expression of asthma symptoms (Marshall, 2004; Wright, 2008). Notably, some of the most reliable psychosocial predictors of asthma expression are family-related stressors (Chen & Schreier, 2008; Kaugars et al., 2004). Furthermore, a growing body of evidence suggests that family stressors might amplify children's immune responses to environmental stimuli (e.g., allergens and pollutants) in a manner that exacerbates asthma symptoms (Chen et al., 2006). Some evidence suggests that insecure attachment is a risk factor for asthma (Cassibba, Van IJzendoorn, Bruno, & Coppola, 2004; Mrazek, Casey, & Anderson, 1987), although investigations of connections between attachment and asthma-relevant measures of inflammatory processes have been lacking.

### Attachment as a Moderator

As we mentioned earlier, we hypothesize that attachment may play an important moderating role in the already established links between stressors (e.g., early adversity) and inflammatory processes. Our central premise for this hypothesis is that the presence of a reliable and sensitive caregiver is known to attenuate stress responses (Adam, Klimes-Dougan, & Gunnar, 2007; Cassidy, Ehrlich, & Sherman, 2013), so, for securely attached individuals, exposure to stressors may be less overwhelming, leading to a less aggressive inflammatory state. Some recent evidence suggests that parents can indeed serve as buffers for children who are exposed to adverse conditions (e.g., Chen et al., 2011; Evans, Kim, Ting, Tesher, & Shanis, 2007; Miller et al., 2011). It will be important to determine the extent to which sensitive parenting can shield children from the inflammatory consequences often associated with adversity.

Even in the absence of extreme adversities, secure attachment may serve a protective function for individuals who experience other acute and chronic stressors. Attachment influences individuals' perceptions, interpretations, and memories of relationship experiences (Dykas & Cassidy, 2011). Securely attached individuals may view stressful experiences (particularly within a relationship context) through a lens that reduces the negative impact. For example, interpersonal conflict might be viewed as a way to resolve differing opinions and reach a mutually beneficial solution for secure individuals, but it might be viewed as a threat to the relationship for insecure individuals. Thus, despite evidence that conflict is associated with inflammation (e.g., Fuligni et al., 2009), this link may not exist or may be attenuated for those who are securely attached.

## Interventions

A compelling body of research suggests that exposure to stressful experiences shapes long-term health outcomes, and systemic inflammation may play an important mediating role in this link (Ehrlich, Miller, & Chen, 2016; Miller et al., 2011). Most of the research supporting this model, however, has been correlational—with many studies relying on cross-sectional designs or retrospective reports—and these study designs rightly come with some criticisms. Researchers' ability to draw conclusions about the causal nature of these links is sharply limited with correlational studies. It is understandable that the bulk of this research would rely on correlational data in light of the concerns about manipulating social experiences, but intervention studies offer a useful avenue for pursuing experimental studies of the causal connections between caregiving experiences and inflammation. As described earlier in this chapter (Miller et al., 2014), there is evidence that family-oriented interventions can reduce inflammation in at-risk children. Additional evidence with a sample of healthy adolescents suggests that an intervention aimed at increasing volunteering was effective at lowering inflammation (Schreier, Schonert-Reichl, & Chen, 2013). Further analyses suggested that these effects may have been partially due to increases in empathy and altruistic behaviors. Researchers with ongoing longitudinal studies aimed at improving attachment security should consider including assessments of physical health and inflammation in order to examine whether the intervention had an effect on these measures. Ideally, new interventions will include baseline measures of inflammation to ensure that the groups do not differ at the outset, but we encourage researchers with existing samples to include measures of inflammation in follow-up assessments as a first step.

## Dyadic Approach

Both parent–child relationships and adult romantic relationships are bidirectional and transactional (i.e., relationship partners reciprocally influence each other). Yet much of the research on attachment (and attachment-related constructs) and immune processes to date has focused on intrapersonal predictors of immune function (i.e., one's own attachment style or report of marital adjustment). Some researchers have already called for a more dyadic approach to studying links between close relationships and health. For example, Pietromonaco, Uchino, and Dunkel Schetter (2013) presented a theoretical model outlining how each partners' adult attachment style and dyadic processes (e.g., each partner's responsiveness) in close adult relationships may influence health behaviors and outcomes. We echo Pietromonaco and colleagues' call for a greater focus on dyadic processes and encourage researchers to test dyadic predictors of inflammation and other immune markers. For example, does a wife's degree of attachment-related avoidance or anxiety predict her husband's inflammatory response to some type of acute stressor, and vice versa? Furthermore, do spouses' attachment styles interact to predict immune markers in each individual? In a sample of married dyads, Gouin and colleagues (2009) did not find evidence for effects of partner attachment style on a spouses' IL-6 production, but additional research on dyadic effects on inflammatory processes is warranted.

This dyadic and transactional approach to studying immune processes can also be extended to parent–child relationships. One study found links between psychological characteristics of parents and inflammation in their children (Wolf, Miller, & Chen, 2008). Specifically, Wolf and colleagues (2008) found that more parental depressive symptoms and greater parental stress predicted increases in children's asthma-related inflammatory processes over time. This finding raises many interesting questions that may be of particular interest to attachment researchers and should be the focus of future research. For example, do children of insecure parents differ from children of secure parents in terms of inflammation? Conversely, do parents of insecure children differ from parents of secure children on immune measures? Furthermore, in two-parent families, do parents' respective attachment styles or states of mind interact to predict child immune outcomes? Finally, the observational methods that have been used to examine inflammatory responses following interactions with a romantic partner (e.g., Kiecolt-Glaser et al., 2005) can be adapted for use with parent–child dyads. For example, how do parent and adolescent attachment style (and the interaction of the two) relate to inflammatory responses following a discussion of a source of conflict in their relationship? In summary, taking a dyadic approach in the study of attachment and inflammatory processes will help to capture the richness and complexity of relationships and will help to provide insight into how attachment, in both parent–child and romantic relationships, relates to immune functioning.

## Developmental and Lifespan Focus

Much of the existing literature on attachment (and attachment-related measures) and immune functioning has been conducted with adults; it will be important to conduct studies across all developmental periods, including studies with infants, children, and adolescents. We acknowledge that this work will not be easy given participant fears of blood draws. But a developmental approach to the study of attachment and immune functioning is critical to understanding how caregiving experiences influence health-relevant biological processes and at what point in development these processes begin to unfold. Furthermore, many biological systems are especially sensitive to environmental effects, particularly in infancy and adolescence, so examination of attachment during these sensitive periods is especially pertinent. Moreover, many biological systems undergo a rapid period of development, expansion, and specialization in early childhood and adolescence, and it may be that caregiving experiences during these developmental periods are especially likely to influence biological systems, with long-term implications.

A truly developmental research approach begins with prenatal studies. The *fetal-programming model* (Lucas, Fewtrell, & Cole, 1999) argues that *in utero* experiences shape infants' development by exposing them to maternal signals about environmental conditions after birth. Pregnancy brings a number of physiological adaptations, including changes to the immune system to reduce the risk of fetal rejection, maintain protection against infection, and prepare for childbirth (Challis et al., 2009; Sacks, Sargent, & Redman, 1999). A growing number of studies have examined the ways that maternal stressful social relationships shape adverse pregnancy outcomes, including preterm birth, preeclampsia, and gestational diabetes, and accumulating evidence suggests that inflammatory processes play a critical role in mediating these links (Christian, 2012; Coussons-Read, 2012). To what extent does maternal attachment insecurity shape inflammatory processes that shape pregnancy outcomes?

Attachment security can be stable across the lifespan, but it can also change as a function of caregiving experiences and changes in the family environment. Another question that will be important to consider is the relative timing of attachment experiences across the lifespan, and how variations in attachment security over time shape inflammatory processes and health. Are there particular sensitive periods (e.g., infancy) during which attachment security is most likely to shape inflammatory processes in the decades to follow? Alternatively, can attachment be viewed from a cumulative risk framework, wherein a dose–response relation exists between the number of years of insecure attachment and inflammation? These questions require large data sets, with many years of assessment of both attachment and inflammation, in order to test competing hypotheses about the nature of attachment–inflammation links (see, e.g., Eisenberger et al., 2010, for discussion of the direction of effects in the link between inflammation and depressive symptoms). Nevertheless, the answers to these questions will help elucidate the role of attachment for immune functioning across the lifespan.

## Conclusions

Because examination of the links between attachment and immune functioning is a new area of research, the number of documented links between these two factors remains quite small. Nevertheless, we believe that the field is reaching a tipping point, and we are eager to see what new insights emerge in our understanding of how attachment experiences shape our immune systems across the lifespan. This interdisciplinary research has the potential to shed light on the varied ways that attachment experiences come to shape development and functioning. We hope that researchers will not be deterred by the complexities of embarking on this program of research, and that they will be motivated to pursue the exciting task of bridging these two fields.

## Acknowledgments

Preparation of this chapter was supported by Grant Nos. HD076563 to Katherine Ehrlich and DA033848 to Jason Jones.

## References

Adam, E. K., Klimes-Dougan, B., & Gunnar, M. R. (2007). Social regulation of the adrenocortical response to stress in infants, children, and adolescents. In D. Coch, G. Dawson, & K. W. Fischer (Eds.), *Human behavior and the developing brain: Atypical development* (2nd ed., pp. 264–304). New York: Guilford Press.

Ader, R. (1980). Presidential address: Psychosomatic and psychoimmunologic research. *Psychosomatic Medicine, 42,* 307.

Ader, R. (2001). Psychoneuroimmunology. *Current Directions in Psychological Science, 10,* 94–98.

Ader, R., & Cohen, N. (1975). Behaviorally conditioned immunosuppression. *Psychosomatic Medicine, 37,* 333–340.

Ainsworth, M. D. S. (1989). Attachments beyond infancy. *American Psychologist, 44,* 709–716.

Ainsworth, M. D. S., Blehar, M., Waters, E., & Wall, S. (1978). *Patterns of attachment: A psychological study of the strange situation.* Hillsdale, NJ: Erlbaum.

Anderson, S. E., Gooze, R. A., Lemeshow, S., & Whitaker, R. C. (2012). Quality of early maternal–child relationship and risk of adolescent obesity. *Pediatrics, 129,* 132–140.

Anderson, S. E., & Whitaker, R. C. (2011). Attachment security and obesity in US preschool-aged children. *Archives of Pediatrics and Adolescent Medicine, 165,* 235–242.

Bertone-Johnson, E. R., Whitcomb, B. W., Missmer, S. A., Karlson, E. W., & Rich-Edwards, J. W. (2012). Inflammation and early-life abuse in women. *American Journal of Preventive Medicine, 43,* 611–620.

Bick, J., Naumova, O., Hunter, S., Barbot, B., Lee, M., Luthar, S. S., et al. (2012). Childhood adversity and DNA methylation of genes involved in the hypothalamus–pituitary–adrenal axis and immune system: Whole-genome and candidate-gene associations. *Development and Psychopathology, 24,* 1417–1425.

Bloom, B., Cohen, R. A., & Freeman, G. (2012). Summary health statistics for U.S. children: National Health Interview Survey, 2011. National Center for Health Statistics. *Vital Health Statistics, 10.*

Bowlby, J. (1973). *Attachment and loss: Vol. 2. Separation.* New York: Basic Books.

Bowlby, J. (1979). *The making and breaking of affectional bonds.* London: Tavistock.

Bowlby, J. (1980). *Attachment and loss: Vol. 3. Loss.* New York: Basic Books.

Bowlby, J. (1982). *Attachment and loss: Vol. 1. Attachment* (2nd ed.). New York: Basic Books. (Original work published 1969)

Bowlby, J. (1988). *A secure base.* New York: Basic Books.

Busse, W. W., & Lemanske, R. F. (2001). Asthma. *New England Journal of Medicine, 344,* 350–362.

Carpenter, L., Gawuga, C. E., Tyrka, A. R., Lee, J. K., Anderson, G. M., & Price, L. H. (2010). Association between plasma IL-6 response to acute stress and early-life adversity in healthy adults. *Neuropsychopharmacology, 35,* 2617–2623.

Cassibba, R., Van IJzendoorn, M. H., Bruno, S., & Coppola, G. (2004). Attachment of mothers and children with recurrent asthmatic bronchitis. *Journal of Asthma, 41,* 419–431.

Cassidy, J., Ehrlich, K. B., & Sherman, L. J. (2013). Child–parent attachment and response to threat: A move from the level of representation. In M. Mikulincer & P. R. Shaver (Eds.), *Nature and development of social connections: From brain to group* (pp. 125–143). Washington, DC: American Psychological Association.

Challis, J. R., Lockwood, C. J., Myatt, L., Norman, J. E., Strauss, J. F., & Petraglia, F. (2009). Inflammation and pregnancy. *Reproductive Sciences, 16,* 206–215.

Chen, E., Hanson, M. D., Paterson, L. Q., Griffin, M. J., Walker, H. A., & Miller, G. E. (2006). Socioeconomic status and inflammatory processes in childhood asthma: The role of psychological stress. *Journal of Allergy and Clinical Immunology, 117,* 1014–1020.

Chen, E., Miller, G. E., Kobor, M. S., & Cole, S. W. (2011). Maternal warmth buffers the effects of low early-life socioeconomic status on pro-inflammatory signaling in adulthood. *Molecular Psychiatry, 16,* 729–737.

Chen, E., & Schreier, H. M. C. (2008). Does the social environment contribute to asthma? *Immunology and Allergy Clinics of North America, 28,* 649–664.

Christian, L. M. (2012). Psychoneuroimmunology in pregnancy: Immune pathways linking stress with maternal health, adverse birth outcomes, and fetal development. *Neuroscience and Biobehavioral Reviews, 36,* 350–361.

Cicchetti, D., Rogosch, F. A., & Toth, S. L. (2006). Fostering secure attachment in infants in maltreating families through preventive interventions. *Development and Psychopathology, 18,* 623–649.

Coan, J. A., Schaefer, H. S., & Davidson, R. J. (2006). Lending a hand: Social regulation of the neural response to threat. *Psychological Science, 17,* 1032–1039.

Coelho, R., Viola, T. W., Walss-Bass, C., Brietzke, E., & Grassi-Oliveira, R. (2013). Childhood maltreatment and inflammatory markers: A systematic review. *Acta Psychiatrica Scandinavica, 129,* 180–192.

Cohen, S., Doyle, W. J., Turner, R. B., Alper, C. M., & Skoner, D. P. (2004). Childhood socioeconomic status and host resistance to infectious illness in adulthood. *Psychosomatic Medicine, 66,* 553–558.

Cole, S. W. (2013). Social regulation of human gene expression: Mechanisms and implications for public health. *American Journal of Public Health, 103,* S84–S92.

Coussons-Read, M. E. (2012). The psychoneuroimmunology of stress in pregnancy. *Current Directions in Psychological Science, 21,* 323–328.

Cyr, C., Euser, E. M., Bakermans-Kranenburg, M. J., & Van IJzendoorn, M. H. (2010). Attachment security and disorganization in maltreating and high-risk families: A series of meta-analyses. *Development and Psychopathology, 22,* 87–108.

Danese, A., Moffitt, T. E., Harrington, H., Milne, B. J., Polanczyk, G., Pariante, C. M., et al. (2009). Adverse childhood experiences and adult risk factors for age-related disease: Depression, inflammation, and clustering of metabolic risk markers. *Archives of Pediatric Adolescent Medicine, 163,* 1135–1143.

Danese, A., Pariante, C. M., Caspi, A., Taylor, A., &

Poulton, R. (2007). Childhood maltreatment predicts adult inflammation in a life-course study. *Proceedings of the National Academy of Sciences, 104*, 1319–1324.

Danesh, J., Collins, R., Appleby, P., & Peto, R. (1998). Association of fibrinogen, C-reactive protein, albumin, or leukocyte count with coronary heart disease: Meta-analyses of prospective studies. *Journal of the American Medical Association, 279*, 1477–1482.

Donoho, C. J., Crimmins, E. M., & Seeman, T. E. (2013). Marital quality, gender, and markers of inflammation in the MIDUS cohort. *Journal of Marriage and Family, 75*, 127–141.

Dozier, M., & Kobak, R. R. (1992). Psychophysiology in attachment interviews: Converging evidence for deactivating strategies. *Child Development, 63*, 1473–1480.

Dykas, M. J., & Cassidy, J. (2011). Attachment and the processing of social information across the life span: Theory and evidence. *Psychological Bulletin, 137*, 19–46.

Ehrlich, K. B., Miller, G. E., & Chen, E. (2016). Childhood adversity and adult physical health. In D. Cicchetti (Ed.), *Developmental psychopathology* (3rd ed., Vol. 4, pp. 1–42). Hoboken, NJ: Wiley.

Eisenberger, N. I., Inagaki, T. K., Mashal, N. M., & Irwin, M. R. (2010). Inflammation and social experience: An inflammatory challenge induces feelings of social disconnection in addition to depressed mood. *Brain, Behavior, and Immunity, 24*, 558-563.

Eisenberger, N. I., Master, S. L., Inagaki, T. K., Taylor, S. E., Shirinyan, D., Lieberman, M. D., et al. (2011). Attachment figures activate a safety signal-related neural region and reduce pain experience. *Proceedings of the National Academy of Sciences USA, 108*, 11721–11726.

Evans, G. W., Kim, P., Ting, A. H., Tesher, H. B., & Shannis, D. (2007). Cumulative risk, maternal responsiveness, and allostatic load among young adolescents. *Developmental Psychology, 43*, 341–351.

Fagundes, C. P., Glaser, R., & Kiecolt-Glaser, J. K. (2013). Stressful early life experiences and immune dysregulation across the lifespan. *Brain, Behavior, and Immunity, 27*, 8–12.

Fluhr, J. W., Feingold, K. R., & Elias, P. M. (2006). Transepidermal water loss reflects permeability barrier status: Validation in human and rodent *in vivo* and *ex vivo* models. *Experimental Dermatology, 15*, 483–492.

Fries, A. B. W., Ziegler, T. E., Kurian, J. R., Jacoris, S., & Pollak, S. D. (2005). Early experience in humans is associated with changes in neuropeptides critical for regulating social behavior. *Proceedings of the National Academy of Sciences USA, 102*, 17237–17240.

Fuligni, A. J., Telzer, E. H., Bower, J., Cole, S. W., Kiang, L., & Irwin, M. R. (2009). A preliminary study of daily interpersonal stress and C-reactive protein levels among adolescents from Latin American and European backgrounds. *Psychosomatic Medicine, 71*, 329–333.

Genero, N. P., Miller, J. B., Surrey, J., & Baldwin, L. M. (1992). Measuring perceived mutuality in close relationships: Validation of the Mutual Psychological Development Questionnaire. *Journal of Family Psychology, 6*, 36–48.

Glaser, R., & Kiecolt-Glaser, J. K. (2005). Stress-induced immune dysfunction: Implications for health. *Nature Reviews Immunology, 5*, 243–251.

Glaser, R., Kiecolt-Glaser, J. K., Marucha, P. T., MacCallum, R. C., Laskowski, B. F., & Malarkey, W. B. (1999). Stress-related changes in proinflammatory cytokine production in wounds. *Archives of General Psychiatry, 56*, 450–456.

Gouin, J. P., Glaser, R., Loving, T. J., Malarkey, W. B., Stowell, J., Houts, C., et al. (2009). Attachment avoidance predicts inflammatory responses to marital conflict. *Brain, Behavior, and Immunity, 23*, 898–904.

Gouin, J. P., Glaser, R., Malarkey, W. B., Beversdorf, D., & Kiecolt-Glaser, J. K. (2012). Childhood abuse and inflammatory responses to daily stressors. *Annals of Behavioral Medicine, 44*, 287–292.

Gunnar, M., & Quevedo, K. (2007). The neurobiology of stress and development. *Annual Review of Psychology, 58*, 145–173.

Heyman, R. E. (2004). Rapid Marital Interaction Coding System (RMICS). In P. K. Kerig & D. H. Baucom (Eds.), *Couple observational coding systems* (pp. 67–94). Mahwah, NJ: Erlbaum.

Hotamisligil, G. S. (2006). Inflammation and metabolic disorders. *Nature, 444*, 860–867.

Jaenisch, R., & Bird, A. (2003). Epigenetic regulation of gene expression: How the genome integrates intrinsic and environmental signals. *Nature Genetics, 33*, 245–254.

Jirtle, R. L., & Skinner, M. K. (2007). Environmental epigenomics and disease susceptibility. *Nature Reviews Genetics, 8*, 253–262.

Jones, J. D., Ehrlich, K. B., Brett, B. E., Gross, J., Mohr, J., Hopper, E., et al. (2015). *African American adolescents' perceptions of parental secure base support predict serum levels of C-reactive protein 20 years later.* Manuscript under review.

Kasle, S., Wilhelm, M. S., McKnight, P. E., Sheikh, S. Z., & Zautra, A. J. (2010). Mutuality's prospective beneficial effects on inflammation in female patients with rheumatoid arthritis. *Arthritis Care and Research, 62*, 92–100.

Kaugars, A. S., Klinnert, M. D., & Bender, B. G. (2004). Family influences on pediatric asthma. *Journal of Pediatric Psychology, 29*, 475–491.

Kidd, T., Poole, L., Leigh, E., Ronaldson, A., Jahangiri, M., & Steptoe, A. (2014). Attachment anxiety predicts IL-6 and length of hospital stay in coronary artery bypass graft surgery (CABG) patients. *Journal of Psychosomatic Research, 77*, 155–157.

Kiecolt-Glaser, J. K. (2009). Psychoneuroimmunology: Psychology's gateway to the biomedical future. *Perspectives on Psychological Science, 4*, 367–369.

Kiecolt-Glaser, J. K., Gouin, J. P., Weng, N. P., Malarkey, W. B., Beversdorf, D. Q., & Glaser, R. (2011). Childhood adversity heightens the impact of later-life caregiving stress on telomere length and inflammation. *Psychosomatic Medicine, 73*, 16–22.

Kiecolt-Glaser, J. K., Loving, T. J., Stowell, J. R., Malarkey, W. B., Lemeshow, S., Dickinson, S. L., & Glaser, R. (2005). Hostile marital interactions, proinflammatory cytokine production, and wound healing. *Archives of General Psychiatry, 62*, 1377–1384.

Kiecolt-Glaser, J. K., Marucha, P. T., Malarkey, W. B., Mercado, A. M., & Glaser, R. (1995). Slowing of wound healing by psychological stress. *Lancet, 346*, 1194–1196.

Kiecolt-Glaser, J. K., McGuire, L., Robles, T. F., & Glaser, R. (2002). Psychoneuroimmunology: Psychological influences on immune function and health. *Journal of Consulting and Clinical Psychology, 70*, 537–547.

Kiecolt-Glaser, J. K., & Newton, T. L. (2001). Marriage and health: His and hers. *Psychological Bulletin, 127*, 472–503.

Kuhns, D. B., DeCarlo, E., Hawk, D. M., & Gallin, J. I. (1992). Dynamics of the cellular and humoral components of the inflammatory response elicited in skin blisters in humans. *Journal of Clinical Investigation, 89*, 1734–1740.

Libby, P., Ridker, P. M., & Hansson, G. K. (2009). Inflammation in atherosclerosis: From pathophysiology to practice. *Journal of the American College of Cardiology, 54*, 2129–2138.

Libby, P., & Theroux, P. (2005). Pathophysiology of coronary artery disease. *Circulation, 111*, 3481–3488.

Lucas, A., Fewtrell, M. S., & Cole, T. J. (1999). Fetal origins of adult disease—the hypothesis revisited. *British Medical Journal, 319*, 245–249.

Main, M. (1990). Cross-cultural studies of attachment organization: Recent studies, changing methodologies, and the concept of conditional strategies. *Human Development, 33*, 48–61.

Main, M., & Hesse, E. (1990). Parents' unresolved traumatic experiences are related to infant disorganized attachment status: Is frightened and/or frightening parental behavior the linking mechanism? In M. Greenberg, D. Cicchetti, & E. M. Cummings (Eds.), *Attachment in the preschool years: Theory, research, and intervention* (pp. 161–184). Chicago: University of Chicago Press.

Marques, A. H., Silverman, M. N., & Sternberg, E. M. (2009). Glucocorticoid dysregulations and their clinical correlates: From receptors to therapeutics. *Annals of the New York Academy of Sciences, 1179*, 1–18.

Marshall, G. D. (2004). Neuroendocrine mechanisms of immune dysregulation: Applications to allergy and asthma. *Annals of Allergy, Asthma, and Immunology, 93*, S11–S17.

Martikainen, P., & Valkonen, T. (1996). Mortality after the death of a spouse: Rates and causes of death in a large Finnish cohort. *American Journal of Public Health, 86*, 1087–1093.

Maseri, A., & Fuster, V. (2003). Is there a vulnerable plaque? *Circulation, 107*, 2068–2071.

McGowan, P. O., Sasaki, A., D'Alessio, A. C., Dymov, S., Labonte, B., Szyf, M., et al. (2009). Epigenetic regulation of the glucocorticoid receptor in human brain associates with child abuse. *Nature Neuroscience, 12*, 342–348.

McWilliams, L. A., & Bailey, S. (2010). Associations between adult attachment ratings and health conditions: Evidence from the National Comorbidity Survey Replication. *Health Psychology, 29*, 446–453.

Mikulincer, M., & Shaver, P. R. (2007). *Attachment in adulthood: Structure, dynamics, and change.* New York: Guilford Press.

Miller, G. E., Brody, G. H., Yu, T., & Chen, E. (2014). A family-oriented psychosocial intervention reduces inflammation in low-SES African American youth. *Proceedings of the National Academy of Sciences USA, 111*, 11287–11292.

Miller, G. E., & Chen, E. (2010). Harsh family climate in early life presages the emergence of proinflammatory phenotype in adolescence. *Psychological Science, 21*, 848–856.

Miller, G. E., Chen, E., Fok, A., Walker, H., Lim, A., Nicholls, E. P., et al. (2009). Low early-life social class leaves a biological residue manifest by decreased glucocorticoid and increased proinflammatory signaling. *Proceedings of the National Academy of Sciences USA, 106*, 14716–14721.

Miller, G. E., Chen, E., & Parker, K. J. (2011). Psychological stress in childhood and susceptibility to the chronic diseases of aging: Moving toward a model of behavioral and biological mechanisms. *Psychological Bulletin, 137*, 959–997.

Miller, G. E., Chen, E., Sze, J., Marin, T., Arevalo, J. M. G., Doll, R., et al. (2008). A genomic fingerprint of chronic stress in humans: Blunted glucocorticoid and increased NF-kappaB signaling. *Biological Psychiatry, 64*, 266–272.

Miller, G. E., Cohen, S., & Ritchey, A. K. (2002). Chronic psychological stress and the regulation of pro-inflammatory cytokines: A glucocorticoid resistance model. *Health Psychology, 21*, 531–541.

Mrazek, D. A., Casey, B., & Anderson, I. (1987). Insecure attachment in severely asthmatic preschool children: Is it a risk factor? *Journal of the American Academy of Child and Adolescent Psychiatry, 26*, 516–620.

Nachmias, M., Gunnar, M., Mangelsdorf, S., Parritz, R. H., & Buss, K. (1996). Behavioral inhibition and stress reactivity: The moderating role of attachment security. *Child Development, 67*, 508–522.

National Institute on Aging. (2010). An introduction to menopause. Retrieved from *www.nia.nih.gov/sites/default/files/menopause_time_for_a_change_0.pdf.*

Picardi, A., Battisti, F., Tarsitani, L., Baldassari, M., Copertaro, A., Mocchegiani, E., et al. (2007). Attachment security and immunity in healthy women. *Psychosomatic Medicine, 69*, 40–46.

Picardi, A., Miglio, R., Tarsitani, L., Battisti, F., Baldassari, M., Copertaro, A., et al. (2013). Attachment style and immunity: A 1-year longitudinal study. *Biological Psychology, 92*, 353–358.

Pietromonaco, P. R., Uchino, B., & Dunkel Schetter, C. (2013). Close relationship processes and health: Implications of attachment theory for health and disease. *Health Psychology, 32*, 499–513.

Pollitt, R. A., Kaufman, J. S., Rose, K. M., Diez-Roux, A. V., Zeng, D., & Hess, G. (2007). Early-life and adult socioeconomic status and inflammatory risk markers in adulthood. *European Journal of Epidemiology, 22*, 55–66.

Puig, J., Englund, M. M., Simpson, J. A., & Collins, W. (2013). Predicting adult physical illness from infant attachment: A prospective longitudinal study. *Health Psychology, 32*, 409–417.

Raison, C. L., & Miller, A. H. (2003). When not enough is too much: The role of insufficient glucocorticoid signaling in the pathophysiology of stress-related disorders. *American Journal of Psychiatry, 160*, 1554–1565.

Rakyan, V. K., Down, T. A., Balding, D. J., & Beck, S. (2011). Epigenome-wide association studies for common human diseases. *Nature Reviews Genetics, 12*, 529–541.

Ridker, P. M. (2003). Clinical application of C-reactive protein for cardiovascular disease detection and prevention. *Circulation, 107*, 363–369.

Ridker, P. M. (2007). Inflammatory biomarkers and risks of myocardial infarction, stroke, diabetes, and total mortality: Implications for longevity. *Nutrition Reviews, 65*, S253–S259.

Robles, T. F., Brooks, K. P., Kane, H. S., & Dunkel Schetter, C. (2013). Attachment, skin deep?: Relationships between adult attachment and skin barrier recovery. *International Journal of Psychophysiology, 88*, 241–252.

Rohleder, N., Marin, T. J., Ma, R., & Miller, G. E. (2009). Biologic cost of caring for a cancer patient: Dysregulation of pro- and anti-inflammatory signaling pathways. *Journal of Clinical Oncology, 27*, 2909–2915.

Sacks, G., Sargent, I., & Redman, C. (1999). An innate view of human pregnancy. *Immunology Today, 20*, 114–118.

Salmon, J. K., Armstrong, C. A., & Ansel, J. C. (1994). The skin as an immune organ. *Western Journal of Medicine, 160*, 146–152.

Sapolsky, R. M., Romero, L. M., & Munck, A. U. (2000). How do glucocorticoids influence stress responses?: Integrating permissive, suppressive, stimulatory, and preparative actions. *Endocrine Reviews, 21*, 55–89.

Sbarra, D. A. (2009). Marriage protects men from clinically meaningful elevations in C-reactive protein: Results from the National Social Life, Health, and Aging Project (NSHAP). *Psychosomatic Medicine, 71*, 828–835.

Schreier, H. M. C., Schonert-Reichl, K. A., & Chen, E. (2013). Effect of volunteering on risk factors for cardiovascular disease in adolescents. *JAMA Pediatrics, 167*, 327–332.

Schultze-Florey, C. R., Martínez-Maza, O., Magpantay, L., Breen, E. C., Irwin, M. R., Gündel, H., et al. (2012). When grief makes you sick: Bereavement induced systemic inflammation is a question of genotype. *Brain, Behavior, and Immunity, 26*, 1066–1071.

Segerstrom, S. C., & Miller, G. E. (2004). Psychological stress and the human immune system: A meta-analytic study of 30 years of inquiry. *Psychological Bulletin, 130*, 601–630.

Shaver, P. R., & Mikulincer, M. (2002). Attachment-related psychodynamics. *Attachment and Human Development, 4*, 133–161.

Sloan, E. K., Capitanio, J. P., Tarara, R. P., Mendoza, S. P., Mason, W. A., & Cole, S. W. (2007). Social stress enhances sympathetic innervation of primate lymph nodes: Mechanisms and implications for viral pathogenesis. *Journal of Neuroscience, 27*, 8857–8865.

Slopen, N., Lewis, T. T., Gruenewald, T. L., Mujahid, M. S., Ryff, C. D., Albert, M. A., et al. (2010). Early life adversity and inflammation in African Americans and Whites in the Midlife in the United States Survey. *Psychosomatic Medicine, 72*, 694–701.

Solomon, G. F., & Moos, R. H. (1964). Emotions, immunity, and disease: A speculative theoretical integration. *Archives of General Psychiatry, 11*, 657–674.

Sroufe, L. A., & Waters, E. (1977). Attachment as an organizational construct. *Child Development, 48*, 1184–1199.

Steinberg, L. (2005). Cognitive and affective development in adolescence. *Trends in Cognitive Sciences, 9*, 69–74.

Sternberg, E. M. (2006). Neural regulation of innate immunity: A coordinated nonspecific host response to pathogens. *Nature Reviews Immunology, 6*, 318–328.

Uchino, B. N., Bosch, J. A., Smith, T. W., Carlisle, M., Birmingham, W., Bowen, K. S., et al. (2013). Relationships and cardiovascular risk: Perceived spousal ambivalence in specific relationship contexts and its links to inflammation. *Health Psychology, 32*, 1067–1075.

Uchino, B. N., Cacioppo, J. T., & Kiecolt-Glaser, J. K. (1996). The relationship between social support and physiological processes: A review with emphasis on underlying mechanisms and implications for health. *Psychological Bulletin, 119*, 488–531.

Weaver, I. C. G., Cervoni, N., Champagne, F. A., D'Alessio, A. C., Sharma, S., Seckl, J. R., et al. (2004). Epigenetic programming by maternal behavior. *Nature Neuroscience, 7*, 847–854.

Whisman, M. A., & Sbarra, D. A. (2012). Marital adjustment and interleukin-6 (IL-6). *Journal of Family Psychology, 26*, 290–295.

Whitelaw, E., & Garrick, D. (2006). Epigenetic mechanisms. In P. Gluckman & M. Hanson (Eds.), *Developmental origins of health and disease* (pp. 62–74). New York: Cambridge University Press.

Wolf, J. M., Miller, G. E., & Chen, E. (2008). Parent psychological states predict changes in inflammatory markers in children with asthma and healthy children. *Brain, Behavior, and Immunity, 22,* 433–441.

Wright, R. J. (2008). Exploring biopsychosocial influences on asthma expression in both the family and community context. *American Journal of Respiratory and Critical Care Medicine, 177,* 129–130.

Yeh, E. T. H., & Willerson, J. T. (2003). Coming of age of C-reactive protein: Using inflammation markers in cardiology. *Circulation, 107,* 370–371.

# Chapter 10

# Attachment and Temperament as Intersecting Developmental Products and Interacting Developmental Contexts Throughout Infancy and Childhood

Brian E. Vaughn
Kelly K. Bost

For developmental scientists, the principal motivations for engaging in developmental research are (1) the desire to describe the emergence of organismic forms in the material, behavioral, psychological, and/or historical realms and (2) the desire to both characterize and explain the progressive transformations of those forms over the lifespan. An additional, but also vital, motivation is to use the information obtained from basic understandings of the emergence and transformation of forms to describe and explain individual, group, and population variability in developmental trajectories, especially with reference to the antecedents of favorable and unfavorable life course outcomes.

Although describing these motivations is easy enough, developmental scientists also acknowledge that studies of emergent forms are complex: Growth trajectories for different forms often intersect and interact to modify initial growth trajectories in ways that cannot be anticipated by knowledge of the phenomena prior to their interaction. Moreover, it is becoming increasingly clear that many life course outcomes thought to be associated with individual differences in specific

developmental trajectories are contingent on the outcomes of the interactions among different trajectories and/or their interactions with the physical and social contexts within which those trajectories are realized. An inevitable consequence of taking the interactions among developmental trajectories and their contexts seriously has been the recognition that current conceptual/theoretical frameworks used to describe specific developmental phenomena and to explain individual differences in developmental trajectories are, at best, incomplete and require expansion, revision, or replacement.

In this chapter, we address these issues for the two most widely accepted and empirically supported developmental frameworks that have been proposed as explanations of individual differences in socioemotional adaptation and the construction of personality, namely, attachment and temperament. In previous editions of this handbook, we have discussed the conceptual foundations of the two theoretical domains, their common (and different) aims and claims, and the results of studies focused on the nature of relations between these domains and on their joint prediction of salient life outcomes for infants and children. In the first major section of this chapter, we reprise themes from previous editions because they ground the arguments that follow.

In the second section, we review studies published since 2007 that have examined the interaction of attachment and temperament constructs in relation to life course outcomes. Among these studies, several have tested for evidence of differential susceptibility to environmental influences. Individuals located within one region of a trait dimension may be especially vulnerable to social environments of lower quality, *but* may benefit from very high-quality social environments to a greater extent than children located at different regions of the same trait dimension. We also consider recent studies that have tested the interaction of temperament and behavioral contexts (usually parenting quality) as a predictor of children's attachment-related outcomes. We then review recent studies that have extended the scope of attachment and temperament research to health-related topics and focus on the pediatric obesity literature as an example. Unfortunately, the joint effects of attachment and temperament or their interactions were not examined in these studies. The chapter concludes with an appeal for more theory-driven research on relations between attachment and temperament domains.

## Attachment and Temperament: Background

### Grounding the Theories

At the core of Bowlby and Ainsworth's attachment theory are questions concerning why and how bonds between children and their primary caregivers are constructed over the early years, as well as how the shared experiences leading to and maintaining attachment relationships shape and guide children's developmental trajectories of behavior, affect, cognition, and the formation of subsequent close relationships. The theory contains both explicit and implicit assumptions concerning socioemotional development and adjustment across the lifespan; nevertheless, attachment *relationships* are social co-constructions, and the central premises of the theory concern the making, maintenance, breaking, and subjective meaning of those relationships.

By way of comparison, modern temperament theory (e.g., Rothbart, 2011) was intended to describe and explain endogenously organized individual differences in action styles, reactivity, and regulation. Temperament theory stipulates that these differences are grounded in neurophysiological mechanisms underlying activity, affect, attention, and the regulation of these domains (e.g., Posner & Rothbart, 2009; Rothbart & Bates, 2006). Temperament dimensions are often (but not always) discussed as "core" aspects of personality (see Rothbart & Bates, 2006). Temperamental differences carry substantial implications for the quality and adaptedness of personality and social behavior over the life course, although the routes of temperamental influence(s) can be both direct and indirect (e.g., Rothbart, Posner, & Hershey, 1995). Unlike attachments, temperamental traits are not construed as products of social interactions or relationships, but some temperament traits may be modified as a result of transactions with the social environment (e.g., Braungart-Rieker, Hill-Soderlund, & Karrass, 2010; Pesonen et al., 2008).

### Attachment

Bowlby (1969/1982, 1973, 1980) borrowed concepts, insights, and empirical findings from several intellectual traditions in formulating attachment theory. Psychoanalytic/object relations theory was a source of insights concerning the nature of the infant–caregiver relationship. For example, the infant–caregiver relationship was viewed as a true love relationship, with all of the emotional implications of a love relationship, and dissolution of this relationship through prolonged separations was thought to precipitate a grief reaction in the child. Moreover, the early child–caregiver relationship served as a model that influenced the ways in which a child's future intimate relationships were constructed. Finally, social and psychological adjustment was conceptualized in terms of the capacities to work, love, affiliate, and play. To the extent that attachments constructed in the context of caregiver–infant interactions constituted the foundation for learning to "love well," they constituted a cornerstone for inter- and intrapersonal adjustment across a lifetime.

Ethological and comparative psychological research provided Bowlby with motivational constructs (e.g., the attachment behavioral system) and the empirical data he needed to explain a child's tendency to seek and maintain proximity to caregivers, without having to appeal to traditional behaviorist or psychoanalytic models. Bowlby (1969/1982) suggested that human infants are equipped with a rudimentary attachment behavioral system at birth that is organized to maintain proximity to the caregiver in the first years of life, and that this behavioral system governs the expression of attachment behavior on a moment-to-moment basis. He explained the presence of this behavioral system as an evolved adaptation that increased the likelihood of infant survival in the environments inhabited by early human populations.

Properties of this behavioral system were characterized using control systems concepts (e.g., proximity to the caregiver is the system's "set-goal," and the degree of proximity is dynamically adjusted through "goal-corrected behavior" that is informed by "feedback" from sensory inputs to the system). Bowlby also coordinated his developmental schedule for the emerging attachment relationship with Piaget's periods of sensorimotor and preoperational intelligence. Like Piaget, Bowlby believed that infants and young children actively participated in their own development, and he saw active participation as a defining difference between attachment theory and both psychoanalytic and behaviorist explanations of the child–caregiver bond.

Bowlby believed that repeated activations of attachment behavior over the early years resulted in the child's constructing an internal (or mental) model of the resulting relationship. He based his concept of "internal working models" (e.g., Bowlby, 1973) on the ideas of Craik (1943), who had suggested that people construct mental models for all kinds of physical and social phenomena as heuristics for explanation of the operation and functioning of those phenomena. Bowlby found the concept attractive because it suggested both a process and a structure for preserving the child's attachment relationship in the absence of overt attachment behavior and also in the absence of the caregiver (see Bretherton & Munholland, Chapter 4, this volume).

## NORMATIVE CLAIMS

From an attachment perspective, the child–caregiver bond is a special sort of relationship (i.e., a love relationship) arising from the operation of an evolved behavioral system acting to promote proximity and contact with the primary caregiver in the service of survival. As the system is activated in both normal and emergency situations (i.e., when the infant is stressed by internal or by external stimuli) and as the set-goal is repeatedly attained (i.e., contact or proximity is achieved), the pattern of individual interactions becomes organized as a recognizable and unique relationship characterizing the child–caregiver dyad (for discussion of connections between interactions and relationships, see Hinde, 1987; Hinde & Stevenson-Hinde, 1987). This relationship is co-constructed with the caregiver over ontogenetic time in a regular, expectable sequence that parallels the growth of sensorimotor intelligence. Further activity of the behavioral system in the context of an attachment relationship provides input for the assembly of the *internal working model* of the relationship and of related models of the attachment figure and of the self. These assumptions constitute the normative, species-specific claims for attachment theory.

## INDIVIDUAL-DIFFERENCE CLAIMS

Another influence on Bowlby's thinking about attachment arose from his association with Mary Ainsworth, whose research focused on the "security" construct (i.e., the feeling of safety and comfort arising from the satisfaction of basic physical and psychological needs and from the knowledge that future satisfaction of needs is not at risk). She recognized that the attachment relationship should be the primary source of security for a young child. That this relationship is a source of security can be inferred from the organization of the child's behavior with reference to the caregiver. As Ainsworth observed, for example, in 1967, the child uses the caregiver as a base for exploring the local environment in both familiar and unfamiliar settings. Furthermore, when distressed, threatened, or simply bored, proximity and contact with the caregiver generally returns the "system" to a more balanced state, allowing the child to continue exploration. She referred to the balance of attachment and exploratory behavior organized around a specific caregiver as the "secure base" and "haven of safety" phenomena (Ainsworth, Blehar, Waters, & Wall, 1978).

Although Bowlby's account of attachment co-construction was normative, he emphasized that attachment had individual-difference implications in the domains of personality and socioemotional adaptation. Security theory provided a means for exploring those implications. Fieldwork convinced Ainsworth (1967; Ainsworth et al., 1978) that differences in the patterns of secure base behavior characterizing different child–mother dyads reflected differences in the effectiveness of the attachment relationship as a source of security. Although differences in the organization of secure base behavior were apparent at home (e.g., Ainsworth et al., 1978; Vaughn & Waters, 1990), they were also distinguished by qualitatively distinct responses of the child to separation and reunion events in the Strange Situation procedure (Ainsworth et al., 1978). Drawing on naturalistic observations of child–mother interactions at home, Ainsworth and colleagues (1978) argued that the differences in secure base behavior seen in the Strange Situation were predictable from qualities of mother–infant interaction over the first year of life. In general, caregivers who typically respond sensitively to their child's communicative signals have securely attached children (De Wolff & Van IJzendoorn, 1997). Thus, individual differences in attachment behavior organization reflect accommodations of the child's attachment behavioral system to characteristic qualities of the interactive environment. Differences in experienced attachment relationships influence personality development and psychosocial adjustment by virtue of their influences on beliefs and expectations concerning the self and the self in relation to others.

## Temperament

For over 15 years, the psychobiological theory of temperament articulated by Rothbart (e.g., Rothbart, Sheese, Rueda, & Posner, 2011) has dominated temperament research. Rothbart defines *temperament* as affective, motivational, and cognitive adaptations based on inherited neuroanatomical and physiological structures that may also be shaped by experience. Individual differences with respect to reactivity and regulation in the domains of attention, emotionality, and motor activity are the phenotypic expressions of temperament. Rothbart and Bates (2006) defined *reactivity* as a person's characteristic mode of responding to changes in stimulation, including responses at behavioral, autonomic, and neuroendocrine levels. *Self-regulation* was defined as the processes operating to adjust the person's characteristic level of reactivity across domains in response to variations in environmental demands (see Block & Block, 1980, for a similar characterization of broader personality constructs that include temperamental traits as subordinate elements, but also incorporate an individual's life history).

Biological mechanisms associated with individual differences in reactivity are active early in life, although reactivity is expressed within motivational systems that develop as individual modules. Regulatory processes depend on maturation of the central nervous system; consequently, they develop on uneven schedules over the early years. For example, regulatory mechanisms controlling autonomic and neuroendocrine functions mature earlier than conscious regulatory processes such as "effortful control," which are thought to modulate reactivity for motor behavior, thought, and emotions (e.g., Rothbart, Sheese, & Posner, 2007). Rothbart and Bates (2006) suggested that the consolidation of regulatory capacity could change a child's characteristic level of reactivity between ages 3 and 6 years. Consequently, long-term rank-order stability of temperament dimensions may be expected to be modest from infancy but should increase after toddlerhood (e.g., Putnam, Rothbart, & Gartstein, 2008).

Rothbart and associates (e.g., Posner & Rothbart, 2009; Rothbart et al., 2007, 2011) have reviewed broad literatures concerning the genetic and neuroanatomical structures supporting both the reactive and the regulatory aspects of temperament. A range of brain structures and asymmetries of brain activation have also been identified as predictors of both approach and inhibitory aspects of temperament (e.g., Hane, Fox, Henderson, & Marshall, 2008; He et al., 2010), although the expected pattern of relations between asymmetry of brain activity and inhibitory temperament dimensions are sometimes counter to prediction (e.g., LoBue, Coan, Thrasher, & DeLoache, 2011).

These kinds of results offer compelling evidence that variations in human action, cognition, and emotion have a material basis, and that the central nervous system participates in these functions in a complex, transactional manner. Moreover, results of these studies support the notion that virtually every physical/physiological "structure" associated with temperamental variability has multiple functions in both development and adaptation, and that these functions may become reorganized as the environments to which the child must adjust change over ontogenetic time. Finally, these studies highlight the interactive nature of this underlying material participation in behavior, cognition, and emotion, insofar as "effects" of temperament and their underlying structures are often mediated and/or moderated by aspects of the physical and social environments (e.g., Davidson & McEwen, 2012).

## NORMATIVE CLAIMS

Rothbart (2011) argues that the underlying neural and physiological structures governing motivation (e.g., approach–withdrawal, avoidance), emotion (e.g., fear, anger, joy), and their regulation are species-specific attributes of humans, and that these structures are assembled according to prescribed developmental schedules over the first years of life. These structures function in support of the organism's viability during infancy and childhood, suggesting that they are evolved adaptations. For example, emotions and affects convey information to the experiencing child about the salience and valence of the surrounding environment, in terms of that environment's support (or threat) to the experiencing infant or child's current well-being (e.g., Campos, Frankel, & Camras, 2004; Campos, Thein, & Owen, 2003), and the behavioral manifestations of affect regulate behavior in both self and others (e.g., Walle & Campos, 2012). Likewise, mechanisms regulating the experience of affects/emotions (as well as thought and action), both in terms of the intensity and duration of the experience and in terms of the frequency with which specific states are experienced, have adaptive consequences (e.g., Diamond & Aspinwall, 2003; Shin et al., 2011). Normatively then, temperament is the nexus of linkages among neuroanatomical, neuroendocrine, and physiological systems that controls the phenotypic expression of system functions at the behavioral, feeling, and mental levels.

## INDIVIDUAL-DIFFERENCE CLAIMS

Of course, temperament concepts refer to individual differences within a population, and variability of phenotypic expression gives rise to notions of temperamental reactivity *dimensions* and their regulation. An infant's temperament is construed as a biological "given" or essence that is, at least potentially, present from conception forward, and it is this essential quality that defines the mode(s) of adaptation possible for a given child in the face of a variable environment.

Because temperament is an essential quality of the child, Rothbart and Bates (2006) argued that temperamental variability necessarily contributes to later variability along dimensions of personality (e.g., Grist & McCord, 2010). Moreover, temperament is linked, both directly and indirectly with adjustment (and maladjustment) over the lifespan (e.g., Bush, Lengua, & Colder, 2010; Chen, Deater-Deckard, & Bell, 2014; Mills et al., 2011; Zalewski, Lengua, Wilson, Tranick, & Bazinet, 2011).

## How Attachment and Temperament Overlap

### Conceptual Overlap and Distinctions

Attachment theory and Rothbart's psychobiological temperament theory are similar in several respects. In both theories, the expression of action, affect, and thought in relevant domains is grounded in neuroanatomical and physiological structures whose functions promote the immediate survival of the individual, and these structures orient the individual's trajectory of future growth and adaptation. Likewise, both describe regulatory mechanisms and processes as central aspects of the theory. In both frameworks, underlying processes related to the phenotypic expression of system function and system regulation are assumed to develop early in life. Finally, both theories propose that aspects of personality and intra- and interpersonal adjustment are influenced by the quality of adaptation within those domains. Given these metatheoretical similarities and the overlap in content between the two theories, perhaps especially with respect to affective experience, it is not surprising that the early research attempting to integrate these approaches emphasized contests over the overlapping content at both conceptual and empirical levels (see Mangelsdorf & Frosch, 1999; Vaughn & Bost, 1999; Vaughn & Shin, 2011). However, by the advent of the current millennium, it was generally accepted that neither attachment nor temperament theory could subsume the other, and researchers began to explore the interactions between domains as predictors to intra- and interpersonal adjustment outcomes (see Vaughn, Bost, & Van IJzendoorn, 2008).

Despite their similarities, attachment and temperament theories are intended to explain very different phenomena. The central problem addressed by attachment theory is the construction and maintenance of interpersonal relationships and their consequences for the developing child over the life course. As such, attachment is a social and psychological phenomenon that cannot be reduced to the activity of central nervous system structures governing proximity and contact seeking. For Bowlby (e.g., 1969/1982), the attachment behavioral system acts to promote proximity and contact between the child and caregiver, and it is the history of experiences in which proximity and contact regulate the child's internal state (e.g., Feldman, Singer, & Zagoory, 2010) that result in the assembly of the attachment relationship. Consequently, it is a social process involving the child and caregiver that determines the outcome of attachment system activation. Temperament theory, on the other hand, assumes that reactivity and regulation of affect, attention, as well as motor activity are determined primarily by "set-points" for neuroanatomical and physiological structures that are internal to the child and variable across children (Rothbart 2011). Rothbart and Bates (2006) acknowledge that the child's characteristic degree of reactivity may be modified internally, as regulatory mechanisms and processes mature, or externally, as a consequence of experience (e.g., Blair et al., 2006), but temperament remains an essential attribute of the child that is not explicitly relational at any developmental period.

Developmental aspects of temperament theory address questions concerning the sources of age-related differences in the trajectories of reactivity and regulation within persons, whereas the developmental aspects of attachment theory address questions concerning the gradual assembly of the attachment relationship between the child and caregiver(s) over the early years. Consequently, normative questions arising from assumptions of attachment theory (e.g., Bowlby's assumption that establishing a primary attachment relationship is a normative developmental accomplishment) do not intersect with the assumptions of temperament theory. However, Rothbart and colleagues (e.g., 2011) and others have drawn attention to the developmental/organizational aspects of temperamental reactivity and the (potentially) reorganizing effects of emergent regulatory mechanisms that mature according to different timetables, as well as the potential effects of external regulators of reactivity, which might include attachment.

## Empirical Overlap

Research examining both attachment and temperament domains has suggested that the caregiving environment supporting the formation of attachment relationships also influences aspects of temperament. Propper and colleagues (2008) reported that genetic risk for suboptimal vagal regulation in response to a stressor was moderated by maternal sensitivity (i.e., when a child with the "risk" allele had a mother with higher maternal sensitivity,

vagal regulation did not differ from that of children with the "low-risk" allele). Similarly, Jahromi, Putnam, and Stifter (2004) reported that maternal interventions regulated distress reactivity in 2- and 6-month-olds, and that multiple modes of intervention were more effective than any single intervention tactic. In another study, Paulussen-Hoogeboom, Stams, Hermanns, Peetsma, and van den Wittenboer (2008) found that parenting style mediated a relation between negative emotionality and internalizing problem behaviors in childhood, such that authoritative parenting style fully mediated the relation between child negative emotionality and internalizing problem behaviors. Braungart-Rieker and colleagues (2010) reported that maternal sensitivity moderated the trajectory of fear reactivity from the first to second year. Infants with more sensitive mothers showed smaller increases in fear reactivity than did infants with less sensitive mothers. Finally, Hane and Fox (2006) studied neural indicators of stress reactivity and emotionality in relation to maternal care behavior. They found elevated indicators of stress reactivity for infants of mothers who provided low-quality care. Most of these studies cannot speak to causal ordering of infant reactivity or regulatory capacity and parental behavior because assessments of both were concurrent. Nevertheless, the findings suggest that reactivity of some physiological and psychological systems underlying temperament is relatively labile during the early years. This conclusion is consistent with Rothbart and Bates's (2006) suggestion that social forces can modify initial levels of reactivity.

In the previous edition of this volume, we reviewed a handful of studies that examined interactions of attachment and temperament and/or interactions of parenting antecedents to attachment and temperament. These studies did not yield to a simple interpretation, in part because much of this research was not directed to attachment or to temperament questions per se; rather, the goals were to explain adjustment (or maladjustment) at some developmental period in terms of being predictable from temperament and attachment security and/or parenting practices. In the next section, we continue our review of studies published since 2007 that test interactions between temperament and attachment variables. We first review research addressing the direct and interactive effects of attachment and temperament on salient outcomes, then consider the question of differential susceptibility (e.g., Belsky & Pleuss, 2009; Pluess & Belsky, 2010), which has become a focus of attachment and temperament research since the previous edition of this handbook appeared.

## Attachment and Temperament Interact to Predict Behavioral, Personality, and Mental Health Outcomes

### Mediating and Moderating Interactions

#### Mediating Interactions

The notion of *mediation* has two somewhat different meanings in developmental research. The traditional meaning (Baron & Kenny, 1986) concerns causal implications of a predictor variable on an outcome that is largely indirect; that is, a predictor (A) does not directly cause the final outcome (C); rather, it is causally antecedent to an intermediate variable (B) that is the causal antecedent to the outcome (C). When C is regressed on both A and B, the intermediate variable is the primary (or only) significant predictor. Models testing this kind of mediation often measure predictors and outcomes that are temporally ordered, such that A is measured before B, which is measured before C. A second kind of statistical mediation analysis uses data collected concurrently and should not presume causal influences of predictors on outcomes. When this sort of analysis is attempted, it is prudent to test multiple models that switch the order of A and B in the prediction of C, to determine whether a mediating interpretation is justified. In our literature review, we found four published papers that tested mediating effects for attachment and temperament. In each study, tests for mediation of an attachment (A) and outcome (C) association by a temperament variable were reported. Two studies used temporally ordered measurements, and two used concurrent (or nearly so) measurements.

Drake, Belsky, and Fearon (2014) tested the hypothesis that a relation between attachment security (Strange Situation procedure classifications) and school engagement in grade 5 was mediated by temperamental regulatory capacity. Significant indirect effects were observed, but only for one (of three) regulation measures. Rispoli, McGoey, Koziol, and Schreiber (2013) tested a model predicting child social competence in kindergarten that included an indirect pathway from attachment security (using an adaptation of Waters's Attachment Q-Sort [AQS], sorted by observers)

through preschool temperament (negative emotionality) to social competence. They failed to find a temperamental mediation, although a significant indirect pathway was observed through parent emotional supportiveness. The model reported did not include direct paths from attachment to social competence, so the degree of mediation is difficult to estimate.

Two studies (i.e., Heikamp, Trommsdorff, Druey, Hübner, & von Suchadoletz, 2013; Panfile & Laible, 2012) tested for mediation effects using concurrent data. They reported that the relation between attachment (Waters's AQS sorted by mothers) and empathy was mediated by emotion regulation. The relation between attachment and empathy was not significant when the pathway from emotion regulation to empathy was included in the model. However, in the Heikamp and colleagues (2013) report, both the indirect pathway (via inhibitory control) and the direct pathway from attachment (maternal AQS sorts) were significant when predicting regulatory capacity. Neither of these studies reported the results of alternative models switching the initial and mediating predictors. Taken together, these results provide weak evidence that effects of attachment on subsequent outcomes are mediated by temperamental differences. However, this conclusion is tempered by the acknowledgment that the studies differ in important ways in terms of both attachment measures and the temperamental variable chosen for testing mediation.

#### Moderated Interactions

Bergman, Sarkar, Glover, and O'Connor (2008) examined relations between prenatal stress and early childhood fearfulness as a function of attachment classification category (4 categories scored using the Cassidy, Marvin, and MacArthur Working Group Strange Situation Procedure Protocol, 1992). Interaction plots suggested that the moderation effect was due to differences between the insecure-resistant (high-positive association) and insecure-avoidant cases (small-negative association), with slopes for other categories suggesting moderate positive relations between prenatal stress and fearfulness. Stevenson-Hinde, Shouldice, and Chicot (2011) also reported a moderating effect of the maternal anxiety × child behavioral inhibition relation that was due to a difference for the insecure-resistant cases. In this instance, however, the association was signed negatively. Although both studies reported moderation, their results are contradictory. In another report, Kochanska and Kim (2013) tested moderation of a relation between toddler anger proneness and subsequent parental power assertion in discipline settings (which, in turn, predicted children's later rule violation and reduced capacity to delay gratification). However, this chain of associations was observed only for insecurely attached children.

Temperamental moderation of attachment to subsequent outcome associations was reported in two studies. In a sample of toddlers (33 months old), McElwain, Holland, Engle, and Wong (2012) found that anger proneness moderated relations between attachment security and child–mother interaction patterns for children with high and low anger proneness. Attachment security (scored on a 9-point scale from the protocol by Cassidy et al., 1992) was positively associated with committed compliance (in challenge tasks) and self-assertion (in play tasks) when children scored higher on anger proneness. However, children with higher security scores engaged in more help-seeking behavior during play if they had low or moderate anger proneness scores. Troxel, Trentacosta, Forbes, and Campbell (2013) found that infant negative emotionality moderated effects of attachment (AQS by observers at 24 months) on sleep problems at 36 months. Children with higher AQS security scores were reported to have fewer sleep problems, but only if they had higher negative emotionality scores at 6 months.

Although these studies suggest that attachment and temperament domains do (sometimes) interact in the prediction of subsequent outcomes, inclusion of measures for both domains in studies of childhood adaptive functioning is relatively rare, at least in comparison to studies relating each domain separately to various outcomes. It is not easy to summarize these results succinctly. Moreover, no two studies used identical measures of attachment and temperament for children at the same ages, and the outcome domains being predicted from attachment and temperament measures varied across studies. Replication studies are sorely needed.

## Differential Susceptibility to Context: Temperament and Attachment

Belsky and associates (e.g., Belsky, 1997; Belsky & Pluess, 2009; Pluess & Belsky, 2010) proposed a special sort of moderation, differential susceptibility, as an alternative to diathesis–stress theories of

risk and vulnerability. According to the diathesis–stress model, the combination of an underlying "risky" genotype *and* exposure to a specific stressor is sufficient to explain the presence of maladaptive outcomes (e.g., problem behaviors) over the life course, whereas differential susceptibility models suggest that both maladaptive and optimally adapted outcomes could be associated with the gene that was inappropriately called "risky"; that is, the combination of what had been considered to be a "risky" genotype and an environmental or social stressor was associated with poor outcomes, but when the inappropriately labeled "risky" genotype was paired with a nurturing environment, the combination would result in an especially positive outcome, making the term *risky* inappropriate (see Ellis & Boyce, 2011). The differential susceptibility hypothesis is consistent with evolutionary logic in that genotypic variability should not reach equilibrium in a population if one allele consistently imposes a great cost without also conferring substantial benefits in some circumstances. Belsky (e.g., 1997) suggested that attachment security might be one of the developmental outcomes that could be understood better if considered from the differential susceptibility perspective.

With regard to attachment security, research examining differential susceptibility has two branches. First, some studies have considered whether parental sensitivity to infant/child communicative signals predicts attachment security during infancy and early childhood equally well at different levels of some temperamental attribute (most often a composite dimension implying negative emotionality or behavioral inhibition/fear, but other dimensions related to temperamental effortful control also have been tested). From the differential susceptibility perspective, high-negative emotionality (or behavioral inhibition/fear) should be associated with insecure attachment when paired with low levels of parental sensitivity but should be positively associated with attachment security when paired with high levels of parental sensitivity. Critical tests involve contrasts between children with high scores for assessments of negative emotionality (or behavioral inhibition/fear) and those with low scores for this dimension. Differential susceptibility models demand that the high–high combination of temperamental quality and parental sensitivity differ significantly in the direction of optimality from the low–high combination of temperament and parental sensitivity, and that both types should differ significantly from the high–low combination of temperament and parenting quality.

A second group of studies has not focused on attachment security as an outcome but rather on the moderating effects of temperament on associations between attachment security and some later outcome variable (e.g., sociability with others, problem behaviors). In other studies, parenting quality and temperament dimensions are considered as predictors of outcomes that have been associated with individual differences in attachment security in the broader attachment literature (e.g., internalizing or externalizing problem behaviors, social competence), but measures of attachment security per se are not included in the analyses.

We summarize the results of the studies investigating attachment security as an outcome in some detail but provide a less detailed summary of representative studies examining moderating effects of temperament on attachment security (or parenting) effects for subsequent outcomes. Some studies included molecular genetics data, as well as, or in lieu of, phenotypic temperament data (see Bakermans-Kranenberg & Van IJzendoorn, Chapter 8, this volume). Only results involving the phenotypic temperament data are reviewed here.

### Differential Susceptibility to Parenting Quality and Attachment Security

Belsky (1997) proposed that infants with specific underlying genotypes might be very sensitive to differences in parenting quality, such that they thrive extremely well when exposed to high-quality parenting but fare quite poorly when exposed to low-quality parenting. He suggested that the association between parenting quality and attachment security should be significant, substantial, and positive for these children. Alternatively, if infants' genotypes rendered them less sensitive to parenting quality, the association between parenting and attachment security would be less substantial and often not significant, even if positive. A number of studies have tested the effects of parenting quality on attachment security for children varying on dimensions of temperamental vulnerability/risk, but relatively few have reported all of the contrasts among groups that would provide strong support for the differential susceptibility hypothesis.

Luijk and colleagues (2011) tested whether infant capacity for stress regulation (negative emotionality) moderated the relation between maternal sensitivity and attachment security (using a continuous security scoring of infant behaviors in the Strange Situation procedure). In their analyses, the interaction of stress reactivity and maternal sensitivity was a significant predictor of attachment security, and the results for children at risk for high stress reactivity conformed to the differential susceptibility hypothesis. That is, when exposed to less sensitively responsive mothers, these children tended to be less secure, but when exposed to more sensitive mothers, they tended to be more secure. For children with markers suggesting low stress reactivity (or better regulatory capacity to cope with stress), the association between maternal sensitivity and attachment security was not significant. De Schipper, Oosterman, and Schuengel (2012) also found that shy/inhibited children in foster care who were paired with more sensitive foster caregivers were more likely to be securely attached than were shy/inhibited children paired with less sensitive foster caregivers. This effect was not observed for those children who were less shy/inhibited. However, in this study, children scoring either higher or lower with respect to shyness did not differ when paired with low-sensitive foster caregivers, which is inconsistent with the differential susceptibility hypothesis.

Klein Velderman, Bakermans-Kranenburg, Juffer, and Van IJzendoorn (2006) reported on an intervention to increase maternal sensitivity in a sample at risk for low sensitivity to child communicative signals and found that mothers of highly reactive infants benefited more than other mothers from the intervention experience. More importantly, their children were more susceptible to maternal *changes* in sensitivity due to the intervention, and changes in maternal sensitivity were more strongly correlated with attachment security for high-reactive infants than for low-reactive infants whose mothers had received the intervention. However, even though the association between maternal sensitivity change and attachment security was significant for high-reactive infants in this study, the absolute levels of attachment security did not differ for high- or low-reactive infants when their mothers received intervention. It is not entirely clear whether these results support the differential susceptibility hypothesis.

Cassidy, Woodhouse, Sherman, Stupica, and Lejuez (2011) also reported on an intervention designed to increase attachment security in a sample at risk for insecure attachment as a consequence of their level of irritability during the neonatal period, and found that the intervention was more effective for infants who had been highly irritable (vs. moderately irritable) as neonates. However, highly and moderately irritable neonates did not differ in the control condition, which is contrary to the differential susceptibility model. The researchers also tested for moderating influences of maternal attachment status (from the Experiences in Close Relationships Questionnaire; Brennan, Clark, & Shaver, 1998) on the differential susceptibility effect and found differences supporting both kinds of differential susceptibility. For highly secure mothers, infants who had been highly irritable showed the greatest benefit from the intervention, but there was no difference between irritability groups in the control condition. However, for more dismissing mothers, positive intervention effects were observed for the highly irritable infants (compared to moderately irritable infants), and highly irritable infants fared less well in the control group than did moderately irritable infants. No evidence favoring the differential susceptibility hypothesis was found for two other attachment status categories (i.e., fearful or preoccupied). These results are complicated, but they do provide support for the differential susceptibility hypothesis for some children, some of the time.

Although some support has been found for the differential susceptibility hypothesis linking attachment security to temperament via effects of parental sensitivity, other studies have failed to find such evidence. De Schipper, Tavecchio, and Van IJzendoorn (2008) tested for moderating effects of temperamental irritability on a relation between caregiving quality (with nonparental caregivers) and attachment security (using observer AQS descriptions) but failed to find a significant effect. Stevenson-Hinde and colleagues (2011) tested the joint influence of child behavioral inhibition and maternal anxiety on child attachment security ratings (based on a modified Strange Situation procedure). The interaction of behavioral inhibition and maternal anxiety was not significant, and only the maternal anxiety variable was a uniquely significant predictor of attachment security when both variables and their interaction term were simultaneously entered as predictors in a regression. Stevenson-Hinde and colleagues did not explicitly address differential susceptibility, and it may be that maternal anxiety levels are not a valid proxy for sensitive caregiving, so conclusions should be drawn cautiously.

## Attachment by Temperament Interactions Suggesting Differential Susceptibility

The studies reviewed here tested the interaction of attachment security and one or another temperamental attribute as a predictor of some adaptive (or not) outcome. Differential susceptibility is inferred when the interaction term is significant and the association between attachment security and the outcome variable differs for children at the opposite extremes of the temperament variable's distribution. However, for some of the studies, explicit tests of the significance of differences between more temperamentally "difficult"/securely attached and less temperamentally "difficult"/securely attached children were not reported.

McElwain and colleagues (2012) tested for differential susceptibility of children high (vs. low) for temperamental anger proneness to the influence of attachment security in relation to children's behavior during mother–child interaction. In this study, child responsiveness, help seeking, self-assertion, and committed compliance were assessed across play, cleanup, and snack tasks. The authors reported significant attachment security × temperament interactions for both self-assertion and committed compliance. Consistent with differential susceptibility hypotheses, plots of the interactions for children with low, intermediate, and high anger proneness showed that children high in anger proneness were the least self-assertive and least committed in compliance when they were less secure, and were the most self-assertive and committed in compliance when they were more secure, whereas children low in anger proneness tended to be more self-assertive when insecure but less self-assertive when securely attached.

Gilissen and associates reported two studies examining children's vagal tone (indicative of stressful arousal) to film clips during early and middle childhood in relation to temperamental fearfulness and parent–child relationship quality. Gilissen, Koolstra, Van IJzendoorn, Bakermans-Kranenburg, and van der Veer (2007) found that 4-year-olds with higher temperamental fear showed the lowest level of distress physiological reactions to fear-inducing film clips if they had a more harmonious relationship with the parent (assessed using Biringen's [2000] Emotional Availability Scales as a proxy for attachment), but they showed the highest level of fearful response to those clips if they had a less harmonious parent–child relationship. This result was replicated by Gilissen, Bakermans-Kranenburg, Van IJzendoorn, and van der Veer (2008) with 4-year-old twins and also with 7-year-old twins (attachment assessed using the Attachment Story Completion Task [Bretherton, Ridgeway, & Cassidy, 1990] for the older children) using skin conductance rather than vagal activity as the index of stress responding. The two age groups were combined for analysis, with an age covariate. Again, the interaction of fearfulness and attachment quality was significant, with the highly fearful, insecure group of children exhibiting the highest level of physiological stress, whereas the highly fearful, secure group of children exhibited the lowest level of physiological stress to the film clips.

Stupica, Sherman, and Cassidy (2011) examined attachment security, neonatal irritability, and their interaction as predictors of toddlers' exploration and sociability with nonparental adults. They suggested that differential susceptibility was a plausible explanation for the sociability outcome but not for exploration (which was more consistent with the diathesis–stress interpretation).

In the Troxel and colleagues (2013) study, discussed previously, the final path model suggested a mediated moderation relation that is at least partially consistent with differential susceptibility. In their model, attachment security predicted sleep problems at 36 months, and sleep problems predicted problem behaviors at 54 months, but only for children with higher negative emotionality as infants. Thus, more negatively emotional children who were securely attached at 36 months had fewer concurrent sleep problems than did their insecurely attached counterparts, and the full indirect path from attachment to problem behaviors via sleep problems was significant for the negatively emotional children. For children low on negative emotionality, no significant pathways were observed. Because the data were not reported in a manner that tested the difference between high negatively emotional/secure children and low negatively emotional/secure children, we are cautious about claiming this study as compelling evidence for differential susceptibility. Nevertheless, the results suggest that high negatively emotional children are responsive to the quality of care they receive in a way that is not the case for low negatively emotional children with respect to sleep problems.

Failure to detect differential susceptibility when relevant analyses were reported was also found. Lickenbrock and colleagues (2013) tested temperament (negative reactivity assessed at 7 months) by attachment security (from the Strange Situation procedure with both mother and father, assessed at 12 and 14 months, respectively) interactions in relation to child compliance in cleanup and delay tasks (assessed at 20 months). Children high with respect to negative reactivity showed neither the lowest levels of compliance when they were insecure nor the highest levels of compliance

when they were secure. Tests including child security with both parents also failed to show evidence of differential susceptibility.

## Parenting Quality/Sensitivity by Temperament Interactions as Predictors of Adjustment Outcomes in Early Childhood

Many studies have examined aspects of parenting quality × temperament interactions in the prediction of a range of positively adaptive and maladaptive outcomes in early childhood (e.g., problem behaviors, self-regulation) that have also been associated with individual differences in attachment security. The results are mixed, and because these studies did not explicitly test for attachment × temperament interactions, we only briefly summarize their results with respect to differential susceptibility. Evidence in favor of the differential susceptibility hypothesis was reported in some studies (e.g., Kim & Kochanska, 2012; Mesman et al., 2009; Pluess & Belsky, 2009; Poehlman et al., 2012). However, other investigators failed to find such evidence (e.g., Chen et al., 2014; Cipriano-Essel, Skowron, Stifter, & Teti, 2013; Kochanska & Kim, 2013). In these latter studies, the data fit more closely to the diathesis–stress or dual-risk models (i.e., low-quality care exacerbated and/or good-quality care ameliorated risk, but negative temperamental traits did not potentiate a superoptimal outcome when children were exposed to high-quality care).

## Attachment, Temperament, and Somatic Health

The contributions of attachment and temperament research to children's development are primarily within the domains of relationship construction, interpersonal functioning, and mental health. However, provocative hypotheses regarding the relevance of attachment and temperament for understanding somatic health outcomes and trajectories arise from studies identifying links between social relationships, personality, and physical health (e.g., Capitanio, 2011; Pietromonaco, Uchino, & Dunkel-Schetter, 2013; Selye, 1956; see Ehrlich, Miller, Jones, & Cassidy, Chapter 9, this volume). This inquiry has been fueled by technological advances and by studies documenting mechanisms through which social experiences become biologically translated in ways that increase or decrease vulnerability for disease (e.g.,

Boyce & Ellis, 2005; Repetti, Robles, & Reynolds, 2011; Slavich & Irwin, 2014).

Although some studies have linked adult attachment—primarily self-reported attachment anxiety—and physical health and/or immune related outcomes (e.g., Jaremka et al., 2013; Maunder, Hunter, & Lancee, 2011), few studies have reported relations between early attachment and/or temperament and physical health outcomes. In this section, we explore attachment and temperament as phenomena that may influence regulatory processes associated with physical health and initiate cascades toward or away from physical illness. We briefly review literature regarding potential biological mechanisms through which attachment and temperament may affect somatic health, then turn to one illustrative example from the pediatric literature, namely, childhood obesity.

Regarding possible biological mechanisms linking attachment, temperament, and physical health, the most relevant frameworks pertain to the complex interactions among social risk, physiological stress responses, biological dysregulation (i.e., allostatic load), and immune system functioning (e.g., Boyce, Sokolowski, & Robinson, 2012; Shonkoff, Garner, & the Psychosocial Aspects of Child and Family Health Committee on Early Childhood Adoption, and Dependent Care Section on Developmental and Behavioral Pediatrics, 2012). It is thought that chronic activation or alteration of adaptive biological regulatory responses to distress result in diminished capacities to mount effective stress responses or to recover quickly from future stress responses. Increased allostatic load also leads to greater deterioration and chronic dysregulation of these biological systems. The links between allostatic processes and health outcomes involve multiple physiological systems, including the sympathetic nervous system (SNS), the HPA axis, and the immune system (e.g., Hostinar, Sullivan, & Gunnar, 2014; Irwin & Cole, 2011; Radtke, MacDonald, & Tacchini-Cottier, 2013).

Recent research on immune system functioning is noteworthy because it is thought that chronic *interpersonal* stress can result in sustained up-regulation of inflammation through proinflammatory cytokines (e.g., Slavich & Irwin, 2014). Importantly, some of the most powerful triggers that increase signaling of proinflammatory transcription control pathways involve social isolation, rejection, evaluation, and conflict (e.g., Kemeny, 2009; Taylor, 2010). Indeed, early childhood "toxic stress", including harsh, unresponsive, and emotionally unavailable parenting, has been associated with increases in inflammation indicative of proinflammatory immune system functioning (e.g., Danese, Pariante, Caspi, Taylor, & Poulton, 2007; Taylor, Lehman, Kiefe, & Seeman, 2006). However, consistent supportive transactions may buffer physiological stress responses, possibly by reducing proinflammatory states (Chen, Miller, Kobor, & Cole, 2011).

Given these associations between social-affective processes and inflammation, we would expect that relational experiences during the early years and biologically based tendencies influencing reactivity and regulation should influence the nature of these associations (Luecken & Lemery, 2004). Attachment system activation and caregiver responses are among the first transactions through which dyadic stress, coping, and resulting regulation of internal states occur. Over time, these experiences may become embodied through programming of neural circuitry governing physiological responses to everyday challenges. Secure attachments could support children's flexible and adaptive biological stress response patterns that act to deter the development of a proinflammatory phenotype. Chronic insensitive parental responding or outright rejection, on the other hand, may elevate interpersonal stress reactivity in children, increase physiological dysregulation, and heighten inflammation risk (Repetti et al., 2011). Existing data demonstrate a link between attachment security and HPA axis functioning (e.g., Gunnar, Brodersen, Nachmias, Buss, & Rigatuso, 1996; Spangler & Grossmann, 1993). Similarly, internal "set-points" with respect to reactivity and regulation (i.e., temperament) could exacerbate or attenuate relations between environmental challenge and physical health through its interface with biological stress responses (Gunnar & Quevedo, 2007) and may interact with attachment quality to determine somatic health outcomes (Gunnar & Donzella, 2002; see Ehrlich, Miller, Jones, & Cassidy, Chapter 9, this volume).

Recent longitudinal data support extension of these hypotheses to somatic health domains. Puig, Englund, Simpson, and Collins (2013) reported that children classified as anxious-resistant in the Strange Situation procedure at 18 months were about six times more likely to report physical illnesses at age 32 than children classified as secure at 18 months. Anxious-avoidant children were approximately three times more likely, and anxious-resistant children were 7.5 times more likely to report *inflammation-related* illnesses at age 32 when compared to secure children. Similar results have been reported in retrospective studies of maternal warmth (e.g., Carroll et al., 2013; Chen et al., 2011). With respect to temperament, multimethod assessments of self-control obtained over the first decade of life predicted scores on a laboratory-based physical health index, including cardiovascular, metabolic, and inflammation assessments, at age 32 (Moffitt et al., 2011). The Moffit and colleagues (2011) and Puig and colleagues studies are, to our knowledge, the only longitudinal studies examining *early* attachment and/or temperament and *adult* physical illness or biological risk. Although more longitudinal studies like these are needed, a growing literature suggests that attachment, temperament, and aspects of physical health in childhood predict subsequent health outcomes. One such outcome is childhood obesity, to which we now turn.

## Attachment/Parenting and Pediatric Obesity

Most studies examining how parents contribute to children's eating behavior and pediatric obesity have focused on general parenting and feeding styles, food access, restriction, and preferences (e.g., Davison & Birch, 2002), but a few studies document associations between attachment and obesity-related outcomes. Anderson and Whitaker (2011) used data from the Early Childhood Longitudinal Study–Birth Cohort (ECLS-B; Bethel, Green, Kalton, & Nord, 2005) to examine attachment security and obesity in preschool-age children. Attachment security at 24 months was measured with an adaptation of Waters's AQS (observer sorts), and children were classified as insecure if their scores were in the lowest quartile and secure otherwise. Children's body mass index (BMI, kg/m$^2$) at age 4.5 years was the obesity index. Maternal responsiveness, child engagement, and *child negativity* coded from mother–child play interactions were used as covariates (as were other parenting practices related to obesity, maternal health measures, and sociodemographic characteristics), but no interactions were tested, nor was child temperament *per se* included. Logistic regressions revealed that after all the covariates were included in the model, for insecure children, the odds of obesity at 4.5 years were significantly higher than those for children with secure attachment. More recently, Anderson, Lemeshow, and Whitaker (2014) examined the relations between 9-month mother–child interaction and

obesity risk at 5.5 years of age using ECLS-B data. Mother–infant interaction quality was coded from videotapes, with scores divided into quartiles. Infant scores did not predict obesity risk, but the incidence of obesity was higher for children in the lowest quartile of maternal interaction quality scores (20.2% compared to 13.9% for children in highest quartile). However, after adjusting for maternal education, income, and race/ethnicity, maternal scores were no longer significantly associated with child obesity.

Anderson Gooze, Lemeshow, and Whitaker (2012) examined early maternal care and adolescent obesity risk using data from the National Institute of Child Health and Human Development (NICHD) Study of Early Child Care and Youth Development (SECCYD; NICHD Early Child Care Research Network, 1994). An "early maternal–child relationship quality " score was created using maternal sensitivity and child security scores at 15, 24, and 36 months. *Low maternal sensitivity* was defined as the lowest quartile for each of the time periods. With respect to child attachment, Strange Situation procedure classifications (secure vs. insecure) were used at 15 and 36 months, and AQS scores were used at 24 months (with *insecurity* defined as the lowest quartile of AQS scores, which was < .16). After adjusting for child gender and birthweight, the odds of adolescent obesity were 2.45 times higher for children with the poorest relationships compared to those with more secure relationships. The odds ratio was reduced when all sociodemographic and maternal obesity controls were entered into the model but still remained significant. Low maternal sensitivity at each time period was associated with increased odds of adolescent obesity, whereas only the 24-month insecurity (AQS observer sorts) assessment was associated with increased odds of adolescent obesity. Nevertheless, at 24 and 36 months, having both low maternal sensitivity and insecure attachment put children at significantly greater risk for adolescent obesity than if either was considered alone (Anderson et al., 2012).

## Temperament and Pediatric Obesity

The focus on the role of child temperament in obesity has emerged in part from the nutrition research showing that *capacities to self-regulate eating* depend on hunger and satiety cues that operate automatically (Birch & Deysher, 1986), but are also affected by distress and emotional factors (Herman & Polivy, 2004), presumably because brain regions governing energy balance are also implicated in emotion regulation and stress responses (Dallman, 2010). Moreover, stress responses and/or emotion dysregulation are associated with metabolic syndrome, with higher energy intake from sweet/salty foods in schoolchildren, and with children's higher BMI (Blissett, Haycraft, & Farrow, 2010; Braet & VanStrien, 1997; Faith, Allison, & Geliebter, 1997; Nguyen-Michel, Unger, & Spruijt-Metz, 2007).

Reviews of studies testing relations between temperament and pediatric obesity suggest that exploring more global self-regulation and reactivity behaviors, beyond those surrounding energy intake, is fruitful. Anzman-Frasca and colleagues (2012) reported on 18 published studies (between 1985 and 2011) examining some aspect of temperamental negative reactivity or self-regulation in infants and young children and child weight-related outcomes. In 12 of the 13 studies reviewed, *temperamental negative reactivity* was measured using a variety of scales or composites from standard parent self-report assessments of temperament (e.g., Infant Behavior Questionnaire—Revised [IBQ-R]; Children's Behavior Questionnaire [CBQ]; Revised Infant Temperament Questionnaire [RITQ]; Emotionality, Activity, and Sociability [EAS] questionnaire; Behavioral Style Questionnaire [BSQ]; Infant Characteristics Questionnaire [ICQ]). Two of the five *self-regulation* studies used behavioral assessments (e.g., inhibitory control tasks), and three used subscales from the CBQ, Colorado Childhood Temperament Inventory (CCTI), and IBQ.

With respect to negative reactivity, all three short-term longitudinal (weight gain from birth to 6 or 8 months or 6–12 months) and three of the four cross-sectional studies (sample ages ranging from birth to 8 years) found significant positive relations between temperamental negativity (especially Distress to Limitations and Negativity Reactivity/Mood) and children's weight outcomes. However, weight status in the short-term longitudinal studies was assessed prior to measures of temperament, so temporal order was an issue (e.g., Anzman-Frasca et al., 2012). The longitudinal evidence was more mixed, with four longitudinal studies having relatively small and homogenous samples reporting significant associations between negative reactivity and child weight status (i.e., Carey, Hegvik, & McDevitt, 1988; Slining, Adair, Goldman, Borja, & Bentley, 2009; Wells et al., 1997; Wu, Dixon, Dalton, Tudiver, & Liu, 2011), but failures to find evidence for such relations in large-scale cohort studies (e.g., Pryor et al., 2011).

With respect to self-regulation, Anzman-Frasca and colleagues (2012) reported that one cross-sectional study ($N = 63$) found no significant associations between inhibitory control and child BMI percentiles (Tan & Holub, 2011), but that all four longitudinal studies revealed significant negative associations between some aspect of regulation (i.e., infant soothability, observations of self-control, and delay of gratification) and subsequent child outcomes, including BMI $z$-scores, weight gain, obesity risk, and measured adiposity (Faith & Hittner, 2010; Francis & Susman, 2009; Graziano, Calkins, & Keane, 2010; Wells et al., 1997). Anzman-Frasca and colleagues (2012) noted that there are mixed findings with respect to soothability (e.g., positive associations with weight outcomes for girls in one sample). In contrast, behavioral assessments of emotion regulation, delay of gratification, and inhibitory control tend to show consistent (negative) associations with subsequent unhealthy weight status. Notably, in a study using NICHD SECCYD data, Francis and Susman (2009) found that children who were less able to self-regulate at age 3 and less able to delay gratification at age 5 had the highest BMI scores and the most rapid BMI gains over six time points from 3 to 12 years of age.

More recently, Rollins, Loken, Savage, and Birch (2014a) examined the interaction between girls' inhibitory control and profiles of maternal controlling feeding practices as a predictor of changes in BMI and eating in the absence of hunger (EAH) from 5 to 7 years of age. The effect of low inhibitory control on BMI and EAH depended on the maternal feeding practice. Children who had highly controlling mothers (i.e., who set limits about eating and restricted all snacks) and low inhibitory control were at the highest risk for EAH, and children of mothers at the very low end of controlling behaviors (i.e., children who had unlimited access to snacks) and low inhibitory control had the highest percent change in BMI across the 2 years (Rollins et al., 2014b). These changes were not seen for children with high inhibitory control.

### Attachment/Parenting Quality, Temperament, and Pediatric Obesity

Wu and colleagues (2011) used data from the NICHD sample to examine the combined effects of child temperament and maternal sensitivity at 6 months on the development of childhood obesity (age 2 years to sixth grade). Maternal reports of infant temperament using the Infant Temperament Questionnaire (ITQ;short version) were used to create an index of "difficultness," which was then used to group children into difficult, average, or easy temperament categories. Maternal sensitivity was based on the composite sums for observed sensitivity to nondistress, intrusiveness (reversed), and positive regard. Mothers were grouped into sensitive or insensitive categories by a median split. Six combinations of child temperament and maternal sensitivity groupings were created, and the easy temperament/sensitive mother category served as the reference group in most analyses.

The total effect of early maternal sensitivity and child temperament on weight status was not significant in early childhood (ages 2–4 years), but was significant at school age (5–12 years). Maternal insensitivity paired with any temperament category (easy, average, and difficult) predicted increased risk for overweight or obese status across the school-age years, with children having difficult temperament *and* insensitive parenting being at greater risk for overweight or obese status in the school-age years (compared to the reference group). Children with more difficult temperaments *and* sensitive parenting, however, were not significantly more likely to be overweight/obese at school age (compared to the reference group). Only children with difficult or average temperament who experienced insensitive care had a significantly higher BMI percentile during school age (compared to the easy/sensitive group). These findings are valuable not only because they suggest that the effects of temperament on the development of pediatric obesity depend on maternal sensitivity and developmental period, but also because difficult temperament in the context of sensitive caregiving environments may result in a more optimal (child weight-related) outcome. This interpretation would be consistent with the differential susceptibility hypothesis.

In a cross-sectional study of 77 obese children (8–16 years of age) and a matched comparison group (N = 69), Zeller, Boles, and Reiter-Purtill (2008) examined differences in parenting style and child temperament between the two groups. A global "difficult temperament" score was created by dichotomizing each subscale of the Revised Dimensions of Temperament Survey (Parent Report) and summing across subscales (resulting in scores ranging from 0 to 6). Maternal reports of their parenting on dimensions of warmth, psychological control, and behavioral control were also used in

the analyses. Mothers of obese children (compared to mothers of nonoverweight children) reported that their children had more difficult temperaments and described their own parenting practices as being lower in behavioral control (than did mothers of nonoverweight children). Difficult temperament, lower behavioral control, and the interaction of low maternal warmth and difficult temperament significantly increased the odds that a child was obese (effect sizes small to medium based on Cohen's *d*). Boles, Reiter-Purtill, and Zellar (2013) reported similar results in longitudinal data for a subsample from the Zeller and colleagues (2008) study (N = 52 persistently obese; 32 nonoverweight comparison cases). They showed that over a 50-month period, persistently obese adolescents who also had difficult temperaments as children were more likely to be parented with pressure to eat practices if their mothers described themselves as lower on psychological control. However, persistently obese children with less difficult temperaments (i.e., < 1 standard deviation below the mean) were parented with pressure to eat if their mothers were higher on psychological control.

In a cross-sectional study of Iranian youth (9–13 years of age) classified as obese, Bahrami, Kelishadi, Jafari, Kaveh, and Isanejad (2013) tested a model suggesting that relations between parent attachment (Inventory of Parent and Peer Attachment—Revised) and perceptions of eating control would be mediated by children's self-reported impulsivity and general self-control. They suggested that eating control, in turn, would predict child BMI. Although the model was supported, it is difficult to draw conclusions because limited information was provided regarding the specific path coefficients and indirect effect sizes. The findings are worth mentioning, however, because Bahrami and colleagues tested potential mechanisms through which attachment and self-regulation might influence obesity-related behavior.

## Summary: Attachment, Temperament, and Health

The findings reviewed here suggest that early attachments and child temperament may have important implications for our understanding of emergent biological risk markers for disease, but several recommendations can be made for further research in this area. First, more studies using early attachment assessments are needed, especially in light of the findings reported by Puig and colleagues (2013) linking both anxious-resistant and anxious-avoidant attachment classifications to inflammation-related illnesses in adulthood, and results showing that continuity of attachment insecurity across the 12- and 18-month time periods increased subsequent physical health risks. The findings are promising, but more and better data are needed to probe further the nature of these relations with respect to anxiety and avoidance dimensions, as well as across different attachment assessments and relationships. In addition, findings from the few studies that combined attachment/parenting and temperament assessments in the prediction of child health outcomes call for more focused studies examining these interactions, especially with respect to the differential susceptibility hypothesis.

## Reflections on the State of Research Relating Attachment and Temperament

Theories of attachment and temperament ground the most generative research programs on socioemotional development during infancy and childhood. The tension between these theories and their respective research programs has stimulated substantial growth in developmental knowledge and continues to stir controversy. However, in most of the research reviewed here, there is little evidence of that controversy. Rather, most of the recent studies have simply appropriated into their own studies measures used by attachment and temperament researchers for studying infant or early childhood prediction of adaptive (or maladaptive) functioning at some later period of development. Thus, most of these studies have rather little to say about attachment or temperament theories per se. Furthemore, when both attachment and temperament measures are included in studies, investigators do not seem to attach much importance to whether one, both, or their interactions (implying mediation or moderation) become statistically significant predictors of the outcome(s) being studied. We also note that replications are rarely reported in this literature. Consequently, the generality of findings remains an open question.

The single exception to this summary statement regarding the state of research and theory about attachment and temperament is the emergence of the differential susceptibility hypothesis and the research it has motivated. The notion that genotypic/phenotypic attributes might *either* put an infant/child "at risk" *or* confer a substantial adaptive benefit, depending on qualities of the environment to which the individual is exposed over the period of development, is provocative and may, as research findings accumulate, require important changes in the ways that development in both attachment and temperament domains are understood. Belsky (1997) suggested that parenting quality (i.e., sensitivity to infant communicative signals) could lead to very different attachment outcomes for children characterized as very emotionally reactive during infancy, depending on whether they were exposed to lower- or higher-quality (i.e., sensitive) parenting. These differences have in fact been reported in several (but not all) studies. What is most provocative, however, is that for *low* emotionally reactive children, the relation between parental sensitivity and attachment outcomes does not appear to be significant in most of these studies. This finding runs counter to most accounts of the nature of secure attachment relationships and demands an explanation. If parental sensitivity is not the foundation for attachment security for low emotionally reactive infants, what accounts for attachment differences among these infants and young children? Answering this question will be an important task for the attachment research community over the coming years.

## Acknowledgments

Preparation of this chapter has been supported in part by National Science Foundation Grant No. BCS 1251322; National Institute of Food and Agriculture (NIFA) Hatch Project Nos. ALA042-1-09042 and ILLU-793-392; and the NIFA under the Illinois Transdisciplinary Obesity Prevention Program Grant No. 2011-67001-30101 to the Division of Nutritional Sciences at the University of Illinois. We gratefully acknowledge Dr. Matthew Ong and Anneliese Feld, MPH, for their assistance and feedback. Errors of commission or omission are the responsibility of the authors.

## References

Ainsworth, M. D. S. (1967). *Infancy in Uganda: Infant care and the growth of love.* Baltimore: Johns Hopkins University Press.

Ainsworth, M. D. S., Blehar, M. C., Waters, E., & Wall, S. (1978). *Patterns of attachment: A psychological study of the strange situation.* Hillsdale, NJ: Erlbaum.

Anderson, S. E., Gooze, R. A., Lemeshow, S., & Whitaker, R. C. (2012). Quality of early maternal–child relationship and risk of adolescent obesity. *Pediatrics*, *129*, 132–140.

Anderson, S. E., Lemeshow, S., & Whitaker, R. C. (2014). Maternal–infant relationship quality and risk of obesity at age 5.5 years in a national cohort. *BioMed Central Pediatrics*, *14*, 54.

Anderson, S. E., & Whitaker, R. C. (2011). Attachment security and obesity in US preschool-aged children. *Archives of Pediatric and Adolescent Medicine*, *165*, 235–242.

Anzman-Frasca, S., Stifter, C., & Birch, L. (2012). Temperament and childhood obesity risk: A review of the literature. *Journal of Developmental and Behavioral Pediatrics*, *33*, 732–745.

Bahrami, F., Kelishadi, R., Jafari, N., Kaveh, Z., & Isanejad, O. (2013). Association of children's obesity with the quality of parent–child attachment and psychological variables. *Acta Paediatricia*, *102*, e321–e324.

Baron, R. M., & Kenny, D. A. (1986). The moderator-mediator variable distinction in social psychological research: Conceptual, strategic and statistical considerations. *Journal of Personality and Social Psychology*, *51*, 1173–1182.

Belsky, J. (1997). Variation in susceptibility to rearing influences: An evolutionary argument. *Psychological Inquiry*, *8*, 182–186.

Belsky, J., & Pluess, M. (2009). Beyond diathesis stress: Differential susceptibility to environmental influences. *Psychological Bulletin*, *135*, 885–908.

Bergman, K., Sarkar, P., Glover, V., & O'Connor, T. G. (2008). Quality of child–parent attachment moderates the impact of antenatal stress on child fearfulness. *Journal of Child Psychology and Psychiatry*, *49*, 1089–1098.

Bethel, J., Green, J. L., Kalton, G., & Nord, C. (2005). Early Childhood Longitudinal Study, Birth Cohort (ECLS-B), sampling (Vol. 2 of the ECLS-B Methodology Report for the 9-month data collection, 2001-02 (NCES 2005-147). Washington, DC: National Center for Education Statistics, Institute of Education Sciences, U.S. Department of Education.

Birch, L. L., & Deysher, M. (1986). Calorie compensation and sensory specific satiety: Evidence for self regulation of food intake by young children. *Appetite*, *7*, 323–331.

Biringen, Z. (2000). Emotional availability: Conceptualization and research findings. *American Journal of Orthopsychiatry*, *70*, 104–114.

Blair, C., Granger, D., Willoughby, M., Kivlighan, K., & The Family Life Project Investigators. (2006). Maternal sensitivity is related to hypothalamic–pituitary–adrenal axis reactivity and regulation in response to emotion challenge in 6-month-old infants. *Annals of the New York Academy of Sciences*, *1094*, 263–267.

Blisset, J., Haycraft, E., & Farrow, C. (2010). Inducing preschool children's emotional eating: Relations with parental feeding practices. *American Journal of Clinical Nutrition*, *92*, 359–365.

Block, J. H., & Block, J. (1980). The role of ego-control and ego-resiliency in the organization of behavior. In W. A. Collins (Ed.), *Development of cognition, affect, and social relations* (Minnesota Symposium on Child Psychology, Vol. 13, pp. 39–101). Hillsdale, NJ: Erlbaum.

Boles, R., Reiter-Purtill, J., & Zeller, M. (2013). Persistently obese youth: Interactions between parenting styles and feeding practices with child temperament. *Clinical Pediatrics*, *52*, 1098–1106.

Bowlby, J. (1982). *Attachment and loss: Vol. 1. Attachment* (2nd ed.). New York: Basic Books. (Original work published 1969)

Bowlby, J. (1973). *Attachment and loss: Vol. 2. Separation: Anxiety and anger*. New York: Basic Books.

Bowlby, J. (1980). *Attachment and loss: Vol. 3. Loss: Sadness and depression*. New York: Basic Books.

Boyce, W. T., & Ellis, B. J. (2005). Biological sensitivity to context: 1. An evolutionary–developmental theory of the origins and functions of stress reactivity. *Development and Psychopathology*, *17*, 271–301.

Boyce, W. T., Sokolowski, M. B., & Robinson, G. E. (2012). Toward a new biology of social adversity. *Proceedings of the National Academy of Sciences*, *109*(Suppl. 2), 17143–17148.

Braet, C., & VanStrien, T. (1997). Assessment of emotional, externally induced and restrained eating behaviour in nine to twelve-year-old obese and nonobese children. *Behaviour Research and Therapy*, *35*, 863–873.

Braungart-Rieker, J. M., Hill-Soderlund, A. L., & Karrass, J. (2010). Fear and anger reactivity trajectories from 4 to 16 months: The roles of temperament, regulation, and maternal sensitivity. *Developmental Psychology*, *46*, 791–804.

Brennan, K. A., Clark, C. L., & Shaver, P. R. (1998). Self-report measurement of adult romantic attachment: An integrative overview. In J. A. Simpson & W. S. Rholes (Eds.), *Attachment theory and close relationships* (pp. 46–76). New York: Guilford Press.

Bretherton, I., Ridgeway, D., & Cassidy, J. (1990). Assessing internal working models of attachment relationships: An Attachment Story Completion Task for 3-year-olds. In M. T. Greenberg, D. Cicchetti, & E. M. Cummings (Eds.), *Attachment in the preschool years: Theory, research, and intervention* (pp. 87–119). Chicago: University of Chicago Press.

Bush, N. R., Lengua, L. J., & Colder, C. R. (2010). Temperament as a moderator of the relation between neighborhood and children's adjustment. *Journal of Applied Developmental Psychology*, *31*, 351–361.

Campos, J. J., Frankel, C. B., & Camras, L. (2004). On the nature of emotion regulation. *Child Development*, *75*, 377–394.

Campos, J. J., Thein, S., & Owen, D. (2003). A Darwinian legacy to understanding human infancy: Emotional expressions as behavior regulators. *Annals of the New York Academy of Sciences*, *1000*, 110–134.

Capitanio, J. P. (2011). Individual differences in emotionality: Social temperament and health. *American Journal of Primatology, 73*, 507–515.

Carey, W. B., Hegvik, R. L., & McDevitt, S. C. (1988). Temperamental factors associated with rapid weight gain and obesity in middle childhood. *Journal of Developmental and Behavioral Pediatrics, 9*, 194–198.

Carroll, J. E., Gruenewald, T. L., Taylor, S. E., Janicki-Deverts, D., Matthews, K. A., & Seeman, T. E. (2013). Childhood abuse, parental warmth, and adult multisystem biological risk in the coronary artery risk development in young adults study. *Proceedings of the National Academy of Science, 110*, 17151–17153.

Cassidy, J., & Marvin, R. S., with the MacArthur Working Group SSP Protocol. (1992). *Attachment organization in preschool children: Procedures and coding manual.* Unpublished manuscript, University of Virginia, Charlottesville, VA.

Cassidy, J., Woodhouse, S. S., Sherman, L. J., Stupica, B., & Lejuez, C. W. (2011). Enhancing infant attachment security: An examination of treatment efficacy and differential susceptibility. *Development and Psychopathology, 23*, 131–148.

Chen, E., Miller, G. E., Kobor, M. S., & Cole, S. W. (2011). Maternal warmth buffers the effects of low early-life socioeconomic status on pro-inflammatory signaling in adulthood. *Molecular Psychiatry, 16*, 729–737.

Chen, N., Deater-Deckard, K., & Bell, M. A. (2014). The role of temperament by family environment interactions in child maladjustment. *Journal of Abnormal Child Psychology, 42*, 1251–1262.

Cipriano-Essel, E., Skowron, E. A., Stifter, C. A., & Teti, D. M. (2013). Heterogeneity in maltreated and non-maltreated preschool children's inhibitory control: The interplay between parenting quality and child temperament. *Infant and Child Development, 22*, 501–522.

Craik, K. (1943). *The nature of exploration.* Cambridge, UK: Cambridge University Press.

Dallman, M. F., (2010). Stress-induced obesity and the emotional nervous system. *Trends in Endocrinology and Metabolism, 21*, 159–165.

Danese, A., Pariante, C. M., Caspi, A., Taylor, A., & Poulton, R. (2007). Childhood maltreatment predicts adult inflammation in a life-course study. *Proceedings of the National Academy of Sciences, 104*, 1319–1324.

Davidson, R. J., & McEwen, B. S. (2012). Social influences on neuroplasticity: Stress and interventions to promote well-being. *Nature Neuroscience, 15*, 689–695.

Davison, K. K., & Birch, L. (2002). Obesigenic families: Parents' physical activity and dietary intake patterns predict girls' risk of overweight. *International Journal of Obesity, 26*, 1186–1193.

De Schipper, J. C., Oosterman, M., & Schuengel, C. (2012). Temperament, disordered attachment, and parental sensitivity in foster care: Differential findings on attachment security for shy children. *Attachment and Human Development, 14*, 349–365.

De Schipper, J. C., Tavecchio, L. W. C., & Van IJzendoorn, M. H. (2008). Children's attachment relationships with day care caregivers: Associations with positive caregiving and the child's temperament. *Social Development, 17*, 454–470.

De Wolff, M. S., & Van IJzendoorn, M. H., (1997). Sensitivity and attachment: A meta-analysis on parental antecedents of infant attachment. *Child Development, 68*, 571–591.

Diamond, L. M., & Aspinwall, L. G. (2003). Emotion regulation across the life span: An integrative perspective emphasizing self-regulation, positive affect, and dyadic processes. *Motivation and Emotion, 27*, 125–156.

Drake, K., Belsky, J., & Fearon, R. M. P. (2014). From early attachment to engagement with learning in school: The role of self-regulation and persistence. *Developmental Psychology, 50*, 1350–1361.

Ellis, B. J., & Boyce, W. T. (2011). Differential susceptibility to the environment: Toward an understanding of sensitivity to developmental experiences and context. *Development and Psychopathology, 23*, 1–5.

Faith, M. S., Allison, D. B., & Geliebter, A. (1997). Emotional eating and obesity: theoretical considerations and practical recommendations. In S. Dalton (Ed.), *Obesity and weight control: The health professional's guide to understanding and treatment* (pp. 439–465). Gaithersburg, MD: Aspen.

Faith, M. S., & Hittner, J. B. (2010). Infant temperament and eating style predict change in standardized weight status and obesity risk at 6 years of age. *International Journal of Obesity, 34*, 1515–1523.

Feldman, R., Singer, M., & Zagoory, O. (2010). Touch attenuates infants' physiological reactivity to stress. *Developmental Science, 13*, 271–278.

Francis, L., & Susman, E. (2009). Self-regulation and rapid weight gain in children from age 3 to 12 years. *Archives of Pediatrics and Adolescent Medicine, 163*, 297–302.

Gilissen, R., Bakermans-Kranenburg, M. J., Van IJzendoorn, M. H., & van der Veer, R. (2008). Parent–child relationship, temperament, and physiological reactions to fear-inducing film clips: Further evidence for differential susceptibility. *Journal of Experimental Child Psychology, 99*, 182–195.

Gilissen, R., Koolstra, C. M., Van IJzendoorn, M. H., Bakermans-Kranenburg, M. J., & van der Veer, R. (2007). Physiological reactions of preschoolers to fear-inducing film clips: Effects of temperamental fearfulness and the parent–child relationship. *Developmental Psychobiology, 49*, 187–195.

Graziano, P., Calkins, S., & Keane, S. P. (2010). Toddler self-regulation skills predict risk for pediatric obesity. *International Journal of Obesity, 34*, 633–641.

Grist, C. L., & McCord, D. M. (2010). Individual differences in preschool children: Temperament or personality? *Infant and Child Development, 19*, 264–274.

Gunnar, M. R., Brodersen, L., Nachmias, M., Buss, K., & Rigatuso, J. (1996). Stress reactivity and attachment security. *Developmental Psychobiology, 29*, 191–204.

Gunnar, M. R., & Donzella, B. (2002). Social regulation of the cortisol levels in early human development. *Psychoneuroendocrinology, 27*, 199–220.

Gunnar, M. [R.], & Quevedo, K. (2007). The neurobiology of stress and development. *Annual Review of Psychology, 58*, 147–173.

Hane, A. A., & Fox, N. A. (2006). Ordinary variations in maternal caregiving influence human infants' stress reactivity. *Psychological Science, 17*, 550–556.

Hane, A. A., Fox, N. A., Henderson, H. A., & Marshall, P. J. (2008). Behavioral reactivity and approach–withdrawal bias in infancy. *Developmental Psychology, 44*, 1491–1496.

He, J., Degnan, K. A., McDermott, J. M., Henderson, H. A., Hane, A. A., & Fox, N. A. (2010). Anger and approach motivation in infancy: Relations to early childhood inhibitory control and behavior problems. *Infancy, 15*, 246–269.

Heikamp, T., Trommsdorff, G., Druey, M. D., Hübner, R., & von Suchadoletz, A. (2013). Kindergarten children's attachment security, inhibitory control, and the internalization of rules of conduct. *Frontiers in Psychology, 4*, 133.

Herman, C. P., & Polivy, J. (2004). The self-regulation of eating: Theoretical and practical problems. In R. F. Baumeister & K. D. Vohs (Eds.), *Handbook of self-regulation: Research, theory, and applications* (pp. 492–508). New York: Guilford Press.

Hinde, R. A. (1987). *Individuals, relationships, and culture.* Cambridge, UK: Cambridge University Press.

Hinde, R. A., & Stevenson-Hinde, J. (1987). Interpersonal relationships and child development. *Developmental Review, 7*, 1–21.

Hostinar, C. E., Sullivan, R. M., & Gunnar, M. R. (2014). Psychobiological mechanisms underlying the social buffering of the hypothalamic–pituitary–adrenocortical axis: A review of animal models and human studies across development. *Psychological Bulletin, 140*, 256–282.

Irwin, M. R., & Cole, S. W. (2011). Reciprocal regulation of the neural and innate immune systems. *Nature Reviews Immunology, 11*, 625–632.

Jahromi, L. B., Putnam, S. P., & Stifter, C. A. (2004). Maternal regulation of infant reactivity from 2 to 6 months. *Developmental Psychology, 40*, 477–487.

Jaremka, L., Glaser, R., Loving, T., Malarkey, W., Stowell, J., & Kiecolt-Glaser, J. (2013). Attachment anxiety is linked to alterations in cortisol production and cellular immunity. *Psychological Science, 24*, 272–279.

Kemeny, M. E. (2009). Psychobiological responses to social threat: Evolution of a psychological model in psychoneuroimmunology. *Brain, Behavior, and Immunity, 23*, 1–9.

Kim, S., & Kochanska, G. (2012). Mothers' power assertion; children's negative, adversarial orientation; and future behavior problems in low-income families:

Early maternal responsiveness as a moderator of the developmental cascade. *Journal of Family Psychology, 29*, 1–9.

Klein Velderman, M. K., Bakermans-Kranenburg, M. J., Juffer, F., & Van IJzendoorn, M. H. (2006). Effects of attachment-based interventions on maternal sensitivity and infant attachment: Differential susceptibility of highly reactive infants. *Journal of Family Psychology, 20*, 266–274.

Kochanska, G., & Kim, S. (2013). Difficult temperament moderates links between maternal responsiveness and children's compliance and behavior problems in low-income families. *Journal of Child Psychology and Psychiatry, 54*, 323–332.

Lickenbrock, D. M., Braungart-Rieker, J. M., Ekas, N. V., Zentall, S. R., Oshio, T., & Planaps, E. M. (2013). Early temperament and attachment security with mothers and fathers as predictors of toddler compliance and noncompliance, *Infant and Child Development, 22*, 580–602.

LoBue, V., Coan, J. A., Thrasher, C., & DeLoache, J. S. (2011). Pre-frontal asymmetry and parent-rated temperament in infant. *PLoS ONE, 6*(7), e22694.

Luecken, L. J., & Lemery, K. S. (2004). Early caregiving and physiological stress responses. *Clinical Psychology Review, 24*, 171–191.

Luijk, M. P. C. M., Tharner, A., Bakermans-Kranenburg, M., Van IJzendoorn, M. H., Maddoe, V. W. V., Hofman, A., et al. (2011). The association between parenting and attachment security is moderated by a polymorphism in the mineralocorticoid receptor gene: Evidence for differential susceptibility. *Biological Psychology, 88*, 37–40.

Mangelsdorf, S. C., & Frosch, C. A. (1999). Temperament and attachment: One construct or two? *Advances in Child Development and Behavior, 27*, 181–220.

Maunder, R., Hunter, J., & Lancee, W. (2011). The impact of attachment insecurity and sleep disturbance on symptoms and sick days in hospital-based healthcare workers. *Journal of Psychosomatic Research, 70*, 11–17.

McElwain, N. L., Holland, A. S., Engle, J. M., & Wong, M. S. (2012). Child anger proneness moderates associations between child–mother attachment security and child behavior with mothers at 33 months. *Journal of Family Psychology, 26*, 76–86.

Mesman, J., Stoel, R., Bakermans-Kranenburg, M. J., Van IJzendoorn, M. H., Juffer, F., Koot, H. M., et al. (2009). Predicting growth curves of early childhood externalizing problems: Differential susceptibility of children with difficult temperament. *Journal of Abnormal Child Psychology, 37*, 625–636.

Mills, R. S., Hastings, P. D., Helm, J., Serbin, L. A., Etezadi, J., Stack, D. M., et al. (2011). Temperamental, parental, and contextual contributors to early-emerging internalizing problems: A new integrative analysis approach. *Social Development, 21*, 229–253.

Moffitt, T., Arseneault, L., Belsky, D., Dickson, N., Hancox, R., Harrington, H., Houts, et al. (2011). A gradient of childhood self-control predicts health, wealth, and public safety. *Proceedings of the National Academy of Sciences USA, 108,* 2693–2609.

Nguyen-Michel, S. T., Unger, J. B., & Spruijt-Metz, D. (2007). Dietary correlates of emotional eating in adolescence. *Appetite, 49,* 494–499.

NICHD Early Child Care Research Network. (1994). Child care and child development: The NICHD Study of Early Child Care. In S. L. Friedman & H. C. Haywood (Eds.), *Developmental follow-up: Concepts, domains, and methods* (pp. 377–396). New York: Academic Press.

Panfile, T. M., & Laible, D. J. (2012). Attachment security and child's empathy: The mediating role of emotion regulation. *Merrill–Palmer Quarterly, 58,* 1–21.

Paulussen-Hoogeboom, M. C., Stams, G. J., Hermanns, J. M., Peetsma, T. T., & van den Wittenboer, G. L. (2008). Parenting style as a mediator between children's negative emotionality and problematic behavior in early childhood. *Journal Genetic Psychology, 169*(3), 209–226.

Pesonen, A.-K., Räikkönen, K., Heinonen, K., Komsi, N., Järvenpää, A. L., & Strandberg, T. (2008). A transactional model of temperamental development: Evidence of a relationship between child temperament and maternal stress over five years. *Social Development, 17,* 326–340.

Pietromonaco, P., Uchino, B., & Dunkel-Schetter, C. (2013). Close relationship processes and health: Implications of attachment theory for health and disease. *Health Psychology, 32,* 499–513.

Pluess, M., & Belsky, J. (2010). Children's differential susceptibility to effects of parenting. *Family Science, 1,* 14–25.

Poehlman, J., Hane, A., Burnson, C., Maleck, S., Hamburger, E., & Shah, P. E. (2012). Preterm infants who are prone to distress: Differential effects of parenting on 36-month behavioral and cognitive outcomes. *Journal of Child Psychology and Psychiatry, 53,* 1018–1025.

Posner, M., & Rothbart, M. K. (2009). Toward a physical basis of attention and self-regulation. *Physics of Life Reviews, 6,* 103–120.

Propper, C., Moore, G. A., Mills-Koonce, W. R., Halpern, C. T., Hill-Soderlund, A. L., Calkins, S. D., et al. (2008). Gene–environment contributions to the development of infant vagal reactivity: The interaction of dopamine and maternal sensitivity. *Child Development, 79,* 1377–1394.

Pryor, L. E., Tremblay, R. E., Boivin, M., Touchette, E., Dubois, L., Genolini, C., et al. (2011). Developmental trajectories of body mass index in early childhood and their risk factors. *Archives of Pediatric and Adolescent Medicine, 165,* 906–912.

Puig, J., Englund, M., Simpson, J., & Collins, A. (2013). Predicting adult physical illness from infant attachment: A prospective longitudinal study. *Health Psychology, 32,* 409–417.

Putnam, S. P., Rothbart, M. K., & Gartstein, M. A. (2008). Homotypic and heterotypic continuity of fine-grained temperament during infancy, toddlerhood, and early childhood. *Infant and Child Development, 17,* 387–405.

Radtke, F., MacDonald, H. R., & Tacchini-Cottier, F. (2013). Regulation of innate and adaptive immunity by Notch. *Nature Reviews Immunology, 13,* 427–437.

Repetti, R., Robles, T., & Reynolds, B. (2011). Allostatic processes in the family. *Development and Psychopathology, 23,* 921–938.

Rispoli, K. M., McGoey, K. E., Koziol, N. A., & Schreiber, J. B. (2013). The relation of parenting, child temperament, and attachment security in early childhood to social competence at school entry. *Journal of School Psychology, 51,* 643–658.

Rollins, B., Loken, E., Savage, J., & Birch, L. (2014a). Effects of restriction on children's intake differ by child temperament, food reinforcement, and parent's chronic use of restriction. *Appetite, 73,* 31–39.

Rollins, B., Loken, E., Savage, J., & Birch, L. (2014b). Maternal controlling feeding practices and girls' inhibitory control interact to predict changes in BMI and eating in the absence of hunger from 5 to 7 years. *American Journal of Clinical Nutrition, 99,* 249–257.

Rothbart, M. K. (2011). *Becoming who we are: Temperament and personality in development.* New York: Guilford Press.

Rothbart, M. K., & Bates, J. E. (2006). Temperament. In N. Eisenberg (Vol. Ed.) & W. Damon & R. M. Lerner (Eds.-in-Chief), *Handbook of child psychology* (Vol. 3, pp. 99–166). New York: Wiley.

Rothbart, M. K., Posner, M. I., & Hershey, K. L. (1995). Temperament, attention, and developmental psychopathology. In D. Cicchetti & D. J. Cohen (Eds.), *Manual of developmental psychopathology* (Vol. 1, pp. 315–340). New York: Wiley.

Rothbart, M. K., Sheese, B. E., & Posner, M. I. (2007). Effortful control: Linking temperament, brain network and genes. *Child Development Perspectives, 1,* 2–7.

Rothbart, M. K., Sheese, B. E., Rueda, M. R., & Posner, M. I. (2011). Developing mechanisms of self-regulation in early life. *Emotion Review, 3,* 207–213.

Selye, H. (1956). *The stress of life.* New York: McGraw-Hill.

Shin, N., Vaughn, B. E., Akers, V., Kim, M., Stevens, S. Krzysik, L., et al. (2011). Are happy children socially successful?: Testing a central premise of positive psychology in a sample of preschool children. *Journal of Positive Psychology, 6,* 366–367.

Shonkoff, J. P., Garner, A. S., & Committee on Psychosocial Aspects of Child and Family Health Committee on Early Childhood Adoption, and Dependent Care Section on Developmental and Behavioral Pediatrics. (2012). The lifelong effects of early childhood adversity and toxic stress. *Pediatrics, 129,* e232–e246.

Slavich, G., & Irwin, M. R. (2014). From stress to inflammation and major depressive disorder: A social signal transduction theory of depression. *Psychological Bulletin, 140,* 774–815.

Slining, M. M., Adair, L., Goldman, B. D., Borja, J., & Bentley, M. (2009). Infant temperament contributes to early infant growth: A prospective cohort of African-American infants. *International Journal of Behavioral Nutrition and Physical Activity, 6,* 51.

Spangler, G., & Grossman, K. E. (1993). Biobehavioral organization in securely and insecurely attached infants. *Child Development, 64,* 1439–1450.

Stevenson-Hinde, J., Shouldice, A., & Chicot, R. (2011). Maternal anxiety, behavioral inhibition, and attachment, *Attachment and Human Development, 13,* 199–215.

Stupica, B., Sherman, L. J., & Cassidy, J. (2011). Newborn irritability moderates the association between infant attachment security and toddler exploration and sociability. *Child Development, 82,* 1381–1389.

Tan, C., & Holub, S. (2010). Children's self-regulation in eating: Associations with inhibitory control and parent's feeding behavior. *Journal of Pediatric Psychology, 36,* 340–345.

Taylor, S. E. (2010). Mechanisms linking early life stress to adult health outcomes. *Proceedings of the National Academy of Sciences, 107,* 8507–8512.

Taylor, S. E., Lehman, B. J., Kiefe, C. I., & Seeman, T. E. (2006). Relationship of early life stress and psychological functioning to adult C-reactive protein in the Coronary Artery Risk Development in Young Adults study. *Biological Psychiatry, 60,* 819–824.

Troxel, W. M., Trentacosta, C. J., Forbes, E. E., & Campbell, S. B. (2013). Negative emotionality moderates associations among attachment, toddler sleep, and later problem behaviors. *Journal of Family Psychology, 27,* 127–136.

Vaughn, B. E., & Bost, K. K. (1999). Attachment and temperament: Redundant, independent, or interacting influences on interpersonal adaptation and personality development? In J. Cassidy & P. R. Shaver (Eds.), *Handbook of attachment: Theory, research, and clinical applications* (pp. 198–225). New York: Guilford Press.

Vaughn, B. E., Bost, K. K., & Van IJzendoorn, M. H. (2008). Attachment and temperament: Additive and interactive influences on behavior, affect, and cognition during infancy and childhood. In J. Cassidy & P. R. Shaver (Eds.), *Handbook of attachment* (2nd ed., pp. 192–216). New York: Guilford Press.

Vaughn, B. E., & Shin, N. (2011). Attachment, temperament, and adaptation: One long argument. In D. Cicchetti & G. I. Roisman (Eds.), *The origins and organization of adaptation and maladaptation: Minnesota Symposia on Child Psychology* (Vol. 36, pp. 55–107). New York: Wiley.

Vaughn, B. E., & Waters, E. (1990). Attachment behavior at home and in the laboratory: Q-Sort observations and strange situation classifications of one-year-olds. *Child Development, 61,* 1965–1973.

Walle, E. A., & Campos, J. J. (2012). Interpersonal responding to discrete emotions: A functionalist approach to the development of affect specificity. *Emotion Review, 4,* 413–422.

Wells, J. C., Stanley, M., Laidlaw, A. S., Day, J. M., Stafford, M., & Davies, P. S. (1997). Investigation of the relationship between infant temperament and later body composition. *International Journal of Obesity-Related Metabolic Disorders, 21*(5), 400–406.

Wu, T., Dixon, W. E., Dalton, W. T., Tudiver, F., & Liu, X. (2011). Joint effects of child temperament and maternal sensitivity on the development of childhood obesity. *Maternal and Child Health, 15,* 469–477.

Zalewski, M., Lengua, L. J., Wilson, A. C., Tranick, A., & Bazinet, A. (2011). Emotion regulation profiles, temperament, and adjustment problems in preadolescents. *Child Development, 82,* 951–966.

Zeller, M. H., Boles, R. E., & Reiter-Purtill, J. (2008). The additive and interactive effects of parenting style and temperament in obese youth seeking treatment. *International Journal of Obesity, 32,* 1474–1480.

# Chapter 11

# Studying the Biology of Human Attachment

Amie A. Hane
Nathan A. Fox

Since the original publication of the *Handbook of Attachment* in 1999, research on the biological aspects of attachment has flourished, providing a more holistic understanding of attachment-related behavior and the physiological substrates that operate in tandem with behavior to affect social relationships. In this updated chapter, we focus specifically on infant physiological responding and expand on the literature reviewed in our chapter in the previous edition in the areas of infant autonomic and neuroendocrine correlates of behavior in the Strange Situation paradigm (Ainsworth & Wittig, 1969). We address the burgeoning enterprise of assessing the dyadic physiology of early caregiving behavior, epigenetics, and infant physiology. We also incorporate research on oxytocin and its role in the affiliative behavior of parents and infants, as well as the emerging field of parental neuroscience. Throughout this chapter, we hope to demonstrate that attachment behaviors are influenced by multiple physiological systems, and that the arbitrary distinction between "nature" and "nurture" has been replaced by a continually growing body of research showing that relationships *both influence and are influenced by* underlying biological processes. Recent work that is drawing attention to the coordination of physiological systems has added an additional layer of depth to this field, pointing to the importance of the inclusion of multiple levels of analysis

simultaneously. New research has also incorporated contextual variables to support cumulative/dual-risk models, whereby child physiological responses to relationship challenges are influenced by factors such as chronic stress and maternal depression. By reviewing the literature demonstrating that behavioral and biological systems are deeply intertwined and embedded within the larger relational ecology of relationship functioning, we hope to elucidate the rich, multisystemic complexity that underlies affiliative behavior and human attachment.

## Psychophysiology

*Psychophysiology* is the study of how physiological processes intersect with and influence psychological processes and behavior. Psychophysiological research includes measurement of physiological systems that are correlated with observed behavioral responses; it examines how individual differences in physiological responding predispose people to certain behavioral responses. Examples of this approach are studies measuring task-elicited autonomic activity; research measuring hormones, including the activity of the hypothalamic–pituitary–adrenocortical (HPA) axis during tasks designed to provoke stress; and research on the role of oxytocin in mediating attachment-related behaviors.

In studies assessing autonomic activity, several measures provide an index of physiological arousal or enhanced sympathetic or parasympathetic activity in response to a task demand (e.g., Phillips, Carroll, Hunt, & Der, 2006). Autonomic measures have also been used to detect different states of attention. For example, heart rate (HR) change has been measured in response to visual or auditory stimuli in preverbal infants. Sustained HR deceleration is viewed as indicating sustained attention (Courage, Reynolds, & Richards, 2006). In the case of research measuring HPA axis activity, the assumption is that changes in the level of activation of the HPA axis reflect the individual's response to stress (Gunnar & Donzella, 2002). Psychologists measure cortisol change as an index of HPA activity and interpret it as an indirect measure of an individual's stress reactivity.

A psychophysiological approach differs from a neuroscience approach in several ways. First, unlike techniques that image or measure brain activity, measures of autonomic or HPA axis activity are indirect assessments of brain–behavior links. Second, the time course of autonomic or HPA axis activity is generally much slower than the time course of brain activity. Third (this is a generalization), psychophysiologists are often more interested in the psychological processes and contextual factors that alter physiology and less interested in identifying brain circuitry underlying behaviors. The psychophysiological approach has been especially useful for studies of infants and young children because it is difficult to apply brain imaging technologies to them.

Both neuroscience and psychophysiology have been used to study the psychological states involved in attachment. In the past, most attachment research was conducted with infants and young children, and most studies involving physiological measures assessed autonomic and HPA reactivity—and these two areas of research continue to move in important new directions. The development of conceptual and methodological approaches for measuring and understanding adult attachment has provided an opportunity to use brain imaging measures. In this chapter, although we focus especially on psychophysiological measures, we review both approaches to the study of psychological states associated with attachment.

Attachment has long been viewed as a biobehavioral state in which multiple physiological and behavioral systems are organized to provide an individual with a sense of security (i.e., safety within an environment) and intimacy with significant others (Bowlby, 1969/1982). Individual differences in the organization of certain behaviors have been well characterized by attachment classifications based on experiences in attachment relationships (Ainsworth, Blehar, Waters, & Wall, 1978). And there is empirical evidence that individual differences in attachment are associated with differences in the processing of perceptual information (Cohen & Shaver, 2004; Mikulincer & Shaver, 2007). Thus, the study of attachment can be approached from a physiological perspective by examining either (1) individual differences in arousal or hormonal changes as a function of differences in attachment classification or (2) individual differences in cognitive and affective brain circuitry associated with attachment classifications.

## Psychophysiology and Attachment

In this section, we review studies of infant attachment that have included measures of either autonomic activity or activity of the HPA axis; both kinds of studies have increased in number since the previous (2008) edition of this volume. The studies can be grouped into two categories: those examining physiological responses of human infants in Ainsworth's Strange Situation paradigm (Ainsworth & Wittig, 1969), and those in which individual differences in infant physiological responses have been measured outside of the Strange Situation. The latter body of research focuses on individual differences in physiological reactivity that may be related to attachment classification or to infant behavior in the Strange Situation. We do not review the literature on correlations between infant electroencephalographic (EEG) responses and attachment in this chapter, but we encourage readers to refer to the previous *Handbook of Attachment* for a review (Fox & Hane, 2008).

We next review animal and human research demonstrating that the quality of early caregiving environments shapes individual differences in physiological and behavioral responses to stress. We then turn to the physiological effects of caregiver variables and focus specifically on two important areas of growth since the publication of the previous edition of this volume: oxytocin and neuroscience approaches to adult attachment behavior. Throughout these reviews, we hope to inform the reader about both the complexity and the benefits of using psychophysiological and imaging methods to study different aspects of infant attachment behavior, and to highlight the most recent advances that point to a more integrated view of brain, genetic expression, physiology, and behavior that operate in tandem to produce attachment-related behavior.

It is important to raise a number of caveats concerning psychophysiological studies, particularly those measuring autonomic or HPA axis activity. The first caveat concerns the multidetermined nature of the response. Despite its simplicity of measurement, HR, for example, is complexly determined; there are both neural and extraneural influences on it. Extraneural influences include hormonal effects that are the result of sympathetic activity or metabolic effects that may be a function of somatic activity, ranging from digestion to muscle movement. There are also mechanical influences on HR, including changes in respiratory activity that affect HR via the stretch receptors in the lungs (Porges & Byrne, 1992). There are intrinsic influences on HR as well; the heart beats at a particular rate as a function of electrical discharge via pacemaker cells at the sinoatrial node. HR responds to changes in other systems, such as fluctuations in blood pressure. Most neural influence on the heart is via the vagus or 10th cranial nerve (Katona & Jih, 1985). The vagus nerve, which originates in the brainstem, has complex interconnections with neural centers regulating respiration and is linked with both afferent and efferent connections to the midbrain and cortical regions of the brain (Porges, 1995). Thus, HR (and HR change) may be the result of multiple physiological factors, only some of which directly affect or reflect psychological state.

Changes in cortisol level are also multidetermined. Cortisol, secreted by the HPA axis, is the hormone of energy; hence, it is released as a result of many aspects of an organism's interaction with its environment, including responses to novelty, appetitive behavior, sexual stimulation, and injury or illness, as well as psychological stressors (Adam, Klimes-Dougan, & Gunnar, 2007). The secretion of cortisol within the HPA system has its own circadian rhythm, and the adrenocortical system is slow to respond; thus, it may take 25–30 minutes before a change in cortisol levels as a function of environmental challenge can be detected.

The multidetermined nature of psychophysiological responses requires, at the very least, careful methodological consideration. The measurement of HR has sometimes been supplemented with measures of somatic activity, to rule out its influences on HR. Attempts have also been made to extract from the HR signal the portion of variance that can be exclusively related to neural influence (e.g., Porges & Bohrer, 1991). Studies of cortisol response should take into account time of day for sample collection because of changes due to circadian rhythms. These precautions and concerns are critical in allowing inferences about psychophysiological responses to be made.

A second caveat regarding the measurement and interpretation of physiological responses such as autonomic and HPA axis activity is the issue of individual differences in the initial level of response. The *law of initial values* states that the initial baseline level of a physiological system will affect the degree to which that system responds to stimulus presentation. For example, people with high levels of basal cortisol and those with more normative levels may respond differently to a stressor. The notion is that there is a ceiling level above which the system usually does not operate. It is important, therefore, that individual differences in baseline level be incorporated into any analysis of phasic responses. The usual approaches include computing change scores between baseline and phasic responses or using analysis of covariance, with baseline level as the covariate.

The issue of baseline level is complicated when researchers are assessing infants and young children. Because these research participants cannot be instructed to sit quietly for a baseline recording, researchers have attempted to devise methods for recording physiological responses when infants are not responding to a strong stimulus challenge. The key is to record "baseline" in a noninvasive experimental condition that may be replicated across children. It is often necessary to record behavior during such "baseline" physiological assessments, to ensure that all children are in the same state.

Baseline differences may also speak to the underlying physiological mechanisms that affect magnitude of response. Porges, Stamps, and Walter (1974) noted, for example, that some infants do not display HR deceleration in response to a visual stimulus. These infants have relatively high HRs. When studying this issue, Porges and colleagues found that the same high-HR group also displayed low HR variability. When subjects were grouped into those displaying high versus low resting HR variability, those with high resting variability were more likely to show the supposedly normative decelerative pattern. In subsequent work, Porges (1991, 1996; Porges, Doussard-Roosevelt, Portales, & Suess, 1994) argued that initial baseline differences in HR are due to vagal control of the heart, and that differences in the degree of this control predict HR responsivity.

## Autonomic Responding and Attachment

### Autonomic Responding within the Strange Situation

The Strange Situation paradigm (Ainsworth & Wittig, 1969) was designed to assess the quality of an infant's attachment to a primary caregiver. (See Solomon & George, Chapter 18, this volume, for a detailed description of the Strange Situation paradigm.)

There are three insecure classifications: "avoidant," "resistant," and "disorganized." Avoidant infants ignore their caregivers' return after an absence and may actively avoid proximity and contact. Resistant infants display proximity- and contact-seeking behaviors, while at the same time displaying resistance to caregiver attempts to soothe distress. Disorganized infants are likely to display contradictory emotions; to appear confused, apprehensive, and hypervigilant; to make incomplete or undirected movements; and to show depressed affect and possibly behavioral stilling. Unlike the disorganized infants, the secure, avoidant, and resistant infants are viewed as having a coherent strategy for coping with separation, although the secure infants are viewed as having the most adaptive strategy.

In the Strange Situation, infants may locomote wherever they please in an unfamiliar laboratory playroom. Some infants run to the door after their caregiver leaves. Others move close to their caregiver when the unfamiliar adult enters, whereas still others play with toys and explore the room. The high mobility within the confines of the experimental setting once placed limits on researchers' ability to measure ongoing physiological activity. Recent advances in ambulatory electrocardiographic (ECG) technology have led to major advances in acquisition of ECG data during the Strange Situation. In our chapter in the previous edition of this volume (Fox & Hane, 2008), we reviewed the earlier literature on HR changes based solely on Strange Situation classification. Here we present more recent work that examines the role of additional influences, such as dyadic interactive behavior, that provide a more nuanced snapshot of infant HR–behavior associations within the Strange Situation.

Spangler and Grossmann (1993) examined the HR of attachment-classified infants during object manipulation and play with their mothers. They found that the avoidant infants did not display HR acceleration when looking at their mothers, whereas the secure and disorganized infants did. The avoidant infants did, however, display acceleration while looking at objects or during object manipulation, whereas the disorganized and secure infants displayed HR deceleration. Because HR is a nonspecific marker of arousal, interpretation of the similar HR patterns seen in disorganized and securely attached infants is difficult. It is plausible that for disorganized infants, HR acceleration when looking to mother may represent fear arousal (Hesse & Main, 2006), whereas HR acceleration in the securely attached infant when looking to mother may represent normative separation anxiety. Spangler and Grossmann stated that "the heightened heart rate when looking to the mother [of secure infants] indicates that visual contact with mother was initiated specifically during episodes of physiological arousal" (p. 1447). In the absence of a precise linkage between measures of gaze behavior and specification of when these behaviors were coded, however, this seems to be a post hoc explanation. Given the clinical significance of disorganized attachment classifications (see Lyons-Ruth & Jacobvitz, Chapter 29, this volume), future research examining the autonomic responding of disorganized infants within the Strange Situation paradigm is an important direction; such research would elucidate both the nature of the disorganized behavior and its impact on the developing systems that underlie stress reactivity.

Bono and Stifter (1995) examined the relations between measures of HR and HR variability assessed immediately before and after the Strange Situation as a function of infant attachment classification at 18 months of age. The authors reported that infants categorized as resistant displayed faster HR and less variability in *heart period* (HP, the interval between heart beats, which is inversely related to HR) than did secure infants. These differences, however, may be due to the extreme degree of upset displayed by resistant infants and their inability to be soothed during reunion. To the extent that resistant infants display behavioral problems in regulating their affect in the Strange Situation and immediately thereafter, autonomic activity will mimic those patterns of dysregulation.

Another study examined the degree of physiological attunement between mothers and infants in a sample of low-socioeconomic-status young women (age 20 or under, M = 17.8; Zelenko et al., 2005). In this report, mean HR was recorded by Mini-Logger monitors that collected and stored HR signals every 10 seconds from mothers and infants as they underwent the Strange Situation paradigm. Forty-one mother–infant dyads participated, of which 23 were classified as securely attached, six were classified as insecure-avoidant, and 12 as insecure-resistant. No mean attachment group differences in HR were detected from the infants at baseline; nor were there significant differences in HR change across separation and reunion episodes between the attachment groups. All infants showed a pattern of HR acceleration during separations and deceleration upon reunion. Mothers showed no significant differences in baseline HR across the groups. However, the pattern of mean HR change for mothers of resistant infants differed significantly from that of mothers of secure and avoidant infants. For mothers of secure and avoidant infants, HR followed a pattern consistent with that of their infants—acceleration during separation and deceleration upon reunion. However, mothers of resistant infants showed HR acceleration during reunion episodes. For securely attached infants, maternal HR slowed after the successful calming of the infant, whereas the HR of mothers of resistant infants remained elevated. This inability of mothers of resistant infants to recover from the stress of separation may be a function of maternal dysregulation that contributed to the insecure attachment of the infant, a by-product of the stress associated with soothing a distress-prone infant, or a combination of these states. Although not statistically significant, the descriptive findings obtained from calculating dyadic consistency (a crude index of physiological attunement) in HR revealed that mothers and their resistant infants scored lower in dyadic consistency than securely attached dyads—an effect necessarily driven by the discrepant profile of the mothers of resistant infants, given the lack of significant HR differences among the infants across attachment groups.

Zelenko and her colleagues (2005) also assessed frequency and intensity of infant crying during the Strange Situation, and noted that resistant infants cried more than the other two attachment groups. Hence, resistant infants showed a discordance between behavioral distress and physiological arousal, which is reminiscent of

the discordance between physiological and behavioral distress of the avoidant infants studied by Spangler and Grossmann (1993), but is discrepant from Bono and Stifter's (1995) findings of increased physiological arousal in resistant infants. It is important to note that Zelenko and colleagues' sample consisted of young, poor mothers and their infants, who were probably at increased risk for poor developmental outcomes. It is unclear whether similar effects would be obtained from a more normative sample. As well, Bono and Stifter measured cardiac functioning before and after but not during the Strange Situation, whereas Zelenko and colleagues' effects were driven by changes in cardiac functioning during the procedure.

Stevenson-Hinde and Marshall (1999) examined the role of attachment security in the relation between behavioral inhibition and cardiac reactivity. Using an extreme groups approach, they selected 126 children (age 4½ years), based on level of behavioral inhibition (high, medium, or low). Behavioral inhibition was assessed via maternal report and behavioral observation in the laboratory, and children underwent the Strange Situation procedure to have their attachment security assessed while cardiac data were recorded from both the mother and the infant via telemetry. HP and HR variability (respiratory sinus arrhythmia [RSA]) was noted during four specific periods in the Strange Situation paradigm: after Episode 3 with the stranger reading a story; at the start of Episode 7, with the examiner playing a recorded story; following a structured self-esteem interview (Harter & Pike, 1984), while another excerpt from the story was played from an audiocassette; and at the end of Episode 9, as mother and child sat quietly alone. Of the children with usable cardiac data, 38 were classified as securely attached, six were classified as insecure-avoidant, and eight as insecure-resistant. No significant inhibition group or attachment group differences were found in child mean HP or RSA (aggregated across all four assessment points). A significant interaction effect indicated that children low in behavioral inhibition who were securely attached had significantly higher mean HP than did securely attached children who were high in behavioral inhibition and insecurely attached children who were low in inhibition. A similar effect was found for RSA (itself highly correlated with mean HP in this sample, $r = .80$), with low-inhibition, securely attached children showing the highest degree of RSA, although the interaction effect was not significant. Securely attached children who were not highly inhibited showed significant increase in HP upon reunion with their mothers. Highly inhibited children, regardless of attachment status, showed no such increase, indicating that attachment security and the absence of behavioral inhibition are requisite for a significant increase in HP upon reunion. Hence, this study provides additional support for the notion that insecurely attached children and inhibited children manifest disorganization in psychophysiological responses to the challenges of the Strange Situation. Notably, this study also provides evidence for the benefit of considering temperament, attachment, and physiological reactivity in concert because there was no relation between attachment status and cardiac reactivity when inhibition was not considered.

## Individual Differences in Autonomic Responding Outside of the Strange Situation Paradigm

Porges and colleagues (1994) conceptualized vagal tone as reflecting the degree to which infants will be reactive and able to self-regulate. Infants with high basal vagal tone are thought to display more mature autonomic regulation and thus may exhibit both greater reactivity and superior self-regulatory strategies. Izard and colleagues (1991) examined the relation between vagal tone measured at 3, 4½, 6, and 9 months of age and attachment status at 13 months of age in 54 infants. Forty infants were classified as securely attached, eight were classified as avoidant, and six as resistant. Measures of vagal tone, HR, and HR variance were collected at each age assessed during the first year of life. A continuous measure of security was used as the dependent measure, and vagal tone scores were computed for each of the different assessment points.

Izard and colleagues (1991) reported that measures of vagal tone measured during early infancy significantly predicted attachment insecurity at 13 months. Specifically, infants with high vagal tone at 3 months and high HR variance at 4½ months were more likely to be classified as insecure at 13 months, although there were no differences between avoidant and resistant infants. Izard and colleagues' findings seem contrary to Porges's (1991) prediction regarding the role of vagal tone in emotion regulation. Porges argues that high basal vagal tone should reflect more mature autonomic regulation and greater regulatory capacity. It is unclear why these autonomic measures at this young age differed in the direction

that they did; nor is it clear why there was a lack of differentiation at each of the other ages assessed.

Fox and colleagues conducted a series of studies aimed at examining relations among individual differences in emotion expression and emotion regulation, and measures of autonomic activity (Fox, 1989; Fox & Gelles, 1984; Stifter & Fox, 1990). Fox and Gelles (1984) found that 3-month-old infants who displayed high HR variability and low HR were more likely to express positive emotions in response to maternal bids than were infants with high HR and low HR variability. *HR variability* was defined in this study as the mean of the successive differences in HR over the recording epoch. HR variability (particularly of the mean successive differences) is highly correlated with measures of RSA, such as vagal tone. The authors reasoned that high HR variability, like vagal tone, should reflect an infant's ability to mount an organized behavioral response. This was confirmed, as they found that infants with high HR variability displayed more positive interactive behavior. In subsequent studies, Fox (1985) found that infants with high vagal tone were more reactive as young infants and also more likely to display positive social behaviors as toddlers. In contrast to Izard and colleagues' (1991) findings, but consistent with Porges's (1991) prediction, these data suggest that high vagal tone is associated with more organized social responsivity. Porges has argued that the level of vagal tone reflects the degree to which the organism will exhibit an organized response to stimulus challenge. The manner of autonomic response is reflected in organized overt behavior. Thus, infants with high vagal tone should display less dysregulated and more organized behavioral responses to novelty and challenge; infants with low vagal tone should display less organized behavioral responses to stimulation.

Fox (1985) related individual differences in HR variability to attachment status within a high-risk (premature) sample of infants. Of the 60 infants in the sample, 43 were classified at 12 months of age as secure, 16 were classified as avoidant, and only one was classified as resistant. Although there were no differences between attachment classification groups (avoidant vs. secure) on any of the autonomic measures, individual differences in behavior in the Strange Situation were related to 3-month HR variability. Specifically, infants who cried during the Strange Situation at 12 months had higher HR variability at 3 months. In addition, infants with high HR variability at 3 months displayed greater regulation at reunion during the

Strange Situation; that is, they resumed playing in a shorter period of time. Fox argued that high HR variability, like vagal tone, reflects better physiological organization, such that children with high variability are not only more reactive but also better able to self-regulate than infants with low variability.

Other evidence suggests that attachment security predicts cardiac reactivity in early childhood (Burgess, Marshall, Rubin, & Fox, 2003). In their study of 172 families, Burgess and colleagues (2003) examined relations between attachment classification at 14 months, behavioral inhibition at 24 months, social behavior at 4 years, and cardiac functioning (HP and RSA) at 14 and 24 months and at 4 years. Cardiac assessments at each age were made during the 3 minutes in which the child quietly attended to a video monitor. No significant group differences were yielded for attachment group on HP or RSA at 14 or 24 months. Also, no significant group differences as a function of inhibition (low, medium, and high) on HP or RSA at 14 or 24 months were found. However, attachment security (and not behavioral inhibition) predicted HP and RSA at 4 years. Specifically, avoidant infants showed significantly higher HP and RSA than did secure and resistant infants.

The association between 14-month attachment status and cardiac reactivity some 3 years thereafter is an impressive demonstration of the potential evocative effects of attachment security on physiological arousal. The predictive association between 14-month attachment and 4-year cardiac reactivity, and the lack of association with contemporaneous (or more proximal) assessment of cardiac reactivity and attachment security, suggest that the avoidant pattern of attachment acquired in infancy may have influenced the development of physiological reactivity. That is, infants who employed a coping strategy characterized by avoidance, or seeming indifference to maternal separation and reunion, may have acquired a generalized pattern of underarousal that continued to develop across late infancy and was not salient until early childhood. In the same study, Burgess and colleagues (2003) found that children who were classified as avoidant in infancy and who were low in inhibition at 24 months scored significantly higher than all other attachment–inhibition groups on externalizing behavior problems on the Child Behavior Checklist (CBCL; Achenbach & Edelbrock, 1991), an effect that was largely carried by high scores on the Aggression subscale of the CBCL.

Raine (1996) proposed a model of physiological underarousal in the development of antisocial behavior, which has been empirically supported (e.g., Raine, Venables, & Williams, 1990). Although three-way interactions involving attachment security, behavioral inhibition, and cardiac reactivity as determinants of childhood behavior problems were not examined in the Burgess and colleagues (2003) report, it seems plausible that avoidant infants who are also uninhibited and who acquire a cardiac profile characterized by underarousal may be at considerable risk for the development of antisocial behavior in early childhood and beyond, which is a worthy topic for future research.

Recent research has examined the physiological correlates of attachment disorganization. Tharner and colleagues (2013) proposed a dual-risk model when examining the physiological responding of disorganized infants in the Strange Situation. In their large sample of 450 mother–infant dyads enrolled in the Generation R Study, they found a significant interaction between maternal postpartum depressive symptoms and attachment disorganization on infant baseline RSA. Specifically, 14-month-olds who were classified as disorganized and whose mothers were depressed showed lower resting RSA, while the same was not true for infants who had only one such risk factor (depressed mother or disorganized attachment). In another study, physiological dysregulation was predictive of later attachment disorganization. In a study of 206 mother–infant dyads drawn from the Durham Child Health Development Study, Holowchwost, Gariépy, Propper, Mills-Koonce, and Moore (2014) examined infant physiological responding during the still-face paradigm (SFP) at infant age 6 months, quality of mother–child interaction during 10 minutes of free-play at 6 months, and attachment security at 12 months. They found that infant physiological responding and maternal interactive style at 6 months jointly predicted attachment disorganization at 12 months. Infants who showed higher levels of RSA during the interactive periods of the SFP and also had mothers who showed more negative and intrusive interactions, showed higher levels of subsequent attachment disorganization in the Strange Situation (Holochwost et al., 2014). Hence, high levels of RSA during interactions that are negative and intrusive may represent a maladaptive behavioral profile that foretells behavioral disorganization under stress. Taken together, this recent evidence supports a dual-risk model for disorganized attachment, whereby contextual/parenting behaviors *and* a maladaptive physiological profile, with lower resting RSA and higher reactive RSA (during stressful interactions marked by negative parenting behavior) being associated with the pattern of fear and comfort seeking seen in disorganized attachment. Future research is warranted to examine this profile.

Holochwost and colleagues (2014) failed to control for baseline RSA in assessing SFP responding, and in light of the lower basal level of RSA found by Tharner and colleagues (2013), it would be premature to draw inferences about the exact nature of the physiological profile that acts in concert with parenting factors to yield disorganized attachment. An important future direction is to examine infant vagal suppression and augmentation (in light of basal levels) under conditions of both social interaction and relationship disruption.

## Cortisol and Attachment

### Cortisol Responding in the Context of the Strange Situation

A number of researchers have measured the cortisol levels of infants assessed in the Strange Situation. The cortisol response takes place over a much longer time course than do other physiological systems. Thus, measuring cortisol in saliva or plasma 15–30 minutes after completion of the Strange Situation may accurately capture an infant's HPA response during the testing procedure. Gunnar, Mangelsdorf, Larson, and Hertsgaard (1989) observed 66 infants in the Strange Situation at 13 months of age. Saliva was obtained from them, first at home prior to coming to the laboratory, then immediately before and immediately after the Strange Situation procedure. Of the 66 infants, 37 were classified as secure, 10 as avoidant, 16 as resistant, and three were classified as disorganized. There were no differences among attachment groups in either cortisol level or the degree of cortisol change. In a follow-up, Gunnar, Colton, and Stansbury (1992) examined differences in salivary cortisol between 47 securely attached infants and 24 insecurely attached infants. Again, saliva was collected immediately prior to and immediately after the Strange Situation paradigm. No differences in salivary cortisol reactivity were found among infants classified as avoidant, resistant, and secure.

Spangler and Grossmann (1993), on the other hand, reported finding differences in salivary

cortisol reactivity between their infant attachment groups. In their study of 41 infants, saliva was collected immediately prior to the Strange Situation paradigm, then 15 and 30 minutes afterward. They found significant cortisol increases in infants categorized as disorganized compared to secure infants 15 minutes after the Strange Situation, as well as significant secure–insecure differences 30 minutes after it. Spangler and Grossmann argued that these data support a cortisol–coping hypothesis, with secure infants being better able than insecure infants to cope with the stress of separation in the Strange Situation. They also commented on the differences between their findings and those of the two studies conducted by Gunnar's group (Gunnar et al., 1989, 1992). They noted that these differences could have resulted from variation in the length of time after the session before saliva was collected. In the studies by Gunnar and colleagues (1989, 1992), saliva was collected 5–10 minutes after the session; in the Spangler and Grossmann study, it was collected at 15 minutes, then again at 30 minutes after the Strange Situation paradigm. Given the slow response time of cortisol, the Gunnar and colleagues data may not have reflected the full effect of the Strange Situation on the insecure infants.

In a subsequent study, Hertsgaard, Gunnar, Erickson, and Nachmias (1995) examined 38 infants from a high-risk population. Unlike other studies, this one did not control for time of day at which saliva was obtained; nor was there any pretest cortisol measurement. Of the 34 subjects with usable data, 17 were classified as secure, five were classified as avoidant, one as resistant, and 11 as disorganized. Results of the analyses revealed that the infants with disorganized classifications had more elevated cortisol levels than all of the other infants combined. Further inspection of the data revealed that the main difference in level was between the avoidant and disorganized infants. That is, avoidant infants displayed the lowest cortisol values, and disorganized infants displayed the highest. The authors argued that these data support the notion that infants categorized as disorganized may have greater vulnerability to stressful situations. It is, of course, also interesting that the infants classified as avoidant did not show elevated cortisol levels. If, in fact, avoidant infants are physiologically stressed during the Strange Situation, one would expect their cortisol levels to be higher than those of secure infants. It is also important to note that the initial level of cortisol was not assessed; therefore, it is unclear whether the cortisol levels represent different responses to the Strange Situation or initial differences between groups in levels of cortisol.

In a subsequent study, Nachmias, Gunnar, Mangelsdorf, Parritz, and Buss (1996) examined 73 children at 18 months of age in the Strange Situation. There were 13 children classified as avoidant, 12 classified as resistant, and 48 classified as secure. Salivary samples were collected immediately prior to the Strange Situation paradigm and 45 minutes after the onset of the testing session. The children had also been observed on a previous occasion responding to several novel events presented as part of assessing behavioral inhibition. *Behavioral inhibition* was defined as the tendency to restrain or restrict one's approach to new people, places, events, and/or objects (Kagan & Snidman, 1991). Although the authors did not find a relation between inhibition and security of attachment, they did find that children with higher behavioral inhibition had higher post-session cortisol levels if they were also insecure. Secure inhibited children did not exhibit significant cortisol reactivity; nor, for that matter, did insecure infants who were low in inhibition. Thus, the degree of cortisol reactivity in response to the Strange Situation in insecure children was heightened among those with higher behavioral inhibition. These results nicely illustrate Gunnar's stress model, in which the security of attachment is viewed as a buffer against stress; in this model, infants who are securely attached should exhibit a reduced stress response. In fact, inhibited infants who were securely attached did show lower cortisol responses.

Bernard and Dozier (2010) examined change in infant cortisol in response to the stress of the Strange Situation. In order to control carefully for baseline measures in assessing change in response specifically to the Strange Situation, the order of a laboratory play task and the Strange Situation was counterbalanced and home saliva samples were collected. The range of ages in the low-risk sample of 32 mother–infant dyads ranged from 11 to 20 months ($M = 15.2$, standard deviation = 2.3). Change in cortisol before and after the free-play and Strange Situation procedures (40, 65, and 80 minutes postarrival to the laboratory) were examined in relation to attachment disorganization. Infants classified as disorganized ($n = 8$) showed a significant increase in salivary cortisol only in the Strange Situation, with no such association found for the free-play condition. As well, no such pattern was found for infants with an organized classification (A, B, or C). Though the sample is small, the findings support the hypothesis that disorganization is associated with more acute stress in response to the Strange Situation. As well, the authors found that cortisol concentrations acquired at home prior to the laboratory visit did not significantly differ from those acquired in the laboratory before the Strange Situation paradigm began. And the comparison of cortisol change in the free play versus the Strange Situation is additionally important, revealing that for disorganized infants, cortisol reactivity to the Strange Situation is specific to the challenge of the paradigm itself.

Consistent with recent trends toward examining cumulative risk factors for physiological dysregulation and attachment, Luijk and colleagues (2010) examined maternal depression (lifetime history of depression, as reported during pregnancy) and infant cortisol responding to the Strange Situation paradigm in a sample of 369 mother–infant dyads drawn from the Generation R Study. Saliva was collected from 14-month-olds at baseline, directly after, and 15-minutes after the Strange Situation paradigm. The distribution of attachment classifications was 413 secure, 136 avoidant, and 166 resistant infants. Across the sample, 162 were classified as disorganized. Infants classified as resistant showed a significant increase in cortisol (over basal levels) relative to secure and avoidant infants, a finding that remained robust when researchers controlled for maternal depression. However, this effect was qualified by an interaction with maternal depression, with resistant children whose mothers reported higher levels of lifetime depression showing the steepest increase in cortisol reactivity. This pattern of cortisol reactivity is consistent with the behaviorally reactive profile of resistant infants, who are unable to use their caregiver as a source of comfort. Furthermore, resistant infants were more likely to show increased stress reactivity if their caregiver reported a previous diagnosis of depression.

Additional evidence in support of the dual-risk model for infant physiological regulation examined the timing of maternal depressive symptoms and infant HPA reactivity in the Strange Situation. Applying a novel approach, Laurent, Ablow, and Measelle (2011) examined infant cortisol responding in the Strange Situation. In an at-risk sample of 86 mothers, symptoms of depression were assessed via questionnaire in the third trimester of pregnancy, 5 months postnatal, and 18 months postnatal. At infant age 18 months, infant saliva samples were collected at baseline, immediately after and 15 minutes after the Strange

Situation. The data were not coded for attachment classification; however, the use of growth curve modeling to document change in cortisol in infants elucidates the nature of infant responding during the Strange Situation. Across the sample, infant cortisol data fit a curvilinear model, with levels increasing from baseline to immediately after the Strange Situation and decreasing 15 minutes later. Higher levels of maternal prenatal depression were associated with a hyporesponsive (blunted) cortisol response in infants, whereas higher depressive symptoms in both postnatal assessments of maternal depression were associated with a hyperresponsive (increased stress) cortisol response in infants. Furthermore, an increase in maternal depressive symptoms from low prenatal levels to higher postnatal levels was associated with hypercorticolism in infants, with a steeper cortisol peak immediately after the Strange Situation and lack of recovery 15 minutes after the Strange Situation. This study expands the study of the biology of attachment by providing evidence that "fetal programming" may impact the physiology underlying relationship functioning. Emergent literature on the effects of fetal programming due to maternal psychopathology (Grant et al., 2009) and teratogenic exposures (Haley, Handmaker, & Lowe, 2006) on infant cortisol responding in the SFP provide additional support for the importance of extending the examination of dual-risk models into the prenatal period. Research that integrates measures of fetal risk, infant physiology, and attachment security will be an important future direction.

## Individual Differences in Cortisol Responding Outside of the Strange Situation

Longitudinal evidence indicates that attachment security foretells subsequent physiological regulation as assessed via salivary cortisol. In a comprehensive examination of biobehavioral organization, attachment security, and behavioral inhibition, Schieche and Spangler (2005) assessed 76 toddlers in the Strange Situation at 12 months; inhibited temperament at 22 months via maternal report; maternal and child behavior during a challenge task (i.e., a series of structured tasks of progressive difficulty, which culminated in the necessary involvement of the mother for successful completion) at 22 months; and salivary cortisol in infants before and 15 and 30 minutes after the challenge paradigm at 22 months. Nineteen infants were classified as insecure-avoidant, 23 as secure, 11 as insecure-resistant, and 23 as disorganized.

Contemporaneous associations between behavior during the challenge task and cortisol showed that elevated cortisol was associated with low task orientation and low exploration in the infants, which in turn were associated with low supportive maternal presence and reduced quality of maternal assistance during the challenge task (although no significant relations between cortisol and maternal behavior during the task were revealed). Across the sample, infants showed a decline in cortisol during the challenge task, and this was particularly evident for infants who were reported by their mothers as low on behavioral inhibition. However, differential levels of cortisol were revealed for highly inhibited children depending on attachment status, with securely attached inhibited infants showing the expected decrease in cortisol from task onset to 30 minutes after the task. Avoidant infants, in contrast, showed a decrease from task onset to 15 minutes after the task, but a modest (nonsignificant) increase in cortisol 30 minutes after the task, suggesting a delayed activation of the HPA axis. This finding was complemented by behavioral findings indicating that avoidant infants manifested less effective coping and an inability to use their mothers as a source of support during the challenge task. Within-group analyses revealed that elevated cortisol was associated with low task orientation and exploration, low help-seeking behavior, and high proximity seeking for the insecure group (A, C, and D combined). No significant correlations involving cortisol within the secure group were obtained.

Recent evidence points to the importance of individual differences in infant diurnal rhythms in cortisol and attachment security. In the large sample previously described, Luijk and colleagues (2010) examined the diurnal rhythms of cortisol prior to the lab visit in which the Strange Situation paradigm was administered. The typical diurnal rhythm of cortisol is one in which cortisol is high shortly after awakening and then declines steadily across the day, though the age at which this pattern is manifest is of some dispute (e.g., see de Weerth & van Geert, 2002; Gunnar & Donzella, 2002). Chronic stress exposure, including painful procedures in the neonatal intensive care unit (Grunau et al., 2005); child maltreatment (Doom, Cicchetti, & Rogosch, 2014); and child poverty (Zalewski, Lengua, Kiff, & Fisher, 2012) are associated with blunted, or less variable, diurnal rhythms in cortisol. Luijk and colleagues collected saliva samples from infants immediately upon awakening, and again 30 minutes later, midafternoon, late afternoon, and at bedtime. Across their large sample, 14-month-olds showed the predicted pattern of high levels at waking and a decline throughout the day. However, this healthy pattern of cortisol secretion was significantly different for infants who showed disorganized behavior in the Strange Situation; they showed a flattened slope, particularly between waking and the next collection, 30 minutes later. This finding provides physiological evidence that is consistent with the body of research linking contextual risk/chronic early-life stress to attachment disorganization.

Taken together, the research findings suggest that the association between early attachment, stress reactivity, and social behavior later in infancy is dependent on an infant's temperamental disposition and chronic stress exposure; and that for an insecurely attached or disorganized infant, physiological reactivity is associated with a corresponding behavioral profile characterized by an inability to use the mother effectively as a source of support in the face of environmental challenge.

## Quality of Caregiving and Infant Physiological Arousal

Quality of maternal caregiving, particularly caregiving that is sensitive (i.e., involving prompt, contingent, and appropriate responsiveness to infant cues and signals; Ainsworth et al., 1978), is the key theoretical antecedent to infant attachment security. An exciting body of research involving both animals and humans is revealing that natural (in the case of animals) or ordinary (for humans) variations in the quality of maternal caregiving shape both neurological systems and the expression of genes that regulate stress reactions.

Meaney and his colleagues (Caldji et al., 1998; Francis, Diorio, Liu, & Meaney, 1999; Liu & Diorio, 1997) have shown that naturally occurring variations in quality of maternal caregiving behavior (MCB) among rat dams shapes the development of the neural substrates that underlie the phenotypic behavioral and endocrine responses to stress in offspring. These researchers noted that the MCB of rat dams in the postnatal period—specifically, in terms of nursing posture (arched-backed vs. lying down) and frequency of licking

and grooming behavior—is normally distributed. They created extreme groups of pups based on the quality of MCB received (low vs. high levels of licking/grooming and arched-backed nursing) and followed these offspring into adulthood. Compared with adult offspring that received high degrees of maternal licking/grooming and arched-backed nursing in the postnatal period, the adult offspring of dams that provided low degrees of maternal licking/grooming and arched-backed nursing showed a behavioral response reflective of heightened levels of stress reactivity, including higher frequencies of startle responses, less open-field exploration, and longer latencies to eat food presented in a novel environment (Caldji et al., 1998; Francis et al., 1999). These differences in behavior were accompanied by a corresponding neuroendocrine profile characteristic of heightened fearfulness (Caldji et al., 1998), such as increased plasma adrenocorticotropic hormone and corticosterone responses to restraint stress, and decreased sensitivity to the inhibitory effects of glucocorticoids during acute stress (Liu & Diorio, 1997). The behavioral differences were also associated with decreased central benzodiazepine receptor density in the central, lateral, and basolateral nuclei of the amygdala and locus ceruleus (Caldji et al., 1998).

In a study based on retrospective self-report, Pruessner, Champagne, Meaney, and Dagher (2004) found that human adults who reported extremely low-quality relationships with their parents evidenced significantly more release of dopamine in the ventral striatum and a higher increase in salivary cortisol during a stressful event than individuals who reported extremely high-quality parental relations. Such an effect suggests that early human caregiving may similarly affect the development of the systems that underlie stress reactivity.

In an effort to extend this provocative set of findings to human infants, we (Hane & Fox, 2006) examined the relation between quality of MCB and behavioral and physiological indices of stress reactivity in 9-month-old infants. The quality of MCB during routine activities in the home (e.g., feeding and changing) was assessed with Ainsworth's (1976) original global scales for rating degree of maternal sensitivity, which included ratings for acceptance, availability, appropriateness of interaction, and delight in the infant, as well as an intrusiveness scale developed by Park, Belsky, Putnam, and Crnic (1997).

We then compared the infants who received low-quality MCB to those who experienced high-quality MCB on indices of stress reactivity, also assessed at age 9 months, and found that infants who experienced low-quality MCB displayed significantly more fearfulness during the presentation of novel stimuli and less sociability with an experimenter. In addition, the infants receiving low-quality MCB showed a pattern of right frontal EEG asymmetry. These infants were not found to differ in terms of earlier temperament from the infants who received high-quality MCB, based on degree of positive and negative reactivity to novelty assessed at age 4 months. However, infants who received low-quality MCB were more likely to express higher levels of negative affect during interactions with their mothers at age 9 months than infants in the high-quality MCB group, which may reflect the influence of infant negative disposition on MCB and/or infant negativity in response to low MCB.

In a longitudinal follow-up to Hane and Fox (2006), we examined whether the effects of the quality of MCB in infancy persist across time and influence social behavior in early childhood (Hane, Henderson, Reeb-Sutherland, & Fox, 2010). We found that, relative to children who experienced high-quality MCB as infants (high MCB children), those who received low-quality MCB (low MCB children) showed increased stress reactivity on measures that parallel those used in our earlier report, including inhibited social behavior with adults and right frontal EEG asymmetry. Low MCB children also manifested more aggression during play with a novel, same-sex peer, and mothers reported that low MCB children tended to show more internalizing problems and more proneness to anger in social situations than high MCB children. As in the 2006 study by Hane and Fox, these effects were not influenced by earlier negative reactivity to novelty.

Parent and colleagues (2005) and Zhang, Parent, Weaver, and Meaney (2004) theorized that low-quality maternal care may forecast the future and thereby prepare offspring for the ecology that is to come. The highly malleable neurobiology of young offspring is accordingly programmed by suboptimal early care, and adapts more readily by mounting defensive responses to stress across the lifespan (Parent et al., 2005; Zhang et al., 2004). One central tenet of this hypothesis is that the experience of low-quality early maternal care yields defensive/stress responding in the early rearing environment. To examine if this model may apply to human infants, Hane and Philbrook (2012) examined the direct experience of low-quality MCB on infant cortisol responding. Mothers and infants were observed in the home, and mothers' quality of maternal care during tub bathing was coded for maternal sensitivity. Salivary cortisol was measured in infants prior to tub bathing and again 15 minutes following removal of the neonate from the bath water. Consistent with earlier MCB work and the animal models, infants of mothers who provided lower quality MCB showed a larger increase in cortisol following the experience of routine care. Hence, the experience of being in a routine, ordinary, regularly occurring care task with an insensitive caregiver is associated with elevated physiological stress responding. Such findings lend support for the notion that the experience of insensitive maternal care in humans results in defensive/stress responding. Consistent with epigenetic models of early maternal care, such elevated stress responding to normative early caregiving routines for infants of insensitive mothers may program the neonate to respond with elevated stress in the future (Hane & Philbrook, 2012).

Exposure to early and pronounced stressors that cause dysregulation of the HPA axis predispose individuals to further problems in dealing with environmental stressors, and persistent difficulty in coping with stress exacerbates risk for behavioral and health problems (Meaney, 2001). The molecular mechanism for these effects is epigenetic in nature, with maternal care leading to alterations of hippocampal glucocorticoid receptor genes (Champagne, 2013). The neuroendocrine changes associated with dysregulation of the HPA axis alter the organism's energy availability and cardiovascular health, which over time may predispose individuals to steroid-induced diabetes, hypertension, and other risk factors for heart disease (Brindley & Rolland, 1989).

Bowlby, Ainsworth, and others have contended that the importance of the quality of the mother–infant relationship is far-reaching. A body of research has documented the association between attachment security and general health outcomes (see Ehrlich, Miller, Jones, & Cassidy, Chapter 9, this volume, for discussion of attachment and psychoneuroimmunology). New evidence indicates a potential link between maternal insensitivity and poorer health. Wendland and colleagues (2014) found that low levels of maternal sensitivity in infancy (age 6 months) predicted higher body mass index in girls at age 4. Prospective longitudinal studies examining the association between maternal sensitivity and health outcomes across the lifespan are critical for identifying the long-term influence of early maternal care in humans.

## The Role of Oxytocin in the Formation of Affiliative Bonds

In our chapter in the previous edition of this handbook (Fox & Hane, 2008), we reviewed the literature on physiology and adult attachment patterns. For this current chapter, we highlight advancements in research on the neuroscience of parenting and the formation of affiliative bonds, focusing on the hormone oxytocin. Using definitions that vary from those of Bowlby and Ainsworth, Feldman (2012a, p. 154) has defined affiliative bonds as "selective and enduring attachments" that are formed by the coordination of physiological and behavioral systems between partners. According to Feldman (2012b), the coordination of the biobehavioral systems underlying affiliative bonding serves as the foundation for healthy functioning in relationships. Oxytocin (OT) is a neuropeptide (neuronal signaling molecules that influence cortical activity), with the major site of genetic expression/synthesis in the magnocellular neurons of the hypothalamus, including paraventricular and supraoptic nuclei. In response to environmental cues such as infant breast feeding, childbirth, and environmental stress, processed OT is released from the posterior pituitary into circulation. OT is closely related to neuroendocrine stress responding (Gimpl & Fahrenholz, 2001). In humans, it can be measured peripherally in blood, saliva, and urine samples. The central actions of OT are numerous, including modulation of neuroendocrine responding, complex social bonds, and factors related to reproduction in both men and women. OT is of particular interest to attachment researchers because it is centrally involved in affiliative behaviors, including sexual activity (Behnia et al., 2014), social cooperation (Feng et al., in press), forgiveness (Yao et al., 2014), and empathy (Bartz et al., 2010). Although the precise mechanisms underlying the function of OT remain underspecified, there is evidence that its role in affiliative behavior may be mediated by reduction in neuroendocrine stress responding, though the anxiolytic and antistress efficacy of OT depends on the nature of the individual's stress response profile, for example, early life stress exposure (Grimm et al., 2014), and adult attachment history and social context (Olff et al., 2013). OT has been found to increase social sensitivity under conditions of social stress (Eckstein et al., 2014); and other research indicates that OT administration allows for more flexibility in shifting attention in the face of threat (Ellenbogen, Linnen, Grumet, Cardoso, & Joober, 2012). There is still much to learn about

the neurological underpinnings and downstream effects of OT, stress, and social behavior.

The role of OT in early parental caregiving and attachment-related behaviors is equally underspecified and complex. In animal models, administration of OT induces parental care, including higher levels of licking and grooming behavior and also aggression in rats (e.g., see Bosch & Neumann, 2012). Recent attention has also shifted to fetal programming and the role of postnatal OT exposure as a buffer against deleterious outcomes associated with prenatal stress exposure and exposure to teratogens. For example, administration of OT to offspring of prenatally stressed dams reverses social incompetence, suggesting that OT may serve a protective function for offspring exposed to high levels of antenatal stress (Lee, Brady, Shapiro, Dorsa, & Koenig, 2007). This rapidly growing animal OT literature cuts across a variety of species, examines a host of outcomes, and indicates that the effects of OT are dependent on timing of exposure and individual differences, such as sex and contextual risk.

The human attachment OT literature is also growing rapidly and reveals similar complexities. Most importantly, although this field is in its infancy, the study of OT in attachment-related behaviors has moved swiftly into integrating multiple physiological systems and behavior. One such example is Feldman's (2012a) biobehavioral synchrony model, which highlights the multiple physiological and behavioral influences that operate in tandem, or synchronously, between the parent and child to influence relationship functioning and stress responding. This approach is holistic, but much like the aforementioned animal and social neuroscience work, poses challenges for interpretation.

Consistent with animal models, plasma OT levels in both human mothers and fathers is associated with affectionate parenting behavior. In a longitudinal study of 160 parents and their firstborn infants, patterns of parent–child interaction were observed, and plasma OT samples were collected in the home in the early neonatal period and again at infant age 6 months (Gordon, Zagoory-Sharon, Leckman, & Feldman, 2010). Plasma levels of OT for mothers and fathers increased across time, and maternal and paternal levels did not differ significantly from each other. Higher levels of maternal OT were associated with more affectionate touch, infant-directed speech, and positive facial affect. Higher levels of paternal OT were associated with an increase in playful stimulatory behavior, including touch and play with objects.

Additional evidence points to an increase in OT following mutually rewarding parent–child exchanges. Feldman, Gordon, Schneiderman, Weisman, and Zagoory-Sharon (2010) measured maternal and paternal plasma and salivary cortisol at baseline and again 15 minutes after a parent–infant play session in the laboratory when infants were 4–6 months of age. Salivary and plasma OT levels were highly interrelated for both mothers and fathers, and maternal and paternal OT were remarkably similar in their levels at both collection points. A significant increase pre- to postplay in OT was revealed only for mothers who showed high levels of affectionate interactions with their infants. For fathers, OT increased only for those who showed a high level of playful stimulation with their infants. Taken together, both studies support the role of OT in underlying caregiving-related behaviors, though this research is limited by the correlational nature of the design.

One major advantage to the use of OT is the methodology allowing for safe administration via nasal spray. This approach to administering doses of OT allows for the development of well-controlled experimental designs to examine the effect of OT on parenting behaviors. Weisman, Zagoory-Sharon, and Feldman (2012) examined whether intranasal OT administration in fathers influenced physiological and behavioral indicators of positive social engagement. In a sample of 35 fathers and 5-month-old infants, fathers were randomized to OT or placebo conditions, and saliva was collected from fathers and infants at baseline (before OT administration), and at 20 and 40 minutes following a father–child interaction, during which ECG data were acquired. Relative to fathers in the placebo condition, fathers who received OT showed increased vagal tone during interaction with their infant and promoted positive social engagement with the infant, including gaze and social reciprocity. Infants of fathers in the OT condition showed parallel increases in OT, vagal tone, and social reciprocity, despite not having any direct exposure to OT manipulation themselves.

In another study of fathers and infants, Feldman's group examined the similar patterns of physiological synchrony in father–infant interactions in terms of cortisol responding during a stress-inducing paradigm (the SFP). Fathers were randomly assigned to an OT or placebo condition, and observed with their 5-month-olds in the SFP twice, in sessions that were 1 week apart. Saliva was collected during each SFP laboratory visit, similar to that in Weisman and colleagues (2012).

Relative to fathers in the placebo group, fathers exposed to OT showed an increase in cortisol responding during the SFP, which is consistent with research showing that OT increases social sensitivity (Eckstein et al., 2014). The effects of OT exposure on infant biobehavioral responses to the SFP depended on the quality of the interaction within the dyad, such that for infants who experienced high social synchrony with fathers, paternal OT exposure was associated with elevated cortisol and increased gazing at the father during the still-face portion of the SFP. For infants embedded in a dyad characterized by asynchronous exchanges, paternal OT was associated with attenuated infant cortisol response to the SFP and less gazing in response to the "still-faced" father. This is consistent with other OT research showing that the effects of OT on stress responding and relationship functioning depend on individual-difference variables (Grimm et al., 2014), and, importantly, extends this work to individual differences in attachment-related behavior.

## Neuroscience Studies of Parenting

The field of neuroimaging has exploded since publication of the previous edition of this handbook. This includes the new field of *parental neuroscience*, or research examining maternal neural responses to infant cues and attachment-related behaviors. A body of imaging research has examined patterns of neural activation in response to familiar versus unfamiliar faces, and in some instances has examined differences in women's responses to faces of their own children versus faces of unfamiliar children. For example, Nitschke and colleagues (2004) showed women photographs of their own infants, unfamiliar infants, and unfamiliar adults. Women also rated their hedonic responses to each of the photographs. Results revealed strong bilateral activation of orbitofrontal cortex when women viewed pictures of their own infants, compared to either unfamiliar infants or unfamiliar adults. Women's ratings of their hedonic response to the pictures revealed heightened positive affect to pictures of their own children versus other children. Interestingly, the brain response to their own versus unfamiliar infants diminished over time. That is, in a second block of exposures, the difference in brain response (but not in the hedonic rating) between their own and unfamiliar infants decreased. The orbitofrontal cortex is a region of the prefrontal cortex that has been implicated in the decoding of the affective valence of a stimulus. It has been implicated in rodent and human work as a brain region that is important for reward processing (Knutson, Westdorp, Kaiser, & Hommer, 2000; Schoenbaum, Chiba, & Gallagher, 1998). Nitschke and colleagues suggest that it may also be involved in attachment-related behaviors, particularly those involved in experiencing positive affect toward an attachment figure.

In similar work, Leibenluft, Gobbini, Harrison, and Haxby (2004) examined women's neural activation while each woman viewed pictures of her own child, a friend's child, an unfamiliar child, or an unfamiliar adult. The design of the study allowed comparison of familiar versus unfamiliar children and women's own children versus familiar children to determine the neural specificity of each comparison. Results revealed that a complex set of brain networks was activated for each of the different types of stimuli. Viewing one's own child versus a familiar child activated amygdala, insula, anterior paracingulate cortex, and superior temporal sulcus. Viewing familiar versus unfamiliar children activated regions similar to those seen in prior studies in which familiar versus unfamiliar adults were viewed. The authors suggested that viewing one's own child (vs. another familiar child) activates emotional responses and cognitions that may reflect attachment, protection, and empathy. Although subjects were asked prior to scanning to rate the stimuli, the questions did not cover the psychological states that are proposed to be associated with activation of these different neural structures.

Additional support for the complexity of the neural circuitry involved in a mother's recognition of her own child, as compared with another, under conditions of distress and nondistress extend this research by adding an additional layer of context. Noriuchi, Kikuchi, and Senoo (2008) scanned mothers as they were asked to view a series of video clips of their own child versus an unfamiliar 16-month-old in both distressing (Strange Situation) and nondistressing (free play) tasks. Distinct neurological profiles of activation were found when mothers viewed their own (vs. another) child, particularly involving the orbitofrontal cortex, periaqueductal gray, anterior insula, and dorsal and ventrolateral parts of the putamen. Higher activity in the right orbitofrontal cortex was associated with increased joy in the play-viewing condition, whereas activation of the right orbitofrontal cortex was associated with anxiety while viewing

the child in the Strange Situation. The inclusion of ratings of maternal feelings marks an import extension to the neuroscience of parenting, allowing an opportunity to examine neurological responses that underlie specific affective responses related to the experience and emotions of mothering.

Another import direction is the incorporation of observed mother–infant interactive behavior and maternal neurological responding to infant distress. Musser, Kaiser-Laurent, and Ablow (2012) observed 22 mothers interacting with their 18-month-old infants and coded maternal sensitivity and intrusiveness. Mothers were later exposed to the sound of their own or another infant crying. More sensitive mothers showed greater neurological activation to their own infant's cry in the right frontal pole and inferior frontal gyrus, regions associated with emotion processing and regulation. The pattern of activation may be consistent with better recognition of their own infant's emotions and the ability to regulate their own negative emotion in order to respond sensitively. Mothers with an intrusive style of responding showed greater activation in the left anterior insula and temporal pole to their own infant's cry, regions that are associated with sensory and emotion processing and empathy, perhaps suggesting that intrusive mothers have a more reactive and acute empathic response to infant discomfort that contributes to intrusive behavior. Mothers who experienced harmonious interactions with their infant displayed greater activation in left hippocampal regions associated with memory and stress regulation. Hence, harmonious interactions may be associated with better maternal representation of the dyad's interactional history and mothers' ability to regulate stress during infant crying. The inclusion of observed mother–infant interactive behavior in the field of parental neuroscience is yet another major advancement that is providing a more complete picture of how maternal brain activation to infant cues is embedded within the larger relational ecology of the dyad.

## Conclusions

Throughout this chapter, we have reviewed contemporary approaches to the study of the biology of human attachment. This vast field is expanding rapidly in new and exciting directions. Here we have focused specifically on psychophysiological and neuroscientific approaches to studying attachment. Each approach involves complex technologies, with its own set of methodological issues and constraints. Current advancements in temporal precision of measurement and designs that integrate multiple biological systems along with the context of care have advanced the field considerably since the previous edition of this handbook.

## References

Achenbach, T., & Edelbrock, C. (1991). *Manual for the Child Behavior Checklist and Revised Child Behavior Profile*. Burlington: University of Vermont, Department of Psychiatry.

Adam, E. K., Klimes-Dougan, B., & Gunnar, M. R. (2007). Social regulation of the adrenocortical response to stress in infants, children, and adolescents: Implications for psychopathology and education. In D. Coch, G. Dawson, & K. W. Fischer (Eds.), *Human behavior, learning, and the developing brain: Atypical development* (pp. 264–304). New York: Guilford Press.

Ainsworth, M. D. S. (1976). *Technical manual for the Systems for Coding Infant Attachment and Reciprocal Maternal Behaviors*. Princeton, NJ: Educational Testing Service.

Ainsworth, M. D. S., Blehar, M. C., Waters, E., & Wall, S. (1978). *Patterns of attachment: A psychological study of the SSP*. Hillsdale, NJ: Erlbaum.

Ainsworth, M. D. S., & Wittig, B. A. (1969). Attachment and exploratory behaviour of one-year-olds in a SSP. In B. M. Foss (Ed.), *Determinants of infant behaviour* (Vol. 4, pp. 113–136). London: Methuen.

Bartz, J. A., Zaki, J., Bolger, N., Hollander, E., Ludwig, N. N., Kolevzon, A., et al. (2010). Oxytocin selectively improves empathic accuracy. *Psychological Science, 21*(10), 1426–1428.

Behnia, B., Heinrichs, M., Bergmann, W., Jung, S., Germann, J., Schedlowski, M., et al. (2014). Differential effects of intranasal oxytocin on sexual experiences and partner interactions in couples. *Hormones and Behavior, 65*(3), 308–318.

Bernard, K., & Dozier, M. (2010). Examining infants' cortisol responses to laboratory tasks among children varying in attachment disorganization: Stress reactivity or return to baseline? *Developmental Psychology, 46*(6), 1771–1778.

Bono, M., & Stifter, C. A. (1995, April). Changes in infant cardiac activity elicited by the SSP and its relation to attachment status. In C. A. Brownell (Chair), *Early development of self-regulation in the context of the mother–child relationship*. Symposium conducted at the biennial meeting of the Society for Research in Child Development, Indianapolis, IN.

Bosch, O. J., & Neumann, I. D. (2012). Both oxytocin and vasopressin are mediators of maternal care and aggression in rodents: From central release to sites of action. *Hormones and Behavior, 61*(3), 293–303.

Bowlby, J. (1982). *Attachment and loss: Vol. 1. Attachment*. New York: Basic Books. (Original work published 1969)

Brindley, D. N., & Rolland, Y. (1989). Possible connections between stress, diabetes, obesity, hypertension, and altered lipoprotein metabolism that may result in atheroselerosis. *Clinical Science, 77*, 453–461.

Burgess, K. B., Marshall, P. J., Rubin, K. H., & Fox, N. A. (2003). Infant attachment and temperament as predictors of subsequent externalizing problems and cardiac physiology. *Journal of Child Psychology and Psychiatry, 6*, 819–831.

Caldji, C., Tannenbaum, B., Sharma, S., Francis, D., Plotsky, P. M., & Meaney, M. J. (1998). Maternal care during infancy regulates the development of neural systems mediating the expression of fearfulness in the rat. *Proceedings of the National Academy of Sciences USA, 95*, 5335–5340.

Champagne, F. A. (2013). Early environments, glucocorticoid receptors, and behavioral epigenetics. *Behavioral Neuroscience, 127*(5), 628–636.

Cohen, M. X., & Shaver, P. R. (2004). Avoidant attachment and hemispheric lateralisation of the processing of attachment- and emotion-related words. *Cognition and Emotion, 18*(6), 799–813.

Courage, M. L., Reynolds, G. D., & Richars, J. E. (2006). Infants' attention to patterned stimuli: Developmental change from 3 to 12 months of age. *Child Development, 77*, 680–695.

de Weerth, C., & van Geert, P. (2002). A longitudinal study of basal cortisol in infants: Intra-individual variability, circadian rhythm and developmental trends. *Infant Behavior and Development, 25*(4), 375–398.

Diamond, L. M. (2001). Contributions of psychophysiology to research on adult attachment: Review and recommendations. *Personality and Social Psychology Review, 5*, 276–295.

Doom, J. R., Cicchetti, D., & Rogosch, F. A. (2014). Longitudinal patterns of cortisol regulation differ in maltreated and nonmaltreated children. *Journal of the American Academy of Child and Adolescent Psychiatry, 53*(11), 1206–1215.

Eckstein, M., Scheele, D., Weber, K., Stoffel-Wagner, B., Maier, W., & Hurlemann, R. (2014). Oxytocin facilitates the sensation of social stress. *Human Brain Mapping, 35*(9), 4741–4750.

Ellenbogen, M. A., Linnen, A. M., Grumet, R., Cardoso, C., & Joober, R. (2012). The acute effects of intranasal oxytocin on automatic and effortful attentional shifting to emotional faces. *Psychophysiology, 49*(1), 128–137.

Feldman, R. (2012a). Bio-behavioral synchrony: A model for integrating biological and microsocial behavioral processes in the study of parenting. *Parenting: Science and Practice, 12*(2–3), 154–164.

Feldman, R. (2012b). Oxytocin and social affiliation in humans. *Hormones and Behavior, 61*(3), 380–391.

Feldman, R., Gordon, I., Schneiderman, I., Weisman, O., & Zagoory-Sharon, O. (2010). Natural variations in maternal and paternal care are associated with systematic changes in oxytocin following parent–infant contact. *Psychoneuroendocrinology*, 35(8), 1133–1141.

Feng, C., Hackett, P. D., DeMarco, A. C., Chen, X., Stair, S., Haroon, E., et al. (in press). Oxytocin and vasopressin effects on the neural response to social cooperation are modulated by sex in humans. *Brain Imaging and Behavior*.

Fox, N. A. (1985). Behavioral and autonomic antecedents of attachment in high-risk infants. In M. Reite & T. Field (Eds.), *The psychobiology of attachment and separation* (pp. 389–414). Orlando, FL: Academic Press.

Fox, N. A. (1989). Psychophysiological correlates of emotional reactivity during the first year of life. *Developmental Psychology*, 25, 364–372.

Fox, N. A., & Gelles, M. (1984). Face-to-face interaction in term and preterm infants. *Infant Mental Health Journal*, 5, 192–205.

Fox, N. A., & Hane, A. A. (2008). Studying the biology of human attachment. In J. Cassidy & P. R. Shaver (Eds.), *Handbook of attachment: Theory, research, and clinical applications* (2nd ed., pp. 217–240). New York: Guilford Press.

Francis, D. D., Diorio, J., Liu, D., & Meaney, M. J. (1999). Nongenomic transmission across generations of maternal behavior and stress response in the rat. *Science*, 286, 1155–1158.

Gimpl, G., & Fahrenholz, F. (2001). The oxytocin receptor system: Structure, function, and regulation. *Physiology Review*, 81(2), 629–683.

Gordon, I., Zagoory-Sharon, O., Leckman, J. F., & Feldman, R. (2010). Oxytocin and the development of parenting in humans. *Biological Psychiatry*, 68(4), 377–382.

Grant, K.-A., McMahon, C., Austin, M.-P., Reilly, N., Leader, L., & Ali, S. (2009). Maternal prenatal anxiety, postnatal caregiving and infants' cortisol responses to the still-face procedure. *Developmental Psychobiology*, 51(8), 625–637.

Grimm, S., Pestke, K., Feeser, M., Aust, S., Weigand, A., Wang, J., et al. (2014). Early life stress modulates oxytocin effects on limbic system during acute psychosocial stress. *Social Cognitive and Affective Neuroscience*, 9(11), 1828–1835.

Grunau, R. E., Holsti, L., Haley, D. W., Oberlander, T., Weinberg, J., Solimano, A., et al. (2005). Neonatal procedural pain exposure predicts lower cortisol and behavioral reactivity in preterm infants in the NICU. *Pain*, 113(3), 293–300.

Gunnar, M. R., Colton, M., & Stansbury, K. (1992, May). *Studies of emotional behavior, temperament, and adrenocortical activity in human infants*. Paper presented at the Eighth International Conference on Infant Studies, Miami, FL.

Gunnar, M. R., & Donzella, B. (2002). Social regulation of the cortisol levels in early human development. *Psychoneuroendocrinology*, 27(1–2), 199–220.

Gunnar, M. R., Mangelsdorf, S., Larson, M., & Herts-

gaard, L. (1989). Attachment, temperament, and adrenocortical activity in infancy: A study of psychoendocrine regulation. *Developmental Psychology*, 25, 355–363.

Haley, D. W., Handmaker, N. S., & Lowe, J. (2006). Infant stress reactivity and prenatal alcohol exposure. *Alcoholism: Clinical and Experimental Research*, 30(12), 2055–2064.

Hane, A. A., & Fox, N. A. (2006). Ordinary variations in maternal caregiving of human infants influence stress reactivity. *Psychological Science*, 17, 550–556.

Hane, A. A., Henderson, H. A., Reeb-Sutherland, B. C., & Fox, N. A. (2010). Ordinary variations in human maternal caregiving in infancy and biobehavioral development in early childhood: A follow-up study. *Developmental Psychobiology*, 52(6), 558–567.

Hane, A. A., & Philbrook, L. E. (2012). Beyond licking and grooming: Maternal regulation of infant stress in the context of routine care. *Parenting: Science and Practice*, 12(2–3), 144–153.

Harter, S., & Pike, R. (1984). The Pictorial Scale of Perceived Competence and Acceptance in Young Children. *Child Development*, 55, 1969–1982.

Hertsgaard, L., Gunnar, M., Erickson, M. F., & Nachmias, M. (1995). Adrenocortical responses to the SSP in infants with disorganized/disoriented attachment relationships. *Child Development*, 66, 1100–1106.

Hesse, E., & Main, M. (2006). Frightened, threatening, and dissociative parental behavior in low-risk samples: Description, discussion, and interpretations. *Development and Psychopathology*, 18(2), 309–343.

Holochwost, S. J., Gariépy, J. L., Propper, C. B., Mills-Koonce, W. R., & Moore, G. A. (2014). Parenting behaviors and vagal tone at six months predict attachment disorganization at twelve months. *Developmental Psychobiology*, 56(6), 1423–1430.

Izard, C. E., Porges, S. W., Simons, R. F., Haynes, O. M., Hyde, C., Parisi, M., et al. (1991). Infant cardiac activity: Developmental changes and relations with attachment. *Developmental Psychology*, 27, 432–439.

Kagan, J., & Snidman, N. (1991). Infant predictors of inhibited and uninhibited profiles. *Psychological Science*, 2, 40–44.

Katona, P. G., & Jih, F. (1985). Respiratory sinus arrhythmia: A noninvasive measure of parasympathetic cardiac control. *Journal of Applied Physiology*, 39, 801–805.

Knutson, B., Westdorp, A., Kaiser, E., & Hommer, D. (2000). FMRI visualization of brain activity during a monetary incentive delay task. *NeuroImage*, 12(1), 20–27.

Laurent, H. K., Ablow, J. C., & Measelle, J. (2011). Risky shifts: How the timing and course of mothers' depressive symptoms across the perinatal period shape their own and infant's stress response profiles. *Development and Psychopathology*, 23(2), 521–538.

Lee, P. R., Brady, D. L., Shapiro, R. A., Dorsa, D. M., & Koenig, J. I. (2007). Prenatal stress generates deficits in rat social behavior: Reversal by oxytocin. *Brain Research, 1156,* 152–167.

Leibenluft, E., Gobbini, M. I., Harrison, T., & Haxby, J. V. (2004). Mothers' neural activation in response to pictures of their children and other children. *Biological Psychiatry, 56,* 225–232.

Liu, D., & Diorio, J. (1997). Maternal care, hippocampal glucocorticoid receptors, and hypothalmic–pituitary–adrenal responses to stress. *Science, 277,* 1659–1663.

Luijk, M. P. C. M., Saridjan, N., Tharner, A., Van IJzendoorn, M. H., Bakermans-Kranenburg, M. J., Jaddoe, V. W. V., et al. (2010). Attachment, depression, and cortisol: Deviant patterns in insecure-resistant and disorganized infants. *Developmental Psychobiology, 52*(5), 441–452.

Meaney, M. J. (2001). Maternal care, gene expression, and the transmission of individual differences in stress reactivity across generations. *Annual Review of Neuroscience, 24,* 1161–1192.

Mikulincer, M., & Shaver, P. R. (2007). *Attachment in adulthood: Structure, dynamics, and change.* New York: Guilford Press.

Musser, E. D., Kaiser-Laurent, H., & Ablow, J. C. (2012). The neural correlates of maternal sensitivity: An fMRI study. *Developmental Cognitive Neuroscience, 2*(4), 428–436.

Nachmias, M., Gunnar, M., Mangelsdorf, S., Parritz, R., & Buss, K. (1996). Behavioral inhibition and stress reactivity: The moderating role of attachment security. *Child Development, 67,* 508–522.

Nitschke, J. B., Nelson, E. E., Rusch, B. D., Fox, A. S., Oakes, T. R., & Davidson, R. J. (2004). Orbitofrontal cortex tracks positive mood in mothers viewing pictures of their newborn infants. *NeuroImage, 21,* 583–592.

Noriuchi, M., Kikuchi, Y., & Senoo, A. (2008). The functional neuroanatomy of maternal love: Mother's response to infant's attachment behaviors. *Biological Psychiatry, 63*(4), 415–423.

Olff, M., Frijling, J. L., Kubzansky, L. D., Bradley, B., Ellenbogen, M. A., Cardoso, C., et al. (2013). The role of oxytocin in social bonding, stress regulation and mental health: An update on the moderating effects of context and interindividual differences. *Psychoneuroendocrinology, 38*(9), 1883–1894.

Parent, C., Zhang, T.-Y., Caldji, C., Bagot, R., Champagne, F. A., Pruessner, J., et al. (2005). Maternal care and individual differences in defensive responses. *Current Directions in Psychological Science, 14*(5), 229–233.

Park, S., Belsky, J., Putnam, S., & Crnic, K. (1997). Infant emotionality, parenting, and 3-year inhibition: Exploring stability and lawful discontinuity in a male sample. *Developmental Psychology, 32,* 218–227.

Phillips, A. C., Carroll, D., Hunt, K., & Der, G. (2006). The effects of the spontaneous presence of a spouse/partner and others on cardiovascular reactions to an acute psychological challenge. *Psychophysiology, 43*(6), 633–640.

Porges, S. W. (1991). Vagal tone: An autonomic mediator of affect. In J. A. Garber & K. A. Dodge (Eds.), *The development of affect regulation and dysregulation* (pp. 111–128). New York: Cambridge University Press.

Porges, S. W. (1995). Orienting in a defensive world: Mammalian modifications of our evolutionary heritage: A polyvagal theory (Presidential address, 1994). *Psychophysiology, 32,* 301–318.

Porges, S. W. (1996). Physiological regulation in high-risk infants: A model for assessment and potential intervention. *Development and Psychopathology, 8,* 43–58.

Porges, S. W., & Bohrer, R. E. (1991). The analysis of periodic processes in psychophysiological research. In J. T. Cacioppo & L. G. Tassinary (Eds.), *Principles of psychophysiology: Physical, social, and inferential elements* (pp. 708–753). New York: Cambridge University Press.

Porges, S. W., & Byrne, E. A. (1992). Research methods for measurement of heart rate and respiration. *Biological Psychology, 34,* 93–130.

Porges, S. W., Doussard-Roosevelt, J. A., Portales, A. L., & Suess, P. E. (1994). Cardiac vagal tone: Stability and relation to difficultness in infants and 3-year-olds. *Developmental Psychology, 27,* 289–300.

Porges, S. W., Stamps, L. E., & Walter, G. F. (1974). Heartrate variability and newborn heart-rate responses to illumination changes. *Developmental Psychology, 10,* 507–513.

Pruessner, J. C., Champagne, F., Meaney, M. J., & Dagher, A. (2004). Dopamine release in response to a psychological stress in humans and its relationship to early maternal care: A positron emission tomography study using [c]raclopride. *Journal of Neuroscience, 24,* 2825–2831.

Raine, A. (1996). Autonomic nervous system activity and violence. In D. M. Stoff & R. B. Cairns (Eds.), *Neurobiological approaches to clinical aggression research* (pp. 145–168). Mahwah, NJ: Erlbaum.

Raine, A., Venables, P. H., & Williams, M. (1990). Relationships between central and autonomic measures of arousal at age 15 years and criminality at age 24 years. *Archives of General Psychiatry, 47,* 1003–1007.

Schieche, M., & Spangler, G. (2005). Individual differences in biobehavioral organization during problem solving in toddlers: The influence of maternal behavior, infant–mother attachment, and behavioral inhibition on the attachment–exploration balance. *Developmental Psychobiology, 46,* 293–306.

Schoenbaum, G., Chiba, A. A., & Gallagher, M. (1998). Orbitofrontal cortex and basolateral amygdala encode expected outcomes during learning. *Nature Neuroscience, 1*(2), 155–159.

Spangler, G., & Grossmann, K. E. (1993). Biobehavioral

organization in securely and insecurely attached infants. *Child Development, 64*, 1439–1450.

Stevenson-Hinde, J., & Marshall, P. J. (1999). Behavioral inhibition: Heart period, respiratory sinus arrhythmia: An attachment perspective. *Child Development, 70*, 805–832.

Stifter, C. A., & Fox, N. A. (1990). Infant reactivity: Physiological correlates of newborn and 5-month temperament. *Developmental Psychology, 26*, 582–588.

Tharner, A., Dierckx, B., Luijk, M. P. C. M., Van IJzendoorn, M. H., Bakermans-Kranenburg, M. J., van Ginkel, J. R., et al. (2013). Attachment disorganization moderates the effect of maternal postnatal depressive symptoms on infant autonomic functioning. *Psychophysiology, 50*(2), 195–203.

Weisman, O., Zagoory-Sharon, O., & Feldman, R. (2012). Oxytocin administration to parent enhances infant physiological and behavioral readiness for social engagement. *Biological Psychiatry, 72*(12), 982–989.

Wells, J. K. K., Stanley, M., Laidlaw, A. S., Day, J. M. E., Staford, M., & Davies, P. S. (1997). Investigation of the relationship between infant temperament and later body composition. *International Journal of Obesity, 21*, 400–406.

Wendland, B. E., Atkinson, L., Steiner, M., Fleming, A. S., Pencharz, P., Moss, E., et al. (2014). Low maternal sensitivity at 6 months of age predicts higher BMI in 48 month old girls but not boys. *Appetite, 82*, 97–102.

Yao, S., Zhao, W., Cheng, R., Geng, Y., Luo, L., & Ken, K. M. (2014). Oxytocin makes females, but not males, less forgiving following betrayal of trust. *International Journal of Neuropsychopharmacology, 17*(11), 1785–1792.

Zalewski, M., Lengua, L. J., Kiff, C. J., & Fisher, P. A. (2012). Understanding the relation of low income to HPA-axis functioning in preschool children: Cumulative family risk and parenting as pathways to disruptions in cortisol. *Child Psychiatry and Human Development, 43*(6), 924–942.

Zelenko, M., Kraemer, H., Huffman, L., Gschwendt, M., Pageler, N., & Steiner, H. (2005). Heart rate correlates of attachment status in young mothers and their infants. *Journal of the American Academy of Child and Adolescent Psychiatry, 44*, 470–476.

Zhang, T. Y., Parent, C., Weaver, I., & Meaney, M. J. (2004). Maternal programming of individual differences in defensive responses in the rat. *Annals of the New York Academy of Sciences, 1032*, 85–103.

# Chapter 12

# Toward a Neuroscience of Attachment

## James A. Coan

Neurobiological studies of attachment are either abundant or scarce, depending on one's research tradition and what, precisely, one means by *attachment*. On the one hand, the past few decades have seen a great deal of nonhuman animal work detailing the neural mechanisms supporting social bonding, familiarity, affiliation, caregiving, and other behaviors that can (and often do) fall under the "attachment" rubric (see Polan & Hofer, Chapter 6, and Suomi, Chapter 7, in this volume). On the other hand, neuroscientific investigations of normative attachment in *humans* have been relatively limited. And the neural circuits supporting attachment *styles* (e.g., secure, anxious or ambivalent, and avoidant, in the social psychology tradition; autonomous, preoccupied, and dismissing, in the clinical and developmental tradition; see Crowell, Fraley, & Roisman, Chapter 27, this volume) are even more mysterious (Coan, 2010). These facts (and a cursory glance at the Contents for this volume) underscore the complexity of attachment as a domain of inquiry and suggest that, at present, any neuroscience of attachment is likely to be limited in both empirical foundation and theoretical scope.

Nevertheless, real progress is being made, and the neuroscience of attachment has much to gain from the integration of multiple research perspectives and traditions (Sokolowski, 2010). Following Bowlby (1969/1982) and Ainsworth (1989), I consider attachment bonds to be characterized by a high frequency of close proximity to putative "attachment figures," especially during times of emotional stress. Moreover, attachment relationships serve regulatory functions, often in relation not only to basic physiological needs but also with respect to many forms of emotional responding. These regulatory functions are *social* insofar as they result from interaction with *conspecifics* (other members of the same species). Some of the regulatory functions of attachment relationships are obvious and fundamental. For example, human infants literally cannot survive without the assistance of an adult caregiver. In later childhood, however, and in adult attachment relationships, emotion may be seen as the primary target of social regulation (Mikulincer & Shaver, Chapter 24, this volume), and social relationships may even regulate primary perceptional systems that mediate emotional responses (Coan & Sbarra, 2015; Gross & Proffitt, 2013). A major interest here is the social regulation of threat vigilance and responding (Carter & DeVries, 1999; Coan, Schaefer, & Davidson, 2006; Edens, Larkin, & Abel, 1992; Hofer, 1995).

A large literature now suggests that a range of interactive social behaviors target physiological systems, temperamental dispositions, and overt behaviors associated with the stress response (DeVries, Glasper, & Detillion, 2003; Sachser, Kaiser, & Hennessy, 2013). For example, supportive social behaviors attenuate stress-related activity in the autonomic nervous system (ANS) and the hypothalamic–pituitary–adrenocortical (HPA) axis (Lewis & Ramsay, 1999; Wiedenmayer, Magarinos, McEwen, & Barr, 2003). Maternal grooming behaviors affect glucocorticoid receptor gene expression underlying hippocampal and HPA axis stress reactivity in rat pups (Turecki & Meaney, 2016). In the context of a novel, mildly stressful environment, rats in the company of a familiar companion engage in more exploration and play-soliciting behavior than do rats in the company of an unfamiliar companion (Terranova, Cirulli, & Laviola, 1999).

Theorists have long argued that social bonding serves the regulatory functions of security provision and distress alleviation with respect to negative affect and arousal (Bowlby, 1973; Mikulincer, Shaver, & Pereg, 2003). Evolutionary theorists dating back to Darwin have even argued that because mammalian emotional responding evolved in a social context, emotional behavior is virtually inextricable from social behavior (Buss & Kenrick, 1998; Darwin, 1872/1998). Recent work in visual perception suggests that proximity to social resources fundamentally alters even our earliest perceptional mechanisms (Gross & Proffitt, 2013; Schnall, Harber, Stefanucci, & Proffitt, 2008). These diverse perspectives and literatures suggest that any robust conception of attachment will include multiple distributed subsystems, including (but probably not limited to) those devoted to perception, memory, emotion, motivation, emotion regulation, and social affiliation.

The promise of an "attachment neuroscience" is at once to provide critical information about how the brain supports attachment behaviors and to forge links among research traditions as diverse as the basic neurosciences, behavioral ecology, and various subdomains of psychology (e.g., developmental, social, and clinical), as well as affective science. In this chapter, the neural systems supporting emotion, motivation, emotion regulation, and social behavior are first reviewed. Following this, the social regulation of emotion and individual differences in attachment behavior are considered from the perspective of behavioral neuroscience. Based on these reviews, I describe a *"social baseline" theory* that integrates the study of social relationships with principles of attachment, behavioral ecology, cognitive neuroscience, and perception science. The social baseline theory borrows heavily from theoretical work on the predictive nature of the brain and the *economy of action*

built into the management of metabolic resources devoted to emotional and social behavior. Finally, recommendations are made for the development of a robust future neuroscience of attachment.

## Attachment as a Neural Construct

Although attachment bonds are widely believed to result from a universal, innate "attachment behavioral system," attempts to locate a single, dedicated attachment circuit is likely to be (to paraphrase Wittgenstein) a bit like trying to find the real artichoke by peeling away all its leaves. Almost any interpretation of the attachment behavioral system reveals it to be a higher-order construct comprising distinct behaviors about which a great deal is known, even at the neural level (see Hane & Fox, Chapter 11, and Polan & Hofer, Chapter 6, this volume). For example, many studies have addressed the neurobiology of social behaviors such as recognition and familiarity, proximity seeking, separation distress, soothing, and maternal caregiving. Thus, one of my goals in this chapter is to introduce the neuroscientific study of attachment from the perspective of what is currently known about its social and emotional *constituents*.

A corollary goal is to move toward bridging two broad, rigorous, productive, and unfortunately disparate literatures. One is a thriving animal literature dedicated to what is variously termed "social bonding," "pair bonding," and "attachment bonding." The other contains a vast body of research on human attachment behavior, including studies of individual differences in internal working models of attachment (reviewed in Mikulincer & Shaver, 2007; Chapter 24, this volume; also see J. A. Feeney, Chapter 21, this volume). These two worlds have had little to say to each other—a reflection of their starkly different assumptions and research strategies as much as their different subject populations. Animal models emphasize discrete social processes in terms of specific causal neural structures, circuits, neurotransmitters, neuropeptides, pheromones, or hormones. Attachment relationships are defined observationally, by the presence of separation distress or physiological soothing as a function of close proximity. By contrast, social, clinical, and developmental psychologists often focus their efforts on assumed "behavioral systems," seeking to understand how humans behave in—and, importantly, what they have to *say* about—relational contexts.

This is not to say that research on attachment in humans has not utilized physiological measurement. On the contrary, attachment researchers have used measures of ANS physiology, electroencephalography (EEG), glucocorticoid levels, and more recently, functional magnetic resonance imaging (fMRI). These measures have provided valuable insights into human social behavior, but they are rarely capable of identifying causal brain–behavior relationships (Norris, Coan, & Johnstone, 2007), and their frequent dependence on self-report measures (including coded interviews) may result in neurobiological correlates that are quite distinct from those of behaviorally defined animal models (Williamson, 2006).

Yet another difficulty presents itself in bridging these literatures. Even if the definitions of attachment were perfectly matched, and if the neural measures applied to humans and nonhuman animals were identical, the neural processes associated with attachment behaviors in nonhuman animals may not generalize perfectly to those in humans. Work on the social communication value of pheromones provides an excellent example of this point. *Pheromones* are chemical substances that convey information between members of the same species (Beny & Kimchi, 2014). It is certain that nearly all animals, including humans, show at least some evidence of two distinct olfactory systems (Shipley, Ennis, & Puche, 2003). The *primary olfactory system* is dedicated to the detection of odors that convey information about food or the presence of predators, and this system is most commonly associated with the sense of smell. By contrast, the *accessory olfactory system* is, in many species, dedicated to the detection of specific pheromonal information. This accessory olfactory system consists of the vomeronasal organ (VNO) and the accessory olfactory bulb (AOB). Pheromones make contact with the VNO, exciting pheromone-specific sensory neurons projecting to the AOB.

In a wide variety of species, this system is capable of providing rapid and powerful information about sex, reproductive capacity, mate location, territorial boundaries, and even social status (Beny & Kimchi, 2014; Insel & Fernald, 2004). Nevertheless, the strongest of these findings derive exclusively from studies of nonprimate animals. After a great deal of initial excitement about the possibility of a human pheromone system, enthusiasm has waned significantly amid evidence that although there does appear to be a human VNO, (1) there is no obvious pheromone-specific sensory

neuron associated with it; (2) vomeronasal receptor genes present in the human genome appear to be *pseudogenes* (genes that have lost their protein-coding ability); and (3) the AOB does not appear to exist at all in the brains of adult humans (Meredith, 2001; Smith, Laitman, & Bhatnagar, 2014). In other words, the VNO—the primary and best-understood mechanism of socially critical pheromonal communication in animals—appears to be vestigial in humans.

Despite these cautions, it is clear that research on animals has yielded invaluable information about the neurobiology of attachment, without which any understanding of human attachment would, at the neural level, be severely impoverished. Moreover, advanced neuroimaging techniques such as EEG, positron emission tomography (PET), transcranial magnetic stimulation (TMS), and fMRI promise access to human neural processes at a level of detail undreamed of until the very end of the 20th century. Hence, the potential for building bridges between animal and human attachment literatures is higher than it has ever been. fMRI studies in particular, by virtue of their rapid proliferation and relative lack of invasiveness, are beginning to supply pieces of the human social-bonding puzzle that will complement anatomical and molecular work in animals. Such advances promise the formation of a more comprehensive neuroscience of attachment.

## The Neural Constituents of Attachment

Neural systems supporting attachment are likely to include, at a minimum, those underlying incentive motivation, emotional responding, emotion regulation, and discrete social behaviors, such as the establishment of familiarity and preference, proximity seeking, separation distress, and social affect regulation. This chapter does not provide an exhaustive treatment of all possible constituent systems underlying attachment. In truth, because so many neural structures are involved one way or another in attachment behavior, it is possible to think of the entire human brain as an attachment system. Auditory, olfactory, and visual sensory systems are heavily implicated for obvious reasons. Memory processes—involving, for example, long-term memory consolidation and retrieval in the hippocampus—underlie familiarity, recognition, and the maintenance of shared histories.

Many different regulatory needs affected by attachment relationships are likely to be related to activity in the hypothalamus. Conflict-monitoring demands will be made on the anterior cingulate cortex (ACC). Each of these systems and more contribute to attachment in a variety of ways. In this chapter, however, I review a smaller number of putatively basic elements.

## Preliminary Considerations

### Behavioral versus Neural Systems

I should first distinguish between what ethologists call "behavioral systems" and what neuroscientists call "neural systems." A *behavioral system* is a set of behaviors associated with a common causal antecedent and resulting, once activated, in a common consequence, which in turn deactivates the system. Bowlby (1969/1982) described several behavioral systems associated with social behavior. When discussing behavioral systems such as these, there is a great temptation to view the behavioral system as having a one-to-one relationship with some underlying neural system. But such tidy correspondences are rare. *Neural systems* are coordinated neural inputs and signaling targets among populations of neurons that form a circuit. Neural systems can be tightly organized in close physical proximity or distributed throughout the brain. The problem is that similar behaviors may be caused by dissimilar neural systems. Moreover, similar neural activations can result in quite distinct behaviors. So the search for specific neural circuits associated with observationally defined behavioral systems is fraught with theoretical and empirical difficulty.

### Bottom-Up versus Top-Down Processing

Although the terms *bottom-up* and *top-down processing* are frequently used in the cognitive neurosciences (and throughout the remainder of this chapter), their meanings may not be immediately obvious. Bottom-up processes begin, more or less, with sensory information, usually within subcortical brain structures, working "up" to more integrative areas within the cortex. The process of receiving sensory inputs from the environment and converting those inputs into neural pulses that are relayed to cortical structures as consciously perceived information about one's surroundings would be an example of this. Top-down processes are essentially the opposite. In this case, integrative,

cortically mediated information is sent "down" to more sensory-oriented subcortical structures, often for some regulatory purpose. One example of a top-down process might be the brain's tendency to impute information from memory and experience into stimuli in the periphery of the visual field, thereby imposing "best guesses" on ambiguous visual information. These distinctions are necessarily simplified, but not unreasonably so. Exceptions and ambiguities are legion, but the difference between top-down and bottom-up processing retains its pragmatic utility both neuroanatomically and conceptually.

## Emotional and Motivational Elements

### Incentive Motivation, Reward, and the Dopamine System

Incentive motivation involves the acquisition of rewarding stimuli. The intensity of incentive motivation varies as a function of the state of the individual and the magnitude of the reward. For example, if a typical Westerner is mildly hungry and is offered a kind of food that is normally undesirable—*uni* (raw sea urchin), for example—there will be little incentive motivation to eat the food. If the individual is extremely hungry, however, the incentive motivation to eat the *uni* will be high. Similarly, if the same individual is again only mildly hungry, but is given a food item that is deemed highly desirable—say, a piece of chocolate cake—the incentive motivation to eat the cake will be high.

Incentive motivation plays a key role in a number of attachment-related processes (e.g., proximity seeking) and is tightly linked to the dopamine projection system of the ventral tegmental area (VTA). Dopamine is produced in the VTA and substantia nigra, and is projected to a variety of distinct networks (Lammel, Lim, & Malenka, 2014). This dopaminergic activity represents a neural substrate for the facilitation of goal-directed behavior (Berridge, 2007; Depue & Collins, 1999). Strongly implicated in this function is the nucleus accumbens, which is a major terminus of dopaminergic projections from the VTA (Tzschentke & Schmidt, 2000). Dopaminergic activity within the VTA and nucleus accumbens has been repeatedly associated with reinforcing stimuli and the experience of pleasure. For example, rats capable of directly stimulating these circuits with a lever press will repeatedly do so, even in lieu of access to food, water, and sex. This preference for lever pressing over food and water will continue even to the point of death (Bozarth & Wise, 1996).

Dopaminergic cells in the VTA are highly responsive to conditioning (Depue & Collins, 1999), especially to cues that predict the receipt of reward (Schultz, Dayan, & Montague, 1997). Importantly, the VTA is also responsive to stimuli that are *unconditioned* (Rolls, 2007). *Unconditioned stimuli* are those that naturally, automatically, and unconditionally trigger a response in an organism. *Positive unconditioned stimuli* act as reinforcers, and include certain flavors, water, sleep, touch, and a variety of social cues. *Negative unconditioned stimuli* act as punishers or negative reinforcers, and include pain, social deprivation, and putrefying odors (Rolls, 2007). With repeated exposure to unconditional reinforcers, dopaminergic neurons in the VTA become sensitive to sensory cues associated with those stimuli. In this way, the VTA begins to activate the nucleus accumbens earlier and earlier in a "chain of cues" that increase the probability of coming into contact with the original unconditioned reinforcer (e.g., an attractive potential mate). Conditioned associations between cues related to desirable unconditioned stimuli and dopaminergic activity in the VTA increase the predictability of those unconditioned stimuli, and hence the opportunities for obtaining them (Depue & Collins, 1999).

### The Amygdala and Hippocampus in Affect and Memory

The amygdala is now one of the most widely recognized brain structures associated with emotion (Johansen, Cain, Ostroff, & LeDoux, 2011). Far from a unitary structure, the amygdala contains many subnuclei, accounting for its involvement in a vast array of emotional responses (Davis & Whalen, 2001). A large body of research now supports the notion that the amygdala is sensitive to both conditioned and unconditioned signs of threat. Moreover, at least two pathways to amygdala activation associated with visual stimuli exist, both of which can mediate fear learning. One is a very rapid and direct route through the thalamus (the thalamoamygdala pathway) that processes obvious or highly specific sensory information (Öhman, 2005; Phelps & LeDoux, 2005). Another pathway processes slower and more complex information in the visual cortex before activating the amygdala. When paired with unconditioned aversive stimuli

(e.g., a loud noise, pain), otherwise meaningless stimuli are quickly associated with the presence of a threat—conditioning dependent to a large degree on the amygdala. The amygdala is also exquisitely sensitive to social signals expressed on the face (Benuzzi et al., 2007; Rolls, 2007). Fearful faces, in particular, reliably activate the amygdala in normal human subjects (Thomas et al., 2001; Whalen et al., 2004). And human patients with impaired amygdala functioning have difficulty processing emotional facial expressions, especially those communicating social emotions (Adolphs, Baron-Cohen, & Tranel, 2002).

The amygdala also plays a major role in the consolidation of long-term memories. Amygdala activity during memory encoding is associated with the recall of emotionally salient information even weeks after testing (Hamann, Ely, Grafton, & Kilts, 1999). The amygdala "tags" sensory experiences as significant or salient, and this tagging is prominently represented in long-term memory consolidation. Importantly, the hippocampus appears to support the formation, storage, and consolidation of associations between internal states and spatial or contextual environmental stimuli (Brasted, Bussey, Murray, & Wise, 2003). Ultimately, both the amygdala and the hippocampus are likely to underlie the identification and consolidation of significant interactions between attachment figures and emotionally salient situations. The amygdala will tag emotionally salient stimuli and will participate, along with the hippocampus, in the consolidation of contextual cues associated with those stimuli in long-term memory. Among those cues will be the behavior of attachment figures.

### Threat Responding, Social Soothing, and the Hypothalamus

The hypothalamus regulates a variety of metabolic and autonomic processes, as well as linking the central nervous system to the endocrine system, most famously in the case of cortisol release via the HPA axis (Dickerson & Kemeny, 2004). The hypothalamus receives inputs from a wide variety of structures implicated in social behavior, emotion, stress, and attachment, including the amygdala, prefrontal cortex (PFC), and hippocampus (McEwen, 2007). The periventricular nucleus of the hypothalamus is capable of synthesizing corticotropin-releasing hormone (CRH) (Aguilera & Liu, 2012). In threat responding, CRH released by the hypothalamus stimulates the release of adrenocorticotropic hormone (ACTH) in the pituitary gland. ACTH causes increased production of cortisol and catecholamines (e.g., epinephrine and norepinephrine) in the adrenal cortex. This cortisol is circulated throughout the body, including the brain. Critically, circulating cortisol in the brain is capable of activating glucocorticoid receptors in the hippocampus that feed back to inhibit the HPA axis (Kemeny, 2003).

Importantly, the hypothalamus is one of the key structures implicated in the regulatory effects of social soothing on neural threat responding, including interactions with attachment figures (Coan, Schaefer, & Davidson, 2006; Conner et al., 2012). The precise mechanisms by which social soothing down-regulates HPA axis activity are unknown, but the hypothalamus is known to coordinate the activity of many behavioral and physiological systems, including those involved in maternal behavior and pair bonding (Kim et al., 2011). Moreover, maternal and pair-bonding behaviors are strongly associated with oxytocin and vasopressin—neuropeptides (reviewed below) that the hypothalamus is capable of synthesizing in abundance (Carter, 1995; Gainer & Wray, 1994).

## The PFC, Emotion, and Emotion Regulation

Many regions of the PFC are implicated in emotion, motivation, and emotion regulation (Coan & Allen, 2004; Ray & Zald, 2012). Indeed, portions of the PFC are strongly connected to the dopaminergic projection system (e.g., nucleus accumbens and VTA), and the PFC shares numerous connections with the amygdala, hippocampus, and hypothalamus. For example, the orbitofrontal region of the PFC assists the amygdala and hippocampus in linking the emotional value of secondary sensory information (e.g., place cues) to primary reinforcers, such as food, water, and social contact (Rolls, 2007).

One of the major functions of the PFC is the regulation of emotion. Prefrontal regions may bias brain circuits responsible for appraising the emotional content of sensory stimuli and instantiating behavior directed toward approach- or avoidance-related goals (Davidson & Irwin, 1999). Different portions of the PFC underlie different emotion regulation strategies (Ochsner, Silvers, & Buhle, 2012). These can include "automatic" forms of emotion regulation, as well as effortful forms related to the cognitive control of attention or stimulus

appraisal (Ellenbogen, Schwartzman, Stewart, & Walker, 2006). Some automatic forms of emotion regulation are conditioning and extinction learning, including instrumental avoidance. These rapid and automatic regulatory functions (especially extinction learning) have been associated with the ventromedial and medial orbital PFC (Milad et al., 2005; Quirk & Beer, 2006; Sierra-Mercado, Corcoran, Lebrón-Milad, & Quirk, 2006). More "effortful" forms of regulation require attention, working memory, and other cognitive operations (Sheppes, Catran, & Meiran, 2009). For example, cognitive reappraisals have been used to alter the meaning of a stimulus, and attentional practices (e.g., meditation) have been used to alter attentional foci associated with affective stimuli. These processes have been associated with more lateral, especially dorsolateral, portions of the PFC—regions also known to support working memory, language, and action planning operations (Kanske, Heissler, Schönfelder, Bongers, & Wessa, 2010).

Thus, the PFC may be associated with attachment processes in at least two ways. First, over time, medial orbital circuits may encode conditioned or "automatic" responses to attachment figures related to excitatory or inhibitory responses to threat cues. Second, dorsolateral circuits may modulate cognitive operations associated with attachment figures in reflective, working memory. In truth, these distinctions are not likely to be as discrete as the previous formulation suggests, but the distinction between medial orbital and dorsolateral circuits of the PFC offers a useful neural heuristic for thinking about the regulatory influences of attachment figures in automatic versus explicit terms, respectively.

## Emotional Constituents in Combination

Because all of the previously described constituent systems are linked, it is possible for them to coordinate in important ways. For example, dopaminergic neurons in the VTA share connections with many regions other than the nucleus accumbens, including the amygdala (in various nuclei, as well as the extended amygdala), the hippocampus, the hypothalamus, and the PFC. In this way, these structures form their own distributed networks of often reciprocal influence. To understand how such a network may function, consider the distribution of activity following an encounter with an unconditionally rewarding stimulus. Dopamine is released from the VTA, which stimulates dopaminergic activity in the nucleus accumbens associated with anticipatory pleasure. The amygdala "tags" sensory properties of the stimulus as significant during the process of long-term memory consolidation via the hippocampus, which also encodes contextual information as part of the consolidation process. The PFC uses this information to effect action plans and regulate subsequent behavior relevant to the stimulus. As experience with the rewarding stimulus increases in frequency (partly as a function of successful regulation and action planning activity in the PFC), the affective "tagging" of cues associated with it proceeds down a "chain of cues," increasing the probability that the rewarding stimulus will be accessed (or avoided in the case of unconditionally negative reinforcers).

More concretely, consider an encounter with an attractive potential mate. In many species, including humans, such an encounter is unconditionally reinforcing. The encounter initially elicits pleasurable feelings and an increase in incentive motivation associated with the partner. The amygdala tags sensory features of the encounter as salient during the process of memory consolidation, in cooperation with the hippocampus; the VTA becomes conditioned to cues associated with (and predictive of) the potential mate, thereby activating incentive motivation circuits early in the "chain of cues" that will increase the likelihood of encountering the potential mate again. With repeated exposures, and a bit of luck, the potential mate may even respond in kind. With this, the complex process of attachment bonding has begun (see Zeifman & Hazan, Chapter 20, this volume). During the attachment bonding process, the PFC utilizes information about the potential mate to adjust its emotion regulation activities, opting in many cases to cede some level of regulatory effort to the potential mate, as discussed below.

## Social Elements

### Familiarity and Preference

A bedrock feature of any social species (as well as any conception of attachment) is the ability to distinguish individuals who are familiar from those who are not—an ability that in turn is yoked to a preference for the familiar. Indeed, the establishment and maintenance of preferences for familiar others (caregivers, peers, one's mate, etc.) form the first necessary condition of attachment bonds. Throughout evolutionary time, familiarity was probably a matter of survival, and so it remains

in the case of infants and their caregivers. One of the striking things about humans (and many other mammals) is how well *designed* we are for affiliation (Depue & Morrone-Strupinsky, 2005). Many stereotyped behaviors, including facial expressions, vocalization, bodily gestures, and so forth, are calibrated to signal social closeness and/or discomfort. These signals are readily recognized by most humans and may in many cases be innate (Laird & Strout, 2007; Rolls, 2007).

More than 40 years ago, Bowlby (1969/1982) suggested that infant–mother bonds, characterized by both the ability to distinguish the caregiver from others and a strong preference for the caregiver, formed very rapidly. This is true of many species (Rilling & Young, 2014). Most researchers who study infants agree that the development of attachment bonds is critical because infants often must survive long periods of early development totally dependent upon their caregivers, even when those caregivers are neglectful or abusive (Simpson & Belsky, Chapter 5, this volume).

Among social species, the most common manifestation of the attachment bond is that between an infant and its mother. Human infants can distinguish their mothers from others within hours after birth (DeCasper & Fifer, 1980). But attachment bonding is a generalized capacity only *very frequently* applied to the actual mother. For example, many birds become bonded within hours to the first moving object they encounter. Interestingly, Lorenz (1935) observed that the geese he reared not only bonded to him (and followed him) as if he was the parent, but also that they "courted" him upon reaching sexual maturity, preferring him even to other geese. These observations raise important questions about the degree to which early sensory objects associated with a caregiver are "etched" into the developing brain, how such a thing could occur, and whether a critical period for bonding formation exists in early development.

### Filial Bonding, the Locus Ceruleus, and the Amygdala

*Filial bonds* are those concerning an offspring and a parent. In humans, strong attachment to the caregiver usually develops by 6 months of age, but behaviors resembling filial bonding appear from birth. Filial bonds may differ from adult affiliation behaviors in important ways, due to the dependent nature of the offspring–parent relationship. Many offspring of social species are totally dependent on a caregiver for survival, and attachments are imperative regardless of the quality of the care (Hofer & Sullivan, 2001). Indeed, nonhuman primates form strong attachments to their mothers even when the mothers are abusive, and this pattern extends to human children (Moriceau & Sullivan, 2005). Rat pups have been observed to form preferences even to stimuli paired with electric shock. This seemingly paradoxical effect prevents pups from aversion learning while being handled roughly by the mother (Hofer, 2006)—an unfortunate predicament, but better than being abandoned. Ultimately, filial bonds form in a context of significant dependence, at least early in development, which may also explain why they occur so rapidly and unconditionally by comparison with attachment formation in adulthood.

Filial bonding also occurs in a context of significant neural development. The human brain grows exponentially during the first year of life and continues to develop rapidly into the second year (Franceschini et al., 2007). Glucose metabolism rises gradually until about the fourth year and, on average, the level of brain glucose metabolism is more than double that of adults until about age 10 (Chugani, 1998). The production of *neurotrophins* (proteins that support neuron survival) depends on neuronal activity and, by extension, environmental stimuli (Berardi & Maffei, 1999; Cancedda et al., 2004). Within the first 2 years of development in humans, the brain's production of axons, dendrites, and synapses far exceeds its needs. Synaptic connections are then "pruned" throughout childhood by lack of use; that is, synaptic connections that go unused are discarded (Reichardt, 2006). In this way, the environment exerts its influence on the otherwise genetically determined development of the brain. At a systems level, neural organization tends to follow functioning—repetitive and patterned activation—during development (Hebb, 1949; Posner & Rothbart, 2007).

During the earliest stages of this process, at least two brain structures, the locus ceruleus and the amygdala, interact to facilitate filial bonding. Although in adults norepinephrine *moderates* memory consolidation and learning (Cahill, Prins, Weber, & McGaugh, 1994), norepinephrine from the locus ceruleus appears to be both necessary and sufficient for learning in human and animal neonates (Sullivan, 2003). And the neonate locus ceruleus releases large amounts of norepinephrine early in development (Nakamura & Sakaguchi, 1990). Combined with the look, sound, and smell of a caregiver, familiarity with that caregiver occurs rapidly. Importantly, this learning is occurring alongside a neonatal amygdala that is not yet fully

functional, making it difficult or impossible for aversive conditioning to occur (Sullivan, 2003). Thus, because the amygdala is immature during early neonatal development, it may not be capable of associating aversive stimuli with alarm or avoidance behavior, which may leave virtually all stimuli to be simply encoded as " 'familiar' or not."

During this developmental period, neural pathways linking amygdala to hippocampus are similarly underdeveloped, as are many regions within the PFC (Herschkowitz, 2000). This suggests that learning in neonates may not involve the PFC, or may do so only in limited ways. In either case, these systems begin to develop rapidly in infancy, leading many to refer to this developmental time as a "critical" or "sensitive" period for neural development. Sensitive periods have been studied extensively in terms of the brain's sensory systems. For example, temporary blockage of visual input to one eye in cats during early development causes irreversible impairment in the visual cortex (Hubel & Wiesel, 1970). Similarly, children born deaf have been observed to cease vocalizations in late infancy, probably due to a lack of auditory stimuli (Schauwers et al., 2004). Interestingly, environments rich in social and cognitive complexity are associated with significantly more synapses per neuron throughout the visual cortex than are simple socially paired housing and individual housing (Briones, Klintsova, & Greenough, 2004). These effects remain even after later environments are changed or reversed, suggesting that plastic changes associated with early experiences are persistent.

In combination, these findings suggest that filial bonding occurs rapidly and unconditionally. Moreover, the filial bond develops in a context of rapid neural development, during what appears to be a sensitive period of learning. As discussed in greater detail below, this process (especially to the extent that it involves developing links between the PFC and affective structures such as the amygdala and nucleus accumbens) may result in the development of different reflexive "assumptions" about the nature of the social world, including the world as it will be encountered in the future. This may set the stage for different broad strategies for engaging (or avoiding) social stimuli, perhaps especially during emotional situations. Indeed, conditions under which the filial bond forms and develops may constitute a kind of rudimentary "preworking model" of interdependence and affect regulation—of attachment—that is either altered or reinforced during the course of development throughout childhood.

## Adult Affiliation, Nucleus Accumbens, and the Social Neuropeptides

Of course, attachment bonds characterized by interdependence and affect regulation extend far beyond the prototypic mother–infant relationship. Adult attachments occur in the context of romantic relationships, especially monogamous ones—but adult attachment is probably not restricted to this. Indeed, relationships that meet attachment criteria have by now been documented between pairs of individuals as diverse as adult romantic partners (Fraley & Shaver, 2000), captive chimpanzee cagemates (Bard, 1983), chimpanzees and their human caretakers (Miller, Bard, Juno, & Nadler, 1990), and domesticated dogs and their owners (Topal, Miklosi, Csanyi, & Doka, 1998). Aspects of attachment seem to occur even between organization members and their leaders (Davidovitz, Mikulincer, Shaver, Ijzak, & Popper, 2007).

Of interest here are neural circuits that support the establishment and maintenance of attachment bonds in later childhood and adulthood. How does the brain facilitate movement from a first encounter through simple familiarity to an attachment bond? A reasonable first step consists of positive, possibly unconditioned social affiliation behaviors (e.g., eye gaze, soothing vocalizations, nonthreatening facial and bodily behaviors). It is clear that some social cues are unconditionally capable of activating neural structures supporting incentive or reward motivation, especially the nucleus accumbens and the VTA (Young & Wang, 2004). Even passively viewed images of female faces activate the VTA and nucleus accumbens unconditionally in heterosexual men (Aharon et al., 2001). In rats, maternal females show an increase in dopamine release in the nucleus accumbens when exposed to pups (Hansen, Bergvall, & Nyiredi, 1993). Depletion of dopamine in the VTA and nucleus accumbens via lesions or dopamine antagonists virtually eliminates rat maternal behavior (Hansen, Harthon, Wallin, Löfberg, & Svensson, 1991). Interestingly, maternal behaviors not directly associated with caregiving, such as nest building, passive nursing, and aggression, are virtually unaffected by these manipulations. Other studies have linked dopamine release in the nucleus accumbens and VTA to the spontaneous establishment of partner preferences (Aragona et al., 2006).

Mating behavior in the absence of partner preference is also associated with dopamine in the nucleus accumbens (Balfour, Yu, & Coolen, 2004), however, suggesting that dopaminergic activity in the nucleus accumbens is insufficient in itself for the establishment of partner preferences. This raises the question of how partner preference is "linked up" to the dopaminergic incentive motivation system. Here the neuropeptides oxytocin and vasopressin appear to play major roles (Depue & Morrone-Strupinsky, 2005; Young & Wang, 2004). Both have been associated with the formation of partner preference regardless of mating behavior, and both, but especially oxytocin, are elicited by positive social behaviors (Carter, 2014). Moreover, both are capable of potentiating dopaminergic activity in the VTA and nucleus accumbens in response to social cues (Shahrokh, Zhang, Diorio, Gratton, & Meaney, 2010).

Perhaps the most celebrated example of the function of these neuropeptides derives from work on pair bonding within monogamous prairie voles (Carter, 1995; Insel & Fernald, 2004; Young & Wang, 2004). When these animals forge a pair bond, they mate, share nests and territory, cooperate in the care of their young, and forcefully reject intruders of either sex. Unlike in nonmonogamous animals—including other variants of voles—the nucleus accumbens in these animals is rich in oxytocin receptors. Moreover, structures such as the VTA and ventral pallidum are rich in receptors for vasopressin (Lim & Young, 2006).

These findings offer clues as to how social cues activate incentive motives associated with dopaminergic activity and in turn the formation of partner preferences and proximity-seeking behavior. Socially sensitive oxytocin and vasopressin synthesized within the medial preoptic area of the hypothalamus project to circuits in the VTA, nucleus accumbens, and ventral pallidum, and probably stimulate dopaminergic activity linked to social incentives. Because activation of this dopaminergic system is frequently associated with positive affect and reward, the degree of oxytocin and vasopressin activity may determine the degree to which a social experience is rewarding, by virtue of the dopaminergic cascade that follows it.

## Proximity Seeking, the Dopamine System, and Endogenous Opioids

One of the natural consequences of familiarity, preference, and bonding is *proximity seeking*, a characteristic of social behavior strongly associated with attachment. Proximity seeking is likely to be an extension of motivational circuits associated with reward and partner preference. Of course, individuals can seek close proximity both as a function of positive affect and reward, and in response to cues of punishment, where the goal is the provision of safety (Depue & Morrone-Strupinsky, 2005). In the case of positive affect, proximity is sought because the attachment figure has become associated with rewarding feelings of pleasure, and close proximity increases the frequency or intensity of these feelings. In the case of negative affect, the attachment figure may serve as a safety cue, eliciting approach behaviors oriented toward the acquisition of security (Beckes, Coan, & Morris, 2013). In this way, proximity seeking can involve both reward-related approach behaviors and approach behaviors associated with active avoidance.

Behaviorally, these motivations may appear to be identical, but they are likely to involve both shared and distinct neural circuits. Moreover, although attachment theory emphasizes the emotion regulation function of proximity seeking due to the need for security, it may be counterproductive to downplay the role of proximity seeking due to reward processes. In addition to the reinforcing nature of dopaminergic activation, for example, consummatory pleasure may play a role in rewarding social interaction. After all, positive social experiences are characterized in everything from semistructured scientific interviews to ancient literature as involving feelings of warmth, closeness, love, affection, and pleasure. Depue and Morrone-Strupinsky (2005) have argued that feelings of consummatory pleasure promote the development of contextual associative memory networks that help both to establish and to maintain social bonds, and that are ultimately responsible for many of the *regulatory* effects associated with the soothing and security provided by attachment relationships. The critical substrate for these feelings, and perhaps for the socioaffective regulatory effects that accompany them, may be the release of endogenous opioids that often follows activation of oxytocin receptors—not only in structures such as the nucleus accumbens and VTA but also within the anterior cingulate cortex and elsewhere.

There is abundant evidence for the role of endogenous opioids in a wide variety of social behaviors (Loseth, Ellingsen, & Leknes, 2014). In humans and other animals, these opioids are released during childbirth, nursing, maternal caregiving, sexual activity, and many modes of tactile stimulation, including grooming and play behavior

(Carter & Keverne, 2002; Keverne, Martensz, & Tuite, 1989). This release may mediate the reward associations that are forged between infants and mothers, as well as between romantic partners and even platonic friends. For example, morphine, an opioid receptor agonist, increases the reinforcing effects of a host of maternal behaviors, mother–infant bonding, time spent by juveniles (rats) with their mothers after a brief separation, grooming, and juvenile play behavior (Agmo, Barreau, & Lemaire, 1997; Nocjar & Panksepp, 2007; Panksepp, Nelson, & Siviy, 1994; Vanderschuren, Niesink, & Van Pee, 1997). By contrast, opioid receptor antagonists such as naltrexone reduce the reward-conditioning effects associated with each of these forms of social contact (Graves, Wallen, & Maestripieri, 2002; Holloway, Cornil, & Balthazart, 2004). In humans, the administration of the opioid antagonist naltrexone was associated with increased voluntary isolation from friends, as well as decreased levels of enjoyment in the company of others (Jamner & Leigh, 1999).

Importantly, tactile stimulation appears to play a particularly powerful role in the activation of affiliative reward conditioning (Melo et al., 2006). In some animals, the affiliative conditioning associated with maternal behavior is attenuated in the absence of tactile stimulation.

## Attachment and Social Affect Regulation

Many evolutionary accounts of the reproductive advantages of infant–caregiver bonds have been proposed, but similar accounts of adult attachment bonds are relatively recent (see Simpson & Belsky, Chapter 5, and Zeifman & Hazan, Chapter 20, this volume). Fraley and Shaver (2000) have proposed that adult attachments represent homologies of the infant–caregiver bond coopted by natural selection to facilitate pair bonding. By this account, adult and infant–caregiver attachment systems entail similar goals (the survival of offspring) and operate according to similar conditions of activation (e.g., presence of a threat) and termination (e.g., regulation of threat responding by the attachment figure). Evolutionary perspectives such as these address *ultimate* functions, in the sense of explaining why attachment bonds and capabilities persist among so many species.

Function can be considered in a more proximal, ontogenetic sense as well, and it is at this level that the regulation of affect may take center stage. Proximal functions of the attachment system are thought primarily to reflect social regulation of emotional responding. Bowlby (1969/1982), following along with Ainsworth, Blehar, Waters, and Wall (1978), argued that a critical function of attachment figures is the provision of a "secure base" from which infants can explore their worlds relatively free of anxiety, and a "safe haven" to which the infants can return when distressed. It was proposed, for example, that the base from which an infant can explore his or her world is secure to the extent that the caregiver is responsive to the infant's distress. Many have since proposed that the quality of the caregiver–infant attachment bond—especially of the caregiver's status as a secure base—holds consequences for child and adult emotional functioning, including styles of interpersonal relating and emotion regulation capabilities. A very large behavioral database now supports this notion with respect to both childhood and adulthood (Beckes & Coan, 2015).

Throughout childhood, and certainly by adulthood, the regulatory effects of attachment relationships are likely to be felt in two broad ways (Coan, 2011). The first is immediate, such as when the attachment figure *mediates* a decrease in emotional responding "online." An example of this may be when a caregiver holds a child's hand during a blood draw at the doctor's office, thus actively soothing the child's anxiety as it occurs. The second is more generalized, where the attachment figure *moderates* the degree of emotional responding through, for example, a "mental representation." These social regulatory moderators may manifest either as internal working models based on procedural and semantic memory, or as declarative, explicitly recalled mental images. Indeed, online regulation experiences are likely to condition mental representations in both implicit and declarative memory. In the sections that follow, immediate, online regulation is considered in contrast to mental representations of a putative attachment figure, often referred to as *internal working models*, that may serve to preempt the level of distress an individual experiences in the face of a potential threat.

## Socially Mediated Regulation

The psychological and physiological impact of everyday stress is offset in part by social buffering (Cohen & Wills, 1985). This social buffering occurs at all levels (e.g., group, caregiver, famil-

iar conspecific), but familiarity, physical contact, and attachment are associated with the strength of social regulation effects (Cohen, 2004; Cohen, Janicki-Deverts, Turner, & Doyle, in press). Even in rats, the presence of familiar conspecifics increases exploration and attenuates HPA axis activity under conditions of threat (Kiyokawa, Kikusui, Takeuchi, & Mori, 2004; Ruis et al., 1999). Familiar conspecifics attenuate emotional stress responding in nonhuman primates during new social group formation and social conflict (Gust, Gordon, Brodie, & McClure, 1996; Weaver & de Waal, 2003). These effects are widely believed to derive from the activity of oxytocin, vasopressin, and endogenous opioids in the VTA, ventral pallidum, nucleus accumbens, anterior cingulate, insular cortex, and portions of the ventromedial PFC (Carter & DeVries, 1999; Kosfeld, Heinrichs, Zak, Fischbacher, & Fehr, 2005; Loseth et al., 2014; Nocjar & Panksepp, 2007).

Increasingly, researchers have sought to identify how neural circuits associated with social affiliation and emotion function in contexts that combine some form of social interaction with externally generated emotional stress. For example, my colleagues and I have collected functional brain images from married women (Coan, Schaefer, & Davidson, 2006) and both male and female platonic friends (Coan, Beckes, & Allen, 2013), as they were subjected to the threat of mild electric shock while alone, and while holding hands with either a relational partner (spouse or friend) or anonymous experimenter. Our results suggest that supportive touch even from strangers can attenuate threat-related neural activity, and that these regulatory effects are moderated in important ways. Higher current relationship quality, for example, corresponds with greater regulation of threat-related neural activity in the right anterior insula, superior frontal gyrus, and hypothalamus during spousal, but not stranger, hand holding (Coan, Schaefer, & Davidson, 2006). And greater perceived *mutuality*—a measure of shared feelings, goals and interests—is associated with less threat-related activation of the lateral prefrontal cortex and supplementary motor cortex whether the relational partner is present or not (Coan, Kasle, Jackson, Schaefer, & Davidson, 2013).

Other work is converging on similar results. For example, in the presence of their mother, the brains of high-anxious children respond to anxiety-provoking words indistinguishably from those of low-anxious children, but high-anxious children show increased threat-related activation of the ventromedial PFC and hypothalamus while alone (Conner et al., 2012). Individuals show reduced pain and pain-related activation of the anterior insula and dorsal ACC when viewing images of a loved one (Eisenberger et al., 2011; Younger, Aron, Parke, Chatterjee, & Mackey, 2010). Indeed, the social regulation of pain is by now a well documented phenomenon (Krahé, Springer, Weinman, & Fotopoulou, 2013), with attachment style emerging as an important moderator (Sambo, Howard, Kopelman, Williams, & Fotopoulou, 2010; Wilson & Ruben, 2011). Even simple reminders of secure attachments reduce activation in the ventral ACC, PFC (lateral and medial), and hypothalamus during threat of social exclusion (Karremans, Heslenfeld, van Dillen, & Van Lange, 2011).

### Socially Moderated Regulation

Thus far, we have primarily considered basic systems supporting "normative" manifestations of attachment behavior, as well as concrete examples of regulatory functions of the attachment system. However, the regulatory effects of caregiving experiences, such as those between infants and caregivers, or even between romantic partners, are likely to extend far beyond online moments of soothing and security provision. Bowlby (1979) thought that early attachment experiences held implications for interpersonal and emotional functioning "from the cradle to the grave" (p. 129), and in the past several decades many researchers have adopted this idea as one way to understand adult interpersonal functioning (Mikulincer & Shaver, 2007).

Unfortunately, much of what is known about links among early social experience, neural development, and subsequent emotional behavior has been derived from studies of low social status, abuse, and neglect. For example, low status, neglectful, or abusive early social environments are associated with risks for heightened stress reactivity, anxiety, depression, and social deviance that extend well into adulthood (Gonzalez, Beckes, Chango, Allen, & Coan, 2015; Teicher, Samson, Polcari, & McGreenery, 2006). In one study, children who had experienced social deprivation and neglect in Romanian orphanages were observed to have lower overall levels of vasopressin, as well as blunted oxytocin responses to physical contact with their caregivers, relative to family-reared children (Wismer-Fries, Ziegler, Kurian, Jacoris, &

Pollak, 2005). Social isolation, generally, is a well-known risk factor for a number of neurodevelopmental, physiological, and psychosocial problems, ranging from anxiety and depression to increased risk of suicide, family discord, poor health behavior, cognitive decline, cardiovascular disease, stress-related dwarfism, increased vulnerability to trauma, and even all-cause death (Barber, Eccles, & Stone, 2001; Cacioppo & Cacioppo, 2014; Henriksen, Torsheim, & Thuen, 2014; House, Landis, & Umberson, 1988; Kawachi & Berkman, 2001; Knox & Uvnäs-Moberg, 1998; Newcomb & Bentler, 1988; Norman, Hawkley, Ball, Berntson, & Cacioppo, 2013; Skuse, Albanese, Stanhope, Gilmour, & Voss, 1996). In nonhuman primates, frequent or prolonged separation of offspring from caregivers (primarily mothers) can result in socially deviant behavior and dysregulated physiology later in life (Mineka & Suomi, 1978; Suomi, Chapter 7, this volume). Among brown capuchin monkeys, patterns of mother–offspring behavior partially determine the postconflict reconciliation styles of offspring during later interactions with nonfamilial conspecifics (Weaver & de Waal, 2003).

### Neural Mechanisms

Researchers have begun to identify neural mechanisms linking early parental care to trait-like individual differences in threat responding over the lifespan (Sachser et al., 2013; Weaver, Diorio, Seckl, Szyf, & Meaney, 2004). For example, in rats, grooming behavior by the mother "sets" or "programs" the degree to which her offspring react to threat cues throughout their lives. This modulation of threat reactivity has been observed both in behavior and in HPA axis activity. Moreover, associations between maternal grooming and offspring threat reactivity have been linked to the molecular regulation of genes that moderate HPA axis functioning. As reviewed earlier, the HPA axis has its own built-in regulatory mechanism in the hippocampus, whereby circulating cortisol activates hippocampal glucocorticoid receptors, which in turn down-regulate the production of CRH in the hypothalamus. Grooming attenuates the methylation of genes that encode for glucocorticoid receptors in the hippocampus, thus enhancing their expression and making the hippocampus more sensitive to circulating cortisol (Meaney & Szyf, 2005). Cross-fostering studies by Meaney and colleagues suggest that lifelong stress reactivity—

and even the subsequent maternal behavior of female rat pups—is attributable more to the degree
of postnatal maternal grooming than to genetic
inheritance (Weaver et al., 2004). More recent
studies suggest that similar patterns may soon be
found with regard to the methylation of genes that
encode for oxytocin receptors (Jack, Connelly, &
Morris, 2012; Kumsta, Hummel, Chen, & Heinrichs, 2013; Puglia, Lillard, Morris, & Connelly,
2015).

### Attachment and Internal Working Models

According to attachment theory (Bowlby,
1969/1982, 1973; Mikulincer & Shaver, 2007),
threat detection capabilities may have coevolved
with the attachment behavioral system, thus increasing the likelihood that humans will seek out
and maintain proximity to attachment figures from
infancy onward. From this perspective, distress alleviation could be considered a vital mechanism
through which attachments are formed (Beckes &
Coan, 2015), and the attachment system could be
considered a dedicated component of the brain's
overall stress response (Taylor et al., 2000, 2004).
Indeed, evidence suggests that even subliminally
presented threats increase access to attachment-
related cognitions and bias attention toward recognizing individuals who could be considered
more responsive to distress (Beckes et al., 2013;
Beckes, Simpson, & Erickson, 2010). Moderating the degree to which proximity to attachment
figures is sought in the context of a threat is "attachment security," which is presumed to be the
product of many attachment-related experiences
involving both threats and attachment figures.
These experiences shape "internal working models" of attachment that guide emotion regulation
throughout life (see Cassidy, 1994; Bretherton &
Munholland, Chapter 4, this volume). According
to Bowlby (1969/1982), internal working models
are mental representations of the responsiveness
and practical utility of attachment figures when
threats arise, and of the self in relationship with
these figures.

Indeed, Hofer (2006) has described a process
by which very early developmental experiences in
interactions with a caregiver may plausibly proceed
from the online regulation of fundamental neural
systems supporting sensorimotor, thermal, and nutritional functions to the shaping of internal working models of attachment security. In this model,
in early development, access to primary reinforcers
(e.g., food, water, warmth, touch) is dependent on
(1) caregiver support and (2) brain circuitry used
to solicit caregiver support via expressed affect.
Over the course of development, what begins as
the regulation of physiological needs via affect becomes the regulation of affect per se (Hofer, 2006).
Throughout this process, the regulatory behavior
of the attachment figure (e.g., the provision of
security, the alleviation of distress) is likely to set
expectations about the availability of attachment
figures during times of stress—the internal working models reflecting attachment security.

Thus, internal working models are likely to
reflect conditioned associations between proximity to attachment figures and both internal needs
and external signs of threat, mediated through the
amygdala, nucleus accumbens, and hippocampus, as well as portions of the PFC. These conditioned associations may remain stable for long
periods of time, especially to the extent that they
continue to be reinforced by internal feelings of
security, prevailing social contingencies, or both.
This process probably allows individuals to adapt
themselves to a variety of environmental conditions (e.g., security-restoring or security-enhancing experiences with attachment figures, frequent
or lengthy absence of the caregiver, abuse by the
caregiver, excessive caregiving). Such adaptations are referred to in various research traditions
as "attachment patterns," "attachment styles," or
"attachment states of mind" (e.g., secure, anxious
or ambivalent, avoidant, preoccupied). These adaptations are thought to be relatively stable when
the individual remains in a stable environment,
and can be measured by observations, self-report
questionnaires, and structured interviews (e.g.,
in this volume, see Crowell, Fraley, & Roisman,
Chapter 27; Kerns & Brumariu, Chapter 17; Solomon & George, Chapter 18).

Behavioral research on the effects of different
adult attachment styles suggests the presence of
two relatively independent axes regarding attachment insecurity—anxiety and avoidance—along
which individuals can vary (J. A. Feeney, Chapter 21 this volume; Mikulincer & Shaver, 2007).
Moreover, different combinations of scores along
these dimensions can result in particular styles
of interpersonal relating. For example, individuals low in attachment anxiety and in attachment
avoidance are considered generally secure in their
attachments to others. Individuals high in both
avoidance and anxiety are thought to avoid attachment relationships out of fear, while those
high in avoidance but low in anxiety are thought
to be dismissing of attachments, compulsively

self-reliant, and unlikely to seek proximity to attachment figures under stress (Bartholomew & Horowitz, 1991; Brennan, Clark, & Shaver, 1998). Finally, individuals low in avoidance but high in anxiety are thought to be preoccupied with the status of their attachment relationships and the availability of attachment figures.

Although a number of researchers are now examining associations between attachment style and neural activity, dedicated circuits that are causally responsible for attachment style remain mysterious, if indeed there are any. In most cases, attachment styles manifest as individual differences in responses among neural circuits that otherwise generally support emotion, emotion regulation, threat vigilance, and social cognition (Vrtička & Vuilleumier, 2012). Early studies suggested that insecurely attached infants of depressed mothers were more likely to show PFC asymmetries lateralized to the right (Dawson et al., 2001). EEG asymmetries in alpha power (8–13 Hz) correspond with emotional reactivity and regulation, with relatively greater left PFC activity indexing an increased probability of approach behavior, and relatively greater right PFC activity indexing an increased probability of avoidance (Coan & Allen, 2004; Coan, Allen, & McKnight, 2006; Steiner & Coan, 2011). Thus, according to Dawson and colleagues (2001), insecurely attached infants of depressed mothers have a trait-like propensity to engage in avoidance behavior. This is consistent with recent observations of greater amygdala volumes in adults who were identified as insecurely attached a full 22 years earlier (Moutsiana et al., 2015). Moreover, individuals who score high in attachment avoidance may have lower cell density within the hippocampus—a condition also associated with clinical conditions such as posttraumatic stress disorder (PTSD) (Quirin, Gillath, Pruessner, & Eggert, 2010). At the genetic level, attachment anxiety and avoidance are associated with polymorphisms in dopaminergic and serotonergic receptor genes, respectively (Gillath, Shaver, Baek, & Chun, 2008), suggesting that insecurity is influenced in part by genetic vulnerabilities to social dysfunction and emotional dysregulation.

Securely attached individuals may be generally less reactive to distress, even in very early attentional processing (Nash, Prentice, Hirsh, McGregor, & Inzlicht, 2014), though security primes have also been associated with *increased* prefrontal, striatal, and parahippocampal activity, probably reflecting increments in self-regulatory motivation and capability (Canterberry & Gillath, 2013;

Eisenberger et al., 2011; Younger et al., 2010). Insecure attachment, by contrast, has been associated with elevated neural activity throughout the brain under conditions of threat, stress, and pain. Indeed, avoidant attachment has been associated with more, not less, activation of prefrontal systems associated with emotion regulation, suggesting that insecure attachment may entail increased regulatory activity attributable either to diminished regulatory efficiency or greater emotional burden (Vrtička, Bondolfi, Sander, & Vuilleumier, 2012), with heightened emotional burden being the most likely explanation. For example, high attachment avoidance is associated with greater laser-evoked N2 and P2 amplitudes—putative EEG measures of threat salience—in the presence of romantic partners (Krahé et al., 2015). This suggests that attachment-related avoidance renders potentially threatening stimuli even more threatening, at least when other people are present. This also raises interesting questions about the function of this kind of avoidance, which may include a desire to avoid additional burdens associated with close relationships. Under ordinary circumstances, time with relational partners may be enjoyable and even relaxing, but for avoidant individuals, stress entails dealing with not only the stressor but also the relational partner. Partners in this case are costs rather than resources. Thus, for such people, it may be best to be alone when stressed.

Attachment anxiety has also been associated with a variety of threat- and pain-related processes in the brain. For example, individuals high in attachment anxiety show increased responding in the dorsal anterior cingulate cortex (dACC)—a region associated with identifying salience and incongruities with expected outcomes—in addition to the right amygdala and parahippocampal areas (Buchheim et al., 2006; DeWall et al., 2012; Gillath, Bunge, Shaver, Wendelken, & Mikulincer, 2005; Vrtička et al., 2012). Importantly, while considering negative relationship scenarios, higher attachment anxiety scores correspond with increased activation within the temporal pole on the one hand and diminished orbitofrontal activity on the other (Gillath et al., 2005). This suggests that individuals high in attachment anxiety have trouble engaging regulatory systems when signs of relationship trouble are present. In summary, these studies suggest that individuals high in attachment anxiety may suffer from greater emotional reactivity, mediated through heightened vigilance for potential threats, especially because of an insecurity about the availability of social resources.

## Social Baseline Theory

Social affect regulation, within the context of attachment theory, can be viewed as a core function of attachment relationships. Social influences on the regulation of affect are sufficiently powerful and unconditioned to suggest that the brain's first and most effective approach to affect regulation is via social proximity and interaction. This is most obvious during infancy, in which very basic physiological needs are regulated first via affect expression, leading to a dynamic of regulating affect per se (Hofer, 2006). For the infant, this is occurring in a context of rapid and expansive neural development—possibly a "critical period" during which a number of expectations about the nature of the infant's future environment are formed. Much of this development is occurring in the PFC, a region of the brain powerfully implicated, among many other things, in affect regulation. Because the PFC is underdeveloped in infancy, the caregiver effectively serves as a kind of surrogate PFC (Gee et al., 2013)—a function that may hold a number of neurodevelopmental consequences for emotion reactivity and regulation throughout life (Gee et al., 2014; Tottenham, 2012).

Social baseline theory (Beckes & Coan, 2011; Coan & Sbarra, 2015) suggests that social affect regulation was long ago adopted as an efficient and cost-effective means of regulating affect. It draws on the "economy of action" principle built into biological systems that requires organisms to consume more energy than they expend if they are to survive to reproduce (Proffitt, 2006). Because all bodily activities (including neural activities) expend energy, energy expenditure must be managed. Proffitt has proposed that one of the ways in which the brain manages energy expenditure is via changes in sensory perception that aid in decision making about the deployment of an organism's resources. For example, Proffitt has observed that donning a heavy backpack causes hills to appear steeper and objects to appear farther away, thus discouraging individuals from using their resources to climb those hills or approach those objects. In this way, the brain can be thought of as a "Bayesian machine," making "bets" at any given time about what resources to deploy and at what level of effort (Clark, 2013; Friston, 2010).

Social baseline theory draws on this Bayesian view of the brain to propose that social species in fact *assume* relatively close proximity to conspecifics because they have adopted social proximity and interaction as an environmental niche (Beckes & Coan, 2011). For humans especially, social proximity and interaction are strategies for economizing energy expenditure in everything from raising children (Burkart, Hrdy, & Van Schaik, 2009) to regulating basal metabolic rates and core body temperatures (Nuñez-Villegas, Bozinovic, & Sabat, 2014). This implies that the absence or loss of conspecifics, in defying this baseline assumption, functionally adds to the perceived cost of interacting with the environment—especially in (but not limited to) threatening contexts (Coan & Sbarra, 2015). Bowlby (1969/1982) held an explicitly similar view of human adaptation, also detailing the emotional damage wrought by a relational partner (parent, romantic partner, friend, even a stranger) who is simply unresponsive in times of need (Beckes & Coan, 2015). Ultimately, both attachment theory and social baseline theory propose that social isolation is, for a social organism, akin to donning a heavy backpack: It alters both the real and perceived costs of survival. In proposing social baseline theory, I do not intend to invalidate or supplant attachment theory. Rather, my interest in social baseline theory is to describe a more generalized and abstracted set of neural and ecological principles—principles that may shed light on mechanisms underlying the attachment dynamics described by Bowlby almost half a century ago. To this end, social baseline theory starts with at least two ways in which the presence of conspecifics may reduce, for social organisms, the actual and perceived cost of engagement with the environment. I call these strategies "risk distribution" and "load sharing."

### Risk Distribution

The first way in which social species, including humans, benefit from close social proximity is via the simple distribution of risk in the environment—colloquially, through safety in numbers. Many species benefit from living in groups, and simple risk distribution strategies are likely to be *plesiomorphic*, or relatively ancient, in evolutionary terms. Although group living incurs resource consumption costs, the benefits may outweigh those costs sufficiently to create conditions under which group cohesion ultimately promotes the survival of each individual in the group. Risk distribution speaks to the amount of risk a given individual carries as a function of the degree to which he or she is alone, and it can manifest in many ways (Davies, Krebs, & West, 2012). For example, any given individual is at substantially reduced risk of personal danger (e.g., predation) when group size increases. Among many species there is a thermal advantage of huddling, a process known as *social thermoregulation* (Canals, Rosenmann, & Bozinovic, 1989). Some social species utilize group size to maximize their performance as predators; this too can be a form of risk distribution, for if contact with prey is maximized by groups of predators, the risk that any one predator will perish from starvation is minimized.

Social species are capable of assessing the distribution of risk and making Bayesian decisions about the cost-effectiveness of a variety of behaviors at any given time. Practically speaking, the presence or absence of conspecifics provides, at the lowest level of social proximity, a heuristic for deploying potentially costly resources. For example, in the presence of conspecifics, ostriches are less vigilant for predators. Indeed, the degree to which ostriches engage in vigilance behavior while searching for food decreases steadily as group members are added—even as the overall vigilance each ostrich benefits from does not change (Bertram, 1980). Insofar as activities such as threat vigilance are effortful—are yoked to perceived bodily resources or opportunity costs—they are deployed only as needed. Resources that are saved by social proximity are either conserved or applied to other valuable purposes.

## Load Sharing

Risk distribution is likely to influence attention—particularly vigilance for potential danger—and this may bring wider implications for cognitive and affective activities that either share attentional circuitry or compete with that circuitry for metabolic resources carried in the blood (see Dietrich, 2009). But the impact of risk distribution on a host of other cortical and behavioral activities is likely to be more limited. This is especially true of prefrontal regions supporting working memory and inhibitory control—including the self-regulation of emotional responses. Interestingly, such prefrontally mediated activities are thought to be particularly costly to deploy for long periods of time, either because they compete with other regions for blood or entail an opportunity cost by limiting other vital functions mediated through the same regions (Dietrich, 2004, 2009; Kurzban, Duckworth, Kable, & Myers, 2013). Evidence for this derives in part from studies of "ego depletion" as a consequence of effortful attention, working memory, and self-control. In this work, individuals who are asked to engage in tasks re-

quiring self-regulation are commonly less capable of similar tasks later on. Importantly, these and similar depletion effects are likely attributable to the way the brain "budgets" its available resources as a function of expected future demands, rather than the literal depletion of currently available fuel within the brain (Job, Dweck, & Walton, 2010; Kurzban, 2010).

Social baseline theory predicts that the PFC and many of the regulatory processes it supports may be particularly affected by the presence of an attachment figure, especially in, but not limited to, the context of a threat. Here the advantage of close proximity extends far beyond simple models of risk distribution: Over and above the probabilistic dilution of risk, a trusted and interdependent associate can be counted on to engage in a number of health- and safety-enhancing behaviors on one's behalf. Such behaviors may include the identification and acquisition of resources, vigilance for future environmental threats, caring for one's needs, and nurturing of one's offspring. These allegiances—these attachments—serve to distribute the cost of many of life's metabolically expensive activities, not least being the regulation of one's own negative affect. Simply put, affect regulation is possible, but more difficult, in isolation. I refer to this second level of social regulation as "load sharing," and I believe it is an essential component of attachment relationships throughout the lifespan. Load sharing is likely to be relatively *apomorphic*, or more specific to social animals, particularly humans. Human brains are highly sensitive to the load-sharing significance of close attachment bonds and adjust their efforts accordingly. For example, individuals in close, trusted relationships will invest less effort in down-regulating their negative affect, leaving them less responsive to threat cues and other signs of possible harm (Coan, Schaefer, & Davidson, 2006; Coan et al., 2013; Edens et al., 1992; Mikulincer & Florian, 1998; Robles & Kiecolt-Glaser, 2003). Indeed, humans will spontaneously down-regulate their efforts in the presence even of strangers if all are engaged in a shared goal (Ingham, Levinger, Graves, & Peckham, 1974). And humans just as spontaneously engage in goal and intention sharing (Tomasello, Carpenter, Call, Behne, & Moll, 2005; Warneken & Tomasello, 2009). Thus, the social brain may be designed to distribute both physical and cognitive effort across social networks as a function of common goal pursuit, and this may be a key process in how attachment relationships facilitate successful affect regulation.

Unlike risk distribution strategies, which are primarily sensitive to numbers alone, load sharing is likely to develop as the brains of individuals in a relationship become familiar with one another, especially in the context of coping with adversity or sharing goals. Over time, individuals in attachment relationships may literally become part of each other's emotional response and regulation strategy. This is not metaphorical, but literal, even at the neural level. For example, we have observed that the brain encodes threats to familiar friends almost as if those threats were directed at the self, but also that threats directed at strangers are encoded quite differently (Beckes, Coan, & Hasselmo, 2013). We, and others before us (most notably Aron and colleagues; cf. Aron & Aron, 1996; Aron & Fraley, 1999; Mashek, Aron, & Boncimino, 2003), have suggested that this reflects an incorporation of the familiar other into the neural representation of the self—that, indeed, this may well be what the subjective feeling of familiarity *is* at the neural level. The self is, after all, not something the brain has so much as *does*. Being a collection of neural circuits tasked with a job, the "self" is likely to be quite flexible, indeed both expandable and collapsible, with implications for how the brain budgets its bioenergetic resources, and always with the corollary goal of economizing those resources if possible. As applied to affect regulation and attachment theory, a man who has been alone for a long period of time may learn to depend heavily on his own prefrontally mediated emotion regulation capabilities, but upon establishing an attachment relationship, the degree to which he perceives his environment to be threatening may diminish in proportion to the perceived increase in resources brought to bear by the attachment figure, and, in turn, his emotion regulatory burden will lighten. The effect should literally reduce the frequency with which he exercises his PFC in the service of emotion regulation. With sufficient experience in the relationship, the level of interdependence associated with emotion regulation needs can become strong. Indeed, a grim reminder of this occurs when one or the other member of an attached pair is suddenly absent due to death or divorce, leaving the partner severely dysregulated (Krietsch, Mason, & Sbarra, 2014; O'Connor & Arizmendi, 2014; Sbarra, Law, & Portley, 2011; Schultze-Florey et al., 2012).

As mentioned above, we have observed this dynamic in vivo using a paradigm that combines supportive touch with the threat of electric shock, all during fMRI. In the first of these studies (Coan,

Schaefer, & Davidson, 2006), married women in an MRI scanner were confronted with the threat of a mild electric shock under each of three conditions: while alone, while holding a stranger's hand, and while holding their spouse's hand. Women in the highest-quality relationships showed the lowest degree of threat-related brain activation, limiting their response to relatively automatic regulation of threat perception via structures such as the ventromedial PFC. When a marital relationship was of relatively poor quality, however, the number of problems confronting a woman's brain under threat increased to include attention to bodily sensory afferents, presumably related to the threat of shock (right anterior insula), task salience (superior frontal gyrus), and release of regulatory stress hormones (hypothalamus). As the hand-holding partner switched from attachment figure to stranger, however, yet more problems presented themselves, with additional threat-related brain activations triggered to solve them. For example, threat-related vigilance increased (e.g., via the superior colliculus); effortful emotion regulation strategies were employed (e.g., via the right dorsolateral PFC); and areas were recruited that indicated increased threat-related avoidance motivation (e.g., the caudate and nucleus accumbens). But when facing the threat alone, the brain appeared to perceive yet more problems requiring attention, adding—to the already enumerated threat responses—increasing bodily arousal (e.g., through the ventral ACC) and the coordination of visceral and musculoskeletal responses (e.g., via the posterior cingulate, supramarginal gyrus, and postcentral gyrus). Since then, we have observed a similar pattern of results when the relational partner was a platonic friend (Coan et al., 2013), and among couples suffering from relationship distress *after*, but not before, 20 weeks of attachment-related emotionally focused couple therapy supervised by Susan Johnson (Johnson et al., 2013; Brassard & Johnson, Chapter 35, this volume).

Importantly, the social affect regulation observed in these studies appears to be a mediated through a relatively bottom-up process, as opposed to solo affect regulation, which is more top-down. When engaging in self-regulation, a person is likely to engage in costly, effortful cognitive and attentional strategies in the service of inhibiting either somatic responses or neural activity supporting the identification of threats. This effortful regulation of affect relies to a great degree on the PFC. In this way, self-regulation frequently occurs in the context of an affective response that has already transpired. By contrast, social affect regulation may be mediated through early perception, decreasing threat sensitivity and obviating the need for any self-regulatory effort at all. Thus, social affect regulation could be characterized as more efficient, or less costly, than self-regulation strategies (cf. Gross & Thompson, 2007) such as the suppression of emotional responses, cognitive reappraisal, or mindfulness meditation. The extent to which this is true awaits further investigation.

### Attachment Styles as Bayesian Priors

Of course, the preceding discussion offers only a simplified, normative, idealized model of social affect regulation. It is likely that superimposed on all of the processes described earlier are trait-like, and to some extent experience-based, assumptions about the function and metabolic cost of social factors in regulating the perception of threats, and hence of affect (Bar-Kalifa & Rafaeli, 2015). Accordingly, one way to conceptualize attachment styles and internal working models is as prior probabilities in a Bayesian decision-making process (Clark, 2013; Friston, 2010), in which the goal is to predict the regulatory cost-effectiveness of potential attachment figures (Coan, 2010). In this way, attachment styles represent strategies, based on prior experience, for making decisions about how to utilize one's own neural resources in the presence or absence of strangers and attachment figures. Indeed, we have observed that individuals who experienced higher levels of (behaviorally coded) maternal support in early adolescence were—12 years later—also less responsive to threat cues in the insula and PFC during supportive hand holding by a friend. Individuals whose childhood neighborhoods were characterized by low social capital and high crime showed the opposite pattern, with supportive hand holding having less of a regulatory effect (Coan et al., 2013).

A secure attachment style presumably disposes a person to make bets closely in accordance with the idealized picture described earlier. By contrast, avoidant and anxious strategies may encourage individuals to make greater use of their own resources even in the presence of social support, or to place themselves outside the reach of social support in the hopes of avoiding additional costs (e.g., having to regulate others as well as self), thus, again, requiring them to rely on their own emotion regulation strategies. At present, this Bayesian conceptualization of attachment style is predominantly a matter of conjecture. I expect that future neuroscientific studies of attachment will provide additional clues to the nature of social affect regulation in the brain.

### Recommendations and Conclusions

In this chapter, I have sought (1) to synthesize a broad array of studies in the service of introducing the reader to the current state of the neurosciences as they pertain to research on attachment, and (2) to propose a plausible model of how what is known about the social brain and affect regulation may eventually be combined with attachment theory. This effort has necessarily included discussions of the neural constituents of attachment, from neural systems supporting emotion and motivation to those supporting emotion regulation, filial bonding, familiarity, proximity seeking, and individual differences in attachment style. What follows is a partial list of recommendations for researchers excited about pursuing the neuroscience of attachment. (Other models and suggestions can be found in other chapters in this volume, especially Simpson & Belsky, Chapter 5; Hane & Fox, Chapter 11; and Polan & Hofer, Chapter 6.)

• *Expand the cognitive and emotional repertoire in laboratory challenges.* Studies of the neural systems underlying attachment should combine the presence or absence of attachment cues (e.g., proximity to attachment figures) with laboratory situations that elicit a range of emotional responses— not only threats but also potential rewards, losses, and even effortful cognitive activity that may be affectively ambiguous (Coan & Maresh, 2014). Many theorists have proposed that the attachment behavioral system is activated during threats to the individual or to the individual's attachment bond, but few researchers of attachment processes at the neural level have actually designed studies with this in mind. Fewer still have sought to identify how social contact influences neural responses to positive affect elicitations. Social baseline theory suggests that attachment figures may offset the cognitive (and indeed physiological) costs of a wide variety of activities (Coan & Sbarra, 2015), and the full range ought to be explored. In my view, much recent work points to the regulatory impact of social relationships in ways that have yet to be framed from the perspective of attachment theory. For example, proximity to social resources may alter visual sensory perception (Gross & Proffitt, 2013), the frequency of supportive interpersonal touch may affect athletic performance (Kraus, Huang, & Keltner, 2010), and collective IQ (the IQ score of a group) may increase more as a function of sensitivity to interpersonal social cues than of individual intelligence (Woolley, Chabris, Pentland, Hashmi, & Malone, 2010). Moreover, the increasing sensitivity and even portability of modern neuroimaging techniques (e.g., functional near-infrared imaging, wireless EEG) offer great creative potential for moving the neuroscience of attachment into more nuanced and comprehensive cognitive and emotional territory.

• *Be sensitive to sex differences.* Little is known about how the sex of an individual under study affects activity in the attachment behavioral system, or indeed the neural constituents of attachment. Self-reported sex differences have been noted in behavioral studies, however. For example, women are more likely to endorse items indicating a preoccupied attachment strategy characterized by worry that their partners will leave them, whereas men are more likely to endorse a dismissive or avoidant strategy characterized by discomfort with interpersonal closeness (Bartholomew & Horowitz, 1991). And many have observed that women are most bothered by their male partners' avoidance, whereas men are most bothered by their female partners' anxiety (Mikulincer & Shaver, 2007). Others have reported sex differences in relationship stability as a function of attachment styles, suggesting that attachment styles may interact in important ways with gender roles (Kirkpatrick & Davis, 1994).

• *Pursue animal models of attachment style.* To date, there are virtually no studies of attachment *styles* in nonhuman animals, despite growing evidence that other personality dimensions are evident in nonhuman animals (Gosling, 2008). The "Big Five" personality structure and distribution are very similar in humans and chimpanzees (King & Figueredo, 1997), and the anxiety and avoidance dimensions of attachment style are somewhat related to the Big Five traits of Neuroticism and Agreeableness, respectively (Noftle & Shaver, 2006). Other personality traits shared to one degree or another with humans have been observed in species as diverse as gorillas, hyenas, domesticated dogs, cats, donkeys, pigs, rats, octopi, and even guppies (Gosling & John, 1999). Attempts to study attachment styles in nonhuman animals would constitute a badly needed step toward bridging the gaps between the human and animal literatures addressing attachment behavior. Indeed, recent work suggests that dogs might be a good place to start looking at animal attachment styles. Dogs are increasingly understood to possess a degree of sensitivity to social cues in humans that may surpass even our nearest genetic relatives (Hare, Brown, Williamson, & Tomasello, 2002; Hare & Tomasello, 2005).

• *Allow for systemic effects in research designs.* Most attachment style research identifies effects of a given participant's attachment style on his or her own attachment behavior. One question of great interest is the degree to which the attachment style of one member of a dyad affects the behavior of the other member. (See J. A. Feeney, Chapter 21, this volume, for examples.) For instance, Coan, Schaefer, and Davidson (2005) presented evidence that in married couples, the husband's preoccupation score corresponded with increased neural threat reactivity throughout the wife's brain if she was holding the hand of a stranger (while her possibly jealous husband looked on). More generally, we know that relationship satisfaction is affected by the attachment style of an individual's relationship partner (Kane et al., 2007). A neuroscience of attachment will benefit from an understanding of how systemic or dyadic effects of attachment style affect current cognitive and emotional functioning.

• *Seek to understand contextual and situational influences.* Nearly a half-century of research makes clear that personality is most stable within classes of situations as opposed to across situations (Mischel, Shoda, & Mendoza-Denton, 2002). Indeed, individual differences in brain activity are more reliable and predictive when evoked by a laboratory challenge than when trying to capture a general trait that is situation-independent, as in the commonly explored "resting" condition (Coan, Allen, et al., 2006; Stewart, Coan, Towers, & Allen, 2014). Applied to attachment theory, we can reasonably ask: Is a particular woman secure in her relationship with her spouse to the same degree that she is in her relationship with her best friend, mother, or sister? Moreover, does her attachment style manifest itself in the same way to a threat to her relationship as to her personal sense of bodily harm? Would she have endorsed the same level of security during a previous relationship that she does in her current one? Some studies suggest that within-person variation in attachment style across different relationships may be substantial (La Guardia, Ryan, Couchman, &

Deci, 2000), even if a stable higher-order attachment style persists across time and situations (Fraley, 2002; Fraley, Vicary, Brumbaugh, & Roisman, 2011). This is likely to be especially true at the neural level, where measures can be very sensitive to small changes in context.

• *Implement longitudinal designs.* One extremely important problem for the neuroscience of attachment is delineating the process by which two individuals progress from not being attached to being attached (for discussion, see Zeifman & Hazan, Chapter 20, this volume). What is the rate at which this typically occurs? How is this affected by attachment style? What is the role of distress and its alleviation (Beckes & Coan, 2015)? With special relevance to this chapter, which neural structures associated with emotional responding, motivation, and emotion regulation are particularly sensitive to this process? For example, at what point, or with what kinds of interpersonal experiences, does a stranger who regulates the brain's autonomic and musculoskeletal response to threat become a partner who regulates additional neural processes related to effortful affect regulation and threat vigilance? How does the ability to regulate one's own emotional responses covary with one's ability to yield to the regulatory efforts of a loved one? Longitudinal studies may also address questions of within-subject variation in attachment style over both time and relationships.

• *Pursue clinical implications.* As I reviewed briefly earlier, and as discussed by scores of other scholars in recent decades (Cacioppo et al., 2007; Holt-Lunstad, Smith, & Layton, 2010; House et al., 1988; *PLoS Medicine* Editors, 2010; Robles & Kiecolt-Glaser, 2003), social relationships hold major implications for health and well-being. As the neural mechanisms supporting these effects become better known, it may be possible to implement clinical interventions that not only emphasize the forging and maintenance of close relationships, but also focus on the use of social affect regulation for clinical purposes.

For example, we have used relationship therapy to transform couples that do not show a strong social regulation effect on neural threat responding into those that do (Johnson et al., 2013). But the inclusion of attachment figures may potentiate the therapeutic effects of individual interventions as well. For example, the presence of a relational partner may reduce the level of attentional disengagement that highly anxious people deploy in stressful situations (Maresh, Beckes, & Coan,

2013). This may at first blush not seem like much of an advantage, but consider that attentional disengagement—an extreme avoidance response to stress—may be implemented because individuals are unable to cope with stressors experienced as too overwhelming. This is why experiential avoidance can be a significant impediment to treatment in disorders such as PTSD, which can require sometimes intense emotional responding during exposure (Badour, Blonigen, Boden, Feldner, & Bonn-Miller, 2012). Indeed, there is a growing interest in providing individual therapy in conjunction with dyadic interventions (Baucom, Belus, Adelman, Fischer, & Paprocki, 2014; Johnson, 2002). It warrants emphasis here that most stress reduction techniques involve highly individualized activities (e.g., cognitive-behavioral therapy, mindfulness meditation) that may be less efficient or more effortful than they would be if done in the context of supportive social networks or attachment relationships. Few or no cognitive or meditation-based interventions are designed with this specifically in mind.

Finally, the careful delineation of neural systems underlying attachment can expand our basic understanding of a wide variety of disorders that implicate social processes. The potential exists for this work to inform research on disorders ranging from autism to fragile X syndrome, Williams syndrome, depression, social anxiety, schizophrenia, and virtually all of the personality disorders (most or all of which are more or less defined in terms of social behaviors).

• *Differentiate behavioral from neural systems.* A major challenge to future neuroscientists interested in the study of attachment will be the temptation to think of the attachment behavioral system as a unitary neural construct, which it almost certainly is not. Numerous neural processes, each with its own unique problems to solve, contribute to what we have come to call the "attachment behavioral system"; indeed, this system may be little more than a convenient rubric for describing the collective social activities of social bonding and social affect regulation. On the other hand, the attachment behavioral system may represent an emergent property of its constituent neural components that is, under some conditions and in some situations, relatively irreducible.

• *Collaborate.* The neuroscience of attachment represents uncommonly fertile ground for a wide variety of researchers, from neuroscientists to psychologists, biologists, physicians, epidemiologists, and others. Individuals from diverse scientific traditions can contribute many essential pieces to this fundamentally important puzzle. Because this area is so necessarily multidisciplinary, researchers interested in these and related questions will do well to explore contacts in related disciplines as their particular research questions call for it (Cacioppo et al., 2007). It is for precisely this reason that collaborations are increasingly the norm among the social, cognitive, and affective neurosciences, as well as among molecular geneticists interested in attachment-related neural functioning (cf. Bakermans-Kranenburg & Van IJzendoorn, 2008; Chapter 8, this volume; Puglia et al., 2015). Such collaborations enrich the science and often richly reward the scientists who take part. When focused on a question as fundamentally important as the neuroscience of attachment, I expect that collaborative efforts will be embraced with great enthusiasm.

## Acknowledgments

I would like to thank Jude Cassidy and Philip R. Shaver for their helpful comments on this chapter.

## References

Adolphs, R., Baron-Cohen, S., & Tranel, D. (2002). Impaired recognition of social emotions following amygdala damage. *Journal of Cognitive Neuroscience*, 14, 1264–1274.

Agmo, A., Barreau, S., & Lemaire, V. (1997). Social motivation in recently weaned rats is modified by opiates. *Developmental Neuroscience*, 19, 505–520.

Aguilera, G., & Liu, Y. (2012). The molecular physiology of CRH neurons. *Frontiers in Neuroendocrinology*, 33(1), 67–84.

Aharon, I., Etcoff, N., Ariely, D., Chabris, C. F., O'Connor, E., & Breiter, H. C. (2001). Beautiful faces have variable reward value: fMRI and behavioral evidence. *Neuron*, 32, 537–551.

Ainsworth, M. D. S. (1989). Attachments beyond infancy. *American Psychologist*, 44, 709–716.

Ainsworth, M. D. S., Blehar, M. C., Waters, E., & Wall, S. (1978). *Patterns of attachment: A psychological study of the strange situation*. Hillsdale, NJ: Erlbaum.

Aragona, D. J., Liu, Y., Yu, Y. J., Curtis, J. T., Detwiler, J. M., Insel, T. R., et al. (2006). Nucleus accumbens dopamine differentially mediates the formation and maintenance of monogamous pair bonds. *Nature Neuroscience*, 9, 134–139.

Aron, A., & Fraley, B. (1999). Relationship closeness as

including other in the self: Cognitive underpinnings and measures. *Social Cognition*, 17, 140–160.

Aron, E. N., & Aron, A. (1996). Love and expansion of the self: the state of the model. *Personal Relationships*, 3, 45–58.

Badour, C. L., Blonigen, D. M., Boden, M. T., Feldner, M. T., & Bonn-Miller, M. O. (2012). A longitudinal test of the bi-directional relations between avoidance coping and PTSD severity during and after PTSD treatment. *Behaviour Research and Therapy*, 50(10), 610–616.

Bakermans-Kranenburg, M. J., & Van IJzendoorn, M. H. (2008). Oxytocin receptor (OXTR) and serotonin transporter (5-HTT) genes associated with observed parenting. *Social Cognitive and Affective Neuroscience*, 3(2), 128–134.

Balfour, M. E., Yu, L., & Coolen, L. M. (2004). Sexual behavior and sex-associated environmental cues activate the mesolimbic system in male rats. *Neuropsychopharmacology*, 29, 718–730.

Bar-Kalifa, E., & Rafaeli, E. (2014). Above and below baselines: The nonmonotonic effects of dyadic emotional support in daily life. *Journal of Social and Personal Relationships*, 32, 161–179.

Barber, B. L., Eccles, J. S., & Stone, M. R. (2001). Whatever happened to the jock, the brain, and the princess?: Young adult pathways linked to adolescent activity involvement and social identity. *Journal of Adolescent Research*, 16(5), 429–455.

Bard, K. A. (1983). The effect of peer separation in young chimpanzees (*Pan troglodytes*). *American Journal of Primatology*, 5, 25–37.

Bartholomew, K., & Horowitz, L. M. (1991). Attachment styles among young adults: A test of a four-category model. *Journal of Personality and Social Psychology*, 61, 226–244.

Baucom, D. H., Belus, J. M., Adelman, C. B., Fischer, M. S., & Paprocki, C. (2014). Couple-based interventions for psychopathology: A renewed direction for the field. *Family Process*, 53(3), 445–461.

Beckes, L., & Coan, J. A. (2011). Social baseline theory: The role of social proximity in emotion and economy of action. *Social and Personality Psychology Compass*, 5(12), 976–988.

Beckes, L., & Coan, J. A. (2015). The distress-relief dynamic in attachment bonding. In V. Zayas & C. Hazan (Eds.), *Bases of adult attachment: From brain to mind to behavior* (pp. 11–33). New York: Springer.

Beckes, L., Coan, J. A., & Hasselmo, K. (2013). Familiarity promotes the blurring of self and other in the neural representation of threat. *Social Cognitive and Affective Neuroscience*, 8, 670–677.

Beckes, L., Coan, J. A., & Morris, J. P. (2013). Implicit conditioning of faces via the social regulation of emotion: ERP evidence of early attentional biases for security conditioned faces. *Psychophysiology*, 50(8), 734–742.

Beckes, L., Simpson, J. A., & Erickson, A. (2010). Of

snakes and succor: Learning secure attachment associations with novel faces via negative stimulus pairings. *Psychological Science*, 21(5), 721–728.

Benuzzi, F., Pugnaghi, M., Meletti, S., Lui, F., Serafini, M., Baraldi, P., et al. (2007). Processing the socially relevant parts of faces. *Brain Research Bulletin*, 74, 344–356.

Beny, Y., & Kimchi, T. (2014). Innate and learned aspects of pheromone-mediated social behaviours. *Animal Behaviour*, 97, 301–311.

Berardi, N., & Maffei, L. (1999). From visual experience to visual function: Roles of neurotrophins. *Journal of Neurobiology*, 41, 119–126.

Berridge, K. C. (2007). The debate over dopamine's role in reward: The case for incentive salience. *Psychopharmacology*, 191, 391–431.

Bertram, B. C. R. (1980). Vigilance and group size in ostriches. *Animal Behaviour*, 28(1), 278–286.

Bowlby, J. (1973). *Attachment and loss: Vol. 2. Separation: Anxiety and anger*. New York: Basic Books.

Bowlby, J. (1979). *The making and breaking of affectional bonds*. London: Tavistock.

Bowlby, J. (1982). *Attachment and loss: Vol. 1. Attachment* (2nd ed.). New York: Basic Books. (Original work published 1969)

Bozarth, M. A., & Wise, R. A. (1996). Toxicity associated with long-term intravenous heroin and cocaine self-administration in the rat. *Journal of the American Medical Association*, 254, 81–83.

Brasted, P. J., Bussey, T. J., Murray, E. A., & Wise, S. P. (2003). Role of the hippocampal system in associative learning beyond the spatial domain. *Brain*, 126, 1202–1223.

Brennan, K. A., Clark, C. L., & Shaver, P. R. (1998). Self-report measurement of adult attachment: An integrative overview. In J. A. Simpson & W. S. Rholes (Eds.), *Attachment theory and close relationships*. (pp. 46–76). New York: Guilford Press.

Briones, T. L., Klintsova, A. Y., & Greenough, W. T. (2004). Stability of synaptic plasticity in the adult rat visual cortex induced by complex environment exposure. *Brain Research*, 1018, 130–135.

Buchheim, A., Erk, S., George, C., Kachele, H., Ruchsow, M., Spitzer, M., et al. (2006). Measuring attachment representation in an FMRI environment: A pilot study. *Psychopathology*, 39(3), 144–152.

Burkart, J. M., Hrdy, S. B., & Van Schaik, C. P. (2009). Cooperative breeding and human cognitive evolution. *Evolutionary Anthropology*, 18, 175–186.

Buss, D. M., & Kenrick, D. T. (1998). Evolutionary social psychology. In D. T. Gilbert, S. T. Fiske, & G. Lindzey (Eds.), *The handbook of social psychology* (pp. 982–1026). New York: McGraw-Hill.

Cacioppo, J. T., Amaral, D. G., Blanchard, J. J., Cameron, J. L., Carter, C. S., Crews, D., et al. (2007). Social neuroscience: Progress and implications for mental health. *Perspectives on Psychological Science*, 2, 99–123.

Cacioppo, J. T., & Cacioppo, S. (2014). Older adults reporting social isolation or loneliness show poorer cognitive function 4 years later. *Evidence-Based Nursing*, 17(2), 59–60.

Cahill, L., Prins, B., Weber, M., & McGaugh, J. L. (1994). Beta-adrenergic activation and memory for emotional events. *Nature*, 371, 702–704.

Canals, M., Rosenmann, M., & Bozinovic, F. (1989). Energetics and geometry of huddling in small mammals. *Journal of Theoretical Biology*, 141(2), 181–189.

Cancedda, L., Putignano, E., Sale, A., Viegi, A., Berardi, N., & Maffei, L. (2004). Acceleration of visual system development by environmental enrichment. *Journal of Neuroscience*, 24, 4840–4848.

Canterberry, M., & Gillath, O. (2013). Neural evidence for a multifaceted model of attachment security. *International Journal of Psychophysiology*, 88(3), 232–240.

Carter, C. S. (1995). Physiological substrates of mammalian monogamy: The prairie vole model. *Neuroscience and Biobehavioral Reviews*, 19, 303–314.

Carter, C. S. (2014). Oxytocin pathways and the evolution of human behavior. *Annual Review of Psychology*, 65, 17–39.

Carter, C. S., & DeVries, A. C. (1999). Stress and soothing: An endocrine perspective. In M. Lewis & D. Ramsay (Eds.), *Soothing and stress* (pp. 3–18). Mahwah, NJ: Erlbaum.

Carter, C. S., & Keverne, E. B. (2002). The neurobiology of social affiliation and pair bonding. *Hormones, Brain and Behavior*, 1, 299–337.

Cassidy, J. (1994). Emotion regulation: Influences of attachment relationships. In N. Fox (Ed.), The development of emotion regulation. *Monographs of the Society for Research in Child Development*, 59, (2–3, Serial No. 240), 228–249.

Chugani, H. T. (1998). A critical period of brain development: Studies of cerebral glucose utilization with PET. *Preventive Medicine*, 27, 184–188.

Clark, A. (2013). Whatever next?: Predictive brains, situated agents, and the future of cognitive science. *Behavioral and Brain Sciences*, 36(3), 181–204.

Coan, J. A. (2010). Adult attachment and the brain. *Journal of Social and Personal Relationships*, 27, 210–217.

Coan, J. A. (2011). The social regulation of emotion. In J. Decety & J. T. Cacioppo (Eds.), *Handbook of social neuroscience* (pp. 614–623). New York: Oxford University Press.

Coan, J. A., & Allen, J. J. B. (2004). Frontal EEG asymmetry as a moderator and mediator of emotion. *Biological Psychology*, 67, 7–49.

Coan, J. A., Allen, J. J. B., & McKnight, P. E. (2006). A capability model of individual differences in frontal EEG asymmetry. *Biological Psychology*, 72, 198–207.

Coan, J. A., Beckes, L., & Allen, J. P. (2013). Childhood maternal support and social capital moderate the regulatory impact of social relationships in adulthood. *International Journal of Psychophysiology*, 88, 224–231.

Coan, J. A., Kasle, S., Jackson, A., Schaefer, H. S., & Davidson, R. J. (2013). Mutuality and the social regulation of neural threat responding. *Attachment and Human Development*, 15, 303–315.

Coan, J. A., & Maresh, E. L. (2014). Social baseline theory and the social regulation of emotion. In J. J. Gross (Ed.), *The handbook of emotion regulation* (2nd ed., pp. 221–236). New York: Guilford Press.

Coan, J. A., & Sbarra, D. A. (2015). Social baseline theory: The social regulation of risk and effort. *Current Opinion in Psychology*, 1, 87–91.

Coan, J. A., Schaefer, H. S., & Davidson, R. J. (2005). Marital adjustment and interpersonal styles moderate the effects of spouse and stranger hand holding on activation of neural systems underlying response to threat. *Psychophysiology*, 42, S44.

Coan, J. A., Schaefer, H. S., & Davidson, R. J. (2006). Lending a hand: Social regulation of the neural response to threat. *Psychological Science*, 17, 1032–1039.

Cohen, S. (2004). Social relationships and health. *American psychologist*, 59, 676–684.

Cohen, S., Janicki-Deverts, D., Turner, R. B., & Doyle, W. J. (in press). Does hugging provide stress-buffering social support?: A study of susceptibility to upper respiratory infection and illness. *Psychological Science*.

Cohen, S., & Wills, T. A. (1985). Stress, social support, and the buffering hypothesis. *Psychological Bulletin*, 98, 310–357.

Conner, O. L., Siegle, G. J., McFarland, A. M., Silk, J. S., Ladouceur, C. D., Dahl, R. E., et al. (2012). Mom—it helps when you're right here!: Attenuation of neural stress markers in anxious youths whose caregivers are present during fMRI. *PloS One*, 7, e50680.

Darwin, C. (1998). *The expression of emotions in man and animals*. Oxford, UK: Oxford University Press. (Original work published 1872)

Davidovitz, R., Mikulincer, M., Shaver, P. R., Ijzak, R., & Popper, M. (2007). Leaders as attachment figures: Their attachment orientations predict leadership-related mental representations and followers' performance and mental health. *Journal of Personality and Social Psychology*, 93, 632–650.

Davidson, R. J., & Irwin, W. (1999). The functional neuroanatomy of emotion and affective style. *Trends in Cognitive Science*, 3(1), 11–21.

Davies, N. B., Krebs, J. R., & West, S. A. (2012). *An introduction to behavioural ecology* (4th ed.). Hoboken, NJ: Wiley-Blackwell.

Davis, M., & Whalen, P. J. (2001). The amygdala: Vigilance and emotion. *Molecular Psychiatry*, 6(1), 13–34.

Dawson, G., Ashman, S. B., Hessl, D., Spieker, S., Frey, K., Panagiotides, H., et al. (2001). Autonomic and brain electrical activity in securely- and insecurely-attached infants of depressed mothers. *Infant Behavior and Development*, 24(2), 135–149.

DeCasper, A. J., & Fifer, W. P. (1980). Of human bonding: Newborns prefer their mothers' voices. *Science*, 208, 1174–1176.

Depue, R. A., & Collins, P. F. (1999). Neurobiology of the structure of personality: Dopamine, facilitation of incentive motivation, and extraversion. *Behavioral and Brain Sciences*, 22, 491–517.

Depue, R. A., & Morrone-Strupinsky, J. V. (2005). A neurobehavioral model of affiliative bonding: Implications for conceptualizing a human trait of affiliation. *Behavioral and Brain Sciences*, 28, 313–395.

DeVries, A. C., Glasper, E. R., & Detillion, C. E. (2003). Social modulation of stress responses. *Physiology and Behavior*, 79, 399–407.

DeWall, C. N., Masten, C. L., Powell, C., Combs, D., Schurtz, D. R., & Eisenberger, N. I. (2012). Do neural responses to rejection depend on attachment style?: An fMRI study. *Social Cognitive and Affective Neuroscience*, 7(2), 184–192.

Dickerson, S. S., & Kemeny, M. E. (2004). Acute stressors and cortisol responses: A theoretical integration and synthesis of laboratory research. *Psychological Bulletin*, 130(3), 355–391.

Dietrich, A. (2004). Neurocognitive mechanisms underlying the experience of flow. *Consciousness and Cognition*, 13(4), 746–761.

Dietrich, A. (2009). The transient hypofrontality theory and its implications for emotion and cognition. In T. McMorris, P. D. Tomporowski, & M. Audiffren (Eds.), *Exercise and cognitive function* (pp. 69–90). Chichester, UK: Wiley.

Edens, J. L., Larkin, K. T., & Abel, J. L. (1992). The effect of social support and physical touch on cardiovascular reactions to mental stress. *Journal of Psychosomatic Research*, 36, 371–382.

Eisenberger, N. I., Master, S. L., Inagaki, T. K., Taylor, S. E., Shirinyan, D., Lieberman, M. D., et al. (2011). Attachment figures activate a safety signal-related neural region and reduce pain experience. *Proceedings of the National Academy of Sciences USA*, 108(28), 11721–11726.

Ellenbogen, M. A., Schwartzman, A. E., Stewart, J., & Walker, C. D. (2006). Automatic and effortful emotional information processing regulates different aspects of the stress response. *Psychoneuroendocrinology*, 31, 373–387.

Fraley, R. C. (2002). Attachment stability from infancy to adulthood: Meta-analysis and dynamic modeling of developmental mechanisms. *Personality and Social Psychology Review*, 6, 123–151.

Fraley, R. C., & Shaver, P. R. (2000). Adult romantic attachment: Theoretical developments, emerging controversies, and unanswered questions. *Review of General Psychology*, 4, 132–154.

Fraley, R. C., Vicary, A. M., Brumbaugh, C. C., & Roisman, G. I. (2011). Patterns of stability in adult attachment: An empirical test of two models of continuity and change. *Journal of Personality and Social Psychology, 101,* 974–992.

Franceschini, M. A., Thaker, S., Themelis, G., Krishnamoorthy, K. K., Bortfeld, H., Diamond, S. G., et al. (2007). Assessment of infant brain development with frequency-domain near-infrared spectroscopy. *Pediatric Research, 61,* 546–551.

Friston, K. (2010). The free-energy principle: A unified brain theory? *Nature Reviews. Neuroscience, 11*(2), 127–38.

Gainer, H., & Wray, S. (1994). Cellular and molecular biology of oxytocin and vasopressin. In E. Knobil & J. Neill (Eds.), *The physiology of reproduction* (pp. 1099–1129). New York: Raven Press.

Gee, D. G., Gabard-Durnam, L. J., Flannery, J., Goff, B., Humphreys, K. L., Telzer, E. H., et al. (2013). Early developmental emergence of human amygdala–prefrontal connectivity after maternal deprivation. *Proceedings of the National Academy of Sciences, 110,* 15638–15643.

Gee, D. G., Gabard-Durnam, L. [J.], Telzer, E. H., Humphreys, K. L., Goff, B., Shapiro, M., et al. (2014). Maternal buffering of human amygdala–prefrontal circuitry during childhood but not during adolescence. *Psychological Science, 25*(11), 2067–2078.

Gillath, O., Bunge, S. A., Shaver, P. R., Wendelken, C., & Mikulincer, M. (2005). Attachment-style differences in the ability to suppress negative thoughts: Exploring the neural correlates. *NeuroImage, 28,* 835–847.

Gillath, O., Shaver, P. R., Baek, J.-M., & Chun, D. S. (2008). Genetic correlates of adult attachment style. *Personality and Social Psychology Bulletin, 34*(10), 1396–1405.

Gonzalez, M. Z., Beckes, L., Chango, J., Allen, J. P., & Coan, J. A. (2015). Adolescent neighborhood quality predicts adult dACC response to social exclusion. *Social Cognitive and Affective Neuroscience, 10*(7), 921–928.

Gosling, S. D. (2008). Personality in non-human animals. *Social and Personality Psychology Compass, 2*(2), 985–1001.

Gosling, S. D., & John, O. P. (1999). Personality dimensions in nonhuman animals: A cross-species review. *Current Directions in Psychological Science, 8*(3), 69–75.

Graves, F. C., Wallen, K., & Maestripieri, D. (2002). Opioids and attachment in rhesus macaque (*Macaca mulatta*) abusive mothers. *Behavioral Neuroscience, 116,* 489–493.

Gross, E. B., & Proffitt, D. (2013). The economy of social resources and its influence on spatial perceptions. *Frontiers in Human Neuroscience, 7,* 772.

Gross, J. J., & Thompson, R. A. (2007). Emotion regulation: Conceptual foundations. In J. J. Gross (Ed.), *Handbook of emotion regulation* (pp. 3–24). New York: Guilford Press.

Gust, D. A., Gordon, T. P., Brodie, A. R., & McClure, H. M. (1996). Effect of companions in modulating stress associated with new group formation in juvenile rhesus macaques. *Physiology and Behavior, 59,* 941–945.

Hamann, S. B., Ely, T. D., Grafton, S. T., & Kilts, C. D. (1999). Amygdala activity related to enhanced memory for pleasant and aversive stimuli. *Nature Neuroscience, 2,* 289–293.

Hansen, S., Bergvall, A. H., & Nyiredi, S. (1993). Interaction with pups enhances dopamine release in the ventral striatum of maternal rats: a microdialysis study. *Pharmacology, Biochemistry and Behavior, 45,* 673–676.

Hansen, S., Harthon, C., Wallin, E., Löfberg, L., & Svensson, K. (1991). The effects of 6-OHDA-induced dopamine depletions in the ventral or dorsal striatum on maternal and sexual behavior in the female rat. *Pharmacology, Biochemistry and Behavior, 39,* 71–77.

Hare, B., Brown, M., Williamson, C., & Tomasello, M. (2002). The domestication of social cognition in dogs. *Science, 298,* 1634–1636.

Hare, B., & Tomasello, M. (2005). Human-like social skills in dogs? *Trends in Cognitive Sciences, 9*(9), 439–444.

Hebb, D. O. (1949). *The organization of behavior.* New York: Wiley.

Henriksen, R. E., Torsheim, T., & Thuen, F. (2014). Loneliness, social integration and consumption of sugar-containing beverages: testing the social baseline theory. *PLoS One, 9*(8), e104421.

Herschkowitz, N. (2000). Neurological bases of behavioral development in infancy. *Brain and Development, 22,* 411–416.

Hofer, M. A. (1995). Hidden regulators: Implications for a new understanding of attachment, separation, and loss. In S. Goldberg, R. Muir, & J. Kerr (Eds.), *Attachment theory: Social, developmental, and clinical perspectives* (pp. 203–230). Hillsdale, NJ: Analytic Press.

Hofer, M. A. (2006). Psychobiological roots of early attachment. *Current Directions in Psychological Science, 15,* 84–88.

Hofer, M. A., & Sullivan, R. M. (2001). Toward a neurobiology of attachment. In C. A. Nelson & M. Luciana (Eds.), *Handbook of developmental cognitive neuroscience* (pp. 599–616). Cambridge, MA: MIT Press.

Holloway, K. S., Cornil, C. A., & Balthazart, J. (2004). Effects of central administration of naloxone during the extinction of appetitive sexual responses. *Behavioural Brain Research, 153,* 567–572.

Holt-Lunstad, J., Smith, T. B., & Layton, J. B. (2010). Social relationships and mortality risk: A Meta-analytic review. *PLoS Medicine, 7,* e1000316.

House, J. S., Landis, K. R., & Umberson, D. (1988). Social relationships and health. *Science, 241*(4865), 540–545.

Hubel, D. H., & Wiesel, T. N. (1970). The period of susceptibility to the physiological effects of unilateral eye closure in kittens. *Journal of Physiology, 206,* 419–436.

Ingham, A. G., Levinger, G., Graves, J., & Peckham, V. (1974). The Ringelmann effect: Studies of group size and group performance. *Journal of Experimental Social Psychology, 10,* 371–384.

Insel, T. R., & Fernald, R. D. (2004). How the brain processes social information: Searching for the social brain. *Annual Review of Neuroscience, 27,* 697–722.

Jack, A., Connelly, J. J., & Morris, J. P. (2012). DNA methylation of the oxytocin receptor gene predicts neural response to ambiguous social stimuli. *Frontiers in Human Neuroscience, 6,* 280.

Jamner, L. D., & Leigh, H. (1999). Repressive/defensive coping, endogenous opioids and health: How a life so perfect can make you sick. *Psychiatry Research, 85,* 17–31.

Job, V., Dweck, C. S., & Walton, G. M. (2010). Ego depletion——is it all in your head?: Implicit theories about willpower affect self-regulation. *Psychological Science, 21*(11), 1686–1693.

Johansen, J. P., Cain, C. K., Ostroff, L. E., & LeDoux, J. E. (2011). Molecular mechanisms of fear learning and memory. *Cell, 147*(3), 509–524.

Johnson, S. M. (2002). *Emotionally focused couple therapy with trauma survivors: Strengthening attachment bonds.* New York: Guilford Press.

Johnson, S. M., Burgess Moser, M., Beckes, L., Smith, A., Dalgleish, T., Halchuk, R., et al. (2013). Soothing the threatened brain: Leveraging contact comfort with emotionally focused therapy. *PloS One, 8*(11), e79314.

Kane, H. S., Jaremka, L. M., Guichard, A. C., Ford, M. B., Collins, N. L., & Feeney, B. C. (2007). Feeling supported and feeling satisfied: How one partner's attachment style predicts the other partner's relationship experiences. *Journal of Social and Personal Relationships, 24*(4), 535–555.

Kanske, P., Heissler, J., Schönfelder, S., Bongers, A., & Wessa, M. (2010). How to regulate emotion?: Neural networks for reappraisal and distraction. *Cerebral Cortex, 21,* 1379–1388.

Karremans, J. C., Heslenfeld, D. J., van Dillen, L. F., & Van Lange, P. A. M. (2011). Secure attachment partners attenuate neural responses to social exclusion: An fMRI investigation. *International Journal of Psychophysiology, 81*(1), 44–50.

Kawachi, I., & Berkman, L. F. (2001). Social ties and mental health . *Journal of Urban Health: Bulletin of the New York Academy of Medicine, 78,* 458–467.

Kemeny, M. E. (2003). The psychobiology of stress. *Current Directions in Psychological Science, 12,* 124–129.

Keverne, E. B., Martensz, N. D., & Tuite, B. (1989). Beta-endorphin concentrations in cerebrospinal fluid of monkeys are influenced by grooming relationships. *Psychoneuroendocrinology, 14,* 155–161.

Kim, P., Feldman, R., Mayes, L. C., Eicher, V., Thompson, N., Leckman, J. F., et al. (2011). Breastfeeding, brain activation to own infant cry, and maternal sensitivity. *Journal of Child Psychology and Psychiatry and Allied Disciplines, 52*(8), 907–915.

King, J. E., & Figueredo, A. J. (1997). The five-factor model plus dominance in chimpanzee personality. *Journal of Research in Personality, 31*(2), 257–271.

Kirkpatrick, L. A., & Davis, K. E. (1994). Attachment style, gender, and relationship stability: A longitudinal analysis. *Journal of Personality and Social Psychology, 66*(3), 502–512.

Kiyokawa, Y., Kikusui, T., Takeuchi, Y., & Mori, Y. (2004). Partner's stress status influences social buffering effects in rats. *Behavioral Neuroscience, 118,* 798–804.

Knox, S. S., & Uvnäs-Moberg, K. (1998). Social isolation and cardiovascular disease: An atherosclerotic pathway? *Psychoneuroendocrinology, 23*(8), 877–890.

Kosfeld, M., Heinrichs, M., Zak, P. J., Fischbacher, U., & Fehr, E. (2005). Oxytocin increases trust in humans. *Nature, 435,* 673–676.

Krahé, C., Paloyelis, Y., Condon, H., Jenkinson, P. M., Williams, S. C. R., & Fotopoulou, A. (2015). Attachment style moderates partner presence effects on pain: A laser-evoked potentials study. *Social Cognitive and Affective Neuroscience, 10*(8), 1030–1037.

Krahé, C., Springer, A., Weinman, J. A., & Fotopoulou, A. (2013). The social modulation of pain: Others as predictive signals of salience—a systematic review. *Frontiers in Human Neuroscience, 7,* 386.

Kraus, M. W., Huang, C., & Keltner, D. (2010). Tactile communication, cooperation, and performance: An ethological study of the NBA. *Emotion, 10*(5), 745–749.

Krietsch, K. N., Mason, A. E., & Sbarra, D. A. (2014). Sleep complaints predict increases in resting blood pressure following marital separation. *Health Psychology, 33*(10), 1204–1213.

Kumsta, R., Hummel, E., Chen, F. S., & Heinrichs, M. (2013). Epigenetic regulation of the oxytocin receptor gene: Implications for behavioral neuroscience. *Frontiers in Neuroscience, 7,* 83.

Kurzban, R. (2010). Does the brain consume additional glucose during self-control tasks? *Evolutionary Psychology, 8,* 245–260.

Kurzban, R., Duckworth, A., Kable, J. W., & Myers, J. (2013). An opportunity cost model of subjective effort and task performance. *Behavioral and Brain Sciences, 36*(6), 661–679.

La Guardia, J. G., Ryan, R. M., Couchman, C. E., & Deci, E. L. (2000). Within-person variation in security of attachment: A self-determination theory perspective on attachment, need fulfillment, and well-being. *Journal of Personality and Social Psychology, 79*(3), 367–384.

Laird, J. D., & Strout, S. (2007). Emotional behaviors as emotional stimuli. In J. A. Coan & J. J. B. Allen

(Eds.), *The handbook of emotion elicitation and assessment* (pp. 54–64). New York: Oxford University Press.

Lammel, S., Lim, B. K., & Malenka, R. C. (2014). Reward and aversion in a heterogeneous midbrain dopamine system. *Neuropharmacology, 76*(Pt. B), 351–359.

Lewis, M., & Ramsay, D. S. (1999). Effect of maternal soothing on infant stress response. *Child Development, 70*(1), 11–20.

Lim, M. M., & Young, L. J. (2006). Neuropeptidergic regulation of affiliative behavior and social bonding in animals. *Hormones and Behavior, 50,* 506–517.

Lorenz, K. (1935). Der kumpan in der umwelt des vogels [The companion in the environment of birds]. *Journal of Ornithology, 83,* 137–413.

Loseth, G. E., Ellingsen, D.-M., & Leknes, S. (2014). State-dependent ?-opioid modulation of social motivation. *Frontiers in Behavioral Neuroscience, 8,* 430.

Maresh, E. L., Beckes, L., & Coan, J. A. (2013). The social regulation of threat-related attentional disengagement in highly anxious individuals. *Frontiers in Human Neuroscience, 7,* 515.

Mashek, D. J., Aron, A., Boncimino, M. (2003). Confusions of self with close others. *Personality and Social Psychology Bulletin, 29,* 382–392.

McEwen, B. S. (2007). Physiology and neurobiology of stress and adaptation: Central role of the brain. *Physiological Reviews, 87,* 873–904.

Meaney, M. J., & Szyf, M. (2005). Environmental programming of stress responses through DNA methylation: Life at the interface between a dynamic environment and a fixed genome. *Dialogues in Clinical Neuroscience, 7*(2), 103–123.

Melo, A. I., Lovic, V., Gonzalez, A., Madden, M., Sinopoli, K., & Fleming, A. S. (2006). Maternal and littermate deprivation disrupts maternal behavior and social-learning of food preference in adulthood: Tactile stimulation, nest odor, and social rearing prevent these effects. *Developmental Psychobiology, 48,* 209–219.

Meredith, M. (2001). Human vomeronasal organ function: A critical review of best and worst cases. *Chemical Senses, 26,* 433–445.

Mikulincer, M., & Florian, V. (1998). The relationship between adult attachment styles and emotional and cognitive reactions to stressful events. In J. A. Simpson & W. S. Rholes (Eds.), *Attachment theory and close relationships* (pp. 143–165). New York: Guilford Press.

Mikulincer, M., & Shaver, P. R. (2007). *Attachment in adulthood: Structure, dynamics, and change.* New York: Guilford Press.

Mikulincer, M., Shaver, P. R., & Pereg, D. (2003). Attachment theory and affect regulation: The dynamics, development, and cognitive consequences of attachment-related strategies. *Motivation and Emotion, 27,* 77–102.

Milad, M. R., Quinn, B. T., Pitman, R. K., Orr, S. P., Fischl, B., & Rauch, S. L. (2005). Thickness of ventromedial prefrontal cortex in humans is correlated with extinction memory. *Proceedings of the National Academy of Sciences, 102,* 10706–10711.

Miller, L. C., Bard, K. A., Juno, C. J., & Nadler, R. D. (1990). Behavioral responsiveness to strangers in young chimpanzees (*Pan troglodytes*). *Folia Primatologica, 55,* 142–155.

Mineka, S., & Suomi, S. J. (1978). Social separation in monkeys. *Psychological Bulletin, 85,* 1376–1400.

Mischel, W., Shoda, Y., & Mendoza-Denton, R. (2002). Situation–behavior profiles as a locus of consistency in personality. *Current Directions in Psychological Science, 11*(2), 50–54.

Moriceau, S., & Sullivan, R. M. (2005). Neurobiology of infant attachment. *Developmental Psychobiology, 47,* 230–242.

Moutsiana, C., Johnstone, T., Murray, L., Fearon, P., Cooper, P., Pliatsikas, C., et al. (2015). Insecure infant attachment predicts greater amygdala volumes in early adulthood. *Journal of Child Psychology and Psychiatry, 56*(5), 540–548.

Nakamura, S., & Sakaguchi, T. (1990). Development and plasticity of the locus coeruleus: A review of recent physiological and pharmacological experimentation. *Progress in Neurobiology, 34,* 505–526.

Nash, K., Prentice, M., Hirsh, J., McGregor, I., & Inzlicht, M. (2014). Muted neural response to distress among securely attached people. *Social Cognitive and Affective Neuroscience, 9*(8), 1239–1245.

Newcomb, M. D., & Bentler, P. M. (1988). Impact of adolescent drug use and social support on problems of young adults: A longitudinal study. *Journal of Abnormal Psychology, 97*(1), 64–75.

Nocjar, C., & Panksepp, J. (2007). Prior morphine experience induces long-term increases in social interest and in appetitive behavior for natural reward. *Behavioural Brain Research, 181,* 191–199.

Noftle, E. E., & Shaver, P. R. (2006). Attachment dimensions and the big five personality traits: Associations and comparative ability to predict relationship quality. *Journal of Research in Personality, 40*(2), 179–208.

Norman, G. J., Hawkley, L., Ball, A., Berntson, G. G., & Cacioppo, J. T. (2013). Perceived social isolation moderates the relationship between early childhood trauma and pulse pressure in older adults. *International Journal of Psychophysiology, 88*(3), 334–338.

Norris, C. J., Coan, J. A., & Johnstone, I. T. (2007). Functional magnetic resonance imaging and the study of emotion. In J. A. Coan & J. J. B. Allen (Eds.), *The handbook of emotion elicitation and assessment* (pp. 440–459). New York: Oxford University Press.

Nuñez-Villegas, M., Bozinovic, F., & Sabat, P. (2014). Interplay between group size, huddling behavior and basal metabolism: An experimental approach in the social degu. *Journal of Experimental Biology, 217,* 997–1002.

O'Connor, M.-F., & Arizmendi, B. J. (2014). Neuropsychological correlates of complicated grief in older spousally bereaved adults. *Journals of Gerontology B: Psychological Sciences and Social Sciences, 69,* 12–18.

Ochsner, K. N., Silvers, J. A., & Buhle, J. T. (2012). Functional imaging studies of emotion regulation: a synthetic review and evolving model of the cognitive control of emotion. *Annals of the New York Academy of Sciences, 1251,* E1–E24.

Öhman, A. (2005). The role of the amygdala in human fear: Automatic detection of threat. *Psychoneuroendocrinology, 30,* 953–958.

Panksepp, J., Nelson, E. E., & Siviy, S. (1994). Brain opioids and mother–infant social motivation. *Acta Paediatrica, 397,* 40–46.

Phelps, E. A., & LeDoux, J. E. (2005). Contributions of the amygdala to emotion processing: from animal models to human behavior. *Neuron, 48,* 175–187.

Posner, M. I., & Rothbart, M. K. (2007). Research on attention networks as a model for the integration of psychological science. *Annual Review of Psychology, 58,* 1–23.

Proffitt, D. R. (2006). Embodied perception and the economy of action. *Perspectives on Psychological Science, 1,* 110–122.

Puglia, M. H., Lillard, T. S., Morris, J. P., & Connelly, J. J. (2015). Epigenetic modification of the oxytocin receptor gene influences the perception of anger and fear in the human brain. *Proceedings of the National Academy of Science USA, 112*(11), 3308–3313.

Quirin, M., Gillath, O., Pruessner, J. C., & Eggert, L. D. (2010). Adult attachment insecurity and hippocampal cell density. *Social Cognitive and Affective Neuroscience, 5,* 39–47.

Quirk, G. J., & Beer, J. S. (2006). Prefrontal involvement in the regulation of emotion: convergence of rat and human studies. *Current Opinion in Neurobiology, 16,* 723–727.

Ray, R. D., & Zald, D. H. (2012). Anatomical insights into the interaction of emotion and cognition in the prefrontal cortex. *Neuroscience and Biobehavioral Reviews, 36,* 479–501.

Reichardt, L. F. (2006). Neurotrophin-regulated signalling pathways. *Philosophical Transactions of the Royal Society of London, 361,* 1545–1564.

Rilling, J. K., & Young, L. J. (2014). The biology of mammalian parenting and its effect on offspring social development. *Science, 345*(6198), 771–776.

Robles, T. F., & Kiecolt-Glaser, J. K. (2003). The physiology of marriage: Pathways to health. *Physiology and Behavior, 79,* 409–416.

Rolls, E. T. (2007). Emotion elicited by primary reinforcers and following stimulus-reinforcement association learning. In J. A. Coan & J. J. B. Allen (Eds.), *The handbook of emotion elicitation and assessment* (pp. 137–157). New York: Oxford University Press.

Ruis, M. A. W., te Brake, J. H. A., Buwalda, B., De Boer, S. F., Meerlo, P., Korte, S. M., et al. (1999). Housing familiar male wildtype rats together reduces the long-term adverse behavioural and physiological effects of social defeat. *Psychoneuroendocrinology,* 285–300.

Sachser, N., Kaiser, S., & Hennessy, M. B. (2013). Behavioural profiles are shaped by social experience: when, how and why. *Philosophical Transactions of the Royal Society of London B: Biological Sciences, 368,* 20120344.

Sambo, C. F., Howard, M., Kopelman, M., Williams, S., & Fotopoulou, A. (2010). Knowing you care: effects of perceived empathy and attachment style on pain perception. *Pain, 151*(3), 687–693.

Sbarra, D. A., Law, R. W., & Portley, R. M. (2011). Divorce and death: A meta-analysis and research agenda for clinical, social, and health psychology. *Perspectives on Psychological Science, 6*(5), 454–474.

Schauwers, K., Gillis, S., Daemers, K., De Beukelaer, C., De Ceulaer, G., Yperman, M., et al. (2004). Normal hearing and language development in a deaf-born child. *Otology and Neurotology, 25,* 924–929.

Schnall, S., Harber, K. D., Stefanucci, J. K., & Proffitt, D. R. (2008). Social support and the perception of geographical slant. *Journal of Experimental Social Psychology, 44,* 1246–1255.

Schultz, W., Dayan, P., & Montague, P. R. (1997). A neural substrate of prediction and reward. *Science, 275,* 1593–1599.

Schultze-Florey, C. R., Martínez-Maza, O., Magpantay, L., Breen, E. C., Irwin, M. R., Gündel, H., & O'Connor, M.-F. (2012). When grief makes you sick: Bereavement induced systemic inflammation is a question of genotype. *Brain, Behavior, and Immunity, 26,* 1066–1071.

Shahrokh, D. K., Zhang, T.-Y., Diorio, J., Gratton, A., & Meaney, M. J. (2010). Oxytocin–dopamine interactions mediate variations in maternal behavior in the rat. *Endocrinology, 151*(5), 2276–2286.

Sheppes, G., Catran, E., & Meiran, N. (2009). Reappraisal (but not distraction) is going to make you sweat: physiological evidence for self-control effort. *International Journal of Psychophysiology, 71,* 91–96.

Shipley, M. T., Ennis, M., & Puche, A. C. (2003). The olfactory system. In P. M. Conn (Ed.), *Neuroscience in medicine* (pp. 579–593). New York: Humana Press.

Sierra-Mercado, D. J., Corcoran, K. A., Lebrón-Milad, K., & Quirk, G. J. (2006). Inactivation of the ventromedial prefrontal cortex reduces expression of conditioned fear and impairs subsequent recall of extinction. *European Journal of Neuroscience, 24,* 1751–1758.

Skuse, D., Albanese, A., Stanhope, R., Gilmour, J., & Voss, L. (1996). A new stress-related syndrome of growth failure and hyperphagia in children, associated with reversibility of growth-hormone insufficiency. *Lancet, 348,* 353–358.

Smith, T. D., Laitman, J. T., & Bhatnagar, K. P. (2014). The shrinking anthropoid nose, the human vomeronasal organ, and the language of anatomical reduction. *Anatomical Record, 297,* 2196–2204.

Sokolowski, M. B. (2010). Social interactions in "simple" model systems. *Neuron, 65*(6), 780–794.

Steiner, A. R. W., & Coan, J. A. (2011). Prefrontal asymmetry predicts affect, but not beliefs about affect. *Biological Psychology*, 88(1), 65–71.

Stewart, J. L., Coan, J. A., Towers, D. N., & Allen, J. J. B. (2014). Resting and task-elicited prefrontal EEG alpha asymmetry in depression: Support for the capability model. *Psychophysiology*, 51(5), 446–455.

Sullivan, R. M. (2003). Developing a sense of safety: The neurobiology of neonatal attachment. *Annals of the New York Academy of Sciences*, 1008, 122–131.

Taylor, S. E., Klein, L. C., Lewis, B. P., Gruenewald, T. L., Gurung, R. A. R., & Updegraff, J. A. (2000). Biobehavioral responses to stress in females: Tend-and-befriend, not fight-or-flight. *Psychological Review*, 107, 411–429.

Taylor, S. E., Sherman, D. K., Kim, H. S., Jarcho, J., Takagi, K., & Dunagan, M. S. (2004). Culture and social support: Who seeks it and why? *Journal of Personality and Social Psychology*, 87, 354–362.

Teicher, M. H., Samson, J. A., Polcari, A., & McGreenery, C. E. (2006). Sticks, stones, and hurtful words: Relative effects of various forms of childhood maltreatment. *American Journal of Psychiatry*, 163, 993–1000.

Terranova, M. L., Cirulli, F., & Laviola, G. (1999). Behavioral and hormonal effects of partner familiarity in periadolescent rat pairs upon novelty exposure. *Psychoneuroendocrinology*, 24, 639–656.

The *PLoS Medicine* Editors. (2010). Social relationships are key to health, and to health policy. *PLoS Medicine*, 7, e1000334.

Thomas, K. M., Drevets, W. C., Whalen, P. J., Eccard, C. H., Dahl, R. E., Ryan, N. D., et al. (2001). Amygdala response to facial expressions in children and adults. *Biological Psychiatry*, 49, 309–316.

Tomasello, M., Carpenter, M., Call, J., Behne, T., & Moll, H. (2005). Understanding and sharing intentions: The origins of cultural cognition. *Behavioral and Brain Sciences*, 28, 675–691; discussion 691–735.

Topal, J., Miklosi, A., Csanyi, V., & Doka, A. (1998). Attachment behavior in dogs (*Canis familiaris*): A new application of Ainsworth's (1969) Strange Situation test. *Journal of Comparative Psychology*, 112, 219–229.

Tottenham, N. (2012). Human amygdala development in the absence of species-expected caregiving. *Developmental Psychobiology*, 54, 598–611.

Turecki, G., & Meaney, M. (2016). Effects of the social environment and stress on glucocorticoid receptor gene methylation: A systematic review. *Biological Psychiatry*, 79(2), 87–96.

Tzschentke, T. M., & Schmidt, W. J. (2000). Functional relationship among medial prefrontal cortex, nucleus accumbens, and ventral tegmental area in locomotion and reward. *Critical Reviews in Neurobiology*, 14, 131–142.

Vanderschuren, L. J. M. J., Niesink, R. J. M., & Van Pee, J. M. (1997). The neurobiology of social play behavior in rats. *Neuroscience and Biobehavioral Reviews*, 21, 309–326.

Vrtička, P., Bondolfi, G., Sander, D., & Vuilleumier, P. (2012). The neural substrates of social emotion perception and regulation are modulated by adult attachment style. *Social Neuroscience*, 7(5), 473–493.

Vrtička, P., & Vuilleumier, P. (2012). Neuroscience of human social interactions and adult attachment style. *Frontiers in Human Neuroscience*, 6, 00212.

Warneken, F., & Tomasello, M. (2009). Varieties of altruism in children and chimpanzees. *Trends in cognitive sciences*, 13, 397-402.

Weaver, A., & de Waal, F. B. M. (2003). The mother–offspring relationship as a template in social development: Reconciliation in captive brown capuchins (cebus apella). *Journal of Comparative Psychology*, 117, 101–110.

Weaver, I. C. G., Diorio, J., Seckl, J. R., Szyf, M., & Meaney, M. J. (2004). Early environmental regulation of hippocampal glucocorticoid receptor gene expression: Characterization of intracellular mediators and potential genomic target sites. In T. Kino, E. Charmandari, & G. P. Chrousos (Eds.), *Glucocorticoid action: Basic and clinical implications* (pp. 182–212). New York: New York Academy of Sciences.

Whalen, P. J., Kagan, J., Cook, R. G., Davis, F. C., Kim, H., Polis, S., et al. (2004). Human amygdala responsivity to masked fearful eye whites. *Science*, 306, 2061.

Wiedenmayer, C. P., Magarinos, A. M., McEwen, B. S., & Barr, G. A. (2003). Mother lowers glucocorticoid levels of preweaning rats after acute threat. *Annals of the New York Academy of Sciences*, 1008, 304–307.

Williamson, A. (2006). Using self-report measures in neurobehavioral toxicology: Can they be trusted? *Neurotoxicology*, 28, 227–234.

Wilson, C. L., & Ruben, M. A. (2011). A pain in her arm: Romantic attachment orientations and the tourniquet task. *Personal Relationships*, 18(2), 242–265.

Wismer-Fries, A. B., Ziegler, T. E., Kurian, J. R., Jacoris, S., & Pollak, S. D. (2005). Early experience in humans is associated with changes in neuropeptides critical for regulating social behavior. *Proceedings of the National Academy of Science*, 102, 17237–17240.

Woolley, A. W., Chabris, C. F., Pentland, A., Hashmi, N., & Malone, T. W. (2010). Evidence for a collective intelligence factor in the performance of human groups. *Science*, 330, 686–688.

Young, L. J., & Wang, Z. (2004). The neurobiology of pair bonding. *Nature Neuroscience*, 7, 1048–1054.

Younger, J., Aron, A., Parke, S., Chatterjee, N., & Mackey, S. (2010). Viewing pictures of a romantic partner reduces experimental pain: involvement of neural reward systems. *PloS One*, 5(10), e13309.

# PART III

# ATTACHMENT IN INFANCY AND CHILDHOOD

# Chapter 13

# Normative Development
## The Ontogeny of Attachment in Childhood

Robert S. Marvin
Preston A. Britner
Beth S. Russell

Whilst especially evident during early childhood, attachment behavior is held to characterize human beings from the cradle to the grave.
—JOHN BOWLBY (1979, p. 129)

During the 1940s and 1950s, a number of emerging studies suggested that very young children, when separated from their mothers for a considerable period of time, proceed through a series of reactions that have become known as protest, despair, and detachment (e.g., Burlingham & Freud, 1944; Robertson, 1953). These or similar reactions were so common, despite variations in the care received by the child, that John Bowlby departed from the contemporary scientific and clinical consensus and decided that the loss of the *specific mother figure* was the most important factor in these reactions. From here, Bowlby went on to develop his "ethological–control systems" theory of the infant's tie, or attachment, to his or her mother or primary caregiver (Bowlby, 1958, 1969/1982, 1973, 1980). In a partnership that went on to span nearly 40 years, Bowlby and Mary Ainsworth (1967; Ainsworth, Blehar, Waters, & Wall, 1978), among others, sought to answer questions such as the following:

Why does the young child become so distressed by the loss of his or her mother?

What processes account for each of the three phases of loss?

What *is* the bond that ties the child to his or her mother?

What are its forms, and how do they emerge?

And ultimately, how do we understand form and functioning "when things go wrong?"

Bowlby and his colleagues decided that answering these questions required a shift to the study of the early development of this bond in normally developing children and their families. They were convinced that only by understanding the normal formation and functioning of an attachment relationship would we be able to understand its malfunctioning. These efforts resulted in some of the most empirically and theoretically significant contributions to the study of children's development in the second half of the 20th century. The theory that emerged was consistent with then-current theories of biology, embryology, cognitive science, and general systems theory. It was at the same time specific enough to incorporate species and cultural differences, and general enough to incorporate species and cultural similarity. It came closer than any other theory to being equally applicable to questions of normative development and of individual differences and maladaptive developmental pathways.

Through the mid-1970s, there was much excitement and controversy about Bowlby's theory of the ontogeny of attachment. However, by the 1980s, the field of attachment research had undergone a significant change: The study of individual differences had come to occupy so much of the focus that exploration of the *ontogeny* of attachment had nearly been abandoned. Ainsworth's identification of three "primary" strategies of attachment (e.g., Ainsworth et al., 1978), Main and Solomon's (1990) discovery of a "disorganized" pattern of attachment, and Main, Goldwyn, and Hesse's (2003) research on adults' attachment patterns have contributed enormously to our understanding of differential strategies within intimate relationships, as well as child and adult psychopathology. Ethological studies of behavioral development, however, point to the obvious but often ignored importance of survival of the individual at each developmental point. This will certainly be no less the case in the study of human attachment. Only by studying individual pathways *through the course of development* will we truly understand the origins, nature, and sequelae of the attachment bond.

Do we think that attachment behavior, and a secure attachment, are developmental tasks only of infancy, to be superseded by later tasks such as self-control and self-reliance (Garon, Longard, Bryson, & Moore, 2012), individuation (Kruse & Walper, 2008), autonomy (Beyers, Goossens, Vansant, & Moors, 2003), or independent and socialized behavior (Baumrind, 1980)? There are theoretical and empirical reasons for rejecting a strong developmental tasks position (Ainsworth, 1990).

Perhaps the most important reason for studying the developing forms of attachment behavior is related to common experience and to one of Bowlby's most fundamental theoretical claims: that the biological function of attachment behavior is protection of the youngster from a variety of dangers. Preschool and even older children, in our present environment and in our "environment of evolutionary adaptedness" (Bowlby, 1969/1982), are vulnerable to a wide range of dangers. How children and their caregivers organize protective proximity and contact, and how they continue to

use their caregivers as a secure base for exploration, remain as important during later periods of development as during the first year of life. Although the frequency of attachment behavior may wane across development, it remains as important when activated in a 4- or 8-year-old as it was during infancy. And how the attachment behavioral system is organized with other behavioral systems of the individual (and of the caregivers), such that the person is protected while exploring other developmental activities, becomes a crucial question for many developmental domains across the lifespan.

Bowlby (1969/1982) placed his theory of the development of attachment squarely within the biological, general systems, and cognitive sciences. The theory is actually an integration and elaboration of several conceptual schemes: general systems theory, including especially communication and control systems theory; cognitive science, much of which can be considered part of systems theory; evolutionary theory; ethology and the study of primate behavior; and descriptive studies of human infants and young children interacting with their caregivers. Our description of the development of attachment in childhood in this chapter presents Bowlby's theory, along with the elaborations provided by several scholars regarding developmental changes during the preschool and early school age years. More detailed descriptions of attachment theory as applied to adolescence and adulthood are presented in the chapters in Part IV of this volume.

## General Systems Perspective

At an abstract information–theoretical level, if a system is to survive, certain invariant conditions must be maintained, both among its constituent elements and in its relationship with its environment (Ashby, 1952, 1956). In particular essential respects, variety must be kept within certain limits or the system will not survive. If a system cannot control input from the environment in a manner that keeps these essential variables within the limits, then it must be "coupled" with another system that can keep the variety in the first system within the limits. In other words, there must be a close coupling, bond, or attachment between the two systems that serves to protect the less "self-reliant" system. This is a formal statement of Bowlby's basic thesis regarding the biological function of child–parent attachment: It protects the child from a wide range of dangers—from either internal changes or environmental inputs—that would push some essential variable(s) beyond the system's (i.e., the child's) limits of survival.

In a system that develops toward increasing self-reliance over time, this coupling can have another aspect. In many biological organisms, the protective bond has a component that facilitates the youngster's tendency to explore and learn (i.e., to develop the skills needed for its autonomous integration into the larger group). Within this protective relationship, the developing organism thus becomes progressively less dependent for protection on the bond with its parent. Eventually, the developing organism obtains the necessary skills, within its coupling with its larger social context, to control internal change and environmental input in ways that stay within the limits necessary for survival. This complex developmental pattern constitutes the crux of Ainsworth's (1967) concept of the child's use of its mother as a haven of safety and secure base for exploration. It emphasizes that at each point in development, the attachment–caregiving interactions between the youngster and his or her attachment figure(s) compensate for, and complement, the lack of motor, cognitive, communication, and social skills on the youngster's part, such that the youngster is always protected while being afforded as much independence as possible to learn those skills. Finally, it suggests that at any given point in development, skills or behavioral systems across developmental domains will fit together in a manner that makes adaptive sense in terms of survival at that point.

## Bowlby's Control Systems Model of Development

Research on both primates and humans indicates that this developmental pattern takes place in the context of a complex network of "affectional bonds," including the close attachment of infant to mother. Ainsworth (1967) defines an *affectional bond* as a relatively long-enduring tie in which the partner is important as a unique individual, and noninterchangeable. Harlow was one of the first to propose distinct affectional systems or bonds (Harlow & Harlow, 1965), with the explicit connotation that different bonds function to achieve different outcomes. Bowlby took this a step further in distinguishing among a number of behavioral systems, each with its own predictable outcome

and biological function (see Cassidy, Chapter 1, this volume). Following on Harlow's early work, a number of distinct affectional bonds have been identified, including the attachment bond; the parent's complementary, caregiving bond; the sexual pair bond; sibling/kinship bonds; and friendship bonds (Ainsworth, 1990; see B. C. Feeney & Woodhouse, Chapter 36, and Zeifman & Hazan, Chapter 20, this volume). In our opinion, the essential contribution of Bowlby's theory is his description of the behavioral systems underlying these bonds, and the developmental changes in those behavioral systems.

### Behavioral Systems

Attachment theory proposes a number of behavioral systems that are species-universal, although there may be (subtle) differences across both individuals and breeding populations (e.g., Freedman & Gorman, 1993). Each behavioral system consists of a set of interchangeable, functionally equivalent behaviors (i.e., behaviors that have the same predictable effect or outcome; Bowlby, 1969/1982). At the same time, each behavior serves more than one behavioral system. For example, locomotion serves, among others, the attachment, exploration, and wariness behavioral systems. It is for this reason that Sroufe and Waters (1977) insisted that the infant's attachment behavior can be fully understood only from an organizational perspective.

A nonexhaustive list of behavioral systems would include those related to feeding, reproduction, caregiving, attachment, exploration, sociability, and fear/wariness. Following ethological theory, Bowlby proposed that the behavior patterns associated with each of these behavioral systems have been selected through evolution because they fulfill a biological function: They help to ensure the survival and reproductive success of the individual and his or her genes. The biological function of attachment behavior, and of wary behavior, is protection of the youngster from a wide range of dangers. The biological function of exploratory and sociable behavior is that of learning the skills necessary for more self-reliant survival, both in terms of individual skills and of smooth integration into the social group.

Behavioral systems include rules for the selection, activation, and termination of behaviors based on the individual's internal state and environmental context. As implied earlier, attachment researchers have focused on three specific behavioral systems: attachment, fear/wariness, and exploration. Ainsworth (1990) and Marvin (1997) have suggested that it is useful to think of a fourth, the sociability behavioral system, which is related to children's friendly interactions.

Attachment theory proposes that in normal development, the operation of these four behavioral systems is affected by specific environmental and organismic events. They also exhibit a complex dynamic balance (Ainsworth, 1967), which has the predictable outcome of ensuring that the youngster develops more sophisticated coping skills, but does so within the protective bond to the attachment figure(s). Specifically, when the youngster's attachment and/or wariness behavioral systems are minimally activated, his or her exploration and/or sociability behavioral systems can easily be activated. Activation of the wariness system serves as a terminating condition for the exploration and/or sociability systems, and coincidently as an activating condition for the attachment behavioral system. Proximity or contact with the attachment figure, then, often serves to minimize activation of the attachment and wariness behavioral systems, which in turn can reactivate the exploration and/or sociability systems. This is part of the underlying control system for what Ainsworth (1967) described as "using the mother as a secure base for exploration." Finally, as many mothers, fathers, babysitters, and child care providers know, a strongly activated exploration system can reduce activation of the attachment system.

There is some evidence that as the youngster develops through the preschool years, the organization among these four behavioral systems changes and becomes more elaborate (e.g., Greenberg & Marvin, 1982). There is also some evidence that in young children raised in environments extremely dissimilar from the "environment of evolutionary adaptedness" (e.g., in a maltreating or institutional setting without consistent caregivers), these four behavioral systems often do not exhibit this equilibrated organization, leading to what could appropriately be called a *developmental disorder* (e.g., O'Connor et al., 2003; Rutter et al., 2012; Zeanah, Smyke, Koga, & Carlson, 2005; see review by Dozier & Rutter, Chapter 30, this volume).

## Complexity of Behavioral Systems

Drawing from ethology, Bowlby (1969/1982) proposed that behavioral systems differ not only in function but also in their structural complexity. The simplest is a *reflex*—a highly stereotyped behavior activated by a stimulus at a specific threshold and carried to completion. A more complex behavior, called a *fixed action pattern* by ethologists, is also a highly stereotyped behavior activated and terminated by specific stimuli, but its threshold for activation varies according to the state of the organism, and it often makes use of some feedback from the environment during its execution. Many of the basic attachment behaviors that Ainsworth (1967) identified, such as grasping, crying, and smiling, might also be considered fixed action patterns.

Although seemingly quite primitive, these simple behavior patterns can assume an elegant complexity when placed in the context in which they evolved. In the case of attachment behavior, the context is one of close proximity to a caregiver who responds with specific behaviors that complement the infant's behavior. The immediate effect of many behaviors is to bring about a change in the environment that serves as an activating condition for another behavior, often forming a lengthy sequence with an eventual outcome that is necessary for the individual's survival. For example, when a hungry neonate cries, that behavior *predictably* activates the maternal behavior of picking the infant up and placing it at the breast. The pick up, or at least the stimulus of the breast or nipple on the infant's face, terminates the cry and activates rooting. This predictably brings the infant's mouth in contact with the nipple, which serves as a terminating condition for rooting and an activating in the baby a condition for grasping the nipple with its lips. The stimulus of the nipple in the mouth, in turn, activates sucking, and finally liquid in the mouth stimulates swallowing. Whereas the complexity and predictability of this sequence might appear purposeful, goal-directed— or to use Bowlby's term *goal-corrected*—on the part of the infant, in fact it is not. Interruption of the sequence at any point would lead to failure of the overall sequence. Instead, Bowlby referred to these behaviors as having a specified "predictable outcome," as long as the behavior is executed in an environment similar to the one in which the behavior evolved. The predictable outcome of attachment behaviors more generally is proximity and/or contact with a caregiver/attachment figure. This construct of a predictable outcome is especially important for at least two reasons. First, it allows us to understand relatively simple forms of behavior as achieving an important outcome without our inferring that the youngster executed the behavior intentionally, despite the fact that the behavior sequence occurs in a predictable way.

Second, it forces us to view these simple behavior patterns as taking place in a dyadic or larger context: They have little meaning if they are not described and understood in the relationship context in which they evolved.

A yet more complicated pattern of behavior is a goal-corrected pattern. As with simpler forms of behavior, goal-corrected behaviors have activating and terminating conditions, as well as predictable outcomes, but they achieve the outcome through a more sophisticated process. In order to engage in goal-corrected behavior, an organism must have an especially complex, dynamic, internal representation of relevant aspects of self, his or her behavior, the environment, and the object or person toward whom the behavior is directed. Bowlby used the term *internal working model* (IWM) for these representations, but he also referred to them as "representational models," which are loosely equivalent to Piagetian "schemes." IWMs are not static images, but flexible models that are used to understand and predict one's relations with the environment, and to construct complex sequences of behavior based on plans that can achieve specific, internally represented outcomes. Studies of the early parent–child relationship have identified crucial moments in the sequence of actions during a goal-directed exchange. Specifically, the moment of repair in a mismatched exchange carries the most crucial information to both parent and child (Kogan & Carter, 1996). For example, when the neonate cries in the night, signaling that she is cold, her distress may increase when she is exposed to check for a soiled diaper, as may her parent's distress at failing to soothe her cry; both experience relief when settled in for a snuggle, warming the cold baby and reassuring the caregiver. When a goal-corrected behavior sequence is activated, the child continuously orients his or her behavior and selects alternative behaviors, based in part on the feedback received from the effects of the behavior. When the set-goal is achieved, the perceived discrepancy between the set-goal and the organism's state is reduced to zero, and the behavioral plan terminates.

Drawing again from the work of the ethologists, Bowlby (1969/1982) proposed that there are variations in how behaviors, and behavioral systems, are coordinated into more complex wholes. Among them are the following:

1. Very simple behaviors can be coordinated in chain-linked sequences, with the terminating condition for one behavior serving as the activating condition for the next.

2. There can be chains with alternative links. In this case, when one link in the chain fails to achieve an outcome that activates the next link in the chain, some other link is activated in a non-goal-corrected manner. For example, studies employing the still-face paradigm describe infants who respond to an unavailable caregiver by switching behavior by similarly increasing their distress cues or by disengaging (Mesman, Van IJzendoorn, & Bakermans-Kranenburg, 2009; Toda & Fogel, 1993).

3. Complex, goal-corrected behavior patterns can themselves be organized together in chain-linked sequences, with the terminating condition for the first goal-corrected pattern serving as the activating condition for the second.

4. An action based on one behavioral system alternates with an action based on another system. Ethologists have found that these complex sequences often form the basis for important social interactions and communicative signals.

5. Partially executed behaviors from one behavioral system can occur simultaneously with partially executed behaviors from another, conflicting behavioral system.

## Ontogeny of Behavioral Systems

The final step in laying the groundwork for Bowlby's model of the ontogeny of attachment is to outline the three processes that he proposed as basic to development in general. First, the early forms of behaviors are sometimes directed toward different objects in the environment than those to which the mature form will be directed later in development. Usually, the range of stimuli that elicit a particular behavior becomes restricted over the course of development. Second, behavioral systems that are functional early in development are often of a very simple type. Over the course of development, these simpler systems tend to become superseded by more complex, sophisticated ones with correspondingly complex IWMs. Third, whereas some behavioral systems are functional in simple form early in development, others start out being executed only partially, in a nonfunctional way, or in an inappropriate place in a behavioral sequence. In this case, the important developmental process is the integration of these nonfunctional components into functional wholes.

One of the most important implications of this third process is that once a behavioral system has become organized, it assumes some inherent stability (Ashby, 1956; Thelen & Ulrich, 1991).

It may maintain the same organization even if it has developed along nonfunctional lines and may persist even in the absence of the conditions in which it developed. This part of the developmental model has clear implications for the study of developmental psychopathology. However, it also has important implications for more adaptive development, in suggesting both that there may be systemic, structurally based sensitive periods in development, and that beyond a certain point in development, it may be especially difficult—albeit not impossible—for a developmental process or outcome to take shape in a "normal" fashion.

## The Ontogeny of Attachment

### Development of Attachment during the First Year of Life

Bowlby proposed four phases in the development of the attachment behavioral system, with the first three occurring during the first year of life, and the fourth beginning sometime around the child's fourth birthday.

### Phase I: Orientation and Signals without Discrimination of Figure

Consistent with much new research of the 1960s, Bowlby proposed that immediately or very soon after birth, the baby's signal and motor systems are especially adept at eliciting interest and caregiving from other humans, such that proximity, physical contact, nutrition, and warmth are the predictable outcomes. In this sense, the development of the infant's attachment behavior cannot be fully understood except as taking place in the context of the complementary behavior of his or her caregivers. An extensive body of research focuses on caregiving-as-context for many domains of development, and thorough consideration of these caregiving behaviors and their developmental changes is beyond the scope of this chapter (but see, e.g., Britner, Marvin, & Pianta, 2005; George & Solomon, 1996; B. C. Feeney & Woodhouse, Chapter 36, this volume).

During this first phase in the development of attachment, baby and caregiver engage in interactions of many types, and from the perspective of the caregiver's behavior, many of these interactions are goal-corrected. From the perspective of the baby's own behavioral organization and control, there are *predictable outcomes*, rather than set-

goals, of the behaviors. Thus, during Phase I, the infant's IWMs are present but primitive and are probably limited to internal "on again, off again" experiences associated with the activation and termination of individual behaviors. In this sense, the functioning of the young infant's IWMs are no more separate from actual behaviors than in Stage I of Piaget's (1952) theory of the sensorimotor period.

At birth or very soon thereafter, every sensory system in the infant is working and continues to improve in functioning. Among the sensory systems especially important in the development of attachment behavior are the auditory and visual systems. At or soon after birth, most infants are capable of visual orientation and tracking, and are especially responsive to contour and pattern, especially if the stimulus is moving slowly. By 4 weeks of age, most infants exhibit a preference for looking at the human face compared to other objects (Wolff, 1969). Very soon after birth, infants tend to quiet and attend to soft auditory stimuli and appear especially responsive to the human voice. Infants, and even full-term fetuses, recognize and prefer their own mother's voice to that of a stranger (Kisilevsky et al., 2003). During this first phase, each of these systems has its own activating and terminating conditions, and there is as yet no "internal" connection between the systems. Reaching, grasping, and clinging are also crucial attachment behaviors in all primates, and they develop relatively late in humans. It is not until after about 2 months of age that the human infant's grasp is highly developed and controlled by anything other than a reflex-like process of activation by stimulation of the palm of the hand. It is at about this same time that the visual system becomes chain-linked with the motor system in a manner allowing the infant to make ballistic-like movements toward an object in the visual field. Finally, smiling and crying are additional, important attachment behaviors displaying a similar developmental course. Smiling tends to be activated, and crying terminated, in a relatively automatic way by a range of specific conditions. These conditions become increasingly selective and integrated within more complex behavioral systems over the first 6 months.

Thus, at first it is largely the caregiver who maintains proximity and protects the infant, although the newborn is equipped to be especially responsive to other humans and to elicit caregiving and affection from them. Over the course of the first weeks of life, these patterns of infant—

caregiver interaction are repeated frequently. If the caregiver's initiations and responses are well attuned to the infant's behaviors (i.e., if the baby's attachment behaviors are predictably terminated by the caregiver's behavior), then stable patterns of interaction are established. These reciprocal patterns of caregiver–infant behaviors ultimately minimize the frequency and intensity of attachment behaviors such as crying, and more readily elicit other behaviors, such as visual orientation and smiling. In this context, the infant is seen as establishing its own behavioral and autoregulatory rhythms (e.g., Stern, 1985), so that stable "internal" and dyadic rhythms are established.

Bowlby (1969/1982) proposed that in the environment of evolutionary adaptedness, Phase I lasts from birth to sometime between 8 and 12 weeks of age, roughly coinciding with early developmental trajectories for crying in human and nonhuman primates and of dramatic neurobehavioral and sensory developments (Brazelton, 1962; Marshall, 2011). He suggested, however, that under unfavorable conditions, this phase can last much longer.

### Phase II: Orientation and Signals Directed toward One or More Discriminated Figures

The shift from Phase I to Phase II is gradual, and it takes place earlier with some attachment behaviors and complex attachment behavior patterns than with others (Ainsworth, 1967; Bowlby, 1969/1982). Three related issues are important in defining this transition.

First, during Phase II, there is an elaboration of simple behavioral systems into more complex ones. The simple behavioral systems of the Phase I infant become integrated within the infant into complex, chain-linked behavioral systems. The primary focus here is on the *control* of the individual systems. Whereas in Phase I, the caregiver provided the conditions for terminating one behavioral link in a chain and activating the next, during Phase II, the infant assumes much of this control. Many of the sensorimotor advances of the 3- to 6-month-old infant illustrate this shift in behavioral control. For example, as early as 3 months of age, perception of the bottle or breast itself serves as an activating stimulus for opening the mouth, and often bringing the hand(s) toward the mouth (Hetzer & Ripin, 1930, as cited in Bowlby, 1969/1982). By 4 months, the infant's visual system begins to activate the motor behavior of reaching for an object. Through a reciprocal

feedback process, the infant alternates its gaze between hand and the object, then grasps the object. By 5 months, the infant is so adept at this that he or she is able to reach out and grasp parts of mother's body and clothing while being held by her, or as she is leaning over him or her. By the end of the first year of life, infants clearly understand the causal mechanism of reaching, grasping, and attaining an object (Sommerville & Woodward, 2005). Other researchers have studied related developmental elaborations using other theoretical models positing self-organization through social interactions with caregivers (e.g., Hsu & Fogel, 2003; Tronick, 2007).

The second defining issue for Phase II is the restriction of range of effective activating and terminating conditions. Bowlby proposed that as infant and caregiver repeat these sequences of interaction, and as the sequences come increasingly under the infant's control in this chain-linked fashion, there is a tendency for the activating and terminating conditions to become restricted to those most commonly part of the behavioral sequence (cf. Thelen & Ulrich's [1991] notion of "attractor states"). Specifically, Phase II is operationally defined in terms of the infant differentiating between the most familiar caregivers and others in directing his or her attachment behavior.

A third and equally important component of Phase II is the infant's increasing tendency to initiate attachment–caregiving and sociable interactions with the principal caregiver(s). Ainsworth (1967) observed that as early as 2 months of age, and increasingly thereafter, infants are active in seeking interaction rather than passively responding to it. Thus, in at least two ways, the infant of Phase II gains responsibility for maintaining contact and interaction with the attachment figure(s): initiating more of the interaction and being able to exert more control over the interaction through increasingly complex chain-linked behaviors.

The elaboration of chain-linked behavioral systems, and the infant's increasingly differential attachment and sociable behavior, may also have important implications for describing the distinct developmental pathways toward the individual differences in patterns of attachment that Ainsworth discovered (e.g., Ainsworth et al., 1978), and found to be applicable to preschoolers (Cassidy & Marvin, 1992; Etzion-Carasso & Oppenheim, 2000), young school-age children (Bohlin, Hagekull, & Andersson, 2005; Main & Cassidy, 1988), and adults (Bakermans-Kranenburg & Van IJzendoorn, 2009; Main, Kaplan, & Cassidy,

1985). There is substantial evidence that the pathways to differential strategies of attachment begin in the first 3 months of life. For example, parents of later-avoidant infants tend to terminate their infants' cries less often and hold them less during the first months of life (Ainsworth et al., 1978). In these cases, the infant is left in a distressed state for considerable periods of time. The context is then ripe for the infant to develop alternative links in its behavioral chains, where behavior on the part of the infant can terminate its distress (e.g., turning its focus in a rather forced manner to exploration). The patterns of infant–parent interaction along this developmental pathway can become stabilized through the same processes at work in the normative, eventually secure, infant, leading to an "avoidant" strategy and a tendency for the infant to contribute to the perpetuation of the pattern. The divergent developmental pathway of the "ambivalent" or "resistant" infant develops according to an analogous process (Ainsworth, 1967; Cassidy & Berlin, 1994).

Finally, these characteristics of Phase II have implications for describing the nature of the infant's IWMs. Most importantly, the infant can increasingly differentiate his or her primary caregiver(s) from others, and in that sense "know" who they are. However, the infant cannot yet conceive of the attachment figure as someone with a separate existence from his or her own experience. Consistent with Piaget's (1952) theory of Stages II and III of the sensorimotor period, Bowlby's theory also implies that this infant's IWMs parallel its chain-linked sequences of behavior: The infant's awareness has expanded to encompass the continuity represented by these sequences, but not yet to the point where he or she can use internal experimentation or manipulation of images, goals, and intentions to devise a plan for achieving a set-goal.

## Phase III: Maintenance of Proximity to a Discriminated Figure by Locomotion and Signals

Phase III, beginning sometime between 6 and 9 months of age, is the phase during which the infant is thought to consolidate attachment to its caregiver(s). It is characterized by a number of important motor, cognitive, and communicative changes, as well as changes in organization among behavioral systems that lead most experts to consider the infant to be "really" attached during this phase.

### NEW ATTACHMENT BEHAVIORS

Locomotion provides the infant with not only a vastly increased ability to control proximity to the attachment figure, to move off to explore, to expand his or her horizons in innumerable ways, but also to place him- or herself in significant danger. In fact, four of the six additional attachment behaviors that Ainsworth (1967) identified are based on this newly developed motor skill. Ainsworth observed these behaviors as differential approach to mother, especially on reunion or when distressed, at 28 weeks; differential following of the mother when she leaves the room at 24 weeks; use of the mother as a secure base for exploration (making exploratory excursions from her, returning to her from time to time, and terminating exploration and attempting to regain proximity if she moves off) at 28 weeks; and flight to the mother as a haven of safety when alarmed at 34 weeks. Two other attachment behaviors to emerge during this same period depend less directly on locomotion (Ainsworth, 1967): differential burying of face (while climbing on the mother; or after an excursion away from her, the infant buries its face in the mother's lap) at 28 weeks; and differential clinging to the mother when alarmed, ill, or distressed at 43 weeks. By 6–8 months, the baby is able to cling to the caregiver in a rather automatic way as its attention is directed elsewhere.

### INFORMATION PROCESSING AND IWMS

A second, revolutionary change associated with the shift to Phase III is an elaboration of the infant's cognitive skills. Some of the systems mediating a child's attachment behavior and many of the earlier, chain-linked behaviors become organized under the infant's intentional control. Bowlby suggested that the Phase III infant has an internal image of a "set-goal" he or she would like to achieve (e.g., physical contact with the attachment figure). The infant can now: operate internally on available behaviors (i.e., a plan) and select behaviors that are likely to achieve that set-goal (e.g., crawl around the sofa to mother); execute the plan; alter it as a function of feedback; then terminate the plan when the discrepancy between the set-goal and the infant's perception of his or her position is reduced to zero.

This describes, in "control systems" terminology, what traditional cognitive theorists have referred to as the infant's newly emerging ability to differentiate means from ends. The ability to organize attachment behavior on a goal-corrected basis also implies that the infant now has an internal image of the attachment figure that is independent of perception (object permanence). In a rather elegant longitudinal study, Bell (1970) demonstrated the parallel (in Piaget's terms, the "horizontal decalage") between the development of object permanence, person (mother) permanence, and the onset of goal-corrected proximity seeking. Consistent with the proposition that children will develop such a general purpose skill first in relationship-based and emotionally salient contexts, Bell found that most infants developed person permanence before object permanence. An active debate endures, however, on the human- or object-first hypotheses (e.g., Bonatti, Frot, Zangl, & Mehler, 2002).

The baby's set-goal in interactions with the attachment figure will vary because sometimes the set-goal will be to maintain some distance from the attachment figure while the infant explores the social and physical world. At other times, it will be mere proximity, or nothing short of close physical contact. What "setting" his or her goal takes at any given time is the result of many factors, including physiological state (e.g., hunger, fatigue); the presence or absence of an alarming event in the environment; assessment of the caregiver's attention to him or her; and whether the caregiver is present, departing/absent, or returning from an absence (Bowlby, 1969/1982). It will also depend on the dyad's history of relatively stable patterns (i.e., individual differences) of attachment–caregiving interactions.

## COMMUNICATION SKILLS

Concurrent with these locomotor and cognitive changes are those in the infant's verbal and nonverbal communication skills. During Phase II, the infant displays increased visual and vocal engagement with others, much of which is of a turn-taking, prelanguage format to which caregivers tend to respond as if it were intentional (Bruner, 1981; Heimann et al., 2006). During Phase III, the infant uses communicative signals in a goal-corrected manner as part of a repertoire of plans for achieving a set-goal that often involves regulating the behavior of others for purposes of requesting or rejecting actions or objects; attracting or maintaining another's attention; and/or establishing/maintaining joint attention for purposes of sharing an experience (Bruner, 1981). At first through the infant's display

and understanding of nonverbal utterances and signals, later through single-word utterances, and still later (18–36 months of age) through complex verbal communication, youngster and caregiver(s) are able to alter each other's behavior indirectly by directly altering each other's set-goals (Marvin, 1977).

All these changes have important implications for the Phase III baby's internal working models. At this point, the baby has separate models of caregiver(s) and of self. These consist of images and plans ordered in some form of a hierarchy—or event schemas or scripts (Stern, 1985)—of self and other. The content of the infant's IWMs are probably derived from some combination of the stable, chain-linked sequences of interaction already developed with the caregiver(s) and the newly stabilizing patterns that emerge with the motor, cognitive, and communication skills that develop during Phase III. The likely more elaborate content of infants' IWMs is also echoed in psychosocial theories of development, as Erikson (1950) proposed that the cumulative sense of trust or mistrust an infant builds across the first year relates to both a sense of confidence in the caregiver and a sense of confidence in the self as an effective agent in social exchanges—the later being a clear parallel to developing schemas or IWM. Indeed, Pittman, Keiley, Kerpelman, and Vaughn (2011) suggest that attachment history—with its foundation in infancy—provides the context for identity formation.

In Phase III, the infant's IWMs remain primitive in at least two ways. First, the infant is limited to thinking about caregiver and self only in terms of caregiver behaviors. The infant has yet to comprehend that the attachment figure has unique perceptions and goals, and that these can differ from his or her own. Second, the infant is unable to think about behaviors in terms of long sequences. The infant's ability to operate in this internal fashion is limited to individual goal-plan hierarchies, or event schemas, with each thought activated and terminated by specific stimuli.

## THE EXPLORATION SYSTEM

The fourth important change that takes place during Phase III is especially related to the changes in the infant's locomotor and cognitive changes (i.e., the elaboration of his exploration behavioral system). The development of locomotion and of object permanence, the more sophisticated understanding of mean–ends relations, the ability increasingly to organize exploration on the basis of goal-corrected behavior, and emerging imitation and conversational skills (e.g., Piaget, 1952) all enhance the infant's ability to learn about the physical and social environment, to test and learn the "rules" that govern those interactions, and to categorize those interactions symbolically and linguistically.

## THE SOCIABILITY SYSTEM

Closely related to the exploration system is the infant's sociability system. Although there appear to be individual differences related to both temperament and relationship history in Phase III infants, infants in this phase are likely to stop exploration when confronted by a strange person, remain wary (or even fearful) for some moments, and either remain stationary or move away from the stranger and toward the attachment figure. After some few moments, if the stranger displays positive affect, is not intrusive, and matches his or her responses to the infant's behavior, the infant is likely to interact sociably, with rapidly decreasing wariness (e.g., Bretherton & Ainsworth, 1974).

## THE WARINESS SYSTEM

The fifth and final major Phase III change involves the infant's wariness behavioral system. Wariness toward novel, and especially sudden, nonhuman events has obvious survival value. What is less obvious is the nature, developmental course, and role played by wariness toward unfamiliar *humans*. Despite the earlier bias toward responding to human stimuli, during the last quarter of the first year, infants increasingly are more wary of unfamiliar adults (Bretherton & Ainsworth, 1974). Although there may be individual and reproductive gene pool differences in temperamental reactivity to strangers (e.g., Kagan, & Fox, 2006), this developmental shift appears to exist whether the infant is raised in a culture in which the norm is single or multiple caregivers (cf. Ainsworth, 1967).

Reciprocal linkages among the older infant's wariness, sociability, and attachment behavioral systems are more obvious and predictable than they were earlier. If the wariness system is highly activated, the infant tends to retreat to the parent as a haven of safety; if it is not, the infant may continue to stare at a nonintrusive stranger, or may initiate or respond sociably. In many cases, one can see a cycling of conflicting behavioral systems, with the infant moving back and forth from parent to stranger, as the distance from each tends to activate one system and terminate the other.

## SENSITIVE PERIODS

That infants become more, rather than less, wary toward unfamiliar humans over the period from 6 to 18–24 months of age, is important for at least two reasons. First, infants *are* vulnerable to danger from other humans, and until they are more able to predict which individuals are dangerous, it is adaptive that their initial reaction be wariness. Second, one of the developmental mechanisms involved in the consolidation of infants' attachment is the reduction in the range of individuals able to activate and terminate infants' attachment behavior (Bowlby, 1969/1982). The infant more and more comes to approach familiar caregiver(s) and to retreat from unfamiliar individuals of the same species. In its general form, this phenomenon is characteristic of many species and is common in the study of "sensitive periods" in development (Bateson, 1976; Knudsen, 2004; Marvin & Britner, 2008).

Bowlby (1969/1982) suggested that the readiness to become quickly attached remains intact at least through the end of the first year. This does not imply that the specific attachment, a more versus less adaptive *form* of attachment, or the lack of an attachment, is completely irreversible after this sensitive period. The results from studies of infants placed in foster care, or raised in East European orphanages and adopted into low-risk homes, suggest that children *can* form discriminating or selective attachments for the first time well after 1 year. However, infants placed in foster care after 12 months of age have been found to be more rejecting toward their new caregivers than younger infants (see Dozier & Rutter, Chapter 30, this volume). And contemporary studies of children adopted from orphanages (e.g., O'Connor et al., 2003; Rutter et al., 2012) increasingly indicate that these children form attachments, but that those attachments are at increased risk of being organized in a significantly less adaptive manner than would be expected given that they are being raised in a low-risk home.

## ORGANIZATION AMONG BEHAVIORAL SYSTEMS

It is during Phase III that the dynamic balance described earlier among the four behavioral systems fully emerges (Ainsworth et al., 1978). For most infants, this balance culminates in organizing the new developments of this phase into what Ainsworth (1990) referred to as the "hallmark" of an attachment—the infant's use of the attachment figure as a secure base for exploration. Stable *variations* in this organization are evident in the different insecure strategies of attachment (Ainsworth et al., 1978; Main & Solomon, 1990). In the case of the "avoidant" strategy, the infant tends, when the attachment system is highly activated, to inhibit attachment behavior and (often) activate the exploration system. In the "resistant" strategy, the infant tends to overamplify the attachment and wariness systems. In the case of infants classified as having a "disorganized" attachment, the simultaneous and/or sequential activation and termination of behavioral systems are especially contradictory and take a form that puts the infant at risk of not being protected (e.g., with activation of the attachment system also serving to activate wary behavior toward the caregiver).

## SUBORDINATE ATTACHMENT FIGURES AND TYPES OF RELATIONSHIPS

Throughout human evolution, children have been raised in families, which themselves are part of larger groups of varied size and composition. Most children have experienced multiple caregivers, giving them the opportunity to form specific attachments to a number of figures. Even in his early writings, Bowlby (e.g., 1958) proposed that infants tend to become attached to a number of caregivers, and that "for a child of 18 months to have only one attachment figure is quite exceptional" (Bowlby, 1969/1982, p. 304).

Several studies across many cultures have suggested that a minority of infants select more than one attachment figure almost as soon as they begin to show any differential attachment behavior, whereas a majority do so by 18 months (e.g., Ainsworth, 1967; Konner, 1976; Schaffer & Emerson, 1964). These and other studies (e.g., Myers, Jarvis, & Creasey, 1987; Umemura, Jacobvitz, Messina, & Hazen, 2013), however, suggest that not all attachment figures are treated by the infant as equivalent. Infants are attached to a range of caregivers; however, attachment behavior, especially when the infant is distressed, hungry, tired, or ill, tends to be focused on a particular person when both that person and other attachment figures are available. Thus, most infants seem to have a network of attachment figures, but the available

data suggest that they may tend to choose one figure as the "primary" attachment figure. Importantly, others may be chosen as the primary figure for play or other types of interactions (see Mesman, Van IJzendoorn, & Sagi-Schwartz, Chapter 37, this volume).

## Development of Attachment during the Toddler and Preschool Years

Most research on social and emotional development during the postinfancy preschool period has focused on issues other than attachment—for example, autonomy, self-control, independence, and socialization. These issues imply a decline in attachment behavior, as the child deals with these later "developmental tasks." Although the framework of developmental tasks can be helpful in guiding our research, it can also lead us astray by restricting the focus to single issues. A full understanding requires viewing development across multiple domains. In fact, while the child *is* becoming more autonomous and self-reliant during the preschool years, he or she remains vulnerable to a range of dangers. The child makes increasingly distant forays from the attachment figure while exploring the environment but is still at an early point in developing the skills needed for self-protection. The close attachment to the caregiver thus remains crucially important to the child's survival and socialization. It is adaptive, rather than "regressive," that attachment behavior remains easily activated.

As we move to the study of attachment in the postinfancy years, we must also be careful not to lose the focus on *behavior* as the child's representational and communicative abilities become increasingly noticeable. Because infants' mental models of attachment cannot possibly be symbolic (i.e., language-based), it must be assumed that those cognitive structures that relate to attachment *behavior* in infancy constitute the mental model (Bretherton, 1993). There is a natural shift in research on attachment past infancy to move to the level of cognitive–emotional representation. The trap is to move to the cognitive level to the relative exclusion of behavior. This would be a terrible error. Bowlby's whole theory—or the cognitive-behavioral part of it—is based on the important linkage between IWMs and behavior. The point is that older children do not move from the level of behavior to the level of internal representation: They become able to process and manipulate plans and goals at that internal level, and increasingly to control behavior with that internal processing. We must remember that the function of an IWM is to organize behavior in more flexible ways.

## Changes in Attachment Behavior during the Toddler/Preschool Years

Although most of our knowledge about the ontogeny of attachment behavior is restricted to the first 12–15 months of life, a few naturalistic studies (e.g., Blurton-Jones, 1972; Konner, 1976; Lyons-Ruth, Connell, Zoll, & Stahl, 1987) and a number of laboratory-based studies (e.g., Main & Cassidy, 1988; Marvin, 1977; Marvin & Greenberg, 1982; Mittal, Russell, Britner, & Peake, 2013; Russell, Londhe, & Britner, 2013) provide a general outline of the normative course of attachment behavior over the preschool and early school years. In reviewing the literature, Bowlby (1969/1982) suggested that during the second and most of the third year of life, attachment behavior is shown neither at less intensity nor less frequency than at the first birthday. In fact, use of attachment figures as a secure base is a critical component of the child's rapidly expanding physical and social world, and attachment behavior therefore remains a major part of his or her behavioral organization.

Overall, 2-year-olds tend to maintain as much, or more, proximity to their mothers as do 1-year-olds. At the same time, they also make more extensive excursions away in order to explore with their more elaborate cognitive and motor abilities. Several studies (e.g., Schaffer & Emerson, 1964) have found that toddlers tend to monitor actively not only the mother's movements but also her attention. When she is not attending to him or her, the child often executes attachment behavior with the set-goal of regaining her attention. This adaptive behavior pattern is sometimes unappreciated in Western cultures, in which it is commonly seen as regressive or controlling "attention seeking" and as frustrating to parents.

Before the third birthday, children are not very adept at maintaining proximity when their attachment figure is moving. The perception of the caregiver moving off is typically a condition that terminates the toddler's exploratory behavior and activates attachment behavior. At this younger age, children can follow the caregiver around the familiar home but find following the caregiver difficult if he or she is moving steadily away from the child. In this situation, one or both members of the dyad initiate physical contact, and the tod-

dler is carried. After the third birthday, with much improved locomotor skills, the child is much less likely to be carried under relaxed circumstances.

When undergoing a separation from the mother that is not of their own initiative, 2-year-olds tend to be as distressed as 1-year-olds, although they are more able to rely on calling and active search behaviors rather than crying. Many 3- and 4-year-olds also become mildly upset by such brief separations, but less so than 2-year-olds, and they are more willing than younger children to be left for brief periods in the company of friendly adults. By the third birthday, it appears that it is being left *alone* that is especially upsetting and likely to elicit strong attachment behavior. If briefly left alone, or if mildly distressed by being left with a friendly adult, most 3- and 4-year-olds are able to wait for the attachment figure's return before executing attachment behavior (Marvin, 1977). For a more detailed review of changes in preschoolers' responses to separations, proximity seeking and contacts with their caregiver, and the organization of the attachment system, see Marvin and Britner (2008).

Research by Marvin (1977; Marvin & Greenberg, 1982) and Cassidy (Cassidy et al., 1992; Main & Cassidy, 1988) suggest the importance of Bowlby's (1969/1982) proposed final phase in the development of attachment, the "goal-corrected partnership." They are also congruent with earlier research suggesting that sometime around age 4, children are much less dependent on physical proximity and contact with their attachment figure(s) to maintain a sense of security and are increasingly comfortable spending appreciable periods of time in the company of nonfamilial peers and adults (Blurton-Jones, 1972; Konner, 1976). In the following sections, we briefly review literature on other developmental domains relevant to the changes in attachment behavior outlined earlier, then review the theoretical and empirical work on the goal-corrected partnership.

## Developmental Changes in Relations among Behavioral Systems

Ainsworth and colleagues (1978) showed how, in 1-year-olds, the attachment, exploration, wariness, and sociability systems function in the dynamic equilibrium described earlier. Observation of young children's behavior when they are introduced to a friendly adult stranger presents an excellent opportunity to study this dynamic balance, and it has yielded some evidence that this organization changes over the preschool years in a way that is consistent with the youngster's gradually increased responsibility for self-protection based on increasingly sophisticated behavioral organization.

Greenberg and Marvin (1982) studied young children's initial reactions to a friendly stranger. The most common response among 3- and 4-year-olds was to (apparently) ignore the stranger and continue exploring, without activation of either the wariness or attachment behavioral systems. The next most common response was the *simultaneous* activation of the wariness and sociability systems (usually in the form of coy expressions) and coincidental activation of the attachment system. No 2-year-olds displayed this more complex pattern. Most children of all three ages eventually played sociably with the stranger. Whereas a few of the younger children remained fearful of the stranger throughout the situation, none of the older children did so. Finally, all 2-year-olds (but none of the 3- or 4-year-olds) who displayed wariness toward the stranger while the mother was gone also displayed attachment behavior toward the mother when she returned. Greenberg and Marvin suggested that this decreased developmental coupling of the wariness and attachment behavioral systems, and the increased developmental coupling of the wariness and sociability systems, could have important implications for children's increasing ability to cope with strangers on their own: The careful approach implied by the coincidental activation of the wariness and sociability systems could provide the basis for strategies of social interaction that could fulfill the same protective function earlier fulfilled by the close physical bond between the child and his or her attachment figure(s).

## Changes in Locomotor and Self-Care Skills

Humans exhibit a developmental organization during the preschool years that suggests the crucial importance of a continuing protective attachment, while at the same time providing the young child with the independence necessary to learn the skills that will be required during the following phase. Milk teeth are completed between ages 2 and 3 years, and by 3 years children are quite independent in feeding themselves. Although Western cultures are now clearly different, in less industrialized cultures, breast feeding tapers off between 3 and 4 years of age. By age 3, the child's locomotor skills have developed to the point that he or she

can assume much of the responsibility for gaining and maintaining proximity to the attachment figure under most conditions, as well as engage in vigorous play with other children and practice many of the social skills he or she will use in a over the next decade. By the beginning of the school-age period, the child is capable of most of the motor skills of older children, although strength, endurance, coordination, etc. continue to improve.

## Changes in Communication Skills

It is during the preschool period that children develop most of the communication skills that will later be required for stable integration into their social group(s), independent of the close physical tie to their attachment figure(s). By 30 months, children increasingly communicate about past and future events and emotional states, and connected narrative discourse emerges as children begin to relate logical sequences of events across many utterances (e.g., Bretherton, 1993; Dunn, 1994). Dunn (1994) found that during the second and third years, children are increasingly able to recognize, understand, and converse about the feelings and behaviors of other family members; they comfort, tease, argue, joke, and blame. She concluded that by 3 years of age, children understand surprisingly complex rules for social interaction, interpret others' feelings and goals, and use such rules to manipulate others' internal states. It now seems clear that by age 4, most children are becoming competent at one of our species' most sophisticated communication skills: thinking and conversing about the feelings, goals, and plans of others with whom they are interacting (see Hughes & Leekham, 2004). This skill, indicative of children's developing theory of mind, should have important implications for the organization of attachment interactions.

Although there has been little recent research on the ontogeny of nonverbal expressions in preschool children, some of the early work in human ethology (Blurton-Jones, 1972; Hinde, 1976) suggested that many of the expressions used to regulate interactions during childhood and adolescence develop during the preschool years. Furthermore, studies of coy expressions (Marvin, 1997) and of posed expressions of happiness, surprise, anger, fear, sadness, and disgust (Lewis, Sullivan, & Vasen, 1987) again suggest that the period between the third and fourth birthdays is especially important in the developmental elaboration and understanding of a range of complex expressions used to regulate interactions.

## Changes in Information-Processing Skills and IWMs

Extensive research, including the work of Bretherton (1993), Callaghan and colleagues (2005), Cassidy and Marvin (1992), Dunn (1994), Stern (1985), and Ziv, Oppenheim, and Sagi-Schwartz (2004), suggests that during the second through sixth years of life, children are developing sophisticated and accurate (in the sense of nonegocentric) IWMs of their own, and of others' behavior and internal experiences. At the same time, they are developing surprisingly sophisticated IWMs of implicit and explicit rules for social behavior and interaction. The reader is referred to the studies listed earlier, and to other chapters in this volume (particularly Bretherton and Munholland, Chapter 4) for information about the *content* of, and individual differences in, these IWMs, and to Marvin and Britner (2008) for details on developmental changes in their underlying *form*.

## Phase IV: Implications of the Partnership for the Organization of Attachment Behavior during the Preschool Years

Although this partnership is certainly a general purpose skill used in interactions with family members, other adults, and peers, it is likely that it will first be applied in emotionally powerful interactions such as attachment–caregiving interactions. Marvin (1977) and Marvin and Greenberg (1982) studied its application to this type of interaction and suggested two important organizational changes. The first is related to the young preschooler's ability to inhibit attachment behavior and insert the caregiver's plans into the child's own plan for proximity, resulting in what might be called the "emergent partnership." The second is related to the older preschooler's ability to operate internally on the goals and plans of self and other simultaneously, to understand objectively (i.e., nonegocentrically) the causal relations between the caregiver's goals/plans and behavior, and to engage in goal-corrected negotiations with the caregiver regarding a shared plan for proximity, forming a goal-corrected partnership.

With regard to the first organizational change, Bowlby (1969/1982) proposed that a toddler's attachment plans vary in the extent to which they are designed to influence the behavior of the

attachment figure. He suggested that the earliest goal-corrected plans for changing the caregiver's behavior are primitive (e.g., pushing her in certain directions, knocking a book off his lap, throwing a tantrum). These early attempts are based either on changing the caregiver's behavior directly through physical means or indirectly, through crying and anger. During this same period, parents rely largely on techniques such as distracting the toddler to influence his or her behavior.

As the dyad's conversational skills become elaborated, and as the child develops self-control, it should become increasingly the case that child and mother are able to change each other's behavior through linguistic communication. Although the child cannot yet negotiate a shared plan with the caregiver in a goal-corrected manner, the child *can* attempt to change the caregiver's goal or plan, inhibit ongoing behavior, insert one of the caregiver's goals into his or her own plan for action, and thus function in an interaction that has the "predictable outcome" of shared goals.

Marvin (1977) provided an initial test of this hypothesis by administering two analogous procedures to a sample of 2-, 3-, and 4-year-old children, one relevant to interaction in a nonattachment context (i.e., a waiting task), and the other in an attachment–caregiving context (i.e., the Strange Situation). The results of both procedures suggest that by 3 years of age, most children are able to inhibit ongoing, goal-corrected behavior across at least two types of interactions, insert one of mother's communicated goals into their own plan, and wait until the circumstances are appropriate for both mother and child before executing their plan.

The results also suggest a further change in the organization of attachment behavior sometime around the fourth birthday. The hierarchical reorganization of the older preschooler's IWMs and information-processing skills that enables the child to operate in a nonegocentric fashion *simultaneously* on the perspectives of self and others, and in a goal-corrected manner to construct shared plans with the caregiver, should have important implications for the organization of attachment behavior. Marvin (1977) suggested that at least five component skills are involved: (1) the ability to recognize that the attachment figure possesses internal events including thoughts, goals, plans, feelings, and so forth; (2) the ability to distinguish between the caregiver's point of view and one's own, especially when they differ; (3) the ability to infer, from logic and/or experience, what factors control the caregiver's goals and plans; (4) the ability to assess the degree of coordination, or match, between their respective points of view; and (5) the ability to influence the caregiver's goals and plans in a goal-corrected manner. On the basis of much research over the past 20 years (e.g., Bretherton, 1993; Dunn, 1994; Mittal et al., 2013), it seems possible that by age 4, most children possess these component skills.

We do not mean to imply that children age 4 years or older do not want, need, or enjoy physical proximity and contact with their attachment figures. Under conditions of distress, illness, and fear, children—even much older children—continue to retreat to their attachment figure(s) as a haven of safety. As suggested by the attachment classification systems developed by Cassidy and Marvin (1992) and Main and Cassidy (1988), preschool and young school-age children also continue to maintain and enjoy this close tie through a range of intimate behaviors. What is implied by the model is that this older preschooler has come to organize attachment behavior in a new way: one that enables the child to realize that he or she and the attachment figure have a continuing relationship whether or not they are in close proximity. This new organization is one in which the child is increasingly responsible for maintaining whatever protective proximity is necessary. In conjunction with the other recently developed locomotor, communication, and information-processing skills, this organization allows the older child to maintain a close tie to the attachment figure(s) while increasingly moving off from them and spending more time with a peer group, teachers, and others.

## Changes in Attachment Behavior beyond the Preschool Years

Bowlby (1969/1982) suggested that the goal-corrected partnership is probably the last phase in the ontogeny of attachment. By this he seems to have meant that there are no further "stage" changes in this behavioral system. The attachment behavioral system, however, remains important throughout the lifespan and does continue to undergo significant changes. These probably include further elaborations at the same "level," as well as changes in the relations between the attachment and other behavioral systems, the higher-order control structures, activating and terminating conditions, and IWMs. Certainly, there are also many instances in which children form new attachments. One clear implication is

that attachment becomes increasingly difficult to measure as it becomes more sophisticated, more abstract, and less dependent on proximity and contact, as the behavioral systems becomes elaborated into more and more complex systems (Bowlby, 1969/1982). For a detailed account of the course of these developmental changes, see Marvin and Britner (2008), as well as the relevant developmental chapters in this volume.

## Conclusion

Attachment theory began with Bowlby's (e.g., 1958) attempt to understand the psychopathological effects of maternal deprivation by studying the normative course of the ontogeny of this earliest relationship. Bowlby's hope was that if we better understood this normative course, we would be in an improved position to understand disruption. We are convinced that Bowlby's attempt to integrate the study of individual differences with that of normative development is as important today as it was six decades ago. The last 20 years have seen contributions to the attachment literature that emphasize descriptions of individual differences across special populations; in particular, there is a trend toward considerations of what might be considered comorbidity or the linkages between processes and outcomes for unique samples (i.e., populations of individuals identified as on the autism spectrum or struggling with attention disorders, or studies that consider connections between attachment quality in early childhood and later conduct disorders and other social or mental health pathologies). Perhaps the largest overarching need this field must address in future work is the current dearth of scholarship on the lifespan nature of normative attachment, across a diversity of populations and sociocultural contexts.

This volume is filled with chapters addressing a variety of populations, relationships, and developmental periods. A full understanding of each of these separate issues will not be possible without considering the organization of the individual's attachment behavioral system in the period under study. In fact, the most powerful design would be to *integrate* normative and differential approaches through the use of developmental pathway models first discussed by Bowlby (1969/1982; based on Waddington, 1957) and supplemented by our growing understanding of the different kinds of relationships that emerge across development.

# References

Ainsworth, M. D. S. (1967). *Infancy in Uganda: Infant care and the growth of love.* Baltimore, MD: Johns Hopkins University Press.

Ainsworth, M. D. S. (1990). Some considerations regarding theory and assessment relevant to attachments beyond infancy. In M. T. Greenberg, D. Cicchetti, & E. M. Cummings (Eds.), *Attachment in the preschool years: Theory, research and intervention* (pp. 463–488). Chicago: University of Chicago Press.

Ainsworth, M. D. S., Blehar, M. C., Waters, E., & Wall, S. (1978). *Patterns of attachment: A psychological study of the Strange Situation.* Hillsdale, NJ: Erlbaum.

Ashby, W. R. (1952). *Design for a brain.* New York: Wiley.

Ashby, W. R. (1956). *An introduction to cybernetics.* New York: Wiley.

Bakermans-Kranenburg, M., & Van IJzendoorn, M. H. (2009). The first 10,000 Adult Attachment Interviews: Distributions of adult attachment representations in clinical and non-clinical groups. *Attachment and Human Development, 11,* 223–263.

Bateson, P. P. G. (1976). Rules and reciprocity in behavioural development. In P. P. G. Bateson & R. A. Hinde (Eds.), *Growing points in ethology* (pp. 401–421). Cambridge, UK: Cambridge University Press.

Baumrind, D. (1980). New directions in socialization research. *American Psychologist, 35,* 639–652.

Bell, S. M. V. (1970). The development of the concept of the object as related to infant–mother attachment. *Child Development, 40,* 291–311.

Beyers, W., Goossens, L., Vansant, I., & Moors, E. (2003). Structural model of autonomy in middle and late adolescence: Connectedness, separation, detachment, and agency. *Journal of Youth and Adolescence, 32,* 351–365.

Blurton-Jones, N. (1972). *Ethological studies of child behavior.* New York: Cambridge University Press.

Bohlin, G., Hagekull, B., & Andersson, K. (2005). Behavioral inhibition as a precursor of peer social competence in early school age: The interplay with attachment and nonparental care. *Merrill–Palmer Quarterly, 51,* 1–19.

Bonatti, L., Frot, E., Zangl, R., & Mehler, J. (2002). The human first hypothesis: Identification of conspecifics and individuation of objects in the young infant. *Cognitive Psychology, 44,* 388–426.

Bowlby, J. (1958). The nature of the child's tie to his mother. *International Journal of Psycho-Analysis, 39,* 350–373.

Bowlby, J. (1973). *Attachment and loss: Vol. II. Separation.* New York: Basic Books.

Bowlby, J. (1979). *The making and breaking of affectional bonds.* London: Tavistock.

Bowlby, J. (1980). *Attachment and loss: Vol. III. Loss.* New York: Basic Books.

Bowlby, J. (1982). *Attachment and loss: Vol. I. Attachment* (2nd ed.). New York: Basic Books. (Original work published 1969)

Brazelton, T. B. (1962). Crying in infancy. *Pediatrics, 29,* 579–588.

Bretherton, I. (1993). From dialogue to internal working models: The coconstruction of self in relationships. In C. A. Nelson (Ed.), *Memory and affect in development: The Minnesota Symposia on Child Psychology* (Vol. 26, pp. 237–263). Hillsdale, NJ: Erlbaum.

Bretherton, I., & Ainsworth, M. D. S. (1974). Responses of 1-year-olds to a stranger in a Strange Situation. In M. Lewis & L. A. Rosenblum (Eds.), *The origins of fear* (pp. 131–164). New York: Wiley.

Britner, P. A., Marvin, R. S., & Pianta, R. C. (2005). Development and preliminary validation of the caregiving behavior system: Association with child attachment classification in the preschool Strange Situation. *Attachment and Human Development, 7,* 83–102.

Bruner, J. (1981). The social context of language acquisition. *Language and Communication, 1,* 155–178.

Burlingham, D., & Freud, A. (1944). *Young children in war-time.* London: Allen & Unwin.

Callaghan, T., Rochat, P., Lillard, A., Claux, M. L., Odden, H., Itakura, S., et al. (2005). Synchrony in the onset of mental state reasoning: Evidence from 5 cultures. *Psychological Science, 16,* 378–384.

Cassidy, J., & Berlin, L. (1994). The insecure/ambivalent pattern of attachment: Theory and research. *Child Development, 65,* 971-991.

Cassidy, J., & Marvin, R. S., with the MacArthur Attachment Working Group. (1992). *Attachment organization in preschool children: Procedures and coding manual.* Unpublished document, University of Virginia.

Dunn, J. (1994). Changing minds and changing relationships. In C. Lewis & P. Mitchell (Eds.), *Children's early understanding of mind: Origins and development* (pp. 297–310). Hillsdale, NJ: Erlbaum.

Erikson, E. H. (1950). *Childhood and society.* New York: Norton.

Etzion-Carasso, A., & Oppenheim, D. (2000). Open mother–preschooler communication: Relations with early secure attachment. *Attachment and Human Development, 2,* 347–370.

Freedman, D. G., & Gorman, J. (1993). Attachment and the transmission of culture: An evolutionary perspective. *Journal of Social and Evolutionary Systems, 16,* 297–329.

Garon, N. M., Longard, J., Bryson, S. E., Moore, C. (2012). Making decisions about now and later: The development of future-oriented self-control. *Cognitive Development, 27,* 314–322.

George, C., & Solomon, J. (1996). Representations of relationships: Links between caregiving and attachment. *Infant Mental Health Journal, 17,* 198–216.

Greenberg, M. T., & Marvin, R. S. (1982). Reactions of preschool children to an adult stranger: A behavioral systems approach. *Child Development, 53,* 481–490.

Harlow, H. F., & Harlow, M. K. (1965). The affectional systems. In A. M. Schrier, H. F. Harlow, & F. Stollnitz (Eds.), *Behavior of nonhuman primates* (Vol. 2, pp. 287–334). New York: Academic Press.

Heimann, M., Strid, K., Smith, L., Tjus, T., Ulvund, S. E., & Meltzoff, A. N. (2006). Exploring the relation between memory, gestural communication, and the emergence of language in infancy: A longitudinal study. *Infant and Child Development, 15*, 233–249.

Hinde, R. A. (1976). On describing relationships. *Journal of Child Psychology and Psychiatry, 17*, 1–19.

Hsu, H.-C., & Fogel, A. (2003). Stability and transitions in mother–infant face-to-face communication during the first 6 months: A microhistorical approach. *Developmental Psychology, 39*, 1061–1082.

Hughes, C., & Leekam, S. (2004). What are the links between theory of mind and social reasoning?: Review, reflections and new directions for studies of typical and atypical development. *Social Development, 13*, 590–619.

Kagan, J., & Fox, N. A. (2006). Biology, culture, and temperamental biases. In N. Eisenberg, W. Damon, & R. M. Lerner (Eds.), *Handbook of child psychology: Vol. 3. Social, emotional, and personality development* (6th ed.; pp. 167–225). Hoboken, NJ: Wiley.

Kisilevsky, B. S., Hains, S. M., Lee, K., Xie, X., Huang, H., Ye, H. H., et al. (2003). Effects of experience on fetal voice recognition. *Psychological Science, 14*, 220–224.

Knudsen, E. I. (2004). Sensitive periods in the development of the brain and behavior. *Journal of Cognitive Neuroscience, 16*, 1412–1425.

Kobak, R. (1994). Adult attachment: A personality or relationship construct? *Psychological Inquiry, 5*, 42–44.

Kogan, N., & Carter, A. S. (1996). Mother–infant reengagement following the still-face: The role of maternal emotional availability in infant affect regulation. *Infant Behavior and Development, 19*, 359–370.

Konner, M. (1976). Maternal care, infant behavior and development among the !Kung. In R. Lee & I. DeVore (Eds.), *Kalahari hunter gatherers: Studies of the !Kung San and their neighbors* (pp. 377–394). Cambridge, MA: Harvard University Press.

Kruse, J., & Walper, S. (2008). Individuation in relation to parents: Predictors and outcomes. *International Journal of Behavioral Development, 32*, 390–400.

Lewis, M., Sullivan, M. W., & Vasen, A. (1987). Making faces: Age and emotion differences in the posing of emotional expressions. *Developmental Psychology, 23*, 690–697.

Lyons-Ruth, K., Connell, D. B., Zoll, D., & Stahl, J. (1987). Infants at social risk: Relations among infant maltreatment, maternal behavior, and infant attachment behavior. *Developmental Psychology, 23*, 223–232.

Main, M., & Cassidy, J. (1988). Categories of response to reunion with the parent at age six: Predictable from infant attachment classifications and stable over a one-month period. *Developmental Psychology, 24*, 415–426.

Main, M., Goldwyn, R., & Hesse, E. (2003). *Adult attachment scoring and classification system.* Unpublished manuscript, University of California, Berkeley.

Main, M., Kaplan, N., & Cassidy, J. (1985). Security in infancy, childhood, and adulthood: A move to the level of representation. In I. Bretherton & E. Waters (Eds.), *Growing points of attachment theory and research. Monographs of the Society for Research in Child Development, 50*(1–2), 66–104.

Main, M., & Solomon, J. (1990). Procedures for identifying infants and disorganized/disoriented during the Ainsworth Strange Situation. In M. T. Greenberg, D. Cicchetti, & E. M. Cummings (Eds.), *Attachment in the preschool years: Theory, research and intervention* (pp. 134–146). Chicago: University of Chicago Press.

Marshall, J. (2011). Infant neurosensory development: Considerations for infant child care. *Early Childhood Education Journal, 39*, 175–181.

Marvin, R. S. (1977). An ethological–cognitive model for the attenuation of mother–child attachment behavior. In T. M. Alloway, L. Krames, & P. Pliner (Eds.), *Advances in the study of communication and affect, Vol. III: Attachment behavior* (pp. 25–60). New York: Plenum Press.

Marvin, R. S. (1997). Ethological and general systems perspectives on child–parent attachment during the toddler and preschool years. In N. Segal, G. Weisfeld, & C. Weisfeld (Eds.), *Genetic, ethological, and evolutionary perspectives on human development* (pp. 189–216). Washington, DC: American Psychological Association.

Marvin, R. S., & Britner, P. A. (2008). Normative development: The ontogeny of attachment. In J. Cassidy & P. Shaver (Eds.), *Handbook of attachment: Theory, research, and clinical applications* (2nd ed., pp. 269–294). New York: Guilford Press.

Marvin, R. S., & Greenberg, M. T. (1982). Preschoolers' changing conceptions of their mothers: A social-cognitive study of mother–child attachment. In D. Forbes & M. T. Greenberg (Eds.), *New directions for child development: Children's planning strategies* (Vol. 18, pp. 47–60). San Francisco: Jossey-Bass.

Mesman, J., Van IJzendoorn, M. H., & Bakermans-Kranenburg, M. J. (2009). The many faces of the still-face paradigm: A review and meta-analysis. *Developmental Review, 29*, 120–162.

Mittal, R., Russell, B. S., Britner, P. A., & Peake, P. K. (2013). Delay of gratification in two- and three-year-olds: Associations with attachment, personality, and temperament. *Journal of Child and Family Studies, 22*, 479–489.

Myers, B. J., Jarvis, P. A., & Creasey, G. L. (1987). Infants' behavior with their mothers and grandmothers. *Infant Behavior and Development, 10*, 245–259.

O'Connor, T. G., Marvin, R. S., Rutter, M., Olrick, J., Britner, P. A., and the English and Romanian Adoptees Study Team. (2003). Child–parent attachment following early severe institutional deprivation. *Development and Psychopathology, 15*, 19–38.

Piaget, J. (1952). *The origins of intelligence in children.* New York: International Universities Press.

Pittman, J. F., Keiley, M. K., Kerpelman, J. L., & Vaughn, B. E. (2011). Attachment, identity, and intimacy: Parallels between Bowlby's and Erikson's paradigms. *Journal of Family Theory and Review, 3,* 32–46.

Robertson, J. (1953). *A two-year-old goes to hospital* [Film]. London: Tavistock Child Development Research Unit.

Russell, B. S., Londhe, R., & Britner, P. A. (2013). Parenting contributions to the delay of gratification in young preschool-aged children. *Journal of Child and Family Studies, 22,* 471–478.

Rutter, M., Beckett, C., Castle, J., Colvert, E., Kreppner, J., Mehta, M., et al. (2012). Effects of profound early institutional deprivation: An overview of findings from a UK longitudinal study of Romanian adoptees. In G. M. Wrobel & E. Neil (Eds.), *International advances in adoption research for practice* (pp. 147–167). Hoboken, NJ: Wiley.

Schaffer, H. R., & Emerson, P. E. (1964). The developments of social attachments in infancy. *Monographs of the Society for Research in Child Development, 29*(3), 1–77.

Sommerville, J. A., & Woodward, A. L. (2005). Pulling out the intentional structure of action: The relation between action processing and action production in infancy. *Cognition, 95,* 1–30.

Sroufe, L. A., & Waters, E. (1977). Attachment as an organizational construct. *Child Development, 48,* 1184–1199.

Stern, D. (1985). *The interpersonal world of the infant.* New York: Basic Books.

Thelen, E., & Ulrich, B. D. (1991). Hidden skills: A dynamic systems analysis of treadmill stepping during the first year of life. *Monographs of the Society for Research in Child Development, 56* (1, Serial No. 223), 1–98.

Toda, S., & Fogel, A. (1993). Infant response to the still-face situation at 3 and 6 months. *Developmental Psychology, 29,* 532–538.

Tronick, E. (2007). *The neurobehavioral and social-emotional development of infants and children.* New York: Springer.

Umemura, T., Jacobvitz, D., Messina, S., & Hazen, N. (2013). Do toddlers prefer the primary caregiver or the parent with whom they feel more secure?: The role of toddler emotion regulation. *Infant Behavior and Development, 36,* 102–114.

Waddington, C. H. (1957). *The strategy of the genes.* London: Allen & Unwin.

Wolff, P. H. (1969). The natural history of crying and other vocalizations in early infancy. In B. M. Foss (Ed.), *Determinants of infant behavior* (Vol. 4; pp. 81–109). New York: Barnes & Noble.

Zeanah, C., Smyke, A., Koga, S., & Carlson, E. (2005) Attachments in institutionalized and community children in Romania. *Child Development, 76,* 1015–1028.

Ziv, Y., Oppenheim, D., & Sagi-Schwartz, A. (2004). Social information processing in middle childhood: Relations to infant–mother attachment. *Attachment and Human Development, 6,* 327–348.

# Chapter 14

# Precursors of Attachment Security

R. M. Pasco Fearon
Jay Belsky

Why do some infants develop secure attachments to their primary caregivers, whereas others establish insecure relationships? This is the central question addressed in this chapter. Even though John Bowlby was deeply concerned with the consequences of variation in the quality of early attachments, Mary Ainsworth brought the topic of the origins of individual differences in infant–parent attachment to center stage. Bowlby (e.g., 1944) originally focused his thinking on evolution, species-typical development, and the effects of major separations from parents early in life, whereas Ainsworth (1973) was the first to devote considerable empirical and theoretical energies to the determinants of secure and insecure attachments in normal, nonclinical populations.

Central to Ainsworth's extension of Bowlby's attachment theory was the contention that a sensitive, responsive caregiver is of fundamental importance to the development of a secure attachment bond during the opening years of life. Thus, a caregiver capable of providing security-inducing, sensitive, responsive care understands the child's individual attributes; accepts the child's behavioral proclivities; and is thereby capable of consistently orchestrating harmonious interactions between self and child, especially, though not exclusively, those in which the soothing of distress is involved. In extending Bowlby's theory,

Ainsworth never expressed the belief that the development of the relationship between infant and caregiver was determined entirely by the caregiver. Nevertheless, she was convinced that the developing relationship was not shaped equally by the two participants. Recognizing the greater maturity and power of the adult, Ainsworth attributed disproportionate influence to the adult caregiver.

Nonetheless, the notion of maternal sensitivity championed by Ainsworth in her efforts to account for individual differences in attachment security was defined at least in part in terms of what the child brought to the relationship and, more specifically, how the child behaved at a particular time (i.e., the child's cues, needs, focus of attention, ongoing activities). By definition, then, care that is sensitive and theorized to promote security in the child does not take exactly the same form for all children. Nor does it take the same form across all situations in the case of a particular child.

The first part of this chapter contains a summary of research on the effects of mothering and mother–infant interaction on attachment security—the issues raised most directly by Ainsworth. Related evidence pertaining to the effects of the quality of fathering and of nonparental caregivers' care on attachment to father and to caregivers, respectively, is also considered. In addition, the issue of whether effects of sensitive care on attachment security are evident outside the Western world is considered, as this is important for understanding how universal or general these developmental processes are.

In the second part of the chapter, the broader social or ecological context of attachment and parental care is considered. An ecological perspective draws attention to the multiple levels of influence affecting care (see Belsky & Jaffee, 2006) and therefore, in principle, affecting attachment security. These influences include the psychological attributes of the mother, her relations with her partner, and the degree to which she has access to other social agents who provide instrumental and emotional support. Thus, whereas the core of attachment theory focuses on the microprocesses of development, emphasizing the daily interactional exchanges between parent and child and the developing internal working model of the child, the ecological/social-contextual perspective highlights the contextual factors and processes likely to influence these microdevelopmental processes.

## The Quality of Maternal and Nonmaternal Care

Soon after Ainsworth (1973) first advanced her ideas and evidence of the role of maternal sensitivity in fostering the development of a secure attachment relationship, what might be regarded as a "cottage industry" developed within the field of developmental psychology, seeking to replicate—or refute—her findings. Child temperament was the major focus of those initially seeking to disconfirm Ainsworth's theory and evidence (Chess & Thomas, 1982; Kagan, 1982), and in this chapter in previous editions (1999 and 2008) it was difficult to consider the role of maternal sensitivity and the quality of maternal care more generally without devoting some attention to the influence of this particular infant characteristic. But the field has moved on from this focus, no doubt because of the absence of evidence—reviewed in earlier editions of this volume—substantiating this claim. In fact, even the proposition that variation in the manifestation of insecurity—resistance versus avoidance—might reflect effects of temperament (Belsky & Rovine, 1987) has not been persuasively supported (Vaughn, Bost, & Van IJzendoorn, 2008). Rather than review the relevant research, we refer the interested reader to Bakermans-

Kranenburg and Van IJzendoorn (2012) and to previous chapters by Belsky and Fearon (2008) and Vaughn and associates (2008) in the preceding edition of this volume (see also Vaughn & Bost, Chapter 10, this volume).

Even if temperament, especially difficult temperament and proneness to distress, has not proven to be a major contributor to attachment security, it would be a mistake to presume that challenges to Ainsworth's sensitivity hypothesis have been abandoned. As the next subsection makes clear, researchers have now turned to the role of genetics in shaping attachment. We consider this new body of research before considering evidence implicating sensitivity and the quality and nature of care that children receive more generally as an important determinant of attachment security.

## The Role of Genes

Two distinct approaches to this issue are considered here, one quantitative-genetic in orientation, relying on twin designs, and the other molecular-genetic in character, focusing on measured genes. A more in-depth treatment of the behavioral genetics of attachment is provided by Bakermans-Kranenburg and Van IJzendoorn, Chapter 8, this volume.

### Twin Studies

Four studies assessing infant–mother attachment in samples of monozygotic (MZ) and dizygotic (DZ) twins have proved strikingly similar in their results. In a sample of 157 MZ and DZ twins seen in the Strange Situation at 12 months, Bokhorst and colleagues (2003) found 60% correspondence in MZ twins and 57% in DZ twins. In genetic modeling, 52% of the variance in attachment security within the organized categories was attributable to shared environmental effects, whereas the remainder was estimated to be due to nonshared environment and measurement error. When disorganization was considered, no genetic or shared environmental effects were detected, and all of the variance was attributable to nonshared environment and measurement error. Broadly convergent results have been reported by O'Connor and Croft (2001) in an older sample of preschoolers using the MacArthur modified Strange Situation (see also Ricciuti, 1992, for an early small-scale study yielding comparable findings). More recently, Roisman and Fraley (2008) reported similar results from a relatively large ($N = 485$) twin study of 2-year-olds, using a shortened version of the observer-reported Attachment Q-Sort (AQS), and found that 53% of the variance in security was attributable to shared environment, 36% to non-shared environment and measurement error, and a nonsignificant 17% to genes. Bucking this trend of limited or no genetic influence is the investigation by Finkel and Matheny (2000), who documented significant genetic effects (25%) and no shared environmental effects on attachment security. This surprising result appeared to be due to the low DZ correspondence (compared to other DZ samples or fraternal siblings) of 48%, rather than a high correspondence among MZ twins (which was 66%). Conceivably, these researchers' reliance on a non-standard separation–reunion procedure originally designed to assess temperament could explain why their results are so different from the other four investigations.

Despite the relatively modest sample sizes of each of these studies, the cumulative picture is quite consistent, suggesting a significant role for shared and nonshared environmental effects and apparently little role for genetics, at least in the low-risk populations studied. This conclusion is buttressed by results from the only genetic study of infant–*father* attachment, which relied on AQS Security scores derived from mother sorts of infant behavior vis-à-vis the father (Bakermans-Kranenburg, Van IJzendoorn, Bokhorst, & Schuengel, 2004): Genetic modeling revealed that attachment was explained virtually exclusively by shared environmental (59%) and unique environmental (41%) factors. Moreover, these results are consistent with data indicating that the attachment security of infants placed in foster care is predictable from the adult attachment status of the genetically unrelated foster caregiver (Dozier, Stovall, Albus, & Bates, 2001), as well as the fact that infants can show different patterns of attachment to their mothers and fathers (e.g., Steele, Steele, & Fonagy, 1996). The apparent preeminence of the environment—and of the shared environment in particular—is a remarkable confirmation of a key hypothesis of attachment theory.

## Molecular Genetics Research

Molecular genetic studies represent an alternative methodology for investigating the role of genes in the development of attachment. Much of this work was stimulated by Lakatos and colleagues' (2000,

2002) groundbreaking investigation linking disorganized attachment with a polymorphism of the *DRD4* dopamine receptor gene (*Exon III 48-bp VNTR*). Twelve of 17 disorganized infants had the 7-repeat allele of this gene (which has been found to confer lower dopamine neurotransmission than the more common 4-repeat allele), compared to 21 of 73 nondisorganized infants. Quite a number of efforts to replicate this genotype–phenotype association have failed to reproduce the finding. Indeed, Bakermans-Kranenburg and Van IJzendoorn's (2007) meta-analysis revealed a weighted effect size for the association of $d = 0.05$ ($N = 542$), which was not significant. And in the time since their report, five additional studies have proven consistent with this early multistudy analysis (Frigerio et al., 2009; Luijk et al., 2011 [involving two independent cohorts]; Raby et al., 2012; Spangler, Johann, Ronai, & Zimmerman, 2009).

Although the association between attachment and the *DRD4* gene has proved unreliable, several other gene variants have been examined in relation to attachment security and insecurity, mostly with respect to gene × environment (G × E) interactions (but see Spangler et al., 2009, for a genotype–phenotype study). Van IJzendoorn and Bakermans-Kranenburg (2006), for example, found that unresolved loss in mothers ($N = 85$) was more strongly associated with disorganized attachment among *DRD4/7+* infants relative to *DRD4/7 –* infants, suggesting greater susceptibility to the effects of unresolved maternal loss in the former. Spangler and colleagues (2009; $N = 106$) examined the *DRD4* gene and parental responsiveness, detecting no G × E interaction (or main effect of *DRD4*), but they did find (in addition to a genetic main effect) an interaction with the *5-HTTLPR* (serotonin transporter) gene: Infants with less responsive maternal care and the short-form of the *5-HTTLPR* gene were more likely to be disorganized. Similar results were reported by Barry, Kochanska, and Philibert (2008; $N = 88$): Overall insecurity in the Strange Situation (rather than disorganization specifically) was predicted by the combination of low responsiveness and the short-form of the *5-HTTLPR* gene. When examining attachment security at both 12 and 18 months, Raby and colleagues (2012; $N = 154$) failed to find a genetic main effect of *5-HTTLPR* (as did Frigerio et al. [2009] and Barry et al. [2008]) or an interaction between the *5-HTTLPR* gene and responsiveness of maternal care, although it is notable that this study did not include codes for disorganized attachment. Perhaps most important are the results of a report from Luijk and colleagues (2011) indicating that no genetic main effects or G × E interactions proved replicable across two large samples, the Dutch Generation R study ($N$ = 506–547) and the U.S. National Institute of Child Health and Development (NICHD) Study of Early Child Care and Youth Development ($N$ = 478–522), especially since all the candidate genes implicated in the attachment literature were considered (*DRD4*, *5-HTTLPR*, two oxytocin receptor genes, and *COMT*), along with their interaction with parental sensitivity in relation to security and disorganization. (Although one genetic main effect—of the *COMT* gene—was significant for disorganization in both samples at the uncorrected 5% level, it would not survive corrections for multiple hypothesis testing.)

A conservative interpretation of all the genetic data reviewed is that environmental effects are well substantiated, but genetic effects are not. It would nevertheless be hasty to exclude the role of genes given the current corpus of evidence. Data from psychiatric genetics clearly indicate that single-gene effects tend to have extremely small, but cumulatively significant, effects on psychopathology (see Kendler, 2013), and the same may prove true for other domains of development, including attachment (see Bakermans-Kranenburg & Van IJzendoorn, Chapter 8, this volume). Larger-scale studies capable of detecting small genetic effects and G × E interactions will be necessary to address these issues in the future. Furthermore, we lack large-scale twin studies of attachment that are properly powered to detect moderate or small genetic effects on disorganized attachment in particular, which is typically present at relatively low frequencies, especially in low-risk samples. Finally, current research has focused almost exclusively on the first 3 years of life. We cannot assume that attachment security measured in later development will show the same profile of environmental influence as that seen in infants and toddlers. Indeed, a recent relatively large twin study of adolescents ($N$ = 551 twin pairs) using a representational measure of attachment, the Child Attachment Interview, found that nearly 40% of the variance in security–insecurity and narrative coherence was attributable to genes, and the influence of the shared environment was estimated to be zero (Fearon, Schmueli-Goetz, Viding, Fonagy, & Plomin, 2014). These striking findings suggest that the causal influences on attachment organization may change with development, perhaps particularly as attachment security shifts from a predominantly behavioral and relational construct in very early childhood to one that is generalized (not relationship-specific) and representational in middle childhood and beyond. Whether similar patterns of heritability will be observed in adulthood remains to be seen.

## The Role of Maternal Care

There can be little doubt, in accord with Ainsworth's (1973) original theorizing and her intensive research on just 26 mother–infant dyads, that variation in observed maternal sensitivity in the first year is linked to security in the Strange Situation. This is revealed in studies of middle-class U.S. (e.g., Braungart-Reiker, Garwood, Powers, & Wang, 2001; Fish & Stifter, 1995 [girls only]; Isabella, 1993; Kochanska, 1998; Teti, Gelfand, Messinger, & Isabella, 1995), Canadian (Pederson & Moran, 1996), and German (Grossmann, Grossmann, Spangler, Suess, & Unzner, 1985) families, as well as economically disadvantaged, often single-parent families (Egeland & Farber, 1984; Krupka, Moran, & Pederson, 1996; Susman-Stillman, Kalkoske, Egeland, & Waldman, 1996). Furthermore, security is associated with prompt responsiveness to distress (Crockenberg, 1981; Del Carmen, Pedersen, Huffman, & Bryan, 1993); moderate appropriate stimulation (e.g., Belsky, Rovine, & Taylor, 1984); and interactional synchrony (Isabella & Belsky, 1991; Isabella, Belsky, & von Eye, 1989), warmth, involvement, and responsiveness (e.g., Bates, Maslin, & Frankel, 1985; NICHD Early Child Care Network, 1997); as well as autonomy support (Bernier, Matte-Gagne, Belanger, & Whipple, 2014) and mutually responsive interactions (e.g., Kochanska, Aksan, & Carlson, 2005). In contrast, insecure-avoidant attachments are related to intrusive, excessively stimulating, controlling interactional styles, and insecure-resistant attachments to an unresponsive, underinvolved approach to caregiving (Belsky et al., 1984; Harel & Scher, 2003; Isabella et al., 1989; Lewis & Fiering, 1989; Malatesta, Grigoryev, Lamb, Albin, & Culver, 1986; Smith & Pederson, 1988; Vondra, Shaw, & Kevinides, 1995).

In addition to such associations from studies using the Strange Situation procedure, similar contemporaneous and time-lagged relations have emerged in North American research using the AQS to assess attachment security (Krupka et al., 1996; Moran, Pederson, Petit, & Krupka, 1992; Pederson et al., 1990; Scholmerich, Fracasso,

Lamb, & Broberg, 1995; note that this latter study used the mother-completed AQS, which appears less valid than those completed by objective raters, see Van IJzendoorn, Vereijken, Bakermans-Kranenburg, & Riksen-Walraven, 2004) and in related research conducted in Japan (Vereijken, Riksen-Walraven, & Kondo-Ikemura, 1997). All this is not to say that there have been no failures to replicate such theoretically anticipated results (e.g., Notaro & Volling, 1999; Schneider-Rosen & Rothbaum, 1993), but rather that the preponderance of evidence is more rather than less consistent with the sensitivity—or at least quality-of-care hypothesis.

It must be noted, however, that the strength of the discerned association between quality of rearing (e.g., sensitivity) and attachment security is not large. De Wolff and Van IJzendoorn (1997), drawing upon data from 66 investigations involving some 4,176 infant–mother dyads, discerned an overall effect size of 0.17 between attachment security and various measures of mothering and of mother–child interaction (e.g., sensitivity, contiguity of maternal response, physical contact, cooperation). These studies collectively produced highly heterogeneous effect sizes, suggesting substantial systematic differences between studies. When the meta-analysis was restricted to only the subset of 30 investigations that measured sensitivity ($n = 1,666$), the effect size was somewhat larger (0.22). And when the 16 studies ($n = 837$) that relied on Ainsworth's original sensitivity rating scales were considered, the effect size was larger still (0.24)—and was no longer heterogeneous; that is, variation in effect sizes produced by these studies was no greater than would be expected by chance. Nevertheless, effect sizes across investigations that relied upon different operationalizations of mothering and mother–infant interaction were more similar than different. And, moreover, the magnitude of the discerned effects was not influenced (i.e., moderated) by the length of observations of mother–child interaction. Whether one regards the magnitude of the effect of maternal care as weak or moderate, it is indisputable that Ainsworth's core theoretical proposition linking maternal sensitivity with attachment security has been empirically confirmed (Belsky, 1997).

Four possibilities might account for why attachment security is less well accounted for by maternal sensitivity than many expected. The first is a "technological" gap, in that the quality, intensity, or context of measurement of sensitivity (or indeed attachment) is suboptimal. The fact that

several recent studies using the Maternal Behavior Q-Set have repeatedly found substantially higher associations between sensitivity and attachment than the earlier meta-analytic average lends some credence to this first argument (Behrens, Parker, & Haltigan, 2011; Pederson, Gleason, Moran, & Bento, 1998; Raval et al., 2001; Tarabulsy et al., 2005; see also Atkinson et al., 2005). The evidence that associations between attachment and sensitivity are stronger when the AQS is used to measure security (average $r = .39$, see Van IJzendoorn et al., 2004) may also point to measurement issues, although the fact that the AQS is typically used with older children than the Strange Situation may also be relevant. Although not measuring child attachment security directly, recent findings by Lindhiem, Bernard, and Dozier (2011) make a critical point: When observational measurements of sensitivity were conducted repeatedly—and composited—the average correlation with maternal representations of attachment (measured with the Adult Attachment Interview [AAI]) rose quite dramatically: from $r = .37$ with just one observation, to $r = .46$ with two, $r = .51$ with four, and $r = .54$ with seven combined observations. Measurement error clearly plays a major—and generally underappreciated—role in the strength of association between observations of sensitivity and attachment-related constructs. Furthermore, it is almost certain that measurements of attachment security are noisier than the adult attachment classifications analyzed in this study (e.g., see Pinquart, Feusner, & Ahnert, 2013); hence, the real effects of error on the sensitivity–security association may be even greater than this research might lead us to infer.

The second possibility—a "moderator" gap—as to why quality of caregiving is not as predictive of attachment security as presumed by theory concerns the fact that unidentified variables may affect the sensitivity–attachment link. If this was the case and such moderation were not taken into account, it would diminish the overall meta-analytic average. This gap is addressed later in this chapter, when we discuss the proposition of differential susceptibility to rearing influences. However, it is worth noting that factors other than the child's susceptibility to rearing influences may also moderate the sensitivity–security association. For example, middle-class samples tend to reveal larger effect sizes than lower socioeconomic status (SES) samples (De Wolff & Van IJzendoorn, 1997; see also Meins et al., 2012). Furthermore, Atkinson and colleagues (2005) have presented suggestive evidence that sensitivity may interact with parental attachment representations—indicating either that sensitive interactions may attenuate, if not eliminate, anticipated effects of parental insecure attachment representations on child–parent attachment organization, or that sensitivity may have differential effects on child security depending on the parent's representations of attachment. Such possibilities highlight the need to consider the role that parental characteristics may play in the extent to which quality of rearing affects child attachment.

The third and fourth possibilities for why effects of sensitivity emerge as small-to-modest in magnitude are that the most predictive elements of parenting behavior have perhaps not been identified and fall outside the definition of sensitivity (i.e., a "domain" gap), and that other factors unrelated to parental behavior contribute to attachment security and mediate the association (a "third-variable" gap) (Belsky, 2005a). We consider some examples of such possibilities later in this chapter, in the discussion of broader ecological influences on attachment security and when we examine personal/psychological resources of mothers—particularly the constructs of "mind-mindedness" and "reflective functioning."

In any event, two recent trends are worthy of note. First, some recent evidence suggests that sensitivity may relate more strongly to attachment security when it is restricted to an assessment of the parent's sensitivity to the child's distress rather than a broader array of cues (Leerkes, 2011; McElwain & Booth-LaForce, 2006). This is a potentially critical insight because although it certainly was the case that Ainsworth defined sensitivity rather broadly, there are good theoretical reasons for expecting that sensitivity to attachment-related—and thus distress—cues and behaviors should be most causally influential. Having said that, the relatively strong associations between attachment and mutuality/synchrony (i.e., not clearly focused on responsiveness to distress cues) found in meta-analytic work (De Wolff & Van IJzendoorn, 1997) would seem to challenge an overly simplistic acceptance of the sensitivity to distress proposition. Either way, what is clear is that current explanatory frameworks for why some children develop secure and others develop insecure attachments are limited in terms of their power to predict such variation in attachment security.

A second notable trend, which in a sense directs attention in the opposite direction, is that investigators have begun to consider domains of parenting that are quite different and even perhaps orthogonal to sensitivity. For example, Bernier and colleagues (2014) recently argued that maternal support for exploration and autonomy may influence attachment organization because it supports the "exploration side" of the secure-base concept. Consistent with that claim, these scholars observed that both traditionally defined sensitivity and maternal autonomy support independently predicted attachment security, as assessed using the observer-completed AQS. Furthermore, these researchers found that, collectively, these two dimensions of maternal behavior fully mediated the association between parental representations of attachment and infant security. The finding, though in need of replication, should lead future investigators to expand their measurement focus when trying to capture parenting behaviors that shape the development of attachment security. In any case, it is clear that the quest to elucidate the causal antecedents of attachment is far from over (De Wolff & Van IJzendoorn, 1997).

### From Correlational to Experimental Evidence

The modesty of the meta-analytically derived correlation between maternal behavior and attachment security, coupled with the logical possibility that this reliably discerned association could be a product of the effect of infant characteristics—even if not apparently temperament or genotype—on maternal interactive style provides a basis for questioning the causal role of maternal care in fostering security or insecurity. Experimental intervention studies are the most compelling source of evidence about causation. In that regard, Van den Boom's (1990) study of 100 highly irritable infants provides perhaps the clearest example. Three home visits designed to foster mothers' "contingent, consistent, and appropriate responses to both positive and negative infant signals" were administered to 50 mothers randomly assigned to an experimental group. The home visitor/intervenor "aimed to enhance mothers' observational skills . . . [and] assisted mothers to adjust their behaviors to their infant's [sic] unique cries" (p. 258). Control group mothers were simply observed in interaction with their babies. Importantly, the two groups of mothers were equivalent in terms of maternal behavior prior to the implementation of the intervention.

Impressively, not only did postintervention observations reveal that maternal sensitivity was greater in the experimental group, but results of Strange Situation evaluations 4 months after the termination of the intervention were strongly consistent with predictions derived from attachment theory: Whereas a full 68% (34 of 50) of the infants in the control group were classified as insecure, this was true of only 28% (14 of 50) of the experimental subjects. No doubt these findings resulted from the fact that "experimental mothers respond[ed] to the whole range of infant signals (during postintervention home observation), whereas control mothers mainly focus[ed] on very negative infant signals" (van den Boom, 1990, p. 256). More specifically, in the insecurity-producing control group,

mildly negative infant behaviors like fussing are ignored for most of the time or are responded to ineffectively. Positively toned attachment behaviors, on the contrary, are ignored for the most part. And infant exploration is either ignored or interfered with. The program mothers' infants' negative actions boost maternal positive actions. Maternal anger is not observed. . . . Positive social infant behaviors are also responded to in a positive fashion. And program mothers are attentive to the infant's exploration, but they do not interfere in the process. (van den Boom, 1990, p. 256)

These findings that chronicle a causal—not just correlational—impact of the quality of maternal care on attachment security are mainly in accord with those of other experimental investigations. In a key meta-analysis on the subject, Bakermans-Kranenburg, Van IJzendoorn, and Juffer (2003) showed that interventions are effective in enhancing maternal sensitivity, and that in particular, short-term interventions (like van den Boom's [1990]) are the most effective in promoting the development of a secure attachment. Indeed, the combined effect size for 10 studies that sought to promote security by focusing specifically on sensitivity was 0.39 (Bakermans-Kranenburg et al., 2003; for additional discussion of attachment-based interventions, see Berlin, Zeanah, & Lieberman, Chapter 32, this volume).

## Parental Behavior and Disorganized Attachment

A related body of work has also sought to illuminate the role, if any, of relational experience in determining whether a child develops a disorganized attachment. Early studies documenting links between child maltreatment and disorganized attachment—which a recent meta-analysis substantiates (Cyr, Euser, Bakermans-Kranenburg, & Van IJzendoorn, 2010)— gave birth to Main and Hesse's (1990) hypothesis that fear in the attachment relationship serves as the driving force behind disorganization. Research testing of this proposition provides the clearest example of the need to move beyond sensitivity in seeking to understand the interactional determinants of attachment. This is because at least 10 independent studies have found that disorganized attachment is associated with disturbances in parenting behavior that may be considered frightening to the infant (rather than insensitive) or in other ways atypical (Abrams, Rifkin, & Hesse, 2006; Goldberg, Benoit, Blokland, & Madigan, 2003; Kelly, Grienenberger, & Slade, 2005; Lyons-Ruth, Bronfman, & Parsons, 1999; Madigan et al., 2011; Madigan, Moran, & Pederson, 2006; Schuengel, Bakermans-Kranenburg, & Van IJzendoorn, 1999; Tomlinson, Cooper, & Murray, 2005; True, Pisani, & Oumar, 2001). In fact, in a 2006 meta-analytic review of the evidence, Madigan and colleagues (2006) revealed the overall association between anomalous parental behavior and disorganized attachment to be equivalent to a correlation of $r = .34$. Intriguingly, meta-analytic evidence also indicates that maternal sensitivity is only very weakly associated with disorganized attachment (Van IJzendoorn, Schuengel, & Bakermans-Kranenburg, 1999), a result that also has emerged in more recent work focused on very preterm/very low birthweight infants (Wolke, Eryigit-Madzwamuse, & Gutbrod, 2014). In fact, three studies chronicle the effects of frightening/atypical maternal behavior on disorganization even when maternal sensitivity is statistically controlled (Moran, Forbes, Evans, Tarabulsy, & Madigan, 2008; Schuengel et al., 1999; True et al., 2001).

A number of researchers have sought to broaden the domain of inquiry from an emphasis on frightening/frightened/dissociative (FR) behavior to disconnected and extremely insensitive parenting (Out, Bakermans-Kranenburg, & Van IJzendoorn, 2009), and to disturbances in parental affective communication (Lyons-Ruth et al., 1999). The latter category subsumes FR behavior but also includes less obviously frightening atypical maternal behavior, such as affective communication errors (e.g., contradictory cues), role confusion (e.g., role reversal or sexualized behavior), and withdrawal (creating physical or verbal distance from the infant; see Lyons-Ruth et al., 1999). Empirically, both of these broader sets of maternal behaviors have been found to be associated with disorganized attachment (Abrams et al., 2006; Goldberg et al., 2003; Lyons-Ruth et al., 1999 [see also Lyons-Ruth, Yellin, Melnick, & Atwood, 2005, on the same sample]; Madigan et al., 2006; Out et al., 2009; see Lyons-Ruth & Jacobvitz, Chapter 29, this volume, for a review of studies of affective communication errors and disorganization).

What currently cannot be discerned from this body of research is whether disrupted affective communication and disconnected or extremely insensitive parenting contribute additional predictive power over and above that accounted for by FR behavior because little research has evaluated this possibility; nor, indeed, has there been any examination of whether there is variable discriminative power within the domains of FR behavior itself. There are hints in the literature that dissociative behavior may be particularly important (Abrams et al., 2006; Madigan et al., 2006; Schuengel et al., 1999) but this is currently based on a limited and mixed evidence base. Quite apart from whether available measures of maternal behavior have greater or lesser predictive power, a critical question that no correlational study has addressed directly is whether any of the associations detected are truly causal, though one investigation has linked *change* in atypical maternal behavior with *change* in attachment disorganization from 12 to 24 months (Forbes, Evans, Moran, & Pederson, 2007). Interestingly, Juffer, Bakermans-Kranenburg, and Van IJzendoorn (2005) presented a reanalysis of data from their earlier sensitivity-based intervention study, reporting that the intervention reduced disorganized attachment. Intriguingly, despite the focus of the intervention, the intervention effect on disorganization was not mediated by changes in sensitivity. The investigators speculated that the intervention may have indirectly reduced FR behavior, perhaps by increasing parents' attention to and awareness of their child's behavior and the impact of their own behavior on the child. In any event, the positive impact of sensitivity-based interventions on disorganized attachment has been confirmed in a meta-analysis of 15 intervention studies, ones not originally designed to reduce FR behavior (Bakermans-Kranenburg, Van IJzendoorn, & Juffer, 2005). Notable, too, are the positive results of the Bernard and colleagues (2012) and the Moss and colleagues (2011) intervention efforts designed to lower rates of disorganized attachment and increase those of secure attachment

in maltreated children by fostering nurturing parental care. Collectively, these results indicate that disorganization is susceptible to environmental remediation, but how these changes take place is an important remaining question for clinicians and scientists alike.

## Cultural Variation

Cross-cultural variation in parenting can shed further light on the nature of the interactional antecedents of attachment security (see also Mesman, Van IJzendoorn, & Sagi-Schwartz, Chapter 37, this volume). One might wonder, for example, whether the association between sensitivity and attachment emerges in non-U.S. or non-European samples, where cultural norms for raising infants may be quite different. To address this issue, Posada, Carbonell, Alzate, and Plata (2004) conducted an intensive investigation of patterns of parenting behavior in 30 Colombian families. Data were gathered via standardized assessments of maternal sensitivity (using the Maternal Behavior Q-Sort [MBQS]) and open-ended ethnographic transcripts of parenting behavior. There was considerable correspondence between the domains of parenting identified through ethnographical analysis and those originally developed by Ainsworth (1973) and refined by Pederson and colleagues (1990). Furthermore, both maternal sensitivity identified by the MBQS and the ethnographically derived parenting parallel to sensitivity correlated significantly with infant attachment security as measured with the AQS. Similar results were obtained by Zevalkink, Riksen-Walraven, and Van Lieshout (1999) with a Sudanese–Indonesian sample and by Peterson and colleagues (2001) in a study of Ugandan mothers and infants. Further evidence demonstrating the expected predictive associations between sensitivity and attachment is provided by Ding, Xiu, Wang, Li, and Wang (2012) in a sample of Chinese dyads and by Jin, Jacobvitz, Hazen, and Jung (2012) in a sample from South Korea. Tomlinson and colleagues (2005) also detected robust associations between attachment and various indices of parenting quality (sensitivity, intrusiveness, coerciveness, remoteness) in a sample of extremely impoverished black South African mother–infant dyads. These authors were also able to show that disorganized attachment was associated with a modified measure of maternal FR behavior administered when the infants were 2 months of age. True and colleagues (2001) further found infant disorganization to be correlated with observed maternal FR behavior in a sample of Malian infants and mothers, whereas broader measures of sensitivity were only marginally correlated with security. Studies also tend to chronicle associations between sensitivity and attachment in samples of differing ethnicity within Western populations (e.g., Candelaria, Teti, & Black, 2011; Dexter, Wong, Stacks, Beeghly, & Barnett, 2013). Notably, using data from the NICHD Study of Early Child Care (Bakermans-Kranenburg, Van IJzendoorn, & Kroonenburg, 2004) examined whether patterns of association between attachment and sensitivity were similar between European American and African American families. The associations proved to be highly consistent across groups, and the significantly lower mean attachment security score (measured via the observer-reported AQS) in the African American group was fully accounted for by differences in SES.

Clearly, then, there is reasonably consistent evidence that the theoretically anticipated relation between quality of parenting and attachment security is observed across a wide range of cultural contexts, which is not to say that culture does not matter. Consider in this regard Carlson and Harwood's (2003) evidence that Puerto Rican mothers used more physically controlling tactics in caregiving than European American mothers, and that more of such behavior was associated with secure attachment in the Puerto Rican group but with greater avoidance in European American infants (see also Huang, Lewin, Mitchell, & Zhang, 2012). Although the small sample size and imperfect matching of the two groups limit interpretation of these findings, they do underscore the need for additional research on culture-specific associations between parenting and attachment. A recent book on the cultural anthropology of attachment provides a number of other intriguing examples of apparently marked differences in childrearing practices, which, while generally not strongly contesting the main thrust of current attachment theory, may help to refine our understanding of the culturally variable and universal aspects of parental behavior involved in the development of secure and insecure attachment (Otto & Keller, 2014).

## Nonmaternal Care

Even though attachment theory is often cast as a theory of the infant–*mother* relationship, most attachment scholars consider attachment to be involved in emotionally close child–*adult* rela-

tionships more generally. Indeed, Bowlby made it clear that in writing about the mother, he was assuming that mothers are usually the primary caregivers. If, as is now widely recognized, infants and young children can establish relationships with more than a single individual (neither Bowlby nor Ainsworth argued otherwise), a theoretically important question is whether the interactional processes highlighted as important to the development of secure relationships with mothers also operate with other adults. The few available studies of fathers and of nonparental caregivers indicate that this is indeed the case.

### Infant–Father Attachment

In fact, even though the majority of investigations that have examined the relation between quality of paternal care and infant–father attachment security have individually failed to document a significant effect of fathering on attachment security (e.g., Belsky, 1983; Braungart-Reiker et al., 2001; Schneider-Rosen & Rothbaum, 1993; Volling & Belsky, 1992), a different picture emerges when the results of studies are subjected to meta-analysis. The most recent meta-analysis of 16 studies ($N$ = 1,355) found an average, highly significant, correlation of $r$ = .12, which was homogeneous and showed little sign of publication bias (Lucassen et al., 2011). The association, though robust, is clearly smaller than that generally found for mothers, although whether methodological or substantive factors account for this difference is unclear; this is clearly a topic warranting more research in the future. One recent report calls attention to the potential utility of taking into account quantity of fathering (i.e., paternal involvement) when evaluating effects of quality of fathering (i.e., sensitivity). Brown, Mangelsdorf, and Neff (2012) found that the anticipated adverse effect of low sensitivity was attenuated when father involvement was high. Indeed, it was when sensitivity and involvement were both low that security vis-à-vis the father was lowest.

### Infant–Caregiver Attachment

Ahnert, Pinquart, and Lamb's (2006) meta-analysis of 40 investigations involving almost 3,000 children (average age = 29.6 months) reveals a great deal about the security of children's relationships with nonparental caregivers. First, attachments to nonparental providers were less likely to be secure than attachments to parents (in studies that measured both) when assessed by means of the Strange Situation, but equally secure attachments were more likely when Q-sort methods were used. Second, the security of children's relationships with their mothers and fathers was significantly related to the security of their attachment to their care providers. Third, secure attachment to caregivers was more likely in home-based than in center-based care, more likely for girls than for boys, and more likely when children had been with particular caregivers for longer periods. The fact that secure attachments to caregivers were more likely to be detected in older than in newer studies across the quarter century of research covered by the meta-analysis suggests that this trend may be the result of the ever-increasing emphasis on education (i.e., literacy, numeracy) in child care, at the expense of emotional development.

Most important from the standpoint of the current chapter was evidence addressing the influence of caregiver sensitivity on security of attachment to caregiver. Making a distinction between sensitivity to individual children (as always investigated in the case of parents) and sensitivity to a group of children, Ahnert and colleagues (2006) found that setting mattered: Whereas care providers' sensitivity to individual children predicted attachment security in the small groups that characterize home-based settings (and more so when the number of children being cared for was smaller), sensitivity to the group as a whole best predicted security of attachment to caregivers in larger groups (i.e., centers), though individual sensitivity was also related to security.

Evidence from an intervention study suggests, at least in the case of home-based care, that the relations detected in the meta-analysis are causal. When Galinsky, Howes, and Kontos (1995) improved the care of home-based caregivers via a training program, security of infant–provider attachments improved. Unfortunately, no such research has been carried out in groups to document either indisputably causal relations or differential effects of individual versus group sensitivity in the development of secure attachment to care provider. These comments notwithstanding, the evidence reviewed suggests that relationship processes somewhat similar to those delineated in studies of parenting appear relevant to the development of secure relationships with others with whom a child is expected to develop a close, affectional bond. (See Howes & Spieker, Chapter 15, this volume, for additional discussion.)

## Summary of the Evidence

When considered in its entirety, the evidence summarized in this section pertaining to mothering, fathering, and the care provided by some other consistent caregiver offers support for Ainsworth's (1973) extension of Bowlby's theory of attachment. Individual differences in attachment security, whether measured with the laboratory-based Strange Situation or the home-based AQS procedure, are systematically related to the quality of the care that an infant or toddler experiences with a particular caregiver; this is true of both the role of sensitivity in fostering security and of FR or atypical parental behavior in fostering disorganization. What makes the former (and some of the latter) evidence particularly convincing is that it is both correlational and experimental in nature; longitudinal as well as cross-sectional; apparently cross-culturally generalizable; and derived from studies of fathers and child care providers ,as well as mothers. Finally, the evidence currently indicates that genes and temperament play a rather limited role in the development of attachment security at least in early childhood.

## Differential Susceptibility

However theoretically important the data linking adult–infant interaction to attachment security may be, the fact remains that associations between rearing and attachment are only modest in magnitude. Recent evolutionary theorizing highlights one possible reason—referred to above as a "moderator" gap—for this less than strong association. Moreover, intriguing evidence is offered that temperament may be important to attachment in ways that have not heretofore been appreciated.

Elsewhere, Belsky (1997; Belsky & Pluess, 2013) notes that because the future is uncertain, it makes biological sense for children to vary, particularly within a family, in their susceptibility to rearing influence (see also Ellis, Boyce, Belsky, Bakermans-Kranenburg, & Van IJzendoorn, 2011). If all children are equally influenced by parental care, then there may be—or would have been in the environment of evolutionary adaptedness—the risk that when the future does not prove consistent with parents' (not necessarily conscious) expectations, presumed to guide (often in unconscious ways) their rearing practices, then all children within a family may be led into a literal or at least a reproductive dead end.

Perhaps one way that natural selection has reduced the likelihood of this pitfall in the course of shaping human development is by increasing the probability that parents will conceive children who vary in their tendencies to be influenced by their rearing experiences, with some being more and others less susceptible. *Fixed strategists* may develop along lines established principally by their biological makeup, whereas *plastic strategists* may navigate the ship of development according to prevailing (rearing) winds (in line with general evolutionary terminology, the term *strategist* in no way implies conscious intent on the part of a child).

If differential susceptibility to rearing represents an evolved characteristic of our species, then research efforts failing to distinguish infants/children along these lines may both over- and underestimate effects of rearing, including studies of rearing influences on attachment security. Research may overestimate rearing influences for fixed strategists and underestimate them for plastic strategists. Evidence (both correlational and experimental) suggest that highly negatively emotional infants/toddlers may be especially susceptible to rearing influence, especially with regard to developmental outcomes related to self-control and socioemotional development (for a review, see Belsky, 2005b); this is also true in the case of studies of parenting and attachment. Consider first the fact that the intervention study documenting perhaps the largest indisputably causal effect of rearing on attachment was carried out on a sample preselected for being highly negatively emotional (van den Boom, 1994). Consider next the fact that when Klein-Velderman, Bakermans-Kranenburg, Juffer, and Van IJzendoorn (2006) formally tested Belsky's (1997) differential susceptibility hypothesis by means of their experimental intervention, they found support for it: Attachment security proved most susceptible to intervention-induced changes in maternal sensitivity among infants who were highly negative. Although a second sensitivity trial failed to replicate this effect (Van Zeijl et al., 2006), a third, more recent intervention trial in the United States did (Cassidy, Woodhouse, Sherman, Stupica, & Lejuez, 2011).

In light of these intriguing results, it is interesting to note that studies of G × E interaction have generally failed to find genetic variants that explain differential susceptibility effects related to attachment, and remarkably few studies have reported on sensitivity × temperament interactions in nonexperimental studies in this domain. It may be that such observational studies have generally failed to find such interactions because of constraints on the range of sensitivity (or temperament) often observed in normative samples, and because sensitivity provides only a partial picture of the key interactional determinants of attachment security. Both these limitations may severely limit statistical power. Intervention studies, by targeting at-risk groups and by experimentally changing sensitivity, may yield greater power to detect differential susceptibility effects and may also induce changes beyond that captured by sensitivity. There is a need for more attachment-focused interventions of sufficient scale and mechanistic focus to deepen our understanding of the causal influences on attachment and the populations of infants (or parents) most amenable to effective intervention.

For further consideration of the contribution of evolutionary theory to thinking about attachment and human development see Simpson and Belsky (Chapter 5, this volume).

## Psychological and Social-Contextual Determinants

Having considered the interactional determinants of attachment security, we now consider the role of more "distal" factors implicated by an ecological perspective: in particular, parental personality and related psychological attributes, excluding parental state of mind regarding attachment, which is addressed in another chapter in this volume (see Hesse, Chapter 26), and the marital/partner relationship.

### Parental Psychological Resources and Personality

Because the provision of security-inducing sensitive care requires the accurate reading of, and timely and empathic responding to a child's affective and behavioral cues, there are theoretical grounds for expecting the caregiver's psychological attributes to be related to the child's security of attachment. Moreover, much theory and evidence indicate that both mothers' and fathers' psychological health and well-being affect the quality of care that parents provide (see Belsky & Jaffee, 2006). Evidence from both normal and clinical samples underscores the importance of parental psychological makeup vis-à-vis infant attachment security.

## Nonselected Samples

Cross-sectional studies and longitudinal ones (in which personality is measured prior to attachment security) indicate that in nonselected populations, secure attachment relationships are more likely to develop when mothers are psychologically healthy. Maslin and Bates (1983) found, for example, that mothers of secure infants scored higher than mothers of insecure infants on a series of personality subscales measuring nurturance, understanding, autonomy, inquisitiveness, and dependence, and lower on a subscale assessing aggressiveness. Subsequently, Del Carmen and colleagues (1993) reported that mothers who scored higher on prenatal anxiety were more likely than their lower-scoring counterparts to have insecure 1-year-olds, and O'Connor (1997) observed that mothers of secure infants were likely to describe themselves as self-confident, independent, cheerful, adaptable, and affectionate. In the largest study to date, involving more than 1,100 infants, maternal personality was assessed when infants were 1 month of age, and it was found that mothers of infants classified as secure at age 15 months scored higher on a composite index of psychological adjustment (Agreeableness + Extraversion – Neuroticism – Depression) than mothers of insecure infants (NICHD Early Child Care Network, 1997). Atkinson and colleagues' (2000) meta-analysis revealed, moreover, that across 13 studies, maternal stress was significantly associated with attachment insecurity (mean effect size = 0.19). It is notable that findings like these are not restricted to economically advantaged families, but also emerge in research on high-risk, low-SES households (Jacobson & Frye, 1991; Sims, Hans, & Cox, 1996), as well as in countries outside North America (Scher & Mayseless, 2000).

Not all relevant investigations, however, provide evidence of statistically significant associations between parental personality and attachment security (e.g., Belsky, Rosenberger, & Crnic, 1995; Levitt, Weber, & Clark, 1986; Zeanah et al., 1993). Perhaps more noteworthy, though, is the lack of any evidence indicating that parents of secure infants are *less* psychologically healthy than other parents.

In addition to focusing on maternal personality and psychological distress, research on attachment has considered other aspects of maternal psychological functioning in an effort to better understand what Van IJzendoorn (1995) has labeled the *transmission gap*—the fact that measured sensitivity does not fully account for the link, as some anticipated it might, between a mother's own state of mind regarding attachment and infant attachment security. Meins, Fernyhough, Fradley, and Tuckey (2001, p. 638) have focused on *mind-mindedness*, which they define as a mother's readiness "to treat her infant as an individual with a mind, rather than merely as a creature with needs that must be satisfied." Support for their hypothesis that mind-mindedness contributes to attachment security comes from work showing that mothers of secure infants are more likely than mothers of insecure infants to make appropriate mind-minded comments when interacting with their infants, an association now multiply replicated (Laranjo, Bernier, & Meins, 2008; Lundy, 2003; Meins et al., 2001, 2012). Meins and colleagues (2001) also found that the effect of mind-mindedness was independent of the significant contribution of maternal sensitivity to the prediction of attachment security, though it has not yet been reported that this fills the "transmission gap." Slade, Grienenberger, Bernbach, Levy, and Locker (2005) reported similar results upon measuring a construct seemingly related to mind-mindedness labeled *reflective functioning* (RF; Fonagy, Steele, Moran, Steele, & Higgitt, 1991), even showing in a pilot study that it mediates some of the effect of adult attachment on infant attachment. Stacks and colleagues (2014) also recently found RF to be predictive of attachment security, an effect partially mediated by maternal sensitivity and negativity. Oppenheim, Koren-Karie, and Sagi (2001), examining a different but closely related construct, found that mothers' insightfulness when discussing their children, particularly coherence, richness, and insight regarding the children's thoughts, feelings, and motives, is associated with secure attachment. Collectively, these studies provide compelling evidence that parental personal characteristics related to the capacity to think coherently and insightfully about the child's feelings and thoughts may be an important factor in determining the security of the child–parent attachment relationship, albeit via parenting behaviors that themselves remain in need of better identification and measurement.

## Clinical Samples

Depression in its various manifestations—unipolar and bipolar—is the clinical disorder most often studied in relation to attachment security. On the basis of evidence linking both unresponsive/detached and intrusive/rejecting mothering with maternal depression (see Belsky & Jaffee, 2006, for a review), there are strong grounds for expecting children of depressed mothers to be at heightened risk of insecure attachment. Perusal of the available evidence reveals seemingly inconsistent findings, however. Whereas some research fails to find the expected significant association between maternal depression and elevated rates of insecurity (Frankel, Maslin-Cole, & Harmon, 1991; Lyons-Ruth, Zoll, Connell, & Grunebaum, 1986; Sameroff, Seifer, & Zax, 1982; Stacks et al., 2014; Tharner et al., 2013), other investigations do document such a link (Campbell, Cohn, Meyers, Ross, & Flanagan, 1993; D'Angelo, 1986; Das Eiden & Leonard, 1996; DeMulder & Radke-Yarrow, 1991; Gaensbauer, Harmon, Cytryn, & McKnew, 1984; Gravener et al., 2012; Hayes, Goodman, & Carlson, 2013; Hopkins, Gouze, & Lavigne, 2013; Lyons-Ruth, 1988; Murray, Fiori-Cowley, Hooper, & Cooper, 1996; Radke-Yarrow, 1991; Radke-Yarrow, Cummings, Kuczynski, & Chapman, 1985; Spieker & Booth, 1988; Teti et al., 1995; Tomlinson et al., 2005).

Martins and Gaffan (2000) conducted a meta-analysis of seven studies that compared rates of attachment insecurity in samples of mothers with a clinical diagnosis of unipolar depression and nondepressed controls. They statistically documented significant variability across studies in the rates of infant–mother attachment insecurity associated with depression. When one study outlier was removed, significantly higher levels of insecurity emerged in depressed samples than controls—although when another outlying sample was removed, this effect was diminished to nonsignificance. For a homogeneous set of studies that broadly found an association with attachment, rates of infant disorganization and avoidance were significantly elevated in depressed populations, but rates of resistance were not.

In a broader meta-analysis of depression and attachment that included 15 studies of clinical and nonclinical samples, Atkinson and colleagues (2000) discerned a significant overall association between depression and attachment (effect size $r = 0.18$), with clinical samples yielding a stronger effect size than nonclinical ones (0.27 vs. 0.09). Like Martins and Gaffan (2000), Atkinson and colleagues also noted significant variability within the group of clinical samples, but they could detect no reliable predictor of effect size. Importantly, further meta-analytic work by Van IJzendoorn and colleagues (1999) indicated that in nonclinical samples, maternal depressive symptoms may have a rather limited association with disorganized attachment, with the overall meta-analytic correlation being $r = -.01$, compared to $r = .13$ in clinical samples.

In summary, the relation between depression and insecurity and, to a lesser extent, disorganization emerges repeatedly, though not in every study, suggesting that it is likely to be dependent upon a variety of factors. Some work raises the prospect that in addition to whether a sample comprises clinical or nonclinical cases, parental attachment security (McMahon, Barnett, Kowalenko, & Tennant, 2006) and degree of exposure to maternal depression may matter for the infant (i.e., chronicity of depression), though this latter prospect was not substantiated in the Atkinson and colleagues (2000) meta-analysis. In any event, evidence linking depression with insecurity and/or disorganization is likely to be driven by the effect of depression on the quality of care that mothers provide, as it is presumably when sensitive behavior is disrupted or FR behavior is manifested that links would be expected to emerge. This analysis is consistent with the mediational thinking informing this entire chapter, which stipulates that even though maternal psychological well-being, as well as a the mother's marital/couple relationship and social support, may directly affect attachment insecurity (through some unspecified process), most of the effect of such distal factors will likely flow through their impact on the quality of care the mother actually provides. Perhaps the best evidence of such a mediational process involving maternal psychological well-being comes from a recent report addressing parental depressive symptoms in relation to attachment security measured with the AQS in a large ($N = 796$) sample of 4-year-olds. It revealed multiple mediating pathways—and most notably ones involving observed insensitivity of interactions and self-reported hostile–coercive parenting (Hopkins et al., 2013; see also Benn, 1986).

## The Marital/Couple Relationship

An abundance of evidence indicates that a supportive relationship with a spouse or partner during the infancy and toddler years is correlated with the very kinds of parenting theorized (and found) to predict attachment security (e.g., Tarabulsy et al., 2005; Tomlinson et al., 2005; for narrative reviews, see Belsky & Jaffee, 2006, and Grych, 2002;

for a meta-analytic review, see Krishnakumar & Buehler, 2000). Given data linking relationship quality with many of the aspects of parenting found to be predictive of attachment security (De Wolff & Van IJzendoorn, 1997), there are strong grounds to expect a relation between marital/couple functioning and infant–parent attachment security. The fact that a mediational perspective leads to such a prediction does not preclude the possibility that relationship quality may affect attachment security directly rather than exclusively via parenting-mediated processes. Not only does Davies and Cummings's (1994) emotional security hypothesis lead to such a prediction, but Owen and Cox's (1997) failure to find evidence of a parent-mediated linkage is also consistent with it. Especially in the case of overt conflict, it is not difficult to imagine how exposure to such aversive interactions between mother and father could foster insecurity directly.

Available evidence is consistent with both mediational and direct-effect theorizing. That is, children growing up with parents who have better functioning couple relationships are more likely to develop secure attachments than those growing up in households where parents are less happy in their relationships. Such results emerge from cross-sectional studies carried out in the United States (Crnic, Greenberg, & Slough, 1986; Goldberg & Easterbrooks, 1984; Howes & Markman, 1989; Jacobson & Frye, 1991; Lindsey, Caldera, & Tankersley, 2009) and in Japan (Durrett, Otaki, & Richards, 1984). Moreover, in work with poor African American mothers and infants, Sims and colleagues (1996) found that when fathers were physically violent with mothers, infants were more likely to be insecurely attached to their mothers.

More important than these results from cross-sectional research are those from several longitudinal studies. In one such investigation, Howes and Markman (1989) found that wives who prenatally reported higher levels of marital satisfaction and lower levels of spousal conflict had children who scored higher on the AQS 1–3 years later. Tracking similar middle-class families across a somewhat shorter time period, Lewis, Owen, and Cox (1988) reported that 1-year-old daughters (but not sons) were more likely to be securely attached to their mothers when marriages were more harmonious during pregnancy. Subsequently, Teti and colleagues (1995) showed that greater marital harmony before a second child was born predicted greater security (via the observer-rated AQS) on the part of the firstborn both in the

last trimester of the mother's pregnancy and up to 2 months following the birth of the younger sibling. In related work, Owen and Cox (1997) found that more marital conflict (observed prenatally and at 3 months postpartum) predicted less secure infant–father attachments and greater disorganization in infant–mother relationships (assessed at 12 months), even after researchers controlled for each parent's psychological maturity. Such findings seem consistent with those reported by Belsky and Isabella (1988), indicating that relationship quality declines more precipitously across the transition to parenthood in the case of infants subsequently classified as insecurely attached to their mothers. Also noteworthy is Spieker's (1988; Spieker & Booth, 1988) research on high-risk mother–infant dyads, showing that the lowest levels of spousal support measured prenatally and at 3 months postpartum characterize the marriages in families in which infants develop disorganized attachments. Especially important given mediational thinking that links distal factors with attachment security is evidence that insecure attachment and reciprocity of parent–child interactions may mediate the association between early marital distress and the child's later peer relationships (Lindsey et al., 2009).

Despite the seeming persuasiveness of the cross-sectional and longitudinal data, it would be a mistake to cite only the aforementioned research and leave the impression that all studies of marital/couple relationships and attachment present such positive and statistically significant results. Not only have a number of investigations failed to find a significant association between some index of relationship quality and infant–parent attachment security (Belsky, 1996; Belsky et al., 1995; Das Eiden & Leonard, 1996; Harrison & Ungerer, 2002; Levitt et al., 1986; Teti, Nakasawa, Das, & Wirth, 1991; Wong, Mangelsdorf, Brown, Neff, & Schoppe-Sullivan, 2009; Zeanah et al., 1993) but one study of an unusual sample—Japanese mothers living in the United States due to their husbands' employment—also produced results showing higher levels of marital quality to be associated with less AQS-rated security (Nakasawa, Teti, & Lamb, 1992).

A number of studies draw attention to the potential importance of indirect effects mediating between parental relationship quality and child attachment, which may help account for the fact that not all studies consistently show the predicted association. In one illuminating piece of work, Isabella (1994) found that even though no direct relation between marital quality (measured prenatally) and attachment security (at 1 year) could be discerned, an indirect pathway of influence did appear to exist, mediated by maternal role satisfaction. Whereas the work of Isabella underscores an indirect (and not typically studied) process by which relationship quality might affect the infant–mother attachment bond, work by Das Eiden, Teti, and Corns (1993) draws attention to the need to study relationship quality in context, and to consider moderators as well as mediators. Although Das Eiden and colleagues found that higher levels of marital quality were related to higher levels of security, as measured via the AQS, further analyses revealed that this relation was restricted to families in which mothers were classified as insecure on the AAI. Also illustrating interactive mechanisms, Finger, Hans, Bernstein, and Cox (2009) studied a group of poor, urban African American mothers, fathers, and their infants. The mothers of disorganized infants reported less father support, and more mother–father conflict, and showed less sensitive and more problematic (i.e., harsh, or passively withdrawn) parenting. Notably, disorganized attachment was particularly prevalent among non-coresiding families that experienced high levels of conflict. These effects were not robustly mediated by parenting, although insensitive and problematic parenting was correlated with mother–father conflict. In a large-scale study of 4-year-olds, using the observer-completed AQS, Hopkins and colleagues (2013) revealed multiple pathways mediating marital conflict and attachment security, particularly via maternal depression and self-reported hostile/coercive parenting behavior. Similarly, Dickstein, Seifer, and Albus (2009) found that couple relationship quality indirectly influenced attachment via the pattern of family interactions and overall family functioning (see also Holland & McElwain, 2013, for similar findings regarding coparenting as a mediator of the marital quality-attachment association). What all these data indicate, in conclusion, is that for a full understanding of the relationship's impact on the development of secure or insecure attachment bonds, additional information about family context and family processes is useful.

One final empirical observation about interparental relations and attachment security merits attention—the potential effects of custody and visitation on attachment in separated families (Lamb & Kelly, 2001). Simply put, how does overnight visitation—typically with noncustodial fathers—affect early attachment, especially with the mother? One longitudinal study of high-risk families that has addressed this issue empirically found that "frequent overnights were significantly associated with attachment insecurity among infants" (Tornello et al., 2013, p. 871). Further work is clearly needed to verify these findings.

## Integration and Conclusions

Evidence considered in the first part of this chapter documented the role played by the quality of maternal and nonmaternal care in fostering secure and insecure attachments to mothers and fathers/other caregivers, respectively, as well as the apparent influence of FR and atypical maternal behavior on attachment disorganization in both Western and non-Western cultural contexts. Importantly, the evidence pertaining to infant–mother attachment security is experimental—and thereby causal—as well as correlational in nature. Also considered was the possibility that effect sizes may be modest because children may vary in their susceptibility to rearing influence, with high levels of negative emotionality perhaps demarcating infants maximally susceptible to such influence. Since the version of this chapter in the previous edition, two key trends have emerged in the literature: First, questions regarding the possibility that specific genes may be implicated in the development of attachment—alone or in interaction with the caregiving environment—have not been borne out by the weight of more, and larger, studies. Recent work continues to attest to the importance of the environment in the development of attachment, as Ainsworth would have predicted. Second, researchers have highlighted the potential importance of shifting the focus of inquiry regarding the interactional determinants of attachment beyond sensitivity, broadening out in some cases (e.g., Bernier et al., 2014), and narrowing down in others (e.g., Leerkes, 2011). Our view of the state of play of the field is that measurement issues (domains of parental behavior, contexts of observation, age-to-age changes in influential parental behaviors, and measurement unreliability) will be critically important if we are to move toward a more comprehensive understanding of the interactional determinants of attachment. Crucially, sophisticated models explaining precisely how parental behavior influences the organization of attachment are largely lacking, and have not moved much in recent years, beyond the rather general internal working models concept. These are critical challenges for the coming decades of attachment research.

In the second half of this chapter, we focused on determinants of attachment suggested by an ecological perspective. Central to the discussion of psychological and contextual factors is the assumption that so-called "distal" influences—be they less distant (e.g., personality) or more distant (e.g., the marital relationship)—exert most of their effects by influencing more proximal processes of parent–child interaction. Although ample evidence provides grounds for concluding that all of the factors we have considered play a role in shaping the development of a secure or insecure attachment bond, inconsistency in the evidence has been repeatedly and purposefully highlighted. Up to this point, however, these factors have themselves not been placed "in context." By organizing the second part of the chapter around various factors, even while emphasizing mediational processes of influence, we have run the risk of leaving the impression that these sources of influence on the parent–child relationship, and thus on the child's attachment to his or her parent, operate in isolation. Nothing could be further from the truth.

Theory and research draw attention to the need simultaneously to consider stresses and supports (Belsky, 1984; Belsky & Isabella, 1988; Belsky & Jaffee, 2006)—or, in the terms of developmental psychopathology, risk and protective factors (Cicchetti, 1983; Sroufe & Rutter, 1984). Central to both of these theoretical orientations are the postulates (1) that risks can be balanced by strengths; and (2) that risks of problematical developmental outcomes, including attachment insecurity, are more likely to be realized as risk factors accumulate and are not balanced by supports or compensatory factors. Consider in this regard, Belsky and Isabella's (1988) finding that the more indications that a family and a specific infant–parent relationship were "at risk"—due to lower levels of parental psychological adjustment, poorer marital/couple relationship quality, more negative and less positive infant temperament, less social support, more work–family stress, and lower SES—the more likely infant–mother and infant–father relationships were to be insecure (Belsky, 1996; Belsky et al., 1995; see also Scher & Mayseless, 2000). Thus, not only do processes of mediation need to be central to our understanding of the origins of individual differences in attachment (distal factors → parent–child interaction → attachment security), but so too do moderational

ones because the impact of one source of influence is highly likely to be contingent on another. As Bronfenbrenner (1979, p. 38) so astutely noted in regard to the ecology of human development, and thus with respect to the etiology of secure and insecure infant–parent attachment bonds, "the principal main effects are likely to be interactions."

## References

Abrams, K. Y., Rifkin, A., & Hesse, E. (2006). Examining the role of parental frightened/frightening subtypes in predicting disorganized attachment within a brief observational procedure. *Development and Psychopathology, 18*, 345–361.

Ahnert, L., Pinquart, M., & Lamb, M. E. (2006). Security of children's relationships with nonparental care providers: A meta-analysis. *Child Development, 74*, 664–679.

Ainsworth, M. D. S. (1973). The development of infant–mother attachment. In B. M. Caldwell & H. N. Ricciuti (Eds.), *Review of child development research* (Vol. 3, pp. 1–94). Chicago: University of Chicago Press.

Atkinson, L., Goldberg, S., Raval, V., Pederson, D., Benoit, D., Moran, G., et al. (2005). On the relation between maternal state of mind and sensitivity in the prediction of infant attachment security. *Developmental Psychology, 41*, 42–53.

Atkinson, L., Paglia, A., Coolbear, J., Niccols, A., Parker, K. C. H., & Guger, S. (2000). Attachment security: A meta-analysis of maternal mental health correlates. *Clinical Psychology Review, 20*, 1019–1040.

Bakermans-Kranenburg, M. J., & Van IJzendoorn, M. H. (2007). Research review: Genetic vulnerability or differential susceptibility in child development: The case of attachment. *Journal of Child Psychology and Psychiatry, 48*(12), 1160–1173.

Bakermans-Kranenburg, M. J., & Van Ijzendoorn, M. H. (2012). Integrating temperament and attachment: The differential susceptibility paradigm. In M. Zentner & R. L. Shiner (Eds.), *Handbook of temperament* (pp. 403–424). New York: Guilford Press.

Bakermans-Kranenburg, M. J., Van IJzendoorn, M. H., Bokhorst, C. L., & Schuengel, C. (2004). The importance of shared environment in infant–father attachment: A behavioral genetic study of the Attachment Q-Sort. *Journal of Family Psychology, 18*, 545–549.

Bakermans-Kranenburg, M. J., Van IJzendoorn, M. H., & Juffer, F. (2003). Less is more: Meta-analysis of sensitivity and attachment interventions in early childhood. *Psychological Bulletin, 129*, 195–215.

Bakermans-Kranenburg, M. J., Van IJzendoorn, M. H., & Juffer, F. (2005). Disorganized infant attachment and preventive interventions: A review and meta-analysis. *Infant Mental Health Journal, 26*, 191–216.

Bakermans-Kranenburg, M. J., Van IJzendoorn, M. H.,

& Kroonenberg, P. M. (2004). Differences in attachment security between African-American and white children: Ethnicity or socio-economic status? *Infant Behavior and Development, 27,* 417–433.

Barry, R. A., Kochanska, G., & Philibert, R. A. (2008). G × E interaction in the organization of attachment: Mothers' responsiveness as a moderator of children's genotypes. *Journal of Child Psychology and Psychiatry, 49*(12), 1313–1320.

Bates, J. E., Maslin, C. A., & Frankel, K. A. (1985). Attachment security, mother–child interaction, and temperament as predictors of behavior-problem ratings at age three years. In I. Bretherton & E. Waters (Eds.), Growing points of attachment theory and research. *Monographs of the Society for Research in Child Development, 50*(1–2, Serial No. 209), 167–193.

Behrens, K. Y., Parker, A. C., & Haltigan, J. D. (2011). Maternal sensitivity assessed during the Strange Situation Procedure predicts child's attachment quality and reunion behaviors. *Infant Behavior and Development, 34*(2), 378–381.

Belsky, J. (1983). *Father–infant interaction and security of attachment: No relationship.* Unpublished manuscript, Pennsylvania State University.

Belsky, J. (1984). The determinants of parenting: A process model. *Child Development, 55,* 83–96.

Belsky, J. (1996). Parent, infant, and social-contextual determinants of attachment security. *Developmental Psychology, 32,* 905–914.

Belsky, J. (1997). Theory testing, effect-size evaluation, and differential susceptibility to rearing influence: The case of mothering and attachment. *Child Development, 64,* 598–600.

Belsky, J. (2005a). The developmental and evolutionary psychology of intergenerational transmission of attachment. In C. S. Carter, L. Ahnert, K. Grossmann, S. Hrdy, M. Lamb, S. Porges, et al. (Eds.), *Attachment and bonding: A new synthesis* (pp. 169–198). Cambridge, MA: MIT Press.

Belsky, J. (2005b). Differential susceptibility to rearing influence: An evolutionary hypothesis and some evidence. In B. J. Ellis & D. F. Bjorklund (Eds.), *Origins of the social mind: Evolutionary psychology and child development* (pp. 139–163). New York: Guilford Press.

Belsky, J., & Fearon, R. M. P. (2008). Precursors of attachment security. In J. Cassidy & P. R. Shaver (Eds.), *Handbook of attachment: Theory, research, and clinical applications* (2nd ed., pp. 295–316). New York: Guilford Press.

Belsky, J., & Isabella, R. (1988). Maternal, infant, and social-contextual determinants of attachment security. In J. Belsky & T. Nezworski (Eds.), *Clinical implications of attachment* (pp. 41–94). Hillsdale, NJ: Erlbaum.

Belsky, J., & Jaffee, S. (2006). The multiple determinants of parenting. In D. Cicchetti & D. Cohen (Eds.), *Developmental psychopathology: Vol. 3. Risk, disorder, and adaptation* (2nd ed., pp. 38–85). Hoboken, NJ: Wiley.

Belsky, J., & Pluess, M. (2013). Beyond risk, resilience and dysregulation: Phenotypic plasticity and human development. *Development and Psychopathology, 25,* 1243–1261.

Belsky, J., Rosenberger, K., & Crnic, K. (1995). Maternal personality, marital quality, social support and infant temperament: Their significance for infant–mother attachment in human families. In C. Pryce, R. Martin, & D. Skuse (Eds.), *Motherhood in human and nonhuman primates* (pp. 115–124). Basel, Switzerland: Karger.

Belsky, J., & Rovine, M. (1987). Temperament and attachment security in the Strange Situation: An empirical rapprochement. *Child Development, 58,* 787–795.

Belsky, J., Rovine, M., & Taylor, D. G. (1984). The Pennsylvania Infant and Family Development Project: III. The origins of individual differences in infant–mother attachment: Maternal and infant contributions. *Child Development, 55,* 718–728.

Benn, R. K. (1986). Factors promoting secure attachment relationships between employed mothers and their sons. *Child Development, 57,* 1224–1231.

Bernard, K., Dozier, M., Bick, J., Lewis-Morrarty, E., Lindhiem, O., & Carlson, E. (2012). Enhancing attachment organization among maltreated children: Results of a randomized clinical trial. *Child Development, 83*(2), 623–636.

Bernier, A., Matte-Gagne, C., Belanger, M. E., & Whipple, N. (2014). Taking stock of two decades of attachment transmission gap: Broadening the assessment of maternal behavior. *Child Development, 85*(5), 1852–1865.

Bokhorst, C. L., Bakermans-Kranenburg, M. J., Fearon, R. M. P., Van IJzendoorn, M. H., Fonagy, P., & Schuengel, C. (2003). The importance of shared environment in mother–infant attachment security: A behavioral genetic study. *Child Development, 74,* 1769–1782.

Bowlby, J. (1944). Forty-four juvenile thieves: Their characters and home life. *International Journal of Psycho-Analysis, 25,* 19–52.

Bowlby, J. (1982). *Attachment and loss: Vol. 1. Attachment.* New York: Basic Books. (Original work published 1969)

Braungart-Rieker, J. M., Garwood, M. M., Powers, B. P., & Wang, X. (2001). Parental sensitivity, infant affect, and affect regulation: Predictors of later attachment. *Child Development, 72,* 252–270.

Bronfenbrenner, U. (1979). *The ecology of human development.* Cambridge, MA: Harvard University Press.

Brown, G. L., Mangelsdorf, S. C., & Neff, C. (2012). Father involvement, paternal sensitivity and father–child attachment security in the first 3 years. *Journal of Family Psychology, 26,* 421–430.

Campbell, S. B., Cohn, J. F., Meyers, T. A., Ross, S., & Flanagan, C. (1993, April). Chronicity of maternal depression and mother–infant interaction. In D. Teti (Chair), *Depressed mothers and their children: Individual differences in mother–child outcome.* Symposium conducted at the biennial meeting of the Society for Research in Child Development, New Orleans, LA.

Candelaria, M., Teti, D. M., & Black, M. M. (2011). Multi-risk infants: Predicting attachment security from sociodemographic, psychosocial, and health risk among African-American preterm infants. *Journal of Child Psychology and Psychiatry, 52*(8), 870–877.

Carlson, V. J., & Harwood, R. L. (2003). Attachment, culture, and the caregiving system: The cultural patterning of everyday experiences among Anglo and Puerto Rican mother–infant pairs. *Infant Mental Health Journal, 24*, 53–73.

Cassidy, J., Woodhouse, S. S., Sherman, L. J., Stupica, B., & Lejuez, C. (2011). Enhancing infant attachment security: An examination of treatment efficacy and differential susceptibility. *Development and Psychopathology, 23*(1), 131–148.

Chess, S., & Thomas, A. (1982). Infant bonding: Mystique and reality. *American Journal of Orthopsychiatry, 5*, 213–222.

Cicchetti, D. (1983). The emergence of developmental psychopathology. *Child Development, 55*, 1–7.

Crnic, K. A., Greenberg, M. T., & Slough, N. M. (1986). Early stress and social support influences on mothers' and high-risk infants' functioning in late infancy. *Infant Mental Health Journal, 7*, 19–33.

Crockenberg, S. B. (1981). Infant irritability, mother responsiveness, and social support influences on the security of infant–mother attachment. *Child Developmental, 52*, 857–869.

Cyr, C., Euser, E. M., Bakermans-Kranenburg, M. J., & Van IJzendoorn, M. H. (2010). Attachment security and disorganization in maltreating and high-risk families: A series of meta-analyses. *Development and Psychopathology, 22*(1), 87–108.

D'Angelo, E. J. (1986). Security of attachment in infants with schizophrenic, depressed, and unaffected mothers. *Journal of Genetic Psychology, 147*, 421–422.

Das Eiden, R., & Leonard, K. (1996). Paternal alcohol use and the mother–infant relationship. *Development and Psychopathology, 8*, 307–323.

Das Eiden, R., Teti, D., & Corns, K. (1993, April). *Maternal working models of attachment, marital adjustment, and the parent–child relationship.* Paper presented at the biennial meeting of the Society for Research in Child Development, New Orleans, LA.

Davies, P., & Cummings, E. M. (1994). Marital conflict and child adjustment: An emotional security hypothesis. *Psychological Bulletin, 116*, 387–411.

Del Carmen, R., Pedersen, F., Huffman, L., & Bryan, Y. (1993). Dyadic distress management predicts security of attachment. *Infant Behavior and Development, 16*, 131–147.

DeMulder, E. K., & Radke-Yarrow, M. (1991). Attachment with affectively ill and well mothers: Current behavioral correlates. *Developmental Psychopathology, 3*, 227–242.

De Wolff, M., & Van IJzendoorn, M. (1997). Sensitivity and attachment: A meta-analysis on parental antecedents of infant attachment. *Child Development, 68*, 571–591.

Dexter, C. A., Wong, K., Stacks, A. M., Beeghly, M., & Barnett, D. (2013). Parenting and attachment among low-income African American and Caucasian preschoolers. *Journal of Family Psychology, 27*(4), 629–638.

Dickstein, S., Seifer, R., & Albus, K. E. (2009). Maternal adult attachment representations across relationship domains and infant outcomes: The importance of family and couple functioning. *Attachment and Human Development, 11*(1), 5–27.

Ding, Y. H., Xiu, X., Wang, Z. Y., Li, H. R., & Wang, W. P. (2012). Study of mother–infant attachment patterns and influence factors in Shanghai. *Early Human Development, 88*(5), 295–300.

Dozier, M., Stovall, K. C., Albus, K., & Bates, B. (2001). Attachment for infants in foster care: The role of caregiver state of mind. *Child Development, 72*, 1467–1477.

Durrett, M. E., Otaki, M., & Richards, P. (1984). Attachment and the mother's perception of support from the father. *International Journal Behavior Development, 7*, 167–176.

Egeland, B., & Farber, E. A. (1984). Infant–mother attachment: Factors related to its development and changes over time. *Child Development, 55*, 753–771.

Ellis, B. J., Boyce, W. T., Belsky, J., Bakermans-Kranenburg, M. J., & Van IJzendoorn, M. H. (2011). Differential susceptibility to the environment: A neurodevelopmental theory. *Development and Psychopathology, 23*, 7–28.

Fearon, P., Shmueli-Goetz, Y., Viding, E., Fonagy, P., & Plomin, R. (2014). Genetic and environmental influences on adolescent attachment. *Journal of Child Psychology and Psychiatry, 55*(9), 1033–1041.

Finger, B., Hans, S. L., Bernstein, V. J., & Cox, S. M. (2009). Parent relationship quality and infant-mother attachment. *Attachment and Human Development, 11*(3), 285–306.

Finkel, D., & Matheny, A. P., Jr. (2000). Genetic and environmental influences on a measure of infant attachment security. *Twin Research, 3*(4), 242–250.

Fish, M., & Stifter, C. (1995). Patterns of mother–infant interaction and attachment. *Infant Behavior and Development, 18*, 435–446.

Fonagy, P., Steele, M., Moran, G., Steele, H., & Higgitt, A. (1991). The capacity for understanding mental states: The reflective self in parent and child and its significance for security of attachment. *Infant Mental Health Journal, 13*, 200–216.

Forbes, L. M., Evans, E. M., Moran, G., & Pederson, D. R. (2007). Change in atypical maternal behavior predicts change in attachment disorganization from 12 to 24 months in a high-risk sample. *Child Development, 78*, 955–971.

Frankel, K., Maslin-Cole, C., & Harmon, R. (1991, April). *Depressed mothers of preschoolers.* Paper presented at the biennial meeting of the Society for Research in Child Development, Seattle, WA.

Frigerio, A., Ceppi, E., Rusconi, M., Giorda, R., Raggi, M. E., & Fearon, P. (2009). The role played by the interaction between genetic factors and attachment in the stress response in infancy. *Journal of Child Psychology and Psychiatry, 50*(12), 1513–1522.

Gaensbauer, T. J., Harmon, R. J., Cytryn, L., & McKnew, D. H. (1984). Social and affective development in infants with a manic–depressive parent. *American Journal of Psychiatry, 141*, 223–229.

Galinsky, E., Howes, C., & Kontos, S. (1995). *The family child care training study.* New York: Families and Work Institute.

Goldberg, S., Benoit, D., Blokland, K., & Madigan, S. (2003). Atypical maternal behavior, maternal representations, and infant disorganized attachment. *Development and Psychopathology, 15*, 239–257.

Goldberg, W. A., & Easterbrooks, M. A. (1984). The role of marital quality in toddler development. *Developmental Psychology, 20*, 504–514.

Goldstein, L., Diener, M., & Mangelsdorf, S. (1996). Maternal characteristics and social support across the transition to motherhood: Associations with maternal behavior. *Journal of Family Psychology, 10*, 60–71.

Gravener, J. A., Rogosch, F. A., Oshri, A., Narayan, A. J., Cicchetti, D., & Toth, S. L. (2012). The relations among maternal depressive disorder, maternal expressed emotion, and toddler behavior problems and attachment. *Journal of Abnormal Child Psychology, 40*(5), 803–813.

Grossmann, K., Grossmann, K. E., Spangler, G., Suess, G., & Unzner, L. (1985). Maternal sensitivity and newborns' orientation responses as related to quality of attachment in northern Germany. In I. Bretherton & E. Waters (Eds.), Growing points of attachment theory and research. *Monographs of the Society for Research in Child Development, 50*(1–2, Serial No. 209), 233–257.

Grych, J. (2002). Marital relationships and parenting. In M. Bornstein (Ed.), *Handbook of parenting: Vol. 4. Social conditions and applied parenting* (2nd ed., pp. 203–225). Mahwah, NJ: Erlbaum.

Harel, J., & Scher, A. (2003). Insufficient responsiveness in ambivalent mother–infant relationships: Contextual and affective aspects. *Infant Behavior and Development, 26*(3), 371–383.

Harrison, L. J., & Ungerer, J. A. (2002). Maternal employment and infant–mother attachment security at 12 months postpartum. *Developmental Psychology, 38*, 758–773.

Hayes, L. J., Goodman, S. H., & Carlson, E. (2013). Maternal antenatal depression and infant disorganized attachment at 12 months. *Attachment and Human Development, 15*(2), 133–153.

Holland, A. S., & McElwain, N. L. (2013). Maternal and paternal perceptions of coparenting as a link between marital quality and the parent–toddler relationship. *Journal of Family Psychology, 27*(1), 117–126.

Hopkins, J., Gouze, K. R., & Lavigne, J. V. (2013). Direct and indirect effects of contextual factors, caregiver depression, and parenting on attachment security in preschoolers. *Attachment and Human Development, 15*(2), 155–173.

Howes, C., & Markman, H. J. (1989). Marital quality and child functioning: A longitudinal investigation. *Child Development, 60*, 1044–1051.

Huang, Z. J., Lewin, A., Mitchell, S. J., & Zhang, J. (2012). Variations in the relationship between maternal depression, maternal sensitivity, and child attachment by race/ethnicity and nativity: Findings from a nationally representative cohort study. *Maternal and Child Health Journal, 16*(1), 40–50.

Isabella, R. A. (1993). Origins of attachment: Maternal interactive behavior across the first year. *Child Development, 64*, 605–621.

Isabella, R. A. (1994). Origins of maternal role satisfaction and its influences upon maternal interactive behavior and infant–mother attachment. *Infant Behavior and Development, 17*, 381–388.

Isabella, R. [A.], & Belsky, J. (1991). Interactional synchrony and the origins of infant–mother attachment: A replication study. *Child Development, 62*, 373–384.

Isabella, R. [A.], Belsky, J., & von Eye, A. (1989). Origins of infant–mother attachment: An examination of interactional synchrony during the infant's first year. *Developmental Psychology, 25*, 12–21.

Jacobson, S. W., & Frye, K. F. (1991). Effect of maternal social support on attachment: Experimental evidence. *Child Development, 62*, 572–582.

Jin, M. K., Jacobvitz, D., Hazen, N., & Jung, S. H. (2012). Maternal sensitivity and infant attachment security in Korea: Cross-cultural validation of the Strange Situation. *Attachment and Human Development, 14*(1), 33–44.

Juffer, F., Bakermans-Kranenburg, M. J., & Van IJzendoorn, M. H. (2005). The importance of parenting in the development of disorganized attachment: Evidence from a preventive intervention study in adoptive families. *Journal of Child Psychology and Psychiatry, 46*, 263–274.

Kagan, J. (1982). *Psychological research on the human infant: An evaluative summary.* New York: W. T. Grant Foundation.

Kelly, K., Grienenberger, J., & Slade, A. (2005). Maternal reflective functioning, mother-infant affective communication, and infant attachment: Exploring the link between mental states and observed caregiving behavior in the intergenerational transmission of attachment. *Attachment and Human Development, 7*(3), 299–311.

Kendler, K. S. (2013). What psychiatric genetics has taught us about the nature of psychiatric illness and what is left to learn. *Molecular Psychiatry, 18*(10), 1058–1066.

Klein Velderman, M. K., Bakermans-Kranenburg, M. J., Juffer, F., & Van IJzendoorn, M. H. (2006). Effects of attachment-based interventions on maternal sensitivity and infant attachment: Differential susceptibility of highly reactive infants. *Journal of Family Psychology*, 20, 266–274.

Kochanska, G. (1998). Mother–child relationship, child fearfulness, and emerging attachment: A short-term longitudinal study. *Developmental Psychology*, 34, 480–490.

Kochanska, G., Aksan, N., & Carlson, J. J. (2005). Temperament, relationships, and young children's receptive cooperation with their parents. *Developmental Psychology*, 41, 648–660.

Krishnakumar, A., & Buehler, C. (2000). Interparental conflict and parenting behaviors: A meta-analytic review. *Family Relations*, 49, 25–44.

Krupka, A., Moran, G., & Pederson, D. (1996, April). *The quality of mother–infant interactions in families at risk for maladaptive behavior: A window on the process of attachment.* Paper presented at the International Conference on Infant Studies, Providence, RI.

Lakatos, K., Nemoda, Z., Toth, I., Ronai, Z., Ney, K., Sasvari-Szekely, M., et al. (2002). Further evidence for the role of the dopamine D4 receptor (*DRD4*) gene in attachment disorganization: Interaction of the exon III 48-BP repeat and the -521 C/T promoter polymorphisms. *Molecular Psychiatry*, 7, 27–31.

Lakatos, K., Toth, I., Nemoda, Z., Ney, K., Sasvari-Szekely, M., & Gervai, J. (2000). Dopamine D4 receptor (*DRD4*) gene polymorphism is associated with attachment disorganization in infants. *Molecular Psychiatry*, 5, 633–637.

Lamb, M. E., & Kelly, J. B. (2001). Using the empirical literature to guide the development of parenting plans for young children. *Family Court Review*, 39, 365–371.

Laranjo, J., Bernier, A., & Meins, E. (2008). Associations between maternal mind-mindedness and infant attachment security: Investigating the mediating role of maternal sensitivity. *Infant Behavior and Development*, 31(4), 688–695.

Leerkes, E. M. (2011). Maternal sensitivity during distressing tasks: A unique predictor of attachment security. *Infant Behavior and Development*, 34(3), 443–446.

Levitt, M., Weber, R., & Clark, M. (1986). Social network relationships as sources of maternal support and well-being. *Developmental Psychology*, 22, 310–316.

Lewis, M., & Feiring, C. (1989). Infant, mother, and mother–infant interaction behavior and subsequent attachment. *Child Development*, 60, 831–837.

Lewis, M., Owen, M. T., & Cox, M. J. (1988). The transition to parenthood: III. Incorporation of the child into the family. *Family Press*, 27, 411–421.

Lindhiem, O., Bernard, K., & Dozier, M. (2011). Maternal sensitivity: Within-person variability and the utility of multiple assessments. *Child Maltreatment*, 16(1), 41–50.

Lindsey, E. W., Caldera, Y. M., & Tankersley, L. (2009). Marital conflict and the quality of young children's peer play behavior: The mediating and moderating role of parent–child emotional reciprocity and attachment security. *Journal of Family Psychology*, 23(2), 130–145.

Lucassen, N., Tharner, A., Van IJzendoorn, M. H., Bakermans-Kranenburg, M. J., Volling, B. L., Verhulst, F. C., et al. (2011). The association between paternal sensitivity and infant–father attachment security: A meta-analysis of three decades of research. *Journal of Family Psychology*, 25(6), 986–992.

Luijk, M. P., Roisman, G. I., Haltigan, J. D., Tiemeier, H., Booth-LaForce, C., Van IJzendoorn, M. H., et al. (2011). Dopaminergic, serotonergic, and oxytonergic candidate genes associated with infant attachment security and disorganization?: In search of main and interaction effects. *Journal of Child Psychology and Psychiatry*, 52(12), 1295–1307.

Lundy, B. L. (2003). Father– and mother–infant face-to-face interactions: Differences in mind-related comments and infant attachment? *Infant Behavior and Development*, 26(2), 200–212.

Lyons-Ruth, K. (1988, April). *Maternal depression and infant disturbance.* Paper presented at the International Conference on Infant Studies, Washington, DC.

Lyons-Ruth, K., Bronfman, E., & Parsons, E. (1999). Maternal frightened, frightening, or atypical behavior and disorganized infant attachment patterns. *Monographs of the Society for Research in Child Development*, 64(3, Serial No. 258), 67–96.

Lyons-Ruth, K., Yellin, C., Melnick, S., & Atwood, G. (2005). Expanding the concept of unresolved mental states: Hostile/helpless states of mind on the Adult Attachment Interview are associated with disrupted mother–infant communication and infant disorganization. *Development and Psychopathology*, 17, 1–23.

Lyons-Ruth, K., Zoll, D., Connell, D. B., & Grunebaum, H. U. (1986). The depressed mother and her one-year-old infant: Environmental context, mother–infant interaction and attachment. In E. Tronick & T. Field (Eds.), *Maternal depression and infant disturbance* (pp. 61–82). San Francisco: Jossey-Bass.

Madigan, S., Benoit, D., & Boucher, C. (2011). Exploration of the links among fathers' unresolved states of mind with respect to attachment, atypical paternal behavior, and disorganized infant-father attachment. *Infant Mental Health Journal*, 32(3), 286–304.

Madigan, S., Moran, G., & Pederson, D. R. (2006). Unresolved states of mind, disorganized attachment relationships, and disrupted interactions of adolescent mothers and their infants. *Developmental Psychology*, 42, 293–304.

Main, M., & Hesse, E. (1990). Parents' unresolved traumatic experiences are related to infant disorganized attachment status: Is frightened and/or frightening parental behavior the linking mechanism? In M. T. Greenberg, D. Cicchetti, & E. M. Cummings (Eds.), *Attachment in the preschool years: Theory, research, and intervention* (pp. 161–182). Chicago: University of Chicago Press.

Malatesta, C. Z., Grigoryev, P., Lamb, C., Albin, M., & Culver, C. (1986). Emotion socialization and expressive development in preterm and full-term infants. *Child Development*, 57, 316–330.

Martins, C., & Gaffan, E. A. (2000). Effects of early maternal depression on patterns of infant–mother attachment: A meta-analytic investigation. *Journal of Child Psychology and Psychiatry, 41*, 737–746.

Maslin, C. A., & Bates, J. E. (1983, April). *Precursors of anxious and secure attachments: A multivariant model at age 6 months.* Paper presented at the biennial meeting of the Society for Research in Child Development, Detroit, MI.

McElwain, N. L., & Booth-LaForce, C. (2006). Maternal sensitivity to infant distress and nondistress as predictors of infant–mother attachment security. *Journal of Family Psychology, 20*(2), 247–255.

McMahon, C. A., Barnett, B., Kowalenko, N. M., & Tennant, C. C. (2006). Maternal attachment state of mind moderates the impact of postnatal depression on infant attachment. *Journal of Child Psychology and Psychiatry, 47*(7), 660–669.

Meins, E., Fernyhough, C., de Rosnay, M., Arnott, B., Leekam, S. R., & Turner, M. (2012). Mind-mindedness as a multidimensional construct: Appropriate and nonattuned mind-related comments independently predict infant–mother attachment in a socially diverse sample. *Infancy, 17*(4), 393–415.

Meins, E., Fernyhough, C., Fradley, E., & Tuckey, M. (2001). Rethinking maternal sensitivity: Mothers' comments on infants' mental processes predict security of attachment at 12 months. *Journal of Child Psychology and Psychiatry, 42*, 637–648.

Moran, G., Forbes, L., Evans, E., Tarabulsy, G. M., & Madigan, S. (2008). Both maternal sensitivity and atypical maternal behavior independently predict attachment security and disorganization in adolescent mother–infant relationships. *Infant Behavior and Development, 31*(2), 321–325.

Moran, G., Pederson, D., Pettit, P., & Krupka, A. (1992). Maternal sensitivity and infant–mother attachment in a developmentally delayed sample. *Infant Behavior and Development, 15*, 427–442.

Moss, E., Dubois-Comtois, K., Cyr, C., Tarabulsy, G. M., St-Laurent, D., & Bernier, A. (2011). Efficacy of a home-visiting intervention aimed at improving maternal sensitivity, child attachment, and behavioral outcomes for maltreated children: A randomized control trial. *Development and Psychopathology, 23*(1), 195–210.

Murray, L., Fiori-Cowley, A., Hooper, R., & Cooper, P. (1996). The impact of postnatal depression and associated adversity on early mother–infant interactions and later infant outcome. *Child Development, 67*, 2512–2526.

Nakasawa, M., Teti, D. M., & Lamb, M. E. (1992). An ecological study of child–mother attachments among Japanese sojourners in the United States. *Developmental Psychology, 28*, 584–592.

National Institute of Child Health and Human Development (NICHD) Early Child Care Network. (1997). The effects of infant child care on infant–mother attachment security: Results of the NICHD Study of Early Child Care. *Child Development, 68*, 860–879.

Notaro, P. C., & Volling, B. L. (1999). Parental responsiveness and infant–parent attachment: A replication study with fathers and mothers. *Infant Behavior and Development, 22*, 345–352.

O'Connor, M. (1997, March). *Maternal personality characteristics on the MMPI and infant attachment.* Paper presented at the biennial meeting of the Society for Research in Child Development, Washington, DC.

O'Connor, T. G., & Croft, C. M. (2001). A twin study of attachment in preschool children. *Child Development, 72*, 1501–1511.

Oppenheim, D., Koren-Karie, N., & Sagi, A. (2001). Mothers' empathic understanding of their preschoolers' internal experience: Relations with early attachment. *International Journal of Behavioral Development, 25*(1), 16–26.

Otto, H., & Keller, H. (2014). *Different faces of attachment: Cultural variations on a universal human need.* Cambridge, UK: Cambridge University Press.

Out, D., Bakermans-Kranenburg, M. J., & Van IJzendoorn, M. H. (2009). The role of disconnected and extremely insensitive parenting in the development of disorganized attachment: Validation of a new measure. *Attachment & Human Development, 11*(5), 419–443.

Owen, M., & Cox, M. (1997). Marital conflict and the development of infant–parent attachment relationships. *Journal of Family Psychology, 11*, 152–164.

Pederson, D., Gleason, K. E., Moran, G., & Bento, S. (1998). Maternal attachment representations, maternal sensitivity, and the infant–mother attachment relationship. *Developmental Psychology, 34*, 925–933.

Pederson, D., & Moran, G. (1996). Expressions of the attachment relationship outside of the Strange Situation. *Child Development, 67*, 915–927.

Pederson, D., Moran, G., Sitko, C., Campbell, K., Ghesqure, K., & Acton, H. (1990). Maternal sensitivity and the security of infant–mother attachment. *Child Development, 61*, 1974–1983.

Peterson, N. J., Drotar, D., Olness, K., Guay, L., & Kiziri-Mayengo, R. (2001). The relationship of maternal and child HIV infection to security of attachment among Ugandan infants. *Child Psychiatry and Human Development, 32*, 3–17.

Pinquart, M., Feusner, C., & Ahnert, L. (2013). Meta-analytic evidence for stability in attachments from infancy to early adulthood. *Attachment and Human Development, 15*(2), 189–218.

Posada, G., Carbonell, O. A., Alzate, G., & Plata, S. J. (2004). Through Colombian lenses: Ethnographic and conventional analyses of maternal care and their associations with secure base behavior. *Developmental Psychology, 40*, 508–518.

Raby, K., Cicchetti, D., Carlson, E. A., Cutuli, J., Englund, M. M., & Egeland, B. (2012). Genetic and caregiving-based contributions to infant attachment: Unique associations with distress reactivity and attachment security. *Psychological Science, 23*(9), 1016–1023.

Radke-Yarrow, M. (1991). Attachment patterns in children of depressed mothers. In C. M. Parkes, J. Stevenson-Hinde, & P. Maras (Eds.), *Attachment across the life cycle* (pp. 115–126). London: Tavistock/Routledge.

Radke-Yarrow, M., Cummings, E. M., Kuczynski, L., & Chapman, M. (1985). Patterns of attachment in two- and three-year olds in normal families and families with parental depression. *Child Development, 56,* 884–893.

Raval, V., Goldberg, S., Atkinson, L., Benoit, D., Myhal, N., Poulton, L., et al. (2001). Maternal attachment, maternal responsiveness and infant attachment. *Infant Behavior and Development, 24,* 281–304.

Ricciuti, A. E. (1992). Child–mother attachment: A twin study (University Microfilms No. 9324873). *Dissertation Abstracts International, 54,* 3364.

Roisman, G. I., & Fraley, R. C. (2008). A behavior-genetic study of parenting quality, infant attachment security, and their covariation in a nationally representative sample. *Developmental Psychology, 44*(3), 831–839.

Sameroff, A. J., Seifer, R., & Zax, M. (1982). Early development of children at risk for emotional disorder. *Monographs of the Society for Research in Child Development, 47*(7), 1–82.

Scher, A., & Mayseless, O. (2000). Mothers of anxious/ambivalent infants: Maternal characteristics and child-care context. *Child Development, 71,* 1629–1639.

Schneider-Rosen, K., & Rothbaum, F. (1993). Quality of parental caregiving and security of attachment. *Developmental Psychology, 29,* 358–367.

Scholmerich, A., Fracasso, M., Lamb, M., & Broberg, A. (1995). Interactional harmony at 7 and 10 months of age predicts security of attachment as measured by Q-sort ratings. *Social Development, 34,* 62–74.

Schuengel, C., Bakermans-Kranenburg, M. J., & Van IJzendoorn, M. H. (1999). Frightening maternal behavior linking unresolved loss and disorganized infant attachment. *Journal of Consulting and Clinical Psychology, 67,* 54–63.

Sims, B., Hans, S., & Cox, S. (1996, April). *Raising children in high-risk environments: Mothers' experience of stress and distress related to attachment security.* Poster presented at the biennial meeting of the International Conference on Infant Studies, Providence, RI.

Slade, A., Grienenberger, J., Bernbach, E., Levy, D., & Locker, A. (2005). Maternal reflective functioning, attachment, and the transmission gap: A preliminary study. *Attachment and Human Development, 7,* 283–298.

Smith, P. B., & Pederson, D. R. (1988). Maternal sensitivity and patterns of infant–mother attachment. *Child Development, 59,* 1097–1101.

Spangler, G., Johann, M., Ronai, Z., & Zimmermann, P. (2009). Genetic and environmental influence on attachment disorganization. *Journal of Child Psychology and Psychiatry, 50*(8), 952–961.

Spieker, S. J. (1988). Patterns of very insecure attachment forward in samples of high-risk infants and toddlers. *Topics in Early Childhood Special Education, 6,* 37–53.

Spieker, S. J., & Booth, C. (1988). Maternal antecedents of attachment quality. In J. Belsky & T. Nezworski (Eds.), *Clinical implications of attachment* (pp. 95–176). Hillsdale, NJ: Erlbaum.

Sroufe, L. A., & Rutter, M. (1984). The domain of developmental psychopathology. *Child Development, 55,* 17–29.

Stacks, A. M., Muzik, M., Wong, K., Beeghly, M., Huth-Bocks, A., Irwin, J. L., et al. (2014). Maternal reflective functioning among mothers with childhood maltreatment histories: Links to sensitive parenting and infant attachment security. *Attachment and Human Development, 16*(5), 515–533.

Steele, M., Steele, H., & Fonagy, P. (1996). Associations amongst Attachment Classifications of Mothers, Fathers and Their Infants. *Child Development, 67,* 541–555.

Susman-Stillman, A., Kalkoske, M., Egeland, B., & Waldman, I. (1996). Infant temperament and maternal sensitivity as predictors of attachment security. *Infant Behavior and Development, 19,* 33–47.

Tarabulsy, G. M., Bernier, A., Provost, M. A., Maranda, J., Larose, S., Moss, E., et al. (2005). Another look inside the gap: Ecological contributions to the transmission of attachment in a sample of adolescent mother–infant dyads. *Developmental Psychology, 41,* 212–224.

Teti, D., Gelfand, D., Messinger, D., & Isabella, R. (1995). Maternal depression and the quality of early attachment. *Developmental Psychology, 31,* 364–376.

Teti, D., Nakasawa, M., Das, R., & Wirth, O. (1991). Security of attachment between preschoolers and their mothers: Relations among social interaction, parenting stress, and mothers' sorts of the attachment Q-set. *Developmental Psychology, 27,* 440–447.

Tharner, A., Dierckx, B., Luijk, M. P., Van IJzendoorn, M. H., Bakermans-Kranenburg, M. J., van Ginkel, J. R., et al. (2013). Attachment disorganization moderates the effect of maternal postnatal depressive symptoms on infant autonomic functioning. *Psychophysiology, 50*(2), 195–203.

Tomlinson, M., Cooper, P., & Murray, L. (2005). The mother–infant relationship and infant attachment in a South African peri-urban settlement. *Child Development, 76,* 1044–1054.

Tornello, S. L., Emery, R., Rowen, J., Potter, D., Ocker, B., & Xu, Y. (2013). Overnight custody arrangements, attachment, and adjustment among very young children. *Journal of Marriage and the Family, 75,* 871–885.

True, M. M., Pisani, L., & Oumar, F. (2001). Infant–mother attachment among the Dogon of Mali. *Child Development, 72,* 1451–1466.

van den Boom, D. (1990). Preventive intervention and the quality of mother–infant interaction and infant exploration in irritable infants. In W. Koops, H. J.

G. Soppe, J. L. van der Linden, C. M. Molenaar, & J. J. F. Schroots (Eds.), *Developmental psychology behind the dikes* (pp. 249–270). Amsterdam: Uitgeverji Eburon.

van den Boom, D. (1994). The influence of temperament and mothering on attachment and exploration. *Child Development, 65*, 1457–1477.

Van IJzendoorn, M. H. (1995). Adult attachment representations, parental responsiveness, and infant attachment: A meta-analysis on the predictive validity of the Adult Attachment Interview. *Psychological Bulletin, 117*, 387–403.

Van IJzendoorn, M. H., & Bakermans-Kranenburg, M. J. (2006). *DRD4* 7-repeat polymorphism moderates the association between maternal unresolved loss or trauma and infant disorganization. *Attachment and Human Development, 8*, 291–307.

Van IJzendoorn, M. H., Schuengel, C., & Bakermans-Kranenburg, M. J. (1999). Disorganized attachment in early childhood: Meta-analysis of precursors, concomitants, and sequelae. *Development and Psychopathology, 11*, 225–249.

Van IJzendoorn, M. H., Vereijken, C. M., Bakermans-Kranenburg, M. J., & Riksen-Walraven, J. (2004). Assessing attachment security with the Attachment Q Sort: Meta-analytic evidence for the validity of the observer AQS. *Child Development, 75*(4), 1188–1213.

Van Zeijl, J., Mesman, J., Van IJzendoorn, M. H., Bakermans-Kranenburg, M. J., Juffer, F., Stolk, M. N., et al. (2006). Attachment-based intervention for enhancing sensitive discipline in mothers of 1- to 3-year-old children at risk for externalizing behavior problems: A randomized controlled trial. *Journal of Consulting and Clinical Psychology, 74*(6), 994–1005.

Vaughn, B. E., Bost, K. K., & Van IJzendoorn, M. H. (2008). Attachment and temperament: Additive and interactive influences on behavior, affect, and cognition during infancy and childhood *Handbook of attachment: Theory, research, and clinical applications* (2nd ed., pp. 192-216). New York: Guilford Press.

Vereijken, C., Riksen-Walraven, J., & Kondo-Ikemura, K. (1997). Maternal sensitivity and infant attachment security in Japan: A longitudinal study. *International Journal of Behavioral Development, 21*, 35–49.

Volling, B. L., & Belsky, J. (1992). Infant, father, and marital antecedents of infant–father attachment security in dual-earner and single-earner families. *International Journal of Behavioral Development, 15*, 83–100.

Vondra, J., Shaw, D., & Kevinides, M. (1995). Predicting infant attachment classification from multiple, contemporaneous measures of maternal care. *Infant Behavior and Development, 18*, 415–425.

Wolke, D., Eryigit-Madzwamuse, S., & Gutbrod, T. (2014). Very preterm/very low birthweight infants' attachment: infant and maternal characteristics. *Archives of Disease in Child: Fetaland Neonatal Edition, 99*(1), F70–F75.

Wong, M. S., Mangelsdorf, S. C., Brown, G. L., Neff, C., & Schoppe-Sullivan, S. J. (2009). Parental beliefs, infant temperament, and marital quality: Associations with infant–mother and infant–father attachment. *Journal of Family Psychology, 23*(6), 828–838.

Zeanah, C., Benoit, D., Barton, M., Regan, C., Hirshberg, L., & Lipsett, L. (1993). Representations of attachment in mothers and their one-year-old infants. *Journal of the American Academy of Child and Adolescent Psychiatry, 32*, 278–286.

Zevalkink, J., Riksen-Walraven, J. M., & Van Lieshout, C. F. M. (1999). Attachment in the Indonesian caregiving context. *Social Development, 8*, 21–40.

# Chapter 15

# Attachment Relationships in the Context of Multiple Caregivers

## Carollee Howes
## Susan Spieker

In his early writings, Bowlby (1969/1982) proposed that a child develops a hierarchy of attachment relationships—usually first with the mother as the primary caregiver. In 1967, Ainsworth wrote that "nearly all the babies in this sample who became attached to their mothers during the period spanned by our observations became attached also to some other familiar figure—father, grandmother, or other adult in the household, or to an older sibling" (p. 315). The Ainsworth sample comprised Ghanda infants in East Africa. Ainsworth's next major work was the Baltimore study of child–mother attachment (Ainsworth, Blehar, Waters, & Wall, 1978). Although this work was concerned with patterns of infant–mother attachment relationships, Ainsworth and colleagues (1978) still acknowledged the possibility of other attachment figures: "The mother figure is, however, the principal caregiver, whether the natural mother or someone else plays that role" (p. 5).

Although, as these quotations show, recognition of alternative attachment figures has been part of attachment theory from the beginning, attachment research involving children has been conducted largely on the child–mother attachment relationship. There are practical reasons to consider children as having a network of attachment figures. In the United States, families outside the dominant culture (particularly people of color, immigrant families, and families living in or close to poverty) have historically used a variety of childrearing configurations involving networks of caregiving adults rather than a single caregiver (Jackson, 1993). As the roles of women and men in family life have changed, and as the two-income family has become an economic necessity, most children are now regularly cared for by more than one adult. Some children who are adopted, and children in foster care, experience multiple attachment relationships not only simultaneously but also sequentially. As research on multiple attachment relationships has become more common, there is little dispute that children form attachment relationships with child care providers, and that child–mother and child–other attachments are independent in antecedents and quality (Ahnert, Pinquart, & Lamb, 2006).

Considering multiple attachment figures raises theoretical issues for attachment theory. Central to the theory is a set of propositions about how attachments are formed and the influence of attachment relationships on subsequent development. Because alternative attachment relationships are formed in different contexts, and often in different developmental periods (i.e., subsequent to maternal attachments), examining antecedents of alternative attachment relationships can inform and expand the theory. Similarly, examining the predictive power of attachment quality with alternative attachment figures for aspects of children's development can expand our understanding of the roles of relationships in development. Moreover, including multiple caregivers as part of a network of attachment figures may expand our understanding of the organization of internal working models of attachment.

While research published in the interval between the second and third editions of the *Handbook of Attachment* has not challenged the assumption that children may establish attachment relationships with their nonparental child care providers, there is some evidence that asking these caregivers for their perceptions of their relationships with particular children may result in relationship descriptions less aligned with attachment theory than observations of child–caregiver attachment behaviors in child care settings (Howes, Fuligni, Hong, Huang & Lara-Cinisomo, 2013; Hughes, 2012; Sabol & Pianta, 2012; Spilt & Koomen, 2009; Thijs & Koomen, 2009). Recent research has placed greater emphasis on child care providers as teachers who are responsible for children's school readiness, and has extended the measurement of teacher–child relationships to older children (prekindergarten, elementary school). In these newer research efforts, caregivers' perceptions of caregiver–child relationships may include perceptions of self-efficacy, particularly in areas of behavior management and academic instruction, as well as perceptions of warmth and closeness. These teacher perception measures, most commonly the Student–Teacher Relationship Scale (Pianta, 2001), appear to refer not only to attachment behaviors but also to sociability and compliance behaviors (Howes et al., 2013; Hughes, 2012; Verschueren & Koomen, 2012). Notably, Howes and colleagues (2013) found less convergence between Attachment Q-Set (Waters, 1987) and Student–Teacher Relationship Scale (Pianta, 2001) scores than had previously been reported (Howes & Ritchie, 1998). Therefore, in this chapter we review only research utilizing observational measures of attachment behaviors.

While research using caregiver perceptions of child–caregiver relationships has raised fundamental questions about measuring multiple attachments to other-than-mother caregivers, a second body of research provides new evidence for the potentially supportive nature of these child–caregiver relationships. Two studies link children's diurnal cortisol profiles to the quality of their child–caregiver relationships (Ahnert, Harwardt-

Heinecke, Kappler, Eckstein-Madry, & Milatz , 2012; Badanes, Dmitrieva, & Watamura, 2012). In both studies children with more secure attachments to caregivers were more likely to show falling cortisol levels across the child care day (Badnes et al., 2012) or week (Ahnert et al., 2012).

Finally, in this chapter of this new edition we review a number of intervention studies designed to improve the quality of child–caregiver attachment security in other-than-mother child dyads. Changing caregiver practices to be more sensitive and responsive, and increasing caregivers' ability to reflect on their practice, are associated with increases in child–caregiver attachment security.

In this chapter, we first consider children's attachments to other-than-mother caregivers (alternative caregivers), then describe, in some detail, child–mother attachment relationship quality when children attend child care and may also develop attachment relationships with nonparental caregivers.

## Attachment to Nonparental Caregivers

### Developmental Issues

Attachment theory assumes that a caregiver and infant will begin to construct their relationship from the moment of birth. Children's repertoires of social signals and their capacities for memory, internal representation, and affective knowledge develop at the same time as first attachments. Children encounter other attachment figures at varying points in their development. For some alternative caregivers—fathers; grandparents and other relatives; adoptive and foster parents with whom a child is placed at birth; and infant child care providers—we can assume that the course of attachment relationship construction is similar from a developmental point of view to that of child–mother attachment relationship construction. However, other relationships between the child and caregivers begin later in the child's life, and regarding these relationships, both developmental considerations and previous relationship history may have shaping influences.

### Simultaneously Formed Attachment Relationships

In two-parent families, children, from birth onward, are assumed to construct attachment relationships simultaneously with both of their parents (Easterbrooks & Goldberg, 1987). However, even when multiple parental attachment relationships are constructed within the same developmental period and within the same household, attachment security with the two parents often differs, suggesting that each attachment relationship is shaped by specific interactions (Fox, Kimmerly, & Shafer, 1991; Grossmann et al., 2002; Van IJzendoorn & De Wolff, 1997).

There is almost no literature on grandparent–child attachment relationships constructed concurrently with child–parent relationships. There is also little research on attachment relationships between children and child care providers when a child is enrolled in child care prior to the formation of an attachment relationship with one or both parents or parental figures. For example, the youngest children in the large ($N = 2,867$) sample used in Ahnert and colleagues' (2006) meta-analysis were toddlers enrolled in child care after establishing parental attachments. In one more recent study, Howes and Wishard Guerra (2009) followed a sample of children born to low-income Mexican immigrant parents and placed in child care by age 2 months. Over the 3 years of the study, children tended to have secure relationships with both mothers and caregivers, but the two kinds of security scores were statistically independent at each assessment period. In this sample, the family circumstances of the mother tended to influence child security scores with mothers but not with caregivers, further suggesting independence of the two relationships.

### Sequentially Formed Attachment Relationships

Most toddlers or older children who encounter alternative attachment figures already have at least one internal working model (IWM) of an attachment relationship because these representations are developed during the first year. In sequentially formed attachments, both the developmental context and the relationship history differ from those affecting infant–mother attachments. In this section, we review literature on the construction of attachment relationships with sequential nonparental caregivers. When we describe the construction of sequential attachment relationships with child care providers, we are concerned with whether these relationships are constructed according to developmental processes similar to

those seen in child–mother attachment relationships. When we describe the construction of sequential attachment relationships to foster and adoptive parents, we are concerned with not only developmental processes but also the issue of prior difficult relationships.

### Forming New Relationships with Child Care Providers

The formation of infant–mother attachment relationships can be observed as children track or follow their mothers, cry to alert the mothers to their distress, or maintain social contact through smiles and vocalizations. Do children use these same behaviors when they are left in the care of a child care provider or a teacher, or is there another developmental process? Three studies have explicitly examined this question in relation to toddlers. Raikes (1993) had center-based providers complete Attachment Q-Sorts (Waters, 1987) for the children in their care. Security scores increased as the toddlers spent more time with the providers, indicating relationship formation. Barnas and Cummings (1997) compared toddlers' attachment behaviors with long-term staff members (3 months or more in the center) and short-term staff members. Children directed more attachment behaviors to the long-term staffers, and long-term staffers were more successful than short-term staffers in soothing distressed children. Howes and Oldham (2001) observed toddlers daily, then weekly, during their first 6 months in child care. The frequency of attachment behavior decreased over the children's first 2 months in child care. However, the initial frequency of attachment behaviors and their rate of decrease over time were unrelated to the children's attachment security by the end of 6 months in child care. Thus, the formation of toddler–child care provider attachment relationships appears to be similar to the formation of an infant–mother attachment. When toddlers begin child care, they direct attachment behaviors to the caregivers, and with increased time in the setting, children's interactions with the caregivers become more organized, similar to attachment organizations found in mother–child dyads.

### Forming New Relationships with Adoptive or Foster Parents

Classic studies of adoptive children indicated that children adopted after the beginning of attachment relationship formation (6–8 months) had difficulty forming positive, trusting relationships with their adoptive parents (Tizard & Rees, 1975; Yarrow, Goodwin, Manheimer, & Milowe, 1973). More recent studies of children adopted before, during, and after the developmental period of initial attachment formation suggest that attachment formation in infants adopted during their first year is similar to child–mother attachment formation and does not have a critical period (Dontas, Maratos, Fafoutis, & Karangelis, 1985; Marcovitch et al., 1997; Singer, Brodzinsky, Ramsay, Steir, & Waters, 1985). (See Dozier & Rutter, Chapter 30, this volume, for further discussion of issues concerning adoption.)

Describing attachment formation in foster care children and children adopted from institutions with severe caregiving deprivation policies is a stringent test of the dual influences of developmental period and prior relationship history on the process of constructing an attachment relationship. Most foster care children have experienced difficult relationships but not necessarily severe deprivation. Researchers question whether these children can form secure attachments with alternative caregivers, and whether the process of attachment formation is similar to attachment formation in typical children. In an early study (Howes & Segal, 1993), almost half of the children (47%) removed from their homes because of maternal abuse or neglect and placed in high-quality shelter care were able to develop secure attachment relationships with shelter caregivers within 2 months of placement. Foster children placed in therapeutic preschool programs are also able to form secure attachments to their caregivers (Howes & Ritchie, 1999). Extensive and long-term follow-up of children in institutional care suggest that while these children may, when adopted, form attachment relationships, indiscriminate behavior persists (Bakermans-Kranenburg et al., 2011). See Dozier and Rutter, Chapter 30, this volume, for more detailed discussion of these issues.

## Pathways to Secure Attachment Relationships with Alternative Caregivers

An important premise of attachment theory and research is that caregiver behavior, specifically, sensitive and responsive behavior, and caregiver attachment representations are important in the construction of secure attachment relationships (Ainsworth et al., 1978; Cassidy et al., 2005; Van IJzendoorn, 1995). Not surprisingly, sensitive and responsive behaviors—and, to a lesser extent, caregiver "states of mind with respect to attachment" assessed in the Adult Attachment Interview (AAI)—have been the topics of research on the antecedents of secure attachments with nonparental caregivers.

### Sensitive and Responsive Caregiver Behaviors

Early studies on child–father and child–caregiver attachments (with the term *caregiver* referring to a nonparental child care provider) revealed that more sensitive previous or current caregiving was linked to more secure attachment relationships (Anderson, Nagel, Roberts, & Smith, 1981; Cox, Owen, Henderson, & Margand, 1992; Easterbrooks & Goldberg, 1987; Goossens & Van IJzendoorn, 1990; Howes & Hamilton, 1992a; Howes & Ritchie, 1998; Howes, Rodning, Galluzzo, & Myers, 1988; Howes & Smith, 1995).

Meta-analytic work suggests that for child–caregiver attachment relationships, the form of child care may influence caregiver sensitivity (Ahnert et al., 2006). Security in child–caregiver relationships in child care centers was best predicted by warm and sensitive care that monitored both individual children's needs and the needs of the entire group of children. Caregivers were, not surprisingly, more successful at this dual focus when the groups of children were smaller. In family-based child care, with smaller groups of children, dyadic responsivity by itself predicted attachment security.

### Caregiver States of Mind

When children in the meta-analysis (Ahnert et al., 2006) had experienced discontinuous care, and perhaps were less trusting of child care providers in general (see Howes & Hamilton, 1993), they were less likely to be secure. This suggests that the average professional caregiver's level of sensitivity may not be sufficient to produce secure attachment relationships with children whose relationship histories have predisposed them to consider adult caregivers unavailable or untrustworthy (Howes & Ritchie, 2002). Caregivers' perceptions of children can influence attachment security, particularly if the children differ from them in ethnic background. If children are ethnically mismatched with caregivers, and if the children evoke negative emotions from these caregivers, the caregivers are more likely to report conflictual child–teacher relationships (Rudasill, Rimm-Kaufman, Justice, & Pence, 2006; Saft & Pianta, 2001; Stuhlman & Pianta, 2002).

Two recent intervention studies involved directing intervention efforts toward each caregiver's state of mind regarding attachment. Biringen and colleagues (2012) combined course work on attachment with coaching onsite in caregiving practices associated with caregiver and child mutual emotional availability. Caregivers from the intervention group and the children for whom they cared increased in both emotional availability and attachment security compared to caregivers and children in the control group. Spilt, Koomen, Thijs, and Van deLeij (2012) more directly addressed caregivers' state of mind regarding attachment. Using relationship-focused reflection, they targeted caregivers' mental representations of relationships with specific children. Caregivers in the experimental group were more likely than caregivers in the control group to report increases in closeness with the children and were observed to be more sensitive in their interactions with them.

## Organization of Child IWMs in Multiple-Caregiver Contexts

Examining attachment in the context of multiple caregivers requires that we consider how representations of multiple attachment relationships are organized in a child's IWMs. According to attachment theory, the child forms internal representations of self and relationships with others based on repeated interactions with attachment figures (Bowlby, 1969/1982). Several different possibilities for the organization of IWMs of multiple attachment relationships have been suggested: "hierarchical," in which the child's representation of the most salient caregiver, most often the mother, is the most influential (Bretherton, 1985); "integrative," in which the child integrates all of his or her attachment relationships into a single representation (Van IJzendoorn, Sagi, & Lambermon, 1992); and "independent," in which the different representations are independent both in quality and in their influence on development (Howes, 1999). To evaluate the empirical support for a model of organization of IWMs, two bodies of literature must be considered. In one body of literature, researchers have examined the concordance in the quality of children's attachments to more than one caregiver. In the second, researchers have compared the predictability of children's developmental outcomes from their attachment security with different caregivers.

### Concordance of Attachment Quality

There have been two major meta-analyses examining concordance of attachment relationship quality across caregivers. Fox and colleagues (1991) conducted a meta-analysis examining the concordance of infant–mother and infant–father attachment security. They concluded that mother and father relationships were modestly concordant; that is, they were not independent. This is consistent with the literature suggesting that the mother may shape father–child interaction and subsequent relationship quality (Steele, Steele, & Fonagy, 1995), and it supports a hierarchical model of organization.

Ahnert and colleagues (2006) examined the concordance of child–mother and child–caregiver attachment security and like Fox and colleagues (1991) concluded that the two relationships were independent. Although children were less likely to be secure with their professional care providers than with their mothers, there is little evidence in the literature suggesting that the child's mother shapes child–caregiver interaction patterns. Therefore, this analysis supports an independent rather than a hierarchical model of organization.

### Prediction of Developmental Outcomes

Relatively few studies have examined the differential prediction of developmental outcomes from attachment quality of relationships with more than one caregiver. As might be expected from the greater amount of time mothers, compared with fathers, spend with their children, child–mother attachment quality is generally (but not always) more predictive of child outcomes than is child–father attachment quality (Main, Hesse, & Kaplan, 2005; Main, Kaplan, & Cassidy, 1985; Suess, Grossmann, & Sroufe, 1992; Volling & Belsky, 1992; but see also Easterbrooks & Goldberg, 1987; Grossmann et al., 2002; Lamb, Hwang, Frodi, & Frodi, 1982; Main & Weston, 1981; Steele et al., 1996). Two longitudinal studies have examined children's developmental outcomes using child–mother and child–caregiver relationships as predictors of children's outcomes. The Haifa longitudinal study examined prediction from quality of child–mother, child–father, and child–*metapelet* relationships in infancy to social and emotional outcomes in early childhood, early and late adolescence, and early adulthood (Sagi-Schwartz & Aviezer, 2005). In early childhood, previous child–*metapelet* attachment security predicted preschool children's social competence with peers better than did child–parent attachment security (Oppenheim, Sagi, & Lamb, 1988). Furthermore, scores based on a network of caregivers (mother, father, and *metapelet*) better predicted general social competence in early childhood than did child–mother attachment security (Van IJzendoorn et al., 1992). Network security in early childhood was also most predictive of child competence with peers in a Dutch sample of children, mothers, and childcare providers (Van IJzendoorn et al., 1992). These findings support an independent or integrative model of IWM organization. By adolescence and adulthood, results from the Haifa study were less conclusive with regard to the organization of IWMs. Beyond early childhood, networks of attachment relationships were not as predictive of outcomes as was early attachment security with mother and father (Sagi-Schwartz & Aviezer, 2005).

The Howes longitudinal study examined the ability of child–mother, child–caregiver, and child–teacher relationships from infancy through middle childhood to predict concurrent and early and late adolescent social and emotional outcomes. In the toddler period, attachment relationships with mother and child care providers predicted behavior with peers, supporting an integrative organization of IWMs (Howes et al., 1988). At preschool, the findings suggested an independent organization, with early security of attachment to a child care provider predicting preschool children's social competence with peers (Howes, Matheson, & Hamilton, 1994). At age 9 (Howes, Hamilton, & Phillipsen, 1998) and at age 14 (Howes & Tonyan, 2000), early attachment security with mother was the best predictor of child–mother relationship quality, and early attachment security with child care providers was the best predictor of child–teacher attachment security. These results argue for an independent organization. However, peer friendships in these last two developmental periods were best predicted by preschool friendship quality, suggesting that whereas early attachment security with child care providers predicted early friendship with peers, peer relation-

ship quality in later developmental periods was independent of early attachments to adults. By late adolescence (Howes & Aikens, 2002) the pattern of relations between early attachments to mothers and caregivers on the one hand, and social and emotional competence on the other, did not fit any of the proposed models of IWM organization. Complex relations were found among adolescent functioning, gender, and early emotion regulation in child care and early relationships with adults.

Far more research than two longitudinal studies is needed to support any of the proposed conceptions of IWM organization resulting from multiple attachment relationships (for further discussion of these issues, see Kobak, Rosenthal, & Serwik, 2005; Thompson & Raikes, 2003). As more and more children develop social and emotional competence through attachment relationships with mothers and other salient caregivers, researchers should consider planning studies that describe relationships with multiple attachment figures across time.

## Relations between Child Care and Maternal Attachment

A dramatic demographic shift in the rearing experiences of infants in the United States occurred in the closing decades of the 20th century. By the mid-1980s, the number of mothers in the paid labor force with infants under 1 year of age reached 50%. Social scientists began to ask whether the experience of repeated separations from mother, and time away from mother during the development of a child's primary attachments, had adverse consequences for the quality of infant–mother attachment.

### Concern That Child Care Was a Risk for Insecure Infant–Mother Attachment

During the 1980s, two multistudy analyses converged on the conclusion that more than 20 hours/ week of child care in the first year of life was associated with elevated rates of insecure infant–mother attachment, as measured by the Strange Situation (Ainsworth & Wittig, 1969; see Solomon & George, Chapter 18, this volume). Belsky and Rovine (1988) and Clarke-Stewart (1989) reported insecurity rates for infants with extensive child care to be 43 and 36%, respectively, compared with rates of 26 and 29% for groups with no or limited early child care experience. These differences were particularly marked for insecure-avoidant classifications. Lamb, Sternberg, and Prodromidis (1992) reanalyzed data from 13 studies and also found that children in exclusive maternal care had higher rates of security than other infants. In contrast to the earlier studies, however, Lamb and colleagues found elevated insecurity and avoidance for infants in any child care exceeding a mere 5 hours/week, and insecurity and avoidance rates for infants receiving this low level of child care were not different from those receiving extensive care of more than 20 hours/week.

The explanation of these effects was a matter of controversy. Barglow, Vaughn, and Molitor (1987) hypothesized that the elevation in the rate of insecure-avoidant attachment indicated that these infants experienced repeated separations from their mothers as rejection. Others wondered whether time away from each other might disrupt the proximal processes of mother–child interaction, affecting a mother's ability to respond to her infant with sensitivity (Brazelton, 1985; Jaeger & Weinraub, 1990; Owen & Cox, 1988) or the infant's expectation of an available and responsive parent (Sroufe, 1988).

Eventually, two interpretations of the data became common in the developmental and popular literature. One was that the experience of extensive child care in the first year of life was indeed a risk factor for the development of insecure infant–mother attachment (Belsky, 1990), although the majority of infants with this early experience did develop secure attachments. The second interpretation focused on the measurement of attachment insecurity itself. Clarke-Stewart (1989) suggested that the two brief separations in the Strange Situation procedure were not stressful enough for infants with extensive child care experience, and that the autonomy and independence displayed by these less distressed infants upon reunion with their mothers was in fact misinterpreted as avoidance. Clarke-Stewart asserted that the Strange Situation may not be a valid measure of attachment for infants with extensive child care experience.

The evidence relevant to these two interpretations was mixed. The results of the 1980s studies were consistent, but Roggman, Langlois, Hubbs-Tait, and Rieser-Danner (1994), studying a small but later-born cohort, found no association between child care experience and infant–mother attachment security. Other researchers found no differences in distress or exploration in the Strange Situation for infants with insecure-avoidant classifications and varying amounts of child care experience (Belsky & Braungart, 1991; McCartney & Galanopoulos, 1988), and Berger, Levy, and Compaan (1995) supplied evidence that the Strange Situation was equally valid for infants with and without extensive child care in the first year. Thus, the "infant day care controversy" (Westman, 1988) was in full swing when the National Institute of Child Health and Human Development (NICHD) initiated the Study of Early Child Care to address these and other questions about the effects of early child care on children's social, emotional, cognitive, and language development.

## The NICHD Study of Early Child Care

The 1,364 participants in the NICHD Study of Early Child Care and Youth Development (NICHD SECCYD; "Youth Development" was added to the title of the study when it was extended in its third phase to follow participants through sixth grade) were recruited throughout 1991 from 31 hospitals in 10 sites across the United States, in accordance with a conditionally random sampling plan designed to ensure that participant families reflected the educational, economic, and ethnic diversity of their respective sites. The corporate author, the NICHD Early Child Care Research Network (NICHD ECCRN), published two articles (1997, 2001) on the effects of early child care on attachment as assessed by the Strange Situation at 15 and 36 months. Subsequent named-author papers (e.g., Huston & Rosenkrantz Aronson, 2005; Tran & Weinraub, 2006), using the same data set, also addressed this question, although the question has not been the focus of inquiry since the previous edition of this volume. Others have used the data to examine predictors of attachment security (e.g., Campbell et al., 2004) or the influence of attachment security on child development (e.g., Fearon & Belsky, 2011; O'Connor, Collins, & Supplee, 2012), regardless of child care experience. And, as the title of the study suggests, the ECCRN has published extensively about the influences of early child care experiences on a wide range of developmental outcomes up to age 15 (e.g., Vandell et al., 2010). Other analyses focus on topics that are not related to early child care, such as afterschool experience, physical activity, family processes, and school environments. Currently, the sample has been followed into early adulthood (e.g., Fraley, Roisman, Booth-LaForce, Owen, & Holland, 2013).

The NICHD SECCYD has considerable methodological strength. The sample size has been nearly as large as the largest of the multistudy analyses in the 1980s (Clarke-Stewart, 1989). The study has been prospective and longitudinal, following children identified at birth, thus reducing selection biases. Parents determined the timing, type, and amount of child care, and presumably considered quality in their choices; the researchers recorded this information regularly and observed the quality of the major arrangements during the first phase of the study at child ages 6, 15, 24, and 36 months. The design of the study used a broad multivariate framework, permitting the effects of child care on infant–mother attachment security to be studied "in context." The examination of effects in context was important because none of the previous studies had indicated that insecurity was inevitable for children with extensive early child care experience—only that rates of insecurity were elevated. Characteristics of the child (e.g., sex, temperament), child care experience (type, amount, age of entry, stability, and quality), and characteristics of the family (including socioemotional processes and economic resources) could all interact with each other to influence child outcomes, including attachment security. Children were not randomly assigned to child care, and complex family selection factors influenced family decisions about the type of child care children would experience. The basic analytic approach of the NICHD ECCRN was to assess the amount of variance of any outcome explained by child care-related variables that was over and above that explained by selection, family, and child factors. The major child care associations with attachment reported in the ECCRN papers are reviewed below.

## The NICHD Study of Early Child Care and Infant–Mother Attachment

The NICHD ECCRN (1997) analyses had two purposes. The first was to explore the validity of the Strange Situation for assessing attachment security of infants with extensive experience in child care by comparing a subsample of infants who experienced more than 30 hours/week of child care from ages 4 to 15 months ($n = 263$) with infants who had fewer than 10 hours/week of child care

during this period ($n = 251$). The validation measures included 5-point ratings of the infants' distress during the separation episodes of the Strange Situation, and the coders' self-rated confidence (5-point scale) with which they assigned the various secure or insecure major classifications. In these validity analyses, the five-category attachment classification (A, B, C, D, U) was used. Results of 2 (high vs. low child care intensity) × 5 (attachment classification) analyses of variance for the distress and confidence ratings provided no support for the hypothesis that the Strange Situation was a less valid measure of attachment for children with extensive child care experience. There was no main effect of child care intensity on either of these ratings.

The second purpose of the 1997 analyses was to examine the main effects of age of entry and child care quantity, stability, and quality on infant attachment security, as well as the interaction of these features of child care with aspects of the family and/or child. Two kinds of interactions were tested. The first set addressed the "dual-risk" hypothesis, namely, that large amounts of child care, poor-quality child care, or frequent changes in care over time would promote insecure infant–mother attachment in the context of other risks, such as difficult temperament, being a male, or residing with a mother who had poor psychological adjustment or was less sensitive and responsive to the infant. A "compensatory" hypothesis was also tested, namely, that when family or child risks were high, child care that began early in life and was stable, extensive, or of high quality would foster the formation of a more secure infant–mother attachment. In a series of logistic regression analyses, the dichotomous dependent attachment variable (secure–insecure or secure–avoidant) was predicted from one of five characteristics of the mother or the child, one of five characteristics of child care, and the interaction between the two selected (mother–child and child care) variables, entered one at a time.

The "main effects" hypotheses for child care received no support. None of the five child care variables (two measures of observed quality of care, the amount of care, the age of entry, and the frequency of care starts), entered after the selection and family–child variables, significantly predicted attachment security. Six of the 25 interaction terms included in the logistic regression analyses were significant predictors of attachment security. A consistent pattern observed across five of the six significant interactions was that the highest rates of insecurity occurred under dual-risk conditions. Infants were less likely to be secure when low maternal sensitivity/responsiveness was combined with poor-quality child care, more than minimal amounts of child care, or more than one care arrangement. In addition, boys experiencing many hours in care were somewhat less likely to be securely attached (and girls experiencing more hours in care were somewhat more likely to be secure). The interaction analyses also provided evidence for compensatory effects. The proportion of attachment security among children with the least sensitive and responsive mothers was higher in high-quality child care than in low-quality care.

Additional detailed analyses of the NICHD SECCYD data set likewise found no evidence of main effects. Booth and colleagues (2002) and Huston and Rosenkrantz Aronson (2005), analyzing detailed data, examined amount of mothers' time with their infants in the first year of life and found no associations with attachment security at 15 or 36 months. Thus, one of the hypothesized mechanisms for earlier findings on attachment security—that extensive child care did not give mothers and children sufficient time to get to know one another—was not supported. Nevertheless, another paper by the NICHD ECCRN (1999), based on longitudinal analyses that controlled for selection, child, and family predictors, reported that more hours of child care predicted less maternal sensitivity and less positive child engagement with the mother. Apparently the effect of hours in child care does not overlap completely with the effect of time with mother. Another failure to replicate prior results completely, using different analyses from the data set, was reported by Tran and Weinraub (2006), who did not find an interaction between maternal sensitivity and stability of child care predicting infant attachment. Tran and Weinraub used a slightly different measure of stability and a somewhat different subset of participants. These instances of lack of replication highlight the relatively small effect sizes of the significant interactions in the 1997 article.

In comparing the results of the NICHD SECCYD with those of earlier studies, considerable weight should be given to the NICHD study because of its size and the quality of the data. But the possibility of cohort effects is real and may be responsible for some of the differences in findings between this and earlier studies. Families in the 1990s that used child care may have differed in important ways from their earlier counterparts. Maternal employment during a child's infancy became an increasingly "mainstream" practice; also, families and child care providers may have been more aware of the child care controversy than were families in the 1970s and 1980s, and so may have worked harder to support the infant–parent relationship.

The limitations of the NICHD SECCYD should not be ignored. The highest-risk families, including those with adolescent mothers or families with vulnerable, ill, or premature newborns were not included in the sample. Although nearly one-fourth of the sample was low-income, low income was almost completely confounded with racial minority status (specifically, African American), making it impossible to examine these factors independently. Finally, the researchers were less likely to be permitted to observe child care arrangements presumed to be of low quality. All of these limitations affect the generalizability of conclusions from the seminal 1997 study about the main and interactive effects of family–child characteristics and child care quality on infant attachment and other outcomes.

## The Haifa Study of Early Child Care and Infant–Mother Attachment

A later Israeli study modeled on the NICHD SECCYD was designed to address some of these issues. The Haifa Study of Early Child Care (Sagi, Koren-Karie, Gini, Ziv, & Joels, 2002), also funded by the NICHD, "was designed to shed further light on issues pertaining to the effects of early child care on the development of the infant–mother attachment relationship in general, and on the published data from the NICHD Early Child Care Research Network in particular" (p. 1167). Because in Israel child care centers are part of a nationwide network, the quality is relatively homogeneous and not confounded with socioeconomic status (SES) because infants from families of all income and education levels are placed in the same centers. The researchers used a randomized, stratified sampling strategy for all healthy, singleton births in the greater Haifa metropolitan area in a 1-year period. The final sample included 758 families at all SES levels. The analytic approach closely followed that reported by the NICHD ECCRN (1997). Like the NICHD SECCYD researchers, the Haifa researchers controlled for selection, family, and child characteristics before testing for main and interaction effects involving features of child care. Sagi and colleagues (2002) found that infants who experienced center care in the first year of life (46% insecure), as compared to those who experienced no child care or care by relatives, paid individuals, or family day care (26% insecure overall), were more likely to be insecurely attached to their mothers. Further analyses implicated the high infant–caregiver ratio (M = 8.01, standard deviation = 1.69) in Israeli centers. Among infants cared for by professional caregivers, those experiencing infant–caregiver ratios of 3:1 or less had a security rate of 72%, compared to 57% for infants experiencing higher infant–caregiver ratios. The researchers also demonstrated that infant–caregiver ratios, not amount of care, were what predicted infant attachment security. When only infants cared for in centers were considered, there was no difference in amount of care experienced by infants who were secure or insecure with their mothers. Finally, eight of 24 interaction terms were significant, most supporting a dual-risk interpretation. Low maternal sensitivity combined with an indicator of low-quality child care always yielded the lowest proportion of securely attached infants. Three interactions with child gender indicated that boys were particularly vulnerable to center care, unstable care, and high infant–caregiver ratios.

Most of the insecure Israeli infants were ambivalent; very few were avoidant, consistent with previous studies of infant attachment in Israel (Scher & Mayseless, 2000; Van IJzendoorn & Sagi, 1999). In contrast, many of the U.S. child care studies found that most of the infants in child care classified as insecure with their mothers were avoidant, and this difference underscores the cultural context in which these studies were conducted. Both the NICHD ECCRN (1997) study and the Haifa study found small effect sizes for child care variables. The results of the two studies are similar and complementary. The Haifa study compensates for one of the limitations of the NICHD SECCYD, which was that observations of quality in the lowest-quality settings were frequently denied. In Israel, the centers were of uniformly very poor quality, and access was readily available. The Haifa study's inclusion of very low-quality center care for infants from a range of SES groups expands the continuum of quality under which the effects of child care have been studied, and has important policy implications for the well-being of infants placed in center care.

In summary, the NICHD SECCYD and the Haifa infant study examined effects of child care experience during the development of primary attachments in infancy on the security of the infant–mother attachment relationship. The 2001

report of the NICHD ECCRN extended the approach of the 1997 article to examine the continued effects of this early experience, and also examined the effects of child care that began after the formation of the infant–mother attachment relationship on children's preschool Strange Situation classifications with mothers at 36 months. Because the 1999 NICHD ECCRN report found that more hours per week in child care was associated with lower maternal sensitivity and less positive engagement of child with mother over the first 3 years of life, main effects of child care on attachment security that were not noted at 15 months might have emerged by 36 months. The 2001 analyses addressed whether child care experience (amount, number of arrangements, age of entry, and quality), alone or in combination with family, maternal, or child factors, was associated with attachment security at 36 months. In addition, analyses examined child, family, and child care correlates of stability–instability of Strange Situation attachment classifications from 15 to 36 months.

## Child Care and Infant–Mother Attachment Stability

Several authors have reported links between early child care experience and attachment stability from infancy to preschool. In a low-risk sample, Howes and Hamilton (1992b) found significant stability in attachment from infancy to the preschool period. In addition, they found instability to be associated with hours per week in child care. Children who entered part-time child care as infants or 3-year-olds had more stable maternal attachment classifications, regardless of quality of attachment, than children who entered full-time care as infants or 3-year-olds. The stability described by Howes and Hamilton is interesting in light of a report by Egeland and Heister (1995). In their high-risk sample from the 1970s, early and extensive child care beginning in the first year seemed to have a negative effect on children who were secure as infants, but a positive effect on those who were insecure. Furthermore, infant attachment security predicted later outcomes only for children who were not in early and extensive child care before 18 months of age. Egeland and Heister speculated that these relations may be mediated by a change in attachment security from infancy to preschool for children in child care, with greater stability of attachment to mother for children who did not experience child care. Egeland

and Heister did not, however, actually assess pre-school security in their study. In contrast, Rauh, Ziegenhain, Muller, and Wijnroks (2000), following a German sample, found that attachment stability in the first 2 years of life was related to maternal sensitivity, but not to variations in child care experience across that time period.

Unlike the 1997 NICHD ECCRN study, the NICHD ECCRN (2001) analyses considered all four attachment classifications (A, B, C, D) using multinomial logistic regression. Results revealed that mothers who exhibited more sensitivity and responsiveness across play assessments between 6 and 36 months were more likely to have children with secure- rather than insecure-controlling classifications, and marginally more likely to have children with insecure-avoidant versus insecure-controlling, insecure-ambivalent versus insecure-controlling, and secure versus insecure-ambivalent classifications. None of the three child care predictors available for the whole sample significantly predicted any attachment classification. That is, variations in the amount of care, the frequency of care arrangements, or age of entry did not increase or decrease a child's chances of being assigned a particular attachment classification, after controls for all selection and mother–family–child variables were imposed. As a direct follow-up of the 15-month interaction findings, four interactions (sensitivity × quality, sensitivity × hours, sensitivity × number of arrangements, and hours × child gender) at 36 months were tested, one at a time, in the multinomial logistic regression models. One interaction term was significant, suggesting that as hours in care increased, children with more sensitive parents were more likely to be classified as secure, and children with less sensitive parents were more likely to be classified as insecure-ambivalent. Thus, overall, findings on the follow-up effects of child care experience were congruent with the findings on earlier effects, and they support the conclusion that the effects of child care experience that begins during the development of primary attachments persist into the preschool years.

The ECCRN (2001) also reported logistic regression analyses predicting security versus insecurity at 36 months within both the initially secure and initially insecure groups. These analyses determined whether child care experience could explain why some children who were initially secure remained that way over time, whereas others did not, and why some children who were initially insecure remained that way, whereas others did

not. There was one effect of child care experience for children who were classified as secure at 15 months: Those whose classification changed from secure to insecure were more likely to have initiated at least 10 hours/week of child care during the interval between 15 and 35 months, compared with children whose classification remained secure. This was a small effect ($r = .09$). These new results for sequential effects of child care after the formation of primary attachments are in contrast to the results for simultaneous child care experiences, described earlier.

In summary, analyses from the NICHD SEC-CYD have consistently found that family influences are stronger than child care effects in determining the quality of child–mother attachment as measured by the Strange Situation at 15 and 36 months. However, some evidence for dual-risk effects has been found at both ages. It seems that for children whose interactions with their mothers are already distressed, long daily separations from mothers increase the likelihood of insecure attachment. Entry into child care after developing a primary attachment also appears to elevate risk for insecurity somewhat. A similar finding was reported by Lamb and colleagues (1992), who found that insecure infant–mother attachments were significantly more common among infants assessed after 15 months of age, and among those who entered care between 7 and 12 months of age rather than earlier.

In both the NICHD SECCYD and the Haifa study, any adverse effects of child care on child–mother attachment were observed more in groups at risk because the quality of maternal care was less sensitive and responsive—that is, because the relationship was already troubled. As an extreme example of this phenomenon, Crittenden (1983) reported on the effects of mandatory protective day care (respite care) for young children of maltreating and neglecting mothers. After 4 years, the outcomes for the two groups were similar except that those placed in day care had earlier removals for foster care than comparable children who could not be placed in day care. Crittenden concluded that mandatory protective day care had hastened, but not caused, the removal of the children. She explained this surprising outcome in terms of attachment theory, citing evidence that both maltreating mothers and their infants could be considered anxiously attached, and that, as such, they would be more vulnerable to experiences of separation. Both mothers and infants reacted to the day care placement with a combination of direct and repressed anger, which exacerbated their already strained relationship and accelerated infants' removal from the home.

The Haifa study complements the NICHD SECCYD by including a range of child care quality that was not confounded by family SES. Together, these studies add to the literature on child–mother attachment in the context of multiple caregiving. Much of child care (especially in infancy, and for some cultural groups more than others) is provided by fathers, grandparents, relatives, friends, and neighbors. The literature suggests little or no impact of these caregiving arrangements on the primary infant–mother attachment relationship. However, there appears to be a threshold effect that is illustrated by results from the Haifa study: More formal group care, with large numbers of children and large child–caregiver ratios, may make the formation of *any* secure attachment—whether to the mother or an alternative caregiver—less likely. This conclusion is supported by the meta-analysis of Ahnert and colleagues (2006) meta-analysis, who found that children's attachments to caregivers in child care were observed to be less secure when group size and child–caregiver ratios were large. It may be that children under these adverse circumstances develop strategies with all of their caregivers that are adapted to increase the probability of protection and survival under threatening conditions, which after all is the evolutionary purpose of attachment.

## Summary and Conclusions

Most children grow and develop within a changing network of attachment relationships, which includes some enduring attachment figures and some that change with time and circumstances. The child is a co-constructor of all of these relationships. Children construct relationships with mothers and residential fathers within the same family. Children come and go between home and child care facilities; the adult caregivers communicate with each other or do not; they collaborate in caring for the child or they do not. However, child–parent and child–caregiver attachment relationships are largely independent in quality and may have different antecedents. The process of forming attachment relationships is similar for parents and alternative caregivers for typical children, particularly children who are very young and/or experiencing positive parental relation-

ships. The construction of secure attachments appears more dependent on particularly skilled and sensitive adult behaviors when children have experienced prior difficult relationships. As with parents, the quality of caregiving may influence attachment formation, but other attributions of the children by the caregivers may also be important.

We know less about the role of alternative caregivers in terms of children's long-term development. Parents, particularly mothers, are undoubtedly the emotionally salient and sustaining attachment figures in most cases. Child care providers are not long-term participants in the social networks of most children. In general, we can draw few conclusions about the importance of early versus later or sustained experiences with alternative attachment figures. We could find no longitudinal studies of long-term alternative attachment relationships—for example, those with grandparents. Far more research than currently exists is needed to support any of the proposed conceptions of the organization of IWMs based on multiple attachment relationships.

## References

Ahnert, L., Harwardt-Heinecke, E., Kappler, G., Eckstein-Madry, T., & Milatz, A. (2012). Student–teacher relationships and classroom climate in first grade: How do they relate to students' stress regulation? *Attachment and Human Development, 14*(3), 249–263.

Ahnert, L., Pinquart, M., & Lamb, M. E. (2006). Security of children's relationships with nonparental care providers: A meta-analysis. *Child Development, 77,* 664–679.

Ainsworth, M. D. S. (1967). *Infancy in Uganda: Infant care and the growth of love.* Baltimore: Johns Hopkins University Press.

Ainsworth, M. D. S., Blehar, M., Waters, E., & Wall, S. (1978). *Patterns of attachment: A psychological study of the Strange Situation.* Hillsdale, NJ: Erlbaum.

Ainsworth, M. D. S., & Wittig, B. (1969). Attachment and exploratory behaviour of one-year-olds in a Strange Situation. In B. Foss (Ed.), *Determinants of infant behaviour* (Vol. 4, pp. 111–173). London: Methuen.

Anderson, C. W., Nagel, P., Roberts, M., & Smith, K. (1981). Attachment in substitute caregivers as a function of center quality and caregiver involvement. *Child Development, 52,* 53–51.

Badanes, L., Dmitrieva, J., & Watamura, S. (2012). Understanding cortisol reactivity across the day at child care: The potential buffering role of secure attachments to caregivers. *Early Childhood Research Quarterly, 27,* 156–165.

Bakermans-Kranenburg, M. J., Steele, H., Zeanah, C. H., Muhamedrahimov, R. J., Vorria, P., Dobrova-Krol, N. A., et al. (2011). III. Attachment and emotional development in institutional care: Characteristics and catch up. *Monographs of the Society for Research in Child Development, 76*, 62–91.

Barglow, P., Vaughn, B. E., & Molitor, N. (1987). Effects of maternal absence due to employment on the quality of infant–mother attachment in a low-risk sample. *Child Development, 58*, 945–954.

Barnas, M. V., & Cummings, E. M. (1997). Caregiver stability and toddlers' attachment-related behaviors towards caregivers in day care. *International Journal of Behavioral Development, 17*, 141–147.

Belsky, J. (1990). Developmental risks associated with infant day care: Attachment insecurity, noncompliance, and aggression? In S. S. Chehrazi (Ed.), *Psychosocial issues in day care* (pp. 37–68). Washington, DC: American Psychiatric Association.

Belsky, J., & Braungart, J. M. (1991). Are insecure-avoidant infants with extensive day-care experience less stressed by and more independent in the Strange Situation? *Child Development, 62*, 567–571.

Belsky, J., & Rovine, M. J. (1988). Nonmaternal care in the first year of life and the security of infant–parent attachment. *Child Development, 59*, 157–167.

Berger, S., Levy, A., & Compaan, K. (1995, March). *Infant attachment outside the laboratory.* Paper presented at the biennial meeting of the Society for Research in Child Development, Indianapolis, IN.

Biringen, Z., Altenhofen, S., Aberle, J., Baker, M., Brosal, A., Bennett, S., et al. (2012). Emotional availability, attachment, and intervention in center-based child care for infants and toddlers. *Development and Psychopathology, 24*, 23–34.

Booth, C. L., Clarke-Stewart, K. A., Vandell, D. L., McCartney, K., & Owen, M. T. (2002). Childcare usage and mother–infant "quality time." *Journal of Marriage and the Family, 64*, 16–26.

Bowlby, J. (1982). *Attachment and loss: Vol. 1. Attachment.* New York: Basic Books. (Original work published 1969)

Brazelton, T. B. (1985). *Working and caring.* New York: Basic Books.

Bretherton, I. (1985). Attachment theory: Retrospect and prospect. In I. Bretherton & E. Waters (Eds.), Growing points of attachment theory and research. *Monographs of the Society for Research in Child Development, 50*(1–2, Serial No. 209), 3–35.

Campbell, S. B., Brownell, C. A., Hungerford, A., Spieker, S. I., Mohan, R., & Blessing, J. S. (2004). The course of maternal depressive symptoms and maternal sensitivity as predictors of attachment security at 36 months. *Development and Psychopathology, 16*, 231–252.

Cassidy, J., Woodhouse, S. S., Cooper, G., Hoffman, K., Powell, B., & Rodenberg, M. (2005). Examining the precursors of infant attachment security: Implications for early intervention and intervention research. In L. J. Berlin, Y. Ziv, L. Amaya-Jackson, & M. T. Greenberg (Eds.), *Enhancing early attachments: Theory, research, intervention, and policy* (pp. 34–60). New York: Guilford Press.

Clarke-Stewart, K. A. (1989). Infant day care: Maligned or malignant? *American Psychologist, 44*, 266–273.

Cox, M. J., Owen, M., Henderson, V. K., & Margand, N. A. (1992). Prediction of infant–father and infant–mother attachment. *Developmental Psychology, 28*, 777–783.

Crittenden, P. M. (1983). The effect of mandatory protective daycare on mutual attachment in maltreating mother–infant dyads. *Child Abuse and Neglect, 7*, 297–300.

Dontas, C., Maratos, O., Fafoutis, M., & Karangelis, A. (1985). Early social development in institutionally reared Greek infants: Attachment and peer interaction. In I. Bretherton & E. Waters (Eds.), Growing points of attachment theory and research. *Monographs of the Society for Research in Child Development, 50*(1–2, Serial No. 209), 135–175.

Easterbrooks, M. A., & Goldberg, W. (1987). Toddler development in the family: Impact of father involvement and parenting characteristics. *Child Development, 55*, 770–752.

Egeland, B., & Heister, M. (1995). The long-term consequences of infant day-care and mother–infant attachment. *Child Development, 66*, 474–485.

Fearon, R. M., & Belsky, J. (2011). Infant–mother attachment and the growth of externalizing problems across the primary-school years. *Journal of Child Psychology and Psychiatry, 52*, 782–791.

Fox, N. A., Kimmerly, N. L., & Schafer, W. D. (1991). Attachment to mother/attachment to father: A meta-analysis. *Child Development, 52*, 210–225.

Fraley, R. C., Roisman, G. I., Booth-LaForce, C., Owen, M. T., & Holland, A. S. (2013). Interpersonal and genetic origins of adult attachment styles: A longitudinal study from infancy to early adulthood. *Journal of Personality and Social Psychology, 104*, 817–838.

Goossens, F. A., & Van IJzendoorn, M. H. (1990). Quality of infants' attachment to professional caregivers: Relation to infant–parent attachment and daycare characteristics. *Child Development, 51*, 832–837.

Grossmann, K., Grossmann, K. E., Fremmer-Bombik, E., Kindler, H., Scheuerer-Englisch, H., & Zimmermann, P. (2002). The uniqueness of the child–father attachment relationship: Fathers' sensitive and challenging play as a pivotal variable in a 16-year longitudinal study. *Social Development, 11*, 307–331.

Howes, C. (1999). Attachment relationships in the context of multiple caregivers. In J. Cassidy & P. R. Shaver (Eds.), *Handbook of attachment: Theory, research, and clinical applications* (pp. 671–687). New York: Guilford Press.

Howes, C., & Aikens, J. W. (2002). Peer relations in the transition to adolescence. In H. W. Reese & R. Kail (Eds.), *Advances in child development and behavior*

(Vol. 30, pp. 195–230). San Diego, CA: Academic Press.

Howes, C., Fuligni, A. S., Hong, S. S., Huang, Y., & Lara-Cinisomo, S. (2013). The preschool instructional context and child—teacher relationships. *Early Education and Development, 24*, 273–291.

Howes, C., & Hamilton, C. E. (1992a). Children's relationships with caregivers: Mothers and child care teachers. *Child Development, 63*, 859–866.

Howes, C., & Hamilton, C. E. (1992b). Children's relationships with child care teachers: Stability and concordance with parental attachments. *Child Development, 63*, 867–878.

Howes, C., & Hamilton, C. E. (1993). The changing experience of child care: Changes in teachers and in teacher–child relationships and children's social competence with peers. *Early Childhood Research Quarterly, 8*, 15–32.

Howes, C., Hamilton, C. E., & Phillipsen, L. C. (1998). Stability and continuity of child–caregiver relationships. *Child Development, 69*, 418–426.

Howes, C., Matheson, C. C., & Hamilton, C. E. (1994). Maternal, teacher, and child care history correlates of children's relationships with peers. *Child Development, 55*, 257–273.

Howes, C., & Oldham, E. (2001). Processes in the formation of attachment relationships with alternative caregivers. In A. Göncü & E. L. Klein (Eds.), *Children in play, story, and school* (pp. 267–287). New York: Guilford Press.

Howes, C., & Ritchie, S. (1998). Changes in child–teacher relationships in a therapeutic preschool program. *Early Education and Development, 4*, 411–422.

Howes, C., & Ritchie, S. (1999). Attachment organizations in children with difficult life circumstances. *Development and Psychopathology, 11*, 254–268.

Howes, C., & Ritchie, S. (2002). *A matter of trust: Connecting teachers and learners in the early childhood classroom.* New York: Teachers College Press.

Howes, C., Rodning, C., Galluzzo, D. C., & Myers, L. (1988). Attachment and child care: Relationships with mother and caregiver. *Early Childhood Research Quarterly, 3*, 703–715.

Howes, C., & Segal, J. (1993). Children's relationships with alternative caregivers: The special case of maltreated children removed from their homes. *Journal of Applied Developmental Psychology, 17*, 71–81.

Howes, C., & Smith, E. W. (1995). Children and their child care caregivers: Profiles of relationships. *Social Development, 4*, 44–61.

Howes, C., & Tonyan, H. A. (2000). Links between adult and peer relations across four developmental periods. In K. A. Kerns, J. Contreras, & A. Neal-Barnett (Eds.), *Examining associations between parent–child and peer relationships* (pp. 85–114). New York: Greenwood.

Howes, C., & Wishard Guerra, A. (2009) Networks of attachment relationships in low-income children of Mexican heritage: Infancy through preschool. *Social Development, 18*, 816–915.

Hughes, J. N. (2012) Teacher–student relationships and school adjustment: Progress and remaining challenges. *Attachment and Human Development, 14*, 319–327.

Huston, A. C., & Rosenkrantz Aronson, S. (2005). Mothers' time with infant and time in employment as predictors of mother–child relationships and children's early development. *Child Development, 76*, 467–482.

Jackson, J. F. (1993). Multiple caregiving among African Americans and infant attachment: The need for an emic approach. *Human Development, 35*, 87–102.

Jaeger, E., & Weinraub, M. (1990). Early maternal care and infant attachment: In search of process. In K. McCartney (Ed.), *Child care and maternal employment: A social ecology* (pp. 71–90). San Francisco: Jossey-Bass.

Kobak, R., Rosenthal, N., & Serwik, A. (2005). The attachment hierarchy in middle childhood: Conceptual and methodological issues. In K. A. Kerns & R. A. Richardson (Eds.), *Attachment in middle childhood* (pp. 71–88). New York: Guilford Press.

Lamb, M. E., Hwang, C.-P., Frodi, A. M., & Frodi, M. (1982). Security of mother- and father-infant attachment and its relation to sociability with strangers in traditional and nontraditional Swedish families *Infant Behavior and Development, 5*, 355–367.

Lamb, M. E., Sternberg, K. J., & Prodromidis, M. (1992). Nonmaternal care and the security of infant–mother attachment: A reanalysis of the data. *Infant Behavior and Development, 15*, 71–83

Main, M., Hesse, E., & Kaplan, N. (2005). Predictability of attachment behavior and representational processes at 1, 6, and 19 years of age: The Berkeley longitudinal study. In K. E. Grossmann, K. Grossmann, & E. Waters (Eds.), *Attachment from infancy to adulthood: The major longitudinal studies* (pp. 245–304). New York: Guilford Press.

Main, M., Kaplan, N., & Cassidy, J. (1985). Security in infancy, childhood, and adulthood: A move to the level of representation. In I. Bretherton & E. Waters (Eds.), Growing points of attachment theory and research. *Monographs of the Society for Research in Child Development, 50*(1–2, Serial No. 209), 66–104.

Main, M., & Weston, D. R. (1981). The quality of toddlers' relationships to mother and to father: Related to conflict and the readiness to establish new relationships. *Child Development, 52*, 932–970.

Marcovitch, S., Goldberg, S., Gold, A., Washington, J., Wasson, C., Krekewich, K., et al. (1997). Determinants of behavioural problems in Romanian children adopted in Ontario. *International Journal of Behavioral Development, 20*, 17–31.

McCartney, K., & Galanopoulos, A. (1988). Child care and attachment: A new frontier the second time around. *American Journal of Orthopsychiatry, 58*, 17–24.

National Institute of Child Health and Human Development (NICHD) Early Child Care Research Network (ECCRN). (1997). The effects of infant child care on infant–mother attachment security: Results of the NICHD Study of Early Child Care. *Child Development, 68,* 860–879.

National Institute of Child Health and Human Development (NICHD) Early Child Care Research Network (ECCRN). (1999). Child care and mother–child interaction in the first 3 years of life. *Developmental Psychology, 35,* 1399–1413.

National Institute of Child Health and Human Development (NICHD) Early Child Care Research Network (ECCRN). (2001). Child-care and family predictors of preschool attachment and stability from infancy. *Developmental Psychology, 37,* 847–862.

O'Connor, E. E., Collins, B. A., & Supplee, L. (2012). Behavior problems in late childhood: The roles of early maternal attachment and teacher–child relationship trajectories. *Attachment and Human Development, 14,* 265–288.

Oppenheim, D., Sagi, A., & Lamb, M. E. (1988). Infant–adult attachments on the kibbutz and their relation to socio-emotional development four years later. *Developmental Psychology, 27,* 727–733.

Owen, M., & Cox, M. (1988). Maternal employment and the transition to parenthood: Family functioning and child development. In A. Gottfried & A. Gottfried (Eds.), *Maternal employment and children's development: Longitudinal research* (pp. 85–119). New York: Plenum Press.

Pianta, R. C. (2001). *Student Teacher Relationship Scale.* Lutz, FL: Psychological Assessement Resources.

Raikes, H. A. (1993). Relationship duration in infant care: Time with a high ability teacher and infant–teacher attachment. *Early Childhood Research Quarterly, 8,* 309–325.

Rauh, H., Ziegenhain, U., Muller, B., & Wijnroks, L. (2000). Stability and change in infant–mother attachment in the second year of life: Relations to parenting quality and varying degrees of day-care experience. In P. M. Crittenden & A. H. Claussen (Eds.), *The organization of attachment relationships: Maturation, culture, and context* (pp. 251–276). New York: Cambridge University Press.

Roggman, L. A., Langlois, J. H., Hubbs-Tait, L., & Rieser-Danner, L. A. (1994). Infant day-care, attachment, and the "file drawer problem." *Child Development, 65,* 1429–1443.

Rudasill, K. M., Rimm-Kaufman, S. E., Justice, L. M., & Pence, K. (2006). Temperament and language skills as predictors of teacher–child relationship quality in preschool. *Early Education and Development, 17,* 271–291.

Sabol, T., & Pianta, R. C. (2012). Recent trends in research on teacher–child relationships. *Attachment and Human Development, 14,* 213–231.

Saft, E., & Pianta, R. C. (2001). Teacher perceptions of their relationships with students: Effects of child age, gender, and ethnicity of teachers and children. *School Psychology Quarterly, 16,* 125–141.

Sagi, A., Koren-Karie, N., Gini, M., Ziv, Y., & Joels, T. (2002). Shedding further light on the effects of various types and quality of early child care on infant–mother attachment relationship: The Haifa Study of Early Child Care. *Child Development, 73,* 1166–1186.

Sagi-Schwartz, A., & Aviezer, O. (2005). Correlates of attachment to multiple caregivers in kibbutz children from birth to emerging adulthood: The Haifa longitudinal study. In K. E. Grossmann, K. Grossmann, & E. Waters (Eds.), *Attachment from infancy to adulthood: The major longitudinal studies* (pp. 165–197). New York: Guilford Press.

Scher, A., & Mayseless, O. (2000). Mothers of anxious/ambivalent infants: Maternal characteristics and child-care context. *Child Development, 71,* 1629–1639.

Singer, L. M., Brodzinsky, D. M., Ramsay, D., Steir, M., & Waters, E. (1985). Infant–mother attachment in adoptive families. *Child Development, 55,* 1573–1551.

Spilt, J., & Koomen, H. (2009). Widening the view on teacher–child relationships: Teachers narratives concerning disruptive versus nondisruptive children. *School Psychology Review, 38,* 86–101.

Spilt, J., Koomen, H., Thijs, J., & Van deLeij, A. (2012). Supporting teachers' relationships with disruptive children: The potential of relationship-focused reflection. *Attachment and Human Development, 14,* 305–318.

Sroufe, L. A. (1988). A developmental perspective on day care. *Early Childhood Research Quarterly, 3,* 51–50.

Steele, H., Steele, M., & Fonagy, R. (1996). Associations among attachment classifications of mothers, fathers, and their infants. *Child Development, 67,* 541–555.

Stuhlman, M., & Pianta, R. C. (2002). Teachers' narratives about their relationships with children: Associations with behaviors in the classroom. *School Psychology Review, 31,* 148–163.

Suess, G. J., Grossmann, K. E., & Sroufe, L. A. (1992). Effects of infant attachment to mother and father on quality of adaptation in preschool: From dyadic to individual organization of self. *International Journal of Behavioral Development, 15,* 73–55.

Thijs, J., & Koomen, H. (2009). Toward a further understanding of teachers' reports of early teacher–child relationships: Examining the roles of behavior appraisals and attributions. *Early Childhood Research Quarterly, 24,* 186–197.

Thompson, R., & Raikes, H. A. (2003). Towards the next quarter century: Conceptual and methodological challenges for attachment theory. *Development and Psychopathology, 15,* 691–718.

Tizard, B., & Rees, J. (1975). The effect of early institutional rearing on the behavior problems and affectional relationships of four-year-old children. *Journal of Child Psychology and Psychiatry, 15,* 51–77.

Tran, H., & Weinraub, M. (2006). Child care effects in context: Quality, stability, and multiplicity in non-maternal child care arrangements during the first 15 months of life. *Developmental Psychology, 42,* 566–582.

Van IJzendoorn, M. H. (1995). Adult attachment representations, parental responsiveness and infant attachment: A meta-analysis on the predictive validity of the Adult Attachment Interview. *Psychological Bulletin, 117,* 387–403.

Van IJzendoorn, M. H., & De Wolff, M. S. (1997). In search of the absent father: Meta-analysis of infant–father attachment: A rejoinder to our discussants. *Child Development, 60,* 71–91.

Van IJzendoorn, M. H., & Sagi, A. (1999). Cross-cultural patterns of attachment: Universal and contextual dimensions. In J. Cassidy & P. R. Shaver (Eds.), *Handbook of attachment: Theory, research, and clinical applications* (pp. 713–734). New York: Guilford Press.

Van IJzendoorn, M. H., Sagi, A., & Lambermon, M. W. E. (1992). The multiple caregiver paradox: Data from Holland and Israel. *New Directions for Child Development, 57,* 5–27.

Vandell, D. L., Belsky, J., Burchinal, M., Vandergrift, N.,

& Steinberg, L. (2010). Do effects of early child care extend to age 15 years?: Results from the NICHD study of early child care and youth development. *Child Development, 81,* 737–756.

Verschueren, K., & Koomen, H. (2012). Teacher–child relationships from an attachment perspective. *Attachment and Human Development, 14,* 205–211.

Volling, B., & Belsky, J. (1992). The contribution of child–mother and father–child relationships to the quality of sibling interaction: A longitudinal study. *Child Development, 53,* 1209–1222.

Waters, E. (1987). *Attachment Behavior Q-Set (Revision 3.0).* Stony Brook: State University of New York at Stony Brook, Department of Psychology.

Westman, J. C. (1988). The infant day care controversy. *American Journal of Psychiatry, 145,* 1177–1178.

Yarrow, L. J., Goodwin, M. S., Manheimer, H., & Milowe, I. D. (1973). Infancy experiences and cognitive and personality development at 10 years. In L. J. Stone, H. T. Smith, & L. B. Murphy (Eds.), *The competent infant: Research and commentary* (pp. 1277–1281). New York: Basic Books.

## Chapter 16

# Early Attachment and Later Development
## *Reframing the Questions*

### Ross A. Thompson

How does the child foreshadow the adult-to-be? Philosophers, spiritualists, playwrights, and, most recently, behavioral scientists have sought to understand how early dispositions and influences provide a foundation for adult personality. Among the answers they have offered is the influence of early, close relationships. This view was eventually crystallized in Freud's (1940/1963, p. 45) famous dictum that the infant–mother relationship is "unique, without parallel, established unalterably for a whole lifetime as the first and strongest love-object and as the prototype of all later love-relations." Drawing on this psychoanalytic heritage, Bowlby (1969/1982, 1973, 1980) enlisted formulations from evolutionary biology, developmental psychology, and control systems theory to argue that a warm and continuous relationship with a caregiver promotes psychological health and well-being throughout life in a manner that accords with the adaptive requirements of the human species. In collaboration with Ainsworth (1967, 1973), he proposed that differences in the security of infant–mother attachment have significant long-term implications for later intimate relationships, self-understanding, and even risk for psychopathology. Bowlby's conceptual integration was provocative, and with the validation of reliable methods for assessing the security of attachment in infants and young children, it could be examined empirically.

There have been three stages to the research that followed on early attachment and later development. The first consisted of studies in the late 1970s, confirming that early attachment relationships *could* be stable over time and predict later aspects of psychosocial functioning, such as peer sociability, positive affect, and cooperativeness (e.g., Matas, Arend, & Sroufe, 1978). These studies were important because they provided initial support for the claims of attachment theory and distinguished this approach from earlier approaches, guided by social learning theory, in which researchers had found little consistency in attachment measures and little prediction of later behavior (see Masters & Wellman, 1974).

The second stage consisted of several decades of subsequent research exploring the breadth of later behavior that was associated with attachment security. Consistent with Bowlby's formulations, developmental researchers explored the association between early security and later relations with parents, peers, friends, and other social partners, as well as with self-concept, competence in preschool and kindergarten, personality development, social cognition, behavior problems, and indicators of emergent psychopathology. Moreover, guided by a general expectation that a secure attachment would predict better later functioning, researchers broadened their inquiry to explore how security predicted later cognitive and language development, exploration and play, curiosity, ego resiliency, math achievement, and even political ideology, extending the range of predictive correlates far beyond what Bowlby originally envisioned. This breadth of documented sequelae was possible, in part, because of the availability of large longitudinal data sets, such as the National Institute of Child Health and Human Development Study of Early Child Care and Youth Development (NICHD SECCYD), even though they had not really been designed to test the later outcomes of attachment security (Thompson, 2008a). Attachment theory was thus stretched to explain a variety of empirical associations between attachment and later behavior, some of which were theoretically unpredicted and may have resulted from unmeasured mediators as well as direct causal influences. To illustrate, a number of studies have documented an association between security of attachment and later measures of cognitive performance and IQ, but more carefully designed mediational studies show that this is because of differences in parental quality of assistance, peer relationships, and children's cooperativeness at school—mediators that are fully consistent with attachment theory (Drake, Belsky, & Fearon, 2014; West, Mathews, & Kerns, 2013).

This has led to a third stage of research characterized by broader analyses of what is reliably known about the consequences of attachment (through meta-analysis and other approaches) and the use of more incisive methodologies to examine direct and indirect outcomes of early security. These methodologies have included growth curve modeling, mediational analyses, and the use of biologically informed designs. In a sense, this third stage involves a thoughtful reconsideration of how and why early attachment security should be associated with later development, and exploration of alternative models for why security might predict later behavior in direct and indirect ways. These studies also draw on samples in which the security of attachment was not stable over time. The discussion of empirical studies that follows includes examples of these approaches to reframing the question of attachment and later behavior in more sophisticated ways.

This chapter begins, therefore, with consideration of alternative explanations for why a secure attachment should be associated with later behavior, with a focus on attachment security in the early years. Following this is a review of the research examining these associations in the developmental domains that have been best studied:

parent–child relationships, close relationships with peers and other partners, personality, emotion regulation, emotion understanding, social cognition, conscience, and self-concept. In a final section, these results are discussed in light of what we can conclude about how attachment security influences later development, which research approaches are most likely to elucidate this association in future studies, and future directions.

## Conceptual Perspectives

To an observer, it might appear surprising that it is necessary to begin this discussion by sorting through the various conceptual explanations for why early attachment security should be associated with later development. After all, wasn't Bowlby clear on this issue?

The challenge facing contemporary attachment researchers is not only Bowlby's theory, but also its generativity. Attachment theory was formulated decades ago, at a time when scientific understanding of infancy and early childhood underestimated the cognitive and behavioral sophistication of the young child and the dynamics of early parent–child relationships. There have also been significant advances in behavioral genetics, evolutionary biology, and developmental neuroscience since Bowlby's time, as well as advances in research methodology. It is natural that Bowlby's heirs would update, elucidate, and expand his formulations in ways that he could not anticipate in their efforts to keep the theory current with advancing knowledge. Furthermore, as would be expected of a conceptually innovative approach, Bowlby's theory provides a conceptual umbrella for broad and narrow constructions of the developmental impact of attachment relationships. Grossmann (1999), for example, has identified at least two different conceptualizations of "internal working models" in Bowlby's theory (and two others are profiled below). The breadth of Bowlby's theory offers room for diverse explanations for the impact of early attachment based on the biologically adaptive qualities of attachment relationships, the quality of parent–child interaction, the dynamics of personality growth, emergent social representations, developing stress neurobiology, and other influences. Beyond theoretical breadth, of course, is the fact that subsequent attachment researchers have had their own ideas about the influence of early attachment security, which they have sought to harmonize with Bowlby's formulations.

These are all signs of a vibrant, generative theory. Indeed, it can be argued that today the proper role of Bowlby's theory is not as a source of orthodoxy for attachment theorists (much as Freud's theory was treated in the early decades of psychoanalysis), but rather as a foundation for new thinking about early parent–child relationships. The problem this presents for contemporary researchers, however, is the proliferation of conceptual explanations for why early attachment might be associated with later development. Beyond the casual post hoc explanations offered by researchers for unexpected empirical findings, in other words, there have grown from the foundation of Bowlby's theory various attachment minitheories, with somewhat different views of the nature of the developmental influences arising from secure or insecure early relationships.

In this section, therefore, the goal is to summarize and evaluate several alternative views of the developmental influence of attachment that have become significant in contemporary attachment research. Each approach is discussed with respect to certain key conceptual questions. For which developmental domains is early security likely to be most important, and at what ages? How much should the effects of early attachment be expected to endure, and what mediators might affect its continuing influence? What are the conditions in which attachment should most influence later development? Although most approaches do not provide clear answers to all of these conceptual questions, the purpose in posing them is to clarify our thinking about why early attachment should be developmentally provocative.

### Internal Working Models

One of Bowlby's most heuristically powerful formulations is the view that attachment security influences psychological growth through children's developing mental representations, or *internal working models* (IWMs), of the social world. IWMs are based on infants' expectations for the accessibility and responsiveness of their caregivers. These expectations develop into broader representations of their attachment figures, interpretations of their relational experiences, guidelines about how to interact with others, and even beliefs about themselves as relational partners. These mental representations initially enable immediate forecasts of the caregiver's responsiveness, and they expand into broader interpretive filters through which children and adults reconstruct their experience

of new relationships in ways that are consistent with past experiences and the expectations arising from secure or insecure attachments. As a consequence, children choose new partners and behave with them in ways that are consistent with, and thus help to confirm, the expectations created from earlier attachments. IWMs therefore constitute the bridge between an infant's experience of sensitive or insensitive care and the development of beliefs and expectations that affect subsequent experience in close relationships. This concept has been theoretically generative: Bretherton and Munholland (Chapter 4, this volume), Crittenden (1990), Main (1991), Sroufe and Fleeson (1988), Thompson (2006), and Dykas and Cassidy (2011) have each offered contemporary extensions of Bowlby's concept of IWMs.

In Bowlby's formulation, therefore, IWMs would be expected to be most directly associated with the child's capacities to create and maintain successful close relationships (with parents, peers, teachers, and others), establish a positive self-image, and develop constructive social representations of people and of relationships. However, because Bowlby used the IWM concept as a kind of conceptual metaphor rather than creating a rigorously defined theoretical construct, its abstraction has enabled this concept to assume wide-ranging explanatory breadth in attachment research. IWMs have been enlisted to "explain" the association between attachment security and a wide range of correlates, causing some to question whether IWMs constitute a "catch-all, post-hoc explanation" for almost anything to which a secure attachment is found to be associated (Belsky & Cassidy, 1994, p. 384). At the least, this use of the IWM concept has led to considerable uncertainty about its defining features, functioning, and measurement.

One solution to this problem of underspecificity is to clarify what IWMs are and how they develop. Unfortunately, theoretical views diverge among attachment researchers. While some researchers view IWMs as primarily unconscious, prelinguistic perceptual–affective processes akin to the Freudian dynamic unconscious, others regard IWMs as consciously accessible cognitive representations (Grossmann, 1999). Attachment researchers also differ in how IWMs function (Thompson, 2008b). To Dykas and Cassidy (2011), for example, IWMs govern information processing, and individuals with secure attachment histories are more likely to process, in an open manner, a broad range of positive and negative information related to attachment concerns in a positively biased manner. By contrast, insecure individuals are more likely to defensively exclude information that is likely to lead to psychological pain, such as the child who "forgets" being abandoned in childhood, but if information does not risk psychological pain, they will process this information in a negatively biased fashion. Thompson (2006, 2010) focuses instead on the content of IWMs, arguing that secure individuals are likely to have more constructive representations of other people, more positive expectations for social interaction, greater social and emotional understanding, more positive self-concept, and more advanced conscience development compared to insecurely attached individuals. In this view, IWMs develop in concert with other allied advances in event representation, social expectations, autobiographical memory, self-awareness, and a variety of other social-cognitive skills. In this view, moreover, IWMs are shaped by not only the child's direct relational experience but also secondary representations through conversational discourse with adult caregivers, reflecting the significance of language for providing young children with insight into others' motivations, thoughts, and feelings, relationships, and the self. Rich, supportive conversational discourse, especially about difficult issues, thus becomes another manner by which parental sensitivity is manifested and contributes to the intergenerational transmission of attachment working models (Thompson, 2010).

These alternative formulations are not necessarily mutually exclusive, although they have different implications for how IWMs influence social behavior, their accessibility, and the factors influencing consistency and change in IWMs over time. However, these alternative views share in common the expectation that IWMs change developmentally with the child's conceptual advances and that social experience is formative to the development and potential revision of early IWMs. The field needs greater theoretical development of the IWM construct, building on Bowlby's theory and subsequent advances in developmental science, to guide thinking about their development, behavioral influences, and measurement.

### Emergent Personality Organization

Another conceptualization of the influence of early attachment on later development is that attachment security shapes emergent personality processes in infancy and early childhood which,

as they mature and become consolidated, exert a continuing influence on subsequent personality growth. Early attachment is important because it inaugurates adaptive or maladaptive organizational processes in personality that render young children more or less competent in facing subsequent challenges in personality growth.

This view is best articulated in the "organizational perspective" that has been advanced by Sroufe (2005; Sroufe, Egeland, Carlson, & Collins, 2005) and others (e.g., Cicchetti, 2006). This neo-Eriksonian perspective portrays personality growth as a succession of developmental challenges around which critical aspects of personality development are organized. During the first year, of course, the development of a secure attachment is central. In successive years, relevant developmental issues include the growth of an autonomous self in toddlerhood, the acquisition of effective peer relationships in preschool, successful adaptation to school, coordination of friendship and group membership in middle childhood, and identity and self-reflection in adolescence. The successful mastery of earlier developmental challenges is believed to provide a stronger psychological foundation for subsequent challenges because of the internal resources in personality organization that have developed and the supportive relationships on which the child can rely. In this view, therefore, the sequelae of early attachment security vary depending on the salient developmental challenges facing the child at subsequent ages, but in each case a secure attachment provides a better foundation for successful adaptation.

The organizational view is an influential and powerful model for attachment researchers, especially its description of the developmental challenges characterizing each stage of life. Moreover, the fact that these challenges tend to be broadly conceived permits attachment researchers to examine a wide variety of potential outcomes during each subsequent period of development. However, research from this perspective sometimes overlooks the continuing influence of supportive parental care, which may also contribute to the child's developmental adaptation at each stage and its association with early attachment security, as described next.

### Consistency and Change in Parent–Child Relationships

In infancy and early childhood, parent–child relationships are described as secure or insecure. By adulthood, security is often viewed as an attribute of the person. Attachment theory seeks to explain how characteristics of relationships become incorporated into personality. In the developmental transition from attachment-as-relationship to attachment-as-personal-attribute, however, the continuing importance of the quality of parent–child relationships should not be overlooked. Stated simply, an early secure attachment provides a stronger foundation for subsequent psychosocial achievements if the sensitive, supportive parental care initially contributing to attachment security is maintained over time (Lamb, Thompson, Gardner, & Charnov, 1985). In that ongoing relationship of parental support, young children continue to enjoy the benefits of parental sensitivity in the rich sharing of parent–child conversation, their cooperative activity in learning and exploration, the emotional understanding and coaching that parents can provide, and in other ways. Children respond to parental support in these ways by becoming increasingly receptive to their parents' influences and socialization incentives as they identify with the adults' goals and behavior (Kochanska, 2002; Waters, Kondo-Ikemura, Posada, & Richters, 1991). However, if the earlier sensitive care that initially inspired a secure attachment is not maintained, there is less reason to anticipate that early attachment security would be associated with later positive behavior. In this view, therefore, the significance of early attachment for later development is contingent, to some extent, on the continuing sensitivity of parental care, especially in a child's early years.

In an empirical assessment of this formulation, Belsky and Fearon (2002) used data from the NICHD SECCYD. Analyzing attachment classifications in the Strange Situation at 15 months and subsequent measures of maternal sensitivity at 24 months, they reported that the children who obtained the highest scores on a broad range of social and cognitive measures at 36 months were those who were securely attached and who subsequently experienced sensitive care. Those performing most poorly at 36 months were insecurely attached in infancy and experienced later insensitive care. Of the two intermediate groups, children who were initially insecurely attached but who subsequently experienced sensitive care scored higher on all outcome measures than did children who were initially secure but later experienced insensitive care. These researchers also found that maternal reports of life stress, depression, social support, and family resources at infant age 24 months helped

to explain why some securely attached infants subsequently experienced insensitive maternal care, and why some initially insecure infants later experienced sensitive care. In each case, declines in maternal sensitivity were associated with the number of negative life events and lack of support that mothers experienced when children were age 2, which were likely to affect children as well as their mothers.

These findings are consistent with those reported by other researchers (e.g., Beijersbergen, Juffer, Bakermans-Kranenburg, & Van IJzendoorn, 2012; Sroufe, Egeland, & Kreutzer, 1990), and with the literature concerning the correlates of stability and change in the security of attachment (see Thompson, 2006, for a review). Taken together, they indicate that early security of attachment interacts with the quality of subsequent experience (particularly sensitive parental care and broader life stresses) in predicting developmental outcomes. Indeed, these findings suggest that later quality of care may be at least as important as early security in predicting later development. The continuing sensitivity of parental care may be especially important in the early years, when IWMs are still rudimentary and personality is taking shape. In this respect, the continuing harmony of the parent–child relationship may constitute a bridge between a secure attachment in infancy and the development of later personality and working models of relationships.

### Biological Processes

Biological processes can mediate the association of early attachment with later developmental outcomes. There are three ways this may occur: through species-typical reproductive strategies, the effects of early experience on stress neurobiology, and genetic and epigenetic processes.

First, attachment was viewed by Bowlby (1969/1982) and his followers as an evolved behavioral system to promote the inclusive fitness of the human species. When infants seek the protective proximity of adults, especially when offspring are distressed, alarmed, or in danger, this behavior promotes survival to maturity and eventual reproductive success. This is most likely to occur when adults are sensitively responsive to the infant's cues and secure attachment develops. But patterns of insecure attachment can also be regarded as evolved adaptations to alternative forms of parental care to enable offspring survival, such as avoidance (and potential search for alternative attachment figures) when the adult is consistently unresponsive, and resistance (and demand for support) when the adult is unreliably responsive (Chisholm, 1999). Viewed in this light, early attachment patterns can be regarded as *ontogenetic adaptations* that function to help individuals to reach maturity but have no necessarily enduring significance.

However, early attachments may instead be *deferred adaptations* that facilitate growth to maturity and also provide a foundation for lifelong behavioral patterns related to reproductive success (Bjorklund, 1997). This view is consistent with life history theory (Chisholm, 1999; Stearns, 1992). In an influential application of life history theory to attachment, Belsky, Steinberg, and Draper (1991) argued that the quality of parental care sensitizes young organisms to the supportiveness or aversiveness of the environment into which the children have been born, and this early experience thus affects not only the security of attachment but other behavioral adaptations related to reproductive success, such as the timing of pubertal maturation, the onset of sexual activity, preferences in pair bonding, and eventual parental investment in their own offspring (see also Simpson & Belsky, Chapter 5, this volume). In essence, children whose early family experiences are characterized by high stress (and consequent insecurity) are likely to develop reproductive strategies that are low-investment and opportunistic, whereas children in low-stress, secure families develop in the opposite manner. This formulation is important, therefore, for defining a somewhat wider range of later outcomes that are affected by early attachment and the quality of parental care. The range of outcomes depends, however, on whether attachment is viewed as an ontogenetic or a deferred adaptation.

Second, whether or not early attachment is viewed in the context of species-typical reproductive strategies, the stress or support of early experiences can have significant biological and behavioral consequences for young children. Several research literatures underscore how early experiences of chronic stress can alter the neurocircuitry of developing stress reactivity and other neurobiological systems, causing children to develop dysregulated patterns of stress responding that can undermine self-regulation, heighten threat vigilance, and blunt attentional focus and cognitive functioning (see review by Thompson, 2015). These early experiences of chronic stress can include enduring maternal depression and an adult's emotional inaccessibility, as well as abusive events, underscoring the reliance of young children on adult solicitude. Consistent with this view, this research literature also shows that social support buffers the effects of stress, and an important manifestation of social support in early childhood is sensitive parental care. Thus one reason that early security or insecurity may be associated with later behavior is that the stress-buffering consequences of a secure attachment, especially for young children in difficult circumstances, enable better emotion regulation, socioemotional, and cognitive functioning. Although there is some evidence that securely attached infants show diminished biological markers of stress responding in the company of their mothers compared to insecurely attached infants (Nachmias, Gunnar, Mangelsdorf, Parritz, & Buss, 1996; Spangler & Grossmann, 1993), more research is needed to determine the biological stress-buffering effects of secure attachment.

Third, genetic characteristics that contribute to a secure or insecure attachment may help to account for the later consequences of that attachment. Thus, for example, a child with a genetic polymorphism associated with impulsive behavior (i.e., the dopamine D4 receptor [*DRD4*] 7-repeat polymorphism) may be more likely to develop an insecure attachment in early childhood and also have later conduct problems. This has, however, proven to be a challenging formulation to study, even in the context of rapid advances in molecular genetics because large samples (typically much larger than those common to attachment research) are required to yield reliable conclusions concerning the association of specific polymorphisms with behavior (Roisman, Booth-LaForce, Belsky, Burt, & Groh, 2013). In light of the failure to confirm significant associations of hypothesized polymorphisms with attachment in at least one large data set (Roisman et al., 2013), and the finding of behavioral genetics research that the genetic component of variability in early attachment is negligible (Roisman & Fraley, 2008), further study is needed to determine whether early attachment is directly associated with specific polymorphisms and, if so, their association with later outcomes.

It is likely, however, that more complex gene × gene and gene × environment interactions characterize the development of attachment security. Moreover, emerging work in behavioral epigenetics suggests that experiential influences may be important to gene expression as they alter the biochemical regulatory system that activates, silences, or changes the transcriptional activity of genes without altering structural DNA (see Bakermans-Kranenburg & Van IJzendoorn, Chapter 8, this volume). As the elegant rat pups studies of Meaney (2010) and his colleagues illustrate, the quality of maternal care is a major influence of early experience associated with gene expression (see Thompson, 2015, for a review). It is therefore possible to hypothesize that one of the consequences of a secure or insecure attachment is its epigenetic effects on gene expression, particularly genes associated with stress reactivity. It remains to be seen whether this is a promising means of understanding the behavioral correlates of early attachment security.

### Interim Conclusion

It is apparent, therefore, that attachment researchers have a variety of conceptual approaches to guide their inquiry into the developmental outcomes of early security. Moreover, these formulations differ in important and meaningful ways. They emphasize different outcomes, for example: Some approaches highlight the relational consequences of early secure or insecure relationships; others, the representational consequences of attachment security; some highlight the influence of attachment on stages of personality growth, whereas others focus on reproductively adaptive strategies. Although some formulations view the continuing influence of parenting practices in childhood as a mediator of the enduring effects of early security, others make no such claim. In several approaches, the consequences of attachment security are developmentally graded—that is, the effects of attachment depend on when security is assessed and when outcomes are evaluated—but others offer more general predictions. Most of these approaches also expect stronger associations between attachment security and its contemporaneous correlates than those in long-term predictive relations, but they differ in the reasons why.

These conceptual differences are important because they have implications for research design (Thompson, 2000; Thompson & Raikes, 2003). If, for example, researchers expect that later behavior arises from an interaction between early security and the continuing quality of parental care, it is important to measure each of these factors in follow-up studies. Likewise, other potential moderators of this association should also be assessed, such as family stress or the child's biological individuality. Furthermore, the association of attachment with the *rate of change* in psychosocial outcomes is a potentially important but underexplored implication of several of the formulations discussed earlier. In the research review that follows, promising examples of research designs such as these are highlighted. Unfortunately, most of the research uses a straightforward pre–post design in which early attachment is associated with outcomes measured later (and sometimes attachment and outcomes are measured contemporaneously) in which potential mediators are unmeasured and causal associations are sometimes obscured. With the current effort to better understand the processes underlying direct and indirect consequences of attachment security, informed by ideas from developmental neurobiology, life history theory, personality theory, and new ideas about the development of representation and relationships from developmental science, we can hope that there will be further advances in the use of research designs that are equal to the conceptual richness of this field.

## Empirical Perspectives

Consistent with these conceptual perspectives, this review of research is organized according to the various outcome domains to which attachment security has been theoretically and empirically associated most strongly. The review begins with the relational outcomes anticipated from a secure attachment (warmer subsequent parent–child relationships, closer relationships with peers and other partners); then moves on to personality outcomes and emotion regulation. It then examines work on the representational correlates and outcomes of a secure attachment—emotion understanding, social cognition, conscience, and finally self-concept. The biological processes associated with attachment security have been studied most recently and this chapter touches on the more limited findings that this work has yielded. The prediction of early attachment relative to risk for psychopathology is also an important outcome domain, but it is not considered in this chapter because it is discussed extensively elsewhere in this handbook (see DeKlyen & Greenberg, Chapter 28, and Lyons-Ruth & Jacobvitz, Chapter 29). In light of the enormous empirical literature in this area, this review should be viewed as a selective, not an exhaustive, overview of the major findings and important new directions for research.

### Parent–Child Relationship

The strongest and most direct outcome of a secure attachment should be more positive parent–child interaction in follow-up assessments. This expectation has been partially confirmed in a series of short-term longitudinal studies in which securely attached children showed greater enthusiasm, compliance, and positive affect—and less frustration and aggression—during shared tasks with their mothers during the second year (e.g., Frankel & Bates, 1990; Matas et al., 1978), although longer-term associations between infant security and parent–child interaction at ages 3 (Youngblade & Belsky, 1992) and 5 (Van IJzendoorn, van der Verr, & van Vliet-Visser, 1987) were inconsistent. These and other studies suggest that securely attached infants tend to maintain more harmonious relations with their mothers, but (as discussed earlier) this likely depends on consistency over time in the quality of mother–child interaction. Consistency in the quality of parent–child interaction over time is often mediated by intervening events, such as family stress, significant changes in family circumstances (such as parental separation or divorce), or other conditions affecting relational harmony (Thompson, 2006). Viewed more broadly, early security seems to inaugurate what Kochanska (2002) describes as a "mutually responsive orientation" between parent and child that, if maintained, contributes to shared cooperation, the socialization of behavior and values, and the child's enthusiastic responsiveness to the parent's incentives.

If this is so, it suggests that the security of attachment is not only a direct predictor of developmental outcomes but also a moderator of other aspects of parent–child relationships that contribute to those outcomes. Parenting stress may, for example, more strongly predict later problem behavior for children who are in insecure relationships with their parents than for secure children (Tharner et al., 2012). Another example comes from a longitudinal study in which parents' observed power assertion with their 2- to 3-year-olds predicted a composite of measures of children's "resentful opposition to parents" at age 4½, which in turn predicted children's antisocial conduct at age 5½. These associations were observed only for children who had been insecurely attached in infancy, however, and they were absent for securely attached children (Kochanska, Barry, Stellern, & O'Bleness, 2009). Similar findings were reported by Kochanska and Kim (2012). In each study,

the direct associations between attachment and later outcomes were weak or nonexistent. Taken together, these findings suggest that early attachment can either contribute to or buffer the development of broader characteristics of the parent–child relationship—cooperativeness, negative reactivity, responsiveness—to which other child and parent characteristics also contribute.

Consistent with attachment theory, moreover, children's secure or insecure representations of their family relationships also mediate the effects of family processes on developmental outcomes. The research program of Cummings, Davies, and their colleagues illustrate these processes. In one longitudinal study, for example, first graders' insecure representations of their parents' marital relationship explained the association between interparental conflict observed 1 year earlier and children's emotional and classroom difficulties in second grade (Sturge-Apple, Davies, Winter, Cummings, & Schermerhorn, 2008). Heightened interparental conflict was associated with greater insecurity a year later, and with school difficulties a year after that. In a similar manner, the effects of parental depressive symptomatology on second graders' externalizing problems were mediated by children's insecure representations of family relationships assessed 1 year earlier (Cummings, Schermerhorn, Keller, & Davies, 2008). It is not easy to assess young children's representations of relationships, but further attention to these representations as mediating and moderating influences on developmental outcomes is clearly warranted, especially with evidence that these representations may emerge very early (at least when studied using visual expectancy paradigms in infancy; see Johnson, Dweck, & Chen, 2007). In therapeutic contexts, for example, it may not be enough to change the behavior of a parent who has been an inadequate or abusive caregiver without also altering the child's mental expectations for the behavior of that adult (see, e.g., Toth, Maughan, Manley, Spagnola, & Cicchetti, 2002).

### Other Close Relationships

Another relational context in which the benefits of early security might be observed is peer relationships. In a meta-analysis, Groh and colleagues (2014) found a robust association between child–mother attachment and peer social competence: Avoidant, resistant, and disorganized children each showed comparably lower levels of peer competence relative to secure children. The association of attachment and social competence with peers did not vary by children's age or the amount of time between attachment and peer assessments. Interestingly, and contrary to earlier meta-analytic findings, the association was *weaker* when social competence with friends was compared to competence with nonfriends (see Pallini, Baiocco, Schneider, Madigan, & Atkinson, 2014, for similar meta-analytic results). It appears, however, that attachment security is important both to the development of peer social competence and of friendships, although different developmental processes may be involved with each.

Building on these findings, attachment researchers have delved into why these associations exist. Raikes, Virmani, Thompson, and Hatton (2013), enlisting the NICHD SECCYD longitudinal sample, used growth curve modeling to show that children decreased in peer conflict from preschool to first grade, but securely attached children (assessed at 24 months) showed a steeper decline over this period and were lower in peer conflict in first grade. Also, children with greater social problem-solving skills and lower hostile attributions showed lower levels and greater declines in peer conflict. Raikes and Thompson (2008a), using the same NICHD SECCYD sample, showed further that children with early secure attachment showed enhanced social problem-solving skills and diminished hostile attribution bias at 54 months and in first grade. Securely attached children were also less lonely than insecure children, reflecting the self-referential elements of peer social competence (see also Berlin, Cassidy, & Belsky, 1995). These social representations may be shaped by aspects of mother–child interaction associated with a secure attachment. McElwain, Booth-LaForce, and Wu (2011) reported that talk about mental states during play with their 24-month-olds was more characteristic of the mothers of secure than insecure children, and that attachment indirectly influenced the quality of children's friendships at 54 months and first grade through maternal mental-state discourse. In another study with the NICHD SECCYD sample, mother–child affective mutuality at 54 months was one avenue by which early attachment security predicted friendship quality in third grade (McElwain, Booth-LaForce, Lansford, Wu, & Dyer, 2008). The emotional catalysts of mother–child interaction and discourse, children's constructive social representations, their social self-confidence, and greater social skills are among several developmental processes by which

early attachment security can influence later peer relationships. Others meriting further exploration include parents' coaching social skills and the opportunities provided by parents to socialize with other children (see Berlin, Cassidy, & Appleyard, 2008).

As young children's social worlds expand, they develop relationships with a broader range of adults and children, with some adults (e.g., care providers and early childhood teachers) assuming a caregiving role. Relationships with these adults are affected, as we would expect, both by the child's relational history (e.g., mother–child attachment security) and by the specific characteristics of that adult, such as his or her sensitivity and responsiveness (see reviews of this research by Ahnert, Pinquart, & Lamb, 2006; Berlin et al., 2008; Howes & Spieker, Chapter 15, and Williford, Carter, & Pianta, Chapter 41, this volume). Throughout these experiences, children with secure attachments are more competent at creating and maintaining more extensive and supportive social networks, and experiencing greater social support as a result (see, e.g., Anan & Barnett, 1999; Booth, Rubin, & Rose-Krasnor, 1998; Bost, Vaughn, Washington, Cielinski, & Bradbard, 1998). These social and emotional resources are likely to offer secure children many benefits in their interactions with others, further underscoring the indirect, as well as direct, avenues by which secure attachment contributes to psychological well-being.

## Personality

The largest and most comprehensive study of early attachment and its developmental consequences is the Minnesota Study of Risk and Adaptation from Birth to Adulthood (Sroufe, 2005; Sroufe et al., 2005). This prospective longitudinal study of children and families in poverty focused on the association between attachment and personality, thus enlisting the "organizational perspective" described earlier. In this study, children were recruited in infancy with their families and followed through age 34 years. Strange Situation observations were conducted at 12 and 18 months; in the years that followed, personality characteristics were assessed regularly through behavioral observations, interviews, observer ratings, self-reports, and semiprojective instruments.

The reports based on this study revealed significant associations between early attachment security and personality characteristics throughout childhood and adolescence, including relations with measures of emotional health, self-esteem, agency and self-confidence, positive affect, ego resiliency, and social competence in interactions with peers, teachers, camp counselors, romantic partners, and others (see Sroufe et al. [2005] for a detailed discussion, including a list of citations to specific research reports). The researchers concluded that the association between attachment security in infancy and emergent personality owed primarily to the continuing quality of care—or, in the authors' words, "continuity at this age is still primarily at the level of the relationship" (Sroufe et al., 2005, p. 110).

As children matured, moreover, the continuing importance of early attachment was in the context of subsequent developmental influences. Sroufe and his colleagues found that the prediction of later personality was enhanced when early attachment measures were supplemented by other indicators of the quality of subsequent care, which could transform as well as sustain the effects of early security (see Carlson, Sroufe, & Egeland, 2004). Moreover, as time progressed between Strange Situation assessments and later personality outcomes, the effects of early security were more likely to be indirect—mediated and/or moderated by subsequent relational influences (Sroufe, Coffino, & Carlson, 2010). In recognizing that personality outcomes are multidetermined and that attachment security is only one of many constituent influences, in other words, these researchers emphasized that both developmental history and current experience are important in shaping personality growth.

The Minnesota study has been an important and provocative contribution to the research on the consequences of early attachment, and it is one of the most important studies to document long-term associations between attachment security and later personality outcomes. Few other studies have sought to replicate the findings reported from this study, however, but in view of some nonreplications (e.g., Bates, Maslin, & Frankel, 1985; Easterbrooks & Goldberg, 1990), continued efforts to confirm and extend these important findings are warranted. Equally important are future studies that are designed, as was the Minnesota study, to view the significance of early attachment security in the context of subsequent developmental influences on multidetermined personality outcomes (see Sroufe, Chapter 43, this volume).

## Emotion Regulation

One of the functions of attachment relationships is to assist in regulating children's emotions, especially emotions that are potentially disturbing or overwhelming (Cassidy, 1994; Thompson, 1994). This is most evident when parents respond sensitively to the distress of their infants, but it is also an ongoing feature of secure relationships, even as children mature and become more capable of emotion self-regulation. Moreover, through the parents' acceptance of children's emotions and willingness to communicate openly about them, parents in secure relationships foster children's developing emotional awareness and scaffold the growth of competent, flexible skills in emotion self-regulation. Thus children in secure relationships are stronger in emotion regulation than are children in insecure relationships, in which parents may be more dismissive, punitive, or critical of the children's emotional expressions (Thompson, 2015).

The relevance of a secure attachment to emotion regulation is apparent from infancy through adolescence, and is observed behaviorally and neurobiologically. In a study of the responses of 18-month-olds to moderate stressors, for example, Nachmias and colleagues (1996) reported that postsession cortisol elevations were found only for temperamentally inhibited toddlers who were in insecure relationships with their mothers. For inhibited toddlers in secure relationships, their mothers' presence helped to buffer the physiological effects of challenging events. Gilliom, Shaw, Beck, Schonberg, and Lukon (2002) reported that boys who were securely attached at age 1½ were observed to use more constructive anger management strategies at age 3½. Securely attached boys were more likely to use distraction, ask questions about the frustration task, and wait quietly than were insecurely attached boys. Contreras, Kerns, Weimer, Gentzler, and Tomich (2000) found that security in middle childhood was significantly associated with children's constructive coping with stress, and that the measure of coping mediated the association between attachment and children's peer competence.

A variety of influences can help to account for the association between secure attachment and more competent emotion regulation skills (Thompson, Virmani, Waters, Meyer, & Raikes, 2013). Securely attached infants can better enact behavioral strategies (e.g., proximity seeking) that are likely to result in greater emotion management by the mother (Leerkes & Wong, 2012). Mothers in secure relationships are likely to perceive and interpret more sensitively their children's emotions as they arise (Waters et al., 2010), and they are more likely to talk with children about their emotion-related experiences in a richly elaborative manner (Laible & Thompson, 2000; Ontai & Thompson, 2002). Perhaps as a consequence, securely attached children have greater depth in their emotion understanding, including their appreciation of effective emotion regulation strategies (Waters & Thompson, 2014). These intervening influences contribute to an awareness of the multiple avenues by which secure and supportive caregiving relationships foster the growth of emotion regulation skills.

### Emotion Understanding

Several attachment researchers have proposed and tested the hypothesis that owing to the greater psychological intimacy they share with the attachment figure, securely attached children should have deeper emotion understanding than insecure children. Several studies have confirmed this to be true in contemporaneous associations with preschoolers using the Attachment Q-Sort (AQS; Laible & Thompson, 1998; Ontai & Thompson, 2002), and in predictive associations with infant Strange Situation classifications (Steele, Steele, Croft, & Fonagy, 1999) or early childhood AQS ratings (Raikes & Thompson, 2006). Secure children are indeed more proficient at identifying emotions in others and, in some cases, empathizing with them (Murphy & Laible, 2013). These studies also indicate that securely attached children are especially skilled at understanding negative emotions and mixed feelings, which are conceptually more complex than positive emotions.

Several studies have sought to understand the relational catalysts of this enhanced emotion understanding. They have drawn on Bowlby's (1973) portrayal of the emotionally more open communication between securely attached children and their caregivers that enables more candid sharing and discussion—particularly of negative emotions, which may be more troubling, disturbing, or confusing to young children (see Bretherton & Munholland, Chapter 4, this volume). Ontai and Thompson (2002) and Laible (2004) found that more secure preschoolers had mothers who, in discussions with them of recent past events and in storybook reading, used a more descriptively rich,

elaborative style of conversation about emotion. These findings are consistent with others indicating that the mothers of secure children use a more elaborative conversation style with offspring, which has also been found to enhance young children's memory representations and autobiographical recall, as well as emotion understanding (Reese, 2002). Mothers in secure relationships have been found to provide greater validation and support of their child's viewpoint and to engage in greater coaching of emotion regulation (Raikes & Thompson, 2008b; Thompson et al., 2013). Indeed, Raikes and Thompson (2006) found that the quality of mother–child conversations about emotion mediated the association between attachment security and emotion understanding in 3-year-olds. In reciprocal fashion, preschool children in secure relationships spontaneously talk about emotions more often in their everyday conversations with their mothers (Raikes & Thompson, 2008b).

When talking about shared events in a rich, interactive, elaborative manner, the mothers of securely attached children are likely to provide them with enhanced understanding of the psychological dimensions of human interaction and of the influence of emotions and other mental phenomena in everyday events (Thompson, Laible, & Ontai, 2003). This is important for at least two reasons. First, as described below, it provides an avenue by which emotion understanding becomes enlisted into other developmental achievements, including social-cognitive understanding and conscience development, in which securely attached children are also more proficient. Second, it promotes in young children the capacity for mentalization that may be at the heart of secure relationships and their intergenerational transmission (see Fonagy Luyten, Allison, & Campbell, Chapter 34, this volume).

### Social Cognition

Enhanced understanding of emotions may contribute to the greater social competence of secure children. In a study by Denham, Blair, Schmidt, and DeMulder (2002), multiple measures of attachment security were obtained when children were age 3, along with several measures of emotional competence (including assessments of emotion understanding, emotion regulation, and anger expression). Children were subsequently studied in their kindergarten classrooms to assess peer social competence. The researchers confirmed a direct pathway from early attachment security to kindergarten social competence and also an indirect pathway through children's emotional competence. The greater emotion understanding of securely attached children benefits their social interactions with peers.

Secure attachment is also associated with other social-cognitive contributors to peer competence. In three studies, Cassidy, Kirsh, Scolton, and Parke (1996) examined the association between attachment and children's attributions concerning peer motivation. Infant attachment classifications were not strongly predictive of preschoolers' responses to story questions concerning the motivations of peer story characters when their negative behavior had ambiguous intent. But when attachment and attributional probes were assessed contemporaneously, securely attached kindergartners and first graders responded as predicted: Secure children were more likely to attribute benign motives to, and insecure children to infer hostile intent in, the story characters. Moreover, these attributions concerning peer motivation were found to mediate the association between attachment security and peer friendship nominations in a sociometric procedure. Ziv, Oppenheim, and Sagi-Schwartz (2004) examined differences in social information processing in Israeli middle schoolers on the basis of infant attachment classifications. Based on children's responses to interview questions after watching a filmed series of peer interaction vignettes, the researchers found that there were no differences on questions concerning the encoding or interpretation of social behavior or generation of alternative responses, but securely attached youth were more likely to believe that peers would respond positively and constructively to competent social initiatives.

Analyzing data from the NICHD SECCYD, Raikes and Thompson (2008a) examined the association between early attachment security (at 15 months in the Strange Situation, 24 months based on the AQS, and 36 months in the modified Strange Situation for preschoolers) and several measures of social cognition when children were 54 months and in first grade. They found that children deemed resistantly attached at 36 months were more likely to make negative motivational attributions to peers as first graders than were secure children (replicating Cassidy et al., 1996). Securely attached children at 24 and 36 months were more likely to identify socially competent and relevant solutions to social problem-solving tasks than were insecure children. This study is noteworthy for several reasons. First, in each of

these predictive outcomes from attachment security, researchers controlled for the influence of parenting (including maternal sensitivity and depressive symptomatology) at multiple assessments to ensure that these were outcomes of early security rather than of continuity in parenting practices. Second, the prediction of these social-cognitive variables was especially strong when children were securely attached at more than one assessment. Finally, infant Strange Situation classifications never predicted later social cognition, perhaps because of the more rudimentary IWMs underlying infant attachments compared to attachments at 24 and 36 months of age (Thompson, 2000).

Taken together, these findings suggest that the enhanced peer social competence of securely attached children derives from a variety of social-cognitive skills related to emotion understanding, attributional tendencies, social problem-solving skills, and social expectations, consistent with Bowlby's IWM construct. But what about social cognition in relation to partners other than peers? There has been much less research on this topic, and existing studies are less clear. With respect to theory of mind, for example, studies of false-belief understanding have yielded a mixed pattern of results, and even when methods were adapted to characteristics of the mother–child relationship, securely attached children have shown no consistent advantage (e.g., Meins, Fernyhough, Russell, & Clark-Carter, 1998; Meins et al., 2002; Ontai & Thompson, 2008). But other social-cognitive capacities may be more relevant to attachment security. In an intriguing study, Corriveau and colleagues (2009) asked whether the security of attachment in infancy would predict children's judgments of the credibility of information provided by the mother compared to an adult stranger more than 3 years later. Three tasks involving ambiguous stimuli were used in which the mother and the stranger offered different interpretations of the stimuli. In two tasks, either adult could plausibly be correct, but in the third task, the stranger was more clearly correct than mother. Securely attached children accepted the mother's judgment when she was plausibly correct but used the stranger's information when it was apparent that the stranger was correct. By contrast, insecure-resistant children relied on the mother's information in all tasks, and insecure-avoidant children did not use the mother's judgments even when she might be accurate. Studies like this underscore the value of further studying both person-specific and generalized social understanding derived from mother–child relationships and the influence of attachment security on this understanding.

## Conscience

Conscience concerns the young child's development and application of generalizable standards of conduct, and is thus viewed as an early foundation of moral development. Kochanska (2002) has argued that one of the motivators of conscience development is the young child's commitment to maintaining a relationship of warm, mutual responsiveness with the caregiver. In this respect, a secure attachment might be expected to be associated with greater compliance and cooperation, and this association has been confirmed (Kochanska, Aksan, & Carlson, 2005; Laible & Thompson, 2000). Kochanska (1995) has also shown that a secure attachment is especially influential for children who are temperamentally relatively fearless; for these children, the emotional incentives of the mother–child relationship (rather than the anxiety provoked by discipline practices) motivate conscience development.

As in research on emotion understanding, researchers have also sought to understand in more depth the role of attachment, in relation to other developmental influences, in the growth of conscience. Kochanska, Aksan, Knaack, and Rhines (2004) reported that for securely attached children (assessed in the Strange Situation at 14 months), the parents' responsiveness and use of gentle discipline (from 14 to 45 months) predicted later conscience (assessed at 56 months in assessments of morally relevant behavior and thinking), but that for insecure children, there was no such association. These findings complement other studies, reviewed earlier, documenting a negative developmental trajectory from parental power assertion to child noncompliance that was observed only for insecurely attached children, and suggest that parental practices have differential emotional impact depending on the security of child–parent attachment. Indeed, there is further longitudinal evidence that a secure attachment helps to amplify the benefits of early, positive parent–child influences for later conscience development (Kochanska et al., 2010). Other research shows that mothers of secure preschoolers are more likely to use justifications and compromise and less likely to aggravate conflict during disputes with their children (Laible, Panfile, & Makariev, 2008).

These findings offer a new perspective on early moral development. Contrary to the tradi-

tional view that young children comply with their parents to avoid negative sanctions, these studies suggest that the positive incentives of mutually cooperative, secure parent–child relationships are motivationally very important in conscience development. Moreover, several studies suggest that when mothers focus attention on people's feelings and needs, rather than rules and the consequences of breaking them, conscience development is enhanced because it enlists young children's capacities for emotion understanding (Laible & Thompson, 2000, 2002; also see Thompson & Winer, 2014). Taken together, these findings suggest that a new approach to early moral development is needed to better recognize the humanistic, relational foundations of early conscience (Thompson, 2012).

## Self-Concept

Bowlby's (1969/1982, 1973, 1980) argument that attachment security influences young children's self-concept, particularly their conceptions of themselves as loved and lovable, has guided several research inquiries into attachment and self-concept. Cassidy (1988) found that securely attached 6-year-olds described themselves in generally positive terms in a puppet interview but were capable of admitting that they were imperfect (i.e., they were flexible or "open"). Insecurely attached children either revealed a more negative self-image or resisted admitting flaws, and similar results were reported by Verschueren, Marcoen, and Schoefs (1996). Clark and Symons (2000) also found that attachment at age 5 (on the AQS) was significantly associated with the positivity and openness of children's responses to a contemporaneous puppet interview, but not with self-esteem, although a previous assessment of attachment at age 2 (also using the AQS) was not associated with either measure. Goodvin, Meyer, Thompson, and Hayes (2008) found that AQS attachment at age 4 predicted the positivity of young children's self-concept at age 5, even when they controlled for contemporaneous attachment security. Secure children also viewed themselves as more agreeable and as expressing less negative affect. Doyle, Markiewicz, Brendgen, Lieberman, and Voss (2000) found that secure attachment was associated with a more positive self-concept in young adolescents.

Each of these studies measured explicit self-concept in young children. Only two studies have measured implicit self-concept. One was by Colman and Thompson (2002), who presented

5-year-olds with both manageable and difficult puzzle tasks. Children with lower AQS security scores spontaneously expressed more self-doubt about their abilities or negative self-appraisals during *both* tasks, such as saying, "This is too hard for me." The second study was by Cassidy, Ziv, Mehta, and Feeney (2003) who examined the association between security and children's preferences for receiving positive or negative feedback about the self. They found that a more secure attachment was associated with seeking more positive feedback about the self, and that this association was mediated by global self-worth.

Thus, research on implicit self-concept is consistent with the findings of young children's explicit self-descriptions in highlighting the more positive self-representations of securely attached children. More research is needed into *why* attachment has these associations with self-concept. One clue comes from the previously described study by Goodvin and colleagues (2008). In this sample, a composite measure of the mother's emotional stress was negatively associated with her child's positive self-concept. In another longitudinal clinical study, maternal depression when children were 20 months old was associated with young children's concurrent attachment insecurity and their insecurity at 36 months, which in turn predicted negative representations of the self at 48 months (Toth, Rogosch, Sturge-Apple, & Cicchetti, 2009). Each study supports a view of more supportive parent–child relationships (and better parental functioning) contributing to more positive self-representations by young children.

## Conclusion

This review does not exhaust the range of correlates and outcomes of early attachment security that have been studied. But by focusing on these, it is possible to evaluate the outcomes most germane to Bowlby's theory and to derive lessons for the future of attachment research.

### What Have We Learned?

In the broadest sense, the picture that this vast empirical literature yields is both encouraging and daunting. On the one hand, there is a broader, more coherent network of correlates and outcomes of early attachment security than has ever before been revealed. This literature indicates,

usually in replicated findings, that children with a secure attachment history are capable of developing and maintaining more supportive relationships, especially with their parents and with peers, than are insecure children; they develop a variety of desirable personality qualities in childhood and adolescence; they are more likely to exhibit constructive forms of emotionality and emotion self-regulation; and they exhibit more positive self-regard in both explicit and implicit assessments of self-concept. Some of the more interesting recent findings come from studies of the representational correlates and outcomes of attachment security. Securely attached children exhibit greater emotion understanding, demonstrate more competent social problem-solving skills, assume more benign attributions for peers' motivations in ambiguous situations, are more advanced in conscience development, and are less lonely than are insecurely attached children.

Early security clearly makes a significant difference for psychological development, but more progress is needed in the design of research to elucidate *why* this difference occurs. There are clues. Early security is more strongly associated with psychological sequelae when children continue to experience sensitive parental care, and security is maintained over time. The content and quality of mother–child conversation may be part of that sensitive parental care, with the mothers of secure children conversing with their offspring in more elaborative and psychologically supportive and informative ways. Attachment security may also mediate the effects of other parenting practices on early psychological development and contribute to trajectories of positive or negative parent–child interaction and child well-being over time. Early secure or insecure attachment may thus be especially predictive of later psychological outcomes when it is considered in the context of broader aspects of parental care and family life. The social-cognitive advantages of children with a secure attachment history are important mediators of their social competence, especially with peers and other relational partners. In addition, how secure and insecure children perceive themselves and their own characteristics may be another significant contributor to their better psychological functioning. Attachment security may be important not only for how young children think but also how they attend to, process, and remember events related to their relational experiences. Finally, research in this field is increasingly examining three potentially important mediators of the influence of attachment on psychological development: the effects of attachment security as a biological buffer of stress, the influence of supportive parental care on the development of self-regulatory capacities, and the value of a secure attachment for the growth of psychological understanding and mentalizing ability.

## Future Directions

These important clues to how early attachment influences later psychological functioning constitute an agenda for future study. Future advances in understanding the association between early attachment and psychological growth will occur as studies are designed to examine more incisively the intervening processes that connect them, consistent with this third stage of research on early attachment and its sequelae. Carefully designed longitudinal research and analytical designs that enable the detection of direct and mediated associations between attachment and later outcomes are likely to be important contributions to that productive future research literature. In addition, consistent with some of the more exciting research insights of this field, exploration of continuing parental influences (e.g., conversational fluency, discipline practices), contextual demands (e.g., family stress and disruption), biological processes (e.g., stress reactivity, genetic and epigenetic influences), representational processes (e.g., self-referential beliefs, motivational influences), and self-regulatory processes mediating attachment and its outcomes will be especially informative. Moreover, the one study that has used growth curve modeling to examine the association of attachment security with the *rate of change* in psychosocial functioning (Raikes et al., 2013) offers a model for how other researchers can exploit the benefits of longitudinal research to elucidate the impact of attachment on psychological development.

Further understanding of these developmental processes will benefit from continued use of meta-analysis to elucidate the strength of the associations between attachment and developmental outcomes, and the various influences that can mediate these associations. Moreover, research in this field will continue to benefit significantly from the secondary analysis of large-sample longitudinal data sets in which attachment measures have been included. Along with this benefit, however, there are two cautions. The first is that the availability of these data sets further encourages attachment researchers to examine atheoretically the predictive association of attachment with any and all possible outcomes (after all, the data are available

for doing so), then to devise post hoc explanations for the significant associations that emerge, often without consideration of whether direct or mediated explanations are best warranted. This data-driven approach is problematic for the construction and clarity of attachment theory. The second caution is that researchers' strong reliance on the NICHD SECCYD data set compels greater attention to replication and confirmation of findings yielded by a single, albeit uniquely informative, data set.

This chapter has devoted comparable attention to theoretical and empirical perspectives because their integration has been generative for attachment research. Theory development remains, therefore, another important future goal. "All good things go together" is not a sophisticated developmental theory, but the ever-widening network of outcomes to which attachment security has become associated and the failure to attend to discriminant validity of the attachment construct combine to undermine the clarity of what a secure attachment means and contributes to early development. If attachment theory does not have a coherent explanation for this variety of outcomes, and cannot provide a clear account of what outcomes should *and should not* be related to early security, the integrity of the attachment construct is in doubt because theory development cannot be bootstrapped by findings of empirical research alone without potentially holding attachment theory accountable for formulations it should not and perhaps cannot embrace. Future research must be designed to examine, therefore, in a theory-driven manner, both the convergent and the discriminant validity of the attachment construct, and the extent to which the associations between attachment and other behaviors derive from theoretically predicted mediators (see also Sroufe, Chapter 43, this volume).

Attachment research continues to be vigorous and exciting decades after Bowlby's theory (Cassidy, Jones, & Shaver, 2013). These new avenues to explore are one reason why.

## References

Ahnert, L., Pinquart, M., & Lamb, M. E. (2006). Security of children's relationships with nonparental care providers: A meta-analysis. *Child Development, 74,* 664–679.

Ainsworth, M. D. S. (1967). *Infancy in Uganda: Infant care and the growth of love.* Baltimore: Johns Hopkins University Press.

Ainsworth, M. D. S. (1973). The development of infant–mother attachment. In B. Caldwell & H. Ricciuti (Eds.), *Review of child development research* (Vol. 3, pp. 1–94). Chicago: University of Chicago Press.

Anan, R., & Barnett, D. (1999). Perceived social support mediates between prior attachment and subsequent adjustment: A study of urban African American children. *Developmental Psychology, 35,* 1210–1222.

Bates, J. E., Maslin, C. A., & Frankel, K. A. (1985). Attachment security, mother–child interaction, and temperament as predictors of behavior-problem ratings at age three years. In I. Bretherton & E. Waters (Eds.), Growing points of attachment theory and research. *Monographs of the Society for Research in Child Development, 50*(Serial No. 209), 167–193.

Beijersbergen, M. D., Juffer, F., Bakermans-Kranenburg, M. J., & Van IJzendoorn, M. H. (2012). Remaining or becoming secure: Parental sensitive support predicts attachment continuity from infancy to adolescence in a longitudinal adoption study. *Developmental Psychology, 48,* 1277–1282.

Belsky, J., & Cassidy, J. (1994). Attachment: Theory and evidence. In M. Rutter & D. Hay (Eds.), *Development through life* (pp. 373–402). Oxford, UK: Blackwell.

Belsky, J., & Fearon, R. M. (2002). Early attachment security, subsequent maternal sensitivity, and later child development: Does continuity in development depend upon continuity of caregiving? *Attachment and Human Development, 4,* 361–387.

Belsky, J., Steinberg, L., & Draper, P. (1991). Childhood experience, interpersonal development, and reproductive strategy: An evolutionary theory of socialization. *Child Development, 62,* 647–670.

Berlin, L. J., Cassidy, J., & Appleyard, K. (2008). The influence of early attachments on other relationships. In J. Cassidy & P. R. Shaver (Eds.), *Handbook of attachment* (2nd ed., pp. 333–347). New York: Guilford Press.

Berlin, L. J., Cassidy, J., & Belsky, J. (1995). Loneliness in young children and infant–mother attachment: A longitudinal study. *Merrill–Palmer Quarterly, 41,* 91–103.

Bjorklund, D. F. (1997). The role of immaturity in human development. *Psychological Bulletin, 122,* 153–169.

Booth, C., Rubin, K., & Rose-Krasnor, L. (1998). Perceptions of emotional support from mother and friend in middle childhood: Links with social–emotional adaptation and preschool attachment security. *Child Development, 69,* 427–442.

Bost, K., Vaughn, B., Washington, W., Cielinski, K. L., & Bradbard, M. (1998). Social competence, social support, and attachment: Demarcation of construct domains, measurement, and paths of influence for preschool children attending Head Start. *Child Development, 69,* 192–218.

Bowlby, J. (1973). *Attachment and loss: Vol. 2. Separation: Anxiety and anger.* New York: Basic Books.

Bowlby, J. (1980). *Attachment and loss: Vol. 3. Loss: Sadness and depression.* New York: Basic Books.

Bowlby, J. (1982). *Attachment and loss: Vol. 1. Attachment.* New York: Basic Books. (Original work published 1969)

Carlson, E., Sroufe, L., & Egeland, B. (2004). The construction of experience: A longitudinal study of representation and behavior. *Child Development, 75,* 66–83.

Cassidy, J. (1988). Child–mother attachment and the self in six-year-olds. *Child Development, 59,* 121–134.

Cassidy, J. (1994). Emotion regulation: Influences of attachment relationships. In N. A. Fox (Ed.), The development of emotion regulation and dysregulation: Biological and behavioral aspects. *Monographs of the Society for Research in Child Development, 59*(2–3, Serial No. 240), 228–249.

Cassidy, J., Jones, J. D., & Shaver, P. R. (2013). Contributions of attachment theory and research: A framework for future research, translation, and policy. *Development and Psychopathology, 25,* 1415–1434.

Cassidy, J., Kirsh, S., Scolton, K., & Parke, R. (1996). Attachment and representations of peer relationships. *Developmental Psychology, 32,* 892–904.

Cassidy, J., Ziv, Y., Mehta, T. G., & Feeney, B. C. (2003). Feedback seeking in children and adolescents: Associations with self-perceptions, attachment representations, and depression. *Child Development, 74,* 612–628.

Chisholm, J. S. (1999). *Death, hope and sex: Steps to an evolutionary ecology of mind and morality.* New York: Cambridge University Press.

Cicchetti, D. (2006). Development and psychopathology. In D. Cicchetti & D. J. Cohen (Eds.), *Developmental psychopathology: Vol. 1. Theory and method* (2nd ed., pp. 1–23). Hoboken, NJ: Wiley.

Clark, S., & Symons, D. (2000). A longitudinal study of Q-sort attachment security and self-processes at age 5. *Infant and Child Development, 9,* 91–104.

Colman, R. A., & Thompson, R. A. (2002). Attachment security and the problem-solving behaviors of mothers and children. *Merrill–Palmer Quarterly, 48,* 337–359.

Contreras, J. M., Kerns, K. A., Weimer, B. L., Gentzler, A. L., & Tomich, P. L. (2000). Emotion regulation as a mediator of associations between mother–child attachment and peer relationships in middle childhood. *Journal of Family Psychology, 14,* 111–124.

Corriveau, K. H., Harris, P. L., Meins, E., Fernyhough, C., Arnott, B., Elliott, L., et al. (2009). Young children's trust in their mother's claims: Longitudinal links with attachment security in infancy. *Child Development, 80,* 750–761.

Crittenden, P. M. (1990). Internal representational models of attachment relationships. *Infant Mental Health Journal, 11,* 259–277.

Cummings, E. M., Schermerhorn, A. C., Keller, P. S., & Davies, P. T. (2008). Parental depressive symptoms, children's representations of family relationships, and child adjustment. *Social Development, 17,* 278–305.

Denham, S., Blair, K., Schmidt, M., & DeMulder, E. (2002). Compromised emotional competence: Seeds of violence sown early? *American Journal of Orthopsychiatry, 72,* 70–82.

Doyle, A. B., Markiewicz, D., Brendgen, M., Lieberman, M., & Voss, K. (2000). Child attachment security and self-concept: Associations with mother and father attachment style and marital quality. *Merrill–Palmer Quarterly, 46,* 514–539.

Drake, K., Belsky, J., & Fearon, R. M. P. (2014). From early attachment to engagement with learning in school: The role of self-regulation and persistence. *Developmental Psychology, 50,* 1350–1361.

Dykas, M. J., & Cassidy, J. (2011). Attachment and the processing of social information across the life span: Theory and evidence. *Psychological Bulletin, 137,* 19–46.

Easterbrooks, M., & Goldberg, W. (1990). Security of toddler–parent attachment: Relation to children's sociopersonality functioning during kindergarten. In M. Greenberg, D. Cicchetti, & E. Cummings (Eds.), *Attachment in the preschool years* (pp. 221–244). Chicago: University of Chicago Press.

Frankel, K., & Bates, J. (1990). Mother–toddler problem solving: Antecedents in attachment, home behavior, and temperament. *Child Development, 61,* 810–819.

Freud, S. (1963). *An outline of psychoanalysis* (J. Strachey, Trans.). New York: Norton. (Original work published 1940)

Gilliom, M., Shaw, D. S., Beck, J. E., Schonberg, M. A., & Lukon, J. L. (2002). Anger regulation in disadvantaged preschool boys: Strategies, antecedents, and the development of self-control. *Developmental Psychology, 38,* 222–235.

Goodvin, R., Meyer, S., Thompson, R. A., & Hayes, R. (2008). Self-understanding in early childhood: Associations with attachment security and maternal emotional risk. *Attachment and Human Development, 10,* 433–450.

Groh, A. M., Fearon, R. P., Bakermans-Kranenburg, M. J., Van IJzendoorn, M. H., Steele, R. D., & Roisman, G. I. (2014). The significance of attachment security for children's social competence with peers: A meta-analytic study. *Attachment and Human Development, 16,* 103–136.

Grossmann, K. E. (1999). Old and new internal working models of attachment: The organization of feelings and language. *Attachment and Human Development, 1,* 253–269.

Johnson, S. C., Dweck, C. S., & Chen, F. S. (2007). Evidence for infants' internal working models of attachment. *Psychological Science, 18,* 501–502.

Kochanska, G. (1995). Children's temperament, mothers' discipline, and security of attachment: Multiple pathways to emerging internalization. *Child Development, 66,* 597–615.

Kochanska, G. (2002). Mutually responsive orientation between mothers and their young children: A context for the early development of conscience. *Current Directions in Psychological Science, 11,* 191–195.

Kochanska, G., Aksan, N., & Carlson, J. J. (2005). Temperament, relationships, and young children's receptive cooperation with their parents. *Developmental Psychology, 41,* 648–660.

Kochanska, G., Aksan, N., Knaack, A., & Rhines, H. (2004). Maternal parenting and children's conscience: Early security as a moderator. *Child Development, 75,* 1229–1242.

Kochanska, G., Barry, R. A., Stellern, S. A., & O'Bleness, J. J. (2009). Early attachment organization moderates the parent–child mutually coercive pathway to children's antisocial conduct. *Child Development, 80,* 1288–1300.

Kochanska, G., & Kim, S. (2012). Toward a new understanding of legacy of early attachments for future antisocial trajectories: Evidence from two longitudinal studies. *Development and Psychopathology, 24,* 783–806.

Kochanska, G., Woodard, J., Kim, S., Koenig, J., Yoon, J., & Barry, R. (2010). Positive socialization mechanisms in secure and insecure parent child dyads: Two longitudinal studies. *Journal of Child Psychology and Psychiatry, 51,* 998–1009.

Laible, D. (2004). Mother–child discourse surrounding a child's past behavior at 30 months: Links to emotional understanding and early conscience development at 36 months. *Merrill–Palmer Quarterly, 50,* 159–180.

Laible, D., Panfile, T., & Makariev, D. (2008). The quality and frequency of mother–toddler conflict: Links with attachment and temperament. *Child Development, 79,* 426–443.

Laible, D., & Thompson, R. A. (1998). Attachment and emotional understanding in preschool children. *Developmental Psychology, 34,* 1038–1045.

Laible, D., & Thompson, R. A. (2000). Mother–child discourse, attachment security, shared positive affect, and early conscience development. *Child Development, 71,* 1424–1440.

Laible, D., & Thompson, R. A. (2002). Mother–child conflict in the toddler years: Lessons in emotion, morality, and relationships. *Child Development, 73,* 1187–1203.

Lamb, M. E., Thompson, R. A., Gardner, W., & Charnov, E. L. (1985). *Infant–mother attachment.* Hillsdale, NJ: Erlbaum.

Leerkes, E. M., & Wong, M. S. (2012). Infant distress and regulatory behaviors vary as a function of attachment security regardless of emotion context and maternal involvement. *Infancy, 17,* 455–478.

Main, M. (1991). Metacognitive knowledge, metacognitive monitoring, and singular (coherent) versus multiple (incoherent) models of attachment: Findings and directions for future research. In C. M. Parkes, J. Stevenson-Hinde, & P. Marris (Eds.), *Attachment across the life cycle* (pp. 127–159). London: Routledge.

Masters, J. C., & Wellman, H. M. (1974). The study of human infant attachment: A procedural critique. *Psychological Bulletin, 81,* 213–237.

Matas, L., Arend, R., & Sroufe, L. (1978). Continuity of adaptation in the second year: The relationship between quality of attachment and later competence. *Child Development, 49,* 547–556.

McElwain, N. L., Booth-LaForce, C., Lansford, J. E., Wu, X., & Dyer, W. J. (2008). A process model of attachment–friend linkages: Hostile attribution biases, language ability, and mother–child affective mutuality as intervening mechanisms. *Child Development, 79*, 1891–1906.

McElwain, N. L., Booth-LaForce, C., & Wu, X. (2011). Infant–mother attachment and children's friendship quality: Maternal mental-state talk as an intervening mechanism. *Developmental Psychology, 47*, 1295–1311.

Meaney, M. J. (2010). Epigenetics and the biological definition of gene × environment interactions. *Child Development, 81*, 41–79.

Meins, E., Fernyhough, C., Russell, J., & Clark-Carter, D. (1998). Security of attachment as a predictor of symbolic and mentalising abilities: A longitudinal study. *Social Development, 7*, 1–24.

Meins, E., Fernyhough, C., Wainwright, R., Das Gupta, M., Fradley, E., & Tuckey, M. (2002). Maternal mind-mindedness and attachment security as predictors of theory of mind understanding. *Child Development, 73*, 1715–1726.

Murphy, T. P., & Laible, D. J. (2013). The influence of attachment security on preschool children's empathic concern. *International Journal of Behavioral Development, 37*, 436–440.

Nachmias, M., Gunnar, M., Mangelsdorf, S., Parritz, R. H., & Buss, K. (1996). Behavioral inhibition and stress reactivity: The moderating role of attachment security. *Child Development, 67*, 508–522.

Ontai, L., & Thompson, R. A. (2002). Patterns of attachment and maternal discourse effects on children's emotion understanding from 3 to 5 years of age. *Social Development, 11*, 433–450.

Ontai, L., & Thompson, R. A. (2008). Attachment, parent–child discourse and theory of mind development. *Social Development, 17*, 47–60.

Pallini, S., Baiocco, R., Schneider, B. H., Madigan, S., & Atkinson, L. (2014). Early child–parent attachment and peer relations: A meta-analysis of recent research. *Journal of Family Psychology, 28*, 118–123.

Raikes, H. A., & Thompson, R. A. (2006). Family emotional climate, attachment security, and young children's emotion understanding in a high-risk sample. *British Journal of Developmental Psychology, 24*, 89–104.

Raikes, H. A., & Thompson, R. A. (2008a). Attachment and parenting quality predict children's problem-solving, attributions, and loneliness with peers. *Attachment and Human Development, 10*, 319–344.

Raikes, H. A., & Thompson, R. A. (2008b). Conversations about emotions in high-risk dyads. *Attachment and Human Development, 10*, 359–377.

Raikes, H. A., Virmani, E. A., Thompson, R. A., & Hatton, H. (2013). Declines in peer conflict from preschool through first grade: Influences from early attachment and social information processing. *Attachment and Human Development, 15*, 65–82.

Reese, E. (2002). Social factors in the development of autobiographical memory: The state of the art. *Social Development, 11*, 124–142.

Roisman, G. I., Booth-LaForce, C., Belsky, J., Burt, K. B., & Groh, A. M. (2013). Molecular-genetic correlates of infant attachment: A cautionary tale. *Attachment and Human Development, 15*, 384–406.

Roisman, G. I., & Fraley, R. C. (2008). A behavior-genetic study of parenting quality, infant attachment security, and their covariation in a nationally representative sample. *Developmental Psychology, 44*, 831–839.

Spangler, G., & Grossmann, K. E. (1993). Biobehavioral organization in securely and insecurely attached infants. *Child Development, 64*, 1439–1450.

Sroufe, L. A. (2005). Attachment and development: A prospective, longitudinal study from birth to adulthood. *Attachment and Human Development, 7*, 349–367.

Sroufe, L. A., Coffino, B., & Carlson, E. A. (2010). Conceptualizing the role of early experience: Lessons from the Minnesota Longitudinal Study. *Developmental Review, 30*, 36–51.

Sroufe, L. A., Egeland, B., Carlson, E. A., & Collins, W. A. (2005). *The development of the person: The Minnesota Study of Risk and Adaptation from Birth to Adulthood.* New York: Guilford Press.

Sroufe, L. A., Egeland, B., & Kreutzer, T. (1990). The fate of early experience following developmental change: Longitudinal approaches to individual adaptation in childhood. *Child Development, 61*, 1363–1373.

Sroufe, L. A., & Fleeson, J. (1988). The coherence of family relationships. In R. A. Hinde & J. Stevenson-Hinde (Eds.), *Relationships within families* (pp. 27–47). Oxford, UK: Clarendon Press.

Stearns, S. C. (1992). *The evolution of life histories.* Oxford, UK: Oxford University Press.

Steele, H., Steele, M., Croft, C., & Fonagy, P. (1999). Infant–mother attachment at one year predicts children's understanding of mixed emotions at six years. *Social Development, 8*, 161–178.

Sturge-Apple, M. L., Davies, P. T., Winter, M. A., Cummings, E. M., & Schermerhorn, A. (2008). Interparental conflict and children's school adjustment: The explanatory role of children's internal representations of interparental and parent–child relationships. *Developmental Psychology, 44*, 1678–1690.

Tharner, A., Luijk, M. P., Van IJzendoorn, M. H., Bakermans-Kranenburg, M. J., Jaddoe, V. W. V., Hofman, A., et al. (2012). Infant attachment, parenting stress, and child emotional and behavioral problems at age 3 years. *Parenting: Science and Practice, 12*, 261–281.

Thompson, R. A. (1994). Emotion regulation: A theme in search of definition. In N. Fox (Ed.), The development of emotion regulation and dysregulation: Biological and behavioral aspects. *Monographs of the Society for Research in Child Development, 59*(2–3, Serial No. 240), 25–52.

Thompson, R. A. (2000). The legacy of early attachments. *Child Development, 71*, 145–152.

Thompson, R. A. (2006). The development of the person: Social understanding, relationships, self, conscience. In W. Damon & R. M. Lerner (Series Eds.) & N. Eisenberg (Vol. Ed.), *Handbook of child psychology: Vol. 3. Social, emotional, and personality development* (6th ed., pp. 24–98). Hoboken, NJ: Wiley.

Thompson, R. A. (2008a). Measure twice, cut once: Attachment theory and the NICHD Study of Early Child Care and Youth Development. *Attachment and Human Development, 10*(3), 287–297.

Thompson, R. A. (2008b). Attachment-related mental representations: Introduction to the special issue. *Attachment and Human Development, 10*(4), 347–358.

Thompson, R. A. (2010). Feeling and understanding through the prism of relationships. In S. D. Calkins & M. A. Bell (Eds.), *Child development at the intersection of emotion and cognition* (pp. 79–95). Washington, DC: American Psychological Association.

Thompson, R. A. (2012). Wither the preconventional child?: Toward a life-span moral development theory. *Child Development Perspectives, 6*(4), 423–429.

Thompson, R. A. (2015). Relationships, regulation, and early development. In R. M. Lerner (Series Ed.) & M. E. Lamb (Vol. Ed.), *Handbook of child psychology and developmental science: Vol. 3. Social and emotional development* (7th ed., pp. 201–246). New York: Wiley.

Thompson, R. A., Laible, D., & Ontai, L. (2003). Early understanding of emotion, morality, and the self: Developing a working model. In R. Kail (Ed.), *Advances in child development and behavior* (Vol. 31, pp. 137–171). San Diego, CA: Academic Press.

Thompson, R. A., & Raikes, H. A. (2003). Toward the next quarter-century: Conceptual and methodological challenges for attachment theory. *Development and Psychopathology, 15*, 691–718.

Thompson, R. A., Virmani, E., Waters, S. F., Meyer, S., & Raikes, A. (2013). The development of emotion self-regulation: The whole and the sum of the parts. In K. Barrett, N. A. Fox, G. A. Morgan, D. J. Fidler, & L. A. Daunhauer (Eds.), *Handbook of self-regulatory processes in development* (pp. 5–26). New York: Taylor & Francis.

Thompson, R. A., & Winer, A. (2014). Moral development, conversation, and the development of internal working models. In C. Wainryb & H. Recchia (Eds.), *Talking about right and wrong: Parent–child conversations as contexts for moral development* (pp. 299–333). New York: Cambridge University Press.

Toth, S. L., Maughan, A., Manly, J. T., Spagnola, M., & Cicchetti, D. (2002). The relative efficacy of two interventions in altering maltreated preschool children's representational models: Implications for attachment theory. *Development and Psychopathology, 14*, 877–908.

Toth, S. L., Rogosch, F. A., Sturge-Apple, M., & Cicchetti, D. (2009). Maternal depression, children's attachment security, and representational development: An organizational perspective. *Child Development, 80*, 192–208.

Van IJzendoorn, M., van der Veer, R., & van Vliet-Visser, S. (1987). Attachment three years later: Relationships between quality of mother–infant attachment and emotional/cognitive development in kindergarten. In L. Tavecchio & M. Van IJzendoorn (Eds.), *Attachment in social networks* (pp. 185–224). Amsterdam: Elsevier.

Verschueren, K., Marcoen, A., & Schoefs, V. (1996). The internal working model of the self, attachment, and competence in five-year-olds. *Child Development, 67*, 2493–2511.

Waters, E., Kondo-Ikemura, K., Posada, G., & Richters, J. E. (1991). Learning to love: Mechanisms and milestones. In M. R. Gunnar & L. A. Sroufe (Eds.), *Minnesota Symposium on Child Psychology: Vol. 23. Self processes and development* (pp. 217–255). Hillsdale, NJ: Erlbaum.

Waters, S., & Thompson, R. A. (2014). *Children's perceptions of anger regulation strategies in two social contexts: Associations with age, gender, and attachment.* Manuscript under review.

Waters, S., Virmani, E., Thompson, R. A., Meyer, S., Raikes, A., & Jochem, R. (2010). Emotion regulation and attachment: Unpacking two constructs and their association. *Journal of Psychopathology and Behavioral Assessment, 32*, 37–47.

West, K. K., Mathews, B. L., & Kerns, K. A. (2013). Mother–child attachment and cognitive performance in middle childhood: An examination of mediating mechanisms. *Early Childhood Research Quarterly, 28*, 259–270.

Youngblade, L., & Belsky, J. (1992). Parent–child antecedents of 5-year-olds' close friendships: A longitudinal analysis. *Developmental Psychology, 28*, 700–713.

Ziv, Y., Oppenheim, D., & Sagi-Schwartz, A. (2004). Social information processing in middle childhood: Relations to infant–mother attachment. *Attachment and Human Development, 6*, 327–348.

# Chapter 17

# Attachment in Middle Childhood

Kathryn A. Kerns
Laura E. Brumariu

Research on children's attachments in middle childhood is a relatively new area of inquiry. The first chapter on the topic appeared in the second edition of the *Handbook of Attachment* (Kerns, 2008). Our goals in this chapter are to provide an update on what we know about attachment in middle childhood (7–12 years of age) and to highlight areas in need of further study. Several themes are highlighted. First, we now have a greater understanding of the key features of attachment in middle childhood. Second, there continue to be clear differences in opinion regarding how to conceptualize and measure attachment in this age period, and still surprisingly thin data on the validity of attachment assessments for this period. Finally, as in other developmental periods, attachment is related to parenting and to children's social, emotional, and cognitive development. Following the elaboration of these themes, we conclude with several recommendations for future research.

## The Nature of Attachment in Middle Childhood

The developmental period of middle childhood can be distinguished from both early childhood and adolescence. In early childhood, children's social worlds are largely oriented around and shaped by family members. Even if young children spend substantial time outside the home (e.g., in day care), parents are clearly the primary social figures in children's lives, and they often function not only as attachment figures but also as teachers and playmates. In middle childhood, children's social worlds expand: They may spend significant time away from parents, and parents may have less control and influence over the environments and social contacts children experience. Entrance to formal schooling places new demands on children and provides an important context for mastery or failure experiences. Peers take on greater salience, and by middle childhood, children have a clear preference for peers rather than parents as playmates (Kerns, Tomich, & Kim, 2006; Seibert & Kerns, 2009). Children become more self-reliant and assume greater responsibility for their behavior both at home and at school. There are also important advances in metacognition, memory, and cognitive flexibility; greater self-awareness, more consideration of psychological traits, and enhanced understanding of others; and a greater capacity to regulate emotions (Raikes & Thompson, 2005). Children also begin to undergo the physical changes associated with puberty (Richardson, 2005). Middle childhood can also be distinguished from adolescence; during the latter period, children gain increasing independence (autonomy from parents, greater decision-making authority). For example, there may be a normative shift toward greater avoidance or a more dismissing attitude toward parental attachments between late middle childhood and early adolescence (Ammaniti, Van IJzendoorn, Speranza, & Tambelli, 2000), and there is an emergence of attachments, including romantic ones, to peers in late adolescence (see Allen & Tan, Chapter 19, this volume).

We believe there are four defining features of attachment in middle childhood. First, Bowlby (1987; cited in Ainsworth, 1990) suggested that the goal of the attachment system changes from *proximity* to the attachment figure in early childhood to *the availability of* the attachment figure in middle childhood. Thus, in contrast to preschoolers, a boy or girl in middle childhood is content with longer separations and increased distance from the attachment figure, as long as he or she knows that it is possible to make contact with the figure (e.g., by telephone) and to reunite with the figure if needed (e.g., following an injury to the child). These changes probably occur partly because of a child's increased self-regulation, and partly because of parents' and children's expectations regarding greater child autonomy. These expectations may in turn be influenced by requirements for children to spend more time away from parents (e.g., because of school attendance and other formal activities, such as clubs and sports). Although children report relying less frequently on attachment figures as they get older (Kerns et al., 2006; Lieberman, Doyle, & Markiewicz, 1999), two longitudinal studies suggest that children's perceptions of caregiver availability and security actually increase in middle childhood (Kerns et al., 2006, Study 2; Verscheueren & Marcoen, 2005).

A second defining feature is that parents are the principal attachment figures for children in middle childhood. When asked about situations likely to invoke the need for an attachment figure (e.g., times when a child is afraid or sad, or specific situations such as separation from home), even 11- to 12-year-old children show a strong preference for parents over peers (Kerns et al., 2006; Kobak, Rosenthal, & Serwik, 2005; Seibert & Kerns, 2009). Interview studies reveal that children report going to parents in a range of situations, including when they are feeling ill or scared, coping with separation from or loss of an attachment figure or pet, and when they are distressed about a social conflict or have performed poorly

at school or in sports (Kerns & Seibert, in press; Vandevivere, Braet, & Bosmans, 2015). Children do spend substantial time with peers, and peers are clearly preferred over parents for companionship (Kerns et al., 2006; Seibert & Kerns, 2009). Children may report going to siblings, grandparents, teachers, and peers in situations in which contact with an attachment figure would be expected (e.g., when the child is sad or ill), but these nonparental figures typically play a secondary role and are more likely to be approached when parents are not immediately available (Seibert & Kerns, 2009). Mayseless (2005) has proposed that the use of peers as temporary attachment figures facilitates the transition to investment in peer relationships that is likely to occur in adolescence.

A third characteristic of attachment in middle childhood is a shift toward greater coregulation of secure base contact between the child and a parental figure. Bowlby (1973) proposed that a fourth phase of attachment, the goal-corrected partnership, emerges sometime after age 3, when a child is better able to understand a parent's desires, communications, and decisions, and is able to take these into consideration when developing plans and goals. Waters, Kondo-Ikemura, Posada, and Richters (1991) proposed that this shift in attachment may emerge later, during middle childhood, which they termed *the emergence of a supervisory partnership*. They suggested that parents may assume responsibility for maintaining contact with the child at younger ages, but in middle childhood, the child increasingly takes responsibility for communicating with the attachment figure (e.g., informing him or her of the child's whereabouts and changes in plans). Consistent with this suggestion is evidence that securely attached children are better about checking in and communicating with parents about their activities and whereabouts (Kerns, Aspelmeier, Gentzler, & Grabill, 2001). Another aspect of coregulation is that children and their parents may jointly work together to solve the child's problems, as a way to prepare a child to be able to cope better on his or her own (Cobb, 1996; Kerns, Brumariu, & Seibert, 2011). Thus, by the end of middle childhood, the attachment between child and parent can be viewed as a collaborative alliance, whereby the child is still relying on the stronger, wiser parental figure but is also beginning to use the parent as a resource rather than relying on the parent to solve the child's problems.

Finally, in middle childhood, attachment figures continue to function both as *safe havens* in times of distress and as *secure bases* that support a child's exploration. This might seem like an obvious restatement of the secure base construct, but at older ages, attachment assessments tend to focus primarily on the safe haven function of attachments (e.g., asking a child what he or she does when upset). By middle childhood, as children's worlds expand, attachment figures also provide support for exploration (e.g., promoting confidence in tackling challenges, showing confidence in the child's abilities). Hence, a marker of secure attachment is the ability of parent–child dyads to coordinate and balance needs for care with needs for exploration (Cobb, 1996; Grossmann, Grossmann, & Kindler, 2005; Kerns, Mathews, Koehn, Williams, & Siener, 2015). Furthermore, consistent with studies of preschoolers (Bretherton, 2010), there is some evidence that mothers provide relatively more safe haven support and fathers provide relatively more secure base support to children in late middle childhood and early adolescence (Kerns et al., 2015).

## Measuring Attachment in Middle Childhood

Due to space limitations, we do not present a thorough review of measurement issues and specific measures of attachment in middle childhood (for a comprehensive review, see Kerns & Seibert, in press; see also Bosmans & Kerns, 2015). Nevertheless, the topic deserves comment to aid readers in evaluating the literature discussed here. Unlike younger age periods, when observational assessments of specific attachments (e.g., to mothers) are universally used, there is currently no dominant conceptual or methodological approach for studies of middle childhood.

Although some studies have used observational assessments of attachment with children 6–8 years of age (e.g., Bureau & Moss, 2010), the vast majority of studies of middle childhood employ what can broadly be termed *representational measures of attachment*. Children develop cognitive (working) models of themselves in relation to their attachment figures, based on their experiences with their primary attachment figures (Bowlby (1969/1982). Working models have often been conceptualized as schemas or scripts that capture relationship rules (see Bretherton & Munholland, Chapter 4, this volume). Given the decline in the frequency and intensity of attachment behaviors

in middle childhood, along with the child's enhanced coping abilities, most studies in middle childhood assess attachment representations rather than a child's secure base behavior toward a caregiver. Representational measures require obtaining reports from the child. There are three important distinctions among these measures. Some measures (e.g., script measures, story stems, autobiographical interviews) require scoring by an outsider who considers not only what the child says but how the information is presented (e.g., whether the narrative is coherent), whereas others (questionnaires) are based on the child's direct reporting about experiences with attachment figures. The former are thought to capture both conscious and unconscious representations, whereas the latter capture only conscious representations. As might be expected, the overlap between these two types of measures is modest (Granot & Mayseless, 2001; Kerns, Abraham, Schlegelmilch, & Morgan, 2007; Kerns, Brumariu, et al., 2011; Kerns, Tomich, Aspelmeier, & Contreras, 2000; Psouni & Apetroaia, 2014). A second important distinction concerns whether the measures are intended to assess the quality of a specific attachment relationship (e.g., to the mother) or more general representations. Relationship-specific measures include separation–reunion measures (Main, Kaplan, & Cassidy, 1985; Moss, Bureau, Béliveau, Zdebik, & Lépine, 2009), story stem interviews (Granot & Mayseless, 2001; Kerns, Brumariu, et al., 2011), ratings of parent safe haven and secure base support from autobiographical interviews (Kerns et al., 2015), and questionnaires (Brenning, Soenens, Braet, & Bosmans, 2011; Kerns et al., 2001). Measures of general attachment representations include script story assessments (Psouni & Apetroaia, 2014) and autobiographical interviews that focus on narrative coherence (e.g., Child Attachment Interview: Shmueli-Goetz, Target, Fonagy, & Datta, 2008; Friends and Family Interview: Kriss, Steele, & Steele, 2012). A third distinction is that some measures assess variations in security, whereas others are designed to assess both secure and specific insecure patterns of attachment.

The diversity of measures, and of the conceptualizations of attachment inherent in the measures, is both a strength and a weakness. On the positive side, multiple measures can be advantageous: With a single measure, there is always a concern that one is studying the measure rather than the underlying construct. The use of multiple measures allows for more thorough assessment of a construct by more broadly sampling the relevant domain. In a new field, it can be helpful to have more than one approach because some measures may ultimately prove to have greater validity than others. By using different measures, the field avoids prematurely relying on a single approach. Unfortunately, several complications can arise when investigators adopt a wide range of approaches. Most measures are closely tied to the secure base and safe haven constructs, but in a few cases, assessments of "attachment" appear to tap other aspects of parent–child relationships (e.g., alienation or social support). Measures that assess global qualities such as social support may fail to be context-sensitive; the mother of a securely attached child would presumably be more sensitive to a child's distress cues than a mother of an avoidantly attached child, but there is no theoretical reason to expect that a mother of an avoidantly attached child would be unsupportive of her child's academic goals or shared interests (in fact, nonsocial activities might be a focus of interaction and could function to allow maintenance of the relationship without emotional engagement). Finally, a number of new measures have been published since the previous edition of this handbook, but most have generated only limited validity data, with the focus so far on testing how a new measure correlates with child adjustment rather than examining how it is related to observational assessments of parenting or even to other measures of attachment (Kerns & Seibert, in press).

What the field needs now is not new representational measures but studies that can shed light on which of the current approaches provide the best assessments. Needed are basic studies that examine the degree to which different measures of either specific relationships or general representations converge with each other; studies of the degree of overlap between relationship-specific and representational measures, which could shed light on how general representations are constructed; and careful consideration of both convergent and discriminant validity of measures. Evidence of convergent validity should include a demonstration that a measure of attachment is associated with the quality of care a child experiences, not just the child's adjustment. As more studies are conducted, meta-analysis could be used to examine the relative magnitude of the correlates of different measures or measurement approaches. Finally, there are some observational procedures that assess attachment behavior in middle childhood. For example, separation–reunion procedures have been developed

for 6- to 8-year-olds to assess attachment patterns and forms of attachment disorganization (Bureau & Moss, 2010; Easterbrooks, Bureau, & Lyons-Ruth, 2012; see Solomon & George, Chapter 18, this volume, for a detailed discussion), and efforts are under way to develop assessments for 10- to 12-year-olds based on parent–child interactions during discussion tasks (e.g., Brumariu, Kerns, Bureau, & Lyons-Ruth, 2014; Cobb, 1996). In this chapter, we have included only studies in which attachment constructs were clearly measured, and we have excluded studies that employed questionnaire measures of perceived parenting (e.g., parental acceptance) or single-item questionnaires. We included studies based on questionnaire, interview, or observational measures, although due to space constraints, we do not separate findings by measurement approach.

## Continuity and Change in Attachment in Middle Childhood

In the absence of disruptions in the quality of caregiving or the loss of attachment figures, one would expect at least moderate continuity in the quality of attachment over time (Fraley, 2002; Pinquart, Feussner, & Abnert, 2013). Several studies have evaluated whether attachment is stable within the middle childhood period (ages 7–12 years), examining intervals ranging from 1 month to 3 years. Most studies find evidence for stability, although there is substantial variability in the magnitude of the estimates (Granot & Mayseless, 2001; Kerns et al., 2000; Kerns, Schlegelmich, Morgan, & Abraham, 2005; Shmueli-Goetz et al., 2008; Verschueren & Marcoen, 2005). Ammaniti and colleagues (2000) found substantial stability in attachment from ages 10 to 14 years, and Grossmann and colleagues (2005) found evidence of continuity from middle childhood to early adulthood. By contrast, studies that examined whether behavioral measures of secure attachment in infancy or early childhood predict representational measures of secure attachment in middle childhood have been mixed (no association: Ammaniti, Speranza, & Fedele, 2005; Aviezier, Sagi, Resnick, & Gini, 2002; Bohlin, Hagekull, & Rydell, 2000; evidence for an association: Dubois-Comtois, Cyr, & Moss, 2011; Grossmann et al., 2002, 2005).

It should also be noted that some studies of stability have related early behavioral measures of specific attachments (e.g., the Strange Situation) to later representational measures of general attachment representations. In addition to differences in methods, weak associations might be expected if the latter are based on experiences in multiple attachment relationships. Longitudinal, multimethod studies are needed to examine stability both within and across measurement approaches (i.e., observational and representational measures; relationship-specific and general measures). The substantial variation in stability estimates suggests that change is also occurring for many children during these years, and that the 8–10 age period may be a time of reorganization in children's models of relationships (e.g., advances in social comparison abilities may lead children to change their evaluations of their attachment figures). Thus, studies examining factors that may account for both continuity and change are warranted.

## Associations with Parenting

One of the strong claims derived from attachment theory is that sensitive and responsive care provided by an attachment figure promotes the development of a secure relationship with that caregiver. Studies of young children have documented an association between maternal sensitivity and secure attachment (Thompson, Chapter 16, this volume). A few studies have examined how attachment is related to parenting for children ages 7–12 years. One set of studies examined secure attachment in relation to global parenting qualities and found that more securely attached children reported greater perceived acceptance by parents (Bosmans, Braet, Koster, & De Raedt, 2009; Kerns, Brumariu, et al., 2011). Such children also tend to have parents who report a greater willingness to serve as a secure base (Kerns, Klepac, & Cole, 1996, Study 2; Kerns et al., 2000). Secure attachment is also associated with observer ratings of maternal acceptance and positive affect (Dubois-Comtois et al., 2011; Kerns, Brumariu, et al., 2011; Scott, Riskman, Woolgar, Humayun, & O'Connor, 2011). In middle childhood, parents not only need to be responsive and available but also to act in ways that support the development of the child's autonomy (Cobb, 1996). Secure attachment is also associated with children's perceptions of parents as supporting autonomy and exerting low psychological control (Bosmans et al.,

2009; Kerns, Brumariu, et al., 2011), and with observer ratings of low levels of psychological control (Kerns, Brumariu, et al., 2011).

A second set of studies examined attachment and specific parenting practices. More securely attached children were more cooperative in monitoring situations and had parents who were more knowledgeable about (who more closely monitored) their children (Kerns et al., 2001; Scott et al., 2011). Attachment is also related to parental emotion socialization, in that parents of more securely attached children report less punitive reactions to child displays of distress (Cummings, George, Koss, & Davies, 2013), express less negative emotion when discussing their child (Scott et al., 2011), and endorse an emotion coaching (rather than a dismissing) meta-emotion philosophy (Chen, Lin, & Lu, 2012).

Some studies have examined associations between parenting and specific forms of insecurity. Children who reported more avoidant coping with mothers perceived their parents to exhibit lower levels of involvement, support, and monitoring of their activities (Karavasilis, Doyle, & Markiewicz, 2003; Yunger, Corby, & Perry, 2005). Children who scored higher on preoccupied coping also reported higher levels of psychological control from their mothers in one study (Yunger et al., 2005), but not another (Karavasilis et al., 2003). These researchers used child questionnaires to assess both parenting and attachment. In another study, avoidant coping was associated negatively with mothers' and fathers' reports of willingness to serve as a secure base (Kerns et al., 2000). Studies using observational assessments find that mothers of securely attached children show the most supportive parenting, whereas mothers of disorganized children show the most problematic parenting, with fewer distinctive associations for ambivalent and avoidant attachment (Kerns et al., 2000; Kerns, Brumariu, et al., 2011; Dubois-Comtois et al., 2011; Scott et al., 2011). In addition, Green, Stanley, and Peters (2007) found that mothers of disorganized children scored high on measures of "expressed emotion" (which generally involved negative or unpleasant emotion).

In summary, although the data are limited in comparison to that for younger age periods, secure attachment in middle childhood is related to sensitive, responsive, and accepting parenting, as well as to greater support for autonomy and low use of psychological control. Relatively few studies have included observational assessments of parenting or focused on parenting correlates of the insecure attachment patterns. Parents of children in middle childhood face many important tasks other than fostering security (e.g., encouraging independence, mastery, politeness, and conformity to rules), but researchers are just beginning to examine how attachment is related to specific parenting practices. In addition, there has been little consideration of how attachment might moderate the influence of parenting practices, as has been examined at younger ages (e.g., Kochanska, Barry, Stellern, & O'Bleness, 2009), or whether attachment and parenting are uniquely related to child adjustment (Scott et al., 2011). Important tasks for future research include investigating these questions, as well as considering how the broader family system interfaces with child–parent attachments (see, e.g., work on attachment and marital conflict; Davies, Harold, Goeke-Morey, & Cummings, 2002).

## Associations with Cognitive, Social, and Emotional Development

An important finding at younger ages is that the formation of a secure attachment to a parent is associated with greater cognitive, emotional, and social competence (see Thompson, Chapter 16, this volume), and researchers have also investigated these links in middle childhood (ages 7–12 years). In one kind of study, assessments of attachment in infancy or preschool have been used to predict children's competence in middle childhood. These studies, reviewed elsewhere (Fearon, Bakermans-Kranenburg, Van IJzendoorn, Lapsley, & Roisman, 2010; Groh, Roisman, Van IJzendoorn, Bakermans-Kranenburg, & Fearon, 2012; Groh et al., 2014; Madigan, Atkinson, Laurin, & Benoit, 2013; Pallini, Baiocco, Schneider, Madigan, & Atkinson, 2014; Schneider, Atkinson, & Tardif, 2001; West, Mathews, & Kerns, 2013; in this volume, see Thompson, Chapter 16, and DeKlyen & Greenberg, Chapter 28), indicate that attachment early in life is associated with greater social, emotional, and cognitive competence and fewer behavior problems in middle childhood. The typical strategy in these studies is to measure attachment in the first few years but not again, in middle childhood. Thus, the studies show the predictive significance of early attachment, although there is ambiguity in the interpretation of the findings. They might demonstrate that early attachment

per se is important for later development, or given that attachment is moderately stable (Fraley, 2002; Pinquart et al., 2013), they might imply that associations between early attachment and later outcomes are mediated by middle childhood attachment. Due to study designs used to date, these two possibilities cannot be distinguished, which indicates the importance of including assessments of attachment in middle childhood.

The following literature review focuses on studies in which both attachment and competence were assessed within middle childhood, and they show that in middle childhood attachment is related in theoretically meaningful ways to children's cognitive, social, and emotional adjustment. Measures of child functioning have included observations of child behavior, maternal reports, teacher reports, and child self-reports. A few studies relied solely on child questionnaires to measure both attachment and child functioning (mostly in the self-concept or behavior problem domains).

### Associations with Cognitive Development and School Adaptation

Does the quality of attachment have implications for a child's cognitive competence and cognitive performance? The available data provide strong evidence for a link between secure attachment and a child's school attitudes and classroom behaviors. Studies show that more securely attached children report greater perceived academic competence and mastery motivation (Bacro, 2012; Diener, Isabella, Behunin, & Wong, 2008; Duchesne & Larose, 2007; Kerns et al., 1996, Study 1; Moss & St.-Laurent, 2001); moreover, they are rated by teachers as showing better classroom adjustment in areas such as participation or academic skills (Aviezer et al., 2002; Diener et al., 2008; Easterbrooks & Abeles, 2000; Easterbrooks, Davidson, & Chazan, 1993; Granot & Mayseless, 2001; Jacobsen & Hofmann, 1997; Kerns et al., 2000). These links have been documented in both longitudinal and cross-sectional studies, using a variety of attachment measures. Other studies have examined how attachment is related to measures of cognitive performance such as achievement test scores and IQ tests. Here the data are more mixed (see West et al., 2013, for a review). Some researchers have found that secure attachment is not related to IQ scores, grade point averages, or achievement test performance (Dubois-Comtois et al., 2011; Granot & Mayseless, 2001; Kerns et al., 1996, Study 1; Moss & St.-Laurent, 2001; Shmueli-Goetz et al., 2008; for mixed evidence, see Aviezer et al., 2002; Bacro, 2012), whereas other studies have found that secure attachment is associated with higher scores on IQ or logic tests (Easterbrooks et al., 1993; Jacobsen, Edelstein, & Hofmann, 1994; Jacobsen & Hofmann, 1997). In some samples, insecure-controlling or disorganized children have been found to have the lowest school grades or performance on tests of cognitive skills (Jacobsen et al., 1994; Moss & St.-Laurent, 2001), suggesting that this group may be especially at risk for problems in cognitive development.

A newer direction in this area involves exploring mechanisms that could explain *why* attachment is related to school attitudes, performance, or IQ. It is possible that the presence of a secure base directly fosters enthusiasm and exploration of the school environment, by providing children with the support and self-confidence needed to tackle challenges. It is also possible that associations between attachment and school outcomes are mediated (best explained) by parenting practices. For example, Moss, St.-Laurent, Dubois-Comtois, and Cyr (2005) found that the link between disorganized attachment and school performance could be explained by the quality of children's collaborative interactions with their caregivers. Other studies suggest that associations between early secure attachment and later school performance or IQ might be due to the quality of teaching assistance parents provide (O'Connor & McCartney, 2007; West et al., 2013; see Williford, Carter, & Pianta, Chapter 41, this volume). Child characteristics such as self-regulation and a cooperative orientation to school demands are other factors that help explain why early attachment is related to later grades or IQ (O'Connor & McCartney, 2007; West et al., 2013).

## Associations with Self-Concept and Social Information Processing

Bowlby (1973) proposed that children who experience responsive and sensitive care are likely to view themselves as worthy of others' affection. In addition, children who form secure attachments are thought to possess a balanced self-view and are able to acknowledge personal limitations (Cassidy, 1988). This leads to the expectation that securely attached children will hold positive but realistic

self-views. In several studies of 8- to 12-year-olds, children who reported more secure attachments to parents also reported higher self-esteem (Cassidy, Ziv, Mehta, & Feeney, 2003; Doyle, Markiewicz, Brengden, Lieberman, & Voss, 2000; Kerns et al., 1996, Study 1; Sharpe et al., 1998; Verschueren & Marcoen, 2002, 2005; Yunger et al., 2005) or social self-efficacy (see Coleman, 2003, for child–father but not child–mother attachment). Secure attachment is also associated with fewer weight concerns, a more positive body image, and more adaptive beliefs and behaviors regarding eating (Goosens, Braet, Bosmans, & Decaluwé, 2011; Goossens, Braet, van Durme, Decaluwé, & Bosmans, 2012; Sharpe et al., 1998). These studies are limited in that both attachment and self-concept were measured with self-report questionnaires, which may overestimate the link between the two. In addition, these studies all tested the hypothesis that secure attachment would be related to higher self-esteem, yet children with an avoidant attachment may provide overly positive reports (Borelli, David, Corwley, Snaevely, & Mayes, 2013; Cassidy, 1988). Thus, studies that assess self-worth on a positivity dimension may not be well suited to testing the hypothesis that securely attached children have a positive but *balanced* view of the self. These problems can be reduced by employing independent assessments of attachment and self-concept. More securely attached children were rated by teachers as having more self-confidence (Jacobsen & Hofmann, 1997), more positive self-views as assessed with a puppet interview (Clark & Symons, 2009), and greater access to self-evaluations (i.e., they discussed the self spontaneously and easily; Easterbrooks & Abeles, 2000), although in two studies, interview or observational measures of attachment were not related to child reports of self-esteem (Bohlin et al., 2000; Easterbrooks & Abeles, 2000).

One reason why more securely attached children are hypothesized to maintain positive self-views is that they are thought to process social information in a positively biased way. Research evaluating this hypothesis has accelerated in the last few years. One set of studies examined social information processing in the context of social problem solving. Securely attached children have shown a positive bias in their attributions about others in two studies (Bauminger & Kimhi-Kind, 2008; Clark & Symons, 2009), but not in a third (Granot & Mayseless, 2012). More securely attached children generated more prosocial solutions (Bauminger & Kimhi-Kind, 2008; Granot &

Mayseless, 2012). Another set of studies examined attention and memory biases in relation to attachment. Cassidy and colleagues (2003) found that more secure 11- to 14-year-olds were more likely to attend selectively to positive information about themselves. Two studies by Bosmans and colleagues (2007, 2009) examined how preferential attention to pictures of their mothers was related to children's attachment. The two studies showed that insecurely attached children focused their attention more narrowly on their mothers, which was interpreted as showing decreased exploration during the task. Another study showed that insecurely attached children were more likely to show biased (increased) recall of negative information about their mothers (Dujardin, Bosmans, Braet, & Goossens, 2014).

In summary, although there are some inconsistent findings, for the most part, the middle childhood literature shows that more securely attached children hold positive but balanced views of the self, show a positive bias in the way they interpret others' actions, and generate more prosocial solutions to peer problems. Most studies in this area have focused on the correlates of security, so it is not clear whether children with different insecure attachment patterns can be differentiated in terms of their self-esteem and social information-processing approaches.

## Associations with Emotion Regulation and Personality

Emotion regulation is an integral aspect of attachment. By definition, emotional distress is addressed effectively in the secure parent–child dyad, with mitigation of distress (i.e., return of positive mood) and the child's return to exploration of the environment. Furthermore, it is hypothesized that securely attached children internalize effective ways to cope with stress and are consequently resilient when coping with problems, even in the absence of the caregiver (Kerns et al., 2007; Sroufe, 1983). By contrast, security of attachment is not hypothesized to be associated strongly with measures of temperament such as emotionality (Vaughn & Bost, Chapter 10, this volume).

In contrast to the situation at the time the previous edition of this handbook was published, there are now several studies that have investigated links between attachment and emotion in middle childhood (Parrigon, Kerns, Abtahi, & Koehn, 2015). Researchers who focus on mood

or the experience of specific emotion states have found that more securely attached children report more positive and less negative mood in daily interactions (Abraham & Kerns, 2013; Kerns et al., 2007) and higher positive emotion on a trait measure of affect (Borelli, Crowley, et al., 2010). The emotional experience of homesickness, by contrast, has not been consistently related to individual differences in attachment (Kerns, Brumariu, & Abraham, 2008; Thurber & Sigman, 1998; Thurber, Sigman, Weisz, & Schmidt, 1999). Securely attached children do report greater awareness of their emotional states (Brumariu, Kerns, & Seibert, 2012). More recently, researchers also tested whether securely attached children show more adaptive patterns of emotion regulation; they found that more securely attached children use more constructive coping strategies, such as seeking support from others or problem solving (Abraham & Kerns, 2013; Colle & Del Giudice, 2011; Contreras, Kerns, Weimer, Gentzler, & Tomich, 2000; Gaylord-Harden, Taylor, Campbell, Kesselring, & Grant, 2009; Kerns et al., 2007; Psouni & Apetroaia, 2014). One study found that avoidance was linked with emotion suppression, whereas ambivalence was linked with emotion dysregulation (Brenning, Soenens, Braet, & Bosmans, 2012). In the one study that assessed all four attachment patterns (secure, avoidant, ambivalent, disorganized), Brumariu and colleagues (2012) discovered that disorganization was related to coping; disorganized children were less likely to use active coping strategies and more often catastrophized when things went wrong. Finally, two studies examined attachment in relation to physiological indicators of emotion regulation. Borelli, David, and colleagues (2010) found that more securely attached children showed a stronger reaction followed by quicker recovery when presented with an aversive stimulus. Gillisen, Bakermans-Kranenburg, Van IJzendoorn, and van der Veer (2008) found that children who were securely attached showed lower electrodermal reactivity during a social stressor task, and this effect was accentuated for children who also had long alleles for a serotonin transporter gene (5-HTT).

Others have examined how attachment is related to personality or temperament. Surprisingly, one study found that secure attachment was not related to ego resilience (Easterbrooks & Abeles, 2000), although other studies suggest that securely attached children can better tolerate frustration and show better emotion control (Kerns et al., 2007; Shmueli-Goetz et al., 2008). Chen and

Chang (2012) found that insecurely attached children were more likely to use coercive strategies to control resources. Researchers have found no association between attachment and temperament in middle childhood when the latter was measured as extraversion (Jacobsen & Hofmann, 1997) or difficult temperament/negative emotionality (Chen, 2012; Contreras et al., 2000), with mixed evidence for behavioral inhibition/shyness (Borelli, David, et al., 2010; Brumariu & Kerns, 2010a).

Collectively, the emerging literature suggests that more securely attached children use more adaptive emotion regulation strategies and experience more positive and less negative mood states. One limitation is that most studies have examined attachment in relation to trait-like patterns of affect and emotion regulation; thus, we know relatively little about attachment and emotion as assessed in real time (for exceptions, see Borelli, David, et al., 2010; Gillisen et al., 2008), when it is possible to capture the dynamics of emotion (e.g., recovery following a stressor). There are also few studies that examined whether specific forms of insecure attachment (e.g., avoidance) are associated with distinct emotion profiles, as Cassidy (1994) and Sroufe (1983) have suggested (exceptions would be Brenning, Soenens, Braet, & Bosmans, 2012; Borelli, Crowley, et al., 2010; Brumariu et al,. 2012). Finally, given the evidence that attachment is linked with emotional competence, it would be worth exploring whether emotion regulation mediates associations between attachment and other aspects of adjustment (for examples in the domain of internalizing symptoms, see Brenning et al., 2012; Brumariu et al., 2012; Brumariu & Kerns, 2013).

## Associations with Peer Relationships and Peer Competence

One of the most extensively investigated questions in middle childhood research is whether attachment predicts the quality of children's peer relationships. There are several reasons for expecting an association between the two. The development of a secure attachment may foster greater exploration, including exploration of peer relationships (Kerns, 1996). In addition, children who form secure attachments to caregivers may show greater interest in and motivation for engaging with other social partners (Sroufe, Egeland, & Carlson, 1999), and may learn socially competent interaction styles from responsive

caregivers (Kerns et al., 1996). Also, more securely attached children may develop more adaptive emotion regulation capacities, which are especially important for peer relationships in middle childhood, when there is an emphasis on controlling one's emotions with peers (Contreras et al., 2000). Meta-analyses, based mostly on studies with younger children, showed that attachment is related to friendship and to social behavior or popularity with peers (Groh et al., 2014; Pallini et al., 2014; Schneider et al., 2001). The review below is more selective than the meta-analyses because it includes only studies of children in middle childhood, but it is more expansive than some meta-analyses that included only studies using behavioral measures of attachment.

In the friendship domain, investigators have examined whether attachment is related to the quantity and quality of children's friendships. Evidence for a link between attachment and the number of children's friendships is mixed (Kerns et al., 1996, Study 1; Lieberman et al., 1999). By contrast, studies consistently find that attachment is related to the quality of children's friendships, as indexed by measures of support, companionship, responsiveness, and conflict (Howes & Tonyan, 2000; Kerns et al., 1996, Study 2; Lieberman et al., 1999; see Abraham & Kerns, 2013, for a discussion of associations for positive friendship quality but not conflict). A second group of studies has examined whether children who form secure attachments to caregivers are more popular (more highly accepted) by their peers. Five studies found that children more securely attached to their mothers were better liked and less likely to be rejected by their peers (Barcons et al., 2012; Bohlin et al., 2000; Chen, 2012; Granot & Mayseless, 2001; Kerns et al., 1996, Study 1). However, two studies found an association between secure attachment and peer popularity for child–father, but not child–mother attachment (Verschueren & Marcoen, 2002, 2005), and another study found no association between peer popularity and attachment to mothers or to fathers (Lieberman et al., 1999). Thus, while the evidence is somewhat mixed, overall, it appears that secure attachment is associated with greater peer popularity.

A final group of studies examined secure child–mother attachment and global ratings of peer competence or observational measures of competent peer interactions. Securely attached children showed greater social engagement and participation with peers (Bohlin et al., 2000; Chen, 2012; Yunger et al., 2005); reported fewer difficulties with peers (Cummings et al., 2013); and were rated higher by parents, teachers, or camp counselors on measures of peer competence (Abraham & Kerns, 2013; Barcons et al., 2014; Contreras et al., 2000; for contrary evidence, see Easterbrooks & Abeles, 2000).

In summary, there is substantial evidence for an association between secure attachment and peer relationships, especially when the *quality* of children's relationships and social behavior is the focus. These associations have been found in studies using a variety of measures of both attachment and peer relationships. In their review of the link between attachment and peer relationships, Schneider and colleagues (2001) concluded that there is not a strong need for additional studies documenting an association between the two. This conclusion also seems to apply to the study of attachment and peer relationships in middle childhood. Rather, we need more studies aimed at explaining why this link is found (e.g., Abraham & Kerns, 2013; Contreras et al., 2000; McElwain, Booth-LaForce, Lansford, Wu, & Dyer, 2008), as well as studies that consider how attachment and peer relationships jointly and uniquely influence children's social development (e.g., Sroufe et al., 1999).

We also note that most studies have focused on the peer correlates of secure attachment and have not examined whether specific insecure attachment patterns are associated with specific peer deficits in middle childhood. Some differences between preschoolers with secure, ambivalent, and avoidant attachments were hypothesized and found in the Minnesota longitudinal project (Sroufe, 1983). In one follow-up study of the Minnesota sample into middle childhood, ambivalent children were found to be least efficacious in their peer relations, whereas avoidant children were the most isolated from peers (Shulman, Elicker, & Sroufe, 1994). Three more recent studies have examined insecure attachment patterns and the specificity of peer difficulties. These studies, which, unlike the Minnesota studies, included disorganized children as a separate group, suggest that both avoidant and disorganized children show the most problems with peers in middle childhood, particularly in the areas of exclusion or aggression (Granot & Mayseless, 2001; Jacobvitz & Hazen, 1999; Seibert & Kerns, 2015). Ambivalent children showed few peer difficulties (Granot & Mayseless, 2001; Seibert & Kerns, 2015). Clearly, research in this area has only just begun to test the specificity hypothesis.

## Associations with Behavior Problems and Clinical Symptoms

A secure attachment provides a healthy foundation for development, whereas an insecure attachment to one's primary attachment figures is likely to be associated with difficulties in personality development and, in some cases, clinical symptoms (see DeKlyen & Greenberg, Chapter 28, this volume). It is therefore not surprising that one of the most frequently investigated topics in middle childhood is whether attachment is related to signs of psychopathology. Almost all of the studies measure clinical symptoms (e.g., externalizing problems) rather than clinical diagnoses. In this section, we focus on studies published since the previous edition of this handbook.

As was found in the review in the previous edition of this handbook (Kerns, 2008), more recent studies show that attachment security is linked to lower levels of externalizing problems in middle childhood (Cummings et al., 2013; Scott et al., 2011). Lyons-Ruth (1996) proposed that disorganized attachment might be the insecure attachment pattern most clearly related to externalizing problems, but evidence for this idea is mixed (Granot & Mayseless, 2001; Jacobsen & Hofmann, 1997; Moss et al., 2009; Scholtens, Rydell, Bohlin, & Thorell, 2014). Interestingly, attention and thought difficulties have been linked to both secure attachment (Abrines et al., 2012) and disorganized attachment (Borelli, David, et al., 2010; Green et al., 2007; Scholtens et al., 2014; Thorell, Rydell, & Bohlin, 2012).

Studies published since the previous edition of the handbook also show that securely attached children experience lower levels of internalizing problems (Brumariu & Kerns, 2010a; Kerns, Brumariu, et al., 2011; Kerns, Siener, & Brumariu, 2011). Other researchers have examined whether specific forms of insecurity are differentially related to internalizing problems. Although there has been speculation that internalizing problems are most likely to be related to ambivalent or preoccupied attachment (Sroufe, Egeland, Carlson, & Collins, 2005; Yunger et al., 2005), studies indicate that measures of internalizing problems to correlate with self-report measures of both avoidance (Brenning et al., 2011, 2012) and ambivalent-preoccupied attachment (Brenning et al., 2011, 2012; Brumariu & Kerns, 2008). Conceptually, there has been little discussion of why disorganization would be related to internalizing problems. We suggest that the lack of a clear strategy to cope with distress and the associated profound emotion dysregulation, combined with feelings of helplessness and vulnerability in the face of frightening situations, may lead disorganized children to experience anxiety and depression (Brumariu et al., 2012; Brumariu, Obsuth, & Lyons-Ruth, 2013). In studies that assessed disorganization, which utilize representational measures of attachment, disorganized attachment was related to internalizing symptoms (Borelli, David, Crowley, & Mayes, 2010; Brumariu & Kerns, 2010a; Brumariu et al., 2012; Moss et al., 2009).

In summary, children who form a secure attachment to their mothers are less likely to experience clinical symptoms in middle childhood, including conduct and attention problems, and internalizing symptoms. There are virtually no data on child–father attachment and children's adjustment because studies have either assessed only child–mother attachment or have aggregated child–mother and child–father attachment measures (see Cummings et al., 2013, for an exception). It is difficult to draw conclusions regarding whether specific insecure patterns place children at risk for specific types of clinical symptom, partly because different studies included different insecure groups for both conceptual and methodological reasons. Some clinically focused studies examined only security and disorganization (e.g., Borelli, David, et al., 2010). Other studies used questionnaires, which can assess avoidance and ambivalence (preoccupation) but are unable to assess disorganization. Existing meta-analyses do not decisively answer questions about relations of attachment to clinical symptoms in middle childhood (Kerns & Brumariu, 2014). Some meta-analyses included only studies that used behavioral measures of attachment (Fearon et al., 2010; Groh et al., 2012; Madigan et al., 2013); as a consequence, the studies included mostly children under the age of 8. It is unclear whether those findings will generalize to older ages because some clinical symptoms (e.g., depression, social anxiety) do not typically emerge until late middle childhood or adolescence. A meta-analysis of attachment and anxiety did include a broad age range (Colonnesi et al., 2011), but a large number of the included studies had only questionnaire data for attachment, and disorganization was not examined. Furthermore, it is important to note that studies of attachment and clinical diagnosis are largely absent from the literature.

Finally, it is important to keep in mind that attachment is likely to be only one of many factors that influence the development of psychopathology; thus, it is not surprising that, when considered in isolation, attachment is only modestly related to signs of psychopathology. Even when attachment predicts psychopathology, it is almost a certainty that other factors (e.g., genes, poverty, abuse, and peer relationships) are also involved and, indeed, attachment is often not the strongest predictor of adjustment. One direction for future research is to study attachment along with other known risk factors to examine the relative importance of attachment for psychopathology. For example, recent studies indicate attachment is related to anxiety, even after researchers control for temperament. Emerging evidence with rodents and young children demonstrates epigenetic consequences of early social interaction, particularly with mothers, with implications for brain development, behavior, and mental health (e.g., Champagne, 2010). An exciting future direction is to investigate epigenetic modifications linked specifically with attachment in middle childhood. Similarly, another direction is to test models that include additional factors that may mediate or explain the links between attachment and clinical symptoms (e.g., Brumariu & Kerns, 2010b; Kerns & Brumariu, 2014).

## Conclusions and Future Directions

This review reveals that there has been an acceleration of research on attachment in middle childhood (see also Bosmans & Kerns, 2015). Progress has been made in characterizing the nature of attachment in middle childhood. The variety of attachment measures that have been developed await further validation. Research on attachment and parenting highlights the need to expand beyond the earlier focus on sensitivity as the only or even the main aspect of parenting that may contribute to the development and maintenance of attachment at older ages, identifying other constructs such as psychological control and support for autonomy as important at this age. Finally, the substantial evidence that has accrued indicates that, similar to what has been found at younger ages, secure attachment in middle childhood is associated with greater social, emotional, and cognitive competence, and less clinical symptomatology.

While there has been substantial progress, a continuing limitation is that the literature often seems to be driven mainly by a desire to retest old findings and questions in a new age period, rather than to take the developmental context of middle childhood into account. Some examples of how a developmental perspective could inform future work include answering the following questions:

- What are the important transformations in child–parent attachment in middle childhood, and what individual or contextual factors help parents and children negotiate these changes?

Although there has been attention to how the manifestation of avoidance, ambivalence, and disorganization may change in early childhood, we know very little about how these patterns may change in middle childhood.

- What are the most developmentally salient challenges in middle childhood, and is secure attachment most strongly linked to these?

There has been speculation regarding gender differences in attachment that may emerge during middle childhood, with girls tending toward ambivalence and boys tending toward avoidance, driven partly by biological changes (Del Giudice, 2009), but to our knowledge there have been few tests of these ideas (see Bakermans-Kranenburg & Van IJzendoorn, 2009, for mixed evidence).

- Children are beginning to spend more time away from parents. How do their experiences with peers or other adults affect a child's attachments to his or her parents?

- When are children able to integrate representations of different relationships into a general representation, and is the timetable for when this occurs affected by experiential factors?

Although at one time there was a lack of attachment measures for middle childhood, the current problem is that there are many measures, most of which have not been very extensively validated (Kerns & Seibert, in press). More attention needs to be paid to validation of measures, including studies examining overlap among measures and associations with parenting. Investigators need to consider their choice of measures carefully, making sure that the chosen measure captures the construct of interest. Self-report questionnaires have been used to assess children's perceptions of attachment, and although their use should not be ruled out a priori, it is important to recognize their limitations, especially when they are correlated only with other questionnaires completed by the children. The most common approach is to examine the correlates of secure attachment,

with some studies examining attachment disorganization. There is actually very little evidence for distinctive correlates of avoidant and ambivalent attachment in middle childhood. Is it that our measures are not adequately capturing these patterns at older ages? Is it that avoidant and ambivalent children are mostly coping adequately at this age, and only disorganized children are failing to show healthy adaptation? As of now, we simply do not know.

Our review shows that there is now substantial evidence that child–mother attachment is related to children's school adaptation, peer relationships, emotion regulation, social information processing, and internalizing and externalizing symptoms. There is not a strong need for additional studies designed solely to document these bivariate associations, but there are still a number of questions to address. Researchers are just beginning to examine specific mechanisms that might account for the documented associations. There could also be greater consideration of factors that might moderate the links between attachment and child adaptation. Another challenge for the field is to understand how attachment and other aspects of social experience operate together to influence children's social development. We need more studies that place attachment within a broader context, considering multiple influences (e.g., Sroufe et al., 2005).

Finally, the vast majority of studies have focused on mother–child attachment with American or European children growing up in traditional family structures (households headed by one or two parents). An important direction for future research to consider is the nature and role of attachment in a variety of circumstances. For example, there may be cultures in which children rely on several "principal" attachment figures that include extended relatives, as well as parents. We know of no studies in middle childhood that have examined attachments for children who have little contact with their parents.

## References

Abraham, M. M., & Kerns, K. A. (2013). Positive and negative emotions and coping as mediators of the link between mother–child attachment and peer relationships. *Merrill–Palmer Quarterly, 59*, 399–425.

Abrines, N., Barcons, N., Marre, D., Brun, C., Fornieles, A., & Fumadó, V. (2012). ADHD-like symptoms and attachment in internationally adopted children. *Attachment and Human Development*, 14(4), 405–423.

Ainsworth, M. D. S. (1990). Epilogue: Some considerations regarding theory and assessment relevant to attachments beyond infancy. In M. T. Greenberg, D. Cicchetti, & E. M. Cummings (Eds.), *Attachment in the preschool years* (pp. 463–488). Chicago: University of Chicago Press.

Ammaniti, M., Speranza, A. M., & Fedele, S. (2005). Attachment in infancy and in early and late childhood: A longitudinal study. In K. A. Kerns & R. A. Richardson (Eds.), *Attachment in middle childhood* (pp. 115–136). New York: Guilford Press.

Ammaniti, M., Van IJzendoorn, M. H., Speranza, A. M., & Tambelli, R. (2000). Internal working models of attachment during late childhood and early adolescence: An exploration of stability and change. *Attachment and Human Development*, 2, 328–346.

Aviezer, O., Sagi, A., Resnick, G., & Gini, M. (2002). School competence in young adolescence: Links to early attachment relationships beyond concurrent self-perceived competence and representations of relationships. *International Journal of Behavioral Development*, 26, 397–409.

Bacro, F. (2012). Perceived attachment security to father, academic self-concept and school performance in language mastery. *Journal of Child and Family Studies*, 21(6), 992–1002.

Bakermans-Kranenburg, M. J., & Van IJzendoorn, M. H. (2009). No reliable gender differences in attachment across the lifespan. *Behavioral and Brain Sciences*, 32(1), 22–23.

Barcons, N., Abrines, N., Brun, C., Sartini, C., Fumadó, V., & Marre, D. (2012). Social relationships in children from intercountry adoption. *Children and Youth Services Review*, 34(5), 955–961.

Barcons, N., Abrines, N., Brun, C., Sartini, C., Fumadó, V., & Marre, D. (2014). Attachment and adaptive skills in children of international adoption. *Child and Family Social Work*, 19(1), 89–98.

Bauminger, N., & Kimhi-Kind, I. (2008). Social information processing, security of attachment, and emotion regulation in children with learning disabilities. *Journal of Learning Disabilities*, 41(4), 315–332.

Bohlin, G., Hagekull, B., & Rydell, A. (2000). Attachment and social functioning: A longitudinal study from infancy to middle childhood. *Social Development*, 9, 24–39.

Borelli, J. L., Crowley, M. J., David, D. H., Sbarra, D. A., Anderson, G. M., & Mayes, L. C. (2010). Attachment and emotion in school-aged children. *Emotion*, 10(4), 475–485.

Borelli, J. L., David, D. H., Crowley, M. J., & Mayes, L. C. (2010). Links between disorganized attachment classification and clinical symptoms in school-aged children. *Journal of Child and Family Studies*, 19(3), 243–256.

Borelli, J. L., David, D. H., Crowley, M. J., Snavely, J. E., & Mayes, L. C. (2013). Dismissing children's percep-

tions of their emotional experience and parental care: Preliminary evidence of positive bias. *Child Psychiatry and Human Development*, 44(1), 70–88.

Bosmans, G., Braet, C., Koster, E., & De Raedt, R. (2009). Attachment security and attentional breadth toward the attachment figure in middle childhood. *Journal of Clinical Child and Adolescent Psychology*, 38(6), 872–882.

Bosmans, G., De Raedt, R., & Braet, C. (2007). The invisible bonds: Does the secure base script of attachment influence children's attention toward their mother? *Journal of Clinical Child and Adolescent Psychology*, 36(4), 557–567.

Bosmans, G., & Kerns, K. A. (2015). Attachment in middle childhood: Progress and prospects. In G. Bosmans & K. A. Kerns (Eds.), Attachment in middle childhood: Theoretical advances and new directions in an emerging field (*New Directions in Child and Adolescent Development*, Serial No. 148, pp. 1–14). San Francisco: Jossey-Bass.

Bowlby, J. (1973). *Attachment and loss: Vol. 2. Separation: Anxiety and anger*. New York: Basic Books.

Bowlby, J. (1982). *Attachment and loss: Vol. 1. Attachment*. New York: Basic Books. (Original work published 1969)

Brenning, K., Soenens, B., Braet, C., & Bosmans, G. (2011). An adaptation of the Experiences in Close Relationships Scale—Revised for use with children and adolescents. *Journal of Social and Personal Relationships*, 28(8), 1048–1072.

Brenning, K. M., Soenens, B., Braet, C., & Bosmans, G. (2012). Attachment and depressive symptoms in middle childhood and early adolescence: Testing the validity of the emotion regulation model of attachment. *Personal Relationships*, 19(3), 445–464.

Bretherton, I. (2010). Fathers in attachment theory and research: A review. *Early Child Development and Care*, 180(1–2), 9–23.

Brumariu, L. E., & Kerns, K. A. (2008). Mother–child attachment and social anxiety symptoms in middle childhood. *Journal of Applied Developmental Psychology*, 29, 393–402.

Brumariu, L. E., & Kerns, K. A. (2010a). Mother–child attachment patterns and different types of anxiety symptoms: Is there specificity of relations? *Child Psychiatry and Human Development*, 41, 663–674.

Brumariu, L. E., & Kerns, K. A. (2010b). Parent–child attachment and internalizing symptomatology in childhood and adolescence: A review of empirical findings and future directions. *Development and Psychopathology*, 22, 177–203.

Brumariu, L. E., & Kerns, K. A. (2013). Pathways to anxiety: Contributions of attachment history, temperament, peer competence, and ability to manage intense emotions. *Child Psychiatry and Human Development*, 44, 504–515.

Brumariu, L. E., Kerns, K. A., Bureau, J.-F., Lyons-Ruth, K. (2014). *Middle Childhood Attachment Strategies*

*Coding System (Version 1)*. Unpublished manual, Harvard University, Cambridge, MA.

Brumariu, L. E., Kerns, K. A., & Seibert, A. C. (2012). Mother–child attachment, emotion regulation, and anxiety symptoms in middle childhood. *Personal Relationships, 19*, 569–585.

Brumariu, L. E., Obsuth, I., & Lyons-Ruth, K. (2013). Quality of attachment relationships and peer relationship dysfunction among late adolescents with and without anxiety disorders. *Journal of Anxiety Disorders, 27*, 116–124.

Bureau, J., & Moss, E. (2010). Behavioural precursors of attachment representations in middle childhood and links with social adaptation. *British Journal of Developmental Psychology, 28*, 657–677.

Cassidy, J. (1988). Child–mother attachment and the self in six-year-olds. *Child Development, 59*, 121–134.

Cassidy, J. (1994). Emotion regulation: Influences of attachment relationships. In N. A. Fox (Ed.), The development of emotion regulation: Biological and behavioral considerations. *Monographs of the Society for Research in Child Development, 59*(2–3, Serial No. 240), 228–249.

Cassidy, J., Ziv, Y., Mehta, T. G., & Feeney, B. C. (2003). Feedback seeking in children and adolescents: Associations with self-perceptions, attachment representations, and depression. *Child Development, 74*, 612–628.

Champagne, F. A. (2010). Epigenetic influence of social experiences across the lifespan. *Developmental Psychobiology, 52*(4), 299–311.

Chen, B. (2012). The association between self-reported mother–child attachment and social initiative and withdrawal in Chinese school-aged children. *Journal of Genetic Psychology, 173*(3), 279–301.

Chen, B., & Chang, L. (2012). Adaptive insecure attachment and resource control strategies during middle childhood. *International Journal of Behavioral Development, 36*(5), 389–397.

Chen, F., Lin, H., & Li, C. (2012). The role of emotion in parent–child relationships: Children's emotionality, maternal meta-emotion, and children's attachment security. *Journal of Child and Family Studies, 21*(3), 403–410.

Clark, S. E., & Symons, D. K. (2009). Representations of attachment relationships, the self, and significant others in middle childhood. *Journal of the Canadian Academy of Child and Adolescent Psychiatry, 18*(4), 316–321.

Cobb, L. H. (1996). Adolescent–parent attachments and family problem-solving styles. *Family Process, 35*, 57–82.

Coleman, P. K. (2003). Perceptions of parent–child attachment, social self-efficacy, and peer relationships in middle childhood. *Infant and Child Development, 12*(4), 351–368.

Colle, L., & Del Giudice, M. (2011). Patterns of attachment and emotional competence in middle childhood. *Social Development, 20*(1), 51–72.

Colonnesi, C., Draijer, E. M., Jan, J. M., Stams, G., Van der Bruggen, C. O., Bögels, S. M., et al. (2011). The relation between insecure attachment and child anxiety: A meta-analytic review. *Journal of Clinical Child and Adolescent Psychology, 40*(4), 630–645.

Contreras, J. M., Kerns, K. A., Weimer, B. L., Gentzler, A. L., & Tomich, P. L. (2000). Emotion regulation as a mediator of associations between mother–child attachment and peer relationships in middle childhood. *Journal of Family Psychology, 14*, 111–124.

Cummings, E., George, M. W., Koss, K. J., & Davies, P. T. (2013). Parental depressive symptoms and adolescent adjustment: Responses to children's distress and representations of attachment as explanatory mechanisms. *Parenting: Science And Practice, 13*(4), 213–232.

Davies, P. T., Harold, G. T., Goeke-Morey, M. C., & Cummings, E. M. (2002). Child emotional security and interparental conflict. *Monographs of the Society for Research in Child Development, 67*(3, Serial No. 270), 1–115.

Del Giudice, M. (2009). Sex, attachment, and the development of reproductive strategies. *Behavioral and Brain Sciences, 32*(1), 1–21.

Diener, M. L., Isabella, R. A., Behunin, M. G., & Wong, M. S. (2008). Attachment to mothers and fathers during middle childhood: Associations with child gender, grade, and competence. *Social Development, 17*(1), 84–101.

Doyle, A., Markiewicz, D., Brendgen, M., Lieberman, M., & Voss, K. (2000). Child attachment security and self-concept: Associations with mother and father attachment style and marital quality. *Merrill–Palmer Quarterly, 46*(3), 514–539.

Dubois-Comtois, K., Cyr, C., & Moss, E. (2011). Attachment behavior and mother–child conversations as predictors of attachment representations in middle childhood: A longitudinal study. *Attachment and Human Development, 13*, 335–357.

Duchesne, S., & Larose, S. (2007). Adolescent parental attachment and academic motivation and performance in early adolescence. *Journal of Applied Social Psychology, 37*(7), 1501–1521.

Dujardin, A., Bosmans, G., Braet, C., & Goossens, L. (2014). Attachment-related expectations and mother-referent memory bias in middle childhood. *Scandinavian Journal of Psychology, 55*(4), 292–302.

Easterbrooks, M. A., & Abeles, R. (2000). Windows to the self in 8-year-olds: Bridges to attachment representation and behavioral adjustment. *Attachment and Human Development, 2*, 85–106.

Easterbrooks, M. A., Bureau, J., & Lyons-Ruth, K. (2012). Developmental correlates and predictors of emotional availability in mother–child interaction: A longitudinal study from infancy to middle childhood. *Development and Psychopathology, 24*, 65–78.

Easterbrooks, M. A., Davidson, C. E., & Chazan, R. (1993). Psychosocial risk, attachment, and behavior problems among school-aged children. *Development and Psychopathology, 5,* 389–402.

Fearon, R., Bakermans-Kranenburg, M. J., Van IJzendoorn, M. H., Lapsley, A., & Roisman, G. I. (2010). The significance of insecure attachment and disorganization in the development of children's externalizing behavior: A meta-analytic study. *Child Development, 81*(2), 435–456.

Fraley, R. (2002). Attachment stability from infancy to adulthood: Meta-analysis and dynamic modeling of developmental mechanisms. *Personality and Social Psychology Review, 6*(2), 123–151.

Gaylord-Harden, N. K., Taylor, J. J., Campbell, C. L., Kesselring, C. M., & Grant, K. E. (2009). Maternal attachment and depressive symptoms in urban adolescents: The influence of coping strategies and gender. *Journal of Clinical Child and Adolescent Psychology, 38*(5), 684–695.

Gilissen, R., Bakermans-Kranenburg, M. J., Van IJzendoorn, M. H., & van der Veer, R. (2008). Parent–child relationship, temperament, and physiological reactions to fear-inducing film clips: Further evidence for differential susceptibility. *Journal of Experimental Child Psychology, 99*(3), 182–195.

Goossens, L., Braet, C., Bosmans, G., & Decaluwé, V. (2011). Loss of control over eating in pre-adolescent youth: The role of attachment and self-esteem. *Eating Behaviors, 12*(4), 289–295.

Goossens, L., Braet, C., Van Durme, K., Decaluwé, V., & Bosmans, G. (2012). The parent–child relationship as predictor of eating pathology and weight gain in preadolescents. *Journal of Clinical Child and Adolescent Psychology, 41*(4), 445–457.

Granot, D., & Mayseless, O. (2001). Attachment security and adjustment to school in middle childhood. *International Journal of Behavioral Development, 25,* 530–541.

Granot, D., & Mayseless, O. (2012). Representations of mother–child attachment relationships and social-information processing of peer relationships in early adolescence. *Journal of Early Adolescence, 32*(4), 537–564.

Green, J., Stanley, C., & Peters, S. (2007). Disorganized attachment representation and atypical parenting in young school age children with externalizing disorder. *Attachment and Human Development, 9,* 207–222.

Groh, A. M., Fearon, R., Bakermans-Kranenburg, M. J., Van IJzendoorn, M. H., Steele, R. D., & Roisman, G. I., (2014). The significance of attachment security for children's social competence with peers: A meta-analytic study. *Attachment and Human Development, 16,* 103–136.

Groh, A. M., Roisman, G. I., Van IJzendoorn, M. H., Bakermans-Kranenburg, M. J., & Fearon, R. (2012). The significance of insecure and disorganized attachment for children's internalizing symptoms: A meta-analytic study. *Child Development, 83*(2), 591–610.

Grossmann, K., Grossmann, K. E., Fremmer-Bombik, E., Kindler, H., Scheuerer-Englisch, H., & Zimmermann, P. (2002). The uniqueness of the child–father attachment relationship: Fathers' sensitive and challenging play as a pivotal variable in a 16-year longitudinal study. *Social Development, 11,* 307–331.

Grossmann, K., Grossmann, K. E., & Kindler, H. (2005). Eraly care and the roots of attachment and partnership representations. In K. E. Grossmann, K. Grossman, & E. Waters (Eds.), *Attachment from infancy to adulthood: The major longitudinal studies* (pp. 98–136). New York: Guilford Press.

Howes, C., & Tonyan, H. (2000). Links between adult and peer relations across four developmental periods. In K. A. Kerns, J. M. Contreras, & A. M. Neal-Barnett (Eds.), *Family and peers: Linking two social worlds* (pp. 85–113). Westport, CT: Praeger.

Jacobsen, T., Edelstein, W., & Hofmann, V. (1994). A longitudinal study of the relation between representations of attachment in childhood and cognitive functioning in childhood and adolescence. *Developmental Psychology, 30,* 112–124.

Jacobsen, T., & Hofmann, V. (1997). Children's attachment representations: Longitudinal relations to school behavior and academic competency in middle childhood and adolescence. *Developmental Psychology, 33,* 703–710.

Jacobvitz, D., & Hazen, N. (1999). Developmental pathways from infant disorganization to childhood peer relationships. In J. Solomon & C. George (Eds.), *Attachment disorganization* (pp. 127–159). New York: Guilford Press.

Karavasilis, L., Doyle, A. B., & Markiewicz, D. (2003). Associations between parenting style and attachment to mother in middle childhood and adolescence. *International Journal of Behavioral Development, 27,* 153–164.

Kerns, K. A. (1996). Individual differences in friendship quality: Links to child–mother attachment. In W. M. Bukowski, A. F. Newcomb, & W. W. Hartup (Eds.), *The company they keep: Friendship in childhood and adolescence* (pp. 137–157). New York: Cambridge University Press.

Kerns, K. A. (2008). Attachment in middle childhood. In J. Cassidy & P. R. Shaver (Eds.), *Handbook of attachment: Theory, research, and clinical applications* (2nd ed., pp. 366–382). New York: Guilford Press.

Kerns, K. A., Abraham, M. M., Schlegelmilch, A., & Morgan, T. A. (2007). Mother–child attachment in later middle childhood: Assessment approaches and associations with mood and emotion regulation. *Attachment and Human Development, 9,* 33–53.

Kerns, K. A., Aspelmeier, J. E., Gentzler, A. L., & Grabill, C. M. (2001). Parent–child attachment and monitoring in middle childhood. *Journal of Family Psychology, 15,* 69–81.

Kerns, K. A., & Brumariu, L. E. (2014). Is insecure parent–child attachment a risk factor for the development of anxiety in childhood or adolescence? *Child Development Perspectives, 8,* 12–17.

Kerns, K. A., Brumariu, L. E., & Abraham, M. M. (2008). Homesickness at summer camp: Associations with the mother–child relationship, social self-concept, and peer relationships in middle childhood. *Merrill–Palmer Quarterly, 52,* 473–498.

Kerns, K. A., Brumariu, L. E., & Seibert, A. C. (2011). Multi-method assessment of mother–child attachment: Links to parenting and child depressive symptoms in middle childhood. *Attachment and Human Development, 13,* 315–333.

Kerns, K. A., Klepac, L., & Cole, A. (1996). Peer relationships and preadolescents' perceptions of security in the child–mother relationship. *Developmental Psychology, 32,* 457–466.

Kerns, K. A., Mathews, B., Koehn, A., Williams, C., & Siener, S. (2015). Assessing both safe haven and secure base support in parent–child relationships. *Attachment and Human Development, 17*(4), 337–353.

Kerns, K. A., Schlegelmilch, A., Morgan, T. A., & Abraham, M. M. (2005). Assessing attachment in middle childhood. In K. A. Kerns & R. A. Richardson (Eds.), *Attachment in middle childhood* (pp. 46–70). New York: Guilford Press.

Kerns, K. A., & Seibert, A. C. (in press). Finding your way through the thicket: Promising approaches to assessing attachment in middle childhood. In E. Waters, B. Vaughn, & H. Waters (Eds.), *Measuring attachment.* New York: Guilford Press.

Kerns, K. A., Siener, S., & Brumariu, L. E. (2011). Mother–child relationships, family context, and child characteristics as predictors of anxiety symptoms in middle childhood. *Development and Psychopathology, 23,* 593–604.

Kerns, K. A., Tomich, P. L., Aspelmeier, J. E., & Contreras, J. M. (2000). Attachment-based assessments of parent–child relationships in middle childhood. *Developmental Psychology, 36,* 614–626.

Kerns, K. A., Tomich, P. L., & Kim, P. (2006). Normative trends in children's perceptions of availability and utilization of attachment figures in middle childhood. *Social Development, 15,* 1–22.

Kobak, R., Rosenthal, N., & Serwik, A. (2005). The attachment hierarchy in middle childhood: Conceptual and methodological issues. In K. A. Kerns & R. A. Richardson (Eds.), *Attachment in middle childhood* (pp. 71–88). New York: Guilford Press.

Kochanska, G., Barry, R. A., Stellern, S. A., & O'Bleness, J. J. (2009). Early attachment organization moderates the parent–child mutually coercive pathway to children's antisocial conduct. *Child Development, 80,* 1288–1300.

Kriss, A., Steele, H., & Steele, M. (2012). Measuring attachment and reflective functioning in early adolescence: An introduction to the Friends and Family Interview. *Research In Psychotherapy: Psychopathology, Process and Outcome, 15*(2), 87–95.

Lieberman, M., Doyle, A., & Markiewicz, D. (1999). Developmental patterns in security of attachment to mother and father in late childhood and early adoles-cence: Associations with peer relations. *Child Development, 70,* 202–213.

Lyons-Ruth, K. (1996). Attachment relationships among children with aggressive behavior problems: The role of disorganized early attachment patterns. *Journal of Consulting and Clinical Psychology, 64,* 64–73.

Madigan, S., Atkinson, L., Laurin, K., & Benoit, D. (2013). Attachment and internalizing behavior in early childhood: A meta-analysis. *Developmental Psychology, 49*(4), 672–689.

Main, M., Kaplan, N., & Cassidy, J. (1985). Security of infancy, childhood, and adulthood: A move to the level of representation. In I. Bretherton & E. Waters (Eds.), Growing points of attachment theory and research. *Monographs of the Society for Research in Child Development, 50*(1–2, Serial No. 209), 66–104.

Mayseless, O. (2005). Ontogeny of attachment in middle childhood: Conceptualization of normative changes. In K. A. Kerns & R. A. Richardson (Eds.), *Attachment in middle childhood* (pp. 1–23). New York: Guilford Press.

McElwain, N. L., Booth-LaForce, C., Lansford, J. E., Wu, X., & Dyer, W. (2008). A process model of attachment-friend linkages: Hostile attribution biases, language ability, and mother–child affective mutuality as intervening mechanisms. *Child Development, 79*(6), 1891–1906.

Moss, E., Bureau, J., Béliveau, M., Zdebik, M., & Lépine, S. (2009). Links between children's attachment behavior at early school-age, their attachment-related representations, and behavior problems in middle childhood. *International Journal of Behavioral Development, 33*(2), 155–166.

Moss, E., & St.-Laurent, D. (2001). Attachment at school age and academic performance. *Developmental Psychology, 37,* 863–874.

Moss, E., St.-Laurent, D., Dubois-Comtois, K., & Cyr, C. (2005). Quality of attachment at school age: Relations between child attachment behavior, psychosocial functioning, and school performance. In K. A. Kerns & R. A. Richardson (Eds.), *Attachment in middle childhood* (pp. 189–211). New York: Guilford Press.

O'Connor, E., & McCartney, K. (2007). Attachment and cognitive skills: An investigation of mediating mechanisms. *Journal of Applied Developmental Psychology, 28*(5–6), 458–476.

Pallini, S., Baiocco, R., Schneider, B. H., Madigan, S., & Atkinson, L. (2014). Early child–parent attachment and peer relations: A meta-analysis of recent research. *Journal of Family Psychology, 28*(1), 118–123.

Parrigon, K. S., Kerns, K. A., Abtahi, M. M., & Koehn, A. (2015). Attachment and emotion in middle childhood and adolescence. *Psychological Topics, 24,* 27–50.

Pinquart, M., Feussner, C., & Ahnert, L. (2013). Meta-analytic evidence for stability in attachments from infancy to early adulthood. *Attachment and Human Development, 15*(2), 189–218.

Psouni, E., & Apetroaia, A. (2014). Measuring scripted attachment-related knowledge in middle childhood: The Secure Base Script Test. *Attachment and Human Development, 16,* 22–41.

Raikes, H. A., & Thompson, R. A. (2005). Relationships past, present, and future: Reflections on attachment in middle childhood. In K. A. Kerns & R. A. Richardson (Eds.), *Attachment in middle childhood* (pp. 255–282). New York: Guilford Press.

Richardson, R. A. (2005). Developmental contextual considerations of parent–child attachment in the later middle childhood years. In K. A. Kerns & R. A. Richardson (Eds.), *Attachment in middle childhood* (pp. 24–45). New York: Guilford Press.

Schneider, B. H., Atkinson, L., & Tardif, C. (2001). Child–parent attachment and children's peer relations: A quantitative review. *Developmental Psychology, 37,* 86–100.

Scholtens, S., Rydell, A., Bohlin, G., & Thorell, L. B. (2014). ADHD symptoms and attachment representations: Considering the role of conduct problems, cognitive deficits and narrative responses in nonattachment-related story stems. *Journal of Abnormal Child Psychology, 42*(6), 1033–1042.

Scott, S., Riskman, J., Woolgar, M., Humayun, S., & O'Connor, T. G. (2011). Attachment in adolescence: Overlap with parenting and unique prediction of behavioural adjustment. *Journal of Child Psychiatry and Psychology, 52,* 1052–1062.

Seibert, A. C., & Kerns, K. A. (2009). Attachment figures in middle childhood. *International Journal of Behavioral Development, 33,* 347–355.

Seibert, A. C., & Kerns, K. A. (2015). Early mother–child attachment: Longitudinal prediction to the quality of peer relationships in middle childhood. *International Journal of Behavioral Development, 39*(2), 130–138.

Sharpe, T. M., Killen, J. D., Bryson, S. W., Shisslak, C. M., Estes, L. S., Gray, N., et al. (1998). Attachment style and weight concerns in preadolescent and adolescent girls. *International Journal of Eating Disorders, 23,* 39–44.

Shmueli-Goetz, Y., Target, M., Fonagy, P., & Datta, A. (2008). The Child Attachment Interview: A psychometric study of reliability and discriminant validity. *Developmental Psychology, 44*(4), 939–956.

Shulman, S., Elicker, J., & Sroufe, L. A. (1994). Stages of friendship growth in preadolescence as related to attachment history. *Journal of Social and Personal Relationships, 11,* 341–361.

Sroufe, L. A. (1983). Infant–caregiver attachment and patterns of adaptation in preschool: The roots of maladaptation and competence. In M. Perlmutter (Ed.), *Minnesota Symposium on Child Psychology: Vol. 16.*

*Development and policy concerning children with special needs* (pp. 41–83). Hillsdale, NJ: Erlbaum.

Sroufe, L. A., Egeland, B., & Carlson, E. A. (1999). One social world: The integrated development of parent–child and peer relationships. In W. A. Collins & B. Laursen (Eds.), *Relationships as developmental contexts* (pp. 241–261). Hillsdale, NJ: Erlbaum.

Sroufe, L. A., Egeland, B., Carlson, E. A., & Collins, W. A. (2005). *The development of the person: The Minnesota Study of Risk and Adaptation from Birth to Adulthood.* New York: Guilford Press.

Thorell, L. B., Rydell, A., & Bohlin, G. (2012). Parent–child attachment and executive functioning in relation to ADHD symptoms in middle childhood. *Attachment and Human Development, 14*(5), 517–532.

Thurber, C. A., & Sigman, M. D. (1998). Preliminary models of risk and protective factors for childhood homesickness: Review and empirical synthesis. *Child Development, 69,* 903–934.

Thurber, C. A., Sigman, M. D., Weisz, J. R., & Schmidt, C. K. (1999). Homesickness in preadolescent and adolescent girls: Risk factors, behavioral correlates, and sequelae. *Journal of Clinical Child Psychology, 28,* 185–196.

Vandevivere, E., Braet, C., & Bosmans, G. (2015). Under what conditions do early adolescents need maternal support? *Journal of Early Adolescence, 35*(2), 162–169.

Verschueren, K., & Marcoen, A. (2002). Perceptions of self and relationship with parents in aggressive and nonaggressive rejected children. *Journal of School Psychology, 40,* 501–522.

Verschueren, K., & Marcoen, A. (2005). Perceived security of attachment to mother and father: Developmental differences and relations to self-worth and peer relationships at school. In K. A. Kerns & R. A. Richardson (Eds.), *Attachment in middle childhood* (pp. 212–230). New York: Guilford Press.

Waters, E., Kondo-Ikemura, K., Posada, G., & Richters, J. E. (1991). Learning to love: Mechanisms and milestones. In M. Gunnar & L. A. Sroufe (Eds.), *Minnesota Symposium on Child Psychology: Vol. 23. Self processes in early development* (pp. 217–255). Hillsdale, NJ: Erlbaum.

West, K., Mathews, B., & Kerns, K. A. (2013). Mother–child attachment and cognitive performance in middle childhood: An examination of mediating mechanisms. *Early Childhood Research Quarterly, 28,* 259–270.

Yunger, J. L., Corby, B. C., & Perry, D. G. (2005). Dimensions of attachment in middle childhood. In K. A. Kerns & R. A. Richardson (Eds.), *Attachment in middle childhood* (pp. 89–114). New York: Guilford Press.

# Chapter 18

# The Measurement of Attachment Security and Related Constructs in Infancy and Early Childhood

Judith Solomon
Carol George

In this chapter we examine the methods of assessing attachment security in infancy and early childhood, at both the level of behavior and the level of representation. Our first goal is to provide an overview and summary of available measures, along with information about their psychometric properties and the ways they have been used in research. Our second goal is to evaluate the current state of infant and early childhood measurement in the field of attachment. How well do the available instruments and protocols actually reflect the construct of attachment security? How useful are these measures for testing core predictions in attachment theory? Discussions of many of these measures have been updated to reflect work since 2008. Readers are referred to earlier editions of this handbook for more complete discussions.

This chapter can be used in several ways. Some readers, especially those new to research in this area, can use the chapter as a source of information to help select measures appropriate to their research. For readers who are familiar with childhood attachment assessment and well grounded in attachment theory, this is an opportunity to examine all of the measures together. This kind of overview is important for understanding the development of the field and providing a sense of new directions and opportunities for theory and research.

## The Domain of Attachment Security

*Attachment security* was defined by Ainsworth, Blehar, Waters, and Wall (1978) as the state of being secure or untroubled about the availability of the attachment figure. As a construct, security can never be directly observed, but must be inferred from what is observable. Furthermore, a construct is "evidenced in a variety of forms of behavior and not perfectly so in any one of them" (Nunnally, 1978, p. 84). How, then, do we determine whether a particular measure of attachment security is a "good" or valid measure of the construct?[1]

In practice, psychologists typically follow a three-step process in constructing a measure. First, they operationalize the construct of interest, either intuitively or with respect to theory or prior research. Second, they establish the reliability of the measure by looking at test–retest or short-term stability and, for measures that are tester-derived and require some judgment, determine whether there is interjudge agreement. Finally, they evaluate how well the measure predicts other theoretically important variables (convergent or construct validity) or is uncorrelated with theoretically unrelated variables (discriminant validity) (Campbell & Fiske, 1959).

Nunnally (1978) pointed out, however, that this approach is based on an inherent circularity in logic. We predict a relation between constructs, we "find" it using measures of the constructs at hand, and we thereby infer that our measures are valid. Optimally, Nunnally suggests three different steps: (1) The domain of relevant indices or variables ("observables") must be specified, indicating which variables are indicative of security and which are not; (2) the intercorrelations among multiple concurrent measures of the construct must be ascertained; and (3) each measure must be cross-validated with respect to a network of other theoretically important constructs that have been similarly validated. Rather than being sequential, these three steps constitute a reflective process in which knowledge gained from one step transforms our understanding of the others.

For attachment researchers, the domain of "observables" for infancy and toddlerhood (12–20 months) is drawn from Bowlby's (1969/1982, 1973, 1980) ethological attachment theory. *Attachment behaviors* are those that increase proximity to or maintain contact with a particular attachment figure. They are understood to be organized with respect to an internal control system (*the attachment system*) that has the adaptive function of protection and the set-goal of physical proximity or felt security A critical feature of this model, with important implications for measurement, must be emphasized: The type of attachment behavior observed depends on the degree to which the attachment system is activated. When a young child is alarmed, he or she can be expected to signal clearly for proximity to and contact with the attachment figure (e.g., crying, approaching, reaching, clinging). Once these goals are achieved, and in the absence of further disturbance, the child can be expected to seek or accept some distance from the attachment figure and return to exploration. Attachment behavior under conditions of low activation, often referred to as *secure-base behavior*, can be difficult to distinguish from friendly, affiliative behavior and may be very much influenced by features of the external environment.

Ainsworth and colleagues (1978) argued that this pattern of shifting between exploration and attachment will appear disturbed or distorted to the extent that the infant perceives the attachment figure to be inaccessible or unresponsive. Thus, Ainsworth's classic measure of attachment in infancy (the Strange Situation) and Waters and Deane's Attachment Q-Sort measure (AQS; Waters, 1995; Waters & Deane, 1985) focus on deviations from this basic pattern as a measure of insecurity in infant–parent attachment.

Attachment theory is less specific regarding appropriate measures of security in the third and fourth year of life and beyond. The attachment system is believed to function throughout this period, and indeed throughout the lifespan, but with diminishing sensitivity. Fewer situations are perceived as threatening, and knowledge of the parent's accessibility (rather than actual proximity or contact) is increasingly effective in terminating attachment behavior. In addition, the broader and more flexible behavioral repertoire of the older child, and the child's capacity to anticipate and coordinate with the parent's behavior, can make it more difficult for scientific observers to perceive the underlying organization of attachment behavior. At the same time, language and symbolic achievements during this period make it feasible to begin assessing attachment security at the representational level.

## Core Theoretical Predictions

Whether one follows Nunnally's model of optimal construct validation or more approximate procedures, the validity (retrodictive, concurrent, predictive) of a measure is a fundamental concern. There are probably as many theoretically interesting relations among constructs in the field of attachment as there are researchers to propose them. Attachment theory, as articulated by Bowlby and Ainsworth, however, provides certain key predictions regarding the relation between security and other variables that are core to the theory itself. The validity of any particular measure of security should be assessed at a minimum with respect to these. Acknowledging that there may be some dispute in the boundary areas, we propose the following core predictions:

1. *Attachment security should be positively related to the caregiver's accessibility and responsiveness to the child.* This prediction is implicit in the definition of security itself—that is, the state of being untroubled (confident) that the attachment figure will be available and will permit proximity and contact to the extent needed. An important corollary to this prediction is that attachment security with one caregiver should be independent of security with the other, insofar as the sensitivity of the two caregivers can be shown to differ. This fol-

lows from the definition of attachment security as a reflection of a particular relationship (Ainsworth et al., 1978) and not a property of the child (e.g., temperament).

Beginning with Ainsworth's pioneering work, maternal responsiveness and accessibility are typically assessed through variables reflecting the mother's prompt and appropriate response to the infant's attachment signals—that is, at the behavioral level. The field has shown increasing interest in the representational aspects of parental (especially maternal) sensitivity, and in the maternal qualities that permit or support sensitivity. By extension, such variables ought to be related to attachment security as assessed through behavior observations and, in turn, provide validity information for attachment measures.

2. *Attachment security in a particular caregiver–child relationship should tend to remain stable over time (continuity).* Although Bowlby (1973, 1980) was well aware of destabilizing influences on infant–caregiver attachment (e.g., repeated separation, life stress) and avoided the doctrine of critical periods, he proposed that the quality of attachment should become increasingly stable and resistant to change as a function of mutual adaptation in interaction patterns, and in each party's expectations about the other and the relationship, which become consolidated at the representational level. Sroufe and Waters (1977) emphasized the organizational quality of attachment; that is, although particular attachment behaviors may show little stability (due to the situation or the child's development), the underlying quality or organization of the relationship is expected to remain stable.

3. *Attachment security should predict other important aspects of development.* Related to but distinct from the notion of continuity is the general hypothesis proposed by Bowlby (1973) and elaborated both theoretically and empirically by Sroufe (1979; Sroufe & Waters, 1977) that attachment security should predict other key aspects of development. Bowlby emphasized the effects of insecurity arising from separation and loss on the development of psychopathology. In contrast, Sroufe articulated the more normative construct of "coherence" in development; that is, successes or failures in one developmental task (e.g., attachment in infancy) should predispose the child (and the caregiver–child dyad) to success or failure in subsequent developmental tasks

(e.g., autonomy, social competence). Sroufe's notion, though perhaps less central to attachment theory proper, parallels in many respects Erikson's (1950) classic formulation of developmental stages and has captured the attention of many researchers. It is important to note that it implies prediction relative to constructs other than attachment security, either concurrently or from one developmental period to another. In contrast, continuity implies prediction from an attachment security measure at one time relative to the same or a different measure of attachment security at another. Demonstration of *coherence* across time does not necessarily establish stability in the attachment relationship.

4. *Attachment security can be assessed by using similar or parallel measures cross-culturally and across attachment figures.* In the first two volumes of his *Attachment and Loss* trilogy, Bowlby (1969/1982, 1973, 1980) painstakingly built a case for the species-specific and therefore universal nature of attachment behavior in the young child. To the degree that a measure is based on ethological attachment theory, it should function similarly across cultures; that is, it should be as effective in describing the range of attachment relationships found in one culture (society, ethnic group, socioeconomic status [SES]) as in any other. In addition, it should be correlated in similar ways with measures of other theoretically important constructs, particularly caregiver behavior. By virtue of the same reasoning, the effectiveness of security measures and the pattern of correlations with caregiver behavior should be similar for all attachment figures (e.g., mother, father, other caregivers).

## Organization of This Chapter

For the period of infancy through early childhood (ages 12 months to approximately 72 months), measures of attachment security are based on observation of behavior. They vary according to whether they focus on attachment behavior directed toward the caregiver or on representational assessment based on the child's linguistic or play behavior. The foundation of attachment assessment is the classification approach to attachment relationships pioneered by Ainsworth and colleagues (1978). This system of multidimensional categories of relationship based on the infant's behavior in a laboratory separation-and-reunion context is both intuitively and theoretically compelling. The majority of measures for the period beyond early toddlerhood have been designed deliberately to capture these same or similar qualitative differences in child–caregiver attachment at both the behavioral and representational levels. An alternative approach is Waters's (1995) AQS method, which permits observers to capture the *dimension* of security in naturalistic circumstances.

We begin by describing Ainsworth's classification system and the subsequent addition of the disorganized/disoriented category. For this "gold standard" measure we review findings for all the validation criteria describe above. This is followed by a description of classification systems for reunion behavior and mental representation of preschool and kindergarten-age children, then by information on the AQS approach. Due to space limitations, our survey of validation studies for these measures is more compressed. Each section includes a brief discussion of unresolved issues in the construct validation of the measure(s) in question. We conclude with some general comments on the state of measurement in the field.[2]

## Attachment Classification in Infancy: The Strange Situation

Attachment classification is based on the behavior of the young toddler (12–20 months of age) in the Strange Situation. (Following Ainsworth's usage, this age child is referred to as an *infant*.) This laboratory procedure was designed to capture the balance of attachment and exploratory behavior under conditions of increasing, though moderate, stress. Full directions for running the session and for classification are presented in Ainsworth and colleagues (1978). Contrary to those instructions, however, experienced users typically do not provide a distraction to the mother (e.g., reading material), and they curtail separations if the infant becomes extremely distressed. An outline of the episodes that make up the Strange Situation is shown in Table 18.1. Infant attachment relationships are classified into one of three main groups: a "secure" group (B) and two "insecure" groups, "avoidant" (A) and "resistant" or "ambivalent" (C). Table 18.2 provides a brief description of classification criteria. Instructions are also available for designating eight subgroups, but the subgroups are rarely examined separately (due to limited sample sizes) and are not considered further here. Classification is based on the infant's behavior toward the caregiver during the two reunion episodes, viewed in the context of behavior in the preceding and intervening episodes and in response to the caregiver's current behavior. The infant's behavior during reunions is also rated on four scales of infant–caregiver interactive behavior that are used in the process of classification: Proximity and Contact Seeking, Contact Maintaining, Avoidance, and Resistance to Contact and Interaction.

About 15% of attachments in normative samples, and much higher percentages in high-risk samples, are difficult to classify with the original ABC criteria (Main & Solomon, 1986, 1990; Van IJzendoorn, Schuengel, & Bakermans-Kranenburg, 1999). Main and Solomon (1986) described the range of behaviors found in such unclassifiable infants and developed guidelines for assignment of most of these insecure infants to a

## TABLE 18.1. Episodes of the Strange Situation

| Episode | Duration | Description |
|---------|----------|-------------|
| 1 | 1 minute | *Parent, infant:* Dyad introduced to room. |
| 2 | 3 minutes | *Parent, infant:* Infant settles in, explores. Parent assists only if necessary. |
| 3 | 3 minutes | *Parent, infant, stranger:* Introduction of a stranger. Stranger plays with infant during the final minute. |
| 4 | 3 minutes | *Infant, stranger:* Parent leaves infant with stranger. *First separation.* |
| 5 | 3 minutes | *Parent, infant:* Parent returns. Stranger leaves quietly. *First reunion.* |
| 6 | 3 minutes | *Infant:* Parent leaves infant alone in room. *Second separation.* |
| 7 | 3 minutes | *Infant, stranger:* Stranger enters room and stays with infant, interacting as necessary. |
| 8 | 3 minutes | *Parent, infant:* Parent returns. Stranger leaves quietly. *Second reunion.* |

**TABLE 18.2. Strange Situation Classification Groups**

| Group | Brief description |
|---|---|
| Secure (B) (Ainsworth et al., 1978) | Uses mother as secure base for exploration. Separation: Signs of missing parent, especially during the second separation. Reunion: Actively greets parent with smile, vocalization, or gesture. If upset, signals or seeks contact with parent. Once comforted, returns to exploration. |
| Avoidant (A) (Ainsworth et al., 1978) | Explores readily, little display of affect or secure-base behavior. Separation: Responds minimally, little visible distress when left alone. Reunion: Looks away from, actively avoids parent; often focuses on toys. If picked up, may stiffen, lean away. |
| Ambivalent or resistant (C) (Ainsworth et al., 1978) | Visibly distressed upon entering room, often fretful or passive; fails to engage in exploration. Separation: Unsettled, distressed. Reunion: May alternate bids for contact with signs of angry rejection, tantrums; or may appear passive or too upset to signal, make contact. Fails to find comfort in parent. |
| Disorganized/disoriented (D) (Main & Solomon, 1990) | Behavior appears to lack observable goal, intention, or explanation—for example, contradictory sequences or simultaneous behavioral displays; incomplete, interrupted movement; stereotypes; freezing/stilling; direct indications of fear/apprehension of parent; confusion, disorientation. Most characteristic is lack of a coherent attachment strategy, despite the fact that the baby may reveal the underlying patterns of organized attachment (A, B, C). |

*Note.* Descriptions in Groups A, B, and C are based on Ainsworth et al. (1978). Descriptions in Group D are based on Main and Solomon (1990).

fourth classification group termed "disorganized/disoriented" (D). Infants classified as Group D show a diverse set of behaviors characterized by a sometimes momentary disruption or contradiction in the smooth flow of behavior, a lack of observable explanation in the immediate situation, a breakdown or violation of the well-recognized sequences of behavior that are characteristic of the attachment groups, or direct signs of fear and confusion. The underlying ABC classification often remains detectable and, in the majority of cases, this underlying pattern matches the mothers' attachment classification (Van IJzendoorn, 1995). Main and Solomon suggested, therefore, that this underlying pattern be noted as part of the classification process.

## Validation of the Measure

Beginning with Ainsworth's seminal work, validation of the infant classification system has been an ongoing priority. Many chapters in this volume reflect this progress and should be consulted accordingly. We begin with a lengthy discussion of reliability issues because the methodology departs substantially from what researchers in other areas of psychology may be familiar with, but we set this issue aside when discussing other measures later in the chapter.

## Reliability

### INTERCODER AGREEMENT

The Ainsworth system and other classification measures that we describe elsewhere in this chapter require extensive training. *Certification*, that is, proof that the researcher can meet a minimum reliability standard (usually 80% or higher) is desirable and typically is a requirement in peer-reviewed publications. Unlike *event coding*, which involves tallies of precisely defined acts, the *classification process* requires matching a particular case to a multidimensional, categorical template or prototype. Manuals for classification are composed mainly of written descriptions of these templates but cannot capture the range and nuance of behavior that is necessary for accurate categorization, which is why training by experts is common practice.

Within-laboratory agreement for trained coders tends to be very high, ranging from 100% to 85% (Ainsworth et al., 1978; Main & Weston, 1981; Waters, 1978). Five expert coders and Ainsworth independently classified all or a subset of 37 cases (videotapes), several of which were chosen because of the classification difficulties they presented (Carlson & Sroufe, 1993). Agreement percentages ranged from 50 to 100%, with the highest agreement (86%) found between Ainsworth and others. The fact that not all coders were trained to identify the disorganized/disoriented group may have lowered average reliability. Studies that made use of coders trained to identify the disorganized/disoriented group report across- and within-laboratory agreement ranging from 80 to 88% (Carlson, 1998; Lyons-Ruth, Repacholi, McLeod, & Silva, 1991).

When classification groups are disproportionately represented in a sample, high overall agreement (between judges or between classifications in stability assessments) may mask poor concordance for one or several of the (less common) groups. This is a particular problem in attachment research because secure classifications usually account for at least 50% of cases in nonclinical samples. Indeed, several investigators have noted that reports of high stability in classification are actually disproportionately due to stability (continuity) in the secure group but not in the insecure groups (e.g., Belsky, Campbell, Cohn, & Moore, 1996; Solomon & George, 1996; Waters, Merrick, Treboux, Crowell, & Albersheim, 2000). It is recommended that researchers report kappa or equivalent statistics that are adjusted for the relative frequencies of categories, along with raw reliability/stability figures. A large discrepancy between the raw (unweighted) concordance statistic and kappa indicates that agreement, stability, and so on, are unevenly distributed in the sample.

### TEST–RETEST (SHORT-TERM) STABILITY

Ainsworth repeated Strange Situation assessments over a 2-week period and found low stability, presumably reflecting sensitization of infants to the separation procedure (Ainsworth et al., 1978). The collapse of avoidant strategies in the second assessment was especially noteworthy: A number of previously avoidant infants on retest showed behavior patterns that we might now classify as disorganized. Separation of assessments by a month or more is recommended, and this practice appears to be the rule for observation-based attachment measures.

## Relation to Other Measures of Security

One of the most compelling aspects of the original work was Ainsworth and colleagues' exceptional effort to validate the classification groups with respect to infant behavior toward the mother in the home. Home observation data for the original sample of 23 babies was based on detailed narrative records of monthly visits over the course of the first year of life. Drawing on this work, Ainsworth was able to develop a rich and complex portrait of each relationship. Well-known findings from the study link classification in the Strange Situation to a set of variables reflecting the frequency and quality of infant attachment behavior in the home. Attachment classifications have also been assessed against home-based measures of attachment security—both a category system developed by Ainsworth and the AQS, which yields a summary security score reflecting the quality of an infant's secure-base behavior in the home. Both approaches show that secure versus insecure laboratory attachment classifications are related to different patterns of infant behavior in the home in ways predicted by theory. The two main insecure groups (A and C), however, were generally less well discriminated from each other in the home (Ainsworth et al., 1978; Vaughn & Waters, 1990).

## Prediction to Core Variables

### MOTHER–CHILD INTERACTION

Ainsworth's original home observations established key differences among mothers of secure, avoidant, and ambivalent infants on four highly intercorrelated variables: *sensitivity* (defined as prompt and appropriate responsiveness to the infant's signals), *acceptance* (vs. rejection), *cooperation*, and *psychological accessibility*. Mothers of secure infants were high on all four dimensions; mothers of avoidant infants provided the infants little positive experience with physical proximity and were rejecting; and mothers of ambivalent infants were inconsistently responsive to infant distress and other signals. These findings were replicated in several studies in both naturalistic and structured situations, although the associations have been weaker in the replications. An often cited meta-analysis concluded that parental sensitivity, although clearly important, does not appear to be the exclusive factor in the development of secure attachment (De Wolff & Van IJzendoorn, 1997). Given the centrality of the sensitivity construct in contemporary attachment theory, this is a radical notion. Failure to replicate Ainsworth's original findings may be due to reliance on limited samples of interaction, or shifts in the operational definition of sensitivity toward an emphasis on theoretically distinct constructs such as warmth, acceptance, and emotional availability. In support of this suggestion, more recent studies demonstrate that maternal sensitivity to distress signals in the early months, rather than sensitivity in general, is the key predictor of attachment security (Leerkes, 2011; McElwain & Booth-LaForce, 2006).

The identification of the disorganized/disoriented category exerts another influence on the strength of the association found between sensitivity and attachment security. Recent studies indicate that two dimensions of maternal behavior are linked to this classification—frightening or frightened/dissociative behavior, and some kinds of atypical, disrupted communication (Lyons-Ruth et al., 2013; Madigan et al., 2006). A growing body of literature also suggests that attachment disorganization may reflect neurological vulnerability (Padrón, Carlson, & Sroufe, 2014; Tharner et al., 2011). The variation reflected in the standard Ainsworth ABC categories, however, is better explained by the history of mother–child interaction than by the direct effect of biological variables (Fearon et al., 2006).

## CONTINUITY

Estimates of continuity depend on the age of the child at time of first and follow-up assessments, and the measures involved. The empirical findings have been mixed. Findings of very high stability of classification (over 70%) have been reported across both short and long time periods (e.g., Hamilton, 2000; Main & Cassidy, 1988; Waters, 1978). Nevertheless, studies showing substantial instability of classification between infancy and early childhood, and between these periods and young adulthood, are accumulating. In their review of longitudinal findings for 1,000 children in the National Institute of Child Health and Human Development Study of Early Child Care and Youth Development (NICHD SECCYD), Groh and colleagues (2014) reported low but significant concordance in secure versus insecure classifications between infants ages 15 and 36 months, and no significant concordance between the 15-month and 18-year assessments. Similarly, Pinquart, Feussner, and Ahnert (2013) in the most comprehensive meta-analysis of stability studies to date, reported lower stability for those originating in the second year of life compared to studies initiated later. Lack of stability of the D group attachment classification within the second year of life may be due to an increase in numbers of disorganized/disoriented infants between ages 12 and 18 months (Lyons-

Ruth, Yellin, Melnick, & Atwood, 2003; Vondra, Shaw, Swearingen, Cohen, & Owens, 2001). Possibly, at infant age 15 months, the Strange Situation captures mother–child dyads at a time when this transition is not yet complete. However, in the NICHD Early Child Care Research Network (2001) study, the greatest instability was in the avoidant, not the disorganized dyads. A critical finding is that in most stability studies, change in classification is systematically related to major shifts in maternal sensitivity or to family events such as loss, divorce, major illness, and poverty (on the negative side) and marriage or new relationships (on the positive side). Thus, findings of low stability do not challenge the bedrock assumption that Strange Situation classifications provide a reasonable reflection of the parent–child relationship and perhaps should be given less weight overall in the evaluation of the validity of measures.

## COHERENCE

Inspired by Sroufe's (1979) early articulation of the coherence of development across developmental tasks, the field has continued to generate a large body of research on the links between early attachment security and later functioning, including those in relationships with parents, peers, and romantic partners (in this volume, see Thompson, Chapter 16; Ehrlich, Miller, Jones, & Cassidy, Chapter 9; Williford, Carter, & Pianta, Chapter 41). Bowlby's seminal predictions about the connections between early parent–child attachment and later psychopathology have borne fruit in the study of the sequelae to disorganized attachment, which predicts both dissociative and externalizing behavior in longitudinal studies and meta-analyses (Carlson, 1998; Fearon & Belsky, 2011; Rutter, Kreppner, & Sonuga-Barke, 2009). In contrast, avoidance appears to be linked to general internalizing symptoms (Carlson, 1998; Groh, Roisman, Van Ijzendoorn, Bakermans-Kranenburg, & Fearon, 2012; Madigan, Atkinson, Laurin, & Benoit, 2013; in this volume, see DeKlyen & Greenberg, Chapter 28; Lyons-Ruth & Jacobvitz, Chapter 29).

## CROSS-CULTURAL PREDICTIONS AND PREDICTIONS RELATIVE TO OTHER CAREGIVERS

Studies of infants from cultures beyond North America in the Strange Situation have mainly been limited to Western Europe, but researchers have also examined infants and their mothers in Israel, Japan, Shanghai in China, Indonesia, Puerto Rico, Mexico, and two sites in Africa. Although secure classifications appear to be normative (modal) cross-culturally, cultural differences have emerged in the proportions of attachment groups. Corresponding observations of maternal behavior in the home suggest that such differences reflect systematic cultural patterns of maternal sensitivity to infant signals and cross-cultural differences in the frequency of separation from their mothers (for a review, see Mesman, Van IJzendoorn, & Sagi-Schwartz, Chapter 37, this volume).

Investigators report no difficulty in classifying infant–father attachment relationships from the Strange Situation. In several, but not all, studies, the modal classification category is secure (e.g., Cox, Owen, Henderson, & Margand, 1992). A recent meta-analysis of attachment to father shows a clear link between attachment to father and paternal sensitivity to the infant's attachment signals (Lucassen et al., 2011). Studies do suggest that in comparison to mothers, fathers' behavior is more closely linked to marital conditions, and to infant temperament and gender (Lickenbrock et al., 2013; Schoppe-Sullivan et al., 2006). The mechanisms by which infants arrive at qualitatively similar attachment strategies given large culture- and parent-related differences in patterns of interaction continues to need further investigation.

## Discussion

There can be little doubt that attachment classification by highly trained judges captures fundamental and far-reaching qualities of the infant–mother relationship. The reliability and predictive validity of Ainsworth's classification measure are well established in U.S. and Western European populations. However, important questions remain about the psychometric properties and meaning of the measure for infant–father relationships, relationships with other caregivers, and attachment relationships in non-Western societies. One of the most significant contributions of the method stems from its recognition of attachment relationship patterns or types, which has permitted researchers to describe and explicate individual differences in early relationships in a simple way that predicts significant developmental outcomes years later.

The ABC groups were based on the study of a middle-class sample of only 23 mothers and infants, observed four decades ago. As described previously, studies using much larger samples have revealed lower levels of stability of attachment between 12 and 18 months than were suggested by earlier, smaller studies (e.g., Waters, 1978). Mothers' work patterns, the degree of fathers' involvement in the lives of very young children, and economic conditions also have changed considerably since the era when early work was undertaken.

The most consequential addition to the original Ainsworth system, the disorganized/disoriented group, would not have been identified had researchers not attempted to replicate early findings in larger and atypical populations, and had they not been open to unexpected variations in behavior (Main & Solomon, 1990). Systematic research following on that original work has revealed the importance of this category for understanding variation at the more insecure and clinical end of the spectrum. The explanatory power of Ainsworth's methodology is increased substantially when this category is included in the study.

Ainsworth's reliance on a categorical approach to qualitative differences in attachment reflected her background in clinical assessment and her conviction that patterns of behavioral constellations, rather than individual differences in particular behaviors, distinguish types of attachment (Ainsworth & Marvin, 1995). Statistically less sensitive than dimensional measures, categorical systems require larger samples to establish reliable group differences. Many researchers who make use of Ainsworth's classification system (or other systems derived from it) are forced to reduce variability to a simple secure–insecure dimension because of inadequate sample size, usually in the insecure groups.

Fraley and Spieker (2003) tested the taxonomic structure of the standard Ainsworth categories. They argued that a very large portion of the variance associated with the ABC classifications can be summarized by two dimensions broadly representing "approach–avoidance" and "resistance–emotional confidence." Researchers interested in avoiding some of the well-known methodological pitfalls of categorical analysis could make use of this approach to dimensional scaling or the early one devised by Richters, Waters, and Vaughn (1988) from Ainsworth's interactive scales. Neither approach taps aspects of behavior relevant to attachment disorganization, but the disorganization scale, usually used as a part of the classification process (Main & Solomon, 1990) can serve this same purpose. (For an example of how these scales intercorrelate, see Groh et al., 2014.) Infant classification procedures have become so closely identified with the construct of security that it is difficult for researchers to conceive that different or additional measures may be necessary or feasible. In part, this reflects the simple brilliance of the Strange Situation procedure: It is hard to imagine another situation that can as reliably and ethically activate attachment behavior in the second year of life. The procedure makes use of a "natural cue to danger" (Bowlby, 1973)—separation from the attachment figure—to activate the attachment system. The use of distinct episodes allows the coder to observe the infant's immediate response to particular events and the coherence of behavior across episodes. Furthermore, the situation appears to provide the "right" amount of stress. Too little stress does not activate the attachment system adequately, judging by the results of home observations (e.g., Ainsworth et al., 1978; Vaughn & Waters, 1990) and therefore may not allow critical distinctions among insecure groups to be revealed. Very high stress, such as that provided by repeating the procedure twice in 2 weeks, appears to result in a breakdown of attachment strategies, again obscuring important differences among groups. Last, given that the primary threat to the child in the Strange Situation is a (transitory) threat to the relationship, the inferential leap from an observed pattern of attachment behavior to the infant's confidence regarding the psychological responsiveness of the caregiver seems to be a relatively modest one.

The validity of the security construct as measured by the Strange Situation requires its cross-validation with one or more other measures of infant security. Researchers often treat adult attachment measures as sources of cross-validation, but this presumes the very theoretical association that Bowlby's theory was designed to test. As we discuss later, the alternative measure of security in early toddlerhood, the AQS, does not reveal distinctions among the insecure groups, although, as we discuss later, some researchers attempt to use it in this way. Strictly speaking, the construct validation for infant attachment classifications technically is incomplete. We hope that this rather unsettling realization inspires researchers to devise alternative measurement approaches.

## Classification of Attachment in the Preschool Period

Investigators have followed two approaches to developing classification systems for children's attachment behavior beyond infancy. The dominant approach is based on an assumption of continuity between infancy and older ages, with allowances for developmental changes in the actual behaviors indicative of one or another type of relationship. In order to develop guidelines for 2-year-olds, Marvin (1977) and Schneider-Rosen (1990) modified Ainsworth's assessment criteria developmentally; for example, the timing and quality of distance interaction (including talking) were used as indices of security instead of the proximity seeking and contact maintenance of very young children. Marvin also considered the quality of parent–child negotiations around departures and reunions as an index of the quality of the goal-corrected partnership that according to attachment theory begins to emerge in an older toddler (Bowlby, 1969/1982, 1973, 1980). Main and Cassidy (1988) developed classification criteria for 6-year-olds by finding lawful continuities in reunion behavior for children whose infant attachment classifications were known. This effort was followed by Cassidy and Marvin, with the MacArthur Attachment Working Group (1992), who adjusted the Main and Cassidy kindergarten system downward for preschool-age children (from 2½ to 4½ years old) based on careful and extensive observations of their reunion behavior

The second approach, called by Crittenden (1992a, 1992b) the "dynamic-maturational model," focuses on dynamic changes in the quality of attachment arising from the interaction between maturation and current experience. Based on the concept of developmental pathways, this approach emphasizes the possibilities for changes in quality of attachment over time. The classification process places greater emphasis on inferences regarding the function of the child's behavior toward the parent, framed in terms of seeking psychological safety. There are strong similarities between the Preschool Assessment of Attachment (PAA; Crittenden, 1992a) system and the Preschool Attachment Classification System (PACS; Cassidy et al., 1992), as well as a number of subtle but significant differences. In both systems, attachment groups are distinguished by the communicative or defensive goals that underlie attachment patterns. In both, for example, the avoidant pattern is viewed as a defensive behavioral strategy organized around the goal of decreasing the probability of emotional involvement or confrontation. In Crittenden's PAA, however, this defensive strategy includes not only cool or neutral avoidance of the parent (as in the Main–Cassidy and Cassidy, Marvin, and MacArthur systems) but also behavior that might be seen as caregiving or hypercompliance. These are linked to neutral avoidance by the fact that in both strategies, the child takes the major initiative in regulating proximity and communication with the parent.

Both approaches use the Strange Situation procedure, especially the two separations and reunions of the original. Some investigators have introduced variations to accommodate the older age of the children, such as slightly longer separations, changes in the role and/or gender of the stranger, changes in the instructions to the caregiver, and blending with other laboratory tasks and procedures. A common approach in recent studies, recommended in the manual (Cassidy et al., 1992), is to omit the stranger episodes entirely, thus leaving the child alone in the room during both separations. We refer to this procedure as a "modified Strange Situation procedure." (The manual also accepts the use of the stranger as it is done for infants. Unfortunately, there has been no systematic determination of whether these variations materially affect the reunion behavior of the children.)

A description of the categories used in systems for the 5- to 6-year-olds and 2- to 3-year-olds is provided in Table 18.3. Although the Main and Cassidy system for 6-year-olds was developed earlier, we present information about the Cassidy, Marvin, and MacArthur system (1992) first because it applies to chronologically younger children. We next consider the Main–Cassidy system. Crittenden's PAA system has seen some increased use in recent years, especially with high-risk samples. It has been adapted to capture precursors in toddlerhood of the more extreme A- and C-type relationships and for school-age children, using representational materials (Crittenden, Kozlowska, & Landini, 2010; Farnfield, Hautamäki, Nørbech, & Sahhar, 2010). The dynamic maturational model also has been elaborated to follow attachment development through adulthood. Due to space limitations, we do not further describe the limited validation information available for the PAA below, but note that despite some overlap in category labels, the two systems do not result in comparable classifications in low risk samples

(Hautamäki, Hautamäki, Neuvonen, & Maliniemi-Piispanen, 2010; Rauh, Ziegenahin, Muller, & Wijnroks, 2000; Spieker & Crittenden, 2010).

## The Cassidy, Marvin, and MacArthur Group Preschool Attachment Classification System for Preschoolers

The PACS provides guidelines for a "secure" group (B) and four "insecure" groups as follows: "avoidant" (A), "ambivalent" (C), "controlling/disorganized" (D), and "insecure/other" (IO). (Main and Cassidy [1988] noted in their kindergarten age sample that the majority of formerly disorganized/disoriented infants showed a pattern of controlling the mother in a negative (D1) or positive (D2) manner, and this is reflected in the combination of these types into a single "D" group in the preschool system.) Classifications are based primarily on the child's behavior toward the mother during both reunions. Researchers report adequate interjudge agreement on these measures.

### Relation to Other Measures of Attachment Security

Classification in the PACS has been shown to be related both to the AQS Security subscale (Waters & Deane, 1985) and to representational measures of attachment. Considering the AQS findings first, a meta-analysis of studies through 2004 showed that secure PACS classification is significantly related to preschoolers' attachment security in the home, but at a more modest level than for infants (combined $r = .26$; range $= .10$ to $-.40$ for children 30 months or older and $r = .31$; range $= .25$ to $-.57$ for children ages 12–18 months; Van IJzendoorn et al., 2004). Subsequently, Moss, Bureau, Cyr, and Dubois-Comtois (2006), found significant differences in AQS security overall among children classified according to the Cassidy and colleagues (1992) system. AQS security was higher for children classified as secure than for those classified as ambivalent or disorganized (but not controlling), but there were no reliable differences between the secure and avoidant or controlling groups. Posada (2006) reported no significant difference among attachment classification groups in the overall AQS security.

Early on, three studies showed links between PACS classifications and the Attachment Story

**TABLE 18.3. Early Childhood Laboratory Separation–Reunion Classification Systems: Major Classification Groups**

| Group | Cassidy, Marvin, & MacArthur (PACS) | Crittenden (PAA) | Main–Cassidy |
|---|---|---|---|
| B | *Secure*: Uses parent as secure base for exploration. Reunion behavior is smooth, open, warm, positive. | *Secure/balanced*: Relaxed, intimate, direct expression of feelings, desires. Able to negotiate conflict or disagreement. | *Secure*: Reunion behavior is confident, relaxed, open. Positive, reciprocal interaction or conversation. |
| A | *Avoidant*: Detached, neutral nonchalance, but does not avoid interaction altogether. Avoids physical or psychological intimacy. | *Defended*: Acts to reduce emotional involvement or confrontation. Focuses on play and exploration at expense of interaction. | *Avoidant*: Maintains affective neutrality; subtly minimizes and limits opportunities for interaction. |
| C | *Ambivalent*: Protests separation strongly. Reunion characterized by strong proximity-seeking, babyish, coy behavior. | *Coercive*: Maximizes psychological involvement with parent; exaggerates problems and conflict. Is coercive, for example, threatening (resistant, punitive) and/or disarming (innocent, coy). | *Ambivalent*: Heightened intimacy and dependency on parent. Reunion characterized by ambivalence, subtle hostility, exaggerated cute or babyish behavior. |
| D | *Controlling/disorganized*: Characterized by controlling behavior (punitive, caregiving) or behaviors associated with infant disorganization. | | *Controlling*: Signs of role reversal: punitive (rejecting, humiliating) or caregiving (cheering, reassuring, falsely positive). |
| A/C | | *Defended/coercive*: Child shows both defended and coercive behaviors, appearing together or in alternation. | |
| A/D | | *Anxious/depressed*: Sad/depressed; stares, extreme distress/panic. | |
| IO or U | *Insecure/other*: Mixtures of insecure indices that do not fit into any of the other groups. | *Insecure/other*: Acts incoherently in relation to parent. | *Unclassifiable*: Mixture of insecure indices that do not fit into any of the other groups including behaviors associated with infant disorganization. |

*Note.* Cassidy–Marvin, Main–Cassidy: Organized groups = A, B, C. PAA: Organized groups = A, B, C, A/C.

Completion Task (ASCT), a representational measure of attachment security (Bretherton, Oppenheim, Buchsbaum, Emde, & the MacArthur Narrative Group, 1990; Bretherton, Ridgeway, & Cassidy, 1990; Shouldice & Stevenson-Hinde, 1992). Preschoolers classified as secure, compared to those classified as insecure, received higher scores for representational security (i.e., they were judged more open to negative feelings and better able to tolerate attachment fears). Finally, Groh and colleagues (2014) report significant negative correlations between security in the PACS and dismissive and preoccupied profile scores generated from the Adult Attachment Interview.

### Prediction to Core Variables

#### MOTHER–CHILD INTERACTION

Clear differences between the secure and insecure groups' quality of interaction have been demonstrated in several studies. Mothers of secure children are rated higher than mothers of insecure children in qualities such as sensitivity, socialization, positive involvement, and scaffolding in cognitively challenging tasks or cleanup in normative families across the full spectrum of incomes (e.g., NICHD Early Childcare Research Network, 1991). Recently, Dexter, Wong, Stacks, Beeghly, and Barnett (2013) investigated low-income African American and European American mothers, and found no effect of ethnicity but a clear link between maternal warmth and responsiveness in secure versus insecure dyads. In contrast, differences between the secure and the various insecure groups, or among the insecure groups, have not uniformly been found. In the previously discussed NICHD study, significant differences between attachment groups were mainly found between the controlling/disorganized and secure classifications. Moss and her colleagues (Humber & Moss, 2005; Moss, Bureau, Cyr, Mongeau, & St.-Laurent, 2004; Moss, Cyr, & Dubois-Comtois, 2004) found overall smoother and more positive interaction during a brief "snack time" in a comparison between secure and insecure dyads with children ages 3 to 7 (note that the Main–Cassidy system was adapted for classifications for children age 6 years and older). The clearest differences in both age periods were between dyads with secure versus disorganized/controlling children. O'Connor, Bureau, McCartney, and Lyons-Ruth (2011) looked in detail at the mother–child interaction variables that best differentiated the disorganized/controlling groups from organized insecure (A, C) and secure groups in the NICHD sample. Maternal hostility was significantly higher for the disorganized groups, whereas maternal support and respect for autonomy was lower for the D group as opposed to the secure and insecure groups. Within the subtypes of the controlling/D-group children, quality of interaction was worst for the controlling/punitive and behaviorally disorganized groups and comparable to secure dyads for the controlling/caregiving group. The dimensional scales used in the study likely were insensitive to the unique qualities of the caregiving group, where positive interaction is supported by the child's rather than the mother's behavior (Main & Cassidy, 1988; Solomon & George, 1999d). Finally, between-group differences in maternal behavior emerged in a study by Britner, Marvin, and Pianta (2005). They developed a classification system and rating scales for maternal behavior in the modified Strange Situation reflecting qualities captured from Ainsworth's original studies and studies of adult attachment representation. Agreement be-tween mother and child classifications was high, though not exact (kappa = .57). Though this system seems to provide strong evidence for distinctions in maternal behavior corresponding to all of the child classifications, the fact that mother and child categories are based on the same sample of behavior is problematic.

Studies in non-normative samples provide indirect evidence that classification reflects differences in maternal behavior. Just to cite relatively recent studies involving, variously, maltreated children, children whose mothers experience domestic violence, and mothers who are adolescent, impoverished, depressed, or anxiety-disordered, fewer relationships are classified as secure and more as "atypical" (e.g., disorganized, controlling, or insecure/other) than comparison children (Barnett et al., 2006; Campbell et al., 2004; Fish, 2004; Levendosky, Bogat, Huth-Bocks, Rosenblum, & von Eye, 2011; Lounds, Borkowski, Whitman, Maxwell, & Weed, 2005; Toth, Rogosch, Manly, & Cicchetti, 2006). Several researchers who studied attachment involving adopted or institutionalized young Romanian or Chinese children found disorganized and atypical behavior to be highly characteristic (Zeanah, Smyke, Koga, & Carlson, 2005). Lower levels of disorganization or atypical behavior and increased security become evident after placement in foster or adoptive homes (McLaughlin, Zeanah, Fox, & Nelson, 2012).

## CONTINUITY

A number of studies provide data on continuity (stability) of classification from toddlerhood. Three studies found significant but very low stability in classifications over time (Levendosky et al., 2011; NICHD Early Child Care Research Network, 2001; Seifer et al., 2004), and two studies with somewhat smaller samples reported no significant stability over the early childhood period (Bar-Haim, Sutton, Fox, & Marvin, 2000; Fish, 2004). Significant but moderate continuity of classification (kappa = approximately .40) is reported in yet other studies (Cassidy, Berlin, & Belsky, 1990; Cicchetti & Barnett, 1991; Lounds et al., 2005; Shouldice & Stevenson-Hinde, 1992). The secure pattern showed the highest consistency over time, but the studies differed on which of the insecure patterns was most likely to shift. Shifts into the secure category were the most common for the unstable insecure infants.

In the only study to date of stability *within* the preschool period of the Cassidy and colleagues

(1992) classifications in a normative population, Moss, Cyr, Bureau, Tarabulsy, and Dubois-Combois (2005) found moderate stability between 3½- and 5½-year-olds in a sample that was heterogeneous with respect to SES. Stability of group assignment was over 60% for all groups except the avoidant group, which shifted considerably. Seventy percent of disorganized 3½-year-olds shifted into the controlling category within this time period, suggesting that this is the point at which disorganized children consolidate their secondary controlling strategies. The level of instability in classification might in itself raise questions about the validity of the Cassidy and colleagues' system, based on the premise that stability will be the norm. Investigators in each of these studies established, however, that shifts between the secure and insecure classification(s) typically were related to corresponding changes in mother–child interaction and/or other key factors (e.g., domestic violence, marital distress, and separation).

## COHERENCE

Differences between secure and insecure children are found in other, theoretically related developmental domains. Several studies show, as would be expected, that secure children are more cooperative with their mothers than insecure ones in brief laboratory tasks (e.g., Cassidy et al., 1992; Moss, Bureau, et al., 2004). A key matter from the point of view of coherence of development, however, is whether group differences can be detected in other relationships and in underlying social or cognitive strengths. Questions along these lines have been addressed in secondary analyses of the findings from the NICHD SECCYD. For example, Raikes and Thompson (2008) found that at 24 months, AQS security and secure versus insecure attachment in the PACS system at 36 months predicted children's social problem-solving skills and lower self-reported loneliness at 54 months of age. Similarly, Drake, Belsky, and Fearon (2014) used latent growth curve analysis to demonstrate effects of secure attachment at 36 months on social self-control and flexibility and task persistence in grade 1. Social self-control, in turn, mediated links between earlier attachment and school engagement in grades 3 and 5 (see also Fish, 2004; Moss & St-Laurent, 2001; Stacks & Oshio, 2009). The NICHD studies did not find similar effects of attachment security measured earlier, at 15 months. Researchers have also found that children classi-

fied as secure in the PACS were less likely than insecure, especially avoidant and/or controlling/disorganized children, to show externalizing behavioral problems (Moss, Cyr, et al., 2004). In a clinical population, children classified as controlling/disorganized were more likely to be diagnosed with conduct disorder (for further information, see Lyons-Ruth & Jacobvitz, Chapter 29, this volume).

## CROSS-CULTURAL STUDIES AND OTHER RELATIONSHIPS

The PACS has been used to study attachment in the United States, England, Canada, and Romania. There is no published information on preschool attachment in countries or cultures other than these.

## The Main–Cassidy Attachment Classification for Kindergarten-Age Children

The Main and Cassidy (1988) attachment classification system for kindergarten-age children was developed on a sample of 33 children whose infant attachment classifications in the Strange Situation (A, B, and D) were known and who had experienced no major change in caretaking relationships. The system was further tested and extended on a new sample of 50 children that afforded enough C children to establish classification guidelines for this group. Classification is based on a child's behavior during the first 3 or 5 minutes of reunion with the parent following a 1-hour separation, rather than on the episodes and timing of the Strange Situation. Guidelines are provided for five major classification groups: "secure" (B), "avoidant" (A), "ambivalent" (C), "controlling" (D), and "unclassifiable" (U). Criteria for subgroup classifications are also provided. Rating scales for security and avoidance have been developed as well. The major criteria for classification are shown in Table 18.3.

### Short-Term Stability

Stability of classification over a 1-month period in Main and Cassidy's (1988) sample of 50 was 62%. Instability was largely due to change involving the controlling group. The authors suggest that instability in part reflects sensitization to the test situation (i.e., the relaxation of defenses under conditions of safety).

## Relation to Other Measures of Security

Main–Cassidy classifications have been shown to be related to secure versus insecure classifications using five different procedures for classifying children's representations of attachments, including picture-based and doll play protocols and family drawings (Barone & Lionetti, 2012; Behrens & Kaplan, 2011; Bureau, Béliveau, Moss, & Lépine, 2006; Gloger-Tippelt, Gomille, Koenig, & Vetter, 2002; Jacobsen & Hofmann, 1997; Solomon, George, & De Jong, 1995). Most systems captured secure versus insecure attachment status or show concordance for some of the A, B, C, and D groups. Only Solomon and George's ADPA differentiated reliably among all of the groups A–D in both a U.S. and a Japanese sample (Kayoko, 2006).

## Prediction to Core Variables

### MOTHER–CHILD INTERACTION

Based on their studies of a French Canadian sample, Moss and colleagues reported that mother–child interaction in secure dyads was more harmonious than that within insecure dyads, with the lowest scores received by mothers of controlling, disorganized, or unclassifiable children of all subtypes (Humber & Moss, 2005; Moss, Gosselin, Parent, Rousseau, & Dumont, 1997; Moss, Rousseau, Parent, St.-Laurent, & Saintonge, 1998). George and Solomon (1990, 1996, 2000) replicated this finding in their U.S. sample. Finally, in a study of Japanese kindergarteners, classification with the Main and Cassidy system was significantly associated with mothers' Adult Attachment Interview classifications (Behrens & Kaplan, 2011).

### CONTINUITY

Main and Cassidy (1988) and Wartner, Grossmann, Fremmer-Bombik, and Suess (1994) reported very high stability (kappa > .76) between 12-month and 6-year A, B, C, and D classifications with mothers. As described previously, Moss and colleagues (2005) recently demonstrated moderate continuity over a 2-year period between Cassidy and Marvin (1992) preschool classifications and adapted Main–Cassidy classifications at age 6.

### COHERENCE

Cohn (1990) and Wartner and colleagues (1994) found that securely attached children were judged to be more socially competent and accepted than the insecurely attached children, although the studies differed as to which insecure group showed the greatest deficit (C or A). Insecure classification, especially in the D group, was linked to externalizing behavioral problems in high- and low-risk samples (Easterbrooks, Biesecker, & Lyons-Ruth, 2000; Lecompte & Moss, 2014; Solomon et al., 1995). Paralleling these findings, Cassidy, Kirsh, Scolton, and Parke (1996, Study 2) found that secure children had more positive representations of peers' intentions and feelings, as assessed from social problem-solving vignettes, than did insecure children. Secure versus insecure Main–Cassidy classifications were also found to be related to representational measures of self-esteem and attachment, with secure children judged to be more open about themselves and about feelings of vulnerability than insecure children (Cassidy, 1988; Slough & Greenberg, 1990). Controlling children were found to depict more themes of conflict on a representational storytelling measure (Moss, Bureau, Béliveau, Zdebik, & Lépine, 2009). Seven year later, children classified controlling–punitive in kindergarten described themselves as higher in externalizing behavior at age 13, and their mothers were more likely to describe themselves as helpless to control the child (Lecompte & Moss, 2014).

### CROSS-CULTURAL STUDIES

The Main–Cassidy system has been used in the United States, Canada, Iceland, Germany, Italy, Australia, and Japan. Fathers' self-reported responsiveness to their child's distress, but not warmth, were associated with child classification group and lower avoidance (George, Cummings, & Davies, 2010).

## Discussion

Based on widespread use and the corresponding state of validation overall, the Cassidy and Marvin (1992) system must now be considered the preferred measure for assessment of attachment of 3- and 4-year-olds, especially for researchers who are interested in differences among the four classification groups. The measure has been investigated with respect to all of the validation criteria described earlier and appears to be related both to other relationship measures and to the core variables in ways that broadly parallel research on infant classifications.

In the 2008 edition of this volume, reports of low or inconsistent continuity between toddler and preschool classifications led us to question the validity of the PAC. Since then, accumulating evidence of limited stability of classifications in the 12- to 15-month range have caused us to rethink this issue. Furthermore, recent analyses of longitudinal data showing that PAC classifications correspond more closely than early classifications to 24 month AQS scores and to later socioemotional development indicate its value (Drake et al., 2014; Raikes & Thompson, 2008). Instability in classification may be a poor marker of the validity of the measure in this age range. Attachments are likely to undergo major change between the third and fifth years of life, reflecting expectable shifts in parent–child relationships and development in the child's capacity for language, representation, goal-corrected behavior, and self-control. Appropriately, studies of parent–child interaction in this period tend to focus on cooperation in cleanup tasks or joint cognitive problem solving rather than parental guidance of play. This may be one reason why researchers have found that preschool classifications show clearer relations to social problem solving and school readiness than do toddler classifications.

Finally, we would like to point out a methodological issue that may not have emerged clearly in earlier discussion. The Main–Cassidy classification system that served as a model for the PACs seems not to have seen much use in recent years. Possibly this is because it covers a transitional age between preschool and elementary school; possibly this is due to a scarcity of formal training opportunities for the Main–Cassidy system. Moss, and researchers trained by her, typically refer to adapting the Main–Cassidy procedure when their participants are 5–6 years of age. It is not always clear what is meant. In some reports, the 1-hour separation is shortened; in others, these investigators report basing classifications on two separations and reunions rather than one. From our own research with the Main–Cassidy system, we know that there can be surprising inconsistencies between first and second reunion behavior, with some children apparently changing from avoidant to ambivalent or the reverse, to provide one example. These adaptations may lead to classification differences between those trained by Moss and others who strictly follow the Main–Cassidy guidelines. There may be sound reasons for adaptations. Nevertheless, it has become something of a tradition for us, as authors of this chapter, to emphasize the need for better standardization and cross-validation of adapted measures, and we do so here again.

## Attachment Measures Based on Symbolic Representation

Bowlby (1969/1982) posited the construct of an internal representational model of attachment that arises from actual experiences and is used to evaluate present circumstances and guide future action. Such models are now conceptualized variously as comprising specific content or scripts, including affect, and information-processing rules that integrate and determine perception and memory (Bretherton, Grossmann, Grossmann, & Waters, 2005; Waters & Waters, 2006). Recent studies suggest that infants as young as 12 months may encode knowledge about their relationships in both representational and sensorimotor forms (Johnson et al., 2010). By the preschool years, symbolic forms of mental representation are readily accessed and therefore have been the subject of considerable research.

Research on children's internal representations of attachment was inspired by work in Main's laboratory in the mid-1980s, which led to the development of the Adult Attachment Interview (AAI; George, Kaplan, & Main, 1984, 1985, 1996). Beginning with Kaplan's (1987) attempts to capture representational processes in family drawings and the Separation Anxiety Test (see below), and Cassidy's (1988) self-esteem and family stories, investigators have gone on to create a wide variety of measures, some original, others adapted from previous efforts. No single measure has been systematically validated according to our criteria. Due to space limitations, we restrict our discussion to a few measures that are currently in use or have accumulated the most validity information. We briefly describe the general procedures for the different types of measures, along with key validation information. We further compare and contrast validation findings as part of a general discussion. We refer readers to the original reports and to previous editions of this book for additional information.

## Picture Response Measures

Two closely related measures (Kaplan, 1987; Slough & Greenberg, 1990) incorporate the procedures of the Separation Anxiety Test (SAT), a picture-response protocol that was first developed for adolescents by Shouldice and Stevenson-Hinde (1992) and modified from Hansburg (1972) for children ages 4–7 by Klagsbrun and Bowlby (1976). The procedure consists of a set of six photographs depicting attachment-related scenes ranging from mild (a parent says goodnight to a child in bed) to stressful (a child watches a parent leave). Each picture is introduced by an adult, and the child is asked to describe how the child in the picture feels and what that child will do. Kaplan (1987) developed a classification system for children's verbal responses to the pictures that differentiates attachment groups on the basis of emotional openness and ability to envision constructive solutions to feelings engendered by separation; this system was significantly related to 6-year-olds' infant attachment classifications. Using Kaplan's procedure or adaptations of it, other researchers find that SAT responses differentiate secure from insecure children's reunion and AQS security scores, self-acceptance, behavioral adjustment, and school and cognitive performance, and foster mothers' emotional investment in the child (Ackerman & Dozier, 2005; Clark & Symons, 2000; Easterbrooks et al., 2000; Jacobsen & Hoffmann, 1997).

## Doll Play

Several different doll-play protocols have been developed, along with major variants in approaches to classification and rating. Bretherton's original approach to studying symbolic representation in the preschool period, the ASCT (Bretherton et al., 1990) is the foundation for most of the work in this area. Here we describe Bretherton's system in some detail along with three commonly used variations: the ASCT Q-Sort Classification System (Miljkovitch, Pierrehumbert, Bretherton, & Halfon, 2004; Miljkovitch, Pierrehumbert, Karmaniola, & Halfon, 2003); the Attachment Doll Play Assessment (ADPA; George & Solomon, 1990, 1996, 2000), and the Manchester Child Attachment Story Task (MCAST; Goldwyn, Stanley, Smith, & Green, 2000). Other similar protocols appearing in the literature include those by Gloger-Tippelt and colleagues (2002), Op-

penheim (1997), and Verschueren, Marcoen, and Schoefs (1996).

The ASCT doll-play procedure was originally designed to assess attachment security in 4-year-olds. The procedure makes use of four stories: child spills juice, child hurts her knee, child "discovers" a monster in the bedroom, and parental separation–reunion. (Three of these four stories can also be found in the MacArthur Story Stem Battery (MSSB), a group of 10 stories reflecting a variety of parent–child interactions, which were developed in collaboration between Bretherton and other members of the MacArthur team (Bretherton et al., 1990). In the ASCT, an adult introduces each story with a story stem that describes what has happened, and the child is asked to enact what happens next using a standardized, four-member family (mother, father, and two siblings of the same gender as the child). Bretherton developed a classification system to identify the four main attachment groups (A, B, C, and D). Detailed transcripts are made of children's verbal behavior and enactment of each story, and classifications are based on summary scores of the children's predominant responses to the stories. Separate criteria for each story were established on a priori grounds based on characteristic reunion behavior for each group and Kaplan's early descriptions of SAT responses. Bretherton reported significant concordance with secure versus insecure classifications on the Cassidy and colleagues (1992) PACS. There was no match, however, for type of insecurity (A, C, D) across the two measures. Doll-play classifications were converted to security scores and were found to be highly correlated with prior AQS security scores at 25 months and marginally correlated with concurrent AQS security scores at 47 months. Variations on Bretherton's security scale in Portuguese samples replicated the finding of significant correspondence with prior AQS security scores of preschoolers (Wong et al., 2011) and demonstrated that security ratings of institutionalized four to eight year olds were lower than those of children in comparison samples and related to teacher and caretaker ratings of aggression (Torres, Maia, Verissimo, & Silva, 2012). Page and Bretherton (2001) developed an expanded assessment that also includes additional stories from the MSSB and an extensive set of categories representing attachment-related themes, scored simply present–absent. This approach does not permit ratings or classification of attachment but has been employed to describe children's representations of family relationships postdivorce (Bretherton et al., 2013; Page & Bretherton, 2001), and in studies of maltreatment and maternal depression (Macfie et al., 1999; Toth, Rogosch, Sturge-Apple, & Cicchetti, 2009; Trapolini, Ungerer, & McMahon, 2007).

Miljkovitch, Pierrehumbert, and colleagues (Miljkovitch et al., 2003, 2004; Pierrehumbert, Ramstein, Karmaniola, & Halfon, 1996) developed a Q-sort rating and classification procedure for children's ASCT narratives that is the basis for several studies by that group. It includes 65 items tapping content and narrative structure in a manner that is meant to parallel ratings for the AAI ratings. Along with the Q-sort, they developed a priori criterion sorts (i.e., profiles) for security, avoidance, ambivalence (hyperactivation), and disorganization (i.e., chaotic, violent events). They report high intercoder reliability for the Q-sort profiles, and researchers have posed interesting questions about non-normative groups; yet results of studies using this system are uneven. For example, with regard to the core variable of parental sensitivity, Miljkovitch and colleagues (2013) reported that maternal unresponsiveness during play at 6 months and low sensitivity at 12 months predicted ASCT disorganization at 42 months, but the positive end of those continua were unrelated to security. When maternal AAIs were used to establish predictive validity, concordance was found only for the ASCT secure and avoidant groups, but not the hypervigilant (ambivalent) or disorganized groups (Miljkovitch et al., 2004). In a similar study with a French sample of single and married parents, predicted concordance between the AAI and ASCT group was found for married but not for single mothers (Miljkovitch, Danet, & Bernier, 2012). Recent studies by Stievenart, Roskam, Meunier, and Van de Moortele (2012) with a Belgian sample show a lack of correspondence between AQS and the ASCT Q-sorts, and an overall increase in security and decrease in disorganization Q-scores between the ages of 3 and 8 among children with externalizing symptoms.

George and Solomon (1990, 1996, 2000; Solomon & George, 2002; Solomon et al., 1995) developed the ADPA using an alternative pattern-based approach to deriving classifications from doll-play responses to the ASCT (Bretherton) story stems. The system originally identified four attachment groups descriptively termed "confident" (B), "casual" (A), "busy" (C), and "frightened" (D). A later revision of this scheme integrated those classification criteria with Bowlby's (1973, 1980) description of defensive processes related to separation and loss. These patterns can also be detected in mothers' internal caregiving representations and in adult responses to projective attachment stimuli (George & West, 2012; Solomon & George, 1999a, 1999c, 1999d). Security is expected to reflect a flexible integration of attachment-related thoughts and feelings, whereas strategies of defensive exclusion of information can be systematically brought into play as responses to anxiety regarding attachment figures. These processes include *deactivation* (prevention of attachment-related thoughts and feelings) associated with avoidant classifications and *cognitive disconnection* (disconnection from awareness of the links between affect and thought), associated with ambivalent classification. When attachment-related distress cannot be contained (assuaged), "dysregulation" of the attachment system (or in Bowlby's [1980] terms, a "segregated system") is likely to be the result. Depiction of uncontained frightening and catastrophic events, as well as persistent constriction (refusal to play), is seen as evidence of dysregulation. Both the original and the revised systems were tested on a sample middle-class kindergartners (ages 5–7). Concordance between the revised representation classifications and attachment classifications based on reunion behavior is 79% (kappa = .70) (Kayoko, 2006; Solomon & George, 2002). Mother–child synchrony in a cooperative task significantly differentiated the secure from each of the insecure groups, with the largest differences occurring between the secure and disorganized groups (George & Solomon, unpublished data). The ADPA has been used successfully with a range of normative and high-risk samples (e.g., Goodman, Bartlett, & Stroh, 2013; Stacks & Oshio, 2009).

The MCAST (Goldwyn et al., 2000) constitutes a third, slightly different approach to classifying doll-play enactments. The procedures and stories differ slightly from the ASCT; most notably, in the MCAST a story about a child getting lost in the mall is substituted for the overnight separation and reunion story stem. The 33 scales devised for the procedure cover attachment behavior, coherence of the narrative, disorganized phenomena (both depicted and displayed by the subject), and mentalization. Protocols are classified into A, B, C, and D groups by comparing scale profiles to a priori profiles. In the original validation study with 4- to 7-year-olds, there was substantial stability of classification over a 5-month period. Children classified secure on the MCAST were also classified as secure on the SAT, but there was no discrimination regarding the insecure classifications. There was low to moderate concordance between secure and insecure child classifications and maternal AAI classifications, with the best match between disorganized child representation and maternal unresolved status. The MCAST has been administered to low-SES primary grade children (Berlin et al., 2011), children with reactive attachment disorder (Minnis et al., 2009), and those with conduct disorder (Pasalich, Dadds, Hawes, & Brennan, 2012). The disorganized classification was overrepresented in both clinical groups. The MCAST protocol has been computerized for ease of group administration (Minnis et al., 2009) and has been used to capture the movement toward security in a study of late adopted children (Pace, Zavattini, & D'Alessio, 2012).

### Family Drawing

Kaplan and Main (Main, Kaplan, & Cassidy, 1985) developed a preliminary classification system for the drawings of children of kindergarten age or older, based on features such as the individuality of family members, groundedness of the drawing, and frightening or overbright content. Some investigators report concordance between this system or adaptations of it and Strange Situation classifications, especially for the secure or disorganized groups (Benoit, Parker, & Zeanah 1997; Fury, Carlson, & Sroufe, 1997; Madigan, Goldberg, Moran, & Pederson, 2004; Madigan, Ladd, & Goldberg, 2003; Main, Kaplan, & Cassidy, 1985; Pianta, Longmaid, & Ferguson, 1999; but see Behrens & Kaplan, 2011). Clarke, Ungerer, Chahoud, Johnson, and Stiefel (2002) reported links among picture drawing classifications, SAT classifications, and Cassidy Puppet Interview classifications (designed to tap self-esteem) for a sample of boys with attention-deficit/hyperactivity disorder (ADHD).

### Discussion

A review of the available literature on measures of young children's representations of attachment reveals a wealth of efforts to capture variation related to security. Investigators find the representational measures to be a rich source of information and a fruitful basis for hypothesis generation. At their best, representational data reveal both the content and the structure of young

children's "state of mind" (Main, 2000) regarding attachment, permitting researchers to explore psychologically important regulatory processes in young children, such as fantasy and defense, and to trace the links between children's and adults' construction of representational models. Given the similarity between these procedures and traditional clinical tools such as doll play and family drawing, it is understandable that they have been readily adopted by researchers with clinical interests. Construct validation for any one measure is incomplete, yet, collectively, it seems that more researchers are attempting to assess their measures with respect to the four core hypotheses we have outlined. We urge investigators to establish the congruence of new measures with reunion or other interaction-based measures of child attachment security. This continues to be necessary because a high level of abstraction is inherent in the construct of an attachment representation, and children's cognitive and language development can influence the quality of their responses to representational stimuli.

Research to date demonstrates direct analogues to well-established qualitative differences in parent–child interaction and to representational processes identified in secure adults. For example, the behavior of the secure infant and kindergartner is characterized by open and direct communication of affect and by active, persistent, and unambivalent expression of attachment behavior. Criteria for representational security in several systems also include direct acknowledgment of affect (sadness, longing, anger) and a clear sense that reassurance or relief is forthcoming. In the ADPA classification system, secure children symbolically depict separation anxiety, as well as confidence, in the favorable resolution of these fears and concerns. Furthermore, the cognitive complexity and narrative structure of their play clearly parallel the coherence and integration of thought characteristic of the attachment representations of secure adults (Main, 2000). Studies focusing on representational processes in high-risk populations show that several of the available measures detect the disorganized end of the continuum in the form of highly aggressive, chaotic, or catastrophic representations of family life typically associated with disorganized attachment. To our knowledge, only the ADPA system places "frozen" or constricted doll play at that end of the continuum as well. The former are associated with controlling–punitive reunion behavior in the Main and Cassidy system, whereas the latter are associated with controlling–caregiving classification (Solomon et al., 1995).

Most of the representational measures show correspondences with either concurrent or prior attachment measures, but none, except the ADPA and, in some studies, the Kaplan SAT classification, differentiates completely or reliably among insecure reunion classifications. This means that most of the systems we described earlier ought not to be used as attachment classification proxies. We speculate that the relative success of the ADPA and Kaplan's SAT stems from a development process that focused on cases with known classification, allowing the developer to home in on the features of greatest importance (see also Main & Cassidy, 1988). The more common approach is to move from theory to a priori categories based on what might appear to be qualitative parallels between behavior and representation.

We briefly note two areas that need special attention as measures continue to be refined. First, we encourage investigators to develop measures directly from the representational material produced by a particular procedure, instead of relying on a priori considerations alone or "borrowing" criteria from one measure and applying them to another. For example, it appears that in response to SAT stimuli, avoidant children often say, "I don't know." In the ADPA, this response is not characteristic of avoidant children when they are responding to doll-play scenarios; when it is repeated or mixed with other "response-avoidant" tactics, it is instead characteristic of some controlling/disorganized children. Transfer of Kaplan's picture-based system to doll-play materials may be one reason why several doll-play-based systems have failed to distinguish among insecure classification groups. Verbal responses to pictures and doll play may well draw on different memory processes (e.g., explicit vs. implicit memory).

Second, we continue to be uneasy with how freely investigators adjust or reinvent coding and rating scales from the originals, borrow scales and operational definitions from other systems, and extend rating and classification systems to older or younger children without clear rationale or revalidation of the new approach. Space limitations have precluded detailed description of all of the methodological variations flying under the same banner, so to speak, but there are certainly many available. Diversity in approach is essential to the joint project of construct validation. Yet standardization of procedures and definitions of variables (e.g., security) is required to replicate findings, understand replication failures, and make punitive progress in general.

On a hopeful note, we are pleased to call attention to a promising new paradigm for assessing mental representations of attachment in infants as young as age 12 months (Johnson & Chen, 2011). Johnson and colleagues (2010) used a visual habituation paradigm and animated video stimuli to test the implicit expectations of 12-month-olds about the responsiveness of mothers. In the simplest protocol, infants were habituated to a video depicting a large, nonrepresentational shape (the mother) moving away from a small one, which then cried. Infants were next shown a test video depicting either the return of the large figure to the small one (responsive mother portrayal) or the further removal of that figure (unresponsive mother portrayal). Results showed that secure infants looked longer at the mother in the unresponsive scenario, implying a violation of their expectations, whereas insecure infants looked longer at the responsive mother video, suggesting that maternal responsiveness violated their expectations. The investigators have focused on contributory hormonal and genetic factors to this phenomenon. Clearly, however, this general paradigm will allow exploration of a host of questions about individual differences in very early representational processes.

## The AQS: Infancy through 5 Years

In contrast to systems of classifying child behavior and representation, the AQS assesses the quality of a child's secure-base behavior in the home. The system was developed by Waters (1995) to provide a practical alternative to the Ainsworth home observation narratives. Within the AQS system, secure-base behavior is defined as the smooth organization of and appropriate balance between proximity seeking and exploration (Posada, Waters, Crowell, & Lay, 1995). The Q-set for the AQS consists of 90 items designed to tap a range of phenomena believed to reflect either the secure-base phenomenon itself or behavior associated with it in children ages 1–5. Items are sorted into one of nine piles, according to whether they are considered characteristic or uncharacteristic of a child's behavior. Sorts can be completed by trained observers or by parents. Waters (1995) recommends that sorts by observers be based on two to three visits, for a total of 2–6 hours of observation in the home, with additional observations if observers disagree.

The AQS permits the salience of a behavior in a child's repertoire to be distinguished from the frequency with which the behavior occurs. In addition, it helps to prevent observer biases and lends itself to an array of qualitative and quantitative analyses. AQS data can be analyzed in terms of individual items or summary scales, or a child's Q-sort profile can be compared to a criterion sort. Waters developed criterion sorts for the construct of attachment security and for several other constructs (social desirability, dependence, sociability) by collecting and averaging the item sorts of experts in the attachment research field. The child's security score is the correlation coefficient between the observer's sort and the criterion sort; it represents the child's placement on a linear continuum with respect to the security construct. Validated sorts for the A, C, or D insecure attachment groups defined by the Strange Situation are not available, although some researchers have developed classifications on a priori grounds for particular purposes (Howes & Wishard Guerra, 2009; Smeekens, Riksen-Walraven, & Van Bakel, 2009). We return to the issue of demarcating classification groups with AQS criterion scores later in this section.

Van IJzendoorn and colleagues (2004) undertook a meta-analysis of 139 AQS studies ($N$ = 13,835 children, ages 12–70 months) for the purpose of establishing the validity of this measure. Below we rely on their findings for parsimony but refer to specific studies in which updated information is available or when specific points require a more fine-grained approach.

## Intercoder Agreement

In comparison to classification systems, reliability on the AQS does not require extensive training or certification of reliability. Studies report interobserver reliability (correlations between sorts) ranging from .72 to .95. The correlation between mothers' and trained observers' sorts tends to be moderate (approximately .40 to .55) in small to medium-size samples but improves considerably as a function of training and supervision of mothers, as well as the degree to which observers have opportunity to see a sufficient range of child behavior (Teti & McGourty, 1996). Tarabulsy and colleagues (2008) found that residual maternal and observer scores result in different patterns of correlation with extraneous factors such as temperament and psychosocial risk, indicating that

multiple observers are preferable for generating reliable data.

## Short-Term Stability

Short-term stability data, representing repeated sorts in close succession, are not reported in the literature.

## Relation to Other Measures of Attachment

AQS security scores differentiate infants classified as secure and insecure in the Strange Situation in several but not all published studies. Average AQS scores for the secure group in the Strange Situation tend to range from about .30 to .50; average scores for the insecure groups tend to be about .25 (Waters & Deane, 1985). Paralleling Ainsworth's original finding that insecure groups are difficult to distinguish on the basis of their behavior in the home, distinctive differences between infants classified as A or C in the Strange Situation typically do not emerge clearly; however, infants classified as disorganized in the Strange Situation are characterized by very low or negative AQS scores.

Van IJzendoorn and colleagues' (2004) meta-analysis reveals significantly lower correlations between the AQS and reunion-based attachment measures for preschoolers than for younger children. Moss and colleagues (2006) found the two measures to be significantly associated overall, with significant differences between the secure and the disorganized and ambivalent classifications, but not between the secure, avoidant or controlling ones. Results from Posada (2006), however, are consistent with the meta-analysis. Links between AQS security and representational measures are also somewhat mixed; there are positive correlations at 25 months and 37 months using the Bretherton ASCT measure, but failure to find a relation in others using different doll-play measures (Oppenheim, 1997; Smeekens et al., 2009; Stievenart et al., 2012).

## Prediction to Core Variables

### Parent–Child Interaction

Across both the infancy and preschool periods, maternal sensitivity scores based on brief home visits are significantly related to AQS security, especially using observer-generated sorts. In contrast to Strange Situation classifications, assessments of temperament, especially negative reactivity, show moderate correlations with AQS security, but, again, less so for observer-generated sorts than for caregiver-generated ones. Some researchers reported moderate concordance between mothers' and fathers' AQS security scores, which might also reflect the effect of temperament, among other factors (Bakermans-Kranenburg, Van IJzendoorn, Bokhorst, & Schuengel, 2004; Caldera & Lindsey, 2006). Van IJzendoorn 's meta-analysis revealed no relation between security with father and AQS scores, or between paternal sensitivity and AQS security. However, a recent, carefully conducted study by Brown, Mangelsdorf, and Neff (2012) revealed significant associations between paternal sensitivity and AQS scores at 36 months.

## Continuity

Using caregiver sorts, Belsky and Rovine (1990) and Teti and McGourty (1996) reported low to moderate long-term stability between ages 1 and 3. Steele and colleagues (2014) demonstrated significant but low continuity between 24-month-olds' AQS scores and secure base script knowledge at age 18.

## Coherence

In Van IJzendoorn and colleagues' (2004) meta-analysis and in more recent studies, AQS security is significantly related to measures of social competence with peers and siblings, to fewer child problem behaviors, and to greater child empathy (Murphy & Laible, 2013). A variety of parental and couple/family variables (e.g., marital/couple relationship quality, social support, parenting stress, SES) also appear to be related to AQS security (Howes & Wishard Guerra, 2009; Moss et al., 2006). Raikes and Thompson (2008) found that AQS security was superior to Strange Situation measures at 15 and 36 months in predicting declines in peer conflict from preschool to first grade.

## Cross-Cultural Studies

In a major study on the cross-cultural validity of the AQS, researchers determined that mothers and experts in a range of countries (China, Japan, Israel, Columbia, Germany, Norway, and the United States) discriminated attachment security from the constructs of dependency and social desirability (Posada et al., 1995). Although the structure of the data was broadly similar cross-culturally, the correlations among maternal sorts across cultures tends to be low. Posada and colleagues (2013) extended this approach by showing broad cross-cultural agreement among experts about the manifestations of secure-base behavior in the home in nine different countries. Mothers' sorts demonstrated both the normative nature of secure-base behavior as assessed with the AQS and unique cultural profiles.

## Discussion

The great promise of the AQS lies in its emphasis on naturalistic observation in ecologically valid contexts. The procedure can be used reliably across a variety of national, cultural, and risk groups. From a practical perspective, it permits researchers to estimate attachment security without the need for laboratory space and equipment or extensive training of observers. For the infancy period (ages 12–18 months), there is a substantial literature demonstrating a reliable though modest correspondence with judgments of security in the Strange Situation and with maternal sensitivity; a more inconsistent picture of the relationships among these variables emerges for the preschool period. The AQS procedure also does not allow reliable distinctions to be made among the insecure groups, although, as would be predicted theoretically, infants and children classified as disorganized are characterized by the lowest security scores (Atkinson et al., 1999; Roskam, Meunier, & Stievenart, 2011).

In versions of this chapter in earlier editions, we commented extensively on possible reasons for this divergence. Given limited space, we refer readers to those earlier discussions and turn instead to recent developments. Somewhat ironically, the first of these is an upsurge in the number of investigators describing their AQS findings in terms of secure versus insecure classifications or even disorganized classifications (Altenhofen, Clyman, Little, Baker, & Biringen, 2013; Bergin & McCollough, 2009; Howes & Wishard Guerra, 2009; Niemann & Weiss, 2011; Smeekens et al., 2009; Stievenart et al., 2012; Steele et al., 2014). For this purpose, the investigators cite previous studies (e.g., Park & Waters, 1989) that used AQS scores in the neighborhood of .33 as a security cutoff score. Most of the previously described studies focus on atypical populations, such as foster care and adopted children, cocaine exposed infants, and immigrant families. It is understandable that authors want to make use of comparisons to the well-established Strange Situation categories, especially when communicating clinical data; the AQS is certainly more portable and "user-friendly" than Strange Situation procedures. We see this practice as an unfortunate expedient, however. There is as yet relatively little empirical information about how high-risk and clinical samples differ from normative ones in the distribution of AQS security scores or how these scores map onto actual Strange Situation classifications. Such data are costly and time-consuming to gather. Until more suitable methodological tools are available, however, we remind researchers that the AQS security criterion represents only one of the many dimensions relevant to classification; the data cannot be "reverse-engineered" to approximate Strange Situation classifications.

In this context, we note with interest some initial attempts to create "user-friendly," brief attachment assessment tools. For example, John, Morris, and Halliburton (2012) asked mothers of intellectually disabled children in India to rate 62 of the AQS items on a scale from 1 (characteristic of her child) to 3 (uncharacteristic of her child). Cronbach's alpha was .77. These Q ratings were modestly but significantly correlated with scores for the mother's Emotional Availability. This technique was adapted from work by Roggman (Coyl, Newland, & Freeman, 2010; Newland, Coyl, & Freeman, 2008), who found that mothers' ratings were highly correlated with their subsequent sorts, following 2 weeks of observation of their child ($r$ = .62). Although one could wish for considerably more validation of the "Q-list," this technique has the merit of simplicity, and further development of this measure and others like it may be promising in future. A different approach is illustrated by Andreassen and West (2007), who described painstaking efforts to create a 45-item Toddler Attachment Q-Sort (TAQS-45) for over 10,000 preschoolers who were part of the Early Childhood Longitudinal Study–Birth Cohort. Preliminary validation on a small sample of preschoolers showed a positive relation between security and dyadic mutuality (Spieker, Nelson, & Condon, 2011). Readers may also be interested in work by Tarabulsy and colleagues (2009) as an example of this kind of adaptation, applied to the validation of shortened version of the Maternal Behavior Q-Sort.

## Conclusions

Our survey of the research in attachment measurement for infants and young children has given us a reasonably good overview of the area and a sense of where the field as a whole seems to be heading. The period since the last edition of this handbook has not seen major development of new measures. Despite unresolved methodological questions, investigators have made use of the available "good-enough" instruments and protocols to press on, focusing in particular on more diverse and high-risk populations, intervention studies, biological mechanisms, and long-term developmental trajectories.

This is a good time to consider whether the available attachment measures and their adaptations (validated or intuitively crafted) are adequate for the questions investigators wish to study, or whether new tools are now required. In our view, there is a need for two kinds of methodological tools. The first may be described as "efficient" measures, that is, observer- or parent-generated, that are suitable for large-scale, multivariate research and intervention studies. Conventional questionnaires have proven difficult to design in this field (but see George and Solomon, 2011). In part, this is because of the difficulty of getting past parents' defensive exclusion of the very information we would like them to report (George & West, 2012). The AQS seems to be the most promising instrument to adapt for this purpose. The full process, however, can take one to several hours to complete. Earlier we described attempts to create short-form AQSs that might be suitable for large samples or subjects with limited time available. To our knowledge, these adaptations have not been validated against Strange Situation classifications, but this should be feasible. These efforts are promising, but we refer researchers to our previous cautions about using Q-sort data as a substitute for attachment classification.

Though less efficient, there is also a need for new or revised measures based on direct observation, the tradition that was so fruitful in the early years of building and testing attachment theory. There is a particular need for improved measurement for the D classification, which is evidently characteristic of a very broad group of infants in high-risk samples but is also in normative samples. The developmental and mental health risks associated with disorganization appear to go beyond the early findings of a link between maltreatment and disorganization, and may include the full range of externalizing disorders (from classroom disruption to callous–unemotional traits), borderline and dissociative disorders, and, possibly, a range of internalizing disorders (see Lyons-Ruth & Jacobvitz, Chapter 29, this volume). As a first step in this process, it might be worthwhile to reexamine the extensive list of D indices that are used for classification, originally delineated by Main and Solomon (1990). The indices are grouped according to classes of conflict behavior, dissociative processes, states of fear and confusion, or heterogeneous varieties of anomalous behavior patterns. The underlying logic of this categorization, naturally enough, presumes a particular causal explanation structure—Main's hypothesis that disorganization reflects irresolvable conflict aroused by a frightening or frightened parent (Hesse & Main, 2000). But there may be other ways to organize the indices to reveal the existence of additional mechanisms or processes. For examples of preliminary approaches to understanding individual differences among the indices, see Forbes, Cox, Moran, and Pederson (2006) and Padrón and colleagues (2014).

In this context, we reprise a concern that we expressed in the second edition of the *Handbook of Attachment*: the assessment of attachment for children who have or are continuing to experience deprivation of attachment figures, disrupted attachments, and major or frequent separations. These children were originally of great interest to Bowlby and other researchers who contributed to our basic knowledge in this area. They are also a population of growing interest to attachment researchers and increasingly fill the caseloads of infant mental health and other clinical practitioners—many of whom use (or would like to use) conventional attachment measures as part of their assessments. It is not clear, however, that our current attachment methodology is sensitive enough for clinical uses or whether there are modifications that might make it so.

We propose that questions such as these require a new look at standard measures and the development of new, ecologically valid ones. Attachment researchers are aware that the interpretation of separation–reunion procedures is questionable when it is uncertain whether a child has developed an attachment to a particular caregiver, or when the child has recently undergone a major separation. Disorganized attachment is very commonly observed in adopted and foster children and in young institutionalized children. The meaning of this "disorganized" attachment behavior cannot be assumed to be the same as it is for typical, home-

reared children. Many of these children show, in addition, what have been termed "anomalous" patterns that are not well described in the literature (see Jacobsen & Haight, 2011; Zeanah et al., 2005). There is clearly a need for further behavioral differentiation among all of these groups of children, including those who merit the "atypical" or "unclassifiable" label (Kreppner, Rutter, Marvin, O'Connor, & Sonuga-Barke, 2011). Careful observation may reveal behavioral variants that discriminate among various etiological conditions. In short, we need a reexamination of the separation–reunion behavior of these children—akin to what was involved originally in detecting disorganization of attachment (Main & Solomon, 1986, 1990). Additional research is equally necessary to explore the nature of attachment under other very adverse conditions (e.g., when parents are severely mentally ill) and to determine whether disorganized attachment behavior in benign circumstances carries much risk at all. The present methodological challenge is to expand our ability to make finer distinctions within the disorganized group, which currently is undifferentiated. We end this chapter, confident that we will see progress in this fertile area.

## Notes

1. It must be emphasized that the construct of security is meaningful only for a relationship in which a child has already developed an attachment to a particular caregiver. In situations where this is in doubt (e.g., in studies involving transitions to foster care), the interpretation of any measure of security is problematic.

2. For this review, we rely mainly on the published, English-language journal literature. This may have the unintended consequence of exaggerating the appearance of a relation between any two variables, but it ensures that studies have undergone peer review and that we ourselves have seen the article.

## References

Ackerman, J. P., & Dozier, M. (2005). The influence of foster parent investment on children's representations of self and attachment figures. *Journal of Applied Developmental Psychology, 26*, 507–520.
Ainsworth, M. D. S., Blehar, M. C., Waters, E., & Wall, S. (1978). *Patterns of attachment: A psychological study of the Strange Situation*. Hillsdale, NJ: Erlbaum.
Ainsworth, M. D. S., & Marvin, R. S. (1995). On the shaping of attachment theory and research: An in-

terview with Mary D. S. Ainsworth (Fall 1994). In E. Waters, B. E. Vaughn, G. Posada, & K. Kondo-Ikemura (Eds.), Caregiving, cultural, and cognitive perspectives on secure-base behavior and working models: New growing points of attachment theory and research. *Monographs of the Society for Research in Child Development* (2–3, Serial No. 244), 3–21.

Altenhofen, S., Clyman, R., Little, C., Baker, M., & Biringen, Z. (2013). Attachment security in three-year-olds who entered substitute care in infancy. *Infant Mental Health Journal, 34*(5), 435–445.

Andreassen, C., & West, J. (2007). Measuring socioemotional functioning in a national birth cohort study. *Infant Mental Health Journal, 28*, 627–646.

Atkinson, L., Chisholm, V. C., Scott, B., Goldberg, S., Vaughn, B. E., Blackwell, J., et al. (1999). Maternal sensitivity, child functional level, and attachment in down syndrome. *Monographs of the Society for Research in Child Development, 64*, 45–66.

Bakermans-Kranenburg, M. J., Van IJzendoorn, M. H., Bokhorst, C. L., & Schuengel, C. (2004). The importance of shared environment in infant–father attachment: A behavioral genetic study of the Attachment Q-Sort. *Journal of Family Psychology, 18*, 545–549.

Bar-Haim, Y., Sutton, D. B., Fox, N. A., & Marvin, R. S. (2000). Stability and change of attachment at 14, 24, and 58 months of age: Behavior, representation, and life events. *Journal of Child Psychology and Psychiatry, 41*, 381–388.

Barnett, D., Clements, M., Kaplan-Estrin, M., McCaskill, J. W., Hunt, K. H., Butler, C. M., et al. (2006). Maternal resolution of child diagnosis: Stability and relations with child attachment across the toddler to preschooler transition. *Journal of Family Psychology, 20*, 100–107.

Barone, L., & Lionetti, F. (2012). Attachment and emotional understanding: A study on late-adopted preschoolers and their parents. *Child: Care, Health and Development, 38*, 690–696.

Behrens, K., & Kaplan, N. (2011). Japanese children's family drawings and their link to attachment. *Attachment and Human Development, 13*, 437–450.

Belsky, J., Campbell, S. B., Cohn, J. F., & Moore, G. (1996). Instability of infant–parent attachment security. *Developmental Psychology, 32*, 921–924.

Belsky, J., & Rovine, M. (1990). Q-sort security and first-year nonmaternal care. *New Directions for Child Development, 49*, 7–22.

Benoit, D., Parker, K. C. H., & Zeanah, C. H. (1997). Mothers' representations of their infants assessed prenatally: Stability and association with infants' attachment classifications. *Journal of Child Psychology and Psychiatry, 38*, 307–313.

Bergin, C., & McCollough, P. (2009). Attachment in substance-exposed toddlers: The role of caregiving and exposure. *Infant Mental Health Journal, 30*, 407–423.

Berlin, L. J., Whiteside-Mansell, L., Roggman, L. A., Green, B. L., Robinson, J., & Spieker, S. (2011). Testing maternal depression and attachment style as

moderators of Early Head Start's effects on parenting. *Attachment and Human Development, 13*, 49–67.

Bowlby, J. (1973). *Attachment and loss: Vol. 2. Separation: Anxiety and anger.* New York: Basic Books.

Bowlby, J. (1980). *Attachment and loss: Vol. 3. Loss: Sadness and depression.* New York: Basic Books.

Bowlby, J. (1982). *Attachment and loss: Vol. 1. Attachment.* New York: Basic Books. (Original work published 1969)

Bretherton, I., Grossmann, K. E., Grossmann, K., & Waters, E. (2005). In pursuit of the internal working model construct and its relevance to attachment relationships. In K. E. Grossmann, K. Grossmann, & E. Waters (Eds.), *Attachment from infancy to adulthood: The major longitudinal studies* (pp. 13–47). New York: Guilford Press.

Bretherton, I., Gullón-Rivera, Á. L., Page, T. F., Oettel, B. J., Corey, J. M., & Golby, B. J. (2013). Children's attachment-related self-worth: A multi-method investigation of postdivorce preschoolers' relationships with their mothers and peers. *Attachment and Human Development, 15*(1), 25–49.

Bretherton, I., Oppenheim, D., Buchsbaum, H., Emde, R., & the MacArthur Narrative Group. (1990). *The MacArthur Story Stem Battery.* Unpublished manuscript, University of Wisconsin–Madison.

Bretherton, I., Ridgeway, D., & Cassidy, J. (1990). Assessing internal working models of the attachment relationship: An attachment story completion task for 3-year-olds. In M. T. Greenberg, D. Cicchetti, & E. M. Cummings (Eds.), *Attachment in the preschool years* (pp. 273–308). Chicago: University of Chicago Press.

Britner, P. A., Marvin, R. S., & Pianta, R. C. (2005). Development and preliminary validation of the caregiving behavior system: Association with child attachment classification in the preschool Strange Situation. *Attachment and Human Development, 7*, 83–102.

Brown, G. L., Mangelsdorf, S. C., & Neff, C. (2012). Father involvement, paternal sensitivity, and father–child attachment security in the first 3 years. *Journal of Family Psychology, 26*, 421–430.

Bureau, J.-F., Béliveau, M.-J., Moss, E., & Lépine, S. (2006). Association entre l'attachement mère-enfant et les récits d'attachement à la période scolaire. [Association between mother–child attachment and attachment narratives during the school-age years]. *Canadian Journal of Behavioural Science, 38*, 50–62.

Caldera, Y. M., & Lindsey, E. W. (2006). Coparenting, mother–infant interaction, and infant–parent attachment relationships in two-parent families. *Journal of Family Psychology, 20*, 275–283.

Campbell, D., & Fiske, D. (1959). Convergent and discriminant validation by the multitrait–multimethod matrix. *Psychological Bulletin, 56*, 81–105.

Campbell, S. B., Brownell, C. A., Hungerford, A., Spieker, S. J., Mohan, R., & Blessing, J. S. (2004). The course of maternal depressive symptoms and maternal sensitivity as predictors of attachment security at 36 months. *Development and Psychopathology,* 16(2), 231–252.

Carlson, E. A. (1998). A prospective longitudinal study of attachment disorganization/disorientation. *Child Development,* 69, 1107–1128.

Carlson, E. A., & Sroufe, L. A. (1993, Spring). Reliability in attachment classification. *Society for Research in Child Development Newsletter,* p. 12.

Cassidy, J. (1988). Child–mother attachment and the self. *Child Development,* 59, 121–134.

Cassidy, J., Berlin, L., & Belsky, J. (1990, April). *Attachment organization at age 3: Antecedent and concurrent correlates.* Paper presented at the biennial meetings of the International Conference on Infant Studies, Montreal, Canada.

Cassidy, J., Kirsh, S. J., Scolton, K. L., & Parke, R. D. (1996). Attachment and representations of peer relationships. *Developmental Psychology,* 32(5), 892–904.

Cassidy, J., & Marvin, R. S., with the MacArthur Attachment Working Group. (1992). *Attachment organization in preschool children: Coding guidelines* (4th ed.). Unpublished manuscript, University of Virginia.

Cicchetti, D., & Barnett, D. (1991). Attachment organization in maltreated preschoolers. *Development and Psychopathology,* 3, 397–411.

Clark, S. E., & Symons, D. K. (2000). A longitudinal study of Q-sort attachment security and self-processes at age 5. *Infant and Child Development,* 9, 91–104.

Clarke, L., Ungerer, J., Chahoud, K., Johnson, S., & Stiefel, I. (2002). Attention deficit hyperactivity disorder is associated with attachment insecurity. *Clinical Child Psychology and Psychiatry,* 7, 179–198.

Cohn, D. A. (1990). Child–mother attachment of six-year-olds and social competence at school. *Child Development,* 61, 152–162.

Cox, M. J., Owen, M. T., Henderson, V. K., & Margand, N. A. (1992). Prediction of infant–father and infant–mother attachment. *Developmental Psychology,* 28, 474–483.

Coyl, D. D., Newland, L. A., & Freeman, H. (2010). Predicting preschoolers' attachment security from parenting behaviours, parents' attachment relationships and their use of social support. *Early Child Development and Care,* 180, 499–512.

Crittenden, P. M. (1992a, 1994). *Preschool Assessment of Attachment.* Unpublished manuscript, Family Relations Institute, Miami, FL.

Crittenden, P. M. (1992b). The quality of attachment in the preschool years. *Development and Psychopathology,* 4, 209–241.

Crittenden, P., Kozlowska, K., & Landini, A. (2010). Assessing attachment in school-age children. *Clinical Child Psychology and Psychiatry,* 15, 185–208.

De Wolff, M., & Van IJzendoorn, M. H. (1997). Sensitivity and attachment: A meta-analysis on parental antecedents of infant attachment. *Child Development,* 6, 571–591.

Dexter, C. A., Wong, K., Stacks, A. M., Beeghly, M.,

& Barnett, D. (2013). Parenting and attachment among low-income African American and Caucasian preschoolers. *Journal of Family Psychology,* 27(4), 629–638.

Drake, K., Belsky, J., & Fearon, R. M. P. (2014). From early attachment to engagement with learning in school: The role of self-regulation and persistence. *Development and Psychology,* 50, 1350–1361.

Easterbrooks, M. A., Biesecker, G., & Lyons-Ruth, K. (2000). Infancy predictors of emotional availability in middle childhood: The roles of attachment security and maternal depressive symptomatology. *Attachment and Human Development,* 2, 170–187.

Erikson, E. H. (1950). *Childhood and society.* New York: Norton.

Farnfield, S., Hautamäki, A., Nørbech, P., & Sahhar, N. (2010). DMM assessments of attachment and adaptation: Procedures, validity and utility. *Clinical Child Psychology and Psychiatry,* 15, 313–328.

Fearon, R. M. P., & Belsky, J. (2011). Infant–mother attachment and the growth of externalizing problems across the primary-school years. *Journal of Child Psychology and Psychiatry,* 52, 782–791.

Fearon, R. M. P., Van IJzendoorn, M. H., Fonagy, P., Bakermans-Kranenburg, M. J., Schuengel, C., & Bokhorst, C. L. (2006). In search of shared and non-shared environmental factors in security of attachment: A behavior-genetic study of the association between sensitivity and attachment security. *Developmental Psychology,* 42, 1026–1040.

Fish, M. (2004). Attachment in infancy and preschool in low socioeconomic status rural Appalachian children: Stability and change and relations to preschool and kindergarten competence. *Development and Psychopathology,* 16, 293–312.

Forbes, L. M., Cox, A., Moran, G., & Pederson, D. R. (2006, July). *Exploring expressions of disorganization in the Strange Situation in a high-risk sample.* Poster presented at the World Association for Infant Mental Health, Paris, France.

Fraley, R. C., & Spieker, S. J. (2003). Are infant attachment patterns continuously or categorically distributed?: A taxometric analysis of strange situation behavior. *Developmental Psychology,* 39, 387–404.

Fury, G. S., Carlson, E. A., & Sroufe, L. A. (1997). Children's representations of attachment in family drawings. *Child Development,* 68, 1154–1164.

George, C., Kaplan, N., & Main, M. (1984, 1985, 1996). *Adult Attachment Interview protocol.* Unpublished manuscript, University of California at Berkeley.

George, C., & Solomon, J. (1990, 1996, 2000). *Six-year attachment doll play classification system.* Unpublished manuscript, Mills College, Oakland, CA.

George, C., & Solomon, J. (2011). Caregiving helplessness: The development of a screening measure for disorganized maternal caregiving. In J. Solomon & C. George (Ed.), *Disorganized attachment and caregiving* (pp. 133–166). New York: Guilford Press.

George, C., & West, M. L. (2012). *The Adult Attachment*

*Projective Picture System: Attachment theory and assessment in adults.* New York: Guilford Press.

George, M., Cummings, E. M., & Davies, P. T. (2010). Positive aspects of fathering and mothering, and children's attachment in kindergarten. *Early Child Development and Care, 180*(1–2), 107–119.

Gloger-Tippelt, G., Gomille, B., Koenig, L., & Vetter, J. (2002). Attachment representations in 6-year-olds: Related longitudinally to the quality of attachment in infancy and mothers' attachment representations. *Attachment and Human Development, 4,* 318–339.

Goldwyn, R., Stanley, C., Smith, V., & Green, J. (2000). The Manchester Child Attachment Story Task: Relationship with the parental AAI, SAT, and child behavior. *Attachment and Human Development, 2,* 71–84.

Goodman, G., Bartlett, R. C., & Stroh, M. (2013). Mothers' borderline features and children's disorganized attachment representations as predictors of children's externalizing behavior. *Psychoanalytic Psychology, 30*(1), 16–36.

Groh, A. M., Roisman, G. I., Booth-LaForce, C., Fraley, R. C., Owen, M. T., Cox, M. J., et al. (2014). The Adult Attachment Interview: Psychometrics, stability and change from infancy, and developmental origins: IV. Stability of attachment security from infancy to late adolescence. *Monographs of the Society for Research in Child Development, 79*(3), 51–66.

Groh, A. M., Roisman, G. I., Van IJzendoorn, M. H., Bakermans-Kranenburg, M. J., & Fearon, P. (2012). The significance of insecure and disorganized attachment for children's internalizing symptoms: A meta-analytic study. *Child Development, 83,* 591–610.

Hamilton, C. E. (2000). Continuity and discontinuity of attachment from infancy through adolescence. *Child Development, 71,* 690–694.

Hansburg, H. G. (1972). *Adolescent separation anxiety: Vol. 1. A method for the study of adolescent separation problems.* Springfield, IL: Charles C Thomas.

Hautamäki, A., Hautamäki, L., Neuvonen, L., & Maliniemi-Piispanen, S. (2010). Transmission of attachment across three generations. *European Journal of Developmental Psychology, 7*(5), 618–634.

Hesse, E., & Main, M. (2000). Disorganized infant, child, and adult attachment: Collapse in behavioral and attentional strategies. *Journal of the American Psychoanalytic Association, 48,* 1097–1127.

Hesse, E., & Main, M. (2006). Frightened, threatening, and dissociative parental behavior in low-risk samples: Description, discussion, and interpretations. *Development and Psychopathology, 18,* 309–343.

Howes, C., & Wishard Guerra, A. G. (2009). Networks of attachment relationships in low-income children of Mexican heritage: Infancy through preschool. *Social Development, 18,* 896–914.

Humber, N., & Moss, E. (2005). The relationship of preschool and early school age attachment to mother–child interaction. *American Journal of Orthopsychiatry, 75,* 128–141.

Jacobsen, T., & Hofmann, V. (1997). Children's at- tachment representations: Longitudinal relations to school behavior and academic competency in middle childhood and adolescence. *Developmental Psychology, 33,* 703–710.

John, A., Morris, A. S., & Halliburton, A. L. (2012). Looking beyond maternal sensitivity: Mother–child correlates of attachment security among children with intellectual disabilities in urban India. *Journal of Autism and Developmental Disorders, 42*(11), 2335–2345.

Johnson, S. C., & Chen, F. S. (2011). Socioemotional information processing in human infants: From genes to subjective construals. *Emotion Review, 3*(2), 169–178.

Johnson, S. C., Dweck, C. S., Chen, F. S., Stern, H. L., Ok, S.-J., & Barth, M. (2010). At the intersection of social and cognitive development: Internal working models of attachment in infancy. *Cognitive Science, 34*(5), 807–825.

Kaplan, N. (1987). *Individual differences in six-year-olds' thoughts about separation: Predicted from attachment to mother at one year of age.* Unpublished doctoral dissertation, University of California at Berkeley.

Kayoko, Y. (2006). Assessing attachment representations in early childhood: Validation of the attachment doll play. *Japanese Journal of Educational Psychology, 54,* 476–486.

Klagsbrun, M., & Bowlby, J. (1976). Responses to separation from parents: A clinical test for young children. *British Journal of Projective Psychology, 21,* 7–21.

Kreppner, J., Rutter, M., Marvin, R., O'Connor, T., & Sonuga-Barke, E. (2011). Assessing the concept of the 'insecure-other' category in the Cassidy–Marvin scheme: Changes between 4 and 6 years in the English and Romanian adoptee study. *Social Development, 20,* 1–16.

Lecompte, V., & Moss, E. (2014). Disorganized and controlling patterns of attachment, role reversal, and caregiving helplessness: Links to adolescents' externalizing problems. *American Journal of Orthopsychiatry, 84,* 581–589.

Leerkes, E. M. (2011). Maternal sensitivity during distressing tasks: A unique predictor of attachment security. *Infant Behavior and Development, 34,* 443–446.

Levendosky, A. A., Bogat, G. A., Huth-Bocks, A. C., Rosenblum, K., & von Eye, A. (2011). The effects of domestic violence on the stability of attachment from infancy to preschool *Journal of Clinical Child and Adolescent Psychology, 40,* 398–410.

Lickenbrock, D. M., Braungart-Rieker, J. M., Ekas, N. V., Zentall, S. R., Oshio, T., & Planalp, E. M. (2013). Early temperament and attachment security with mothers and fathers as predictors of toddler compliance and noncompliance. *Infant and Child Development, 22,* 580–602.

Lounds, J. J., Borkowski, J. G., Whitman, T. L., Maxwell, S. E., & Weed, K. (2005). Adolescent parenting and attachment during infancy and early development. *Parenting: Science and Practice, 5,* 91–118.

Lucassen, N., Tharner, A., Van IJzendoorn, M. H., Bakermans-Kranenburg, M. J., Volling, B. L., Verhulst, F. C., et al. (2011). The association between paternal sensitivity and infant–father attachment security: A meta-analysis of three decades of research. *Journal of Family Psychology, 25,* 986–992.

Lyons-Ruth, K., Bureau, J.-F., Easterbrooks, M. A., Obsuth, I., Hennighausen, K., & Vulliez-Coady, L. (2013). Parsing the construct of maternal insensitivity: Distinct longitudinal pathways associated with early maternal withdrawal. *Attachment and Human Development, 15*(5–6), 562–582.

Lyons-Ruth, K., Repacholi, B., McLeod, S., & Silva, E. (1991). Disorganized attachment behavior in infancy: Short-term stability, maternal and infant correlates, and risk-related subtypes. *Development and Psychopathology, 3,* 377–396.

Lyons-Ruth, K., Yellin, C., Melnick, S., & Atwood, G. (2003). Childhood experiences of trauma and loss have different relations to maternal unresolved and hostile-helpless states of mind on the AAI. *Attachment and Human Development, 5,* 330–352.

Macfie, J., Toth, S. L., Rogosch, F. A., Robinson, J., Emde, R. N., & Cicchetti, D. (1999). Effect of maltreatment on preschoolers' narrative representations of responses to relieve distress and of role reversal. *Developmental Psychology, 35,* 460–465.

Madigan, S., Atkinson, L., Laurin, K., & Benoit, D. (2013). Attachment and internalizing behavior in early childhood: A meta-analysis. *Developmental Psychology, 49*(4), 672–689.

Madigan, S., Bakermans-Kranenburg, M. J., Van IJzendoorn, M. H., Moran, G., Pederson, D. R., & Benoit, D. (2006). Unresolved states of mind, anomalous parental behavior, and disorganized attachment: A review and meta-analysis of a transmission gap. *Attachment and Human Development, 8,* 89–111.

Madigan, S., Goldberg, S., Moran, G., & Pederson, D. R. (2004). Naïve observers' perceptions of family drawings by 7-year-olds with disorganized histories. *Attachment and Human Development, 6,* 223–239.

Madigan, S., Ladd, M., & Goldberg, S. (2003). A picture is worth a thousand words: Children's representations of family as indicators of early attachment (Vol. 5, pp. 19–37). London: Taylor & Francis.

Main, M. (1990). Cross-cultural studies of attachment organization: Recent studies, changing methodologies, and the concept of conditional strategies. *Human Development, 33,* 48–61.

Main, M. (2000). The organized categories of infant, child, and adult attachment: Flexible vs. inflexible attention under attachment-related stress. *Journal of the American Psychoanalytic Association, 48,* 1055–1096.

Main, M., & Cassidy, J. (1988). Categories of response to reunion with the parent at age 6: Predictable from infant attachment classifications and stable over a 1-month period. *Developmental Psychology, 24,* 415–426.

Main, M., Kaplan, N., & Cassidy, J. (1985). Security in infancy, childhood, and adulthood: A move to the level of representation. In I. Bretherton & E. Waters (Eds.), Growing points of attachment theory and research. *Monographs of the Society for Research in Child Development, 50*(1–2, Serial No. 209), 66–104.

Main, M., & Solomon, J. (1986). Discovery of a new, insecure disorganized/disoriented attachment pattern. In T. B. Brazelton & M. Yogman (Eds.), *Affective development in infancy* (pp. 95–124). Norwood, NJ: Ablex.

Main, M., & Solomon, J. (1990). Procedures for identifying infants as disorganized/disoriented during the Ainsworth Strange Situation. In M. T. Greenberg, D. Cicchetti, & E. M. Cummings (Eds.), *Attachment in the preschool years* (pp. 121–160). Chicago: University of Chicago Press.

Main, M., & Weston, D. R. (1981). The quality of the toddler's relationship to mother and to father: Related to conflict behavior and the readiness to establish new relationships. *Child Development, 52,* 932–940.

Marcovitch, S., Goldberg, S., Gold, A., Washington, J., Wasson, C., Krekewich, K., et al. (1997). Determinants of behavioral problems in Romanian children adopted in Ontario. *International Journal of Behavioral Development, 20,* 17–31.

Marvin, R. S. (1977). An ethological–cognitive model of the attenuation of mother–child attachment behavior. In T. Alloway, L. Krames, & P. Pilner (Eds.), *Advances in the study of communication and affect: Vol. 3. Attachment behavior* (pp. 25–60). New York: Plenum.

McElwain, N. L., & Booth-LaForce, C. (2006). Maternal sensitivity to infant distress and nondistress as predictors of infant–mother attachment security. *Journal of Family Psychology, 20*(2), 247–255.

McLaughlin, K. A., Zeanah, C. H., Fox, N. A., & Nelson, C. A. (2012). Attachment security as a mechanism linking foster care placement to improved mental health outcomes in previously institutionalized children. *Journal of Child Psychology and Psychiatry, 53*(1), 46–55.

Meehl, P. E. (1973). *Psychodiagnosis: Selected papers.* Minneapolis: University of Minnesota Press.

Miljkovitch, R., Danet, M., & Bernier, A. (2012). Intergenerational transmission of attachment representations in the context of single parenthood in France. *Journal of Family Psychology, 26*(5), 784–792.

Miljkovitch, R., Moran, G., Roy, C., Jaunin, L., Forcada-Guex, M., Pierrehumbert, B., et al. (2013). Maternal interactive behaviour as a predictor of preschoolers' attachment representations among full term and premature samples. *Early Human Development, 89*(5), 349–354.

Miljkovitch, R., Pierrehumbert, B., Bretherton, I., & Halfon, O. (2004). Associations between parental and child attachment representations. *Attachment and Human Development, 6*(3), 305–325.

Miljkovitch, R., Pierrehumbert, B., Karmaniola, A., & Halfon, O. (2003). Les représentations d'attachement du jeune enfant. Développement d'un système de codage pour les histoires à compléter [Preschoolers' attachment representations: Development of a coding system for the story completion task]. *Devenir*, 15(2), 143–177.

Minnis, H., Green, J., O'Connor, T. G., Liew, A., Glaser, D., Taylor, E., et al. (2009). An exploratory study of the association between reactive attachment disorder and attachment narratives in early school-age children. *Journal of Child Psychology and Psychiatry*, 50, 931–942.

Moss, E., Bureau, J.-F., Béliveau, M.-J., Zdebik, M., & Lépine, S. (2009). Links between children's attachment behavior at early school-age, their attachment-related representations, and behavior problems in middle childhood. *International Journal of Behavioral Development*, 33, 155–166.

Moss, E., Bureau, J.-F., Cyr, C., & Dubois-Comtois, K. (2006). Is the maternal Q-set a valid measure of preschool child attachment behavior? *International Journal of Behavioral Development*, 30, 488–497.

Moss, E., Bureau, J.-F., Cyr, C., Mongeau, C., & St.-Laurent, D. (2004). Correlates of attachment at age 3: Construct validity of the preschool attachment classification system. *Developmental Psychology*, 40, 323–334.

Moss, E., Cyr, C., Bureau, J., Tarabulsy, G. M., & Dubois-Combois, K. (2005). Stability of attachment during the preschool period. *Developmental Psychology*, 41, 773–783.

Moss, E., Cyr, C., & Dubois-Comtois, K. (2004). Attachment at early school age and developmental risk: Examining family contexts and behavior problems of controlling-caregiving, controlling-punitive, and behaviorally disorganized children. *Developmental Psychology*, 40, 519–532.

Moss, E., Gosselin, C., Parent, S., Rousseau, D., & Dumont, M. (1997). Attachment and joint problem-solving experiences during the preschool period. *Social Development*, 6, 1–17.

Moss, E., Rousseau, D., Parent, S., St.-Laurent, D., & Saintonge, J. (1998). Correlates of attachment at school age: Maternal reported stress, mother–child interaction, and behavior problems. *Child Development*, 69, 1390–1405.

Moss, E., & St-Laurent, D. (2001). Attachment at school age and academic performance. *Developmental Psychobiology*, 37(6), 863–874.

Murphy, T. P., & Laible, D. J. (2013). The influence of attachment security on preschool children's empathic concern. *International Journal of Behavioral Development*, 37, 436–440.

National Institute of Child Health and Human Development (NICHD) Early Child Care Research Network. (2001). Child-care and family predictors of preschool attachment and stability from infancy. *Developmental Psychology*, 31, 847–862.

Newland, L. A., Coyl, D. D., & Freeman, H. (2008). Predicting preschoolers' attachment security from fathers' involvement internal working models, and use of social support. *Early Child Development and Care*, 178, 785–801.

Niemann, S., & Weiss, S. (2011). Attachment behavior of children adopted internationally at six months post adoption. *Adoption Quarterly*, 14(4), 246–267.

Nunnally, J. C. (1978). *Psychometric theory*. New York: McGraw-Hill.

O'Connor, E., Bureau, J. F., McCartney, K., & Lyons-Ruth, K. (2011). Risks and outcomes associated with disorganized/controlling patterns of attachment at age three years in the National Institute of Child Health and Human Development Study of Early Child Care and Youth Development. *Infant Mental Health Journal*, 32, 450–472.

Oppenheim, D. (1997). The attachment doll-play interview for preschoolers. *International Journal of Behavioral Development*, 20, 681–697.

Ostler, T., & Haight, W. L. (2011). Viewing young foster children's responses to visits through the lens of maternal containment: Implications for attachment disorganization. In J. Solomon & C. George (Eds.), *Disorganized attachment and caregiving* (pp. 269–291). New York: Guilford Press.

Pace, C. S., Zavattini, G. C., & D'Alessio, M. (2012). Continuity and discontinuity of attachment patterns: A short-term longitudinal pilot study using a sample of late-adopted children and their adoptive mothers. *Attachment and Human Development*, 14, 45–61.

Padrón, E., Carlson, E. A., & Sroufe, L. A. (2014). Frightened versus not frightened disorganized infant attachment: Newborn characteristics and maternal caregiving. *American Journal of Orthopsychiatry*, 84(2), 201–208.

Page, T., & Bretherton, I. (2001). Mother- and father-child attachment themes in the story completions of preschoolers from post-divorce families: Do they predict relatioinships with peers and teachers? *Attachment and Human Development*, 3, 1–29.

Park, K. A., & Waters, E. (1989). Security of attachment and preschool friendships. *Child Development*, 60, 1076–1081

Pasalich, D. S., Dadds, M. R., Hawes, D. J., & Brennan, J. (2012). Attachment and callous-unemotional traits in children with early-onset conduct problems. *Journal of Child Psychology and Psychiatry*, 53, 838–845.

Pederson, D. R., Moran, G., Sitko, C., Campbell, K., Ghesquire, K., & Acton, H. (1990). Maternal sensitivity and the security of infant–mother attachment: A Q-sort study. *Child Development*, 61, 1974–1983.

Pianta, R. C., Longmaid, K., & Ferguson, J. E. (1999). Attachment-based classifications of children's family drawings: Psychometric properties and relations with children's adjustment in kindergarten. *Journal of Clinical Child Psychology*, 28, 244–255.

Pierrehumbert, B., Ramstein, T., Karmaniola, A., & Halfon, O. (1996). Child care in the preschool years: Attachment, behaviour problems and cognitive development. *European Journal of Psychology of Education*, 11(2), 201–214.

Pinquart, M., Feussner, C., & Ahnert, L. (2013). Meta-analytic evidence for stability in attachments from infancy to early adulthood. *Attachment and Human Development, 15,* 189–218.

Posada, G. (2006). Assessing attachment security at age three: Q-sort home observations and the MacArthur Strange Situation adaptation. *Social Development, 15,* 644–658.

Posada, G., Lu, T., Trumbell, J., Kaloustian, G., Trudel, M., Plata, S. J., et al. (2013). Is the secure base phenomenon evident here, there, and anywhere?: A cross-cultural study of child behavior and experts' definitions. *Child Development, 84,* 1896–1905.

Posada, G., Waters, E., Crowell, J. A., & Lay, K.-L. (1995). Is it easier to use a secure mother as a secure base?: Attachment Q-Sort correlates of the adult attachment interview. In E. Waters, B. E. Vaughn, G. Posada, & K. Kondo-Ikemura (Eds.), *Caregiving, cultural, and cognitive perspectives on secure-based behavior and working models: New growing points of attachment theory and research. Monographs of the Society for Research in Child Development, 60*(2–3, Serial No. 244), 133–145.

Raikes, H. A., & Thompson, R. A. (2008). Attachment security and parenting quality predict children's problemsolving, attributions, and loneliness with peers. *Attachment and Human Development, 10,* 319–344.

Rauh, H., Ziegenhain, U., Muller, B., & Wijnroks, L. (2000). Stability and change in infant–mother attachment in the second year of life. In P. M. Crittenden & A. H. Claussen (Eds.), *The organization of attachment relationships: Maturation, culture, and context* (pp. 251–276). New York: Cambridge University Press.

Richters, J. E., Waters, E., & Vaughn, B. E. (1988). Empirical classification of infant–mother relationships from interactive behavior and crying during reunion. *Child Development, 59,* 512–522.

Roskam, I., Meunier, J.-C., & Stievenart, M. (2011). Parent attachment, childrearing behavior, and child attachment: Mediated effects predicting preschoolers' externalizing behavior. *Journal of Applied Developmental Psychology, 32*(4), 170–179.

Rutgers, A. H., Van IJzendoorn, M. H., Bakermans-Kranenburg, M. J., & Swinkels, S. H. N. (2007). Autism and attachment: The Attachment Q-Sort. *Autism, 11,* 187–200.

Rutter, M., Kreppner, J., & Sonuga-Barke, E. (2009). Emanuel Miller lecture: Attachment insecurity, disinhibited attachment, and attachment disorders: Where do research findings leave the concepts? *Journal of Child Psychology and Psychiatry, 50*(5), 529–543.

Schneider-Rosen, K. (1990). The developmental reorganization of attachment relationships: Guidelines for classification beyond infancy. In M. T. Greenberg, D. Cicchetti, & E. M. Cummings (Eds.), *Attachment in the preschool years* (pp. 185–220). Chicago: University of Chicago Press.

Schoppe-Sullivan, S. J., Diener, M. L., Mangelsdorf, S. C., Brown, G. L., McHale, J. L., & Frosch, C. A. (2006). Attachment and sensitivity in family context: The roles of parent and infant gender. *Infant and Child Development, 15,* 367–385.

Seifer, R., LaGasse, L. L., Lester, B., Bauer, C. R., Shankaran, S., Bada, H. S., et al. (2004). Attachment status in children prenatally exposed to cocaine and other substances. *Child Development, 75,* 850–868.

Shouldice, A. E., & Stevenson-Hinde, J. (1992). Coping with security distress: The Separation Anxiety Test and attachment classification at 4.5 years. *Journal of Child Psychology and Psychiatry, 33,* 331–348.

Slough, N. M., & Greenberg, M. T. (1990). Five-year olds' representations of separation from parents: Responses from the perspective of self and other. *New Directions for Child Development, 48,* 67–84.

Smeekens, S., Riksen-Walraven, J. M., & Van-Bakel, H. J. A. (2009). The predictive value of different infant attachment measures for socioemotional development at age 5 years. *Infant Mental Health Journal, 30,* 366–383.

Smyke, A. T., Zeanah, C. H., Fox, N. A., Nelson, C. A., & Guthrie, D. (2010). Placement in foster care enhances quality of attachment among young institutionalized children. *Child Development, 81,* 212–223.

Solomon, J., & George, C. (1996). Defining the caregiving system: Toward a theory of caregiving. *Infant Mental Health Journal, 17,* 3–17.

Solomon, J., & George, C. (1999a). The caregiving system in mothers of infants: A comparison of divorcing and married mothers. *Attachment and Human Development, 1,* 171–190.

Solomon, J., & George, C. (1999b). The effects on attachment of overnight visitation in divorced and separated families: A longitudinal follow-up. In J. Solomon & C. George (Eds.), *Attachment disorganization* (pp. 243–264). New York: Guilford Press.

Solomon, J., & George, C. (1999c). The measurement of attachment security in infancy and childhood. In J. Cassidy & P. R. Shaver (Eds.), *Handbook of attachment: Theory, research, and clinical applications* (pp. 287–316). New York: Guilford Press.

Solomon, J., & George, C. (1999d). The place of disorganization in attachment theory: Linking classic observations with contemporary findings. In J. Solomon & C. George (Eds.), *Attachment disorganization* (pp. 3–32). New York: Guilford Press.

Solomon, J., & George, C. (2000). Toward an integrated theory of maternal caregiving. In J. Osofsky & H. E. Fitzgerald (Eds.), *WAIMH handbook of infant mental health: Vol. 3. Parenting and child care* (pp. 323–368). New York: Wiley.

Solomon, J., & George, C. (2002, April). *Understanding children's attachment representations in terms of defensive process.* Paper presented at the 4th Annual Conference of the International Academy of Family Psychology, Heidelberg, Germany.

Solomon, J., & George, C. (2006). Intergenerational transmission of dysregulated maternal caregiving:

Mothers describe their upbringing and childrearing. In O. Mayseless (Ed.), *Parenting representations: Theory, research, and clinical implications* (pp. 265–295). Cambridge, UK: Cambridge University Press.

Solomon, J., & George, C. (2011). The disorganized attachment-caregiving system: Dysregulation of adaptive processes at multiple levels. In J. Solomon & C. George (Eds.), *Disorganized attachment and caregiving* (pp. 3–24). New York: Guilford Press.

Solomon, J., George, C., & De Jong, A. (1995). Children classified as controlling at age six: Evidence of disorganized representational strategies and aggression at home and at school. *Development and Psychopathology, 7,* 447–463.

Spieker, S., & Crittenden, P. M. (2010). Comparing two attachment classification methods applied to preschool strange situations. *Clinical Child Psychology and Psychiatry, 15,* 97–120.

Spieker, S., Nelson, E. M., & Condon, M.-C. (2011). Validity of the TAS-45 as a measure of toddler-parent attachment: Preliminary evidence from Early Head Start families. *Attachment and Human Development, 13,* 69–90.

Sroufe, L. A. (1979). The coherence of individual development: Early care, attachment, and subsequent developmental issues. *American Psychologist, 34,* 834–841

Sroufe, L. A., & Waters, E. (1977). Attachment as an organizational construct. *Child Development, 48,* 1184–1199.

Stacks, A. M., & Oshio, T. (2009). Disorganized attachment and social skills as indicators of Head Start children's school readiness skills. *Attachment and Human Development, 11,* 143–164.

Stams, G.-J. J. M., Juffer, F., Van IJzendoorn, M. H., & Hoksbergen, R. A. C. (2001). Attachment-based intervention in adoptive families in infancy and children's development at age 7: Two follow-up studies. *British Journal of Developmental Psychology, 19,* 159–180.

Steele, R. D., Waters, T. A., Bost, K. K., Vaughn, B. E., Truitt, W., Waters, H. S., et al. (2014). Caregiving antecedents of secure base script knowledge: A comparative analysis of young adult attachment representations. *Developmental Psychology, 50,* 2526–2538.

Stevenson-Hinde, J., & Shouldice, A. (1995). Maternal interactions and self-reports related to attachment classifications at 4.5 years. *Child Development, 66,* 583–596.

Stievenart, M., Roskam, I., Meunier, J. C., & Van de Moortele, G. (2012). Assessment of Preschoolers' attachment security using the Attachment Q-set and the Attachment Story Completion Task. *The International Journal of Educational and Psychological Assessment, 12,* 62–80.

Strayer, F. F., Verissimo, M., Vaughn, B. E., & Howes, C. (1995). A quantitative approach to the description and classification of primary social relationships. In E. Waters, B. E. Vaughn, G. Posada, & K. Kondo-Ikemura (Eds.), Caregiving, cultural, and

cognitive perspectives on secure-based behavior and working models: New growing points of attachment theory and research. *Monographs of the Society for Research in Child Development, 60*(2–3, Serial No. 244), 49–70.

Tarabulsy, G. M., Provost, M. A., Bordeleau, S., Trudel-Fitzgerald, C., Moran, G., Pederson, D. R., et al. (2009). Validation of a short version of the maternal behavior Q-set applied to a brief video record of mother–infant interaction. *Infant Behavior and Development, 32,* 132–136.

Tarabulsy, G. M., Provost, M. A., Larose, S., Moss, E., Lemelin, J.-P., Moran, G., et al. (2008). Similarities and differences in mothers' and observers' ratings of infant security on the Attachment Q-Sort. *Infant Behavior and Development, 31,* 10–22.

Teti, D. M., & McGourty, S. (1996). Using mothers versus trained observers in assessing children's secure base behavior: Theoretical and methodological considerations. *Child Development, 67,* 597–605.

Tharner, A., Herba, C. M., Luijk, M., Van IJzendoorn, M. H., Bakermans-Kranenburg, M. J., Govaert, P. P., et al. (2011). Subcortical structures and the neurobiology of infant attachment disorganization: A longitudinal ultrasound imaging study. *Social Neuroscience, 6,* 336–347.

Thorell, L. B., Rydell, A.-M., & Bohlin, G. (2012). Parent–child attachment and executive functioning in relation to ADHD symptoms in middle childhood. *Attachment and Human Development, 14,* 517–532.

Torres, N., Maia, J., Verissimo, M., & Silva, F. (2012). Attachment security representations in institutionalized children and children living with their families: Links to problem behavior. *Clinical Psychology and Psychotherapy, 19,* 25–36.

Toth, S. L., Rogosch, F. A., Manly, J. T., & Cicchetti, D. (2006). The efficacy of toddler–parent psychotherapy to reorganize attachment in the young offspring of mothers with major depressive disorder: A randomized preventive trial. *Journal of Consulting and Clinical Psychology, 74,* 1006–1016.

Toth, S. L., Rogosch, F. A., Sturge-Apple, M., & Cicchetti, D. (2009). Maternal depression, children's attachment security, and representational development: An organizational perspective. *Child Development, 80*(1), 192–208.

Trapolini, J. A., Ungerer, A., & McMahon, C. A. (2007). Maternal depression and children's attachment representatons during the preschool years. *British Journal of Developmental Psychology, 25,* 247–261.

van Bakel, H. J. A., & Riksen-Walraven, J. M. (2004). AQS security scores: What do they represent?: A study in construct validation. *Infant Mental Health Journal, 25,* 175–193.

Van IJzendoorn, M. (1995). Adult attachment representations, parental responsiveness, and infant attachment: A meta-analysis on the predictive validity of the Adult Attachment Interview. *Psychological Bulletin, 117,* 387–403.

Van IJzendoorn, M. H., Rutgers, A. H., Bakermans-Kranenburg, M. J., van Daalen, E., Dietz, C., Buitelaar, J. K., et al. (2007). Parental sensitivity and attachment in children with autism spectrum disorder: Comparison with children with mental retardation, with language delays, and with typical development. *Child Development, 78*, 597–608.

Van IJzendoorn, M. H., Schuengel, C., & Bakermans-Kranenburg, M. J. (1999). Disorganized attachment in early childhood: Meta-analysis of precursors, concomitants, and sequelae. *Development and Psychopathology, 11*, 225–249.

Van IJzendoorn, M. H., Vereijken, C. M. J. L., Bakermans-Kranenburg, M. J., & Riksen-Walraven, J. M. (2004). Assessing attachment security with the Attachment Q-Sort: Meta-analytic evidence for the validity of the observer AQS. *Child Development, 75*, 1188–1213.

Vaughn, B. E., Strayer, F. F., Jacques, M., Trudel, M., & Seifer, R. (1991). Maternal descriptions of 2- and 3-year-old children: A comparison of Attachment Q-Sorts in two socio-cultural communities. *International Journal of Behavioral Development, 14*, 249–271.

Vaughn, B. E., & Waters, E. (1990). Attachment behavior at home and in the laboratory: Q-sort observations and Strange Situation classifications of one-year-olds. *Child Development, 61*, 1965–1973.

Venet, M., Bureau, J. F., Gosselin, C., & Capuano, F. (2007). Attachment representation in a sample of neglected preschool age children. *School Psychology International, 28*, 264–293.

Verschueren, K., Marcoen, A., & Schoefs, V. (1996). The internal working model of the self, attachment, and competence in five-year olds. *Child Development, 67*, 2493–2511.

Vondra, J. I., Shaw, D. S., Swearingen, L., Cohen, M., & Owens, E. B. (2001). Attachment stability and emotional and behavioral regulation from infancy to preschool age. *Development and Psychopathology, 13*, 13–33.

Wartner, U. G., Grossmann, K., Fremmer-Bombik, E., & Suess, G. (1994). Attachment patterns at age six in south Germany: Predictability from infancy and implications for preschool behavior. *Child Development, 65*, 1010–1023.

Waters, E. (1978). The reliability and stability of individual differences in infant–mother attachment. *Child Development, 49*, 483–494.

Waters, E. (1995). The Attachment Q-Set (Version 3.0). In E. Waters, B. E. Vaughn, G. Posada, & K. Kondo-Ikemura (Eds.), Caregiving, cultural, and cognitive perspectives on secure-base behavior and working models: New growing points of attachment theory and research. *Monographs of the Society for Research in Child Development, 60*(2–3, Serial No. 244), 234–246.

Waters, E., & Beauchaine, T. P. (2003). Are there really patterns of attachment?: Comment on Fraley and Spieker (2003). *Developmental Psychology, 39*, 417–422.

Waters, E., & Deane, K. E. (1985). Defining and assessing individual differences in attachment relationships: Q-methodology and the organization of behavior in infancy and early childhood. In I. Bretherton & E. Waters (Eds.), Growing points of attachment theory and research. *Monographs of the Society for Research in Child Development, 50*(1–2, Serial No. 209), 41–65.

Waters, E., Merrick, S., Treboux, D., Crowell, J., & Albersheim, L. (2000). Attachment security in infancy and early adulthood: A twenty-year longitudinal study. *Child Development, 71*, 684–689.

Waters, H. S., Rodrigues, L. M., & Ridgeway, D. (1998). Cognitive underpinnings of narrative attachment assessment. *Journal of Experimental Child Psychology, 71*, 211–234.

Waters, H. S., & Waters, E. (2006). The attachment working models concept: Among other things, we build script-like representations of secure base experiences. *Attachment and Human Development, 8*, 185–198.

Webster, L., & Hackett, R. (2011). An exploratory investigation of the relationships among representation security, disorganization, and behavior in maltreated children. In J. Solomon & C. George (Eds.), *Disorganized attachment and caregiving* (pp. 292–317). New York: Guilford Press.

Wilkins, D. ( 2012). Disorganised attachment indicates child maltreatment: How is this link useful for child protection social workers? *Journal of Social Work Practice:Psychotherapeutic Approaches in Health, Welfare and the Community, 26*, 15–30.

Wong, M., Bost, K., Shin, N., Veríssomo, M., Maia, J., Monteiro, L., et al. (2011). Preschool children's mental representations of attachment: Antecedents in their secure base behaviors and maternal attachment scripts. *Attachment Human Development, 13*, 489–502.

Zeanah, C. H., Smyke, A. T., Koga, S. F., & Carlson, E. (2005). Attachment in institutionalized and community children in Romania. *Child Development, 76*, 1015–1028.

# PART IV

# ATTACHMENT IN ADOLESCENCE AND ADULTHOOD

# Chapter 19

# The Multiple Facets
# of Attachment in Adolescence

Joseph P. Allen
Joseph S. Tan

The psychosocial development that takes place across adolescence brings profound changes in the meaning and expression of attachment-related cognition, behavior, and affect. Our understanding of the changing and multifaceted nature of the adolescent attachment system has advanced greatly since the previous edition of this handbook was published. Previously, we had argued that research should begin to focus not simply on adolescents' internal states of mind regarding attachment but also on their attachment *relationships*. Several prescriptions followed, including the need to assess caregiver relationships *both* historically and currently, to begin to take into account peer relationships, and to recognize the role of broader physical and cognitive factors influencing attachment processes. The field has recently made remarkable strides in addressing each of these needs: We have developed promising measures of qualities of adolescent attachment relationships with parents, including assessments of the ways these change over time. We have documented the gradual emergence of attachment-like qualities in peer and romantic relationships. And we have learned about the ways in which attachment states of mind intersect both with physiological states and perceptual biases to help explain qualities of both current and future relationships.

The study of adolescent attachment has now moved productively back toward its origins—as a means to understand *relationship* qualities and behaviors. This movement inevitably shifts our conceptualization of attachment in adolescence away from a unitary focus on internal states of mind and toward a multifaceted view recognizing the constellation of relational, behavioral, and affective elements at play. This shift in turn has profound implications for our understanding of both the meaning of attachment in adolescence and the continuities with attachment at other points in the lifespan. Below we consider our advances in understanding of these multiple facets of attachment in adolescence, first in terms of normative development, then in terms of individual differences in attachment processes and their relation to adolescent psychosocial functioning. We then conclude with a discussion of the implications of this multifaceted perspective on adolescent attachment for the study of continuities with attachment in other phases of the lifespan, and for our understanding of the broader nature of the attachment system during this period.

# Normative Development of the Attachment System in Adolescence

## Transformations in Attachment Relationships with Caregivers

One of the defining social challenges of adolescence is that in seeking to establish emotional self-sufficiency, adolescents must often work *not* to need to turn to their primary caregivers to meet attachment needs. During adolescence, rapidly developing competencies decrease the need for dependence on parental attachment figures, and the strong need to explore and master new environments promotes healthy growth in the exploratory system. These changes necessitate a new balance between attachment behaviors and exploratory needs, with exploration taking an increasingly central role.

In principle, this process is analogous to the competing influences of the exploratory and attachment systems in infancy, although the press for autonomy in adolescence may be more relentless and more directly in competition with the press of the attachment system (Allen, Moore, & Kuperminc, 1997). These changes, however, may change the *threshold* at which the attachment system activates and drives behavior, although, by themselves, they are not likely to fundamentally alter the dynamics at play. Parents continue to be used as attachment figures even into young adulthood (Rosenthal & Kobak, 2010), and the attachment system is still likely to activate and be readily observable under conditions of danger or separation distress (Rosenthal & Kobak, 2010). Adolescents may be on the verge of tears far less often than infants, but when they are highly distressed, their likelihood of turning to parents for help is still likely to increase dramatically. In this respect, the attachment system operates much as it always has, albeit with a different and rapidly changing balance between attachment and exploratory behaviors.

Yet this balancing act is more challenging than it first appears because at the same time that adolescents are seeking to develop greater emotional self-sufficiency vis-à-vis their attachment figures, they are also negotiating often contentious issues of behavioral autonomy (i.e., who controls the teens' behavior) with these same figures. Whereas the goal-corrected partnership in infancy might be described as reflecting a coordinated effort between parent and child, in adolescence it seems more appropriate to consider this as a *negotiated* effort, and the negotiations will almost inevitably be challenging. To a degree unparalleled elsewhere in development (with the possible exception of early toddlerhood), the adolescent struggle for behavioral autonomy becomes an omnipresent background against which attachment processes must play out. The many years of prior operation of the attachment system—and the habitual patterns of responding that have become established—are likely at times to be perceived by the adolescent as a potential threat to efforts to establish behavioral autonomy. Put simply, it can be difficult at times for a teen to fiercely oppose his or her parents' control efforts while feeling pulled by both habit and the attachment system to retain their shoulders to cry on.

Kobak and Duemmler (1994) suggested that a potential saving grace in this process is a subtle but important shift in the goal of goal-corrected partnership: The partnership with caregivers ideally becomes less about the caregiver meeting most or all of the adolescents' attachment needs, and more about helping the adolescent develop a capacity to meet attachment needs autonomously, in ways that do not solely depend on interactions with a caregiver. As an adolescent gains communication and perspective-taking skills, it becomes possible for both teen and parent to modify (or correct) their attachment-related behavior when necessary, to meet the teen's evolving attachment needs appropriately, while balancing other needs as well. Even the shared goal of seeing the adolescent gradually achieve autonomy from and even occasional opposition to parental desires can become something onto which both parties can hold. This shared goal can then become an extension of the adolescent's internal representation of the parent as a secure base supporting the adolescent's exploration of evolving independence (Sroufe, Egeland, Carlson, & Collins, 2005). In this way, the attachment bond can remain strong, at least for secure teens, even if at times teens say they do not necessarily want to feel attached.

A further critical change as adolescence progresses is that the attachment hierarchy—implied by teens giving consistent preference to certain individuals over others when the attachment system is activated (Bowlby, 1969/1982)—becomes more flexible and even multidimensional. First peers, then romantic partners, begin to enter into this hierarchy. Although the stress of severe illness likely would still cause an adolescent to turn to parents, as in the original attachment hierarchy, peer-related stressors, which can also be severe and distressing, might well result in a close peer or romantic partner moving temporarily into the primary position in the attachment hierarchy (Markiewicz, Lawford, Doyle, & Haggart, 2006). Parent gender also matters, with mothers being more likely than fathers to remain at the top of the attachment hierarchy through the transition from adolescence to young adulthood (Rosenthal & Kobak, 2010).

One might question whether this constellation of changes might lead teens to become more dismissing of attachment. A comparison of the distribution of teen AAI classifications with adult AAI classifications finds that teens' states of mind regarding attachment are more likely to be classified as insecure-dismissing of attachment than adults' states of mind (Bakermans-Kranenburg & Van IJzendoorn, 2009). This finding may be somewhat misleading as a marker of teens' overall status, however, stemming in part from the primary focus of the Adult Attachment Interview (AAI) on early childhood memories of attachment to *parents*. The most healthy and adaptive approach appears to be a gradual, somewhat intentional shift in the focus of the adolescent's attachment system from parents to peers and/or to romantic partners. Even for secure adolescents, this shift may require directing attention away from childhood memories of dependency on parents and toward both emotional independence and stronger peer bonds. Assessing attachment states of mind primarily with regard to the one type of relationship that adolescents are most likely to be trying to deemphasize is likely to yield a portrait of adolescent attachment that overidentifies dismissing states of mind. Indeed, the intense adolescent preoccupation with establishing deep, emotionally engaging peer relationships—in part around attachment and dependency needs—suggests that even if the adolescent is deemphasizing the attachment relationship *with parents*, this is not at all the same as being dismissive of attachment more generally.

## Transformations in Intrapsychic Processes

As an individual moves into adolescence, the intrapsychic roots of the attachment system (in representations of early experience with caregivers) begin to grow, enriched by the rapidly developing functional independence and cognitive capacity of the adolescent. These developing capacities allow an adolescent to begin to construct, from

experiences with multiple caregivers, a more integrated and generalized state of mind regarding attachment experiences (Hesse, 2008; Main, Kaplan, & Cassidy, 1985). Moreover, by adolescence the attachment system can be assessed in terms of a single overarching attachment state of mind that displays stability over time (Allen, McElhaney, Kuperminc, & Jodl, 2004; Hesse, 2008; Zimmermann & Becker-Stoll, 2002). In adolescence, the domains in which attachment-relevant experiences occur, and the ways in which these can be evaluated, have grown and broadened, with significant implications for the development of an internalized attachment state of mind. The adolescent continues to have attachment relationships with caregivers, although these are changing as described earlier. In addition, the adolescent is able to integrate diverse attachment-relevant experiences (e.g., past and present, with multiple caregivers, and in new relationships) and to begin to reevaluate cognitions, memories, and affective reactions related to attachment. The resulting adolescent state of mind is not so much a mirror of past experiences as an *outgrowth* of those experiences that is also influenced by current relationship qualities, as well as growing cognitive and emotional capacities.

The factors that drive the development of adolescent internal states of mind regarding attachment are both emotional and cognitive. Emotionally, the adolescent is not simply moving away from reliance on parents; rather, he or she is continuing the lifelong process of learning to self-soothe and regulate emotional reactions. An important secondary effect of this growing self-soothing capacity in adolescence is an increase in the adolescent's capacity to reevaluate the nature of his or her attachment relationship with parents. As the adolescent comes to need caregivers less to maintain a sense of emotional equilibrium and felt security, he or she is freed up to evaluate more critically the caregiver relationships. Main, Goldwyn, and Hesse (2002) refer to this cognitive and emotional freedom as "epistemic space," and suggest that it allows individuals to evaluate their parents as attachment figures more objectively.

Similarly, the adolescent's developing cognitive capacity aids in integrating a history of diverse experiences with individual caregivers into a single overall state of mind regarding attachment. The development of formal operational reasoning ability and dramatic increases in cognitive differentiation of self and other that characterize this period (Keating, 1990) also allow the teen to begin to establish a more consistent view of the self as existing apart from interactions with specific caregivers. The advent of formal operational thinking also allows an adolescent to contemplate abstract and counterfactual possibilities. This in turn allows him or her to compare relationships with different attachment figures both to one another and to hypothetical ideals. Adolescents therefore not only demonstrate a capacity to think about attachment in a general way, which extends beyond any single relationship, but they also have the capacity to operate metacognitively on this thinking. As a result, they can begin to reconstruct (or at least tinker with) their own states of mind regarding attachment. The adolescent therefore gains the capacity to "deidealize" parents—to see them in both positive and negative ways (Steinberg, 2005). This capacity to evaluate past attachment experiences coherently is one of the hallmarks of a state of mind regarding attachment, labeled "autonomous, yet valuing of attachment." Indeed, adolescent deidealization in the context of an overall positive relationship with parents has been strongly associated with greater security (Allen et al., 2003). This potential for reevaluation is one of the prime reasons why adolescents' states of mind are neither bound nor even likely to mirror exactly the qualities of their past attachment experiences.

## Transformations in Peer Relationships

In the midst of changing parental relationships and growing cognitive and emotional capacities, adolescents are beginning a major lifelong task: learning to establish supportive peer bonds. By midadolescence, interactions with peers have begun to take on many of the functions they will serve for the remainder of the lifespan—providing important sources of intimacy; feedback about social behavior, social influence, and information; and ultimately attachment, sexual relationships, and lifelong partnerships (Collins & Laursen, 2004; Collins, Welsh, & Furman, 2009). These developments create important challenges for our efforts to understand the operation of the attachment system during this period.

One key question is: When do peer relationships become attachment relationships? Alternatively, this question can be more fruitfully, though less conventionally, phrased: How do peer relationships *gradually* take on attachment functions? A continuum perspective seems necessary to understand this process and, indeed, such an

approach is increasingly being adopted within the research literature. We now know that there is a broad array of neural, physiological, and psychological systems underlying attachment behavior (see Coan, Chapter 12, this volume). These include systems that manage physiological arousal, establish a sense of emotional security, and deactivate primitive centers of the brain that support "flight" under conditions of stress (Coan, 2010; Hofer, 2006; Sbarra & Hazan, 2008).

We also know that by late adolescence, long-term relationships can be formed in which peers (either romantic partners or close friends) potentially serve as attachment figures in all senses of the term (Hazan & Shaver, 1987). Main (1999) has posited that the attachment system evolved partly because of the value for humans, as vulnerable members of a ground-living species, of associating with others as a source of safety. Indeed, the absence of positive social connections in adulthood creates as great a risk for illness and even early death as widely recognized risk factors such as obesity and cigarette smoking (Holt-Lunstad, Smith, & Layton, 2010). The implication of these findings is that the task of learning to form supportive attachment relationships may be nearly as much a survival skill in adolescence as it is in infancy.

But is this about attachment, or are these new relationships something different? If we are interested in identifying a relationship process identical to what is seen in infancy, the answer is clearly that what is seen in adolescence is something different. Attachment relationships, as they exist in infancy, appear in many ways unique to that phase of life. Given the infant's extreme vulnerability, limited capacities for self-help, and intense, completely dependent relationships with caregivers, an array of attachment-related emotions, cognitions, physiological reactions, and behaviors all come together simultaneously and powerfully under conditions of stress, creating a fully functioning attachment system. In adolescence, in contrast, it is not clear whether the more primitive neural circuits in the brain (e.g., the amygdala and the caudate/nucleus accumbens) responsible for detecting and physically responding to threat are activated in quite the same way by the psychosocial stressors that adolescents typically experience. In addition, the change that is occurring is not just a gradual transition from one class of attachment figures (parents) to another (peers). A relationship among equals, in which each person may serve at different times in both the care-seeking and caregiving roles, may be a context that fundamentally alters the meaning and expression of attachment behaviors that were previously directed toward a caregiver.

With these differences comes the likelihood that the multiple functions and features of the attachment system—which often operate powerfully and in unison during infancy—may begin to operate less synchronously in adolescence, particularly in interactions with peers. In addition, with the adolescent's increased cognitive capacity comes increased flexibility in directing attachment behavior. Adolescents gradually gain the capacity to be "opportunistic" in seeking out a potential attachment figure, whether it be a fellow camper at a 6-week summer camp or a close-in-age sibling to whom a teen turns as his or her parents go through a divorce. Rather than wading into the semantic quagmire of delineating the precise conditions under which a given relationship beyond infancy becomes an "attachment relationship," it may make more sense to recognize that adolescent relationships increasingly take on critical attachment functions, even if such functions are neither as synchronous nor as intense as they were in earlier relationships with caregivers.

Recent research has produced significant gains in our understanding of how this process grows and unfolds. Zeifman and Hazan (2008) conducted pioneering work in developing the WHOTO interview, which assesses the extent to which adolescents learn to turn to peers to meet the various attachment functions outlined by Ainsworth. Similarly, Rosenthal and Kobak (2010) brought these conceptualizations together in developing the Important People Interview. These two lines of work have established that adolescents do indeed establish hierarchies of attachment that include persons other than primary caregivers. They also show that the relative positioning of peers, romantic partners, and caregivers in these hierarchies depends not only on the developmental stage of the adolescent but also the particular stressor facing the adolescent. In nonemergency situations of stress, peers are often preferred over parents for support (Zeifman & Hazan, 2008). Peers are also increasingly sought out in adolescence when parents are not available (Kobak, Rosenthal, Zajac, & Madsen, 2007). General peer support-seeking is not the same as full-blown attachment behavior, however (Waters & Cummings, 2000). Finding that peers are increasingly preferred for support seeking does not mean that peer relationships have become full attachment relationships (Rosenthal & Kobak, 2010). Furman (2001) has suggested, for example, that friendships serve proximity-seeking and safe-haven functions but lack other qualities of attachment relationships, such as separation distress and enduring commitment. Although peers are often sources of support, parents overwhelmingly are found at the top of the attachment hierarchy under conditions in which adolescents are likely to need to draw strongly on the attachment system (i.e., situations involving danger or separation distress; Rosenthal & Kobak, 2010). Understanding which stressors and responses can be clearly labeled as attachment processes, which are "merely" support seeking, and which are in the hazy middle as peer relationships gradually develop in intensity, is a work in progress.

Yet, there is a clear developmental progression in whom adolescents turn to in stressful situations. Peers, for example, steadily increase in primacy from early into mid- to late-adolescence. This evolution then continues, with friends gradually receding somewhat in primacy as romantic partners take increasingly primary roles, eventually even in comparision with primary caregivers (Markiewicz et al., 2006; Rosenthal & Kobak, 2010). The length of a romantic partner relationship is one of the primary determinants of whether this relationship becomes a clearly identified full attachment bond because such bonds take time to develop (Rosenthal & Kobak, 2010). These romantic relationships do not, of course, result solely from developing interests in forming attachments with peers. They also reflect the operation of a sexual/reproductive system that is at least as biologically rooted and critical to species survival as the attachment system (Collins et al., 2009; Hazan & Shaver, 1987). The sexual and attachment systems both push toward the establishment of romantic relationships, characterized by sufficient intensity, shared interests, and strong affect, to begin to take over some of the functions of prior parent–child relationships.

## Individual Differences in the Attachment System in Adolescence

### Individual Differences in Relationships with Primary Caregivers

The potential tension between adolescents' developmental push to gain autonomy and the operation of the attachment system is central to understanding individual differences in adolescents' attachment relationships with primary caregivers. The negotiation of attachment and autonomy issues is normatively challenging for virtually all families at some point, but it may be especially difficult for the family of an adolescent with an insecure state of mind or an insecure ongoing attachment relationship with one or both parents. The combined stress of new peer and academic challenges, changing relationships, and growing emotional and behavioral independence from parents tend to activate the attachment system repeatedly and increase the impact of insecurity on an adolescent's behavior. In addition, insecure adolescents (and parents) may be overwhelmed by the affect brought on by disagreements that are part of the autonomy-development process (Kobak, Cole, Ferenz-Gillies, Fleming, & Gamble, 1993), and may perceive these disagreements as threats to already shaky relationships. An insecure adolescent may have a history of less than positive experiences with attachment figures in times of need, which is likely to further color attachment-related interactions during adolescence.

Just as the balance of exploration from a secure base has been highly informative with respect to individual differences in infant attachments, the balance of autonomy and attachment processes in adolescence is a robust indicator of the quality of an adolescent's state of mind regarding attachment (Allen et al., 2003). A secure, goal-corrected partnership potentially allows both parent and teen to recognize the teen's autonomy strivings and to support these while maintaining the relationship. Prematurely disengaging from this partnership and transferring attachment behavior to peers, in contrast, has been associated with risk for difficulties ranging from susceptibility to peer influence, to aggressive and delinquent behavior (Markiewicz et al., 2006; Rosenthal & Kobak, 2010). For a secure partnership to be maintained, two key ingredients are required: a strong capacity to communicate across the increasingly divergent perspectives and needs of the parent and teen, and a willingness on both sides to manage conflict in a way that allows the adolescent to seek autonomy while maintaining the parent–teen relationship.

## Communication

Qualities of parent–teen communication and concordance between key parent and teen perceptions in interactions now appear to be among the most consistent and strongest correlates of both the adolescent's state of mind regarding attachment and the current quality of the parent–teen attachment relationship. If a parent knows his or her teen well, and perceives the teen's current state similarly to the way the teen perceives it, communication processes are clearly functioning well. This concordance in perceptions turns out to be one of the best predictors both of an autonomous/valuing adolescent state of mind and of a secure, ongoing parent–teen relationship. For example, a mother's accuracy in predicting her teen's responses on a self-perception inventory has been robustly linked to adolescent security in the AAI (Allen et al., 2003). The correlation of security with this marker of sensitivity is even somewhat higher ($r = .35$) than is typically found in studies of parental sensitivity toward infants (De Wolff & Van IJzendoorn, 1997). Similarly, coherence in the AAI is linked to the degree of parent–teen synchrony regarding the teens' internalizing symptoms, externalizing behaviors, and perceptions of family conflict (Berger, Jodl, Allen, McElhaney, & Kuperminc, 2005; Ehrlich, Cassidy, & Dykas, 2011). Beyond the AAI, adolescent reports of lower avoidance in current relationships with parents using the Experiences in Close Relationships (ECR) scale have been linked to fewer discrepancies in parent and teen reports regarding parenting behavior (Ehrlich, Cassidy, Lejuez, & Daughters, 2014).

Two possible mechanisms can account for the relation between security and parent–teen concordance in perceptions: First, more secure adolescents may *allow* parents to be more sensitive because the teens communicate their emotional states to their parents more accurately. Becker-Stoll, Fremmer-Bombik, Wartner, Zimmermann, and Grossmann (2001) reported a reliable association between adolescents' security and the degree to which they were affectively communicative in a discussion task. Other evidence links teen attachment insecurity to broader perceptual biases and asynchronies between teens and their *peers* (Berger et al., 2005; Dykas, Woodhouse, Ehrlich, & Cassidy, 2012; Ehrlich et al., 2013). These findings, discussed in greater detail below, suggest that the security–concordance link in teen–parent relationships at least partly reflects a stable property that resides in the teen—perhaps accuracy of communication in reporting internal states.

A second mechanism accounting for the relation between insecurity and parent–teen concordance in perceptions is a relative lack of difficulty among secure (compared to insecure) individuals in accurately recalling past emotional experiences (Allen & Manning, 2007; Hesse, 2008). In laboratory tasks, parents and teens with insecure-dismissing states of mind display reduced memory for childhood emotional stimuli (Dykas, Woodhouse, Jones, & Cassidy, 2014), a pattern that has also been observed at other points in the lifespan (Dykas & Cassidy, 2011). This is at best only a partial explanation of the discordance–insecurity link, however, as a preoccupied state of mind was related to heightened recall of childhood experiences in this paradigm. Lack of parent–teen concordance may also be a result of *biases* in memories that are recalled. Six weeks after an observed mother–teen interaction, teens with autonomous/valuing states of mind in the AAI recalled less negativity in interactions with their mothers than they had initially perceived, although no such changes for insecure teens were observed (Dykas, Woodhouse, Ehrlich, & Cassidy, 2010). With fathers, conversely, it was insecure teens who changed in taking on less positive memories of interactions over time; no change was observed for secure teens. Although somewhat inconsistent, these findings provide evidence of memory biases operating in ways that would bolster positive feelings about relationships for secure teens, while undermining them for insecure teens. Notably, teen insecurity was also linked to increased *maternal* negativity in recall over time in this paradigm, suggesting just how tightly interwoven family systems processes and attachment systems are during this period.

Some evidence suggests that particular types of miscommunication and dyadic asynchrony are associated with particular types of insecure states of mind regarding attachment. For teens with a dismissing attachment state of mind, parent–teen concordance regarding adolescents' internalizing symptoms was generally poor and discrepancies were not directional in nature (i.e., there was not a consistent pattern of over- or underreporting symptoms by either party relative to the other; Berger et al., 2005). The tendency for individuals with dismissing states of mind to avoid or resist discussing emotionally distressing events that activate the attachment system may account for their generally poor communication regarding their internal states. This notion is consistent with long-standing evidence that avoidance restricts communication (Mikulincer & Nachshon, 1991).

For teens with a preoccupied attachment state of mind, a specific form of bias in communication was found: Adolescents with preoccupied states of mind consistently reported the presence of symptoms at levels that were significantly high-er than those recognized and reported in the adolescents by either their parents or peers. For preoccupied individuals, symptom reports may be seen as cries of distress (e.g., as attachment behaviors) (Allen, Moore, Kuperminc, & Bell, 1998). From this perspective, we see that insecure-preoccupied adolescents are behaving in a way that might reflect hyperactivation of their attachment system. They are reporting their distress to a high degree, although they do not find that these reports are heard (or fully believed) by the people closest to them.

## Conflict Resolution

One of the more consistent findings in the adolescent attachment literature is that teens with secure attachment states of mind tend to handle conflicts with parents by engaging in productive, problem-solving discussions that balance autonomy strivings with efforts to preserve relationships (Allen et al., 2003, 2004; Allen, Porter, McFarland, McElhaney, & Marsh, 2007; Zimmermann, Mohr, & Spangler, 2009). Similar findings have been observed with regard to self-reported security, as well as with interview-based assessments of the security of current family relationships (Steinberg, Davila, & Fincham, 2006). In particular, relationship-maintaining behaviors in the midst of conflict are most consistently linked to adolescent security and, typically, the behavior of the adolescent (rather than the parents) is most predictive. In some sense, these relationship-supporting behaviors may be viewed as "secure-base" behaviors, in which the secure adolescent revisits and refreshes the attachment bond even in the midst of exploring verbal autonomy from parents. This process can be observed even very early in adolescence. Attachment security in current relationships with parents, assessed via the Late Childhood Attachment Interview (Zimmermann & Scheuerer-Englisch, 2000) is related to more agreeable and less hostile autonomy displays among 12-year-olds (Zimmermann et al., 2009). Although much of the research in this area has been done with mothers, research with fathers is consistent with the operation of a similar process in which paternal use of harsh, relationship-undermining conflict tactics is linked to adolescent insecurity (Allen et al., 2007).

Security within the current relationship with parents also appears to moderate effects of preexisting genetic dispositions on the autonomy process. The short allele of the serotonin transporter gene, 5-HTTLPR, for example, has been associated with greater emotionality and sensitivity to emotional stimuli in the environment. Secure adolescents with this short allele have been found to have greater agreeability in handling autonomy issues with parents, whereas insecure adolescents with this same short allele displayed more hostile autonomy in interactions with parents (Zimmermann et al., 2009). The results suggest that security may aid the adolescent in handling preexisting temperamental emotionality and sensitivity. Notably, no main effects of this short allele on attachment security were found.

In terms of specific types of insecure states of mind, dismissing adolescents show the least autonomy and relatedness of all attachment groups observed in interactions with parents (Becker-Stoll et al., 2008). This suggests that a dismissing individual's characteristic withdrawal from engagement with attachment experiences may particularly hinder the task of renegotiating parent–adolescent relationships. Families of dismissing adolescents also tend, in turn, to be less responsive to their adolescents, at least as compared to families of preoccupied adolescents (Reimer, Overton, Steidl, Rosenstein, & Horowitz, 1996).

For adolescents with dismissing states of mind, research on a physiological marker of stress—heart rate interbeat interval reactivity—suggests that difficulty in managing the stress of autonomy-based conflicts with parents may partially explain the link between attachment insecurity and adolescent autonomy and relatedness struggles. Dismissing adolescents displayed less interbeat interval reactivity (i.e., appeared *less* stressed) during the AAI than secure adolescents, perhaps reflecting their general success in minimizing attention paid to stressful aspects of attachment memories. However, during a conflict interaction task with their mothers, dismissing adolescents displayed significantly greater interbeat interval reactivity, thus appearing significantly more stressed than adolescents with secure states of mind (Beijersbergen, Bakermans-Kranenburg, Van IJzendoorn, & Juffer, 2008). These results are consistent with the idea that dismissing adolescents avoid emotionally charged discussions but then struggle when such discussions cannot be avoided. This finding in many ways is consistent with the earlier suggestion that insecure adolescents with the short allele of the 5-HTTLPR gene may struggle more with emotionality in handling autonomy discussions (Zimmermann et al., 2009).

Insecure preoccupation, in contrast, appears to be most strongly associated with heightened and unproductive overengagement with parents in arguments that ultimately undermine an adolescent's autonomy (Allen & Hauser, 1996). This overengagement appears to extend well into late adolescence because adolescents with insecure-preoccupied states of mind appear more likely to have difficulty leaving home successfully for college, displaying higher levels of both conflict and contact with parents during the transition (Bernier, Larose, & Whipple, 2005). These effects were not observed for adolescents who were not leaving for college, suggesting that these attachment dynamics are activated mainly in the presence of the significant stress of leaving home on the attachment system.

### Individual Differences in Peer Relationships

A large, rapidly growing body of research suggests a fairly tight link between a secure adolescent attachment organization and competence in close friendships. Secure adolescents are more comfortable with the intimate emotional interactions common in close friendships (Allen et al., 2007; Sroufe et al., 2005; Weimer, Kerns, & Oldenberg, 2004; Zimmermann, 2004). Security has also been consistently associated with higher quality friendships and lower stress in peer relationships in general (Seiffge-Krenke, 2006; Shomaker & Furman, 2009). Observational data suggest that this competence is a result of generalized comfort in handling emotional reactions in challenging situations (Zimmermann, Maier, Winter, & Grossmann, 2001). Conversely, using Hazan and Shaver's (1987) three-category prototype measure of attachment style, anxious-ambivalent adolescents are found to be more prone to interpersonal hostility (Cooper, Shaver, & Collins, 1998). Preoccupied states of mind similarly are associated with greater stress in peer relationships (Seiffge-Krenke, 2006). Although some research suggests that security is more relevant to functioning in close relationships than in broader peer relationships, and that representations of different types of relationships at times display only modest concordance with one another (Furman, Stephenson, & Rhoades, 2014; Lieberman, Doyle, & Markiewicz, 1999), adolescent security has been linked to broader measures of social competence, such as popularity and social acceptance, as well as to generally more prosocial behavior and less shy or aggressive behavior with peers (Allen et al., 1998, 2007; Dykas, Ziv, & Cassidy, 2008). Conversely, more dismissing (vs. secure) states of mind have been associated more generally with poorer focus on problem discussions and weaker communication skills with friends, even after accounting for gender differences and current parent–adolescent relationship qualities (Shomaker & Furman, 2009).

Similar to the previously discussed findings with parents, significant communication and perceptual difficulties appear as one potential explanation for the problematic peer relationships of insecure adolescents. Using the ECR scale, for example, avoidant attachment styles in adolescence have been associated with absolute discrepancies between adolescent and peer perceptions of the adolescent's peer relationships (Ehrlich et al., 2014). In addition, teens with avoidant styles report more negative self-perceptions of peer relationships (even compared to their peers' reports), suggesting a specific negative attentional bias on the part of the avoidant adolescent. At least in part, this bias appears to be linked to difficulties in trying to recall and evaluate past relationship experiences. For example, although adolescents classified as secure and insecure on the AAI did not differ in how they perceived unfamiliar peers initially, attachment-related differences emerged over time. Two weeks after the interaction, insecure adolescents remembered the interactions as less positive and more negative and also recalled being treated with greater hostility than they had initially reported. In contrast, secure adolescents' memories of the negative aspects of the interaction and of hostile treatment remained stable, although, like insecure adolescents, they recalled the conflicts as being less positive than initially reported (Dykas et al., 2012).

These findings are important as a potential explanation of the origin of hostile attributional biases in adolescents. These attributional biases, in which individuals interpret ambiguous behaviors of others as likely to be hostile in nature, have proven to be one of the best explanatory mechanisms identified to date to account for adolescent aggression toward peers (Dodge, 1993). The perceptual and recall bias findings cited earlier—tying together insecurity, perceptual biases, and hostility—suggest that the origin of hostile attributional biases may lie within qualities of attachment relationships and attachment memories. These findings are also consistent with the long-standing finding that hostility, as observed by close friends, is linked to late

adolescents' insecure attachment states of mind (Kobak & Sceery, 1988).

A second mechanism to explain the peer-relational difficulties of insecure adolescents relates to their potential difficulty in handling the intensity of close relationships. Discomfort with attachment-related affect and experiences may lead adolescents with dismissing attachment strategies to push away peers, particularly those who could become close friends (Larose & Bernier, 2001; Spangler & Zimmermann, 1999). Anxious attachment styles assessed via the Measure of Attachment Quality have similarly been related to stronger physiological reactions, in the form of higher blood pressure, to peer interactions and to conflict situations (Gallo & Matthews, 2006). This suggests that one reason insecure adolescents may push away peers who could become close friends is to prevent being overwhelmed by the emotionality engendered by close relationships.

Strong connections have also been found between security and the ability to seek emotional support from a peer (Allen et al., 2007). Linkages between AAI security and adaptive support seeking have even been found when adolescents are asked to interact with unfamiliar peers (Feeney, Cassidy, & Ramos-Marcuse, 2008). The use of unfamiliar peers makes clear that the observed linkages are unlikely to be solely a result either of qualities of current peer interactions influencing attachment or of peer selection effects. In some cases, adaptive support-seeking behavior with peers is more strongly linked with adolescent attachment states of mind than are some of the best markers of maternal and paternal relationship qualities (Allen et al., 2007). This is not necessarily surprising given that mastering the realm of peer relationships may be the single greatest social-developmental challenge faced by most adolescents, and that the nexus of energy in developing attachment behaviors is gradually shifting from parent to peer relations during adolescence.

Individual differences in attachment are also consistently linked to behavior in romantic and sexual relationships in adolescence. Qualities of adolescents' representations of relationships with romantic partners display substantial similarities to representations of relationships with parents and friends (Furman, 2001). Similarly, positive adolescent secure-base scripts from interactions with parents have been linked to romantic attachment styles characterized by less avoidance and anxiety (Dykas, Woodhouse, Cassidy, & Waters, 2006). Notably, both attachment states of mind from the

AAI and attachment representations from the Current Relationship Interview have been found to predict qualities of current romantic relationships, with each of these indices accounting for unique variance in current relationship qualities (Haydon, Collins, Salvatore, Simpson, & Roisman, 2012; Roisman, Madsen, Hennighausen, Sroufe, & Collins, 2001): These constructs are clearly not redundant, but rather are each capturing important aspects of adolescent attachment processes linked to future behavior.

In terms of attachment within romantic relationships, assessments of self-reported insecurity in these relationships has been linked both to greater anxiety among relationship partners and to greater incidence of (but less enjoyment derived from) sexual intercourse (Tracy, Shaver, Albino, & Cooper, 2003). Current social-environmental factors appear to moderate these effects. Adolescents with preoccupied states of mind whose mothers appeared overbearing in interactions were more likely to engage in early sexual activity, whereas preoccupied adolescents whose mothers were less overbearing had strikingly lower rates of early sexual activity (Marsh, McFarland, Allen, McElhaney, & Land, 2003). Similarly, preoccupied females who also had problematic interactions with teachers were at heightened risk of precocious sexual involvement (Kobak, Herres, Gaskins, & Laurenceau, 2012). Of course, in thinking about qualities of romantic relationships, *partners'* attachment organization will also be important to consider because even later in adulthood, only modest evidence of assortative mating with respect to attachment exists (Treboux, Crowell, & Waters, 2004).

## Attachment and Adolescent Mental Health

A number of recent studies suggest substantial links between adolescent states of mind and mental health. As described below, both preoccupied and dismissing strategies have been implicated in problems of psychosocial functioning, although the two are associated with somewhat different patterns of problematic functioning. Recently, insecurity in measures of both current attachment styles and qualities of current attachment relationships have also been linked to mental health difficulties.

Adolescents' use of preoccupied strategies has been most closely linked to internalizing problems, including self-reports of depression, anxiety disorders, internalizing symptoms, and stress during transitions (Bakermans-Kranenburg & Van IJzendoorn, 2009; Bernier et al., 2005; Cole-Detke & Kobak, 1996; Larose & Bernier, 2001). In addition, preoccupied attachment states of mind may interact with a wide array of psychosocial and environmental factors to predict critical outcomes. When preoccupied teens are confronted with intrapsychic states or environments that are confusing or enmeshing, higher levels of internalizing symptoms are found. For example, Adam, Sheldon-Keller, and West (1996) reported that suicidality in adolescence was associated with a combination of preoccupied and unresolved attachment status. Similarly, preoccupied adolescents who had mothers who could not exercise their own autonomy in discussions (i.e., were passive and enmeshed) displayed higher levels of depression (Marsh et al., 2003).

Preoccupied teens also display risk for at least some externalizing behaviors, tending to increase over time in levels of sexual risk-taking and aggressive behavior (Dawson, Allen, Marston, Hafen, & Schad, 2014; Kobak, Zajac, & Smith, 2009). This risk for externalizing behavior also appears to be moderated by social-environmental factors. For example, when preoccupied teens are exposed to positive friendships, they appear at lower risk for delinquent behavior (McElhaney, Immele, Smith, & Allen, 2006). When exposed to effective maternal behavioral control strategies, both preoccupied and secure teens have lower levels of delinquent behavior than do dismissing teens exposed to the same maternal behavior (Allen et al., 1998). In contrast, in unresponsive environments, such as when mothers who display extremely high levels of their own (maternal) autonomy in discussions, perhaps asserting themselves to the point of ignoring their adolescents, preoccupied teens have higher levels of drug use and delinquent behavior over the following year (Marsh et al., 2003).

One potential explanation for this effect in female adolescents may be that that an insecure-anxious attachment style is linked to the presence of higher cortisol levels upon awakening and a diminished cortisol awakening response indicative of a degree of dysregulation in physiological stress mediation processes (Oskis, Loveday, Hucklebridge, Thorn, & Clow, 2011). This potential dysregulation, and the need to manage it, may in turn lead preoccupied and anxiously attached adolescents to be particularly sensitive to their social environments. It should be noted, however, that a hyperactivated attachment system, although clearly problematic, is nonetheless a system that continues to function; in cases where it brings the adolescent into contact with positive social interactions, it appears to at least potentially leave the teen responsive to these as well (Allen et al., 1998).

In contrast to preoccupied adolescents, adolescents with dismissing strategies appear more likely to take on externalizing behaviors, which may serve to distract attention from attachment-related cues (Bakermans-Kranenburg & Van IJzendoorn, 2009; Kobak & Cole, 1994). Dismissing attachment states of mind have been found predictive of increasing delinquency and externalizing behavior over both shorter and longer spans of adolescence (Allen et al., 2002, 2007), although not all studies reveal such an effect (Kobak & Zajac, 2011). In addition, dismissing attachment strategies have been linked to difficulty getting assistance from peers and teachers, as well as to peer-reported social withdrawal during the transition to college (Larose & Bernier, 2001). Consistent with this finding, insecurity that manifests itself primarily as dismissal of attachment in early adolescence has been linked to relative *decreases* in social skills over time (Allen et al., 2002) and to less active coping strategies (Seiffge-Krenke & Beyers, 2005). Cole-Detke and Kobak (1996) also reported that in a college population, individuals with an eating disorder were more likely to use dismissing strategies; the attention given to their eating behaviors was hypothesized to distract from internal states of emotional distress. Unlike preoccupied adolescents, dismissing adolescents do not appear to be particularly sensitive to parental behaviors. For example, a factor such as parental control of adolescent behavior, which is well established as a buffer against delinquency, does not appear to serve this role for dismissing teens (Allen et al., 1998).

Unresolved states of mind have been the subject of far less psychopathology research than dismissing or preoccupied states. Unresolved states have been linked to prior negative experiences including poor early attachments in infancy and the preschool years, problematic middle school teacher–child relationships, and friendship difficulties in early adolescence (Aikins, Howes, & Hamilton, 2009; Madigan, Moran, & Pederson, 2006). Experiences of trauma and childhood sexual abuse have also been linked to an unresolved attachment state of mind in adolescence (Bailey, Moran, & Pederson, 2007; Madigan, Vaillancourt, McKibbon, & Benoit, 2012). In turn, these states

of mind have been significantly related to dissociative thought problems in adolescence (Madigan et al., 2012). Among adolescents requiring residential treatment, a heightened prevalence of insecure-unresolved attachment status has been repeatedly observed (Allen, Hauser, & Borman-Spurrell, 1996; Wallis & Steele, 2001).

Beyond the AAI, insecurity assessed via a number of other attachment measures has been linked to problems in functioning. Using the Childhood Attachment Interview (Target, Fonagy, & Shmueli-Goetz, 2003), patterned after the AAI's approach to assessing states of mind, adolescent insecurity has been linked to oppositional defiant disorder and teacher ratings of behavioral adjustment difficulties at school (Scott, Briskman, Woolgar, Humayun, & O'Connor, 2011). Both effects were observed, over and above those obtained from careful observations of qualities of parenting behavior (Scott et al., 2011). Using the Experiences in Close Relationships measure, Lee and Hankin (2009) found that both anxious and avoidant attachment styles predicted increases in anxiety and depressive symptoms over time.

We also now have evidence of specific parent–adolescent attachment relationship qualities linked to adolescent mental health. Adolescents' perceptions of parents as a secure base are associated with lower parent reports of adolescent internalizing and externalizing symptoms (Woodhouse, Dykas, & Cassidy, 2009). Maternal attachment states of mind have been found to predict sons' military adjustment, even over and above sons' states of mind, suggesting continued potential influence of mother–son attachment processes (Scharf, Mayseless, & Kivenson-Baron, 2012). Higher levels of security in adolescents' current attachment styles also predict lower levels of substance abuse, an effect that appears to be mediated by higher levels of maternal monitoring of adolescent behavior (Branstetter, Furman, & Cottrell, 2009).

When long-term predictions to adolescence from earlier periods were examined in the Minnesota Study of Risk and Adaptation, stable patterns (as opposed to occasional instances) of insecurity were the strongest predictors of a variety of problematic functional outcomes (Van Ryzin, Carlson, & Sroufe, 2011). Relatedly, predictions from infancy appear to be mediated partly by problematic peer relationships in the intervening period (Bosquet & Egeland, 2006). Together, these findings suggest that in terms of future predictions, enduring patterns of problematic attachment and social relationship functioning may be of greater importance than occasional instances of apparent insecurity.

Attachment theory is also beginning to serve as an underpinning for interventions with disturbed adolescents. Pilot work on the Connect Program, an attachment-focused, manualized intervention for parents and teens at risk for aggressive behavior, has found decreases in levels of conduct problems, as well as depression and anxiety over time, among participating teens (Moretti & Obsuth, 2009). Within long-term residential treatment, security has been found to predict adolescents' secure base use with therapists, although this effect was not seen in short-term treatment (Zegers, Schuengel, Van IJzendoorn, & Janssens, 2006). This suggests that only long-term treatment may have been able to create a sufficiently intense relationship between teen and therapist to call attachment states of mind strongly into play.

## Lifespan Continuity, Discontinuity, and an Organizational Perspective on Attachment in Adolescence

A fundamental challenge for lifespan theories of attachment is the finding that adolescent attachment processes display only modest continuity with qualities of attachment relationships earlier in the lifespan (Hamilton, 2000; Weinfield, Whaley, & Egeland, 2004), even though the AAI appears to produce relatively stable classifications across adolescence (Allen et al., 2004; Zimmermann & Becker-Stoll, 2002). Adolescent security assessed with the AAI also displays very modest concurrent correlations with maternal security and none with paternal security (Allen et al., 2004; Scharf et al., 2012). Some concordances have been observed between specific adolescent state-of-mind scales within the AAI and both maternal and paternal state-of-mind scales, although even these are quite modest in size (Scharf et al., 2012). The low absolute magnitude of these continuities is consistent with the notion that as AAI states of mind develop, inputs beyond early caregiver relationship qualities and parents' current states of mind play a prominent role.

Research is now beginning to identify qualities of the ongoing parent–adolescent relationship that may influence adolescent attachment security. For example, when autonomy-undermining, enmeshed behavior between mothers and adolescents is observed at age 16, it predicts relative decreases in security in adolescent states of mind from ages 16 to 18 (Allen et al., 2004). Conversely, the presence of adolescent *secure-base scripts*—adolescents' expectations that attachment relationships will provide a secure base from which to explore the larger environment—has been linked to security in adolescent states of mind (Dykas et al., 2006). Also, parents' self-reported secure attachment styles have now been found to predict adolescents' use of parents as a secure base while discussing a disagreement, with consistent mediation of adolescent security via parents' lack of hostile behavior toward the adolescent (Jones & Cassidy, 2014).

Genetic factors have also been examined as potential sources of continuity and discontinuity in attachment processes across time and generations. With attachment as assessed via a Child Attachment Interview, designed to closely follow the principles of the AAI (Shmueli-Goetz, Target, Fonagy, & Datta, 2008), substantial heritability is found along with significant nonshared environment effects and virtually no shared environmental effects (Fearon, Shmueli-Goetz, Viding, Fonagy, & Plomin, 2014). These authors suggest that as children develop, heritable traits gradually influence their interactions with caregivers in ways that then shape their attachment states of mind, but do so uniquely for each child within a family. Conversely, evidence of strong environmental influences on attachment is found among youth exposed to extremes in poor parenting during early childhood. Among these youth, about half are secure in Child Attachment Interview assessments of their relationships with foster parents, whereas almost all are insecure in relationship to birth parents (Joseph, O'Connor, Briskman, Maughan, & Scott, 2014).

Perhaps the most important explanation for the lack of strong continuity between infant Strange Situation status and adolescent AAI security, however, lies in the fundamental difference in the nature of these two constructs. If we simply examine the origin of the AAI and the validation research that led to its rapid adoption in the field, it is difficult to avoid the conclusion that the AAI is most directly tapping not the *attachment* system of the individual, but the *caregiving* system, although clearly the two are closely connected (Allen & Manning, 2007). Just as with adults, the AAI coding system predicts adolescent parents' success as caregivers in raising a secure infant far more strongly than it predicts any other single outcome (Ward & Carlson, 1995)—as indeed it was primarily designed to do (Main et al., 1985). This may well explain why the AAI is more strongly related to current peer relationships than to parental relationships: Teens rarely serve as caregivers to parents but may at times meet needs of peers. Observed continuities between infant attachment status and adolescent management of autonomy struggles with parents also make clear that infant attachment status has implications for future adolescent relationship qualities, even if not directly for adolescent states of mind (Grossmann et al., 2005; Zimmermann et al., 2001). Infant security with mothers has even been found to be more predictive of observed qualities of autonomy and relatedness in adolescent–mother interactions than it is of adolescent states of mind regarding attachment (Becker-Stoll et al., 2008). Together, these findings suggest that continuity from infant attachment security to the qualities of an adolescent attachment *relationship* can be observed, even in the absence of continuity from infant security to the adolescent's later internalized *state of mind* regarding attachment.

Recognition of the multifaceted nature of the attachment system in adolescence can help make sense of these findings. Prior to recent advances, researchers often had only the AAI to rely on in assessing adolescent attachment. The temptation to squeeze myriad constructs (e.g., current relationship security, representations of current and past relationships, attachment styles) under the umbrella of the AAI was understandable, although it made explaining inconsistent continuity findings nearly impossible. Recently, however, the field has advanced to the point that we now have the means to assess directly many facets of the attachment system independently, and to gain greater precision in our terminology and understanding of attachment as an organizational construct.

In understanding what these developments mean for the relation of adolescent attachment to attachment at other stages, a botanical metaphor perhaps best captures the organic and complex nature of the phenomena at hand. We can view the attachment system as analogous to a tree with strong roots in infant–caregiver attachment as seen in the Strange Situation. By adolescence, those roots remain and support the health of the tree, but they have now given rise to a highly complex organism with multiple facets, each distinct, yet each part of the same organic whole: We now can and must attend not only to historical and ongoing attachment relationships to caregivers (the roots and tree trunk) but also to the beginnings of new attachment relationships with close peers and romantic partners (the branches), to patterns of information processing relative to attachment that are affected by and affect each of these (the shape of the tree), and to the emergence of a caregiving system (flowers) that ultimately will affect attachment processes in the next generation (seeds). In addition, *each* of these facets is influenced by environmental factors such as exposure to severe stressors and new peer relationships.

Understanding continuities between the infant Strange Situation and the adolescent AAI remains a worthy endeavor, but this botanical metaphor suggests that this task is in many ways analogous to trying to find the similarities between the roots and the flowers of a tree. There are likely to be not only multiple areas of continuity but also multiple areas of divergence and, indeed, branching among distinct yet related attachment constructs. The search for simple "stability" in attachment from infancy to adolescence becomes logically problematic because measuring stability requires the existence of the same construct at both points. Even the search for exceptionally strong continuities over time between fundamentally different facets of an organic system may well lead to disappointment. Links are likely to exist, but they are likely to be more complex than straightforward, as befits any truly developmental process. To put it most simply, the growing complexity of the adolescent social, emotional, and cognitive world necessitates a growing complexity of our understanding of the role of the attachment system as an organic factor within it.

## Acknowledgment

This chapter was completed with the assistance of grants from the National Institute of Child Health and Human Development.

## References

Adam, K. S., Sheldon-Keller, A. E., & West, M. (1996). Attachment organization and history of suicidal behavior in clinical adolescents. *Journal of Consulting and Clinical Psychology, 64*, 264–272.

Aikins, J. W., Howes, C., & Hamilton, C. (2009). Attachment stability and the emergence of unresolved representations during adolescence. *Attachment and Human Development, 11*(5), 491–512.

Allen, J. P., & Hauser, S. T. (1996). Autonomy and relatedness in adolescent–family interactions as predictors of young adults' states of mind regarding attachment. *Development and Psychopathology, 8*(4), 793–809.

Allen, J. P., Hauser, S. T., & Borman-Spurrell, E. (1996). Attachment theory as a framework for understanding sequelae of severe adolescent psychopathology: An 11-year follow-up study. *Journal of Consulting and Clinical Psychology, 64*(2), 254–263.

Allen, J. P., & Manning, N. (2007). From safety to affect regulation: Attachment from the vantage point of adolescence. *New Directions in Child and Adolescent Development, 117*, 23–39.

Allen, J. P., Marsh, P., McFarland, C., McElhaney, K. B., Land, D. J., Jodl, K. M., et al. (2002). Attachment and autonomy as predictors of the development of social skills and delinquency during midadolescence. *Journal of Consulting and Clinical Psychology, 70*(1), 56–66.

Allen, J. P., McElhaney, K. B., Kuperminc, G. P., & Jodl, K. M. (2004). Stability and change in attachment security across adolescence. *Child Development, 75*, 1792–1805.

Allen, J. P., McElhaney, K. B., Land, D. J., Kuperminc, G. P., Moore, C. M., O'Beirne-Kelley, H., et al. (2003). A secure base in adolescence: Markers of attachment security in the mother–adolescent relationship. *Child Development, 74*, 292–307.

Allen, J. P., Moore, C. M., & Kuperminc, G. P. (1997). Developmental approaches to understanding adolescent deviance. In S. S. Luthar & J. A. Burack (Eds.), *Developmental psychopathology: Perspectives on adjustment, risk, and disorder* (pp. 548–567). New York: Cambridge University Press.

Allen, J. P., Moore, C. [M.], Kuperminc, G. [P.], & Bell, K. (1998). Attachment and adolescent psychosocial functioning. *Child Development, 69*(5), 1406–1419.

Allen, J. P., Porter, M. R., McFarland, F. C., McElhaney, K. B., & Marsh, P. A. (2007). The relation of attachment security to adolescents' paternal and peer relationships, depression, and externalizing behavior. *Child Development, 78*, 1222–1239.

Bailey, H. N., Moran, G., & Pederson, D. R. (2007). Childhood maltreatment, complex trauma symptoms, and unresolved attachment in an at-risk sample of adolescent mothers. *Attachment and Human Development, 9*(2), 139–161.

Bakermans-Kranenburg, M. J., & Van IJzendoorn, M. H. (2009). The first 10,000 adult attachment interviews: Distributions of adult attachment representations in clinical and non-clinical groups. *Attachment and Human Development, 11*(3), 223–263.

Becker-Stoll, F., Fremmer-Bombik, E., Wartner, U., Zimmermann, P., & Grossmann, K. E. (2008). Is attachment at ages 1, 6 and 16 related to autonomy and relatedness behavior of adolescents in interaction towards their mothers? *International Journal of Behavioral Development, 32*(5), 372–380.

Beijersbergen, M. D., Bakermans-Kranenburg, M. J., Van IJzendoorn, M. H., & Juffer, F. (2008). Stress

regulation in adolescents: Physiological reactivity during the Adult Attachment Interview and conflict interaction. *Child Development, 79*(6), 1707–1720.

Berger, L. E., Jodl, K. M., Allen, J. P., McElhaney, K. B., & Kuperminc, G. P. (2005). When adolescents disagree with others about their symptoms: Differences in attachment organization as an explanation of discrepancies between adolescent-, parent-, and peer-reports of behavior problems. *Development and Psychopathology, 17*, 489–507.

Bernier, A., Larose, S., & Whipple, N. (2005). Leaving home for college: A potentially stressful event for adolescents with preoccupied attachment patterns. *Attachment and Human Development, 7*(2), 171–185.

Bosquet, M., & Egeland, B. (2006). The development and maintenance of anxiety symptoms from infancy through adolescence in a longitudinal sample. *Development and Psychopathology, 18*(2), 517–550.

Bowlby, J. (1982). *Attachment and loss, Vol. 1.* New York: Basic Books. (Original work published 1969)

Branstetter, S. A., Furman, W., & Cottrell, L. (2009). The influence of representations of attachment, maternal–adolescent relationship quality, and maternal monitoring on adolescent substance use: A 2-year longitudinal examination. *Child Development, 80*(5), 1448–1462.

Coan, J. A. (2010). Adult attachment and the brain. *Journal of Social and Personal Relationships, 27*(2), 210–217.

Cole-Detke, H., & Kobak, R. (1996). Attachment processes in eating disorder and depression. *Journal of Consulting and Clinical Psychology, 64*(2), 282–290.

Collins, W. A., & Laursen, B. (2004). Changing relationships, changing youth: Interpersonal Contexts of adolescent development. *Journal of Early Adolescence, 24*(1), 55–62.

Collins, W. A., Welsh, D. P., & Furman, W. (2009). Adolescent romantic relationships. *Annual Review of Psychology, 60*(1), 631–652.

Cooper, M. L., Shaver, P. R., & Collins, N. L. (1998). Attachment styles, emotion regulation, and adjustment in adolescence. *Journal of Personality and Social Psychology, 74*(5), 1380–1397.

Dawson, A. E., Allen, J. P., Marston, E. G., Hafen, C. A., & Schad, M. A. (2014). Adolescent insecure attachment as a predictor of maladaptive coping and externalizing behaviors in emerging adulthood: The mediating role of maladaptive coping. *Attachment and Human Development, 16*(5), 462–478.

De Wolff, M., & Van IJzendoorn, M. H. (1997). Sensitivity and attachment: A meta-analysis on parental antecedents of infant attachment. *Child Development, 68*(4), 571–591.

Dodge, K. A. (1993). Social-cognitive mechanisms in the development of conduct disorder and depression. *Annual Review of Psychology, 44*, 559–584.

Dykas, M. J., & Cassidy, J. (2011). Attachment and the processing of social information across the life span:

Theory and evidence. *Psychological Bulletin, 137*(1), 19–46.

Dykas, M. J., Woodhouse, S. S., Cassidy, J., & Waters, H. S. (2006). Narrative assessment of attachment representations: Links between secure base scripts and adolescent attachment. *Attachment and Human Development, 8*(3), 221–240.

Dykas, M. J., Woodhouse, S. S., Ehrlich, K. B., & Cassidy, J. (2010). Do adolescents and parents reconstruct memories about their conflict as a function of adolescent attachment? *Child Development, 81*(5), 1445–1459.

Dykas, M. J., Woodhouse, S. S., Ehrlich, K. B., & Cassidy, J. (2012). Attachment-related differences in perceptions of an initial peer interaction emerge over time: Evidence of reconstructive memory processes in adolescents. *Developmental Psychology, 48*(5), 1381–1389.

Dykas, M. J., Woodhouse, S. S., Jones, J. D., & Cassidy, J. (2014). Attachment-related biases in adolescents' memory. *Child Development, 85*(6), 2185–2201.

Dykas, M. J., Ziv, Y., & Cassidy, J. (2008). Attachment and peer relations in adolescence. *Attachment and Human Development, 10*(2), 123–141.

Ehrlich, K. B., Cassidy, J., & Dykas, M. J. (2011). Reporter discrepancies among parents, adolescents, and peers: Adolescent attachment and informant depressive symptoms as explanatory factors. *Child Development, 82*(3), 999–1012.

Ehrlich, K. B., Cassidy, J., Lejuez, C. W., & Daughters, S. B. (2014). Discrepancies about adolescent relationships as a function of informant attachment and depressive symptoms. *Journal of Research on Adolescence, 24*(4), 654–666.

Fearon, P., Shmueli-Goetz, Y., Viding, E., Fonagy, P., & Plomin, R. (2014). Genetic and environmental influences on adolescent attachment. *Journal of Child Psychology and Psychiatry, 55*(9), 1033–1041.

Feeney, B. C., Cassidy, J., & Ramos-Marcuse, F. (2008). The generalization of attachment representations to new social situations: Predicting behavior during initial interactions with strangers. *Journal of Personality and Social Psychology, 95*(6), 1481–1498.

Furman, W. (2001). Working models of friendships. *Journal of Social and Personal Relationships, 18*(5), 583–602.

Furman, W., Stephenson, J. C., & Rhoades, G. K. (2014). Positive interactions and avoidant and anxious representations in relationships with parents, friends, and romantic partners. *Journal of Research on Adolescence, 24*(4), 615–629.

Gallo, L. C., & Matthews, K. A. (2006). Adolescents' attachment orientation influences ambulatory blood pressure responses to everyday social interactions. *Psychosomatic Medicine, 68*(2), 253–261.

Grossmann, K., Grossmann, K. E., Kindler, H., & Waters, E. (2005). Early care and the roots of attachment and partnership representations. In K. Grossman, K. E. Grossman, & H. Kindler (Eds.), *Attachment from infancy to adulthood: The major longitudinal studies* (pp. 98–136). New York: Guilford Press.

Hamilton, C. E. (2000). Continuity and discontinuity of attachment from infancy through adolescence. *Child Development, 71*, 690–694.

Haydon, K. C., Collins, W. A., Salvatore, J. E., Simpson, J. A., & Roisman, G. I. (2012). Shared and distinctive origins and correlates of adult attachment representations: The developmental organization of romantic functioning. *Child Development, 83*(5), 1689–1702.

Hazan, C., & Shaver, P. (1987). Romantic love conceptualized as an attachment process. *Journal of Personality and Social Psychology, 52*, 511–524.

Hesse, E. (2008). The Adult Attachment Interview: Protocol, method of analysis, and empirical studies. In J. Cassidy & P. R. Shaver (Eds.), *Handbook of attachment: Theory, research, and clinical applications* (2nd ed., pp. 552–598). New York: Guilford Press.

Hofer, M. (2006). Psychobiological roots of early attachment. *Current Directions in Psychological Science, 15*(2), 84–88.

Holt-Lunstad, J., Smith, T. B., & Layton, J. B. (2010). Social relationships and mortality risk: A meta-analysis. *PLoS Medicine, 7*(7), 1–20.

Jones, J. D., & Cassidy, J. (2014). Parental attachment style: Examination of links with parent secure base provision and adolescent secure base use. *Attachment and Human Development, 16*(5), 437–461.

Joseph, M. A., O'Connor, T. G., Briskman, J. A., Maughan, B., & Scott, S. (2014). The formation of secure new attachments by children who were maltreated: An observational study of adolescents in foster care. *Development and Psychopathology, 26*(1), 67–80.

Keating, D. P. (1990). Adolescent thinking. In S. S. Feldman & G. R. Elliott (Eds.), *At the threshold: The developing adolescent* (pp. 54–89). Cambridge, MA: Harvard University Press.

Kobak, R., Herres, J., Gaskins, C., & Laurenceau, J. P. (2012). Teacher–student interactions and attachment states of mind as predictors of early romantic involvement and risky sexual behaviors. *Attachment and Human Development, 14*(3), 289–303.

Kobak, R., Rosenthal, N. L., Zajac, K., & Madsen, S. D. (2007). Adolescent attachment hierarchies and the search for an adult pair-bond. *New Directions for Child and Adolescent Development, 2007*(117), 57–72.

Kobak, R., & Zajac, K. (2011). Rethinking adolescent states of mind. In D. Cicchetti & G. I. Roisman (Eds.), *Minnesota Symposia on Child Psychology: The origins and organization of adaptation and maladaptation* (Vol. 4, pp. 185–229). New York: Wiley.

Kobak, R., Zajac, K., & Smith, C. (2009). Adolescent attachment and trajectories of hostile–impulsive behavior: Implications for the development of personality disorders. *Development and Psychopathology, 21*(3), 839–851.

Kobak, R. R., & Cole, H. (1994). Attachment and meta-monitoring: Implications for adolescent autonomy and psychopathology. In D. Cicchetti & S. L. Toth (Eds.), *Disorders and dysfunctions of the self: Rochester Symposium on Developmental Psychopathology* (Vol. 5, pp. 267–297). Rochester, NY: University of Rochester Press.

Kobak, R. R., Cole, H., Ferenz-Gillies, R., Fleming, W., & Gamble, W. (1993). Attachment and emotion regulation during mother-teen problem-solving: A control theory analysis. *Child Development, 64,* 231–245.

Kobak, R. R., & Duemmler, S. (1994). Attachment and conversation: Toward a discourse analysis of adolescent and adult security. In K. Bartholomew & D. Perlman (Eds.), *Attachment processes in adulthood: Advances in personal relationships* (Vol. 5, pp. 121–149). London: Jessica Kingsley.

Kobak, R. R., & Sceery, A. (1988). Attachment in late adolescence: Working models, affect regulation and representations of self and others. *Child Development, 59,* 135–146.

Larose, S., & Bernier, A. (2001). Social support processes: Mediators of attachment state of mind and adjustment in late adolescence. *Attachment and Human Development, 3*(1), 96–120.

Lee, A., & Hankin, B. L. (2009). Insecure attachment, dysfunctional attitudes, and low self-esteem predicting prospective symptoms of depression and anxiety during adolescence. *Journal of Clinical Child and Adolescent Psychology, 38*(2), 219–231.

Lieberman, M., Doyle, A.-B., & Markiewicz, D. (1999). Developmental patterns in security of attachment to mother and father in late childhood and early adolescence: Associations with peer relations. *Child Development, 70*(1), 202–213.

Madigan, S., Moran, G., & Pederson, D. R. (2006). Unresolved states of mind, disorganized attachment relationships, and disrupted interactions of adolescent mothers and their infants. *Developmental Psychology, 42*(2), 293–304.

Madigan, S., Vaillancourt, K., McKibbon, A., & Benoit, D. (2012). The reporting of maltreatment experiences during the Adult Attachment Interview in a sample of pregnant adolescents. *Attachment and Human Development, 14*(2), 119–143.

Main, M. (1999). Attachment theory: Eighteen points. In J. Cassidy & P. R. Shaver (Eds.), *Handbook of attachment: Theory, research, and clinical applications* (pp. 845–887). New York: Guilford Press.

Main, M., Goldwyn, R., & Hesse, E. (2002). *Adult attachment scoring and classification systems, Version 7.1.* Unpublished manuscript, University of California at Berkeley.

Main, M., Kaplan, N., & Cassidy, J. (1985). Security in infancy, childhood, and adulthood: A move to the level of representation. In I. Bretherton & E. Waters (Eds.), Growing points in attachment theory and research. *Monographs of the Society for Research in Child Development, 50*(Serial No. 209), 66–104.

Markiewicz, D., Lawford, H., Doyle, A. B., & Haggart, N. (2006). Developmental differences in adolescents' and young adults' use of mothers, fathers, best friends, and romantic partners to fulfill attachment needs. *Journal of Youth and Adolescence, 35*(1), 121–134.

Marsh, P., McFarland, F. C., Allen, J. P., McElhaney, K. B., & Land, D. J. (2003). Attachment, autonomy, and multifinality in adolescent internalizing and risky behavioral symptoms. *Development and Psychopathology, 15*(2), 451–467.

McElhaney, K. B., Immele, A., Smith, F. D., & Allen, J. P. (2006). Attachment organization as a moderator of the link between peer relationships and adolescent delinquency. *Attachment and Human Development, 8,* 33–46.

Mikulincer, M., & Nachshon, O. (1991). Attachment styles and patterns of self-disclosure. *Journal of Personality and Social Psychology, 61*(2), 321–331.

Moretti, M. M., & Obsuth, I. (2009). Effectiveness of an attachment-focused manualized intervention for parents of teens at risk for aggressive behaviour: The Connect Program. *Journal of Adolescence, 32*(6), 1347–1357.

Oskis, A., Loveday, C., Hucklebridge, F., Thorn, L., & Clow, A. (2011). Anxious attachment style and salivary cortisol dysregulation in healthy female children and adolescents. *Journal of Child Psychology and Psychiatry, 52*(2), 111–118.

Reimer, M. S., Overton, W. F., Steidl, J. H., Rosenstein, D. S., & Horowitz, H. (1996). Familial responsiveness and behavioral control: Influences on adolescent psychopathology, attachment, and cognition. *Journal of Research on Adolescence, 6*(1), 87–112.

Roisman, G. I., Madsen, S. D., Hennighausen, K. H., Sroufe, L. A., & Collins, W. A. (2001). The coherence of dyadic behavior across parent–child and romantic relationships as mediated by the internalized representation of experience. *Attachment and Human Development, 3*(2), 156–172.

Rosenthal, N. L., & Kobak, R. (2010). Assessing adolescents' attachment hierarchies: Differences across developmental periods and associations with individual adaptation. *Journal of Research on Adolescence, 20*(3), 678–706.

Sbarra, D. A., & Hazan, C. (2008). Coregulation, dysregulation, self-regulation: An integrative analysis and empirical agenda for understanding adult attachment, separation, loss, and recovery. *Personality and Social Psychology Review, 12*(2), 141–167.

Scharf, M., Mayseless, O., & Kivenson-Baron, I. (2012). Intergenerational concordance in Adult Attachment Interviews with mothers, fathers and adolescent sons and subsequent adjustment of sons to military service. *Attachment and Human Development, 14*(4), 367–390.

Scott, S., Briskman, J., Woolgar, M., Humayun, S., & O'Connor, T. G. (2011). Attachment in adolescence: Overlap with parenting and unique prediction of behavioural adjustment. *Journal of Child Psychology and Psychiatry, 52*(10), 1052–1062.

Seiffge-Krenke, I. (2006). Coping with relationship stressors: The impact of different working models of attachment and links to adaptation. *Journal of Youth and Adolescence, 35*(1), 25–39.

Seiffge-Krenke, I., & Beyers, W. (2005). Coping trajectories from adolescence to young adulthood: Links to attachment state of mind. *Journal of Research on Adolescence, 15*(4), 561–582.

Shmueli-Goetz, Y., Target, M., Fonagy, P., & Datta, A. (2008). The Child Attachment Interview: A psychometric study of reliability and discriminant validity. *Developmental Psychology, 44*(4), 939–956.

Shomaker, L. B., & Furman, W. (2009). Parent–adolescent relationship qualities, internal working models, and styles as predictors of adolescents' observed interactions with friends. *Journal of Social and Personal Relationships, 26*(5), 579.

Spangler, G., & Zimmermann, P. (1999). Attachment representation and emotion regulation in adolescents: A psychobiological perspective on internal working models. *Attachment and Human Development, 1*(3), 270–290.

Sroufe, L. A., Egeland, B., Carlson, E. A., & Collins, W. A. (2005). *The development of the person: The Minnesota Study of Risk and Adaptation from Birth to Adulthood.* New York: Guilford Press.

Steinberg, L. (2005). *Adolescence.* New York: McGraw-Hill.

Steinberg, S. J., Davila, J., & Fincham, F. (2006). Adolescent marital expectations and romantic experiences: Associations with perceptions about parental conflict and adolescent attachment security. *Journal of Youth and Adolescence, 35*(3), 333–348.

Target, M., Fonagy, P., & Shmueli-Goetz, Y. (2003). Attachment representations in school-age children: The development of the Child Attachment Interview (CAI). *Journal of Child Psychotherapy, 29*(2), 171–186.

Tracy, J. L., Shaver, P. R., Albino, A. W., & Cooper, M. L. (2003). Attachment styles and adolescent sexuality. In P. Florsheim (Ed.), *Adolescent romantic relations and sexual behavior: Theory, research, and practical implications* (pp. 137–159). Mahwah, NJ: Erlbaum.

Treboux, D., Crowell, J. A., & Waters, E. (2004). When "new" meets "old": Configurations of adult attachment representations and their implications for marital functioning. *Developmental Psychology, 40*(2), 295–314.

Van Ryzin, M. J., Carlson, E. A., & Sroufe, L. A. (2011). Attachment discontinuity in a high-risk sample. *Attachment and Human Development, 13*(4), 381–401.

Wallis, P., & Steele, H. (2001). Attachment representations in adolescence: Further evidence from psychiatric residential settings. *Attachment and Human Development, 3*(3), 259–268.

Ward, M. J., & Carlson, E. A. (1995). Associations among adult attachment representations, maternal sensitivity, and infant–mother attachment in a sample of adolescent mothers. *Child Development, 66,* 69–79.

Waters, E., & Cummings, E. M. (2000). A secure base from which to explore close relationships. *Child Development, 71*(1), 164–172.

Weimer, B. L., Kerns, K. A., & Oldenberg, C. M. (2004). Adolescents' interactions with a best friend: Associations with attachment style. *Journal of Experimental Child Psychology, 88*(1), 102–120.

Weinfield, N. S., Whaley, G. J. L., & Egeland, B. (2004). Continuity, discontinuity, and coherence in attachment from infancy to late adolescence: Sequelae of organization and disorganization. *Attachment and Human Development, 6*(1), 73–97.

Woodhouse, S. S., Dykas, M. J., & Cassidy, J. (2009). Perceptions of secure base provision within the family. *Attachment and Human Development, 11*(1), 47–67.

Zegers, M. A., Schuengel, C., Van IJzendoorn, M. H., & Janssens, J. M. (2006). Attachment representations of institutionalized adolescents and their professional caregivers: Predicting the development of therapeutic relationships. *American Journal of Orthopsychiatry, 76*(3), 325–334.

Zeifman, D., & Hazan, C. (2008). Pair bonds as attachments: Reevaluating the evidence. In J. Cassidy & P. R. Shaver (Eds.), *Handbook of attachment: Theory, research, and clinical applications* (2nd ed., pp. 438–455). New York: Guilford Press.

Zimmermann, P. (2004). Attachment representations and characteristics of friendship relations during adolescence. *Journal of Experimental Child Psychology, 88*(1), 83–101.

Zimmermann, P., & Becker-Stoll, F. (2002). Stability of attachment representations during adolescence: The influence of ego-identity status. *Journal of Adolescence, 25*(1), 107–124.

Zimmermann, P., Maier, M. A., Winter, M., & Grossmann, K. E. (2001). Attachment and adolescents' emotion regulation during a joint problem-solving task with a friend. *International Journal of Behavioral Development, 25*(4), 331–343.

Zimmermann, P., Mohr, C., & Spangler, G. (2009). Genetic and attachment influences on adolescents' regulation of autonomy and aggressiveness. *Journal of Child Psychology and Psychiatry, 50*(11), 1339–1347.

Zimmermann, P., & Scheuerer-Englisch, H. (2000). *Late Childhood Attachment Interview coding manual.* Unpublished manuscript, Regensburg University, Regensburg, Germany.

# Chapter 20

# Pair Bonds as Attachments

## Mounting Evidence in Support of Bowlby's Hypothesis

### Debra M. Zeifman
### Cindy Hazan

When Bowlby (1979) made his often-cited claim that attachment is an integral part of human existence "from the cradle to the grave," it was more a hypothesis than an empirically established fact. In spite of limited empirical proof, from the time adult romantic relationships were first conceptualized as attachments (Ainsworth, 1989; Hazan & Shaver, 1987), investigations of adult attachment have proliferated, based largely on the assumption that pair-bond relationships are the prototypical adult instantiation of attachment (Ainsworth, 1991). In this chapter, we examine the basis for the assumption that romantic relationships qualify as attachment bonds and therefore constitute the appropriate context for investigating adult attachment phenomena. We review a growing body of evidence that infant–caregiver and adult romantic relationships share unique psychological properties, are subserved by many of the same hormonal and neurophysiological mechanisms, and serve similar functions from an evolutionary standpoint. In doing so, we critically examine a corollary of attachment theory: that attachments confer benefits that are distinct from those associated with other relationships. Throughout the chapter, we present findings from diverse disciplines supporting Bowlby's original hypothesis.

One reason for questioning the assumption that romantic relationships are genuine attach-ments concerns the presumed function of attachment bonds. In theory, the attachment behavioral system evolved in response to selection pressures in the "environment of evolutionary adaptedness" (EEA) that made it advantageous for infants to maintain proximity to protectors (Bowlby, 1958, 1969/1982). Few would argue with the adaptive benefits of a system that led vulnerable young to seek protection from their more mature and competent guardians, or with the necessity of such a system for human infant survival. It is considerably less apparent that attachment might contribute to *adult* survival (Kirkpatrick, 1998) or why enduring bonds between sexual partners is the norm in our species (Quinlan, 2008). It cannot simply be assumed that adult attachment serves the same function as infant attachment. Attachment to a romantic partner is not necessary for survival; nor is a pair bond necessary for survival of offspring. If, however, having an attachment to a romantic partner enhances individuals' chances of survival and/or the survival of joint offspring, it can be said to serve a similar function in adulthood as it does in infancy.

Do pair-bond partners replace parents in their roles as principal attachment figures, and if so, by what processes does the transition occur? Is there compelling evidence that the attachment system is operative in adult romantic relationships? What are the unique features of attachment relationships that distinguish them from other kinds of relationships? Are adult attachment relationships the ideal mating context, or are short-term sexual pairings equally advantageous for producing and rearing offspring? Are sexual/romantic partnerships unique in the fitness advantages they confer or can the same benefits be gleaned from friendships? These are some of the questions addressed in this chapter.

In our research, we started by investigating the process by which attachments are transferred from parents to peers. We briefly summarize our findings and review literature that supports the idea that pair bonds are attachments in the technical sense. Throughout the chapter, we address issues related to the function and evolutionary significance of the attachment system in adulthood, paying particular attention to how the attachment system relates to other behavioral systems. Within our broad overview of the literature, we integrate recent evidence suggesting that many of the same brain regions implicated in infant attachment are also involved in forming adult attachments. Finally, we consider alternative evolutionary and sociological theories of relationships, and address contradictions with attachment theory.

## From Parental Attachment to Pair Bonds

### How Attachment Is Defined

Bowlby (1969/1982) defined the specific socioemotional bond to which his theory applied, and distinguished it from other kinds of social ties. Attachment bonds have four defining features: *proximity maintenance*, *separation distress*, *safe haven*, and *secure base*. Once an attachment bond has formed, these features are readily observable in the overt behavior of an infant in relation to a primary caregiver (usually the mother). She serves as a secure base from which the infant (hereafter called "he" for convenience) ventures forth and interacts with the social and physical world. He continuously monitors her proximity and availability. If he senses danger or feels anxious for any reason, he retreats to her as a source of comfort and a haven of safety. Because separations from her signal potential danger, he will object to and be distressed by them. As long as she is perceived to be sufficiently near and responsive, he will be motivated to explore his environment.

In theory, this dynamic balance between attachment and exploration is an integral part of behavior throughout the lifespan, and the four essential features of attachment relationships are characteristic of adult attachments as well. Nevertheless, changes as a function of maturation are expected. One predictable change concerns the time and distance from the attachment figure that can be comfortably tolerated. A typical 12-month-old will exhibit greater distress (and more disrupted exploration) as the result of even brief separations from a caregiver than will a 36-month-old (Marvin, Britner, & Russell, Chapter 13, this volume). By late childhood or early adolescence, longer separations are usually negotiated without undue upset, and separation distress is less apparent except in the case of unexpected and/or extended caregiver unavailability. One basis for growth in children's ability to tolerate separations is cognitive—older children can conjure a mental representation of an attachment figure, comprehend the circumstances of her absence (e.g., "Mommy is at work"), and imagine and await an impending reunion. Adults begin their relationships with a well-developed ability to mentally represent (and fantasize about) others, which leads to important differences between infant and adult attachment dynamics.

Two other changes in attachments across development are their degree of mutuality and the integration of sexuality with other aspects of the emotional bond. The asymmetrical (complementary) attachments of early life—in which infants seek and derive security from caregivers but do not provide security in return—are hypothesized to be replaced by more symmetrical (reciprocal) attachments. And, whereas infants initially seek out caregivers because caregivers tend to basic needs, such as hunger and the need for contact comfort, sexual attraction is often the precipitating force bringing adult partners into intimate contact in adulthood. According to Bowlby and others, the pair-bond relationship—in which sexual partners *mutually* derive and provide security—is the prototype of attachment in adulthood. Thus, in the typical course of relationship development, the sexual mating, caregiving, and attachment systems often become integrated (Fraley & Shaver, 2000; Hazan & Shaver, 1994; Mikulincer & Goodman, 2006; Shaver, Hazan, & Bradshaw, 1988). And although these interrelated behavioral systems can operate independently of one another, especially in the early stages of relationships (Diamond, 2004; Fisher, Aron, Mashek, Li, & Brown, 2002), the three systems are often integrated in pair-bond relationships that endure (O'Leary, Acevedo, Aron, Huddy, & Mashek, 2012).

## The Ontogeny of Infant Attachment

Given the opportunity, all normal human infants become attached to their primary caregivers, typically within the first 8 months of life. Attachment formation proceeds through a series of phases, beginning in the first weeks of life and culminating with the establishment of a "goal-corrected partnership" toward the middle of the third year (Bowlby, 1969/1982). The process begins with close physical proximity, which is initially maintained by intentional actions of the caregiver and reflexive behavior on the part of the infant (e.g., crying, sucking, clinging). In time, the infant learns to associate the caregiver with comfort and alleviation of distress (i.e., with viewing her as a safe haven). Typically, by about 8 months of age, and concurrent with the onset of self-produced locomotion and stranger wariness, the infant begins to protest separations and to use the caregiver as a base of security while exploring. Separation distress is an accepted indicator that an attachment bond is fully formed. Note that the components, which together define attachment, do not emerge simultaneously but rather in sequence, and full-blown attachments take a period of time to develop.

Although multiple attachments are the norm, not all attachment figures are equivalent. An infant shows clear discrimination among caregivers and a consistent preference for the principal caregiver (Colin, 1985, 1987; Cummings, 1980). Even if several caregivers are regularly available, an infant reliably seeks and maintains proximity to one, especially when distressed (Ainsworth, 1967, 1982). The infant also exhibits more intense protest upon being separated from the principal attachment figure compared to others (Schaffer & Emerson, 1964) and in unfamiliar settings is most reassured by this figure's presence (Ricciuti, 1974; Shill, Solyom, & Biven, 1984). Therefore, the principal attachment figure is not simply one among a coterie of possible protectors, but the individual with whom the infant has a privileged relationship. Bowlby (1958, 1969/1982) referred to this tendency to form one special attachment as "monotropy," and he considered it a crucial aspect of the survival-enhancing function of attachment (see also Cassidy, Chapter 1, this volume).

Over the course of development, the composition and structure of individuals' attachment hierarchies change. According to Ainsworth (1989), parental figures tend to be permanent members of the attachment hierarchy, but they eventually assume a position secondary in importance to the pair-bond partner. We explored the timing and processes of the transition from complementary (parental) to reciprocal (peer) attachment in two related studies (see Hazan & Zeifman, 1994).

## The Transfer of Attachment from Parents to Peers

Peer relationships during childhood and adolescence are usually characterized as *affiliative*, that is, functionally distinct from parental attachments and presumably regulated by a different behavioral system. Although there is obvious overlap in the behaviors that typify these two kinds of social bonds, affiliative relationships at this age primarily provide stimulation and increase arousal, in contrast to the arousal-moderating and security-enhancing provisions of attachment bonds. Yet *some* components of attachment may be present in peer relationships in childhood.

One aspect of attachment—proximity seeking—seems to be typical of peer relationships by childhood, although such relationships would not qualify as attachments in the full sense of the term. By age 3, children are capable of sustaining complex social interactions with agemates and show a growing interest in doing so (Gottman, 1983; Rubin, 1980). During middle childhood, youngsters develop more intimate relationships with their peers (Buhrmester & Furman, 1987) and increasingly turn to them for comfort. By late adolescence, peers come to be preferred over parents as sources of emotional support (Steinberg & Silverberg, 1986). The confiding and support-seeking aspects of peer relationships appear to be functionally similar to the parent-directed safe-haven behavior of infancy and early childhood.

Based on these developmental shifts in the *target* of attachment behaviors, we reasoned that a key to understanding the transfer of attachment from parents to peers might lie in an analysis of attachment at the component level. We used an interview measure of attachment's four components and administered it to over 100 children and adolescents ranging in age from 6 to 17. For each of the components, participants were asked to name the single *most preferred* person in several representative situations.

We found that nearly all children and adolescents in the sample were peer-oriented in terms of proximity seeking; they preferred to spend time in the company of peers rather than parents. Regarding the safe-haven component, there was an apparent shift between ages 8 and 14, with peers coming to be preferred over parents as sources of comfort and emotional support. For the majority, however, parents continued to serve as bases of security and as the primary sources of separation distress. Only among the oldest adolescents (the 15- to 17-year-old group) did we find full-blown attachments to peers—relationships containing all four components. Of this minority that considered peers to be their primary attachment figure, the overwhelming majority named a boyfriend or girlfriend (i.e., a *romantic* partner).

In a second study, we explored the time course of adult attachment formation. Research on romantic relationship formation suggests that whether and which attachment features are present may depend on how long a couple has been together. For example, romantic couples typically experience an especially strong desire for physical proximity and contact in the initial stages of a relationship (Berscheid, 1984), whereas the provision of mutual support and care becomes more important in later stages (Reedy, Birren, & Schaie, 1981; Sternberg, 1986). Thus, in adult as well as infant attachments, the presence or absence of attachment components may depend on the stage of relationship development.

We administered the same interview used in our child and adolescent study to a diverse sample of over 100 adults ranging in age from 18 to 82, but this time we grouped subjects by *stage* of relationship development rather than age. Three relationship status groups were identified: "not in a romantic relationship," "in a romantic relationship for less than 2 years," and "in a romantic relationship for 2 or more years." The majority of participant responses to questions about the target of attachment behaviors were captured by the following categories: parent, adult sibling, friend, and romantic partner.

We found that adults were clearly peer-oriented in both proximity-seeking and safe-haven behaviors. Nearly all adult respondents preferred spending time with and seeking emotional support from their friends and/or partners rather than their parents. But findings for the other two components varied as a function of relationship status. Participants in romantic relationships of at least 2 years' duration overwhelmingly named partners as

the individuals whose absence was most distressing and whose presence served as a base of security. Those in shorter-term romantic relationships and those without partners tended to name parents.

The results of these studies (and a replication by Fraley & Davis, 1997) are consistent with Bowlby's hypothesis that attachment behavior typically becomes redirected toward a sexual partner in adulthood. Full-blown attachments (with all four components) were observed almost exclusively in two kinds of social relationships—with parents or romantic partners. Furthermore, and just as Bowlby predicted, pair-bond partners did assume the status of principal attachment figures (by being preferred over parents). Finally, it appears that romantic relationships require approximately 2 years to become full-blown attachments. Individuals in shorter-term romantic relationships and those without partners tended to look to parents to satisfy some attachment needs.

Since the time of our original studies, neuroimaging research has strengthened two of our claims: that romantic partners provide emotional support distinct from the variety provided by friends or strangers, and that romantic relationships take a period of time to gel. In one study, volunteers who were deeply in love with their long-term romantic partners viewed photographs of their partners and of a friend with whom they were equally well acquainted. Compared to photographs of friends, photographs of romantic partners evoked a different pattern of neural activity, implicating regions involved in pair bonding and attachment (Bartels & Zeki, 2000). In another study, women who held their spouses' hands while being subjected to the threat of electrical shock showed less activation of regions indicative of perceived threat than married women who held the hand of an unfamiliar male experimenter. The effect was also dose-dependent: Women who reported the highest levels of marital satisfaction had the greatest reduction in activation associated with perceived threat (Coan, Schaefer, & Davidson, 2006). These results, together with our initial finding that romantic relationships uniquely display the four characteristic features of attachments, suggest that romantic partners may provide emotional security in adulthood that is not typically provided by other relationships.

Neuroimaging studies also strengthen the claim that attachments take a period of time to develop. In the earliest stages of romance, individuals who are "in love" show increased activation in dopamine-rich regions of the brain associated with reward when viewing the photograph of a romantic partner compared to the photograph of a close friend (Xu et al., 2011). In the more advanced stages of romantic relationships, when viewing photos of their romantic partners, individuals also show activation in opioid-rich regions associated with maternal attachment and pair bonding (Acevedo, Aron, Fisher, & Brown, 2012a, 2012b). These differences in brain activity produced by imagining a short- versus long-term partner are consistent with differences we documented in the targets of attachment behavior depending on the length of a relationship. Romantic partners begin as sources of arousal and positive, often sexual, stimulation; it is only after a period of time that romantic partners become attachment figures capable of providing not only stimulation but also emotional security.

## The Nature of the Bond in Pair Bonds

So far, we have presented evidence that pair-bond relationships are characterized by the same features as infant–caregiver attachments and develop according to the same process, at least in terms of the sequence in which various components come into play. If the attachment system is operative in pair bonds, its effects should also be conspicuous in other aspects of relationship functioning. In fact, the congruencies are far-reaching. They include the nature of physical contact that typifies and distinguishes attachment bonds, the factors that influence the selection of attachment figures, reactions to attachment disruption and loss, and the centrality of attachment to physical health and psychological well-being. We discuss each of these in turn.

### Physical Contact

Freud was among the first to write about the striking similarities in the physical intimacy that typifies lovers and mother–infant pairs. Like caregivers and their infants, adult sexual partners (at least initially) spend much time engaged in mutual gazing, cuddling, nuzzling, sucking, and kissing in the context of prolonged face-to-face, skin-to-skin, belly-to-belly contact, and the touching of body parts otherwise considered "private." It is noteworthy that these most intimate of human interpersonal exchanges are, in virtually every

culture, limited to parent–infant and pair-bond relationships (Eibl-Eibesfeldt, 1975). Although some forms of intimate contact may occur in isolation within other social relationships (e.g., kissing among friends), their collective occurrence is more restricted. When friends violate these social norms by engaging in intimate physical contact, they label themselves "friends with benefits" to denote the provision of benefits not usually associated with mere friendship (Carey, 2007).

Nearly universal prohibitions against physical intimacy outside recognized pair bonds (at least for females) has generally been attributed to the fact that copulations outside such bonds reduce confidence in paternity. Such restrictions may also reflect an implicit understanding that close physical contact with another could lead to a subsidiary emotional bond that would jeopardize the principal one. In subcultures where extrapair sexual contact is permitted, efforts to avoid emotional involvement are common. For example, prostitutes commonly refuse to engage in kissing and other forms of intimate face-to-face contact with their clients (Nass & Fisher, 1988). If an emotional bond is not desired in the context of a physically intimate relationship, special steps must be taken to protect against its formation. Research on "friends with benefits" indicates that these relationships often become strained when one party becomes more attached than the other (Carey, 2007).

There is evidence that the chemical basis for the effects of close physical contact may be the same for lovers and mother–infant pairs. Oxytocin, a peptide released during suckling/nursing interactions and thought to induce infant attachment and maternal bonding, is also released at sexual climax and has been implicated in the cuddling that often follows sexual intercourse (i.e., "afterplay"; Carter, 1992, 2003).

Esch and Stefano (2007) have noted a similarity in the contexts in which physical contact between attachment partners typically takes place. In the case of infants, emotional distress (in the form of crying) typically precipitates caregiver interventions that involve intimate physical contact, such as breast feeding. In the case of adults, sexual desire or need, which can be described as stressful (Marazziti & Canale, 2004), precedes physical contact, and, typically, sexual intercourse. In both cases, an uncomfortable state of arousal leads an individual to seek social contact with another person who is a source of comfort and relief. Repeated sequences in which physical contact with a potential attachment figure serves to relieve overarousal are likely to recruit the hypothalamic–pituitary–adrenal (HPA) axis and other physiological means of coping with stress. The HPA axis, in turn, may trigger the release of opioids and neuropeptides, such as oxytocin, known to induce feelings of well-being and contentment (Esch & Stefano, 2007). It is through intimate physical contact, therefore, that an attachment figure becomes not only a source of pleasure and stimulation but also a source of calm and contentment.

Similarities in the nature and context of physical contact that typify pair-bond and infant–caregiver relationships differentiate them from other classes of social relationships.

Although it is the sexual system that motivates intimate contact in the initial stages of adult romantic relationships, and the attachment system that motivates contact in infant–caregiver relationships, repeated intimate physical contact fosters the development of an attachment.

### Selection Criteria

If pair–bond relationships involve the attachment system, one might expect some overlap between infants and adult romantic partners in terms of the criteria on which selections are based. However, the qualities that make one a good mother or father are not necessarily the same qualities that make one appealing as a sexual partner. There is the additional complication of well-documented sex differences in mate selection criteria, attributed to differences in parental investment that are present and influential even before conception.

Differential parental investment theory (Trivers, 1972) holds that sexual encounters may have vastly different consequences for males and females, resulting in different optimal mating strategies and different mate selection criteria. Males have an abundant supply of small sperm cells that is constantly replenished, whereas females have a far more limited supply of large egg cells, produced at a rate of about one per month. Added to this are the female burdens of gestation and lactation, requiring years of investment. Because the male contribution to offspring can be so limited, the most effective reproductive strategy for males may be to take advantage of all mating opportunities with fertile partners. Females, for whom every sexual encounter is potentially quite costly, might benefit from being choosier and limiting sexual encounters to males who possess and appear willing to share valuable resources. Research confirms

that females are in fact "choosier" than males, though they employ different strategies depending on the phase of their menstrual cycle—selecting men with "good genes" in the most fertile phase, and men with "good character," or a tendency to invest in offspring, during the less fertile phase of the cycle (Gangestad, Garver-Apgar, Simpson, & Cousins, 2007).

Numerous studies have found sex differences in mate selection criteria consistent with male–female differences in parental investment. For example, in a survey of 37 cultures, Buss (1989) found that males generally assign greater importance than females to the physical appearance of potential mates, preferring partners who look youthful and healthy—both of which may have at one time been reasonably good indices of fertility (Buss, 1989; Symons, 1979). In contrast, females typically care more than males about the social status and earning power of potential partners; this is a sensible mate selection strategy for ensuring that offspring are themselves well provided for and reproductively fit.

Sex differences are negligible, however, when it comes to evaluating potential partners for long- versus short-term relationships (Kenrick, Groth, Trost, & Sadalla, 1993). Given that humans tend to reproduce in the context of long-term relationships, it is this context that is most relevant to understanding mate selection in our species. Moreover, although sex differences in the relative importance of traits such as physical appearance and social status are reliable, *neither* trait is assigned highest priority by *either* sex. For both men and women, the most highly valued qualities in a potential mate are "kind/understanding" and "intelligent" (Buss, 1989). In choosing among potential reproductive partners, males *and* females prefer those who are responsive and competent, and these traits matter more to them than wealth or beauty.

Men and women also tend to prefer partners who are similar to themselves on numerous dimensions, including socioeconomic status and physical attractiveness (Berscheid, 1984; Hinsz, 1989). This may reflect the more general tendency to prefer what is familiar. In the case of mating, preexisting similarities draw potential partners into the same activities and social circles, thereby increasing familiarity. The English word *familiar* comes from the Latin *familia*, which connotes "family" or "household." Others who are similar can seem like family, and may be especially appealing partners for romantic relationships.

It is noteworthy that the factors found to exert the greatest influence on the selection of pair-bond partners are similar to those used by infants in "choosing" among potential attachment figures. In the case of infants, "preference" is given to individuals who are kind, responsive, competent, and familiar—especially in the context of distress alleviation. The one who most consistently and most competently reduces discomfort and provides a safe haven (i.e., the *principal* caregiver) is the one to whom an infant is most likely to become attached (Bowlby, 1958, 1969/1982). Adults are sensitive to these same cues and care more about these qualities than about cues of fertility or resources, suggesting that reproductive partners are evaluated as potential attachment figures. Because pair-bond relationships are relatively enduring, attachment-relevant criteria are taken into account when mates are selected.

Prototypical pair bonds involve the integration of three social-behavioral systems: sexual mating, caregiving, and attachment. Attachment-relevant qualities consistently top the list of mate-selection criteria for both genders across cultures (Shackelford, Schmitt, & Buss, 2005). These qualities are relevant to mating because we humans need to select reproductive partners who will also be good companions and parents.

### Reactions to Separation and Loss

Additional evidence that attachment is integral to pair-bond relationships comes from research on bereavement and routine marital separation. The original inspiration for Bowlby's theory came from his observations of infants and children separated from their principal caregivers. He found it remarkable (and indeed in conflict with prevailing secondary drive theories) that the separations were so distressing, given that nutritional and hygienic needs were being met by surrogates. Even more striking were the similarities across children in how they responded. Bowlby identified what appeared to be a universal pattern of reactions, which he labeled the "protest–despair–detachment" sequence. The initial reaction is characterized by agitation, hyperactivity, crying, resistance to others' offers of comfort, and extreme anxiety, often to the point of panic. Eventually, this active protest subsides, only to be replaced by a period of lethargy, inactivity, and disrupted sleeping and eating behavior. In time, a degree of emotional detachment from the lost attachment figure fa-

cilitates the resumption of normal, preseparation activities and functioning.

If the attachment system is operative in pair bonds, adult reactions to the loss of a partner should be similar to those of infants separated from their caregivers. Several studies have documented essentially the same sequence in adults grieving for the loss of a spouse: initial anxiety and panic, followed by lethargy and depression, and eventually recovery through emotional detachment (Hazan & Shaver, 1992; Parkes & Weiss, 1983; Weiss, 1975) or reorganization (Fraley & Shaver, 1999; Chapter 3, this volume). Even brief, routine separations are enough to trigger this pattern of response in some married individuals (Vormbrock, 1993).

The protest–despair–detachment (or reorganization) sequence is observed almost exclusively in two social-relational contexts: infant– and child–caregiver relationships and pair bonds. The death of a relative or the decision of a friend to move away may cause sadness, but such events do not normally evoke panic. The profound separation reactions of infants and adult lovers may reflect the mutual reliance of attachment partners on one another to regulate internal physiological states (Hofer, 1994). It makes good adaptive sense to react with anxiety and protest to even the temporary "loss" of an individual who serves as a primary source of emotional and/or physical security. The fact that this reaction is the norm among adults separated from their long-term partners, and *not* the normal reaction to the loss of other kinds of social ties, is another indication that the attachment system is active in pair bonds.

### Physical and Psychological Health Effects

The notion that attachment meets a very real biological need, at least early in life, was established in studies of infants reared in orphanages and other institutional settings (Robertson, 1953; Spitz, 1946). Although adults are clearly less dependent on social bonds for basic survival, there is ample evidence that they incur health benefits from having one, and suffer health decrements as a consequence of the absence or loss of such bonds. Relationship disruption (especially divorce) makes one more susceptible to a wide range of physical and psychological ills, including disease, impaired immune functioning, accidents, substance abuse, suicide, and various other forms of psychopathology (e.g., Bloom, Asher, & White, 1978; Goodwin, Hurt, Key, & Sarret, 1987; Lynch, 1977; Uchino,

Cacioppo, & Kiecolt-Glaser, 1996; and several chapters in Part V of this volume).

Among the most common life stressors, attachment-related losses cause the most subjective distress. Death of a spouse is the leading stressful event on the Social Readjustment Rating Scale, followed by divorce and marital separation (Holmes & Rahe, 1967). Weiss (1973) found that loneliness takes at least two distinct forms, depending on whether social deprivation is due to the absence of an intimate companion (which he labeled "emotional loneliness") or a lack of friends ("social loneliness"). Consistent with Weiss's theory, a national survey indicated that the loss or absence of a pair-bond relationship was associated with feelings of "desperation" and anxiety, whereas lack of friendships was associated with feelings of "restless boredom" (Rubenstein & Shaver, 1982). Social support in the form of friendship does not help alleviate the distress of losing or being separated from a spouse (Stroebe, Stroebe, Abakoumkin, & Schut, 1996). Vormbrock's (1993) review of the literature on war- and job-related routine marital separations led to a similar conclusion: The social provisions of pair bonds are sufficiently distinctive that most social relationships cannot compensate for their loss. Interestingly, Vormbrock found that renewing relationships with parental *attachment* figures was helpful in moderating the anxiety caused by spousal absence.

If attachment bonds have exceptional effects on physical and psychological functioning, such effects should be absent not only in other types of relationships but also in the kinds of relationships that typically develop into attachments but have yet to achieve that status. In fact, early maternal deprivation is associated with long-term developmental consequences *only* if it occurs *after* an attachment bond between infant and mother has been established (Bowlby, 1958). Separations prior to 8 months of age do not increase the probability of poor developmental outcomes. Similarly, Weiss (1988) found that widows and widowers married for less than 2 years did not show the same (protest–despair–detachment/reorganization) sequence of reactions as those grieving for the loss of longer-term bonds.

In summary, the results of a number of studies indicate that bonds between adult partners and infant–caregiver pairs are similarly and uniquely powerful in their impact on physical and psychological well-being. Other kinds of interpersonal relationships offer valuable social provisions, but emotional security does not appear to be one of

them. Otherwise, disruptions would give rise to acute anxiety, which they do not. If separation distress is a marker of attachment, bonds between long-term adult partners clearly qualify.

## The Function of Attachment in Adult Life

Bowlby (1969/1982) argued that the attachment system is a species-typical characteristic that evolved to serve a protective, survival-enhancing function. Infants who became attached to and then stayed close to protectors had significantly better chances of living to reproductive age than infants who failed to develop such bonds. The survival value and evolutionary origins of adult attachment are less obvious and therefore are subject to debate.

Some theorists (e.g., Kirkpatrick, 1998) reject the notion that the attachment system is integral to pair bonds on the grounds that reflexive proximity seeking in the face of danger would be maladaptive for adults. According to this line of reasoning, a propensity to seek protection from a mate, rather than aiding in the fight against some external threat, would be more likely to jeopardize adult survival than enhance it. Because females are, on average, smaller and weaker than their male counterparts, it is particularly doubtful that men could gain a survival advantage by turning to their female partners for assistance. Furthermore, given the unlikelihood that an entire system would be retained yet undergo a qualitative change in its function, pair bonds cannot involve the attachment system. There are several flaws in this line of reasoning, however.

One major shortcoming of this argument is its limited conceptualization of the protective function of attachment. Although the risk of predation in the EEA was undoubtedly reduced for infants who became attached to their caregivers, the benefits of the bond would have extended far beyond physical protection, even in infancy. Attachments also ensure that infants receive adequate care in the form of food, warmth, shelter, guidance, and monitoring—all of which enhance survival. By relying on a narrow definition of *protection*, the argument fails to take into account normative developmental changes in the behavioral manifestations of attachment. As children mature and become more competent, primitive forms of attachment behavior, such as reflexive proximity seeking, decline. Older children and adolescents, however, continue to depend on parents for many aspects of care, and continue to benefit from having someone who is deeply invested in their welfare and reliably available to help if needed. The fact that a behavior is transformed across development is insufficient proof of divergent function (Tinbergen, 1963). Feeding behavior also changes dramatically from infancy to adulthood, but the basic function—procuring nutrition—remains essentially the same.

To evaluate whether attachment serves the same protective function in adulthood as in infancy requires that *protection* be defined in a manner that encompasses its full meaning and acknowledges normative developmental change. Furthermore, to address the question of function, it must be established that such protection affords adaptive advantage by translating reliably into enhanced survival and reproductive success in the EEA. Hence, a key to understanding the function of attachment in adulthood lies in an examination of the circumstances in which pair bonding evolved.

### The Evolution of Pair Bonds

If human reproductive success required nothing more than conception, reproductive partners could part ways as soon as a viable pregnancy was achieved. In actuality, however, the vast majority of human males and females opt to remain with the same partner for a more extended period of time (Eibl-Eibesfeldt, 1989; Mellen, 1981). This trend is thought to have followed a birthing crisis in which the infant's large head, housing a more fully developed brain, could not easily pass through the birth canal of our bipedal female ancestors (Trevathan, 1987). Infants who were born prematurely, with less developed brains and smaller heads, were more likely to survive (as were their mothers). Immaturity at birth also offered the added advantage of a longer period of learning during a time of heightened neural plasticity. This would have been a distinct advantage in a species with complex social organization as our own. The benefits of premature birth, however, brought new risks and challenges. The effort required to care adequately for exceedingly dependent offspring during a protracted period of immaturity, along with the major tasks of socialization, made paternal investment an advantage, if not a necessity. Exceptionally helpless and vulnerable offspring would have had poor chances of surviving to re-

productive age or developing the necessary skills for mating and parenting without a strong force to keep fathers around and involved.

Many unique features of human sexuality appear to have evolved for the purpose of fostering an enduring bond between reproductive partners. Most mammals mate only during the short estrus periods of the female, but human sexual desire and activity are not so restricted. Women can be sexually receptive during any phase of their menstrual cycle, despite the fact that conception is possible only during a small fraction of it. This physiological adaptation enables a couple to maintain a continuous tie on the basis of sexual reward (Eibl-Eibesfeldt, 1975). Concealed ovulation may also increase the costs of straying. Males of many diverse species guard their mates during periods of sexual receptivity so as to ensure paternity. If ovulation is hidden, as it is in humans, it is difficult for the male to determine when fertilization is possible, and the optimal male strategy may shift toward guarding and remaining with the same sexual partner for longer periods of time (Alcock, 1989).

When the adaptive problem of immature offspring and the corresponding need for paternal investment arose in the course of human evolution, our species—by virtue of its altricial nature—already had available a well-designed, specialized, flexible, but reliable mechanism for ensuring that two individuals would be highly motivated to stay together and vigorously resist being separated. The mechanism was attachment. In light of the generally conservative tendencies of evolution and natural selection, it is highly probable that this preexisting mechanism would have been exploited for the purpose of keeping reproductive partners together. Pair bonds are primarily reproductive relationships, but sex serves more than a reproductive function in our species. The unique features of human reproductive physiology and anatomy help to ensure that partners will engage in the kinds of intimate exchanges known to foster attachment formation.

### Reproductive Advantages of Pair Bonds

In our species, reproductive success requires negotiation of at least three adaptive challenges: surviving to reproductive age, mating, and providing adequate care to offspring so that they too will survive to reproduce. We have argued that the relative immaturity of human newborns created a situation in the EEA in which survival depended on not only infants forming a strong bond to protectors but also a mechanism that would hold reproductive partners together for an extended period of time. The attachment system, which had evolved to ensure an enduring bond between infants and caregivers, was exploited for this additional purpose. But the advantages of pair bonding extend beyond its role in offspring survival. Benefits include enhanced survival and reproductive fitness for mates, as well as the intergenerational transmission of reproductive strategies that confer further advantage to offspring (see Simpson & Belsky, Chapter 5, this volume).

There is mounting evidence that offspring mating strategies may depend critically on the pair-bond status of parents, especially mothers. Adolescents from father-absent homes show precocious sexual interest, earlier sexual maturation, more negative attitudes toward potential mates, and less interest in long-term relationships than do their counterparts reared in father-present homes (Belsky, 1999; Draper & Belsky, 1990; Draper & Harpending, 1982; Ellis, McFayden-Ketchum, Dodge, Pettit, & Bates, 1999; Surbey, 1990). Girls in father-absent homes are at increased risk for early sexual activity and teenage pregnancy (Ellis et al., 2003). In other words, if parents choose not to remain together, their children are more likely to adopt approaches to mating that emphasize quantity over quality. Parental divorce has also been found to affect offspring mating strategies and behavior (Barber, 1998). Female children of divorce tend to fear closeness and abandonment, whereas male children show a lack of achievement orientation and a greater likelihood of abandoning relationships (Henry & Holmes, 1998; Wallerstein, 1994). Thus, the failure of reproductive partners to maintain long-term bonds may have a negative effect on the mating success of their offspring.

Whether opportunistic, short-term mating strategies are less advantageous than stable, long-term strategies is the source of an ongoing debate (e.g., Belsky, 1999; Buss, 1997; Schmitt, 2005). According to life history theory (Stearns, 1992), organisms possess finite resources that must be allocated to various challenges, including survival, growth, mating, and parenting. Local circumstances determine the balance of time and energy an individual devotes to each. Adolescents from unstable families may benefit from adopting a strategy of mating early and often so as to ensure the survival of at least some offspring in an unpredictable environment. Both long- and short-term strategies can be viewed as reasonable and comparably adaptive responses to different ecologies, and these strategies can shift within an individual's lifetime in response to changing life circumstances.

We have argued that although it is clearly advantageous for humans to be capable of facultative mating adaptations that take account of varying ecological conditions (Buss & Schmitt, 1993; Gangestad & Simpson, 2000), the correlates of short- and long-term mating strategies are not supportive of the view that they are different but equal (for alternative viewpoints, see Belsky, 1999; Simpson & Belsky, Chapter 5, this volume). The ability to adjust behavior to nonoptimal circumstances is clearly important, but such adjustments are unlikely to produce optimal results. In many cultures, infant mortality rates are higher among children without an investing father (Hill & Hurtado, 1995). Infants raised by both parents are weaned at a later age than those who are raised by single mothers, suggesting one avenue through which infant health and parental fitness may be enhanced by the presence of strong pair bonds (Quinlan & Quinlan, 2008). In the currency of evolution, a superior strategy is one that enhances reproductive success. Pair bonds not only contribute to the survival of offspring but also leave offspring better equipped to attract and retain mates of their own, which in turn improves overall reproductive fitness.

In addition to the direct and indirect benefits that accrue to the progeny of stable pair bonds, there are advantages for the mates themselves. Women ovulate more regularly if they are in a stable sexual relationship (e.g., Cutler, Garcia, Huggins, & Preti, 1986; Veith, Buck, Getzlaf, Van Dalfsen, & Slade, 1983), and they reach menopause significantly later if sexual activity is consistent (Kaczmarek, 2007). The quality of attachments also influences reproductive success. Women suffering from infertility of unknown etiology tend to have an avoidant attachment style (Justo, Maia, Ferreira-Diniz, Santos, & Moreira, 1997). Earlier we cited evidence that partners in long-term relationships enjoy more robust physical and mental health. More fit individuals would be better able to protect and provide for themselves and loved ones. As for the protective aspects of attachment, adults, too, need someone to look out for them—someone to search for them if they fail to show up at the expected time, take care of them when they are sick, help defend them against external threats, and reassure them.

One reason pair bonds may enhance fitness is that sexual partners are equally and uniquely genetically related to their joint offspring and are therefore highly motivated to work together to ensure their survival. Although it is widely acknowledged that mates share genetic interests in offspring, it is generally assumed that this shared genetic investment is not as binding as the shared genetic interests of blood relatives because sexual loyalties can be easily reversed as in the case of infidelity (Daly & Wilson, 1996). This assumption, however, may underestimate the degree of relatedness of sexual partners. In fact, with the exception of first-degree relatives, a high degree of inbreeding has been the norm in our species (Thornhill, 1991). The low incidence of interracial marriage and the prevalence of look-alike partners (Hinsz, 1989) indicate that individuals tend to select mates from their own genetic pool. Although mates will not typically be first-degree relatives, they are still more likely to be "related" than two randomly selected individuals from the population at large.

The symmetry in degree of genetic relatedness of parents to their joint offspring may explain fathers' unique motivation to provide adequately when a mother is engaged in the energetically costly practice of breast feeding. In a survey of diverse traditional societies, stable pair bonds were strongly associated with later infant weaning ages (Quinlan & Quinlan, 2008). The presence of adult relatives other than the child's father in the household, in contrast, had the opposite effect on the duration of breast feeding, hastening weaning. One reason fathers may be uniquely positioned to support lactation is that a father and mother are the only two adults who share 50% of their genes with their child. Even in an extended-kin household, other relatives share at most only 25% of their genes with the offspring of a single mother, as in the case of a grandmother living with her daughter and grandchild. Although mothers may benefit from the contributions of relatives other than the child's father, they may also feel obligated to wean offspring sooner, so that they can contribute to a household in ways that benefit the whole family. Some authors have therefore suggested that pair bonds evolved in order to support lactation (Quinlan & Quinlan, 2008), or that lactation is a "critical period" for paternal investment (Marlowe, 2003).

Sexual partners share an interest in having their offspring survive and thrive. Although there are multiple pathways to reproductive success, and

optimal reproductive strategies depend on local ecologies, there is substantial evidence that the survival and fitness of humans is enhanced by the presence of both strong pair bonds and investing fathers. On the basis of the evidence, we would argue that the attachment system serves to cement an enduring emotional bond between sexual partners that translates today, as it did in the EEA, into differential survival of offspring and reproductive success under many environmental conditions.

## A Model of Adult Attachment Formation

Bowlby (1969/1982) identified four phases in the development of infant–caregiver attachments: preattachment, attachment in the making, clearcut attachment, and goal-corrected partnership (see Marvin, Britner, & Russell, Chapter 13, this volume). We have proposed a corresponding fourphase model of adult attachment using Bowlby's model as a provisional guide (Hazan, Gur-Yaish, & Campa, 2004; Zeifman & Hazan, 1997). We have likened the adult counterpart of the infant preattachment phase to what Eibl-Eibesfeldt (1989) called the "proceptive program." Males and females of reproductive age are inherently interested in social interaction with potential mates and display flirtatious signals somewhat indiscriminately. It is likely that these playful, sexually charged exchanges continue when partners first become involved and that they are more characteristic of partners' interactions than attachment behaviors per se.

In contrast, as described earlier, the behaviors of partners in the throes of romantic infatuation show many resemblances to infant–caregiver interactions (Shaver et al., 1988), including prolonged mutual gazing, cuddling, nuzzling, and "baby talk." We have suggested that these types of exchanges may be indicative of the second phase, "attachment in the making." This is consistent with Bowlby's (1979) view that "in terms of subjective experience, the formation of a bond is described as falling in love" (p. 69). In infancy, the onset of the third phase, "clear-cut attachment," is indicated by the emergence of new attachment behaviors—and, specifically, by their organization around a single caregiver who has become the reliably preferred target of proximity maintenance and safe-haven behaviors, and elicitor of securebase and separation-distress behaviors.

The childhood indicators of the fourth phase, "goal-corrected partnership," primarily reflect cognitive-developmental changes over the first 3 years of life. We have hypothesized that there nevertheless may be a comparable final phase in adult attachment formation, characterized by a decline in overt displays of attachment behavior and a redirection of attention to other aspects of life (e.g., work, hobbies, and friendships). In a goal-corrected partnership, a romantic partner has achieved the status of an attachment figure and serves as a secure base, emboldening the individual to explore his or her environment with a greater sense of security (Feeney & Thrush, 2010).

The concept of stages in establishing an adult attachment has gained support empirically. As noted earlier, it is now clear that individuals display different patterns of neural activity in response to viewing photos of their romantic partners depending on how long they have been in a relationship (e.g., Xu et al., 2011). Fisher and her colleagues (2002; Fisher, Aron, & Brown, 2005) have proposed three stages of romantic relationship development that correspond to the behavioral systems recruited sequentially, and that serve somewhat independent functions. In the first stage, lust, driven by sex hormones, triggers interest in *any* potential partner. This nonspecific sexual interest is replaced by romantic attraction to a *specific* person, a stage Fisher and colleagues associate with the mating system and hypothesize is undergirded by neurotransmitters, such as dopamine, that are central to reward and arousal. The ultimate value of the mating system is that focusing attention on one specific individual conserves mating effort and reproductive energy. Finally, the attachment system is recruited in relationships that progress to the next stage in order to ensure that couples stay together long enough to provide and care for offspring. Although Fisher and colleagues (2002) do not explicitly propose a time frame, this three-stage framework might be seen as corresponding to the preattachment, attachment in the making, and clear-cut attachment phases that we have proposed.

## Attachment versus Other Perspectives on Mating

The attachment theory (AT) perspective on human mating has at times been misunderstood. For example, AT is mischaracterized as claiming that there is only one adaptive mating strategy, monogamous pair bonding (e.g., Schmitt, 2005). In this section, we address some of these misconceptions and explain areas of difference and complementarity among various evolutionary perspectives on human mating. In particular, we address two prominent theories: sexual strategies theory (SST; Buss & Schmitt, 1993), which emphasizes between-gender differences in preference for long-term versus short-term mating strategies; and strategic pluralism theory (SPT; Gangestad & Simpson, 2000), which emphasizes within-gender variability in the adoption of short- versus long-term mating strategies as a function of ecological factors.

AT posits that attachment is one of three interrelated behavioral systems operating in a pair bond, alongside the sexual/mating and caregiving systems. We have reviewed evidence that these three systems are distinct in their neurobiological underpinnings, behavioral manifestations, and psychological dynamics (Fisher, 2000; Fisher et al., 2002). It is understood that relationships can engage these systems somewhat independently (e.g., sexual behavior in the absence of attachment; Diamond, 2004). In the typical pair bond, however, the three systems become integrated. In adults, sexual attraction motivates the kind of physical interactions that over time tend to foster mutual attachment and caregiving. If a pair bond results in the birth of a child, then caregiving is extended to offspring (Hazan & Zeifman, 1994).

AT, SST, and SPT differ in which or how many of the various behavioral systems they address. SST focuses almost exclusively on the sexual/mating system, in which there are well-documented sex differences. For example, compared to females, college-age males report greater desire for short-term matings (Buss & Schmitt, 1993). AT, in contrast, is not concerned with hypothetical mating behavior or short-term matings; attachments are, by definition, *enduring* emotional bonds. SPT, like SST, focuses on the sexual/mating system but also indirectly on the caregiving system, in the form of parental investment, and especially on tradeoffs in the effort afforded to each. The balance of effort allocated to mating versus caregiving is hypothesized to vary within gender as a function of various ecological factors. For example, in highly unstable environments, both males and females show increased interest in short-term strategies (Gangestad & Simpson, 2000). SPT acknowledges that long-term mating is the behavioral norm, but it does not address the nature of the bond that develops between long-term mates. AT is unique in that it focuses on the dynamics of a pair bond as an integration of the sexual mating, caregiving, and attachment systems.

Another common misconception regarding AT is that an enduring bond or an attachment implies sexual monogamy (Schmitt, 2005). We adopt the view common among animal researchers that *monogamy* refers to a broader constellation of social behaviors between sexual partners, such as nonsexual proximity maintenance, joint territory, prolonged association, and shared parenting (Dewsbury, 1987; Moller, 2003). Although human mating could not be described as monogamous if monogamy were synonymous with sexual fidelity, most human mating systems qualify for less constrained definitions of monogamy (Dewsbury, 1987). Indeed, many animals that are viewed as monogamous because they show a reliable preference for a specific mate engage in copulations outside pair bonds, as evidenced by genetic investigations of paternity (Carter et al., 1997; Mendoza & Mason, 1997). And, across the animal kingdom, one of the characteristics that best predicts monogamy is having immature young in need of extensive parental care for a protracted maturation period, as humans do (Dewsbury, 1987; Moller, 2003).

We have argued here and elsewhere that long-term pair bonds confer reproductive benefits relative to other mating strategies. This does not mean that other reproductive strategies are not also adaptive. It is important to distinguish between optimal adaptations and optimal outcomes. Ainsworth, Blehar, Waters, and Wall (1978) described three attachment styles among infants: secure, insecure-avoidant, and insecure-ambivalent. Whereas the secure attachment style is considered optimal as both an adaptation and an outcome, the two insecure attachment styles are also considered optimal adaptations to particular caregiving environments—a rejecting caregiver in the case of an avoidant infant, and an inconsistent one in the case of an ambivalent one (Ainsworth et al., 1978)—but not optimal outcomes. Similarly, short-term mating strategies may be adaptive in that they optimize existing resources, particularly when resources are scarce and environments are unpredictable (Belsky, Steinberg, & Draper, 1991; Gangestad & Simpson, 2000); at the same time, they may be nonoptimal in terms of outcome when compared to the long-term strategies typically adopted in more stable environments.

Another source of confusion is the relation between attachment style and mating strategy.

Whereas *attachment style* concerns an individual's expectations regarding the availability and responsiveness of mates, *mating strategy* concerns how mates are obtained, whether for the long or the short term. Avoidant individuals have low expectations regarding the availability and responsiveness of partners (Hazan & Shaver, 1994; Mikulincer & Shaver, 2007), and are more apt than secure individuals to adopt a short-term mating strategy (Schachner & Shaver, 2004; Simpson & Gangestad, 1991). However, in spite of negative expectations, many avoidant individuals marry (a long-term strategy), as evidenced by the significant proportion of individuals in studies of attachment style and marriage who are classified as avoidant (e.g., Feeney, Noller, & Callan, 1994; Fuller & Fincham, 1995; Kobak & Hazan, 1991). Having a particular attachment style may predispose one toward a particular mating strategy, but it is by no means determinative.

One reason attachment style and mating strategy do not necessarily follow a single developmental trajectory (e.g., from secure attachment to monogamous, long-term mating strategy) is that each is responsive to environmental conditions at different points in development. AT locates the critical "decision point" shaping attachment style in childhood (in response to the local caregiving environment), whereas SPT locates the "decision point" for mating strategy in adulthood (in response to the local mating environment). However, neither attachment styles nor mating strategies are static entities; both accommodate ongoing events and existing resources and can change across the lifespan (Bowlby, 1980; Fuller & Fincham, 1995).

Schmitt (2005) has criticized the AT view that long-term pair bonds are adaptive, on the grounds that self-reported preferences for short-term mating strategies are associated in a college-age population with such adaptive personality traits as self-esteem, extraversion, and emotional stability. If, for the sake of argument, we accept the premise that an adaptive mating strategy is one that is associated with other adaptive personality traits, we have to consider whether the sexual behaviors of college students qualify as mating or reproductive strategies in the evolutionary sense. Insofar as mating strategies in evolutionary terms are strategies for producing and rearing offspring, sexual behavior that is intentionally uncoupled from that goal might not qualify as a mating strategy at all. In our current culture, birth control and the loosening of restrictions on premarital sex allow college-age adults to make conscious decisions about engaging in a period of sexual experimentation. This freedom from the potential consequences of sexual behavior was impossible in our EEA or in previous generations, and it may represent a behavioral *neophenotype*—a new pattern of behavior that was not commonly observed or that did not exist before in nature (Kuo, 1967).

Given modern means of avoiding pregnancy, preferring a short-term mate or an uncommitted sexual relationship during college or early adulthood may be distinct from adopting a similar mating strategy in the postcollege years, when decisions about long-term mates and children are often made in our culture. In fact, among men who are slightly older than college age and married, short-term mating strategies are not related to positive personality traits (Schmitt, 2005). This suggests that conclusions about mating strategies based on college-age samples may generalize poorly to marital and familial relationships—the typical contexts in which reproduction occurs.

In addition to the problem of basing conclusions about mating strategies on college-age samples, one of the weaknesses of SST is that the preponderance of SST research is based on expressed preferences or hypothetical behavior rather than actual behavior (e.g., Buss, 1989). For example, typical short-term mating measures ask respondents to indicate the number of sexual partners desired across various time frames and/or the likelihood of engaging in sexual intercourse with desirable partners after knowing them for various time intervals (Buss & Schmitt, 1993; Schmitt, Shackelford, Duntley, Tooke, & Buss, 2001). Although such preferences may tell us about the motivational systems underlying behavior, they do not tell the complete story of the behavior itself or of its effect on outcomes. For example, although humans evolved a preference for foods high in sugar and fat content when food was scarce, this preference in our current environment contributes to obesity, disease, and premature morbidity. Similarly, a robust libido and sexual imagination in and of themselves may be associated with positive outcomes because social, cultural, religious, and demographic constraints limit the expression of sexual behavior in most societies. The impact of restricted versus unrestricted sexual practices on various outcomes is, on the other hand, somewhat independent of the impact of restricted and unrestricted sexual desire.

When studies examine the personality profiles of those who actually engage in behavior that is typical of short-term strategies, rather than those who merely express a preference for doing so, the results paint a less sanguine portrait of short-term strategists. In fact, Paul, McManus, and Hayes (2000) found that individuals who reported experiencing "hookups" (i.e., casual sexual encounters with relative strangers), especially hookups involving sexual intercourse, had lower self-esteem than those who did not. The emphasis of SST on the correlates of expressed preferences rather than actual practices also downplays the negative mental health consequences of short-term strategies, which are apparent from an extensive clinical literature on the harmful effects of emotional loneliness, breakups, divorce, and sexual infidelity (Hall & Fincham, 2006; Weber, 1998; Weiss, 1975). These damaging effects of relationship disruption and dissolution, coupled with growing evidence of therapeutic effects of relationship endurance, suggest that although diverse reproductive strategies exist, long-term strategies are likely to continue to be the norm.

## Are Attachment Relationships Truly Unique?

One premise of attachment theory that has been challenged in recent years is the notion that attachment relationships confer unique benefits that are not readily available in other close relationships such as sibling relationships or friendships (DePaulo & Morris, 2005). DePaulo has coined the term *singlism* to refer to the fact that public policy discriminates against singles, and that singles are often subjected to harsh judgment and negative stereotypes simply by virtue of remaining uncoupled in a society that values pair bonds and marriage. Included in her case for the stigmatization of singles are psychologists' claims that marriage promotes health and well-being and that singlehood is detrimental to health and well-being (Seligman, 2002). In their critique of AT and of our work in particular, De Paulo and Morris (2005, p. 75) fault us for failing to consider that nonsexual relationships might count as attachments, and having a "dreamy" or idealized view of sexual unions that fails to take quality into account. In the next section, we clarify our position in relation to three of DePaulo and Morris's assertions.

First, the debate over who qualifies as a principal attachment figure in a modern culture like our own, in which many individuals elect to remain single well into adulthood, in some ways mirrors earlier challenges to Bowlby's claim that mothers are typically at the apex of the attachment hierarchy in childhood even in extended-kin homes or in the era of day care. In our view, DePaulo and Morris (2005) are right to call into question exactly which relationships ought to be viewed as full-blown or principal attachments in adulthood. In fact, that question was at the heart of our original study of the transfer of attachment from parents to peers, and bears on the larger question of how attachment hierarchies change over time in the normal course of development and maturation. Although we do not preclude the possibility of adults being principally attached to siblings, other relatives, or close friends, we have found, as have others, that this is not the case for the majority of adults. Typically, although some types of attachment behaviors may be preferentially directed toward friends and relatives, the majority of adults view a romantic partner as their *principal* attachment figure (Pitman & Scharfe, 2010; Trinke & Bartholomew, 1997). We would contend that just as most infants form a principal attachment to a mother-like figure, most adults form a principal attachment to a sexual or romantic partner.

Second, DePaulo and Morris (2005) question the assumption that the health benefits of being pair bonded are restricted to those who are married or cohabiting with a sexual partner. There again, our position is based on empirical evidence and stresses the ultimate outcome that interests evolutionarily minded psychologists most: reproductive fitness. Married people do enjoy better physical and mental health than do singles or even cohabiting adults (Horwitz, White, & Howell-White, 1996), although the reasons for this effect are far from clear and continue to be the subject of intense debate (Musick & Bumpass, 2012). More importantly for reproductive fitness, children reared in homes of married mothers enjoy enriched environments, better health, more stable finances, and greater emotional security than their counterparts reared in the homes of single or cohabiting mothers (Bzostek & Beck, 2011; Rosenkrantz Aronson, & Huston, 2004). One study published in an obstetrics journal concludes that marriage protects pregnancy and is associated with lower rates of numerous adverse birth outcomes, including prematurity and low birthweight. The authors note that in their examination of birth records from the 1990s in a Finnish teaching hospital, this marital-context advantage persisted even after cohabitation and single parenthood had become less stigmatized (Raatikainene, Heiskanen, & Heinonen, 2005). Indeed, from our own evolutionary standpoint, it is surprising that cohabitation does not confer benefits on par with marriage, and may reflect the instability of cohabitation relative to marriage (Lichter, Qian, & Mellott, 2006) or a lower level of commitment from the outset among those who cohabitate rather than marry.

Third, DePaulo and Morris (2005) and others have argued that psychologists' claims regarding the benefits of marriage often fail to take into account the quality of marriage, and are based largely on comparisons between happily married couples and singles rather than singles and all marrieds, happy and otherwise. Indeed, it is clear that research comparing the health and well-being of both adults and children in conflict-ridden marriages to those in stable, happy marriages strongly support the contention that marriage is not a panacea and can be detrimental to one's health (Bzostek & Beck, 2011; Musick & Bumpass, 2012). We agree with DePaulo and Morris's assertion that relationship quality must be taken into account in any study of the health benefits or costs of being coupled. We would argue, however, that AT has, if anything, emphasized the impact of individual differences in relationship quality (i.e., attachment style) on relationship dynamics and outcomes, sometimes to the neglect of normative processes.

## Conclusions

The evidence reviewed in this chapter indicates that pair bonds are similar in many respects to the one type of interpersonal tie that most researchers agree does involve the attachment system—infant–caregiver bonds. Furthermore, the similarities extend far beyond the superficial to include fundamental features, functions, dynamics, and processes. From this extensive evidence, we conclude that attachment is indeed integral to pair bonds and that, conversely, pair bonds are the prototypical (if not the only) instantiation of attachment in adulthood.

As for the functions of attachment in adult life, we have argued that there is significant overlap with those of attachment in infancy. The attachment system helps to ensure the development of an enduring bond that enhances survival and reproductive fitness in direct, as well as indirect, ways. Pair bonds are not simply mutually beneficial alliances based on the principles of reciprocal altruism. Instead, they involve such a profound psychological and physiological interdependence that the absence or loss of one partner can be literally life threatening for the other.

Bowlby's original hypotheses concerning pair-bond attachment were based on little more than his formidable powers of observation and deep insights into human affectional behavior. In the time since their formulation, a substantial body of empirical data on relationships has been amassed—one that, on the whole, supports his initial speculations. The evidence indicates that attachment needs persist from the cradle to the grave. And, just as Bowlby surmised, in adulthood, such needs are typically satisfied by pair bonds.

## References

Acevedo, B. P., Aron, A., Fisher, H. E., & Brown, L. L. (2012a). Neural correlates of long-term intense romantic love. *Social Cognitive and Affective Neuroscience, 7*(2), 145–159.

Acevedo, B. P., Aron, A., Fisher, H. E., & Brown, L. L. (2012b). Neural correlates of marital satisfaction and well-being: Reward, empathy, and affect. *Clinical Neuropsychiatry, 9*(1), 20–31.

Ainsworth, M. D. S. (1967). *Infancy in Uganda: Infant care and the growth of attachment.* Baltimore: Johns Hopkins University Press.

Ainsworth, M. D. S. (1982). Attachment: Retrospect and prospect. In C. M. Parkes & J. Stevenson-Hinde (Eds.), *The place of attachment in human behavior* (pp. 3–30). New York: Basic Books.

Ainsworth, M. D. S. (1989). Attachments beyond infancy. *American Psychologist, 44*(4), 709–716.

Ainsworth, M. D. S. (1991). Attachments and other affectional bonds across the life cycle. In C. M. Parkes, J. Stevenson-Hinde, & P. Marris (Eds.), *Attachment across the life cycle* (pp. 33–51). New York: Tavistock/Routledge.

Ainsworth, M. D. S., Blehar, M. C., Waters, E., & Wall, S. (1978). *Patterns of attachment: A psychological study of the Strange Situation.* Hillsdale, NJ: Erlbaum.

Alcock, J. (1989). *Animal behavior: An evolutionary approach.* Boston: Sinauer.

Barber, N. (1998). Sex differences in disposition toward kin, security of adult attachment, and sociosexuality as a function of parental divorce. *Evolution and Human Behavior, 19,* 125–132.

Bartels, A., & Zeki, S. (2000). The neural basis of romantic love. *NeuroReport, 11*(17), 3829–3834.

Belsky, J. (1999). Modern evolutionary theory and patterns of attachment. In J. Cassidy & P. R. Shaver (Eds.), *Handbook of attachment: Theory, research, and clinical applications* (pp. 141–161). New York: Guilford Press.

Belsky, J., Steinberg, L., & Draper, P. (1991). Childhood experience, interpersonal development, and reproductive strategy: An evolutionary theory of socialization. *Child Development, 62,* 647–670.

Berscheid, E. (1984). Interpersonal attraction. In G. Lindzey & E. Aronson (Eds.), *Handbook of social psychology* (3rd ed., pp. 413–484). Reading, MA: Addison-Wesley.

Bloom, B. L., Asher, S. J., & White, S. W. (1978). Marital disruption as a stressor: A review and analysis. *Psychological Bulletin, 85,* 867–894.

Bowlby, J. (1958). The nature of the child's tie to his mother. *International Journal of Psycho-Analysis, 39,* 350–373.

Bowlby, J. (1979). *The making and breaking of affectional bonds.* London: Tavistock/Routledge.

Bowlby, J. (1980). *Attachment and loss: Vol. 3. Loss: Sadness and depression.* New York: Basic Books.

Bowlby, J. (1982). *Attachment and loss: Vol. 1. Attachment* (2nd ed.). New York: Basic Books. (Original work published 1969)

Buhrmester, D., & Furman, W. (1987). The development of companionship and intimacy. *Child Development, 58,* 1101–1113.

Buss, D. M. (1989). Sex differences in human mate preferences: Evolutionary hypotheses tested in 37 cultures. *Behavioral and Brain Sciences, 12,* 1–49.

Buss, D. M. (1997). The emergence of evolutionary social psychology. In J. A. Simpson & D. T. Kenrick (Eds.), *Evolutionary social psychology* (pp. 387–400). Mahwah, NJ: Erlbaum.

Buss, D. M., & Schmitt, D. P. (1993). Sexual strategies theory: An evolutionary perspective on human mating. *Psychological Review, 100,* 204–232.

Bzostek, S. H., & Beck, A. N. (2011). Familial instability and young children's physical health. *Social Science and Medicine, 73*(2), 282–292.

Carey, B. (2007, October 2). Friends with benefits, and stress too. Retrieved from *www.nytimes.com/2007/10/02/health/02sex.html.*

Carter, C. S. (1992). Oxytocin and sexual behavior. *Neuroscience and Biobehavioral Reviews, 16,* 131–144.

Carter, C. S. (2003). Developmental consequences of oxytocin. *Physiology and Behavior, 79,* 383–397

Carter, C. S., DeVries, A. C., Taymans, S. E., Roberts, R. L., Williams, J. R., & Getz, L. L. (1997). Peptides, steroids, and pair bonding. *Annals of the New York Academy of Sciences, 807,* 260–272.

Coan, J. A., Schaefer, H. S., & Davidson, R. J. (2006). Lending a hand: Social regulation of the neural response to threat. *Psychological Science, 17,* 1032–1039.

Colin, V. (1985). *Hierarchies and patterns of infants' attachments to parents and day caregivers: An exploration.* Unpublished doctoral dissertation, University of Virginia.

Colin, V. (1987). *Infants' preferences between parents before and after moderate stress activates behavior.* Paper presented at the biennial meeting of the Society for Research in Child Development, Baltimore, MD.

Cummings, E. M. (1980). Caregiver stability and attachment in infant day care. *Developmental Psychology, 16,* 31–37.

Cutler, W. B., Garcia, C. R., Huggins, G. R., & Preti, G. (1986). Sexual behavior and steroid levels among gynecologically mature premenopausal women. *Fertility and Sterility, 45,* 496–502.

Daly, M., & Wilson, M. (1996). Evolutionary psychology and marital conflict. In D. M. Buss & N. M. Malamuth (Eds.), *Sex, power, conflict: Evolutionary and feminist perspectives* (pp. 9–28). New York: Oxford University Press.

DePaulo, B. M., & Morris, W. L. (2005). Singles in society and in science. *Psychological Inquiry, 16*(2–3), 57–83.

Dewsbury, D. A. (1987). The comparative psychology of monogamy. In D. W. Leger (Ed.), *Nebraska Symposium on Motivation* (Vol. 35, pp. 6–43). Lincoln: University of Nebraska Press.

Diamond, L. M. (2004). Emerging perspectives on distinctions between romantic love and sexual desire. *Current Directions in Psychological Science, 13,* 116–119.

Draper, P., & Belsky, J. (1990). Personality development in evolutionary perspective. *Journal of Personality, 58,* 141–161.

Draper, P., & Harpending, H. (1988). A sociobiological perspective on the development of human reproductive strategies. In K. MacDonald (Ed.), *Sociobiological perspectives on human development* (pp. 340–372). New York: Springer-Verlag.

Eibl-Eibesfeldt, I. (1975). *Ethology: The biology of behavior.* New York: Holt, Rinehart & Winston.

Eibl-Eibesfeldt, I. (1989). *Human ethology.* New York: Aldine de Gruyter.

Ellis, B. J., Bates, J. E., Dodge, K. A., Fergusson, D. M., Horwood, L. J., Pettit, G. S., et al. (2003). Does father absence place daughters at special risk for early sexual activity and teenage pregnancy? *Child Development, 74,* 801–821.

Ellis, B. J., McFadyen-Ketchum, S., Dodge, K. A., Pettit, G. S., & Bates, J. E. (1999). Quality of early family relationships and individual differences in the timing of pubertal maturation in girls: A longitudinal test of an evolutionary model. *Journal of Personality and Social Psychology, 77,* 387–401.

Esch, T., & Stefano, G. B. (2007). The neurobiology of love. *Activitas Nervosa Superior, 49*(1–2), 1–18.

Feeney, J. A., Noller, P., & Callan, V. J. (1994). Attachment style, communication and satisfaction in the early years of marriage. In K. Bartholomew & D. Perlman (Eds.), *Advances in personal relationships: Vol. 5. Attachment processes in adulthood* (pp. 269–308). London: Jessica Kingsley.

Feeney, B. C., & Thrush, R. L. (2010). Relationship influences on exploration in adulthood: The characteristics and function of a secure base. *Journal of Personality and Social Psychology, 98*(1), 57–76.

Fisher, H., Aron, A., & Brown, L. L. (2005). Romantic love: An fMRI study of a neural mechanism for mate choice. *Journal of Comparative Neurology, 493,* 58–62.

Fisher, H. E. (2000). Lust, attraction, attachment: Biology and evolution of the three primary emotion systems for mating, reproduction, and parenting. *Journal of Sex Education and Therapy, 25*(1), 96–104.

Fisher, H. E., Aron, A., Mashek, D., Li, H., & Brown, L. L. (2002). Defining the brain systems of lust, romantic attraction, and attachment. *Archives of Sexual Behavior, 31*(5), 413–419.

Fraley, R. C., & Davis, K. E. (1997). Attachment formation and transfer in young adults' close friendships and romantic relationships. *Personal Relationships, 4,* 131–144.

Fraley, R. C., & Shaver, P. R. (1999). Loss and bereavement: Attachment theory and recent controversies concerning "grief work" and the nature of detachment. In J. Cassidy & P. R. Shaver (Eds.), *Handbook of attachment: Theory, research, and clinical implications* (pp. 735–759). New York: Guilford Press.

Fraley, R. C., & Shaver, P. R. (2000). Adult romantic attachment: Theoretical developments, emerging controversies, and unanswered questions. *Review of General Psychology, 4,* 132–154.

Fuller, T. L., & Fincham, F. D. (1995). Attachment style in married couples: Relation to current marital functioning, stability over time, and method of assessment. *Personal Relationships, 2,* 17–34.

Gangestad, S. W., Garver-Apgar, C. E., Simpson, J. A., & Cousins, A. J. (2007). Changes in women's mate preferences across the ovulatory cycle. *Journal of Personality and Social Psychology, 92,* 151–163

Gangestad, S. W., & Simpson, J. A. (2000). The evolution of human mating: Trade-offs and strategic pluralism. *Behavioral and Brain Sciences, 23,* 573–644.

Goodwin, J. S., Hurt, W. C., Key, C. R., & Sarret, J. M. (1987). The effect of marital status on stage, treatment and survival of cancer patients. *Journal of the American Medical Association, 258,* 3125–3130.

Gottman, J. M. (1983). How children become friends. *Monographs of the Society for Research in Child Development, 48*(3, Serial No. 201), 1–86.

Hall, J. H., & Fincham, F. D. (2006). Relationship dissolution following infidelity. In M. A. Fine & J. H. Harvey (Eds.), *Handbook of divorce and relationship dissolution* (pp. 153–168). Mahwah, NJ: Erlbaum.

Harlow, H. F. (1958). The nature of love. *American Psychologist, 13,* 673–685.

Hazan, C., Gur-Yaish, N., & Campa, M. (2004). What does it mean to be attached? In W. S. Rholes & J. A. Simpson (Eds.), *Adult attachment: Theory, research, and clinical implications* (pp. 55–85). New York: Guilford Press.

Hazan, C., & Shaver, P. R. (1987). Romantic love conceptualized as an attachment process. *Journal of Personality and Social Psychology, 52,* 511–524.

Hazan, C., & Shaver, P. R. (1992). Broken attachments. In T. L. Orbuch (Ed.), *Close relationship loss: Theoretical approaches* (pp. 90–108). Hillsdale, NJ: Erlbaum.

Hazan, C., & Shaver, P. R. (1994). Attachment as an organizational framework for research on close relationships. *Psychological Inquiry, 5*, 1–22.

Hazan, C., & Zeifman, D. (1994). Sex and the psychological tether. In K. Bartholomew & D. Perlman (Eds.), *Advances in personal relationships: Vol. 5. Attachment processes in adulthood* (pp. 151–177). London: Jessica Kingsley.

Henry, K., & Holmes, J. G. (1998). Childhood revisited: The intimate relationships of individuals from divorced and conflict-ridden families. In J. A. Simpson & W. S. Rholes (Eds.), *Attachment theory and close relationships* (pp. 280–316). New York: Guilford Press.

Hill, K., & Hurtado, M. (1995). *Demographic/life history of Ache foragers*. New York: Aldine de Gruyter.

Hinsz, V. B. (1989). Facial resemblance in engaged and married couples. *Journal of Social and Personal Relationships, 6*, 223–229.

Hofer, M. A. (1994). Hidden regulators in attachment, separation and loss. *Monographs of the Society for Research in Child Development, 59*(2–3), 192–207, 250–283.

Holmes, T. H., & Rahe, R. H. (1967). The Social Readjustment Rating Scale. *Journal of Psychosomatic Research, 11*, 213–218.

Horwitz, A. V., White, H. R., & Howell-White, S. (1996). Becoming married and mental health: A longitudinal study of a cohort of young adults. *Journal of Marriage and the Family, 58*(4), 895–907.

Justo, J. M. R. M., Maia, C. B., Ferreira-Diniz, F., Santos, C. L., & Moreira, J. M. (1997, June). *Adult attachment style among women with infertility of unknown biological cause.* Paper presented at the International Network on Personal Relationships Conference, Miami University, Oxford, OH.

Kaczmarek, M. (2007). The timing of natural menopause in Poland and associated factors. *Maturitas, 57*(2), 139–153.

Kenrick, D. T., Groth, G. E., Trost, M. R., & Sadalla, E. K. (1993). Integrating evolutionary and social exchange perspectives on relationships: Effects of gender, self-appraisal, and involvement level on mate selection criteria. *Journal of Personality and Social Psychology, 64*, 951–969.

Kirkpatrick, L. A. (1998). Evolution, pair-bonding, and reproductive strategies: A reconceptualization of adult attachment. In J. A. Simpson & W. S. Rholes (Eds.), *Attachment theory and close relationships* (pp. 353–393). New York: Guilford Press.

Kobak, R. R., & Hazan, C. (1991). Attachment in marriage: Effects of security and accuracy of working models. *Journal of Personality and Social Psychology, 60*, 861–869.

Kuo, Z. Y. (1967). *The dynamics of behavior development: An epigenetic view*. New York: Random House.

Lichter, D. T., Qian, Z., & Mellott, L. M. (2006). Marriage or dissolution?: Union transitions among poor cohabiting women. *Demography, 43*(2), 223–240.

Lynch, J. J. (1977). *The broken heart: The medical consequences of loneliness*. New York: Basic Books.

Marazziti, D., & Canale, D. (2004). Hormonal changes when falling in love. *Psychoneuroendocrinology, 29*(7), 931–936.

Marlowe, F. W. (2003). A critical period for provisioning by Hadza men: Implications for pair bonding. *Evolution and Human Behavior, 24*(3), 217–229.

Mellen, S. L. W. (1981). *The evolution of love*. Oxford, UK: Freeman.

Mendoza, S. P., & Mason, W. A. (1997). Attachment relationships in new world primates. *Annals of the New York Academy of Sciences, 807*, 203–209.

Mikulincer, M., & Goodman, G. S. (Eds.). (2006). *Dynamics of romantic love: Attachment, caregiving, and sex*. New York: Guilford Press.

Mikulincer, M., & Shaver, P. R. (2007). *Attachment in adulthood: Structure, dynamics, and change*. New York: Guilford Press.

Moller, A. P. (2003). The evolution of monogamy: Mating relationships, parental care and sexual selection. In U. H. Reichard & C. Boesch (Eds.), *Monogamy: Mating strategies and partnerships in birds, humans and other mammals* (pp. 29–41). Cambridge, UK: Cambridge University Press.

Musick, K., & Bumpass, L. (2012). Reexamining the case for marriage: Union formation and changes in well-being. *Journal of Marriage and Family, 74*(1), 1–18.

Nass, G. D., & Fisher, M. P. (1988). *Sexuality today*. Boston: Jones & Bartlett.

O'Leary, K. D., Acevedo, B. P., Aron, A., Huddy, L., & Mashek, D. (2012). Is long-term love more than a rare phenomenon?: If so, what are its correlates? *Social Psychological and Personality Science, 3*(2), 241–249.

Parkes, C. M., & Weiss, R. S. (1983). *Recovery from bereavement*. New York: Basic Books.

Paul, E. L., McManus, B., & Hayes, A. (2000). "Hookups": Characteristics and correlates of college students' spontaneous and anonymous sexual experiences. *Journal of Sex Research, 37*, 76–88.

Pitman, R., & Scharfe, E. (2010). Testing the function of attachment hierarchies during emerging adulthood. *Personal Relationships, 17*(2), 201–216.

Quinlan, R. J. (2008). Human pair-bonds: Evolutionary functions, ecological variation, and adaptive development. *Evolutionary Anthropology, 17*, 227–238.

Quinlan, R. J., & Quinlan, M. B. (2008). Human lactation, pair-bonds, and alloparents: A cross-cultural analysis. *Human Nature, 19*(1), 87–102.

Raatikainen, K., Heiskanene, N., & Heinonen, S. (2005). Marriage still protects pregnancy. *BJOG: An International Journal of Obstetrics and Gynaecology, 112*, 1411–1416.

Reedy, M. N., Birren, J. E., & Schaie, K. W. (1981). Age and sex differences in satisfying love relationships across the adult life span. *Human Development, 24*, 52–66.

Ricciuti, H. N. (1974). Fear and the development of social attachments in the first year of life. In M. Lewis & L. Rosenblum (Eds.), *Origins of fear* (pp. 73–106). New York: Wiley.

Robertson, J. (1953). Some responses of young children to the loss of maternal care. *Nursing Times, 49,* 382–386.

Rosenkrantz Aronson, S., & Huston, A. C. (2004). The mother–infant relationship in single, cohabiting, and married families: A case for marriage? *Journal of Family Psychology, 18*(1), 5–18.

Rubenstein, C., & Shaver, P. R. (1982). *In search of intimacy.* New York: Delacorte.

Rubin, Z. (1980). *Children's friendships.* Cambridge, MA: Harvard University Press.

Schachner, D. A., & Shaver, P. R. (2004). Attachment dimensions and motives for sex. *Personal Relationships, 11,* 179–195.

Schaffer, H. R., & Emerson, P. E. (1964). The development of social attachments in infancy. *Monographs of the Society for Research in Child Development, 29*(3, Serial No. 94).

Schmitt, D. P. (2005). Sociosexuality from Argentina to Zimbabwe: A 48-nation study of sex, culture, and strategies of human mating. *Behavioral and Brain Sciences, 28,* 247–311.

Schmitt, D. P., Shackelford, T. K., Duntley, J., Tooke, W., & Buss, D. M. (2001). The desire for sexual variety as a key to understanding basic human mating strategies. *Personal Relationships, 8,* 425–455.

Seligman, M. E. P. (2002). *Authentic happiness: Using the new positive psychology to realize your potential for lasting fulfillment.* New York: Free Press.

Shaver, P. R., Hazan, C., & Bradshaw, D. (1988). Love as attachment: The integration of three behavioral systems. In R. J. Sternberg & M. L. Barnes (Eds.), *The psychology of love* (pp. 68–99). New Haven, CT: Yale University Press.

Shackelford, T. K., Schmitt, D. P., & Buss, D. M. (2005). Universal dimensions of human mate preferences. *Personality and Individual Differences, 39*(2), 447–458.

Shill, M. A., Solyom, P., & Biven, C. (1984). Parent preference in the attachment exploration balance in infancy: An experimental psychoanalytic approach. *Child Psychiatry and Human Development, 15,* 34–48.

Simpson, J. A., & Gangestad, S. W. (1991). Individual differences in sociosexuality: Evidence for convergent and discriminant validity. *Journal of Personality and Social Psychology, 60,* 870–883.

Spitz, R. A. (1946). Anaclitic depression. *Psychoanalytic Study of the Child, 2,* 313–342.

Stearns, S. (1992). *The evolution of life histories.* New York: Oxford University Press.

Steinberg, L., & Silverberg, S. B. (1986). The vicissitudes of autonomy in early adolescence. *Child Development, 57,* 841–851.

Sternberg, R. J. (1986). A triangular theory of love. *Psychological Review, 93,* 119–135.

Stroebe, W., Stroebe, M., Abakoumkin, G., & Schut, H. (1996). The role of loneliness and social support in adjustment to loss: A test of attachment versus stress theory. *Journal of Personality and Social Psychology, 70,* 1241–1249.

Surbey, M. (1990). Family composition, stress, and human menarche. In F. Bercovitch & T. Zeigler (Eds.), *The socioendocrinology of primate reproduction* (pp. 71–97). New York: Liss.

Symons, D. (1979). *The evolution of human sexuality.* New York: Oxford University Press.

Thornhill, N. W. (1991). An evolutionary analysis of rules regulating human inbreeding and marriage. *Behavioral and Brain Sciences, 14,* 247–281.

Tinbergen, N. (1963). On aims and methods of ethology. *Zeitschrift für Tierpsychologie, 20,* 410–433.

Trevathan, W. (1987). *Human birth.* New York: Aldine de Gruyter.

Trinke, S. J., & Bartholomew, K. (1997). Hierarchies of attachment relationships in young adulthood. *Journal of Social and Personal Relationships, 14*(5), 603–625.

Trivers, R. L. (1972). Parental investment and sexual selection. In B. Campbell (Ed.), *Sexual selection and the descent of man* (pp. 1871–1971). Chicago: Aldine.

Uchino, B. N., Cacioppo, J. T., & Kiecolt-Glaser, J. K. (1996). The relationship between social support and physiological processes: A review with emphasis on underlying mechanisms and implications for health. *Psychological Bulletin, 119,* 488–531.

Veith, J. L., Buck, M., Getzlaf, S., Van Dalfsen, P., & Slade, S. (1983). Exposure to men influences the occurrence of ovulation in women. *Physiology and Behavior, 31,* 313–315.

Vormbrock, J. K. (1993). Attachment theory as applied to war-time and job-related marital separation. *Psychological Bulletin, 114,* 122–144.

Wallerstein, J. S. (1994). Children after divorce: Wounds that don't heal. In L. Fenson & J. Fenson (Eds.), *Human development, 94/95* (pp. 160–165). Guilford, CT: Dushkin.

Weber, A. L. (1998). Losing, leaving, and letting go: Coping with nonmarital breakups. In B. H. Spitzberg & W. R. Cupach (Eds.), *The dark side of close relationships* (pp. 267–306). Mahwah, NJ: Erlbaum.

Weiss, R. S. (1973). *Loneliness: The experience of emotional and social isolation.* Cambridge, MA: MIT Press.

Weiss, R. S. (1975). *Marital separation.* New York: Basic Books.

Weiss, R. S. (1988). Loss and recovery. *Journal of Social Issues, 44,* 37–52.

Xu, X., Aron, A., Brown, L., Cao, G., Feng, T., & Weng, X. (2011). Reward and motivation systems: A brain mapping study of early-stage intense romantic love in Chinese participants. *Human Brain Mapping, 32*(2), 249–257.

Zeifman, D., & Hazan, C. (1997). A process model of adult attachment formation. In S. Duck (Ed.), *Handbook of personal relationships* (2nd ed., pp. 179–195). Chichester, UK: Wiley.

# Chapter 21

# Adult Romantic Attachment

## Developments in the Study
## of Couple Relationships

### Judith A. Feeney

My partner is extremely affectionate, which suits me down to the ground.
I've always, always craved affection all my life, mainly through parental—bad
parental—relationships. So, I don't know, but I put it down to that. And she's
the only person I've ever gone out with that's actually given me the affection
I've wanted.

—RESEARCH PARTICIPANT

It is not unusual for people, in describing their couple relationships, to emphasize the impact of early experiences with caregivers; such an emphasis is reflected in this brief quotation from a research participant. This focus on the legacy of early social experiences is consistent with Bowlby's (1969/1982, 1973, 1980) theory of attachment, which recognizes the vital role of attachment behavior throughout the life cycle, and the enormous importance for later relationships of the bonds formed between children and their caregivers. This chapter examines the proposition that romantic love can be conceptualized as an attachment process, influenced in part by experiences with caregivers. The aim is to present the original theoretical and empirical work on which this proposition is based, to outline the considerable advances that have since occurred in this research area, and to explore some unresolved issues and likely future directions.

## The First Studies of Romantic Love as Attachment

Although Bowlby's attachment theory dealt primarily with the bonds that form between infants and their caregivers, theoretical work dating from the early 1980s argued for the relevance of attachment principles to adults' close relationships as well. These arguments centered on the functions of attachment bonds. Specifically, infant attachment bonds involve "proximity maintenance" and "separation protest" (seeking proximity to an attachment figure and resisting separation; see Cassidy, Chapter 1, this volume), and establishment of a "secure base" (using the attachment figure as a base from which to explore the environment) and a "safe haven" (turning to the attachment figure for comfort in times of threat). According to Weiss (1982, 1991), these attachment functions apply to most committed

435

couple relationships: Adults derive comfort and security from their partners, want to be with them (especially in times of stress), and protest when partners' availability is threatened. Similarly, Ainsworth (1989) described sexual pair bonds as the prime example of adult attachments.

Attachment theory also suggests a link between the *quality* of infant attachment relationships and subsequent adult attachment relationships. Bowlby proposed that during the years of "immaturity" (infancy to adolescence), individuals gradually develop expectations of attachment figures, based on experiences with these individuals. Expectations about the availability and responsiveness of attachment figures are incorporated into "internal working models," which guide perceptions and behavior in later relationships (see Bretherton & Munholland, Chapter 4, this volume, for an extensive discussion of working models).

Despite claims of continuity between childhood and adult relationships, the attachment perspective on romantic relationships did not become an active topic of research until Hazan and Shaver reported their seminal studies (Hazan & Shaver, 1987; Shaver & Hazan, 1988; Shaver, Hazan, & Bradshaw, 1988). In these papers, Hazan and Shaver proposed that romantic love could be conceptualized as an attachment process. Furthermore, because variations in early social experience produce relatively lasting differences in relationship styles, the three major attachment styles described in the infant literature (Ainsworth, Blehar, Waters, & Wall, 1978) should be manifested in romantic love. (Following Hazan and Shaver's terminology, I use the terms *secure*, *avoidant*, and *anxious-ambivalent* to refer to these styles in adults.)

In support of these arguments, Hazan and Shaver presented theoretical analyses of love and attachment, integrated with new empirical data. Their theoretical analyses (Shaver & Hazan, 1988) addressed several issues, including the conceptualization of adult love as an integration of behavioral systems (attachment, caregiving, and sex), and compared the attachment perspective with previous theories of love. These issues are briefly discussed later in this chapter.

The empirical studies (Hazan & Shaver, 1987) assessed the link between attachment style and aspects of childhood and adult relationships. Hazan and Shaver developed a forced-choice, self-report measure of adult attachment consisting of three paragraphs, designed to capture the main features of the three infant attachment patterns described by Ainsworth and colleagues (1978). Participants were asked to choose the paragraph most descriptive of their feelings in close relationships. This measure was used with a large sample of respondents to a questionnaire printed in a local newspaper, and in a separate study with an undergraduate sample. Participants completed questions assessing general attitudes toward close relationships, together with experiences specific to their "most important romance." Results showed that the frequencies of the three styles were similar to those observed among American infants from middle-class families: Just over half the adults described themselves as "secure," and of the remainder, slightly more classified themselves as "avoidant" than as "anxious-ambivalent." In line with predictions based on attachment theory, the three attachment groups differed in their reports of early family relationships, working models of attachment, and love experiences.

In reporting their results, Hazan and Shaver (1987) noted the limitations of their initial studies. Because of constraints on data collection, the measures were brief and simple, and focused on participants' experience of a single romantic relationship. Although this focus might seem to imply a trait approach, the authors recognized that relationship qualities are influenced by "factors unique to particular partners and circumstances" (Hazan & Shaver, 1987, p. 521). This important point is addressed again later in this chapter.

## Early Studies of Romantic Attachment: Replications and Extensions

Despite the limitations of their initial research, Hazan and Shaver succeeded in providing both a *normative* account of romantic love (i.e., an account of the typical processes of romantic attachment) and an understanding of *individual differences* in adult relationship styles. Providing a bridge between infant attachment theory and theories of romantic love, their work generated intense interest among relationship researchers, who soon set out to replicate and extend the initial findings. Two questions addressed by these early studies were the conceptual links between love and attachment, and the salience of attachment issues to individuals in romantic relationships. (Some early studies also assessed attachment-related differences in affect regulation; see Mikulincer & Shaver, 2015; Chapter 24, this volume.)

## Conceptualizing Love and Attachment

The first two studies discussed here addressed the conceptualization of love and attachment. Shaver and Hazan (1988) proposed that previous theories of love (theories of "love styles"; of "anxious" love; and of separate components of love) could be integrated within the attachment perspective. To test this proposition, Levy and Davis (1988) assessed the links between attachment style and measures of the love styles described by Lee (1973, 1988) and the components of love discussed by Sternberg (1986; for further discussion of these theories, see Sternberg & Weis, 2006.)

The love styles described by Lee are *eros* (passionate love), *ludus* (game-playing love), *storge* (friendship love), *mania* (possessive, dependent love), *pragma* (logical, "shopping-list" love), and *agape* (selfless love). Shaver and Hazan (1988) argued that this typology could be reduced to the three attachment styles: Their formulation linked secure attachment to a combination of eros and agape, avoidant attachment to ludus, and anxious-ambivalent attachment to mania (storge and pragma were not seen as forms of romantic love). Levy and Davis's (1988) results, based on ratings of each attachment and love style, largely supported this formulation. Furthermore, all three components of Sternberg's (1986) model of love (intimacy, passion, commitment) were related positively to secure attachment and negatively to avoidant and anxious-ambivalent attachment, highlighting the

link between secure attachment and better relationship functioning.

Like Levy and Davis (1988), we (J. A. Feeney & Noller, 1990) were interested in the interrelations among theories of love (Table 21.1 summarizes the findings of these two studies). In particular, we queried the assertion that theories of "anxious love" are unidimensional, and equivalent to anxious-ambivalent attachment (Shaver & Hazan, 1988). Using factor analysis, we assessed the structure of a broad set of measures: self-esteem, loving, love styles, and anxious love (e.g., "limerence"; Tennov, 1979). Of particular interest was the fact that measures of anxious love were multidimensional. The limerence measure, for example, yielded four factors: "obsessive preoccupation," "self-conscious anxiety with partners," "emotional dependence," and "idealization." Four higher-order factors emerged from the set of measures: "neurotic love" (preoccupation, dependence, and idealization); "circumspect love" (friendship, pragma); "self-confidence" (self-esteem, lack of self-conscious anxiety); and "avoidance of intimacy" (high scores on ludus; low scores on loving, eros, and agape). All four factors strongly differentiated the attachment groups. Secure participants' experience of love was self-confident and neither neurotic nor intimacy-avoiding. Both insecure groups lacked self-confidence, but whereas avoidant participants reported avoiding intimacy, anxious-ambivalent individuals reported a desperate, impetuous approach to love. Although these results generally supported Shaver and Hazan's formulation, it seems that one aspect of anxious love ("self-conscious anxiety") characterizes both insecure groups, rather than being specific to anxious-ambivalence.

**TABLE 21.1. Measures of Love Associated with the Three Major Attachment Styles as of 1990**

| Measure | Secure | Avoidant | Anxious-ambivalent |
|---|---|---|---|
| Love styles | Eros (passionate love), agape (selfless love) | Ludus (game-playing love) | Mania (possessive love) |
| Components of love | High on intimacy, passion, and commitment | Low on intimacy, passion, and commitment | Low on intimacy, passion, and commitment |
| Higher-order factors | High on self-confidence (high on self-esteem and low on self-conscious anxiety with partners); low on avoidance of intimacy; low on neurotic love | High on avoidance of intimacy (high on ludus and low on eros, agape, and loving); low on self-confidence; low on neurotic love | High on neurotic love (high on preoccupation, dependence, and idealization); low on circumspect love (friendship, pragma); low on self-confidence; low on avoidance of intimacy |

*Note.* Data from J. A. Feeney and Noller (1990) and Levy and Davis (1988).

### Salience of Attachment Issues to Perceptions of Romantic Relationships

The studies reported so far point to meaningful relations between romantic attachment style and love experiences. However, these studies relied on closed-ended, self-report measures. Because such structured measures may lead to response sets such as experimenter demand and social desirability, we (J. A. Feeney & Noller, 1991) argued that these studies had not established the *salience* of attachment issues to individuals' evaluations of their romantic relationships; that is, attachment issues may not be very important to individuals, except when they are introduced by measurement procedures.

To address this problem, we asked participants in dating relationships to provide open-ended verbal descriptions of their relationships, and later, to complete Hazan and Shaver's (1987) measure of attachment style. Using content analysis, we examined whether participants spontaneously referred to issues that are central to working models of attachment: openness, closeness, dependence, commitment, and affection. Supporting the salience of attachment themes, we found that 89% of the sample referred to at least one of these issues; on average, one-fifth of the content of the transcripts was devoted to these issues. The three attachment groups also differed markedly in the content of their reports, as illustrated by the extracts in Table 21.2. Secure participants described mutual support but advocated a balance between intimacy and autonomy. Both secure and avoidant participants described their relationships as friendship-based; unlike secure participants, however, avoidant individuals preferred clear limits to closeness, dependence, commitment, and displays of affection. Anxious-ambivalent participants, in contrast, preferred unqualified closeness, commitment and affection, and tended to idealize their partners. These results fit with findings based on structured measures of relationship experiences.

## Advances in Conceptualization and Measurement

Understanding recent studies of romantic attachment requires us to consider the advances in conceptualization and measurement on which they are based. In terms of measurement, Hazan and Shaver's (1987) forced-choice item had clear limitations (as they themselves noted). Reliance on a single item required assumptions about the number of attachment styles and raised concerns about reliability of measurement. Given these problems, researchers soon sought more refined measures. Before these refinements are discussed, however, two points should be noted.

First, the three-group measure continues to be used by some researchers, and offers both ease of

---

**TABLE 21.2. Extracts from Open-Ended Reports of Romantic Relationships Supplied by Participants from Three Attachment Groups**

**Secure:** "We're really good friends, and we sort of knew each other for a long time before we started going out—and we like the same sort of things. Another thing which I like a lot is that he gets on well with all my close friends. We can always talk things over. Like if we're having any fights, we usually resolve them by talking it over—he's a very reasonable person. I can just be my own person, so it's good, because it's not a possessive relationship. I think that we trust each other a lot."

**Avoidant:** "My partner is my best friend, and that's the way I think of him. He's as special to me as any of my other friends. His expectations in life don't include marriage, or any long-term commitment to any female, which is fine with me, because that's not what my expectations are as well. I find that he doesn't want to be overly intimate, and he doesn't expect too much commitment—which is good. . . . Sometimes it's a worry that a person can be that close to you, and be in such control of your life."

**Anxious-ambivalent:** "So I went in there . . . and he was sitting on the bench, and I took one look, and I actually melted. He was the best-looking thing I'd ever seen, and that was the first thing that struck me about him. So we went out and we had lunch in the park. . . . So we just sort of sat there—and in silence—but it wasn't awkward . . . like, you know, when you meet strangers and you can't think of anything to say, it's usually awkward. It wasn't like that. We just sat there, and it was incredible—like we'd known each other for a real long time, and we'd only met for about 10 seconds, so that was—straightaway my first feelings for him started coming out."

*Note.* Data from J. A. Feeney and Noller (1991).

administration and a strong conceptual link with infant attachment theory. Furthermore, it has shown consistent links with relationship variables. Thus, the question is not whether that measure produces meaningful and valid results, but rather, how it might be improved psychometrically.

Second, it should be noted that Hazan and Shaver were not the first researchers to measure adult attachment. The Adult Attachment Interview (AAI; George, Kaplan, & Main, 1984) taps memories of childhood relationships with parents, and respondents' evaluations of the effects of these experiences on their adult personality. Interview transcripts can be used to identify three attachment patterns ("secure," "dismissing," and "preoccupied"), based on the content and coherence of the accounts. The validity of this measure is supported by links between parents' attachment classification, assessed by the AAI, and their children's attachment classification, assessed by observers (Main & Goldwyn, 1984; Main, Goldwyn, & Hesse, 2003). AAI classifications have also been related to couple relationship quality, as noted later in this chapter. Most of the measures discussed in this chapter differ from the AAI in two key respects: They focus on adult romantic attachment (as opposed to current state of mind regarding childhood attachment), and they require less in-depth training to administer and score. (For more details concerning the AAI, see Crowell, Fraley, & Roisman, Chapter 27, and Hesse, Chapter 26, this volume.)

## Typologies of Attachment: Three or Four Styles?

Hazan and Shaver's (1987) original measure described three styles, based on extrapolation from studies of the major infant attachment styles. Bartholomew (1990; Bartholomew & Horowitz, 1991) subsequently proposed a four-group model of adult attachment, based on Bowlby's claim that attachment patterns reflect working models of self and others. Bartholomew argued that models of self can be dichotomized as positive or negative (the self is seen as worthy of love and attention, or as unworthy). Similarly, models of others can be positive or negative (others are seen as available and caring, or as unreliable or rejecting). Working models of self and others jointly define four attachment styles, including two avoidant styles (see Figure 21.1). "Dismissing-avoidant" individuals emphasize achievement and self-reliance, maintaining a sense of self-worth at the expense of intimacy. "Fearful-avoidant" individuals desire intimacy but distrust others, avoiding close involvements that may entail loss or rejection.

Self-report prototypes of the four attachment styles were developed (similar in form to Hazan and Shaver's three descriptions), together with interview schedules that yield ratings on the four prototypes (Bartholomew & Horowitz, 1991). Substantial convergence has been established between Bartholomew's interview and self-report measures, and between classifications from Bar-

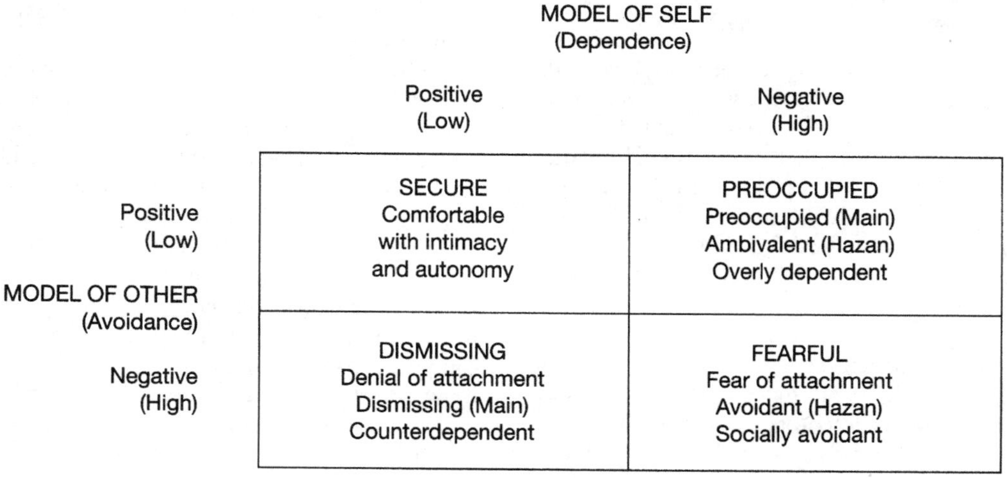

MODEL OF SELF
(Dependence)

|  | Positive (Low) | Negative (High) |
|---|---|---|
| Positive (Low)<br><br>MODEL OF OTHER (Avoidance) | SECURE<br>Comfortable<br>with intimacy<br>and autonomy | PREOCCUPIED<br>Preoccupied (Main)<br>Ambivalent (Hazan)<br>Overly dependent |
| Negative (High) | DISMISSING<br>Denial of attachment<br>Dismissing (Main)<br>Counterdependent | FEARFUL<br>Fear of attachment<br>Avoidant (Hazan)<br>Socially avoidant |

**FIGURE 21.1.** The four adult attachment styles defined by Bartholomew in terms of working models of self and others. From Bartholomew (1990). Copyright 1990 by Sage Publications, Inc. Reprinted by permission.

tholomew's interview schedule and those based on the AAI (Bartholomew & Shaver, 1998), although this continues to be disputed (see Crowell et al., Chapter 27, this volume). The three-group and four-group measures also show meaningful relations with each other (Brennan, Shaver, & Tobey, 1991). Participants who choose the secure category of Bartholomew's measure also tend to choose the secure category of the other, and those choosing the preoccupied category tend to choose the original anxious-ambivalent category. Most fearful-avoidant individuals endorse Hazan and Shaver's description of avoidance (which emphasizes discomfort with closeness), but dismissing-avoidant individuals are drawn from both secure and avoidant groups.

The four-group model is validated by empirical support for two distinct types of avoidance. For example, the interpersonal problems of fearful-avoidant individuals involve social insecurity and lack of assertiveness, whereas those of dismissing-avoidant individuals involve excessive coldness (Bartholomew & Horowitz, 1991; J. A. Feeney, Noller, & Hanrahan, 1994). As a result, researchers have increasingly adopted the four-group model of adult attachment. This model is consistent with reports of a fourth infant attachment style, marked by characteristics of both avoidance and anxious ambivalence (e.g., Crittenden, 1985; Main & Solomon, 1990), in that fearful-avoidant adults tend to endorse both avoidant and anxious-ambivalent prototypes (Brennan et al., 1991).

### From Categorical to Dimensional Measures

Questions have been raised not only about the number of adult attachment styles, but also about the appropriate form of measurement. Categorical measures have several limitations: They fail to capture individual differences within a particular attachment style; they seem to imply that attachment styles are mutually exclusive; and they assume that the themes within each attachment description form a consistent whole. To address these issues, researchers began breaking each description into its component statements and using factor-analytic methods to investigate the structure. Although item content varied slightly across studies, findings generally suggested two major dimensions, "avoidance" (discomfort with closeness) and "attachment anxiety" (J. A. Feeney, Noller, & Callan, 1994; J. A. Feeney, Noller, & Hanrahan, 1994; Simpson, Rholes, & Nelligan, 1992).

Avoidance contrasts elements of the original secure and avoidant descriptions (e.g., "I find it easy to trust others" vs. "I am nervous when anyone gets too close"). Attachment anxiety taps themes central to anxious-ambivalent attachment, such as fear of rejection and desire for extreme closeness (e.g., "I often worry that my partner doesn't really love me," "I find that others are reluctant to get as close as I would like").

Similarly, a comprehensive study of all available self-report items (Brennan, Clark, & Shaver, 1998) yielded two higher-order factors: "anxiety" (about relationship issues) and "avoidance" (discomfort with closeness and interdependence). These dimensions are related to the four groups of Bartholomew's model: Dismissing and fearful groups report more avoidance of intimacy than secure and preoccupied groups, suggesting that avoidance is linked to working models of others; preoccupied and fearful groups report more anxiety about rejection and unlovability than secure and dismissing groups, suggesting that anxiety is linked to working models of self (J. A. Feeney, 1995). The Experiences in Close Relationships Scale (ECR), developed by Brennan and colleagues (1998), has been widely used, and many studies have supported its validity. Short forms of the measure have also been proposed, using either the first half of the full item set (Mikulincer, Shaver, Gillath, & Nitzberg, 2005) or a subset of items selected on the basis of item response theory (e.g., Lafontaine, Brassard, Lussier, Valois, Shaver, & Johnson, 2015). One full-length version, the revised ECR (ECR-R; Fraley, Waller, & Brennan, 2000) was designed to yield better discrimination at the "secure" ends of each scale (anxiety and avoidance).

Griffin and Bartholomew (1994) advocated a "prototype" approach to the assessment of adult attachment: This regards the four types as important predictors of relationship outcomes (adding to the predictive power of the two dimensions) but recognizes that the boundaries between them are "fuzzy." However, Fraley and Waller (1998) rejected this conclusion, noting that the question of whether individual differences should be viewed in terms of categories (latent types) or dimensions cannot be resolved by cluster analysis, by examining the distributions of attachment variables, or by considerations of convenience. Taxometric techniques, designed specifically to evaluate evidence of "groups" versus "dimensions," suggest that differences in adult attachment are best understood in terms of dimensions (Fraley & Waller, 1998).

Although considerable consensus exists concerning the utility and structure of dimensional self-report measures of romantic attachment, reducing this complex construct to two dimensions inevitably loses some information. In a study employing the Attachment Style Questionnaire (ASQ; J. A. Feeney, Noller, & Hanrahan, 1994) with Italian clinical and nonclinical samples (Fossati et al., 2003), use of the minimum partial statistic to estimate the correct number of factors confirmed the five factors proposed earlier (J. A. Feeney, Noller, & Hanrahan, 1994): "confidence in self and others," "need for approval," "preoccupation with relationships," "discomfort with closeness," and "relationships as secondary" (to achievement). Furthermore, discomfort with closeness was related to sample (clinical, nonclinical), but relationships as secondary was not; yet when only two factors are extracted from the ASQ, items from both these scales load on the same primary dimension (avoidance). Similarly, in later research (Fossati et al., 2009), impulsive aggression was predicted by preoccupation with relationships but not by need for approval; yet items from both these scales define the primary dimension of anxiety. Hence, in some contexts, measures with more complex structures may offer important advantages.

## Working Models and Romantic Attachment

Theoretical and empirical work on the structure and function of working models highlights their importance to relationship experiences. With regard to structure, Collins and Read (1994) argued that individuals develop a hierarchy of working models, with a set of generalized models lying at the top, models for particular classes of relationships (e.g., family members, peers) at an intermediate level, and models for particular relationships (e.g., father, spouse) at the lowest level. Research suggests that models higher in the hierarchy apply to a wide range of others but are less predictive for any specific situation (Fraley, Heffernan, Vicary, & Brumbaugh, 2011; Overall, Fletcher, & Friesen, 2003.) Furthermore, there is evidence that the effects of general working models may be moderated by relationship-specific models, as assessed by perceptions of partner responsiveness and supportiveness (Collins, Guichard, Ford, & Feeney, 2004).

Collins and colleagues (2004; Collins & Read, 1994) further suggested that working models include four components: memories of attachment-related experiences; beliefs, attitudes, and expectations of self and others in relation to attachment; attachment-related goals and needs; and strategies and plans for achieving these goals. These components vary across attachment groups, as summarized in Table 21.3 (the three-group model is used here because many experimental studies of affect regulation are based on it).

With regard to memory, for example, secure individuals tend to remember their parents as warm and affectionate; avoidant individuals remember their mothers as cold and rejecting; and anxious-ambivalent individuals remember their fathers as unfair (e.g., J. A. Feeney & Noller, 1990; Priel & Besser, 2000; Rothbard & Shaver, 1994). These findings from retrospective reports fit with attachment theory (although not with the link in AAI research between dismissing avoidance and idealization of parents), but we cannot be sure to what extent the memories are affected by more recent experiences. Attachment avoidance and anxiety are also linked to faster associative responses between exposure to the name of mother or romantic partner and negative personal attributes, implying the existence of negative representations of close others in an associative memory network (Zayas & Shoda, 2005). Furthermore, recent studies (e.g., Selcuk, Zayas, Gunaydin, Hazan, & Kross, 2012) suggest that although the negative affect elicited by upsetting memories can be reduced by activating mental representations of attachment figures, these benefits are weaker for insecure adults (especially those high in avoidance).

In terms of functions, working models shape our cognitive, emotional, and behavioral responses to others (Collins & Read, 1994; Collins et al., 2004; Mikulincer & Shaver, 2015, Chapters 6 and 7). Working models affect cognitive responses by directing us to pay attention to certain aspects of social stimuli (particularly goal-related stimuli), by creating biases in memory encoding and retrieval, and by affecting explanation processes. For example, secure adults show faster recognition of positive-outcome words set in an interpersonal context, whereas avoidant adults show faster recognition of negative-outcome words (Baldwin, Fehr, Keedian, Siedel, & Thomson, 1993). Furthermore, secure adults' explanations of relationship events reflect their stronger sense of security and confidence in partners' availability (Collins, 1996; Gallo & Smith, 2001), and their appraisals of rela-

**TABLE 21.3. Attachment Group Differences in Working Models**

| Secure | Avoidant | Anxious-ambivalent |
|---|---|---|
| Memories | | |
| Parents warm and affectionate | Mothers cold and rejecting | Fathers unfair |
| Attachment-related beliefs, attitudes | | |
| Few self-doubts; high in self-worth and self-efficacy | Suspicious of human motives | Others complex and difficult to understand |
| Generally liked by others | Others intrusive; not trustworthy or dependable | People have little control over own lives |
| Thinks others are generally well-intentioned and good-hearted | Doubts honesty and integrity of parents and others | Relational ambivalence |
| Thinks others are generally trustworthy, dependable, and altruistic | Lacks confidence in social situations; expects relationship failure | Unrealistic expectations of partners and relationships |
| Interpersonally oriented | Not interpersonally oriented | Hungry for love and support |
| Attachment-related goals and needs | | |
| Desires intimate relationships and interdependence | Desires to maintain physical and emotional distance | Desires extreme intimacy and validation from partners |
| Seeks balance of closeness and autonomy in relationships | Limits intimacy to satisfy needs for autonomy; averse to commitment | Seeks lower levels of autonomy |
| Mutual care and support | Places greater weight on goals such as impersonal achievement | Fears rejection and abandonment |
| Plans and strategies | | |
| Acknowledges distress | Manages distress by cutting off negative affect | Heightened displays of distress and anger |
| Modulates negative affect in constructive way | Minimizes distress-related emotional displays; denies vulnerability | Solicitous and compliant at times; also demanding and coercive |
| Invests in relationship development and maintenance | Compulsive self-reliance; withholds intimate disclosure | Focuses on own emotional needs |

tionship partners are more stable over time (Alfasi, Gramzow, & Carnelley, 2010), and less contingent on recent partner behavior (J. A. Feeney, 2002; Pietromonaco & Feldman Barrett, 2006).

With regard to emotional responses, working models affect both primary and secondary appraisals of relational events (Collins et al., 2004). *Primary appraisal* refers to the immediate emotional reaction to a situation. In *secondary appraisal*, cognitive processing may maintain, amplify, or lessen the initial emotional response, depending on how the individual interprets the experience. For example, individuals who are anxious about attachment feel more immediate distress in the face of hurtful partner behavior; furthermore, they often interpret this behavior as intentional and undeserved, which tends to amplify the distress (J. A. Feeney, 2004, 2005). Many studies have linked attachment anxiety and avoidance with difficulties in emotion regulation, and research also points to differences in brain responses to stressful events (see Shaver & Mikulincer, 2013, for a review).

Working models affect behavioral responses through the activation of stored plans and strategies, and the construction of new plans and strategies (Collins & Read, 1994). An example of a stored strategy that may have developed in childhood is an individual "running to Mother" whenever conflict with the spouse arises. In the absence of an available existing strategy, new strategies may be devised for current situations. Hence, working models may affect decisions about whether to avoid conflict issues or discuss them openly with one's spouse (J. A. Feeney, 2003). Research has linked attachment insecurity to a range of maladaptive relational behaviors, including unselective responses during speed dating (McClure, Lydon, Baccus, & Baldwin, 2010), less synchronization with partners' behavior (Gabriel, Kawakami, Bartak, Kang, & Mann, 2010), and less honesty and authenticity (Gillath, Sesko, Shaver, & Chun, 2010).

## Stability, Change and the Conceptualization of Attachment

Although studies have shown reasonable stability of attachment patterns across the early childhood years, the extent of stability remains an issue both for developmental researchers and for investigators of romantic attachment. Attachment theory supports both the tendency toward stability and the possibility of change. Several factors promote the stability of working models (Bowlby, 1980). First, individuals tend to select environments that fit their beliefs about self and others. Second, the information-processing biases outlined earlier lead people to perceive social events in ways that support existing models. Third, working models may be self-perpetuating; for example, someone who believes that others are untrustworthy may approach them defensively, eliciting further rejection.

Despite these forces promoting stability, change in working models is clearly possible. For example, becoming involved in a stable, satisfying relationship may disconfirm negative expectations based on earlier experiences. The high percentage of secure respondents generally found in samples of stable couples supports this effect (J. A. Feeney, Noller, & Callan, 1994; Senchak & Leonard, 1992), as does the following comment made by a research participant:

> I had a real problem trusting anyone at the start of any relationship. A couple of things happened to me when I was young, which I had some emotional difficulties getting over. At the start of our relationship, if P. had been separated from me, I would have been constantly thinking: "What was he doing?"; "Was he with another girl?"; "Was he cheating on me?"; all that would have been running through my head. Over a 3-year period of going out, you look at it in a different light; you learn to trust him.

Similarly, a secure person who is involved in a particularly negative relationship may become insecure as a result, as suggested by another research participant:

> Before I started seeing T., I was in another long relationship with another fellow . . . and the last couple of months were really bad. I was always really confident about myself and secure about myself, but he made me feel in 2 months—just seemed to ruin everything I'd ever felt good about myself, and I felt bad about everything I did, and he made me feel bad. And so I've got this constant thing in the back of my head that maybe that might happen again.

Quantitative research has assessed the stability of adult romantic attachment over intervals ranging from 1 week to 27 years. Given the large number of studies addressing this topic, a consideration of the individual findings is beyond the scope of this chapter; however, broad conclusions can be drawn (Mikulincer & Shaver, 2015). With forced-choice (three- or four-group) measures, approximately one-fourth of participants show a change in attachment type across assessments (Baldwin & Fehr, 1995). This figure varies little with the time lag between assessments. Ratings of attachment prototypes are moderately stable, as are multiple-item scales (e.g., J. A. Feeney, Noller, & Callan, 1994; J. A. Feeney, Passmore, & Peterson, 2007); when the limited reliability of multiple-item scales is considered, their stability is quite high. And interview measures (whether forced-choice or ratings) tend to be even more stable than self-reports or peer reports (Scharfe & Bartholomew, 1994).

Given that adult attachment measures are not perfectly stable (even accounting for unreliability), researchers have considered the meaning of "change over time" (Davila & Cobb, 2004). Some have posited individual differences in the stability of attachment, whereby adverse early experiences render certain individuals more prone to change (Davila, Burge, & Hammen, 1997), but longitudinal studies provide mixed support for this claim ( J. A. Feeney et al., 2007; Scharfe & Cole, 2006). Others have debated whether attachment style should be conceptualized as an enduring, trait-like characteristic, or as reflecting recent experiences in particular relationships. Stability data (outlined earlier) support both positions. Stability estimates are moderately high; indeed, some data suggest that attachment style is more stable than relationship status (Kirkpatrick & Hazan, 1994).

However, other studies highlight the role of recent experiences, linking change in attachment to the formation and dissolution of couple bonds (e.g., Kirkpatrick & Hazan, 1994; Scharfe & Cole, 2006) and to first-time parenthood (J. A. Feeney, Alexander, Noller, & Hohaus, 2003).

Importantly, "traits" and "relationships" are intertwined rather than mutually exclusive (Fraley & Brumbaugh, 2004). For example, by choosing particular partners, individuals may find themselves in situations that confirm their relational expectations. Supporting this claim, studies of romantic attachment reveal a degree of "partner matching." Although the form of this matching remains contentious (are we attracted to secure partners, or to those with a similar or a complementary style?), most studies of hypothetical partners and of real couples find links between partners' attachment characteristics (Holmes & Johnson, 2009; Strauss, Morry, & Kito, 2012). In particular, there is substantial evidence that secure individuals tend to be paired with secure, responsive partners—a situation that should confirm positive working models. Hence, attachment is both trait-like and somewhat contextually fluid.

A related controversy regarding change in attachment contrasts the role of major relational events versus the role of short-term fluctuations. According to the first perspective, change is most likely in the face of significant relationship experiences. As noted earlier, several studies have supported this position; however, others have failed to do so (see Mikulincer & Shaver, 2015, for a review). The second perspective proposes that adults have multiple attachment orientations, derived from their varied relational experiences; at any given time, attachment measures reflect the orientation elicited by situational factors. This perspective is supported by evidence that priming adults to think about a particular kind of relationship influences perceptions of partners (Baldwin, Keelan, Fehr, Enns, & Koh-Rangarajoo, 1996). Furthermore, relatively simple manipulations involving exposure to security-priming words or to mental representations of responsive attachment figures influence working models and associated responses: Positive effects of priming extend to affect (Selcuk et al., 2012), perceptions of romantic partners (Carnelley & Rowe, 2007), forgiveness of partner transgressions (Karremans & Aarts, 2007), and responses to partners' hurtful behavior (Cassidy, Shaver, Mikulincer, & Lavy, 2009).

Fraley and Brumbaugh (2004) have advanced the debate over stability and change by clarifying issues related to attachment organization. These researchers argued that once a developmental pathway becomes established, it is less likely to change: Social environments are usually relatively stable, and intraindividual processes (e.g., assimilation of new information) operate to maintain expectations. Nevertheless, external events exert a nontrivial influence. Fraley and Brumbaugh further noted that simply studying the stability of attachment across two time points tells us little about attachment organization. Data regarding *patterns* of stability (rather than just the *degree* of stability) are needed to evaluate two contrasting positions: the *prototype perspective* (which assumes that although attachment patterns can change, a stable factor underlies them and promotes continuity), and the *contextual or revisionist perspective* (which views working models as fluid structures, sensitive to changes in social environments). Two intensive longitudinal studies of attachment, assessing the magnitude and patterns of correlations over time, supported the prototype model (Fraley, Vicary, Brumbaugh, & Roisman, 2011). As the researchers noted, this support for a latent, enduring factor raises important questions about the persistence of changes induced by security priming; perhaps enduring change in attachment also requires other major change, such as change in the attachment network.

On a related note, Xu and Shrout (2013) discussed the suitability of measures of adult attachment for capturing the dynamics of attachment change. They argued that researchers need to consider the within-person reliability of different measures (as well as the traditional between-person reliability). In particular, within-person change is important in evaluating whether attachment has been influenced by priming manipulations over a limited period of time, before the new experiences are likely to have been integrated into working models.

## Romantic Attachment Security and Relationship Quality

A huge body of research attests to the link between romantic attachment security (whether assessed in terms of styles or dimensions) and the quality of couple relationships (see Mikulincer & Shaver, 2015, Chapter 10). Again, a complete presentation of individual findings is beyond the scope of this chapter; however, the following sections provide an overview of the major issues, together with illustrative findings.

Early studies of dating relationships (Levy & Davis, 1988; Simpson, 1990) linked secure attachment with high levels of trust, commitment, satisfaction, and interdependence. By contrast (and consistent with attachment theory), avoidant and anxious-ambivalent attachment were negatively related to trust and satisfaction, and avoidant attachment was also related to low levels of interdependence and commitment.

Since then, many studies (increasingly employing longitudinal designs and multiple assessment methods) have confirmed the link between attachment security and the quality of dating relationships. For example, a recent prospective study (Holland, Fraley, & Roisman, 2012; Holland & Roisman, 2010) assessed attachment using both the ECR and the AAI, scoring the latter along two dimensions: security versus insecurity and deactivation (dismissing) versus hyperactivation (preoccupation). Using the ECR, anxiety (but not avoidance) predicted poor relationship quality, both self-reported and observer-rated, a year later. The AAI measure of deactivation–hyperactivation yielded few results, but higher security prospectively predicted perceived and observed relationship quality, even when researchers controlled for prior levels of interpersonal functioning.

Attachment measures also predict the quality of marital relationships. In an early study of attachment and marriage (Kobak & Hazan, 1991), spouses completed measures of working models and marital satisfaction, and engaged in interaction tasks that involved confiding and problem solving. Accuracy of working models (extent of agreement with the spouse about one's own working models) was related to marital satisfaction and to observers' ratings of marital interaction. Furthermore, secure working models were related to higher marital satisfaction and to ratings of less rejection and more supportiveness during problem solving.

Again, subsequent research has confirmed the link between attachment security and marital quality (e.g., Banse, 2004; J. A. Feeney, 2002; Meyers & Landsberger, 2002). In an innovative approach to this topic, Roberts and Greenberg (2002) developed an interaction task that required spouses to discuss times when they had experienced positive feelings toward one another. Coding of the interactions revealed that all spouses in highly satisfying marriages shared feelings related to at least one of the attachment functions de-

scribed earlier (proximity seeking, separation protest, secure base, and safe haven). Most referred to three or four of these functions, supporting the importance of "felt security" and of the specific themes outlined by attachment theory.

More recent longitudinal research (Clark, Lemay, Graham, Pataki, & Finkel, 2010) has also linked attachment security to endorsement of a communal norm in marriage, reflecting concern for the partner's welfare. Specifically, attachment anxiety premarriage was linked concurrently to lower adherence to a communal norm and lower perceptions of partners' adherence to a communal norm; attachment avoidance showed both concurrent and prospective links with adherence to an exchange (reciprocity-based) norm. These results are important given that couples generally reported valuing and striving toward the communal norm.

Collectively, these studies of dating and marital relationships highlight robust links between individuals' own insecurity and poor relationship functioning (dyadic effects are addressed shortly). It is worth noting that some early studies of dating couples suggested that the implications of attachment dimensions for relationship quality might be gender-specific; that is, women's attachment anxiety was a strong correlate of their negative relationship evaluations, whereas for men, comfort with closeness was the crucial attachment dimension (Collins & Read, 1990; Kirkpatrick & Davis, 1994). However, subsequent research has generally failed to replicate these gender differences; rather, both avoidance and anxiety predict reduced relationship satisfaction for both genders (Mikulincer & Shaver, 2015). Further, these findings extend to men's and women's same-sex relationships (Mohr, Selterman, & Fassinger, 2013).

Recent meta-analyses of studies of dating and marriage have confirmed adult attachment as an important predictor of multiple dimensions of relationship quality. A major contribution of one meta-analysis (Li & Chan, 2012) was to highlight the differential correlates of avoidance and anxiety. Specifically, avoidance is more strongly related to low levels of connectedness, support and general relationship satisfaction, whereas anxiety is more strongly related to conflict. These findings fit with attachment theory: Avoidance involves deactivation of the attachment system, marked by physical and emotional distancing, whereas anxiety involves hyperactivation, manifested in needy and demanding behavior (Mikulincer & Shaver, 2015). This meta-analysis also established that gender has little effect on these associations. In another meta-analysis, Hadden, Smith, and Webster (2014) suggest that the negative associations of anxiety and avoidance with relationship functioning are stronger in longer than in shorter relationships, within cross-sectional samples. This finding raises intriguing alternative explanations that require further investigation; for example, the negative effects of insecurity may accumulate over time, or they may become unmasked as the initial novelty of new relationships fades, or may become stronger as expectations of intimacy increase (Hadden et al., 2014).

## Attachment and Relationship Quality: The Role of Communication

In evaluating the implications of attachment security for relationship quality, it is important to consider the role of communication. Communication is the main avenue through which attachment relationships are maintained (Bretherton, 1990; Kobak & Duemmler, 1994), and conflict-centered communication in particular involves attachment-related processes such as affect regulation (Pietromonaco, Greenwood, & Barrett, 2004). As I discuss next, many researchers have studied attachment and couple communication, using a range of research methods.

In one of the first studies of this topic, Pistole (1989) investigated attachment and conflict resolution styles, using a questionnaire methodology, in a sample of students involved in love relationships. Secure individuals were more likely to use an integrating (problem solving) strategy than those who were insecure, and also compromised more than anxious-ambivalent individuals. Anxious-ambivalent participants were more likely to oblige their partners than were avoidant participants. Subsequently, O'Connell Corcoran and Mallinckrodt (2000) related conflict resolution styles to the ASQ (J. A. Feeney, Noller, & Hanrahan, 1994). Confidence in self and others was related positively to integrating and compromising, and negatively to avoiding; discomfort with closeness showed the reverse pattern of associations. These findings suggest that secure persons' use of more constructive conflict strategies reflects their concern both for supporting their own interests and for enhancing their relationships.

In another study of conflict-centered communication, Gaines, Work, Johnson, Youn, and Lai (2000) examined reported responses to "accommodative dilemmas"—that is, situations in which

an intimate partner behaves negatively. Secure attachment was inversely related to the destructive responses of neglect (passively allowing the situation to deteriorate) and exit (actively harming the relationship). Similarly, studies by Creasey and colleagues (Creasey & Hesson-McInness, 2001; Creasey, Kershaw, & Boston, 1999) linked attachment anxiety and avoidance to questionnaire reports of negative escalation, poorer conflict management skills, and fewer positive conflict tactics. (The link between attachment and responses to severe conflict is addressed later; see "Attachment and Couple Relationships under Stress.")

Recent research (Baptist, Thompson, Norton, Hardy, & Link, 2012) also supports the role of attachment in the intergenerational transmission of relationship difficulties. This study examined avoidance and anxiety as moderators of the association between emotional disengagement in the family of origin and young adults' conflict styles (assessed by responses to scenarios depicting validating, volatile, hostile and conflict-avoiding behaviors). Reports of family disengagement interacted with attachment to predict conflict styles: Anxiety exacerbated the effects of family disengagement on hostile responses, whereas low avoidance buffered its effects on volatile responses.

Patterns of self-disclosure (another key aspect of communication) have also been linked with attachment style (Keelan, Dion, & Dion, 1998; Mikulincer & Nachshon, 1991). In general, secure and anxious-ambivalent individuals report more self-disclosure than avoidant individuals. Security is also associated with greater ability to elicit disclosure from relationship partners, with *topical reciprocity* (discussing the particular topics raised by partners), and with *flexibility* (adapting the extent of self-disclosure to the target and the situation). Similarly, secure individuals report more open expression of feelings (both positive and negative) to their romantic partners (Caldwell & Shaver, 2012; J. A. Feeney, 1995, 1999a).

Research continues to clarify the nature of attachment-related effects on disclosure. Observing dating and married couples as they conversed about routine aspects of their daily life, Tan, Overall, and Taylor (2012) found that the negative link between disclosure and insecurity (both avoidance and anxiety) was specific to the disclosure of thoughts and feelings about the couple relationship. Highlighting the importance of this finding, relationship-focused disclosure was positively associated with relationship quality over time. Furthermore, in a student sample, Garrison, Kahn, Sauer, and Florczak (2012) measured both generalized disclosure tendencies and daily diary reports of "emotional disclosure" regarding unpleasant events. Avoidance was negatively linked to both measures of disclosure. Overall, anxiety showed only weak associations with disclosure measures; however, highly anxious individuals engaged in more emotional disclosure when the emotional intensity of events was high, consistent with their vulnerability to stress and their reliance on others to help regulate affect.

In a comprehensive study of couple communication, we (J. A. Feeney, Noller, & Callan, 1994) followed newlywed couples for 2 years, assessing attachment (comfort with closeness, attachment anxiety) and three aspects of communication: the quality of daily interactions (via diary reports), nonverbal accuracy (via the standard content paradigm), and conflict style (via questionnaires). In daily interactions, husbands' comfort with closeness predicted their greater involvement, disclosure, and satisfaction, whereas wives' attachment anxiety predicted their ratings of domination, conflict, and dissatisfaction. Furthermore, husbands low in attachment anxiety and wives high in comfort showed more nonverbal accuracy. The key correlate of conflict style was attachment anxiety; highly anxious spouses rated their conflicts as coercive and distressing. Longitudinal analyses showed bidirectional relations between attachment and communication, supporting the claim that working models and relationship experiences influence one another. Consistent with these widespread links between attachment and communication variables, subsequent research has linked avoidance and anxiety to less *communication competence* (a composite measure of assertiveness, interpersonal sensitivity, and self-disclosure; Anders & Tucker, 2000).

## Relationship Quality and Communication: Dyadic Effects

Many of the studies reported to this point have employed both members of couples, allowing researchers to assess whether perceptions of relationship quality are related to the attachment characteristics of the partner, as well as those of the reporter. As noted earlier, Hazan and Shaver (1987) argued that relationship quality is shaped by both partners; recognition of the dyadic nature of attachment effects has been a hallmark of recent research.

Early work on this topic used one of two methods, either comparing "couple types" or correlating the attachment scores of one partner with the relationship functioning of the other. Using the former approach, Senchak and Leonard (1992) compared three types: "secure" (in which both spouses chose the secure description of the three-group attachment measure), "insecure" (in which both spouses chose insecure descriptions), and "mixed" (in which one spouse chose the secure description and the other endorsed an insecure description). They found that secure couples reported better marital adjustment (e.g., more intimacy, positive responses to conflict) than mixed and insecure couples did. Cohn, Silver, Cowan, Cowan, and Pearson (1992) linked observers' ratings of marital quality to couple types assessed with the AAI. In contrast to Senchak and Leonard's (1992) findings, mixed couples in this study were rated as similar to secure couples, and as functioning better than insecure couples. Given these conflicting findings regarding the adjustment of mixed couples, it remains unclear whether (or when) a secure partner can buffer the negative effects of insecurity on relationship quality.

Using the correlational approach, early studies of dating relationships (Collins & Read, 1990; Simpson, 1990) suggested that evaluations of dating relationships were linked to partners' attachment ratings, in ways that paralleled the effects of individuals' own attachment ratings: Negative evaluations were made by the partners of men who were uncomfortable with closeness and women who were anxious about relationships. Early studies of attachment and marriage also reported partner effects. Kobak and Hazan (1991) found that wives of less secure husbands were more rejecting and less supportive than other wives, and that husbands of secure wives listened more effectively during problem solving. Similarly, we (J. A. Feeney, Noller, & Callan, 1994) found that communication patterns and marital satisfaction in newlyweds were related to both partners' attachment dimensions. Furthermore, for couples sampled across the life cycle of marriage, marital satisfaction was again related to the comfort and anxiety levels of both partners (J. A. Feeney, 1994).

Given that relationship quality is linked to both partners' attachment characteristics, a further question arises: Do attachment styles of individuals and their partners *interact* to predict relationship quality? This idea is implied by studies of couple types: For example, a secure person may behave differently, depending on the security of the partner. However, comparing three couple types gives limited information because it fails to distinguish between different forms of insecurity.

As outlined next, interactive effects have been addressed more fully by studies using dimensional attachment measures.

In one of the first studies to explore this issue (J. A. Feeney, 1994), couples sampled across the marital life cycle completed measures of attachment and marital satisfaction. As noted earlier, satisfaction was related to both partners' attachment dimensions (main effects). In addition, moderated regression analyses revealed interaction effects for couples married for 10 years or less. Specifically, wives' anxiety was linked with dissatisfaction for both spouses, only if husbands were low in comfort with closeness; by contrast, husbands' anxiety was linked with dissatisfaction, regardless of wives' comfort (see Figure 21.2). It seems that in more recent marriages, anxious husbands' dependent behavior is destructive, perhaps because it violates the male sex role stereotype. Anxious wives' dependent (and stereotype-confirming) behavior may be less harmful except when husbands struggle with intimacy, and hence provide insufficient support.

Using a similar method, reanalyses of data from the study of newlyweds cited earlier (J. A. Feeney, Noller, & Callan, 1994) revealed that husbands' and wives' anxiety levels interacted to predict women's reports of conflict behaviors, both concurrently and longitudinally (J. A. Feeney, 2003). Interestingly, this effect varied in form. For example, wives reported most conflict avoidance when both spouses were anxious, suggesting that their avoidance was driven by both partners' insecurities. However, anxious wives with nonanxious husbands reported *more* coercion than those with anxious husbands; if anxious wives perceive nonanxious husbands as failing to understand their concerns, power struggles may result. Other studies confirm the gender-specific nature of some dyadic attachment effects. For example, Gallo and Smith (2001) found that husbands reported low levels of marital support when they themselves were avoidant but their partners were not. Furthermore, in a study incorporating ratings of the four attachment styles delineated by Bartholomew (1990), the positive effects of security and the negative effects of insecurity were either amplified or attenuated in specific dyadic configurations (Banse, 2004). The most consistent finding concerned husbands' dismissing attachment, which attenuated the effects of wives' preoccupied and dismissing tendencies.

Recent studies of dyadic attachment have used more sophisticated statistical techniques.

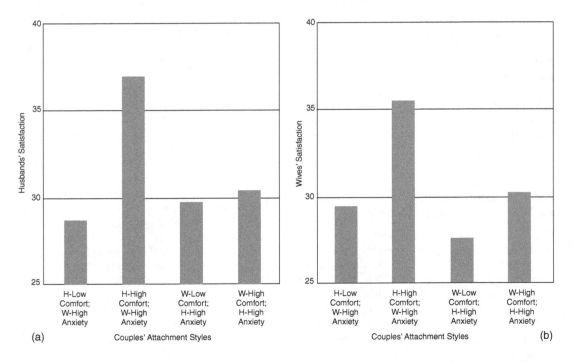

**FIGURE 21.2.** Relationships between couples' attachment styles on the one hand, and husband's satisfaction (a) and wives' satisfaction (b) on the other. H, husband; W, wife.

In particular, the actor–partner interdependence model (APIM; Kashy & Kenny, 2000) recognizes that in couple relationships, partners' scores on the variables of interest are likely to be correlated. The model tests for *actor effects* (e.g., the effect of an individual's anxiety on his or her coercion), *partner effects* (e.g., the effect of an individual's anxiety on the partner's coercion), and interactions between these effects. In a study of disclosure patterns in dating couples (Bradford, Feeney, & Campbell, 2002), this approach yielded actor and partner effects but no interactions. For example, actors' avoidance predicted their questionnaire reports of low levels of disclosure; diary records of daily interactions showed consistent negative effects of anxiety (especially partner effects). In another APIM study, Campbell, Simpson, Kashy, and Rholes (2001) reported that both actor and partner avoidance interacted with level of relationship dependence to predict responses to a stressful situation. For instance, avoidant participants who showed little dependence on their relationships were especially prone to displaying negative behavior, and to eliciting such behavior from their partners.

The APIM model (or multilevel modeling more generally) is now widely used in attachment research and continues to yield important findings. Lavy, Mikulincer, and Shaver (2013) conducted a 14-day diary study showing that own anxiety and partner's avoidance were robust predictors of self-reported intrusive behaviors (e.g., invading the partner's privacy). These findings presumably reflect anxious individuals' needs for control, and avoidant individuals' distancing tendencies, which may prompt partners to resort to intrusiveness in order to achieve closeness. Other dyadic studies highlight the utility of multimethod research. For example, a recent study of marital conflict identified several interaction effects of spouses' attachment dimensions, noting that the combination of an avoidant and an anxious spouse generally predicted more physiological reactivity and less effective caregiving. However, some findings were specific to self-reports or to observed behavior (Beck, Pietromonaco, DeBuse, Powers, & Sayer, 2013). Furthermore, Seedall and Wampler (2012) examined the impact of attachment avoidance on *emotional incongruence*, defined as the difference between physiological arousal and self-reports of in-the-moment feelings toward the partner during conflict discussions. Own avoidance and in-the-moment-feelings interacted to predict arousal: More positive feelings for the partner were linked to less physiological arousal

at low levels of avoidance but to *more* physiological arousal (i.e., incongruence) at high levels of avoidance. These results suggest that avoidant people respond to intense arousal by distracting themselves or repressing negative affect, tendencies that may jeopardize long-term satisfaction (Seedall & Wampler, 2012).

Dyadic studies are also important in highlighting attachment-related differences in partners' perceptions of their interactions. In one recent experiment, Beck, Pietromonaco, DeVito, Powers, and Boyle (2014) videotaped newlywed couples during a conflict-resolution discussion, then asked them to rate their own and their partners' responsiveness during the conflict. Observers also coded both partners' responsive behaviors during the conflict. As compared to observers' ratings, more avoidant participants underestimated both their own and their partner's responsiveness. In another study, Overall, Fletcher, Simpson, and Fillo (2015) assessed participants' perceptions of partners' emotions and partners' actual emotions during couple conflict discussions and during daily interactions over a 3-week period. Using partners' reports of their own emotions as the accuracy benchmark, they found that more avoidant participants overestimated the intensity of their partner's negative emotion. Moreover, they exhibited more hostile and defensive responses to the partner's expression of emotions during the recorded interactions.

In summary, research has linked insecurity in self and partner to negative relationship evaluations; anxious attachment in an individual seems particularly likely to erode the partner's satisfaction, irrespective of gender (Mikulincer & Shaver, 2015). Some studies also point to interactive effects, further indicating that attachment can be fully understood only at the level of the dyad. Dyadic attachment effects are varied and complex, however, and sometimes specific to one gender or one research method (Barry & Lawrence, 2013; Beck et al., 2013).

## Mediating Variables: Exploring the Mechanisms Linking Security to Relationship Quality

The robust link between attachment security and relationship quality raises questions about the *mechanisms* involved in this association. That is, what do secure people do differently that enhances relationship quality? This question has clear implications for interventions; distressed couples may be helped not only by interventions that target working models directly but also by approaches that address intervening (mediating) variables.

One of the first studies to address this issue was our study of newlyweds (J. A. Feeney, Noller, & Callan, 1994). Given that attachment security predicted both communication and marital satisfaction, we suggested that communication patterns (e.g., conflict style, nonverbal accuracy) might mediate the link between attachment security and satisfaction. Our results did not support this hypothesis; rather, in these early marriages, attachment and communication exerted independent effects on satisfaction. However, different findings emerged from the study of attachment and conflict across the marital life cycle (J. A. Feeney, 1994). In this study, the links between attachment dimensions and marital satisfaction were mediated by mutual negotiation of conflict, although for husbands, the mediation was only partial.

In the following decade, studies revealed other mediators of the association between security and relationship quality. Specifically, full or partial mediation was reported for variables such as emotional expressiveness (J. A. Feeney, 1999a), self-disclosure (Keelan et al., 1998), overall communication competence (Anders & Tucker, 2000), benign (relationship-maintaining) attributions for negative partner behavior (Gallo & Smith, 2001; Pearce & Halford, 2008; Sumer & Cozzarelli, 2004), tendency to forgive transgressions (Kachadourian, Fincham, & Davila, 2004), low levels of psychological distress (Meyers & Landsberger, 2002), and perceptions of available support from family and friends (Meyers & Landsberger, 2002).

Mediation models have been another major focus of recent research. In a dating sample, making sacrifices for the partner based on avoidance motives (e.g., fearing partner disapproval) mediated between attachment anxiety and relationship dissatisfaction (Mattingly & Clark, 2012). In a study of married couples in Portugal, the negative links of attachment avoidance with relationship functioning were mediated, for women, by less investment in family rituals (Crespo, Davide, Costa, & Fletcher, 2008). Furthermore, among expectant first-time parents, lack of relationship regulation (behaviors designed to enhance the relationship) mediated between own avoidance and anxiety and relationship dissatisfaction, and between males' avoidance and anxiety and females' dissatisfaction (Pepping & Halford, 2012). Importantly, in an empirical test of *double mediation* effects grounded

in attachment theory, Karantzas, Feeney, Goncalves and McCabe (2014) found substantial support for the hypothesized model, in which anxiety and avoidance predicted low levels of partner support and trust, which in turn were linked with poor conflict management and lack of intimacy, and hence, with relationship dissatisfaction.

In short, studies suggest that secure individuals display a more open and positive interpersonal style, as indicated by a range of affective, cognitive, and behavioral variables; these variables promote positive relationship outcomes (Table 21.4 summarizes these findings). However, mediation effects have often been specific to one gender, to relationship type (dating or married), and to attachment dimension (avoidance or anxiety), again highlighting the complexity of attachment-related dynamics.

## Relationship Quality: Integrating Attachment, Caregiving, and Sexuality

Shaver and colleagues (1988) argued that sexuality and caregiving are independent behavioral systems that are integrated with the attachment system in romantic love. Furthermore, because the attachment system appears very early in the course of development and shapes relational expectations, it plays a pivotal role in influencing the expression of caregiving and sexuality (Hazan & Shaver, 1994). What support exists for these propositions? Empirical studies clearly support the separate importance of each of the proposed components of love (see reviews by Shaver & Mikulincer, 2006, and the volume on romantic love edited by Mikulincer & Goodman, 2006). I have already discussed the robust link between attachment and relationship quality. Support is also emerging for the influence of attachment on caregiving and sexuality, which I discuss next.

### Attachment and Caregiving

In a study of romantic couples, Carnelley, Pietromonaco, and Jaffe (1996) assessed the link between attachment and caregiving, and the implications of these variables for relationship satisfaction. Individuals' attachment security was linked to the provision of more "beneficial" (engaged and reciprocal) care to romantic partners. Moreover, individuals' and partners' attachment security, and partners' provision of beneficial care, all contributed to relationship satisfaction.

**TABLE 21.4. Key Aspects of Relationship Quality Associated with Attachment Dimensions**

| Avoidance (discomfort with closeness) | Relationship anxiety |
|---|---|
| Relationship dissatisfaction | Relationship dissatisfaction |
| Distrust of partners | Distrust of partners |
| Low commitment | Jealousy |
| Low closeness, interdependence, and connection | High levels of conflict |
| Low supportiveness | Distress and hurt in the face of conflict |
| +Low emotional expressiveness | +Coercive and dominating conflict tactics |
| +Low levels of self-disclosure, including flexibility and reciprocity of disclosure | +Maladaptive (distress-maintaining) attributions for negative partner behavior |
| +Low tendency to forgive | +Low tendency to forgive |
| +Low interpersonal competence | +Low interpersonal competence |
| +Low investment in family rituals | +Avoidance motives for sacrificing |
| +Low relationship regulation | +Low relationship regulation |

*Note.* + indicates there is evidence that this variable mediates the association between security and better relationship functioning.

Additional support for the link between attachment and caregiving comes from the work of Kunce and Shaver (1994), who developed self-report scales assessing the quality of caregiving in intimate dyads: Proximity, Sensitivity, Cooperation, and Compulsive Caregiving. In a student sample, these scales showed theoretically meaningful links with attachment style. For example, secure persons reported more proximity and sensitivity than dismissing persons; consistent with their need for approval, preoccupied and fearful individuals reported more compulsive (but less sensitive) caregiving. In a study using these scales with a sample of married couples (J. A. Feeney, 1996), secure attachment was linked to beneficial caregiving to the spouse. Specifically, comfort with closeness and low attachment anxiety were related to more Responsive Caregiving (a composite scale assessing proximity, sensitivity, and cooperation) and to less compulsive caregiving. In addition, marital satisfaction was higher for secure spouses, and for those whose partners reported more responsive caregiving.

The importance of both partners' attachment characteristics is highlighted by a two-part study of spousal caregiving (J. A. Feeney & Hohaus, 2001). Each spouse first provided a semistructured account of the time when he or she had most needed to give the other spouse extra care and support. Next, spouses completed questionnaires assessing attachment dimensions, caregiving style, attachment strength (reliance on the spouse for attachment needs), anticipated caregiving burden, and willingness to provide ongoing spousal care in the future. Content analysis of the semistructured accounts linked attachment dimensions to perceptions of the caregiving process. For example, as caregivers, anxious wives used less problem-focused coping and more escape/avoidance, and husbands high in discomfort used less support seeking. In addition, insecurity in either partner was linked to caregivers' tendency to belittle their spouses' needs ("tedious," "tragedy queen"). In the second part of the study, spouses' willingness to provide ongoing care was related negatively to their own and their partners' discomfort and anxiety; these effects involved relatively complex paths through caregiving style, attachment strength, and anticipated burden.

In an ongoing research program, B. C. Feeney and Collins (2004) have broadened the conceptualization of caregiving by distinguishing between two caregiving processes relevant to couples (see Collins, Guichard, Ford, & Feeney, 2006, for a review). *Safe-haven caregiving* involves responding to the partner's distress, and was the focus of most research until recently. In contrast, *secure-base caregiving* involves supporting the partner's personal growth and exploration activities. From Bowlby's (1988) work on attachment and exploration, B. C. Feeney and Collins (2004) developed an integrated model of these processes that recognizes the complementary roles of caregiver and care receiver. Subsequently, this research program has yielded important findings. For example, attachment dimensions are linked to the motivations for providing (or not providing) secure-base support (B. C. Feeney, Collins, van Vleet, & Tomlinson, 2013): Attachment anxiety is linked to motives reflecting perceived obligation and desire for connection; avoidance is negatively linked to the desire to make the spouse feel good; and both dimensions are linked to perceiving the spouse as needy. Furthermore, these motives predict secure-base behavior; for instance, perceiving the spouse as needy is related to observers' ratings of less effective support.

Consistent with the increasing focus on "positive caregiving," Gosnell and Gable (2013) examined reports of situations in which one partner had shared a success or other positive experience with the other. Avoidant individuals reported feeling embarrassed by partners' support, whereas anxious individuals reported feeling misunderstood. Multilevel modeling also showed that insecure adults tended to react more negatively to perceived partner responsiveness (e.g., with less increase in thankfulness and less reduction in sadness), suggesting a failure to capitalize on positive events.

## Attachment and Sexuality

Support has also emerged for the link between attachment style and sexual attitudes and behaviors. In an early but comprehensive study of this topic, Hazan, Zeifman, and Middleton (1994) asked adults to complete measures of attachment style and the frequency and enjoyment of various sexual behaviors. Three distinct sexual styles were identified, consistent with the three major attachment styles. Secure individuals were less likely to be involved in one-night stands or extradyadic sex, and more likely to report mutual initiation and enjoyment of sex. Avoidant individuals tended to report activities reflecting low psychological intimacy (one-night stands, casual sex), as well as less enjoyment of physical contact. Anxious-ambivalent females reported involvement in exhibitionism, voyeurism, and bondage, whereas anxious-ambivalent males were more sexually reticent. For both sexes, anxious-ambivalence was related to enjoyment of holding and caressing, but not of more clearly sexual behaviors.

Although relatively few studies have focused on long-term couple relationships, research continues to support the link between specific forms of insecurity and the expression of sexuality, and

has paid increasing attention to sexual goals and motivations (see Shaver & Mikulincer, 2012, for a review). Gentzler and Kerns (2004) found that avoidance was related to attitudinal and behavioral measures of *unrestricted sexuality*—that is, feeling comfortable in short-term sexual relationships involving little commitment or emotional closeness. Similarly, avoidant individuals have more accepting attitudes toward casual sex than other attachment groups (Brennan & Shaver, 1995; J. A. Feeney, Noller, & Patty, 1993). Avoidance has also been linked to young people rating their sexual encounters as having relatively little importance (Tracy, Shaver, Cooper, & Albino, 2003) and reporting that they engage in sex in order to impress their peers (Schachner & Shaver, 2004). A study of dating couples (Impett, Gordon, & Strachman, 2008) established both actor and partner effects of avoidance on sexual goals: Avoidant individuals were less focused on enhancing intimacy, expressing love, or pleasing the partner, and more focused on avoiding conflict. The strongest partner effect linked avoidance to partners' reports of focusing on one's own pleasure. Recent research has also clarified the motives behind the robust link between attachment avoidance and extradyadic sex (Beaulieu-Pelletier, Philippe, Lecours, & Couture, 2011): Avoidance predicted concerns about partners' desire for engagement, and these concerns in turn predicted involvement in extradyadic sex; thus, this behavior seems to reflect avoidant individuals' desire to distance themselves in the face of partner demands.

Attachment anxiety also shows a unique set of sexuality correlates, particularly for women. Women's anxiety has been linked to sexual promiscuity, extradyadic sex, and number of sexual partners (Bogaert & Sadava, 2002; Gangestad & Thornhill, 1997). These high rates of sexual activity may reflect anxious women's desire for intense closeness and fears that failure to oblige partners may drive them away (Schachner & Shaver, 2004; Tracy et al., 2003). For both sexes, anxious attachment has also been linked to difficulty in negotiating sexual encounters (J. A. Feeney, Peterson, Gallois, & Terry, 2000) and to unsafe sexual practices (J. A. Feeney, Kelly, Gallois, Peterson, & Terry, 1999): Given their fear of rejection, anxious individuals may be reluctant to risk alienating partners by discussing sexual practices or resisting pressure for unprotected sex (J. A. Feeney & Noller, 2004). Indeed, in the study by Impett and colleagues (2008), anxiety was related to engaging in sex to please the partner, as well as to enhance intimacy and express love.

### Integrating Attachment, Caregiving, and Sexuality

Little empirical work has assessed all three components of romantic bonds, despite the theoretical appeal of such integrative work. One exception is a study of the transition to parenthood (J. A. Feeney, Hohaus, Noller, & Alexander, 2001), which followed couples through pregnancy and the first 6 months of parenthood, and included a comparison sample of couples who were not planning to have children in the near future. Couples were interviewed and completed questionnaires assessing attachment (comfort, anxiety), caregiving (responsive and compulsive care), and sexuality (sexual desire, satisfaction with sexual communication). Results supported the influence of attachment on caregiving and sexuality, for both transition and comparison couples: Security predicted later reports of better sexual functioning and more adaptive caregiving (although only the "anxiety" dimension predicted compulsive care and low sexual desire). Additional analyses identified two trajectories of marital satisfaction among new parents: One group of couples showed stable levels of satisfaction, whereas the other reported declines. These two groups were similar in terms of initial psychological adjustment and coping resources but differed in terms of husbands' attachment and caregiving patterns. The strongest finding was that husbands in couples with declining satisfaction reported more attachment anxiety at the start of the study; these husbands also provided less responsive care to their wives. These findings support the pivotal role of the attachment system and suggest that husbands who enter parenthood with unresolved relationship anxieties put pressure on both partners, perhaps by becoming overly dependent and by responding negatively to conflict.

More recently, Peloquin, Brassard, Delisle, and Bedard (2013) tested an integrative model in which attachment dimensions and caregiving style predicted motives for engaging in sexual intercourse, which in turn predicted sexual satisfaction. Data from a sample of individuals in committed relationships provided substantial support for the model. For example, attachment anxiety was linked to controlling care, which predicted using sex to increase one's own power. In addition, both anxiety and avoidance predicted less sensitive care, leading to less focus on sex as a way of valuing the partner, and hence to less relationship satisfaction. Again, this study reflects the increasing emphasis on integrating attachment-related motives and behaviors.

At the same time, the caution raised by Mikulincer and Shaver (2015) regarding our understanding of the three behavioral systems is warranted; namely, that the available evidence of interrelations among these systems does little to clarify key theoretical issues: Is the attachment system primary? To what extent do the interrelations reflect the common influence of temperament or personality? And do caregiving and sex have recursive influences on attachment security?

## Attachment and Couple Relationships under Stress

Although much of the early research on couple attachment assessed global relationship functioning and suggested pervasive differences between attachment styles, there are compelling reasons for focusing on stressful situations. In infancy, the attachment system regulates the balance between proximity-seeking and exploratory behavior. When attachment figures are nearby and the setting is familiar, infants tend to engage in exploratory activity, but in the face of threat (environmental stressors; conditions in the attachment relationship, such as caregivers' absence; and internal conditions, such as pain), attachment behavior is likely to be evident (Bowlby, 1969/1982). By analogy, similar situations should activate adults' attachment behavior, making attachment-style differences more pronounced (Simpson & Rholes, 1994). Because conditions that threaten attachment relationships are directly relevant to couple functioning, the research I discuss next focuses on these conditions: specifically, partner absence (separation and reunion behavior) and severe instances of relationship conflict.

### Partner Absence

Attachment-related differences in separation and reunion dynamics have been studied in various ways. Mikulincer, Florian, Birnbaum, and Malishkevich (2002) studied responses to "separation reminders" by asking participants to imagine being separated from a relationship partner. For individuals high in attachment anxiety, this manipulation led to heightened accessibility of death-related thoughts, especially when long-term or final separations were imagined. This finding suggests that anxious individuals experience separation as catastrophic, and adopt a hypervigilant attitude to preventing such an outcome (Mikulincer et al., 2002).

Researchers have also studied romantic partners' responses to actual separation episodes. For instance, Cafferty, Davis, Medway, O'Hearn, and Chappell (1994) studied reunion dynamics among couples in which the husbands were deployed overseas during the 1990–1991 Gulf War. Four months after reunion, the men and their wives completed questionnaires assessing attachment style, marital satisfaction, conflict, and affect during reunion. For both deployed men and their wives, secure attachment was related to higher marital satisfaction and less postreunion conflict; preoccupied individuals showed particularly low satisfaction and high conflict. Links between attachment style and affect during reunion were confined to men, perhaps because of the more stressful nature of their separation experience.

Fraley and Shaver (1998) conducted an innovative study of airport separations, finding that women who were anxious about attachment reported greater separation distress. In addition, observers' ratings indicated that when separation was imminent, highly avoidant women were less supportive and more distant, and highly anxious men were less likely to maintain contact with their partners. These associations differed from those among nonseparating couples, supporting the assertion that stressful conditions amplify the negative effects of insecurity.

Another study (J. A. Feeney, 1998) investigated three aspects of partner absence and distancing. The first aspect (physical separation) is considered here, and the others (discouraging of proximity, closeness–distance struggles) are considered in the next section. In one part of the study, participants provided open-ended reports of their experiences of being physically separated from their current dating partners. Content analyses linked attachment security with less separation distress, with more constructive coping, and with perceptions that the experience had strengthened the couple bond. Avoidance was strongly predictive of males' separation behavior, being related to less support seeking and more emotion-focused coping (including substance use); anxiety was associated, for both genders, with less diverse coping strategies, and, for women, with reports of failing to discuss relationship issues on reunion.

More recently, Diamond, Hicks and Otter-Henderson (2008) assessed affect, physiology, and behavior linked to travel-related separations among cohabiting and married couples. Both members of the couples showed significant changes from preseparation to separation, and from separation to reunion, in the quality of daily interactions, positive and negative affect, sleeping problems, and cortisol levels. These changes were not moderated by relationship length or satisfaction, but they were greater for those high in attachment anxiety. Furthermore, upon reunion, declines in subjective stress were less pronounced for those high in avoidance, suggesting that they may find reunions quite stressful, given their preference for interpersonal distance.

## Severe Relationship Conflict

Like long-term or unexpected separations, severe conflict may threaten the couple bond. A laboratory study of dating couples (Simpson, Rholes, & Phillips, 1996) addressed this issue by randomly assigning couples to discuss either a minor or a major relationship conflict. Anxious participants reported feeling greater distress and hostility during the discussions; observers rated them as showing more anxiety, and also rated avoidant men as engaging in lower-quality interactions. These effects were stronger for couples discussing *major* problems, highlighting the impact of relational stress. Anxious participants who discussed major problems also perceived their relationships more negatively after the discussion than before (when researchers controlled for interaction quality). Interestingly, however, diary reports of everyday interactions (Pietromonaco & Barrett, 1997) suggest that preoccupied individuals perceive high-conflict interactions as more satisfying than do other individuals, presumably because these interactions often involve high levels of partner attention and mutual disclosure.

In the second part of the J. A. Feeney (1998) study, couples engaged in three conflict-centered interactions. One interaction involved conflict over a specific issue (use of leisure time); the other two were designed to elicit attachment-related anxiety by having one partner rebuff the other's attempts to maintain closeness (the role of the distant partner was adopted by the male in one interaction, and by the female in the other). Secure attachment was positively related to self-reported expectations and satisfaction for all three interactions. However, secure attachment was unrelated to observers' ratings of responses to issue-based conflict but predicted less negative affect, less withdrawal, and more constructive conversation in response to partners' distancing. These results integrate two key findings: Attachment exerts pervasive effects on *global perceptions* of relationships but is most evident in *observable behavior* in challenging situations.

Attachment is also relevant to closeness–distance struggles. Closeness–distance (or autonomy–connection) is a core relational dilemma: Intimate partners must forgo some autonomy in order to forge a connection, but too much connection stifles their individual identities. Proximity seeking is a key function of attachment behavior; hence, conflict about closeness and distance is likely to activate the attachment system, and may prove intractable if partners have different attachment goals (Byng-Hall, 1999; Pistole, 1994). The final part of the J. A. Feeney (1998) study addressed this issue. Participants discussed their current relationships, and the transcripts were coded for content relevant to closeness–distance (J. A. Feeney, 1999b). Almost all participants (92%) referred to the closeness–distance theme, but ongoing struggles over this issue were more common when the male was avoidant or the female was anxious. Some couples with two insecure partners reported highly distressing cycles of pursuing–distancing, attesting to the difficult emotional climate of these relationships. Similarly, Bartholomew and Allison (2006) suggested that pursuing–distancing cycles often reflect incompatible attachment needs (usually involving one anxious and one avoidant partner), whereas pursuer–pursuer struggles may arise when both partners are high in attachment anxiety. With both these patterns, failure to achieve distance regulation may result in escalating conflict and couple violence.

The role of attachment processes in couple aggression is supported by a dyadic study of empathy and psychological aggression (Peloquin, Lafontaine, & Brassard, 2011). Psychological aggression was linked to actors' anxiety (for both genders), actors' avoidance (for women), and male partners' anxiety. Lack of empathy was also generally related to attachment insecurity, although there was an unexpected positive link between men's anxiety and empathy. Furthermore, women's lack of empathy mediated the association between their insecurity and psychological aggression.

The relevance of attachment issues to the course of couple conflict is further evidenced by

studies of hurt feelings. Content analysis of victims' retrospective reports of hurtful events, together with ratings by expert judges, support the proposition that hurt feelings are elicited by relational transgressions that threaten positive working models (J. A. Feeney, 2005); that is, the sense of personal injury that is a distinctive feature of hurt feelings reflects damage to core beliefs about self-worth and/or partners' dependability. In addition, individual differences in attachment security predict the long-term outcomes of hurtful events (J. A. Feeney, 2004). As already noted, individuals who are highly anxious respond to hurtful partner behavior with more distress and self-blame, which exacerbates their fears and self-doubts. Moreover, avoidant individuals tend to perceive their partners as lacking remorse for hurtful behavior, which fuels further conflict.

In a recent study, Overall, Girme, Lemay, and Hammond (2014) focused on a specific strategy—guilt induction—that anxiously attached people may use in response to relational transgressions, to express frustration and hurt while at the same time retaining closeness to the transgressive partner. Findings indicated that in situations that create relational tension (e.g., criticism and conflict), attachment anxiety was related to exaggerated expressions of hurt feelings and more guilt-inducing verbal and nonverbal responses (as coded by independent observers). Importantly, partners of more anxious participants reported higher levels of guilt, and more anxious individuals appraised their partner and relationship more positively when their partner felt more guilt. However, partners of anxious participants also reported more relationship dissatisfaction. These results suggest that the manipulative stance adopted by anxiously attached people in response to relational tension may foster intimacy and commitment in the short term (due to partners' compensatory efforts to reduce guilt feelings) but can erode partners' satisfaction in the long term.

Additional support for the role of attachment processes in psychological hurt comes from evidence that security-priming manipulations affect recall of hurtful events. Specifically, priming weakens the associations of attachment anxiety with negative affect, feelings of rejection, and destructive behavioral reactions. Conversely, priming strengthens the associations of attachment avoidance with feelings of rejection and weakens associations with defensive reactions, suggesting increased openness to the painful experience (Shaver, Mikulincer, Lavy, & Cassidy,

2009). In addition, an intervention study involving a couples' workshop, focused on principles of attachment and forgiveness, produced increased relationship satisfaction at 6-month follow-up for females in insecure dyads, in contrast to females in secure dyads or control dyads (J. A. Feeney & Fitzgerald, 2012).

## Attachment and Relationship Quality: Further Comments

It is important to note that although attachment measures seem to tap relatively enduring individual differences, attachment style is *not* redundant with basic dimensions of personality. Relations between measures of attachment and personality tend to be modest in size (J. A. Feeney, Noller, & Hanrahan, 1994; Fraley et al., 2011; Noftle & Shaver, 2006; Shaver & Brennan, 1992). In addition, relationship outcomes such as satisfaction and commitment are better predicted by attachment measures than by personality measures (Noftle & Shaver, 2006; Shaver & Brennan, 1992).

Furthermore, although some studies of romantic attachment have simply correlated various self-report measures, this is by no means the only methodology that has been used. Many studies have related attachment measures to independent ratings of behavior (e.g., Barry & Lawrence; 2013; Simpson et al., 1996) or to interview and diary-based reports of relationship functioning (e.g., Bradford et al., 2002; Lavy et al., 2013). Others have gathered corroborative reports from friends (Bartholomew & Horowitz, 1991) or romantic partners (Kobak & Hazan, 1991), or have demonstrated the ability of attachment measures to predict relationship outcomes prospectively (e.g., J. A. Feeney et al., 2001; Holland et al., 2012). Further attesting to the validity of self-reports of romantic attachment, these measures have been linked to indices of unconscious processes, including cognitive processing of relational information (Mikulincer, Gillath, & Shaver, 2002; see Mikulincer & Shaver, Chapter 24, this volume) and physiological processes related to arousal and affect regulation (e.g., Diamond & Hicks, 2005; Diamond et al., 2008; Fraley & Shaver, 1997). Finally, studies have supported specific predictions concerning the relative strength of association between attachment measures and particular behaviors—for example, responses to major versus minor conflicts (Simpson et al., 1996) and to relationship-based versus issue-based conflicts (J.

A. Feeney, 1998). These studies are sufficient in number and diversity to indicate that measures of romantic attachment do not simply tap a generalized tendency to perceive or report events more or less favorably.

## Summary and Future Directions

The proposition that couple relationships can be understood in terms of attachment principles has generated immense interest, and by late 2013, approximately 2,700 authors had cited Hazan and Shaver's (1987) groundbreaking studies. The attachment perspective has important strengths, as noted by Shaver and Hazan (1988) and others (e.g., Clark & Reis, 1988). Attachment theory addresses a range of relationship issues, including anxiety, loneliness, and grief; it explains healthy and unhealthy forms of love in terms of the same principles; and it is developmental in focus (the concept of working models can account both for the continuity of early relational patterns, and for the possibility of change).

Attachment theory seems to be especially useful in addressing certain key issues in the study of couple relationships, such as conflict. This theory helps to explain both the sources of relationship conflict and individual differences in conflict behavior. Research suggests that attachment anxiety is of particular importance here. Highly anxious individuals report more relationship conflict, which suggests that much of this conflict is driven by basic insecurities about love and loss. Those who are highly anxious also respond with coercion and negative escalation, which tend to alienate partners.

The studies discussed in this chapter illustrate major advances in adult attachment research, including the move to dimensional measures that provide more complete description of attachment patterns, the development of analytic strategies for testing dyadic effects, and the identification of mediated pathways from security to relationship functioning. There has also been an increased focus on positive relationship processes and outcomes, such as empathy and forgiveness. Together, these studies shed light on the complex ways in which security and insecurity are played out in couple relationships, and have vital implications for enhancing relationships.

Despite these advances, important issues remain unresolved. One issue raised in this chapter concerns the need to clarify patterns of stability and change in attachment organization, including the intraindividual and relational processes that shape these patterns. This issue may be clarified by longitudinal studies that follow individuals as their first romantic relationships develop—and, equally important, that track individuals who move from relationship to relationship. We are also some way from understanding the interrelations among the behavioral systems of attachment, caregiving and sexuality. In addition, it is important for researchers to integrate findings emerging from studies of couple relationships and from studies of the "individual mind" (see Mikulincer & Shaver, Chapter 24, this volume). Initiatives such as these will broaden the contribution made by the attachment perspective on couple relationships.

# References

Ainsworth, M. D. S. (1989). Attachments beyond infancy. *American Psychologist, 44,* 709–716.

Ainsworth, M. D. S., Blehar, M. C., Waters, E., & Wall, S. (1978). *Patterns of attachment: A psychological study of the Strange Situation.* Hillsdale, NJ: Erlbaum.

Alfasi, I., Gramzow, R. H., & Carnelley, K. B. (2010). Adult attachment patterns and stability in esteem for romantic partners. *Personality and Individual Differences, 48,* 607–611.

Anders, S. L., & Tucker, J. S. (2000). Adult attachment style, interpersonal communication competence, and social support. *Personal Relationships, 7,* 379–389.

Baldwin, M. W., & Fehr, B. (1995). On the instability of attachment style ratings. *Personal Relationships, 2,* 247–261.

Baldwin, M. W., Fehr, B., Keedian, E., Seidel, M., & Thomson, D. W. (1993). An exploration of the relational schemata underlying attachment styles: Self-report and lexical decision approaches. *Personality and Social Psychology Bulletin, 19,* 746–754.

Baldwin, M. W., Keelan, J. P. R., Fehr, B., Enns, V., & Koh-Rangarajoo, E. (1996). Social-cognitive conceptualization of attachment working models: Availability and accessibility effects. *Journal of Personality and Social Psychology, 71,* 94–109.

Banse, R. (2004). Adult attachment and marital satisfaction: Evidence for dyadic configuration effects. *Journal of Social and Personal Relationships, 21,* 273–282.

Baptist, J. A., Thompson, D. E., Norton, A. M., Hardy, N. R., & Link, C. P. (2012). The effects of the intergenerational transmission of family emotional processes on conflict styles: The moderating role of attachment. *American Journal of Family Therapy, 40,* 56–73.

Barry, R. A., & Lawrence, E. (2013). "Don't stand so close to me": An attachment perspective of disengagement and avoidance in marriage. *Journal of Family Psychology, 27,* 484–494.

Bartholomew, K. (1990). Avoidance of intimacy: An attachment perspective. *Journal of Social and Personal Relationships, 7,* 147–178.

Bartholomew, K., & Allison, C. J. (2006). An attachment perspective on abusive dynamics in intimate relationships. In M. Mikulincer & G. S. Goodman (Eds.), *Dynamics of romantic love: Attachment, caregiving, and sex* (pp. 102–127). New York: Guilford Press.

Bartholomew, K., & Horowitz, L. M. (1991). Attachment styles among young adults: A test of a four-category model. *Journal of Personality and Social Psychology, 61,* 226–244.

Bartholomew, K., & Shaver, P. R. (1998). Methods of assessing adult attachment: Do they converge? In J. A. Simpson & W. S. Rholes (Eds.), *Attachment theory and close relationships* (pp. 25–45). New York: Guilford Press.

Beaulieu-Pelletier, G., Philippe, F. L., Lecours, S., & Couture, S. (2011). The role of attachment avoidance in extradyadic sex. *Attachment and Human Development, 13,* 293–313.

Beck, L. A., Pietromonaco, P. R., DeBuse, C. J., Powers, S. I., & Sayer, A. G. (2013). Spouses' attachment pairings predict neuroendocrine, behavioral, and psychological responses to marital conflict. *Journal of Personality and Social Psychology, 105,* 388–424.

Beck, L. A., Pietromonaco, P. R., DeVito, C. C., Powers, S. I., & Boyle, A. M. (2014). Congruence between spouses' perceptions and observers' ratings of responsiveness: The role of attachment avoidance. *Personality and Social Psychology Bulletin, 40,* 164–174.

Bogaert, A. F., & Sadava, S. (2002). Adult attachment and sexual behavior. *Personal Relationships, 9,* 191–204.

Bowlby, J. (1973). *Attachment and loss: Vol. 2. Separation: Anxiety and anger.* New York: Basic Books.

Bowlby, J. (1980). *Attachment and loss: Vol. 3. Loss.* New York: Basic Books.

Bowlby, J. (1982). *Attachment and loss: Vol. 1. Attachment.* New York: Basic Books. (Original work published 1969)

Bowlby, J. (1988). *A secure base.* New York: Basic Books.

Bradford, S. A., Feeney, J. A., & Campbell, L. (2002). Links between attachment orientations and dispositional and diary-based measures of disclosure in dating couples: A study of actor and partner effects. *Personal Relationships, 9,* 491–506.

Brennan, K. A., Clark, C. L., & Shaver, P. R. (1998). Self-report measurement of adult attachment: An integrative overview. In J. A. Simpson & W. S. Rholes (Eds.), *Attachment theory and close relationships* (pp. 46–76). New York: Guilford Press.

Brennan, K. A., & Shaver, P. R. (1995). Dimensions of adult attachment, affect regulation, and romantic relationship functioning. *Personality and Social Psychology Bulletin, 21,* 267–283.

Brennan, K. A., Shaver, P. R., & Tobey, A. E. (1991). Attachment styles, gender and parental problem drinking. *Journal of Social and Personal Relationships*, 8, 451–466.

Bretherton, I. (1990). Open communication and internal working models: Their role in the development of attachment relationships. In R. A. Thompson (Ed.), *Nebraska Symposium on Motivation: Vol. 36. Socioemotional development* (pp. 59–113). Lincoln: University of Nebraska Press.

Byng-Hall, J. (1999). Family couple therapy: Toward greater security. In J. Cassidy & P. R. Shaver (Eds.), *Handbook of attachment: Theory, research, and clinical applications* (pp. 625–645). New York: Guilford Press.

Cafferty, T. P., Davis, K. E., Medway, F. J., O'Hearn, R. E., & Chappell, K. D. (1994). Reunion dynamics among couples separated during Operation Desert Storm: An attachment theory analysis. In K. Bartholomew & D. Perlman (Eds.), *Advances in personal relationships: Vol. 5. Attachment processes in adulthood* (pp. 309–330). London: Jessica Kingsley.

Caldwell, J. G., & Shaver, P. R. (2012). Exploring the cognitive–emotional pathways between adult attachment and ego-resiliency. *Individual Differences Research*, 10, 141–152.

Campbell, L., Simpson, J. A., Kashy, D. A., & Rholes, W. S. (2001). Attachment orientations, dependence, and behaviour in a stressful situation: An application of the actor–partner interdependence model. *Journal of Social and Personal Relationships*, 18, 821–843.

Carnelley, K. B., Pietromonaco, P. R., & Jaffe, K. (1996). Attachment, caregiving, and relationship functioning in couples: Effects of self and partner. *Personal Relationships*, 3, 257–277.

Carnelley, K. B., & Rowe, A. C. (2007). Repeated priming of attachment security influences later views of self and relationships. *Personal Relationships*, 14, 307–320.

Cassidy, J., Shaver, P. R., Mikulincer, M., & Lavy, S. (2009). Experimentally induced security influences responses to psychological pain. *Journal of Social and Clinical Psychology*, 28, 463–478.

Clark, M. S., Lemay, E. P., Jr., Graham, S. M., Pataki, S. P., & Finkel, E. J. (2010). Ways of giving benefits in marriage: Norm use, relationship satisfaction, and attachment-related variability. *Psychological Science*, 21, 944–951.

Clark, M. S., & Reis, H. T. (1988). Interpersonal processes in close relationships. *Annual Review of Psychology*, 39, 609–672.

Cohn, D. A., Silver, D. H., Cowan, C. P., Cowan, P. A., & Pearson, J. (1992). Working models of childhood attachment and couple relationships. *Journal of Family Issues*, 13, 432–449.

Collins, N. L. (1996). Working models of attachment: Implications for explanation, emotion, and behavior. *Journal of Personality and Social Psychology*, 71, 810–832.

Collins, N. L., Guichard, A. C., Ford, M. B., & Feeney, B. C. (2004). Working models of attachment: New developments and emerging themes. In W. S. Rholes & J. A. Simpson (Eds.), *Adult attachment: Theory, research, and clinical implications* (pp. 196–239). New York: Guilford Press.

Collins, N. L., Guichard, A. C., Ford, M. B., & Feeney, B. C. (2006). Responding to need in intimate relationships: Normative processes and individual differences. In M. Mikulincer & G. S. Goodman (Eds.), *Dynamics of romantic love: Attachment, caregiving, and sex* (pp. 149–189). New York: Guilford Press.

Collins, N. L., & Read, S. J. (1990). Adult attachment, working models, and relationship quality in dating couples. *Journal of Personality and Social Psychology*, 58, 644–663.

Collins, N. L., & Read, S. J. (1994). Cognitive representations of attachment: The structure and function of working models. In K. Bartholomew & D. Perlman (Eds.), *Advances in personal relationships: Vol. 5. Attachment processes in adulthood* (pp. 53–90). London: Jessica Kingsley.

Creasey, G., & Hesson-McInness, M. (2001). Affective responses, cognitive appraisals, and conflict tactics in late adolescent romantic relationships: Associations with attachment orientations. *Journal of Counseling Psychology*, 48, 85–96.

Creasey, G., Kershaw, K., & Boston, A. (1999). Conflict management with friends and romantic partners: The role of attachment and negative mood regulation expectancies. *Journal of Youth and Adolescence*, 28, 523–543.

Crespo, C., Davide, I. N., Costa, M. E., & Fletcher, G. J. O. (2008). Family rituals in married couples: Links with attachment, relationship quality, and closeness. *Personal Relationships*, 15, 191–203.

Crittenden, P. (1985). Social networks, quality of child-rearing, and child development. *Child Development*, 56, 1299–1313.

Davila, J., Burge, D., & Hammen, C. (1997). Why does attachment style change? *Journal of Personality and Social Psychology*, 73, 826–836.

Davila, J., & Cobb, R. J. (2004). Predictors of change in attachment security during adulthood. In W. S. Rholes & J. A. Simpson (Eds.), *Adult attachment: Theory, research, and clinical implications* (pp. 133–156). New York: Guilford Press.

Diamond, L. M., & Hicks, A. M. (2005). Attachment style, current relationship security, and negative emotions: The mediating role of physiological regulation. *Journal of Social and Personal Relationships*, 22, 499–518.

Diamond, L. M., Hicks, A. M., & Otter-Henderson, K. D. (2008). Every time you go away: Changes in affect, behavior, and physiology associated with travel-related separations from romantic partners. *Journal of Personality and Social Psychology*, 95, 385–403.

Feeney, B. C., & Collins, N. L. (2004). Interpersonal safe haven and secure base caregiving processes in adulthood. In W. S. Rholes & J. A. Simpson (Eds.),

*Adult attachment: Theory, research, and clinical implications* (pp. 300–338). New York: Guilford Press.

Feeney, B. C., Collins, N. L., van Vleet, M., & Tomlinson, J. M. (2013). Motivations for providing a secure base: Links with attachment orientation and secure base support behavior. *Attachment and Human Development, 15,* 261–280.

Feeney, J. A. (1994). Attachment style, communication patterns, and satisfaction across the life cycle of marriage. *Personal Relationships, 1,* 333–348.

Feeney, J. A. (1995). Adult attachment and emotional control. *Personal Relationships, 2,* 143–159.

Feeney, J. A. (1996). Attachment, caregiving, and marital satisfaction. *Personal Relationships, 3,* 401–416.

Feeney, J. A. (1998). Adult attachment and relationship-centered anxiety: Responses to physical and emotional distancing. In J. A. Simpson & W. S. Rholes (Eds.), *Attachment theory and close relationships* (pp. 189–218). New York: Guilford Press.

Feeney, J. A. (1999a). Adult attachment, emotional control, and marital satisfaction. *Personal Relationships, 6,* 169–185.

Feeney, J. A. (1999b). Issues of closeness and distance in dating relationships: Effects of sex and attachment style. *Journal of Social and Personal Relationships, 16,* 571–590.

Feeney, J. A. (2002). Attachment, marital interaction, and relationship satisfaction: A diary study. *Personal Relationships, 9,* 39–55.

Feeney, J. A. (2003). The systemic nature of couple relationships: An attachment perspective. In P. Erdman & T. Caffery (Eds.), *Attachment and family systems: Conceptual, empirical and therapeutic relatedness* (pp. 139–163). New York: Brunner/Mazel.

Feeney, J. A. (2004). Hurt feelings in couple relationships: Toward integrative models of the negative effects of hurtful events. *Journal of Social and Personal Relationships, 21,* 487–508.

Feeney, J. A. (2005). Hurt feelings in couple relationships: Exploring the role of attachment and perceptions of personal injury. *Personal Relationships, 12,* 253–271.

Feeney, J. A., Alexander, R., Noller, P., & Hohaus, L. (2003). Attachment insecurity, depression, and the transition to parenthood. *Personal Relationships, 10,* 475–493.

Feeney, J. A., & Fitzgerald, J. R. (2012). Relationship education. In P. Noller & G. C. Karantzas (Eds.), *The Wiley-Blackwell handbook of couples and family relationships* (pp. 289–304). Oxford, UK: Wiley-Blackwell.

Feeney, J. A., & Hohaus, L. (2001). Attachment and spousal caregiving. *Personal Relationships, 8,* 21–39.

Feeney, J. A., Hohaus, L., Noller, P., & Alexander, R. (2001). *Becoming parents: Exploring the bonds between mothers, fathers, and their infants.* Cambridge, UK: Cambridge University Press.

Feeney, J. A., Kelly, L., Gallois, C., Peterson, C., & Terry, D. J. (1999). Attachment style, assertive communication, and safer-sex behavior. *Journal of Applied Social Psychology, 29,* 1964–1983.

Feeney, J. A., & Noller, P. (1990). Attachment style as a predictor of adult romantic relationships. *Journal of Personality and Social Psychology, 58,* 281–291.

Feeney, J. A., & Noller, P. (1991). Attachment style and verbal descriptions of romantic partners. *Journal of Social and Personal Relationships, 8,* 187–215.

Feeney, J. A., & Noller, P. (2004). Attachment and sexuality in close relationships. In J. H. Harvey, A. Wenzel, & S. Sprecher (Eds.), *Handbook of sexuality in close relationships* (pp. 183–201). Mahwah, NJ: Erlbaum.

Feeney, J. A., Noller, P., & Callan, V. J. (1994). Attachment style, communication and satisfaction in the early years of marriage. In K. Bartholomew & D. Perlman (Eds.), *Advances in personal relationships: Vol. 5. Attachment processes in adulthood* (pp. 269–308). London: Jessica Kingsley.

Feeney, J. A., Noller, P., & Hanrahan, M. (1994). Assessing adult attachment: Developments in the conceptualization of security and insecurity. In M. B. Sperling & W. H. Berman (Eds.), *Attachment in adults: Theory, assessment, and treatment* (pp. 128–152). New York: Guilford Press.

Feeney, J. A., Noller, P., & Patty, J. (1993). Adolescents' interactions with the opposite sex: Influence of attachment style and gender. *Journal of Adolescence, 16,* 169–186.

Feeney, J. A., Passmore, N. L., & Peterson, C. C. (2007). Adoption, attachment and relationship concerns: A study of adult adoptees. *Personal Relationships, 14,* 129–147.

Feeney, J. A., Peterson, C., Gallois, C., & Terry, D. J. (2000). Attachment style as a predictor of sexual attitudes and behavior in late adolescence. *Psychology and Health, 14,* 1105–1122.

Fossati, A., Acquarini, E., Feeney, J. A., Borroni, S., Grazioli, F., Giarolli, L., et al. (2009). Alexithymia and attachment insecurities in impulsive aggression. *Attachment and Human Development, 11,* 165–182.

Fossati, A., Feeney, J. A., Donati, D., Donini, M., Novella, L., Bagnato, M., et al. (2003). On the dimensionality of the Attachment Style Questionnaire in Italian clinical and nonclinical participants. *Journal of Social and Personal Relationships, 20,* 55–79.

Fraley, R. C., & Brumbaugh, C. C. (2004). A dynamical systems approach to conceptualizing and studying stability and change in attachment security. In W. S. Rholes & J. A. Simpson (Eds.), *Adult attachment: Theory, research, and clinical implications* (pp. 86–132). New York: Guilford Press.

Fraley, R. C., Heffernan, M. E., Vicary, A. M., & Brumbaugh, C. C. (2011). The Experiences in Close Relationships—Relationship Structures Questionnaire: A method for assessing attachment orientations across relationships. *Psychological Assessment, 23,* 615–625.

Fraley, R. C., & Shaver, P. R. (1997). Adult attachment

and the suppression of unwanted thoughts. *Journal of Personality and Social Psychology, 73*, 1080–1091.

Fraley, R. C., & Shaver, P. R. (1998). Airport separations: A naturalistic study of adult attachment dynamics in separating couples. *Journal of Personality and Social Psychology, 75*, 1198–1212.

Fraley, R. C., Vicary, A. M., Brumbaugh, C. C., & Roisman, G. I. (2011). Patterns of stability in adult attachment: An empirical test of two models of continuity and change. *Journal of Personality and Social Psychology, 101*, 974–992.

Fraley, R. C., & Waller, N. G. (1998). Adult attachment patterns: A test of the typological model. In J. A. Simpson & W. S. Rholes (Eds.), *Attachment theory and close relationships* (pp. 77–114). New York: Guilford Press.

Fraley, R. C., Waller, N. G., & Brennan, K. A. (2000). An item response theory analysis of self-report measures of adult attachment. *Journal of Personality and Social Psychology, 78*, 350–365.

Gabriel, S., Kawakami, K., Bartak, C., Kang, S. J., & Mann, N. (2010). Negative self-synchronization: Will I change to be like you when it is bad for me? *Journal of Personality and Social Psychology, 98*, 857–871.

Gaines, S. O., Work, C., Johnson, H., Youn, M. S. P., & Lai, K. (2000). Impact of attachment style and self-monitoring on individuals' responses to accommodative dilemmas across relationship types. *Journal of Social and Personal Relationships, 17*, 767–789.

Gallo, L. C., & Smith, T. W. (2001). Attachment style in marriage: Adjustment and responses to interaction. *Journal of Social and Personal Relationships, 18*, 263–289.

Gangestad, S. W., & Thornhill, R. (1997). The evolutionary psychology of extrapair sex: The role of fluctuating asymmetry. *Evolution and Human Behavior, 18*, 69–88.

Garrison, A. M., Kahn, J. H., Sauer, E. M., & Florczak, M. A. (2012). Disentangling the effects of depression symptoms and adult attachment on emotional disclosure. *Journal of Counseling Psychology, 59*, 230–239.

Gentzler, A. L., & Kerns, K. A. (2004). Associations between insecure attachment and sexual experiences. *Personal Relationships, 11*, 249–265.

George, C., Kaplan, N., & Main, M. (1984). *Adult Attachment Interview protocol*. Unpublished manuscript, University of California at Berkeley.

Gillath, O., Sesko, A. K., Shaver, P. R., & Chun, D. S. (2010). Attachment, authenticity, and honesty: Dispositional and experimentally induced security can reduce self- and other-deception. *Journal of Personality and Social Psychology, 98*, 841–855.

Gosnell, C. L., & Gable, S. L. (2013). Attachment and capitalizing on positive events. *Attachment and Human Development, 15*, 281–302.

Griffin, D. W., & Bartholomew, K. (1994). The metaphysics of measurement: The case of adult attachment. In K. Bartholomew & D. W. Perlman (Eds.),

*Advances in personal relationships: Vol. 5. Attachment processes in adulthood* (pp. 17–52). London: Jessica Kingsley.

Hadden, B. W., Smith, C. V., & Webster, G. D. (2014). Relationship duration moderates associations between attachment and relationship quality: Meta-analytic support for the temporal adult romantic attachment model. *Personality and Social Psychology Review, 18*(1), 42–58.

Hazan, C., & Shaver, P. R. (1987). Romantic love conceptualized as an attachment process. *Journal of Personality and Social Psychology, 52*, 511–524.

Hazan, C., & Shaver, P. R. (1994). Attachment as an organizational framework for research on close relationships. *Psychological Inquiry, 5*, 1–22.

Hazan, C., Zeifman, D., & Middleton, K. (1994, July). *Adult romantic attachment, affection, and sex*. Paper presented at the 7th International Conference on Personal Relationships, Groningen, The Netherlands.

Holland, A. S., Fraley, R. C., & Roisman, G. I. (2012). Attachment styles in dating couples: Predicting relationship functioning over time. *Personal Relationships, 19*, 234–246.

Holland, A. S., & Roisman, G. I. (2010). Adult attachment security and young adults' dating relationships over time: Self-reported, observational and physiological evidence. *Developmental Psychology, 46*, 552–557.

Holmes, B. M., & Johnson, K. R. (2009). Adult attachment and romantic partner preference: A review. *Journal of Social and Personal Relationships, 26*, 833–852.

Impett, E. A., Gordon, A., & Strachman, A. (2008). Attachment and daily sexual goals: A study of dating couples. *Personal Relationships, 15*, 375–390.

Kachadourian, L. K., Fincham, F., & Davila, J. (2004). The tendency to forgive in dating and married couples: The role of attachment and relationship satisfaction. *Personal Relationships, 11*, 373–393.

Karantzas, G. C., Feeney, J. A., McCabe, M., & Goncalves, C. V. (2014). Towards an integrative attachment-based model of relationship functioning. *British Journal of Psychology, 105*(3), 413–434.

Karremans, J. C., & Aarts, H. (2007). The role of automaticity in the inclination to forgive close others. *Journal of Experimental Social Psychology, 43*, 902–917.

Kashy, D. A., & Kenny, D. A. (2000). The analysis of data from dyads and groups. In H. T. Reis & C. M. Judd (Eds.), *Handbook of research methods in social and personality psychology* (pp. 451–477). New York: Cambridge University Press.

Keelan, J. P. R., Dion, K. K., & Dion, K. L. (1998). Attachment style and relationship satisfaction: Test of a self-disclosure explanation. *Canadian Journal of Behavioural Science, 30*, 24–35.

Kirkpatrick, L. E., & Davis, K. E. (1994). Attachment style, gender, and relationship stability: A longitudinal analysis. *Journal of Personality and Social Psychology*, 66, 502–512.

Kirkpatrick, L. E., & Hazan, C. (1994). Attachment styles and close relationships: A four-year prospective study. *Personal Relationships*, 1, 123–142.

Kobak, R. R., & Duemmler, S. (1994). Attachment and conversation: Toward a discourse analysis of adolescent and adult security. In K. Bartholomew & D. Perlman (Eds.), *Advances in personal relationships: Vol. 5. Attachment processes in adulthood* (pp. 121–149). London: Jessica Kingsley.

Kobak, R. R., & Hazan, C. (1991). Attachment in marriage: Effects of security and accuracy of working models. *Journal of Personality and Social Psychology*, 60, 861–869.

Kunce, L. J., & Shaver, P. R. (1994). An attachment-theoretical approach to caregiving in romantic relationships. In K. Bartholomew & D. Perlman (Eds.), *Advances in personal relationships: Vol. 5. Attachment processes in adulthood* (pp. 205–237). London: Jessica Kingsley.

Lafontaine, M.-F., Brassard, A., Lussier, Y., Valois, P., Shaver, P. R., & Johnson, S. M. (2015). Selecting the best items for a short-form Experiences in Close Relationships Questionnaire. *European Journal of Psychological Assessment*. [Epub ahead of print]

Lavy, S., Mikulincer, M., & Shaver, P. R. (2013). Intrusiveness from an attachment theory perspective: A dyadic diary study. *Personality and Individual Differences*, 55, 972–977.

Lee, J. A. (1973). *The colors of love: An exploration of the ways of loving.* Don Mills, ON, Canada: New Press.

Lee, J. A. (1988). Love-styles. In R. J. Sternberg & M. Barnes (Eds.), *The psychology of love* (pp. 38–67). New Haven, CT: Yale University Press.

Levy, M. B., & Davis, K. E. (1988). Lovestyles and attachment styles compared: Their relations to each other and to various relationship characteristics. *Journal of Social and Personal Relationships*, 5, 439–471.

Li, T., & Chan, D. K. (2012). How anxious and avoidant attachment affect romantic relationship quality differently: A meta-analytic review. *European Journal of Social Psychology*, 42, 406–419.

Main, M., & Goldwyn, R. (1984). *Adult attachment scoring and classification system.* Unpublished manuscript, University of California at Berkeley.

Main, M., Goldwyn, R., & Hesse, E. (2003). *Adult attachment scoring and classification system.* Unpublished manuscript, University of California at Berkeley.

Main, M., & Solomon, J. (1990). Procedures for identifying infants as disorganized/disoriented during the Ainsworth Strange Situation. In M. T. Greenberg, D. Cicchetti, & E. M. Cummings (Eds.), *Attachment in the preschool years: Theory, research, and intervention* (pp. 121–160). Chicago: University of Chicago Press.

Mattingly, B. A., & Clark, E. M. (2012). Weakening relationships we try to preserve: Motivated sacrifice, attachment, and relationship quality. *Journal of Applied Social Psychology*, 42, 373–386.

McClure, M. J., Lydon, J. E., Baccus, J. R., & Baldwin, M. W. (2010). A signal detection analysis of chronic attachment anxiety at speed dating: Being unpopular is only the first part of the problem. *Personality and Social Psychology Bulletin*, 36, 1024–1036.

Meyers, S. A., & Landsberger, S. A. (2002). Direct and indirect pathways between adult attachment style and marital satisfaction. *Personal Relationships*, 9, 159–172.

Mikulincer, M., Florian, V., Birnbaum, G., & Malishkevich, S. (2002). The death–anxiety buffering function of close relationships: Exploring the effects of separation reminders on death-thought accessibility. *Personality and Social Psychology Bulletin*, 28, 287–299.

Mikulincer, M., Gillath, O., & Shaver, P. R. (2002). Activation of the attachment system in adulthood: Threat-related primes increase the accessibility of mental representations of attachment figures. *Journal of Personality and Social Psychology*, 83, 881–895.

Mikulincer, M., & Goodman, G. S. (Eds.). (2006). *Dynamics of romantic love: Attachment, caregiving, and sex.* New York: Guilford Press.

Mikulincer, M., & Nachshon, O. (1991). Attachment styles and patterns of self-disclosure. *Journal of Personality and Social Psychology*, 61, 321–331.

Mikulincer, M., & Shaver, P. R. (2015). *Attachment in adulthood: Structure, dynamics, and change* (2nd ed.). New York: Guilford Press.

Mikulincer, M., Shaver, P. R., Gillath, O., & Nitzberg, R. A. (2005). Attachment, caregiving, and altruism: Boosting attachment security increases compassion and helping. *Journal of Personality and Social Psychology*, 89, 817–839.

Mohr, J. J., Selterman, D., & Fassinger, R. E. (2013). Romantic attachment and relationship functioning in same-sex couples. *Journal of Counseling Psychology*, 60, 72–82.

Noftle, E. E., & Shaver, P. R. (2006). Attachment dimensions and the Big Five personality traits: Associations and comparative ability to predict relationship quality. *Journal of Research in Personality*, 40, 179–208.

O'Connell Corcoran, K., & Mallinckrodt, B. (2000). Adult attachment, self-efficacy, perspective taking, and conflict resolution. *Journal of Counseling and Development*, 78, 473–483.

Overall, N. C., Fletcher, G. J. O., & Friesen, M. D. (2003). Mapping the intimate relationship mind: Comparisons between three models of attachment representations. *Personality and Social Psychology Bulletin*, 29, 1479–1493.

Overall, N. C., Fletcher, G. J., Simpson, J. A., & Fillo, J. (2015). Attachment insecurity, biased perceptions of romantic partners' negative emotions, and hostile relationship behavior. *Journal of Personality and Social Psychology*, 108, 730–749.

Overall, N. C., Girme, Y., Lemay, E. P., Jr., & Hammond, M. D. (2014). Attachment anxiety and reactions to relationship threat: The benefits and costs of inducing guilt in romantic partners. *Journal of Personality and Social Psychology, 106*, 235–256.

Pearce, Z. J., & Halford, W. K. (2008). Do attributions mediate the association between attachment and negative couple communication? *Personal Relationships, 15*, 155–170.

Peloquin, K., Brassard, A., Delisle, G., & Bedard, M.-M. (2013). Integrating the attachment, caregiving and sexual systems into the understanding of sexual satisfaction. *Canadian Journal of Behavioural Science, 45*, 185–195.

Peloquin, K., Lafontaine, M.-F., & Brassard, A. (2011). A dyadic approach to the study of romantic attachment, dyadic empathy, and psychological partner aggression. *Journal of Social and Personal Relationships, 28*, 915–942.

Pepping, C. A., & Halford, W. K. (2012). Attachment and relationship satisfaction in expectant first-time parents: The mediating role of relationship enhancing behaviors. *Journal of Research in Personality, 46*, 770–774.

Pietromonaco, P. R., & Barrett, L. F. (1997). Working models of attachment and daily social interactions. *Journal of Personality and Social Psychology, 73*, 1409–1423.

Pietromonaco, P. R., & Feldman Barrett, L. (2006). What can you do for me?: Attachment style and motive underlying esteem for partners. *Journal of Research in Personality, 40*, 313–338.

Pietromonaco, P. R., Greenwood, D., & Barrett, L. F. (2004). Conflict in adult close relationships: An attachment perspective. In W. S. Rholes & J. A. Simpson (Eds.), *Adult attachment: Theory, research, and clinical implications* (pp. 267–299). New York: Guilford Press.

Pistole, M. C. (1989). Attachment in adult romantic relationships: Style of conflict resolution and relationship satisfaction. *Journal of Social and Personal Relationships, 6*, 505–510.

Pistole, M. C. (1994). Adult attachment styles: Some thoughts on closeness–distance struggles. *Family Process, 33*, 147–159.

Priel, B., & Besser, A. (2000). Adult attachment styles, early relationships, antenatal attachment, and perceptions of infant temperament: A study of first-time mothers. *Personal Relationships, 7*, 291–310.

Roberts, L. J., & Greenberg, D. R. (2002). Observational "windows" to intimacy processes in marriage. In P. Noller & J. A. Feeney (Eds.), *Understanding marriage: Developments in the study of couple interaction* (pp. 118–149). Cambridge, UK: Cambridge University Press.

Rothbard, J. C., & Shaver, P. R. (1994). Continuity of attachment across the life span. In M. B. Sperling & W. H. Berman (Eds.), *Attachment in adults: Theory, assessment, and treatment* (pp. 31–71). New York: Guilford Press.

Schachner, D. A., & Shaver, P. R. (2004). Attachment dimensions and sexual motives. *Personal Relationships, 11*, 179–195.

Scharfe, E., & Bartholomew, K. (1994). Reliability and stability of adult attachment patterns. *Personal Relationships, 1*, 23–43.

Scharfe, E., & Cole, V. (2006). Stability and change of attachment representations during emerging adulthood: An examination of mediators and moderators of change. *Personal Relationships, 13*, 363–374.

Seedall, R. B., & Wampler, K. S. (2012). Emotional congruence within couple interaction: The role of attachment avoidance. *Journal of Family Psychology, 26*, 948–958.

Selcuk, E., Zayas, V., Gunaydin, G., Hazan, C., & Kross, E. (2012). Mental representations of attachment figures facilitate recovery following upsetting autobiographical memory recall. *Journal of Personality and Social Psychology, 103*, 362–378.

Senchak, M., & Leonard, K. E. (1992). Attachment styles and marital adjustment among newlywed couples. *Journal of Social and Personal Relationships, 9*, 51–64.

Shaver, P. R., & Brennan, K. A. (1992). Attachment styles and the "Big Five" personality traits: Their connections with each other and with romantic relationship outcomes. *Personality and Social Psychology Bulletin, 18*, 536–545.

Shaver, P. R., & Hazan, C. (1988). A biased overview of the study of love. *Journal of Social and Personal Relationships, 5*, 473–501.

Shaver, P. R., Hazan, C., & Bradshaw, D. (1988). Love as attachment: The integration of three behavioral systems. In R. J. Sternberg & M. Barnes (Eds.), *The psychology of love* (pp. 68–99). New Haven, CT: Yale University Press.

Shaver, P. R., & Mikulincer, M. (2006). A behavioral systems approach to romantic love relationships: Attachment, caregiving, and sex. In R. J. Sternberg & K. Weis (Eds.), *The new psychology of love* (pp. 35–64). New Haven, CT: Yale University Press.

Shaver, P. R., & Mikulincer, M. (2012). Adult attachment and sexuality. In P. Noller & G. C. Karantzas (Eds.), *The Wiley-Blackwell handbook of couples and family relationships* (pp. 161–174). Oxford, UK: Wiley-Blackwell.

Shaver, P. R., & Mikulincer, M. (2013). Adult attachment and emotion regulation. In J. J. Gross (Ed.), *Handbook of emotion regulation* (2nd ed., pp. 237–250). New York: Guilford Press.

Shaver, P. R., Mikulincer, M., Lavy, S., & Cassidy, J. (2009). Understanding and altering hurt feelings: An attachment-theoretical perspective on the generation and regulation of emotions. In A. L. Vangelisti (Ed.), *Feeling hurt in close relationships* (pp. 92–119). New York: Cambridge University Press.

Simpson, J. A. (1990). Influence of attachment styles on romantic relationships. *Journal of Personality and Social Psychology, 59*, 971–980.

Simpson, J. A., & Rholes, W. S. (1994). Stress and secure base relationships in adulthood. In K. Bartholomew & D. Perlman (Eds.), *Advances in personal relationships: Vol. 5. Attachment processes in adulthood* (pp. 181–204). London: Jessica Kingsley.

Simpson, J. A., Rholes, W. S., & Nelligan, J. S. (1992). Support seeking and support giving within couples in an anxiety-provoking situation: The role of attachment styles. *Journal of Personality and Social Psychology, 62,* 434–446.

Simpson, J. A., Rholes, W. S., & Phillips, D. (1996). Conflict in close relationships: An attachment perspective. *Journal of Personality and Social Psychology, 71,* 899–914.

Sternberg, R. J. (1986). A triangular theory of love. *Psychological Review, 93,* 119–135.

Sternberg, R. J., & Weis, K. (Eds.). (2006). *The new psychology of love.* New Haven, CT: Yale University Press.

Strauss, C., Morry, M. M., & Kito, M. (2012). Attachment styles and relationship quality: Actual, perceived, and ideal partner matching. *Personal Relationships, 19,* 14–36.

Sumer, N., & Cozzarelli, C. (2004). The impact of adult attachment on partner and self-attributions and relationship quality. *Personal Relationships, 11,* 355–371.

Tan, R., Overall, N. C., & Taylor, J. K. (2012). Let's talk about us: Attachment, relationship-focused disclo-sure, and relationship quality. *Personal Relationships, 19,* 521–534.

Tennov, D. (1979). *Love and limerence: The experience of being in love.* New York: Stein & Day.

Tracy, J. L., Shaver, P. R., Cooper, M. L., & Albino, A. W. (2003). Attachment styles and adolescent sexuality. In P. Florsheim (Ed.), *Adolescent romance and sexual behavior: Theory, research, and practical implications* (pp. 137–159). Mahwah, NJ: Erlbaum.

Weiss, R. S. (1982). Attachment in adult life. In C. M. Parkes & J. Stevenson-Hinde (Eds.), *The place of attachment in human behavior* (pp. 171–184). New York: Basic Books.

Weiss, R. S. (1991). The attachment bond in childhood and adulthood. In C. M. Parkes, J. Stevenson-Hinde, & P. Marris (Eds.), *Attachment across the life cycle* (pp. 66–76). London: Tavistock/Routledge.

Xu, J. H., & Shrout, P. E. (2013). Assessing the reliability of change: A comparison of two measures of adult attachment. *Journal of Research in Personality, 47,* 202–208.

Zayas, V., & Shoda, Y. (2005). Do automatic reactions elicited by thoughts of romantic partner, mother, and self relate to adult romantic attachment? *Personality and Social Psychology Bulletin, 31,* 1011–1025.

# Chapter 22

# Attachment and Sexual Mating

*The Joint Operation
of Separate Motivational Systems*

## Gurit E. Birnbaum

Sex is a fundamental aspect of many adult attachment relationships. Sexual urges and emotional attachments, however, are not necessarily connected. For example, sexual acts often occur outside the context of romantic relationships (e.g., one-night stands, short-term extradyadic copulations) and, as such, they may be devoid of affectional bonding and be used for relationship-irrelevant reasons (e.g., physical gratification, self-enhancement, stress relief). Moreover, affectional bonding between adults does not always entail sexual desire or sexual acts, as in the case of long-term partners who have lost sexual desire for each other and ceased having sex but are still deeply attached to each other. These examples align with the view that sexual mating and attachment are governed by separate motivational systems; that is, the processes underlying sexual desire and affectional bonding are functionally distinct (motivating reproductive acts, maintaining proximity to a caregiver, respectively; Bowlby, 1982; Diamond, 2003; Fisher, 1998; Fisher, Aron, Mashek, Li, & Brown, 2002).

Nevertheless, joint involvement of the sexual and attachment systems is typical of ongoing romantic relationships in which intimates function as both attachment figures and sexual partners (Birnbaum, 2010; Hazan & Zeifman, 1994). Thus, within the context of romantic relationships, these two behavioral systems mutually influence each other and operate together to affect relationship quality and longevity (Birnbaum, 2010, 2014). In this chapter, I review published evidence that points to a reciprocal relationship between these two systems. I first provide an overview of the contribution of attachment orientations to the appraisal of sexual interactions in adolescence and adulthood, and to our understanding the sex–relationship link. In doing so, I discuss the subordination of the sexual system to attachment processes under relationship-threatening circumstances. I then consider the reverse causal direction, focusing on the role of sex as a promoter of emotional bonds. I conclude by presenting the relationship stage model of sexual desire and suggesting directions for future research on the dual potential of sexual desire for both relationship promotion and deterioration.

## The Contribution of Attachment Orientations to the Appraisal of Sexual Interactions

The attachment system, which is the earliest developing social-behavioral system in humans, evolved because it increased infants' survival chances and future reproductive success by maintaining proximity to supportive figures (Bowlby, 1969/1982, 1973). Over the course of development, the quality of repeated interactions with these attachment figures gradually shapes chronic patterns of relational cognitions and goals. Interactions with attachment figures who are responsive to one's bids for proximity facilitate optimal functioning of the attachment system, promote a sense of attachment security (i.e., confidence that one is lovable and that significant others are supportive when needed), and lead to consolidation of interpersonal goals aimed at forming nurturing intimate relationships. In contrast, recurrent failure to attain the primary goal of "felt security" results in the adoption of alternative regulatory strategies for dealing with the ensuing insecurity: hyperactivation of the attachment system, which characterizes anxious attachment, and deactivation of the attachment system, which characterizes avoidant attachment.

Each of these two defensive attachment strategies is associated with particular constellations of interpersonal goals and mental representations of self and others. Attachment anxiety is associated with extreme abandonment fears, wishes for merger, negative models of the self as needy and helpless, and positive expectations of others as affectionate and warmhearted (Bartholomew & Horowitz, 1991; Mikulincer & Shaver, 2007a). Avoidant attachment, by comparison, is associated with wishes for distance and self-reliance in close relationships, negative models of others as unsupportive, and positive models of self as powerful and controlling (Bartholomew & Horowitz, 1991; Mikulincer & Shaver, 2007a). These early-developing attachment strategies guide interpersonal interactions over the lifespan by affecting desired levels of intimacy and interdependence with adult romantic partners. Accordingly, they are likely to influence the regulatory functioning of the sexual system, which matures later in life (Shaver, Hazan, & Bradshaw, 1988). This theorizing has been widely supported by research showing that attachment orientations help explain variations in the way in which adolescents and adults construe their sexual interactions (see Birnbaum, 2010; Mikulincer & Shaver, 2007b).

## Attachment and Sex in Adolescence

The contribution of attachment processes to the construal and experience of sexual encounters can first be discerned in late adolescence (e.g., Cooper et al., 2006), when attachment needs are increasingly met through intimates, and sexual and romantic explorations become key developmental tasks (see reviews by Collins, Welsh, & Furman, 2009; Tolman & McClelland, 2011; also see Zeifman & Hazan, Chapter 20, this volume). An in-depth look at the sexual dynamics during this period may therefore be particularly informative about how early interpersonal experiences determine the development of sexuality in a relationship context, including the kinds of desires adolescents wish to satisfy, the types of relationships they seek, and what they perceive to be sexually desirable in potential and current partners.

Research has generally indicated that smooth functioning of the attachment system facilitates relaxed engagement in sexual activities and encourages the channelling of sexual desires into a committed intimate relationship, even as early as adolescence. In contrast, negative attachment experiences in childhood and the consolidation of insecure patterns of attachment are likely to impair the functioning of the sexual system in close relationships during this period and later on. Indeed, if a person feels chronically insecure about being loved, whether this is reflected in relational worries or in being uncomfortable with intimacy, it is unlikely that this person's sexual system will function without interference. The nature of interference, however, is different between anxious and avoidant adolescents (Birnbaum, 2010; Mikulincer & Shaver, 2007b).

A more detailed examination of the dynamics of attachment in the sexual realm reveals that, consistent with the idea that attachment security furthers a confident approach to sexuality (Mikulincer & Shaver, 2007b), secure adolescents report lower levels of erotophobia than their less secure peers (i.e., they experience fewer negative affective–evaluative responses to sexual cues). This relaxed approach seems to serve the developmental needs characterizing late adolescence. Indeed, secure adolescents neither tend to delay the onset of intercourse, as avoidant adolescents do, nor engage in sexual intercourse rarely, as anxious adolescent men and avoidant adolescent women do (Cooper, Shaver, & Collins, 1998; Feeney, Noller, & Patty, 1993; Feeney, Peterson, Gallois, & Terry, 2000). Rather, secure adolescents are more likely than insecure adolescents to be involved in long-term romantic relationships, explore their sexual aspects, and enjoy them (Tracy, Shaver, Albino, & Cooper, 2003).

More specifically, secure adolescents differ from their less secure peers in the reasons for engaging in sex and in the circumstances in which they choose to have sex (Cooper et al., 2006). They prefer sexual relationships that involve affection (Potard, Courtois, Réveillère, Bréchon, & Courtois, in press) and, accordingly, are more likely to have sex to promote emotional bonding (e.g., to express love for their partner; Tracy et al., 2003). Secure adolescents are also less likely to have sex because of abandonment fears, and are therefore less likely to defer to their partners' desires and to engage in risky behavior during sex (e.g., having intercourse without birth control or while being intoxicated) or in sexual acts that are otherwise unwanted (Feeney et al., 2000; Paulk & Zayac, 2013; Tracy et al., 2003). This, together with their intimacy goals, may explain why they are less accepting of casual sex and are less likely to engage in it (Feeney et al., 1993; Tracy et al., 2003). Overall, secure adolescents' sexual behavior is one way in which they express their growing commitment to a relationship, promoting the establishment of a satisfying intimate bond with a romantic partner.

Whereas a secure state of mind enables constructive exploration of the sexual realm, attachment insecurities may lead to self-defeating behavior patterns. Attachment-anxious adolescents engage in sex to meet their intense needs for security and love. Tragically, however, their chronic insecurity encourages dysfunctional behavior that confirms their worst fears. In particular, they are more likely than their less anxious agemates to have sex to avoid a partner's rejection (Tracy et al., 2003). Because they wish to avoid partner disapproval and tend to hold onto a partner through sexual acquiescence (Tracy et al., 2003), they find themselves engaging in sexual acts with which they are not comfortable and in which they otherwise would not engage (e.g., Szielasko, Symons, & Price, 2013). Some of these activities (e.g., lack of contraceptive use, alcohol and drug consumption; Feeney et al., 2000; Paulk & Zayac, 2013) expose them to risky situations and result in unwelcome consequences (e.g., sexually transmitted disease; unplanned pregnancies; Cooper et al., 1998, 2006). Their insecurity may also lead them to impose sexual contact on their partners as a way of gaining reassurance or reestablishing connectedness (Szielasko et al., 2013). Such destructive tendencies, which are not satisfying alternatives to genuine intimacy, decrease the likelihood of sustaining mutually gratifying relationships.

Avoidant adolescents, compared to their secure and anxious peers, have a significantly lower preference for sexual relationships that involve affection (Potard et al., in press), probably because they devalue the importance of emotional ties, at least consciously (Fraley & Shaver, 1997), and are threatened by the closeness implied by sex (Birnbaum, 2010). This discomfort with the intimate aspects of sex has many manifestations. Avoidant virgin adolescents report higher levels of erotophobia and fewer noncoital sexual behaviors (e.g., making out, petting) than their less avoidant virgin counterparts (Tracy et al., 2003). When avoidant adolescents do start having sexual intercourse, they do so at an older age (e.g., Bogaert & Sadava, 2002; Gentzler & Kerns, 2004), with lower frequently, and for reasons of self-enhancement and prestige (e.g., being relieved or happy to have lost their virginity) rather than intimacy-promoting ones (e.g., expressing love for their partner; Tracy et al., 2003).

Avoidant adolescents are less likely to enjoy sexual experience and tend to drink or use drugs prior to engaging in sex (Tracy et al., 2003). At the same time, their willingness to forgo intimacy may have health-promoting benefits, leading them to be more likely to use condoms (Feeney et al., 2000). Interestingly, the same motive, intimacy aversion, that leads avoidant adolescents to date rarely and to avoid intimate sexual experience during adolescence takes another form when they move into young adulthood. In particular, they tend to engage in a short-term mating strategy that involves emotionless, uncommitted sexual activities (Cooper et al., 2006; Del Giudice, 2009; Jackson & Kirkpatrick, 2007).

### Attachment and Sex in Adulthood

The patterns of regulating intimacy and emotions and of relating to others that were established in infancy and continued through adolescence seem to affect the functioning of the sexual system in adult romantic and marital relationships (e.g., Cooper et al., 2006). Secure individuals pursue committed intimate relationships, and their sense of sexual confidence, comfort with sexual intimacy, and enjoyment of mutually rewarding sexual interactions contribute to maintaining satisfying romantic relationships (Birnbaum, 2010; Mikulincer & Shaver, 2007a). In particular, secure people are motivated by relationship-promoting goals (Mikulincer & Shaver, 2007b) and are therefore less likely than insecure people to engage in casual sex. Instead, they tend to seek fulfilment of their sexual needs and desires within committed intimate relationships (e.g., Brennan & Shaver, 1995; Paul, McManus, & Hayes, 2000; Stephan & Bachman, 1999).

Their secure state of mind is reflected not only in comfort with intimacy but also in positive sexual self-schemas (e.g., viewing the sexual self as passionate, powerful, and open; Cyranowski & Andersen, 1998). This self-assured approach to sexuality allows secure individuals to experience positive emotions during sexual activity (e.g., Birnbaum, Reis, Mikulincer, Gillath, & Orpaz, 2006) and to respond to their partner's sexual needs without compromising their own preferences. Being free of attachment concerns and sexual performance anxieties also contributes to a "letting go" state of mind that enables them to enjoy exploratory sexual activities with their long-term partner, thereby fostering mutual sexual and relational satisfaction (Mikulincer & Shaver, 2007b; Shaver et al., 1988).

In contrast, preoccupation with attachment concerns keeps interfering with comfortable sexuality for attachment-anxious adults (Bartholomew & Horowitz, 1991; Mikulincer & Shaver, 2007a). Specifically, they use sex to try to achieve attachment goals (e.g., Davis, Shaver, & Vernon, 2003, 2004). For example, they tend to sexualize their desire for affection and are likely to have sex for reasons such as gaining a partner's reassurance and manipulating him or her to reduce the possibility of abandonment (Birnbaum, Mikulincer, & Austerlitz, 2013; Cooper et al., 2006; Davis et al., 2004; Impett, Gordon, & Strachman, 2008; Schachner & Shaver, 2004). They tend to prefer the affectionate aspects of sex (e.g., holding, cuddling, kissing) rather than sex per se (Hazan, Zeifman, & Middleton, 1994). This sexualization of attachment needs is reflected in anxious individuals' "sexting" behavior: They are more likely than less anxious individuals to send texts that solicit sexual activity, possibly in the hope that it will seduce a partner into a more reliable relationship (Weisskirch & Delevi, 2011).

Attachment anxious people are inclined to be attracted to partners who seem willing to provide the sense of reassurance they covet (Birnbaum & Reis, 2012; Holmes & Johnson, 2009; Wei, Mallinckrodt, Larson, & Zakalik, 2005). They fantasize about giving and receiving affection during sexual activity and desire emotional involvement, warmth, and attention from their partners during sexual intercourse (Birnbaum,

Mikulincer, & Gillath, 2011; Birnbaum et al., 2006). Their sexual fantasies also involve submission themes that serve their desire to be irresistibly desired. At the same time, such themes may temporarily satisfy their need to feel that their partner is a stronger, wiser caregiver (Birnbaum, 2007b; Birnbaum, Mikulincer et al., 2011). Unfortunately, attachment-anxious individuals channel not only their relational hopes into the sexual domain but also excessive performance anxieties and relational worries (Birnbaum, Mikulincer, Szepsenwol, Shaver, & Mizrahi, 2014; Birnbaum et al., 2006). In particular, they are threatened by sexual performance failure and the possibility of disappointing their partner (Birnbaum et al., 2014). As a result, they tend to try to please their partners during sexual intercourse, while inhibiting the expression of their own sexual desires (e.g., Davis et al., 2006), often succumbing to unwanted sexual advances (Gentzler & Kerns, 2004; Impett & Peplau, 2002).

Overall, the most conspicuous feature of highly anxious people's construal of sexuality is its ambivalent nature. On the one hand, their erotophilic tendencies (Bogaert & Sadava, 2002) seem to intensify the pleasurable aspects of sex (Birnbaum et al., 2006). On the other hand, doubts about being loved generate negative emotions during sexual intercourse (Birnbaum, 2007a; Birnbaum et al., 2006). Such intruding thoughts and aversive feelings apparently impair anxiously attached people's ability to enjoy sexual interactions freely and frustrate their unrealistic expectations for the ultimate physical and emotional merger. It is therefore hardly surprising that anxiously attached people are prone to suffer from not only relational disillusionment (Mikulincer & Shaver, 2007b) but also sexual disappointment and difficulties (Birnbaum, 2007a; Birnbaum et al., 2006; Burri, Schweitzer, & O'Brien, 2014; Stefanou & McCabe, 2012). In fact, because they rely so heavily on the sexual features of their relationship when appraising their partner's regard for them, their sexual difficulties are likely to be misinterpreted as a sign of rejection and have further negative implications for their relationship (Birnbaum, 2007a; Birnbaum et al., 2006).

Ironically, avoidant individuals use sex, which can be one of the most intimate human interactions, to avoid emotional intimacy. This aversion to emotional intimacy is manifested in approaching sex in a variety of distancing ways. Avoidant people typically dismiss sexual motives that are associated with the promotion of emotional closeness (e.g., expressing affection for a partner; Davis et al., 2004; Impett at al., 2008; Schachner & Shaver, 2004). Instead, they pursue opportunistic, self-serving goals, such as having sex to affirm self-worth, to cope with negative emotions, and to impress peers (Cooper et al., 2006; Schachner & Shaver, 2004). Such self-enhancing motives may account for avoidant people's tendency to engage in one-night stands and short-term extradyadic copulations (Cooper et al., 2006).

Indeed, avoidant people tend to be promiscuous and nonexclusive in intimate relationships. They hold permissive attitudes about casual sex (Brennan & Shaver, 1995; Gentzler & Kerns, 2004; Simpson & Gangestad, 1991) and are less likely to experience sexual fantasies that involve romantic themes and intimate interactions with their partner (Birnbaum, 2007b). These tendencies are reflected in real life in the form of engaging in uncommitted sex with a variety of partners (Bogaert & Sadava, 2002; Gangestad & Thornhill, 1997; Paul et al., 2000; Stephan & Bachman, 1999). In addition, avoidant people are likely to respond favorably to mate-poaching attempts (i.e., attempts to lure them away from their current partners) in a short-term context, but of course, not when the poaching is for the long-term goal of establishing a committed relationship (Schachner & Shaver, 2002). As might be expected, avoidant people's low commitment to their primary relationship explains such extradyadic desires and affairs (DeWall et al., 2011). Ironically, this pattern of extradyadic involvement is reinforced by a primary partner's desire for intimacy, which causes the avoidant individual to back further away (Beaulieu-Pelletier, Philippe, Lecours, & Couture, 2011).

The goal of intimacy aversion may also explain avoidant people's initial attraction to partners with similar needs for independence and their sexual disinterest in potential partners who seem to crave closeness (Birnabum & Reis, 2012; Holmes & Johnson, 2009). Interestingly, although avoidant people express greater willingness to engage in consensual non-monogamous relationships, they are less likely to actually engage in such relationships (Moors, Conley, Edelstein, & Chopik, 2014). They may have a positive attitude toward consensual, nonmonogamous relationships because these relationships offer an opportunity to dilute emotional closeness with a primary partner. At the same time, however, avoidant individuals generally lack the levels of trust and intimacy needed to sustain extradyadic relationships (e.g., Barker, 2005; Moors et al., 2014).

Avoidant people employ other strategies to distance themselves from their primary partner and impede the experience of genuine intimacy. In line with their extreme self-reliance (Mikulincer & Shaver, 2007a), they often masturbate (Bogaert & Sadava, 2002) rather than having frequent sex with their partners (Brassard, Shaver, & Lussier, 2007). When avoidant people do have sex with their partners, they focus on their own sexual needs and are less likely to express physical affection and to attend to their partners' needs. Nevertheless, they are less likely to satisfy their own needs because they tend to experience aversive feelings of estrangement and alienation during sexual interactions, as well as intruding thoughts (Birnbaum & Reis, 2006; Birnbaum et al., 2006). This detached stance even enters into their sexual fantasies, where they play out themes of interpersonal distance and hostility (Birnbaum, 2007b; Birnbaum, Mikulincer, et al., 2011). Such strategies are obviously not conducive to optimal sexual functioning, and like attachment-anxious people, avoidant individuals are inclined to have sexual difficulties (e.g., Birnbaum, 2007a; Burri et al., 2014; Cohen & Belsky, 2008).

## Gender Differences in the Sexual Expressions of Attachment Insecurities

Attachment dynamics in the sexual realm may differ for men and women (e.g., Birnbaum & Laser-Brandt, 2002). Although evolutionary models (e.g., Buss & Schmitt, 1993; Ellis & Symons, 1990) and social-psychological conceptions (DeLamater, 1987; Gagnon & Simon, 1973) attribute these differences to distinct sources of influence (i.e., evolutionary vs. cultural), both perspectives agree that women develop a more emotional–interpersonal orientation toward sexuality than do men. For example, women are more likely to associate sex with receiving and expressing love and are therefore more concerned with their romantic relationships during sexual intercourse. For this reason, they also tend to be more affectionate and nurturing than men during sexual interaction. Men, in contrast, are relatively more motivated by physical release and tend to adopt a more individualistic–recreational orientation toward sexuality. For example, they are more likely to be active, to take the initiator role, and to not only focus on satisfying their partner during sexual activity but also be concerned about experiencing sexual variety (Birnbaum & Laser-Brandt, 2002; Byers & Heinlein, 1989; Carroll, Volk, & Hyde, 1985; Hatfield, Sprecher, Traupmann-Pillemer, Greenberger, & Wexler, 1988; O'Sullivan & Byers, 1992).

Men and women's different approaches to sexuality seem to affect how their attachment insecurities are manifested in the sexual arena. Specifically, although both avoidant men and women strive to minimize expressions of intimacy in sexual interactions (e.g., Birnbaum et al., 2006; Cooper et al., 2006), avoidance is more marked in men's sexuality than in women's. Avoidant men, for example, are more inclined to approve of casual sex, to engage in extradyadic sex, and to use sex for relationship-irrelevant reasons (e.g., coping with upset feelings) as compared with avoidant women (e.g., Birnbaum, Hirschberger, & Goldenberg, 2011; Cooper et al. 2006; Sprecher, 2013).

Sexual fantasies provide another medium in which avoidant men can become remarkably disengaged from their current partner. Indeed, avoidant men, but not avoidant women, are less likely to fantasize sexually about romantic themes (Birnbaum, 2007b). Avoidant men are also inclined to objectify women and casual partners. In particular, they are more likely to view pornography (Szymaski & Stewart-Richardson, 2014) and to sexually coerce women in casual dating situations (e.g., pickups, first dates; Davis, 2006). This extreme pattern of divorcing sex from emotions suggests that male sex role norms, which emphasize sexual conquest and inhibit expressions of vulnerability, exacerbate the destructive effects of avoidance: the negative view of others, the feelings of sexual entitlement, and the blindness to partners' wishes. Women's habitual nurturing tendencies, in contrast, may mitigate these effects.

Gender differences in the sexual manifestations of attachment anxiety are more noticeable. Because of their insecurity, attachment-anxious men may be overtaxed by the burden of the traditional gender role of male as sexual initiator (O'Sullivan & Byers, 1992). The resulting tension and wariness may interfere with sexual desire, especially in situations that involve vulnerability, for example, when initiating sex with a new partner. Anxious men tend to begin having sex at an older age and are less likely to view casual sex positively or to cheat on their partners. As a result, they have fewer sex partners overall compared with less attachment-anxious men (Allen & Baucom, 2004; Cooper et al., 2006; Gentzler & Kerns 2004). As might be expected, their tendency to suppress extradyadic desires is especially pronounced under relationship-threatening conditions (Birnbaum,

Weisberg, & Simpson, 2011) that probably intensify their insecurity. Hence, attachment anxiety may not only lead men to invest resources in their ongoing relationship but also prevent them from using sex as a source of self-worth (Cooper et al., 2006).

To the extent that fantasies create a safer channel for sexual exploration, one might expect that anxiously attached men's sexual fantasies would compensate for their insecurities; at least in that fantasy realm, they might engage in sex to feel better about themselves. Instead, attachment anxiety colors their fantasy world with desires to satisfy their partners and focus on pleasing them (Birnbaum, 2007b). They do, however, tend to substitute pornography for authentic intimacy, probably because it allows them to gratify themselves, if only partially, without having to risk interpersonal rejection. Unfortunately, choosing this source of sexual outlet is associated with sexual dissatisfaction and poorer relationship quality (Szymanski & Stewart-Richardson, 2014). The most destructive manifestation of attachment anxiety in men is a proclivity toward using coercive sex (Brassard et al., 2007), which reflects their desperate wish to regain proximity to a partner who is perceived as unresponsive.

Attachment-anxious women cope differently with their attachment-related insecurities. Their tendency to conflate sex and love (Birnbaum, 2007a; Birnbaum et al., 2006) can paradoxically increase the likelihood of engaging in unrestricted and risky sexual behavior. Consistent with this reasoning, anxious women begin having sex at a younger age than secure or avoidant women, hold positive attitudes toward uncommitted sex, and are inclined to engage in extradyadic affairs (Allen & Baucom, 2004; Bogaert & Sadava, 2002; Gangestad & Thornhill, 1997; Gentzler & Kerns, 2004). Their tendency to defer to their partners' sexual needs (Davis et al., 2006) often leads them to engage in unprotected and consensual unwanted sex and to have higher frequencies of unintended pregnancies (e.g., Cooper, Shapiro, & Powers, 1998; Impett & Peplau, 2002). It therefore seems that anxious women's relational worries create difficulties in negotiating sexual encounters and motivate them to secure alternatives to their current partners, in both the real and virtual worlds. Indeed, their sexual fantasies are marked by unrestricted sexual themes (i.e., scenes involving a variety of sexual partners, along with less intimate copulatory positions and emotionless sex; Birnbaum, 2007b).

## The Joint Contribution of Attachment and Sex to Relationship Quality

Regardless of whether gender-specific construal of sexuality exacerbates or mitigates some of the detrimental sexual implications of attachment insecurities, both kinds of insecurity are associated with aversive sexual experiences and poor relationship quality among men and women (Birnbaum, 2010; Mikulincer & Shaver, 2007a). Their paths of influence are, however, notably different: Attachment anxiety seems to amplify the impact of sexual experiences on the quality of a relationship, whereas avoidance reduces the impact. Attachment-anxious individuals are particularly attuned to cues that indicate whether their partner still has positive regard for them, and they tend to use sexual interactions as a prominent means of such impressions (Birnbaum, 2007a; Davis et al., 2004). Gratifying sexual experiences are likely to instill a sense of being loved and be interpreted as a sign of a good romantic relationship. Conversely, experiencing negative sexual experiences is likely to be taken as a sign of rejection and a symptom of serious relational difficulties. Avoidant people, by comparison, tend to isolate sexuality from psychological intimacy and are thus less likely to associate sexual activity with relationship well-being. Their relationships may therefore neither suffer the adverse effects of frustrating sexual experiences nor benefit from positive sexual experiences.

These findings imply that optimal functioning of the attachment system, as in the case of securely attached partners, involves neither high nor low levels of interdependence between sexual and emotional aspects of a relationship. Rather, intermediate levels of interdependence between these aspects allow sexual interactions to contribute to relationship quality and stability, but not everything depends on the quality of partners' sex lives at a particular point in a relationship. Other aspects of the relationship, such as intimacy, support, communication, and commitment, may be equally or more important to relationship quality in the long run (Birnbaum, 2010, 2014; Birnbaum et al., 2006).

Several dyadic studies have supported this conceptualization. In one study (Birnbaum et al., 2006), both members of heterosexual cohabiting couples reported on their attachment orientations and provided daily diary measures of relationship quality and sexual activity for 42 consecutive days. In addition, each time they had sex, participants reported their feelings and thoughts during that sexual episode (e.g., "During sexual intercourse, I felt bored and apathetic," "During sexual intercourse, my partner made me feel desired"). The findings indicated that, as expected, sexual experiences were associated with relationship quality among couples with an anxiously attached partner, but were uncorrelated with relationship quality among couples with an avoidant partner. These findings imply that sex might not only be most beneficial but also most detrimental to the relationships of anxiously attached intimates.

A more recent diary study of newlywed couples revealed that under nonthreatening relational conditions, sexual activity might benefit not only the relationships of couples with an anxiously attached partner but also those of couples with an avoidant partner (Little, McNulty, & Russell, 2010). In particular, engaging in highly frequent and satisfying sexual activity may lead insecure partners to expect to be more satisfied with the levels of affection and trust in their relationship, thereby mitigating the adverse relational effects of attachment insecurities. In other words, gratifying sex can cause both anxiously and avoidantly attached partners to feel more satisfied in their relationships, as long as it helps them perceive their partners as more available and responsive to their needs and alleviates the fears that typically damage their relationships.

Unfortunately, in the long run, not only can the relationships of avoidant partners benefit from gratifying sexual activity but they can also be adversely affected by sexual difficulties, as demonstrated in a recent longitudinal study (Szepsenwol, Mizrahi, & Birnbaum, 2015). This study examined how chronic deactivation strategies in the sexual and attachment systems interacted within emerging relationships to affect relationship satisfaction over an 8-month period. At the beginning of the study, both members of newly dating couples completed a measure of attachment orientation. They also completed an instrument for assessing *sexual hyperactivation*, which is a predisposition that involves intense but anxious expressions of sexual desire (e.g., "During sexual activity, I worry about my sexual performance"), and *sexual deactivation*, which involves inhibition of sexuality (e.g., "Thoughts about sex do not especially excite or interest me"). In addition, they reported their relationship satisfaction three times during the study period. We found that sexual deactivation had detrimental effects on relationship satisfaction. Unsurprisingly, partners' attachment-related avoidance perpetuated the sexual deactivation effects over time.

## The Coordination of Attachment and Sex in Distress Regulation

The sexual system is particularly susceptible to being subordinated to attachment processes under relationship-threatening circumstances (e.g., insecurity regarding a partner's love, possible mate poaching, prospective separation). Such situations call for distress regulation and activate attachment behaviors such as proximity seeking (e.g., Davis et al., 2003; Mikulincer, Gillath, & Shaver, 2002; Simpson, Rholes, & Phillips, 1996). Because sex is a prominent way for adults to seek physical consolation, under such circumstances, the sexual system may be activated as well to provide the needed closeness and reassurance (Davis et al., 2004). Along with the normative activation of attachment needs, these anxiety-provoking situations are likely to elicit insecurely attached individuals' attachment concerns and related defensive strategies (e.g., Mikulincer & Shaver, 2007a; Simpson & Rholes, 1994). To the extent that sexual behaviors serve the goals of attachment system deactivation or hyperactivation (e.g., limiting intimacy during sexual activity to maintain distance, engaging in sex to avoid rejection, respectively; Birnbaum, 2010; Davis et al., 2006), it is reasonable to expect that under relationship-threatening conditions, the sexual manifestations of these strategies will be especially pronounced.

This theorizing has gained support from several studies that explored sexual responses to a variety of relationship-threatening conditions (e.g., hypothetical relationship threat scenarios, actual troubled interactions). For example, in two series of experiments, participants imagined relationship-threatening scenes (e.g., a partner who considers breaking up, a partner's infidelity), non-relationship-threatening scenes (failure on an examination), or nonthreatening scenarios (e.g., a partner going to a grocery store). Following this procedure, participants rated or described their desire to have sex, reasons for engaging in sex (Birnbaum, Weisberg, et al., 2011), and their sexual fantasies (Birnbaum, Svitelman, Bar-Shalom, & Porat, 2008). We found that anxiously attached people reacted to relationship threat with a mix of insecurity and anger. Specifically, they expressed an intense desire to satisfy partners sexually in their fantasies, but at the same time, they represented themselves in these fantasies as alienated and hostile (Birnbaum et al., 2008).

Relationship threats obviously exacerbate anxiously attached people's habitual insecurity, motivating them to respond with relationship-maintaining behaviors while forgoing their own sexual preferences and satisfaction. The resulting frustration provokes anger toward the threatening partner and amplifies their habitual negative self-representations (e.g., Campbell & Marshall, 2011; Mikulincer & Shaver, 2007a). The ambivalent reaction that relationship threat invokes in anxiously attached people impedes their ability to pursue sexual gratification, as indicated by their reduced hedonistic motivation (Birnbaum, Weisberg, et al., 2011). This intense emotional reaction is also manifested in relationship-damaging behaviors (e.g., recurring bouts of uncontrollable anger, excessive partner surveillance; Guerrero, 1998; Mikulincer & Shaver, 2005) that eventually sabotage their attempts to repair the threatened relationship, confirming their worst fears of relationship loss (e.g., Campbell & Marshall, 2011; Campbell, Simpson, Boldry, & Kashy, 2005; Simpson et al., 1996). Strangely enough, although anxiously attached people have trouble enjoying sex when being flooded with relationship worries, they seem to change their outlook and adopt a "seize the day" approach when death, the final separation, is salient (Birnbaum, Hirschberger, et al., 2011). It is possible that death awareness releases their fears, allowing them to focus on erotic pleasure, as they are less likely to be threatened by something they will inevitably lose.

Unlike anxiously attached people, who use sex to repair their threatened relationships, avoidant people react to threats by withdrawing sexually from their partners and using sex opportunistically. In particular, relationship threat lessened avoidant people's desire to have sex with their partners (Birnbaum, Weisberg, et al., 2011). Furthermore, reminders of death increased the tendency of avoidant people to have sex for self-affirmation reasons, and that of avoidant men to engage in emotion-free, casual sex (Birnbaum, Hirschberger, et al., 2011). These findings suggest that avoidant people attempt to protect themselves against mortality and attachment concerns by engaging in compensatory self-enhancement, as well as defensive distancing from a potentially rejecting partner.

A similar pattern of intensification of habitual defensive tendencies in the face of threat emerged in a fantasy study, which was conducted in a more natural context (Birnbaum, Mikulincer, et al., 2011). In this study, both members of heterosexual cohabiting couples reported their attachment orientations, then provided daily diary measures of their relationship interactions for 21 consecutive days. In addition, immediately after every sexual fantasy during the study period, participants described it in narrative form. The findings showed that distressful relationship events led anxiously attached people to switch from fantasizing about attachment themes, in which they expressed a desire for intimacy and represented the object of their fantasies as warm and affectionate, to fantasizing about submission themes that accentuated their neediness (e.g., portrayal of the self as weak and helpless). Avoidant people, by comparison, reacted to troubled real-world interactions with enhancement fantasies (e.g., portrayal of the self as strong and powerful) and distance-related wishes (escaping reality).

These findings demonstrate the involvement of sexual mental imagery in handling attachment-related stressful events and imply that such events induce compensatory processes that amplify typical attachment-related wishes and self-representations. Among avoidant people, threatening events heighten rejection concerns that trigger a self-regulatory mechanism designed to defend the self against rejection. These mechanisms include compensatory self-enhancement (Andersen & Chen, 2002; Bartz & Lydon, 2004) and defensive distancing from the potentially rejecting partner (Murray, Derrick, Leder, & Holmes, 2008; Murray, Holmes, & Collins, 2006). Among anxiously attached people, the same rejection concerns lead to self-minimization, and even humiliation, in the hope of eliciting caregiving from a powerful partner (Birnbaum, 2007b; Davis et al., 2004). These compensatory relational restoration strategies are intended to protect, at all costs, the threatened relationships.

The studies reviewed earlier indicate that reactions to threat are not necessarily uniform because threats may challenge different goals in different people (i.e., goals associated with different attachment orientations). Situations like the ones examined in these studies (Birnbaum et al., 2008; Birnbaum, Weisberg, et al., 2011), in which a partner explicitly considers ending a relationship or engaging in extradyadic affairs, are likely to challenge both relationship-promoting and self-image goals. As such, they may elicit reactions in the individual aimed at fighting for the specific threatened relationship, along with reactions intended to protect oneself from further losses of self-esteem (e.g., Birnbaum, Weisberg, et al., 2011). Still, reactions to threat may become uniform under certain circumstances, depending on the type of threat and the goals most likely to be challenged by a specific threat. For example, threatening circumstances that bypass the conscious evaluation of attachment-relevant experiences may produce general rejection concerns (e.g., feeling insecure about being loved). These rejection concerns may in turn lead to prioritization of self-protection goals over connectedness goals (Bartz & Lydon, 2004; Cavallo, Fitzsimons, & Holmes, 2010), which resembles the goals that typically motivate avoidant people (Mikulincer & Shaver, 2007a).

This point has been illustrated in a series of studies that examined the effects of activated attachment insecurity on the content of sexual fantasies. In two of these studies (Birnbaum, Simpson, Weisberg, Barnea, & Assulin-Simhon, 2012), participants were subliminally exposed to either a security or an insecurity picture prime (pictorial representations of either maternal caring or maternal rejection), after which they described a sexual fantasy narratively (Study 2) or completed a fantasy checklist (Study 3). The results showed that subliminally activated attachment insecurity exerted a uniformly avoidant effect on the content of sexual fantasies. Specifically, regardless of dispositional attachment orientations, implicit insecurity priming inhibited attachment themes (e.g., portrayal of the self and fantasy partners as affectionate and pleasing) and aroused fantasies that involved interpersonal distance and hostility themes (e.g., portrayal of the self and partners as aggressive and distant). These findings suggest the involvement of unconscious processes in which rejection concerns automatically activate self-protective fantasy responses. Such fantasies entail avoidance motivation that is geared toward protecting the self from further pain of rejection, while inhibiting relationship-promotion goals.

## The Contribution of Partner's Attachment Orientation to Sexual Dynamics

Although sex may involve a solitary act of pleasure, sexual experiences are often integrated into a relational context that influences their construal. Hence, sexual responses to both threatening and unthreatening circumstances may be determined, not only by each individual's characteristics, desires, and experiences, but also by those of her or his partner, as illustrated by several studies. These studies indicate, for example, that partners of anxiously attached people do not report greater levels of sexual dissatisfaction compared to partners of less anxiously attached people, at least in nonclinical samples (Butzer & Campbell, 2008; Impett & Peplau, 2002; but see Brassard, Péloquin, Dupuy, Wright, & Shaver, 2012, for different results in couples seeking marital therapy).

Given that anxiously attached people are oriented toward pleasing their partners during sexual interactions and complying with their wishes (e.g., Davis et al., 2006), it is hardly surprising that their partners are satisfied with their sexual lives. This is not to say that an anxiously attached partner's behavior may not cause sexual and relational difficulties, but rather that their conduct in the sexual domain may compensate for some of their relationship deficiencies. To take one example, men with anxiously attached partners do experience relational distress following negative sexual interactions, probably due to the destructive behavior that such experiences trigger in their partners. However, anxiously attached partners' compensatory behavior seems to offset the negative reaction that their behavior initially evokes, at least inside the bedroom (Birnbaum et al., 2006). In contrast, and as might be expected, partners of avoidant people are generally less satisfied with their sex lives compared to partners of less avoidant people (e.g., Butzer & Campbell, 2008). Moreover, unlike partners of anxiously attached men, partners of avoidant men are unlikely to exhibit less relationship-damaging behaviors following sexual interactions and are less likely to gain overall from such interactions, possibly because sex with an avoidant man is unlikely to meet their emotional needs and to console them (Birnbaum et al., 2006).

This dynamic is even more accentuated when couples face a relationship conflict, as illustrated in a recent study exploring the effects of relationship conflict on sexual motivation (Birnbaum et al., 2013). Couples who attended a laboratory session were randomly assigned to one of two conditions: Half were videotaped as they discussed a major problem in their relationship, whereas the others served as a control group and discussed their daily routine. After the discussion, both partners independently completed measures of perceived partner sexual attractiveness and sexual motives. We found that conflict discussions inhibited certain sexual motives (e.g.,

experiencing pleasure, obtaining stress reduction, feeling emotionally valued by partner) among people with avoidant partners but increased the likelihood of engaging in sex to feel better among people with less avoidant partners. These findings imply that people are unlikely to turn to avoidant partners for sexual consolation in what is sometimes "make-up sex." Indeed, avoidant people are inclined to dismiss their partner's sexual and nonsexual needs, as well as to distance themselves during conflictual interactions (Birnbaum et al., 2006; Mikulincer & Shaver, 2007a; Reis, 2007; Simpson et al., 1996). Therefore, they are less likely to be perceived by their partners as responsive, stress-relieving figures, either inside or outside the bedroom.

The studies demonstrate that a dyadic perspective may offer valuable insight into expressions of attachment dynamics in everyday sexual experience. Still, to uncover fully the interactive nature of couples' sexuality, research should take into account the unique configuration of both partners' attachment orientations. The predictive power of this approach has been described in a study in which both members of established couples reported their attachment orientations and sexual experiences (Brassard et al., 2007). This study highlighted a dyadic interaction pattern in which avoidant men were likely to avoid sexual activities in their current relationships, experience sexual difficulties, or have sex less often if their female partner was also avoidantly attached. This is likely the case because intimacy fears, which apparently burden both partners in this case, keep them from resolving their sexual and relationship problems.

Another dyadic pattern demonstrating that avoidant men are more threatened by intimacy than by its loss is that of avoidant men and anxiously attached women. These couples also report having sex less frequently, probably because anxiously attached women's needs for reassurance collide with their avoidant partners' negative stance toward expressions of intimacy. In addition, anxiously attached men have sex less often if their female partner is less anxiously attached. It is possible that anxiously attached men's efforts to have sex deter less anxiously attached partners, who may view such excessive demands as draining and exasperating. Yet the same sexual advances may be well received by partners with similar intimacy needs, as indicated by the finding that two anxiously attached partners have a relatively high rate of sexual intercourse.

## The Contribution of Sex to the Development of Attachment Bonds

The literature reviewed thus far shows how attachment processes influence the construal of sexual interactions in various relational contexts. Other studies suggest that influences in the reverse direction, from sexual to attachment processes, are also possible, such that sex can affect the attachment bond during its development. Indeed, although the sexual behavioral system evolved to motivate reproductive acts (Buss & Kenrick, 1998), impregnation was frequently not sufficient in ancestral environments for the survival of human offspring, who have a long period of development and vulnerability. This prolonged altriciality rendered biparental caregiving an adaptive reproductive strategy. That is, selection pressures have produced mechanisms that keep human sexual partners attached to each other so that the two of them can jointly care for their offspring and increase the offspring's chances of survival and reproduction (Birnbaum & Reis, 2006; Eastwick, 2009; Fisher, 1998; Hazan & Zeifman, 1994; see also Zeifman & Hazan, Chapter 20, this volume).

Such mechanisms presumably foster behaviors that promote proximity and affectionate contact (e.g., prolonged eye contact, cuddling, kissing), which distinguish attachment bonds from other types of social relationships (e.g., affiliative relationships) and other types of sexual connections (e.g., one-night stands). This complex constellation of proximity and affectionate contact is crucial for the formation of attachment bonds at any age (Acevedo & Aron, 2014; Hazan & Zeifman, 1994). However, the predominant motivations that enhance closeness frequently differ in infancy and adulthood: Security needs motivate proximity seeking and bond development in both phases of life, whereas sexual needs (or, more specifically, sexual desire) motivate proximity seeking and bond development only in adulthood (Berscheid, 1988; Diamond, 2004; Hazan & Zeifman, 1994).

### Unique Features of Human Sexuality and Emotional Bonding

Support for the notion that the sexual system has been "exploited" by evolutionary processes to promote enduring bonds between sexual partners comes from a closer look at the constellation of characteristics that distinguish human sexual-

ity from that of other mammals. Humans tend, for example, to have sex in private and to sleep together afterward (Ford & Beach, 1951). Humans also frequently have sex in the "missionary position" (Ford & Beach, 1951; Reinisch & Beasley, 1991), which, in contrast to the typical sexual positions of most mammals (e.g., canines), enables partners to maintain face-to face, belly-to-belly contact and look into each other's eyes during sexual intercourse. Such behavioral tendencies increase the likelihood of experiencing extended intimate contact and may therefore strengthen the emotional connection between sexual partners (e.g., Birnbaum, 2014; Hazan & Zeifman, 1994).

Additional suggestive evidence for the sex–attachment link derives from neuroimaging research that indicates certain brain regions activated during the experience of sexual desire (e.g., the caudate, insula, putamen) are also activated during experiences of romantic love (see Diamond & Dickenson, 2012, for a review). This overlap in neurological response suggests the existence of a neurobiological pathway through which sexual desire can affect the experience of love and attachment (and vice versa). Neuropeptides that are involved in both sexual and attachment behaviors modulate the functional connectivity between some of these brain regions (Bethlehem, van Honk, Auyeung, & Baron-Cohen, 2013). In particular, oxytocin and vasopressin—which are secreted in humans during foreplay, sexual intercourse, and the moments preceding orgasm (e.g., Carmichael et al., 1987; Carter, 1992; Filippi et al., 2003; Murphy, Seckl, Burton, Checkley, & Lightman, 1987)—facilitate bonding among both humans and other mammals (e.g., Acevedo & Aron, 2014; Carter et al., 2005; Ditzen et al., 2009).

This research suggests that sexual interactions activate the hormone-mediated mechanisms underlying attachment processes in both humans and other species. Still, distinctive characteristics of human sexuality may further increase the release of oxytocin during sexual intercourse and amplify its emotional bonding effects. For example, humans are the only species in which females show permanent breast enlargement that is independent of lactation. This sexually attractive feature furthers nipple stimulation during sexual activity, thereby reinforcing the release of oxytocin. Moreover, humans are rare among mammals in that they experience an extended exposure to oxytocin and vasopressin due to their tendency to have sex throughout the menstrual cycle rather than just prior to ovulation. Overall, the tendency to engage in regular sexual activity that often involves nipple stimulation may enhance sexual bonding in humans and, over time, promote enduring attachment bonds between sexual partners (Young & Wang, 2004).

## Mental Representations of the Sex–Attachment Link

Another line of evidence for the theorized link between sex and emotional bonding comes from phenomenological accounts of sexual experiences. In these studies, participants have been asked to describe the meanings they attach to sexual intercourse (Birnbaum, 2003) and their feelings, expectations, and beliefs about sexual activity (Birnbaum & Gillath, 2006; Birnbaum & Reis, 2006). The results indicate that both men and women commonly mention that sexual activity fosters intimacy between partners (e.g., "To me, sex is an important part of becoming really close to my partner") and nurtures their emotional bond (e.g., "To me, sexual activity is a way of forming an affectionate relationship").

A similar picture has emerged in research exploring people's descriptions of sexual motives. A broad array of potential goals motivates people to engage in sex (e.g., Cooper, Shapiro, et al., 1998; Hill & Preston, 1996; Meston & Buss, 2007). These goals vary across individuals, contexts, and partners (e.g., Birnbaum et al., 2013; Birnbaum, Weisberg, et al., 2011). For example, reasons for engaging in sex with an extradyadic partner (e.g., the desire for novelty and sexual variety) may differ from those that motivate sex in the context of an ongoing romantic relationship (e.g., deterring the partner from seeking sexual gratification elsewhere). Still, some of the most frequently endorsed reasons for having sex among both men and women reflect relationship-based motivation, such as the desire for emotional closeness and for intensifying the relationship (e.g., Meston & Buss, 2007). Viewed together, these phenomenological accounts of sexual experiences, meanings, and motives illustrate that people habitually associate sex with relationship promotion.

Subsequent research has extended these studies by providing evidence for the proposed causal pathway from activation of the sexual system to attachment formation and maintenance. In one series of experiments, participants were subliminally exposed to erotic words or pictures (vs. neutral words or pictures), then completed measures of willingness to initiate a relationship (e.g., self-disclosing to a potential romantic partner) or to engage in activities that increase the likelihood of maintaining an existing romantic relationship (e.g., sacrificing for one's partner). The findings indicate that subliminal exposure to sexually arousing stimuli (vs. neutral stimuli) increases willingness both to self-disclose intimate information to a potential new partner and to engage in relationship-promoting behaviors with current partners (Gillath, Mikulincer, Birnbaum, & Shaver, 2008). Hence, merely thinking about sex, even without being aware of it, may amplify relationship-promoting goals that encourage the use of strategies that allow people to get closer to potential new partners or to intensify a relationship with an existing partner.

## The Relationship Stage Model of Sexual Desire

Building on the argument that the sexual behavioral system has been altered by evolutionary forces to promote enduring bonds between sexual partners, Birnbaum and Finkel (2015a, 2015b) developed a model that delineates the functional significance of sexual desire in relationship development. The central tenet of this model is that sexual desire is among the most important contributors to the initiation, development, and maintenance of attachment bonds in adult romantic relationships. In particular, sexual desire for one's partner (or for a potential partner) serves the functions of assessing gut-level compatibility and determining relationship persistence at all stages. The dominance of these functions, however, varies substantially from one stage to the next. This model clarifies for whom, under which circumstances, and at which relationship stage sexual desire is most likely to influence the bonding process and the fate of the relationship.

When considering how the effects of sexual desire on relationship dynamics vary across relationship stages, the model delineates five such stages. In *the unilateral awareness stage*, A is aware of and forms some evaluative attitudes about B, but the two have not interacted (e.g., A has seen B's online dating profile). In *the surface contact stage*, A and B have interacted, but their level of interdependence is very limited (e.g., A and B have met for a cup of coffee). In *the emerging re-*

*lationship stage*, A's behaviors and experiences are becoming influenced by B's behaviors and experiences, and vice versa (e.g., A and B have started spending several nights a week together). In *the established relationship stage*, A's behaviors and experiences have become strongly influenced by B's behaviors and experiences and vice versa (e.g., A and B have bought a condo together and recently adopted a puppy). In *the fiery limbo stage*, A and B have broken up, but they continue to experience sexual desire for each other (e.g., A and B have broken up and live in separate residences, but they remain attracted to each other).

Of course, the desire for sex, in a general sense, can encourage relationship initiation even before A is aware of the existence of any particular partner. For example, if A is romantically unattached, she might be more likely to go out to a bar if she is experiencing strong rather than low sexual desire (Birnbaum, 2014, 2015). In this case, her desire is not directed toward any person in particular. Instead, the desire for sex functions to facilitate the pursuit of a potential partner who might serve (among other things) as a short-term or long-term sexual outlet (e.g., Fisher et al., 2002). In this way, these sexual urges increase A's tendency to put herself in contexts where she might meet such a partner. The following more detailed discussion of functional value of sexual desire across the five relationship stages focuses exclusively on sexual desire that is directed toward a specific person.

## Unilateral Awareness

In this stage, which represents the minimal definition of a relationship, one individual becomes cognizant of the other individual's existence under any of a wide range of possible circumstances (e.g., an online dating profile, a college course, a local dance club). At this stage, several factors influence how likely the individual is to initiate contact with the other individual to explore the possibility of a romantic connection (e.g., assessment of this individual's romantic availability and interest in him or her). According to the relationship stage model of sexual desire, one of the key predictors of the willingness to exert effort to meet a prospective partner (e.g., sending a first contact message) is the extent to which the individual experiences sexual desire for this person. In other words, the likelihood of initiating potentially romantic contact with a specific person is much higher if he or she arouses one's sexual desire.

## Surface Contact

In this stage, which represents a slightly less minimal definition of a relationship, the two individuals have interacted at least once but are only marginally interdependent. When the individual encounters the other person, he or she assesses the extent to which this prospective partner meets the standards required for further exploring the possibility of a romantic liaison (e.g., Li et al., 2013). In this mate-selection context, the desire to have sex with a potential partner may serve as a means of evaluating this partner's mate value and relationship compatibility (Birnbaum & Reis, 2006). As such, it functions as a gatekeeper that ensures that only compatible partners will be pursued (see also Bredow, Cate, & Huston, 2008). Increased sexual desire for a new acquaintance may signal high mate value or compatibility and is therefore likely to motivate the individual to exert effort to start pursuing a relationship with this desirable person (e.g., asking for a follow-up date). A lack of sexual desire, by contrast, may signify incompatibility and therefore motivate withdrawal from future interactions with this person (Birnbaum & Reis, 2006, 2012).

If so, partner traits that signal mate value, such as those that are theorized to promote reproductive success via parental investment or "good genes" (e.g., warmth-trustworthiness, attractiveness-vitality; Eastwick & Finkel, 2008; Fletcher, Simpson, Thomas, & Giles, 1999) may heighten sexual interest in pursuing individuals who have these traits and increase the desire to bond with them (Fletcher, Kerr, Li, & Valentine, 2014; Lemay, Clark, & Greenberg, 2010). Nevertheless, potential partners are likely to arouse sexual interest only as long as their demeanor indicates that they are compatible mates who will support one's goals (see also Holmes & Johnson, 2009). Support for this claim comes from research that explored sexual responses to a potential partner's provision of responsiveness (Birnbaum & Reis, 2012). Although perceiving a prospective partner as responsive to one's needs may signal that this partner is willing to invest resources in the relationship, not all people react to such expressions of intimacy in the same way. In particular, partner responsiveness heightens sexual interest in this person among less avoidant people, but decreases sexual interest among more avoidant people. Hence, people who typically pursue intimacy goals are likely to view responsiveness as an asset in a potential partner, whereas people who pursue the goal of independence rather than intimacy are likely to be threatened by the emotional closeness imposed by responsiveness.

## Emerging Relationship

Once a suitable partner is found, sexual desire for this partner may motivate a person to exert effort to build a deeply intimate relationship (e.g., spend more meaningful time together; Birnbaum & Gillath, 2006; Gillath et al., 2008). Then, as the relationship progresses from initial encounters to steady dating, partners ordinarily exhibit a rise in relationship maintenance behaviors and in their love for each other (e.g., Berg & McQuinn, 1986). At this stage of relationship emergence, sexual desire and the resulting sexual activity may function as one such ties-strengthening tool. Specifically, the more people desire their partners, the less they are likely to think about ending their relationship and beginning a new one (Regan, 2000). Although these findings imply that desiring one's partner helps a person focus resources on this partner, they do not indicate the emotional processes by which sexual desire contributes to consolidating attachment to a partner in the early stages of dating.

A recent longitudinal study has pointed to such mechanisms (Mizrahi, Hirschberger, Mikulincer, Szepsenwol, & Birnbaum, in press). In this study, both members of couples who had been dating for less than 4 months completed measures of sexual desire, frequency of sexual intercourse, and relationship-specific attachment anxiety and avoidance three times over an 8-month period. We found that relationship-specific attachment insecurities declined over time, but only among individuals who reported relatively high levels of sexual desire and high frequency of sexual intercourse. These findings imply that sexual activity carries the potential to reduce attachment defenses in the early phases of dating, which are inherently characterized by relationship insecurity (Eastwick & Finkel, 2008). By doing so, it produces a relationship environment conductive to the formation of genuine intimacy (see also Rubin & Campbell, 2012).

## Established Relationships

Once the attachment between partners has become well consolidated, sexual desire may still help to maintain the relationship (e.g., Bell, Daly, & Gonzalez, 1987; Birnbaum et al., 2006), but may become less important to its quality than other aspects of the relationship (e.g., Kotler, 1985; Sternberg, 1986). However, sex may turn out to be especially beneficial to the relationship of most people in relationship-threatening situations, when attachment-related goals of proximity seeking are particularly salient. In these situations, people may use sex to restore their endangered relationships (e.g., Birnbaum, 2014; Birnbaum et al., 2008). Frequent sexual activity can also buffer against the detrimental relational consequences of more chronic relationship deficiencies (e.g., neuroticism, poor communication; Litzinger & Gordon, 2005; Russell & McNulty, 2011). Such findings suggest that the intimacy inherent in sexual contact offers a compensatory route for satisfying the otherwise unmet attachment needs for security and love.

## Fiery Limbo

Relationship restoration is not always feasible and partners may drift apart. Following a relationship breakup, ex-partners may never see each other. However, ex-partners frequently stay in touch over the course of days, weeks, or longer, and can still experience deep emotional intimacy. Moreover, they may continue to experience sexual desire for each other and even have sex (Davis et al., 2003; Mason, Sbarra, Bryan, & Lee, 2012; Spielmann, Joel, MacDonald, & Kogan, 2013). The fiery limbo stage is this postbreakup state. One of the most important predictors of the willingness to consider getting back together rather than solidifying the breakup is sexual desire: If sexual desire is weak during this period, then the partners are likely either to become friends or to part ways altogether. If, in contrast, sexual desire is strong, then the partners are likely either to return to their established relationship or hover in fiery limbo and exert effort to continue experiencing intimate contact, pending a decision about whether they are willing to get back together.

## Concluding Comments and Future Directions

Sex has the potential to motivate intensely meaningful experiences whose nature and quality may vary across individuals and contexts. Sex may evoke both positive and negative affect, and it can affirm one's desirability or threaten one's self-worth. Sex may serve as a binding force that encourages emotional bonding between sexual partners. Yet sex may be what causes partners to grow apart, such as when sexual indifference motivates them to look for partners who are more desirable or compatible. As indicated in this chapter, attachment processes may explain some of the individual differences in such sexual experiences. Specifically, mental representations of self and other, developed from early interpersonal experiences that each individual carries forward into adult interactions, apparently determine what people want out of sexual encounters, how they get their needs met, and the functional significance of sex in their close relationships.

Obviously, other forces influence the underlying functions of sex and its contribution to relationship development. The person × context × time interactive framework offered in this chapter can clarify for whom, under what circumstances, and at which relationship stage sex is likely to affect relationship development. As discussed earlier, sex may serve attachment-based goals and assuage attachment insecurities when the relationship is relatively vulnerable, such as in the early stages of emerging relationships, and in partners who have certain negative characteristics or undergo relationship-threatening events. In such cases, sex is most needed as a relationship promoter and is therefore most likely to function as such.

Authors of most chapters in this volume were asked to say how research has developed and theory has changed since 2008, the year the second edition of this handbook was published. In the case of attachment and sexuality, most of the published research has appeared since that date. This new chapter is being included because the subject matter is theoretically and clinically important, and because the groundwork has now been laid for future theoretical and empirical developments. More research is needed to specify mechanisms through which sex influences emotional bonding and to further clarify how early attachment experiences interact with current experiences (e.g., provision of responsiveness, safe-haven caregiving) to affect the construal of sexuality during relationship development. Future studies should also explore the dual potential of the sexual system—on the one hand, to serve as a potent relationship maintenance mechanism and, on the other, as a force motivating people to pursue alternative partners in a world of changing societal trends (e.g., new patterns of sexual communication and "advertis-ing," and an increase in the social acceptability of alternative lifestyles, such as open relationships and polyamory). This is a topic area in which researchers have barely scratched the surface.

## References

Acevedo, B. P., & Aron, A. P. (2014). Romantic love, pair-bonding, and the dopaminergic reward system. In M. Mikulincer & P. R. Shaver (Eds.), *Mechanisms of social connection: From brain to group* (pp. 55–70). Washington, DC: American Psychological Association.

Allen, E. S., & Baucom, D. H. (2004). Adult attachment and patterns of extradyadic involvement. *Family Process, 43,* 467–488.

Andersen, S. M., & Chen, S. (2002). The relational self: An interpersonal social-cognitive theory. *Psychological Review, 109,* 619–645.

Barker, M. (2005). This is my partner, and this is my . . . partner's partner: Constructing a polyamorous identity in a monogamous world. *Journal of Constructivist Psychology, 18,* 75–88.

Bartholomew, K., & Horowitz, L. M. (1991). Attachment styles among young adults: A test of a four-category model. *Journal of Personality and Social Psychology, 61,* 226–244.

Bartz, J. A., & Lydon, J. E. (2004). Close relationships and the working self-concept: Implicit and explicit effects of priming attachment on agency and communion. *Personality and Social Psychology Bulletin, 30,* 1389–1401.

Beaulieu-Pelletier, G., Philippe, F., LeCours, S., & Couture, S. (2011). The role of attachment avoidance in extradyadic sex. *Attachment and Human Development, 13,* 293–313.

Bell, R. A., Daly, J. A., & Gonzalez, C. (1987). Affinity-maintenance in marriage and its relationship to women's marital satisfaction. *Journal of Marriage and the Family, 49,* 445–454.

Berg, J. H., & McQuinn, R. D. (1986). Attraction and exchange in continuing and noncontinuing dating relationships. *Journal of Personality and Social Psychology, 50,* 942–952.

Berscheid, E. (1988). Some comments on love's anatomy: Or, whatever happened to old-fashioned lust? In R. J. Sternberg & M. L. Barnes (Eds.), *The psychology of love* (pp. 359–374). New Haven, CT: Yale University Press.

Bethlehem, R. A., van Honk, J., Auyeung, B., & Baron-Cohen, S. (2013). Oxytocin, brain physiology, and functional connectivity: A review of intranasal oxytocin fMRI studies. *Psychoneuroendocrinology, 38,* 962–974.

Birnbaum, G. E. (2003). The meaning of heterosexual intercourse among women with female orgasmic disorder. *Archives of Sexual Behavior, 32,* 61–71.

Birnbaum, G. E. (2007a). Attachment orientations, sexual functioning, and relationship satisfaction in a community sample of women. *Journal of Social and Personal Relationships, 24,* 21–35.

Birnbaum, G. E. (2007b). Beyond the borders of reality: Attachment orientations and sexual fantasies. *Personal Relationships, 14,* 321–342.

Birnbaum, G. E. (2010). Bound to interact: The divergent goals and complex interplay of attachment and sex within romantic relationships. *Journal of Social and Personal Relationships, 27,* 245–252.

Birnbaum, G. E. (2014). Sexy building blocks: The contribution of the sexual system to attachment formation and maintenance. In M. Mikulincer & P. R. Shaver (Eds.), *Mechanisms of social connection: From brain to group* (pp. 315–332). Washington, DC: American Psychological Association.

Birnbaum, G. E. (2015). On the convergence of sexual urges and emotional bonds: The interplay of the sexual and attachment systems during relationship development. In J. A. Simpson & W. S. Rholes (Eds.), *Attachment theory and research: New directions and emerging themes* (pp. 170–194). New York: Guilford Press.

Birnbaum, G. E., & Finkel, E. J. (2015a). *The fragile spell of desire: A functional perspective on changes in sexual desire across relationship development.* Manuscript submitted for publication.

Birnbaum, G. E., & Finkel, E. J. (2015b). The magnetism that holds us together: Sexuality and relationship maintenance across relationship development. *Current Opinion in Psychology, 1,* 29–33.

Birnbaum, G. E., & Gillath, O. (2006). Measuring subgoals of the sexual behavioral system: What is sex good for? *Journal of Social and Personal Relationships, 23,* 675–701.

Birnbaum, G. E., Hirschberger, G., & Goldenberg, J. L. (2011). Desire in the face of death: Terror management, attachment, and sexual motivation. *Personal Relationships, 18,* 1–19.

Birnbaum, G. E., & Laser-Brandt, D. (2002). Gender differences in the experience of heterosexual intercourse. *Canadian Journal of Human Sexuality, 11,* 143–158.

Birnbaum, G. E., Mikulincer, M., & Austerlitz, M. (2013). A fiery conflict: Attachment orientations and the effects of relational conflict on sexual motivation. *Personal Relationships, 20,* 294–310.

Birnbaum, G. E., Mikulincer, M., & Gillath, O. (2011). In and out of a daydream: Attachment orientations, daily relationship quality, and sexual fantasies. *Personality and Social Psychology Bulletin, 37,* 1398–1410.

Birnbaum, G. E., Mikulincer, M., Szepsenwol, O., Shaver, P. R., & Mizrahi, M. (2014). When sex goes wrong: A behavioral systems perspective on individual differences in sexual attitudes, motives, feelings, and behaviors. *Journal of Personality and Social Psychology, 106,* 822–842.

Birnbaum, G. E., & Reis, H. T. (2006). Women's sexual working models: An evolutionary-attachment perspective. *Journal of Sex Research, 43,* 328–342.

Birnbaum, G. E., & Reis, H. T. (2012). When does responsiveness pique sexual interest?: Attachment and sexual desire in initial acquaintanceships. *Personality and Social Psychology Bulletin, 38,* 946–958.

Birnbaum, G. E., Reis, H. T., Mikulincer, M., Gillath, O., & Orpaz, A. (2006). When sex is more than just sex: Attachment orientations, sexual experience, and relationship quality. *Journal of Personality and Social Psychology, 91,* 929–943.

Birnbaum, G. E., Simpson, J. A., Weisberg, Y. J., Barnea, E., & Assulin-Simhon, Z. (2012). Is it my overactive imagination?: The effects of contextually activated attachment insecurity on sexual fantasies. *Journal of Social and Personal Relationships, 29,* 1131–1152.

Birnbaum, G. E., Svitelman, N., Bar-Shalom, A., & Porat, O. (2008). The thin line between reality and imagination: Attachment orientations and the effects of relationship threats on sexual fantasies. *Personality and Social Psychology Bulletin, 34,* 1185–1199.

Birnbaum, G. E., Weisberg, Y. J., & Simpson, J. A. (2011). Desire under attack: Attachment orientations and the effects of relationship threat on sexual motivations. *Journal of Social and Personal Relationships, 28,* 448–468.

Bogaert, A. F., & Sadava, S. (2002). Adult attachment and sexual behavior. *Personal Relationships, 9,* 191–204.

Bowlby, J. (1973). *Attachment and loss: Vol. 2. Separation: Anxiety and anger.* New York: Basic Books.

Bowlby, J. (1982). *Attachment and loss: Vol. 1. Attachment* (2nd ed.). New York: Basic Books. (Original work published 1969)

Brassard, A., Péloquin, K., Dupuy, E., Wright, J., & Shaver, P. R. (2012). Romantic attachment predicting sexual satisfaction in couples seeking marital therapy. *Journal of Sex and Marital Therapy, 38,* 245–262.

Brassard, A., Shaver, P. R., & Lussier, Y. (2007). Attachment, sexual experience, and sexual pressure in romantic relationships: A dyadic approach. *Personal Relationships, 14,* 475–494.

Bredow, C. A., Cate, R. M., & Huston, T. L. (2008). Have we met before?: A conceptual model of first romantic encounters. In S. Sprecher, A. Wenzel, & J. Harvey (Eds.), *Handbook of relationship initiation* (pp. 3–28). New York: Psychology Press.

Brennan, K. A., & Shaver, P. R. (1995). Dimensions of adult attachment, affect regulation, and romantic relationship functioning. *Personality and Social Psychology Bulletin, 21,* 267–283.

Burri, A., Schweitzer, R., & O'Brien, J. (2014). Correlates of female sexual functioning: Adult attachment and differentiation of self. *Journal of Sexual Medicine, 11*(9), 2188–2195.

Buss, D. M., & Kenrick, D. T. (1998). Evolutionary social psychology. In D. T. Gilbert, S. T. Fiske, & G. Lindzey (Eds.), *The handbook of social psychology* (3rd ed., Vol. 2, pp. 982–1026). New York: McGraw-Hill.

Buss, D. M., & Schmitt, D. P. (1993). Sexual strategies theory: An evolutionary perspective on human mating. *Psychological Review, 100*, 204–232.

Butzer, B., & Campbell, L. (2008). Adult attachment, sexual satisfaction, and relationship. satisfaction: A study of married couples. *Personal Relationships, 15*, 141–154.

Byers, E. S., & Heinlein, L. (1989). Predicting initiations and refusals of sexual activities in married and cohabiting heterosexual couples. *Journal of Sex Research, 26*, 210–231.

Campbell, L., & Marshall, T. (2011). Anxious attachment and relationship processes: An interactionist perspective. *Journal of Personality, 79*, 917–947.

Campbell, L., Simpson, J. A., Boldry, J. G., & Kashy, D. (2005). Perceptions of conflict and support in romantic relationships: The role of attachment anxiety. *Journal of Personality and Social Psychology, 88*, 510–531.

Carmichael, M. S., Humbert, R., Dixen, J., Palmisano, G., Greenleaf, W., & Davidson, J. M. (1987). Plasma oxytocin increases in the human sexual response. *Journal of Clinical Endocrinology and Metabolism, 64*, 27–31.

Carroll, J. L., Volk, K. D., & Hyde, J. S. (1985). Differences between males and females in motives for engaging in sexual intercourse. *Archives of Sexual Behavior, 14*, 131–139.

Carter, C. S. (1992). Oxytocin and sexual behavior. *Neuroscience and Biobehavioral Reviews, 16*, 131–144.

Carter, C. S., Ahnert, L., Grossmann, K. E., Hrdy, S. B., Lamb, M. E., Porges, S. W., et al. (2005). *Attachment and bonding: A new synthesis.* Cambridge, MA: MIT Press.

Cavallo, J. V., Fitzsimons, G. M., & Holmes, J. G. (2010). When self-protection overreaches: Relationship-specific threat activates domain-general avoidance motivation. *Journal of Experimental Social Psychology, 46*, 1–8.

Cohen, D., & Belsky, J. (2008). Avoidant romantic attachment and female orgasm: Testing an emotion-regulation hypothesis. *Attachment and Human Development, 10*, 1–11.

Collins, W. A., Welsh, D. P., & Furman, W. (2009). Adolescent romantic relationships. *Annual Review of Psychology, 60*, 631–652.

Cooper, M. L., Pioli, M., Levitt, A., Talley, A., Micheas, L., & Collins, N. L. (2006). Attachment styles, sex motives, and sexual behavior: Evidence for gender specific expressions of attachment dynamics. In M. Mikulincer & G. S. Goodman (Eds.), *Dynamics of love: Attachment, caregiving, and sex* (pp. 243–274). New York: Guilford Press.

Cooper, M. L., Shapiro, C. M., & Powers, A. M. (1998). Motivations for sex and risky sexual behavior among adolescents and young adults: A functional perspective. *Journal of Personality and Social Psychology, 75*, 1528–1558.

Cooper, M. L., Shaver, P. R., & Collins, N. L. (1998). Attachment styles, emotion regulation, and adjustment in adolescence. *Journal of Personality and Social Psychology, 74*, 1380–1397.

Cyranowski, J. M., & Andersen, B. L. (1998). Schemas, sexuality, and romantic attachment. *Journal of Personality and Social Psychology, 74*, 1364–1379.

Davis, D. (2006). Attachment-related pathways to sexual coercion. In M. Mikulincer & G. Goodman (Eds.), *Dynamics of romantic love: Attachment, caregiving, and sex* (pp. 293–336). New York: Guilford Press.

Davis, D., Shaver, P. R., & Vernon, M. L. (2003). Physical, emotional, and behavioral reactions to breaking up. *Personality and Social Psychology Bulletin, 29*, 871–884.

Davis, D., Shaver, P. R., & Vernon, M. L. (2004). Attachment style and subjective motivations for sex. *Personality and Social Psychology Bulletin, 30*, 1076–1090.

Davis, D., Shaver, P. R., Widaman, K. F., Vernon, M. L., Follette, W. C., & Beitz, K. (2006). "I can't get no satisfaction": Insecure attachment, inhibited sexual communication, and sexual dissatisfaction. *Personal Relationships, 13*, 465–483.

Del Giudice, M. (2009). Sex, attachment, and the development of reproductive strategies. *Behavioral and Brain Sciences, 32*, 1–67.

DeLamater, J. D. (1987). Gender differences in sexual scenarios. In K. Kelley (Ed.), *Females, males, and sexuality* (pp. 127–140). Albany: State University of New York Press.

DeWall, C., Lambert, N., Slotter, E., Pond, R., Deckman, T., Finkel, E., et al. (2011). So far away from one's partner, yet so close to romantic alternatives: Avoidant attachment, interest in alternatives, and infidelity. *Journal of Personality and Social Psychology, 101*, 1302–1316.

Diamond, L. M. (2003). What does sexual orientation orient?: A biobehavioral model distinguishing romantic love and sexual desire. *Psychological Review, 110*, 173–192.

Diamond, L. M. (2004). Emerging perspectives on distinctions between romantic love and sexual desire. *Current Directions in Psychological Science, 13*, 116–119.

Diamond, L. M., & Dickenson, J. (2012). The neuroimaging of love and desire: Review and future directions. *Clinical Neuropsychiatry, 9*, 39–46.

Ditzen, B., Schaer, M., Gabriel, B., Bodenmann, G., Ehlert, U., & Heinrichs, M. (2009). Intranasal oxytocin increases positive communication and reduces cortisol levels during couple conflict. *Biological Psychiatry, 65*, 728–731.

Eastwick, P. W. (2009). Beyond the Pleistocene: Using phylogeny and constraint to inform the evolutionary psychology of human mating. *Psychological Bulletin, 135*, 794–821.

Eastwick, P. W., & Finkel, E. J. (2008). The attachment system in fledgling relationships: An activating role for attachment anxiety. *Journal of Personality and Social Psychology, 95,* 628–647.

Ellis, B. J., & Symons, D. (1990). Sexual differences in sexual fantasy: An evolutionary psychological approach. *Journal of Sex Research, 27,* 527–555.

Feeney, J. A., Noller, P., & Patty, J. (1993). Adolescents' interactions with the opposite sex: Influence of attachment style and gender. *Journal of Adolescence, 16,* 169–186.

Feeney, J. A., Peterson, C., Gallois, C., Terry, D. J. (2000). Attachment style as a predictor of sexual attitudes and behavior in late adolescence. *Psychology and Health, 14,* 1105–1122.

Filippi, S., Vignozzi, L., Vannelli, G. B., Ledda, F., Forti, G., & Maggi, M. (2003). Role of oxytocin in the ejaculatory process. *Journal of Endocrinological Investigation, 26,* 82–86.

Fisher, H. E. (1998). Lust, attraction, and attachment in mammalian reproduction. *Human Nature, 9,* 23–52.

Fisher, H. E., Aron, A., Mashek, D., Li, H., & Brown, L. L. (2002). Defining the brain systems of lust, romantic attraction, and attachment. *Archives of Sexual Behavior, 31,* 413–419.

Fletcher, G. J. O., Kerr, P. S. G., Li, N. P., & Valentine, K. A. (2014). Predicting romantic interest and decisions in the very early stages of mate selection: Standards, accuracy, and sex differences. *Personality and Social Psychology Bulletin, 40,* 540–550.

Fletcher, G. J. O., Simpson, J. A., Thomas, G., & Giles, L. (1999). Ideals in intimate relationships. *Journal of Personality and Social Psychology, 76,* 72–89.

Ford, C. S., & Beach, F. A. (1951). *Patterns of sexual behavior.* New York: Harper & Row.

Fraley, R. C., & Shaver, P. R. (1997). Adult attachment and the suppression of unwanted thoughts. *Journal of Personality and Social Psychology, 73,* 1080–1091.

Gagnon, J. H., & Simon, W. (1973). *Sexual conduct: The social sources of human sexuality.* Chicago: Aldine.

Gangestad, S. W., & Thornhill, R. (1997). The evolutionary psychology of extra-pair sex: The role of fluctuating asymmetry. *Evolution and Human Behavior, 18,* 69–88.

Gentzler, A. L., & Kerns, K. A. (2004). Associations between insecure attachment and sexual experiences. *Personal Relationships, 11,* 249–265.

Gillath, O., Mikulincer, M., Birnbaum, G. E., & Shaver, P. R. (2008). When sex primes love: Subliminal sexual priming motivates relational goal pursuit. *Personality and Social Psychology Bulletin, 34,* 1057–1069.

Guerrero, L. K. (1998). Attachment-style differences in the experience and expression of romantic jealousy. *Personal Relationships, 5,* 273–291.

Hatfield, E., Sprecher, S., Traupmann-Pillemer, J., Greenberger, D., & Wexler, P. (1988). Gender differences in what is desired in the sexual relationship. *Journal of Psychology and Human Sexuality, 1,* 39–52.

Hazan, C., & Zeifman, D. (1994). Sex and the psycho-logical tether. In K. Bartholomew & D. Perlman (Eds.), *Advances in personal relationships: Vol. 5. Attachment processes in adulthood* (pp. 151–177). London: Jessica Kingsley.

Hazan, C., Zeifman, D., & Middleton, K. (1994, July). *Adult romantic attachment, affection, and sex.* Paper presented at the 7th International Conference on Personal Relationships, Groningen, The Netherlands.

Hill, C. A., & Preston, L. K. (1996). Individual differences in the experience of sexual motivation: Theory and measurement of dispositional sexual motives. *Journal of Sex Research, 33,* 27–45.

Holmes, B. M., & Johnson, K. R. (2009). Adult attachment and romantic partner preference: A review. *Journal of Social and Personal Relationships, 26,* 33–52.

Impett, E. A., Gordon, A. M., & Strachman, A. (2008). Attachment and daily sexual goals: A study of dating couples. *Personal Relationships, 15,* 375–390.

Impett, E. A., & Peplau, L. A. (2002). Why some women consent to unwanted sex with a dating partner: Insights from attachment theory. *Psychology of Women Quarterly, 26,* 359–369.

Jackson, J. J., & Kirkpatrick, L. A. (2007). The structure and measurement of human mating strategies: Towards a multidimensional model of sociosexuality. *Evolution and Human Behavior, 28,* 382–391.

Kotler, T. (1985). Security and autonomy within marriage. *Human Relations, 38,* 299–321.

Lemay, E. P., Jr., Clark, M. S., & Greenberg, A. (2010). What is beautiful is good because what is beautiful is desired: Physical attractiveness stereotyping as projection of interpersonal goals. *Personality and Social Psychology Bulletin, 36,* 339–353.

Li, N. P., Yong, J. C., Tov, W., Sng, O., Fletcher, G. J. O., Valentine, K. A., et al. (2013). Mate preferences do predict attraction and choices in the early stages of mate selection. *Journal of Personality and Social Psychology, 105,* 757–776.

Little, K. C., McNulty, J. K., & Russell, V. M. (2010). Sex buffers intimates against the negative implications of attachment insecurity. *Personality and Social Psychology Bulletin, 36,* 484–498.

Litzinger, S., & Gordon, K. C. (2005). Exploring relationships among communication, sexual satisfaction, and marital satisfaction. *Journal of Sex and Marital Therapy, 31,* 409–424.

Mason, A. E., Sbarra, D. A., Bryan, A. E., & Lee, L. A. (2012). Staying connected when coming apart: The psychological correlates of contact and sex with an ex-partner. *Journal of Social and Clinical Psychology, 31,* 488–507.

Meston, C. M., & Buss, D. M. (2007). Why humans have sex. *Archives of Sexual Behavior, 36,* 477–507.

Mikulincer, M., Gillath, O., & Shaver, P. R. (2002). Activation of the attachment system in adulthood: Threat-related primes increase the accessibility of mental representations of attachment figures. *Journal of Personality and Social Psychology, 83,* 881–895.

Mikulincer, M., & Shaver, P. R. (2005). Attachment theory and emotions in close relationships: Exploring the attachment-related dynamics of emotional reactions to relational events. *Personal Relationships, 12,* 149–168.

Mikulincer, M., & Shaver, P. R. (2007a). *Attachment in adulthood: Structure, dynamics, and change.* New York: Guilford Press.

Mikulincer, M., & Shaver, P. R. (2007b). A behavioral systems perspective on the psychodynamics of attachment and sexuality. In D. Diamond, S. J. Blatt, & J. D. Lichtenberg (Eds.), *Attachment and sexuality* (pp. 51–78). New York: Analytic Press.

Mizrahi, M., Hirschberger, G., Mikulincer, M., Szepsenwol, O., & Birnbaum, G. E. (in press). Reassuring sex: Can sexual desire and intimacy repair attachment insecurities? *European Journal of Social Psychology.*

Moors, A. C., Conley, T. D., Edelstein, R. S., & Chopik, W. J. (2014). Attached to monogamy?: Avoidance predicts willingness to engage (but not actual engagement) in consensual non-monogamy. *Journal of Social and Personal Relationships, 32*(2), 222–240.

Murphy, M. R., Seckl, J. R., Burton, S., Checkley, S. A., & Lightman, S. L. (1987). Changes in oxytocin and vasopressin secretion during sexual activity in men. *Journal of Clinical Endocrinology and Metabolism, 65,* 738–742.

Murray, S. L., Derrick, J. L., Leder, S., & Holmes, J. G. (2008). Balancing connectedness and self-protection goals in close relationships: A levels-of-processing perspective on risk regulation. *Journal of Personality and Social Psychology, 94,* 429–459.

Murray, S. L., Holmes, J. G., & Collins, N. L. (2006). Optimizing assurance: The risk regulation system in relationships. *Psychological Bulletin, 132,* 641–666.

O'Sullivan, L. F., & Byers, E. S. (1992). College students' incorporation of initiator and restrictor roles in sexual dating interactions. *Journal of Sex Research, 29,* 435–446.

Paul, E. L., McManus, B., & Hayes, A. (2000). "Hookups": Characteristics and correlates of college students' spontaneous and anonymous sexual experiences. *Journal of Sex Research, 37,* 76–88.

Paulk, A., & Zayac, R. (2013). Attachment style as a predictor of risky sexual behavior in adolescents. *Journal of Social Sciences, 9,* 42–47.

Potard, C., Courtois, R., Réveillère, C., Bréchon, G., & Courtois, A. (in press). The relationship between parental attachment and sexuality in early adolescence. *International Journal of Adolescence and Youth.*

Regan, P. C. (2000). The role of sexual desire and sexual activity in dating relationships. *Social Behavior and Personality, 28,* 51–59.

Reinisch, J. M., & Beasley, R. (1991). *The Kinsey Institute new report on sex.* London: Penguin.

Reis, H. T. (2007). Steps toward the ripening of relationship science. *Personal Relationships, 14,* 1–23.

Rubin, H., & Campbell, L. (2012). Day-to-day changes in intimacy predict heightened relationship passion, sexual occurrence, and sexual satisfaction: A dyadic diary analysis. *Social Psychological and Personality Science, 3,* 224–231.

Russell, V. M., & McNulty, J. K. (2011). Frequent sex protects intimates from the negative implications of neuroticism. *Social Psychological and Personality Science, 2,* 220–227.

Schachner, D. A., & Shaver, P. R. (2002). Attachment style and human mate poaching. *New Review of Social Psychology, 1,* 122–129.

Schachner, D. A., & Shaver, P. R. (2004). Attachment dimensions and motives for sex. *Personal Relationships, 11,* 179–195.

Shaver, P. R., Hazan, C., & Bradshaw, D. (1988). Love as attachment: The integration of three behavioral systems. In R. J. Sternberg & M. Barnes (Eds.), *The psychology of love* (pp. 68–99). New Haven, CT: Yale University Press.

Simpson, J. A., & Gangestad, S. W. (1991). Individual differences in sociosexuality: Evidence for convergent and discriminant validity. *Journal of Personality and Social Psychology, 60,* 870–883.

Simpson, J. A., Rholes, W. S., & Phillips, D. (1996). Conflict in close relationships: An attachment perspective. *Journal of Personality and Social Psychology, 71,* 899–914.

Spielmann, S. S., Joel, S., MacDonald, G., & Kogan, A. (2013). Ex appeal current relationship quality and emotional attachment to ex-partners. *Social Psychological and Personality Science, 4,* 175–180.

Sprecher, S. (2013). Attachment style and sexual permissiveness: The moderating role of gender. *Personality and individual differences, 55,* 428–432.

Stefanou, C., & McCabe, M. P. (2012). Adult attachment and sexual functioning: A review of past research. *Journal of Sexual Medicine, 9,* 2499–2507.

Stephan, C. W., & Bachman, G. F. (1999). What's sex got to do with it?: Attachment, love schemas, and sexuality. *Personal Relationships, 6,* 111–123.

Sternberg, R. J. (1986). A triangular theory of love. *Psychological Review, 93,* 119–135.

Szepsenwol, O., Mizrahi, M., & Birnbaum, G. E. (2015). Fatal suppression: The detrimental effect of sexual and attachment deactivation within emerging romantic relationships. *Social Psychological and Personality Science, 6,* 504–512.

Szielasko, A. L., Symons, D. K., & Price, E. L. (2013). Development of an attachment-informed measure of sexual behavior in late adolescence. *Journal of Adolescence, 36,* 361–370.

Szymanski, D. M., & Stewart-Richardson, D. N. (2014). Psychological, relational, and sexual correlates of pornography use on young adult heterosexual men in romantic relationships. *Journal of Men's Studies, 22,* 64–82.

Tolman, D. L., & McClelland, S. I. (2011). Normative sexuality development in adolescence: A decade in review, 2000–2009. *Journal of Research on Adolescence, 21*, 242–255.

Tracy, J. L., Shaver, P. R., Albino, A. W., & Cooper, M. L. (2003). Attachment styles and adolescent sexuality. In P. Florsheim (Ed.), *Adolescent romance and sexual behavior: Theory, research, and practical implications* (pp. 137–159). Mahwah, NJ: Erlbaum.

Wei, M., Mallinckrodt, B., Larson, L. A., & Zakalik, R. A. (2005). Attachment, depressive symptoms, and validation from self versus others. *Journal of Counseling Psychology, 52*, 368–377.

Weisskirch, R., & Delevi, R. (2011). "Sexting" and adult romantic attachment. *Computers in Human Behavior, 27*, 1697–1701.

Young, L. J., & Wang, Z. (2004). The neurobiology of pair-bonding. *Nature Neuroscience, 7*, 1048–1054.

# Chapter 23

# Same-Sex Romantic Attachment

Jonathan J. Mohr
Skyler D. Jackson

Without warning as a whirlwind swoops on an oak love shakes my heart.
—Sappho

Same-sex romantic relationships appear to have existed in most cultures throughout recorded history, regardless of prevailing attitudes toward homosexuality and bisexuality (Vasey & Vander-Laan, 2014). The scientific study of same-sex couples has evolved over the past several decades from an early emphasis on atheoretical, descriptive research to application of theories that were originally developed to explain different-sex relationship functioning (Kurdek, 1995). The emerging empirical literature on sexual orientation and romantic relationships provides strong evidence that the similarities between different-sex and same-sex relationships far outweigh the differences (Fingerhut & Peplau, 2013).

This chapter provides a basis for applying John Bowlby's attachment theory to same-sex love relationships. The now substantial body of research using attachment theory as a framework for investigating adult romantic relationships has shown not only that romantic love may be profitably conceptualized as part of an attachment-related process but also that diverse aspects of relationship functioning can be reliably predicted by differences in the ways individuals internally represent their attachment relationships (i.e., differences in their working models of attachment; for a review of this literature, see J. A. Feeney, Chapter 21, this volume).

The vast majority of work on adult romantic attachment has focused on different-sex relationships. Although strong arguments have been made concerning the ethical importance of including lesbian, gay male, and bisexual (LGB) individuals in mainstream psychological research (Herek, Kimmel, Amaro, & Melton, 1991), relatively few publications have acknowledged the potential relevance of attachment theory to LGB people or included empirical investigations focusing on this population. Conducting research with same-sex couples may be more challenging than that with other-sex couples (e.g., may require more effort in recruiting participants) and may seem unnecessary to some, given the small numbers of same-sex couples relative to other-sex couples—particularly in light of evidence of similarities between couple types. However, we believe including same-sex partnerships in attachment research can deepen understanding of adult attachment processes. For example, the study of same-sex attachments may help to illuminate ways gender and attachment interact in the dynamics of relationship functioning.

Furthermore, relationship difficulties associated with the enduring societal intolerance of same-sex partnerships may provide an opportunity to understand the role of attachment in how couples manage chronic stress and stigma.

This chapter first explores the evolutionary basis for same-sex attraction and provides an argument for the relevance of the attachment system for LGB adults. The current empirical literature on same-sex couples is then reviewed, with an emphasis on results suggestive of attachment-related processes. Finally, Bowlby's work on fear and loss is used to illustrate ways in which the study of same-sex couples may provide fertile ground for exploring points of intersection between cultural and intrapersonal forces.

## Evolution, Sexual Orientation, and Same-Sex Attachment

Perhaps one of the cleverest challenges to confront evolutionary theory is homosexuality. Homosexuality seems to be a tailor-made rebuttal of the great evolutionary credo—survival of the fittest. How do we explain what is often a lifelong preference for nonreproductive sex?
—JIM MCKNIGHT (1997, p. x)

At the core of Bowlby's (1969/1982) theory is the idea that the human propensity for establishing affectional bonds is adaptive from an evolutionary perspective: The infant–caregiver bond, the romantic partnership, and the intimate friendship all ultimately serve to enhance reproductive success. From an evolutionary perspective, the survival of an infant is usually in the best interests of both infants and their parents because they all have a stake in passing along their genes. Bowlby reviewed evidence that the attachment system in infants is activated most strongly in situations that are potentially threatening to the infant's well-being. The infant, at such times, engages in attachment behaviors that increase proximity to the parent—a figure who could provide protection in dangerous or novel situations. Attachment relationships in adulthood may serve the same adaptive function that they do in infancy. West and Sheldon-Keller (1994) argued that the "function of attachment, the provision of safety and security, remains constant throughout the life span, although the mechanisms of achieving this function change and develop with maturation" (p. 22). Thus, from an attachment perspective, romantic attachments provide adults with reliable

relationships upon which they can depend for protection, care, and support during times of greatest need (e.g., sickness, economic hardship, violent attack). Such protection increases the likelihood that adults will live longer lives, reproduce and raise children into their healthy adulthood, and possibly even provide care for the children's children. From this viewpoint, the establishment of stable romantic attachments may increase the likelihood of surviving into old age and enjoying the reproductive advantage this affords. Furthermore, the reciprocal attachments that characterize adult romantic relationships may serve to discourage dissolution and therefore provide a more secure environment for children.

The existence of same-sex romantic relationships and homoerotic attraction and behavior has long posed a vexing problem for evolutionary theorists. As one writer put it, "Homosexuals were with us through antiquity and, if recent history is any guide, are a robust minority within society. So why hasn't male homosexuality died out as a less reproductive strain of humanity?" (McKnight, 1997, p. 1). Some of the earliest uses of evolutionary theory to address same-sex attractions appeared in the medical literature of the late 19th century (Gibson, 1997). At that time, a common explanation for mental disorders was degeneration theory, which proposed that weakness of the nervous system caused individuals to be especially vulnerable to the primitive impulses constituting our evolutionary legacy. Individuals unable to resist the "beast within" were thought to fall several notches on the evolutionary ladder. Homosexuality was almost always viewed as a form of degeneration in which the original "bi-sexuality of the ancestors of the race, shown in the rudimentary female organs of the male, could not fail to occasion functional, if not organic, reversions when mental or physical manifestations were interfered with by disease or congenital defect" (Kiernan, 1888, quoted in Gibson, 1997, p. 115). Although such reversions were viewed in quite negative terms (and, as demonstrated below, were often linked with masturbation), some doctors recognized the existence of genuine romantic attachments between members of the same sex:

[Sexual perversions are] frequently produced on the neurotic soil of the male and female masturbator. The female masturbator of this type usually becomes excessively prudish, despises and hates the opposite sex, and frequently forms a furious attachment for another woman, to whom she unselfishly devotes herself. (Kiernan, 1888, quoted in Gibson, 1997, p. 116)

It is likely that this form of "furious" attachment was no more intense than those exhibited in other 19th-century sexual relationships. By focusing on same-sex love as a form of deviant sexuality, doctors were unable to recognize that such love was much more than a pitiable and loathsome expression of primitive sexual instincts. Although the outdated language of this example may make its absurdity evident, one does not need to look far to find similar examples from our own time. For example, same-sex couples are sometimes accused of flaunting their sexuality when exhibiting normative attachment or courting behavior, such as holding hands in public (Herek, 1991).

Bowlby also discussed homosexuality from an evolutionary perspective, but his thinking was markedly different from that of the degeneration theorists. Whereas 19th-century doctors viewed same-sex attraction as a lapse into brutish instinctive behavior, Bowlby appeared to think of homosexuality as the product of an efficient but functionally ineffective behavioral apparatus. In the first volume of his trilogy, he observed that the sexual behavioral system in same-sex dyads works perfectly well, in that the predictable outcome of orgasm is routinely achieved (Bowlby, 1969/1982). The puzzle, according to Bowlby (1969/1982), is why the sexual system would ever be organized in a way that runs explicitly counter to intuitive notions of reproductive fitness: "What makes it [same-sex attraction] functionally ineffective is that for some reason the system has developed in such a way that its predictable outcome is unrelated to function" (pp. 130–131). He illustrated this notion of misguided behavior by comparing homosexual sex to an antiaircraft gun that works perfectly, except that it consistently destroys friendly planes rather than enemy ones. This analogy may lack appeal for individuals in same-sex relationships, but it conveys Bowlby's idea that the sexual behavioral system of homosexuals is not serving its functional goal of reproduction.

Although Bowlby clearly saw homosexual desire as evidence of a functional mistake in the evolutionary sense, his limited discussion of the topic at no time denied that legitimate, psychologically healthy same-sex romantic attachments exist. Indeed, his writings about same-sex sexual behavior in a variety of animals primarily reveal his curiosity about the degree to which the sexual behavioral system is environmentally labile. He did not explicitly discuss same-sex couples, but it is likely that he viewed their relationships as subject to the same psychological principles as different-sex romantic attachment relationships. Bowlby maintained that the attachment behavioral system is active from "the cradle to the grave" (1988, p. 82), and he never gave any indication that he believed this to be true only for individuals in different-sex couples. In her initial writings about adult attachment, Mary Ainsworth, Bowlby's collaborative partner, noted that same-sex romantic attachments are likely to function in the same manner as different-sex attachments (Ainsworth, 1985, 1989). She stated that one of the main differences between these two kinds of romantic attachment is that only one of them (i.e., different-sex attachment) is sanctioned by society. This observation points to the importance of context in the development of attachment bonds—a topic discussed later in this chapter.

Bowlby's (1969/1982) discussion of homosexuality was based on his understanding of evolutionary theory, which was not informed by the currently accepted notion that evolutionary success is focused on the survival of the gene (Dawkins, 1976; Kirkpatrick, 1998). As noted below, evolutionary theorists have described possible scenarios wherein homosexuality may contribute to reproductive fitness even when lesbians and gay men do not have children themselves.

If homosexuality is indeed "one of the cleverest challenges to confront evolutionary theory" (McKnight, 1997, p. 1), then it is not surprising that attempts to explain it in terms of reproductive fitness have created such controversy. Bowlby (1969/1982) himself noted that the "task of determining precisely what the function of a certain piece of instinctive behavior is may be considerable" (p. 133). Within the past several decades, a number of interesting and provocative propositions have been made regarding the evolutionary basis of homosexuality (e.g., McKnight, 1997; Miller, 2000), and these have been met with strident opposition and critique (Dickemann, 1995; Santtila et al., 2009, Weinrich, 1995). A complete discussion of recent evolutionary theories of homosexuality is beyond the scope of this chapter, but a few of the most frequently noted theories are mentioned here.

Evolutionary theorists, faced with the puzzle of explaining the continued appearance of same-sex attraction throughout history, have assumed that there is a genetic component to same-sex sexuality (an assumption that has been supported by several twin studies; Hill, Dawood, & Puts, 2013). Although many specific theories have been advanced to address this issue, a number of them come down to the proposition that "gay genes" might offer a direct reproductive advantage to women and men who engage in different-sex relations. Hutchinson (1959) was one the first theorists to offer a scientifically grounded discussion of this possibility (McKnight, 1997). He applied then-current ideas about the adaptive value of the sickle-cell mutation prevalent in some African and Asian populations to evolutionary explanations of homosexuality. The sickle-cell mutation was found to increase resistance to malaria. Although homozygous sickle-cell children (i.e., children with two sickle-cell genes) exhibited strong resistance to malaria, they would often die of severe anemia before reaching puberty. Heterozygous children (i.e., children with one sickle-cell gene and one "normal" gene) would gain a measure of protection from malaria without developing the lethal anemia. These children therefore had an advantage over both the children with two sickle-cell genes and those with two non-sickle-cell genes. Arguments regarding homosexuality can, at least in theory, be made along similar lines: In this case, the assumption is that there exists genetic material that when present to a limited extent, increases the chances a person will have children, but, when present to an even greater extent, increases the chances that a person will have same-sex attractions. Thus, even if homosexuality itself reduces a person's odds of having children (and is thus disadvantageous from a reproductive fitness perspective), the person's biological relatives should produce a higher than average number of children.

Despite the potential for this perspective to explain the persistence of nonheterosexuality in humans over time, no "gay gene" has been identified—though several have been proposed and continue to be investigated (for a review of research on the biology of sexual orientation, see Hill et al., 2013). Some behavioral research, however, has tested hypotheses regarding genetically based characteristics that could both increase reproductive fitness among heterosexuals and increase the expression of same-sex desire in other family members. For example, Zietsch and colleagues (2008) used data from a large community data set of twins to investigate gender atypicality (i.e., the extent to which one possesses physical and behavioral characteristics associated with a different sex). The study was based on the notion that genetic material associated with gender atypicality may both increase a person's attractiveness to potential different-sex partners, and, when present to an even greater extent, increase a person's like-

lihood of having same-sex attractions. Zietsch and colleagues viewed this scenario as plausible given empirical evidence (largely correlational) of links between gender atypicality, attractiveness, and sexual orientation. Statistical modeling of twin data revealed that sex-atypical gender identity (i.e., the tendency to view oneself as having characteristics of a different sex) was positively linked both with nonheterosexuality and, among heterosexuals, with the lifetime estimated number of different-sex sexual partners. Analyses also suggested that these associations were driven partly by genetic material common to the characteristics. Data from female, but not male, participants supported the hypothesis that heterosexuals with a nonheterosexual twin would report a higher than average number of lifetime different-sex sexual partners.

Kin selection theory is the evolutionary perspective that has dominated much of the discourse on sexual orientation (Hill et al., 2013). Kin selection is an evolutionary strategy favoring behavior that improves the reproductive fitness of an organism's biological relatives, even if that behavior comes at a cost to the organism's own reproductive fitness. Wilson (1975) proposed that kin selection may explain the regular presence of homosexuality among humans, offering a view that might well be called the "helpful gay uncle and lesbian auntie" hypothesis. From this perspective, "the homosexual members of primitive societies may have functioned as helpers.... Freed from the special obligations of parental duties, they could have operated with special efficiency in assisting close relatives" (p. 555). The help provided to relatives would presumably increase the number of children who survive to reproductive age, have their own children, and pass along genetic material related to homosexuality. Empirical support for kin-selective explanations for homosexuality has been equivocal at best, with some studies aligning with the theory (e.g., Vasey, Pocock, & VanderLaan, 2007) and others casting doubt on its utility (Bobrow & Bailey, 2001; Santtila et al., 2009). These mixed results have challenged the kin selection hypothesis as an organizing theory of sexual orientation, and have led some scientists to draw on cultural and anthropological perspectives to explain mixed findings across samples and between cultures. For example, VanderLaan, Ren, and Vasey (2013) highlighted the potential importance of considering the cultural context in which kin-directed altruism may have originally evolved, and provided some evidence that humans' ancestral cultures may have featured socially sanctioned male transgender roles consistent with the kin selection hypothesis.

Another theory regarding the adaptive nature of homosexuality stems from a surprisingly consistent finding related to birth order. Many studies have indicated that a man's likelihood of having same-sex attractions is directly related to the number of older biological male siblings he has (for a review, see Bogaert & Skorska, 2011). This finding is clearly sex specific because it has emerged only with respect to men and their older male siblings. Moreover, research has suggested that a similar finding does not emerge when considering older male siblings who are not genetically related. The currently favored explanation for the fraternal birth order effect is based on the idea that in childbirth, mothers come in contact with their son's blood and produce antibodies to male-specific antigens. In subsequent pregnancies with a male fetus, the antibodies cross the placental barrier and somehow influence the developing fetus in a way that increases the likelihood of future homosexuality. Although intriguing, this hypothesis remains speculative (Bogaert & Skorska, 2011). Regardless of the biological processes underlying this birth order effect, how might the link between number of older biological male siblings and same-sex desire be adaptive from an evolutionary perspective? Some scientists have proposed that homosexuality in younger male siblings may decrease the extent to which they compete with their older male siblings for female mates, as well as for the familial resources, such as property and wealth, that may increase their chances of securing mates (Apostolou, 2013; Miller, 2000). However, this hypothesis has received little direct support. Instead, proponents of this theory generally base its validity on the fact that it explains various patterns in reproduction related to homosexuality (e.g., presence of a birth order effect among men but not women).

Despite uncertainty regarding the reproductive advantages associated with the hypothesized "gay" gene or genes, many evolutionary theorists agree on the mechanisms that maintain this genetic material in the gene pool (McKnight, 1997). A form of natural selection called *balance selection* is thought to favor a heterozygous genetic blend, in which men and women possess some homosexual genetic material, but not so much that they will favor homosexual relationships. Balance selection acts to harmonize the forces of *diversifying selection*, which creates great variation in the genetic code related to sexual orientation, and

*directional selection*, which removes genes of lesser overall adaptive value (i.e., homosexual genes). The existence of a continuum of sexual preference among humans is considered to be evidence of diversifying selection, whereas the greater number of different-sex partnerships compared to same-sex partnerships is taken as evidence of directional selection (McKnight, 1997). According to this general approach, evolution performs a balancing act in which so-called "gay genes" are actively maintained in the gene pool, while minimizing the extent to which individuals engage in exclusively same-sex sexual behavior. The potentially adaptive nature of same-sex sexual behavior has been suggested by its occurrence even in many nonhuman animals (for a review, see Bailey & Zuk, 2009), including evidence of enduring same-sex sexual pair bonding among nonhuman primates (Pavelka, 1995).

Most evolutionary theories of same-sex attraction tend to focus on the sexual behavioral system and do not explicitly address the formation of same-sex romantic attachments. What is clear from studies of love, satisfaction, and commitment, however, is that adult same-sex romantic attachments exist (Fingerhut & Peplau, 2013). Although the sexual attractions that precede or follow the formation of same-sex attachments may be the by-products of functional "mistakes" in the evolutionary sense (Bowlby, 1969/1982), no evidence exists to suggest that same-sex romantic attachment functions in inherently different ways than different-sex attachment (see the next section for a review of this empirical literature). Regardless of the precise evolutionary significance of same-sex attractions, it is apparent that LGB individuals have made important contributions to their families, to their communities, and to society. The attachment system offers these individuals the capacity to enjoy greater safety and security through intimate bonds, and thus increase their chances of surviving into old age and making contributions to others' lives over time. Also, given the great variability in sexual behavior among LGB-identified individuals, as well as developments in artificial insemination and family structures, significant numbers of LGB people have children (Patterson, 2013). Thus, romantic attachments may also increase these individuals' ability to provide for their children, as appears to be the case for different-sex couples (Weiss, 1982).

This discussion suggests that an evolutionary perspective on same-sex romantic couples must account for two separate but related phenomena: (1) sexual attraction toward a person of the same sex, and (2) pair bonding with a person of the same sex. Diamond (2003) has provided considerable evidence to support the idea that distinct evolutionary and biobehavioral processes underlie sexual desire and romantic love (see also Birnbaum, Chapter 22, this volume). The main evolutionary function of the sexual system seems clear: to increase inclusive fitness by orienting individuals toward potential reproductive mates. Perhaps the clearest evidence for this proposition is the rather pedestrian observation that most sexual behavior occurs between individuals of different genders (i.e., between individuals who, in principle, are capable of having offspring). Thus, the sexual system has evolved to encourage different-sex attractions. In contrast, as noted earlier, the romantic attachment system is thought to have evolved so as to encourage long-lasting relationships that can serve a protective function in childrearing. Unlike reproduction, which requires partners of different genders, the provision of protection is not tied to gender. An implication of this fundamental difference between the sexual system and romantic attachment system is that the two systems have different evolutionary roots.

Diamond (2003) described a number of studies suggesting that romantic attachment has much more in common with the infant–caregiver attachment system than with the sexual system. Her review indicates that there are substantial parallels between the emotional, biological, and behavioral processes underlying infant attachment and the corresponding processes in romantic attachment. Also, it is generally believed that the capacity for adult pair bonding evolved from the infant attachment system (Fraley, Brumbaugh, & Marks, 2005). Diamond (2003) argued that if these two manifestations of attachment do in fact operate similarly, then, just as the attachment system is not gender-specific for infants, the romantic bonding system should not be gender-specific among adolescents and adults. From this perspective, the tendency to form romantic attachments should not be limited to partners of different genders, and fundamental attachment-related processes should not vary according to the gender composition of a romantic dyad.

Furthermore, because the romantic attachment system is functionally distinct from the sexual system, it should be possible for same-sex attachments to be formed in the absence of sexual desire. In fact, as Diamond (2003) noted, nonsexual attachments between people of the same sex have been documented across diverse cultures

and historical periods. These passionate friendships appear to function similarly to attachment relationships that include a sexual component, featuring basic attachment behaviors such as proximity seeking in stressful situations and separation protest. Some of these nonsexual attachment relationships can even begin with the feelings of infatuation that are often associated with the early phases of traditional romantic courtships. The fact that nonsexual relationships can be "romantic," whereas sexual liaisons can occur in the absence of love, highlights the functional independence of the attachment and sexual systems.

Adding further complexity to this picture is the reality that sex and love are not altogether unrelated. Diamond (2003) offers an interesting discussion of processes through which love may lead to sex and vice versa. Examples of the former are found in Diamond's (2000) longitudinal study of women, all of whom self-identified as lesbian, bisexual, or "questioning" when the research first began. Some participants shared that their only experiences of same-sex attractions were in relation to emotionally intense friendships with specific women. Five years after the first interview, several participants had assumed a heterosexual identity. In these cases, the end of the passionate friendship marked the end of same-sex attractions. In contrast, a few of the lesbian-identified participants shared that they had become sexually involved with a close male friend with whom they had fallen in love, despite remaining mostly sexually attracted to women. Such examples underscore the importance of examining the effects of both intimate friendships and sexual attractions on the development of same-sex romantic relationships, all while keeping in mind the biological, interpersonal, and cultural influences on both sexual orientation and attachment bonds.

Charles Darwin (quoted in Rosario, 1997, p. 9) may not have guessed how long same-sex attractions would remain a mystery when he wrote, "We do not even in the least know the final cause of sexuality: The whole subject is hidden in darkness." Although the evolutionary significance of sexual orientation is still unknown, there appears to be no reason to assume that same-sex romantic attachments operate according to a set of different principles (e.g., set-goals, functions) from those operating in different-sex attachments. However, the unique cultural, interpersonal, and societal dynamics that differentially affect same- and different-sex romantic relationships (e.g., gender power dynamics, social stigma, history of HIV-related loss) may mean that, at times, attachment manifests differently and predicts distinct outcomes among these different populations. Much of the remainder of this chapter, then, compares current knowledge regarding different-sex romantic couples to emerging scholarship on male and female same-sex couples—highlighting areas of convergence, points of divergence, and areas ripe for future research.

## Attachment and Same-Sex Relationship Quality

We have been together 40 years and in these 40 years we were waiting for this.
—EIGEL AXGIL (quoted in Rule, 1989, p. A8)

This statement was made by a 67-year-old Danish citizen after marrying his longtime partner, Axel Axgil, 74, in 1989. They were the first officially registered same-sex couple in modern history. Perhaps the most remarkable feature of the modern same-sex romantic partnership is its resilience in the face of widespread societal condemnation. Despite recent victories in the fight for legalization of same-sex marriage and a broader trend toward the acceptance of LGB relationships in the United States, many same-sex couples still experience stigma, discrimination, and challenges to their legitimacy (McVeigh & Maria-Elena, 2009). In spite of this hostile climate, many LGB individuals manage to forge long-term intimate relationships and enjoy the sense of security afforded by growing older with a person who is invested in one's well-being over time (Fingerhut & Peplau, 2013).

The study of romantic relationships from an attachment perspective was stimulated by the seminal work of Hazan and Shaver (1987; Shaver & Hazan, 1988), who demonstrated that the patterns of attachment found in studies of infant behavior could be profitably applied to investigations of adult love experiences. Since that time, a considerable amount of research has investigated romantic attachment and suggested that it is best conceptualized in terms of two dimensions: attachment avoidance and attachment anxiety (Brennan, Clark, & Shaver, 1998; Mikulincer & Shaver, 2007). Individuals who rely on avoidant strategies minimize their attachment needs due to expectations of rebuff or rejection by romantic partners, especially in times of stress. Thus, high avoidance is associated with discomfort with closeness and interdependence. In contrast, anxious attachment

strategies are conceptualized as a hyperactivation of the attachment system, wherein one's expression of and vulnerability to distress are exaggerated to gain the attention of partners who are believed to be inconsistently available (Pietromonaco & Barrett, 2000). High attachment anxiety is characterized by fear of abandonment, a desire to merge with one's partner, and chronic frustration with what is perceived as a lack of closeness. A sizable body of research indicates the relevance of these attachment strategies in predicting indices of relationship quality such as satisfaction and commitment (e.g., Collins & Read, 1990; Hazan & Shaver, 1987; Kirkpatrick & Davis, 1994), as well as secure-base behavior in stressful situations (e.g., Simpson, Rholes, & Nelligan, 1992; Simpson, Rholes, & Phillips, 1996; for extensive reviews, see J. A. Feeney, Chapter 21, this volume; Mikulincer & Shaver, 2007).

Little empirical work on same-sex romantic relationships has been conducted from an attachment perspective. In what may be the first such study, Ridge and Feeney (1998) collected data from individuals associated with LGB organizations in Australian universities on attachment, romantic and sexual relationships, and—to be discussed later in this chapter—self-disclosure of sexual orientation. A main goal of the study was to replicate basic attachment findings from studies on different-sex couples among a sample of individuals in same-sex relationships. As a whole, results were consistent with findings based on different-sex samples, adding to the considerable evidence that same-sex couples and different-sex couples function similarly (Fingerhut & Peplau, 2013). Attachment security was positively associated with current romantic relationship satisfaction among participants in dating relationships. Individuals endorsing an attachment pattern of high anxiety and low avoidance were more likely than others to report a history of intense love experiences—a finding compatible with the view that anxious strategies involve hyperactivation of the attachment system. The opposite was true for individuals endorsing a pattern of low anxiety and high avoidance, consistent with the view that avoidant strategies involve suppression of intense attachment-related feelings.

Other researchers have provided data on similar links between attachment patterns and romantic relationship variables in LGB individuals. These studies have found associations between attachment security and relationship quality (Elizur & Mintzer, 2003; Kurdek, 2002; Mohr, Selterman,

& Fassinger, 2013), likelihood of being partnered (Brown & Trevethan, 2010), commitment (Kurdek, 1997, 2002; Mohr et al., 2013), communication patterns (Gaines & Henderson, 2002; Mohr et al., 2013; Starks & Parsons, 2014), and partner violence (Craft, Serovich, McKenry, & Lim, 2008). These studies indicate that attachment anxiety and avoidance are linked with less positive relationship evaluations and experiences, mirroring research on different-sex couples.

A few attachment studies have directly compared heterosexual and LGB-identified individuals. Ridge and Feeney (1998) addressed the basic question of whether the relative prevalence of attachment patterns differs in LGB individuals and heterosexuals. Using both dimensional and categorical measures of attachment style, the researchers found no differences between their samples of LGB and heterosexual college students. Kurdek (1997, 2002) examined links between dimensions of attachment and relationship functioning in samples of same-sex and different-sex couples. In neither of the studies did these associations differ for the two couple types. In short, those engaging in same- and different-sex relationships have been found to be similar both in attachment style and in relational correlates of attachment style.

The development and quality of romantic relationships is believed to be a function of not only a person's own attachment pattern but also the corresponding pattern of his or her partner (J. A. Feeney, 2003). Studies of different-sex couples have suggested that people may tend to seek relationships with partners who confirm their attachment-related schemas. For example, individuals with high attachment anxiety have been found to be involved with avoidantly attached partners, who corroborate their belief that they want more closeness than their partners do (Collins & Read, 1990; Kirkpatrick & Davis, 1994). Data from a large community sample of same-sex couples suggest that this may also be true for individuals in same-sex romantic relationships (Mohr et al., 2013). Results provided evidence of partner similarity on attachment anxiety and, to a lesser extent, avoidance. Moreover, people who were highly anxious over relationships tended to have partners who reported higher-than-average levels of avoidance. These partner-matching effects were equally strong for female and male couples, and remained significant even after researchers controlled for relationship length, suggesting that similarity was not due to mutual influence over time.

For different-sex couples, there is ample evidence that partner attachment plays a role in shaping individuals' relationship experiences and evaluations; this speaks to the value of viewing attachment-related processes as part of a dynamic and potentially complex system of mutual influence in romantic relationships (J. A. Feeney, 2003). Mohr and colleagues (2013) provided evidence of similar dynamics in same-sex couples. Results were particularly robust for attachment anxiety: Both own anxiety and partner anxiety were negatively associated with indicators of relationship quality (satisfaction, commitment, trust, intimate everyday discussion), and positively associated with indicators of relationship difficulties (intensity of relationship problems, communication problems). Similar results were obtained for own avoidance, although it was unrelated to relationship satisfaction and commitment. Contrary to hypothesis, partner avoidance was negatively related to ratings of aversive communication and unrelated to all other relationship variables.

Increasingly, research is examining the intersection of attachment and sexual behavior among LGB people. In one example, Ridge and Feeney (1998) found that dismissing participants were most likely to endorse casual sex and view sex solely in terms of its physical rewards, just as has been found in studies of heterosexuals (see J. A. Feeney, Chapter 21, this volume). Findings in a similar vein emerged in a study of male couples (Starks & Parsons, 2014), which found that avoidant men and their partners were more likely than others to report having unprotected anal intercourse with casual sex partners. Another recent study investigated links between sexual exclusivity and same-sex romantic relationship quality, examining the possibility that these links are influenced by attachment security (Mohr et al., 2013). As hypothesized, exclusivity and relationship quality were unrelated for secure participants but positively related in dyads in which either partner was high in attachment anxiety. Thus, although LGB people are less likely than their heterosexual counterparts to prefer exclusivity (Fingerhut & Peplau, 2013), high levels of attachment anxiety may increase the likelihood that outside sexual partners are viewed as threats to the primary relationship.

Several investigations of attachment and relationship satisfaction in different-sex couples have uncovered ways in which gender and attachment interact in predicting satisfaction. Probably the most robust result is that participants' and partners' ratings of relationship quality are best predicted by females' levels of abandonment anxiety and males' levels of avoidance (J. A. Feeney, Chapter 21, this volume). It has been hypothesized that these effects may be due to processes related to gender role socialization, such as a "wife demands, husband withdraws" style of conflict that has been linked with relationship dissatisfaction (Heavey, Layne, & Christensen, 1993). This relational dynamic is strongly suggestive of a female anxious and male avoidant pairing, and couples with this combination of attachment styles are precisely those that have been found to give the lowest ratings of relationship satisfaction in some studies (J. A. Feeney, 1994; Kirkpatrick & Davis, 1994). In addition to gender differences in the links between attachment and relationship functioning, differences have been found in ratings of attachment itself. For example, a study of romantic attachment across 62 cultures indicated that men reported higher levels of dismissing avoidance than women in virtually all regions sampled (Schmitt et al., 2003).

Do similar gender-related patterns emerge in same-sex couples? Even for those acquainted with the sexual orientation literature, it is difficult to make an educated guess about the answer to this question. One might guess that there would be fewer gender-related patterns in same-sex couples given evidence that same-sex couples are less likely than different-sex couples to base their relationships on traditional gender roles (Peplau & Fingerhut, 2007). However, research has indicated that lesbians and gay men differ in ways that are consistent with gender socialization processes (Fassinger & Arseneau, 2007), which might suggest that attachment-related dynamics in same-sex couples may be influenced by traditional gender patterns. Given these opposing perspectives, it is perhaps fitting that the limited empirical data on this topic offer an unclear answer to the question of gender. Contrary to gender stereotypes, studies have provided evidence of higher levels of attachment anxiety in gay and bisexual men than in lesbian and bisexual women (Mohr et al., 2013; Ridge & Feeney, 1998). Fear of abandonment may be especially high in male same-sex partners for a variety of reasons, including greater prevalence of nonmonogamy in male couples (Fingerhut & Peplau, 2013), expectations of lack of intimacy based on restrictive male gender roles (Brown, 1995), and exposure to the particularly negative attitudes and stereotypes associated with male homosexuality and bisexuality (Kite & Whitley, 1996). Findings from one study indicate that the general patterns of results regarding attachment and relationship functioning tend to be quite similar for female and male same-sex couples (Mohr et al., 2013). The main gender difference was the stronger relation for men between attachment security and indicators of relationship quality.

Dynamics reminiscent of traditional gender norms emerged in one study that examined attachment strength—as opposed to attachment style—in a sample of heterosexual and LGB youth (Diamond & Dubé, 2002). Each participant named individuals with whom he or she was most likely to exhibit four classes of attachment behavior: proximity seeking, separation distress, safe-haven, and secure-base behavior. The individual who was named in relation to the most classes of attachment behavior was viewed as the participant's principal attachment figure. Strength of attachment to the attachment figure was measured as a function of the number of classes of attachment behavior in which the participant engaged with the attachment figure. When the principal attachment figure was a romantic partner (as opposed to a platonic friend), the strength of attachment was significantly higher for lesbian and bisexual women than for their gay and bisexual male counterparts. For male participants, attachment strength was somewhat higher for heterosexual youth than for sexual minority youth when the attachment figure was a romantic partner, but somewhat lower when the attachment figure was a friend. For female participants, attachment strength was somewhat higher for sexual minority youth than for heterosexual youth when the attachment figure was a romantic partner. Diamond and Dubé (2002) speculated that these differences in strength of attachment may reflect gender role socialization practices, wherein expression of tender feelings and intimacy needs is discouraged in males and encouraged in females. Restrictive male gender role norms may explain why attachment strength was lowest in romantic relationships with two men and highest in relationships with two women. Of course, research is needed to determine the degree to which these gender differences were in part a function of the age group studied.

One unexplored area in which attachment-related gender differences may be expected in same-sex couples is sexual exclusivity. Male same-sex couples have been found to be more likely than any other type of couple to engage in sexual activities outside the couple relationship, and no significant differences in relationship satisfaction have been found among male couples based on sexual exclusivity (Fingerhut & Peplau, 2013; Kurdek, 1995). This finding suggests a few interesting hypotheses about the possible moderating role of gender in links between nonmonogamy and attachment. First, sex outside of the relationship may be more likely to be perceived as a threat to the attachment relationship in different-sex and female couples than in male couples. If this is true, then nonmonogamy should be more likely to activate the attachment system in different-sex and female couples than in male couples. Second, although attachment security has been linked to sexual exclusivity in a primarily different-sex sample (Hazan, Zeifman, & Middleton, 1994), this connection may not be as strong for men in same-sex relationships (Ramirez & Brown, 2010). Of course, the extent to which these hypotheses are confirmed may depend on cultural norms regarding monogamy, particularly given evidence that cultures vary substantially in views about and engagement in sex outside of a primary relationship (Munsch, 2012).

In short, these findings suggest that basic propositions regarding attachment dynamics in romantic relationships have been supported for same-sex couples, as well as for different-sex couples. Individuals in same-sex couples who are able to establish closeness with their partners and have trust in their partners' availability tend to be more satisfied with their relationships and to report more positive communication patterns. Furthermore, individuals' reports of relationship quality appear to be related to their partners' capacity for closeness and trust. A curious mixture of results has been found regarding the interplay between gender and attachment—some consistent with traditional gender roles, and others inconsistent. Greater clarity may be gained through couple research including assessment of variables that may moderate gender effects, such as adherence to gender role norms, adherence to traditional relationship values, and belief in negative stereotypes about same-sex couples. Differences between male and female same-sex couples with regard to sexual exclusivity may prove to be an area worthy of investigation from an attachment–theoretical perspective. Also, although it seems likely that attachment patterns play a role in the trajectory of same-sex romantic relationships (as has been found for different-sex couples; see J. A. Feeney, Chapter 21, this volume), longitudinal studies of same-sex couples are needed to confirm this proposition. Finally, caregiving dynamics in same-sex couples have been little studied, and would be valuable to examine from an attachment–theoretical perspective, as suggested by research on caregiving in different-sex couples (e.g., B. C. Feeney & Collins, 2001; see also B. C. Feeney & Woodhouse, Chapter 36, this volume).

## Fear, Safety, and Same-Sex Relationships

There were too many of them and they just knocked me to the floor. I couldn't get up and then they started kicking me in the back and the head. There was a group of people nearby who just stood there and did nothing, that's the worst thing about it.
—TONY MINION (who, with his same-sex partner, was attacked by five youth; quoted in James, 2012)

LGB individuals have achieved substantial political and social gains in the past several decades, but institutional oppression and social stigma toward the expression of same-sex desire remain realities throughout much of the world (Ahmad & Bhugra, 2010). Clinical theory and empirical research suggests that the climate of intolerance does indeed affect same-sex couple functioning, despite the movement toward greater acceptance of homosexuality and bisexuality. For example, clinical writings have suggested that both external manifestations of anti-LGB prejudice (e.g., violence, discrimination, rejection) and the internalization of negative views of same-sex attraction (e.g., internalized homonegativity, discrimination expectations) can lead to diminished satisfaction and greater conflict in same-sex couples (Brown, 1995), especially when partners differ with regard to their levels of internalized homonegativity and comfort with being "out of the closet" (Brown, 1995; Patterson & Schwartz, 1994). Such propositions are beginning to receive empirical support: Research findings have suggested that same-sex relationship quality is inversely related to perceived discrimination and stigma sensitivity (Mohr & Fassinger, 2006; Otis, Rostosky, & Riggle, 2006), internalized homonegativity (Balsam & Szymanski, 2005; Elizur & Mintzer, 2003), parental disapproval of individuals' sexual orientation (Smith & Brown, 1997), and chronic nondisclosure of sexual orientation (Berger, 1990).

Understanding the context of LGB individuals' lives is a prerequisite to articulating the unique ways in which attachment variables may play roles in determining same-sex romantic relationship functioning. The LGB identity development process often involves confusion, anxiety, and internal conflict. Many adolescents experiencing same-sex attractions hide this aspect of their lives and thereby suffer from a profound sense of emotional isolation (Savin-Williams, 1995). Those who do openly express their sexual orientation run the risk of ridicule, rejection, and threat. Data from large-scale studies in public high schools provide evidence that LGB youth experience higher levels of bullying, sexual harassment, coercive sex, dating violence, and threat or injury involving a weapon than do heterosexual youth (Goodenow, Szalacha, & Westheimer, 2006; Williams, Connolly, Pepler, & Craig, 2005). Not surprisingly, these studies also indicate that LGB youth are more likely to skip school due to feeling unsafe, as well as to report poor psychosocial functioning and little social support. The climate for LGB individuals is, to a great extent, a function of formal policies regarding homosexuality. Although a number of countries have introduced LGB-affirming policies over the past several years, same-sex sexual activity is criminalized in over 70 countries globally (Itaborahy, 2012). In some counties, homosexuality or same-sex sexual behavior is punished by flogging or death. The accumulated findings of studies such as these provide a sobering view of the difficult circumstances faced by many LGB individuals.

Given these precarious conditions, LGB individuals must learn to identify potential sources of threat and to manage the fear, shame, and anger associated with pervasive anti-LGB stigma and hostility (de Monteflores, 1993; Troiden, 1993). The process of learning to identify sources of possible danger is an important component of the fear behavioral system. Bowlby (1973) wrote extensively about humans' predisposition to react in a self-protective fashion to certain natural or innately recognized clues to danger (e.g., darkness, sudden noise, aloneness), as well as to cultural clues to danger that are learned by observation or personal experience. According to Bowlby, fear reactions are activated both by threatening stimuli (e.g., the approach of a hostile peer) and by inaccessibility of attachment figures (including perceived threats to the accessibility of attachment figures). An individual's total fear reaction at a given time is thought to be an additive function of all the fear stimuli present in the situation. Bowlby identified three behavioral outcomes of fear reactions: immobility (i.e., freezing), increased distance from the feared situation (i.e., fleeing), and increased proximity to one's attachment figure (i.e., seek-

ing). Individuals who are able to use their attachment figures as a secure base for exploration are believed to be less susceptible to fear stimuli than those with insecure attachments.

How might the attachment and fear systems come into play in the process of LGB identity development? If LGB identity development is conceptualized as an exploratory process, then attachment insecurity "may increase susceptibility to fear with regard to the tasks of identity development and curtail the exploration that is often critical in forging a positive LGB identity" (Mohr & Fassinger, 2003, p. 483). Support for this hypothesis has been found in a number of studies indicating that attachment insecurity is linked to negative identity and nondisclosure of sexual orientation (Jellison & McConnell, 2003; Mohr & Fassinger, 2003; Wells & Hansen, 2003). Although the data from these studies did not provide a means of exploring causal relations between attachment and LGB identity variables, the results suggest that attachment insecurity is associated with heightened fear and anxiety about behaviors that are thought to reflect acceptance and openness regarding one's sexual orientation. Responses to this fear and anxiety may involve actively "fleeing" the challenging tasks of LGB identity development, as well as "freezing" one's identity formation process.

The developmental tasks faced by LGB individuals may present what, from an attachment perspective, might be considered double-bind situations. For example, the process of *coming out* (i.e., disclosing one's sexual orientation) to one's parents may involve risking rejection from the very figures to whom one turns in times of distress. Although disclosure to parents is probably challenging for most LGB individuals, the difficulty of the coming-out process is probably even greater to the extent that the parent and child have insecure attachment patterns. Attachment insecurity could exert this effect not only through the poorer interpersonal skills associated with higher levels of anxiety and avoidance but also diminished capacity to negotiate intergroup contact (such as that between LGB youth and their heterosexual parents). This latter possibility is underscored by research suggesting that attachment insecurity is associated with higher levels of outgroup devaluation and threat appraisal (Mikulincer & Shaver, 2001). Few data are available on parent and child attachment dynamics in the coming-out process. However, research suggests that perceptions of early parental caregiving style are linked to likelihood of coming out and degree of parental rejection for one's sexual orientation (Carnelley, Hepper, Hicks, & Turner, 2011; Mohr & Fassinger, 2003). Parents with anti-LGB values may reject their children, regardless of the degree to which they provided a good early caregiving environment. This may help to explain research suggesting that LGB adults are less likely than their heterosexual counterparts to see their parents as a defining feature of their self-concept (Wilson, Zeng, & Blackburn, 2011).

An interesting implication of this possibility is that parent reactions to an LGB youth's coming-out process may alter his or her working models of attachment. A study of gay and bisexual men supported a model in which the association between memories of childhood gender nonconformity and current attachment security was explained by degree of anti-LGB rejection from parents and peers (Landolt, Bartholomew, Saffrey, Oram, & Perlman, 2004). The impact of parental reactions to coming out on LGB individuals' working models of attachment need not be only negative: LGB children may actually come to view their parents as more responsive and reliable as a result of a positive coming-out experience. Such changes may then broaden into a more positive general working model of attachment. Indeed, Carnelley and colleagues (2011) demonstrated that among sexual minorities, positive reactions from one's mother were negatively associated with romantic anxiety among adult gay men. Similarly, our work has indicated that parental support for one's LGB sexual orientation is related to current romantic attachment security, identity, and outness—even when we controlled for memories of early caregiving environment (Mohr & Fassinger, 2003). Although these models have yet to be tested through longitudinal research, the cross-sectional data are consistent with Bowlby's (1988) assertion that working models of attachment can change—for better or for worse—in response to significant experiences with caregivers throughout the lifespan. Regardless of the direction of causal influence between working models and experiences with caregivers, there is little question that LGB youth benefit from parental support. Hershberger and D'Augelli (1995) provided evidence that perceived familial support can serve as a buffer against the deleterious effects of victimization, particularly in regard to more threatening acts of violence.

Just as in the parent–child relationship, same-sex romantic relationships are not immune from double-bind situations. Consider, for example, the case in which one or both partners in a same-sex couple have internalized societal anti-LGB values and attitudes (i.e., have high internalized homonegativity). Such individuals are in the position of desiring romantic attachment relationships that go against their own value systems. Those who develop romantic relationships with same-sex partners may experience a push–pull dynamic, in which they simultaneously desire same-sex intimacy while wishing for distance from partners whose sex embodies the very opposite of what they view as acceptable. As noted earlier, indirect evidence for this proposition has been provided by studies showing that internalized homonegativity is a risk factor for romantic relationship difficulties in same-sex couples. The potential complexity of stigma-related dynamics is underscored by evidence that stigma functions at the dyadic level in same-sex romantic relationships (Mohr & Fassinger, 2006).

Such findings, taken together with attachment research, suggest ways in which attachment and stigma-related variables may be intertwined in determining same-sex relationship functioning. For example, as noted earlier, several studies have found an association between attachment insecurity and internalized homonegativity. One interpretation of this association is that internalized homonegativity may discourage the formation of same-sex bonds in which intimate closeness and trust can be tolerated. Although this proposition has not been tested directly, one study indicated that internalized homonegativity predicted decreases in closeness and commitment over a 2-month period among college students in same-sex dating relationships (Mohr & Daly, 2008). The irony of such a state of affairs is that the inability to use a partner as a secure base for exploration of an LGB identity may prevent an individual from gaining the experiences necessary to decrease levels of internalized homonegativity.

Acute stressors, such as the experience of anti-LGB violence or threats of violence, may also serve to activate the attachment behavioral system. The attachment system is believed to have evolved to ensure individuals' safety at times of greatest threat (Bowlby, 1973). Individual differences in attachment representations are expected to lead to differences in responses to threat (Simpson & Rholes, 1994). Research on responses to acute stress suggests that avoidant victims of anti-LGB violence may be expected to minimize both the impact of such an event and the need for support, whereas anxious victims may be expected to focus on their distress, to blame themselves, and to experience an intense need for soothing from their attachment figures (Mikulincer, Florian, & Weller, 1993; Simpson et al., 1992). Secure victims, however, may be expected to seek direct support for their distress (i.e., to use their partners as a safe haven) and to experience less symptomatology than their insecure counterparts. These different attachment-related strategies for coping may directly affect relationship functioning, or they may affect relationship functioning indirectly through the degree to which they maintain levels of symptomatology resulting from the traumatic stressor. For example, increased use of avoidant behaviors after an incident of anti-LGB violence may affect relationship quality directly through greater avoidance of intimacy and interdependence, and indirectly by maintaining depression levels, which in turn affect couple functioning.

A recent study, however, did not support the hypothesis that attachment security mitigates the negative effects of stigma on same-sex relationship quality (Mohr et al., 2013). Specifically, attachment security did not moderate links between minority stressors (e.g., experiences of anti-LGB violence and discrimination, internalized stigma) and relationship functioning. Similarly, another study failed to support the hypothesis that attachment security buffers the impact of perceived discrimination on distress among LGB people (Zakalik & Wei, 2006). Taken together, these two studies suggest that attachment and minority stress may influence well-being independently rather than interactively. That said, both studies had design elements limiting their ability to provide a strong test of the security-as-buffer hypothesis, including low levels of minority stress and omission of significant sources of minority stress (e.g., chronic self-concealment of sexual orientation). Perhaps most notably, reports of prejudice and discrimination in both studies were retrospective and focused on events that may have occurred many months or years prior to participation. Attachment may reduce the negative impact of specific stressors on psychosocial functioning at the time of the events rather than a substantial time after their occurrence. This possibility seems theoretically plausible because the attachment system itself is a dynamic system that is activated in response to perceived threat.

Finally, the relative invisibility of committed same-sex couples may make LGB individuals more vulnerable to negative societal messages regarding prospects for long-term relationships (Brown, 1995). For example, individuals may internalize the message that same-sex partnerships are primarily defined by sex, and are therefore under continual jeopardy of dissolution due to sexual temptations outside of the relationship or to sexual boredom. Individuals may also believe that same-sex relationships are less legitimate than different-sex relationships because of the relative lack of public, legal, and, in many cases, familial recognition of such relationships (Ainsworth, 1985; Brown, 1995). For LGB people with high levels of attachment anxiety, these beliefs may pose serious threats to their sense of security and lead to chronic activation of the attachment behavioral system. Avoidantly attached people, on the other hand, may respond to such beliefs by maintaining even greater distance than usual from attachment figures. Brown speculated that individuals who have internalized these types of societal messages may be vulnerable to romantic jealousy because they typically view same-sex partnerships as inherently less stable than different-sex relationships. Evidence that insecurely attached individuals are more susceptible to romantic jealousy (Collins & Read, 1990) and to maladaptive responses to jealousy (Sharpsteen & Kirkpatrick, 1997) suggests that the forces of societal heterosexism and attachment may be intertwined in complex ways.

Although the focus of this discussion has been on attachment, it is worth noting that similar dynamics may occur with respect to caregiving processes in same-sex couples. Research on different-sex couples has indicated that avoidant individuals tend to demonstrate lower levels of emotional support and responsiveness compared to others, particularly when their partners are viewed as distressed and needy (B. C. Feeney & Collins, 2001). There is no reason to believe that this basic dynamic would differ in same-sex couples. However, such dynamics would be expected to emerge not only in the stressful situations that all couples face but also in the manifestations of minority stress that are specific to same-sex couples (e.g., anti-LGB rejection, discrimination, violence).

This section has featured examples of attachment-related issues that are common among same-sex couples through their association with the enduring invisibility and hostility faced by LGB individuals. These examples may have given the impression that societal heterosexism, internalized homonegativity, and romantic attachment insecurity weave a web so pervasive and formidable that no same-sex couple can escape a miserable fate. As noted earlier, however, same-sex couples appear to be as satisfied and well adjusted as different-sex couples (Fingerhut & Peplau, 2013). Brown (1995) observed that all same-sex couples must face heterosexism and internalized homonegativity, even couples that have long and happy histories: "I ... know firsthand the challenges that an oppressive reality can throw in the faces of the most happy and well-functioning couples, even when both partners are skillful communicators with a strong commitment to the functioning and health of the relationship" (p. 276). Perhaps, as Simpson and Rholes (1994) have suggested, successfully facing adversity may actually strengthen such a couple's functioning. Learning with one's same-sex partner to negotiate the challenges posed by heterosexism and internalized homonegativity may provide a basis for revising and improving working models of attachment.

Despite such possible benefits of facing adversity, same-sex couples would probably benefit even more from systematic efforts to reduce sources of adversity through legal recognition of same-sex romantic relationships. Public legitimization of same-sex couples may strengthen relationship functioning in a number of ways (e.g., through larger support networks for couples, greater visibility of couple role models, and increased valuing of same-sex relationships). Legal recognition may also create structural barriers to relationship dissolution by increasing the seriousness with which partners take their commitment and requiring more effort of partners who wish to end a relationship. Indeed, evidence suggests that, for same-sex partners, legal recognition is associated with greater investment in the relationship (Fingerhut & Maisel, 2010) and increased relationship continuity (Balsam, Beauchaine, Rothblum, & Solomon, 2008).

Such findings raise the possibility that legal recognition may even lessen the effects of insecure attachment on risk of breakup. Legislation granting same-sex couples legal recognition has been passed in approximately 30 countries, starting with Denmark in 1989 ("Timeline of same-sex marriage," 2014). At this writing, 19 states in the United States provide some type of mechanism for same-sex couples to receive all or most of the state-level rights associated with different-sex marriage (CNN Library, 2014). Despite these developments, it is worth noting that same-sex couples are not given any legal recognition in most parts of the world.

## Loss in Same-Sex Relationships

Several weeks later I was cleaning the garage and found one of his old shirts tossed in a corner. It still smelled like him—that light orange odor. I also found our old beach ball, but I could not let the air out—his breath was in it.
—KENNETH MCCREARY (1991, p. 144)

Bowlby was deeply concerned with the psychological repercussions of losing one's attachment figure—a fact that is not surprising given the central role he accorded to achieving a sense of security and safety through attachment bonds. The final volume of his *Attachment and Loss* trilogy, *Loss: Sadness and Depression*, is devoted to the study of loss and mourning. Bowlby (1980) attempted to explain the process of bereavement from an ethological perspective, and therefore to normalize the intense affective, cognitive, and behavioral shifts that commonly accompany loss. He suggested that reactions to loss can be viewed as part of a broader category of separation from one's attachment figure. From an attachment perspective, the specific sequence of numbing, protest, despair, and reorganization found in infants following a prolonged separation is evidence of an innate behavioral system that has evolved to maximize proximity to caregivers (Bowlby, 1980); this cycle has been amply documented among infants, children, and heterosexual adults (Bowlby, 1980; Fraley & Shaver, Chapter 3, this volume).

Working models of attachment are viewed as moderators of the bereavement process. Anxious attachment, for example, has been linked to chronic mourning in adults (Bowlby, 1980). A person with high attachment anxiety who has lost a romantic partner through either death or relationship dissolution is likely to experience an extended period of yearning for the missing partner, characterized by high levels of anxiety and depression, as well as by unusual difficulty in resuming normal daily routines (Fraley & Shaver, Chapter 3, this volume). Conversely, an avoidant individual is likely to have minimal grief reactions to loss. Although Bowlby believed the suppression of grief to be associated with problems adjusting to loss, debate still continues about the degree to which this is the case (Fraley & Shaver, Chapter 3, this volume).

The attachment literature on loss and bereavement has not yet included reference to same-sex couples, but results from empirical studies of relationship dissolution can be interpreted from an attachment perspective. For example, one study of adjustment to dissolution of romantic relationships indicated that male and female same-sex couples did not differ from different-sex couples with regard to reasons for separation or levels of separation distress (Kurdek, 1997). The finding of no difference in distress levels among types of couples suggests that the attachment system may operate similarly for same-sex and different-sex couples in the context of relationship dissolution. Kurdek also found that predissolution levels of neuroticism (a correlate of attachment anxiety; Noftle & Shaver, 2006) predicted postdissolution levels of separation distress. This result is consistent with the notion that high attachment anxiety is associated with especially difficult recovery from loss and prolonged separation. In an earlier study of relationship dissolution, Kurdek (1991) found that participants who reported experiencing few postdissolution adjustment difficulties placed a low value on dyadic attachment and reported low levels of psychological distress. Given that avoidance is associated with devaluing attachment needs and underreporting symptomatology (Dozier & Lee, 1995), this result may suggest that avoidant LGB individuals tend to report low levels of adjustment problems after ending a romantic relationship. Similar findings have emerged in research with individuals in different-sex relationships. For example, Simpson (1990) found that avoidant men reported especially low levels of emotional distress 6 months after ending a romantic relationship.

The AIDS epidemic forced many gay male couples to confront issues of death and bereavement prematurely. The literature that has emerged from this epidemic provides ample evidence of loss and grieving in the context of same-sex romantic love. Folkman, Chesney, Collette, Boccellari, and Cooke (1996) conducted one of the most intensive studies of AIDS-related bereavement. This study examined preloss predictors of the course of postloss depression in 110 gay men whose partners died of AIDS-related complications. Each man was assessed bimonthly for a 10-month period, starting 3 months before the partner's death. The findings, described below, are consistent with many of Bowlby's assertions regarding loss.

First, although not surprising, the levels and persistence of depression found in this study were comparable to those found in bereaved partners of different-sex married couples, suggesting that few differences exist in the degree to which bereaved

partners in same- and opposite-sex couples experience despair. Folkman and colleagues (1996) constructed a predictive model of postloss depression that included variables representing a variety of domains: demographic, mental health, physical health, stress, resources, and coping. The only significantly predictive demographic variable was length of relationship. Interestingly, caregiver burden did not predict the course of postloss depression. However, the ability to view caregiving in positive terms was linked with faster recovery from postloss depression, consistent with the idea that people who are compulsive or anxious caregivers may be especially vulnerable to chronic mourning (Bowlby, 1980).

One important finding of Folkman and colleagues (1996) is that participants who reported high levels of preloss depression were more likely to have a rapid recovery from postloss depression than those who reported low levels of preloss depression. Interview data indicated that the caregivers were largely preoccupied with the ongoing losses associated with their partners' illness. Depressive mood in response to these losses may indicate a process wherein individuals were beginning to disengage from their partners in preparation for the impending death. This process of beginning bereavement prior to the loss of a partner may be viewed as an early phase of what Bowlby (1980) referred to as the stage of "reorganization." According to Bowlby, healthy recovery from loss requires an acknowledgment that the deceased is no longer available, combined with the ability to maintain a continuing secure bond with the deceased. Thus, beginning to disengage from one's partner before the partner's death may facilitate the process of reorganizing one's life and working models of the partner after the loss. Evidence of continuing bonds with deceased partners is found in such important symbols as the AIDS Memorial Quilt, commemorating those who have died of AIDS-related causes in the United States through panels created by the bereaved (Shelby, 1994).

Folkman and colleagues (1996) also found that levels of depression in bereaved partners who were HIV-positive did not decrease over the 7-month period following the loss. Similar results were found in another longitudinal study, wherein gay male participants who were both bereaved and HIV-positive reported the highest levels of distress (Martin & Dean, 1991). From an attachment perspective, these HIV-positive caregivers may have felt the need to serve as strong, reliable figures for their partners, while simultaneously experiencing attachment distress related to their own illness and the unavailability of their partners as caregivers for them. Thus, HIV-positive caregivers may feel compelled to hide their own attachment distress, which may subsequently lead to difficulties in processing the impending loss.

It is worth noting that what little scholarship exists on same-sex partner bereavement disproportionately focuses on partner loss due to HIV-related illnesses. A number of scholars have highlighted the inappropriateness of generalizing such results to other experiences of same-sex romantic loss (e.g., Bent & Magilvy, 2006; Hornjatkevyc & Alderson, 2011). For example, theoretical and qualitative scholarship has begun to explore the unique bereavement needs and barriers faced by lesbians (e.g., Broderick, Birbilis, & Steger, 2008; Jenkins, Edmundson, Averett, & Yoon, 2013). Lesbians typically do not face HIV-related stigma upon the loss of a partner and are theorized to construct relationship dynamics that differ from gay male relationships in emotional intimacy and balance of power, all of which may influence the experience of loss (Broderick et al., 2008). Gay men who have lost their partners to non-HIV-related causes are also theorized to face unique concerns, such as a lack of resources or support groups for gay men dealing with non-HIV-related bereavement (Hornjatkevyc & Alderson, 2011). They may face stigma due to the erroneous assumption that their partner died of HIV-related causes (and that they, therefore, are likely HIV-positive) and may feel compelled to distinguish their loss from HIV-related losses.

Finally, it is important to highlight the potential role of normative stigma-related hardships (e.g., peer rejection, social discrimination) in the bereavement process of LGB people who have lost a same-sex partner. Facing these hardships may help LGB people build resilience and resources for coping with a traumatic loss (Grossman, D'Augelli, & Dragowski, 2007); however, such challenges also may present unique barriers in the bereavement process. For example, some writers have suggested that loss of a same-sex partner may trigger feelings associated with earlier losses due to sexual orientation stigma (e.g., family and peer rejection, disconnection from racial/ethnic roots; Broderick et al., 2008). Also, being LGB and bereaved may be complicated given the potential for encountering prejudice (Almack, Seymour, & Bel-

lamy, 2010; Fenge & Fannin, 2009). For example, individuals may choose to meet their bereavement needs by accessing social support, which generally requires a disclosure of one's sexual minority status and may lead to invalidation or rejection as an LGB person. Indeed, qualitative research has suggested it is not unusual for bereaved LGB elders to find that heterosexual peers, family members, and mental health service providers fail to recognize the significance of their partnership—or, in some cases, serve as sources of anti-LGB condemnation. A grieving individual from a same-sex couple may attempt to preempt such experiences by concealing or minimizing their bereavement from people to whom they would otherwise disclose their loss. Those who either trivialize or distort the nature of their same-sex partnership (e.g., referring to a partner as a roommate) may experience decreased support during bereavement (Hornjatkevyc & Alderson, 2011). LGB people who choose to completely hide their bereavement may be at risk for *disenfranchised grief*, which refers to "a loss that is not or cannot be openly acknowledged, publically mourned or socially supported" (Doka, 1989, p. 4). Disenfranchised grief has a growing presence in the literature on same-sex partner loss and bereavement because it is theorized to compound the difficulties of the grief process.

Although research is equivocal on the relation between social support and bereavement symptomatology (Stroebe, Folkman, Hansson, & Schut, 2006), theoretical work and empirical studies on same-sex bereavement suggest that lacking support or facing rejection may prolong or complicate the grieving process (Bent & Magilvy, 2006; Jenkins et al., 2013). Of course, opportunities for receiving support are naturally influenced by the extent to which LGB persons have revealed their sexual minority status to others. When individuals facing a loss are not "out" to those from whom they would seek support, then they must make a difficult decision: Conceal the loss and relinquish opportunities for support, or disclose their sexual orientation at what is already a distressing time. Differences in disclosure have been linked with attachment avoidance level (Mohr & Fassinger, 2003) and sociocultural variables associated with environmental support for LGB people, such as age cohort (Almack et al., 2010) and race/ethnicity (Moradi et al., 2010). Such findings highlight the potentially complex interplay between attachment and culture in the bereavement process for those who have lost a same-sex partner.

## Looking Back, Looking Ahead: Summary and Conclusions

Our purpose in this chapter has been to articulate ways in which attachment theory may both contribute to and profit from the study of same-sex romantic relationships. Attachment-relevant research in this area has progressed in a slow but steady fashion in recent years. This gradual and incremental progress is evident when comparing this version of the chapter with the version in the 2008 edition of the *Handbook of Attachment*. Little has changed, for example, in research and theory on the evolutionary basis of sexual orientation, aside from new evidence that cultures vary widely in the extent to which the social roles of homosexual men are consistent with the kin selection hypothesis. New research on romantic relationship functioning has continued to support the view that attachment functions similarly in same-sex and mixed-sex relationships, broadening knowledge through the study of intimate partner violence, relationship status, communication patterns, and partner effects on relationship quality. To a lesser extent, new research in this area has provided insight regarding issues that differentiate same-sex couples from mixed-sex couples, such as work testing attachment security as a relational resilience factor with respect to effects of nonmonogamy and minority stress on relationship quality. The empirical literature on attachment and stigma now features additional findings consistent with the view that parental rejection based on a child's LGB orientation can influence the child's romantic attachment security. New work also raises questions about whether attachment security can mitigate the adverse effects of LGB minority stressors. Finally, this updated chapter features new work on loss and grief in same-sex couples, reflecting an increase in research on loss unrelated to HIV (including a welcome greater focus on female couples). New research and theory in this area has illuminated ways anti-LGB stigma may give rise to the experience of "disenfranchised grief" among people who have lost a same-sex partner.

The relatively slow pace of progress in these research areas is likely due to multiple factors, some of which may differ across specific areas of investigation. However, in no case is the slow pace due to a lack of potential new directions for research. For example, although scholarly interest in the evolutionary basis of homosexuality is not new, nearly all the literature on this topic prior to 2004 has been described as "overwhelmingly theo-

retical and speculative, with no grounding in any quantitative data whatsoever" (Vasey & Vander-Laan, 2014, p. 369). Genetic and cross-cultural research on sexual orientation over the past decade has highlighted potentially useful future directions and may generate greater enthusiasm for this area of scholarship. Beyond the methods explored to date, we believe cross-species research methods have potential for testing hypotheses regarding the evolutionary function of homosexuality and bisexuality. Fraley and colleagues (2005) used comparative and phylogenetic methods to identify characteristics of species exhibiting adult attachment, and to determine whether those species-level associations were due to shared ancestry or convergent evolution (the latter indicating a functional relation). Similar methods could be used to provide an entirely new perspective on kin selection processes and other characteristics hypothesized to accompany same-sex desire and pair bonding.

The study of same-sex couples promises to illuminate points of intersection between attachment processes and stigma, stress, and societal oppression in the functioning of romantic relationships. We believe longitudinal and macro-level research can contribute to understanding in this area of scholarship. For example, although recent research has indicated that attachment is related to variables associated with the LGB identity formation process, it is unclear whether attachment insecurity increases difficulties in the identity process, whether identity difficulties lead to changes in working models of attachment, or whether a third variable influences both attachment and identity. It is equally unclear what implications this may have for the formation, maintenance, and dissolution of same-sex couples. Furthermore, gender differences may contribute to the complexity of this picture. For example, research has indicated that women and men differ with regard to whether same-sex dating relationships begin via certain routes. One older study found that lesbians were more likely to have met their partners in work settings, and gay men were more likely to have met their partners in bars (Bryant & Demian, 1994). Such potential differences in the contexts of romantic relationship formation for lesbians and gay men suggest the possibility that the role and salience of working models of attachment in the early stages of LGB identity formation are moderated by gender. Also, the considerable variation among states and countries in legal status of same-sex couples—from jurisdictions that recognize same-sex marriage to those in which homosexuality is punishable through imprisonment or murder—offers a unique opportunity to examine ways institutional discrimination may influence romantic attachment, romantic relationship quality, and even the extent to which romantic attachment is linked to relationship functioning.

Why have such potentially rich areas for inquiry regarding same-sex couples received relatively little attention by scholars? We suspect the answer to this question may be related to both the continuing lack of interest in sexual minority issues among behavioral scientists and the growing acceptance of same-sex couples. On the one hand, the body of research on same-sex couples is still surprisingly small, a state of affairs made evident by a recent content analysis of 18 journals that publish scholarship on couples and family therapy (Hartwell, Serovich, Grafsky, & Kerr, 2012). The study revealed that 173 articles with significant focus on LGB issues had been published between 1996 and 2010, which reflects an average of less than one article per year in each of the 18 journals studied. Although this number reflects substantial growth in the study of LGB issues (an increase of over 200% in LGB-related publications relative to a similar content analysis covering the years 1975–1995), it is still relatively small. In short, the slow pace of attachment research on same-sex couples is not surprising in light of the slow pace in the greater literature on same-sex couples. Moreover, the small set of scholars who conduct research on same-sex couples may not be well acquainted with attachment theory and research.

On the other hand, we wonder whether the apparent lack of motivation to conduct attachment research with same-sex couples may also be driven by the increasing acceptance of same-sex couples and empirical findings of similarity between same-sex and different-sex couples. These trends may suggest to scholars that any findings for different-sex couples should translate to same-sex couples and therefore no need exists to test for differences or investigate the applicability of theories of romantic relationship functioning to same-sex couples. However, as described earlier, recent research has demonstrated ways that studying same-sex couples can enhance understanding of attachment processes. Despite the clear value of such studies, the modest amount of attachment research on same-sex couples suggests that the potential contributions of such research are not yet viewed by attachment scholars as sufficiently compelling to divert their attention from the many interesting questions that can be more

easily studied in different-sex couples. We suspect romantic attachment researchers often recruit or retain only different-sex couples for their studies because of an unexamined assumption of similarity between couple types, combined with a sense of unease about mixing couple types. One interesting question raised by this practice is whether different-sex and same-sex couples should be combined within the same study. In cases where differences between couple types are not expected, perhaps a case could be made for eliminating couple type as an inclusion or exclusion criterion. After all, participants diverse in race, ethnicity, and age are often combined within a single sample. However, in cases in which a scholar feels reluctant to combine the two couple types into a single sample, this may suggest that the area of inquiry is one in which the study of same-sex couples may be of particular interest to attachment researchers. It is our hope that awareness of such research areas increases among romantic attachment scholars, and motivates scholars to broaden their focus to same-sex romantic partners.

The examples offered in this chapter constitute a first step in identifying some possibilities for future study, but the list is hardly exhaustive. For example, longitudinal research on relationships between lesbian ex-lovers (a little-studied but much-discussed phenomenon; see Weinstock & Rothblum, 2004) may contribute to the growing literature on jealousy and attachment. Furthermore, knowledge about the interplay among the attachment, affiliative, and sexual systems may benefit from intensive study of the considerable diversity in the arrangements that LGB adults create to satisfy their emotional, romantic, and sexual needs (for an interesting discussion of such arrangements, see Rust, 1996). Another potentially interesting line of investigation may be to study the ability of LGB communities to promote secure romantic attachments through their role as a safe haven for LGB individuals and same-sex couples, particularly given evidence that individuals experience anxiety and avoidance in relation to their group attachments that are distinct from the corresponding dimensions of attachments to romantic partners (Smith, Murphy, & Coats, 1999). Furthermore, with a growing number of same-sex couples becoming parents, researchers may profit from examining existing theories of parent–child attachment among same-sex couples engaged in childrearing, due to the unique gender makeup of such families and the controversy that has historically surrounded same-sex parenthood (Goldberg,

2010). These examples, along with those discussed earlier, indicate that the study of same-sex couple functioning provides a rich forum for exploring the complex interplay of forces at the individual, dyadic, and societal levels—an interplay that potentially involves the attachment, fear, sex, and exploration behavioral systems. Mapping of this uncharted territory will both enhance attachment theory and provide much-needed data on same-sex romantic relationships.

## Acknowledgments

We would like to thank Jude Cassidy, Henry Hogue, Phillip R. Shaver, and Susan Woodhouse for their helpful comments on an earlier draft of this chapter.

## References

Ahmad, S., & Bhugra, D. (2010). Homophobia: An updated review of the literature. *Sexual and Relationship Therapy, 25*, 447–455.

Ainsworth, M. D. S. (1985). Attachments across the lifespan. *Bulletin of the New York Academy of Medicine, 61*, 792–812.

Ainsworth, M. S. (1989). Attachments beyond infancy. *American Psychologist, 44*, 709–716.

Almack, K., Seymour, J., & Bellamy, G. (2010). Exploring the impact of sexual orientation on experiences and concerns about end of life care and on bereavement for lesbian, gay and bisexual older people. *Sociology, 44*, 908–924.

Apostolou, M. (2013). Interfamily conflict, reproductive success, and the evolution of male homosexuality. *Review of General Psychology, 17*, 288–296.

Bailey, N. W., & Zuk, M. (2009). Same-sex sexual behavior and evolution. *Trends in Ecology and Evolution, 24*, 439–446.

Balsam, K. F., Beauchaine, T. P., Rothblum, E. D., & Solomon, S. E. (2008). Three-year follow-up of same-sex couples who had civil unions in Vermont, same-sex couples not in civil unions, and heterosexual married couples. *Developmental Psychology, 44*, 102–116.

Balsam, K. F., & Szymanski, D. M. (2005). Relationship quality and domestic violence in women's same-sex relationships: The role of minority stress. *Psychology of Women Quarterly, 29*, 258–269.

Bent, K. N., & Magilvy, J. K. (2006). When a partner dies: Lesbian widows. *Issues in Mental Health Nursing, 27*, 447–459.

Berger, R. M. (1990). Passing: Impact of the quality of same-sex couple relationships. *Social Work, 35*, 328–332.

Bobrow, D., & Bailey, J. M. (2001). Is male homosexuality maintained via kin selection?. *Evolution and Human Behavior, 22*, 361–368.

Bogaert, A. F., & Skorska, M. (2011). Sexual orientation, fraternal birth order, and the maternal immune hypothesis: A review. *Front Neuroendocrinology, 32*, 247–254.

Bowlby, J. (1973). *Attachment and loss: Vol. 2. Separation: Anxiety and anger.* New York: Basic Books.

Bowlby, J. (1980). *Attachment and loss: Vol. 3. Loss: Sadness and depression.* New York: Basic Books.

Bowlby, J. (1982). *Attachment and loss: Vol. 1. Attachment.* New York: Basic Books. (Original work published 1969)

Bowlby, J. (1988). *A secure base: Parent–child attachment and healthy human development.* New York: Basic Books.

Brennan, K. A., Clark, C. L., & Shaver, P. R. (1998). Self-report measurement of adult attachment: An integrative overview. In J. A. Simpson & W. S. Rholes (Eds.), *Attachment theory and close relationships* (pp. 46–76). New York: Guilford Press.

Broderick, D. J., Birbilis, J. M., & Steger, M. F. (2008). Lesbians grieving the death of a partner: Recommendations for practice. *Journal of Lesbian Studies, 12*, 225–235.

Brown, J., & Trevethan, R. (2010). Shame, internalized homophobia, identity formation, attachment style, and the connection to relationship status in gay men. *American Journal of Men's Health, 4*, 267–276.

Brown, L. S. (1995). Therapy with same-sex couples: An introduction. In N. S. Jacobson & A. S. Gurman (Eds.), *Clinical handbook of couple therapy* (pp. 274–294). New York: Guilford Press.

Bryant, A. S., & Demian, N. (1994). Relationship characteristics of American gay and lesbian couples: Findings from a national survey. In L. A. Kurdek (Ed.), *Social services for gay and lesbian couples* (pp. 101–117). New York: Haworth Press.

Carnelley, K. B., Hepper, E. G., Hicks, C., & Turner, W. (2011). Perceived parental reactions to coming out, attachment, and romantic relationship views. *Attachment and Human Development, 13*, 217–236.

CNN Library. (2014, July). Same-sex marriage fast facts. Retrieved August 19, 2014, from *www.cnn.com/2013/05/28/us/same-sex-marriage-fast-facts/index.html*.

Collins, N. L., & Read, S. J. (1990). Adult attachment, working models, and relationship quality in dating couples. *Journal of Personality and Social Psychology, 58*, 644–663.

Craft, S. M., Serovich, J. M., McKenry, P. C., & Lim, J. Y. (2008). Stress, attachment style, and partner violence among same-sex couples. *Journal of GLBT Family Studies, 4*, 57–73.

Crespi, L. (1995). Some thoughts on the role of mourning in the development of a positive lesbian identity. In T. Domenici & R. C. Lesser (Eds.), *Disorienting sexuality: Psychoanalytic reappraisals of sexual identities* (pp. 19–32). New York: Routledge.

Dawkins, R. (1976). *The selfish gene.* New York: Oxford University Press.

de Monteflores, C. (1993). Notes on the management of difference. In L. D. Garnets & D. C. Kimmel (Eds.), *Psychological perspectives on lesbian and gay male experiences* (pp. 218–247). New York: Columbia University Press.

Diamond, L. M. (2000). Sexual identity, attractions, and behavior among young sexual-minority women over a 2-year period. *Developmental Psychology, 36,* 241–250.

Diamond, L. M. (2003). What does sexual orientation orient?: A biobehavioral model distinguishing romantic love and sexual desire. *Psychological Review, 110,* 173–192.

Diamond, L. M., & Dubé, E. M. (2002). Friendship and attachment among heterosexual and sexual-minority youths: Does the gender of your friend matter? *Journal of Youth and Adolescence, 31,* 155–166.

Dickemann, M. (1995). Wilson's Panchreston: The inclusive fitness hypothesis of sociobiology re-examined. *Journal of Homosexuality, 28,* 147–183.

Doka, K. (1989). *Disenfranchised grief: Recognizing hidden sorrow.* Lexington, MA: Lexington Books.

Dozier, M., & Lee, S. W. (1995). Discrepancies between self- and other-report of psychiatric symptomatology: Effects of dismissing attachment strategies. *Development and Psychopathology, 7,* 217–226.

Elizur, Y., & Mintzer, A. (2003). Gay males' intimate relationship quality: The roles of attachment security, gay identity, social support, and income. *Personal Relationships, 10,* 411–435.

Fassinger, R. E., & Arseneau, J. R. (2007). "I'd rather get wet than be under that umbrella": Differentiating the experiences and identities of lesbian, gay, bisexual, and transgender people. In K. J. Bieschke, R. M. Perez, & K. A. DeBord (Eds.), *Handbook of counseling and psychotherapy with lesbian, gay, bisexual, and transgender clients* (2nd ed., pp. 19–49). Washington: American Psychological Association.

Feeney, B. C., & Collins, N. L. (2001). Predictors of caregiving in adult intimate relationships: An attachment theoretical perspective. *Journal of Personality and Social Psychology, 80,* 972–994.

Feeney, J. A. (1994). Attachment style, communication patterns, and satisfaction across the life cycle of marriage. *Personal Relationships, 1,* 333–348.

Feeney, J. A. (2003). The systemic nature of couple relationships: An attachment perspective. In P. Erdman & T. Caffery (Eds.), *Attachment and family systems: Conceptual, empirical, and therapeutic relatedness* (pp. 139–163). New York: Brunner-Routledge.

Fenge, L. A., & Fannin, A. (2009). Sexuality and bereavement: Implications for practice with older lesbians and gay men. *Practice: Social Work in Action, 21,* 35–46.

Fingerhut, A. W., & Maisel, N. C. (2010). Relationship formalization and individual and relationship well-being among same-sex couples. *Journal of Social and Personal Relationships, 27,* 956–969.

Fingerhut, A. W. & Peplau, L. A. (2013). Same-sex romantic relationships. In C. J. Patterson & A. R.

D'Augelli (Eds.), *Handbook of psychology and sexual orientation* (pp. 165–178). New York: Oxford University Press.

Folkman, S., Chesney, M., Collette, L., Boccellari, A., & Cooke, M. (1996). Postbereavement depressive mood and its prebereavement predictors in HIV+ and HIV– gay men. *Journal of Personality and Social Psychology, 70,* 336–348.

Fraley, R. C., Brumbaugh, C. C., & Marks, M. J. (2005). The evolution and function of adult attachment: A comparative and phylogenetic analysis. *Journal of Personality and Social Psychology, 89,* 731–746.

Gaines, S. O., & Henderson, M. C. (2002). Impact of attachment style on responses to accommodative dilemmas among same-sex couples. *Personal Relationships, 9,* 89–93.

Gibson, M. (1997). Clitoral corruption: Body metaphors and American doctors' constructions of female homosexuality. In V. A. Rosario (Ed.), *Science and homosexualities* (pp. 108–132). New York: Routledge.

Goldberg, A. E. (2010). *Lesbian and gay parents and their children: Research on the family life cycle.* Washington, DC: American Psychological Association.

Goodenow, C., Szalacha, L., & Westheimer, K. (2006). School support groups, other school factors, and the safety of sexual minority adolescents. *Psychology in the Schools, 43,* 573–589.

Grossman, A. H., D'Augelli, A. R., & Dragowski, E. A. (2007). Caregiving and care receiving among older lesbian, gay, and bisexual adults. *Journal of Gay and Lesbian Social Services, 18,* 15–38.

Hartwell, E., Serovich, J. M., Grafsky, E. L., & Kerr, Z. (2012). Coming out of the dark: Content analysis of articles pertaining to gay, lesbian, and bisexual issues in couple and family therapy journals. *Journal of Marital and Family Therapy, 38,* 227–243.

Hazan, C., & Shaver, P. (1987). Romantic love conceptualized as an attachment process. *Journal of Personality and Social Psychology, 52,* 511–524.

Hazan, C., Zeifman, D., & Middleton, K. (1994, July). *Adult romantic attachment, affection, and sex.* Paper presented at the 7th International Conference on Personal Relationships, Groningen, The Netherlands.

Heavey, C. L., Layne, C., & Christensen, A. (1993). Gender and conflict structure in marital interaction: A replication and extension. *Journal of Consulting and Clinical Psychology, 64,* 16–27.

Herek, G. M. (1991). Stigma, prejudice, and violence against lesbians and gay men. In J. C. Gonsiorek & J. D. Weinrich (Eds.), *Homosexuality: Research implications for public policy* (pp. 60–80). Newbury Park, CA: Sage.

Herek, G. M., Kimmel, D. C., Amaro, H., & Melton, G. B. (1991). Avoiding heterosexist bias in psychological research. *American Psychologist, 46,* 957–963.

Hershberger, S. L., & D'Augelli, A. R. (1995). The impact of victimization on the mental health and suicidality of lesbian, gay, and bisexual youths. *Developmental Psychology*, *31*, 65–74.

Hill, A. K., Dawood, K., & Puts, D. A. (2013). Biological foundations of sexual orientation. In C. J. Patterson, A. R. D'Augelli (Eds.), *Handbook of psychology and sexual orientation* (pp. 55–68). New York: Oxford University Press.

Hornjatkevyc, N. L., & Alderson, K. G. (2011). With and without: The bereavement experiences of gay men who have lost a partner to non-AIDS-related causes. *Death Studies*, *35*, 801–823.

Hutchinson, G. E. (1959). A speculative consideration of certain possible forms of sexual selection in man. *American Naturalist*, *93*, 81–91.

Itaborahy, L. P. (2012, May). State-sponsored homophobia: A world survey of laws criminalising same-sex sexual acts between consenting adults. Retrieved September 27, 2014, from *www.refworld.org/cgi-bin/texis/vtx/rwmain?docid=50ae380e2*.

James, B. (2012, December 17). Brighton couple devastated by homophobic attack. Retrieved from *www.theargus.co.uk*.

Jellison, W. A., & McConnell, A., R. (2003). The mediating effects of attitudes toward homosexuality between secure attachment and disclosure outcomes among gay men. *Journal of Homosexuality*, *46*, 159–177.

Jenkins, C. L., Edmundson, A., Averett, P., & Yoon, I. (2013). Older lesbians and bereavement: Experiencing the loss of a partner. *Journal of Gerontological Social Work*, *57*, 273–287.

Kirkpatrick, L. A. (1998). Evolution, pair-bonding, and reproductive strategies: A reconceptualization of adult attachment. In J. A. Simpson & W. S. Rholes (Eds.), *Attachment theory and close relationships* (pp. 353–393). New York: Guilford Press.

Kirkpatrick, L. A., & Davis, K. E. (1994). Attachment style, gender, and relationship stability: A longitudinal analysis. *Journal of Personality and Social Psychology*, *66*, 502–512.

Kite, M. E., & Whitley, B. E. (1996). Sex differences in attitudes toward homosexual persons, behaviors, and civil rights: A meta-analysis. *Personality and Social Psychology Bulletin*, *22*, 336–353.

Kurdek, L. A. (1991). The dissolution of gay and lesbian couples. *Journal of Social and Personal Relationships*, *8*, 265–278.

Kurdek, L. A. (1995). Lesbian and gay couples. In A. R. D'Augelli & C. J. Patterson (Eds.), *Lesbian, gay, and bisexual identities over the lifespan: Psychological perspectives* (pp. 243–261). New York: Oxford University Press.

Kurdek, L. A. (1997). Relation between neuroticism and dimensions of relationship commitment: Evidence from gay, lesbian, and different-sex. *Journal of Family Psychology*, *11*, 109–124.

Kurdek, L. A. (2002). On being insecure about the assessment of attachment styles. *Journal of Social and Personal Relationships*, *19*, 803–826.

Landolt, M. A., Bartholomew, K., Saffrey, C., Oram, D., & Perlman, D. (2004). Gender nonconformity, childhood rejection, and adult attachment: A study of gay men. *Archives of Sexual Behavior*, *33*, 117–128.

Martin, J. L., & Dean, L. (1991). Effects of AIDS-related bereavement and HIV-related illness on psychological distress among gay men: A 7-year longitudinal study, 1985–1991. *Journal of Personality and Social Psychology*, *61*, 94–103.

McCreary, K. (1991). Remembrance. In E. Hemphill (Ed.), *Brother to brother: New writings by black gay men*. Boston: Alyson.

McKnight, J. (1997). *Straight science?: Homosexuality, evolution, adaptation*. London: Routledge.

McVeigh, R., & Maria-Elena, D. D. (2009). Voting to ban same-sex marriage: Interests, values, and communities. *American Sociological Review*, *74*, 891–915.

Mikulincer, M., Florian, V., & Weller, A. (1993). Attachment styles, coping strategies, and posttraumatic psychological distress: The impact of the Gulf War in Israel. *Journal of Personality and Social Psychology*, *64*, 817–826.

Mikulincer, M., & Shaver, P. R. (2001). Attachment theory and intergroup bias: Evidence that priming the secure base schema attenuates negative reactions to outgroups. *Journal of Personality and Social Psychology*, *81*, 97–115.

Mikulincer, M., & Shaver, P. R. (2007). *Attachment in adulthood: Structure, dynamics, and change*. New York: Guilford Press.

Miller, E. M. (2000). Homosexuality, birth order, and evolution: Toward an equilibrium reproductive economics of homosexuality. *Archives of Sexual Behavior*, *29*, 1–34.

Mohr, J. J., & Daly, C. A. (2008). Sexual minority stress and changes in relationship quality in same-sex couples. *Journal of Social and Personal Relationships*, *25*, 989–1007.

Mohr, J. J., & Fassinger, R. E. (2003). Self-acceptance and self-disclosure of sexual orientation in lesbian, gay, and bisexual adults: An attachment perspective. *Journal of Counseling Psychology*, *50*, 482–495.

Mohr, J. J., & Fassinger, R. E. (2006). Sexual orientation identity and romantic relationship quality in same-sex couples. *Personality and Social Psychology Bulletin*, *32*, 1085–1099.

Mohr, J. J., Selterman, D., & Fassinger, R. E. (2013). Romantic attachment and relationship functioning in same-sex couples. *Journal of Counseling Psychology*, *60*, 72–82.

Moradi, B., Wiseman, M. C., DeBlaere, C., Goodman, M. B., Sarkees, A., Brewster, M. E., et al. (2010). LGB of color and white individuals' perceptions of heterosexist stigma, internalized homophobia, and outness: Comparisons of levels and links. *Counseling Psychologist*, *38*, 397–424.

Munsch, C. L. (2012). The science of two-timing: The state of infidelity research. *Sociology Compass*, *6*, 46–59.

Noftle, E. E., & Shaver, P. R. (2006). Attachment dimensions and the Big Five personality traits: Associations and comparative ability to predict relationship quality. *Journal of Research in Personality, 40,* 179–208.

Otis, M. D., Rostosky, S. S., & Riggle, E. D. B. (2006). Stress and relationship quality in same-sex couples. *Journal of Social and Personal Relationships, 23,* 81–99.

Patterson, C. J. (2013). Sexual orientation and family lives. In C. J. Patterson & A. R. D'Augelli (Eds.), *Handbook of psychology and sexual orientation* (pp. 223–236). New York: Oxford University Press.

Patterson, D. G., & Schwartz, P. (1994). The social construction of conflict in intimate same-sex couples. In D. D. Cahn (Ed.), *Conflict in personal relationships* (pp. 3–26). Hillsdale, NJ: Erlbaum.

Pavelka, M. S. (1995). Sexual nature: What can we learn from a cross-species perspective? In P. R. Abramson & S. D. Pinkerton (Eds.), *Sexual nature, sexual culture* (pp. 17–36). Chicago: University of Chicago Press.

Peplau, L. A., & Fingerhut, A. W. (2007). The close relationships of lesbians and gay men. *Annual Psychological Review, 58,* 405–424.

Pietromonaco, P. R., & Barrett, L. F. (2000). Attachment theory as an organizing framework: A view from different levels of analysis. *Review of General Psychology, 4,* 107–110.

Ramirez, O. M., & Brown, J. (2010). Attachment style, rules regarding sex, and couple satisfaction: A study of gay male couples. *Australian and New Zealand Journal of Family Therapy, 31,* 202–213.

Ridge, S. R., & Feeney, J. A. (1998). Relationship history and relationship attitudes in gay males and lesbians: Attachment style and gender differences. *Australian and New Zealand Journal of Psychiatry, 32,* 848–859.

Rosario, V. A. (1997). Homosexual bio-histories: Genetic nostalgias and the quest for paternity. In V. A. Rosario (Ed.), *Science and homosexualities* (pp. 1–26). New York: Routledge.

Rule, S. (1989, October 2). Rights for gay couples in Denmark. *New York Times,* p. A8.

Rust, P. C. (1996). Monogamy and polyamory: Relationship issues for bisexuals. In B. A. Firestein (Ed.), *Bisexuality: The psychology and politics of an invisible minority* (pp. 127–148). Thousand Oaks, CA: Sage.

Santtila, P., Högbacka, A. L., Jern, P., Johansson, A., Varjonen, M., Witting, K., et al. (2009). Testing Miller's theory of alleles preventing androgenization as an evolutionary explanation for the genetic predisposition for male homosexuality. *Evolution and Human Behavior, 30,* 58–65.

Savin-Williams, R. C. (1995). Lesbian, gay male, and bisexual adolescents. In A. R. D'Augelli & C. J. Patterson (Eds.), *Lesbian, gay, and bisexual identities over the lifespan: Psychological perspectives* (pp. 165–189). New York: Oxford University Press.

Schmitt, D. P., Alcalay, L., Allensworth, M., Allik, J., Ault, L., Austers, I., et al. (2003). Are men universally more dismissing than women?: Gender differences in romantic attachment across 62 cultural regions. *Personal Relationships, 10,* 307–331.

Sharpsteen, D. J., & Kirkpatrick, L. A. (1997). Romantic jealousy and adult romantic attachment. *Journal of Personality and Social Psychology, 72,* 627–640.

Shaver, P. R., & Hazan, C. (1988). A biased overview of the study of love. *Journal of Social and Personal Relationships, 5,* 473–501.

Shelby, R. D. (1994). Mourning within a culture of mourning. In S. A. Cadwell, R. A. Burnham, Jr., & M. Forstein (Eds.), *Therapists on the front line: Psychotherapy with gay men in the age of AIDS* (pp. 53–79). Washington, DC: American Psychiatric Press.

Simpson, J. A. (1990). Influence of attachment styles on romantic relationships. *Journal of Personality and Social Psychology, 59,* 971–980.

Simpson, J. A., & Rholes, W. S. (1994). Stress and secure base relationships in adulthood. In K. Bartholomew & D. Perlman (Eds.), *Advances in personal relationships: Vol. 5. Attachment processes in adulthood* (pp. 181–204). London: Jessica Kingsley.

Simpson, J. A., Rholes, W. S., & Nelligan, J. S. (1992). Support seeking and support giving within couples in an anxiety-provoking situation: The role of attachment styles. *Journal of Personality and Social Psychology, 62,* 434–446.

Simpson, J. A., Rholes, W. S., & Phillips, D. (1996). Conflict in close relationships: An attachment perspective. *Journal of Personality and Social Psychology, 71,* 899–914.

Smith, E. R., Murphy, J., & Coats, S. (1999). Attachments to groups: Theory and measurement. *Journal of Personality and Social Psychology, 77,* 94–110.

Smith, R. B., & Brown, R. A. (1997). The impact of social support on gay male couples. *Journal of Homosexuality, 33,* 39–61.

Starks, T. J., & Parsons, J. T. (2014). Adult attachment among partnered gay men: Patterns and associations with sexual relationship quality. *Archives of Sexual Behavior, 43,* 107–117.

Stroebe, M. S., Folkman, S., Hansson, R. O., & Schut, H. (2006). The prediction of bereavement outcome: development of an integrative risk factor framework. *Social Science and Medicine, 63,* 2440–2451.

Timeline of same-sex marriage. (2014, August 11). Retrieved August 19, 2014, from *http://en.wikipedia.org/wiki/timeline_of_same-sex_marriage*.

Troiden, R. R. (1993). The formation of homosexual identities. In L. D. Garnets & D. C. Kimmel (Eds.), *Psychological perspectives on lesbian and gay male experiences* (pp. 191–217). New York: Columbia University Press.

VanderLaan, D. P., Ren, Z., & Vasey, P. L. (2013). Male androphilia in the ancestral environment. *Human Nature, 24,* 375–401.

Vasey, P. L., Pocock, D. S., & VanderLaan, D. P. (2007). Kin selection and male androphilia in Samoan fa'afafine. *Evolution and Human Behavior, 28,* 159–167.

Vasey, P. L., & VanderLaan, D. P. (2014). Evolutionary perspectives on male androphilia in humans. In V. A. Weekes-Shackelford & T. K. Shackelford (Eds.), *Evolutionary perspectives on human sexual psychology and behavior* (pp. 369–391). New York: Springer.

Weinrich, J. D. (1995). Biological research on sexual orientation: A critique of the critics. *Journal of Homosexuality, 28,* 197–213.

Weinstock, J. S., & Rothblum, E. D. (Eds.). (2004). *Lesbian ex-lovers: The really long-term relationships.* New York: Haworth Press.

Weiss, R. S. (1982). Attachment in adult life. In C. M. Parkes & J. Stevenson-Hinde (Eds.), *The place of attachment in human behavior* (pp. 171–184). New York: Basic Books.

Wells, G. B., & Hansen, N. D. (2003). Lesbian shame: Its relationship to identity integration and attachment. *Journal of Homosexuality, 45,* 93–110.

West, M. L., & Sheldon-Keller, A. E. (1994). *Patterns of relating: An adult attachment perspective.* New York: Guilford Press.

Williams, T., Connolly, J., Pepler, D., & Craig, W. (2005). Peer victimization, social support, and psychosocial adjustment of sexual minority adolescents. *Journal of Youth and Adolescence, 34,* 471–482.

Wilson, E. O. (1975). *Sociobiology: The new synthesis.* Cambridge, MA: Harvard University Press.

Wilson, G. A., Zeng, Q., & Blackburn, D. G. (2011). An examination of parental attachments, parental detachments and self-esteem across hetero-, bi-, and homosexual individuals. *Journal of Bisexuality, 11,* 86–97.

Zakalik, R. A., & Wei, M. (2006). Adult attachment, perceived discrimination based on sexual orientation, and depression in gay males: Examining the mediation and moderation effects. *Journal of Counseling Psychology, 53,* 302–312.

Zietsch, B. P., Morley, K. I., Shekar, S. N., Verweij, K. J., Keller, M. C., Macgregor, S., et al. (2008). Genetic factors predisposing to homosexuality may increase mating success in heterosexuals. *Evolution and Human Behavior, 29,* 424–433.

# Chapter 24

# Adult Attachment and Emotion Regulation

Mario Mikulincer
Phillip R. Shaver

The titles of the second and third volumes of Bowlby's (1973, 1980) trilogy on attachment—*Separation: Anxiety and Anger* and *Loss: Sadness and Depression*—make clear that emotions were among his central concerns. He was interested in the causes and consequences of emotions aroused by attachment to, and reunion with, attachment figures (e.g., love, tenderness, joy); separation from them (anxiety, anger); and permanent loss of them (grief, sadness, despair). Attachment theory is an attempt to explain how secure attachments develop; how they help people survive temporary bouts of pain, fear, discomfort, and distress; and how they help people emerge from distress and reestablish confidence, hope, optimism, and emotional balance. It also explains how various forms of attachment insecurity develop and interfere with emotion regulation, social adjustment, and mental health—as explained in this and several other chapters in this volume.

Especially in early childhood, but also later in life ("from the cradle to the grave," in Bowlby's frequently quoted words; 1979, p. 129), human beings rely on attachment figures (e.g., parents, spouses/partners, mentors, therapists) for help with emotion regulation. When a security-providing mother reassuringly touches her anxious child or holds the child's hand in a novel or worrisome situation, the child's previously heightened autonomic arousal subsides (e.g., Field, 2002). When a loving husband holds his wife's hand in a painful or anxiety-provoking medical situation, fMRI images of the wife's brain reveal that her physiological arousal is lower than in control conditions (e.g., Coan, Schaefer, & Davidson, 2006; see also Coan, Chapter 12, this volume). (Interestingly, less caring, less supportive husbands' hands do not have as strong a beneficial effect.)

In this chapter, we summarize our model of attachment-system activation and dynamics in adulthood—a model based on what we call "adult attachment theory," which has inspired a large body of research (for more extensive reviews, see Mikulincer & Shaver, 2003, 2013, 2016). The goal of this revised and updated version of our 2008 chapter is to use concepts and findings from attachment research, which originally focused primarily on the mother–child relationship and on children's attachment orientations (as explained in Part III in this volume), to understand the role of emotion regulation in adult attachment relationships and mental representations of attachment experiences. To accomplish this goal, we rely mainly on the large research literature created by social/personality psychologists who use self-report measures of attachment-figure hierarchies and "adult attachment styles," combined with a variety of other measures and experimental research methods, to uncover and illuminate the dynamics of the attachment behavioral system in adulthood (Mikulincer & Shaver, 2016; Shaver & Mikulincer, 2002a, 2002b). There are parallel studies based on interview measures of adult "states of mind with respect to attachment" (the Adult Attachment Interview [AAI]; see Hesse, Chapter 26, and Crowell, Fraley, & Roisman, Chapter 27, this volume), many of which we review in our comprehensive book on adult attachment (Mikulincer & Shaver, 2016). But here, to comply with page limits and focus on our own theoretical model and related research, we review mainly research conducted by social/personality psychologists, occasionally referring to corroborative AAI studies.

Research by social/personality psychologists on dyadic, relational processes related to attachment (and also to caregiving) is reviewed in this volume by J. A. Feeney, Chapter 21; B. C. Feeney and Monin, Chapter 40; B. C. Feeney and Woodhouse, Chapter 36; and Shaver, Mikulincer, Gross, Stern, and Cassidy, Chapter 38. Here we consider mainly the individual psychology of attachment-related emotion regulation processes in adulthood, which are a joint product of previous experiences in attachment relationships and current cognitive and social contexts, including contexts that can be systematically manipulated in a laboratory. (There is presumably also a role for genes in the processes we examine, but there is not enough space here to consider it here. For examples and references, see, e.g., Crawford et al., 2007; Donnellan, Burt, Levendosky, & Klump, 2008; see also Bakermans-Kranenburg & Van IJzendoorn, Chapter 8, this volume.)

The concept of "adult attachment style" explored in this chapter emerged from research by Hazan and Shaver (1987, 1990, 1994), who applied attachment theory to the study of adolescent and adult romantic and marital relationships. In their early studies, Hazan and Shaver employed a simple three-category measure of attachment style based conceptually on Ainsworth's descriptions of three major attachment patterns in infancy (Ainsworth, Blehar, Waters, & Wall, 1978). In an influential 1991 article, Bartholomew and Horowitz argued for a more complete four-category typology based on two dimensions suggested by Bowlby's (1969/1982) analysis of internal working models of self and other. (Bartholomew and Horowitz divided each of these two dimensions, model of self and model of others, into two regions: positive models and negative models, thereby creating four types.)

Bartholomew and Horowitz's theory and measures (Bartholomew & Horowitz, 1991; Griffin & Bartholomew, 1994) inspired numerous other measures and studies, which in 1998 led Brennan, Clark, and Shaver (1998) to factor-analyze all of the self-report items written up to that time. Based on their analyses and on Bartholomew and Horowitz's (1991) findings, Brennan and colleagues (1998) created two 18-item self-report scales (the Experiences in Close Relationships [ECR] scales) to measure attachment-related *anxiety* and *avoidance*. The two dimensions are similar to the two that defined Ainsworth's infant attachment categories (see Ainsworth et al., 1978, Figure 10, p. 102). The ECR scales allow researchers to place adolescent and adult research participants into a two-dimensional attachment-style space defined by attachment anxiety and avoidance. Thousands of studies (summarized and reviewed in Mikulincer & Shaver, in press) have used this approach to study adult attachment phenomena, including many issues related to emotion regulation. (Several alternative measures have been developed along the lines of the ECR and are discussed by Crowell et al., Chapter 27, this volume.)

We begin our review of theory and research with a description of our model of attachment-system activation and functioning in adulthood. Next, we focus on the self- and emotion-regulatory function of attachment-system activation. We review studies of preconscious activation of attachment-related mental representations under threatening conditions and the associated use of support seeking as an emotion regulation strategy. We then review studies concerning the beneficial effects of attachment security on emotion regulation and mental health, as well as the psychological mechanisms that sustain these effects. We consider the distinction between anxious/hyperactivating and avoidant/deactivating strategies that are put into play when no security-providing figure is available or responsive, and we summarize evidence regarding the implications of these strategies (which are associated with attachment anxiety and avoidance, respectively) for emotion regulation and mental health. We also explain briefly how these two kinds of insecurity can be beneficial at a social-group level, even though they are generally troublesome for individuals and for couple relationships. At the end of the chapter, we briefly summarize developments that have occurred since 2008, when the previous version of this handbook appeared, and we outline some future directions.

## A Model of Attachment System Activation and Functioning in Adulthood

In 2003, based on a review of adult attachment studies, we (Mikulincer & Shaver, 2003) proposed a three-phase model of attachment-system activation and dynamics (Figure 24.1). The model comprises three main components or modules. The first involves the monitoring and appraisal of threatening events, which often activate the attachment system (see Cassidy, Chapter 1, this vol-

ume). This component includes the major normative (i.e., pan-human, cross-culturally universal), biologically functional (i.e., adaptive) features of the attachment system as conceptualized by Bowlby (1969/1982), who proposed that the attachment system evolved because it increased infants' chances of survival and eventual reproduction by making it likely that vulnerable infants would seek and maintain proximity to stronger and wiser attachment figures, thereby receiving protection, emotional support, encouragement, guidance, and help with emotion regulation—especially when

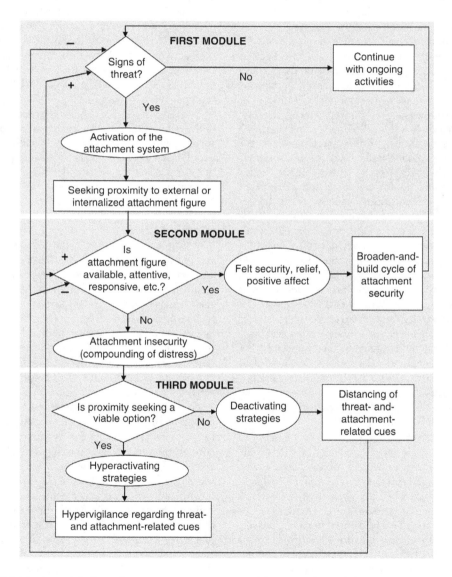

**FIGURE 24.1.** A model of attachment system activation and functioning in adulthood. From Mikulincer and Shaver (2007, p. 31). Copyright 2007 by The Guilford Press. Reprinted by permission.

confronting threats, stressors, or pain. Bowlby believed that the attachment system continues to develop while operating in conceptually similar ways across the lifespan.

The second component of the model deals with the monitoring and appraisal of attachment figure availability and responsiveness. This component is responsible for individual differences in the sense of attachment security ("felt security"; Sroufe & Waters, 1977), which is shaped by repeated experiences with primary attachment figures, whose effective or ineffective caregiving behavior causes a child to become more or less secure. By the time a person reaches adulthood, this component of the attachment system is highly elaborated, based on thousands of experiences. It includes a vast store of conscious and unconscious memories related to encounters with threats and experiences with attachment figures, as well as schematic, script-like mental representations of those experiences—the "internal working models" referred to by Bowlby (1969/1982) and discussed by Bretherton and Munholland in Chapter 4, this volume. Repeated security-restoring and security-enhancing experiences with attachment figures create a dispositional (i.e., fairly stable) sense of felt security, which sustains what we call a "broaden-and-build" cycle of security (following Fredrickson, 2013; see Mikulincer & Shaver, 2016). This cycle influences many aspects of emotion regulation, mental health, personal growth, and social adjustment.

The third component of the model concerns the monitoring and appraisal of the likely utility of seeking proximity to an attachment figure (either a particular figure or such figures in general) as a way of coping with threats to safety and well-being. This component is responsible for individual differences in attachment style and in corresponding strategies of emotion regulation, which can be characterized as secure, hyperactivating, or deactivating (Cassidy & Kobak, 1988).

Hyperactivating strategies are thought to derive from previous experiences in which inattentive, self-preoccupied, or anxious attachment figures were perceived by a child as more likely to respond favorably if the normative strategies of calling, crying, contacting, and clinging were upregulated to the point of demanding a response (a behavior pattern that Bowlby, 1969/1982, called "protest"). Because such behavior, when addressed to a less than fully sensitive and responsive caregiver, is sometimes effective in relieving distress and sometimes not, according to an unpredict-

able partial reinforcement schedule, it is highly resistant to extinction. When consolidated over months and years, hyperactivating strategies and their effects on subjective experience and observable behavior amount to an *anxious*, *anxious-ambivalent*, or *anxious-resistant* pattern of attachment (Ainsworth et al., 1978), which in adolescents and adults we refer to simply as an *anxious* attachment style.

Deactivating strategies are thought to derive from previous experiences in which emotionally cool, distant, rejecting, or hostile caregivers reacted to normative bids for help and support by withdrawing, disapproving, or reacting with anger. This kind of behavior, if common and persistent, makes it likely that a child will inhibit, suppress, or deactivate normal attachment behavior, resulting in an *avoidant* attachment pattern (Ainsworth et al., 1978), which Bowlby (1969/1982) called "compulsive self-reliance."

It is possible for a person to score high on both anxiety and avoidance, a pattern that Bartholomew and Horowitz, 1991, called "fearful avoidance." This is conceptually similar, although not identical, to what is called "disorganized attachment" in the child literature (as discussed by Lyons-Ruth & Jacobvitz, Chapter 29, this volume), but we do not have space here to explain this idea in detail.

Our model includes hypothesized excitatory and inhibitory feedback loops (shown as upward arrows on the left-hand side of Figure 24.1), which result from recurrent use of hyperactivating or deactivating strategies. These loops affect the monitoring of threats and the appraisal of attachment figures' availability or unavailability. In particular, hyperactivating strategies lead to persistent vigilance to threats; being exceptionally expressive of fears, needs, and doubts; and being continually worried about attachment figures' availability and responsiveness. These tendencies predispose a person to engage in excessively dependent behavior, intense and frequent proximity seeking and contact maintenance, and clinginess (Ainsworth et al., 1978; Fraley & Shaver, 1998). Deactivating strategies, in contrast, lead to dismissal or downplaying of potential threats; suppression or denial of worries, needs, and vulnerabilities; and disavowal of the need for an attachment figure's presence or support. These processes sometimes cause a person to ignore attachment figures, reject their offers of assistance, and reduce expressions of affection and intimacy (Edelstein & Shaver, 2004).

## Scripts as Components of Working Models

Theoretically, individual differences in the activation and functioning of the attachment system, as described in Figure 24.1, depend on the extent to which attachment figures are (or were) sensitive and responsive to bids for protection and support. During such interactions, people develop expectations (working models) about the self as lovable and about others as harboring goodwill. Moreover, these interactions provide valuable information about the effectiveness of support seeking as an emotion-regulation device and therefore facilitate the consolidation of procedural knowledge in the form of mental scripts concerning how to deal with threats and adversities. These mental scripts, once activated in a threatening situation, shape a person's reactions to the situation and allow him or her to forecast how the situation will develop and whether the threat will or will not be removed. Depending on the details of a particular individual's script, activation of the script can be beneficial or detrimental to emotion regulation in a particular situation.

### The Secure-Base Script

According to Waters and Waters (2006) and Mikulincer, Shaver, Sapir-Lavid, and Avihou-Kanza (2009), secure adults' interactions with responsive attachment figures and the resulting positive working models of self and others are organized around a relational prototype or *secure-base script*, containing something like the following if–then propositions (which are not necessarily articulated consciously): "If I encounter an obstacle and/or become distressed, then I can approach a significant other for help; he or she is likely to be available and supportive; I will experience relief and comfort as a result of proximity to this person; I can then return to other activities." Once activated, this script, by itself, can mitigate distress, promote optimism and hope, and help a person cope effectively with stressors.

Mikulincer, Florian, and Tolmacz (2009) found that young adults who scored lower on the two self-report scales of the ECR (Brennan et al., 1998)—Attachment Anxiety and Avoidance—were more likely to include elements of the secure-base script (support seeking, support provision, and distress relief) when writing a story about a fictional person under threat (Studies 1 and 2).

Moreover, the two kinds of insecurity—anxiety and avoidance—were associated with different gaps in the secure-base script. People who scored relatively high on attachment anxiety tended to omit or deemphasize the final step in the script (relief and return to other activities), whereas those who scored relatively high on avoidance tended to omit the part about seeking and benefiting from others' support. That is, whereas anxious participants in the studies more often wrote about a threatened or injured protagonist who was seeking support and not achieving relief, avoidant participants more often wrote about a person achieving relief without seeking or receiving support.

Mikulincer and colleagues (2009, Studies 3–8) also reported evidence concerning the cognitive properties of the secure-base script and the ways in which it organizes expectations, memories, and judgments, thereby affecting emotion elicitation and regulation. For example, more secure individuals had greater access to the secure-base script when dreaming about distressing events (Study 4), and they expected to find more secure-base script components (support seeking, support availability) in an imagined story that began with a distressing experience (Study 3). They were also more likely to go beyond the script-relevant information they received and generate additional security-supporting inferences and conjectures (Study 5). This tendency was evident even 5 days after being exposed to the information (Study 7) and was not affected by the depletion of cognitive resources caused by an effortful task—a sign that secure-base-script information was processed easily and automatically (Study 8). Moreover, relatively secure participants were quicker and more confident in making judgments concerning secure-base-script-related information (Studies 6–7). Overall, the findings indicated that secure individuals are experts in the use of the secure-base script for coping with threatening events, which can be of considerable help when they are attempting to maintain emotional balance in threatening situations.

This conclusion is reinforced by findings that attachment security is positively associated with the degree to which the secure-base script underlies dreams in general (Mikulincer, Shaver, & Avihou-Kanza, 2011), dreams about romantic partners (Selterman, Apetroaia, & Waters, 2012), narratives about current relationships (McLean, Bailey, & Lumley, 2014), and interpersonal stories that research participants create based on word prompts (Steele et al., 2014).

## Attachment Insecurity and the "Sentinel" and "Rapid Fight–Flight" Scripts

Besides having gaps in their secure-base scripts, anxious and avoidant individuals possess scripts that guide emotion regulation and coping behavior in threatening situations (Ein-Dor, Mikulincer, & Shaver, 2011a). We call them *sentinel* and *rapid fight–flight* scripts (typical of anxious and avoidant adults, respectively). Attachment anxiety is associated with ready access to a sentinel script (e.g., noticing danger before other people do, warning others about the danger) when writing a story about a threatening event (Ein-Dor et al., 2011a, Study 1), and with better memory for recently encountered sentinel-script information (Study 3). Participants who scored higher on attachment anxiety were also more likely to process sentinel-script information in a deep way and to generate more inferences and conjectures (Study 4). They also had poorer and shallower recall of information that was congruent with the (avoidant) rapid fight–flight schema (Studies 2 and 5), suggesting that they do not possess or use that script.

More avoidant participants proved to have ready access to a rapid fight-flight script of emotion regulation (e.g., escaping a dangerous situation without helping others, acting rapidly without depending on others' actions, not deliberating or cooperating with others) when thinking and writing a story about threatening events (Study 1). Moreover, avoidance was associated with better memory for information relevant to the rapid fight–flight script (Study 3) and with processing this information in a deep way (Study 5). More avoidant participants also exhibited poorer memory for information congruent with the (more anxious) sentinel script (Study 4).

The hypothesis that the sentinel and rapid fight–flight scripts might exist was based originally on thinking about ways in which anxious and avoidant individuals can sometimes benefit the groups to which they belong, despite the usual negative characterizations (including ours) of anxious and avoidant mental emotion regulation strategies and associated coping behavior. In one study, Ein-Dor, Mikulincer, and Shaver (2011b) examined behaviors associated with the two kinds of scripts in a group context. A total of 46 groups of three participants each were unobtrusively observed in a threatening laboratory situation: The room gradually filled with smoke, apparently because of a malfunctioning computer. Group members' attachment anxiety was associated with quicker detection of the danger, and group members who scored higher on avoidance more quickly devised and executed escape responses to the danger, and other group members were quick to follow.

Ein-Dor and colleagues have collected additional evidence for anxious adults' reliance on the sentinel script. For example, Ein-Dor and Perry (2014) studied deceit detection: Attachment anxiety predicted more accurate detection of deceitful statements made during social interactions and also with winning more money while playing poker—a game based on one's ability to detect bluffing. In another study, Ein-Dor and Orgad (2012) focused on the "warning others about danger" component of the sentinel script. Study participants were led to believe they had accidently activated a computer virus, and they were asked to alert the department's computer technicians in another part of the building. On the way to the technicians' office, they encountered various obstacles that might have caused them to delay or give up. But, as expected, more anxious individuals were less willing to be delayed on their way to deliver a warning message.

Regarding avoidance and the associated rapid fight-flight script, Ein-Dor, Reizer, Shaver, and Dotan (2012) examined two domains in which avoidant people might be especially likely to succeed: professional singles tennis tournaments (requiring travel away from home and competing alone) and computer science. These fields reward self-reliance, independence, and the ability to work without emotional expressions and interpersonal closeness—core components of the rapid fight-flight script. As expected, avoidance predicted higher standing in a series of singles tennis tournaments, and also predicted greater career choice satisfaction among computer science students.

For present purposes, the most important implication of the script findings is that attachment security, anxiety, and avoidance are associated with mental representations—scripts of various kinds—that affect emotion-related appraisals of situations and different kinds of behavior following threats. In many situations, being overly vigilant and sensitive to threats (which in some cases may merely be imagined), or overly self-reliant and uncommunicative about feelings, is stressful for the individual in question and damaging to his or her relationships, but in other situations these examples of hyperactivation and deactivation of the attachment system can benefit a person's groups. This is worth keeping in mind when characterizing anxious and avoidant attachment as suboptimal, and when considering why the existence of these insecure patterns was not eliminated during human evolutionary history.

## The Attachment System and Support Seeking

A core contention of attachment theory (Bowlby, 1969/1982) is that reactions to perceived threats and dangers include not only the traditionally emphasized "fight-or-flight" responses (Cannon, 1939) but also seeking proximity to a "stronger and wiser," supportive, and protective attachment figure as a way of protecting and emotionally calming oneself. Main (1990) called this the "primary" attachment strategy. In adulthood (and probably in childhood as well, although our concern here is adulthood), people can seek proximity to and support from an attachment figure either by requesting actual support from a real, flesh-and-blood, physically present relationship partner or by calling on mental images, prototypes, schemas, or specific memories of interactions with human or nonhuman attachment figures (e.g., pets, spiritual beings). Adults can also engage in self-soothing routines learned in interactions with attachment figures (Mikulincer & Shaver, 2004).

In constructing a model of attachment system functioning, we (Mikulincer & Shaver, 2003) postulated a two-stage process by which threat appraisals lead to activation of the primary attachment strategy. In the first stage, threat appraisals trigger preconscious activation of the system, which brings about an automatic increase in the accessibility of attachment-related mental representations in an associative memory network. In the second stage, this preconscious activation, if sufficiently robust, results in conscious thoughts about seeking proximity to attachment figures, behavioral intentions to seek proximity and support, and actual seeking of proximity and support.

We believe that preconscious activation of the attachment system involves heightened access to mental representations (not necessarily conscious) of available and responsive attachment figures; episodic memories of supportive and comforting interactions with these figures; thoughts and images related to closeness, love, comfort, relief, and support; and proximity-seeking goals. These mental processes and contents become automatically available for use in further information processing and can color a person's state of mind and influence his or her behavioral intentions and

actual behaviors, even before they are consciously formulated. This model fits with many findings from more general social-cognitive research, which indicates that accessible cognitive-affective mental contents shape a person's state of mind before they appear in the stream of consciousness (Bargh & Morsella, 2010).

Both stages of attachment-system activation can be affected by a person's dispositional attachment style, which reflects long-term experiences with attachment figures (Mikulincer & Shaver, 2003, 2016; Zayas, Mischel, Shoda, & Aber, 2011). A secure person's history of interactions with available and responsive attachment figures and the resulting secure-base script make it more likely that support seeking will occur in times of need as the default means for emotion regulation. In contrast, insecure people have learned through painful experiences with unavailable or unresponsive attachment figures that the primary attachment strategy (proximity seeking) often fails to accomplish its emotion regulation goal. As a result, insecure individuals rely on alternative ways of regulating emotion rather than directly and confidently seeking proximity to an attachment figure. Avoidant adults are likely to deactivate their attachment system, forgo support seeking, and rely on themselves to deal with threats. Anxious adults are likely to regulate their emotions by signaling or expressing needs and fears, exaggerating their distress, and presenting themselves as extremely vulnerable to pain and injury (Shaver & Mikulincer, 2002a).

### Preconscious Activation of the Attachment System in Adulthood

Preconscious activation of the attachment system was first studied in two series of experiments (Mikulincer, Birnbaum, Woddis, & Nachmias, 2000; Mikulincer, Gillath, & Shaver, 2002) in which young adults were subliminally primed with threat-related words (e.g., *death*, *failure*) or neutral words (e.g., *table*, *hat*). The mental accessibility of cognitive and affective elements related to attachment was assessed with two well-validated cognitive techniques: a lexical decision task (deciding quickly whether particular strings of letters are or are not words), and the Stroop color-naming task (naming, as quickly as possible, the color in which a particular word is printed on a computer screen, which requires inhibiting the overlearned tendency to read the word and activate its associations in memory). These tasks allow researchers to gauge the accessibility of particular mental contents at a given moment, even if these contents are not experienced consciously. Researchers can therefore examine the effects of threatening words on the availability of attachment-related concepts, without research participants knowing what is being examined.

In Mikulincer and colleagues' (2000) studies, young adults performed a lexical decision task in which the letter strings they saw included proximity-related words (e.g., *love*, *hug*), separation-related words (e.g., *separation*, *rejection*), neutral words (e.g., *office*, *table*), positive non-attachment-related words (e.g., *honesty*, *efficacy*), negative non-attachment-related words (e.g., *cheat*, *lazy*), and nonwords (created by scrambling the letters of actual words—e.g., "btale" [*table*], "vleo" [*love*]). Before each letter string was presented, a threating word (e.g., *failure*, *illness*) or a neutral word (*hat*) was flashed on the screen for 20 milliseconds—too short a time to allow a participant to perceive the stimulus consciously. (This procedure is called *subliminal priming* because it operates below the level of consciousness and is analogous to priming a pump to stimulate the flow of water.) Reaction times (RTs) serve as a measure of the accessibility of thoughts related to the target words: The quicker the RT, the greater the accessibility.

In the Mikulincer and colleagues (2000) studies, subliminal threat stimuli resulted in faster identification (implying greater mental availability) of proximity-related words, and the effect did not extend to neutral words or positive words with no obvious attachment-related connotations. Moreover, this heightened accessibility occurred regardless of attachment style (although individual differences in attachment style also had effects, as explained below), suggesting that everyone is subject to preconscious activation of the attachment system, as would be expected if such activation is a species-universal, biologically functional mental process.

Extending these studies, we (Mikulincer et al., 2002) conducted three experiments focused on mental access to the names of attachment figures, with names being, we assume, only small but central parts of the mental representations of these figures. Each study participant completed the WHOTO questionnaire (Hazan & Zeifman, 1994), which identifies people to whom one turns for proximity and support (e.g., "Whom do you like to spend time with?"), a safe haven (e.g., "To whom do you turn for comfort when you're feeling down?"), and a secure base (e.g., "Whom do you

feel you can always count on?"). Each participant also named potentially close others who were not viewed as attachment figures (e.g., father, sibling, friend—if not mentioned in the WHOTO questionnaire). And they named acquaintances who were not emotionally close (e.g., coworkers, casual friends). They also selected names that did not apply to anyone they knew personally. Each participant then performed either a lexical decision task or a Stroop color-naming task. In the lexical decision task, they were presented with the names of their own attachment figures, names of close people who were not attachment figures, names of acquaintances, names of unknown persons, and nonword letter strings. They were asked in each case to indicate as quickly as possible whether each string of letters was or was not a person's name. In the Stroop task, participants were exposed to the same four categories of names, each printed in one of several colors, and were asked to indicate the color in which each name was printed. Before each trial, a threat stimulus (the word *failure* or *separation*) or a neutral word (*hat*, *umbrella*) was presented subliminally for 20 milliseconds.

Across the three experiments, participants reacted to subliminal threats with heightened mental access to attachment figures' names. As compared with emotionally neutral words, subliminal threat words resulted in (1) faster identification of the names of attachment figures in the lexical decision task, and (2) slower color designations of attachment figures' names in the Stroop task. In both cases, short lexical decision RTs and slow color-naming RTs were interpreted as indicating heightened activation of mental representations of attachment figures' names in threatening contexts. Subliminal threat words had no effect on mental representations of close others or acquaintances who were not mentioned in the WHOTO questionnaire. Thus, heightened accessibility of mental representations of a particular person under threatening conditions depended on the extent to which the person was viewed as a safe haven and a secure base (i.e., an attachment figure).

### Individual Differences in Preconscious Activation of the Attachment System

In addition to obtaining the predicted overall effects, we found that more secure adults had readier access to thoughts about proximity and to the names of their attachment figures, *but only in a threatening context* (Mikulincer et al., 2000, 2002);

that is, secure adults were not chronically or continually preoccupied with attachment-related themes or particular attachment figures. Rather, attachment-related cognitions were activated only by signals that protection might be needed. In addition, Mikulincer and colleagues (2000) found that more secure individuals' reactions to subliminal threats were limited to attachment themes with positive connotations; they displayed relatively little activation of words related to separation or rejection. We interpret these results as indicating that secure adults' favorable attachment histories resulted in a distinction in their memories between attachment system activation on the one hand, and worries about rejection on the other.

Attachment-anxious individuals' pattern of attachment-system activation was essentially the opposite of the secure individuals' pattern (Mikulincer et al., 2000, 2002). First, the more anxious people (as indicated by their scores on the ECR Attachment Anxiety scale) displayed heightened mental access to attachment-related themes and attachment figures' names *in both threatening and nonthreatening contexts*. Second, they also displayed readier access to words related to separation and rejection. We interpret these findings as indicating hyperactivation of attachment-related thoughts, which seems to occur even in nonthreatening contexts (or perhaps alters the threshold for perceiving a situation as threatening).

Avoidant individuals produced a more complicated set of results. In general, their pattern of access to attachment-related mental contents resembled that of secure people. However, there were important differences. For avoidant people, thoughts about rejection and separation were relatively inaccessible, even following subliminal exposure to the word *death*, which is usually a potent activator of attachment-related fears (Kalish, 1985). Moreover, these worries suddenly became accessible to avoidant individuals in response to subliminal threats if a "cognitive load" was added to the lexical decision task; that is, when avoidant adults had to engage in an additional cognitively demanding task (rehearsing and remembering a long series of digits), they seemed to lack the resources necessary to maintain their usual defensive exclusion of attachment-related concerns. These results support the theoretical notion that avoidant people are insecure, like anxiously attached people, but are generally using defensive means to suppress or deny their insecurity.

We (Mikulincer et al., 2002) also found that when the threat word was *separation*, secure individuals exhibited enhanced access to the names of their attachment figures, whereas avoidant individuals exhibited *decreased* access. There was no such difference when the subliminal threat word was *failure*, which is not as closely related to attachment. It therefore seems that the attachment system is preconsciously activated under attachment-unrelated threatening conditions in both avoidant and nonavoidant people, but is preconsciously inhibited or deactivated under attachment-related threatening conditions (or at least following the threat of separation) if a person is avoidant. It seems likely that avoidant adults have learned not to appeal to attachment figures when these figures threaten to leave. This result is compatible with Ainsworth and colleagues' (1978) statement that "avoidance short circuits direct expression of anger to the attachment figure, which might be dangerous, and it also protects the baby from re-experiencing the rebuff that he has come to expect when he seeks close contact with his mother" (p. 320). We believe this might be the main reason for avoidant individuals' persistent attempts to divert or suppress feelings of vulnerability and negative emotions when attempting to regulate distress and inner pain.

### Individual Differences in Support-Seeking Tendencies and Behavior

Several studies have confirmed the predicted link between attachment insecurities and lower scores on self-report scales that tap support seeking (see Mikulincer & Shaver, 2016, for a comprehensive review). These attachment-related differences have also been noted in observational studies of the actual seeking of support from relationship partners. In two studies, one member of a dating couple (women in Simpson, Rholes, & Nelligan, 1992; men in Simpson, Rholes, Oriña, & Grich, 2002) was told that she or he would undergo a painful laboratory procedure after waiting with a partner for 5 minutes. During this period, participants' behavior was unobtrusively videotaped, and raters later coded the extent to which each participant sought his or her partner's support. Among women, avoidance inhibited support seeking mainly when their level of distress was high. In such cases, avoidant women often attempted to distract themselves by reading magazines instead of asking for support. For men, however, there was no association between attachment and support seeking. Simpson and colleagues (2002) attributed this lack of association to social norms that inhibit men's seeking of support from women or to men's tendency to perceive the experimental tasks as less threatening. Similar findings have been obtained using the AAI or a secure-base script methodology (e.g., Crowell et al., 2002; Waters, Brockmeyer, & Crowell, 2013).

Two other observational studies provide additional evidence for avoidant and anxious people's problematic attitudes toward support seeking. Fraley and Shaver (1998) unobtrusively coded expressions of desire for proximity and support when romantic or marital partners were about to separate from each other at a metropolitan airport, and Collins and Feeney (2000) coded support-seeking behavior while members of seriously dating couples talked about a personal problem in the laboratory. In both studies, avoidance was associated with less frequent seeking of proximity or support. In addition, although attachment anxiety did not affect direct requests for partner support, more anxious people were more likely to use indirect methods of support seeking, such as asking for help through nonverbal distress signals (crying, pouting, or sulking).

Several other studies using self-report attachment measures have shown that more avoidant, compared with less avoidant, individuals are less likely to benefit from imagined or actual support when coping with stress (e.g., Bodie et al., 2011; Mikulincer & Florian, 1997; Milyavskaya, McClure, Ma, Koestner, & Lydon; 2012). Using the AAI as a measure of security, Simpson, Winterheld, Rholes, and Oriña (2007) found that the specific type of support is critical for understanding the problems insecure people encounter when involved in potentially supportive interactions. Dating couples were videotaped while trying to resolve their most important relationship problem. At peak distress points during each discussion, coders rated the extent to which one partner displayed emotional or instrumental support behaviors, and the other partner was calmed by the partner's support attempts. Whereas securely attached individuals were rated as calmed when their partners provided either emotional or instrumental support, avoidant individuals were rated as calmed when their partners delivered less emotionally imbued and more instrumental support (e.g., giving concrete advice or suggestions concerning how to solve the problem). Similar findings were obtained by Girme, Overall, Simpson, and Fletcher (2015) in an analysis of avoidant adults' reactions to instrumental support offered by their romantic partner during support-related discussions and in daily life. These findings suggest that in order to be effective, supportive efforts need to be tailored to the specific concerns and defenses of avoidant people.

Secure individuals' reliance on supportive interactions has been noted in a series of studies of attachment-style differences in heart rate and blood pressure in a stressful situation (e.g., performing a stressful arithmetic task) in the presence of or in response to the supportiveness of a relationship partner (Carpenter & Kirkpatrick, 1996; B. Feeney & Kirkpatrick, 1996). These studies indicated that the physiological responses of avoidant and anxious women were heightened rather than mitigated by the presence of their romantic partner (compared with a no-partner condition). In another study, Meuwly and colleagues (2012) found that a partner's supportiveness lowered the intensity of cortisol responses to a public speaking task only among relatively secure participants, not among more attachment-anxious participants. This is an example of the role of attachment-related experiences and resulting differences in attachment security in being able, or not, to enlist others in efforts to regulate negative emotions.

## Regulation of Stressful Events and Attachment-Related Threats

In this section, we review evidence concerning ways in which attachment style shapes a person's appraisal and coping strategies for dealing with distressing events, which influence the experience and expression of negative emotions. We also review studies concerning attachment-related differences in (1) the regulation of distress caused specifically by separation or loss, and (2) emotional and physiological reactions to attachment-relevant and attachment-irrelevant stressful events.

### Appraisal of Distress-Eliciting Events

Attachment orientations are related to people's beliefs and expectations about threatening events and their ability to avoid stress or cope effectively with it. With regard to threat appraisals, studies have shown that attachment security is associated with appraising potentially stressful events in less threatening ways. With regard to what Lazarus and Folkman (1984) called "secondary appraisal," there is evidence that secure attachment is related to appraising oneself as able to cope effectively with threats. Specifically, attachment security is associated with higher scores on scales measuring ego resilience, perceived coping resources, and stress-resistant hardy attitudes (e.g., Caldwell & Shaver, 2012; Jones, Brett, Ehrlich, Lejuez, & Cassidy, 2014; Karreman & Vingerhoets, 2012). Attachment security is also associated with more positive expectations about regulating negative moods, and more optimistic and hopeful attitudes toward confronting adversities (e.g., Carnelley, Hepper, Hicks, & Turner, 2011; Han & Pistole, 2014; Jankowski & Sandage, 2011). For example, Jones and colleagues (2014) found that mothers who reported greater attachment-related avoidance and anxiety reported having greater difficulties with emotion regulation 1 year later, and these difficulties, in turn, predicted more distressed, harsher, and less supportive maternal responses to adolescents' negative emotions the following year.

In contrast, people scoring higher on attachment anxiety tend to appraise potentially stressful events in amplified, sometimes catastrophic ways, overemphasizing the imagined danger, and perceiving themselves as unable to cope effectively (see Mikulincer & Shaver, 2016, for a review). For avoidant individuals the findings are more complex. With regard to appraising one's own coping abilities, most studies have found that avoidant people's appraisals are similar to those of secure people (appraising coping resources as adequate). With regard to threat appraisals, however, most studies have found that avoidant attachment, like attachment anxiety, is associated with appraising stressful events as highly threatening. Such appraisals have been noted mainly when avoidant people confronted undeniable and prolonged stressful events, such as impending divorce or caring for a child with a congenital heart defect (e.g., Berant, Mikulincer, & Florian, 2001a, 2001b; Birnbaum, Orr, Mikulincer, & Florian, 1997). These findings have been replicated in longitudinal studies. For example, Berant and colleagues (2001b) found that avoidance predicted increasingly pessimistic appraisals of stressful events over a 1-year period.

## Ways of Coping with Distress-Eliciting Events

Several studies have included assessments of participants' use of particular coping strategies (e.g., problem solving, emotion-focused coping, reappraisal, distancing coping). With regard to prob-lem-focused coping, some researchers have found that secure people are more likely than insecure ones to use this generally effective strategy (e.g., Bazzarian & Besharat, 2012; Deniz & Işik, 2010; Raskin, Kummel, & Bannister, 1998), but other studies have not found a significant association between attachment style and problem-focused coping (e.g., Berant et al., 2001a; Mikulincer & Florian, 1995; Mikulincer, Florian, & Weller, 1993). Some of the latter studies focused on stressful events for which people received extensive problem-solving instructions, such as media information about what to do in case of missile attacks or officers' instructions about how to solve problems during combat training. This may have caused most study participants, regardless of attachment style, to deal with the stressful events in a problem-focused way.

Several studies have found links between avoidant attachment and reliance on distancing coping strategies, such as stress denial, diversion of attention, and behavioral or cognitive disengagement (e.g., Holmberg, Lomore, Takacs, & Price, 2011; Marshall Serran, & Cortoni, 2000; Shapiro & Levendosky, 1999). Also compatible with theory, avoidance has been associated with repression (e.g., Gjerde, Onishi, & Carlson, 2004; Mikulincer & Orbach, 1995; Vetere & Myers, 2002). Moreover, Turan, Osar, Turan, Ilkova, and Damci (2003) found that diabetic persons scoring higher on avoidance relied more on cognitive distancing and passive resignation as coping strategies, which in turn were associated with poor adherence to medical regimens.

Relations between attachment style and distancing coping were also examined in two longitudinal investigations. In a 31-year study, Klohnen and Bera (1998) found that women with an avoidant attachment style at age 52 had scored higher on repressive defensiveness at ages 21 and 43 than women who exhibited a secure style at age 52. Similarly, Zhang and Labouvie-Vief (2004) conducted a 6-year longitudinal study of people ranging in age from late adolescence to late adulthood, and found that although attachment style was relatively stable over the 6-year period, there was some fluidity associated with variations in coping strategies and mental health. An increase in attachment security over the 6-year period covaried with decreased use of distancing coping and increased use of constructive, flexible, and reality-oriented coping strategies. These findings fit well with the theoretical notion that felt security is a resilience resource that helps people maintain emotional balance without having to use avoidant defenses.

In only one study (Berant et al., 2001a, 2001b) were secure individuals more likely than their avoidant peers to rely on distancing coping. Secure mothers of both healthy infants and infants with a mild coronary heart defect (CHD) relied on support seeking and problem solving, but secure mothers of infants with a severe CHD tended to rely on distancing strategies. This suggests that secure mothers can employ distancing coping when thoughts about the stressful condition might impair effective functioning. Suppression of painful thoughts about their infants' illness might have allowed secure women to maintain a positive appraisal of motherhood. As a result, the overwhelming demands of the infants' illness might not have been so discouraging, allowing mothers to mobilize internal and external resources for taking care of their babies. Consistent with this reasoning, Schmidt, Nachtigall, Wuethrich-Martone, and Strauss (2002) and Cohen and Katz (2015) found that attachment security is associated with greater coping flexibility.

Most of the studies that involved the assessment of emotion-focused coping (e.g., wishful thinking, self-blame, rumination) have found that attachment-anxious adults are more likely than secure ones to direct their attention toward their own distress rather than focusing on possible solutions to the problem at hand. For example, several studies have established that people scoring higher on attachment anxiety are more likely to engage in distress-exacerbating mental rumination—moody pondering or thinking anxiously or gloomily about life events (e.g., Caldwell & Shaver, 2012; Garrison, Kahn, Miller, & Sauer, 2014; Reynolds, Searight, & Ratwik, 2014). There is also evidence that anxious attachment is associated with higher levels of worrying about the causes and consequences of threatening events (e.g., Consedine, Tuck, & Fiori, 2013; Warren et al., 2010). For example, Mikulincer and Florian (1998) assessed worrying in the laboratory and found that experimentally induced failure evoked more worries mainly among attachment-anxious people. In addition, more anxiously attached adults scored higher on a scale assessing crying proneness (Denckla, Fiori, & Vingerhoets, 2014) and actually cried more in response to sad music and reported more negative emotions during these crying episodes (Laan, van Assen, & Vingerhoets, 2012).

Anxious people's tendency to direct attention toward distress was also noted in an experiment conducted by Silva, Soares, and Esteves (2012). Participants were asked to search for a target image, while ignoring a previously presented neutral or distress-eliciting prime. The distress prime interfered with image search (lower accuracy), but this interference was stronger among participants who scored higher on attachment anxiety; that is, anxious peoples' attention was automatically directed toward distress, which in turn interfered with task performance.

Interestingly and unexpectedly, some studies have yielded associations between avoidance and emotion-focused coping (e.g., Berant et al., 2001a, 2001b; Birnbaum, Orr, Mikulincer, & Florian, 1997; Lussier, Sabourin, & Turgeon, 1997). These findings suggest that there are limits to deactivating strategies. For example, Berant and colleagues (2001a, 2001b) found that avoidant mothers of newborns tended to rely on distancing coping if their infant was born healthy or with only a mild CHD, but they used emotion-focused coping if their infant was diagnosed with a life-threatening CHD, and they showed a notable increase in the use of this coping strategy a year after the diagnosis. Thus, avoidant defenses, which may be sufficient for dealing with minor stressors, can fail when people encounter severe and persistent stressors. This conclusion is consistent with Bowlby's (1980) idea that avoidant people's segregated mental systems cannot be hidden from conscious awareness indefinitely, and that traumatic events can resurrect distress that had been sealed off from consciousness.

## The Regulation of Attachment-Related Distress

Attachment orientations are particularly relevant for understanding individual differences in the ways in which people experience and react to attachment-related sources of distress (separation, loss). With regard to attachment anxiety, there is consistent evidence for a pattern of hyperactivation of attachment-related painful emotions and thoughts that exacerbate rather than mitigate distress. Using functional magnetic resonance imaging (fMRI) to observe brain processes while recalling a painful separation, Gillath, Bunge, Shaver, Wendelken, and Mikulincer (2005) found that attachment anxiety was associated with higher activation of the left anterior temporal pole and left hippocampus, areas associated with the recall of sad thoughts, and lower activation of the orbitofrontal cortex, an area associated with emotional control. That is, anxious people seemed unable to control the reactivation of separation memories. This conclusion is reinforced by findings from Bailey, Paret, Battista, and Xue (2012), who used a Stroop task and found that attachment anxiety was associated with greater interference in naming the color in which separation-related words were printed—indicating a lack of control over intrusions by separation-related thoughts.

Neural signs of distress hyperactivation by attachment-anxious adults have also been reported by DeWall and colleagues (2012). They found that in response to a simulated experience of social exclusion while lying in an MRI scanner, self-reports of anxious attachment were related to heightened activity in regions involved in distress activation: the dorsal anterior cingulate cortex (dACC) and the anterior insula. Importantly, these brain reactions to social exclusion were attenuated by asking people to reflect on their security-providing attachment figure (Karremans, Heslenfeld, van Dillen, & Van Lange, 2011).

For avoidant people, the main method of dealing with separation-related thoughts is to suppress them. In a pair of experimental studies, Fraley and Shaver (1997) asked participants to write about whatever thoughts and feelings they experienced while being asked to suppress thoughts about a romantic partner leaving them for someone else. The ability to suppress these thoughts was assessed by the number of times they appeared in participants' stream of consciousness following the suppression period and by the level of physiological arousal (skin conductance) during the suppression task. As expected, more avoidant people were more able to suppress separation-related thoughts, as indicated by less frequent thoughts of loss following the suppression task and lower skin conductance during the task. In accord with this finding, Edelstein and Gillath (2008) used a Stroop task and found that avoidance was associated with reduced interference (faster RTs) in naming the color in which separation-related words were printed, reflecting avoidant people's tendency to block access to separation-related thoughts.

Mikulincer, Dolev, and Shaver (2004) replicated and extended Fraley and Shaver's (1997) findings while assessing, in a Stroop task, the cognitive activation of previously suppressed thoughts about a painful separation. Avoidant individuals were able to suppress thoughts related to the breakup; for them, such thoughts were relatively inaccessible, and their own positive self-traits became more accessible than usual (presumably for defensive reasons). However, their ability to maintain this defensive stance was disrupted when a cognitive load—remembering a seven-digit number—was added to the experimental task. Under high cognitive load, avoidant individuals suddenly evinced high availability of thoughts of separation and negative self-traits; that is, the suppressed material resurfaced in experience and behavior when a high cognitive demand was imposed. This fragility of avoidant defenses has been further documented in more recent studies. Kohn, Rholes, and Schmeichel (2012) found that whereas avoidant attachment was associated with less access to early memories of negative attachment experiences in a neutral condition, a cognitive-depletion induction led to heightened access to these memories among more avoidant people. Similarly, Chun, Shaver, Gillath, Mathews, and Jorgensen (2015) found that more avoidant participants' ability to disengage attention from contemptuous faces was impaired (compared to the ability of less avoidant participants) when they were asked to rehearse a seven-digit number while performing the attention task.

While probing further into the regulatory mechanisms underlying avoidant defenses, Fraley, Garner, and Shaver (2000) asked whether they function in a preemptive manner (directing attention away from the information or encoding it in a shallow way) or in a "postemptive" manner (repressing material that has already been encoded). Participants listened to an interview about the loss of a relationship partner and were asked later to recall details of the interview, either soon after hearing them (Study 1) or at various delays ranging from half an hour to 21 days (Study 2). An analysis of forgetting curves revealed that (1) avoidant people initially encoded less information about the interview, and (2) people differing in attachment styles forgot encoded information at the same rate. Thus, avoidant defenses sometimes act preemptively by blocking threatening material from being encoded. In a subsequent study, Fraley and Brumbaugh (2007) found that more avoidant individuals performed worse on tasks assessing both explicit and implicit memories of information about the loss of a sister.

These findings imply that avoidant people are likely to be vigilant to attachment-related information so that its encoding can be blocked. In support of this idea, Maier and colleagues (2005) found that avoidant attachment (assessed with the AAI) was associated with lower identification thresholds (less exposure time needed to identify a picture) for pictures depicting emotion-laden human faces and social interactions. In a more direct test of avoidant people's preemptive vigilance, Zheng, Zhang, and Zheng (2015) found that avoidant people (assessed with the ECR) tended to allocate more cognitive resources when encoding emotional faces at an early stage (170 miliseconds) during an old/new evoked-related potentials task. Similarly, Chun and colleagues (2015) found that more avoidant people (based on the ECR) were more vigilant toward contemptuous faces when the faces were presented for 100 milliseconds but quickly disengaged from them when the faces were presented for 750 milliseconds. Thus, avoidant defenses seem to demand perceptual vigilance to emotional stimuli at an early stage of information processing, in order to keep them from being processed further. We suspect that this is the default avoidant defense. Postemptive strategies are likely to be called upon only if the preemptive approach fails or when a threatening memory is aroused by association.

### Emotional Reactions to Stressful Events

Several researchers have collected participants' reports of psychological distress during stressful events. Across these studies, attachment security has been associated with lower levels of distress, whereas attachment insecurities—anxiety, avoidance, or both—have been associated with heightened distress (see Mikulincer & Shaver, 2016, for a review). The link between attachment security and adaptive emotional reactions to stress has also been validated in experimental studies showing that temporarily activating mental representations of available and responsive attachment figures (a process we call *security priming*) can augment a person's emotional balance, even under fairly stressful circumstances (e.g., Mikulincer, Gillath, et al., 2001; Mikulincer, Hirschberger, Nachmias, & Gillath, 2001; Mikulincer & Shaver, 2001). In these experiments, mental representations of supportive attachment figures have been activated by well-validated social-cognitive techniques, such as subliminally presenting pictures suggestive of attachment figures' availability (e.g., a Picasso drawing of a mother lovingly cradling an infant, a couple holding hands and gazing into each other's eyes), names of people who were designated by participants as security-enhancing attachment figures, positive attachment-related words (e.g.,

*love, closeness, hug*), guided images of available and supportive attachment figures, and visualization of security-enhancing attachment figures' faces. In all of these studies, portrayals of attachment figures' availability led to more positive moods than priming with attachment-unrelated stimuli, even ones suggesting positive emotion (e.g., the word *success*).

Mikulincer, Hirschberger, and colleagues (2001) also found that priming with representations of supportive attachment figures infused formerly neutral stimuli with positive qualities, even when the priming was done subliminally. For example, subliminal presentation of the names of people who were designated by participants as security-enhancing attachment figures, compared with the names of close others or mere acquaintances who were not designated as attachment figures, led to greater liking of previously unfamiliar Chinese ideographs. Moreover, subliminally priming mental representations of available attachment figures induced more positive evaluations of neutral stimuli, even in threatening contexts, and eliminated the detrimental effects that threats otherwise had on liking for neutral stimuli. Thus, priming with mental representations of security-enhancing attachment figures has a calming, soothing effect, similar to the effects of actual interactions with available and responsive relationship partners.

There is also evidence that avoidance can be associated with negative emotional reactions to stressful events. For example, Berant and colleagues (2001b) and Berant, Mikulincer, and Shaver (2008) found that avoidance in mothers of infants with severe forms of CHD was a stronger predictor of deteriorated mental health 1 and 7 years later than was attachment anxiety. Similarly, Reizer, Possick, and Ein-Dor (2010) found that avoidance was associated with heightened distress among couples living in life-endangering areas of Israel (Jewish settlements in the West Bank) but not among couples living in less threatening areas. That is, under chronic, demanding stressful conditions, avoidant deactivating strategies seem to collapse, causing avoidant people to have as high or even higher levels of distress than anxious people. This is reminiscent of laboratory studies showing that avoidant defenses collapse under an experimentally imposed cognitive load (Mikulincer et al., 2004).

The vulnerability of avoidant defenses to collapse has also been noticed in studies assessing physiological responses to stressful events. For example, in two studies, avoidant people (assessed with the AAI) had increased levels of physiological arousal (heightened electrodermal activity) when talking about painful childhood memories or during exposure to infant crying (e.g., Ablow, Marks, Feldman, & Huffman, 2013; Roisman, Tsai, & Chiang, 2004). Similarly, higher self-reported avoidant attachment was associated with heightened physiological reactivity—decreased heart-rate variability (Maunder, Lancee, Nolan, Hunter, & Tannenbaum, 2006), increased skin conductance (Diamond, Hicks, & Otter-Henderson, 2006), and heightened diastolic blood pressure (Kim, 2006) —in response to various laboratory stressors (e.g., recalling a stressful situation, performing demanding tasks, discussing relationship problems with a dating partner). In addition, Kim (2006) found that avoidance was associated with a decrease in *rate-pressure product* (pulse rate multiplied by systolic blood pressure) during a couple discussion, indicating an inability to supply oxygen to cardiac muscles while coping with stress that can "heighten the risk for hypertension and other cardiovascular diseases" (p. 111).

Interestingly, Maunder and colleagues (2006) found that attachment-anxious people's responsiveness to stressors was manifested in higher levels of reported distress but not in heart rate measures, again suggesting that anxious people exaggerate their distress. In Kim's (2006) study, anxious participants' physiological reactivity was observed only when they also reported high levels of distress. This tendency contrasts with avoidant individuals' dissociation between subjective reports of lack of distress and heightened physiological reactivity.

Several studies have assessed attachment-related differences in the activity of the hypothalamic–pituitary–adrenal (HPA) axis—indexed by salivary cortisol levels during and following laboratory-induced stressors. Two studies indicated that avoidant attachment was associated with increased levels of salivary cortisol (Kidd, Hamer, & Steptoe, 2011; Pierrehumbert, Torrisi, Ansermet, Borghini, & Halfon, 2012), two studies (Pierrehumbert et al., 2009; Quirin, Pruessner, & Kuhl, 2008) found a positive association between attachment anxiety and heightened cortisol reactivity, and two studies found no significant attachment–cortisol link (Ditzen et al., 2008; Smeets, 2010). These inconsistencies might have been due in part to variations in the stressors (e.g., aversive noise, the Trier Social Stress Test) and participants' ages (young adults, midlife adults). More research is needed to determine the link between attachment insecurities and HPA dysregulation.

Kidd, Hamer, and Steptoe (2013) went beyond examining acute cortisol responses to stress and assessed cortisol levels across the day. Attachment anxiety was associated with both increased stress perceptions and higher levels of cortisol throughout the day. In addition, anxious attachment was related to heightened bedtime cortisol levels. It seems that anxious attachment strategies not only elevate cortisol levels during waking hours but also interfere with the inability to reduce levels of arousal when preparing to sleep (Maunder, Hunter, & Lancee, 2011).

There is also some evidence concerning attachment-related differences in brain responses to stressful events. Using event-related fMRI, Lemche and colleagues (2006) found that self-reports of attachment anxiety or avoidance were associated with heightened activation in bilateral amygdalae to a stressful stimulus; that is, less secure people tended to react to stress with increased amygdala activity—a neural indication of distress-related arousal.

More information about the brain mechanisms underlying insecure people's regulatory strategies was provided by Vrtička, Bondolfi, Sander, and Vuilleumier (2012), who scanned the brains of people who were asked to attend naturally or cognitively reappraise their emotional responses to unpleasant scenes. Avoidant participants showed increased prefrontal and anterior cingulate activation in response to unpleasant scenes and exhibited increases in dorsolateral prefrontal cortex and left amygdala activity during reappraisal. These results suggest that avoidant people may be less efficient in using reappraisal strategies and need to engage in more effortful control for dealing with distress. Anxious participants showed increases in the right amygdala across the conditions—another sign of their heightened reactivity.

In a recent fMRI study, Moutsiana and colleagues (2014) provided evidence that infant attachment assessed at 18 months predicts neural responses to positive affect inductions at age 22 years. Specifically, adults who had been insecurely attached as infants showed greater activation in prefrontal regions and lower co-activation of nucleus accumbens with prefrontal cortex than adults who had been securely attached as infants. That is, attachment insecurity during infancy seems to be associated with relative inefficiency in the neural regulation of positive emotions during adulthood, and with the need to devote more effortful control during positive emotion inductions.

Considering longer-term neural effects of attachment insecurities, Quirin, Gillath, Pruessner, and Eggert (2010) found that self-reports of attachment anxiety and avoidance were associated with reduced hippocampal cell density, which was associated with poorer emotion regulation. Whereas avoidance was associated with bilateral hippocampal cell reduction, anxiety was related to reduced cell concentration in the left hippocampus. These findings are compatible with a neurotoxic model of stress-induced cell reduction in the hippocampus, contributing to poorer emotion regulation abilities in individuals with insecure attachment orientations. In addition, Moutsiana and colleagues (2015) found that attachment insecurity at 18 months was associated with larger amygdala volumes at 22 years. However, they did not find evidence linking infant attachment status and hippocampal volume in young adulthood.

Attachment strategies are also manifested in emotional reactions to physical illnesses. There is evidence that attachment insecurities, mainly of the anxious kind, are associated with heightened distress among people suffering from physical illness (e.g., Bazzarian & Besharat, 2012; Vilchinsky et al., 2010; Vilchinsky, Dekel, Asher, Leibowitz, & Mosseri, 2013). However, in a prospective 6-month study of patients with acute coronary syndrome, Vilchinsky and colleagues (2010) found that a partner's supportiveness can buffer the observed link between attachment anxiety and distress. Attachment anxiety predicted heightened distress only when spouses did not actively support the patients. This detrimental effect of anxiety evaporated when spouses engaged in more supportive behavior, thereby providing a greater sense of security for the anxious patient.

Overall, data support the hypothesis that secure adults' optimistic appraisals of situations and reliance on constructive ways of coping mitigate distress during periods of stress. They also indicate that attachment anxiety or avoidance can interfere with effective coping and increase distress intensity. In the long run, this means that attachment insecurities increase people's risk for developing serious emotional and physical health problems.

## Cognitive Access to and Structure of Emotional Experiences

Theoretically, attachment strategies should influence a person's access to emotion-related information, that is, the ways in which he or she attends to,

encodes, retrieves, understands, and reacts to such information; and the extent to which he or she is aware of emotional states and their fluctuations. In this section, we review some of the studies that have examined attachment-related individual differences in cognitive access to and architecture of emotional experiences, which is likely to be important for both personal understanding and regulation of one's emotions and the ability to discuss such emotions with relationship partners.

### Access to Emotional Memories

In an early study of emotional memories, Mikulincer and Orbach (1995) noted attachment-related differences in the ways people retrieve early memories of specific emotions. Participants were asked to recall early experiences of anger, sadness, anxiety, or happiness, and their memory retrieval latencies were recorded as indicators of cognitive accessibility. Participants also rated the intensity of emotions in each recalled event.

Avoidant individuals exhibited the poorest access (longest latencies) to sad and anxious memories; anxious people had the quickest access to such memories; and secure people fell in between. Secure people took less time to retrieve positive than negative emotional memories, whereas anxious people had quicker access to negative than to positive memories. Moreover, avoidant people rated focal emotions (e.g., sadness when instructed to retrieve a sad memory) and nonfocal emotions (e.g., anger when instructed to retrieve a sad memory) as less intense than secure people. Anxious people reported experiencing very intense focal and nonfocal emotions when asked to remember instances of anxiety, sadness, and anger. In contrast, secure people rated focal emotions as much more intense than nonfocal emotions.

The findings suggest that secure people rely on more constructive and effective emotion regulation strategies. They acknowledge distress, retain access to negative memories, and process these experiences fully. However, they also have better access to positive memories and tend not to suffer from a spread of activation from one negative memory to another. Van Emmichoven, Van IJzendoorn, de Ruiter, and Brosschot (2003) noted this open attitude toward distress-eliciting information even in a sample of patients with anxiety disorders. It is possible that this open and adaptive pattern of emotion regulation explains Behringer, Reiner, and Spangler's (2011) finding that secure new mothers (as assessed by interviews during pregnancy) displayed heightened sadness and anxiety 2 weeks postpartum and following a return to baseline following 2, 4, and 6 months. Insecure mothers exhibited a stable increase in negative emotions after delivery that did not return to baseline even after 6 months. That is, attachment security seems to help new mothers express and recover from negative emotions.

Mikulincer and Orbach (1995) found that avoidant people's reduced access to negative emotional memories is another indication of their attempts to inhibit the cognitive processing of distress-eliciting outer or inner stimuli. This finding was replicated by Dykas, Woodhouse, Jones, and Cassidy (2014) using the AAI to assess adolescents' state of mind with respect to attachment. Edelstein and colleagues (2005) also found evidence for avoidant people's poor access to negative memories (with avoidance being measured by the ECR) in a study of a sample of child sexual abuse (CSA) survivors. More avoidant people were less accurate in recalling specific, well documented, severe CSA incidents that had occurred approximately 14 years earlier. Interestingly, these memory problems were reduced among avoidant people who reported relatively high levels of maternal support after the abuse, highlighting the buffering effect of security-enhancing interactions.

In a related study, Haggerty, Siefert, and Weinberger (2010) instructed adults to freely recall childhood experiences before the age of 14 years, without explicitly asking them to remember a particular emotionally laden memory. Whereas both attachment anxiety and avoidance were linked to remembering more negative childhood experiences, only avoidance was associated with reduced emotional intensity of these memories, a finding similar to that reported by Mikulincer and Orbach (1995). Other studies have shown that avoidance is associated with less coherent memories of interactions with romantic partners (Sutin & Gillath, 2009) and lower levels of narrative elaboration of both childhood and adolescent memories (McCabe & Peterson, 2011). Interestingly, Sutin and Gillath (2009) found that exposure to insecurity primes (i.e., thinking about a nonresponsive relationship partner) led to less coherent memories.

Mikulincer and Orbach's (1995) finding that attachment anxiety is linked to easy access to negative emotional memories and impaired control of the spread of activation from focal emotions to nonfocal emotions suggests that attachment-anxious people have a somewhat undifferentiated, unregulated organization of emotional memories. This fits with Roisman and colleagues' (2004) findings about people's facial expressions during the AAI. Whereas secure people's facial expressions were congruent with the valence of the childhood events they were describing, anxious people exhibited angry or anxious facial expressions while speaking about neutral or positive childhood experiences. According to Roisman and colleagues, these discrepancies reflect anxious individuals' confusion and emotional dysregulation when being asked to talk about emotionally charged experiences.

Pereg and Mikulincer (2004) studied the cognitive effects of induced negative mood, providing further evidence of insecure people's problems in processing emotional experiences. In two studies, participants were assigned to a negative mood condition or to a control condition, then incidental recall of positive and negative information (Study 1) or causal attributions of a negative event (Study 2) were assessed. The negative mood condition (as compared to the control condition) led secure participants to recall more positive information and less negative information, and to attribute a negative event to less global and stable causes. This mood-incongruent pattern of cognition is likely to inhibit the spread of negative emotions and activate competing positive cognitions (positive recalled information, attributions that maintain a positive view of a partner). As a result, secure people are able to work against the pervasive effects of the negative mood induction and maintain or restore emotional equanimity. In contrast, more anxious participants reacted to the induced negative mood with heightened recall of negative information and an increased tendency to attribute a negative event to more global and stable causes. This mood-congruent pattern of cognition favors the spread of negative emotions in memory and heightens access to distress-eliciting thoughts. These negative cognitions can exacerbate anxious people's chronic distress and negative views of others, and therefore contribute to continued activation of the attachment system.

Findings from Pereg and Mikulincer's (2004) studies also indicated that the memories and causal attribution patterns of avoidant people were not significantly affected by induced negative mood. Avoidant people seemed to exclude negative emotions from awareness and were therefore less likely to use it in cognitive processing.

## Cognitive and Brain Reactions to Emotional Stimuli

There is growing evidence that attachment strategies are manifested in the ways people react to emotional stimuli. Atkinson and colleagues (2009) examined mothers' attention to emotional information using a Stroop task and reported that insecure mothers (assessed with the AAI) showed greater Stroop interference for negative emotion words, reflecting heightened difficulty in disengaging attention from these emotions. Similarly, using data from participants who completed a Stroop task during fMRI, Warren and colleagues (2010) found that attachment insecurities are associated with heightened color-naming interference for negative emotional words and increased activity in prefrontal cortical regions associated with emotion regulation (e.g., right orbitofrontal cortex) and cognitive control (e.g., left dorsolateral prefrontal cortex) during exposure to these words. Again, it seems that attachment insecurities involve vulnerability to distraction by negative emotional clues, and that greater cognitive control is required to attend to task-relevant, nonemotional information.

However, the kind of insecurity, anxious or avoidant, influences the specific ways in which people react to this vulnerability. Whereas avoidant individuals attempt to control the expression of emotion and distance themselves from it, anxious individuals' physiological and behavioral reactions exacerbate difficulties in disentangling attention from the emotional experience. For example, Rognoni, Galati, Costa, and Crini (2008) assessed electroencephalographic (EEG) frontal asymmetry while participants watched video clips inducing happiness, fear, or sadness. Whereas more avoidant people showed no fluctuation in frontal asymmetry in response to depictions of negative emotions, more anxious people exhibited wider frontal right activation in response to these emotions—a sign of threat-related activation in the brain. Similarly, Zilber, Goldstein, and Mikulincer (2007) found that more anxious participants (assessed with the ECR) showed greater brain-related late positive potential (LPP) amplitudes to distress-eliciting pictures—another sign of persistent attention. This response was not observed for positive or neutral pictures.

Avoidant people's tendency to control attention has been observed in a series of studies by Gillath, Giesbrecht, and Shaver (2009). They examined associations between ECR scores and performance on attachment-unrelated attention tasks—a psychological refractory period (PRP) task assessing ability to switch attention rapidly from one stimulus to another and a flanker task assessing ability to resist distracters. As expected, avoidant attachment predicted better performance on both tasks, and the effects remained significant even after the researchers controlled for other personality traits. However, findings also revealed that thinking about a past attachment-related injury eliminated avoidant participants' superior attentional performance. In summary, avoidant people are generally skilled at regulating their attention, but their performance can be hampered by reminders of episodes of rejection, separation, or loss.

There is also evidence that avoidant people's attentional control includes the ability to inhibit brain and cognitive responses to distress-eliciting stimuli. For example, Suslow and colleagues (2009) used fMRI to examine differences in automatic brain reactivity to sad and happy faces as a function of attachment-related avoidance. As expected, avoidance was inversely associated with activity in the amygdala, the insula, and the primary somatosensory cortex (Brodmann area 3 [BA 3]) to sad faces. Subsequently, Suslow, Dannlowski, Arolt, and Ohrmann (2010) found that avoidant attachment was associated with inhibition of affective priming effects of subliminal presentations of sad faces on liking of neutral faces; that is, avoidant defenses seemed to block access to sadness-inducing information, thereby preventing the transfer of negative affect to a neutral stimulus.

## Avoidant Attachment and Lack of Psychobiological Coherence

Avoidant people's reduced access to emotions is also evident in studies examining the coherence between self-reports of emotional experiences and less conscious, more automatic indicators of these experiences. (We assume that higher concordance between these measures implies greater access to emotional experience.) For example, avoidant people score relatively low on self-reports of death anxiety or anger but implicitly reveal these emotions in Thematic Apperception Test (TAT) stories or measured heart rate (Mikulincer, 1998; Mikulincer et al., 1990). Three related studies examined access to emotions during the AAI, and all found that avoidant people verbally expressed few negative feelings during the interview but at the same time exhibited higher levels of physiological arousal (heightened electrodermal activity; Dozier & Kobak, 1992; Roisman et al., 2004) and more intense facial expressions of negative emotions (Zimmermann, Wulf, & Grossmann, 1996).

Spangler and Zimmermann (1999) examined attachment-related differences (based on the AAI) in the coherence of facial muscle reactions (measured with electromyography of the smile and frown muscles) and subjective reactions (pleasantness ratings) to 24 film fragments. For each study participant, they computed the correlation between muscular and subjective reactions across the 24 scenes, with higher positive correlations reflecting higher psychobiological coherence. Attachment security was positively associated with psychobiological coherence, but avoidance was associated with less accurate awareness of physiological states. Zimmermann, Maier, Winter, and Grossmann (2001) extended these findings to the experience of emotions during a problem-solving task: Avoidant people were characterized by a greater discrepancy between self-reported anger and sadness and congruent facial expressions. Similar findings were reported by White and colleagues (2012), who found that avoidant adolescents (in the Child Attachment Interview) reported relatively low levels of distress during a rejection episode, although their brains showed a strong negative reaction to this episode (stronger negative left-frontal slow wave).

Sonnby-Borgstrom and Jonsson (2004) provided further evidence of avoidant individuals' lack of psychobiological coherence when undergoing negative emotions. In their study, people were exposed to pictures of happy and angry faces at three different exposure times (17, 56, and 2,350 milliseconds), and their facial muscle reactions were continuously assessed. When the pictures were presented subliminally and participants could not recognize the faces (at exposure times of 17 or 53 milliseconds), both avoidant and secure individuals activated muscles involved in negative emotional displays (corrugator or "frowning" muscles) when they were presented with angry faces. However, when participants were able to recognize the faces (at an exposure time of 2,350 milliseconds), avoidant participants evinced lower levels of corrugator activity and increased zygomaticus muscle responses (a "smiling" reaction) when exposed to angry faces. In contrast, secure people reacted to these pictures by mimicking them (heightened corrugator activity). Avoidant people's heightened corrugator reaction to sublim-inal exposure to angry faces seems to indicate that these pictures had automatically elicited negative emotions. Therefore, the avoidant participants' tendency to smile when they consciously saw the angry faces suggests a defensive attempt to block cognitive access to and visible expression of negative emotions.

A subsequent study extended these findings to interpersonal interactions. Seedall and Wampler (2012) videotaped couples during a seminatural conversation and an interaction with a therapist, and assessed physiological signs of distress (skin conductance) and the type of affect they expressed to their partner during the interactions. More secure participants showed signs of adequate psychobiological coherence: They expressed more negative feelings toward their partners mainly when they showed increased levels of skin conductance. However, those higher in avoidance expressed more positive feelings toward their partner mainly when they showed increased skin conductance—another possible sign of lack of psychobiological coherence.

## Insecure People's Problems in Identifying and Differentiating Emotions

Pursuing the hypothesis that avoidant people tend to exclude emotions from consciousness, several studies have found positive associations between avoidant attachment and scores on the Toronto Alexithymia Scale, indicating difficulties in identifying and describing emotions (e.g., Barbasio & Granieri, 2013; Hesse & Floyd, 2011; Keating, Tasca, & Hill, 2013). Avoidant attachment (assessed with either self-report scales or the AAI) is also related to inattention to feelings (e.g., Kim, 2005), less emotional awareness (e.g., Monti & Rudolph, 2014), and less recall and more dismissal of dreams (e.g., Contelmo, Hart, & Levine, 2013). More avoidant people are also less likely to use emotion words and reflect on emotional themes while speaking about their childhood experiences in the AAI (e.g., Borelli et al., 2013). In addition, they score lower on tests of emotional intelligence (e.g., Cherry, Fletcher, & O'Sullivan, 2013, Delhaye, Kempenaers, Stroobants, Goossens, & Linkowski, 2013; Lanciano, Curci, Kafetsios, Elia, & Zammuner, 2012; but see Kafetsios, 2004, for an unexpected positive association between avoidant attachment and emotion understanding).

Interestingly, most of the studies that have examined attachment-related differences in alexithymia indicate that attachment-anxious people may also have difficulty identifying and describing their feelings. According to Mallinckrodt and Wei (2005), higher alexithymia scores reflect not only lack of emotional awareness but also difficulties in differentiating between specific emotions and communicating specific feelings to others. It seems possible, therefore, that anxious strategies, which are associated with an undifferentiated, somewhat chaotic emotional architecture, create difficulties in differentiating and identifying specific feelings. In support of this view, Stevens (2014) found that, although attachment-anxious people reported having increased emotional awareness, they struggled to identify their feelings and manage emotion-related responses. Moreover, Hill and colleagues (2013) found that more anxious people (assessed with the ECR) were less likely to report dreams during psychodynamic psychotherapy.

Attachment-anxious individuals' problems in differentiating and identifying specific feelings may be a result of the intensity of their reactions to threatening events. Several studies have indicated that people who score high on attachment anxiety also score high on measures of emotional reactivity or intensity (e.g., Gratz et al., 2015; Wei, Russell, Mallinckrodt, & Vogel, 2007; Wei, Vogel, Ku, & Zakalik, 2005). Some of these studies also indicated that avoidant attachment is associated with lower emotional intensity and expression of both positive emotions (e.g., love, pride) and negative emotions (e.g., anger and sadness). This fits with our idea that even positive emotions play a role in strengthening attachment bonds—something that avoidant people generally do not wish to do. This conclusion was recently supported by Goodall (2015), who found that avoidant people have difficulty regulating positive emotions. Specifically, self-reports of avoidant attachment were associated with lower levels of *savoring strategies* (enhancing or prolonging a positive emotion in order to maximize its effect) and higher levels of *dampening strategies* (limiting or reducing the effect of a positive emotion through a variety of means, e.g., suppression or changing focus away from the positive emotion).

Anxious and avoidant individuals' problems in identifying their feelings are also evident in studies examining individual differences in *mindfulness*—the capacity to maintain mindful attention and awareness to "here and now" stimuli, sensations, feelings, and thoughts without any judgmental attitude. In all of these studies, self-reports of attachment anxiety and avoidance have been inversely associated with self-reports of mindfulness (e.g., Bourne, Berry, & Jones, 2014; Pepping, Davis, & O'Donovan, 2013; Walsh, Balint, Smolira, Frederickson, & Madsen, 2009). Pepping and colleagues (2013) also found that difficulties in emotion regulation fully mediated the negative association between attachment insecurities and mindfulness.

## Conclusions

An enormous body of research—larger than we can cover here—supports an attachment–theoretical approach to understanding emotion regulation in adults. Many creative hypotheses based on the theory have been formulated and tested since 1990, using a variety of research methods—including behavioral observations, interviews, questionnaires, physiological and neuroimaging assessments, subliminal priming, implicit measures of cognitive and emotional processes, and systematic manipulations of threatening contexts and social situations. The findings are coherent, mutually reinforcing, and compatible with the model of attachment system activation and functioning presented here.

When we compare the literature available when we wrote the 2008 version of this chapter with what has been published since, we see that the literature has more than doubled in size. In general it has supported both attachment theory and our model of attachment system functioning, while adding an enormous number of details based on new methods and hypotheses. Especially impressive is the use of experimental methods, including subliminal priming, to probe the mechanisms underlying previous observations and test causal, rather than merely correlational, hypotheses. Also impressive are the revolutionary developments in the study of physiological underpinnings of attachment-related processes, including the expanding use of fMRI, candidate gene methods, and both the assessment and administration of hormones. These new developments are useful for not only the additional light they shed on attachment processes but also the suggestions they offer concerning possible interventions to enhance security (e.g., through security "priming," couple counseling, and therapeutic targeting of particular mediating processes, e.g., avoidant suppression of negative emotions and the use of effective coping skills). These gains in research make possible parallel gains in psychological interventions and, perhaps, in greater self-understanding.

Despite these substantial gains over the period of 8 years since the previous handbook, there are still important issues to be resolved. Most of the social-psychological studies of adults, including our own studies, have involved samples of normal college students and have relied on self-report measures of attachment style. As explained in this volume by Crowell, Fraley, and Roisman (Chapter 27) and by Hesse (Chapter 26), these measures often do not converge well with the AAI, which means that more research is needed to clarify the meaning of the various measures and their associations with emotion regulation. Interestingly, many of the connections between one kind of measure and an outcome or mediational processes are mirrored in studies using the other kind of measure, so the use of the two kinds of measures together might provide a more complete explanation of various outcomes and mediational processes. Additionally, many studies now suggest that some of the individual-difference variance in attachment anxiety (although perhaps not in avoidance) is attributable to genetic factors. If so, it will have implications for both theory and clinical applications. Equally important are epigenetic processes that are just barely beginning to be understood. Finally, we confess that social psychologists who study normal adults (often college students) take the substantial developmental literature on attachment more or less for granted, rarely studying actual links between attachment-related childhood experiences that can help us understand adult emotion regulation. This means that the actual childhood roots of some of the specific phenomena we have studied in adulthood remain to be fully identified. Fortunately, there are now several very long-term longitudinal studies that are beginning to shed a powerful light on these matters, as indicated in several chapters in this volume.

Whatever the final story turns out to be, attachment theory has already advanced the study of emotion regulation in adulthood. Most of the findings summarized here (and in our more comprehensive treatment in Mikulincer & Shaver, 2016) are highly replicable, and many have now been replicated in different countries, using stimulus materials and measures in different languages. Most of the findings are not likely to be challenged or revised in the future. Only their final, complete, and correct interpretation and integration remain to be established.

## References

Ablow, J. C., Marks, A. K., Feldman, S., & Huffman, L. C. (2013). Associations between first-time expectant women's representations of attachment and their physiological reactivity to infant cry. *Child Development, 84*, 1373–1391.

Ainsworth, M. D. S., Blehar, M. C., Waters, E., & Wall, S. (1978). *Patterns of attachment: A psychological study of the Strange Situation*. Hillsdale, NJ: Erlbaum.

Atkinson, L., Leung, E., Goldberg, S., Benoit, D., Poulton, L., Myhal, N., et al. (2009). Attachment and selective attention: Disorganization and emotional Stroop reaction time. *Development and Psychopathology, 21*, 99–126.

Bailey, H. N., Paret, L., Battista, C., & Xue, Y. (2012). Attachment anxiety and attentional control predict immediate and delayed emotional Stroop interference. *Emotion, 12*, 376–383.

Barbasio, C., & Granieri, A. (2013). Emotion regulation and mental representation of attachment in patients with systemic lupus erythematosus: A study using the adult attachment interview. *Journal of Nervous and Mental Disease, 201*, 304–310.

Bargh, J. A., & Morsella, E. (2010). Unconscious behavioral guidance systems. In C. Agnew, D. E. Carlston, W. G. Graziano, & J. R. Kelly (Eds.), *Then a miracle occurs: Focusing on behavior in social psychological theory and research* (pp. 89–118). New York: Oxford University Press.

Bartholomew, K., & Horowitz, L. M. (1991). Attachment styles among young adults: A test of a four-category model. *Journal of Personality and Social Psychology, 61*, 226–244.

Bazzazian, S., & Besharat, M. A. (2012). An explanatory model of adjustment to type I diabetes based on attachment, coping, and self-regulation theories. *Psychology, Health, and Medicine, 17*, 47–58.

Behringer, J., Reiner, I., & Spangler, G. (2011). Maternal representations of past and current attachment relationships, and emotional experience across the transition to motherhood: A longitudinal study. *Journal of Family Psychology, 25*, 210–219.

Berant, E., Mikulincer, M., & Florian, V. (2001a). The association of mothers' attachment style and their psychological reactions to the diagnosis of infants' congenital heart disease. *Journal of Social and Clinical Psychology, 20*, 208–232.

Berant, E., Mikulincer, M., & Florian, V. (2001b). Attachment style and mental health: A 1-year follow-up study of mothers of infants with congenital heart disease. *Personality and Social Psychology Bulletin, 27*, 956–968.

Berant, E., Mikulincer, M., & Shaver, P. R. (2008). Mothers' attachment style, their mental health, and their children's emotional vulnerabilities: A seven-year study of children with congenital heart disease. *Journal of Personality, 76*, 31–66.

Birnbaum, G. E., Orr, I., Mikulincer, M., & Florian, V.

(1997). When marriage breaks up: Does attachment style contribute to coping and mental health? *Journal of Social and Personal Relationships, 14,* 643–654.

Bodie, G. D., Burleson, B. R., Gill-Rosier, J. N., McCullough, J. D., Holmstrom, A. J., & Rack, J. J. (2011). Explaining the impact of attachment style on evaluations of supportive messages: A dual-process framework. *Communication Research, 38,* 228–247.

Borelli, J. L., David, D. H., Rifkin-Graboi, A., Sbarra, D. A., Mehl, M. R., & Mayes, L. C. (2013). Language use in the Adult Attachment Interview: Evidence for attachment-specific emotion regulation. *Personal Relationships, 20,* 23–37.

Bourne, K., Berry, K., & Jones, L. (2014). The relationships between psychological mindedness, parental bonding and adult attachment. *Psychology and Psychotherapy: Theory, Research and Practice, 87,* 167–177.

Bowlby, J. (1973). *Attachment and loss: Vol. 2. Separation: Anxiety and anger.* New York: Basic Books.

Bowlby, J. (1979). *The making and breaking of affectional bonds.* London: Tavistock.

Bowlby, J. (1980). *Attachment and loss: Vol. 3. Sadness and depression.* New York: Basic Books.

Bowlby, J. (1982). *Attachment and loss: Vol. 1. Attachment.* New York: Basic Books. (Original work published 1969)

Brennan, K. A., Clark, C. L., & Shaver, P. R. (1998). Self-report measurement of adult romantic attachment: An integrative overview. In J. A. Simpson & W. S. Rholes (Eds.), *Attachment theory and close relationships* (pp. 46–76). New York: Guilford Press.

Caldwell, J. G., & Shaver, P. R. (2012). Exploring the cognitive–emotional pathways between adult attachment and ego-resiliency. *Individual Differences Research, 10,* 141–152.

Cannon, W. B. (1939). *The wisdom of the body* (2nd ed.). New York: Norton.

Carnelley, K. B., Hepper, E. G., Hicks, C., & Turner, W. (2011). Perceived parental reactions to coming out, attachment, and romantic relationships views. *Attachment and Human Development, 13,* 227–236.

Carpenter, E. M., & Kirkpatrick, L. A. (1996). Attachment style and presence of a romantic partner as moderators of psychophysiological responses to a stressful laboratory situation. *Personal Relationships, 3,* 351–367.

Cassidy, J., & Kobak, R. R. (1988). Avoidance and its relationship with other defensive processes. In J. Belsky & T. Nezworski (Eds.), *Clinical implications of attachment* (pp. 300–323). Hillsdale, NJ: Erlbaum.

Cherry, M. G., Fletcher, I., & O'Sullivan, H. (2013). Exploring the relationships among attachment, emotional intelligence and communication. *Medical Education, 47,* 317–325.

Chun, D. S., Shaver, P. R., Gillath, O., Mathews, A., & Jorgensen, T. D. (2015). Testing a dual-process model of avoidant defenses. *Journal of Research in Personality, 55,* 75–83.

Coan, J. A., Schaefer, H. S., & Davidson, R. J. (2006). Lending a hand: Social regulation of the neural response to threat. *Psychological Science, 17,* 1032–1039.

Cohen, O., & Katz, M. (2015). Grief and growth of bereaved siblings as related to attachment style and flexibility. *Death Studies, 39,* 158–164.

Collins, N. L., & Feeney, B. C. (2000). A safe haven: An attachment theory perspective on support seeking and caregiving in intimate relationships. *Journal of Personality and Social Psychology, 78,* 1053–1073.

Consedine, N. S., Tuck, N. L., & Fiori, K. L. (2013). Attachment and health care utilization among middle-aged and older African-descent men: Dismissiveness predicts less frequent digital rectal examination and prostate-specific antigen screening. *American Journal of Men's Health, 7,* 382–393.

Contelmo, G., Hart, J., & Levine, E. H. (2013). Dream orientation as a function of hyperactivating and deactivating attachment strategies. *Self and Identity, 12,* 357–369.

Crawford, T. N., Livesley, W. J., Jang, K. L., Shaver, P. R., Cohen, P., & Ganiban, J. (2007). Insecure attachment and personality disorder: A twin study of adults. *European Journal of Personality, 21,* 191–208.

Crowell, J. A., Treboux, D., Gao, Y., Fyffe, C., Pan, H., & Waters, E. (2002). Assessing secure base behavior in adulthood: Development of a measure, links to adult attachment representations, and relations to couples' communication and reports of relationships. *Developmental Psychology, 38,* 679–693.

Delhaye, M., Kempenaers, C., Stroobants, R., Goossens, L., & Linkowski, P. (2013). Attachment and socio-emotional skills: A comparison of depressed inpatients, institutionalized delinquents and control adolescents. *Clinical Psychology and Psychotherapy, 20,* 424–433.

Denckla, C. A., Fiori, K. L., & Vingerhoets, A. J. (2014). Development of the Crying Proneness Scale: Associations among crying proneness, empathy, attachment, and age. *Journal of Personality Assessment, 96,* 619–631.

Deniz, M. E., & Işik, E. (2010). Positive and negative affect, life satisfaction, and coping with stress by attachment styles in Turkish students. *Psychological Reports, 107,* 480–490.

DeWall, C. N., Masten, C. L., Powell, C., Combs, D., Schurtz, D. R., & Eisenberger, N. I. (2012). Do neural responses to rejection depend on attachment style?: An fMRI study. *Social Cognitive and Affective Neuroscience, 7,* 184–192.

Diamond, L. M., Hicks, A. M., & Otter-Henderson, K. D. (2006). Physiological evidence for repressive coping among avoidantly attached adults. *Journal of Social and Personal Relationships, 23,* 205–229.

Ditzen, B., Schmidt, S., Strauss, B., Nater, U. M., Ehlert, U., & Heinrichs, M. (2008). Adult attachment and social support interact to reduce psychological but not cortisol responses to stress. *Journal of Psychosomatic Research, 64,* 479–486.

Donnellan, M. B., Burt, S. A., Levendosky, A. A., &

Klump, K. L. (2008). Genes, personality, and attachment in adults: A multivariate behavioral genetic analysis. *Personality and Social Psychology Bulletin, 34,* 3–16.

Dozier, M., & Kobak, R. (1992). Psychophysiology in attachment interviews: Converging evidence for deactivating strategies. *Child Development, 63,* 1473–1480.

Dykas, M. J., Woodhouse, S. S., Jones, J. D., & Cassidy, J. (2014). Attachment-related biases in adolescents' memory. *Child Development, 85,* 2185–2201.

Edelstein, R. S., Ghetti, S., Quas, J. A., Goodman, G. S., Alexander, K. W., Redlich, A. D., et al. (2005). Individual differences in emotional memory: Adult attachment and long-term memory for child sexual abuse. *Personality and Social Psychology Bulletin, 31,* 1537–1548.

Edelstein, R. S., & Gillath, O. (2008). Avoiding interference: Adult attachment and emotional processing biases. *Personality and Social Psychology Bulletin, 34,* 171–181.

Edelstein, R. S., & Shaver, P. R. (2004). Avoidant attachment: Exploration of an oxymoron. In D. Mashek & A. Aron (Eds.), *Handbook of closeness and intimacy* (pp. 397–412). Mahwah, NJ: Erlbaum.

Ein-Dor, T., Mikulincer, M., & Shaver, P. R. (2011a). Attachment insecurities and the processing of threat-related information: Studying schemas involved in insecure people's coping strategies. *Journal of Personality and Social Psychology, 101,* 78–93.

Ein-Dor, T., Mikulincer, M., & Shaver, P. R. (2011b). Effective reaction to danger: Attachment insecurities predict behavioral reactions to an experimentally induced threat above and beyond general personality traits. *Social Psychological and Personality Science, 2,* 467–473.

Ein-Dor, T., & Orgad, T. (2012). Scared saviors: Evidence that people high in attachment anxiety are more effective in alerting others to threat. *European Journal of Social Psychology, 42,* 667–671.

Ein-Dor, T., & Perry, A. (2014). Full house of fears: Evidence that people high in attachment anxiety are more accurate in detecting deceit. *Journal of Personality, 82,* 83–92.

Ein-Dor, T., Reizer, A., Shaver, P. R., & Dotan, E. (2012). Standoffish perhaps, but successful as well: Evidence that avoidant attachment can be beneficial in professional tennis and computer science. *Journal of Personality, 80,* 749–768.

Feeney, B. C., & Kirkpatrick, L. A. (1996). Effects of adult attachment and presence of romantic partners on physiological responses to stress. *Journal of Personality and Social Psychology, 70,* 255–270.

Field, T. (2002). Infants' need for touch. *Human Development, 45,* 100–103.

Fraley, R. C., & Brumbaugh, C. C. (2007). Adult attachment and preemptive defenses: Converging evidence on the role of defensive exclusion at the level of encoding. *Journal of Personality, 75,* 1033–1050.

Fraley, R. C., Garner, J. P., & Shaver, P. R. (2000). Adult attachment and the defensive regulation of attention and memory: Examining the role of preemptive and postemptive defensive processes. *Journal of Personality and Social Psychology, 79,* 816–826.

Fraley, R. C., & Shaver, P. R. (1997). Adult attachment and the suppression of unwanted thoughts. *Journal of Personality and Social Psychology, 73,* 1080–1091.

Fraley, R. C., & Shaver, P. R. (1998). Airport separations: A naturalistic study of adult attachment dynamics in separating couples. *Journal of Personality and Social Psychology, 75,* 1198–1212.

Fredrickson, B. L. (2013). Positive emotions broaden and build. In E. Ashby Plant & P. G. Devine (Eds.), *Advances in experimental social psychology* (Vol. 47, pp. 1–53). New York: Elsevier.

Garrison, A. M., Kahn, J. H., Miller, S. A., & Sauer, E. M. (2014). Emotional avoidance and rumination as mediators of the relation between adult attachment and emotional disclosure. *Personality and Individual Differences, 70,* 239–245.

Gillath, O., Bunge, S. A., Shaver, P. R., Wendelken, C., & Mikulincer, M. (2005). Attachment-style differences in the ability to suppress negative thoughts: Exploring the neural correlates. *NeuroImage, 28,* 835–847.

Gillath, O., Giesbrecht, B., & Shaver, P. R. (2009). Attachment, attention, and cognitive control: Attachment style and performance on general attention tasks. *Journal of Experimental Social Psychology, 45,* 647–654.

Girme, Y. U., Overall, N. C., Simpson, J. A., & Fletcher, G. J. O. (2015). "All or nothing": Attachment avoidance and the curvilinear effects of partner support. *Journal of Personality and Social Psychology, 108,* 450–475.

Gjerde, P. F., Onishi, M., & Carlson, K. S. (2004). Personality characteristics associated with romantic attachment: A comparison of interview and self-report methodologies. *Personality and Social Psychology Bulletin, 30,* 1402–1415.

Goodall, K. (2015). Individual differences in the regulation of positive emotion: The role of attachment and self-esteem. *Personality and Individual Differences, 74,* 208–213.

Gratz, K. L., Kiel, E. J., Latzman, R. D., Moore, S. A., Elkin, T. D., Megason, G. C., et al. (2015). Complex interrelations of trait vulnerabilities in mothers and their infants. *Infancy, 20,* 306–338.

Griffin, D. W., & Bartholomew, K. (1994). Models of the self and other: Fundamental dimensions underlying measures of adult attachment. *Journal of Personality and Social Psychology, 67,* 430–445.

Haggerty, G., Siefert, C., & Weinberger, J. (2010). Examining the relationship between current attachment status and freely recalled autobiographical memories of childhood. *Psychoanalytic Psychology, 27,* 27–41.

Han, S., & Pistole, M. C. (2014). College student binge eating: Insecure attachment and emotion regulation. *Journal of College Student Development, 55,* 16–29.

Hazan, C., & Shaver, P. R. (1987). Romantic love conceptualized as an attachment process. *Journal of Personality and Social Psychology, 52*, 511–524.

Hazan, C., & Shaver, P. R. (1990). Love and work: An attachment–theoretical perspective. *Journal of Personality and Social Psychology, 59*, 270–280.

Hazan, C., & Shaver, P. R. (1994). Attachment as an organizational framework for research on close relationships. *Psychological Inquiry, 5*, 1–22.

Hazan, C., & Zeifman, D. (1994). Sex and the psychological tether. In K. Bartholomew & D. Perlman (Eds.), *Advances in personal relationships: Attachment processes in adulthood* (Vol. 5, pp. 151–177). London: Jessica Kingsley.

Hesse, C., & Floyd, K. (2011). Affection mediates the impact of alexithymia on relationships. *Personality and Individual Differences, 50*, 451–456.

Hill, C. E., Gelso, C. J., Gerstenblith, J., Chui, H., Pudasaini, S., Burgard, J., et al. (2013). The dreamscape of psychodynamic psychotherapy: Dreams, dreamers, dream work, consequences, and case studies. *Dreaming, 23*, 1–45.

Holmberg, D., Lomore, C. D., Takacs, T. A., & Price, E. L. (2011). Adult attachment styles and stressor severity as moderators of the coping sequence. *Personal Relationships, 18*, 502–517.

Jankowski, P. J., & Sandage, S. J. (2011). Meditative prayer, hope, adult attachment, and forgiveness: A proposed model. *Psychology of Religion and Spirituality, 3*, 115–131.

Jones, J. D., Brett, B. E., Ehrlich, K. B., Lejuez, C. W., & Cassidy, J. (2014). Maternal attachment style and responses to adolescents' negative emotions: The mediating role of maternal emotion regulation. *Parenting: Science and Practice, 14*, 235–257.

Kafetsios, K. (2004). Attachment and emotional intelligence abilities across the life course. *Personality and Individual Differences, 37*, 129–145.

Kalish, R. A. (1985). *Death, grief, and caring relationships.* New York: Cole.

Karreman, A., & Vingerhoets, A. J. (2012). Attachment and well-being: The mediating role of emotion regulation and resilience. *Personality and Individual Differences, 53*, 821–826.

Karremans, J. C., Heslenfeld, D. J., Van Dillen, L. F., & Van Lange, P. A. M. (2011). Secure attachment partners attenuate neural responses to social exclusion: An fMRI investigation. *International Journal of Psychophysiology, 81*, 44–50.

Keating, L., Tasca, G. A., & Hill, R. (2013). Structural relationships among attachment insecurity, alexithymia, and body esteem in women with eating disorders. *Eating Behaviors, 14*, 366–373.

Kidd, T., Hamer, M., & Steptoe, A. (2011). Examining the association between adult attachment style and cortisol responses to acute stress. *Psychoneuroendocrinology, 36*, 771–779.

Kidd, T., Hamer, M., & Steptoe, A. (2013). Adult attachment style and cortisol responses across the day in older adults. *Psychophysiology, 50*, 841–847.

Kim, Y. (2005). Emotional and cognitive consequences of adult attachment: The mediating effect of the self. *Personality and Individual Differences, 39*, 913–923.

Kim, Y. (2006). Gender, attachment, and relationship duration on cardiovascular reactivity to stress in a laboratory study of dating couples. *Personal Relationships, 13*, 103–114.

Klohnen, E. C., & Bera, S. (1998). Behavioral and experiential patterns of avoidantly and securely attached women across adulthood: A 31-year longitudinal perspective. *Journal of Personality and Social Psychology, 74*, 211–223.

Kohn, J. L., Rholes, W. S., & Schmeichel, B. J. (2012). Self-regulatory depletion and attachment avoidance: Increasing the accessibility of negative attachment-related memories. *Journal of Experimental Social Psychology, 48*, 375–378.

Laan, A. J., van Assen, M. A., & Vingerhoets, A. J. (2012). Individual differences in adult crying: The role of attachment styles. *Social Behavior and Personality, 40*, 453–472.

Lanciano, T., Curci, A., Kafetsios, K., Elia, L., & Zammuner, V. L. (2012). Attachment and dysfunctional rumination: The mediating role of emotional intelligence abilities. *Personality and Individual Differences, 53*, 753–758.

Lazarus, R. S., & Folkman, S. (1984). *Stress, appraisal, and coping.* New York: Springer.

Lemche, E., Giampietro, V. P., Surguladze, S. A., Amaro, E. J., Andrew, C. M., Williams, S. C., et al. (2006). Human attachment security is mediated by the amygdala: Evidence from combined fMRI and psychophysiological measures. *Human Brain Mapping, 27*, 623–635.

Lussier, Y., Sabourin, S., & Turgeon, C. (1997). Coping strategies as moderators of the relationship between attachment and marital adjustment. *Journal of Social and Personal Relationships, 14*, 777–791.

Maier, M. A., Bernier, A., Pekrun, R., Zimmermann, P., Strasser, K., & Grossmann, K. E. (2005). Attachment state of mind and perceptual processing of emotional stimuli. *Attachment and Human Development, 7*, 67–81.

Main, M. (1990). Cross-cultural studies of attachment organization: Recent studies, changing methodologies, and the concept of conditional strategies. *Human Development, 33*, 48–61.

Mallinckrodt, B., & Wei, M. (2005). Attachment, social competencies, social support, and psychological distress. *Journal of Counseling Psychology, 52*, 358–367.

Marshall, W. L., Serran, G. A., & Cortoni, F. A. (2000). Childhood attachments, sexual abuse, and their relationship to adult coping in child molesters. *Sexual Abuse: Journal of Research and Treatment, 12*, 17–26.

Maunder, R. G., Hunter, J. J., & Lancee, W. J. (2011). The impact of attachment insecurity and sleep disturbance on symptoms and sick days in hospital-based health-care workers. *Journal of Psychosomatic Research, 70*, 11–17.

Maunder, R. G., Lancee, W. J., Nolan, R. P., Hunter, J. J., & Tannenbaum, D. W. (2006). The relationship of attachment insecurity to subjective stress and autonomic function during standardized acute stress in healthy adults. *Journal of Psychosomatic Research, 60,* 283–290.

McCabe, A., & Peterson, C. (2011). Predictors of adult narrative elaboration: Emotion, attachment, and gender. *Imagination, Cognition and Personality, 31,* 327–344.

McLean, H. R., Bailey, H. N., & Lumley, M. N. (2014). The secure base script: Associated with early maladaptive schemas related to attachment. *Psychology and Psychotherapy, 87,* 425–446.

Meuwly, N., Bodenmann, G., Germann, J., Bradbury, T. N., Ditzen, B., & Heinrichs, M. (2012). Dyadic coping, insecure attachment, and cortisol stress recovery following experimentally induced stress. *Journal of Family Psychology, 26,* 937–947.

Mikulincer, M. (1998). Adult attachment style and individual differences in functional versus dysfunctional experiences of anger. *Journal of Personality and Social Psychology, 74,* 513–524.

Mikulincer, M., Birnbaum, G., Woddis, D., & Nachmias, O. (2000). Stress and accessibility of proximity-related thoughts: Exploring the normative and intraindividual components of attachment theory. *Journal of Personality and Social Psychology, 78,* 509–523.

Mikulincer, M., Dolev, T., & Shaver, P. R. (2004). Attachment-related strategies during thought suppression: Ironic rebounds and vulnerable self-representations. *Journal of Personality and Social Psychology, 87,* 940–956.

Mikulincer, M., & Florian, V. (1995). Appraisal of and coping with a real-life stressful situation: The contribution of attachment styles. *Personality and Social Psychology Bulletin, 21,* 406–414.

Mikulincer, M., & Florian, V. (1997). Are emotional and instrumental supportive interactions beneficial in times of stress?: The impact of attachment style. *Anxiety, Stress and Coping: An International Journal, 10,* 109–127.

Mikulincer, M., & Florian, V. (1998). The relationship between adult attachment styles and emotional and cognitive reactions to stressful events. In J. A. Simpson & W. S. Rholes (Eds.), *Attachment theory and close relationships* (pp. 143–165). New York: Guilford Press.

Mikulincer, M., Florian, V., & Tolmacz, R. (1990). Attachment styles and fear of personal death: A case study of affect regulation. *Journal of Personality and Social Psychology, 58,* 273–280.

Mikulincer, M., Florian, V., & Weller, A. (1993). Attachment styles, coping strategies, and posttraumatic psychological distress: The impact of the Gulf War in Israel. *Journal of Personality and Social Psychology, 64,* 817–826.

Mikulincer, M., Gillath, O., Halevy, V., Avihou, N., Avidan, S., & Eshkoli, N. (2001). Attachment theory and reactions to others' needs: Evidence that activation of the sense of attachment security promotes empathic responses. *Journal of Personality and Social Psychology, 81,* 1205–1224.

Mikulincer, M., Gillath, O., & Shaver, P. R. (2002). Activation of the attachment system in adulthood: Threat-related primes increase the accessibility of mental representations of attachment figures. *Journal of Personality and Social Psychology, 83,* 881–895.

Mikulincer, M., Hirschberger, G., Nachmias, O., & Gillath, O. (2001). The affective component of the secure base schema: Affective priming with representations of attachment security. *Journal of Personality and Social Psychology, 81,* 305–321.

Mikulincer, M., & Orbach, I. (1995). Attachment styles and repressive defensiveness: The accessibility and architecture of affective memories. *Journal of Personality and Social Psychology, 68,* 917–925.

Mikulincer, M., & Shaver, P. R. (2001). Attachment theory and intergroup bias: Evidence that priming the secure base schema attenuates negative reactions to out-groups. *Journal of Personality and Social Psychology, 81,* 97–115.

Mikulincer, M., & Shaver, P. R. (2003). The attachment behavioral system in adulthood: Activation, psychodynamics, and interpersonal processes. In M. P. Zanna (Ed.), *Advances in experimental social psychology* (Vol. 35, pp. 53–152). San Diego, CA: Academic Press.

Mikulincer, M., & Shaver, P. R. (2004). Security-based self-representations in adulthood: Contents and processes. In W. S. Rholes & J. A. Simpson (Eds.), *Adult attachment: Theory, research, and clinical implications* (pp. 159–195). New York: Guilford Press.

Mikulincer, M., & Shaver, P. R. (2007). *Attachment in adulthood: Structure, dynamics, and change.* New York: Guilford Press.

Mikulincer, M., & Shaver, P. R. (2013). The role of attachment security in adolescent and adult close relationships. In J. A. Simpson & L. Campbell (Eds.), *Oxford handbook of close relationships* (pp. 66–89). New York: Oxford University Press.

Mikulincer, M., & Shaver, P. R. (2016). *Attachment in adulthood: Structure, dynamics, and change* (2nd ed.). New York: Guilford Press.

Mikulincer, M., Shaver, P. R., & Avihou-Kanza, N. (2011). Individual differences in adult attachment are systematically related to dream narratives. *Attachment and Human Development, 13,* 105–123.

Mikulincer, M., Shaver, P. R., Sapir-Lavid, Y., & Avihou-Kanza, N. (2009). What's inside the minds of securely and insecurely attached people?: The secure-base script and its associations with attachment-style dimensions. *Journal of Personality and Social Psychology, 97,* 615–633.

Milyavskaya, M., McClure, M. J., Ma, D., Koestner, R., & Lydon, J. (2012). Attachment moderates the effects of autonomy-supportive and controlling interpersonal primes on intrinsic motivation. *Canadian Journal of Behavioral Science, 44,* 278–287.

Monti, J. D., & Rudolph, K. D. (2014). Emotional awareness as a pathway linking adult attachment to subsequent depression. *Journal of Counseling Psychology*, 61, 374–382.

Moutsiana, C., Fearon, P., Murray, L., Cooper, P., Goodyer, I., Johnstone, T., & Halligan, S. (2014). Making an effort to feel positive: Insecure attachment in infancy predicts the neural underpinnings of emotion regulation in adulthood. *Journal of Child Psychology and Psychiatry*, 55, 999–1008.

Moutsiana, C., Johnstone, T., Murray, L., Fearon, P., Cooper, P., Pliatsikas, C., et al. (2015). Insecure attachment during infancy predicts greater amygdala volumes in early adulthood. *Journal of Child Psychology and Psychiatry*, 56, 540–548.

Pepping, C. A., Davis, P. J., & O'Donovan, A. (2013). Individual differences in attachment and dispositional mindfulness: The mediating role of emotion regulation. *Personality and Individual Differences*, 54, 453–456.

Pereg, D., & Mikulincer, M. (2004). Attachment style and the regulation of negative affect: Exploring individual differences in mood congruency effects on memory and judgment. *Personality and Social Psychology Bulletin*, 30, 67–80.

Pierrehumbert, B., Torrisi, R., Ansermet, F., Borghini, A., & Halfon, O. (2012). Adult attachment representations predict cortisol and oxytocin responses to stress. *Attachment and Human Development*, 14, 453–476.

Pierrehumbert, B., Torrisi, R., Glatz, N., Dimitrova, N., Heinrichs, M., & Halfon, O. (2009). The influence of attachment on perceived stress and cortisol response to acute stress in women sexually abused in childhood or adolescence. *Psychoneuroendocrinology*, 34, 924–938.

Quirin, M., Gillath, O., Pruessner, J. C., & Eggert, L. D. (2010). Adult attachment insecurity and hippocampal cell density. *Social Cognitive and Affective Neuroscience*, 5, 39–47.

Quirin, M., Pruessner, J. C., & Kuhl, J. (2008). HPA system regulation and adult attachment anxiety: Individual differences in reactive and awakening cortisol. *Psychoneuroendocrinology*, 33, 581–590.

Raskin, P. M., Kummel, P., & Bannister, T. (1998). The relationship between coping styles, attachment, and career salience in partnered working women with children. *Journal of Career Assessment*, 6, 403–416.

Reizer, A., Possick, H., & Ein-Dor, T. (2010). Environmental threat influences psychological distress and marital satisfaction among avoidantly attached individuals. *Personal Relationships*, 17, 585–598.

Reynolds, S., Searight, H. R., & Ratwik, S. (2014). Adult attachment style and rumination in the context of intimate relationships. *North American Journal of Psychology*, 16, 495–506.

Rognoni, E., Galati, D., Costa, T., & Crini, M. (2008). Relationship between adult attachment patterns, emotional experience, and EEG frontal asymmetry. *Personality and Individual Differences*, 44, 909–920.

Roisman, G. I., Tsai, J. L., & Chiang, K. H. (2004). The emotional integration of childhood experience: Physiological, facial expressions, and self-reported emotional response during the Adult Attachment Interview. *Developmental Psychology*, 40, 776–789.

Schmidt, S., Nachtigall, C., Wuethrich-Martone, O., & Strauss, B. (2002). Attachment and coping with chronic disease. *Journal of Psychosomatic Research*, 53, 763–773.

Seedall, R. B., & Wampler, K. S. (2012). Emotional congruence within couple interaction: The role of attachment avoidance. *Journal of Family Psychology*, 26, 948–958.

Selterman, D., Apetroaia, A., & Waters, E. (2012). Script-like attachment representations in dreams containing current romantic partners. *Attachment and Human Development*, 14, 501–515.

Shapiro, D. L., & Levendosky, A. A. (1999). Adolescent survivors of childhood sexual abuse: The mediating role of attachment style and coping in psychological and interpersonal functioning. *Child Abuse and Neglect*, 23, 1175–1191.

Shaver, P. R., & Mikulincer, M. (2002a). Attachment-related psychodynamics. *Attachment and Human Development*, 4, 133–161.

Shaver, P. R., & Mikulincer, M. (2002b). Dialogue on adult attachment: Diversity and integration. *Attachment and Human Development*, 4, 243–257.

Silva, C., Soares, I., & Esteves, F. (2012). Attachment insecurity and strategies for regulation: When emotion triggers attention. *Scandinavian Journal of Psychology*, 53, 9–16.

Simpson, J. A., Rholes, W. S., & Nelligan, J. S. (1992). Support seeking and support giving within couples in an anxiety-provoking situation: The role of attachment styles. *Journal of Personality and Social Psychology*, 62, 434–446.

Simpson, J. A., Rholes, W. S., Orina, M., & Grich, J. (2002). Working models of attachment, support giving, and support seeking in a stressful situation. *Personality and Social Psychology Bulletin*, 28, 598–608.

Simpson, J. A., Winterheld, H. A., Rholes, W. S., & Oriña, M. M. (2007). Working models of attachment and reactions to different forms of caregiving from romantic partners. *Journal of Personality and Social Psychology*, 93, 466–477.

Smeets, T. (2010). Autonomic and hypothalamic–pituitary–adrenal stress resilience: Impact of cardiac vagal tone. *Biological Psychology*, 84, 290–295.

Sonnby-Borgstrom, M., & Jonsson, P. (2004). Dismissing-avoidant pattern of attachment and mimicry reactions at different levels of information processing. *Scandinavian Journal of Psychology*, 45, 103–113.

Spangler, G., & Zimmermann, P. (1999). Attachment representation and emotion regulation in adolescents: A psychobiological perspective on internal working models. *Attachment and Human Development*, 1, 270–290.

Sroufe, L. A., & Waters, E. (1977). Attachment as an

organizational construct. *Child Development, 48,* 1184–1199.

Steele, R. D., Waters, T. E. A., Bost, K. K., Vaughn, B. E., Truit, W., Waters, H. S., et al. (2014). Caregiving antecedents of secure base script knowledge: A comparative analysis of young adult attachment representations. *Developmental Psychology, 50,* 2526–2538.

Stevens, F. L. (2014). Affect regulation styles in avoidant and anxious attachment. *Individual Differences Research, 12,* 123–130.

Suslow, T., Dannlowski, U., Arolt, V., & Ohrmann, P. (2010). Adult attachment avoidance and automatic affective response to sad facial expressions. *Australian Journal of Psychology, 62,* 181–187.

Suslow, T., Kugel, H., Rauch, A. V., Dannlowski, U., Bauer, J., Konrad, C., et al. (2009). Attachment avoidance modulates neural response to masked facial emotion. *Human Brain Mapping, 30,* 3553–3562.

Sutin, A. R., & Gillath, O. (2009). Autobiographical memory phenomenology and content mediate attachment style and psychological distress. *Journal of Counseling Psychology, 56,* 351–364.

Turan, B., Osar, Z., Turan, J. M., Ilkova, H., & Damci, T. (2003). Dismissing attachment and outcome in diabetes: The mediating role of coping. *Journal of Social and Clinical Psychology, 22,* 607–626.

Van Emmichoven, I. A., Van IJzendoorn, M. H., de Ruiter, C., & Brosschot, J. F. (2003). Selective processing of threatening information: Effects of attachment representation and anxiety disorder on attention and memory. *Development and Psychopathology, 15,* 219–237.

Vetere, A., & Myers, L. B. (2002). Repressive coping style and adult romantic attachment style: Is there a relationship? *Personality and Individual Differences, 32,* 799–807.

Vilchinsky, N., Dekel, R., Asher, Z., Leibowitz, M., & Mosseri, M. (2013). The role of illness perceptions in the attachment-related process of affect regulation. *Anxiety, Stress and Coping, 26,* 314–329.

Vilchinsky, N., Haze-Filderman, L., Leibowitz, M., Reges, O., Khaskia, A., & Mosseri, M. (2010). Spousal support and cardiac patients' distress: The moderating role of attachment orientation. *Journal of Family Psychology, 24,* 508–512.

Vrtička, P., Bondolfi, G., Sander, D., & Vuilleumier, P. (2012). The neural substrates of social emotion perception and regulation are modulated by adult attachment style. *Social Neuroscience, 7,* 473–493.

Walsh, J. J., Balint, M. G.. Smolira, D. R., Frederickson, L. K., & Madsen, S. (2009). Predicting individual differences in mindfulness: The role of trait anxiety, attachment anxiety and attentional control. *Personality and Individual Differences, 46,* 94–99.

Warren, S. L., Bost, K. K., Roisman, G. I., Silton, R. L., Spielberg, J. M., Engels, A. S., et al. (2010). Effects of adult attachment and emotional distractors on brain mechanisms of cognitive control. *Psychological Science, 21,* 1818–1826.

Waters, H. S., & Waters, E. (2006). The attachment working models concept: Among other things, we build script-like representations of secure base experiences. *Attachment and Human Development, 8,* 185–198.

Waters, T. E. A., Brockmeyer, S. L., & Crowell, J. A. (2013). AAI coherence predicts caregiving and care seeking behavior: Secure base script knowledge helps explain why. *Attachment and Human Development, 15,* 316–331.

Wei, M., Russell, D. W., Mallinckrodt, B., & Vogel, D. L. (2007). The Experiences in Close Relationship Scale (ECR)–Short Form: Reliability, validity, and factor structure. *Journal of Personality Assessment, 88,* 187–204.

Wei, M., Vogel, D. L., Ku, T. Y., & Zakalik, R. A. (2005). Adult attachment, affect regulation, negative mood, and interpersonal problems: The mediating roles of emotional reactivity and emotional cutoff. *Journal of Counseling Psychology, 52,* 14–24.

White, L. O., Wu, J., Borelli, J. L., Rutherford, H. J. V., David, D. H., Kim-Cohen, J., et al. (2012). Attachment dismissal predicts frontal slow-wave ERPs during rejection by unfamiliar peers. *Emotion, 12,* 690–700.

Zayas, V., Mischel, W., Shoda, Y., & Aber, J. L. (2011). Roots of adult attachment: Maternal caregiving at 18 months predicts adult peer and partner attachment. *Social Psychological and Personality Science, 2,* 289–297.

Zhang, F., & Labouvie-Vief, G. (2004). Stability and fluctuation in adult attachment style over a 6-year period. *Attachment and Human Development, 6,* 419–437.

Zheng, M., Zhang, Y., & Zheng, Y. (2015). The effects of attachment avoidance and the defensive regulation of emotional faces: Brain potentials examining the role of preemptive and postemptive strategies. *Attachment and Human Development, 17,* 96–110.

Zilber, A., Goldstein, A., & Mikulincer, M. (2007). Adult attachment orientations and the processing of emotional pictures: ERP correlates. *Personality and Individual Differences, 43,* 1898–1907.

Zimmermann, P., Maier, M. A., Winter, M., & Grossmann, K. E. (2001). Attachment and adolescents' emotion regulation during a joint problem-solving task with a friend. *International Journal of Behavioral Development, 25,* 331–343.

Zimmermann, P., Wulf, K., & Grossmann, K. E. (1996). *Attachment representation: You can see it in the face.* Poster presented at the biennial meeting of the Internal Society for the Study of Behavioral Development, Quebec City, Canada.

# Chapter 25

# Attachment in Middle and Later Life

Carol Magai
María Teresa Frías
Phillip R. Shaver

Bowlby's formulations about the origins and nature of human attachments (Bowlby, 1969/1982, 1973, 1980) have provided a rich corpus of theory about important aspects of close relationships and their development over time. The theory has stimulated an enormous body of research on attachment during infancy, childhood, and early adulthood, as demonstrated in this handbook. But research on relationships in later life, viewed from an attachment–theoretical perspective, has been relatively limited (Magai & Consedine, 2004). Moreover, there are no longitudinal studies of the stability of attachment styles from early adulthood to middle age and later life, nor is there any research on how attachment patterns established earlier in life influence attitudes and behaviors later in life. Nevertheless, longitudinal research on the relation between early family circumstances (broadly construed) and later-life functioning indicates that early familial conditions predict health and illness, psychological well-being, and even mortality (Duncan, Kalil, & Ziol-Guest, 2013; Preston, Hill, & Drevenstedt, 1998; Weisner, 2005; see Ehrlich, Miller, Jones, & Cassidy, Chapter 9, this volume). This research suggests that there may indeed be long-term consequences of attachment-related bonds formed earlier in life, and that their impact may be of great consequence.

In early life, attachment bonds ensure that the infant maintains proximity to the caregiver under conditions of uncertainty or threat and develops internal working models of this figure's availability and sensitivity. As the child matures, the exploratory or exploration behavioral system, which provides the scaffolding for growth and development of various skills through exploration of the environment, becomes activated; the child ventures further and further away from the caregiver, although the caregiver retains the function of a "safe haven" if the child experiences distress. The process of exploration, development, and individuation evolves over time, and a sense of autonomy is normally achieved by early adulthood. However, it is assumed that because of internal working models, the attachment figure retains his or her power to serve as a real or virtual safe haven when the individual encounters challenges in adult life. The theory also predicts that the internal working models of caregivers generalize to other people in the adult's social networks and that attachment styles are relatively enduring, although they are also responsive to new inputs (Bowlby, 1973; Fraley & Brumbaugh, 2004; Mikulincer & Shaver, 2007). There is now a significant literature on younger adults to support these formulations. However, it is important to assess the viability of these formulations as applied to later life, given the age-graded and role-linked unique challenges that occur across the adult lifespan.

In this chapter, we consider the subject of attachments in middle adulthood and later life in the context of normative adult developmental transitions and challenges. Themes that loom large for middle-aged adults include monitoring the health of aging parents; often taking responsibility for parents' care, sometimes while still providing care to adolescent or young adult offspring (Perrig-chiello & Hoepflinger, 2005); and eventually dealing with the loss of these primary attachment figures. Themes that loom large for later-life adults include increased social, emotional, physical, and financial dependency; dealing with bereavement of spouse and friends; facing issues of encroaching mortality; and finding personal meaning as the end of life approaches.

In the context of this literature review, we explore the questions of (1) whether attachment styles remain relatively stable in later life and (2) under what conditions they might be altered. We also examine how differences in attachment style may inform adult developmental issues. And we explore whether patterns of social exchange and identity of the most common attachment figures in late life are different from those in young adulthood.

Because the literature on affectional bonds in later life is so limited in terms of testing derivations from attachment theory, this review necessarily draws on other literatures that are not grounded in attachment theory but nevertheless speak to attachment issues, in particular, the literature on the nature and quality of affectional bonds in middle and later adulthood and the influence of these bonds on caring for elderly relationship partners. Finally, we focus on issues of loss and bereavement. We restrict our focus to reactions of adult children to the loss of their parent because of space limitations, and because this literature is better developed than the literature on other kinds of affectional bonds (e.g., those between siblings). (For a review of the broader literature on loss and bereavement, see Fraley and Shaver, Chapter 3, this volume.)

## The Distribution and Stability of Attachment Styles in Later Life

One might expect the distribution of attachment styles to be different in later life than in childhood and young adulthood given that attachment bonds are forged not only in relational but also in cultural and historical contexts (Weisner, 2005). We also need to revisit the thesis that attachment styles are relatively stable, for it is conceivable

that the unique challenges of the latter part of the lifespan create differential instability.

## Distribution of Attachment Styles in Older Adults

Studies of younger adults indicate a distribution of attachment styles that resembles the one found in studies of infants and children. About 55–65% of samples studied with self-report attachment measures have been found to be secure, 22–30% are avoidant (or dismissing), and 15–20% are anxious (or ambivalent or preoccupied; e.g., J. A. Feeney & Noller, 1990; Hazan & Shaver, 1987). Bakermans-Kranenburg and Van IJzendoorn (2009) conducted a meta-analysis of studies using the Adult Attachment Interview (AAI) in different countries and languages. They found that in a combined sample of 748 nonclinical North American mothers, 16% were classified as dismissing, 56% were secure-autonomous, 9% were insecure-preoccupied, and 18% were unresolved with respect to trauma or losses. Bakermans-Kranenburg and Van IJzendoorn found a similar distribution in a sample of nonclinical fathers: 24% were classified as dismissing, 50% were secure-autonomous, 11% were insecure-preoccupied, and 15% were unresolved.

These distributions have not been replicated in the few studies of older respondents. In brief, avoidant or dismissing attachment appears to increase or to become more common in older adults, and there are low base rates of ambivalent and/or preoccupied attachment (Van Assche et al., 2013). For example, one cross-sectional study of urban adults with a mean age of 63 years (Magai, Hunziker, Mesias, & Culver, 2000) found that security of attachment, as assessed by the AAI, was negatively correlated with age, and that dismissing attachment was positively correlated. Another study (Diehl, Elnick, Bourbeau, & Labouvie-Vief, 1998) assessed attachment styles in a sample of young (mean age = 30 years), middle-aged (50 years), and older adults (70 years) from a relatively affluent Midwestern suburb; the results indicated that whereas 18% of the young adults were dismissing, 22% of the middle-aged adults were dismissing, and the figure for the oldest sample was 40%. In a study of attachment style and the preparedness of middle-aged adults to provide care to older adults, 56% were classified as secure, 31% were dismissive, 4% were preoccupied, and 9% were fearful (Soerensen, Webster, & Roggman, 2002).

A study of patients with dementia (mean age = 76 years; Magai & Cohen, 1998), in which caregivers were asked to rate their family members' attachment style before the patients became ill, found that 56% were rated as secure, 37% as avoidant, and 6% as ambivalent. In a large, randomly drawn sample of urban elders living in an economically disadvantaged community, 78% were rated as avoidant, with most of the remainder being rated as secure (Magai et al., 2001). In a study of major life events in later life, 39% of participants were classified as secure, 42% as avoidant, and 19% as anxious (Hobdy et al., 2007). In a study of emotion regulation in older adults, 13% of participants were classified as secure, 83% were avoidant, and 4% were preoccupied (Consedine, Fiori, & Magai, 2012). Finally, in a study of emotional experience of adults 50–70 years of age, 12.8% were classified as secure, 77.6% were avoidant, and 9.6% were preoccupied (Consedine & Fiori, 2009).

Although the proportion of avoidant or dismissing and secure individuals varies across samples and appears to have something to do with participants' economic background, the data clearly show that the distribution of attachment styles in older adult samples is distinctly different from the distribution in samples of younger adults. Some authors (Diehl et al., 1998) have suggested that the higher proportion of avoidant older adults may be due to a greater number of losses experienced by older persons. For example, Cicirelli (2010) found that attachment styles in a group of older adult respondents varied as a function of marital status, with the widowed showing greater avoidance.

Magai and colleagues (2001) suggested that these differences may be due to cohort effects. In a test of this hypothesis, the authors subdivided their sample into a younger cohort born between 1922 and 1932, and an older cohort born between 1911 and 1921. The younger cohort had significantly lower numbers of persons with secure attachment than did the older cohort. However, there was no difference between the two age cohorts in terms of the number of close relatives or friends who had died within the past 5 years. Magai and colleagues suggested that the differential proportions of secure attachment in the two cohorts might represent the influence of Watsonian behaviorism, which advocated the withholding of affection from children and would have reached the height of its influence between the 1920s and 1930s, thus affecting the younger cohort.

Certain socialization practices that are thought to lead to the development of dismissive attachment can also be particularly common in certain cultural groups. For example, Consedine, Magai, Horton, and Brown (2012) found that *socialization of repressive coping*, a style of affect regulation in which negative emotions are ignored, downplayed, or dissociated, is more common among African Americans. Alternatively, this effect might be due to intraindividual changes in levels of dismissing, secure, ambivalent, and fearful attachment in response to age-graded developmental challenges. Finally, it is possible that higher rates of avoidant attachment among older adults are due to the way in which avoidant attachment is measured. Studies with older populations typically employ self-report measures originally designed for use with young adults, in which attachment-related avoidance is operationalized as a preference for autonomy and independence. Given that loss of autonomy is a normative threat for older adults due to deteriorating health, it is possible that high rates of attachment-related avoidance reflect autonomy concerns that are normative among older adults rather than changes in the way they experience and behave in close relationships.

In any event, the apparent existence of high rates of avoidant or dismissing attachment in older adults is grounds for concern. Grossmann (1996) advanced the thesis that attachment relations maintained within the larger family system contribute to the survival of family members. His work, as well as that of his colleagues, suggests that particular attachment styles might confer adaptive advantage over other styles later in life. Wensauer and Grossmann (1995), for example, found that grandparents with a secure attachment orientation had larger social networks, named more supportive family members, and received and gave more help, whereas avoidant individuals were significantly more self-reliant. In a related prospective, 10-year longitudinal study of older Australians, Giles, Glonek, Luscza, and Andrews (2005) found that social networks conferred an adaptive advantage over and above those provided by demographic, health, and lifestyle variables. In that study, better networks with friends (and, to a lesser extent, networks with confidants) were protective against mortality over the following decade. Somewhat surprisingly, the effects of social networks with children and relatives were not significant with respect to survival; however, it is important to note that this study did not assess *quality of attachment* to children and other relatives—an important dimension to consider from an attachment–theoretical perspective.

It is possible that the positive effects of attachment security on older adults' subjective well-being and survival are due in part to the fact that they are more skilled at managing and optimizing their social networks. Gillath, Johnson, Selcuk, and Teel (2011) compared a group of older adults who had recently become caregivers of their spouse with a group of college freshmen and examined their responses to their respective life transitions, assuming that both involved changes in social networks. The results showed that although the social network size of the older adults was significantly smaller, they did not differ in the number of close others. Although older adults reported less contact with their network members, maintaining social relationships was easier for secure older adults. Gillath and colleagues interpreted these results as evidence that secure older adults are more skilled at optimizing their social networks to buffer the negative consequences of late-life transitions (e.g., losses) than their less secure counterparts. It appears that by decreasing social contact with peripheral network members, secure older adults can focus on interacting with emotionally close members (Fung, Carstensen, & Lang, 2001).

Fiori, Consedine, and Merz (2011) suggested that attachment styles are also associated with types of social network and patterns of social exchange in later life. They found that greater attachment security was associated with larger kin and non-kin social networks, reciprocal exchange in both kinds of social networks, and fewer kin relationships that involved primarily giving support. In contrast, dismissing attachment was associated with smaller non-kin social networks and fewer non-kin relationships that involved primarily giving support. The authors interpreted the larger size of both kin and non-kin social networks among secure individuals as an indication that they had more people from whom to receive support and the ability to engage in behaviors that preserve social ties. Their ability to form reciprocal relationships may reflect their flexibility and ability to balance the complementary roles of caregiver and care seeker. Fiori and colleagues argued that the smaller size of non-kin networks that characterizes dismissing attachment can be explained by a tendency to distrust others, which decreases willingness to invest dwindling resources in relationships.

Older adults also differ in the identity of their attachment figures and the strength of their relationships with them (Cicirelli, 2010; Van Assche et al., 2013). In a study of a community-based sample of older adults, it was found that participants' attachment figures had changed from those of earlier adult life to adult children, as well as intangible figures, such as deceased loved ones and God. Moreover, participants reported having fewer full-blown attachments (ones in which the same person serves all the attachment functions: proximity, secure base, and safe haven) but a greater variety of attachment figures, including in-laws, caregivers, doctors, and animals (Van Assche et al., 2013). According to Carstensen (1995), the reduced number of full-blown attachments is explained by *socioemotional selectivity theory*, according to which, with age, people become increasingly selective in their relationships and reduce the number of people with whom they maintain closeness.

## Stability and Change in Attachment Styles

Although attachment styles are thought to be relatively stable, with some research even indicating that attachment styles are trait-like (e.g., Banai, Weller, & Mikulincer, 1998), Bowlby's model of attachment patterns was quite accommodating of change (Bowlby, 1973; Fraley & Brumbaugh, 2004). A review of the child development literature by Campos, Barrett, Lamb, Goldsmith, and Stenberg (1983) indicated that, averaged over seven studies, 32% of infants and toddlers showed a change in classification over time. Similar rates have been reported in young adult samples (Baldwin & Fehr, 1995), and rates as high as 46% have been reported in studies of adults undergoing particularly acute stress (Cozzarelli, Karafa, Collins, & Tagler, 2003).

The literature on stability and change in later adulthood is far more limited. Indeed, at this point there are only two longitudinal studies that address this issue, both of which examined changes in attachment over a 6-year period. One study involved a sample of 370 relatively affluent, highly educated, predominantly European American men and women between ages 15 and 87 years (Zhang & Labouvie-Vief, 2004). The other involved 415 less affluent, less well-educated older adults (60% African American, 40% European American) who were 72 years old at the first time of measurement and 78 years old at the second (Consedine & Magai, 2006). The former study indicated that both secure and dismissing attachment increased over time; the latter study indicated that both decreased over time. The discrepancy in findings is probably related to the pronounced demographic differences between the two samples, including the age ranges studied. It may also be due to the fact that the first study relied on simple paragraph measures of attachment style, whereas the latter used the 30-item Relationship Scales Questionnaire (Bartholomew & Horowitz, 1991). In the case of the exclusively later-life sample, Consedine and Magai (2006) suggested that the unexpected decrease in both security and dismissiveness (compared with previous cross-sectional studies) relates to sample-specific changes in the purposes served by attachment figures in later life and changes in patterns of social network engagement and composition. That is, the decrease in security may reflect the loss of key members of social networks due to mortality. Conversely, decreases in dismissiveness may reflect a tendency in this sample, or age group, to place increasing value on intimate, emotionally rewarding relationships when one's expected remaining time with them was limited.

## Attachment and Well-Being in Later Life

As could be expected based on research involving young adults, attachment security in older adults is associated with physical and psychological health and well-being (Bodner & Cohen-Fridel, 2010; Consedine, Fiori, & Merz, 2013). Consedine and colleagues (2013) analyzed responses of 1,118 older adults to health and personality-related self-report measures and found that fearful attachment predicted greater physical impairment, presumably because fearful individuals' tendency to experience greater negative affect (another finding of their study) may contribute to experiencing physical symptoms more negatively.

Effects of adverse childhood experiences with caregivers also seem to affect older adults' sleep cycle. Poon and Knight (2011) found an association, in a sample of older adults, between self-reports of child abuse and neglect, on one hand, and sleep complaints on the other. The authors maintained that abusive or neglectful child–parent interactions may impair individuals' confidence in their ability to cope with stress. Those who experience child abuse are more likely to develop cognitive schemas involving harm, shame, and self-sacrifice (Wright, Crawford, & Castillo, 2009), all of which contribute to hypervigilance, which is physiologically incompatible with sleep. Similarly, Verdecias, Jean-Louis, Zizi, Casimir, and Browne (2009) found an association between a preoccupied attachment style and daytime napping, use of sleep-inducing

medications, and a tendency to sleep less, whereas a secure attachment style was associated with little difficulty initiating sleep.

A chronic sense of attachment insecurity could also cause changes in the functioning of the endocrine system. In adolescence and young adulthood, fearful attachment is associated with high activation of the hypothalamic–pituitary–adrenal (HPA) axis (Dewitte, De Houwer, Goubert, & Buysse, 2010), responsible for increases in cortisol. However, among older adults, cortisol levels of fearful individuals seem to be lower than the levels for other attachment styles (Kidd, Hamer, & Steptoe, 2013). Kidd and colleagues (2013) suggested that chronic activation of the HPA axis may occur in younger individuals who score high on fearful attachment, but over time, the HPA axis loses its resilience as a consequence of chronic dysfunctional activation.

In later life, some of the main causes of activation of the attachment system are losses of valued roles related to one's self-definition. Hobdy and colleagues (2007) studied two groups of older adults, one of individuals who had recently lost their jobs and the other of individuals whose last child had recently moved out of the family home. Perhaps because the job losses were generally unexpected, they were perceived as more threatening than having a grown child leave home. In both loss groups, secure individuals showed less of a drop in well-being than their insecure counterparts, but these results were qualified by gender. Among individuals scoring high on comfort with closeness (one dimension of secure attachment, as measured in this study), greater coping efforts were observed among men experiencing unemployment and among women experiencing an empty nest, each of which is a core aspect of the male or female gender role.

## Attachments between Parents and Children in Later Life

Arguably, the most powerful affectional bonds are the bidirectional ones that develop between children and their parents. In this section, we examine what the literature has to say about the nature and quality of these bonds during later life.

As Ainsworth (1989) noted, there is no reason to think that a child's attachment to his or her parent wanes once adulthood is reached, or that a parent does not continue to offer a safe haven to his or her adult offspring when needed. Although this proposition is intuitively reasonable, the attachment literature with respect to it is not well developed. Interestingly, there is much better-developed theory and research relevant to the parent–child relationship in the sociological literature. In the following paragraphs, we organize the findings about affectional bonds in later life into two categories: (1) attachment of older parents to their adult children, and (2) attachment of adult children to their aging parents. In each section, we attend first to the attachment literature, then to the sociological literature.

## The Attachment of Aging Parents to Their Adult Children

### Findings Based on an Attachment–Theoretical Perspective

In an interview-based assessment of attachment among older adult mothers (mean age = 72 years), Barnas, Pollina, and Cummings (1991) identified three general patterns of attachment to adult children: insecure-avoidant, insecure-mixed (secure–insecure), and secure. Interestingly, an anxious or preoccupied pattern did not appear in this older cohort—a pattern that mirrors research on the distribution of attachment styles in later adulthood (largely based on self-report measures) reviewed earlier. What is especially interesting about this study is that although the majority of women had secure attachments to at least one child, the quality of relationships varied across children for older adults who had more than one child. Half of the mothers had insecure attachments to at least one of their children, with 31% also having very insecure attachments to at least one child. Twenty percent had insecure-avoidant attachments to all of their children, 40% had insecure-mixed attachments to all of their children, and 40% had secure attachments to all their children.

There is a similarly sparse literature on the impact of early rearing experiences on adult patterns of attachment, although researchers suggest that relationship patterns forged early in life have a bearing on attachment relations in adulthood, at least as assessed by retrospective accounts. In a nationally representative sample of people between 15 and 54 years of age, Mickelson, Kessler, and Shaver (1997) found that an array of reported childhood experiences, including abuse and neglect, were associated with attachment in adulthood. Secure attachment was negatively associat-

ed with reports of physical abuse, serious neglect, and being threatened with a weapon; avoidant attachment was positively associated with serious assault, physical abuse, serious neglect, and being threatened with a weapon, rape, and sexual molestation. These interpersonal traumas, with the exception of serious assault, were also positively associated with anxious attachment.

Another study (Diehl et al., 1998) examined the reported early family climate of adults ranging in age from 20 to 87 years. A positive climate in the family of origin was indexed by the extent to which participants reported family members' supporting each other and being allowed to express their feelings freely; a negative family climate was one in which the family members emphasized rules and enforced rules with punishment. Higher ratings on secure attachment were associated with a more positive evaluation of the family of origin. Higher scores on fearful attachment were associated with lower scores on satisfaction with the family of origin and with the current family, and with higher scores on current negative family climate. Higher scores on preoccupied attachment were positively associated with current negative family climate and negatively associated with current positive family climate. Finally, there were no significant associations between dismissing attachment and any of the family-related variables. This research indicates that childhood maltreatment of various kinds, including physical abuse, negatively influences adult attachment representations and adult attachment organization (Cicchetti, Toth, & Lynch, 1995).

### Insights from the Sociological Literature

#### INTERGENERATIONAL SOLIDARITY

Despite the limited literature on parent–child attachment in later life as viewed from an attachment perspective, there is a fair amount of sociological literature on *intergenerational solidarity* (Silverstein & Bengtson, 1997). The term *solidarity* denotes the cohesion among members of families and is defined by three dimensions: "opportunity" (frequency of contact and residential propinquity between generations), "function" (flows of instrumental assistance between generations), and "affinity" (emotional closeness and perceived agreement of opinions). Although there are generally affectional ties between parents and their adult children, the extent of these ties appears to be moderated by the gender of the parent and the child (Rossi & Rossi, 1990). Affectional ties between mothers and their adult daughters appear to be among the strongest and most enduring of intergenerational bonds (Fingerman, 1996; Rossi & Rossi, 1990, 1991).

Using another index of relationship quality, Fingerman (1996) found that 75% of the mothers indicated that their daughters were among the three most important people in their lives; the corresponding percentage of daughters who nominated their mothers as such was 58%. A mother was also more likely to name a daughter as the person she got along with best, and the person with whom she was most likely to speak when upset, than a daughter was to name a mother. Fingerman speculated that this imbalance in relationship quality from the perspectives of mothers and daughters was probably a function of the older women's narrower social networks. As networks shrink in later life, the people who remain in the network tend to become more important as sources of emotional support and gratification (Carstensen, 1995).

Affectional ties between the generations conceivably have an impact on the nature of the social and instrumental support members provide each other in times of need. Two reviews of the literature on the factors that influence intergenerational support (Davey, Janke, & Savla, 2004; Swartz, 2009) indicate that the quality of relationship history is one of several dyadic characteristics that affect a parent's tendency to supply support to his or her adult children, but it is neither a necessary nor a sufficient condition. Support exchanges between the generations, particularly instrumental exchanges, are not entirely dependent on the quality of relations between parents and children. When both the parents and their adult children are healthy and self-sufficient, intergenerational support tends to remain dormant. However, when the child is in need of emotional, instrumental, or financial support, parents tend to provide it even if their relationship is insecure, suggesting that the strongest predictor of intergenerational support is need (Davey et al., 2004; Swartz, 2009).

## INTERGENERATIONAL AMBIVALENCE

Although the theoretical interest in intergenerational ambivalence has increased in recent years, the empirical literature is not yet well developed. In one study based on a sample of mothers 60 years of age and older (Pillemen & Suitor, 2002), about one-third of the mothers were "torn" in

their ties to their oldest child and felt conflicted about the relationship. One source of conflict was the tension between desires for autonomy and dependency. For example, mothers were concerned about encroachments on their autonomy when adult children failed to achieve and maintain normative adult statuses and financial independence. An analysis of the Iowa Youth and Families Project (Shuey, Wilson, & Elder, 2003), which also focused on mothers' experiences of ambivalence with respect to their children, found that a mother's own dependency increased her level of ambivalence.

In another study (Fingerman, 2001), older mothers were interviewed regarding both the pleasures and problems in their relationships, and one of the salient sources of tension was daughters' unsolicited advice or help. Interestingly, Fingerman also found that different mothers resolved the inherent tensions in their relationships in different ways. Three main styles were discerned: constructive, destructive, and avoidant. This distinction in styles of resolving tension finds a parallel in another study (Smith & Goodnow, 1999) of how adults responded to unasked-for support. Three styles were described: assertively ignoring or rejecting the help, active discounting, and accommodating. Although attachment styles were not measured in either study, the tripartite distinction among styles of resolving tensions and conflicts would seem to be compatible with attachment theory.

In another study of intergenerational ambivalence in a sample of 75 men and women above age 65 (Spitze & Gallant, 2004), participants were interviewed in focus groups. One salient theme was ambivalence about the extent to which children involved themselves in their parents' affairs and health. Parents expressed annoyance at children's overprotectiveness and controllingness; at the same time, they were appreciative of the concern these behaviors expressed. Parents tended to deal with their children's overprotectiveness in one of three ways: by withholding information and confiding in others, by ignoring the overprotectiveness, or by simply accepting it. The material also revealed a desire to be independent, coupled with a potentially conflicting desire for connection to children. This raises a particularly important issue with respect to the measurement of attachment in older samples. Dismissing attachment is often rated on the basis of emphasis on self-reliance and autonomy. If assertion of preference for autonomy is related to aging individuals' fears of becoming incapacitated and being burdensome to their children, measures that rely too heavily on evidence of older adults' preference for autonomy and independence will confound attachment with developmentally normative trends. This is an issue to which we return later.

Intergenerational ambivalence has also been examined in a study in which participants of different ages indicated the quality of their relationships with a range of individuals in their social networks (Fingerman, Hay, & Birditt, 2004). Participants were asked to name social partners to whom they felt very close and people who bothered them. Participants could name any or all of their relationships in both circles. From the data, the researchers identified relationships that were solely close, solely problematic, and ambivalent. Fingerman and colleagues (2004) found that the young-old (60–69 years) and the old-old ( >80 years) were more likely to describe both sets of relationships as solely close than were adolescents, young adults, and middle-aged adults. In fact, among the oldest-old, 92% rated their family relationships as close, 8% rated them as ambivalent, and none rated their relationships as solely problematic.

This apparent decline in conflicted relationships with age is consistent with *socioemotional selectivity theory* (Carstensen, 1995), which proposes that older adults deliberately shed their more peripheral and least emotionally gratifying social relationships in the service of regulating emotion and avoiding conflict. In terms of specific relations, the young-old—the oldest group who still had living parents—were more likely to rate the relationships with their parents as close (70%), with none rating parental relations as problematic. In the young adult sample, however, 43% rated their relationships with their parents as close, and 54% rated them as ambivalent. Sixty-three percent of the middle-aged adults rated their relationships with their parents as close, and 31% rated them as ambivalent. As in the case of the oldest-old adults, none of the parental relationships were rated as solely problematic.

Although the study was cross-sectional, the data could be taken as suggesting that people become less ambivalent about their parents as they age, perhaps reconciling differences as they confront the prospects of their own mortality. It should also be noted, however, that in some ways, the data from this study would seem to be at variance with the literature on attachment style distributions in later life; as reported earlier, this literature indicates that dismissiveness tends to increase with age. The difference between the two sets of data may be attributable to the fact that in the Carstensen (1995) study, individuals were describing *specific* relationships rather than a general style of relating to others, which is tapped by self-report measures of adult attachment. It may simply be that when older adults think of peripheral relationships, they downplay their significance (thereby expressing dismissive attitudes); when they think of particular family relationships, they may focus on their positive nature, especially since close relations in later life are more fundamental to their survival and well-being (and thus less likely to be probed for negative content).

Alternatively, the less ambivalent ratings of the older adults in the Carstensen (1995) study may indicate their placing a premium on avoiding negative interactions. Indeed, several studies indicate that older adults tend to shun occasions where negative affect may be aroused, and that they report higher levels of positive emotion, less interpersonal friction, lower levels of negative emotion overall, and less conflict in their close relationships than younger family members do (e.g., Lefkowitz & Fingerman, 2003; Stimpson, Tyler, & Hoyt, 2005). Finally, another alternative explanation may be that children's behaviors toward their parents may become more positive as their parents become older because as parents enter late life, children may become more solicitous toward them and may protect their parents by not raising issues that upset them (Fingerman & Birditt, 2003).

## The Attachment of Adult Children to Their Aging Parents

### The Attachment Perspective

Early in development, the often fairly exclusive child–mother attachment broadens to include the father, siblings, grandparents, and other relatives. In a study involving a representative sample of Japanese and American individuals ranging in age from 8 to 93 years, Antonucci, Akiyama, and Takahashi (2004) examined social networks to determine how social ties are distributed at different ages. The findings were remarkably similar across the two cultures, with only slight variations. In the innermost ring (depicting closest relationships), 8- to 12-year-old children named their mothers first, followed by fathers and siblings. Adults ages 21–39 still mentioned their mothers first, but the next most frequently mentioned persons were spouses. Among 40- to 59-year-olds, spouses were the most frequently nominated as the closest relationships, with children mentioned next, and only then were mothers likely to be named. Among 60- to 79-year-olds, the closest relationships were spouses and children, with mothers no longer being nominated. Finally, among 80- to 93-year-olds, the pattern seen in 60- to 79-year-olds continued, but with the addition of grandchildren. In Japan, grandchildren were sometimes even nominated as being very close.

We note from this study the prominence of the mother as the main attachment figure in early life. Although she is often displaced by a spouse later in adulthood, the mother persists as a close attachment figure through middle age. Her disappearance from the circle of closest relations later in life is likely to be due to her death.

## Insights from the Sociological Literature

### INTERGENERATIONAL SOLIDARITY

There is a fairly sizable literature on solidarity with respect to adult children and their parents, and this literature supplies much evidence of mutual support and value consensus (Bengtson, Rosenthal, & Burton, 1996; Davey et al., 2004). One of the most methodologically sound studies, a nationally representative survey of cross-generational relationships as reported by adult children (Silverstein & Bengtson, 1997), found that 73% of the sample described themselves as very close to their mothers (vs. somewhat close or not close at all) and 57% described themselves as being very close to their fathers. However, feelings of emotional closeness, while common, did not fully capture the range of intergenerational patterns. The same researchers (Bengtson et al., 1996) also applied a latent class analysis to six dimensions of intergenerational solidarity derived from the broader dimensions of opportunity, function, and affinity. The six dimensions were emotional closeness, similarity of opinions, geographic distance, frequency of contact, providing instrumental assistance, and receiving instrumental assistance. Five types of intergenerational relations emerged. The "tight-knit" type was indicated by relations in which adult children reported being engaged with their parents on all six indicators of solidarity. The "sociable" type was characterized by a high degree of emotional closeness and similarity of opinion, close geographic proximity, and frequent contact, but low levels of instrumental exchange. Adult children characterized as "intimate but distant" were engaged with their parents in terms of emotional closeness

and similarity, but not geographic proximity, frequency of contact, or instrumental exchange. The "obligatory" type was characterized by geographical proximity and frequent contact but was low on emotional closeness, similarity, and instrumental exchange. Finally, adult children characterized as "detached" were not engaged with their parents on any of the six indicators of solidarity.

### INTERGENERATIONAL AMBIVALENCE

Earlier we described a study of close, ambivalent, and problematic relationships (Fingerman et al., 2004) based on the ratings of older adults. That same study also gathered data on how young and middle-aged adults rated their relationships with their parents, among other family members and nonfamily individuals. In this case, there was more evidence for ambivalence. Whereas for the oldest group of adults the proportion of relationships with children characterized as ambivalent was quite low (only 6%), 56% of the young adults and 31% of the middle-aged adults rated their relationships with their parents as ambivalent. The corresponding proportions of "close" relationships were 43 and 63%, respectively. Another study (Wilson, Shuey, & Elder, 2003), using data from the Iowa Youth and Families Project, focused on adult children's ambivalent feelings toward their parents and in-laws. The authors found that children were more ambivalent in female dyads, in relations with in-laws, in relations with parents in poor health, and in cases where a daughter was serving as a caregiver to a parent.

## Continuity of Relations over Time

Based on what we know about the intergenerational transmission of attachment styles between mothers and their young infants (e.g., Benoit & Parker, 1994; Fonagy, Steele, & Steele, 1991), one would expect differential patterns of solidarity both to be linked to individuals' relational histories and to affect current functioning. Indeed, there is much evidence to support these expectations. The bulk of literature on intergenerational solidarity and intergenerational ambivalence suggests that the history of early parent–child relationships, such as experiences with rejection (Stimpson et al., 2005; Whitbeck, Hoyt, & Huck, 1994), divorce, and other family problems (Webster & Herzog, 1995), may affect current solidarity in various ways. These include exchanges of help and support (Parrott & Bengtson, 1999), conflict (Clarke, Preston, Raskin, & Bengtson, 1999; Whitbeck et al., 1994), strain (Whitbeck et al., 1994), depression (Stimpson et al., 2005; Whitbeck, Hoyt, & Tyler, 2001), and reciprocity (Silverstein, Conroy, Wang, Giarrusso, & Bengtson, 2002).

## Giving and Seeking Care: Relations to Attachment

Changes in family structure and economics have contributed to generations of a family being more interdependent in many cases, which can both challenge and strengthen family ties. Due to increases in the time devoted to education and the complexity of young families (e.g., involving divorce and children born outside of marriage), middle-aged parents in contemporary families may continue to provide financial support to their young adult children more than parents did in previous decades. Moreover, due to demographic shifts in the population of most Western countries related to reduced mortality and longer lifespans, there is an unprecedented lengthening of the overlap between the lifespans of adult children and their parents (Perrig-chiello & Hoepflinger, 2005). Because of this overlap, elderly parents are nowadays providing child care for their grown children's children (Swartz, 2009). This has become especially important given the increased rates of divorce and single parenting (Bengston, 2001).

An occasion for conflict resides in the changing nature of relationships over developmental time, due to differential engagement of two different behavioral systems—attachment (care seeking) and caregiving. We typically think of the child as the care seeker and the parent as the caregiver, but these roles often change in later life. Despite the extension of disability-free life expectancies within the older adult population, the last phase of the lifespan is often accompanied by physical infirmity and the resulting assumption of substantial burdens of care by middle-aged children. It has been estimated (Perrig-chiello & Hoepflinger, 2005) that approximately 50% of all women (who tend to be the caregivers in families) will need to deal with dependent parents during middle age, and men and women both will need to reengage psychologically with their parents in ways that activate attachment-related feelings and motivations.

Given these demographic changes, both children and parents are faced with adding new roles to their lives. As the parent becomes infirm or incapacitated and becomes a care seeker, the middle-aged adult may need to step in and provide care—generally a new role for the child. These role accretions in the parent–offspring relationship would seem to engender one of the most common sources of intergenerational ambivalence: the role reversal entailed in the transition from adult child to adult caregiver, and in the gradual, unhappy relinquishment of autonomy by the aged parent (Diehl et al., 1998).

### Caregiver: A New Role for the Child

Caring for an elderly parent seems to be a nearly normative task for today's middle-aged adults, which may have negative consequences for both parties of the relationship. Merz, Consedine, Schulze, and Schuengel (2009) examined questionnaire responses of 1,456 Dutch dyads and found that, on the adult child's side, providing support to a parent was associated with feelings of burden that were not affected by relationship quality.

Although the quality of the child–parent bond does not seem to affect the sense of burden of caring for an elderly parent, it may well affect the kind of care aged parents receive from their children (Diehl et al., 1998). The researchers found that empathy and social responsibility—traits associated with the inclination to help others—were positively associated with attachment security and negatively associated with fearful avoidance. Dismissing attachment was negatively associated with empathy, and preoccupied attachment was negatively associated with responsibility. Compatible experimental work (Mikulincer, Shaver, Gillath, & Nitzberg, 2005) has shown that increasing individuals' felt security through both implicit and explicit security priming fosters compassion and altruistic behavior.

Research indicates that concern for aging parents' health is highly salient in the minds of adult children, and that dealing with this concern is a pervasive aspect of relationships with parents (Cicirelli, 2000). Theoretical sociologists provided some of the earliest formulations concerning the motives and means by which adult children provide help to aging parents. From a sociological standpoint, helping behavior is seen as one aspect of intergenerational solidarity, and helping behavior itself is viewed as a function of a particular elderly person's dependency needs, residential propinquity to an adult child, filial obligations, and gender roles. The Longitudinal Study of Generations (Silverstein, Parrott, & Bengtson, 1995) assessed parent–child dyads participating in three waves of data collection. The results indicated that intergenerational affection was the factor that most motivated daughters to provide support, whereas for sons the predominant factors were filial obligation, legitimation of inheritance, and frequency of contact. Data from the same study indicated that a history of affection was also associated with equitable and reciprocal exchange of support, as well as with a greater likelihood of giving and receiving various forms of support and help (Parrott & Bengtson, 1999).

Operating within an attachment perspective, Cicirelli (1983, 1993) proposed that caregiving by adult children is motivated by enduring affectional ties between children and their parents, and by protective motives on the part of children. That is, an adult child, who may still come to an elderly parent for instrumental or emotional support during times of stress (e.g., childrearing, job difficulties, divorce), is motivated to preserve and/or restore the threatened existence of the attachment figure as long as possible, and this may involve becoming a caregiver when the parent is ill. However, the quality of the child's attachment to the parent may influence the quality of his or her caregiving.

In the literature on caregiving in dating and marital relationships (i.e., in young adult samples), secure individuals have been found to report and display more sensitive and responsive care and less controlling caregiving than avoidant and ambivalent individuals (Collins, Guichard, Ford, & Feeney, 2006; B. C. Feeney & Collins, 2001). Attachment-oriented studies of caregiving in the context of adult children providing care to elderly parents are quite limited in number, but the findings are consistent in showing that secure attachment can ameliorate anticipated or experienced caregiver burden. In one of the first studies of its kind, Cicirelli (1983) proposed that affectional ties between children and their parents might be a better predictor of helping than filial obligation. He studied a sample of middle-aged adults with mothers age 60 and above. Attachment was measured by an index of feelings of closeness and perceived similarity through identification; attachment behaviors were assessed by a composite of residential proximity, frequency of visits, and frequency of telephone contacts. Path analysis revealed that caregiving behaviors were predicted by feelings of attachment, maternal dependency, and filial obligation. Current helping behaviors were a direct effect of only two variables, attachment feelings and greater dependency on the part of the parent, whereas feelings of attachment and filial obligation had indirect effects, acting through their effect on what Cicirelli described as "attachment behavior" (defined as communication over distance to maintain psychological closeness). Future help was predicted by attachment behavior, feelings of attachment, low conflict, and parental dependency; filial obligation had no direct effect on commitment to provide future help.

A more recent study assessed the degree to which middle-aged children were prepared to face the challenge of future caregiving responsibilities as a function of attachment style (Soerensen et al., 2002). This study found that security of attachment was a significant and positive predictor of feeling prepared to provide care, whereas both anxious-ambivalent and avoidant attachment predicted lower levels of feeling prepared. Three other studies have examined the actual caregiving experience and its impact on *caregiver burden* (defined as subjective experiences of stress and strain). One study assessed attachment and obligation in daughters caring for elderly mothers (Cicirelli, 1993). The data indicated that although both variables were related to the help provided by the daughters, stronger (or more secure) attachment was associated with less subjective burden, whereas stronger obligation was associated with greater burden. In another study, Crispi, Schiaffino, and Berman (1997) found that secure (vs. insecure) attachment of middle-aged children to a parent diagnosed with dementia was associated with lower "caregiving difficulty" (a measure of subjective and objective burden) and with lower psychological distress.

Another study hinted at the possibility that the attachment style of the older parent and his or her behavior may influence the experience of caregiver burden in the child (Magai & Cohen, 1998). In this study, patients with dementia who were rated as having an anxious attachment style before they became ill displayed more anxious and depressed symptoms than did patients with secure or avoidant attachment styles. Patients with the avoidant style displayed more activity disturbance than patients with the anxious style, and more paranoid symptoms than those with a secure style. Relatedly, caregivers of patients with a secure style reported lower caregiver burden than those caring for patients with avoidant or anxious attachment styles. Thus, there are likely to be reciprocal and dynamic aspects of the care experience at the level of the dyad; this feature is alluded to in a recently published multicomponent conceptual model, with both caregivers' and care recipients' characteristics and behaviors affecting the relationship dynamic (B. C. Feeney & Collins, 2004).

There is evidence of intergenerational transmission of attachment and caregiving patterns. Longitudinal data from a Swiss study, Transitions and Life Perspectives in Middle Age (Perrig-chiello & Hoepflinger, 2005), indicate that *filial autonomy* (a measure of successful coping with normative developmental tasks in adulthood) was negatively correlated with filial helpfulness and with secure relations with the adults' own children. These findings suggest that a strong sense of separateness between middle-aged individuals and their parents was mirrored in a less secure relationship with their own children. Moreover, the strength (or security) of attachment to parents was positively associated with the strength of relationships with the middle-aged participants' own children. Another set of investigators (Wilson et al., 2003), using data from the Iowa Youth and Families Project and focusing on adult children's ambivalent feelings toward their parents and in-laws, found that there is greater ambivalence when there were poor relations during childhood.

Compatible results were found by Klaus (2009), who analyzed the effect of secure attachment and history of supportive interactions on social support provision of German adult children to an elderly parent. In this study, secure attachment was assumed to be expressed by the child's propensity to feel close to the parent. The results showed that children tended to provide more support if they had received more support from the parent in the past and if they were securely attached. Similarly, Swartz (2009) reported that children whose parents had invested more time and emotional and financial support in them tended to provide more support 27 years later. Klaus interpreted the tendency of more securely attached children to be supportive as a result of early parental caregiving behavior and as an effort to keep the parent alive and preserve the emotional bond.

Chen and colleagues (2013) examined adults' attachment representations and the task of caring for elderly parents with dementia. They found that individuals who indicated having a secure base script for caring for an elderly parent also reported less criticism, hostility, and emotional overinvolvement in their relationships with their elderly parents. Moreover, their results showed that such script knowledge has a stronger effect when the caregiving task is perceived as more difficult. Based on these findings, Chen and colleagues argued that the value of knowledge from a secure base script lies more in providing a motivational framework and a goal structure (to be a good, secure base) than in specific skills. Chen and colleagues' results also suggest that a certain amount of stress is required for script knowledge to have an impact on caregiver behavior. It may be that in the context of caring for a parent with dementia, stress represents a signal that allows adult children to recognize the need, then shift into their role as caregivers.

### Help Seeking in Later Life: A New Role for the Parent

Despite older adults' clear preference for retaining their autonomy in later life, most people cannot realistically hope to avoid an increase in dependency if they live long enough. Among the potential elicitors of care seeking are (1) the various forms of chronic illness with which persons are afflicted in late life that require constant monitoring and/or care (e.g., diabetes, poor vision, and kidney disease); (2) growing limitation of activities and greater physical dependency caused by illnesses such as arthritis and circulatory disease; and (3) anxiety and depression resulting from bereavements of various kinds and the individual's own looming death.

Threats and illness are innate elicitors of attachment behavior in early life. In later life, after decades of successful autonomy, encroaching dependency can seem a cruel denouement; as already noted, this newly emerging threat appears to elicit an internal approach–avoidance struggle between autonomy and dependence. Conceivably, this struggle is more difficult for insecurely attached individuals. Anxiously attached people are sometimes too eager to seek care and reassurance from attachment figures in general, which may cause the caregivers to distance themselves, generating even more insecurity in their needy older adult dependents. Avoidant individuals, who are likely to deny their distress, are therefore unlikely to seek help. In both kinds of cases, the insecure elderly parents may perceive less social support, as has been found in studies of younger adults (Vogel & Wei, 2005).

Merz and colleagues (2009) analyzed data from 1,456 dyads data from the Netherlands Kinship Panel Study to investigate emotional experiences in older adults receiving support from and adult children. They found that older adult parents tend to experience negative emotions related to their loss of autonomy, but such reactions are buffered by good relationship quality. As mentioned earlier, secure individuals seem to be better able to deal with the growing dependency that arises in late life.

## Grieving the Death of a Parent

One of the most common attachment-related challenges of adulthood is coming to terms with the death of one's parents. According to the National Survey of Family Households (2003), among 9,230 adults age 45 or older who were interviewed, 58.3% had lost their mother and 75.7% had lost their father. Around 12 million American adults, 5% of the population, lose a parent each year. Demographic data indicate that maternal and paternal deaths are most likely to occur when children are between 45 and 64 years of age and between 35 and 54 years of age, respectively (Winsborough, Bumpass, & Aquilino, 1991). Attachment theory suggests that these losses elicit profound feelings. Yet the literature on this subject is somewhat limited. This seems especially odd given that all of us—if we live long enough—will experience the loss of first one parent and then the other. Once both parents are deceased, feelings of being an "orphan" are common (Stroebe, Schut, & Stroebe, 2005).

What limited literature exists indicates that the death of an aged parent can cause changes in an adult child's marital relationship, sibling relationships, and relationship with the surviving parent. Although the marital relationship can be a source of support when the spouse's parent dies, and can strengthen the relationship (Moss & Moss, 1983–1984), a parent's death may also have deleterious effects. In one prospective study, Umberson (1995) found that recent maternal death was associated with a decline in reported social support from the adult child's marital partner, a reduction in marital harmony, and an increase in the partner's negative behaviors and relationship strain and conflict. Barner and Rosenblatt (2008) also examined how couple relationships are affected by the death of a parent. They found that death of a parent led to changes in both frequency and content of communications between partners and seemed to foster discussion, negotiation, and role transition.

The death of a parent in middle adulthood also has an impact on sibling relationships. Khodyakov and Carr (2009) tested this hypothesis using data from the Wisconsin Longitudinal Survey (WLS) and found a modest negative effect of parental death on adult siblings' perceived relationship closeness, suggesting that living parents unite their children. The authors also found a further negative effect on sibling relationships of having a remaining, widowed parent to care for. One sibling may feel resentment toward the other, if the latter is perceived as not having contributed a fair share to caring for either parent (Cicirelli, 1993) or if they disagree about how well they performed their caregiving roles (Brody, 1990). Finally, in another study, Lee, Dwyer, and Coward (1993) found that father–daughter relationships deteriorated significantly after the mother's death, but that this effect was much weaker for the father–son relationship.

It appears that there are only two attachment-oriented studies of parental bereavement in later life, although in neither case were standard measures of attachment employed. One of the studies (Scharlach, 1991) tested the thesis that resolution of grief depends on the bereaved adult's attachment status relative to the parent who has died. Scharlach considered both initial and residual grief reactions in 35- to 60-year-olds. Results of the study indicated that two of the strongest predictors of initial and residual grief were the expectedness of the parent's death and the level of the adult child's personal autonomy. The latter effect was interpreted as indexing a secure attachment, inasmuch as successful functioning as an autonomous adult is thought to be the result of a healthy separation from one's parents.

In the other study, Popek and Scharlach (1991) used interview and questionnaire data to examine the responses of adult daughters to the deaths of their elderly mothers. The authors found that a daughter's ability to resolve her grief 1–5 years after the mother's death was significantly affected by the kind of relationship they had when the mother was still alive. Coders assessed the nature of each relationship (close or distant) and whether each participant's feelings regarding the mother's death were relatively resolved or unresolved. Thirty-seven percent were classified as close and resolved, 35% were close and unresolved, and 26% were distant and unresolved; one participant's relationship (0.02%) was classified as distant and resolved. Based on the authors' descriptions of other key characteristics of the groupings, the first category probably reflected a secure daughter–mother relationship, the second a preoccupied and/or fearful-avoidant relationship, and the third a dismissing relationship.

Despite the physical departure of the parents from adult children's lives, there is evidence of their continued influence. In fact, one study suggests that internalized representations of parents function as "silent" attachment partners even after the parents' deaths, at least as studied within the context of dementia research (see also Fraley & Shaver, Chapter 3, this volume). The belief among many elderly patients with dementia that one or both of their parents is still alive—called *parent fixation*—has been reported as fairly common (Miesen, 1992).

In a study of the relation between level of cognitive functioning and the expression of various forms of attachment behavior in a psychogeriatric nursing home in the Netherlands, observations of attachment behavior were made with the Standard Visiting Procedure, akin to Ainsworth's Strange Situation, in which the person with dementia was first alone in a room, then with the researcher, and finally with a family member. A critical point in this procedure occurred when the family member suddenly announced that he or she had to leave, thus creating a potentially threatening moment that should activate the attachment system. Individuals who were more cognitively intact exhibited less parent fixation and more overt forms of attachment behavior directed at a family member, such as turning toward or calling after the person. Those who were functioning at a lower level displayed more parent fixation and fewer overt attachment behaviors of any other kind.

Miesen (1992) hypothesized that the invocation of deceased parents by patients with dementia represents an attempt to regulate the fear and uncertainty that accompanies loss of cognitive function. In this view, parent fixation is an attachment behavior expressing the need for safety and security. In the early stages of dementia, he theorized, parent fixation is not observed because other, more organized forms of attachment behavior are still possible, and because of the security provided by available living attachment figures. As the illness progresses, however, the "strange situation" that is dementia becomes a more permanent condition, with the now pervasive experience of feeling un-

safe being increasingly managed internally, as reflected in parent fixation.

Similar conclusions were drawn by Osborne, Stokes, and Simpson (2010), who studied parent fixation in a group of 51 older adults with dementia living in the community or in a nursing home. They interviewed target participants and had one relative of each complete measures of the participant's cognitive impairment and executive functioning, behavioral consequences of parent fixation, premorbid personality, and attachment style. Surprisingly, parent fixation was negatively associated with attachment anxiety, especially among participants living in a nursing home. Osborne and colleagues suggested that "parent fixation may therefore act as a process by which individuals seek symbolic representation of a good, consistent attachment figure" (p. 934).

## What Is New Since 2008? And Where Might Research Go from Here?

One requirement is that authors of this volume say briefly how the literature in a given area has changed since the previous edition of this handbook was published in 2008. In general, the new publications largely converge with and add to the ones that existed before 2008. There is more evidence for the relative frequency of the different attachment patterns later in life, confirming that attachment-related avoidance seems more prevalent in older adults than in younger adults. There is also more evidence for the smaller size of older adults' social networks, a phenomenon that occurs without noticeably reducing the number of very close relationships. There is more evidence for the normative changes in attachment hierarchies, with parents (especially mothers) being important through childhood and peers becoming more important in adolescence and beyond, and with romantic or marital partners being especially important in adulthood. In late life, many adults begin to view one or more of their adult children as attachment figures, causing substantial adjustments in relationship patterns. Many older adults also maintain psychological relationships with deceased members of their attachment hierarchies, and with religious personages, such as God. There is more evidence concerning physiological and health factors in late life, with fearfully avoidant individuals seeming to have more symptom complaints. There is evidence that child abuse, experienced decades before the later years, continues to affect people in numerous ways—a topic that deserves more research attention. Also important is the influence of changing family structures and economics in relations between adult children and their parents. New research indicates that "secure-base scripts" are important in later adulthood, as they were already known to be in childhood and early adulthood. Finally, there is new evidence, although still sparse, for the effects of caring for an elderly parent on the caregivers' marital and sibling relationships.

As the lifespans of older adults in developed societies continue to grow longer, the issues discussed in this chapter will become more important. The proportion of the population that comprises older adults in many of these societies has grown and will continue to grow, placing a greater burden of care on adult children. The gradual erosion of the expectations for marriage is likely to continue, creating new needs for care of children and grandchildren, as well as declining older adults. There will be many opportunities for attachment researchers to examine these social developments.

One issue that was important in the 2008 version of this chapter, and which continues to be important today, is measurement. In particular, researchers should explore alternative measures of attachment patterns in older adults. The existing literature suggests that attachment-related avoidance increases later in life, but no one knows whether this is actually happening or the measures created originally to assess young adults with respect to romantic relationships are less appropriate for older adults. Similarly, the measures of caregiving that have been developed for research on couple relationships need to be reconsidered for extension to the study of other kinds of caregiving—for example, in relation to older adult parents.

In future research, it will be important to differentiate among forms of dependency based on a social environment that elicits and/or reinforces dependent behavior; insecurity-based dependency (similar to anxious, preoccupied attachment); and reasonable, self-accepted dependency, which may be a beneficial stance used to conserve energy and resources in late life (Parks & Pilisuk, 1991). The field would be well served if future research on caregiving and attachment in later adulthood were directed at assessing types of caregiving, types of dependency, and their interactions and long-term consequences.

Little is known about which child in the family becomes the caregiver and what might motivate acceptance of the role. If, as Cicirelli (1983, 1993) proposes, caregiving is motivated in part by children wanting to protect their attachment figures so as to assuage their own "fear of abandonment," we might expect more anxiously attached adult children to rise to the occasion.

We know that innate tendencies to provide care to others in need can be overridden or suppressed by attachment insecurity (B. C. Feeney & Collins, 2001; Mikulincer et al., 2005). At such times, anxiously attached individuals are likely to be focused on their own needs rather than those of their distressed relationship partners. We also know that avoidantly attached individuals tend to be disapproving of other people's vulnerabilities, weaknesses, and needs (Collins & Read, 1994), and therefore cannot be expected to be sensitive to others' distress. This raises questions about the quality of care that insecure adult children will provide, perhaps especially in the presence of the original cause of attachment insecurity (i.e., a parent's insecurity-arousing behavior).

Finally, our review of the literature has brought to the fore the continuing neglect of bereavement following the loss of one or both parents as a midlife experience with potentially profound personal and family significance. Writing about the passing of his own parents, Levy (1999) suggested that when one parent dies, there may be changes in the relationship with the remaining parent; that when either parent or both parents die, there may be changes in other interpersonal relationships or changes in identity that provoke identity reorganization; and that the death of a parent refocuses an adult's sense of time.

An important paper by Stroebe and colleagues (2005) offers a conceptual model—the *dual-process model of coping with bereavement*—that integrates coping theory and attachment theory in a very promising way. The model suggests that there is an array of successful and unsuccessful coping styles, as well as attachment styles, some of which are loss-oriented and others of which are restoration-oriented. Furthermore, Stroebe and colleagues suggest that these coping orientations, when considered jointly with attachment styles, may enable researchers to understand when and for whom the process of continuing or loosening the attachment bonds with a lost loved one are likely to be adaptive or maladaptive. There is a great deal of interesting and important research to be done in this area.

# References

Ainsworth, M. S. (1989). Attachments beyond infancy. *American Psychologist, 44*(4), 709–716.

Antonucci, T. C., Akiyama, H., & Takahashi, K. (2004). Attachment and close relationships across the life span. *Attachment and Human Development, 6,* 353–370.

Bakermans-Kranenburg, M. J., & Van IJzendoorn, M. H. (2009). The first 10,000 Adult Attachment Interviews: Distributions of adult attachment representations in clinical and non-clinical groups. *Attachment and Human Development, 11*(3), 223–263.

Baldwin, M. W., & Fehr, B. (1995). On the instability of attachment style ratings. *Personal Relationships, 2,* 247–261.

Banai, E., Weller, A., & Mikulincer, M. (1998). Interjudge agreement in evaluation of adult attachment style: The impact of acquaintanceship. *British Journal of Social Psychology, 37,* 95–109.

Barnas, M. V., Pollina, L., & Cummings, E. M. (1991). Life-span attachment: Relations between attachment and socioemotional functioning in adult women. *Genetic, Social, and General Psychology Monographs, 117,* 175–202.

Barner, J., & Rosenblatt, P. (2008). Giving at loss: Couple exchange after the death of a parent. *Mortality, 13,* 318–334.

Bartholomew, K., & Horowitz, L. M. (1991). Attachment styles among young adults: A test of a four-category model. *Journal of Personality and Social Psychology, 61,* 226–244.

Bengston, V. L. (2001). Beyond the nuclear family: The increasing importance of multigenerational bonds. *Journal of Marriage and Family, 63,* 1–16.

Bengtson, V. L., Rosenthal, C. J., & Burton, L. (1996). Paradoxes of families and aging. In R. H. Binstock & L. K. George (Eds.), *Handbook of aging and the social sciences* (4th ed., pp. 253–282). San Diego, CA: Academic Press.

Benoit, D., & Parker, K. (1994). Stability and transmission of attachment across three generations. *Child Development, 65,* 1444–1456.

Bodner, E., & Cohen-Fridel, S. (2010). Relations between attachment styles, ageism, and quality of life in late life. *International Psychogeriatrics, 22,* 1353–1361.

Bowlby, J. (1973). *Attachment and loss: Vol. 2. Separation: Anxiety and anger.* New York: Basic Books.

Bowlby, J. (1980). *Attachment and loss: Vol. 3. Loss: Sadness and depression.* New York: Basic Books.

Bowlby, J. (1982). *Attachment and loss: Vol. 1. Attachment.* New York: Basic Books. (Original work published 1969)

Brody, E. M. (1990). *Women in the middle: Their parent care years.* New York: Springer-Verlag.

Campos, J. J., Barrett, K. C., Lamb, M. E., Goldsmith, H. H., & Stenberg, C. (1983). Socioemotional development. In M. M. Haith (Ed.), *Handbook of child psychology: Infancy and developmental psychobiology* (Vol. 2, pp. 783–917). New York: Wiley.

Carstensen, L. L. (1995). Evidence for a life-span theory of socioemotional selectivity. *Current Directions in Psychological Science, 4,* 151–156.

Chen, C. K., Waters, H. S., Hartman, M., Zimmerman, S., Miklowitz, D. J., & Waters, E. (2013). The secure base script and the task of caring for elderly parents: Implications for attachment theory and clinical practice. *Attachment and Human Development, 15,* 332–348.

Cicchetti, D., Toth, S. L., & Lynch, M. (1995). Bowlby's dream comes full circle: The application of attachment theory to risk and psychopathology. *Advances in Clinical Child Psychology, 17,* 1–75.

Cicirelli, V. G. (1983). Adult children's attachment and helping behavior to elderly parents: A path model. *Journal of Marriage and the Family, 45,* 815–825.

Cicirelli, V. G. (1993). Attachment and obligation as daughters' motives for caregiving behavior and subsequent effect on subjective burden. *Psychology and Aging, 8,* 144–155.

Cicirelli, V. G. (2000). An examination of the trajectory of the adult child's caregiving for an elderly parent. *Family Relations, 49,* 169–175.

Cicirelli, V. G. (2010). Attachment relationships in old age. *Journal of Social and Personal Relationships, 27,* 191–199.

Clarke, E. J., Preston, M., Raskin, J., & Bengtson, V. L. (1999). Types of conflicts and tensions between older parents and adult children. *Gerontologist, 39,* 261–270.

Collins, N. L., Guichard, A. C., Ford, M. B., & Feeney, B. C. (2006). Responding to need in intimate relationships: Normative processes and individual differences. In M. Mikulincer & G. S. Goodman (Eds.), *Dynamics of romantic love: Attachment, caregiving, and sex* (pp. 149–189). New York: Guilford Press.

Collins, N. L., & Read, S. J. (1994). Cognitive representations of attachment: The structure and function of working models. In K. Bartholomew & D. Perlman (Eds.), *Advances in personal relationships: Vol. 5. Attachment processes in adulthood* (pp. 53–92). London: Jessica Kingsley.

Consedine, N. S., & Fiori, K. L. (2009). Gender moderates the associations between attachment and discrete emotions in late middle age and later life. *Aging and Mental Health, 13,* 847–862.

Consedine, N. S., Fiori, K. L., & Magai, C. (2012). Regulating emotion expression and regulating emotion experience: Divergent associations with dimensions of attachment among older women. *Attachment and Human Development, 14,* 477–500.

Consedine, N. S., Fiori, K. L., & Merz, E. M. (2013). Attachment, activity limitation, and health symptoms in later life: The mediating roles of negative (and positive) affect. *Journal of Aging and Health, 25,* 56–79.

Consedine, N. S., & Magai, C. (2006, July). *Patterns of attachment and attachment change in later life: Prelimi-*

*nary results from a longitudinal study of 415 older adults.* Paper presented at the third biennial conference of the International Association for Relationship Research, Rethymnon, Crete, Greece.

Consedine, N. S., Magai, C., Horton, D., & Brown, W. M. (2012). The affective paradox: An emotional regulatory account of ethnic differences in self-reported anger. *Journal of Cross-Cultural Psychology, 43,* 723–741.

Cozzarelli, C., Karafa, J. A., Collins, N. L., & Tagler, M. J. (2003). Stability and change in adult attachment styles: Associations with personal vulnerabilities, life events, and global construals of self and others. *Journal of Social and Clinical Psychology, 22,* 315–346.

Crispi, E. L., Schiaffino, K., & Berman, W. H. (1997). The contribution of attachment to burden in adult children of institutionalized parents with dementia. *Gerontologist, 38,* 52–60.

Davey, A., Janke, M., & Savla, J. (2004). Antecedents of intergenerational support: Families in context and families as context. *Annual Review of Gerontology and Geriatrics, 24,* 29–54.

Dewitte, M., De Houwer, J., Goubert, L., & Buysse, A. (2010). A multi modal approach to the study of attachment related distress. *Biological Psychology, 85,* 149–162.

Diehl, M., Elnick, A. B., Bourbeau, L. S., & Labouvie-Vief, G. (1998). Adult attachment styles: Their relations to family context and personality. *Journal of Personality and Social Psychology, 74,* 1656–1669.

Duncan, G. J., Kalil, A., & Ziol-Guest, K. M. (2013). Early childhood poverty and adult achievement, employment and health. *Family Matters, 93,* 27–35.

Feeney, B. C., & Collins, N. L. (2001). Predictors of caregiving in adult intimate relationships: An attachment theoretical perspective. *Journal of Personality and Social Psychology, 80,* 972–994.

Feeney, B. C., & Collins, N. L. (2004). Interpersonal safe haven and secure base caregiving processes in adulthood. In W. S. Rholes & J. A. Simpson (Eds.), *Adult attachment: Theory, research, and clinical implications* (pp. 300–338). New York: Guilford Press.

Feeney, J. A., & Noller, P. (1990). Attachment style as a predictor of adult romantic relationships. *Journal of Personality and Social Psychology, 38,* 281–291.

Fingerman, K. L. (1996). Sources of tension in the aging mother and adult daughter relationship. *Psychology and Aging, 11,* 591–606.

Fingerman, K. L. (2001). *Aging mothers and their adult daughters: A study in mixed emotions.* New York: Springer.

Fingerman, K. L., & Birditt, K. S. (2003). Do age differences in close and problematic family ties reflect the pool of available relatives? *Journals of Gerontology B: Psychological Sciences, 58,* 80–87.

Fingerman, K. L., Hay, E. L., & Birditt, K. S. (2004). The best of ties, the worst of ties: Close, problematic, and ambivalent social relationships. *Journal of Marriage and the Family, 66,* 792–808.

Fiori, K. L., Consedine, N. S., & Merz, E. M. (2011). Attachment, social network size, and patterns of social exchange in later life. *Research and Aging, 33,* 465–493.

Fonagy, P., Steele, H., & Steele, M. (1991). Maternal representations of attachment during pregnancy predict the organization of infant–mother attachment at one year of age. *Child Development, 62,* 891–905.

Fraley, R. C., & Brumbaugh, C. C. (2004). A dynamical systems approach to conceptualizing and studying stability and change in attachment security. In W. S. Rholes & J. A. Simpson (Eds.), *Adult attachment: Theory, research, and clinical implications* (pp. 86–132). New York: Guilford Press.

Fung, H. H., Carstensen, L. L., & Lang, F. R. (2001). Age-related patterns in social networks among European Americans and African Americans: Implications for socioemotional selectivity across the life span. *International Journal of Aging and Human Development, 52,* 185–206.

Giles, L. C., Glonek, G. F. V., Luszca, M. A., & Andrews, R. (2005). Effect of social networks on 10 year survival in very old Australians: The Australian longitudinal study of aging. *Journal of Epidemiology and Community Health, 59,* 574–579.

Gillath, O., Johnson, D. K., Selcuk, E., & Teel, C. (2011). Comparing old and young adults as they cope with life transitions: The links between social network management skills and attachment style to depression. *Clinical Gerontologist, 34,* 251–265.

Grossmann, K. E. (1996). Ethological perspectives on human development and aging. In C. Magai & S. McFadden (Eds.), *Handbook of emotion, adult development, and aging* (pp. 43–66). San Diego, CA: Academic Press.

Hazan, C., & Shaver, P. R. (1987). Romantic love conceptualized as an attachment process. *Journal of Personality and Social Psychology, 52,* 511–524.

Hobdy, J., Hayslip, B., Kaminski, P. L., Crowley, B. J., Riggs, S., et al. (2007). The role of attachment style in coping with job loss and the empty nest in adulthood. *International Journal of Aging and Human Development, 65,* 335–371.

Khodyakov, M., & Carr, D. (2009). The impact of late-life parental death on adult sibling relationships: Do parent's advance directives help or hurt? *Research on Aging, 31,* 495–519.

Kidd, T., Hamer, M., & Steptoe, A. (2013). Adult attachment style and cortisol responses across the day in older adults. *Psychophysiology, 50,* 841–847.

Klaus, D. (2009). Why do adult children support their parents? *Journal of Comparative Family Studies, 40,* 227–241.

Lee, G., Dwyer, J., & Coward, R. (1993). Gender differences in parent care: Demographic factors and same-gender preferences. *Journals of Gerontology B: Psychological Sciences and Social Sciences, 48,* S9–S16.

Lefkowitz, E. S., & Fingerman, K. L. (2003). Positive and negative emotional feelings and behaviors in mother–daughter ties in late life. *Journal of Family Psychology, 17,* 607–617.

Levy, A. (1999). *The orphaned adult: Understanding and coping with grief and change after the death of our parents.* Cambridge, MA: Perseus.

Magai, C., Cohen, C., Milburn, N., Thorpe, B., McPherson, R., & Peralta, D. (2001). Attachment styles in older European American and African American adults. *Journals of Gerontology B: Psychological Sciences and Social Sciences, 56,* 28–35.

Magai, C., & Cohen, C. I. (1998). Attachment style and emotion regulation in dementia patients and their relation to caregiver burden. *Journals of Gerontology B: Psychological Sciences and Social Sciences, 53,* P147–P154.

Magai, C., & Consedine, N. S. (2004). Introduction to the special issue: Attachment and aging. *Attachment and Human Development, 6,* 349–351.

Magai, C., Hunziker, J., Mesias, W., & Culver, L. C. (2000). Adult attachment styles and emotional biases. *International Journal of Behavioral Development, 24,* 301–309.

Merz, E. M., Consedine, N. S., Schulze, H. J., & Schuengel, C. (2009). Wellbeing of adult children and ageing parents: Associations with intergenerational support and relationship quality. *Ageing and Society, 29,* 783–802.

Mickelson, K. D., Kessler, R. C., & Shaver, P. R. (1997). Adult attachment in a nationally representative sample. *Journal of Personality and Social Psychology, 73,* 1092–1106.

Miesen, B. (1992). Attachment theory and dementia. In B. M. L. Miesen (Ed.), *Care-giving in dementia: Research and applications* (pp. 38–56). London: Routledge/Tavistock.

Mikulincer, M., & Shaver, P. R. (2007). *Attachment in adulthood: Structure, dynamics, and change.* New York: Guilford Press.

Mikulincer, M., Shaver, P. R., Gillath, O., & Nitzberg, R. A. (2005). Attachment, caregiving, and altruism: Boosting attachment security increases compassion and helping. *Journal of Personality and Social Psychology, 89,* 817–839.

Moss, M. S., & Moss, S. Z. (1983–1984). The impact of parental death on middle-aged children. *Omega: Journal of Death and Dying, 14*(1), 65–75.

National Survey of Family Households. (2003). *Wave 3 field report.* Madison: University of Wisconsin Survey Center.

Osborne, H., Stokes, G., & Simpson, J. (2010). A psychosocial model of parent fixation in people with dementia: The role of personality and attachment. *Aging and Mental Health, 14,* 928–937.

Parks, S. H., & Pilisuk, M. (1991). Caregiver burden: Gender and the psychological costs of caregiving. *American Journal of Orthopsychiatry, 61,* 501–509.

Parrott, T. M., & Bengtson, V. L. (1999). The effects of earlier intergenerational affection, normative expectations and family conflict on contemporary exchanges of help and support. *Research on Aging, 21,* 73–105.

Perrig-chiello, P., & Hoepflinger, F. (2005). Aging parents and their middle-aged children: Demographic and psychosocial challenges. *European Journal of Aging, 2,* 183–191.

Pillemen, K., & Suitor, J. J. (2002). Explaining mothers' ambivalence toward their adult children. *Journal of Marriage and the Family, 64,* 602–613.

Poon, C. Y. M., & Knight, B. G. (2011). Impact of childhood parental abuse and neglect on sleep problems in old age. *Journals of Gerontology B: Psychological Sciences and Social Sciences, 66,* 307–310.

Popek, P., & Scharlach, A. E. (1991). Adult daughters' relationships with their mothers and reactions to the mothers' deaths. *Journal of Women and Aging, 3,* 79–96.

Preston, S. H., Hill, M. E., & Drevenstedt, G. L. (1998). Childhood conditions that predict survival to advanced ages among African-Americans. *Social Science and Medicine, 47,* 1231–1246.

Rossi, A. S., & Rossi, P. H. (1990). *Of human bonding: Parent–child relations across the life course.* New York: Aldine de Gruyter.

Rossi, A. S., & Rossi, P. H. (1991). Normative obligations and parent–child help exchange across the life course. In K. McCartney (Ed.), *Parent–child relationships throughout life* (pp. 201–223). Hillsdale, NJ: Erlbaum.

Scharlach, A. E. (1991). Factors associated with filial grief following the death of an elderly parent. *American Journal of Orthopsychiatry, 61,* 307–313.

Shuey, K. M., Wilson, A. E., & Elder, G. H., Jr. (2003, August). *Ambivalence in the relationship between aging mothers and their adult children: A dyadic analysis.* Paper presented at the annual meeting of the American Sociological Association, Atlanta, GA.

Silverstein, M., & Bengtson, V. L. (1997). Intergenerational solidarity and the structure of adult child–parent relationships in American families. *American Journal of Sociology, 103,* 429–460.

Silverstein, M., Conroy, S. J., Wang, H., Giarrusso, R., & Bengtson, V. L. (2002). Reciprocity in parent–child relations over the adult live course. *Journals of Gerontology B: Psychological Sciences and Social Sciences, 57,* S3–S13.

Silverstein, M., Parrott, T. M., & Bengtson, V. L. (1995). Factors that predispose middle-aged sons and daughters to provide social support to older parents. *Journal of Marriage and the Family, 57,* 465–475.

Smith, J., & Goodnow, J. J. (1999). Unasked-for support and unsolicited advice: Age and the quality of social experience. *Psychology and Aging, 14,* 108–121.

Soerensen, S., Webster, J. D., & Roggman, L. A. (2002). Adult attachment and preparing to provide care for older relatives. *Attachment and Human Development, 4,* 84–106.

Spitze, G., & Gallant, M. P. (2004). "The bitter with the sweet": Older adults' strategies for handling ambivalence in relations with their adult children. *Research on Aging, 26,* 387–412.

Stimpson, J. P., Tyler, K. A., & Hoyt, D. R. (2005). Effects of parental rejection and relationship quality on depression among older rural adults. *International Journal of Aging and Human Development, 61,* 195–210.

Stroebe, M., Schut, H., & Stroebe, W. (2005). Attachment in coping with bereavement: A theoretical integration. *Review of General Psychology, 9,* 48–66.

Swartz, T. T. (2009). Intergenerational family relations in adulthood: Patterns, variations, and implications in the contemporary United States. *Annual Review of Sociology, 35,* 191–212.

Umberson, D. (1995). Marriage as support or strain?: Marital quality following the death of a parent. *Journal of Marriage and the Family, 57,* 709–723.

Van Assche, L., Luyten, P., Bruffaerts, R., Persoons, P., van de Ven, L., & Vandenbulcke, M. (2013). Attachment in old age: Theoretical assumptions, empirical findings, and implications for clinical practice. *Clinical Psychology Review, 33,* 67–81.

Verdecias, R. N., Jean-Louis, G., Zizi, F., Casimir, G. J., & Browne, R. C. (2009). Attachment styles and sleep measures in a community-based sample of older adults. *Sleep Medicine, 10,* 664–667.

Vogel, D. L., & Wei, M. (2005). Adult attachment and help-seeking intent: The mediating roles of psychological distress and perceived social support. *Journal of Counseling Psychology, 52,* 347–357.

Webster, P. S., & Herzog, A. R. (1995). Effects of parental divorce and memories of family problems on relationships between adult children and their parents. *Journals of Gerontology B: Psychological Sciences and Social Sciences, 50,* S24–S94.

Weisner, T. S. (2005). Attachment as a cultural and ecological problem with pluralistic solutions. *Human Development, 48,* 89–94.

Wensauer, M., & Grossmann, K. E. (1995). Quality of attachment representations, social integration, and use of network resources in old age. *Zeitschrift für Gerontologie und Geriatrie, 28,* 444–456.

Whitbeck, L. B., Hoyt, D. R., & Huck, S. M. (1994). Early family relationships, intergenerational solidarity, and support provided to parents by their adult children. *Journals of Gerontology B: Psychological Sciences and Social Sciences, 49,* S85–S94.

Whitbeck, L. B., Hoyt, D. R., & Tyler, K. A. (2001). Family relationship histories, intergenerational relationship quality, and depressive affect among rural elderly people. *Journal of Applied Gerontology, 20,* 214–229.

Wilson, A. E., Shuey, K. M., & Elder, G. H., Jr. (2003). Ambivalence in the relationship of adult children to aging parents and in-laws. *Journal of Marriage and the Family, 65,* 1055–1077.

Winsborough, H. H., Bumpass, L. L., & Aquilino, W. S. (1991). *The death of parents and the transition to old age* (Working Paper No. NSFH-39). Madison: University of Wisconsin, Center for Demography and Ecology.

Wright, M. O., Crawford, E., Castillo, D. D. (2009). Childhood emotional maltreatment and later psychological distress among college students: The mediating role of maladaptive schemas. *Child Abuse and Neglect, 33,* 59–68.

Zhang, F., & Labouvie-Vief, G. (2004). Stability and fluctuation in adult attachment style over a 6-year period. *Attachment and Human Development, 6,* 419–437.

# Chapter 26

# The Adult Attachment Interview
## Protocol, Method of Analysis, and Selected Empirical Studies: 1985–2015

### Erik Hesse

## Beginnings

Thirty years ago, in an article entitled "Security in Infancy, Childhood, and Adulthood: A Move to the Level of Representation," Main, Kaplan, and Cassidy (1985) reported the results of a 6th-year follow-up study of 40 San Francisco Bay Area children who had been seen with each parent in the Ainsworth Strange Situation (Ainsworth, Blehar, Waters, & Wall, 1978) at 12 (or 18) months of age. In this study, special emphasis was given to verbatim transcriptions taken from a structured interview protocol used with the parents—namely, the Adult Attachment Interview (AAI), developed by Main and her students in the early 1980s (George, Kaplan, & Main, 1984, 1985, 1996). This hour-long interview was unusual in that the *coherence* and *clarity* with which the speaker described early relationships and their effects were examined across the conversation with the interviewer and ultimately became the chief focus of analysis (Main & Goldwyn, 1984a; Main, Goldwyn, & Hesse, 2003). This emphasis on conversational properties stood in sharp contrast to interview formats in which the speaker's direct report and evaluation of various family experiences were simply being recorded as stated (e.g., positive vs. negative), and taken as the target of study.

The protocol for the AAI emerged in conjunction with the Berkeley Social Development Project's longitudinal study of families. Two of Main's graduate students, Carol George and Nancy Kaplan, had asked whether something "further" might be added to their (doctoral and master's) theses (see Hesse, 1999). In response, Main had suggested that each parent be interviewed about his or her family background, and an initial set of queries was assembled, with a particularly well-known question being Kaplan's "Could you give me five adjectives to describe your relationship with each parent in childhood—and then tell me why you chose each adjective?" As the Berkeley studies progressed, the initial brief and somewhat casual (originally half-page) series of questions was extended and elaborated into what ultimately became the formal "Adult Attachment Interview" protocol (George et al., 1994, 1995, 1996; see Table 26.1 below). And, from the first, the AAI protocol was transcribed verbatim for both speakers.

A formal scoring and classification system for the AAI was not originally intended or anticipated, but rather was serendipitously initiated when Main became intrigued by a particular interview in which the speaker's responses to the AAI queries appeared to her to be surprisingly reminiscent of the behavior

**TABLE 26.1. Brief Précis of the Adult Attachment Interview (AAI) Protocol Excerpted from George, Kaplan, and Main (1996)**

1. To begin with, could you just help me to get a little bit oriented to your family—for example, who was in your immediate family, and where you lived?

2. Now I'd like you to try to describe your relationship with your parents as a young child, starting as far back as you can remember.

5. To which parent did you feel closer, and why?

7. Could you describe your first separation from your parents?

10. How do you think your overall early experiences have affected your adult personality? Are there any aspects you consider a setback to your development?

11. Why do you think your parents behaved as they did during your childhood?

15. What is your relationship with your parents like for you currently?

*Note.* The AAI cannot be conducted on the basis of this brief, modified précis of the protocol, which omits a number of questions, as well as the critical follow-up probes. The most recent AAI protocol (George, Kaplan, & Main, 1996; 72 manuscript pages) is available from Naomi Gribneau Bahm (*ngbreliability@gmail.com*). Copyright 1996 by the authors. Adapted by permission.

of B4 infants. B4 is a subcategory of infant secure (B) Strange Situation responses to parental leave-taking and return in which—as compared to Ainsworth's prototypical B3 babies—expressions of distress upon separation are somewhat exaggerated, as is proximity seeking and contact maintaining on reunion (Ainsworth et al., 1978).

But how was it that Main was able to "tell" from a speaker's verbatim AAI text that he would have been the parent of a B4 infant? Although the speaker was clearly essentially coherent and collaborative, Main noted that he went to slightly unusual lengths in describing tender, emotionally affecting aspects of his life, lingering in somewhat lengthy descriptions of his loss of a beloved family member. Thus, like a B4 infant, this speaker to a slightly unusual degree seemed to be attempting to draw and maintain the interviewer's attention, and (not untowardly) to evoke a sympathetic response (see Hesse, 1999, p. 400).

As first reported in 1985, it was soon discovered that differences among transcribed verbatim responses regarding relationships with parents, as discussed within the AAI, could be systematically placed into one of three adult attachment categories—secure, dismissing, or preoccupied (Main, 1985, 2001; Main & Goldwyn, 1984a, 1989; Main et al., 1985, 2003). The fourth ("unresolved for loss or abuse experiences") and fifth ("cannot classify") categories were added later (see Hesse, 1996; Hesse & Main, 2000). Remarkably, both of these latter categories were also found to be systematically associated with offspring who had been classified as *disorganized* in the Strange Situation 5 years previously.

In this current contribution to the third edition of the *Handbook of Attachment*, I focus once more on a brief description of the queries used in the AAI, as well as the associated coding scales and classification system. Although the methods of analyzing AAI transcripts have grown increasingly sophisticated over the years (e.g., Main & Goldwyn, 1984a; Main et al., 2003), from the outset, the scoring procedure focused on the overall coherence of the text. Potential indices of insecure states of mind, are observed via any major contradictions and inconsistencies in the narrative, as well as passages that are exceptionally short, long, irrelevant, or difficult to follow. Thus, once systematized, differences in speakers' language use while responding to queries regarding their attachment history and its effects have consistently been the basis of AAI analysis, and the source of its predictive power.

Over time, the AAI has been increasingly applied in conjunction with clinical, developmental and, most recently, psychophysiological, genetic, and neuroscience research. In "The First 10,000 Adult Attachment Interviews: Distributions of Adult Attachment Representations in Clinical and Non-Clinical Groups," Marian Bakermans-Kranenburg and Marinus Van IJzendoorn (2009) reported that at least 200 adult attachment representation studies, comprising more than 10,500 AAI classifications, had been conducted in the preceding 25 years (1984–2009). In that analysis, Bakermans-Kranenburg and Van IJzendoorn had employed the Web of Science and PsycLIT search engines to locate AAI studies utilizing the system of analysis that ultimately emerged as the Main, Goldwyn, and Hesse classification and scoring system (2003; see Main & Goldwyn, [1984a] for the first version of this system).

Critically, in conjunction with their 2009 analysis, Bakermans-Kranenburg and Van IJzendoorn reported that AAI interviews administered to clinical participants, compared to nonclinical participants, were more frequently classified as insecure (dismissing, preoccupied, or unresolved). Disorders with an internalizing dimension (e.g., borderline personality disorders) were found to be associated with more preoccupied and unresolved AAI classifications, whereas disorders with an externalizing dimension (e.g., antisocial personality disorders) were associated with dismissing and preoccupied classifications. Depressive symptomatology was associated with organized insecurity (e.g., dismissing or preoccupied) but not with the category identifying unresolved loss or abuse. In contrast, adults with identifiable abuse experiences or posttraumatic stress disorder (PTSD) were mostly unresolved. Finally, these authors suggested that use of the AAI coding scales, in addition to the categories, might lead to more reliable associations with clinical symptoms and disorders.

For the purposes of this chapter, a comparable report has been compiled by Sarah Foster at Northumbria University, similarly utilizing Web of Science and PsycLIT search engines. Foster's search has revealed that between 2008 and 2015, more than 130 additional adult attachment representation studies were published, comprised of ~7,800 AAIs. This means that, on average, approximately eight attachment representation studies were published each year between 1985 and 2008, while approximately 16 studies each year were published between 2008 and 2015.

Thus, there has been more than a twofold increase in the last 7 years in empirical AAI representation studies. Relatedly, a notable number of case studies, reviews, and theoretical papers have been published as well.

Given the volume of this literature, space limitations necessarily preclude the same type of extensive review of AAI research contained in the 1999 and 2008 editions of this chapter. I therefore mention some studies only by brief references to topic and author. An emerging empirical literature on the AAI as utilized in conjunction with studies in psychophysiology, genetics, and neuroscience is presented in somewhat more detail. This topical area is selected for somewhat greater elaboration because it is largely new and, I believe, will be of special interest to the majority of readers. A paper devoted to a comprehensive review of empirical AAI studies from 1984 to 2016 is being planned

by Robbie Duschinsky, Sarah Foster, Mary Main, and myself.

The remainder of this chapter is organized into four sections, and is followed by Appendix 26.1, which provides a description of, and the means to accessing, training in AAI analysis. The first section, "The AAI Protocol and The Original Three "Organized" AAI Categories" describes the protocol, and then the secure (F), dismissing (Ds) and preoccupied (E) response patterns first identified by Main and Goldwyn (1984). Thereafter, I discuss the ways in which the organized classifications can be understood in terms of both *attentional* and—separately, albeit relatedly—linguistic (*conversational or discourse*) mechanisms. I conclude this first section by presenting some prototypical responses to an AAI query that are common among the three classifications of "organized" speakers. The unresolved (U) and cannot classify (CC) categories are not discussed until the end of the second section because, by nature, they involve speech characteristics and attentional processes not directly comparable to the organized categories.

In the second section, "The AAI Scoring and Classification System," I describe how trained coders systematically approach the analysis of an AAI transcript. I note that beyond placement into the five major classifications there are two additional means of analyzing the AAI (i.e., via scales and 12 subclassifications). These latter two approaches have drawn less attention in the literature, despite the fact that, in some contexts, they may reveal information not captured by examining results for the F, Ds, E, U, and CC categories alone.

In the third section, "Earned or Evolved Security," I provide a historical and theoretical overview of this topic, especially as it relates to central issues involving conceptualizations of AAI coherence.

In the fourth section, "Selected Empirical Studies Involving the AAI," I review a group of studies based on the AAI, beginning with Main's original investigation of a San Francisco Bay Area sample (Main & Goldwyn, 1984b, 1988, 2008). Here I discuss the best-replicated findings regarding the AAI (including investigations of its psychometric properties), as well as a necessarily select group of studies (with apologies to many excellent investigators whose work is not reviewed) in a variety of other salient domains, such as intervention and longitudinal studies. I conclude with a section on studies—almost exclusively conducted since 2008—involving use of the AAI in conjunction with studies in psychophysiology, genetics, and neuroscience.

Before beginning the descriptive portion of this chapter, I underscore that although self-reported measures of romantic attachment produce many exciting and intriguing results (see, in this volume, Crowell , Fraley, & Roisman, Chapter 27, and J. A. Feeney, Chapter 21; Mikulincer & Shaver, 2016), they show little relation to attachment status as assessed in the AAI (e.g., Roisman et al., 2007).

## The AAI Protocol and the Original Three "Organized" AAI Categories

The AAI protocol, devised as noted by Mary Main and her graduate students at Berkeley (George et al., 1984, 1985, 1996) utilizes a prespecified format, with questions asked in a set order, accompanied by specific follow-up probes. The protocol is deliberately arranged to bring forward structural variations in the presentation of a life history, and interviewers must make certain that their own part of the conversation serves only to highlight, not to alter, participants' usual tendencies to respond in particular ways.

The AAI normally takes approximately an hour to administer and currently (George et al., 1996) consists of 20 questions. The entire interview, including all spoken contributions by both the interviewer and the interviewee, is transcribed verbatim, including (timed) pauses, dysfluencies, and restarts. Cues to intonation, prosody, and nonverbal behavior are omitted.

The AAI opens with a call for a general description of relationships with parents during the speaker's childhood, followed by a request for five adjectives that best represent the relationship with each parent. After the adjectives describing each parent are requested (first for the mother), the speaker is probed for specific episodic memories that illustrate why each descriptor was chosen. This process is then repeated for the father and, when applicable, for any other significant attachment figure (e.g., stepfather or nanny). The interviewer asks which parent the speaker felt closer to and why; what the speaker did when emotionally upset, physically hurt, or ill; and how the parents responded at such times. The participant is then asked about salient separations, possible experiences of rejection, and any threats regarding discipline. Next, the speaker is queried regarding the effects of these experiences on his

or her adult personality; whether any of these experiences constituted a setback in development; why parents are believed to have behaved as they did during childhood; and whether there were any persons who did not serve as parenting figures, yet were thought of as parent-like during childhood. The latter might, for example, include a special teacher or uncle.

An especially important feature of the AAI protocol is the section addressing experiences of loss of significant persons through death. Here, significant losses occurring at any point in the speaker's lifetime are addressed. Speakers are asked to describe how the death occurred, their reactions to the loss at the time, any funeral or memorial service attended, changes in feelings over time, effects on adult personality, and (where relevant) effects on their behavior with their own children. In the case of persons with multiple losses, interviewers restrict their queries to those three or four that seem most significant. Descriptions of any abuse experiences (and, indeed, any overwhelmingly frightening experiences throughout a speaker's lifetime) are also sought.

Toward the close of the interview, participants are queried regarding the nature of current relationships with any living parents. In addition, they are questioned as to how they feel about being separated from their child (or imagined child), and if they are ever worried about their child (or think they would worry about an imagined child). Finally, participants are invited to speculate regarding wishes for their real or imagined child in 20 years, as well as to reflect on anything they feel they have learned or gained from their own experiences growing up. Last, participants are asked what they hope their child (or imagined child) will have learned from experiences of being parented by them.

Table 26.1 offers examples of some of the questions taken from the AAI protocol (George et al., 1985, 1986, 1996) but omits their follow-up probes. The current 72-page protocol is available (see Appendix 26.1), and administering the AAI requires practice with feedback from experienced interviewers.

The central task the interview presents to participants is that of (1) producing and reflecting on memories related to attachment, while *simultaneously* (2) maintaining coherent, collaborative discourse with the interviewer (Hesse, 1996). This is not as easy as it might appear, and George et al. (1985, 1986, 1996) have remarked on the potential of the protocol to "surprise the unconscious."

As indicated earlier, the interview requires the speaker to reflect on and answer a multitude of complex questions regarding his or her life history, the great majority of which the speaker will never have been asked before. In contrast to the pace and content of ordinary conversations, in which each speaker has time for planning what to say, the AAI moves at a relatively rapid pace, so that usually all questions and probes have been presented within an hour's time. However, ample opportunities are provided for speakers to contradict themselves, to find themselves unable to answer clearly, and/or to be drawn into excessively lengthy or digressive discussions of particular topics.

To maintain a consistent and collaborative narrative, a speaker must not only address the question at hand but also be able to remember (and potentially reflect on) what he or she has already said, in order to integrate the overall presentation as it unfurls. It is striking that although the interviewee is always informed in some detail regarding the overall topic of the interview prior to its administration, actually engaging in the process often appears to be a far more powerful experience than anticipated. For some speakers, this leads to notable (and often ultimately systematic and repeated) incoherencies in linguistic aspects of the presentation in that at times the interviewee may not be able to maintain his or her usual degree of control over how the spoken story unfolds.

Given these possibilities, one can readily note that the AAI protocol is structured to bring into relief individual differences in what are presumed to be deeply internalized strategies for regulating emotion and attention when speakers are discussing attachment-related experiences. This is achieved despite the fact that although the interview transcripts contain the full verbatim exchange, including silences and dysfluencies, they are devoid of references to body movement, facial expression, or intonation. It is remarkable, then, that on the basis of language use alone, trained AAI coders are able to score and classify AAI texts such that they predict significantly how speakers will behave with others, including offspring, partners, friends, and even those to whom they have been newly introduced.

Finally, I should emphasize that the claim that for most speakers the interview is able to elicit a particular (usually singular; i.e., "classifiable" as opposed to "unclassifiable") state of mind with respect to attachment is based on the assumption that, by adulthood, what were originally independent attachments to mother and to father (e.g.,

in infant Strange Situation behavior; see Main & Weston, 1981) will have coalesced.

An initial exploration of this assumption was undertaken by Furman and Simon (2004), who administered the AAI twice to 56 young adults. One interview focused only on the mother, and the other, only on the father. As would be expected if a single attachment-related state of mind does eventually predominate in most individuals, despite the independence of Strange Situation classifications observed in infancy, Furman and Simon found that state of mind with respect to the father was significantly related to state of mind with respect to the mother.

## Attentional and Linguistic Processes Involved in Distinguishing among the Organized AAI Categories

This section introduces two ways in which some of the underlying mechanisms that may be responsible for the individual differences in discourse forms characteristic of secure, dismissing, and preoccupied speakers as elicited by the AAI protocol have been conceptualized. I begin with Main's (1990) consideration of attentional flexibility versus inflexibility, and then turn to a discussion of Grice's (1975, 1989) maxims for adherence to, versus violations of, the requirements of conversational coherence and collaboration. The dovetailing of Grice's conversational maxims and the state-of-mind scales that Main and Goldwyn had devised—several years prior to Main's first reading of Grice—has been, and remains, striking. Grice's work has been highly useful heuristically, and references to Grice's maxims have appeared in all but the earliest versions of the AAI scoring and classification system.

## The Organized Categories of the AAI Considered in Terms of Attentional Flexibility

The AAI scoring and classification system was initially grounded in the relation between the three central or organized forms of parental responses to the AAI queries (secure-autonomous, dismissing, or preoccupied) and the three central or organized forms of infant response to that same parent in the Strange Situation (respectively, secure, avoidant, ambivalent/resistant), as first uncovered in Main's San Francisco Bay Area study (Main & Goldwyn, 1984b, 1988, 2008; Main et al., 1985). The term *organized* is rooted in Main's (1990) contention that infants in the original three Strange Situation categories differ in flexibility versus inflexibility of attention to (1) the parent and (2) the inanimate environment—differences that are revealed in the Ainsworth separation-and-reunion procedure. Main has ascribed the capacity for attentional flexibility to secure babies because they readily alternate between attachment and exploratory behavior as the Strange Situation procedure unfolds, exploring in their mothers' presence, and exhibiting attachment behavior (e.g., crying, calling) in the mothers' absence and again upon reunion (this time in the form of seeking proximity and contact), most often followed by return to exploration. Correspondingly, differing forms of attentional *inflexibility* have been ascribed to avoidant and resistant/ambivalent infants.

Main later proposed that the organized AAI categories can also be viewed in terms of attentional flexibility (Main, 1993, 2000; Main, Hesse, & Kaplan, 2005). Thus, attentional flexibility is seen in secure-autonomous parents as they fluidly shift between presenting their attachment-related experiences and responding to the request to evaluate the influences of these experiences (Hesse, 1996). In contrast, differing forms of attentional *inflexibility* are observed in dismissing and preoccupied AAI texts.

## The Organized Categories of the AAI Considered in Terms of Grice's Maxims

Before I discuss further the current methods of analyzing AAI transcripts, I provide a brief review of Grice's (1975, 1989) work. My aim in this section is to facilitate an understanding of differing "organized" language usages within the AAI, and to thereby convey what is actually being assessed when coherence versus incoherence of a given text is considered.

Although the AAI interviewer adheres to the interview questions and their probes as faithfully as possible, there are, of course, two speakers involved in the exchange. This means that, at heart, the interview is a conversation, as well as a response to a request for a spoken autobiography, permitting its analysis in terms of the extent to which the participant's responses approach the "Gricean" requirements for an ideally rational, coherent, and cooperative conversation. Grice (1975, 1989) proposed that these requirements are met insofar as speakers adhere to four specific

"maxims" or principles. To the degree that these maxims are "violated," the conversation strays from the cooperative, rational ideal, but, in fact—as Grice stressed in his later work (1989)—complete and continual adherence is not expected. For a text to be classified as *secure-autonomous*, coherent, cooperative discourse must simply be *relatively* well maintained, as compared to that of insecure conversationalists (defined below) observed in this context.[1] The four maxims are as follows:

1. *Quality: "Be truthful, and have evidence for what you say."* This maxim is violated when, for example, a speaker's parent is described in highly favorable, general terms (e.g., highly positive adjectives), but the specific biographical episodes recounted subsequently contradict (or simply fail to support) the interviewee's adjectival choices. An interview of this kind can also be considered internally inconsistent. Internal inconsistency of the kind just described appears most frequently in the texts of individuals classified as *dismissing.*

2. *Quantity: "Be succinct, and yet complete."* This maxim demands conversational turns of reasonable length—neither too short nor too long. By requiring speakers to be sufficiently "complete," Grice was articulating that incomplete, excessively short answers are not acceptable. This occurs when, for example, "I don't remember" becomes the response to several queries in sequence, cutting off further inquiry. Excessively terse responses occur most frequently in the texts of individuals classified as *dismissing.*

In terms of quantity, Grice also requires that so long as they are complete, responses should be reasonably succinct; consequently, the maxim of (appropriate) quantity can also be violated when a speaker takes excessively long conversational turns. Here, the interviewee may hold the floor for several minutes, perhaps providing increasingly unnecessary (and not infrequently pejorative) details. Excessively lengthy responses occur most frequently in the texts of individuals classified as *preoccupied.*

3. *Relation: "Be relevant to the topic as presented."* The maxim of relation or relevance is violated when, for example, queries regarding the childhood relationship with the speaker's mother are irrelevantly addressed with discussions of current interactions with the mother or descriptions of the speaker's relationship with his or her own children. As might be expected, violations of relevance occur most frequently in the texts of individuals classified as *preoccupied.*

4. *Manner:* "*Be clear and orderly.*" This maxim is violated when, for example, speech becomes grammatically entangled, psychological "jargon" is used, vague terms appear repeatedly, or the speaker does not finish sentences that have been fully started. Violations of manner appear most often in *preoccupied* texts.

Having concluded this discussion of Grice's conversational maxims,[2] I present one representative interview query and provide examples of responses that would be typically associated with each of the three organized AAI classifications. Where relevant, I discuss violations of specific maxims.

### Examining Differing Interview Query Responses as They Relate to the Organized AAI Categories

One question that is especially useful for characterizing individual differences in response to AAI queries, and perhaps also the best-known of all the AAI protocol questions, is question 3, in which the participant is addressed as follows:

> "Now what I'd like you to do is to think of five adjectives, words, or phrases that would best describe your relationship with your mother during childhood—say, between the ages of 5 and 12, but even earlier if you can remember. Take a minute to think, and then I'm going to ask you why you chose them."

Notice that this question includes two parts that operate at different "mental levels": a *semantic* level (the descriptors, or adjectives themselves, devoid of space–time particulars) and an *episodic* level (what happened and, if possible, roughly when), which suggests that there will be a rationale for the adjectival choice. By implication, of course, the interviewer is requesting that any particular adjective selected will be accompanied by an illustrative account.

In essence, the adjectival constellation that the speaker is asked to provide for his or her relationship with a given parent during childhood requires the person (whether consciously or unconsciously, accurately or inaccurately) to produce "on the spot" a fairly complex and incisive synopsis of the general nature of the childhood relationship. Once the adjectival constellation has been provided, the speaker has in effect "taken a stance" as to the kind of relationship he or she had with this particular parent. The adjectival constellation can vary from a set of extremely negative to a set of extremely positive descriptors, but, of course, it can include mixed assessments as well. For example, with respect to the mother, if the choice of adjectives include "loving, caring, supportive, trustworthy, and warm," the speaker is obviously attempting to convey that he or she had a highly positive experience with mother during childhood. However, an adjectival constellation such as "caring, interfering, warm, sort of unpredictable, and rule maker" conveys a more mixed impression.

Next, the participant is systematically probed for a specific memory that would illustrate why each particular word or adjective was selected. This is the portion of the "adjectival" question in which the participant is implicitly asked to begin drawing on episodic memory. Note that even if the adjectives provided by two different speakers were identical, the narrative that emerged in the two cases could have entirely different forms.

Let us consider the "loving . . . " constellation noted earlier. The interviewer is now required to probe as follows:

> "OK, the first word you gave to describe your relationship with your mother during childhood was *loving*. Can you think of a memory or incident that would illustrate why you chose that word?"

The range of potential responses to this request is virtually infinite, yet it will yield information that can be approached with a view toward assigning scores and ultimately a state-of-mind classification. Thus, it is likely that the speaker's response bears deeply on the degree of his or her own self-awareness, and in some cases—whether or not the person is conscious of it—on the motivation to convey a particular impression to the interviewer. Consider as an example the following, and not at all uncommon, response to the interviewer's probe for any memories or incidents that could illustrate why the speaker chose *loving*.

INTERVIEWEE: I don't remember . . . (*5-second pause*). Well, because she was caring and supportive.[3] [Notice that here the speaker is simply using similar words to describe the previous words. In essence, the speaker is repeating the word rather than answering the question.]

INTERVIEWER: Well, this can be difficult because a lot of people haven't thought about these things for a long time, but take a minute and see if you can think of an incident or example.

INTERVIEWEE: (*10-second pause*) Well . . . (*5-second pause*), I guess like, well, you know, she drove me to school, and I was always really proud of her, I mean, she was really pretty, and she took a lot of care with her appearance.

Here it is impossible, of course, to know whether the speaker is aware that she has not answered the question. What can be readily inferred, however, is that (a) an attempt is being made to convey a positive impression of her childhood that (b) in fact does not provide believable support for the adjectives chosen. Clearly, something psychologically quite complex is taking place here, despite the brevity of the response. Although convincingly loving interactions may be recounted later in the interview, at this point, we can say that if the speaker continues along these lines—that is, seeming to attempt to create a positive (but unsupported) picture of her childhood experiences with her mother—it is likely that the transcript as a whole will be classified as dismissing.

Thus, dismissing speakers (dismissing would be the best-fitting classification for the previous speaker if only this interview extract was available) violate Grice's quality/truthfulness maxim by failing to provide evidence for what they have claimed. The responses are frequently also excessively succinct, violating of quantity and perhaps involving (whether deliberate or unconscious) restrictions in attention that lead *away from* rather than participating in a discussion of the topic of childhood experiences with the mother.

I now turn to a second speaker who also describes the mother as "loving."

INTERVIEWEE: Loving . . . (*5-second pause*). My mom would stick up for me to the teacher, or to a kid's parents, or . . . anybody, really. I could put it another way, too. I just knew where I stood with her, and that she'd be comforting if I was upset or crying or something.

INTERVIEWER: Thank you (*interrupted*).

INTERVIEWEE: (*interrupting and continuing*) Oh, maybe you wanted a specific example. Um, that time I set fire to the garage, using my brother's chemistry set, I absolutely positively wasn't supposed to use . . . came running when the neighbors phoned the fire department about the smoke. I expected to get the life lectured out of me, but she just ran straight for me and picked me up and hugged me real hard. Guess

she was so scared and so glad to see me, she just forgot the lecture.

If the discussion of childhood parenting continues steadily in this vein, with well-supported (whether positive or negative) statements regarding parenting and clear responses similar to this one,[4] the trained coder will begin to suspect that the transcript is likely to be classified secure-autonomous.[5] In terms of the Gricean maxims, the speaker I presented here had kept to the maxim of *quality* or truthfulness providing evidence for "loving," which Grice at times called the "overriding principle" for cooperative, rational discourse. There are no violations of manner or relevance (the speaker is easy to follow and stays on topic). The passage is too brief to illustrate attentional flexibility, but no inflexibility is evident.

Finally, here is an example of a third participant, who has also chosen "loving" to describe his mother:

INTERVIEWEE: Uh, yeah, sort of very loving at times, like people were in the old days—uh, my youth, lot of changes since then. I remember home, and home was good and that. And uh, loving, my wife is loving with [child]—taking him out to the movies tonight, special thing he's been wanting to see all week, dadadada. Actually, it's more like a month, that turtle movie, don't like it too much myself. Too many turtles—where are they from, outer space? Saw it, though, now, when was it, um, maybe 6 months ago. Yeah, she's very loving with [child].

INTERVIEWER: Mm-hm. OK, well, what things come to mind when you describe your childhood relationship with your mother as "very loving at times"?

INTERVIEWEE: Really great things, felt really special, really grateful to her for that. My childhood, I remember just sitting on the porch, rocking, rocking back and forth, watching my parents, or maybe having some lemonade—or, you know, this, that, and the other. Special sorts of things, just me and her. I wasn't easy, my temperament was hard on her, kind of hard. Me and my cousins from [Town 1] going down soon—really big birthday, she's gonna be 80, gives my age away. (*Continues.*)

Although speech of this kind is not common, it provides a good example of one of the subclassifications of the preoccupied category ("passively preoccupied," subcategory E1). The speaker is unable to stay with the question, which was about his childhood relationship with his mother, and veers to the relationship his wife has with their child. Other than drinking lemonade together, examples of how the mother was loving during childhood are not provided, since, for whatever reason, the speaker moves into topics irrelevant to the request to support "loving" (e.g., his mother's upcoming birthday). In addition, vague and/or incomprehensible speech is inserted into a number of sentences (e.g., dadadada).

Notice, then, that as in the earlier case of the dismissing (first) speaker, the question asked of this preoccupied speaker is not answered. However, this failure to answer appears in a very different form. These are violations of Grice's maxim of relevance (e.g., moving into topics irrelevant to the question, and lack of clarity).

Thus, while the AAI asks the same questions of each participant, as shown here, very different responses appear not only regarding the same questions but also in illustrating the same adjectives. The essence of the AAI scoring and classification system (Main et al., 2003) amounts to a systematization of the different language uses seen in response to the set questions of the protocol. Unfortunately, space limitations preclude reviewing examples involving a negative adjectival descriptor (see Hesse, 2008).

## The AAI Scoring and Classification System

As noted earlier, the AAI scoring and classification system initially focused only on the original three "organized" classifications and their 12 subclassifications, together with an accompanying set of continuous rating scales (Main & Goldwyn, 1984a). The earliest rules for classifying and scoring AAI transcripts were based on interviews with parents (both mothers and fathers) who were visiting Main's Social Development Project laboratory at the University of California at Berkeley, together with their 6-year-old children. Five years earlier, when the children were between 12 and 18 months of age, each had been seen in the Strange Situation conducted separately with each parent. Scores for reunion behavior (e.g., avoidance or resistance), as well as major classifications and their associated subclassifications (Ainsworth et al., 1978), had been assigned at that time.

Out of the available sample of 103 dyads, Main and Goldwyn had selected a development sample of 36[6] for intensive study. Within this initial sample, they searched for differences and commonalities in the ways the parents of infants who had been judged secure, avoidant, or ambivalent/resistant with them in the Strange Situation 5 years earlier conversed about and described their own attachment histories and their effects. (The U and CC categories were developed later.)

The most notable characteristics of each transcript were recorded, including and especially regarding the speaker's probable experiences with each parent during childhood, together with the speaker's state of mind with respect to his or her attachment history. A speaker's "state of mind" was captured by gradually developed continuous rating scales used to assign secure-autonomous, dismissing, or preoccupied classifications. Both coders used their knowledge of attachment to "guess" the status of each transcript, before "de-blinding" themselves to the Strange Situation classification and subclassification of the speaker's infant. The development sample of 36 texts was subsequently discarded, and—with no further feedback from Main—Goldwyn then continued alone through the remaining 67 texts. The results of this study are described later in this chapter (see also Main & Goldwyn, 1988, 2008).

Later, the scoring and classification system came to include a chapter concerning the identification of speech and reasoning irregularities in the parents of infants judged as disorganized (Main, DeMoss, & Hesse, 1989). The 1989 guidelines were used by Ainsworth and Eichberg (1991) and Fonagy, Steele, and Steele (1991) in the initial parent–infant replication studies.

Over the ensuing years, feedback from studies of parent–infant dyads in other samples (including high-risk and clinical samples) has allowed the system to continue to evolve. Consequently (see Main et al., 2003), the system now includes several means of identifying texts that cannot be classified within the original three-part system (leading to U, CC, or both; e.g., when characteristics of both preoccupied and dismissing texts are present and/or speech patterns are anomalous in themselves).

## The Organized Categories of the AAI

The organized categories of the AAI—secure-autonomous, insecure-dismissing, and insecure-preoccupied—are those in which the speaker shows a definitive, essentially singular "strategy" for getting through the interview, whether by "simply answering the questions" (as secure-autonomous speakers have been informally said to do); by untowardly cutting the discourse short (e.g., " I don't remember") whether within or outside of awareness, together with blocking discussion of potentially distressing aspects of experiences (as speakers whose transcripts are assigned to the insecure-dismissing category tend to do); or by manifesting a confused, unrelenting focus on varying incidents, feelings, and relationships aroused by the interview questions (as insecure-preoccupied speakers tend to do). So long as a single one of these strategies seems to be at work throughout the interview, uninterrupted by a collapse of discourse or reasoning during the discussion of potentially frightening experiences, the transcript is considered organized.

As first noted in my discussion of the AAI protocol, each of the organized states of mind with respect to attachment stand—albeit at the discourse level—in parallel to the secure, avoidant, and resistant forms of attachment behavior seen in the Strange Situation conducted with infants (first termed the *organized* infant attachment strategies by Main, 1990).[7] It is intriguing, then, that parents producing inflexible, insecure-dismissing AAI texts, in which queries are often avoided, tend to have infants who avoid them, essentially "dismissing" the fact of their comings and goings during the Strange Situation. Parents who produce insecure-preoccupied AAI texts, remaining on topics to excessive lengths—often particularly in describing failings of the parents—tend to have infants who are seen as ambivalently (angrily or passively) preoccupied with them rather than attending to the available toys or other aspects of the surroundings. Finally, parents who are flexible in their responses to the AAI queries, neither attempting to bypass them or becoming entangled with or by them, produce secure-autonomous AAI transcripts ("valuing of attachment, but seemingly able to objectively evaluate any particular attachment relationship or experience"), tend to have infants whose attention in the Strange Situation is also flexible, alternating between attachment and exploratory behavior as the parents remain within the room (exploration predominates), leave (attachment behavior eventually predominates) and then return to the room (attachment behavior followed by return to exploration).

AAI coders begin their work with the "experience scales" by deriving scores for central aspects of inferred loving versus unloving behavior of each parenting figure during the interviewee's childhood. Next, continuous scores on the scales for "overall state of mind with respect to attach-

ment" are assigned, including the scale eventually recognized to be of primary importance (i.e., the scale for "coherence of transcript"). Finally, using a "feature" analysis, the coder assigns a best-fitting organized classification and associated subclassification, even if later the text will additionally be found to be primarily unresolved or even unclassifiable (in this latter case, two disparate classifications may have been assigned).

### Scales Estimating a Speaker's Probable Experiences with Each Parent during Childhood

A 9-point continuous scale is provided for the coder's estimation of the degree of "loving behavior" exhibited by each parent during childhood, supported by examples and not to be confused with the speaker's love for the parent or unsupported statements that the parent was loving. Evidence of four kinds of unloving behavior is also assessed (rejecting of the child's attachment; role-inverting/heightening of attachment—or, at the high end, demanding of care; neglecting; and pressuring to achieve). Every other point of each scale (i.e., 1, 3, 5, 7, and 9) is well defined, and each scale includes a lengthy introduction explaining what is meant by the construct. Behavioral examples that may be found in the transcript are offered as well. As is evident, the higher the scores for inferred negative experiences, the necessarily lower the score for loving. Finally, it should be noted that the coder selecting the score may assign a score far different from that which the speaker might have assigned— a fact most obvious when the speaker has provided extremely positive adjectives for the relationship with the mother during childhood, but when asked what the speaker did when hurt or upset during childhood has responded, "I hid. Once I had a broken arm that hurt a lot, but I didn't tell my mother; she would have been real angry." The form taken by the five scales resembles that of Ainsworth and colleagues' (1978) four "sensitivity" scales (available on the Everett Waters website at *www.johnbowlby.com*): a long, well-worked-out introduction followed by alternating point definitions that allow for interpolation by the coder.

### Scales Delineating a Speaker's State of Mind with Respect to Attachment

Once a coder has scored the five scales for loving and unloving behavior, he or she moves to scoring the speaker on eight scales describing state of mind with respect to attachment. Correct scores on the state-of-mind scales cannot be assigned without careful prior assignment of scores for experience. For example, the extent to which the childhood relationship with the mother is "idealized" in the speaker's descriptions and evaluations cannot be determined until the coder has decided how "loving" she probably was. Thus, the eventual assignment to an "overall organized state of mind with respect to attachment" usually depends on the speaker's probable experiences with the parents during childhood only to the extent that experiences are needed to determine state of mind score. This should be clear from the fact that speakers with unfavorable childhoods can be readily assigned to the secure-autonomous category, based on the coherence of their text. (Note, however, that some category placements do not require experience scores for derivation).

In summary, the assignment of a speaker to any given organized category depends on scores on the continuous scales identifying states of mind with respect to attachment, and a feature analysis—not described here—that follows upon it, rather than on the scales for inferred childhood experiences of parenting. The general criteria for assignment to the state-of-mind scales are displayed in Table 26.2.

Although I will soon attend to the striking associations between the original state-of-mind scales and Grice's (1975, 1989) maxims, here I briefly take a historical approach and consider our early definitions and findings. As is clear from Table 26.2, the scale most closely identified with adult (and infant) security from our first efforts onward has been the scale for "coherence of transcript." In *Webster's New International Dictionary* (1959, p. 520), the term *coherence* is derived from the Latin, meaning approximately "a sticking together or uniting of parts." Further regarding this definition, Main and Goldwyn (1988, p. 42) noted that *coherence* may be identified as "a connection or congruity arising from some common principle or relationship; consistency; [or] connectedness of thought, such that the parts of the discourse are clearly related, form a logical whole, or are suitable or suited and adapted to context."

From this point of view, coherence involves more than simply internal consistency. In other words, even if an individual speaks in a manner that is plausible and internally consistent, thereby adhering to the first aspect of the criterion, he or she may still discuss a topic at excessive length or make obscure analogies, thus failing to shape speech in a manner suitable to the discourse ex-

change. Thus, conversational cooperation, as well as internal consistency, was an important component in Main and Goldwyn's (1984a, 1984b) original conceptualization of coherence.

## Recognizing Relations between the State-of-Mind Scales and Grice's Maxims

As noted earlier, in general, discourse is judged to be coherent when a speaker appears able to access and evaluate memories while *simultaneously* remaining plausible (consistent or implicitly truthful) and collaborative (Hesse, 1996). When the discussion and evaluation of attachment-related experiences are in fact reasonably consistent, clear, relevant, and succinct, this leads to relatively high AAI coherence scores and placement in the secure-autonomous category. Notably, from the inception of the AAI onward, scores for overall coherence of AAI transcripts have proven vital to analyses of the text and have been associated with infant security of attachment (see the description of the original San Francisco Bay Area study, below).

As shown in Table 26.2, dismissing speakers had already been identified in the early Main and Goldwyn (1984a) scoring system as having high scores on "idealization of the parent(s)," which pointed to a violation of Grice's maxim of quality ("Be truthful, and have evidence for what you say"). Many dismissing speakers had also been described as excessively succinct, violating the quantity maxim by cutting short the conversational exchange with statements such as "I don't remember." These latter speech habits had been quantified as "insistence on lack of memory." Preoccupied speakers had been identified primarily as violating Grice's maxims of relevance, quantity, and manner, which can be termed the *maxims of collaboration*. Violation of each of these maxims is taken into consideration in the scales for "angrily preoccupied discourse," as well as "passive/vague discourse." For example, with respect to relevance, and as seen in these scales, some preoccupied speakers wander from topic to topic or move away from the context of the query (e.g., discussing current relations with parents when asked about childhood experiences), whereas others become embroiled in excessively lengthy descriptions of past or current problems with parents. Still others do both. Violations of manner also typify preoccupied speakers, as seen especially in vague speech ("sort of, sort of . . . and that"), excessive use of psychological jargon ("My mother had a lot of

**TABLE 26.2. "State-of-Mind" Scales Used in the AAI, Related to the Three Major Categories**

Scales associated with the secure-autonomous adult attachment category

*Coherence of transcript.* For the highest rating, the speaker exhibits a "steady and developing flow of ideas regarding attachment." The person may be reflective and slow to speak, with some pauses and hesitations, or speak quickly, with a rapid flow of ideas; overall, however, the speaker seems at ease with the topic, and his or her thinking has a quality of freshness. Although verbatim transcripts never look like written narratives, there are few significant violations of Grice's maxims of quantity, quality, relation, and manner. The reader has the impression that, on the whole, this text provides a "singular" as opposed to a "multiple" model of the speaker's experiences and their effects (see Main, 1991).

*Metacognitive monitoring* (scale presently under development). For the highest rating, evidence of active monitoring of thinking and recall is evident in several places within the interview. Thus, the speaker may comment on logical or factual contradictions in the account of his or her history, possible erroneous biases, and/or the fallibility of personal memory. Underlying metacognitive monitoring (Forguson & Gopnik, 1988) is active recognition of an appearance–reality distinction (the speaker acknowledges that experiences may not have been as they are being presented), representational diversity (e.g., a sibling may not share the same view of the parents), and representational change (e.g., the speaker remarks that what is said today might not have been said yesterday). This scale is included here because it does identify one of the principal aspects of speech found in secure-autonomous speakers; however, the scale needs further work at present, since criteria for high scores are overly stringent, leading to insufficient range.

Scales associated with the dismissing adult attachment category

*Idealization of the speaker's primary attachment figure(s).* This scale assesses the discrepancy between the overall view of the parent taken from the subject's speech at the abstract or semantic level and the reader's inferences regarding the probable behavior of the parent. Since the reader has no knowledge of the speaker's actual history, any discrepancies come from within the transcript itself. For the highest rating, there is an extreme lack of unity between the reader's estimate of the speaker's probable experience with the primary attachment figure(s) and the speaker's positive to highly positive generalized or "semantic" description. Despite inferred experiences of, for example, extreme rejection or even abuse, the portrait of the parent is consistently positive, and gratuitous praise of the parents may be offered (e.g., references to "wonderful" or "excellent" parents).

*Insistence on lack of memory for childhood.* This scale assesses the speaker's insistence upon the inability to recall his or her childhood, especially as this insistence is used to block further queries or discourse. The scale focuses on the subject's direct references to lack of memory ("I don't remember"). High ratings are given to speakers whose first response to numerous interview queries is "I don't remember," especially when this reply is repeated or remains firmly unelaborated. Low scores are assigned when speakers begin a response with a reference to lack of memory, then actively and successfully appear to recapture access to the experience they have been asked to describe.

*Active, derogating dismissal of attachment-related experiences and/or relationships.* This scale deals with the cool, contemptuous dismissal of attachment relationships or experiences and their import, giving the impression that attention to attachment-related experiences (e.g., a friend's loss of a parent) or relationships (those with close family members) is foolish, laughable, or not worth the time. High ratings are assigned when a speaker makes no effort to soften or disguise his or her dislike of the individual or of the topic, so that—in keeping with the apparent intent of casting the individual (or topic) aside ("My mother? A nobody. No relationship. Next question?")—the sentences used are often brief, and the topic is quickly dropped. However, only low scores are given for "gallows" humor: "Oh hell, I didn't mind another separation, I guess that one was #13." (*Note.* Speakers receiving high scores on this scale are assigned to a relatively rare adult attachment subcategory, Ds2, in which attachment figures are derogated rather than idealized.)

Scales associated with the preoccupied adult attachment category

*Involved/involving anger expressed toward the primary attachment figure(s).* Accurate ratings on this scale depend on close attention to the form of the discourse in which anger toward a particular attachment figure is implied or expressed. Direct descriptions of angry episodes involving past behavior ("I got so angry I picked up the soup bowl and threw it at her") or direct descriptions of current feelings of anger ("I'll try to discuss my current relationship with my mother, but I should let you know I'm really angry at her right now") do not receive a rating on the scale. High ratings are assigned to speech that includes, for example, run-on, grammatically entangled sentences describing situations involving the offending parent; subtle efforts to enlist interviewer agreement; unlicensed, extensive discussion of surprisingly small recent parental offenses; extensive use of psychological jargon (e.g., "My mother had a lot of material around that issue"); angrily addressing the parent as though the parent were present; and, in an angry context, slipping into unmarked quotations from the parent.

*Passivity or vagueness in discourse.* High scores are assigned when, throughout the transcript, the speaker seems unable to find words, seize on a meaning, or focus on a topic. The speaker may, for example, repeatedly use vague expressions or even nonsense words; add a vague ending to an already completed sentence ("I sat on his lap, and that"); wander to irrelevant topics; or slip into pronoun confusion between the self and the parent. In addition, as though absorbed into early childhood states or memories, the subject may inadvertently (not through quotation) speak as a very young child ("I runned very fast") or describe experiences as they are described to a young child ("My mother washed my little feet"). Vague discourse should not be confused with restarts, hesitations, or dysfluency.

material around that issue"), and use of nonsense words ("dadadada"). Phenomena conforming to these violations (hence, pointing to the preoccupied classification) have been quantified in continuous scales identifying passivity or vagueness of discourse (manner) and involved/involving anger (relevance, quantity, and manner). (Brief examples of speech typical of secure, dismissing, and preoccupied speakers were provided earlier.)

Table 26.2 provides an overview of the present continuous scoring systems for states of mind (Main & Goldwyn, 1998; Main et al., 2003). I now return, however, to the remaining work of the AAI coder as he or she reviews the text.

As a close look at Table 26.2 indicates, *an AAI coder's first estimate of category placement is based entirely on the configuration of the continuous scores for the state-of-mind scales.* "Expectable configurations" are given in the AAI scoring and classification manual, where, for example (ignoring the still-under-development metacognition scale), high scores on coherence and low scores on idealization, derogation, involved/involving anger, passivity of discourse, and insistence on lack of memory point to a secure–autonomous transcript, whereas low scores on coherence and high scores on (either or both) involved/involving anger or passivity of discourse point to a preoccupied speaker. An acceptable range for the configuration of scores is given for each AAI classification, and coders record their first estimate of classification from these scores. Where scores point to conflicting major classifications, the coder may begin to consider the likelihood that the text is unorganized (unclassifiable). However, importantly, it is only after recording the classification(s) emerging from the configuration of state-of-mind scores (which is termed the "bottom-up" or "score-to-classification" analysis) that the coder will turn to the "top-down" or (classificatory) feature analysis of the text, as delineated below.

### The Application of a Feature Analysis to Classify, and Subclassify a Respondent's State of Mind

First, it should be underscored that the three organized categories of the AAI are ultimately divided into 12 subclassifications. This is in keeping with Ainsworth's division of her three organized infant Strange Situation classifications into eight subclassifications, which she predicted would "in time prove even more useful than classification into the

three major groups themselves" (Ainsworth et al., 1978, p. 251). Parents' AAI subclassifications and their infants' Strange Situation subclassifications have now been found to be significantly related in four different investigations (as noted in and including Behrens, Hesse, & Main, 2007) but nonetheless remain underutilized.

Second, from its inception, the AAI scoring system has included a set of (9-point) continuous rating scales that assess the speaker's current "state of mind with respect to attachment," whether with respect to a given parent (e.g., idealizing the father) or with respect to discourse patterning in general (e.g., overall coherence of transcript, overall passivity). As researchers from several laboratories have correctly emphasized, use of these scales releases the restriction of range imposed by the presentation of findings only in terms of classifications, hence substantially increasing statistical power (Fyffe & Waters, 1997; Roisman, Fraley, & Belsky, 2007). This section brings together all three current methods of AAI text analysis.

In the final step of interview analysis, a coder determines the applicability of all *features* associated with each major classification (and subclassification) to the transcript in hand. Insofar as possible, this step is carried forward independently of the continuous scores assigned to the scales for states of mind. Table 26.3 elaborates (1) scale score configurations; (2) Gricean discourse characteristics; (3) some of the features that point to particular AAI classifications; and (4) the associated infant Strange Situation classifications.

For reasons of space, I do not elaborate on the particular features pointing to each of the three organized classifications here. Instead, examples of these features are placed in Table 26.3.

### The 12 Subclassifications of the AAI Briefly Noted

As the scales and features developed for the analysis of the AAI were being created, Main and Goldwyn (1984b) began to note what at times were striking differences between transcripts that had been placed in a given major classification category. Thus, for example, within the dismissing classification as a whole (which was associated with the infant avoidant classification devised by Ainsworth et al., 1978), there were four distinct subtypes of transcripts. This indicates at once that the AAI system differs from Ainsworth's in important ways because her infant system contained

**TABLE 26.3. Scale Score Configurations, Feature Analyses, and Their Relations to the Organized Categories of Infant Strange Situation Behavior**

Adult states of mind with respect to attachment

Secure-autonomous (F): Predictive of secure (B) Strange Situation behavior

*Scale score configuration.* Moderate to high scores for coherence. Low to low-moderate scores on scales indicative of insecure states of mind.

*Discourse characteristics.* Coherent, collaborative discourse. Descriptions and evaluations of attachment-related experiences and their effects are reasonably consistent, whether the experiences appear to have been favorable or unfavorable. Discourse does not notably violate any of Grice's maxims.

*Features predominating with respect to attitudes toward attachment.* Avows missing, needing, and depending on others. Seems open and "free to explore" interview topic, indicating a ready flexibility of attention. States that attachment-related experiences have affected his or her development and functioning. Seems at ease with imperfections in the self. Explicit or implicit forgiveness of or compassion for parents. Can flexibly change view of person or event, even while interview is in progress, suggesting autonomy and ultimate objectivity. Sense of balance, proportion, or humor. Ruefully cites untoward flawed behavior of self as appearing at times despite conscious intentions or efforts.

Dismissing (Ds): Predictive of avoidant (A) Strange Situation behavior

*Scale score configuration.* Low scores on coherence; high scores on idealization or derogation of one or both parents, often accompanied by high scores on insistence on lack of memory for childhood.

*Discourse characteristics.* Not coherent. Violates the maxim of quality (consistency/truthfulness), in that positive generalized representations of history are unsupported or actively contradicted by episodes recounted. Violates the maxim of quantity—either via repeated insistence on absence of memory; or via brief contemptuous derogation of, or active contemptuous refusal to discuss, a particular event or figure.

*Features predominating with respect to attitudes toward attachment.* Self positively described as being strong, independent, or normal. Little or no articulation of hurt, distress, or feelings of needing or depending on others. Minimizes or downplays descriptions of negative experiences; may interpret such experiences positively, in that they have made the self stronger. May emphasize fun or activities with parents, or presents and other material objects. Attention is inflexibly focused away from discussion of attachment history and/or its implications: Responses are abstract and/or seem remote from present or remembered feelings or memories, and topic of interview seems foreign. May express contempt for other person(s), or, relatedly, for events usually considered sorrowful (e.g., loss or funerals).

Preoccupied (E): Predictive of resistant/ambivalent Strange Situation behavior

*Scale score configuration.* Low scores for coherence; high scores for either passive or angry preoccupation with experiences of being parented (rarely, preoccupied with frightening experiences).

*Discourse characteristics.* Violates manner, quantity, and/or relevance, while quality/truthfulness may not be violated. In regard to quantity, sentences or conversational turns taken are often excessively long. In regard to manner, responses may be grammatically entangled or filled with vague usages ("dadadada," "and that"). In regard to relevance, the present may be brought into responses to queries regarding the past (or vice versa), or persons or events not the objects of inquiry may be brought into the discussion.

*Features predominating with respect to attitudes toward attachment.* Responses to interview are persistently closely and inflexibly tied to experiences with and influences of the parents, even when these are not the objects of inquiry. May attempt to involve the interviewer in agreement regarding parents' faults; may seem to weakly, confusedly praise parents, but with oscillations suggestive of ambivalence; and/or (rare) may relate frightening experiences involving them. Topic of interview is addressed, but seems inflexible and closed so that interview responses may seem memorized or unconsciously guided, as if the attachment-related history is "an old story." Unbalanced, excessive blaming of either parents or self. Indecisive—for example, evaluative oscillations ("Great mother. Well, not really, actually pretty awful. No, I mean actually, really good mother, except when she ..?. "). May be unusually psychologically oriented, offering authoritative "insights" into motives of self or others. The lexicon of "pop" psychology may appear with excessive frequency.

Infant Strange Situation behavior

*(continued)*

## Secure (B)

*Flexibility of attention*: Explores or plays in parent's presence, changes attentional focus to parent on at least one separation, and seeks parent during at least one reunion. In preseparation episodes, explores room and toys with interest, with occasional returns to or checks with parent ("secure-base phenomenon"). Shows signs of missing parent during separation, often crying by the second separation. Greets parent actively, usually initiating physical contact. Usually some contact maintaining by second reunion, but then settles and returns to play.

## Avoidant (A)

*Little flexibility of attention*: Focuses on toys or environment, and away from parent, whether present, departing, or returning. Explores toys, objects, and room throughout the procedure. Fails to cry on separation from parent. Actively avoids and ignores parent on reunion (i.e., by moving away, turning away, or leaning out of arms when picked up). Little or no proximity or contact seeking, distress, or expression of anger. Response to parent appears unemotional. Focuses on toys or environment throughout procedure.

## Resistant or ambivalent (C)

*Little flexibility of attention*: Focuses on parent throughout much or all of procedure; little or no focus on toys or environment. May be wary or distressed even prior to separation. Preoccupied with parent throughout procedure; may seem angry or passive. Fails to settle and take comfort in parent on reunion, and usually continues to focus on parent and cry. Signs of anger toward parent are mixed with efforts to make contact, or are markedly weak. Fails to return to exploration after reunion, as well as during separation, and often preseparation as well (i.e., preoccupied by parent, does not explore).

*Note.* Descriptions of the adult attachment classification system are summarized from Main et al. (1985, 2003). Descriptions of infant A, B, and C categories are summarized from Ainsworth et al. (1978).

only two subclassifications for avoidant infants (A1 and A2).

As an example, two types of transcripts of speakers who were highly dismissing of attachment—and most frequently having highly avoidant babies (A1)—differed sharply in their characteristics. In the first (Ds1), speakers were remarkably *idealizing* of one or both parents, whereas in the second (rare) subtype (Ds2), speakers were contemptuously *derogating* of one or both parents (or of attachment-related experiences; e.g., making fun of displays of grief following a loss). In a prison population, the Ds2 subclassification has been found with unusual frequency among murderers and prisoners who are otherwise violent toward persons (Hobson et al., 2016). Among mothers, it has been found to be associated with frightening behavior toward offspring (Evans, 2008).

Likewise, five subclassifications of the AAI were developed for secure-autonomous parents, of which four corresponded directly to Ainsworth's four secure infant subclassifications. A fifth subclassification was created for parents who seemed somewhat conflicted or resentful and/or mildly angrily preoccupied regarding their parents (F5). These speakers, however, often somewhat humorously indicated acceptance of the anger and involvement, which had characterized their relationship with their parents and, they concluded,

would probably continue to do so. Interestingly, this subclassification of security was inductively found to predict a prototypically secure (B3) Strange Situation response in offspring.

Finally, three AAI subclassifications were found to predict resistant/ambivalent infant Strange Situation behavior, parallel to two of Ainsworth's Strange Situation subclassifications. Thus, angrily and passively preoccupied speakers were found to have angrily and passively ambivalent babies, respectively. In addition, a third subclassification, E3, *fearfully* preoccupied, was developed for AAI texts. Interestingly, it was developed in order to characterize just one of the 103 Bay Area transcripts. However, this subclassification was later found to be predominant in a study of patients with borderline personality disorder (Patrick, Hobson, Castle, Howard, & Maughan, 1994).

For an extensive description of the AAI and Strange Situation subclassifications, which in several studies have shown a significant parent-to-infant match, see Hesse (2008).

## The Unresolved/Disorganized and Cannot Classify Categories: Breakdowns in Discourse Strategy

The unresolved/disorganized (unresolved, U) and cannot classify (,CC) categories (see Table 26.4) were delineated only some years following the inception of the AAI, most likely because their subtlety and complexity could not be recognized until a firm grounding in the three organized categories had been established. Thus it seems likely that, as is generally true with taxonomic endeavors, an awareness of these "exceptions to the rule" was revealed in systematic ways only after much experience with the more basic entity under consideration had been acquired.

### Delineating and Refining the Unresolved Attachment Category

As early as 1984, Main and Goldwyn had informally noted that the parents of unclassifiable infants, many of whom would later become classified as disorganized/disoriented, sometimes spoke in unusual ways about loss experiences. Unresolved or "disordered" mourning had most commonly been understood as falling into two general categories: (1) "chronic mourning," a continuing strong grief reaction that does not abate over an extended period of time (see Fraley & Shaver, Chapter 3, this volume); or (2) "failed mourning," in which expectable grief is substantially minimized or does not occur (see Bowlby, 1980). As the analysis of discussions of loss experiences within the AAI development sample proceeded, however, it became evident that the linguistic indicators of "unresolved" attachment status in adults that predicted disorganized attachment in infants did not appear as explicit manifestations of either chronic or failed mourning.

Over time, it became increasingly clear that what the parents of disorganized infants had in common were various indications of what was ultimately termed "lapses in the monitoring of reasoning or discourse" during discussions of potentially traumatic experiences (Hesse & Main, 1999, 2000). More specifically, the AAI transcripts of these individuals were distinguished by the appearance of (ordinarily) brief slips in the apparent monitoring of reasoning or of the discourse context during the discussion of loss or (discovered later) other potentially traumatic events (see Table 26.4). Such discourse/reasoning lapses were considered to be suggestive of temporary alterations in consciousness or working memory and are believed to represent either interference from normally dissociated memory or belief systems or unusual absorptions involving memories triggered by the discussion of traumatic events (Hesse & Main, 1999, 2006; Hesse & Van IJzendoorn, 1998, 1999).

Lapses in the monitoring of *reasoning* are manifested in statements that suggest the speaker is temporarily expressing ideas that violate our usual understanding of physical causality or time–space relations. Marked examples of reasoning lapses are seen when speakers make statements indicating that a deceased person is believed simultaneously dead and not dead in the physical sense—for example, "It was almost better when she died because then *she could get on with being dead* and I could get on with raising my family" (Main & Goldwyn, 1998, p. 118, emphasis added). This statement implies a belief, operative at least in that moment, that the deceased remains alive in the physical sense. Statements of this kind may indicate the existence of incompatible belief and memory systems, which, normally dissociated, have intruded into consciousness simultaneously as a result of queries regarding the nature of the loss experience and its effects. Lapses in the monitoring of *discourse* would seem to suggest that the topic has triggered a "state shift" indicative of considerable absorption, appearing to involve entrance into peculiar, compartmentalized, states of mind in which discourse is not appropriately regulated (Hesse, 1996; Hesse & Main, 2006; Hesse & Van IJzendoorn, 1999). Thus, for example, an abrupt alteration or shift in speech register inappropriate to the discourse context occurs when a subject moves from his or her ordinary conversational style into a eulogistic or funereal manner of speaking, or provides excessive detail. (In addition, albeit rarely, individuals experiencing major trauma can also be assigned to the unresolved category on the basis of reports of extreme responses to traumatic events, such as suicide attempts.)

Both sudden state shifts and the abrupt appearance of incompatible ideas suggest momentary but qualitative changes in consciousness. Thus, they appear to represent temporary/local as opposed to global breakdowns in the speaker's discourse strategy. Discourse/reasoning lapses of the kinds just described often occur in high-functioning individuals and are normally not representative of such a speaker's overall conversational style. For this reason, among others, transcripts assigned to the unresolved category are given a best-fitting alternate classification (e.g., unresolved/dismissing [U/Ds]).

Early discoveries regarding the relation between secure, dismissing, and preoccupied parental AAI status and secure, avoidant, and resistant/ambivalent attachment status have already been

**TABLE 26.4. Scale Scores, Discourse Characteristics, and Features Associated with the Disorganized and Unorganized/"Cannot Classify" Categories of the AAI, and Corresponding Infant Strange Situation Categories**

Adult states of mind with respect to attachment

Unresolved/disorganized (U)

*Scale scores.* Scores above 5 on either unresolved loss or unresolved abuse (the distinctions between these are retained) lead to category placement. At scale point 5, the coder must decide whether the transcript fits the unresolved/disorganized classification.

*Discourse characteristics.* During discussions of loss or abuse, individual shows striking lapse in the monitoring of reasoning or discourse. For example, individual may briefly indicate a belief that a dead person is still alive in the physical sense, or that this person was killed by a childhood thought. Individual may lapse into prolonged silence or eulogistic speech. The speaker will ordinarily otherwise fit Ds, E, or F categories.

*Features predominating with respect to attitudes toward attachment.* No particular features beyond lapse. May fit the descriptors for Ds, E, or F.

Unorganized/"cannot classify" (CC)

*Scale score configuration.* Scale scores may point to contradictory insecure classifications (e.g., strong idealizing and strong involved/involving anger are seen within the same transcript) as in the "original" form of CC. Alternatively, all state-of-mind scores are low, none moving fully to midlevel (e.g., below midpoint for all scores indicative of insecure states of mind, as well as for coherence; see Hesse, 1996). Finally, some CC texts cannot be determined by scale scores and rely on the use of feature analysis (Main et al., 2003).

*Discourse characteristics.* The early "contradictory strategies" discourse forms seen in CC texts are described below. In newer forms of CC, violations of Grice's maxims do not necessarily take the forms ordinarily seen in insecure speakers. Coherence violations are not necessarily limited to particular locations in the text, or particular persons or events. In rare and extreme cases, the transcript as a whole may be so incoherent as to be difficult to follow.

*Features.* In the "original" form of CC, features sufficient to fit the text to two directly contrasting classifications (e.g., dismissing and preoccupied) are observable. In one newer form of CC (Main et al., 2003), the transcript is incoherent without elevated scores for insecure states of mind. Transcripts may also now be considered unclassifiable if (1) the speaker seems to attempt to frighten the listener (e.g., with the sudden, unintroduced, detailed discussion of a murder) or (2) refuses to speak during the interview, without responding that memories are unavailable or are too painful to discuss. Finally, transcripts are considered unclassifiable if they seem to fit equally well to both a secure and insecure classification (e.g., CC/Ds/F or CC/F/E).

Infant Strange Situation behaviors

Disorganized/disoriented (D)

The infant displays disorganized and/or disoriented behaviors in the parent's presence, suggesting a temporary collapse of behavioral strategy. For example, the infant may freeze with a trance-like expression, hands in air; may rise at parent's entrance, then fall prone and huddled on the floor; or may cling while crying hard and leaning away with gaze averted. Infant will ordinarily otherwise fit A, B, or C categories. At 6 years of age, previously disorganized infants in several samples have been found to be role-inverting or "disorganized/controlling" with the parent, being either punitive or caregiving/solicitous.

Cannot classify (CC)

The infant displays aspects of more than one classification, without necessarily being primarily or even notably otherwise disorganized/disoriented. For example, the infant may fit well to the avoidant category on the first reunion, and to the resistant category on the second. Alternatively, the infant's Strange Situation behavior may be so diffuse throughout the procedure that it cannot via any single reunion or separation response be found to fit to any single category.

*Note.* Descriptions of the U and CC categories of the adult attachment classification system are summarized from Hesse and Main (2000) and from Main et al. (2003). The description of the infant D category is summarized from Main and Solomon (1990); the description of the child D category is based on Main and Cassidy (1988); and the still new infant/child CC category has been utilized in publications by Abrams et al. (2006) and Behrens et al. (2007).

described. The next discovery regarding the AAI (Main & Hesse, 1990) was based on the identification of a fourth infant Strange Situation classification: disorganized/disoriented (hereafter, disorganized or D; Main & Solomon, 1990). Infants were placed in this fourth category when they failed to maintain the behavioral organization characteristic of those classified as secure, avoidant, or ambivalent-resistant. Although this failure to maintain organization had previously been described as "unclassifiable" Strange Situation behavior by Main and Weston (1981), a review of unclassifiable babies in the large Bay Area sample had indicated that most displayed disorganized and/or disoriented behaviors in the Strange Situation (Main & Solomon, 1986, 1990). Thus, the "unclassifiable" babies were observed engaging in unusual displays such as approaching the parent with head averted, putting hand to mouth in a gesture indicative of apprehension immediately upon reunion with the parent, or rising to approach the parent and then falling prone to the floor. Infants were also labeled disorganized if they froze all movement with arms elevated, or if they held still for many seconds with a trance-like expression.

A follow-up review of Strange Situation videotapes taken from several samples of somewhat to markedly troubled parent–infant dyads led to expansion of this infant system, which was finalized (above) in 1990. Disorganized attachment has now been observed in the majority of infants in maltreatment samples (e.g., Carlson, Cicchetti, Barnett, & Braunwald, 1989; Lyons-Ruth, Connell, Zoll, & Stahl, 1987), whereas in low-risk samples, it has been found associated with both externalizing and internalizing disorders (Fearon, Bakermans-Kranenburg, Van IJzendoorn, Lapsley, & Roisman, 2010; Groh et al., 2012; Van IJzendoorn, Schuengel, & Bakermans-Kranenburg, 1999; see Solomon, George, & De Jong, 1995, for initial findings).

By 1990, it had been shown that unresolved AAI status in a parent predicted disorganized attachment in the infant (Main & Hesse, 1990; see Table 26.4). Specifically, in conjunction with a 6th-year follow-up study, Mary Main and I found that 5 years earlier, 91% (11 of 12) of mothers with unresolved loss or trauma, as identified in the AAI, had had babies who were disorganized with them in the Strange Situation, while only 16% of mothers who were not considered unresolved had had disorganized infants 5 years earlier. Thus, there was now an AAI category corresponding to and predictive of

each of the four Strange Situation categories in use at the time. Since this original study, 9-point scales for both indices of unresolved loss and abuse (e.g., Main et al., 2003) were developed, while as noted similar 9-point scales for scoring infant disorganized behavior had already been developed (Main & Solomon, 1990). Finally, by 2006 an analysis of a subset ($n = 36$) of parents and infants drawn from the Bay Area sample had confirmed a significant correlation between parental lapses of monitoring in the AAI surrounding loss or other trauma and infant disorganized/disoriented behavior in Strange Situations conducted with the parent (phi = .56, $p < .001$; Abrams, Rifkin, & Hesse, 2006).

### Emergence of the Cannot Classify Adult Attachment Category

A fifth interview category, "cannot classify" (CC), emerged in the early 1990s as Mary Main and I began noticing a small percentage of transcripts that failed to meet criteria for placement in any of the three central or organized attachment categories, and additionally did not fit to placement as Unresolved. This was first observed in transcripts in which, for example, an unsupported positive description of one or both of the parents led to a relatively high idealization score, whereas, in direct contradiction to the expected global patterning for dismissing speakers, highly angrily preoccupied speech was also found. Thus, the high idealization score called for placement in the dismissing category, whereas other portions of the transcript called for preoccupied category placement. Main and I (see Hesse, 1996) therefore concluded that these transcripts were unclassifiable and should be placed in a separate group. Because both this "contradictory strategies CC" and other CC subtypes involve low coherence, they are necessarily defined as insecure.

## Earned or Evolved Security

In 1989, "earned" security was suggested as a new (sub)classification of security within the AAI manual, including instructions to coders that this taxonomic placement should be applied to transcripts in which the participant, *although speaking coherently and collaboratively*, either "(a) appeared to have had difficult childhood relationships with parents, and/or (b) another untoward experience such as loss or separation" (Main & Goldwyn,

1989, p. 119). This additional subcategory of security placed greater emphasis on the overriding import of coherence than had appeared in previous coding manuals. Thus, it was now formally proposed that (1) coders should stipulate when a transcript indicated that an individual's experiences had been notably unfavorable, while (2) the individual simultaneously maintained his or her "secure" status via the coherence of his or her narrative. Emphasizing the similarity between "earned" and what was to be called "continuous" security, "earned-secure" speakers have recently been found as likely to have secure infants as those secure speakers who described favorable early experiences (Saunders, Jacobvitz, Zaccagnino, Beverung, & Hazen, 2011).

For clinicians, the concept of "earned" security has had special relevance because it clearly bears directly on the nature of their work. The fact that AAI texts could be found coherent and collaborative even when the speaker's childhood experiences appeared to have been highly unfavorable underscored long-held views that a secure state of mind can be achieved despite early adversity. It was reasoned, then, that so long as clients could be successfully assisted in becoming coherent regarding their experiences via favorable new relationships with a therapist, they might expectably be enabled to attain a secure state of mind. This had already been, of course, the position taken by Bowlby (1988) and many others working in the field of mental health.

Early on, then, Bowlby had suggested that "working models" of the self, relationships, and the self within relationships formed in early childhood—although resistant to change—nonetheless most likely retain the potential for change within the context of new experiences with other persons (see, e.g., Bowlby, 1988). Of course, these changes could be for better or worse, but as a therapist Bowlby's emphasis was on the enduring possibility of positive reorganization within an individual's working models of the self and interpersonal relationships. And, in the same year, Egeland, Jacobvitz, and Sroufe (1988) had reported that within a sample of mothers who had experienced abuse in childhood, those who had received emotional support from a nonabusive adult, participated in therapy, or had an emotionally satisfying supportive partner were markedly less likely to become abusive than those abused mothers who had not had the advantage of such experiences. Other evidence for the possibility of such change was provided shortly thereafter by Rutter, Quinton, and Hill (1990), who, in their longitudinal study of institutionally reared children, found that many became competent parents following warm and confiding marital experiences. Finally, the success of therapists in assisting clients classified insecure on the AAI to attain a secure state of mind with respect to attachment has been empirically documented in two longitudinal studies, as I note below (Buchheim et al., 2016; Levy et al., 2006).

Before going further, I should note that despite my own interest and that of others in retrospectively identified "earned security" I had stated earlier that

> we must leave open the possibility that because the AAI does not necessarily provide valid information about an individual's actual experiences, we do not know whether those who appear to be "earned-secure" have in fact—and, of course, in contradiction to what they "remember" during the AAI—had substantially positive early experiences that are now, ironically, coherently misrepresented. (Hesse, 1999, p. 426)

Thus, it seemed conceivable that *some* individuals considered earned-secure on the basis of their coherent recounting of a harsh childhood may have been secure with at least one parent specifically during the early years of life—a fact that, depending on child age, might well not be readily consciously accessible (Hesse, 1999, p. 426; Hesse, 2008, p. 588). Indeed, early loving experiences with at least one parent could somehow be aiding the speaker in a coherent reconstruction of experiences, despite the fact that later experiences had in fact been unfavorable. These and other important questions regarding the role of early experiences can be addressed only via longitudinal studies (Hesse, 1999). Fortunately, two such studies have been undertaken by Glen Roisman and his colleagues, both in Minnesota: one by Roisman, Padron, Sroufe, and Egeland (2002), and (more recently) the other in conjunction with the National Institute of Child Health and Human Development (NICHD) study of families and children (Roisman, Haltigan, Haydon, & Booth-LaForce, 2014), as discussed below.

I should note here that with increasing time, it has become clear that the term *earned-secure* is not an ideal taxonomic label for this fairly unusual form of AAI security. First, the term implies that the coherence and collaboration of such texts should be seen as a product of a (conscious or unconscious) *effort* to reorganize attachment-related representational states constructively. Of course, some individuals could have reorganized their state of mind *sans* any conscious personal effort; hence, the term *discontinuous secure* might initially seem preferable. Unfortunately, the term *discontinuous secure* still leaves a problem, since it might reference either lost or gained security.

Consequently, given the aforementioned difficulties, I now suggest that both the terms *discontinuous secure* and *earned secure* be replaced with the term *evolved secure*, which implies a forward and positive directional shift, without implying a necessarily conscious and/or active process. And fortuitously, the frequently used initials, ES, can be retained.

I now discuss the unfortunate complications that initially arose because no precise cutoff criteria for scoring earned security were provided before 1998, when Main and Goldwyn set earned-secure criteria: The text must include loving scores of 2.5 or below on the 9-point scale for *both* parents (Main & Goldwyn, 1998). Note that given this restricted guideline, the coder may still have judged the parents to have provided some attention and instrumental assistance during childhood. But, even so, parenting would still have been absent indices of actively loving behavior (e.g., reliable physical affection, the forgiving of the child's misbehavior, or [when appropriate] defending the child to others, such as teachers or overly strict relatives).

Prior to 1998, however, many researchers had of course been eager to explore the topic of earned security and in doing so created early criteria that were markedly less stringent (i.e., earned security was identified in texts in which at least *one* parent scored less than 5 on the 9-point Loving scale, and *either* of the parents also scored 5 or higher on rejecting, neglecting, pressure to achieve and/or role reversal [commonly referred to as the Pearson criteria; see Pearson, Cohn, Cowan, & Cowan, 1994]).

Recently, Roisman and colleagues (2014) attempted to address this issue by examining data using both the less stringent pre-1998 Pearson criteria informally employed by most researchers at that time, as well as the more stringent 1998 Main and Goldwyn criteria for earned secure. Additionally, where comparisons to continuous secure were to be made, Roisman and colleagues have offered analyses additional to the Pearson criteria (i.e.,

analyses that follow Main and Goldwyn's stipulation that only those texts where the average parental Loving scale score was 6.5 or above should be utilized for the "continuous secure" assignment, and each parent scoring 2.5 or below on the Loving scale for "earned secure").

Although these criteria are likely to be met by some individuals interviewed in adulthood, the current criteria for earned-secure AAI status (again, a coherent transcript, despite both parents scoring at 2.5 or below for loving) was not met by any of the 19-year-old participants in the Bay Area follow-up study (Main, Hesse, & Kaplan, 2005), and it was met only infrequently in two other studies of participants averaging 19 years of age (Roisman, Fortuna, & Holland, 2006; Roisman et al., 2002). The fact that so few adolescents are judged to be earned secure is probably not surprising, given that increased potential for introspection normally develops in adulthood. Furthermore, this suggests that future studies of retrospectively identified "earned security" (i.e., identified via apparent remembrances of AAI participants) will be most productive if undertaken within samples of postcollege-age adults.

A number of investigations of earned security within postadolescent samples have now been completed, each utilizing a cross-sectional design. For example, Caspers, Yucuis, Troutman, and Spinks (2006) have reported that continuous secure adults (identified through Loving scores of 5 or above for both parents) were less likely than *both* insecure and earned-secure adults to abuse alcohol or other substances. However, earned-secure adults ($N = 25$, identified as both parents scoring at 2.5 or below on loving) were more likely to have entered psychotherapy than either dismissing or continuous secure participants. Strikingly, like Caspers and her colleagues, Jacobvitz (2008; Jacobvitz, Booher, & Hazen, 2001; see also Saunders et al., 2011) also found that earned-secure adults (both parents scoring at 3 or below on loving) had spent more time in therapy than either continuous secure or insecure participants.

As discussed earlier, before the implementation of the Main and Goldwyn guidelines, most investigators studying earned security had essentially divided their secure participants into two groups: those inferred to have had "more" versus "less" loving parents, with the latter usually being identified by one of the parents having received a loving score either below the sample median or below a score of 5 on the 9-point scale.

In the majority of these studies, mean scores for the mothers' loving behavior during childhood for participants termed *earned secure* have been above 5, with many scores falling well above 5. Although, ideally, these might therefore best have been termed studies of participants with parents inferred to have been "more" versus "less" loving, rather than studies examining continuous secure versus earned-secure participants, they have yielded interesting results.

For example, in a pioneering study in 1994, Pearson and colleagues found that although earned-secure participants scored higher on a depression inventory than did their continuous-secure counterparts, they were equally warm toward their 42-month-old offspring and equally providing of structure. A few years later, Phelps, Belsky, and Crnic (1998) found that self-reported "daily hassles" were not higher for earned-secure than for other mothers, helping to rule out a possible "depressogenic" hypothesis that earned-secure mothers tended simply to report their experiences as being worse than did others. In addition, they found that earned-secure mothers' sensitivity to offspring held up even under high-stress conditions. And perhaps surprisingly, Paley, Cox, Burchinal, and Payne (1999) found that earned-secure wives were no less positive and no more negative than continuous-secure wives during marital interactions.

Beginning on a series investigating the "earned-secure" subclassification, Roisman and colleagues (2002) inspected longitudinal data from 19-year-olds in a Minnesota high-risk sample ($N$ = 170). In this study utilizing the pre-1998 criteria, transcripts in which either parent (usually the father) fell below 5 on the 9-point loving scale were defined as earned-secure. The mean loving scores for mothers of participants identified as earned-secure was 5.46, whereas for continuous-secure participants the mean loving score for mothers was one point higher, 6.50. In sharp contrast, mean *fathers'* loving scores for the two groups differed substantially, being 2.56 for earned-secure and 5.73 for continuous-secure participants. Thus identified (i.e., given the obviously average loving scores of "earned-secure" participants' mothers) it does not seem surprising that earned-secure status in this study was not significantly associated with either (1) having been insecure with mother in the Strange Situation at either 12 or 18 months or (2) significantly less positive observed interactions with mother at 24 months, 42 months, or 13

years of age. Since earned-secure mothers' loving scores *averaged* 5.46 in this study, neither significantly less positive nor significantly less negative outcomes should have been expected.

It would, then, clearly be premature to conclude from this study that AAI scores for parental loving are unrelated to childhood experiences, thereby making retrospective earned/evolved-secure assignments invalid. This is because (1) security or insecurity in infancy was identified on the basis of Strange Situation classification with *mother*, yet (2) retrospective insecurity appears to have been determined mainly on the basis of inferred early insecurity with *father*. For the same reason, observations of father–child interactions would have been necessary to decide whether earned-secure status did or did not correspond significantly with observed early experience.

In a further study aimed at untangling the "meaning" (and reality basis of) the earned-secure classification, Roisman and colleagues (2006) attempted to induce sad or happy moods just before administering the AAI, with a view toward ascertaining whether context could alter reports regarding experience with the parents. In this study, participants were asked to focus for 10 minutes on an autobiographical memory relevant to achieving a sad (or happy) state, although whether the memory needed to relate to interpersonal relationships was not specified. Sad (or happy) music was played during this period, and participants were urged to achieve a mood state as intense and as real as possible. The participants were identified as earned-secure in keeping with the "early" and less stringent earned-secure criteria described above (i.e., if they were coherent during the AAI, and if one of the two parents had received a loving score below 5, as well as a score above 5 for rejecting or neglecting behavior). The remaining coherent participants were regarded as continuous-secure.

With the earned- versus continuous-secure categories defined via the less strict criteria, placement in the earned- versus continuous-secure categories was impressively related to induced mood. Thus, a cross-tabulation of experimental condition among secure participants revealed that participants were overrepresented as earned-secures in the sad condition, and as continuous-secures in the happy condition. The mood induction procedures did not, however, affect insecure speakers, and in interpreting this finding, Roisman and colleagues (2006, p. 61; see also Sroufe & Waters, 1977) suggested that perhaps only secure speakers have the ability to "tune behavior and emotion properly to contextual demands." Importantly, however, and as the investigators emphasize, coherence scores—the heart of the AAI scoring procedure—were *not* affected by induced mood.

It is crucial to note, however, that induced sad moods in this study did not in fact lead to placement in the earned-secure group using Main and Goldwyn's (1988) criteria (i.e., Loving scale scores of 2.5 or below for *both* parents). In the sad condition, fathers' mean loving scores for secure participants were at 4.45 (*SD* = 1.74) and mothers' mean loving scores were 5.52 (which is, again, considered adequate parenting [see Main et al., 2003], and ranged to above 7 (*SD* = 1.66). Thus, even in the sad condition, mothers' loving scores for secure participants remained at the average for most samples, with many secure participants' mothers scoring well above average. As such, the findings of this study cannot be taken to indicate that concurrent sad mood can lead to placement in the earned-secure group.

Roisman and colleagues' (2014) more recent efforts to address the topic of earned security were via longitudinal observations of adolescents participating in the Study of Early Child Care and Youth Development (SECCYD). Contrary to my expectations, even using the strict Main and colleagues (2003) criteria, earned/evolved secure individuals did not appear to have suffered the degree of adversity in parenting relationships throughout as much of their youth as I would have anticipated. Roisman and colleagues found that overall, "earned secures" in the NICHD sample appeared to have had better experiences of parenting during childhood and adolescence than those classified as insecure.

There is a notable exception, however: Using the Main and Goldwyn definition, "earned secures" were observed to have had *below*-average sensitivity from the mother between the early period of 5–64 months (Roisman et al., 2014, p.105), indeed, insensitivity comparable to insecures (earned-secure = –.16, insecure = –.29) existed during this period. In striking contrast, maternal sensitivity scores for continuous-secures during the same period was .56. Thus, impressive differences were observed between 6 months and 5.3 years. This is an intriguing finding, and it warrants further investigation. It is not unreasonable to speculate, as I had in 1999 and 2008, that early insensitivity may be especially influential.

In addition to reduced early maternal sensi-

tivity, using either the earlier or the more stringent criteria, "earned secures" were found to have lower family income relative to needs than "continuous secures," as well as parents who had more depressive symptoms. Finally, in keeping with speculations that earned security could be associated with parental loss or abandonment, and in striking contrast to 5% father absence for continuous secures, father absence was recorded for 28% of earned-secures (31% for those judged insecure). While untoward parental absence is, of course, a potential stressor in its own right, it was specifically noted by Main and Goldwyn (1989, p.119) as one of the experiential factors stipulated as a difficulty which, noted in a coherent transcript, could lead to the assignment of earned-secure. Later versions of the AAI scoring and classification system rely on scores and features devoid of emphasis on specific unfavorable experiences (see Main et al., 2003). Although the other stressors identified among earned-secures in this 2014 study—greater financial difficulties, higher parental depressive symptoms—are not directly related to parental insensitivity (and are also not quantifiable on the existing AAI scales), it is indeed possible that these stressors did in fact lead some "earned-secure" speakers to experience important aspects of parenting as adverse. Put another way, these particular kinds of negative experience may not have been expressed overtly but rather "showed up" in ways that were somehow quantifiable on the existing AAI inferred experience scales. This would, of course, lead to a mismatch between these scales and the negative variables that Roisman and colleagues (2014) were investigating. Thus, some "earned secures" could have had difficult childhoods involving depression or parental absence that are not incisively quantified within the current AAI system. In addition, as in the case of the stability analysis of this sample (Groh et al., 2014), it would be premature to make generalizations regarding evolved security from this study alone.

Thus, whereas in 2008 the degree to which earned-secure status reflected actual (observable) adverse experiences in childhood remained, as previously (Hesse, 1999), an open question, more recent studies have nonetheless failed to provide conclusive evidence to counter the proposition that, strictly defined, earned/evolved-secure status will be found to represent a coherent AAI description of what may ultimately be confirmed as an insecure childhood. Another currently unanswered question is whether the induction of sad moods in persons with secure-autonomous status can reduce parental loving scores sufficiently to ensure that loving behavior on the part of both of the participant's parents would appear inadequate.

The first of these issues will ultimately be resolved by prospective or longitudinal studies of normative samples (including assessments of security with each parent at multiple time points) that follow participants *beyond late adolescence*, so that individuals who are insecure in adolescence will have had the opportunity to form a coherent representation of their lives despite early adverse experiences with parents. The second might be addressed by new mood induction studies, perhaps optimally by asking adult participants to focus on sad versus happy (nonautobiographical) prospective events rather than elements from their autobiographies. However, many other approaches to the investigation of earned security (using the Main and Goldwyn guidelines) should be undertaken as well, and will likely continue to provide interesting outcomes, as demonstrated in several recent cross-sectional studies of adult populations described earlier (e.g., Caspers et al., 2006: Jacobvitz, 2008).

It should also be noted that pre- to posttherapy studies that show moves from insecure to secure-autonomous attachment status (see Levy et al., 2006; see also Buchheim et al., 2016)—both utilizing Kernberg's transference-based therapy (e.g., Yeomans, Clarkin, & Kernberg, 2015)—may eventually allow us to trace one developmental pathway to earned security within adulthood, and therefore may also make an important contribution to our understanding of this intriguing topic. Case studies carefully documenting representational change in states of mind with respect to attachment across the course of therapy may also be useful, and some especially well-described studies are available (see Ammaniti, Dazzi, & Muscetta, 2008; see also Muscetta, Dazzi, DeCoro, Ortu, & Speranza, 1999).

In closing, although Roisman and colleagues' (2014) important study raises critical questions about retrospective accounts of earned security, it nonetheless leaves a significant need for further investigation. Because the 2014 NICHD study utilizes an adolescent sample with an overrepresentation of white and higher-educated families, the distribution is skewed toward security (59%) and, relatedly, both the preoccupied (3%) and unresolved (3%) classifications are significantly underrepresented with respect to global norms (Van IJzendoorn & Bakermans-Kranenberg, 2014). First, more studies utilizing more extensive and carefully implemented measures of parental sensi-

tivity are urgently needed. In addition, the Saunders and colleagues (2011) study suggests that by following Bowlby (1988) theoretically and Rutter and colleagues (1990) empirically, tapping into real experiences may in some cases have indeed led to actual change in the reorganization and coherence of representational processes, which in turn would increase the likelihood of internal consistency in an AAI narrative. Roisman and colleagues' ambitious and admirable report leads me to conclude that until further studies are conducted, utilizing samples with more *normative distributions, and at later ages,* caution is warranted in the interpretation of retrospective accounts of earned or evolved security.

## Selected Empirical Studies Involving the AAI

This section opens with a discussion of Main and Goldwyn's original parent–infant study,[9] which differed from most succeeding studies (except Fonagy et al., 1991) in its emphasis on AAI state-of-mind scale scores, as well as its report of a significant AAI to Strange Situation match in subclassifications (replicated by Behrens et al., 2007). The just-mentioned emphasis on subclassification can be seen as comparable to the emphasis on scales or "dimensions" emphasized elsewhere (e.g., Groh et al., 2014; Roisman et al., 2007) in that it tests the ability of the instrument at fine-grained levels. Additional reviewed AAI studies include topics such as psychometric properties, parent-to-offspring matches, clinical populations, and, as noted earlier, psychophysiology, genetics, and neuroscience.

### *The Bay Area Study: Linking Parental AAI Responses to Infant Attachment Status*

The initial Bay Area study establishing relations between parental AAIs and infant Strange Situation responses to the speaker 5 years earlier involved 32 mothers and 35 fathers, and was conducted by Main and Goldwyn (1988, 2008 [see Note 9]; see also Main et al., 1985; Main & Goldwyn, 1984b; Main et al., 2005). In this randomly selected sample of 67 dyads (sample sizes varied slightly across analyses), 48% of parents were classified as secure, 39% as dismissing, and 13% as preoccupied. The central findings were not only the remarkable correspondence between the three then-existing organized states of mind with respect to attachment based on a parent's AAI and the infant's response to that parent in the Strange Situation, but also the significant match between adult and infant *subclassifications* (briefly mentioned earlier), and finally, significant matches between parental state-of-mind scores and continuous dimensions of the infant's Strange Situation behaviors. As mentioned earlier, at the time the AAI texts were analyzed (Main & Goldwyn, 1982), the infant disorganized attachment category (Main & Solomon, 1986, 1990) had yet to be developed, and anomalous Strange Situation behavior was simply termed "unclassifiable" (Main & Weston, 1981). All unclassifiable infants were moved to their best-fitting organized classification for purposes of analysis, and a single coder, unaware of infant Strange Situation behavior (R. Goldwyn), worked through all interviews. Interjudge agreement with two undergraduate coders was high.

• *Transcripts of interviews with the parents of children who had been secure with them in the Strange Situation 5 years before.* Infant Strange Situation security was assessed with a 3-point scale, in which very secure (B3) infants scored a 3, and insecure infants a 1. With respect to scores for the then-existing state-of-mind scales (later elaborated), *the strongest correlate of infant security of attachment for both mothers and fathers was the coherence observed in the AAI text overall (r = .48 for mothers, r = .53 for fathers).* Finally, a majority of parents of both sexes were matched to their infants in terms of secure versus insecure attachment status. The effect size was d = 1.50 for mother–infant dyads and d = 0.78 for fathers (d = 0.80 marks a strong effect). Interestingly, three of the 18 secure infants (17%) had mothers—also judged secure on the AAI—whose own parents had both scored *below a 3* on the Loving scale. Moreover, for fathers, there was no significant relation between infant security and either of the parents' loving scores on the AAI, and both parents of one father whose infant was judged secure with him had loving scores of 1. Thus a "grandchild's" security with a parent appeared not to be solely a function of the parent's security with his or her own parents. This finding is pertinent, of course, to the topic of "earned/evolved" security, described earlier.

• *Transcripts of interviews with the parents of children who had been avoidant of them in the Strange*

*Situation 5 years before.* To explore relations between infant avoidance and parental state-of-mind characteristics, Ainsworth and colleagues' (1978) 7-point scales for infant avoidance of proximity to the parent during the two 3-minute reunion episodes of the Strange Situation 5 years previously were used. For both mothers and fathers, their infants' avoidance under stress was significantly correlated with their own insistence on lack of memory for childhood (r = .41 for mothers, r = .47 for fathers). For mothers, idealization of their own mothers (r = .47) and fathers (r = .43) were also significantly related to infant avoidance. For fathers, relations between infant avoidance and idealization of their mothers (r = .53) and their fathers (r = .64) were even stronger.[8] At the level of classifications, the effect sizes for the relation between parental dismissing classification and infant avoidant classifications in this sample were d = 1.22 for mothers and d = 0.68 for fathers.

• *Transcripts of interviews with the parents of children who had been resistant with them in the Strange Situation 5 years before.* Scores for infant resistance to the parent on reunion were expected to be correlated with the parent's preoccupied anger toward his or her own parents. For the mother–infant sample (six infants were classified as resistant), preoccupied anger expressed in the AAI regarding both the mother's mother (r = .56) and the mother's father (r = .47) were significantly related to infant angry resistance 5 years earlier. Only two infants were resistant with their fathers.

Transcripts taken from the parents of resistant infants had most commonly been judged preoccupied. Two of the infants of the three preoccupied fathers had been resistant, as were five of the infants of the six preoccupied mothers. The effect size linking maternal preoccupied attachment status to the infant resistant/ambivalent classification was d = 1.75, whereas the link between paternal preoccupied status and infant resistant attachment was d = 1.08.

The observed three-way agreement between AAI status and infant Strange Situation behavior for mother–infant dyads was 75%, whereas the agreement expected by chance was 37% (kappa = .61, p < .001). The three-way agreement for fathers was 69%, whereas the agreement expected by chance was 46% (kappa = .41, p < .01). The match between the 12 AAI "organized" subclassifications and the eight infant Strange Situation subclassifications was 46%, with a 17% match having been expected by chance (see Hesse, 2008, for elaboration).

## Properties of the AAI

In 1996, Van IJzendoorn and Bakermans-Kranenburg reported that in a combined (meta-analytic) sample of 584 nonclinical mothers, 24% were classified as dismissing, 58% as secure-autonomous, and 18% as preoccupied. With the unresolved category considered, a four-way analysis of the available 487 nonclinical mothers showed the following distribution: 16% dismissing, 55% secure-autonomous, 9% preoccupied, and 19% unresolved. The combined distribution of nonclinical fathers was highly similar. A meta-analysis published 12 years later by these same authors (Van IJzendoorn & Bakermans-Kranenburg, 2008) yielded very similar proportions, although the combined sample size was much larger (1,012 nonclinical mothers).

AAI distributions in adolescent samples did not differ significantly from distributions in the nonclinical adult samples. However, combined samples from very low-socioeconomic-status (SES) samples ($N$ = 995) did differ significantly from nonclinical mother samples, with the unresolved and dismissing categories being overrepresented, and the secure-autonomous category correspondingly underrepresented in these samples. The AAI was found to be unrelated to social desirability (Bakermans-Kranenburg & Van IJzendoorn, 1993; Crowell et al., 1996; Sagi et al., 1994), and showed only a modest association with social adjustment (Crowell et al., 1996). Although the AAI in general has been found only weakly related to content-based retrospective parenting style measures and appears to be independent of general personality measures (Van IJzendoorn, 1995), persons classified as preoccupied have been found to report more symptoms on the Minnesota Multiphasic Personality Inventory, whereas dismissing individuals report fewer (Pianta, Egeland, & Adam, 1996).

By 1996 the AAI had been subjected to a series of rigorous psychometric tests of stability and discriminant validity (Van IJzendoorn, 1995). Stability studies typically employ different interviewers across the time period in question, with coders unaware of one another's classifications. With interviews conducted two months apart ($N$ = 83), Bakermans-Kranenburg and Van IJzendoorn (1993) found 78% stability (kappa = .63) across the three organized attachment categories (the

unresolved category was less stable), and an Israeli study of 59 college students in which AAIs were conducted 3 months apart yielded 90% test–retest stability (kappa = .79; Sagi et al., 1994). The mean interjudge agreement for this latter study was 95%. Both studies indicated that category placement could not be attributed to the influence of a particular interviewer.

Benoit and Parker (1994) found 90% three-category stability between a prebirth interview and interviews conducted at 11 months of infant age ($n$ = 84). Stability has also been tested across 18 months in New York (86% three-category stability, kappa = .73; Crowell et al., 1996) and 4 years in Rome (95% secure–insecure correspondence, 70% three-category correspondence; Ammaniti, Speranza, & Candelori, 1996). Steele and Steele (2007) reported striking 5-year stability in a group of 51 mothers interviewed during pregnancy and again when their children were 5 years of age. The interviews were classified by independent teams of coders, and no individuals were considered "cannot classify" at either time period. Remarkably, 86% stability was found within the remaining four major classifications (F/Ds/E/U), across the 5-year period.[9]

Because of the weight given to coherence scores when AAI transcripts are being assigned to secure versus insecure attachment status, it has been important to establish that in five out of six studies conducted by 2008, secure versus insecure adult attachment status had been found to be unrelated to intelligence, including assessments specific to verbal fluency (Van IJzendoorn, 1995). Moreover, because insistence on lack of memory for childhood is associated with the dismissing category, it has been necessary to assess individuals' general abilities involving memory. Thus, if persons assigned to the dismissing category suffer from overall difficulties with childhood memories, their insistence on lack of recall for early relationships and interactions might not pertain to state of mind specific to attachment history. This question was first examined by Bakermans-Kranenburg and Van IJzendoorn (1993), who found the AAI categories to be independent of non-attachment-related memory. In an Israeli study, Sagi and colleagues (1994) used an even broader range of memory tests. Here the accuracy of memories for childhood events was ingeniously assessed, and subjects were also examined for "immediate" memory skills in a test of (non-attachment-related) paired associates. No differences were found across the categories.

One of the most important questions pertaining to the discriminant validity of the AAI stems from its reliance on individual differences in discourse characteristics. If these characteristics were found to generalize to non-attachment-related topics, the inability of the parents of insecure infants to produce coherent and collaborative AAI narratives could not readily be attributed to an (insecure) state of mind arising specifically from a request for a review and evaluation of their attachment history.

This question was addressed by Crowell, Waters and colleagues (1996), using an Employment Experience Interview, which followed the form of the AAI protocol but focused instead on technical aspects of the speaker's work history. Although transcripts of the Employment Experience Interview could be reliably classified as secure-autonomous, dismissing, or preoccupied, these classifications were orthogonal to the secure-autonomous, dismissing, and preoccupied classifications assigned to the same 53 mothers based on the AAI. Thus, it appears that the attachment-related queries within the AAI protocol do in fact have a direct influence on the linguistic form manifested in the interview transcript.

## Further Establishing the Link between Adult (AAI) and Child Attachment Status

Within approximately a decade following the publication of Main and colleagues (1985), the remarkable relation between a parent's AAI classification and his or her infant's Strange Situation classification uncovered in Berkeley had been well replicated, and the association between a parent's discussion of his or her own attachment history and infant Strange Situation behavior was found to be robust. In succeeding years, AAI–Strange Situation matches were found in both high-risk samples (e.g., based on an inner-city Hispanic and African American sample; Ward & Carlson, 1995) and in other languages (German: Grossmann, Fremmer-Bombik, Rudolph, & Grossmann, 1988; Hebrew: Sagi et al., 1997, and Japanese: Behrens et al., 2007; Kazui, Endo, Tanaka, Sakagami, & Suganuma, 2000).

In 1995, Van IJzendoorn used meta-analytic techniques to examine a total of 18 AAI samples, including 854 parent–infant pairs from six different countries. This overview revealed that when the three-way analysis was used, there was a 75%

secure–insecure correspondence between parental and offspring security—a finding that held even when the interview was conducted prior to the birth of the first child (in Toronto: Benoit & Parker, 1994; in London: Fonagy et al., 1991; Steele, Steele, & Fonagy, 1996; in inner-city New York: Ward & Carlson, 1995). The combined effect size of the secure–insecure parent-to-infant match across samples (inclusive of mother–infant and father–infant dyads) was $d = 1.06$ ($r = .47$, biserial $r = .59$), which is considered very large ($d = .80$ is considered large). The explained variation on the basis of $r$ was 22%, and for biserial $r$, it was 35%. Using a statistic devised by Rosenthal (1991), Van IJzendoorn calculated that it would take 1,087 studies with null results to diminish the combined one-tailed $p$ level to insignificance.

Turning to more specific parent-to-infant matches in Van IJzendoorn's (1995) meta-analysis, the combined effect size for the match between the dismissing adult and infant avoidant classifications was $d = 1.02$ (equivalent to $r = .45$), and the match between the preoccupied adult and infant resistant/ambivalent classifications was $d = 0.92$ ($r = .42$). Correspondence for the three-way infant and AAI classifications across the 13 samples for which it could be calculated was 70%. It is interesting as well (Van IJzendoorn's [1995] Table 2, p. 393), however, that in this analysis, 82% (304/369) of secure-autonomous mothers had secure offspring, and 64% of dismissing mothers had insecure-avoidant offspring; however, only 35% of preoccupied mothers had insecure-resistant/ambivalent infants.

As noted earlier, with respect to parent–child dyads, both cannot classify and unresolved interviews are associated with the "disorganized infant" Strange Situation classification (Main & Solomon, 1986, 1990). Both of these AAI categories have been found to predominate in clinical samples (Van IJzendoorn & Bakermans-Kranenburg, 1996, 2008), and infants' disorganized attachment with their mothers has been associated with psychopathology assessed in the same individuals in young adulthood (Carlson, 1998), especially when intervening trauma was present (Ogawa, Sroufe, Weinfield, Carlson, & Egeland, 1997).

In his 1995 meta-analysis, of the nine studies that included unresolved AAI status (548 dyads), Van IJzendoorn calculated $d = 0.65$ (equivalent to $r = .31$) for the relation between normally very brief lapses in speech surrounding traumatic experiences during the AAI and similarly minimal disorganized disruptions in Strange Situation behavior. The fleeting and difficult-to-identify nature of *both* phenomena suggests that the association between adult unresolved status and infant disorganized status may have been attenuated in this calculation—and not only by instability in the appearance of the phenomena but also by the need for extensive training in identifying them.

Consistent with the above, Van IJzendoorn (1995) found that *amount of training* was very strongly related to differences in effect sizes ($z$ = 5.59, $p$ = 1.30E-08), especially when researchers attempt to link unresolved and/or unclassifiable AAI texts to infant disorganization, with less training being associated with markedly smaller effects. For example, the effect size relating unresolved AAI status in 45 mothers to infant disorganized attachment status for Ainsworth and Eichberg's (1991) study (with AAIs coded by Ainsworth following her establishment of reliability across 50 [as opposed to the usual 30] AAI transcripts, and Strange Situations coded by N. Kaplan and D. Weston following training across 75 Strange Situations) was extremely large, or $d$ = 2.32.

As another example of a study in which unresolved parental status was compared to offspring disorganized/controlling behavior (D-controlling is the midchildhood equivalent of infant disorganized attachment), Behrens and colleagues (2007) studied 43 mother–child dyads in Sapporo, Japan. Two experts (E. Hesse and M. Main) in the sixth-year system of coding mother–child reunion classifications (see Main & Cassidy, 1988) coded the reunion behavior of the Japanese children, and Behrens coded the mothers' AAIs. Overall AAI to 6-year reunion matches were strong, and the effect size for mother's unresolved/cannot classify AAI status and her child's status as controlling or cannot classify reunion behavior was $d$ = 1.50 (equivalent to $r$ = .60).

Hughes, Turton, Hopper, McGauley, and Fonagy (2001) provided another illustration of the relation between maternal unresolved AAI status and infant disorganized attachment. This study focused on the effects of stillbirth of a first infant when mothers ($N$ = 53) were seen in the Strange Situation with their next-born infant. The overall association between maternal unresolved status with respect to the stillbirth loss and disorganized attachment as identified in the succeeding offspring was $r$ = .50 ($p$ < .0001). Importantly, the association between stillbirth experience and disorganization in the next infant was not significant once unresolved maternal attachment was excluded from the model.

Twenty years after Van IJzendoorn's 1995 meta-analysis revealing a remarkably strong relation between parental AAI classification and offspring Strange Situation behavior, a new meta-analysis addressing the same issues ("Narrowing the Transmission Gap: A Synthesis of three decades of research on Intergenerational Transmission of Attachment") was published by eight authors from four countries (Verhage et al., 2015). Here, space limitations preclude the article's report of advances made toward narrowing the "transmission gap" that Van IJzendoorn had identified in 1995. I therefore confine myself to summarizing parent–infant concordance from 95 samples ($N$ = 4,819), based on studies conducted "all over the globe" (Verhage et al., 2015, p. 1). To begin with, according to Verhage and colleagues' (2015) conclusion, and somewhat astonishingly, all analyses confirmed the intergenerational transmission of attachment.

A first point made by the authors is that the evidence fails to support a "genetic" account of cross-generational continuity on the basis of either behavioral or molecular genetic studies. Rather, "attachment theory provides a psychological and environmental account of intergenerational transmission" (Verhage et al., 2015, p. 1). Studies were intended to be included only if the AAI coders had received training from a certified AAI trainer (see *attachment-training.com* for a list of certified trainers), and only a few investigators did not provide this information (responding "no information" or "not applicable"). However, investigators were not queried as to whether their coders had successfully completed the available 30-case AAI reliability check (see Appendix 26.1). Studies reporting extreme results (specifically, Ainsworth & Eichberg, 1991, for the remarkable strength reported for the unresolved AAI-disorganized–Strange Situation link, and Solomon & George, 2011, for the absence of any significant AAI–Strange-Situation associations in all four categories) were "winsorized" [transformed to the next largest or smallest value in the distribution]) as extreme outliers.

Verhage and colleagues' (2015) study is extraordinarily thorough; I regret that I can mention only a few additional results here. Using the four-way analysis of the AAI, the autonomous parent to secure infant classification ($k$ = 59, $N$ = 3, 226) yielded a significant combined effect size of $r$ = .31. However, there was a significant difference in effect size between published data ($k$ = 32, $r$ = .40) and unpublished data ($k$ = 27, $r$ = .21). Unresolved status on the AAI also showed an overall significant combined effect size of $r = .21$ ($r = .31$ in the 1995 report), while again, effect sizes for published data were larger and closer to the 1995 report ($r = .28$).

The report by Verhage and colleagues (2015) is monolithic and, indeed, magnificent, covering many more analyses than can be touched on in this chapter. In closing, the authors state: "The association between caregiver attachment representations and child–caregiver attachment has been confirmed as a robust and universal effect by this new series of meta-analyses, albeit smaller than in the initial studies" (p. 23). The authors noted that the smaller "effect sizes were moderated by risk status of the sample, biological relatedness of child–caregiver dyads, and age of the children" (p. 1). Additionally, the effect sizes in this study were no doubt influenced by the fact that AAI coder certification was not available and hence was not a prerequisite for study inclusion.

## Unresolved States of Mind and Frightening/ Disruptive Behavior toward Offspring

In 1990, Mary Main and I first put forward the hypothesis that parents judged to be unresolved on the AAI would exhibit frightened (from facial expressions of fright to direct apprehensive flight from the infant), frightening (and surprisingly, not infrequently predator-like), and/or dissociative behavior toward or in the presence of their offspring. Consequently, by 1991 we had developed an initial coding system for identifying frightened/ frightening/dissociative (FR) parental behavior from videotapes. Our thinking was that if, as we believed, lapses in the monitoring of reasoning or discourse surrounding the discussion of potentially traumatic events during the AAI occurred in conjunction with intrusions from the speaker's partially dissociated frightening experiences (Hesse & Main, 1999, 2006), such intrusions might also occur in the presence of and/or during the parent's interactions with the infant.

The classic manifestations of primitive fear include attack, flight, fainting (e.g., falling to the floor as though "playing dead"), and freezing. Such indices of parental fear, we reasoned, could expectably alarm an infant and place it in a disorganizing paradox similar to that created by direct maltreatment. Thus, as in the case of maltreatment, the haven of safety and the source of alarm would be in the same location, placing the infant in an inherently disorganizing position. Our coding

system identifying FR behavior (Main & Hesse, 1991, 1998) was forwarded to Karlen Lyons-Ruth, to assist in her development of "AMBIANCE," a system identifying parental disruptive behaviors more generally (see Lyons-Ruth, Bronfman, & Parsons, 1999). Unresolved status on the AAI has now been found to predict both frightening and atypical parental behavior in several independent samples (e.g., Abrams et al., 2006; Hesse, 1999; Jacobvitz, Leon, & Hazen, 2006; Lyons-Ruth et al., 1999; Madigan, Moran, & Pederson, 2006; see also Madigan, Bakermans-Kranenburg, et al., 2006).

It should be noted, however, that in a pioneering study of 80 dyads in the Netherlands (Schuengel, Bakermans-Kranenburg, & Van IJzendoorn, 1999), substantially frightening parental behavior was linked to infant disorganization, but—interestingly—only if the unresolved mother had a secondary classification as insecure. Citing the work of Stevenson-Hinde, who had emphasized that sensitive caregiving requires an outward-directed attention, Schuengel et al. suggested that an underlying secure-autonomous state of mind—quite likely via an ability to maintain focus on the immediate surround while overriding intrusions from untoward memories—might be protective in the context of unresolved/*secure* as opposed to unresolved/*insecure* status.

Jacobvitz and colleagues (2006) partially replicated the "protective effect" of underlying security uncovered in Schuengel and colleagues' 1999 study, as would Heinicke and colleagues (2006) in an intervention study. In Jacobvitz and colleagues' (2006) study, 116 prospective first-time mothers were administered the AAI during pregnancy and were videotaped at 8 months of infant age in their homes. As expected, women classified as unresolved with respect to loss and/or abuse displayed substantially higher levels of FR behavior during interactions with their infant than did other mothers, including extended trance-like stilling and anomalous aggressive actions. However, in keeping with Schuengel and colleagues' findings, levels of FR behavior in the Jacobvitz and colleagues study were lower if an unresolved mother's underlying AAI classification was secure. In addition, unresolved responses to loss in the AAI were found in this latter study to fully mediate the association between loss of an attachment figure other than the parent and FR behavior.

Thus, as discussed above, in 1990, Main and Hesse suggested that parental FR behavior would mediate the relation between unresolved lapses in speech in the AAI and infant disorganized behavior in the Strange Situation. Given the fleeting nature of all three of the phenomena under examination—(1) lapses in the monitoring of speech or reasoning during the AAI (Main & Hesse, 1990); (2) FR behavior in parents (Abrams et al., 2006; Hesse & Main, 2006; Main & Hesse, 1990) or, similarly, atypical parental behaviors (Lyons-Ruth et al., 1999); and (3) disorganized infant behavior (Main & Solomon, 1986, 1990)—it is striking that a first meta-analysis of five samples testing the Main–Hesse hypothesis and using investigators at differing levels of training found even a partial (although still incomplete) mediation that accounted for 42% of the variance between parental FR behavior and infant disorganization (Madigan, Bakermans-Kranenburg, et al., 2006). By 2008, Canadian coders highly trained in the Main–Hesse system for assessing parental FR behavior found that maternal FR behavior accounted for over 50% of the variance in the association between maternal unresolved attachment status on the AAI and infant disorganized Strange Situation behavior (Evans, 2008). Still more recently, Jacobvitz, Hazen, Zaccagnino, Messina, and Beverung (2011) reported full mediation between unresolved AAI status and disorganized Strange Situation behavior in offspring via a coding of maternal FR behavior extended to include verbal FR behavior.

## Studies Comparing AAI Classifications in Clinical and Nonclinical Populations

As already noted, the central categories of the AAI were developed and refined in the mid-1980s with respect to a 1-year-old's (secure vs. insecure) response to the speaker in a stressful situation, using a middle- to upper-middle-class sample from the San Francisco Bay Area. It was therefore initially surprising that—without adjustment—this system for assessing adult attachment status was later shown to discriminate between clinical and nonclinical populations (Van IJzendoorn & Bakermans-Kranenburg, 1996, 2008; see also Bakermans-Kranenburg & Van IJzendoorn, 2009). Moreover, in 1996 Van IJzendoorn and Bakermans-Kranenburg showed that the effect size discriminating clinical from nonclinical populations ($d = 1.03$) was virtually identical to that discriminating the parents of secure infants from the parents of insecure infants ($d = 1.06$). Ultimately, in a four-way analysis (secure-autonomous, dismissing,

preoccupied, unresolved/cannot classify), only 8% of members of clinical samples were judged secure. (I note that *clinical samples* as used here indicates persons with specific diagnoses, not those simply electing to enter psychotherapy.)

By the mid-1990s, many studies of clinically distressed adolescents and adults were conducted, and the predominance of the unresolved (as well as the preoccupied) classification was striking. For example, a study of 24 closely comparable female subjects (12 with borderline personality disorder and 12 with dysthymia, none comorbid) was conducted at the Tavistock Clinic, using a coder who was unaware of either the participants' diagnoses or the aims of the investigation (Patrick et al., 1994). Patients with borderline personality disorder were selected for having met at least seven of the eight criteria in the third, revised edition of the *Diagnostic and Statistical Manual of Mental Disorders* (DSM-III-R; American Psychiatric Association, 1987). All of the 12 borderline patients—but only four of the dysthymic patients—were classified as preoccupied (Fisher's exact test, two-tailed; $p = .001$). Moreover, 10 of the 12 patients with borderline personality disorder were classified specifically as fitting to a rare subcategory of preoccupation, termed E3 "fearfully preoccupied with traumatic events and experiences." Importantly, however, whereas the overall *rates* of experiences of loss (and trauma, as defined in AAI manuals) did not differ between the patients with borderline personality disorder and dysthymia, all nine of the borderline subjects reporting loss or trauma were classified as primarily unresolved (e.g., U/E3), as compared with only two of the 10 patients with dysthymia reporting loss or trauma (Fisher's exact test, two-tailed; $p = .0007$). This suggestion of greater sensitivity to loss or trauma in patients with borderline personality disorder as opposed to dysthymia is an important finding, although it likely has more than one possible interpretation.

Two years after Patrick and colleagues' (1994) report, Fonagy and his colleagues (1996) undertook a large study of 82 clinically distressed young adults at a national center for the inpatient treatment of severe personality disorders in London, comparing interviews to those of 85 well-matched controls. The category most strongly differentiating the groups was unresolved (76% inpatients vs. 7% controls) and—as in an earlier study of subjects with anxiety disorders conducted by Manassis, Bradley, Goldberg, Hood, and Swinson (1994; 14 of 18, or 78% unresolved)—subjects with anxiety disorders were found to be especially likely to be unresolved (38 of 44, or 86%). Among the subclassifications, the E3 subcategory of preoccupation was again found to be unexpectedly common in the psychiatric group (28 vs. 1%). Replicating the earlier outcomes of Patrick and colleagues, 47% of the patients with borderline personality disorder had also been classified E3.

A different and highly informative investigation was conducted by administering the AAI to 66 young adults (mean age = 26 years) who had been hospitalized 11 years earlier in adolescence, together with 76 matched (nonhospitalized) controls (Allen, Hauser, & Borman-Spurrell, 1996). Both groups came from upper-middle-class families, and individuals suffering from psychosis or organic impairment were excluded from the hospitalized sample. Any information that could provide evidence of previous hospitalization was carefully removed from the transcripts, so that the coder (Hesse) successfully remained unaware of group status. The proportion of secure-autonomous transcripts among individuals hospitalized 11 years earlier (7.6%) was exceptionally low. Moreover, the interview transcripts of 25.8% of the hospitalized group were judged as "cannot classify," as compared with 6.6% of the comparison group. Speakers who had been hospitalized were more likely to express contempt or derogation for attachment-related experiences and attachment figures, and received higher scores for unresolved responses to abuse experiences. The state-of-mind scale for derogation was also found to be related to criminal behavior and to hard drug use. Given the success of this original study, it is perhaps not surprising that Hauser, Golden, and Allen (2006) concluded that with the development of the AAI, narrative studies have begun to come (or, one might add, to come again) into their own in psychiatry and psychoanalysis.

As explained earlier, speakers are assigned to the "cannot classify" category whenever contradictory discourse strategies (e.g., both elevated indices of dismissal and preoccupation) appear within the AAI. With this in mind, two early case studies are of special interest. In the first, a mother described as "cannot classify" (Minde & Hesse, 1996; the coder was unaware that the transcript was taken from a patient in therapy) successfully demanded to have her child removed by cesarean section 1 month early, and then insisted on staying with the infant in intensive care for periods that far exceeded usual hospital practices. At later times, she was observed to alternate between periods of overinvolvement and periods of neglect.

In the second case study, home observations of a mother judged "cannot classify" by Hughes and McGauley (1997) indicated marked neglect and carelessness to a degree inviting external injury, alternating with sudden trips to the hospital occasioned by (an apparently unsubstantiated) fear of germs. In keeping with the hypothesis that discourse usage in the AAI should be predictive of caregiving, then, these two case studies of unclassifiable (CC), contradictory discourse were reflected in contradictory behavior toward the offspring.

In 2008, the AAI status of adolescents living in the streets of Mexico City with their infants were studied by Gojman de Millán and Millán. These included two individuals coded as "cannot classify," and one—whose behavior and outcome appeared far more promising—coded as "unresolved/secure." Another case study describes a patient classified as "unresolved/preoccupied" on the AAI who suffered from both narcissistic and borderline personality disorders; this case is discussed in terms of both her AAI and her therapist's reflections (Buchheim & Kachele, 2003). Finally, a particularly impressive set of case studies has traced change over the course of psychoanalysis, considering especially the movement from "unresolved/cannot classify" status to organized insecurity over time (Ammaniti et al., 2008).

Ward, Lee, and Polan (2006) investigated a *nonclinical* New York sample of 60 adult women, who were administered the AAI and seen in a diagnostic setting. Using the organized (F/Ds/E) attachment categories in the analysis, the researchers found that a majority of women with insecure attachment classifications were diagnosed with some psychopathology. However, when the unresolved category was included, unresolved participants whose alternative placement was secure-autonomous—while experiencing some difficulties with daily functioning, such as marital discord or physical symptoms—were significantly less likely to be diagnosed with psychopathology than were participants with unresolved/insecure classifications.

In a review of 61 clinical samples, Van IJzendoorn and Bakermans-Kranenburg (2008) used a correspondence analysis to ascertain possible patterning of AAI classifications in relation to clinical diagnoses. All clinical groups with psychiatric diagnoses tended toward insecurity, although clinical status in general was not related to a specific organized insecure AAI category. However, when the three-way analysis was used, individuals with borderline personality disorder and those experiencing more internalizing disorders tended toward the preoccupied classification, as had been indicated earlier in the study conducted by Patrick and colleagues (1994). In contrast, for more externalizing problems and disorders as identified in this study, such as antisocial personality disorder and conduct disorder, there was an overrepresentation of the dismissing classification. (See also Frodi, Dernevik, Sepa, Philipson, & Bragesjö [2001] for a study that revealed an unusual proportion of dismissing transcripts among incarcerated males with psychopathy.) When unresolved and unclassifiable transcripts were taken into account in a four-way analysis, an "extremely strong" association was found among borderline personality disorder, abuse, or suicide. (See also Adshead & Bluglass [2005] for a first study of maternal factitious illness by proxy, in which 60% of these mothers were found to have unresolved transcripts.)

In a follow up study of 111 middle-class Australian mothers with postnatal depression and their infants (McMahon, Barnett, Kowalenko, & Tennant, 2006), chronically depressed mothers were found to be more likely to have infants who were insecurely attached. However, the relation between maternal depression and infant insecurity was moderated by maternal response to the AAI, with secure mothers with postpartum depression being less likely to have insecure infants.

## Applications of the AAI to New Populations

By the second edition of this volume (Hesse, 2008), the AAI had been used to determine (1) whether, among adults, rates of AAI security are decreased by disadvantages such as deafness or blindness (they are not; Van IJzendoorn & Bakermans-Kranenburg, 2008; see also McKinnon, Moran, & Pederson, 2004); (2) whether the daughters of Holocaust survivors in Israel are significantly more likely than daughters of control participants to be insecure on the AAI (they are not; see Sagi-Schwartz et al., 2003); (3) whether concordance rates of attachment are similar between identical twins, when compared to each other as well as to their non-twin siblings (they are, indicating preliminary evidence for shared environmental influence; Constantino et al., 2006; see also Torgerson, Grova, & Sommerstad [2007] for monozygotic vs. dizygotic twins); and (4) whether foster infants' Strange Situation categories were correlated with their foster mothers' AAI classifications

(they are; Dozier, Stovall, Albus, & Bates, 2001; see also M. Steele, Hodges, Kaniuk, Hillman, & Henderson [2003] for associations between adoptive mothers' AAIs and emotional themes in their previously neglected/abused 4-to-6-year olds' doll play). In addition, the attachment status of infertile couples seeking to adopt was examined, and a majority were secure on the AAI (see Santona & Zavattini, 2005). The ways in which older adult mothers with dementia responded to reunion with their adult daughters acting as caregivers was also explored. Indices of reunion security were found to be significantly correlated with daughters' AAI coherence, with more pleasure being exhibited with coherent daughters (H. Steele, Phibbs, & Woods, 2004).

Attachment in relation to religious/spiritual groups has also been investigated. Granqvist, Ivarsson, Broberg, and Hagekull (2007) found that 46% of participants drawn from religious/spiritual groups were secure on the AAI. As expected, scores for mothers' loving behavior during childhood were linked to an image of a loving God. In contrast, New Age spirituality, which can include beliefs in personal contact with the dead, was associated specifically with the unresolved, cannot classify, and preoccupied AAI categories. Finally, strong majorities of devout Catholic laypeople and nuns have been found to be secure on the AAI (Cassibba, Granqvist, Costantini, & Gatto, 2008).

## Intervention Studies

The AAI has also been increasingly utilized in clinical studies, both with individuals in therapy and with those in intervention studies focusing on parents and caregivers. I provide some examples of the latter first.

Heinicke and colleagues (2006; see also Heinicke & Levine, 2008) used the AAI as a prebirth assessment for 57 high-risk mothers in an intervention project involving multiple forms of assistance, including weekly home visits for the first 2 years of life. A regression analysis showed that a combined unresolved trauma/coherence scale from the prebirth AAI was the best predictor of toddler security assessed by the Attachment Q-Sort 2 years later. Additionally, as in Korfmacher, Adam, Ogawa, and Egeland (1997), a mother's coherence on the prebirth AAI predicted her involvement in the work of intervention.

In conjunction with Dozier's Attachment and Biobehavioral Catch-Up Program, Bick and

Dozier (2008) administered the AAI to 200 foster parents, just over half of whom were classified as secure. During the intervention, as in their AAIs, foster mothers with secure-autonomous transcripts were cooperative and collaborative, and were open to discussing potentially painful or sensitive topics. Foster mothers with dismissing transcripts tended to avoid discussing both relationship difficulties and the children's need for nurturance. In contrast, those classified as preoccupied seemed relatively comfortable discussing their attachment-related pasts but were described as fluctuating between seeking reassurance from the intervener and displaying annoyance. Finally, caregivers who were unresolved with regard to loss or trauma were described as seeming to (1) have trouble developing trust in their interveners, (2) have difficulties discussing having been frightened as children, and (3) have difficulty during sessions behaving in non-threatening ways toward children—all findings that accord well with our expectations that individuals with unresolved trauma exhibit frightening behavior toward their children.

Zegers, Schuengel, Van IJzendoorn, and Janssens (2006) administered AAIs both to professional caregivers in institutions and to seriously emotionally and/or behaviorally troubled adolescents placed in their care. Over time, more secure mentors were increasingly perceived as being available as a secure base, and more secure adolescents were perceived as increasing their secure-base use of their mentors.

The AAI has also been increasingly utilized in clinical studies to ascertain, for example, whether AAIs administered to psychoanalytic patients at the beginning and during the later course of psychotherapy can yield not only an increase in scores assigned for coherence of transcript over time but also eventual moves from insecure to secure AAI classifications (Ammaniti et al., 2008). As another example, Levy and colleagues (Levy et al., 2006) administered a preintervention AAI to patients with borderline personality disorder, and a second following 1 year of therapy. Ninety participants were randomly assigned to three different treatment conditions, one of which was Kernberg's (1984; see also Yeomans et al., 2015) transference-focused therapy. Transference-focused therapy revealed significant change in AAI status, specifically, increases in coherence of transcript and a more than threefold increase in secure-autonomous classifications.

More recently, Buchheim and colleagues (2016) have completed a study once more indicat-

ing the success of Kernberg's transference-focused therapy (as compared to therapy administered by experienced community therapists) with patients with borderline personality disorder. At entrance, 50% of the104 borderline patients were identified on the AAI with unresolved trauma: Of interest, this subgroup of borderline patients was found to be especially impaired with respect to psychopathology. However, a significant shift from unresolved to organized attachment status was identified following the year of transference-focused treatment. Finally, patient scores on the AAI Coherence scale improved strongly in the transference-focused group ($d = 1.27$) and just moderately following treatment with experienced community therapists ($d = 0.32$). (For additional discussion of intervention studies, see Hesse, 1999, 2008.)

### Longitudinal Studies

Many kinds of longitudinal studies predictive of eventual AAI status may, of course, be conducted. As one example, Beckwith, Cohen, and Hamilton (1999) found that maternal insensitivity to a child in the early months predicted dismissing AAI status at age 18. With one exception, I focus here on studies that have compared infant Strange Situation behavior with the mother to AAI status determined for the same individuals in young adulthood, and I confine even the majority of these descriptions to a secure–insecure analysis. Many of these studies were reviewed earlier (Hesse, 1999, 2008).

Four U.S. longitudinal studies have been undertaken, each indicating significant infancy-to-adulthood links. Waters, Merrick, Treboux, Crowell, and Albersheim (2000) conducted AAIs with 50 lower- to middle-class young adults seen in Ainsworth's Strange Situation at 12 months. For 72% of participants (kappa = .44, $p < .001$), secure versus insecure infant Strange Situation behavior was predictive of secure versus insecure AAI texts 19–21 years later. This correspondence was somewhat higher (78%; kappa = .52) when participants experiencing intervening trauma were eliminated. In the same year, Hamilton (2000) reported on the predictability of AAI responses in a sample of 30 adolescents (ages 17–19) who had been raised in unconventional settings (e.g., communal living groups). The two-way (secure vs. insecure) correspondence in this study was 77% (kappa = .49).

Using a sample of 42 participants, Main (2001; Main et al., 2005) compared Strange Situation classifications with mothers at 12–18 months of age to AAI status as assessed at age 19. As in Waters and colleagues' (2000) original study, a highly significant secure–insecure match was found across the 18-year period. As predicted in advance, among the 12 participants coded as *disorganized/secure* during infancy, not one was secure on the AAI at age 19. Intriguingly, although most avoidant infants had become dismissing, about half of the previously disorganized infants had become dismissing as well (for a much expanded description of this study, see Main et al., 2005).

In the Minnesota Study of Risk and Adaptation from Birth to Adulthood, a significant 18-month Strange Situation to 26-year AAI secure–insecure match has been reported ($p < .001$; $N = 125$), although the match from 12 months appears to remain insignificant[10] (Sroufe, 2005). Interestingly, as in the Bay Area study of middle-class dyads, in this low-income sample, disorganized/secure infants were only rarely found to be secure in adulthood.

One study conducted in the United States and three outside the United States have yielded insignificant relations between Strange Situation responses and AAI status in young adulthood. The latter include both the Regensburg and Bielefeld longitudinal studies (in which, however, disorganized/secure infants were coded as secure), as described by Grossmann, Grossmann, and Kindler (2005), and the Haifa longitudinal study (Sagi-Schwartz & Aviezer, 2005), in which the infant disorganized category at the time apparently also had yet to be coded. Although it should be noted that only the three-way infant analysis was available to Waters and colleagues (2000) and to Hamilton (2000) as well, it would be prudent to await a four-way analysis including disorganized codings of infant Strange Situation responses before drawing final conclusions regarding the German and Israeli studies.

The SECCYD, a study utilizing the NICHD subsample of 857 adolescents (mean age 17.5 years) reported "evidence for weak stability in attachment security and disorganization" (Groh et al., 2014, p. 63). In this report, the Strange Situation distribution appears reasonably typical for community samples. At the level of the AAI response, however, Van IJzendoorn and Bakermans-Kranenburg (2014) point to the pervasive limitations entailed in the nonresponse bias that the researchers encountered. The nonresponse rate may be what led to the startling underrepresentation of both preoccupied and unresolved catego-

ries (the preoccupied and unresolved categories were each assigned to just 3% of participants, in sharp contrast to the 11% preoccupied and 11% unresolved more usually uncovered in such samples). The study was further complicated by an overrepresentation of dismissing interviews. Finally, 21% of the AAIs were completed by phone (an approach that is not recommended by the originators of the instrument). Thus, although intriguing, the NICHD/SECCYD findings do stand in sharp contrast to the studies listed earlier, and as noted, are in need of replication in a context absent the sample bias encountered by the unusual distribution of consenting participants in this study.

Finally, one highly original longitudinal study of 26 dyads employed mothers' perceptions of their newborns to predict subsequent secure versus insecure AAI classification (Broussard & Cassidy, 2010). Here, Broussard's (1979; Broussard & Hartner, 1970) Neonatal Perception Inventory was used to identify mothers who had positive versus negative perceptions of their offspring. It was hypothesized that as adults, newborns perceived negatively by their mothers would be more likely to be classified insecure on the AAI than infants whose mothers had a positive perception of them. As expected, negative maternal perception of an infant at 1 month of age was associated with subsequent insecure AAI status, as assessed 27–43 years later. Whereas 86% (12 of 14) of positively perceived newborns were classified as secure on the AAI, only 25% (3 of 12) of the negatively perceived infants were secure on the AAI (Fisher's exact test, $p = .001$). Also of interest are findings that adults viewed negatively by their mother as infants were idealizing of the mother, whom AAI coders also identified as less loving and more rejecting.

## Selected Recent Studies

Before turning to a closing section that reviews use of the AAI in conjunction with psychophysiology, genetics, and neuroscience, I very briefly summarize nine of the many important studies involving some of the interesting topical areas and issues currently being explored. I apologize for a majority of studies that could not be included here.

- Individuals prone to overuse of (addiction to) computer games involving role playing are largely classified as unresolved for loss or abuse (Schimmenti, Guglielmucci, Barbasio, & Granieri, 2012).

- In contrast to some folk beliefs regarding the likelihood of disproportionate emotional instability among artists, 88% of performing artists are secure in terms of three-way classifications in the AAI (Thomson & Jacque, 2012a, 2012b).
- A substantial portion of men who have post-traumatic stress disorder following war experience are coded as unresolved/secure (U/F), suggesting that even in the face of extreme trauma, an underlying security can remain (see Nye et al., 2008; also see a replication and extension by Harari et al., 2009).
- Sixty-five percent of individuals with scores equal to or above 4 (on an 10-point scale) on the Adverse Childhood Experiences (ACE) questionnaire are found to be unresolved/cannot classify on the AAI (Murphy et al., 2014).
- Among adult offspring whose parents divorced during their childhood, those who were classified as secure on the AAI prior to their weddings were less likely to divorce in the early years of marriage than their insecure counterparts (Crowell, Treboux, & Brockmeyer, 2009). However, parental divorce increased the likelihood of insecure adult attachment status.
- During a 15-minute conflict interchange, couples in which both members were classified as unresolved for trauma displayed more problematic interactions than partners with any other AAI configurations (Creasey, 2014).
- Two weeks after a 10-minute laboratory task completed with a peer whom they did not know, adolescents insecure (vs. secure) on the AAI remembered their interactions as less positive and more negative (and inclusive of greater hostility) than they had at the time (Dykas, Woodhouse, Ehrlich, & Cassidy, 2012).
- A four-category (secure, dismissing, preoccupied, unresolved) projective, picture-based system entitled the Adult Attachment Projective (AAP) described as providing strong *four-category* agreement with the AAI (George & West, 2011, 2012), has recently been found to have no relation either to AAI classifications themselves or to several of the well-known correlates of the AAI across a sample of 101 interviews. In this study, the AAP was coded by its originator (Jones-Mason, Allen, Hamilton & Weiss, 2015).
- Finally, based on 673 adolescents from the NICHD/SECCYD study, Harriet Waters' Attachment Script Assessment (ASA; Waters & Waters, 2006), which examines the degree to which participants are able to produce a "secure-base" attachment script from a series of attachment-related prompt-words, has yielded a .42 correlation with coherence of mind as assessed in the AAI (Steele et al., 2014). The ASA is designed to provide a continuous, single-scale assessment of security, however, and does not identify varying forms of insecure attachment.

### Psychophysiology, Genetics, and Neuroscience

In an early study, Gribneau (2006; see also Bahm, Simon-Thomas, Main, & Hesse, 2016) presented four categories of images (social positive, nature positive, blatant death/dying, and cemetery images) to young women who had experienced loss, half of whom (16/31) had been coded on the AAI as unresolved. The aim of the study was to examine physiological responses to subtle "generic" reminders of death (cemetery images). As predicted, electroencephalogram (EEG) event-related potentials (ERPs) demonstrated increased physiological responses to cemetery images specific to unresolved women, with the anterior N2 component arguably indicating fearful alerting, as well as involuntary attention. A right-sided asymmetrical posterior P3 component toward all images suggested continuing vigilance/arousal, also specifically for unresolved women. Bahm and colleagues (2016) suggest that

> the early alerting to symbolic images of death via increased cemetery-evoked N2s for unresolved participants may be due to preconscious arousal of aversive implicit memories (Amini, Lewis, Lannon, & Louie, 1996). Such preconscious arousal of fright in response to distal reminders of loss suggests potential linkages to the production of FR behaviors, and may at the least partially explain the connection between unresolved states and such behaviors.

At least 14 studies examining psychophysiology, genetics, and neuroscience in relation to the AAI have been published since the 2008 edition of this handbook and are summarized below.

In recent years, researchers have begun investigating factors related to unresolved trauma beyond the individual's direct experiential domain. In 2009, Caspers and colleagues reported that their multivariate regression analysis indicated a relation between the short version of the serotonin transporter allele (5-HTTLPR) and an increased risk for unresolved trauma in 186 participants. Relatedly, in a pioneering article published in *Biological Psychiatry* concerning epigenetics and unresolved trauma as identified via the AAI, Van IJzendoorn, Caspers, Bakermans-Kranenburg, Beach, and Philibert (2010) reported that in a sample of 143 adopted participants, higher levels of methylation of the 5-HTT promoter-associated C-phosphate-G (CpG) island were associated with increased risk of unresolved responses to loss or other trauma. At the same time, the s/s variant of 5-HTTLPR predicted more unresolved loss or trauma, but only in the case of lower levels of methylation. The authors concluded that associations between 5-HTTLPR polymorphisms and psychological problems are significantly altered by environmentally induced methylation patterns, and that methylation may at times serve positively as an interface between an adverse environment and the developing organism.

One year later, consistent with earlier findings regarding the genetics of differential susceptibility, Bakermans-Kranenburg, Van IJzendoorn, Caspers, and Philibert (2011) reported that among 124 adopted adults, parental problems experienced in childhood (e.g., maternal depression and marital discord) were associated with different outcomes. Participants with the (dopamine receptor) *DRD4-7-r* allele had the highest scores for unresolved loss or trauma. In contrast, those with the *DRD4-7-r* allele who had not experienced parental problems showed the lowest ratings.

Rifkin-Graboi (2008; see also Colizzi, Costa, Pace, & Todarello, 2013; Pierrehumbert et al., 2009; Pierrehumbert, Torrisi, Ansermet, Borghini, & Halfon, 2012) examined emotional regulation via cortisol output in college-age men. Home assays showed little relation to overall AAI security. In the laboratory, participants were presented with both cognitive and attachment-related challenges, the latter presenting hypothetical situations involving separation, loss, and abandonment. As expected, AAI scores for idealization of the parents (a frequent correlate of parental rejection) were associated with a significant rise in cortisol specific to the attachment-related challenge. For further discussion of studies examining links between the AAI and emotion regulation, see Hesse (2008).

Three studies have examined a critical issue within parenting: adult response to infant cries. In a first study of adult response specific to infant crying, which employed functional magnetic resonance imaging (fMRI; Riem et al., 2012), amygdala activation, feelings of irritation, and force, as indicated by a handgrip dynamometer were el-

evated in individuals insecure on the AAI during exposure to infant crying (compared to scrambled control sounds) in 21 women without children. In a related article, Ablow, Marks, Feldman, and Huffman (2013) examined physiological responses to recorded cries among 53 expectant primiparous women. Women secure on the AAI exhibited respiratory sinus arrhythmia (RSA) declines in response to recorded cries, consistent with approach-oriented responses, while insecure-dismissing women displayed RSA and electrodermal increases consistent with behavioral inhibition, and additionally rated the cries as more aversive. Nine months postpartum, the secure women were observed as being more sensitive to infant distress. Finally, using videotapes of crying infants, Leerkes and colleagues (2015) looked for predictors of maternal sensitivity to infant distress among 269 primiparous mothers who had been administered the AAI and found overall coherence of mind directly associated with higher maternal sensitivity to infant distress.

Ammaniti and his colleagues (Lenzi et al., 2013) conducted an especially innovative AAI/fMRI study with nulliparous young adult women, 11 classified as secure and 12 as dismissing. During the fMRI, subjects viewed pictures of infant eye gaze (gleaned from videotaped interactions with their mothers). Infant expressions were: joyous, distressed, and neutral. It was anticipated that individuals classified as secure would show greater empathic responses via greater activation of mirror and limbic brain areas than would individuals classified as insecure. Counterintuitively, viewing the pictures of infants, dismissing subjects activated motor, mirror, and limbic brain areas (including medial orbitofrontal and perigenual anterior cingulate cortex) to a significantly greater extent than those classified as secure. These results were interpreted as indicating that the young women classified as dismissing on the AAI may have shown hyperactivation (as opposed to hypoactivation, which had been expected) as a result of *dysregulation* caused by the arousal of the attachment system. Deactivation in the cortical areas might, in contrast, reflect an expression of the inhibition of attachment behavior, which would, of course, be consistent with the dismissing stance.

In their fMRI study, Galynker and colleagues (2012) found that distinct but overlapping neural networks subserve depression and insecurity on the AAI, which suggests that these interactions might explain the greater difficulty of treating depression in insecure patients.

Farina and colleagues (2014) evaluated cortical connectivity modifications via an EEG lagged coherence analysis following the AAI with 13 patients with dissociative disorders and 13 age- and sex-matched controls. An intriguing new finding was that cortical connectivity *increased* following the AAI in the control subjects but not in the dissociative subjects. In a later report (Farina, Speranza, Imperatori, Quintiliani, & Marca, 2015), again following the AAI, dissociative (but not control) subjects were observed to undergo unfavorable changes indicative of heart rate dysregulation. These results were interpreted as originating in the AAI's demand for a review of childhood attachment experiences impacting dissociative subjects differently.

## Conclusions

The AAI is a unique research tool with the power to tap into multiple psychological and social domains, a point that has been made amply clear by the massive expansion in research since 2008. Nevertheless, there is room for further exploration utilizing the AAI in new areas, including linguistics, cognitive psychology, and, as just illustrated, biology and neuroscience (see Coan, Chapter 12, and Bretherton & Munholland, Chapter 4, this volume). In ending, I remain in agreement with my conclusion in the 1999 edition of this volume:

> Within the AAI, the organization of language pertaining to attachment appears to be a manifestation of the "dynamics" of cognition and emotion as mediated by attention. Individual differences in attentional flexibility may therefore influence patterns of caregiving, which in turn may shape responses in the offspring that influence the organization of its own developing propensities. This has no doubt permanently altered the way language will be considered within the context of clinical and developmental research. (Hesse, 1999, pp. 427–428)

## Appendix 26.1. The Adult Attachment Interview: Administration and Training

### Protocol

The most recent AAI protocol (George, Kaplan, & Main, 1996; 72 manuscript pages) is available from Naomi Gribneau Bahm (ngbreliability@gmail.com).

### Training in the Scoring and Classification of AAI Transcripts

Training in the analysis of the AAI takes place during 2-week institutes, involving one or two certified trainers and 10–20 participants. Usually about seven institutes focused on the Main, Goldwyn, and Hesse system of interview analysis are offered per year. These are taught only by the 10 individuals who have become certified to train by Mary Main and myself. As of 2016, these trainers are Anders Broberg, Nino Dazzi, Sonia Gojman de Millán, Erik Hesse, Tord Ivarsson, Deborah Jacobvitz, Mary Main, David and Deanne Pederson, and June Sroufe. Trainings are frequently offered in North America, Europe, and Mexico, and 10 new trainers from Australia, Austria, Canada, Japan, Sweden, and the United States (East and West Coast) are expected to be certified to train via 2-week training-to-train institutes by December 2016. For dates of upcoming institutes and information, including certified trainer contacts, please see June Sroufe's website (*attachment-training.com*).

It should be noted that having attended an institute held by a certified AAI trainer does not qualify individuals as certified coders. Those wishing to become certified in the analysis of AAI transcripts not only must attend an AAI institute with a certified trainer but also pass a reliability check in which agreement is established with Main and myself across 30 transcripts.

Finally, unfortunately, some individuals who are neither certified in AAI coding nor have attended an AAI institute are (1) claiming certification as AAI coders and/or (2) holding training institutes in the AAI. Some anomalous results will inevitably be incurred when individuals neither trained nor certified in the instrument attempt to implement it in empirical work. As one example, a recent study undertaken and published by untrained, uncertified coders reported a failure to find any link between parental AAI transcripts and infant attachment status as assessed in their offspring. This problem was first identified by Van IJzendoorn (1995), who noted that the extent of an individual's training in the AAI was very strongly related to the ability to predict infant disorganized attachment from parental AAI transcripts.

### Acknowledgments

Parts of this chapter have been adapted from Main, Hesse, and Goldwyn (2008). Copyright 2008 by The Guilford Press. Adapted by permission. I am grateful to Mary Main for her critical input regarding central organizational and substantive aspects of this and earlier editions of this chapter. David and Deanne Pederson made valuable suggestions regarding earlier editions of this presentation, as did Nino Dazzi, Avi Sagi-Schwartz, and Marinus Van IJzendoorn. Early empirical contributions by (listed alphabetically) Ainsworth and Eichberg; Bakermans-Kranenburg and Van IJzendoorn; Crowell and Waters; Fonagy, Steele, and Steele; Main, Kaplan, & Cassidy; Sagi-Schwartz and colleagues; and Ward and Carlson were invaluable to the continuing development of the AAI and inspired many of the researchers who followed upon their work.

With respect to this third (2016) edition of this chapter, I am grateful to Sarah Foster (Northumbria University, United Kingdom), a new and brilliant entrant into the field of attachment, for her extraordinary and meticulous assistance with identifying works suitable for this updated review of the AAI literature. I also thank the Wellcome Trust for supporting Sarah's work in this endeavor via Award No. WT103343AI to Robbie Duschinsky. Finally, I thank Naomi Gribneau Bahm for her invaluable and extensive feedback and assistance in the preparation of this manuscript.

## Notes

1. Violations of these maxims are permitted when "licensed" by the speaker (Grice, 1989). An excessively long speech turn can, for example, be licensed if the speaker begins with "Well, I'm afraid this is going to be quite a long story," whereas a very short turn can be licensed by "I'm really sorry, but I don't feel able to discuss this right now."

2. In the 1999 edition of this volume, I described an Italian study in which coders attempted to apply Grice's four maxims to AAI interview transcripts (Dazzi, DeCoro, Ortu, & Speranza, 1999). Following Gricean maxims as closely as possible, but adding where necessary from the AAI manual (e.g., "passivity" indicators were added directly as violations of manner), these investigators found that, as stated in this chapter, violations of quantity (via excessive brevity) were most pronounced in dismissing texts, and violations of quantity (via excessive length), relevance, and manner were most pronounced in preoccupied texts, whereas relatively few violations of Grice's maxims occurred in secure-autonomous texts. However, more recently, a group of investigators in Leiden who have developed a Coherence Q-Sort have found that attachment-trained sorters place emphasis on different maxims than do naive sorters or linguists; this means that training in AAI institutes remains a necessary prerequisite to identifying the kinds of coherence most relevant to AAI texts (Beijersbergen, Bakermans-Kranenburg, & Van IJzendoorn, 2006).

3. I have composed the quotations in this chapter to preserve confidentiality. Nonetheless, they closely approximate actual quotations from AAI transcripts, and none would seem unusual to an experienced AAI coder.

4. This response is more elaborated than usual, but it has been seen in some interviews and is provided here for heuristic purposes.

5. This does not mean that the same speaker might not also be unresolved.

6. Within AAI manuals the development sample has been accurately described as consisting of 44 participants. However, Main and Goldwyn (1988) had referenced only the initial 36.

7. Notice that, as is the case for infant Strange Situation coding, interview transcripts are always approached first to determine the best-fitting organized category. If the first AAI category placement will ultimately be unresolved or unorganized (cannot classify), the coder must nonetheless designate the organized category that the transcript may secondarily fit (e.g., unresolved/dismissing). The same holds for the Strange Situation, in which an infant judged primarily to be disorganized is also assigned to a best-fitting organized category (e.g., disorganized/avoidant).

8. For both mothers and fathers, as would be expected, coherence of transcript was significantly negatively related to infant avoidance, as was angry preoccupation with either parent, except fathers' preoccupation with their mothers.

9. In a high-risk clinical sample of 37 participants followed across 13 years by Crowell and Hauser (2008), secure–insecure stability was 84%; however, all but two participants were insecure at both time periods, and there was considerable movement among the insecure AAI categories.

10. In an earlier edition of this chapter (Hesse, 2008), I included a first report (57 subjects; Weinfield, Sroufe, & Egeland, 2000). The researchers had used the traditional three-way analysis of behavior in the Strange Situation (disorganized/secure infants were considered secure), and no significant relation between 12-month attachment status and AAI status at age 19 was found. In the more recent report (Sroufe, 2005), disorganized/secure infants had been placed in the insecure infant group, more participants had been seen in the AAI, and the sample had been followed to age 26.

## References

Ablow, J. C., Marks, A. K., Feldman, S. S., & Huffman, L. C. (2013). Associations between first-time expectant women's representations of attachment and their physiological reactivity to infant cry. *Child Development, 84,* 1373–1391.

Abrams, K. Y., Rifkin, A., & Hesse, E. (2006). Examining the role of parental frightened/frightening subtypes in predicting disorganized attachment within a brief observational procedure. *Development and Psychopathology, 18,* 345–361.

Adshead, G., & Bluglass, K. (2005). Attachment representations in mothers with abnormal illness behaviour by proxy. *British Journal of Psychiatry, 187,* 328–333.

Ainsworth, M. D. S. (1967). *Infancy in Uganda: Infant care and the growth of love.* Baltimore: Johns Hopkins University Press.

Ainsworth, M. D. S., Bell, S. M., & Stayton, D. J. (1971). Individual differences in Strange Situation behaviour of one-year-olds. In H.R. Schaffer (Ed.), *The origins of human social relations* (pp. 17–57). New York: Academic Press.

Ainsworth, M. D. S., Blehar, M. C., Waters, E., & Wall, S. (1978). *Patterns of attachment: A psychological study of the Strange Situation.* Hillsdale, NJ: Erlbaum.

Ainsworth, M. D. S., & Eichberg, C. G. (1991). Effects on infant–mother attachment of mother's unresolved loss of an attachment figure or other traumatic experience. In C.M. Parkes, J. Stevenson-Hinde, & P. Marris (Eds.), *Attachment across the life cycle* (pp. 160–183). London: Routledge.

Allen, J. P., Hauser, S. T., & Borman-Spurrell, E. (1996). Attachment theory as a framework for understanding sequelae of severe adolescent psychopathology: An eleven-year follow-up study. *Journal of Consulting and Clinical Psychology, 64,* 254–263.

American Psychiatric Association. (1987). *Diagnostic and statistical manual of mental disorders* (3rd ed., rev.). Washington, DC: Author.

Amini, S., Lewis, T., Lannon, R., & Louie, A. (1996). Affect, attachment, memory: Contributions toward psychobiologic integration. *Psychiatry: Interpersonal and Biological Processes, 59*(3), 213–239.

Ammaniti, M., Dazzi, N., & Muscetta, S. (2008). The AAI in a clinical context: Some experiences and illustrations. In H. Steele & M. Steele (Eds.), *Clinical applications of the Adult Attachment Interview* (pp. 236–269). New York: Guilford Press.

Ammaniti, M., Speranza, A. M., & Candelori, C. (1996). Stability of attachment in children and intergenerational transmission of attachment. *Psichiatria dell'Infanzia e dell'Adolescenza, 63,* 313–332.

Bahm, N. I. G., Simon-Thomas, E. R., Main, M., & Hesse, E. (2016). Unresolved loss predicts event-related potential responses to death-related imagery. *Developmental Psychology.* Manuscript under review.

Bakermans-Kranenburg, M. J., & Van IJzendoorn, M. H. (1993). A psychometric study of the Adult Attachment Interview: Reliability and discriminant validity. *Developmental Psychology, 29,* 870–879.

Bakermans-Kranenburg, M. J., & Van IJzendoorn, M. H. (2009). The first 10,000 Adult Attachment Interviews: Distributions of adult attachment representations in clinical and non-clinical groups. *Attachment and Human Development, 11,* 223–263.

Bakermans-Kranenburg, M. J., Van IJzendoorn, M. H., Caspers, K., & Philibert, R. (2011). DRD4 genotype moderates the impact of parental problems on unresolved loss or trauma. *Attachment and Human Development, 13,* 253–269.

Beckwith, L., Cohen, S. E., & Hamilton, C. E. (1999). Maternal sensitivity during infancy and subsequent life events relate to attachment representation at early adulthood. *Developmental Psychology, 35,* 693–700.

Behrens, K. Y., Hesse, E., & Main, M. (2007). Mothers' attachment status as determined by the Adult Attachment Interview predicts their 6-year-olds' reunion responses: A study conducted in Japan. *Developmental Psychology, 43,* 1553–1567.

Beijersbergen, M. D., Bakermans-Kranenburg, M. J., & Van IJzendoorn, M. H. (2006). The concept of coherence in attachment interviews: Comparing attachment experts, linguists, and non-experts. *Attachment and Human Development, 8,* 353–369.

Benoit, D., & Parker, K. C. H. (1994). Stability and transmission of attachment across three generations. *Child Development, 65,* 1444–1456.

Bick, J., & Dozier, M. (2008). Helping foster parents change: The role of parental state of mind. In H. Steele & M. Steele (Eds.), *Clinical applications of the Adult Attachment Interview* (pp. 452–470). New York: Guilford Press.

Bowlby, J. (1980). *Attachment and loss: Vol. 3. Loss: Sadness and depression.* New York: Basic Books.

Bowlby, J. (1988). Attachment, communication, and the therapeutic process. In J. Bowlby (Ed.), *A secure base: Parent–child attachment and healthy human development* (pp. 137–157). New York: Basic Books.

Broussard, E. R. (1979). Assessment of the adaptive potential of the mother–infant system: The Neonatal Perception Inventories. *Seminars in Perinatology, 3,* 91–100.

Broussard, E. R., & Cassidy, J. (2010). Maternal perception of newborns predicts attachment organization in middle adulthood. *Attachment and Human Development, 12,* 159–172.

Broussard, E. R., & Hartner, M. (1970). Maternal perception of the neonate as related to development. *Child Psychiatry and Human Development, 1,* 16–25.

Buchheim, A., & Kachele, H. (2003). Adult Attachment Interview and psychoanalytic perspective: A single case study. *Psychoanalytic Inquiry, 23,* 81–101.

Buchheim, A., Doering, S., Horz, S., Rentrop, M., Schuster, P., Pokorny, D., et al. (2016). *Change of attachment status in Borderline Personality Disorder: RCT study of transference-focused psychotherapy.* Manuscript submitted for publication.

Carlson, E. A. (1998). A prospective longitudinal study of attachment disorganization/disorientation. *Child Development, 69,* 1107–1128.

Carlson, V., Cicchetti, D., Barnett, D., & Braunwald, K. (1989). Disorganized/disoriented attachment relationships in maltreated infants. *Developmental Psychology, 25,* 525–531.

Caspers, K. M., Paradiso, S., Yucuis, R., Troutman, B., Arndt, S., & Philibert, R. (2009). Association between the serotonin transporter promoter polymorphism (5-HTTLPR) and adult unresolved attachment. *Developmental Psychology, 45,* 64–76.

Caspers, K., Yucuis, R., Troutman, B., & Spinks, R. (2006). Attachment as an organizer of behavior: Implications for substance abuse problems and willingness to seek treatment. *Substance Abuse Treatment, Prevention, and Policy, 1,* 1–10.

Cassibba, R., Granqvist, P., Costantini, A., & Gatto, S. (2008). Attachment and God representations among lay Catholics, priests, and religious: A matched comparison study based on the Adult Attachment Interview. *Developmental Psychology, 44*(6), 1753–1763.

Colizzi, M., Costa, R., Pace, V., & Todarello, O. (2013). Hormonal treatment reduces psychobiological distress in gender identity disorder, independently of the attachment style. *Journal of Sexual Medicine, 10,* 3049–3058.

Constantino, J. N., Chackes, L. M., Wartner, U. G., Gross, N., Brophy, S. L., Vitale, J., et al. (2006). Mental representations of attachment in identical female twins with and without conduct problems. *Child Psychiatry and Human Development, 37,* 65–72.

Creasey, G. (2014). Conflict-management behavior in dual trauma couples. *Psychological Trauma: Theory, Research, Practice, and Policy, 6,* 232–239.

Crowell, J. A., & Hauser, S. T. (2008). AAIs in a high-risk sample: Stability and relation to functioning from adolescence to 39 years. In H. Steele & M. Steele (Eds.), *Clinical applications of the Adult Attachment Interview* (pp. 341–370). New York: Guilford Press.

Crowell, J. A., Treboux, D., & Brockmeyer, S. (2009). Parental divorce and adult children's attachment representations and marital status. *Attachment and Human Development, 11,* 87–101.

Crowell, J. A., Waters, E., Treboux, D., O'Connor, E., Colon-Downs, C., Feider, O., et al. (1996). Discriminant validity of the Adult Attachment Interview. *Child Development, 67,* 2584–2599.

Dazzi, N., DeCoro, A., Ortu, F., & Speranza, A. M. (1999). L'intervista sull'attacamento in preadolescenza: Un'analisi della dimensione della coerenza [The Adult Attachment Interview in pre-adolescence: An analysis of dimensions of coherence]. *Psicologia Clinico dello Sviluppo, 31,* 129–153.

De Wolff, M. S., & Van IJzendoorn, M. H. (1997). Sensitivity and attachment: A meta-analysis on parental antecedents of infant attachment. *Child Development, 68,* 571–591.

Dozier, M., Stovall, K. C., Albus, K. E., & Bates, B. (2001). Attachment for infants in foster care: The role of caregiver state of mind. *Child Development, 72,* 1467–1477.

Dykas, M. J., Woodhouse, S. S., Ehrlich, K. B., & Cassidy, J. (2012). Attachment-related differences in perceptions of an initial peer interaction emerge over time: Evidence of reconstructive memory processes in adolescents. *Developmental Psychology, 48,* 1381–1389.

Egeland, B., Jacobvitz, D., & Sroufe, L. A. (1988). Breaking the cycle of abuse. *Child Development, 59*(4), 1080–1088.

Evans, E. M. (2008). *Understanding maternal trauma: An investigation of the attachment representations, psychological symptomatology, and interactive behaviour of mothers with a trauma history.* Unpublished doctoral dissertation, University of Western Ontario, London, ON, Canada.

Farina, B., Speranza, A. M., Dittoni, S., Gnoni, V., Trentini, C., Vergano, C. M., et al. (2014). Memories of attachment hamper EEG cortical connectivity in dissociative patients. *European Archives of Psychiatry and Clinical Neuroscience, 264*(5), 449–458.

Farina, B., Speranza, A. M., Imperatori, C., Quintiliani, M. I., & Marca, G. D. (2015). Change in heart rate variability after the Adult Attachment Interview in dissociative patients. *Journal of Trauma and Dissociation, 16,* 170–180.

Fearon, R. P., Bakermans-Kranenburg, M. J., Van IJzendoorn, M. H., Lapsley, A. M., & Roisman, G. I. (2010). The significance of insecure attachment and disorganization in the development of children's externalizing behavior: a meta?analytic study. *Child Development, 81*(2), 435–456.

Fonagy, P., Leigh, T., Steele, M., Steele, H., Kennedy, G., Mattoon, M., et al. (1996). The relation of attachment status, psychiatric classification, and response to psychotherapy. *Journal of Consulting and Clinical Psychology, 64,* 22–31.

Fonagy, P., Steele, H., & Steele, M. (1991). Maternal representations of attachment during pregnancy predict the organization of infant–mother attachment at one year of age. *Child Development, 62,* 891–905.

Forguson, L., & Gopnik, A. (1988). The ontogeny of common sense. In J. W. Astington, P. L. Harris, & D. R. Olson (Eds.), *Developing theories of mind* (pp. 226–243). New York: Cambridge University Press.

Frodi, A., Dernevik, M., Sepa, A., Philipson, J., & Bragesjö, M. (2001). Current attachment representations of incarcerated offenders varying in degree of psychopathy. *Attachment and Human Development, 3,* 269–283.

Furman, W., & Simon, V. A. (2004). Concordance in attachment states of mind and styles with respect to fathers and mothers. *Developmental Psychology, 40,* 1239–1247.

Fyffe, C. E., & Waters, E. (1997, April). *Empirical classification of adult attachment status: Predicting group membership.* Paper presented at the biennial meeting of the Society for Research in Child Development, Washington, DC.

Galynker, I. I., Yaseen, Z. S., Katz, C., Zhang, X., Jennings-Donovan, G., Dashnaw, S., et al. (2012). Distinct but overlapping neural networks subserve depression and insecure attachment. *Social Cognitive and Affective Neuroscience, 7,* 896–908.

George, C., Kaplan, N., & Main, M. (1984). *Adult Attachment Interview protocol.* Unpublished manuscript, University of California at Berkeley.

George, C., Kaplan, N., & Main, M. (1985). *Adult Attachment Interview protocol* (2nd ed.). Unpublished manuscript, University of California at Berkeley, Berkeley, CA.

George, C., Kaplan, N., & Main, M. (1996). *Adult Attachment Interview protocol* (3rd ed.). Unpublished manuscript, University of California at Berkeley, Berkeley, CA.

George, C., & West, M. (2011). The Adult Attachment Projective Picture System: Integrating attachment into clinical assessment. *Journal of Personality Assessment, 93*(5), 407–416.

George, C., & West, M. L. (2012). *The Adult Attachment Projective Picture System: Attachment theory and assessment in adults.* New York: Guilford Press.

Gojman de Millán, S., & Millán, S. (2008). The AAI and its contribution to a therapeutic intervention project for violent, traumatized, and suicidal cases. In H. Steele & M. Steele (Eds.), *Clinical applications of the Adult Attachment Interview* (pp. 297–319). New York: Guilford Press.

Granqvist, P., Ivarsson, T., Broberg, A.G., & Hagekull, B. (2007). Examining relations among attachment, religiosity, and New Age spirituality using the Adult Attachment Interview. *Developmental Psychology, 43,* 590–601.

Gribneau, N. I. (2006). *Event-related potentials to cemetery images distinguish electroencephalogram recordings for women unresolved for loss on the Adult Attachment Interview.* Unpublished doctoral dissertation, Department of Integrative Biology, University of California at Berkeley, Berkeley, CA.

Grice, H. P. (1975). Logic and conversation. In P. Cole & J. L. Moran (Eds.), *Syntax and semantics: Vol. 3. Speech acts* (pp. 41–58). New York: Academic Press.

Grice, H. P. (1989). *Studies in the way of words.* Cambridge: Harvard University Press.

Groh, A. M., Roisman, G. I., Booth-La Force, C., Fraley, R. C., Owen, M. T., Cox, M. J., et al. (2014). IV. Stability of attachment security from infancy to late adolescence. *Monographs of the Society for Research in Child Development, 79*(3), 51–66.

Groh, A. M., Roisman, G. I., Van IJzendoorn, M. H., Bakermans-Kranenburg, M. J., & Fearon, R. (2012).

The significance of insecure and disorganized attachment for children's internalizing symptoms: A meta-analytic study. *Child Development, 83*(2), 591–610.

Grossmann, K., Fremmer-Bombik, E., Rudolph, J., & Grossmann, K. E. (1988). Maternal attachment representations as related to patterns of infant–mother attachment and maternal care during the first year. In R.A. Hinde & J. Stevenson-Hinde (Eds.), *Relationships within families: Mutual influences* (pp. 241–260). Oxford, UK: Clarendon Press.

Grossmann, K., Grossmann, K. E., & Kindler, H. (2005). Early care and the roots of attachment and partnership representations: The Bielefeld and Regensburg longitudinal studies. In K. E. Grossmann, K. Grossmann, & E. Waters (Eds.), *Attachment from infancy to adulthood: The major longitudinal studies* (pp. 98–136). New York: Guilford Press.

Hamilton, C. E. (2000). Continuity and discontinuity of attachment from infancy through adolescence. *Child Development, 71,* 690–694.

Harari, D., Bakermans-Kranenburg, M. J., de Kloet, C., Geuze, E., Vermetten, E., Westenberg, H., et al. (2009). Attachment representations in Dutch veterans with and without deployment-related PTSD. *Attachment and Human Development, 11*(6), 515–536.

Hauser, S. T., Golden, E., & Allen, J. P. (2006). Narrative in the study of resilience. *Psychoanalytic Study of the Child, 61,* 205–227.

Heinicke, C. M., Goorsky, M., Levine, M., Ponce, V., Ruth, G., Silverman, M., et al. (2006). Pre- and postnatal antecedents of a home visiting intervention and family developmental outcome. *Infant Mental Health Journal, 27,* 91–119.

Heinicke, C. M., & Levine, S. M. (2008). The AAI anticipates the outcome of a relation-based early intervention. In H. Steele & M. Steele (Eds.), *Clinical applications of the Adult Attachment Interview* (pp. 99–125). New York: Guilford Press.

Hesse, E. (1996). Discourse, memory, and the Adult Attachment Interview: A note with emphasis on the emerging cannot classify category. *Infant Mental Health Journal, 17,* 4–11.

Hesse, E. (1999). The Adult Attachment Interview: Historical and current perspectives. In J. Cassidy & P. R. Shaver (Eds.). *Handbook of attachment: Theory, research, and clinical applications* (pp. 395–433). New York: Guilford Press.

Hesse, E. (2008). The Adult Attachment Interview: Protocol, method of analysis, and empirical studies. In J. Cassidy & P. R. Shaver (Eds.), *Handbook of attachment: Theory, research, and clinical applications* (2nd ed., pp. 552–598). New York: Guilford Press.

Hesse, E., Hobson, R. P., Patrick, M., Maughan, B., & Main, M. (2011, April). *The AAI in a prison population: High scores for unresolved loss in psychopaths, while derogation predicts murder and bodily harm.* Poster presented at the biennial meeting of the Society for Research in Child Development, Montreal, Canada.

Hesse, E., & Main, M. (1999). Second-generation effects of unresolved trauma in non-maltreating parents: Dissociated, frightened, and threatening parental behavior. *Psychoanalytic Inquiry*, 19, 481–540.

Hesse, E., & Main, M. (2000). Disorganized infant, child, and adult attachment: Collapse in behavioral and attentional strategies. *Journal of the American Psychoanalytic Association*, 48, 1097–1127.

Hesse, E., & Main, M. (2006). Frightened, threatening, and dissociative parental behavior in low-risk samples: Description, discussion, and interpretations. *Development and Psychopathology*, 18, 309–343.

Hesse, E., & Van IJzendoorn, M. H. (1998). Parental loss of close family members and propensities towards absorption in offspring. *Developmental Science*, 1, 299–305.

Hesse, E., & Van IJzendoorn, M. H. (1999). Propensities towards absorption are related to lapses in the monitoring of reasoning or discourse during the Adult Attachment Interview: A preliminary investigation. *Attachment and Human Development*, 1, 67–91.

Hobson, R. P., Patrick, M., Maughan, B., Shine, J., MacKeith, J., Main, M., et al. (2016). *Psychopathology and criminal violence: The Adult Attachment Interview in a prison setting.* Manuscript in preparation.

Hughes, P., & McGauley, G. (1997). Mother–infant interaction during the first year with a child who shows disorganization of attachment. *British Journal of Psychotherapy*, 14, 147–158.

Hughes, P., Turton, P., Hopper, E., McGauley, G. A., & Fonagy, P. (2001). Disorganized attachment behavior among infants born subsequent to stillbirth. *Journal of Child Psychology and Psychiatry*, 42, 791–801.

Jacobvitz, D. (2008). Afterword. In H. Steele & M. Steele (Eds.), *Clinical applications of the Adult Attachment Interview* (pp. 471–486). New York: Guilford Press.

Jacobvitz, D., Booher, C., & Hazen, N. (2001, February). *Communication within the dyad: An attachment-theoretical perspective.* Paper presented at the meeting of the Society of Social and Personality Psychologists, San Antonio, TX.

Jacobvitz, D., Hazen, N., Zaccagnino, M., Messina, S., & Beverung, L. (2011). Frightening maternal behavior, infant disorganization and risks for psychopathology. In D. Cicchetti & G. I. Roisman (Eds.), The Minnesota Symposium on Child Psychology: The origins and organization of adaptation and maladaptation (pp. 283–291). Hoboken, NJ: Wiley.

Jacobvitz, D., Leon, K., & Hazen, N. (2006). Does expectant mothers' unresolved trauma predict frightened/frightening maternal behavior?: Risk and protective factors. *Development and Psychopathology*, 18, 363–379.

Jones-Mason, K., Allen, I., Hamilton, S., & Weiss, S. (2015). Comparative validity of the Adult Attachment Interview and the Adult Attachment Projective. *Attachment and Human Development*, 17(5), 429–447.

Kazui, M., Endo, T., Tanaka, A., Sakagami, H., & Suganuma, M. (2000). Intergenerational transmission of attachment: Japanese mother–child dyads. *Japanese Journal of Educational Psychology*, 48, 323–332.

Kernberg, O. F. (1984). *Severe personality disorders: Psychotherapeutic strategies.* New Haven, CT: Yale University Press.

Korfmacher, J., Adam, E., Ogawa, J., & Egeland, B. (1997). Adult attachment: Implications for the therapeutic process in a home intervention. *Applied Developmental Science*, 1, 43–52.

Leerkes, E. M., Supple, A. J., O'Brien, M., Calkins, S. D., Haltigan, J. D., Wong, M. S., et al. (2015). Antecedents of maternal sensitivity during distressing tasks: Integrating attachment, social information processing, and psychobiological perspectives. *Child Development*, 86, 94–111.

Lenzi, D., Trentini, C., Pantano, P., Macaluso, E., Lenzi, G. L., & Ammaniti, M. (2013). Attachment models affect brain responses in areas related to emotions and empathy in nulliparous women. *Human Brain Mapping*, 34, 1399–1414.

Levy, K. N., Meehan, K. B., Kelly, K. M., Reynoso, J. S., Weber, M., Clarkin, J. F., et al. (2006). Change in attachment patterns and reflective function in a randomized control trial of transference-focused psychotherapy for borderline personality disorder. *Journal of Consulting and Clinical Psychology*, 74, 1027–1040.

Lyons-Ruth, K., Bronfman, E., & Parsons, E. (1999). Chapter IV. Maternal frightened, frightening, or atypical behavior and disorganized infant attachment patterns. *Monographs of the Society for Research in Child Development*, 64(3, Serial No. 258), 67–96.

Lyons-Ruth, K., Connell, D. B., Zoll, D., & Stahl, J. (1987). Infants at social risk: Relations among infant maltreatment, maternal behavior, and infant attachment behavior. *Developmental Psychology*, 23, 223–232.

Madigan, S., Bakermans-Kranenburg, M. J., Van IJzendoorn, M. H., Moran, G., Pederson, D. R., & Benoit, D. (2006). Unresolved states of mind, anomalous parental behavior, and disorganized attachment: A review and meta-analysis of a transmission gap. *Attachment and Human Development*, 8, 89–111.

Madigan, S., Moran, G., & Pederson, D. R. (2006). Unresolved states of mind, disorganized attachment relationships, and disrupted interactions of adolescent mothers and their infants. *Developmental Psychology*, 42, 293–304.

Main, M. (Chair). (1985, April). *Attachment: A move to the level of representation.* Symposium conducted at the meeting of the Society for Research in Child Development, Toronto, Canada.

Main, M. (1990). Cross-cultural studies of attachment organization: Recent studies, changing methodologies, and the concept of conditional strategies. *Human Development*, 33, 48–61.

Main, M. (1991). Metacognitive knowledge, metacognitive monitoring, and singular (coherent) vs. multiple (incoherent) models of attachment: Findings and directions for future research. In C. M. Parkes, J. Stevenson-Hinde, & P. Marris (Eds.), *Attachment across the life cycle* (pp. 127–159). London: Routledge.

Main, M. (1993). Discourse, prediction, and recent studies in attachment: Implications for psychoanalysis. *Journal of the American Psychoanalytic Association, 41*(Suppl.), 209–244.

Main, M. (1999). Mary D. Salter Ainsworth: Tribute and portrait. *Psychoanalytic Inquiry, 19,* 682–736.

Main, M. (2000). The organized categories of infant, child, and adult attachment: Flexible vs. inflexible attention under attachment-related stress. *Journal of the American Psychoanalytic Association, 48,* 1055–1096.

Main, M. (2001, April). *Attachment to mother and father in infancy, as related to the Adult Attachment Interview and a self-visualization task at age 19.* Poster presented at the biennial meeting of the Society for Research in Child Development, Minneapolis, MN.

Main, M., & Cassidy, J. (1988). Categories of response to reunion with the parent at age six: Predicted from infant attachment classifications and stable over a one-month period. *Developmental Psychology, 24,* 415–426.

Main, M., DeMoss, A., & Hesse, E. (1989). *Unresolved (disorganized/disoriented) state of mind with respect to experiences of loss.* Unpublished manuscript, University of California, Berkeley, Berkeley, CA.

Main, M., & Goldwyn, R. (1984a). *Adult attachment scoring and classification system.* Unpublished manuscript, University of California, Berkeley, Berkeley, CA.

Main, M., & Goldwyn, R. (1984b). Predicting rejection of her infant from mother's representation of her own experience: Implications for the abused–abusing intergenerational cycle. *International Journal of Child Abuse and Neglect, 8,* 203–217.

Main, M., & Goldwyn, R. (1988). *Interview-based attachment classifications: Related to infant–mother and infant–father attachment.* Unpublished manuscript, University of California, Berkeley, Berkeley, CA.

Main, M., & Goldwyn, R. (1989). *Adult attachment rating and classification system.* Unpublished manuscript, University of California, Berkeley, Berkeley, CA.

Main, M., & Goldwyn, R. (2008). [Parental states of mind and infant attachment in the Bay Area sample]. Unpublished raw data, University of California, Berkeley, Berkeley, CA.

Main, M., Goldwyn, R., & Hesse, E. (2003). *Adult Attachment Scoring and Classification System, Version 7.2.* Unpublished manuscript, University of California, Berkeley, Berkeley, CA.

Main, M., & Hesse, E. (1990). Parents' unresolved traumatic experiences are related to infant disorganized attachment status: Is frightened and/or frightening parental behavior the linking mechanism? In M. T. Greenberg, D. Cicchetti, & E. M. Cummings (Eds.), *Attachment in the preschool years: Theory, research, and intervention* (pp. 161–182). Chicago: University of Chicago Press.

Main, M., & Hesse, E. (1991). *Frightening, frightened, dissociated, deferential, sexualized and disorganized parental behavior: A coding system for frightening parent–infant interactions.* Unpublished manuscript, University of California, Berkeley, Berkeley, CA.

Main, M., & Hesse, E. (1998). *Frightening, frightened, dissociated, deferential, sexualized and disorganized parental behavior: A coding system for frightening parent–infant interactions.* Unpublished manuscript, University of California, Berkeley, Berkeley, CA.

Main, M., Hesse, E., & Kaplan, N. (2005). Predictability of attachment behavior and representational processes at 1, 6, and 19 years of age: The Berkeley longitudinal study. In K. E. Grossmann, K. Grossmann, & E. Waters (Eds.), *Attachment from infancy to adulthood: The major longitudinal studies* (pp. 245–304). New York: Guilford Press.

Main, M., Kaplan, N., & Cassidy, J. (1985). Security in infancy, childhood, and adulthood: A move to the level of representation. In I. Bretherton & E. Waters (Eds.), Growing points of attachment theory and research. *Monographs of the Society for Research in Child Development, 50*(1–2, Serial No. 209), 66–104.

Main, M., & Solomon, J. (1986). Discovery of an insecure-disorganized/disoriented attachment pattern. In T. B. Brazelton & M. W. Yogman (Eds.), *Affective development in infancy* (pp. 95–124). Norwood: Ablex.

Main, M., & Solomon, J. (1990). Procedures for identifying infants as disorganized/disoriented during the Ainsworth Strange Situation. In M. T. Greenberg, D. Cicchetti, & E. M. Cummings (Eds.), *Attachment in the preschool years: Theory, research, and intervention* (pp. 121–160). Chicago: University of Chicago Press.

Main, M., & Weston, D. (1981). The quality of the toddler's relationship to mother and to father: Related to conflict behavior and the readiness to establish new relationships. *Child Development, 52,* 932–940.

Manassis, K., Bradley, S., Goldberg, S., Hood, J., & Swinson, R. P. (1994). Attachment in mothers with anxiety disorders and their children. *Journal of the American Academy of Child and Adolescent Psychiatry, 33,* 1106–1113.

McKinnon, C. C., Moran, G., & Pederson, D. (2004). Attachment representations of deaf adults. *Journal of Deaf Studies and Deaf Education, 9,* 366–386.

McMahon, C. A., Barnett, B., Kowalenko, N. M., & Tennant, C. C. (2006). Maternal attachment state of mind moderates the impact of post-natal depression on infant attachment. *Journal of Child Psychology and Psychiatry, 47,* 660–669.

Mikulincer, M., & Shaver, P. R. (2016). *Attachment in adulthood: Structure, dynamics, and change* (2nd ed.). New York: Guilford Press.

Minde, K., & Hesse, E. (1996). The role of the Adult Attachment Interview in parent–infant psychotherapy: A case presentation. *Infant Mental Health Journal, 17,* 115–126.

Murphy, A., Steele, M., Dube, S. R., Bate, J., Bonuck, K., Meissner, P., et al. (2014). Adverse Childhood Experiences (ACEs) Questionnaire and Adult Attachment Interview (AAI): Implications for parent child relationships. *Child Abuse and Neglect, 38,* 224–233.

Muscetta, S., Dazzi, N., Decoro, A., Ortu, F., & Speranza, A. M. (1999). "States of mind with respect to attachment" and change in a psychotherapeutic relationship: A study of the coherence of transcript in a short-term psychotherapy with an adolescent. *Psychoanalytic Inquiry, 19*(5), 885–921.

Nye, E., Katzman, J., Bell, J., Kilpatrick, J., Brainard, M., & Haaland, K. (2008). Attachment organization in Vietnam combat veterans with posttraumatic stress disorder. *Attachment and Human Development, 10*(1), 41–57.

Ogawa, J. R., Sroufe, L. A., Weinfield, N. S., Carlson, E. A., & Egeland, B. (1997). Development and the fragmented self: Longitudinal study of dissociative symptomatology in a nonclinical sample. *Development and Psychopathology, 9,* 855–879.

Paley, B. J., Cox, M. J., Burchinal, M. R., & Payne, C. C. (1999). Attachment and marital functioning: Comparison of spouses with continuous-secure, earned-secure, dismissing, and preoccupied attachment stances. *Journal of Family Psychology, 13,* 580–597.

Patrick, M., Hobson, R. P., Castle, D., Howard, R., & Maughan, B. (1994). Personality disorder and the mental representation of early social experience. *Development and Psychopathology, 6,* 375–388.

Pearson, J. L., Cohn, D. A., Cowan, P. A., & Cowan, C. P. (1994). Earned- and continuous-security in adult attachment: Relation to depressive symptomatology and parenting style. *Development and Psychopathology, 6,* 359–373.

Phelps, J. L., Belsky, J., & Crnic, K. (1998). Earned security, daily stress, and parenting: A comparison of five alternative models. *Development and Psychopathology, 10,* 21–38.

Pianta, R. C., Egeland, B., & Adam, E. K. (1996). Adult attachment classification and self-reported psychiatric symptomatology as assessed by the Minnesota Multiphasic Personality Inventory–2. *Journal of Consulting and Clinical Psychology, 64,* 273–281.

Pierrehumbert, B., Torrisi, R., Ansermet, F., Borghini, A., & Halfon, O. (2012). Adult attachment representations predict cortisol and oxytocin responses to stress. *Attachment and Human Development, 14,* 453–476.

Pierrehumbert, B., Torrisi, R., Glatz, N., Dimitrova, N., Heinrichs, M., & Halfon, O. (2009). The influence of attachment on perceived stress and cortisol response to acute stress in women sexually abused in childhood or adolescence. *Psychoneuroendocrinology, 34,* 924–938.

Riem, M. M. E., Bakermans-Kranenburg, M. J., Van IJzendoorn, M. H., Out, D., & Rombouts, S. A. R. B. (2012). Attachment in the brain: Adult attachment representations predict amygdala and behavioral responses to infant crying. *Attachment and Human Development, 14,* 533–551.

Rifkin-Graboi, A. (2008). Attachment status and salivary cortisol in a normal day and during simulated interpersonal stress in young men. *Stress, 11,* 210–224.

Roisman, G. I., Fortuna, K., & Holland, A. (2006). An experimental manipulation of retrospectively defined earned and continuous attachment security. *Child Development, 77,* 59–71.

Roisman, G. I., Fraley, R. C., & Belsky, J. (2007). A taxometric study of the Adult Attachment Interview. *Developmental Psychology, 43,* 675–686.

Roisman, G. I., Haltigan, J. D., Haydon, K. C., & Booth-LaForce, C. (2014). VI. Earned-security in retrospect: Depressive symptoms, family stress, and maternal and paternal sensitivity from early childhood to mid-adolescence. *Monographs of the Society for Research in Child Development, 79*(3), 85–107.

Roisman, G. I., Holland, A., Fortuna, K., Fraley, R. C., Clausell, E., & Clarke, A. (2007). The Adult Attachment Interview and self-reports of attachment style: An empirical rapprochement. *Journal of Personality and Social Psychology, 92,* 678–697.

Roisman, G. I., Padrón, E., Sroufe, L. A., & Egeland, B. (2002). Earned-secure attachment status in retrospect and prospect. *Child Development, 73,* 1204–1219.

Rosenthal, R. (1991). *Meta-analytic procedures for social research* (rev. ed.). Newbury Park, CA: Sage.

Rutter, M., Quinton, D., & Hill, J. (1990). Adult outcome of institution-reared children: Males and females compared. In L. N. Robins & M. Rutter (Eds.), *Straight and devious pathways from childhood to adulthood* (pp. 135–157). Cambridge, UK: Cambridge University Press.

Sagi, A., Van IJzendoorn, M. H., Scharf, M. H., Joels, T., Koren-Karie, N., Mayseless, O., et al. (1997). Ecological constraints for intergenerational transmission of attachment. *International Journal of Behavioral Development, 20,* 287–299.

Sagi, A., Van IJzendoorn, M. H., Scharf, M. H., Koren-Karie, N., Joels, T., & Mayseless, O. (1994). Stability and discriminant validity of the Adult Attachment Interview: A psychometric study in young Israeli adults. *Developmental Psychology, 30,* 771–777.

Sagi-Schwartz, A., & Aviezer, O. (2005). Correlates of attachment to multiple caregivers in kibbutz children from birth to emerging adulthood: The Haifa longitudinal study. In K. E. Grossmann, K. Grossmann, & E. Waters (Eds.), *Attachment from infancy to adulthood: The major longitudinal studies* (pp. 165–197). New York: Guilford Press.

Sagi-Schwartz, A., Van IJzendoorn, M. H., Grossmann, K. E., Joels, T., Grossmann, K., Scharf, M., et al. (2003). Attachment and traumatic stress in female Holocaust child survivors and their daughters. *American Journal of Psychiatry, 160,* 1086–1092.

Santona, A., & Zavattini, G. C. (2005). Partnering and parenting expectations in adoptive couples. *Sexual and Relationship Therapy, 20,* 309–322.

Saunders, R., Jacobvitz, D., Zaccagnino, M., Beverung, L. M., & Hazen, N. (2011). Pathways to earned-security: The role of alternative support figures. *Attachment and Human Development, 13,* 403–420.

Schimmenti, A., Guglielmucci, F., Barbasio, C., & Granieri, A. (2012). Attachment disorganization and dissociation in virtual worlds: A study on problematic internet use among players of online role playing games. *Clinical Neuropsychiatry, 9*(5), 195–202.

Schuengel, C., Bakermans-Kranenburg, M. J., & Van IJzendoorn, M. H. (1999). Frightening maternal behavior linking unresolved loss and disorganized infant attachment. *Journal of Consulting and Clinical Psychology, 67,* 54–63.

Solomon, J., & George, C. (2011). Disorganization of maternal caregiving across two generations: The origins of caregiving helplessness. In J. Solomon & C. George (Eds.), *Disorganized attachment and caregiving* (pp. 25–51). New York: Guilford Press.

Solomon, J., George, C., & De Jong, A. (1995). Children classified as controlling at age six: Evidence of disorganized representational strategies and aggression at home and at school. *Development and Psychopathology, 7,* 447–463.

Sroufe, L. A. (2005). Attachment and development: A prospective, longitudinal study from birth to adulthood. *Attachment and Human Development, 7*(4), 349–367.

Sroufe, L. A., & Waters, E. (1977). Attachment as an organizational construct. *Child Development, 48,* 1184–1199.

Steele, H., Phibbs, E., & Woods, R. (2004). Coherence of mind in daughter caregivers of mothers with dementia: Links with their mothers' joy and relatedness on reunion in a Strange Situation. *Attachment and Human Development, 6,* 439–450.

Steele, H., & Steele, M. (2007, July). *Intergenerational patterns of attachment: From pregnancy in one generation to adolescence in the next.* Paper presented at the International Attachment Conference, Changing Troubled Attachment Relations: Views from Research and Clinical Work, Braga, Portugal.

Steele, H., Steele, M., & Fonagy, P. (1996). Associations among attachment classifications of mothers, fathers, and their infants. *Child Development, 67,* 541–555.

Steele, M., Hodges, J., Kaniuk, J., Hillman, S., & Henderson, K. (2003). Attachment representations and adoption: Associations between maternal states of mind and emotional narratives in previously maltreated children. *Journal of Child Psychotherapy, 29,* 187–205.

Steele, R. D., Waters, T. E. A., Bost, K. K., Vaughn, B. E., Truitt, W., Waters, H. S., et al. (2014). Caregiving antecedents of secure base script knowledge: A comparative analysis of young adult attachment representations. *Developmental Psychology, 50,* 2526–2538.

Thomson, P., & Jaque, S. V. (2012a). Dissociation and the Adult Attachment Interview in artists and performing artists. *Attachment and Human Development, 14,* 145–160.

Thomson, P., & Jaque, S. V. (2012b). Holding a mirror up to nature: Psychological vulnerability in actors. *Psychology of Aesthetics, Creativity, and the Arts, 6,* 361–369.

Torgerson, A. M., Grova, B. K., & Sommerstad, R. (2007). A pilot study of attachment patterns in adult twins. *Attachment and Human Development, 9,* 127–138.

Van IJzendoorn, M. H. (1995). Adult attachment representations, parental responsiveness, and infant attachment: A meta-analysis on the predictive validity of the Adult Attachment Interview. *Psychological Bulletin, 117,* 387–403.

Van IJzendoorn, M. H., & Bakermans-Kranenburg, M. J. (1996). Attachment representations in mothers, fathers, adolescents, and clinical groups: A meta-analytic search for normative data. *Journal of Consulting and Clinical Psychology, 64,* 8–21.

Van IJzendoorn, M. H., & Bakermans-Kranenburg, M. J. (2008). The distribution of adult attachment representations in clinical groups: A meta-analytic search for patterns of attachment in 105 AAI studies. In H. Steele & M. Steele (Eds.), *Clinical applications of the Adult Attachment Interview* (pp. 69–96). New York: Guilford Press.

Van IJzendoorn, M. H., & Bakermans-Kranenburg, M. J. (2014). Invited commentary: Confined quest for continuity: The categorical versus continuous nature of attachment. *Monographs of the Society for Research in Child Development, 79*(3), 157–167.

Van IJzendoorn, M. H., Caspers, K., Bakermans-Kranenburg, M.J., Beach, S. R. H., & Philibert, R. (2010). Methylation matters: Interaction between methylation density and serotonin transporter genotype predicts unresolved loss or trauma. *Biological Psychiatry, 68,* 405–407.

Van IJzendoorn, M. H., Schuengel, C., & Bakermans-Kranenburg, M. J. (1999). Disorganized attachment in early childhood: Meta-analysis of precursors, concomitants, and sequelae. *Development and Psychopathology, 11*(02), 225–250.

Verhage, M. L., Schuengel, C., Madigan, S., Fearson, R. M. P., Oosterman, M., Cassibba, R., et al. (2015). Narrowing the transmission gap: A synthesis of three decades of research on intergenerational transmission of attachment. *Psychological Bulletin.* [Epub ahead of print] *http//dx.doi.org/10.1037/bul0000038*

Ward, M. J., & Carlson, E. A. (1995). Associations among adult attachment representations, maternal sensitivity, and infant–mother attachment in a sample of adolescent mothers. *Child Development, 66,* 69–79.

Ward, M. J., Lee, S. S., & Polan, H. J. (2006). Attachment and psychopathology in a community sample. *Attachment and Human Development, 8,* 327–340.

Waters, E., Merrick, S., Treboux, D., Crowell, J., & Albersheim, L. (2000). Attachment security in infancy and early adulthood: A twenty-year longitudinal study. *Child Development, 71,* 684–689.

Waters, H. S., & Waters, E. (2006). The attachment working models concept: Among other things, we build script-like representations of secure-base experiences. *Attachment and Human Development, 8,* 185–197.

*Webster's New International Dictionary of the English Language.* (1959). (A. Neilson, Ed., 2nd ed., unabridged). Springfield, MA: C. & G. Merriam.

Weinfield, N. S., Sroufe, L. A., & Egeland, B. (2000). Attachment from infancy to adulthood in a high-risk sample: Continuity, discontinuity and their correlates. *Child Development, 71,* 695–7021.

Yeomans, F. E., Clarkin, J. F., & Kernberg, O. F. (2015). *Transference-focused psychotherapy for personality disorder: A clinical guide.* Arlington, VA: American Psychiatric Publishing.

Zegers, M. A., Schuengel, C., Van IJzendoorn, M. H., & Janssens, J. M. (2006). Attachment representations of institutionalized adolescents and their professional caregivers: Predicting the development of therapeutic relationships. *American Journal of Orthopsychiatry, 76,* 325–334.

# Chapter 27

# Measurement of Individual Differences in Adult Attachment

Judith A. Crowell
R. Chris Fraley
Glenn I. Roisman

Human attachments play a vital role . . . from the cradle to the grave.
—John Bowlby (1969/1982, p. 208)

**B**owlby and Ainsworth both addressed the importance of the attachment system across the lifespan, and beginning in the mid-1980s, research in adult attachment began to emerge from the theoretical and empirical groundwork laid with respect to the attachment system in infancy. Following an interest in attachment representations, George, Kaplan, and Main (1984, 1985, 1996) created the Adult Attachment Interview (AAI) "to assess the security of the adult's overall working model of attachment, that is, the security of the self in relation to attachment in its generality rather than in relation to any particular present or past relationship" (Main, Kaplan, & Cassidy, 1985, p. 78). Around the same time the AAI was being developed, Hazan and Shaver (1987; Shaver & Hazan, 1988) began to consider the applicability of attachment theory in general, and of Ainsworth's infant classification scheme in particular, to the study of feelings and behavior in romantic relationships.

Given the independence of these groups of investigators, and their different domains of interest and varied professional backgrounds, the lines

of research they initiated developed in different ways. Each inspired variations and offshoots, so that today there are a number of measures of adult attachment. Given their diverse origins, there has been confusion about what these assessments measure, what they are *intended* to measure, and how they are related to each other. In this chapter we aim to identify advances in the measurement literature in recent years, and to continue to provide up-to-date guidelines for researchers undertaking studies of adult attachment. There is a good deal of evidence that different measures of adult attachment do not necessarily converge empirically (e.g., Haydon, Roisman, Marks, & Fraley, 2011; Roisman, Holland, et al., 2007), even though they were all inspired by attachment theory and sometimes relate similarly to outcome variables. As such, not all measures can be used interchangeably in research, and choosing an appropriate measure requires careful thought about the goals of one's study and its foundation in the literature.

We present in the first section of the chapter a brief discussion of attachment theory, especially elements that are key to understanding the attachment system in adults and to assessing it. We discuss the AAI and other narrative measures derived from the developmental tradition, such as the Attachment Script Assessment and the Current Relationship Interview, in the second section. In the third section we describe advances in our understanding of the self-report measures of attachment that grew out of Hazan and Shaver's (1987) efforts to apply Ainsworth's discoveries to the study of romantic relationships, and include some discussion of priming assessments. In the final section we summarize the overlap and distinctions among measures developed in different lines of research on adult attachment.

Before beginning, we note that in the previous two editions of this handbook, this chapter reviewed a variety of self-report measures that have been used to assess attachment to parents and peers, and attachment history more generally. In the interest of conserving space, we have omitted those reviews in this edition. We refer interested readers to previous editions for further information about the Attachment History Questionnaire by Pottharst (1990), the Inventory of Parent and Peer Attachment by Armsden and Greenberg (1987), and the Reciprocal Attachment Questionnaire for Adults and the Avoidant Attachment Questionnaire for Adults (e.g., West, Sheldon, & Reiffer, 1987; West & Sheldon-Keller, 1994).

## Adult Attachment: Theoretical Issues

Two themes from attachment theory are critical to measurement. The first is that the attachment system is *normative*—that is, relevant to the development of all people, and active and important in adult life. The second idea is that there are individual differences in attachment behavior and associated cognitive and emotional elements.

### Adult Attachment

Although some of Bowlby's original inspiration for attachment theory came from his work as a clinician, he primarily drew from research in ethology, observations of animal behavior, and the cognitive psychology of his day. He described the attachment behavioral system as an evolutionarily adaptive motivational–behavioral control system.

The attachment system promotes safety in infancy and childhood through the child's relationship with an attachment figure or caregiver (Bowlby, 1969/1982). Attachment behavior is activated in times of danger, stress, and novelty, with the goal of gaining and maintaining proximity and contact with an attachment figure. Hence, the behavioral manifestations are context-specific (evident in times of danger or anxiety), although elements of the attachment system are active at all times via continuous monitoring of the environment and the availability of attachment figures (Ainsworth, Blehar, Waters, & Wall, 1978; Bretherton, 1985). A child can confidently explore the environment with the active support of a caregiver, secure in the knowledge that this attachment figure is available if a significant need or question should arise. Ainsworth and colleagues (1978) termed this interaction between child and caregiver the "secure base phenomenon," a concept central to attachment theory.

Ainsworth (1991) highlighted the function of the attachment behavioral system in adult relationships, be they parent and child, partner and partner, or adult child caring for aging parent, and emphasized the secure-base phenomenon as the critical element. She stated that a secure attachment relationship is one that facilitates functioning and competence outside of the relationship: There is "a seeking to obtain an experience of security and comfort in the relationship with the partner. If and when such security and comfort are available, the individual is able to move off from the secure base provided by the partner, with the confidence to engage in other activities" (p. 38). Attachment relationships are distinguished from other adult relationships in that they provide feelings of security and belonging, and without them there is loneliness and restlessness (Weiss, 1973, 1991). This function is distinguished from aspects of relationships that provide guidance or companionship; sexual gratification; opportunities to feel needed or to share common interests or experiences, feelings of competence, or alliance and assistance (Ainsworth, 1985; Weiss, 1974). Behavioral elements of attachment in adult life are similar to those observed in infancy: a desire for proximity to the attachment figure when stressed, increased comfort in the presence of the attachment figure, and anxiety when the attachment figure is inaccessible (Shaver & Hazan, 1988; Weiss, 1991). Grief is experienced following the loss of an attachment figure (Bowlby, 1980; Fraley & Shaver, Chapter 3, this volume).

## Individual Differences and Mental Representations or Working Models

The study of adult attachment processes has not tended to emphasize adult attachment relationships and the normative developmental aspects of the attachment system (yet see Zeifman & Hazan, Chapter 20, this volume). Rather, the field has focused largely on individual differences in the organization of attachment behavior and cognitions, and in expectations regarding attachment relationships. The idea of individual differences emerged from the work of Ainsworth and her colleagues (1978), who broadly characterized the infant patterns of attachment as "secure" and "insecure" (which she sometimes called "anxious"). In addition to the security–insecurity distinction, Ainsworth and colleagues drew a second distinction between "avoidance and conflict relevant to close bodily contact" (p. 298)—the avoidant and resistant behaviors that distinguish two of the major insecure patterns. It is important to note that individual differences in attachment security represent differences in the quality of the attachment relationship: "The most conspicuous dimension that has emerged so far is not strength of attachment but security vs. anxiety in the attachment relationship. This does not imply substitution of degree of security for degree of strength" (p. 298). These dimensional aspects of attachment are increasingly relevant to our understanding of adult attachment (Fraley & Roisman, 2014; Fraley & Spieker, 2003b).

Differences among attachment patterns are thought to develop primarily from different experiences with an attachment figure, rather than being directly influenced by genetics, child temperament, or other child characteristics (Ainsworth et al., 1978; Luijk et al., 2011; Roisman, Booth-LaForce, Belsky, Burt, & Groh, 2013; Roisman & Fraley, 2008; Vaughn & Bost, Chapter 10, this volume). The secure pattern characterizes the infant who seeks and receives protection, reassurance, and comfort when stressed. Confident exploration is optimized because of the support and availability of the caregiver. The child comes to feel secure with the attachment figure; hence, the behavioral system corresponds closely with cognitions and emotions in the context of attachment-related experiences. The two major insecure patterns ("avoidant" and "resistant") develop when attachment behavior is met by rejection, inconsistency, or threat from the attachment figure, leaving the infant "anxious" about the caregiver's responsiveness. To reduce this anxiety, the infant's behavior adapts to fit or complement the attachment figure's behavior in the service of minimizing psychological and/or physical distance from a nonoptimal caregiver; in other words, it is strategic within the context of that relationship (Main, 1981, 1990). However, attention to the caregiver in this anxious, strategic way compromises both direct approaches for help and exploratory behavior, and thus is potentially maladaptive outside of that particular relationship.

Current theory and research on adult attachment draw heavily on Bowlby's concept of attachment representations. Importing ideas from cognitive psychology, Bowlby (1973, 1980) hypothesized that individuals develop representations of the functioning and significance of close relationships that make early experiences "portable" to other interpersonal contexts, possibly into the years of maturity. These representations consist of a person's beliefs and expectations about how attachment relationships operate and what he or she gains from them. These cognitive–affective connections mirror the behavioral patterns that emerge in the context of behavioral interactions between an infant/child and parents (Bowlby, 1980).

These cognitions are variably called working models, representations, or states of mind because they are the basis for action in attachment-related situations. They are hypothesized to be relatively stable and can operate automatically, without the need for conscious appraisal; they guide behavior in relationships with parents, and influence expectations, strategies, and behavior in later relationships (Bretherton, 1985; Bretherton & Munholland, Chapter 4, this volume; Main et al., 1985). Nevertheless, at least some aspects are open to revision as a function of significant attachment-related experiences (Booth-LaForce et al., 2014; Crowell, Treboux, & Waters, 2002).

Bowlby's incorporation of mental representations into attachment theory allowed for a lifespan perspective on the attachment system, providing a way of understanding developmental change in the expression of attachment and its ongoing influence on development and behavior in relationships. Bowlby (1973, 1980) also wrote about the problems that arise when a child is presented with a negative view of self and other, and/or with incompatible data about his or her experiences—that is, when the child's firsthand experience of the attachment figure is in opposition to what the parent tells the child about the meaning of the parental behavior. Because information relevant to characterizing an attachment relationship comes from multiple sources (Bowlby, 1973), a child may receive conflicting information that challenges the development of a coherent or efficient representation. Bowlby (1973) and Main (1981, 1990, 1991), among others, have described the strategies required to maintain cognitive organization in the face of stress and conflicting information. These "secondary" strategies (as opposed to the primary strategy of approach, contact seeking, and contact maintenance when the attachment system is activated) require "manipulating the level of output usually called for by the [attachment] system—[and, in addition, manipulating cognitive processes to maintain] a given attachment organization" (Main, 1990, p. 48). Such strategies develop because there are inconsistencies, incompatibilities, and a lack of internal connectedness in the elements of the attachment representation (Bowlby, 1973; Main, 1990, 1991). Strategies may include avoidance of the attachment figure in stressful situations (Main, 1981), oscillation between the two viewpoints (i.e., "child good, parent bad," "child bad, parent good"), and/or acceptance of the parent's view while denying one's own experience (Bowlby, 1973).

A central idea in attachment theory is that early parent–child relationships are prototypes of later love relationships (Roisman, Collins, Sroufe, & Egeland, 2005; Waters, Kondo-Ikemura, Posada, & Richters, 1991). Bowlby hypothesized that early experiences are very influential, and there is a strong tendency toward continuity in parent–child interactions, which affects the continuing development of the attachment system. That is, in addition to having effects on individual personality characteristics, child–parent relationships influence subsequent patterns of family organization and therefore play a role in the intergenerational transmission of family attachment patterns. Much of adult attachment research has been based on the assumption that there are parallel individual differences in infant and adult patterns of attachment and attachment representations (e.g., Hazan & Shaver, 1987; Main et al., 1985; Mikulincer & Shaver, 2007).

Bowlby (1969/1982) also discussed change in attachment patterns. In childhood, if an attachment pattern changes, it is assumed to have been caused by a corresponding change in the quality of parent–child interactions. Bowlby also hypothesized that change in attachment patterns can occur in later life through the influence of new

attachment relationships and the development of formal operational thought. This combination of events would allow the individual to reflect on and reinterpret the meaning of past and present experiences (Bowlby, 1973, 1980, 1988)—for example, within a marriage or as a consequence of psychotherapy. In a couple's relationship, partners can co-construct new attachment representations that take into account both partners' attachment representations, as well as other elements of the relationship (Crowell, Treboux, & Waters, 2002; Haydon, Collins, Salvatore, Simpson, & Roisman, 2012; Oppenheim & Waters, 1995; Owens et al., 1995; Treboux, Crowell, & Waters, 2004). Furthermore, individuals may draw conscious conclusions about their romantic relationships, and their general or specific behaviors or feelings in these relationships.

In general, researchers have attributed the development of adult attachment patterns to three broad sources, although the relative importance and influence of the three sources has been an important research question (see, e.g., Fraley, 2002; Owens et al., 1995; Waters et al., 1991). These sources are: (1) parent–child attachment relationships; (2) peer and romantic relationship experiences, including exposure to one's parents' marriage; and (3) a current adult attachment relationship (Crowell, Treboux, Gao, et al., 2002; Crowell, Treboux, & Waters, 2002; Fraley, Roisman, Booth-LaForce, Owen, & Holland, 2013; Treboux et al., 2004; Zeifman & Hazan, Chapter 20, this volume).

In summary, two core propositions in attachment theory are key to understanding attachment in adulthood and to evaluating existing measures of adult attachment: (1) The attachment system is active in adults, and (2) there are individual differences in adult attachment behavior that have their foundations in attachment experiences and are embodied in both conscious and subconscious mental processes.

## Narrative Assessments of Adult Attachment

The measures described in the following sections are based on the concept of *attachment security*, defined as the effectiveness of an individual's use of an attachment figure as a *secure base* from which to explore and a *safe haven* in times of distress or danger (secure). The use of narratives to assess attachment started with the idea that "mental processes vary as distinctively as do behavioral processes" (Main et al., 1985, p. 78), and that organized behavioral, cognitive, and affective processes are reflected in coherent, organized language. Narrative assessments have derived their validity from observations of attachment behavior in natural settings, and secondarily from their associations with each other.

## The Adult Attachment Interview

In what Main and colleagues (1985) called "a move to the level of representation" (in contrast to the focus on behavior in parent–child attachment relationships), they developed a semistructured interview for adults about childhood attachment experiences and the meaning currently assigned by an individual to past attachment-related experiences (George et al., 1984, 1985, 1996). This AAI and its scoring systems are based on several key ideas about attachment, including the ideas that working models operate at least partially outside of awareness; that they are based on attachment-relevant experiences; that infants begin to develop models that guide behavior in attachment relationships in the first year of life; that representations provide guidelines for behavior and affective appraisal of experience; that formal operational thought allows the individual to observe and assess a given relationship system and, hence, the model of the relationship can be altered without an actual change in experiences in the relationship; and that the models are not templates but are mental structures that serve to "obtain or to limit access to information" (Main et al., 1985, p. 77). In some ways, the "working model" assessed by the AAI can be considered to be an attachment script, developing and elaborating in the context of experience, and serving as a guide for attachment-relevant behavior (see Roisman, 2009). In addition, the AAI scoring system is linked to Bowlby's and Main's ideas about secondary strategies and incompatible models described earlier.

During an AAI, the adult is interviewed about his or her general view of the relationship with parents; ordinary experiences with parents in which the attachment system is presumed to be activated (upset, injury, illness, separation); experiences of loss and/or abuse; and finally the meaning that the adult attributes to these experiences in terms of the parents' behavior and the development of the interviewee's adult personality and behavior. The resulting narrative is transcribed

verbatim, and the transcript is examined for material directly expressed, as well as for unintended qualities of discourse, such as incoherence and inconsistency. Scoring is based on (1) the coder's assessment of the individual's childhood experiences with parents; (2) the language used by the individual; and (3) most importantly, the individual's ability to give an integrated, believable account of experiences and their meaning. The speaker's discourse is considered a reflection of the current "*state of mind* with respect to attachment" (Hesse, Chapter 26, this volume; Main et al., 1985; Main & Goldwyn, 1984; Main, Goldwyn, & Hesse, 2003).

## Main and Goldwyn's Scoring System

The AAI scoring system (e.g., Main & Goldwyn, 1985; Main et al., 2003) was developed by examining parental interviews for which the Strange Situation procedure classifications of the interviewees' infants were already known, and identifying qualities of content and discourse that distinguished among them. Hence, the AAI was expressly developed to capture the issues tapped by the Strange Situation, especially an individual's ability to use an attachment figure as a secure base. The system has been refined over the past 30 years, but it has not yet been published. Extensive training is required to administer and score the interview.

Scoring is done from a transcript, and there are two sets of scales used to sort participants inductively into the primay attachment classifications described below: maternal and paternal *inferred childhood experience* scales and *state of mind* scales. Parental behavior is rated by the coder from the specific memories and descriptions given of parental behavior, not from the assessment of the parenting given by the individual. These inferred childhood experience scales, rated separately for mother and father, include the following: Loving, Rejecting, Neglecting, Involving (i.e., role reversal), and Pressuring to Achieve. The state of mind scales assess discourse style and particular forms of coherence and incoherence: Idealization, Insistence on Lack of Recall, Active Anger, Derogation, Fear of Loss, Metacognitive Monitoring, and Passivity of Speech. Using these ratings and the overall coherence of the transcript, the coder also assigns scores for coherence of transcript and of mind. The concept of *coherence* is based on Grice's (1975) maxims regarding discourse: High coherence means that the narrative adheres to

Grice's maxims of *quality* (it is believable, without contradictions or illogical conclusions), *quantity* (enough, but not too much, information is given to permit the coder to understand the narrative), *relevance* (the individual answers the questions asked), and *manner* (the individual uses fresh, clear language rather than jargon, canned speech, or nonsense words).

Patterns of scale scores are used to assign an adult to one of three major classifications: a secure category ("autonomous") or one of two insecure categories ("dismissing" or "preoccupied"), with the coherence scales being used to make the secure–insecure distinction. The categories parallel the three infant attachment patterns identified by Ainsworth and colleagues (1978), and the discourse style reflects the behavioral elements in infant attachment patterns. Indeed, a recent analysis of coding of narrative secure-base content of the AAI indicated that the correlation between AAI coherence and a laboratory caregiving and care seeking assessment was largely (80%) accounted for by secure-base script knowledge (T. E. Waters, Brockmeyer, & Crowell, 2013).

Individuals classified as secure/autonomous maintain a balanced view of early relationships, value attachment relationships, and view attachment-related experiences as influential in their development. In parallel to the direct approach of the secure infant, the autonomous adult's approach to the interview is open, direct, and cooperative, regardless of how difficult the memories reported are to discuss. The interview itself contains consistent, believable reports of behavior by parents; simply put, the adult's general descriptions of the parenting he or she received correspond well to the specific memories given of parental behavior. Because security is inferred from coherence, any kind of childhood experience may be associated with being classified as autonomous, although in many cases parental behavior is indeed summarized as loving, and there are clear and specific memories given of loving behavior by the parents.

The two major insecure classifications are associated with incoherent accounts, which means that interviewees' assessment of experience are not matched by their descriptions of parental behavior. There is little support provided for a parent's serving as a secure base; and discourse, whether dismissing or preoccupied, mirrors the lack of exploration and inflexibility of insecure infants. Corresponding to the behavior of avoidant infants in the Strange Situation, adults classified as dismissing are uncomfortable with the topic of the interview, deny the impact of early attachment relationships on their personality development, have difficulty recalling specific events, and characteristically idealize experiences. The classification is associated with descriptions of rejection in the coder's opinion (pushing a child away in attachment-activating situations) in the context of an adult's giving an overarching assessment of having loving parents. Just as resistant infants are ambivalent/resistant in the Strange Situation, adults classified as preoccupied display confusion or evaluative oscillation about past experiences, and descriptions of relationships with parents are marked by active anger and/or passivity. The preoccupied classification is associated with involving, even role-reversing parenting, in which the child needed to be alert to parental needs rather than the reverse.

Individuals may be classified as "unresolved," in addition to being assigned one of the three major classifications. Unresolved adults report attachment-related traumas of loss and/or abuse, and manifest confusion and disorganization in the discussion of that topic. The unresolved classification may be given precedence over the major classification in categorizing the individual, and in some analyses, it is considered an insecure classification. A "cannot classify" designation is assigned when the transcript does not fit any of the major classification categories, most commonly when scale scores reflect the co-occurrence of indicators typical of dismissing and preoccupied states of mind (e.g., high idealization of one parent and high active anger toward the other) (Hesse, 1996).

### Kobak's Q-Sort Scoring System

The Adult Attachment Q-Sort is an alternative method of scoring the AAI and was derived from the original scoring system (Kobak, 1993; Kobak, Cole, Ferenz-Gillies, Fleming, & Gamble, 1993). Its latent structure, at least as originally conceptualized (see Kobak et al., 1993), parallels the Strange Situation and Main and Goldwyn scoring systems, but it emphasizes the relation between emotion regulation and attachment representations. Using Kobak's Q-sort, the AAI is scored from a transcript according to a forced distribution of descriptors, and yields scores for two conceptual dimensions: security–anxiety and deactivation–hyperactivation (although largely orthogonal dismissing and preoccupied state of mind prototype scores are also available to the analyst; see below). Security is inferred from coherence and cooperation within the interview and often (although not necessarily) from memories of supportive attachment figures (in the coder's opinion). Deactivation corresponds to dismissing strategies, whereas hyperactivation corresponds to the excessive detail and active anger seen in the transcripts of many preoccupied subjects. These strategies lie at opposite ends of a single dimension, which was originally assumed to be orthogonal to the secure–anxious (insecure) dimension. The AAI transcript is rated by two or more coders, using 100 Q-sort items and instructions that impose a forced normal distribution along a 9-point continuum (Kobak et al., 1993). The sort is correlated with an expert-based prototypical sort for each dimension. The dimensional scores can be used to classify the adult into the categories of the original system, and Kobak and colleagues reported that approximately 80% of individuals receive the same classification with the Q-sort system as with the original system (kappa = .65). The scoring system was created without an attempt to include the "unresolved" or the "cannot classify" categories.

### Fonagy, Steele, Steele, Moran, and Higgitt's Reflective Functioning Scoring System

Building on the idea reflected in the Main and Goldwyn (1984) coding system that security in adulthood in part reflects metacognitive monitoring, Fonagy and colleagues' (1991) system for coding AAI transcripts assesses *reflective functioning*—that is, an adult's quality of understanding his or her own and another's intentions, motivations, and emotions. In a study of 200 parents, the AAI self-reflection function correlated highly with AAI coherence and was a stronger predictor of infant security. Evidence for the validity and utility of measures of reflective function are reviewed by Fonagy, Luyten, Allison, and Campbell (Chapter 34, this volume).

### Distribution of Classifications

In the most recent meta-analysis of AAI classifications (Bakermans-Kranenburg & Van IJzendoorn, 2009), the distribution of AAI classifications in nonclinical samples of women, men, and adolescents was 58% autonomous (secure), 23% dismissing, and 19% preoccupied, with about 18% of individuals also receiving an unresolved classification in association with a major classification. Not surprisingly, the base rate of insecurity in clinical

and at-risk samples was much higher. Although this meta-analysis found no gender differences in distribution of classifications (Bakermans-Kranenburg & Van IJzendoorn, 2009), other large-scale studies relying on the dimensional scoring described below reveal evidence that women score higher on preoccupied states of mind and men score higher on dismissing states of mind (Haydon, Roisman, Owen, Booth-LaForce, & Cox, 2014).

### Stability and Discriminant Validity

High stability of attachment classifications (78–90% for three classification groups across periods ranging from 2 weeks to 13 years) has been observed in a number of studies using the original scoring system (e.g., kappa = .73, 86%, over 21 months; Crowell, Treboux, & Waters,, 2002; see also Allen, McElhaney, Kuperminc, & Jodl, 2004; Bakermans-Kranenburg & Van IJzendoorn, 1993; Benoit & Parker, 1994; Crowell & Hauser, 2008; Sagi et al., 1994.) The secure classification is especially stable, but the unresolved classification often is not. Change from insecure to secure status across the transition to marriage has been associated with positive feelings and coherent cognitions about the relationship with the partner and living away from the family of origin (Crowell, Treboux, & Waters, 2002).

Because the ability to speak coherently about attachment could conceivably be based on non-attachment-related cognitive abilities such as intelligence or memory, the discriminant validity of the original AAI scoring system has been investigated. Security is weakly associated with intelligence in most studies (but see Haydon et al., 2014) and is not significantly associated with memory, social desirability, or discourse style on an unrelated topic (Bakermans-Kranenburg & Van IJzendoorn, 1993; Crowell et al., 1996; Sagi et al., 1994).

### A New Look at the Latent Structure of the AAI

Since the publication of the second edition of the *Handbook of Attachment*, a number of fundamental measurement issues have arisen that should be considered if the AAI is being used as an assessment method. In short—and in some contrast to the conceptualization of the primary coding systems for the AAI that dismissing and preoccupied states of mind are mutually exclusive and rarely co-occur—there is increasing evidence that coherent discourse during the AAI may in fact be distributed along *two relatively independent dimensions* (Roisman, 2009). According to this view, first, the coherent speaker is *internally consistent* when he or she discusses childhood attachment experiences during the AAI. Individuals who do not produce internally consistent discourse during the AAI often idealize their caregivers (e.g., are unable to provide specific memories that support their overly positive descriptions of their relationships with parents) or normalize objectively harsh childhood experiences. Second—and distinctively—the coherent speaker is able to discuss his or her early experiences without becoming emotionally overwrought while doing so, as reflected either in passive discussion of childhood memories (e.g., wandering off into irrelevancies) or, more commonly, by becoming actively upset while recounting early life experiences. A number of recent studies demonstrate the distinctive origins, correlates, and consequences of these individual differences (Fortuna, Roisman, Haydon, Groh, & Holland, 2011; Haydon, Collins, et al., 2012; Haydon et al., 2014; Whipple, Bernier, & Mageau, 2011).

Work supporting this updated conceptualization of the AAI began with path-finding exploratory factor analyses of the AAI state-of-mind scales reported in publications by Bernier and her colleagues (Bernier, Larose, Boivin, & Soucy, 2004; Larose, Bernier, & Soucy, 2005), which were replicated and extended in the context of two large sample studies (Haydon et al., 2012; Roisman, Fraley, & Belsky, 2007). In the first of these investigations, Roisman, Fraley, and Belsky (2007) examined the latent structure of individual differences in adult attachment via analysis of the rating scales used by AAI coders to index adults' states of mind regarding their childhood attachment experiences, scales that are used to sort participants inductively into attachment categories. Specifically, the study combined data from three publications (total N = 504) drawn from the literature on earned-security (Pearson, Cohn, Cowan, & Cowan, 1994; Roisman & Haydon, 2011).

Using principal components analysis, Roisman, Fraley, and Belsky (2007) found evidence that two- and three-component solutions accounted for the variation in AAI state-of-mind scales reasonably well. The two-component solution suggested that variation in AAI state-of-mind scales could be explained by components reflecting (1) scales used to differentiate secure from dismissing adults (i.e., mother idealization, father idealization, coherence of mind, lack of recall,

and metacognitive monitoring); and (2) scales used to identify both preoccupied and unresolved status (i.e., mother anger, father anger, passivity, unresolved abuse, unresolved loss, fear of loss, and overall derogation). The three-component solution suggested that variation in AAI state-of-mind scales could be explained by components reflecting scales used to differentiate secure from dismissing adults, as in the two-component solution, and an additional set of components that suggested two distinct forms of preoccupied discourse, one involving an active, traumatic enmeshment in earlier experiences (i.e., father and mother anger, derogation, and unresolved trauma) and the other a passive, loss-related preoccupation (i.e., unresolved loss, fear of loss, and passivity). This latter finding of two distinct forms of preoccupied discourse was somewhat surprising given that scholars might reasonably have expected separate preoccupied and unresolved sources of variation paralleling the preoccupied and unresolved classifications that can be assigned using the Main and Goldwyn (1984) approach to scoring the AAI. Complicating things further, in both the two- and three-factor solutions, two of the scales that are viewed by Main and Goldwyn as evidence of a dismissing state of mind (i.e., derogation and fear of loss) actually loaded with indicators of preoccupation/unresolved discourse.

In an extension of this work to a larger sample of college student and community participants (N = 842), Haydon, Roisman, and Burt (2012) examined the latent structure of Kobak's (1993) AAI Q-sort. Again using a principal components analysis—this time applied to item-level Q-sort data—Haydon, Roisman, and Burt found that a four-component solution best accounted for the variation in the data. Two of these components reflected relatively independent attachment states of mind (dismissing and preoccupied; note that when items that loaded highly and uniquely on each component were composited, they were correlated very strongly with their identically named Kobak Q-sort prototype scores) and two additional components reflecting inferred experiences with maternal and paternal caregiving figures (for replication of this finding, see Kobak & Zajac, 2011).

All of the factor-analytic research we just described has relied on exploratory techniques. Nonetheless, two publications based on large samples—the National Institute of Child Health and Human Development (NICHD) Study of Early Child Care and Youth Development (SEC-CYD; Haltigan, Roisman, & Haydon, 2014) and a sample of African American and European American mothers in North Carolina (Haltigan, Leerkes, et al., 2014)—have recently provided *confirmatory* factor-analytic evidence that what is commonly referred to as secure/autonomous states of mind actually blends two *empirically distinct* aspects of attachment-related discourse—variation in the degree to which adults can freely evaluate their childhood experiences or are relatively dismissing of those experiences (dismissing states of mind) and variation in preoccupation (preoccupied states of mind; see Roisman & Booth-LaForce, 2014, for more detailed discussion). Haltigan, Leerkes, and colleagues (2014) demonstrated partial measurement equivalence of these factor structures across ethnic groups, as well as in associations between dismissing states of mind and lower levels of observed sensitivity (replicating work by Whipple et al., 2011).

Factor analysis does not address the empirically distinct question of whether individual differences in adult attachment are categorically or continuously distributed (Fraley & Roisman, 2014; Fraley & Spieker, 2003a; Fraley & Waller, 1998; Roisman, Holland, et al., 2007). However, results from taxometric analyses of some of the same data sets described earlier (i.e., Fraley & Roisman, 2014; Roisman, Fraley, & Belsky, 2007) suggest that the primary distinction made by AAI coders between secure and dismissing states of mind within the Main and Goldwyn (1984) coding system is more consistent with an underlying *dimensional* rather than categorical model. (Analyses of the indicators of preoccupation were indeterminate; see Fraley & Roisman, 2014, for discussion.) Both of these reports also examined the inferred-experience scales within the Main and Goldwyn system, and relevant analyses suggested that the quality of caregiving experiences, as recalled by participants and scored by trained observers, is continuously distributed. In short, it does not appear to be the case that there are subsets of individuals who have qualitatively different experiences, as is often assumed in research on retrospectively defined earned security (Roisman & Haydon, 2011).

## Research with the AAI

The AAI had its origins in investigations of the child–parent attachment relationship, and many of the studies based on the AAI have used it for this purpose. There is a consistent link among AAI classifications/dimensions, parenting behav-

ior, and child attachment status. The AAI has also been used to examine attachment between adult romantic partners.

## Studies of Adults as Individuals: Prospective Longitudinal Studies

To examine the idea that early attachment patterns correspond to attachment patterns in adult life, several studies have assessed the relation between infant attachment security and AAI classifications in late adolescence and young adulthood. Although some small sample studies found a substantial degree of correspondence between Strange Situation procedure and AAI security–insecurity in late adolescents and young adults who participated as infants in studies of attachment (e.g., kappa = .44, Waters, Merrick, Treboux, Crowell, & Albersheim, 2000; see also Hamilton, 2000), the two largest studies in this area have produced test–retest stability coefficients that are more modest in magnitude in both a high- and normative-risk cohort ($r$'s ranging from .10 to .15; Groh et al., 2014; Weinfield, Sroufe, & Egeland, 2000).

Precise explanations of cross-study differences in observed continuity remain to be tested and replicated, but it seems likely that the effort to explain stability and instability will be successful (i.e., that discontinuity will turn out to be "principled" or lawful rather than mysterious or haphazard; for a recent example, see Booth-LaForce et al., 2014). In addition, it is important to emphasize that although the rank-order stability of security in the first two decades of life is relatively modest in larger sample studies, significant and fairly substantial proportions of the variance in AAI states of mind (10–20% of the total variance in the state of mind dimensions) were accounted for in the recent age 18 follow-up of the large NICHD SECCYD cohort ($N = 857$) by leveraging data on a range of key developmental assets and interpersonal risk factors (Haydon et al., 2014).

## The Dismissing Strategy

Adults classified as dismissing use strategies that minimize, dismiss, devalue, or deny the impact of negative attachment experiences. During the AAI, college students who used dismissing strategies showed an increase in skin conductance (Dozier & Kobak, 1992; Roisman, Tsai, & Chiang, 2004). Despite efforts to minimize negative aspects of childhood and the importance of early relationships, they showed signs of physiological distress when challenged with these topics. Indeed, adults classified as dismissing underreport distress, psychological symptoms, or problems in interpersonal relationships, compared with the reports of others who know them well (Dozier & Lee, 1995; Kobak & Sceery, 1988).

## Adjustment and Psychopathology

Consistent relations have been found between security and ratings of social adjustment, social support, stress, and depression; the effect sizes have varied depending on ecological and methodological factors (Atkinson et al., 2000; Crowell, Trebous, & Waters, 1999; Kobak & Sceery, 1988; for a review, see Fearon, Groh, Bakermans-Kranenburg, Van IJzendoorn, & Roisman, in press). Clinical populations have a higher proportion of insecure classifications than the general population, but few specific relations between the "organized" AAI types and psychopathology have emerged (Riggs & Jacobvitz, 2002; Van IJzendoorn & Bakermans-Kranenburg, 1996; Van IJzendoorn et al., 1997; Wallis & Steele, 2001; Ward et al., 2001). The unresolved group, however, is overrepresented in clinical samples, and this has led to suggestions that it is more pathological than "organized" insecure classifications (Van IJzendoorn & Bakermans-Kranenburg, 2009). We do not discuss this complex area of investigation further here, but as Lyons-Ruth and Jacobvitz explain in Chapter 29, this volume, it has led to important efforts to expand the AAI coding system to address a variety of trauma-related variations in AAI narratives.

## "Earned" Security

The subset of individuals classified as secure (because they value attachment and are coherent in their discussion of attachment relationships), despite coders rating their parents as unloving, have been termed "earned" secure. Data from both the Minnesota Longitudinal Study of Risk and Adaptation (Roisman, Padron, Sroufe, & Egeland, 2002) and the NICHD SECCYD (Roisman, Haltigan, Haydon, & Booth-LaForce, 2014) demonstrate that such retrospectively defined "earned" secure individuals paradoxically experienced average or better early caregiving during childhood and adolescence, but due to a range of factors, including mood-related biases in their retrospective recall of early caregiving experiences, coders'

tend to rate their parents as relatively unloving (Roisman, Fortuna, & Holland, 2006; Roisman et al., 2002, 2014). Although some scholars disagree with this interpretation (Hesse, 2008), to the best of our knowledge, they have yet to offer an alternative model that explains why (1) both normative-risk (Roisman et al., 2014) and high-risk (Roisman et al., 2002) longitudinal cohorts have provided evidence that the observed maternal and (in the SECCYD) paternal caregiving of retrospectively defined earned secures is average or better (regardless of how earned secure status is defined retrospectively) and (2) experimental mood manipulations can shift ratings on the inferred experience scales (even if not the coherence rating) (Roisman et al., 2006).

## Studies of Child–Parent Attachment Classifications across Generations

Some of the first AAI investigations indicated high correspondence between parental AAI classifications and infant attachment assessed with the Strange Situation (kappa = .46 for three classifications; kappa = .44 for four classifications) and preschoolers' attachment assessed with home observations (Cassibba, Van IJzendoorn, Bruno, & Coppola, 2004; Fonagy, Steele, & Steele, 1991; Posada, Waters, Crowell, & Lay, 1995; Sagi et al., 1992; Steele, Steele, & Fonagy, 1996; Van IJzendoorn, 1992; see the meta-analysis by Van IJzendoorn, 1995). Mother–infant correspondence is greater than father–infant correspondence (Main et al., 1985; Miljkovitch, Pierrehumbert, Bretherton, & Halfon, 2004; Steele et al., 1996; Van IJzendoorn, 1992).

## Studies of Parents' AAI Classifications and Parental Behavior toward Children

Mothers classified as autonomous on the AAI are observed to be more responsive, perceptive, sensitive, and attuned to their infants in the first year of life (Adam, Gunnar, & Tanaka, 2004; DeOliveira, Moran, & Pederson, 2005; Goldberg, Benoit, Blokland, & Madigan, 2003; Grossmann, Fremmer-Bombik, Rudolph, & Grossmann, 1988; Haft & Slade, 1989; Macfie, McElwain, Houts, & Cox, 2005; Slade, Belsky, Aber, & Phelps, 1999; Ward & Carlson, 1995; Zeanah et al., 1993). Similarly, parental security of attachment is associated with parents' sensitivity with their preschool children, and providing help and support during observed tasks and separations in both normative and clinical samples (Cohn, Cowan, Cowan, & Pearson, 1992; Crowell & Feldman, 1988, 1991; Crowell, O'Connor, Wollmers, Sprafkin, & Rao, 1991; Das Eiden, Teti, & Corns, 1995; Oyen, Landy, & Hilburn-Cobb, 2000). Marital functioning appears to have moderating effects (Cohn et al., 1992; Das Eiden et al., 1995). Ratings of child symptoms by parents, teachers, and children themselves indicate that children of insecure parents have higher ratings of problem behavior and child distress (Cowan, Cohn, Pearson, & Cowan, 1996; Crowell et al., 1991). Adolescents classified as secure in the AAI are observed to have secure base relationships with their mothers and are more socially skilled than those classified as insecure (Allen et al., 2002, 2004; Kobak et al., 1993; for a review, see Allen & Tan, Chapter 19, this volume).

### Romantic Relationships

A meta-analysis of AAI attachment classifications of 226 couples showed modest concordance (50–60%, equivalent to a kappa of .20, for three major classifications) between partners for attachment status, accounted for by the secure–secure pairs (Van IJzendoorn & Bakermans-Kranenburg, 1996). Not surprisingly, this finding suggests that factors other than attachment security are active in partner selection and maintenance, although a recent analysis of a comparable number of couples assessed in the meta-analysis demonstrated somewhat more correspondence between *preoccupied* states of mind than dismissing states of mind within couple pairs (Haydon, Roisman, & Burt, 2012), a pattern of results that was also apparent among adult siblings in a study by Fortuna and colleagues (2011).

Little direct relation between the broad construct of marital satisfaction and AAI classification has been found, but reports of feelings of intimacy are related (Benoit, Zeanah, & Barton, 1989; Cohn, Silver, Cowan, Cowan, & Pearson, 1992; O'Connor, Pan, Waters, & Posada, 1995; Zeanah et al., 1993). In addition, feelings about the relationship are related to interactions among AAI status, representations of the adult partnership, marital behavior, and stressful events (Paley, Cox, Harter, & Margand, 2002; Treboux et al., 2004). Associations between attachment security and the use of physical aggression in couples' relationships are consistently obtained (Crittenden, Partridge, & Claussen, 1991; O'Connor et al., 1995; Treboux

et al., 2004). As we discuss later in this chapter, there is little correspondence between the AAI and self-reports of attachment (Roisman, Holland, et al., 2007; Waters, Crowell, Elliott, Corcoran, & Treboux, 2002).

### Couples' Interactions

Studies have found associations between the AAI and attachment/secure-base behaviors in couples' interactions in samples of both late adolescents and adults (Cohn et al., 1992; Creasey, 2002; Creasey & Ladd, 2004, 2005; Crowell, Treboux, Gao, et al., 2002; Curran, Hazen, Jacobvitz, & Feldman, 2005; Furman, Simon, Shaffer, & Bouchey, 2002; Paley, Cox, Burchinal & Payne, 1999; Roisman, Madsen, Hennighausen, Sroufe, & Collins, 2001; Simpson, Rholes, Oriña, & Grich, 2002; Wampler, Riggs, & Kimball, 2004; Wampler, Shi, Nelson, & Kimball, 2003). These studies, combined with recent longitudinal evidence that predictive associations between AAI states of mind and observed relationship quality obtain even after researchers adjust statistically for the association between these variables at baseline (Holland & Roisman, 2010), provide compelling support for the AAI as an assessment of a generalized representation of attachment rather than being specific to a particular type of attachment relationship.

### Relationship Interviews

Several interviews have been developed to assess attachment representations within romantic partnerships (e.g., Bartholomew & Horowitz, 1991; Cowan, Cowan, Alexandrov, Lyon, & Heming, 1999; Crowell & Owens, 1996; Dickstein, Seifer, Albus, & Magee, 2004; Furman & Simon, 2006). Most are rooted in the AAI tradition of examining coherence of discourse, and the findings of relations among these interviews, the AAI, self-reports of the relationship, and observed couples' behavior are similar (Alexandrov, Cowan, & Cowan, 2005; Dickstein et al., 2004; Furman & Simon, 2006; Owens et al., 1995). Of these, the Current Relationship Interview (CRI) is the most well established (Crowell & Owens, 1996; Crowell et al., 2002a; Crowell, Treboux, & Waters, 2002; Furman et al., 2002; Owens et al., 1995; Roisman et al., 2005; Treboux et al., 2004). The CRI investigates the representation of attachment within an adult partnership. It was developed as a way to examine the prototype hypothesis—the hypothesis that adult close relationships are similar in organization to parent–child attachment relationships. More specifically, it has been used to explore the process by which a new attachment relationship may be integrated into an already existing representation of attachment, or by which a new representation develops.

As a narrative assessment, the CRI is intended to examine an individual's representation of attachment and ideas regarding the partner's and his or her own attachment behavior. The interview asks the adult for descriptions of the relationship and for instances of the use of and giving of secure-base support in the relationship. The interview is scored from a transcript, and the subject is classified into one of three groups according to the profile of scores on a variety of rating scales. Rating scales are used to characterize (1) the participant's behavior and thinking about attachment-related issues (e.g., valuing of intimacy and independence); (2) the partner's behavior; and (3) the subject's discourse style (e.g., anger, derogation, idealization, and overall coherence). The CRI and its scoring system parallel the AAI in structure. The secure–insecure dimension is based on coherent reports of being able to use the partner as a secure base and to act as a secure base, or the coherently expressed desire to do so. Individuals who cannot coherently discuss secure-base use and support in the interview are divided between those who avoid discussion of these behaviors or dismiss their significance, and those who appear to heighten or control the attachment elements of the relationship. CRI scoring is based on state of mind regarding attachment, as well as individuals' reports of their own specific attachment behaviors of secure-base support and use. These factors are given primacy in the determination of attachment security rather than the individual's reported feelings about the relationship or the behaviors of the partner.

The secure CRI interview is characterized by coherence; that is, the subject convincingly describes his or her own and the partner's secure-base behavior, or can coherently discuss negative partner behavior. The subject expresses the idea that an adult attachment relationship should provide support for the individuals involved and for their joint development, whether or not the relationship is actually providing these elements. The dismissing CRI classification is given when there is little evidence that the individual views attachment, support, and comfort within the relationship as important, even if the partner is convincingly described as loving. The relationship may be "normalized." A need for autonomy and separateness within the relationship may be emphasized, and there may be a focus on concrete or material aspects of the relationship (e.g., buying a house, going on vacations). The preoccupied CRI classification is given when the subject expresses strong dependence on the partner or attempts to control the partner. The individual may be dissatisfied or anxious about the partner's ability to fulfill his or her needs, and may express ambivalence or confusion about the relationship, the partner, and/or the self, regardless of the descriptions of partner behavior.

## Distribution and Concordance of Classification in Couples

Empirical evidence suggests that the distribution of classifications may vary with the developmental stage of the participants and the relationship (e.g., Alexandrov, Cowan, & Cowan, 2005; Furman et al., 2002). For example, 46% of CRI transcripts were classified as secure in a sample of young engaged adults (Owens et al., 1995), whereas in a married sample with children, 71% were classified as secure with the Couple Attachment Interview (CAI; Alexandrov et al., 2005). Concordance between partners for CRI classifications was 63% premaritally (kappa = .29) and 65% after 15 months of marriage (kappa = .30); for the CAI, the concordance was 69%.

## Stability and Discriminant Validity

Security on the CRI is unrelated to intelligence, education, gender, duration of relationship, or the endorsement of symptoms of depression (Owens et al., 1995). Unlike the AAI, the CRI draws on a current relationship and is subject to life events and partner behaviors. Hence the CRI classifications are expected to be less stable than those of the AAI, especially in the early phases of relationship development (Crowell & Waters, 1997).

## Research with Relationship Interviews

### Reports of Relationships and Marital Satisfaction

Individuals classified as secure with relationship interviews (RIs) report greater satisfaction with their relationship, greater commitment and feelings of love overall, and fewer problems in the relationship than insecure individuals (Alexandrov et al., 2005; Owens et al., 1995; Roisman et al., 2005; Treboux et al., 2004). Investigations consistently reveal that security assessed with RIs is positively related to attachment behavior in couples' interactions (Alexandrov et al., 2005; Crowell, Treboux, Gao, et al., 2002; Furman & Simon, 2006; Roisman et al., 2005).

## Correspondence with the AAI

The correlation of the security scores from concurrently obtained AAIs and CRIs in a normative risk cohort was $r = .51$ (Crowell, Treboux, & Waters, 2002); however, in the higher risk Minnesota Longitudinal Study of Risk and Adaptation (MLSRA) cohort, CRI and AAI classification were not significantly associated (Haydon, Collins, et al., 2012). Evidence suggests that the configuration of the AAI and the CRI within an individual is especially predictive of marital functioning, including divorce rates early in marriage (Dickstein et al., 2004; Treboux et al., 2004). Treboux and colleagues reported that individuals classified as secure on both the AAI and the CRI reported more positive feelings about the relationship, low observed and reported aggression, and divorce rates consistent with the overall mean. They appeared to tolerate stressful life events without marked change in these parameters. Individuals classified as insecure on both the AAI and the CRI are the most aggressive group, by observation and self-report. The behaviors and negative feelings about the relationship escalate in association with stressful events. Individuals classified as AAI insecure/CRI secure reported the *most positive* feelings about their relationships and had a significantly lower divorce rate in early marriage than other configurations. However, when stressed, such individuals report negative feelings about their relationships, and their conflict behavior is more aggressive. Last, individuals classified as AAI secure/CRI insecure report the *most negative* feelings about their relationships and have significantly higher divorce rates than the other configurations. They do not engage in aggressive conflict behaviors, however, even when stressed. These results were supported in the MLSRA study (Haydon, Collins, et al., 2012) in which AAI secure/CRI insecure individuals engaged in more conflict with partners than those with secure CRIs.

Furthermore, Haydon, Collins, and colleagues (2012) addressed the question of whether representations assessed with the AAI and the CRI had shared developmental origins, or whether they were independent. Analyses indicated that these representations have shared origins in some early experiences and shared links to romantic behavior. However, romantic representations assessed with the CRI had distinctive roots in early development, as well as independent links to adult romantic behavior.

## The Attachment Script Assessment

Borrowing from the cognitive literatures on narrative and memory, and based on seminal theoretical work by Bretherton (1987, 1990), developmental psychologists have recently taken another approach to the assessment of attachment representations in adolescents and adults by measuring individual differences in attachment-relevant *scripts* (Waters & Rodrigues, 2001; Waters & Waters, 2006). Cognitive scientists such as Schank (1999) argue that as we encounter similar experiences over time, we begin to summarize commonalities (e.g., the main character(s), causal chain of events, and resolution or ending) across those events and form a script for how those events typically unfold. Waters and Waters (2006) proposed that an individual's history of care and secure-base support is represented in memory as a *secure-base script*.

To assess individual differences in access to this secure-base script (i.e., secure-base script knowledge), H. Waters and colleagues developed the Attachment Script Assessment (ASA), although coding of secure-base script knowledge is also possible based on the autobiographical narratives produced within the AAI. The ASA uses a word-prompt outline in which participants generate short stories with attachment-related themes from a set of words. Ultimately, *secure-base script knowledge* is operationally defined in terms of the degree to which an individual produces narratives in which attachment-relevant events are encountered, a clear need for assistance is communicated, competent help is provided and accepted, and the problem is resolved. In an adult version of the ASA, four word-prompt stories are generated by each participant (two focused on adult–adult and two on adult–child scenarios; Waters & Rodrigues, 2001). In an adolescent version of the measure (see Dykas, Woodhouse, Cassidy, & Waters, 2006; Steiner, Arjomand, & Waters, 2003), participants use developmentally tailored word prompts specific to caregivers.

In the last few years, studies of the ASA examining the developmental significance of individual differences in secure-base script knowledge have provided evidence that the ASA has attractive psychometric properties, including adequate test–retest reliability ($r = .54$, $n = 53$; Vaughn et al., 2006) and convergent validity with coherence of mind as assessed by the AAI (meta-analytic $r = .53$, $n = 87$; Coppola, Vaughn, Cassibba, & Constantini, 2006; Waters & Rodrigues, 2001). Secure-base script knowledge is positively associated with high-quality parenting, as well as attachment security in the next generation (e.g., Bost et al., 2006; Coppola et al., 2006; Veríssimo & Salvaterra, 2006). Although such studies address critical questions regarding the reliability and validity of the ASA as an assessment of secure-base script knowledge, less is known at present about the developmental origins of secure-base script knowledge. However, in the SECCYD, ASA secure-base script knowledge was as strongly associated with earlier infant–mother attachment and maternal sensitivity, as were AAI states of mind measured in the same cohort around age 18 years. Indeed, ASA secure-base script knowledge was actually *more* strongly associated with antecedent paternal sensitivity than were AAI state-of-mind scores (R. Steele et al., 2014).

## Behavioral Assessments of Attachment

A number of investigators have developed systems of observing attachment behaviors between adult partners, many using a standard marital interaction task as the stressor that provokes attachment behavior (Alexandrov et al., 2005; Creasey, 2002; Creasey & Ladd, 2005; Crowell, Treboux, Gao, et al., 2002; Furman & Simon, 2006; Roisman et al., 2005; Wampler et al., 2004). An external anxiety-inducing stressor has also been employed (Simpson, Rholes, Oriña, & Grich, 2002). These assessments focus on support seeking and provision rather than positive and negative communication styles. There is evidence that the more specifically attachment behavior is assessed, as opposed to communication behaviors, the more likely it is to relate to narrative assessments of attachment (Crowell, Treboux, Gao, et al., 2002; Paley et al., 1999).

The Secure Base Scoring System (SBSS) is an example of one such behavioral assessment. Couples are assessed using a standard couples' interaction task that was videotaped and scored with the SBSS (Crowell, Treboux, Gao, et al., 2002). When a partner introduces a concern into the discussion, their secure-base use is scored on four subscales ranging from high quality to low quality. Subscales indicate (1) the clarity of *initial signal* or expression of distress, (2) *maintenance of the signal* as needed, (3) *approach* to the partner for help, and (4) the *ability to be comforted*. Based on these subscales and the general overview of the individual's behavior, the coder assigns a score on the Summary of Secure Base Use scale. *Secure base support* is scored for the partner who is presented with the concern raised by the other. It is scored on four subscales: (1) *interest in the partner*, (2) *recognition of distress or concern*, (3) *interpretation of distress*, and (4) *responsiveness to distress*. A Summary of Secure Base Support scale encompasses the overall support provided by the individual. Because the summary scales are often very highly correlated (women: $r = .86$, men: $r = .88$; Crowell, Treboux, Gao, et al., 2002), the average of the summary scales may be used to represent overall quality of secure-base behavior.

## Self-Report Measures of Romantic Attachment

The study of romantic attachment began in the late 1970s and early 1980s in an attempt to understand the nature and etiology of adult loneliness and the various ways that people experience love. It had been noticed that many lonely adults report troubled childhood relationships with parents and either distant or overly enmeshed romantic relationships, suggesting that attachment history might play a role in the experience of adult loneliness (Rubenstein & Shaver, 1982; Weiss, 1973). Also, social psychologists and anthropologists had observed that there is considerable variability in the way people approach love relationships (ranging from intense preoccupation to psychological distance), and they were developing individual-difference taxonomies to capture this variability (see Sternberg & Barnes, 1988, for examples). Despite these rich descriptions, there was no compelling theoretical framework within which to organize or explain the observed individual differences (Hazan & Shaver, 1994).

In an attempt to address this issue, Hazan and Shaver (1987) published an article in which they conceptualized romantic love as an attachment process, involving the interplay among attachment, caregiving, and sexual behavioral systems. They noted that many of the emotional and behavioral dynamics characteristic of infant–mother attachment relationships also characterize adult romantic relationships. For example, both kinds of relationships involve caressing, ventral–ventral contact, and "baby talk." More importantly, in each case, an individual feels safest and most secure when the other is nearby, accessible, and responsive. Under such circumstances, the partner may be used as a "secure base" from which to explore the environment. When an individual is feeling distressed, sick, or threatened, the partner is used as a "safe haven"—a source of safety, comfort, and protection.

Hazan and Shaver (1987; Shaver & Hazan, 1988) argued that the various approaches to love described by social psychologists reflect individual differences in the organization of the attachment system in adulthood. Specifically, they argued that the major patterns of attachment described by Ainsworth and colleagues (1978)—secure, anxious-resistant, and avoidant—are conceptually similar to the romantic attachment patterns observed among adults. Although Bowlby and Ainsworth had discussed the role of attachment in romantic relationships, no one had actually attempted to assess the individual differences noted among infants by Ainsworth and colleagues in the adult pair-bond context.

## Attachment Style Questionnaires

When Hazan and Shaver (1987) began their work on romantic attachment, they adopted Ainsworth's threefold typology from the Strange Situation paradigm as a framework for organizing individual differences in the ways adults think, feel, and behave in romantic relationships. In their initial studies, Hazan and Shaver developed brief multisentence descriptions of the three proposed attachment types—avoidant, secure, and anxious-resistant. The descriptions were based on an extrapolation of the three infant patterns summarized in the final chapter of Ainsworth and colleagues' (1978) book. Research participants are asked to think back across their history of romantic relationships and indicate which of the three descriptions best captured the way they *generally* experience and act in romantic relationships. They refer to a person's characteristic desires, feelings, and behaviors, and to comments made by relationship partners.

In their initial studies, Hazan and Shaver (1987) found that people's self-reported roman-

tic attachment patterns related to a number of theoretically relevant variables, including beliefs about love and relationships (working models of romantic relationships) and recollections of early experiences with parents. With respect to their romantic relationships, secure people reported higher levels of happiness and trust. People endorsing the avoidant description perceived their mothers as cool and rejecting and, in their romantic relationships, reported a fear of intimacy, difficulty in accepting their partners, and a general belief that romantic love does not last. Anxious-ambivalent adults also reported conflicted relationships with parents and were more likely to report feelings of obsession and jealousy in romantic relationships. Not surprisingly, many researchers adopted Hazan and Shaver's categorical, forced-choice measure because of its novelty, brevity, face validity, and ease of administration.

In 1990, Bartholomew published an important article that challenged researchers to reconsider the three-category model of individual differences in adult attachment. Integrating ideas from a variety of perspectives, Bartholomew argued that people hold separate representational models of themselves (Model of Self) and their social world (Model of Others)—models that have distinct consequences for the way attachment behavior is organized. The Model of Others reflects the expectations, beliefs, and strategies that people have concerning close others in general, and attachment figures in particular. Individuals with a positive Model of Others view attachment figures as trustworthy, reliable, and dependable. Individuals with negatively valenced Models of Others lack confidence in peoples' trustworthiness and dependability. The Model of Self reflects the valence of peoples' views of themselves. People with a positive Model of Self see themselves as competent, autonomous, and worthy of love. People with a negative Model of Self lack confidence, harbor self-doubts, and are vulnerable to psychological distress.

Bartholomew argued that when these two kinds of representational models are crossed with valence (i.e., the models' positivity or negativity), it is possible to derive four, rather than three, major attachment patterns. She borrowed names for the four patterns from a mixture of the Ainsworth and colleagues' (1978), Hazan and Shaver's (1987), and Main and colleagues' (1985) typologies, calling the positive–positive group "secure," the negative–positive group "preoccupied," the positive–negative group "dismissing," and the negative–negative group "fearful" (see Figure 27.1). Following Hazan and Shaver's lead, Bartholomew and Horowitz (1991) developed the Relationship Questionnaire (RQ), a short instrument containing multisentence descriptions of each of the four types.

The wording of three of the four type descriptions (secure, preoccupied, and fearful-avoidant) is very similar to the wording of the three Hazan and Shaver (1987) descriptions (secure, anxious-ambivalent, and avoidant). In fact, Bartholomew (1990) essentially equated the secure categories between the two systems, as well as the anxious-ambivalent pattern. In Bartholomew's model, however, the avoidant type is split into two distinct types. The first kind of avoidance, *fearful-avoidance*, captures the vulnerable, insecure form of avoidance reflected in the Hazan and Shaver avoidant category. These individuals are avoidant of intimacy because they fear being hurt by someone they love. The second type, *dismissing-avoidance*, is not represented in the Hazan and Shaver system. These kinds of individuals avoid intimacy, not because they consciously fear being hurt, but because they value independence and autonomy.

The RQ was more fully developed by Griffin and Bartholomew (1994a) to form the Relationship Styles Questionnaire (RSQ), a 30-item inventory with content from both the Hazan and Shaver (1987) descriptions and the RQ descriptions. The RSQ can be scaled to create a score for each person on each of the four attachment patterns. Due to its multi-item nature, the RSQ exhibits somewhat higher reliability than the RQ ($r$'s of about .65 for the brief scales assessing each of the four attachment patterns; Fraley & Shaver, 1997). Also, the RSQ can be used to score people on the two dimensions (Model of Self and Model of Other) that underlie these patterns. Roisman, Holland, and colleagues (2007) analyzed several alternative scoring systems and recommended one based on Simpson, Rholes, and Nelligan (1992) that provided a better fit to the data than some alternatives (see also Kurdek, 2002).

## The Evolution of Measurement Systems

By the mid-1990s, there was some consensus in the social–personality literature that the Bartholomew

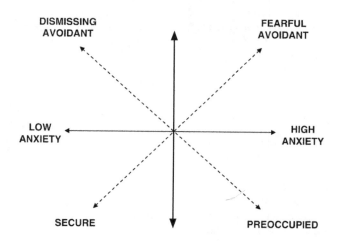

**FIGURE 27.1.** Two-dimensional model of individual differences in adult attachment, per the social–personality tradition.

model was better suited for capturing individual differences than the original Hazan and Shaver model. But there was still lingering concern over whether it was ideal to classify people or to scale them with respect to one or more dimensions. The classification system was potentially valuable because it provided a parallel to the developmental literature and the SSP and AAI attachment patterns. The classification system was also useful because it made it relatively easy to conceptualize the psychological dynamics underlying the various attachment styles.

Nonetheless, a number of limitations began to emerge with the categorical system. First, the classifications were not highly stable. For example, Baldwin and Fehr (1995) observed that the test–retest stability of the categorical measure was only 70% (equivalent to a Pearson's $r$ of approximately .40). Some researchers began to wonder whether some of that instability was due to attempting to assign people to categories who might, in fact, be somewhere near the boundaries in a dimensional space. Second, the categorical system treated the four categories as if they were mutually exclusive, but data from continuous measurements suggested that they were not. Finally, the categorical system disregarded within-category variance that, in practice, seemed useful for predicting outcomes.

As a result of these tensions, some researchers began to use the ratings as a way to scale people in a dimensional space. This led to two problems. First, there was no principled reason for moving from categories to continua. Second, for each self-report measure that was developed and used, there was a different set of scales that varied in number and their interpretation. We discuss each of these problems in turn.

### Types versus Dimensions

Although the gradual move from classifications to ratings was an important step toward improving the measurement of adult attachment, these shifts begged a larger theoretical question: Do people vary continuously or categorically with respect to attachment? This question, sometimes referred to as the "types versus dimensions" question, is a critical one for the study of adult attachment. If people actually vary continuously in attachment organization, but researchers assign people to categories, then important information about individual differences is lost. This loss can have deleterious effects on the study of continuity and change; on mapping of the developmental ante-

cedents and consequences of attachment experiences; on understanding whether certain experiences affect attachment organization; and on bridging the gaps between attachment research in social, personality, clinical, and developmental psychology.

How can one determine whether variation in an unobservable construct, such as attachment organization, is continuous or categorical? Historically, researchers relied on clustering techniques to identify groupings in data (e.g., Collins & Read, 1990; Feeney, Noller, & Hanrahan, 1994). One of the limitations of clustering techniques, such as cluster analysis or latent profile analysis, however, is that they reveal groupings in data regardless of whether natural groupings actually exist. Fortunately, Meehl and his colleagues (e.g., Meehl & Yonce, 1996; Waller & Meehl, 1998) developed a suite of techniques that allow one to uncover the latent structure of a domain and rigorously test taxonic (i.e., typological) conjectures. Fraley and Waller (1998) adopted two of Meehl's techniques, MAXCOV and MAMBAC, to address the types vs. dimensions question in the study of adult attachment. Taxometric analyses of the data from Griffin and Bartholomew's (1994a) RSQ from over 600 undergraduates provided no evidence for a categorical model of attachment, but were consistent with a dimensional model of individual differences (see also Fraley, Hudson, Heffernan, & Segal, 2015).

### What Are the Fundamental Dimensions Underlying Adult Attachment?

In the 1990s, a number of investigators began creating multi-item inventories of adult attachment that could be used to produce continuous attachment scores. Although rooted in Bowlby and Ainsworth's attachment theory, the designers emphasized different constructs and used different methods of test development. Some researchers simply decomposed the items in the original Hazan and Shaver (1987) paragraphs. For example, Collins's (Collins & Read, 1990) Adult Attachment Scale (AAS) was developed by taking the individual sentence fragments in the original Hazan and Shaver descriptions and creating 18 distinct items, each of which was rated on a continuous scale. Based on her psychometric analyses of the items, Collins (Collins & Read, 1990) derived three composites: close, depend, and anxiety. Feeney and colleagues (1994) developed new items designed to capture themes in attachment theory, such as trust, dependence, and self-reliance. A factor analysis of responses to their items uncovered five factors: self-confidence, discomfort with closeness, need for approval, preoccupation with relationships, and the belief that relationships are of secondary importance. Brennan and Shaver (1995) followed a similar approach, generating a large pool of items, which they then factor analyzed. Brennan and Shaver reported seven factors: ambivalence, anxious clinging to partners, jealous and fear of abandonment, frustration with partners, proximity seeking, self-reliance, and trust.

By the mid- to late 1990s, researchers were likely to be overwhelmed by the sheer number of self-report instruments in the literature. To address this problem, Brennan, Clark, and Shaver (1998) gathered all known self-report measures of adult attachment and administered the nonredundant items to 1,086 undergraduates. Factor analyses of the responses revealed two major factors that they labeled attachment-related *anxiety* and attachment-related *avoidance*. The anxiety factor was defined by items such as "I worry that my partner won't want to stay with me" and "I don't think my partner loves me." The avoidance factor was defined at one end by items such as "I am uncomfortable depending on others," and at the opposite end, "I turn to my partner for assurance."

The Brennan report was a substantial advance for three reasons. First, the analyses revealed that the diverse pool of self-report measures of adult attachment was essentially tapping two fundamental domains. Second, it showed how measures originally developed with different objectives could be mapped onto a common dimensional framework. Finally, Brennan and her colleagues (1998) used their data to produce a new questionnaire, the Experiences in Close Relationships (ECR) inventory—a 36-item questionnaire based on the items that best tapped the dimensions of anxiety and avoidance. Brennan and colleagues showed that the 18 items for each subscale hung together well (alphas > .90) and the scales predicted a number of potentially relevant outcomes, such as emotions experienced in an intimate context. The ECR and its derivatives (e.g., the revised ECR [ECR-R]; Fraley, Waller, & Brennan, 2000) are currently the most commonly used self-report measures of adult attachment and are recommended as the primary self-report instruments for assessing adult attachment. The ECR-R is based on an item response theory

analysis of the original item pool used by Brennan and colleagues and produces scores that are highly correlated with those from the ECR. The ECR-S is a shorter version of the original ECR using 12 items instead of 36 items (Wei, Russell, Mallinckrodt, & Vogel, 2007). Each of these measures has excellent psychometric properties (e.g., Cronbach alphas of .85 or higher) and are in widespread use in contemporary research in social and personality psychology.

What do these two dimensions represent theoretically? Within Bartholomew's framework, individual differences are conceptualized in terms of a person's cognitive representations of the self and others. But most self-report instruments appear to be more explicitly concerned with motivations, thoughts, and feelings in close relationships rather than the valence of the cognitions they hold about themselves or others (e.g., Fraley & Shaver, 2000). Thus, in this chapter in the previous edition, we suggested that the dimensions be interpreted within the framework of behavioral–motivational systems rather than models of self–other per se. The distinction between these alternatives might be viewed as pedantic, but we have found that the behavioral–motivational system framing is helpful for situating the study of individual differences within normative models of how the attachment system operates. According to Hazan and Shaver (1994), individual differences in attachment patterns are attributable to two different components of the attachment system. One component involves monitoring of the psychological proximity and availability of the attachment figure. When either the attachment figure is perceived as being available and responsive (the "secure" stance), or the attachment figure's availability is not viewed as relevant to or useful in attaining personal safety, an individual can focus on other issues and goals (e.g., exploration). Stable variation in these states is reflected in individual differences on the attachment anxiety dimension (Fraley & Shaver, 2000). The second component of the system concerns the regulation of attachment behavior with respect to attachment-related concerns. For example, to regulate attachment-related anxiety, people can either seek contact with an attachment figure (i.e., use the figure as a safe haven) or withdraw and attempt to handle the threat alone. The propensity to engage in secure-base strategies versus deactivating the system is reflected in individual differences on the avoidance dimension (see Mikulincer & Shaver, 2007).

### The Nomological Network and Construct Validity

As explained earlier, the AAI coding system was initially developed empirically to maximize the prediction of an *infant's* classification in the Strange Situation paradigm. In this sense, there was an obvious "gold standard" for the AAI's validity—the categories of the Strange Situation paradigm that are based on extensive home and laboratory observations of infants' behavior. In contrast, the self-report instruments in the Hazan and Shaver tradition were not designed to predict any single criterion. Instead, their validity and the value of the research tradition from which they derive rest on their ability to reproduce empirically the network of covariates postulated by the theory (Cronbach & Meehl, 1955). In this section, we discuss the construct validity of measures of adult romantic attachment, focusing on relationship processes, the dismissing strategy in particular, and general adjustment and psychopathology (for more detailed reviews, see this chapter in previous editions of this volume; Mikulincer & Shaver, 2007).

### The Rationale for Assessing Adult Romantic Attachment with Self-Report Methods

There are several reasons why self-report instruments are useful tools for investigating individual differences in adult attachment. First, according to Bowlby, attachment dynamics play an important role in people's emotional experience. Thus, in many respects, assessing those experiences is an important step in studying the implications of attachment dynamics. Self-reports are an obvious means for doing so, although we recognize that rating scales per se represent only one of many ways in which researchers can study experience. Second, most adults have sufficient experience in close relationships to recount how they behave in such relationships and the kinds of things their partners have said to them about their behavior. We do not assume that such reports are error free or that they are not subject to various motivated biases (e.g., Simpson, Rholes, & Winterheld, 2010), but they are useful for studying statistical relations among constructs.

Some scholars have wondered whether self-reports can be useful to assess attachment dynamics when some of these dynamics are likely to be relatively inaccessible or unconscious. Indeed, some people may report that they are not anxious when actually they are; others may simply lack insight into their true motives and behavior. Nonetheless, it is possible to use attachment theory to derive the kinds of beliefs that prototypically avoidant or dismissing people may hold about themselves. For example, a dismissing person should believe that he or she is "independent" and "self-sufficient," does not "worry about abandonment," and maybe even does not "need close relationships." Holding such beliefs is an important part of defensively excluding unwanted thoughts and emotions. It is a separate question—and an important one—whether people endorsing such statements in a questionnaire actually do or do not function well without others. Although self-reports are frequently used to assess individual differences in attachment security, they are rarely used alone to investigate the dynamics of attachment. To probe these deeper issues, researchers often pair self-reports with a variety of behavioral, cognitive, and psychophysiological tasks (see Mikulincer & Shaver, 2007, for a review).

### Attraction and Relationship Formation

Cross-cultural studies suggest that the secure pattern of attachment in infancy is universally considered the most desirable pattern by mothers. Similarly, adults seeking long-term relationships identify responsive caregiving qualities, such as attentiveness, warmth, and sensitivity, as most "attractive" in potential dating partners (e.g., Chappell & Davis, 1998; Frazier, Byer, Fischer, Wright, & DeBord, 1996).

Despite the attractiveness of secure qualities, however, not everyone is paired with a secure partner. Some evidence suggests that people end up in relationships with partners who confirm their existing beliefs about attachment relationships (Collins & Read, 1990; Frazier et al., 1996). In research that has employed social-cognitive methods for studying transference processes, Brumbaugh and Fraley (2006) found that people who held negative representations of significant others (parental or romantic) from their pasts were more likely to feel insecure with novel relationship partners. This suggests that although most people would prefer a supportive partner if given a choice, people tend to reexperience thoughts and feelings in new relationships due to the ways in which existing representations shape new experiences.

Recently researchers have attempted to explain how attachment-related anxiety may compromise relationship opportunities. McClure and

Lydon (2014), for example, studied the behavior of individuals who were engaged in a speed-dating task. Their analyses revealed that people who were high in attachment-related anxiety were more likely to feel conflicted in speed-dating contexts, and that their insecurities spilled over into their behavior (e.g., verbal dysfluencies and interpersonal awkwardness). As a result of these displays, individuals high in attachment-related anxiety were considered less desirable by other speed-daters, which reinforced the negative expectations that they held.

### Relationship Maintenance: Implications for Secure-Base and Safe-Haven Behavior

Overall, secure adults tend to be more satisfied in their relationships than insecure adults. Their relationships are characterized by greater longevity, trust, commitment, and interdependence (e.g., Simpson, 1990), and they are more likely to use romantic partners as a secure base from which to explore the world (Feeney & Thrush, 2010; Fraley & Davis, 1997; see also B. C. Feeney & Woodhouse, Chapter 36, this volume). A large proportion of research on adult attachment has been devoted to uncovering the behavioral and psychological mechanisms that promote security and secure-base behavior in adults. There have been two major discoveries thus far. First, and similar to the developmental attachment tradition, secure adults are more likely than insecure adults to seek support from their partners when they are distressed and to provide support to their distressed partners. Second, the attributions that insecure individuals make concerning their partners' behavior during and following relational conflicts exacerbate, rather than alleviate, their insecurities.

Concerning the first dynamic, Simpson and colleagues (1992) found that overtly distressed secure women were more likely than insecure women to seek emotional support from their partners. Also, secure men were more likely than insecure men to provide support to their distressed partners. Fraley and Shaver (1998) found that secure women who were separating from their partners in an airport were more likely than insecure women to express their anxiety, seek comfort from their partners, and provide comfort for their partners. In contrast, avoidant women were more likely to pull away or withdraw from their partners. Collins and Feeney (2000) found that secure individuals were more likely to offer care and support to their partners during a laboratory discussion of a stressful event.

These findings suggest that part of the reason why some individuals feel more secure in their relationships is that they openly express their worries and receive reassurance and support (B.C. Feeney, 2007). Furthermore, the data suggest that some people feel insecure in their relationships because they cannot turn to their partners for comfort and support. There are at least two explanations for this. First, it may be that having a responsive partner influences the way an individual comes to think and behave in a relationship. Second, individuals who enter relationships with secure expectations are more likely to seek support from others and to elicit responsive behavior from them.

In support of the first interpretation, Simpson, Rholes, and Phillips (1996) observed partners who were instructed to discuss and resolve a major issue in their relationship. They found that anxious adults were more likely to view their partners in a negative light after a major conflict. These adults felt more anger and hostility toward their partners than less anxious individuals, and viewed their relationship as involving less love, commitment, and mutual respect. In contrast, secure individuals viewed their partners in a more positive light after discussing a conflictual topic. Thus conflictual relationship events, despite their negative valence, may provide an opportunity for secure individuals to build their trust in each other. In contrast, such conflicts appear to magnify insecure partners' insecurities and doubts.

Research also suggests that the beliefs and expectations people hold prior to entering a relationship affect secure-base behavior and relationship development. Collins (1996) conducted an experiment in which participants were instructed to read hypothetical scenarios depicting a partner behaving in ambiguous ways (e.g., losing track of the partner at a party). She found that anxious participants inferred hostile and rejecting intentions, whereas secure participants inferred more positive intentions.

### Attachment Styles and Parenting Behavior

Although most of the early research on parent–child interactions was conducted in the developmental tradition using the AAI to assess parents' state of mind with respect to attachment, a growing number of investigators have begun to explore the association between self-reported attachment style and parenting behavior. In one of the earliest studies on this topic, for example, Rholes, Simpson, and Blakely (1995) found that adults who were relatively avoidant were less likely than those who were secure to be sensitive and supportive in their interactions with their children. Jones, Cassidy, and Shaver (2015), who recently reviewed over 60 empirical studies on attachment styles and parenting, found that self-reported attachment was related to a variety of parenting outcomes, including parenting behavior (e.g., the provision of support), feelings about parenting and parenthood (e.g., the desire to have children, ambivalence about parenthood), and expectations and attitudes concerning parenting (e.g., perceptions of the child's difficulty). As Jones and his colleagues note, this kind of work is valuable for a number of reasons. For one, it demonstrates that attachment styles, as they are typically studied in the social-psychological tradition, have implications not only for romantic relationship functioning, but also for parenting. This helps make more explicit the interrelations among attachment and caregiving that have been central to the attachment–theoretical tradition but often are overlooked among social psychologists. This work also provides a point of contact between developmentally informed research and research in social psychology—a common ground that may be useful for understanding how alternative ways of assessing individual differences converge and where they diverge.

## Continuity and Change

Researchers studying continuity and change typically focus on both *normative continuity* (i.e., continuity in mean-levels across time) and rank-order stability (i.e., preservation in the ordering of individual differences across time). With regard to normative continuity and change, large-scale cross-sectional research by Chopik, Edelstein, and Fraley (2013) indicates that attachment-related anxiety is highest among younger adults and lowest among middle-aged and older adults. Attachment-related avoidance shows less dramatic age differences but is lowest in younger adults and highest in middle-aged adults. In addition, across the lifespan, people who are involved in romantic relationships report lower levels of anxiety and avoidance than do single individuals.

With respect to rank-order stability, research suggests that self-report measures of attachment are relatively stable across time. For example, Sibley, Fisher, and Liu (2005) reported that test–retest measures of anxiety and avoidance, measured with the ECR-R, were approximately .90 over a period of 3 weeks. Using a derivative of the ECR-R (to

be discussed in more detail below), Fraley, Vicary, Brumbaugh, and Roisman (2011) found that the test–retest stability of attachment styles was relatively constant whether the test–retest interval was 6 months or 1 year. This pattern of associations implies that there is a stable component to measures of adult attachment that underlies the occasion-to-occasion changes observed across interim assessments.

## Developmental Antecedents

A number of longitudinal studies that have emerged in recent years investigated the developmental antecedents of self-reported attachment styles. For example, in an analysis of data from 15 individuals followed longitudinally, Zayas, Mischel, Shoda, and Aber (2011) found associations between maternal caregiving assessed when infants were 18 months old and self-reported romantic avoidance at age 22. In a larger study involving 1,070 individuals followed from age 10 to age 21 and 27, Salo, Jokela, Lehtimäki, and Keltikangas-Järvinen (2011) found that early maternal nurturance was negatively prospectively related to avoidant attachment. Dinero, Conger, Shaver, Widaman, and Larsen-Rife (2008) found that the quality of observed interactions between adolescents and their parents predicted self-reported attachment at age 25. Chopik, Moors, and Edelstein (2014) found that individuals who had highly nurturing caregivers at age 3 experienced the largest decreases in avoidance over 20 years. Fraley and colleagues (2013) found that features of the caregiving environment, social competence, and the quality of peer relationships predicted some aspects of self-reported attachment at age 18. A variety of nonlongitudinal studies also suggests that variation in self-reported attachment is related to retrospectively recalled experiences, such as the quality of the parent–child relationship (e.g., Hazan & Shaver, 1987), parental divorce (e.g., Fraley & Heffernan, 2013), and the experience of parental abuse and neglect (e.g., Muller, Sicoli, & Lemieux, 2000).

A few broad conclusions can be drawn from this work, although we acknowledge that these conclusions are tentative given the relative dearth of large-scale, longitudinal research. First, although some research suggests that individual differences in attachment, as assessed via self-reports, may have their origins in early caregiving experiences, there is little compelling evidence to suggest that early experiences per se (i.e., independent of caregiving experiences that come later) play a direct role in shaping those differences. The work by Fraley and colleagues (2013), for example, suggests that understanding variation in attachment requires attention to developmental history (e.g., changes in parental sensitivity or the quality of peer relationships) writ large and not merely what transpires in the early years of life (see also Steele et al., 2014). Second, self-reported attachment styles are likely multidetermined. Some investigators, for example, have found that the mere recall of different kinds of relationship experiences may affect the attachment style that people report (Baldwin, Keelan, Fehr, Enns, & Koh-Rangarajoo, 1996). Fraley (2007) suggested that attachment styles might represent an aggregation of people's attachment-related experiences, potentially with the most accessible experiences being those that are most recent or those that are chronically activated.

### The Dismissing Strategy

According to attachment theory, people differ in the strategies they adopt to regulate the distress associated with nonoptimal caregiving. Following a separation and reunion, for example, some insecure children approach, but with ambivalence and resistance; others withdraw, apparently minimizing attachment-related feelings and behavior (Main & Weston, 1981). These different strategies have been referred to as "hyperactivating" or "maximizing" strategies and "deactivating" or "minimizing" strategies, respectively (Cassidy & Kobak, 1988; Fraley, Davis, & Shaver, 1998; Main, 1990). Researchers studying romantic attachment have attempted to illuminate some of the mechanisms underlying these behavioral strategies. In an experimental task in which adults were instructed to discuss losing their partners, Fraley and Shaver (1997) found that dismissing individuals were just as physiologically distressed (as assessed by skin conductance measures) as other individuals. When instructed to suppress their thoughts and feelings, however, dismissing individuals were able to do so effectively. That is, they could deactivate their physiological arousal to some degree and minimize the attention they paid to attachment-related thoughts. (Interestingly, preoccupied adults experienced an increase in arousal, relative to control conditions, when trying to suppress attachment-related anxiety.) Fraley and Shaver argued that such deactivation is possible because avoidant individuals (1) have less complex networks of attachment-related representations, (2) can effectively redirect their attention away from anxiety-provoking stimuli, and (3) can keep their interpersonal world structured so as to minimize attachment-related experiences.

In support of these propositions, Mikulincer and Orbach (1995) found that when asked to recall emotional childhood memories, avoidant adults recalled memories that were characterized by emotional discreteness. That is, when asked to recall a sad memory, avoidant individuals recalled memories that contained only elements of sadness and not elements of anger and anxiety, which tended to be present in the sad memories of secure and especially of preoccupied individuals. Fraley, Garner, and Shaver (2000) found that these recall processes were partly attributable to the way information is encoded rather than the way it is retrieved per se. Indeed, using both explicit and implicit tests of memory, Fraley and Brumbaugh (2007) found that highly avoidant individuals had difficulty remembering attachment-relevant information—even when they were offered financial incentives to recall as much of the information to which they had been exposed as possible.

Research has shown that highly dismissing individuals are less likely to engage in attachment behaviors with their partners (Fraley & Davis, 1997) and are less likely to engage in behaviors thought to promote affectional bonding, such as eye-to-eye contact, kissing, and open communication about feelings (Fraley et al., 1998). In summary, highly dismissing individuals organize their interpersonal behavior in a way that functions to minimize attention to and the experience of attachment-related thoughts and feelings (Fraley et al., 1998).

It should be noted, however, that these strategies can be undermined. Mikulincer, Dolev, and Shaver (2004) utilized a thought suppression paradigm similar to that used by Fraley and Shaver (1997) and found that highly avoidant people did not show even implicit indications of vulnerability after having thought about a relationship breakup; however, when they were placed under a cognitive load (having to remember a seven-digit number), concepts related to breaking up, as well as each avoidant person's own negative traits, became much more available, suggesting that avoidance can be broken down (as is the case with avoidant infants who are overstressed). These studies and others (Berant, Mikulincer, & Shaver, 2008) suggest that strategies used by avoidant individuals require cognitive effort.

## General Adjustment and Psychopathology

In general, individuals who are secure with respect to attachment have high self-esteem and are considered well adjusted, nurturing, and warm by their peers (Bartholomew & Horowitz, 1991). As found in studies using the AAI, this kind of self-esteem is also meaningfully related to attachment organization. For example, although autonomous and dismissing adults typically report high levels of self-esteem, Brennan and Morris (1997) found that secure adults were more likely to derive their self-esteem from internalized positive regard from others, whereas dismissing adults were more likely to derive their self-esteem from various abilities and competencies.

Not surprisingly, adults with a variety of clinical disorders are more likely to report themselves as insecure (see Mikulincer & Shaver, 2007). Depressed adults are more likely to report themselves as insecure (Carnelley, Pietromonaco, & Jaffe, 1994), as are individuals with eating disorders (Brennan & Shaver, 1995; Burge et al., 1997). College students who felt their parents had drinking problems were more likely to rate themselves as insecure (Brennan, Shaver, & Tobey, 1991) and reported they were more likely to "drink to cope" (Brennan & Shaver, 1995).

Brennan and Shaver (1998) examined the structure of self-report measures of 13 personality disorders (e.g., schizoid, paranoid, avoidant, obsessive–compulsive) and discovered that two of the three dimensions underlying these scales are the now-familiar dimensions underlying adult romantic attachment patterns (see Crawford et al., 2006). Woike, Osier, and Candella (1996) examined the association between self-reported attachment and the use of violent imagery in the Thematic Apperception Test (TAT). They found that anxious individuals were the most likely to use violent imagery, and they suggested that such imagery may stem from frustration with romantic partners who thwart attachment needs. Consistent with this line of reasoning, Dutton, Saunders, Starzomski, and Bartholomew (1994) found a high incidence of fearful and preoccupied men (i.e., the two groups highest on the anxiety dimension) within a sample that had been referred for treatment for wife assault.

## Discriminant Validity

Evidence for the construct validity of self-report measures of adult attachment comes from the no-

mological network (Cronbach & Meehl, 1955) of correlations between attachment measures and theoretically relevant variables. And the network corresponds with Bowlby's (1980) belief that attachment orientation is related to many aspects of a person's life. Still, the validity of self-report attachment measures would be called into question if they overlapped too much with measures of constructs viewed as theoretically distant from attachment. Some writers have expressed concern over the possibility that self-report measures of adult attachment are simply assessing relationship satisfaction (Bartholomew, 1994). Although security is correlated with relationship satisfaction, whether assessed with the AAI or with self-report attachment measures, the average magnitude of the correlation in the case of self-report attachment measures is only about .30 (see Mikulincer & Shaver, 2007, for a review). Thus, the correlation is not high enough to suggest that self-report measures of attachment and measures of satisfaction assess the same construct.

Research on adult personality has pointed to a five-factor model of personality (John, 1990; McCrae & Costa, 1990), with the factors being Neuroticism, Extraversion, Openness to Experience, Agreeableness, and Conscientiousness. Thus, questions arise concerning how the two major attachment dimensions fit into this structure and whether they are redundant with one or more of the five factors. Noftle and Shaver (2006) examined associations between the five traits and the attachment dimensions in over 8,000 students; they found that the anxiety dimension was correlated about .42 with Neuroticism, and that avoidance was correlated approximately −.22 with Agreeableness. Thus, the attachment dimensions, when assessed via self-reports, share variance with some of the major personality traits, but are not redundant with those traits. In fact, experimental studies of attachment processes (e.g., Mikulincer, Gillath, & Shaver, 2002) indicate associations between the attachment dimensions and theoretically predicted outcome variables, including behavior, when, for example, Neuroticism is statistically partialed out. Even in concurrent survey research, the attachment variables predict relationship outcomes better than the "Big Five" trait variables (e.g., Noftle & Shaver, 2006). Self-report measures of adult attachment are largely independent of verbal intelligence and social desirability response set (Fraley et al., 1998; Kunce & Shaver, 1994; Mikulincer & Orbach, 1995).

# Current Issues in the Measurement of Adult Romantic Attachment with Self-Reports

The field continues to evolve in new directions, and this growth has led to new challenges and opportunities. In the sections below, we highlight briefly two new issues that have become particularly salient since the previous edition of this volume.

## Hierarchical Models

For the most part social–personality psychologists have conceptualized and assessed adult attachment orientations as if they were domain-general interpersonal constructs. In other words, attachment styles are typically viewed as being relatively general cognitive structures that represent the history of a person's experiences in attachment relationships, and that have relevance for a broad array of contexts, including interpersonal relationships, mental health, and emotion regulation. Collins and Read (1994), however, suggested that there may be value in considering multiple working models in adult attachment research. Specifically, they noted that people hold not only global representations of attachment, but also relationship-specific models. Moreover, they argued that these attachment representations are hierarchically organized. People hold relatively global attachment representations of attachment relationships. But, nested within those, are representations of increasing specificity, including broad representations concerning parents and peers, and, nested within those, representations concerning specific individuals, for example, one's partner, one's mother (see Figure 27.2). Overall, Fletcher and Friesen (2003) provided empirical evidence in support of a hierarchical model by demonstrating that separate measures of attachment across multiple relational domains conformed to the predictions of a hierarchical model. Specifically, they showed that although a single latent variable could partially capture the associations among various relationship-specific measures of attachment, a hierarchical ordering in particular provided a better account of the data.

This hierarchical model has a number of implications for assessment and research (Overall et al., 2003). First, the stability of attachment representations may vary considerably as a function of the specificity of the representation (global vs. relationship-specific). Research has shown that the test–retest stability of global representations in romantic relationships is larger than the stability of relationship-specific representations of partners. For example, the test–retest stability of scores on the ECR-R—a general measure of romantic attachment—is close to .90 over 3 weeks (Sibley et al., 2005), whereas the test–retest stability of attachment toward a specific romantic partner is .65 (Fraley, Vicary, et al., 2011).

The stability of self-reported attachment in different types of relationship contexts may vary, too. Fraley, Vicary, and colleagues (2011) found that relationship-specific self-reports of attachment in romantic relationships ($r \cong .65$) were weaker than those of relationship-specific measures of attachment in people's current relationships with their parents ($r \cong .80$). They speculated that this differential stability may be due to people having more established histories with their parents relative to their romantic partners. Because many adults do not interact with their parents as frequently as they interact with their romantic partners, there may be less room for people's cognitions of their partners to be updated in light of ongoing experiences. Regardless, estimates of stability can vary at different points in the hierarchy, and this can matter greatly for efforts to understand continuity and change in attachment organization.

A second implication of the hierarchical model is that different kinds of attachment representations may be differentially relevant for predicting outcomes. Cozzarelli, Hoekstra, and Bylsma (2000) modified Bartholomew's RQ measure to assess separately people's general thoughts and feelings about others and their thoughts and feelings about their current partner. They found that partner-specific attachment had stronger and more numerous associations with relational outcomes than did general working models. General attachment, however, was strongly associated with broad measures of psychological well-being (see also Pierce & Lydon, 2001).

## Assessment

How should individual differences in attachment be assessed within the framework of a hierarchical model? For the most part, research on these issues has been improvised on a study-by-study basis. Some investigators, for example, have adopted Bartholomew and Horowitz's (1991) RQ and framed it in different ways to tap the desired level

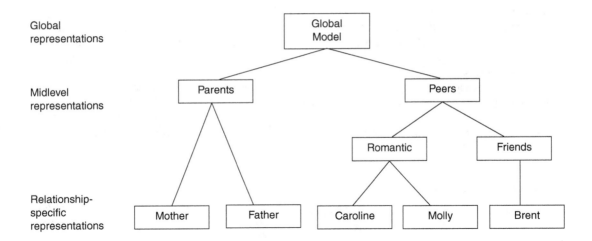

**FIGURE 27.2.** The hiearchical organization of attachment representations within the Collins and Read (1994) framework. The ECR and the ECR-R tends to focus on romantic representations within the midlevel tier. The ECR-RS tends to focus on relationship-specific representations. The RQ is typically used in a more general fashion or may be used to separately target parents and peers at the midlevel tier.

of generality (e.g., Cozzarelli et al., 2000). Other researchers have used measures such as the ECR (e.g., Brumbaugh & Fraley, 2006). The limitation of using different assessment strategies across laboratories, however, should be clear: Doing so makes it challenging to build a cumulative base of knowledge on the issues of interest.

Fraley, Heffernan, Vicary, and Brumbaugh (2011) attempted to solve this problem through the development of the Experiences in Close Relationships—Relationships Structures (ECR-RS), a self-report inventory modeled after the ECR and the ECR-R. They identified nine items that could be used to assess anxiety and avoidance separately in different relationship contexts (e.g., mother, father, partner, and friend). By using the same items but administering them separately across different relationship contexts, it is possible to study the convergence and divergence in attachment across domains without also conflating method with domain. The ECR-RS has been used with increasing frequency in the literature, and studies indicate that people who are relatively secure in one relationship domain also tend to be secure in another. However, there are noteworthy discrepancies. For example, Fraley, Heffernan, and colleagues reported that attachment-related avoidance with respect to how people felt about their mothers correlated only .15 with attachment-related avoidance in the romantic domain.

One limitation of the original ECR-RS is that it does not explicitly assess global attachment representations. It can be averaged across domains to estimate global attachment, which is useful strategy if one is simply trying to obtain a global measure as an end, in and of itself, but it complicates research if researchers are explicitly interested in modeling variation in an outcome as a function of both global and relationship specific models because the global models are fully linearly related to the specific models in such contexts. As such, Fraley and colleagues (2015) have more recently recommended assessing global models separately, but using the same ECR-RS item pool.

### State-Based Assessment and Priming Individual Differences

A growing body of work has focused on experimentally manipulating attachment orientations as a means for testing conceptual models of how variation in attachment may shape thoughts, feelings, and behavior. Of course, there are no clear and obvious means to manipulate a person's attachment style experimentally in any kind of deep and fundamental way, but one way to gain insight into attachment dynamics is by manipulating situations in ways that temporarily lead to increases in experienced security or insecurity.

This reasoning has led to two new and exciting developments in the social-psychological study of adult attachment. First, researchers have developed methods for temporarily priming attachment styles in ways consistent with theoretical models of individual differences. Second, researchers have developed ways to assess attachment-related states separately from the more dispositional representations that people hold of themselves and their attachment figures. These measures allow for a more nuanced understanding of how various contextual and psychological manipulations may lead to temporary changes in attachment functioning.

## Manipulating Individual Differences

Efforts to manipulate individual differences in attachment quality have their origins in social-psychological manipulations of context. For example, in their classic research, Simpson and colleagues (1992) exposed couples to a potentially distressing situation designed to activate their attachment orientations. As several investigators later realized, manipulating the situational context also provides an indirect way to manipulate components of the attachment system itself (e.g., Mikulincer et al., 2002). That is, placing a person in a situation in which the availability and responsiveness of his or her partner is called into question is comparable to manipulating the appraisals that people make regarding the availability and responsiveness of their partners. As such, these kinds of manipulations provide a potential means to probe the operation of the attachment system at a deeper level.

Mikulincer and his colleagues (2002) have utilized this strategy most overtly. For example, in one set of studies, they attempted to prime individual differences in insecurity by exposing people subliminally to threat- or neutral-word primes. They found that threat primes led to increased accessibility of representations of attachment figures as inferred from more rapid lexical decisions to the names of attachment figures.

This kind of strategy has been an influential way of probing the dynamics of the attachment system in the social-personality literature. But, unfortunately, there is not a *standard* way of probing the attachment system at the moment. Some researchers focus on using primes that are presented below the threshold of awareness (e.g., Mikulincer at al., 2002), whereas others use supraliminal primes and manipulations, and guided imagery tasks (e.g., Rowe & Carnelley, 2003). As a consequence of this diversity, it is unclear at the moment whether

some distinctions (e.g., sub- vs. supraliminal) matter for most purposes, which individual difference dimensions are most strongly affected by various manipulations, and which methods are more effective than others. To be clear: This kind of diversity is natural and expected when researchers are charting new empirical territory. But we believe that one of the core challenges for the field over the next few years will be to nail down these issues and create standard methods.

Another complication is that it is not clear which elements of the attachment system should be primed or what the appropriate reference group is. On the one hand, it seems straightforward to prime people's sense of insecurity with respect to anxiety. When people are asked to recall episodes in which they felt insecure about the availability or accessibility of their partners, such a manipulation is face valid with respect to its relevance for understanding variation in the extent to which people are concerned about the accessibility and responsiveness of their partners. But what about *security* priming? Some methods focus on priming security in particular, in part for ethical reasons (it is more defensible to attempt to experimentally manipulate something positive) and in part for theoretical reasons (e.g., to test the hypothesis that temporarily increasing security may lead to increases in prosocial behavior, such as compassion and altruism (e.g., Carnelley & Rowe, 2007; Mikulincer, Shaver, Gillath, & Nitzberg, 2005). Such primes may involve exposing people to security-related words (e.g., *love*, *support*) or having people retrieve from memory episodes in which they felt loved and supported by attachment figures. Do existing security primes influence the anxiety dimension, the avoidance dimension, or both? Our guess is that many existing security primes create more movement on the anxiety axis than on the avoidance axis. But, ultimately, this is an empirical question. Based on an analysis of postpriming written protocols, Carnelley and Rowe (2010) suggested that security priming leads to increases in felt security, positive care, and a sense of merging with another, suggesting that such primes may move people through both dimensions of the two-dimensional space.

What is the optimal way of conceptualizing these issues? We do not have definitive answers, but we do offer two thoughts in the hope that they will be helpful for moving future research forward. First, in many respects, the core issue in the social-psychological tradition in attachment research is whether people feel safe, secure, loved, and accepted. Having a secure base, both literally and symbolically, enables people to explore the world in a less inhibited manner. Theoretically, this is what the anxiety dimension is designed to capture: individual differences in the extent to which people are concerned with the availability and responsiveness of close others. This may be the most natural variable to manipulate in an experimental context. Our guess is that current security primes manipulate the anxiety dimension in one direction and insecure primes manipulate it in the other, but that none of the existing priming procedures are manipulating avoidance in a way that is as direct as the way they are manipulating anxiety. More importantly, however, it might be the case that manipulating attachment-related anxiety is more theoretically central than manipulating avoidance, at least for most purposes.

Second, manipulating avoidance seems like a challenging task given the way avoidance is conceptualized in most theoretical models. In the process models typically depicted in the adult attachment literature (e.g., Fraley & Shaver, 2000; Mikulincer & Shaver, 2007), avoidance reflects a secondary strategy. Specifically, when a person's attachment system is activated (as may be reflected in a temporary boost in attachment-related anxiety), the person may attempt to regulate that anxiety by seeking proximity and comfort from attachment figures or withdrawing from others (i.e., engaging in deactivating strategies). Thus, the activation of anxiety fuels movement along the avoidance dimension and in a direction that is biased toward the person's habitual strategy for regulating attachment-related concerns. This suggests that it might not be possible to manipulate anxiety without also nudging people toward their prototypical strategies for regulating anxiety.

Nonetheless, Fraley and Shaver (1997), for example, attempted to manipulate deactivating strategies by instructing people to inhibit the expression of attachment-related concerns. They also attempted to manipulate anxiety separately by instructing people to imagine the loss of their partner. Mikulincer and colleagues (2004) used a similar procedure but attempted to disrupt the potential efficacy of deactivating strategies by depleting people's cognitive resources. That is, if fewer cognitive resources are available to the person, the strategies are less likely to be effective. This work suggests two possibilities: It might be possible to manipulate avoidance via explicit task instructions to avoid or suppress specific thoughts, feelings, or behaviors. In addition, if avoidance is

resource demanding, deleting a person's cognitive resources may provide an indirect means also to manipulate avoidance experimentally (more so than anxiety).

In summary, there are diverse methods that researchers have used to attempt to temporarily manipulate people's attachment orientations. In our opinion, most of these methods target variation in the anxiety dimension. However, we are not aware of systematic work that clearly maps these manipulations onto changes in attachment. We think future progress can be made by (1) creating standard or commonly used procedures for priming attachment, (2) delineating exactly which components of the attachment system are being varied with those manipulations, and (3) finding ways to vary attachment-related anxiety and avoidance separately to the extent to which it is feasible and useful.

### State-Based Measures

The emerging interest in security priming in the social–personality tradition has led to a need to measure people's state-like thoughts and feelings with respect to attachment. State-based measures are designed to probe people about their momentary feelings, regardless of how they might feel in other moments. One recent measure that is proving useful in this regard is the State Adult Attachment Measure (SAAM; Gillath, Hart, Noftle, & Stockdale, 2009), which is based on a three-factor solution and provides state-based assessments of people feel in the moment. Research by Xu and Shrout (2013) suggests that the SAAM offers a highly reliable means for assessing state-based changes in attachment.

## Discussion

From a topic area that hardly existed before 1985, the study of adult attachment has grown over the past three decades to become one of the most active and visible areas in developmental, social, personality, and clinical psychology. In general, the findings obtained by adult attachment researchers have been interesting, consistent, and compatible with Bowlby's and Ainsworth's theories. Nevertheless, the issue of measurement continues to present intriguing and important challenges. One problem is the lack of convergence among different measures of adult attachment. A number of studies have included more than one measure of some aspect of adult attachment, including measures that tap different relational domains (e.g., relationships with parents or romantic partners) and embody different methods (e.g., interviews, self-reports). In the initial version of this chapter in first edition of the *Handbook of Attachment*, we reported an informal meta-analysis of such studies. The results indicated that the correlation between any two measures of adult attachment were affected both by domain (i.e., whether the measures were designed to assess some aspect of romantic relationships or some aspect of relationships with parents) and method (i.e., whether the measures were based on interviews or self-report). The correlation between different measures of security tended to be greater when there was a match between the method used (e.g., both measures based on self-report or both based on interviews) and the domain (e.g., both measures focused on parental representations or both measures focused on romantic representations).

One important example of this patterning is that the two most commonly used measures of adult attachment (i.e., self-reports of the attachment dimensions and the AAI classifications) have only a very weak association, despite the fact that the two kinds of measures sometimes have similar correlations with other variables (e.g., Granqvist & Kirkpatrick, Chapter 39, this volume; Simpson et al., 2002). Roisman, Holland, and colleagues (2007; see Haydon et al., 2011) published a meta-analysis of all available studies that included both the AAI and some self-report attachment style measure. Aggregating data from over 900 individuals, they found a correlation of only .09, which is a small association by the frequently used standards proposed by Cohen (1992). Moreover, in those particular studies, they found that although both measures predicted important aspects of close relationship functioning in adulthood, they did not necessarily predict the same outcomes in the same ways.

For example, AAI security seems to function as a general personal and interpersonal asset; highly autonomous or secure individuals were more likely to be collaborative in their laboratory interactions with their partners—just as scoring of the AAI itself addresses, in part, the ability and willingness of an interviewee to collaborate with an interviewer (see Hesse, Chapter 26, this volume). The attachment dimensions, in contrast, functioned more like what would be expected from a diathesis–stress perspective on attachment dynamics (e.g., Simpson & Rholes, 1998). Anxiety and avoidance were related to less collaborative interactions, but only among individuals who appraised the interaction as stressful or threatening (and, we suppose, were more likely to have their attachment systems activated).

Although we still do not fully understand how the different measures work and why, or precisely what they measure (as inferred from their broad and largely different nomothetic networks), it is clear that they should not be viewed as substitutes for each other in particular kinds of research. We therefore encourage researchers to use assessment techniques that are most relevant to the kind of relationship or attachment-related processes they wish to study. For example, if a researcher is interested in studying romantic attachment dynamics, he or she should use either one of the multi-item self-report measures (e.g., the ECR or ECR-R) or one of the romantic interview techniques (Crowell and Owen's [1996] CRI or Cowan and colleagues' [1999] CAI). If the researcher is interested in the coherence with which one describes early experiences with attachment figures, he or she should use the AAI. If the focus is on relationship-related emotions and behavior under stressful circumstances, especially as experienced and reported by the person him- or herself, the self-report measures may be more relevant. If the focus is on all of these things at once, it is possible that two kinds of measures will produce both useful findings and insights. Investigators interested in assessing the common variance underlying adolescents' and adults' various attachment orientations will have to assess attachment variation across multiple relationship domains (e.g., parents, close friends, romantic partners), preferably using a variety of methods (e.g., self-reports, interviews) and latent structural modeling techniques (see Griffin & Bartholomew, 1994b).

As we have explained throughout this chapter, each measure was developed for a particular purpose. Therefore, in determining which one or more instruments to use for a particular study, a researcher should consider the theoretical assumptions underlying each instrument. AAI coding is meant to tap an adult's generalized representation of attachment based on his or her current "state of mind with respect to attachment," as inferred from narrative measures of experiences with parents during childhood. Its focus on discourse is based on the assumption that the ability to describe secure-base experiences reflects the nature of those experiences. It is a rich and well-validated measure that provides considerable information about perceived childhood experiences that may shape attachment patterns. Nevertheless, the AAI is expensive and difficult to score.

In contrast, the self-report attachment measures were designed under the assumption that the patterns Ainsworth described would reflect variation in the organization of the attachment system at any age. The self-report measures assume that people can accurately describe some of their thoughts, feelings, and behaviors in romantic or other close relationships. Such measures are not ideal for investigating mechanisms and strategies per se, but they have been effectively used in conjunction with other techniques (e.g., psychophysiological, behavioral, and cognitive procedures) to uncover important aspects of intrapsychic processes and behavior in close relationships.

In summary, before choosing a measure to assess adult attachment, researchers should consider (1) the assumptions underlying each technique, and the conceptual connection between a technique and the concepts and propositions of attachment theory, and (2) the relationship domain to be investigated (e.g., parents, close friends, romantic partners). In light of the substantial differences among adult attachment measures, we urge that considerable caution be taken in how researchers present their findings, and in how they generalize across measures with respect to attachment theory. Furthermore, we encourage researchers to continue to investigate the many measurement issues inherent in the study of adult attachment. There is still a great deal of work to be done before we understand relations and nonrelations among the various instruments and the best ways to assess normative development and individual differences in adult attachment organization. We hope this overview provides a useful basis for further exploration.

## References

Adam, E. K., Gunnar, M. R., & Tanaka, A. (2004). Adult attachment, parent emotion, and observed parenting behavior: Mediator and moderator models. *Child Development, 75,* 110–122.

Ainsworth, M. D. S. (1985). Attachments across the life span. *Bulletin of the New York Academy of Medicine, 61,* 792–811.

Ainsworth, M. D. S. (1991). Attachments and other affectional bonds across the life cycle. In C. M. Parkes, J. Stevenson-Hinde, & P. Marris (Eds.), *Attachment across the life cycle* (pp. 33–51). London: Routledge.

Ainsworth, M. D. S., Blehar, M., Waters, E., & Wall, S. (1978). *Patterns of attachment: A psychological study of the Strange Situation.* Hillsdale, NJ: Erlbaum.

Alexandrov, E. O., Cowan, P. A., & Cowan, C. P. (2005). Couple attachment and the quality of marital relationships: Method and concept in the validation for the new couple attachment interview and coding system. *Attachment and Human Development, 7,* 123–152.

Allen, J. P., Marsh, P., McFarland, C., McElhaney, K. B., Land, D. J., Jodl, K. M., et al. (2002). Attachment and autonomy as predictors of the development of social skills and delinquency during mid-adolescence. *Journal of Consulting and Clinical Psychology, 70,* 56–66.

Allen, J. P., McElhaney, K. B., Kuperminc, G. P., & Jodl, K. M. (2004). Stability and change in attachment security across adolescence. *Child Development, 75,* 1792–1805.

Allen, J. P., McElhaney, K. B., Land, D. J., Kuperminc, G. P., Moore, C. W., O'Beirne-Kelly, H., et al. (2003). A secure base in adolescence: Markers of attachment security in the mother–adolescent relationship. *Child Development, 74,* 292–307.

Armsden, G. C., & Greenberg, M. T. (1987). The Inventory of Parent and Peer Attachment: Relationships to well-being in adolescence. *Journal of Youth and Adolescence, 16,* 427–454.

Atkinson, L., Paglia, A., Coolbear, J., Niccols, A., Parker, K. C. H., & Guger, S. (2000). Attachment security: A meta-analysis of maternal mental health correlates. *Clinical Psychology Review, 20,* 1019–1040.

Bakermans-Kranenburg, M. J., & Van IJzendoorn, M. H. (1993). A psychometric study of the Adult Attachment Interview: Reliability and discriminant validity. *Developmental Psychology, 29,* 870–879.

Bakermans-Kranenburg, M. J., & Van IJzendoorn, M. H. (2009). The first 10,000 Adult Attachment Interviews: Distributions of adult attachment representations in clinical and non-clinical groups. *Attachment and Human Development, 11,* 223–263.

Baldwin, M. W., & Fehr, B. (1995). On the instability of attachment style ratings. *Personal Relationships, 2,* 247–261.

Baldwin, M. W., Keelan, J. P. R., Fehr, B., Enns, V., & Koh-Rangarajoo, E. (1996). Social-cognitive conceptualization of attachment working models: Availability and accessibility effects. *Journal of Personality and Social Psychology, 71,* 94–109.

Bartholomew, K. (1990). Avoidance of intimacy: An attachment perspective. *Journal of Social and Personal Relationships, 7,* 147–178.

Bartholomew, K. (1994). Assessment of individual differences in adult attachment. *Psychological Inquiry, 5,* 23–27.

Bartholomew, K., & Horowitz, L. (1991). Attachment styles among young adults: A test of a four category model. *Journal of Personality and Social Psychology, 61,* 226–244.

Benoit, D., & Parker, K. C. H. (1994). Stability and transmission of attachment across three generations. *Child Development, 65,* 1444–1456.

Benoit, D., Zeanah, C., & Barton, M. (1989). Maternal attachment disturbances in failure to thrive. *Infant Mental Health Journal, 10,* 185–202.

Berant, E., Mikulincer, M., & Shaver, P. R. (2008). Mothers' attachment style, their mental health, and their children's emotional vulnerabilities: A 7-year study of children with congenital heart disease. *Journal of Personality, 76,* 31–66.

Bernier, A., Larose, S., Boivin, M., & Soucy, N. (2004). Attachment state of mind: Implications for adjustment to college. *Journal of Adolescent Research, 19,* 783–806.

Booth-LaForce, C., Groh, A. M., Burchinal, M. R., Roisman, G. I., Owen, M. T., & Cox, M. J. (2014). Caregiving and contextual sources of continuity and change in attachment security from infancy to late adolescence. In C. Booth-LaForce & G. I. Roisman (Eds.), The Adult Attachment Interview: Psychometrics, stability and change from infancy, and developmental origins. *Monographs of the Society for Research in Child Development, 79*(3), 67–84.

Bost, K. K., Shin, N., McBride, B. A., Brown, G. L., Vaughn, B. E., Coppola, G., et al. (2006). Maternal secure base scripts, children's attachment security, and mother–child narrative styles. *Attachment and Human Development, 8,* 241–260.

Bowlby, J. (1973). *Attachment and loss: Vol. 2. Separation: Anxiety and anger.* New York: Basic Books.

Bowlby, J. (1980). *Attachment and loss: Vol. 3. Loss: Sadness and depression.* New York: Basic Books.

Bowlby, J. (1982). *Attachment and loss: Vol. 1. Attachment.* New York: Basic Books. (Original work published 1969)

Brennan, K. A., Clark, C. L., & Shaver, P. R. (1998). Self-report measurement of adult attachment: An integrative overview. In J. A. Simpson & W. S. Rholes (Eds.), *Attachment theory and close relationships* (pp. 46–76). New York: Guilford Press.

Brennan, K. A., & Morris, K. A. (1997). Attachment styles, self-esteem, and patterns of seeking feedback from romantic partners. *Personality and Social Psychology Bulletin, 23,* 23–31.

Brennan, K. A., & Shaver, P. R. (1995). Dimensions of adult attachment, affect regulation, and romantic relationship functioning. *Personality and Social Psychology Bulletin, 21,* 267–283.

Brennan, K. A., & Shaver, P. R. (1998). Attachment styles and personality disorders: Their connections to each other and to parental divorce, parental death, and perceptions of parental caregiving. *Journal of Personality, 66,* 835–878.

Brennan, K. A., Shaver, P. R., & Tobey, A. E. (1991). Attachment styles, gender, and parental problem drinking. *Journal of Social and Personal Relationships, 8,* 451–466.

Bretherton, I. (1985). Attachment theory: Retrospect and prospect. In I. Bretherton & E. Waters (Eds.), Growing points of attachment theory and research. *Monographs of the Society for Research in Child Development, 50*(1–2, Serial No. 209), 3–35.

Bretherton, I. (1987). New perspectives on attachment relations: Security, communication, and working models. In J. Osofsky (Ed.), *Handbook of infant development* (2nd ed., pp. 1061–1100). New York: Wiley.

Bretherton, I. (1990). Open communication and internal working models: Their role in the development of attachment relationships. In R. Thompson (Ed.), *Nebraska Symposium on Motivation: Vol. 36. Socioemotional development* (pp. 57–113). Lincoln: University of Nebraska Press.

Brumbaugh, C. C., & Fraley, R. C. (2006). Transference and attachment: How do attachment patterns get carried forward from one relationship to the next? *Personality and Social Psychology Bulletin, 32,* 552–560.

Burge, D., Hammen, C., Davila, J., Daley, S. E., Paley, B., Lindberg, N., et al. (1997). The relationship between attachment cognitions and psychological adjustment in late adolescent women. *Development and Psychopathology, 9,* 151–167.

Carnelley, K. B., Pietromonaco, P. R., & Jaffe, K. (1994). Depression, working models of others, and relationship functioning. *Journal of Personality and Social Psychology, 66,* 127–140.

Carnelley, K. B., & Rowe, A. C. (2007). Repeated priming of attachment security influences later views of self and relationships. *Personal Relationships, 14,* 307–320.

Carnelley, K. B., & Rowe, A. C. (2010). Priming a sense of security: What goes through people's minds? *Journal of Social and Personal Relationships, 27,* 253–261.

Cassibba, R., Van IJzendoorn, M. H., Bruno, S., & Coppola, G. (2004). Attachment of mothers and children with recurrent asthmatic bronchitis. *Journal of Asthma, 41,* 419–431.

Cassidy, J., & Kobak, R. R. (1988). Avoidance and its relation to other defensive processes. In J. Belsky & T. Nezworski (Eds.), *Clinical implications of attachment* (pp. 300–323). Hillsdale, NJ: Erlbaum.

Chappell, K. D., & Davis, K. E. (1998). Attachment, partner choice, and perceptions of romantic partners: An experimental test of the attachment-security hypothesis. *Personal Relationships, 5,* 327–342.

Chopik, W. J., Edelstein, R. S., & Fraley, R. C. (2013). From the cradle to the grave: Age differences in attachment from early adulthood to old age. *Journal of Personality, 81,* 171–183.

Chopik, W. J., Moors, A. C., & Edelstein, R. S. (2014). Maternal nurturance predicts decreases in attachment avoidance in emerging adulthood. *Journal of Research in Personality, 53,* 47–53.

Cohen, J. (1992). A power primer. *Psychological Bulletin, 112,* 155–159.

Cohn, D. A., Cowan, P. A., Cowan, C. P., & Pearson, J. (1992). Mothers' and fathers' working models of childhood attachment relationships, parenting styles, and child behavior. *Development and Psychopathology,* 4, 417–431.

Cohn, D. A., Silver, D. H., Cowan, C. P., Cowan, P. A., & Pearson, J. (1992). Working models of childhood attachment and couple relationships. *Journal of Family Issues, 13*(4), 432–449.

Collins, N. L. (1996). Working models of attachment: Implications for explanation, emotion, and behavior. *Journal of Personality and Social Psychology, 71,* 810–832.

Collins, N. L., & Feeney, B. C. (2000). A safe haven: an attachment theory perspective on support seeking and caregiving in intimate relationships. *Journal of Personality and Social Psychology, 78,* 1053–1073.

Collins, N. L., & Read, S. J. (1990). Adult attachment, working models, and relationship quality in dating couples. *Journal of Personality and Social Psychology, 58,* 644–663.

Collins, N. L., & Read, S. J. (1994). Cognitive representations of attachment: The structure and function of working models. In K. Bartholomew & D. Perlman (Eds.), *Attachment processes in adulthood: Advances in personal relationships* (Vol. 5, pp. 53–90). London: Jessica Kingsley.

Coppola, G., Vaughn, B. E., Cassibba, R., & Costantini, A. (2006). The attachment script representation procedure in an Italian sample: Associations with Adult Attachment Interview scales and with maternal sensitivity. *Attachment and Human Development, 8,* 209–219.

Cowan, P., Cohn, D., Cowan, C., & Pearson, J. (1996). Parents' attachment histories and children's externalizing and internalizing behavior: Exploring family systems models of linkage. *Journal of Consulting and Clinical Psychology, 64,* 53–63.

Cowan, P. A., Cowan, C. P., Alexandrov, E. O., Lyon, S., & Heming, H. (1999) Couples' Attachment Interview. Unpublished manuscript, University of California, Berkeley.

Cozzarelli, C., Hoekstra, S. J., & Bylsma, W. H. (2000). General versus specific mental models of attachment: Are they associated with different outcomes? *Personality and Social Psychology Bulletin, 26,* 605–618.

Crawford, T. N., Shaver, P. R., Cohen, P., Pilkonis, P. A., Gillath, O., & Kasen, S. (2006). Self-reported attachment, interpersonal aggression, and personality disorder in a prospective community sample of adolescents and adults. *Journal of Personality Disorders, 20,* 331–351.

Creasey, G. (2002). Associations between working models of attachment and conflict management behavior in romantic couples. *Journal of Counseling Psychology, 49,* 365–375.

Creasey, G., & Ladd, A. (2004). Negative mood relations expectancies and conflict behaviors in late adolescent college student romantic relationships: The moderating role of generalized attachment representations. *Journal of Research on Adolescence, 14,* 235–255.

Creasey, G., & Ladd, A. (2005). Generalized and specific attachment representations: Unique and interactive roles in predicting conflict behaviors in close relationships. *Personality and Social Psychology Bulletin, 31,* 1026–1038.

Crittenden, P., Partridge, M., & Claussen, A. (1991). Family patterns of relationships in normative and dysfunctional families. *Development and Psychopathology, 3,* 491–512.

Cronbach, L. J., & Meehl, P. E. (1955). Construct validity in psychological tests. *Psychological Bulletin, 52,* 281–302.

Crowell, J. A., & Feldman, S. S. (1988). Mothers' internal models of relationships and children's behavioral and developmental status: A study of mother–child interaction. *Child Development, 59,* 1273–1285.

Crowell, J. A., & Feldman, S. S. (1991). Mothers' working models of attachment relationships and mother and child behavior during separation and reunion. *Developmental Psychology, 27,* 597–605.

Crowell, J. A., & Hauser, S. (2008). AAIs in a high-risk sample: Stability and relation to functioning from adolescence to 39 years. In H. Steele & M. Steele (Eds.), *Clinical applications of the Adult Attachment Interview* (pp. 341–370). New York: Guilford Press.

Crowell, J. A., O'Connor, E., Wollmers, G., Sprafkin, J., & Rao, U. (1991). Mothers' conceptualizations of parent–child relationships: Relation to mother–child interaction and child behavior problems. *Development and Psychopathology, 3,* 431–444.

Crowell, J. A., & Owens, G. (1996). *Current Relationship Interview and scoring system.* Unpublished manuscript, State University of New York at Stony Brook.

Crowell, J. A., Treboux, D., Gao, Y., Fyffe, C., Pan, H., & Waters, E. (2002). Assessing secure base behavior in adulthood: Development of a measure, links to adult attachment representations, and relations to couples' communication and reports of relationships. *Developmental Psychology, 38,* 679–693.

Crowell, J. A., Treboux, D., & Waters, E. (1999). The Adult Attachment Interview and the Relationship Questionnaire: Relations to reports of mothers and partners. *Personal Relationships, 6,* 1–18.

Crowell, J. A., Treboux, D., & Waters, E. (2002). Stability of attachment representations: The transition to marriage. *Developmental Psychology, 38,* 467–479.

Crowell, J. A., & Waters, E. (1997, April). *Couples' attachment representations: Stability and relation to marital behavior.* Paper presented at the biennial meeting of the Society for Research in Child Development, Washington, DC.

Crowell, J. A., Waters, E., Treboux, D., O'Connor, E., Colon-Downs, C., Feider, O., et al. (1996). Discriminant validity of the Adult Attachment Interview. *Child Development, 67,* 2584–2599.

Curran, M., Hazen, N., Jacobvitz, D., & Feldman, A. (2005). Representations of early family relationships predict marital maintenance during the transition to parenthood. *Journal of Family Psychology, 19,* 189–197.

Das Eiden, R., Teti, D., & Corns, K. (1995). Maternal working models of attachment, marital adjustment, and the parent–child relationship. *Child Development, 66,* 1504–1518.

DeOliveira, C. A., Moran, G., & Pederson, D. R. (2005). Understanding the link between maternal adult attachment classifications and thoughts and feelings about emotions. *Attachment and Human Development, 7,* 153–170.

Dickstein, S., Seifer, R., Albus, K. E., & Magee, K. D. (2004). Attachment patterns across multiple family relationships in adulthood: Associations with maternal depression. *Developmental Psychopathology, 16,* 735–751.

Dinero, R. E., Conger, R. D., Shaver, P. R., Widaman, K. F., & Larsen-Rife, D. (2008). Influence of family of origin and adult romantic partners on romantic attachment security. *Journal of Family Psychology, 22,* 622–632.

Dozier, M., & Kobak, R. R. (1992). Psychophysiology in attachment interviews: Converging evidence for deactivating strategies. *Child Development, 63,* 1473–1480.

Dozier, M., & Lee, S. W. (1995). Discrepancies between self and other-report of psychiatric symptomatology: Effects of dismissing attachment strategies. *Development and Psychopathology, 7,* 217–226.

Dutton, D. G., Saunders, K., Starzomski, A., & Bartholomew, K. (1994). Intimacy–anger and insecure attachment as precursors of abuse in intimate relationships. *Journal of Applied Social Psychology, 24,* 1367–1386.

Dykas, M. J., Woodhouse, S. S., Cassidy, J., & Waters, H. S. (2006). Narrative assessment of attachment representations: Links between secure base scripts and adolescent attachment. *Attachment & Human Development, 8,* 221–240.

Fearon, R. M. P., Groh, A. M., Bakermans-Kranenburg, M. J., Van IJzendoorn, M. H., & Roisman, G. I. (in press). Attachment and developmental psychopathology. In D. Cicchetti (Ed.), *Developmental psychopathology* (3rd ed.). New York: Wiley.

Feeney, B. C. (2007). The dependency paradox in close relationships: Accepting dependence promotes independence. *Journal of Personality and Social Psychology, 92,* 268–285.

Feeney, B. C., & Thrush, R. L. (2010). Relationship influences on exploration in adulthood: The characteristics and function of a secure base. *Journal of Personality and Social Psychology, 98,* 57–76.

Feeney, J. A., Noller, P., & Hanrahan, M. (1994). Assessing adult attachment: Developments in the conceptualization of security and insecurity. In M. B. Sperling & W. H. Berman (Eds.), *Attachment in adults: Clinical and developmental perspectives* (pp. 128–152). New York: Guilford Press.

Fonagy, P., Steele, H., & Steele, M. (1991). Maternal

representations of attachment during pregnancy predict the organization of infant–mother attachment. *Child Development, 62,* 891–905.

Fonagy, P., Steele, M., Steele, H., Moran, G. S., & Higgitt, A. C. (1991). The capacity for understanding mental states: The reflective self in parent and child and its significance for security of attachment. *Infant Mental Health Journal, 12,* 201–218.

Fortuna, K., Roisman, G. I., Haydon, K. C., Groh, A. M., & Holland, A. S. (2011). Attachment states of mind and the quality of young adults' sibling relationships. *Developmental Psychology, 47,* 1366–1373.

Fraley, R. C. (2002). Attachment stability from infancy to adulthood: Meta-analysis and dynamic modeling of developmental mechanisms. *Personality and Social Psychology Review, 6,* 123–151.

Fraley, R. C. (2007). A connectionist approach to the organization and continuity of working models of attachment. *Journal of Personality, 75,* 1157–1180.

Fraley, R. C., & Brumbaugh, C. C. (2007). Adult attachment and preemptive defenses: Converging evidence on the role of defensive exclusion at the level of encoding. *Journal of Personality, 75,* 1033–1050.

Fraley, R. C., & Davis, K. E. (1997). Attachment formation and transfer in young adults' close friendships and romantic relationships. *Personal Relationships, 4,* 131–144.

Fraley, R. C., Davis, K. E., & Shaver, P. R. (1998). Dismissing-avoidance and the defensive organization of emotion, cognition, and behavior. In J. A. Simpson & W. S. Rholes (Eds.), *Attachment theory and close relationships* (pp. 249–279). New York: Guilford Press.

Fraley, R. C., Garner, J. P., & Shaver, P. R. (2000). Adult attachment and the defensive regulation of attention and memory: Examining the role of preemptive and postemptive defensive processes. *Journal of Personality and Social Psychology, 79,* 816–826.

Fraley, R. C., & Heffernan, M. E. (2013). Attachment and parental divorce: A test of the diffusion and sensitive period hypotheses. *Personality and Social Psychology Bulletin, 39,* 1199–1213.

Fraley, R. C., Heffernan, M. E., Vicary, A. M., & Brumbaugh, C. C. (2011). The experiences in close relationships—Relationship Structures Questionnaire: A method for assessing attachment orientations across relationships. *Psychological Assessment, 23,* 615–625.

Fraley, R. C., Hudson, N. W., Heffernan, M. E., & Segal, N. (2015). Are adult attachment styles categorical or dimensional? A taxometric analysis of general and relationship-specific attachment orientations. *Journal of Personality and Social Psychology, 109,* 354–368.

Fraley, R. C., & Roisman, G. I. (2014). Categories or dimensions?: A taxometric analysis of the Adult Attachment Interview. In C. Booth-LaForce & G. I. Roisman (Eds.), The Adult Attachment Interview: Psychometrics, stability and change from infancy, and developmental origins. *Monographs of the Society for Research in Child Development, 79*(3), 36–50.

Fraley, R. C., Roisman, G. I., Booth-LaForce, C., Owen, M. T., & Holland, A. S. (2013). Interpersonal and genetic origins of adult attachment styles: A longitudinal study from infancy to early adulthood. *Journal of Personality and Social Psychology, 104,* 817–838.

Fraley, R. C., & Shaver, P. R. (1997). Adult attachment and the suppression of unwanted thoughts. *Journal of Personality and Social Psychology, 73,* 1080–1091.

Fraley, R. C., & Shaver, P. R. (1998). Airport separations: A naturalistic study of adult attachment dynamics in separating couples. *Journal of Personality and Social Psychology, 75,* 1198–1212.

Fraley, R. C., & Shaver, P. R. (2000). Adult romantic attachment: Theoretical developments, emerging controversies, and unanswered questions. *Review of General Psychology, 4,* 132–154.

Fraley, R. C., & Spieker, S. J. (2003a). Are infant attachment patterns continuously or categorically distributed?: A taxometric analysis of Strange Situation behavior. *Developmental Psychology, 39,* 387–404.

Fraley, R. C., & Spieker, S. J. (2003b). What are the differences between dimensional and categorical models of individual differences in attachment?: Reply to Cassidy (2003), Cummings (2003), Sroufe (2003), and Waters and Beauchaine (2003). *Developmental Psychology, 39,* 423–429.

Fraley, R. C., Vicary, A. M., Brumbaugh, C. C., & Roisman, G. I. (2011). Patterns of stability in adult attachment: An empirical test of two models of continuity and change. *Journal of Personality and Social Psychology, 101,* 974–992.

Fraley, R. C., & Waller, N. G. (1998). Adult attachment patterns: A test of the typological model. In J. A. Simpson & W. S. Rholes (Eds.), *Attachment theory and close relationships* (pp. 77–114). New York: Guilford Press.

Fraley, R. C., Waller, N. G., & Brennan, K. A. (2000). An item response theory analysis of self-report measures of adult attachment. *Journal of Personality and Social Psychology, 78,* 350–365.

Frazier, P. A., Byer, A. L., Fischer, A. R., Wright, D. M., & DeBord, K. A. (1996). Adult attachment style and partner choice: Correlational and experimental findings. *Personal Relationships, 3,* 117–136.

Furman, W., & Simon, V. A. (2006). Actor and partner effects of adolescents' romantic working models and styles on interactions with romantic partners. *Child Development, 77,* 588–604.

Furman, W., Simon, V. A., Shaffer, L., & Bouchey, H. A. (2002). Adolescents' representations of relationships with parents, friends and romantic partners. *Child Development, 73,* 241–255.

George, C., Kaplan, N., & Main, M. (1984). *Adult Attachment Interview protocol.* Unpublished interview, University of California, Berkeley.

George, C., Kaplan, N., & Main, M. (1985). *Adult Attachment Interview protocol* (2nd ed.). Unpublished interview, University of California, Berkeley.

George, C., Kaplan, N., & Main, M. (1996). *Adult At-*

*tachment Interview protocol* (3rd ed.). Unpublished interview, University of California, Berkeley.

Gillath, O., Hart, J., Noftle, E. E., & Stockdale, G. D. (2009). Development and validation of a state adult attachment measure (SAAM). *Journal of Research in Personality, 43,* 362–373.

Goldberg, S., Benoit, D., Blokland, K., & Madigan, S. (2003). Atypical maternal behavior, maternal representations, and infant disorganized attachment. *Developmental Psychopathology, 15,* 239–257.

Grice, P. (1975). Logic and conversation. In P. Cole & J. L. Moran (Eds.), *Syntax and semantics III: Speech acts* (pp. 41–58). New York: Academic Press.

Griffin, D. W., & Bartholomew, K. (1994a). The metaphysics of measurement: The case of adult attachment. In K. Bartholomew & D. Perlman (Eds.), *Advances in personal relationships: Vol. 5. Attachment processes in adulthood* (pp. 17–52). London: Jessica Kingsley.

Griffin, D. W., & Bartholomew, K. (1994b). Models of the self and other: Fundamental dimensions underlying measures of adult attachment. *Journal of Personality and Social Psychology, 67,* 430–445.

Groh, A. M., Roisman, G. I., Booth-LaForce, C., Fraley, R. C., Owen, M. T., Cox, M. J., et al. (2014). Stability of attachment security from infancy to late adolescence. In C. Booth-LaForce & G. I. Roisman (Eds.), *The Adult Attachment Interview: Psychometrics, stability and change from infancy, and developmental origins. Monographs of the Society for Research in Child Development, 79*(3), 51–66.

Grossmann, K., Fremmer-Bombik, E., Rudolph, J., & Grossmann, K. E. (1988). Maternal attachment representations as related to patterns of infant–mother attachment and maternal care during the first year. In R. A. Hinde & J. Stevenson-Hinde (Eds.), *Relationships within families: Mutual influences* (pp. 241–260). Oxford, UK: Clarendon Press.

Haft, W., & Slade, A. (1989). Affect attunement and maternal attachment: A pilot study. *Infant Mental Health Journal, 10,* 157–172.

Haltigan, J. D., Leerkes, E. M., Wong, M. S., Fortuna, K., Roisman, G. I., Supple, A. J., et al. (2014). Adult attachment states of mind: Measurement invariance across ethnicity and associations with maternal sensitivity. *Child Development, 85,* 1019–1035.

Haltigan, J. D., Roisman, G. I., & Haydon, K. C. (2014). The latent structure of the Adult Attachment Interview: Exploratory and confirmatory evidence. In C. Booth-LaForce & G. I. Roisman (Eds)., The Adult Attachment Interview: Psychometrics, stability and change from infancy, and developmental origins. *Monographs of the Society for Research in Child Development, 79*(3), 15–35.

Hamilton, C. E. (2000). Continuity and discontinuity of attachment from infancy through adolescence. *Child Development, 71,* 690–694.

Haydon, K. C., Collins, W. A., Salvatore, J. E., Simpson, J. A., & Roisman, G. I. (2012). Shared and distinctive origins and correlates of adult attachment representations: The developmental organization of romantic functioning. *Child Development, 83,* 1689–1702.

Haydon, K. C., Roisman, G. I., & Burt, K. B. (2012). In search of security: The latent structure of the Adult Attachment Interview revisited. *Development and Psychopathology, 24,* 589–606.

Haydon, K. C., Roisman, G. I., Marks, M.J., & Fraley, R.C. (2011). An empirically derived approach to the latent structure of the Adult Attachment Interview: Additional convergent and discriminant validity evidence. *Attachment and Human Development, 13,* 503–524.

Haydon, K. C., Roisman, G. I., Owen, M. T., Booth-LaForce, C., & Cox, M. J. (2014). Shared and distinctive antecedents of Adult Attachment Interview state-of-mind and inferred experience dimensions. In C. Booth-LaForce & G. I. Roisman (Eds)., The Adult Attachment Interview: Psychometrics, stability and change from infancy, and developmental origins. *Monographs of the Society for Research in Child Development, 79*(3), 108–125.

Hazan, C., & Shaver, P. R. (1987). Romantic love conceptualized as an attachment process. *Journal of Personality and Social Psychology, 52,* 511–524.

Hazan, C., & Shaver, P. R. (1994). Attachment as an organizational framework for research on close relationships. *Psychological Inquiry, 5,* 1–22.

Hesse, E. (1996). Discourse, memory and the Adult Attachment Interview: A note with emphasis on the emerging cannot classify category. *Infant Mental Health Journal, 17,* 4–11.

Hesse, E. (2008). The Adult Attachment Interview: Protocol, method of analysis, and empirical studies. In J. Cassidy & P. R. Shaver (Eds.), *Handbook of attachment: Theory, research, and clinical applications* (2nd ed., pp. 552–598). New York: Guilford Press.

Holland, A. S., & Roisman, G. I. (2010). Adult attachment security and young adults' dating relationships over time: Self-reported, observational, and physiological evidence. *Developmental Psychology, 46,* 552–557.

Jacoby, L. L., Toth, J. P., Lindsay, D. S., & Debner, J. A. (1992). Lectures for a layperson: Methods for revealing unconscious processes. In R. F. Bornstein & T. S. Pittman (Eds.), *Perception without awareness* (pp. 81–120). New York: Guilford Press.

John, O. P. (1990). The "Big Five" factor taxonomy: Dimensions of personality in the natural language and in questionnaires. In L. A. Pervin (Ed.), *Handbook of personality: Theory and research* (pp. 67–100). New York: Guilford Press.

Jones, J. D., Cassidy, J., & Shaver, P. R. (2015). Parents' self-reported attachment styles: A review of links with parenting behaviors, emotions, and cognitions. *Personality and Social Psychology Review, 19,* 44–76.

Kobak, R. R. (1993). *The Attachment Interview Q-Set.* Unpublished manuscript, University of Delaware.

Kobak, R. R., Cole, H., Ferenz-Gillies, R., Fleming, W.,

& Gamble, W. (1993). Attachment and emotional regulation during mother-teen problem solving: A control theory analysis. *Child Development, 64,* 231–245.

Kobak, R. R., & Sceery, A. (1988). Attachment in late adolescence: Working models, affect regulation, and representations of self and others. *Child Development, 59,* 135–146.

Kobak, R. R., & Zajac, K. (2011). Rethinking adolescent states of mind: A relationship/lifespan view of attachment and psychopathology. In D. Cicchetti & G. I. Roisman (Eds.), *The origins and organization of adaptation and maladaptation: Minnesota Symposia on Child Psychology* (Vol. 36). New York: Wiley.

Kunce, L. J., & Shaver, P. R. (1994). An attachment-theoretical approach to caregiving in romantic relationships. In K. Bartholomew & D. Perlman (Eds.), *Advances in personal relationships: Vol. 5. Attachment processes in adulthood* (pp. 205–237). London: Jessica Kingsley.

Kurdek, L. A. (2002). On being insecure about the assessment of attachment styles. *Journal of Social and Personal Relationships, 19,* 811–834.

Larose, S., Bernier, A., & Soucy, N. (2005). Attachment as a moderator of the effect of security in mentoring on subsequent perceptions of mentoring and relationship quality with college teachers. *Journal of Social and Personal Relationships, 22,* 399–415.

Luijk, M. P. C. M., Roisman, G. I., Haltigan, J. D., Tiemeier, H., Booth-LaForce, C., Van IJzendoorn, M.H., et al. (2011). Dopaminergic, serotonergic, and oxytonergic candidate genes associated with infant attachment security and disorganization?: In search of main and interaction effects. *Journal of Child Psychology and Psychiatry, 52,* 1295–1307.

Macfie, J., McElwain, N. L., Houts, R. M., & Cox, M. J. (2005). Intergenerational transmission of role reversal between parent and child: Dyadic and family systems internal working models. *Attachment and Human Development, 7,* 51–65.

Main, M. (1981). Avoidance in the service of attachment: A working paper. In K. Immelman, G. Barlow, M. Main, & L. Petrinovitch (Eds.), *Behavioral development: The Bielefeld interdisciplinary project* (pp. 651–693). New York: Cambridge University Press.

Main, M. (1990). Cross-cultural studies of attachment organization: Recent studies, changing methodologies, and the concept of conditional strategies. *Human Development, 33,* 48–61.

Main, M. (1991). Metacognitive knowledge, metacognitive monitoring, and singular (coherent) versus multiple (incoherent) models of attachment: Findings and directions for future research. In C. M. Parkes, J. Stevenson-Hinde, & P. Marris (Eds.), *Attachment across the life cycle* (pp. 127–159). London: Routledge.

Main, M., & Goldwyn, R. (1984). *Adult attachment scoring and classification system.* Unpublished manuscript, University of California, Berkeley.

Main, M., Goldwyn, R., & Hesse, E. (2003). *Adult at-*

*tachment scoring and classification system.* Unpublished manuscript, University of California, Berkeley.

Main, M., Kaplan, N., & Cassidy, J. (1985). Security of infancy, childhood, and adulthood: A move to the level of representation. In I. Bretherton & E. Waters (Eds.), Growing points of attachment theory and research. *Monographs of the Society for Research in Child Development, 50*(1–2, Serial No. 209), 66–106.

Main, M., & Weston, D. R. (1981). The quality of the toddler's relationship to mother and to father: Related to conflict behavior and the readiness to establish new relationships. *Child Development, 52*, 932–940.

McClure, M. J., & Lydon, J. E. (2014). Anxiety doesn't become you: How attachment anxiety compromises relational opportunities. *Journal of Personality and Social Psychology, 106*, 89–111.

McCrae, R. R., & Costa, P. T. (1990). *Personality in adulthood.* New York: Guilford Press.

Meehl, P. E., & Yonce, L. J. (1996). Taxometric analysis: II. Detecting taxonicity using covariance of two quantitative indicators in successive intervals of a third indicator (MAXCOV procedure). *Psychological Reports, 78*, 1091–1227.

Mikulincer, M., Dolev, T., & Shaver, P. R. (2004). Attachment-related strategies during thought-suppression: Ironic rebounds and vulnerable self-representations. *Journal of Personality and Social Psychology, 87*, 940–956.

Mikulincer, M., Gillath, O., & Shaver, P. R. (2002). Activation of the attachment system in adulthood: Threat-related primes increase the accessibility of mental representations of attachment figures. *Journal of Personality and Social Psychology, 83*, 881–895.

Mikulincer, M., & Orbach, I. (1995). Attachment styles and repressive defensiveness: The accessibility and architecture of affective memories. *Journal of Personality and Social Psychology, 68*, 917–925.

Mikulincer, M., & Shaver, P. R. (2007). *Attachment in adulthood: Structure, dynamics, and change.* New York: Guilford Press.

Mikulincer, M., Shaver, P. R., Gillath, O., & Nitzberg, R. A. (2005). Attachment, caregiving, and altruism: boosting attachment security increases compassion and helping. *Journal of Personality and Social Psychology, 89*, 817–839.

Miljkovitch, R., Pierrehumbert, B., Bretherton, I., & Halfon, O. (2004). Associations between parental and child attachment representations. *Attachment and Human Development, 6*, 305–325.

Muller, R. T., Sicoli, L. A., & Lemieux, K. E. (2000). Relationship between attachment style and post-traumatic stress symptomatology among adults who report the experience of childhood abuse. *Journal of Traumatic Stress, 13*, 321–332.

Noftle, E. E., & Shaver, P. R. (2006). Attachment dimensions and the big five personality traits: Associations and comparative ability to predict relationship quality. *Journal of Research in Personality, 40*, 179–208.

O'Connor, E., Pan, H., Waters, E., & Posada, G. (1995,

March). *Attachment classification, romantic jealousy, and aggression in couples.* Poster presented at the biennial meeting of the Society for Research in Child Development, Indianapolis, IN.

Oppenheim, D., & Waters, E. (1995). Narrative processes and attachment representations: Issues of development and assessment. In E. Waters, B. Vaughn, G. Posada, & K. Kondo-Ikemura (Eds.), Caregiving, cultural, and cognitive perspectives on secure-base behavior and working models: New growing points of attachment theory and research. *Monographs of the Society for Research in Child Development, 60*(2–3, Serial No. 244), 197–215.

Overall, N. C., Fletcher, G. J., & Friesen, M. D. (2003). Mapping the intimate relationship mind: Comparisons between three models of attachment representations. *Personality and Social Psychology Bulletin, 29*, 1479–1493.

Owens, G., Crowell, J., Pan, H., Treboux, D., O'Connor, E., & Waters, E. (1995). The prototype hypothesis and the origins of attachment working models: Adult relationships with parents and romantic partners. In E. Waters, B. Vaughn, G. Posada, & K. Kondo-Ikemura (Eds.), Caregiving, cultural, and cognitive perspectives on secure-base behavior and working models: New growing points of attachment theory and research. *Monographs of the Society for Research in Child Development, 60*(2–3), 216–233.

Oyen, A.-S., Landy, S., & Hilburn-Cobb, C. (2000). Maternal attachment and sensitivity in an at-risk sample. *Attachment and Human Development, 2*, 203–217.

Paley, B., Cox, M., Burchinal, M., & Payne, C. (1999). Attachment and marital functioning: Comparison of spouses with continuous secure, earned secure, dismissing, and preoccupied stances. *Journal of Family Psychology, 13*, 580–597.

Paley, B., Cox, M. J., Harter, K. M., & Margand, N. A. (2002). Adult attachment stance and spouses' marital perceptions during the transition to parenthood. *Attachment and Human Development, 4*, 340–360.

Pearson, J., Cohn, D., Cowan, P., & Cowan, C. P. (1994). Earned- and continuous-security in adult attachment: Relation to depressive symptomatology and parenting style. *Development and Psychopathology, 6*, 359–373.

Pearson, J., Cowan, P., Cowan, C., & Cohn, D. (1993). Adult attachment and adult child–older parent relationships. *American Journal of Orthopsychiatry, 63*, 606–613.

Pierce, T., & Lydon, J. (2001). Global and specific relational models in the experience of social interactions. *Journal of Personality and Social Psychology, 80*, 613–631.

Pistole, M. C. (1989). Attachment in adult romantic relationships: Style of conflict resolution and relationship satisfaction. *Journal of Social and Personal Relationships, 6*, 505–510.

Posada, G., Waters, E., Crowell, J., & Lay, K. (1995).

Is it easier to use a secure mother as a secure base?: Attachment Q-sort correlates of the Adult Attachment Interview. In E. Waters, B. Vaughn, G. Posada, & K. Kondo-Ikemura (Eds.), Caregiving, cultural, and cognitive perspectives on secure-base behavior and working models: New growing points of attachment theory and research. *Monographs of the Society for Research in Child Development, 60*(2–3, Serial No. 244), 133–145.

Pottharst, K. (Ed.). (1990). *Explorations in adult attachment.* New York: Peter Lang.

Rholes, W. S., Simpson, J. A., & Blakely, B. S. (1995). Adult attachment styles and mothers' relationships with their young children. *Personal Relationships, 2,* 35–54.

Riggs, S. A., & Jacobvitz, D. (2002). Expectant parents' representations of early attachment relationships: Association with mental health and family history. *Journal of Consulting and Clinical Psychology, 70,* 195–204.

Roisman, G. I. (2009). Adult attachment: Toward a rapprochement of methodological cultures. *Current Directions in Psychological Science, 18,* 122–126.

Roisman, G. I., & Booth-LaForce, C. (2014). General discussion. In C. Booth-LaForce & G. I. Roisman (Eds.), The Adult Attachment Interview: Psychometrics, stability and change from infancy, and developmental origins. *Monographs of the Society for Research in Child Development, 79*(3), 126–137.

Roisman, G. I., Booth-LaForce, C., Belsky, J., Burt, K. B., & Groh, A. M. (2013). Molecular-genetic correlates of infant attachment: A cautionary tale. *Attachment and Human Development, 15,* 384–406.

Roisman, G. I., Collins, W. A., Sroufe, L. A., & Egeland, B. (2005). Predictors of young adults' representations of and behavior in their current romantic relationship: Prospective tests of the prototype hypothesis. *Attachment and Human Development, 7,* 105–121.

Roisman, G. I., Fortuna, K., & Holland, A. (2006). An experimental manipulation of retrospectively defined earned and continuous attachment security. *Child Development, 77,* 59–71.

Roisman, G. I., & Fraley, R. C. (2008). A behavior-genetic study of parenting quality, infant attachment security, and their covariation in a nationally representative sample. *Developmental Psychology, 44,* 831–839.

Roisman, G. I., Fraley, R. C., & Belsky, J. (2007). A taxometric study of the Adult Attachment Interview. *Developmental Psychology, 43,* 675–686.

Roisman, G. I., Haltigan, J. D., Haydon, K. C., & Booth-LaForce, C. (2014). Earned-security in retrospect: Depressive symptoms, family stress, and maternal and paternal sensitivity from early childhood to mid-adolescence. In C. Booth-LaForce & G. I. Roisman (Eds.), The Adult Attachment Interview: Psychometrics, stability and change from infancy, and developmental origins. *Monographs of the Society for Research in Child Development, 79*(3), 85–107.

Roisman, G. I., & Haydon, K. C. (2011). Earned-security in retrospect: Emerging insights from longitudinal, experimental, and taxometric investigations. In D. Cicchetti & G. I. Roisman (Eds.), *The origins and organization of adaptation and maladaptation: Minnesota symposia on child psychology* (Vol. 36, pp. 109–154). New York: Wiley.

Roisman, G. I., Holland, A., Fortuna, K., Fraley, R. C., Clausell, E., & Clarke, A. (2007). The Adult Attachment Interview and self-reports of attachment style: An empirical rapprochement. *Journal of Personality and Social Psychology, 92,* 678–697.

Roisman, G. I., Madsen, S. D., Hennighausen, K. H., Sroufe, L. A., & Collins, W. A. (2001). The coherence of dyadic behavior across parent–child and romantic relationships as mediate by the internalized representation of experience. *Attachment and Human Development, 3,* 156–172.

Roisman, G. I., Padrón, E., Sroufe, L. A., & Egeland, B. (2002). Earned-secure status in retrospect and prospect. *Child Development, 73,* 1204–1219.

Roisman, G. I., Tsai, J. L., & Chiang, K. H. (2004). The emotional integration of childhood experience: Physiological, facial expressive, and self-reported emotional response during the Adult Attachment Interview. *Developmental Psychology, 40,* 776–789.

Rowe, A., & Carnelley, K. B. (2003). Attachment style differences in the processing of attachment-relevant information: Primed-style effects on recall, interpersonal expectations, and affect. *Personal Relationships, 10,* 59–75.

Rubenstein, C., & Shaver, P. R. (1982). *In search of intimacy.* New York: Delacorte.

Sagi, A., Aviezer, O., Joels, T., Korne-Karje, N., Mayseless, O., Scharf, M., et al. (1992, July). *The correspondence of mother's attachment with infant–mother attachment relationship in traditional and non-traditional kibbutzim.* Paper presented at the 25th International Congress of Psychology, Brussels, Belgium.

Sagi, A., Van IJzendoorn, M., Scharf, M., Korne-Karje, N., Joels, T., & Mayseless, O. (1994). Stability and discriminant validity of the Adult Attachment Interview: A psychometric study in young Israeli adults. *Developmental Psychology, 30,* 771–777.

Salo, J., Jokela, M., Lehtimäki, T., & Keltikangas-Järvinen, L. (2011). Serotonin receptor 2A gene moderates the effect of childhood maternal nurturance on adulthood social attachment. *Genes, Brain and Behavior, 10,* 702–709.

Schank, R. (1999). *Dynamic memory revisited.* Cambridge, UK: Cambridge University Press.

Shaver, P. R., & Hazan, C. (1988). A biased overview of the study of love. *Journal of Social and Personal Relationships, 5,* 473–501.

Sibley, C. G., Fischer, R., & Liu, J. H. (2005). Reliability and validity of the Revised Experiences in Close Relationships (ECR-R) self-report measure of adult romantic attachment. *Personality and Social Psychology Bulletin, 31,* 1524–1536.

Simpson, J. A. (1990). The influence of attachment styles on romantic relationships. *Journal of Personality and Social Psychology, 59*, 971–980.

Simpson, J. A., & Rholes, W. S. (1998). Attachment in adulthood. In J. A. Simpson & W. S. Rholes (Eds.), *Attachment theory and close relationships* (pp. 3–21). New York: Guilford Press.

Simpson, J. A., Rholes, W. S., & Nelligan, J. S. (1992). Support- seeking and support-giving within couple members in an anxiety-provoking situation: The role of attachment styles. *Journal of Personality and Social Psychology, 62*, 434–446.

Simpson, J. A., Rholes, W. S., Oriña, M. M., & Grich, J. (2002). Working models of attachment, support giving, and support seeking in a stressful situation. *Personality and Social Psychology Bulletin, 28*, 598–608.

Simpson, J. A., Rholes, W. S., & Phillips, D. (1996). Conflict in close relationships: An attachment perspective. *Journal of Personality and Social Psychology, 71*, 899–914.

Simpson, J. A., Rholes, W. S., & Winterheld, H. A. (2010). Attachment working models twist memories of relationship events. *Psychological Science, 21*, 252–259.

Slade, A., Belsky, J., Aber, J. L., & Phelps, J. L. (1999). Mothers' representations of their relationships with toddlers: Links to adult attachment and observed mothering. *Developmental Psychology, 35*, 611–619.

Steele, H., Steele, M., & Fonagy, P. (1996). Associations among attachment classifications of mothers, fathers, and their infants. *Child Development, 67*, 541–555.

Steele, R. D., Waters, T. E. A., Bost, K. K., Vaughn, B. E., Truitt, W., Waters, H. S., et al. (2014). Caregiving antecedents of secure base script knowledge: A comparative analysis of young adult attachment representations. *Developmental Psychology, 50*, 2526–2538.

Steiner, M. C., Arjomand, M., & Waters, H. S. (2003, April). *Adolescents' representations of close relationships.* Paper presented at the Biennial Meetings of the Society for Research in Child Development, Tampa, FL.

Sternberg, R. J., & Barnes, M. (Eds.). (1988). *The psychology of love.* New Haven, CT: Yale University Press.

Treboux, D., Crowell, J., & Waters, E. (2004). When "new" meets "old": Configurations of adult attachment representations and their implications for marital functioning. *Developmental Psychology, 40*, 295–314.

Van IJzendoorn, M. H. (1992). Intergenerational transmission of parenting: A review of studies in non-clinical populations. *Developmental Review, 12*, 76–99.

Van IJzendoorn, M. H. (1995). Adult attachment representations, parental responsiveness, and infant attachment: A meta-analysis on the predictive validity of the Adult Attachment Interview. *Psychological Bulletin, 117*, 387–403.

Van IJzendoorn, M. H., & Bakermans-Kranenburg, M. (1996). Attachment representations in mothers, fathers, adolescents and clinical groups: A meta-ana-

lytic search for normative data. *Journal of Clinical and Consulting Psychology, 64*, 8–21.

Van IJzendoorn, M. H., & Bakermans-Kranenburg, M. (2009). Attachment security and disorganization in maltreating families and orphanages. In R. E. Tremblay, M. Boivin, R. Peters (Eds.), *Encyclopedia on early childhood development.* Montreal: Centre of Excellence for Early Childhood Development and Strategic Knowledge Cluster on Early Child Development. Retrieved October 6, 2015, from www.child-encyclopedia.com/documents/van_IJzendoorn-Bakermans-KranenburgANGxp-Attachment.pdf.

Van IJzendoorn, M. H., Feldbrugge, J., Derks, F., de Ruiter, C., Verhagen, M., Philipse, M., et al. (1997). Attachment representations of personality disordered criminal offenders. *American Journal of Orthopsychiatry, 67*, 449–459.

Vaughn, B. E., Veríssimo, M., Coppola, G., Bost, K. K., Shin, N., McBride, B., et al. (2006). Maternal attachment script representations: Longitudinal stability and associations with stylistic features of maternal narratives. *Attachment & Human Development, 8*, 199–208.

Veríssimo, M., & Salvaterra, F. (2006). Maternal secure-base scripts and children's attachment security in an adopted sample. *Attachment and Human Development, 8*, 261–273.

Waller, N. G., & Meehl, P. E. (1998). *Multivariate taxometric procedures: Distinguishing types from continua.* Beverly Hills, CA: Sage.

Wallis, P., & Steele, H. (2001). Attachment representations in adolescence: Further evidence from psychiatric residential settings. *Attachment and Human Development, 3*, 259–268.

Wampler, K. S., Riggs, B., & Kimball, T. G. (2004). Observing attachment behavior in couples: The Adult Attachment Behavior Q-Set (AABQ), *Family Processes, 43*, 315–335.

Wampler, K. S., Shi, L., Nelson, B. S., & Kimball, T. G. (2003). The Adult Attachment Interview and observed couple interaction: Implications for an intergenerational perspective on couple therapy. *Family Processes, 42*, 497–515.

Ward, A., Ramsay, R., Turnbull, S., Steele, M., Steele, H., & Treasure, J. (2001). Attachment in anorexia nervosa: A transgenerational perspective. *British Journal of Medicine and Psychology, 74*, 497–505.

Ward, M. J., & Carlson, E. A. (1995). Associations among adult attachment representations, maternal sensitivity, and infant–mother attachment in a sample of adolescent mothers. *Child Development, 66*, 69–79.

Waters, E., Crowell, J., Elliott, M., Corcoran, D., & Treboux, D. (2002). Bowlby's secure base theory and the social/personality psychology of attachment styles: Work(s) in progress. *Attachment and Human Development, 4*, 230–242.

Waters, E., Kondo-Ikemura, K., Posada, G., & Richters, J. (1991). Learning to love: Mechanisms and milestones. In M. Gunnar & L. A. Sroufe (Eds.), *Self processes and development* (pp. 217–255). Hillsdale, NJ: Erlbaum.

Waters, E., Merrick, S., Treboux, D., Crowell, J., & Albersheim, L. (2000). Attachment security from infancy to early adulthood: A 20-year longitudinal study. *Child Development, 71,*<B> <B*>684–689.

Waters, H. S., & Rodrigues, L. M. (2001, April). *Are attachment scripts the building blocks of attachment representations?* Paper presented at the biannual meeting of the Society for Research in Child Development, Minneapolis, MN.

Waters, H. S., Rodrigues, L. M., & Ridgeway, D. (1998). Cognitive underpinnings of narrative attachment assessment. *Journal of Experimental Child Psychology, 71,* 211–234.

Waters, H. S., & Waters, E. (2006). The attachment working models concept: Among other things, we build script-like representations of secure base experiences. *Attachment and Human Development, 8,* 185–197.

Waters, T. E., Brockmeyer, S. L., & Crowell, J. A. (2013). AAI coherence predicts caregiving and care seeking behavior: secure base script knowledge helps explain why. *Attachment and Human Development, 15,* 316–331.

Wei, M., Russell, D. W., Mallinckrodt, B., & Vogel, D. L. (2007). The Experiences in Close Relationship Scale (ECR)–Short Form: Reliability, validity, and factor structure. *Journal of Personality Assessment, 88,* 187–204.

Weinfield, N. S., Sroufe, L. A., & Egeland, B. (2000). Attachment from infancy to early adulthood in a high-risk sample: Continuity, discontinuity, and their correlates. *Child Development, 71,* 695–702.

Weiss, R. (1973). *Loneliness: The experience of emotional and social isolation.* Cambridge, MA: MIT Press.

Weiss, R. (1974). The provisions of social relationships. In Z. Rubin (Ed.), *Doing unto others* (pp. 17–26). Englewood Cliffs, NJ: Prentice-Hall.

Weiss, R. (1991). Attachment in adult life. In C. M. Parkes, J. Stevenson-Hinde, & P. Marris (Eds.), *Attachment across the life cycle* (pp. 171–184). London: Routledge.

West, M. L., & Sheldon-Keller, A. E. [R.] (1994). *Patterns of relating: An adult attachment perspective.* New York: Guilford Press.

West, M. [L.], Sheldon, A. E. R., & Reiffer, L. (1987). An approach to the delineation of adult attachment: Scale development and reliability. *Journal of Nervous and Mental Disease, 175,* 738–741.

Whipple, N., Bernier, A., & Mageau, G. A. (2011). A dimensional approach to maternal attachment state of mind: Relations to maternal sensitivity and maternal autonomy support. *Developmental Psychology, 47,* 396–403.

Woike, B. A., Osier, T. J., & Candella, K. (1996). Attachment styles and violent imagery in thematic stories about relationships. *Personality and Social Psychology Bulletin, 22,* 1030–1034.

Xu, J. H., & Shrout, P. E. (2013). Assessing the reliability of change: A comparison of two measures of adult attachment. *Journal of Research in Personality, 47,* 202–208.

Zayas, V., Mischel, W., Shoda, Y., & Aber, J. L. (2011). Roots of adult attachment: Maternal caregiving at 18 months predicts adult peer and partner attachment. *Social Psychological and Personality Science, 2,* 289–297.

Zeanah, C., Benoit, D., Barton, M., Regan, C., Hirshberg, L., & Lipsett, L. (1993). Representations of attachment in mothers and their one-year-old infants. *Journal of the American Academy of Child and Adolescent Psychiatry, 32,* 278–286.

# PART V

# PSYCHOPATHOLOGY AND CLINICAL APPLICATIONS

# Chapter 28

# Attachment and Psychopathology in Childhood

Michelle DeKlyen
Mark T. Greenberg

The parent–child relationship has long been considered central to personality development (Bowlby, 1969/1982; Erikson, 1963; Freud, 1965; Greenspan, 1981). Numerous empirical findings link secure parent–child attachment with sociability, compliance, and effective emotion regulation, and insecure attachment to poor peer relations, anger, and poor behavioral self-control (Sroufe, Egeland, Carlson, & Collins, 2005).

The idea that social relationships both affect and are affected by developing psychopathology in childhood is fundamental to most theories of development. Object relations theorists (Mahler, Pine, Bergman, 1975; Winnicott, 1965) and ego psychologists (Freud, 1965) hypothesized that a child's earliest relationships have great impact on the development of mental health. However, despite Bowlby's (1969/1982, 1973) interest in psychopathology, early attachment research focused almost entirely on normative infant development. Although scattered projects in the 1970s and 1980s examined at-risk populations of children and adults with disorders, only recently have researchers seriously attempted to fulfill Bowlby's legacy by utilizing attachment theory to enhance our understanding and treatment of disorder (Cicchetti, Toth, & Lynch, 1995).

Over the last few decades, attachment theory has made major contributions beyond infancy, and

beyond its own proponents. Attachment theory provides a critical developmental frame for understanding *how* caregiving relationships influence processes central to emerging psychopathology— for example, the construction of cognitive–affective expectancies, the capacity for emotional and behavioral regulation, and strategies for coping with stress. In particular, the regulation of emotion—particularly negative emotions such as anxiety, anger, and sadness—plays a critical role in many forms of psychopathology (Izard, Youngstrom, Fine, Mostow, & Trentacosta, 2006).

This chapter reviews what is currently known about the association between attachment and psychopathology in childhood. We focus on *disorder*—that is, behavior serious enough to warrant clinical attention. We begin by briefly describing principles of developmental psychopathology and risk models. We next review research involving attachment, first as a risk factor, then as a central aspect of disorder. We address two fundamental questions: How do attachment constructs contribute to our understanding of childhood disorders, and how might the study of childhood psychopathology enrich the study of attachment? We then reflect on the current state of the field, noting where advances have been made and some of the barriers to further progress.

## Developmental Psychopathology and Models of Risk and Protection

Most of the research linking attachment with psychopathology has considered attachment as a potential risk or protective factor, examining associations between attachment measures and maladaptive behavior in populations ranging from convenience samples to individuals with clinical diagnoses. As we have previously noted, the enthusiasm to utilize attachment theory has at times led to a fruitless search for a "Holy Grail" of psychopathology, seeking main effects of infant attachment on later psychopathology. Although meta-analyses demonstrate that attachment predicts both externalizing and internalizing problems when other factors are not controlled (Fearon, Bakermans-Kranenburg, Van IJzendoorn, Lapsley, & Roisman, 2010; Groh, Roisman, Van IJzendoorn, Bakermans-Kranenburg, & Fearon, 2012), it generally appears to exert its influence *in the context of other risk factors* (Cicchetti & Rogosch, 1997; Greenberg, Speltz, DeKlyen, & Jones, 2001; Keller, Spieker, & Gilchrist, 2005). A short digression will provide a frame for considering the role of attachment in the etiology of psychopathology.

### Risk Factors

Research on risk factors for disorder leads to five general conclusions. First, a single cause is unlikely to be either a necessary or a sufficient cause for most pathology (Greenberg, Speltz, & DeKlyen, 1993); even disorders with established biological mechanisms are potentiated or buffered by other biological or environmental factors. Thus, it is doubtful that attachment insecurity alone will lead to disorder (Sroufe, 1990), although it may increase its likelihood. As a corollary of this principle, few childhood disorders will be eliminated by treating only causes that lie within the child (Rutter, 1982). Even when a powerful biological cause is implicated (e.g., autism), the parent–child relationship is often an appropriate focus for treatment.

A second tenet of developmental psychopathology states that *multiple pathways* exist to and from disorder (Cicchetti & Rogosch, 1997). Different risk factors may lead to the same disorder (*equifinality*), and a given risk factor may contribute to multiple disorders (*multifinality*). For example, poverty, family violence, and parental psycho-

pathology have all been associated with conduct problems, and attachment is a risk factor for both internalizing and externalizing problems. Also, a variable that confers risk for one problem may reduce risk for others (e.g., avoidant attachment may contribute to conduct disorder but decrease the risk of suicide; Adam, Sheldon-Keller, & West, 1995). Of particular importance, the influence of a risk factor may be moderated by other factors (e.g., gender, ethnicity, genetic allele variants). This is central to notions of *differential susceptibility* (Ellis, Boyce, Belsky, Bakermans-Kranenburg, & Van IJzendoorn, 2011), which may explain some mixed findings in past research and show a way forward to understanding the developmental processes leading to pathology.

Third, risk factors occur at multiple levels, including the individual, the caregiver, and the broader ecological context (Bronfenbrenner, 1979; Kobak, Cassidy, Lyons-Ruth, & Ziv, 2006). At each level, some factors have implications for attachment (social support may affect sensitive caregiving), but others may not (e.g., peer deviance, school quality).

Fourth, associations between risk and outcome may be nonlinear. Although one risk factor may not predict poor outcomes, the likelihood of disorder may increase rapidly with additional risks (Greenberg et al., 2001). It is as yet unclear whether certain risk factors or combinations of risks matter more than others.

A fifth guiding principle is that risk factors may differentially influence outcomes in different developmental periods. Attachment might have its greatest influence in early development, while cognitive ability becomes more critical in middle childhood, and peer relationships and parental monitoring are especially influential during adolescence. Although attachment theorists do not claim that there is a critical period with respect to attachment, early experience models suggest that infant attachment is particularly important and may influence later adaptation beyond what environmental continuity can explain (Fraley, 2002).

### Protective Factors

Protective factors reduce the likelihood of poor outcomes under conditions of risk. These include characteristics of the individual (e.g., temperament and intelligence); the quality of relationships (e.g., attachment); and ecological factors (e.g., school quality, neighborhood safety, and laws that support children and families).

Considerable controversy exists regarding whether specific factors should be designated as risks or as protective (Masten, 2001; Stouthamer-Loeber et al., 1993). Socioeconomic status, attachment security, and peer group status may be conceptualized as risks in some studies and as protective in others, depending on the population being studied, the range of variation, and the investigator's theoretical bent. Attachment insecurity has been described as a risk factor (Sroufe, 1983), whereas secure attachment can be viewed as conferring protection under conditions of risk (Morisset, Barnard, Greenberg, Booth, & Spieker, 1990).

Coie and colleagues (1993) suggest that protective factors operate in several ways. They may directly decrease dysfunction, prevent the occurrence of a risk factor, buffer the effect of a risk factor, or disrupt the mediational chain by which risk leads to disorder. Well-planned prospective longitudinal studies are needed to identify the risk factors that predict psychopathology, the dynamic relation between risk and protective factors at different ages, and the factors most likely to serve as buffers against negative outcomes for persons with multiple risks.

## A Proposed Risk Factor Model

On the basis of these principles, we proposed a model for conceptualizing the early onset of disruptive behavior problems, incorporating four risk domains for which considerable evidence has accumulated: (1) child characteristics; (2) quality of attachment; (3) parental management; and (4) family ecology (Greenberg et al., 1993, 2001). This model may apply to other forms of child psychopathology as well, although some domains are likely more important to certain disorders. Ineffective parenting may contribute more to externalizing than to internalizing disorders (Patterson, DeBaryshe, & Ramsey, 1989), whereas child trauma may especially relate to dissociative disorders (Liotti, 1995). Also, it is likely that different aspects of these risks predict different disorders. For example, reactive temperament may be associated with externalizing, and inhibited temperament with internalizing difficulties. Similarly, parental punitiveness and underinvolvement may create risk for conduct problems (Patterson et al., 1989), and overcontrol and the absence of autonomy pro-

motion may predict anxiety or depression (Kobak, Sudler, & Gamble, 1991). The type of insecurity has also been predicted to determine what type of disorder emerges. Finally, different risk factor combinations (e.g., insecure attachment and family adversity vs. difficult temperament and poor parent management) may lead to differing behaviors and require different treatments.

Here are a few examples: Assessing biological vulnerability, insecure attachment, poor parent management, and adverse family circumstances in a comparison of clinic-referred preschoolers and normally behaving children, we found that children with risk in all four domains were far more likely to receive diagnoses of oppositional defiant disorder (Greenberg et al., 2001). Child characteristics, parent management, and attachment security all uniquely differentiated the two groups, but family adversity did not. Person-oriented analyses demonstrated that increasing the number of risks substantially increased the likelihood of disorder: Clinic-referred children were 34 times more likely than comparison children to be at risk in all four domains. Relative improvement over chance (RIOC) was elevated for one pattern involving child characteristics, poor parenting, and family adversity, and for another including poor parenting, insecure attachment, and family adversity. Disorder occurred in individuals with other patterns, but those patterns were no more common among clinic-referred than comparison boys. Clinic-referred children rarely had risk in fewer than two domains.

Behavior problems are not always associated with insecure attachment, as evidenced by case studies of securely attached children with externalizing problems (Campbell, 1990; Greenberg, Speltz, DeKlyen, & Endriga, 1991). Symptoms may be triggered by recent stressors; in other cases, biological vulnerability or family disorder may be apparent. This is likely true for other forms of psychopathology as well.

In a study testing this model, Keller and colleagues (2005) found that risk in a single domain is insufficient to predict disorder. In two-domain analyses, insecurely attached children with high infant negativity were more likely to display the high-problem-behavior trajectory, whereas securely attached children with high negativity did not. In three-domain analyses, the high-problem-behavior trajectory was most likely when insecure attachment and high-risk parenting were combined with multiproblem family ecology or high infant negativity.

## Process Models and the Contribution of Attachment to Disorder

Models are most likely to be useful when they specify linkages between *types* of insecurity and later disorder and describe mechanisms by which attachment is expected to influence development. Theory-based process models are essential to establish child attachment as causal. We have suggested four interrelated mechanisms that may link attachment to psychopathology: observed behavior, emotion regulation, cognitive–affective structures, and motivational processes.

Attachment may contribute to maladaptation through its direct effect on behavior. Behaviors labeled disruptive have considerable power to regulate caregiving, especially when other strategies are ineffective or unavailable (Greenberg et al., 1993). Thus, whining, noncompliance, and other negative forms of attention seeking may be viewed as attachment strategies that, although effective in the short-term (e.g., caregiver attention may be either increased or reduced by child negativity), serve as a setting condition for maladaptive interactions (e.g., coercive processes; Patterson, Reid, & Dishion, 1992). Similarly, the immature, angry, or dependent behaviors of the ambivalently attached child may maintain a caregiver's attention but become problematic in the wider environment (Cassidy & Berlin, 1994). Main and Hesse (1990) hypothesized that in the absence of a coherent and predictable environment, the disorganized infant may take control of aspects of the parent–child relationship during the preschool years. This role reversal, while maintaining a connection to the parent, may lead to maladaptive behaviors (e.g., bossiness, parentification).

Attachment may also affect later disorder through the emotion regulatory processes that develop within the parent–child dyad. Theory and research affirm the importance of emotion regulation in the etiology and maintenance of diverse disorders (Chaplin & Cole, 2005; Izard et al., 2006). Self-regulation strategies are believed to evolve from early interactions that shape subsequent responses to challenging situations (for a review of relevant research, see Calkins & Leerkes, 2011). Guttmann-Steinmetz and Crowell (2006) elaborate how securely attached infants' experiences enhance their capacity to tolerate and manage affect, whereas the strategies of avoidant and ambivalent infants (minimization and exaggeration of emotion, respectively) interfere with effective regulation. Dyadic interactions in early childhood may influence emotion regulation via neural organization and conditioning (Galynker et al., 2012; Greenberg & Snell, 1997; Hane & Fox, 2006; LeDoux, 1995; Olsavsky et al., 2013; Schore, 2005), and associations between attachment and cortisol, heart rate, and vagal tone suggest mechanisms common to emotion, the attachment system, and various disorders (Gunnar, 2000; Hertsgaard, Gunnar, Erickson, & Nachmias, 1995; Lyons-Ruth, Dutra, Schuder, & Bianchi, 2006; Spangler & Schieche, 1998; see also Hane & Fox, Chapter 11, this volume). However, empirical evidence regarding how attachment moderates the neural processes involved in emotion regulation is still preliminary (Coan, 2008; see, in this volume, Coan, Chapter 12, and Polan & Hofer, Chapter 6). Given the degree to which emotion regulation is central to both attachment and diverse psychopathological conditions, it is surprising that there has not been more research in this area.

A third mechanism involves developing social cognitions. Parenting is thought to shape the infant's cognitive–affective schema or "working model" of the self and others (Bowlby, 1973). This working model then biases perceptions of the actions and desires of others, influences behavior, and sets into motion a pattern of interactions that reinforce and stabilize these biases (Bretherton & Munholland, Chapter 4, this volume; Main, Kaplan, & Cassidy, 1985). Attachment patterns are therefore expected to be associated with social information processing. When a secure and trusting bond forms between parent and child, both develop positive working models of the relationship, which include attributions of responsiveness, warmth, and trust, setting the stage for cooperative interactions. Insecure attachment may crystallize working models characterized by anger, mistrust, anxiety, and/or fear. Dykas and Cassidy (2011) propose that insecure individuals either suppress painful information or process it according to negative schemas. They review evidence that attachment working models influence memory, theory of mind, attributional biases, emotional understanding, and coping strategies. For example, several studies have provided support for Dodge's (1991) hypothesis that children with insecure attachments are more likely to report hostile attributions when presented with hypothetical peer dilemmas (e.g., Cassidy, Kirsh, Scolton, & Parke, 1996; Raikes & Thompson, 2008), which may result in hypervigilance and anger and increase the likelihood of reactive aggression. Similarly, Zaccagnino and colleagues (2013) found that children with disorganized attachments had more hostile attributions, and both disorganized and ambivalently attached children reported more aggressive responses to social situations.

Attachment also is likely to contribute to maladaptation through motivational processes. Attachment may promote either a generalized positive or a resistant social orientation, providing differential levels of readiness for socialization (Richters & Waters, 1991). Children with warm, contingent relations are more likely to comply with parent control and to develop a prosocial orientation in early and middle childhood (Kochanska et al., 2010; Maccoby & Martin, 1983; Waters, Kondo-Ikemura, Posada, & Richters, 1991). Secure attachment might then deter children from deviance and facilitate the formation of positive bonds with other adults and institutions that protect against delinquency and social destructiveness, as explicated in social control theories (Hawkins, Arthur, & Catalano, 1995).

## Theory and Research Linking Attachment to Childhood Psychopathology

Attachment theory and research have informed the study of child psychopathology in two major ways. First, a body of work has considered how attachment relationships influence disorder by increasing risk or buffering the effects of other risk factors. Second, in extreme cases, atypical attachment patterns can themselves be considered disorders (Lieberman & Zeanah, 1995)—for example, when caregiving is seriously disrupted or is pathogenic due to severe maltreatment or institutionalization. Each of these approaches is considered below.

Our task is complicated by the many ways in which researchers have assessed attachment and psychopathology, often making comparisons between studies difficult. Some studies use attachment classifications, and others use dimensional ratings. When using categorical measures, some report only secure versus insecure attachment, whereas others apply the three-category system, and still others include the fourth (disorganized or controlling) category. Some assess infant attachment, and others measure attachment later in childhood, often concurrent with the outcome of interest. Some use behavioral observations (e.g.,

separation–reunions), whereas others use parent- or observer-reported behavior descriptions (e.g., the Q-sort), and still others use representational measures (e.g., projective pictures, story stem narratives, or self-descriptive questionnaires). Which measure is appropriate depends to some degree on the subject's developmental age, but little research has examined how measures conducted at different ages and with different methodologies relate to each other over time. To what extent various measures assess equivalent constructs is an open question.

With respect to psychopathology, some researchers report on broad categories (externalizing and internalizing), and others assess specific disorders. Still others use dimensional measures of behavior, assuming that higher scores are worse—but sometimes few, if any, of the subjects have scored at clinical levels, and measures may not be linearly related to well-being (e.g., too little behavior may be as maladaptive as too much). Comparing studies within such diversity presents a challenge.

In our view, reliance on the secure–insecure dichotomy runs the risk of reducing analyses to little more than a comparison of generally good versus generally bad caregiving environments. It lacks the specificity that attachment theory can provide, and to the degree that there are meaningful differences between insecure categories, these may cancel each other out. Furthermore, the association between insecurity and psychopathology is often weak and clinically not very useful (Rutter, Kreppner, Sonuga-Barke, et al., 2009). Therefore, after briefly reviewing early findings, we focus on studies that assess specific categories of insecurity. For consistency and ease of reading, we generally use the terms *avoidant*, *ambivalent*, *disorganized*, and/or *controlling* to refer to the basic insecure classifications, although some authors use different terms for analogous categories. A strong association has been found between infant disorganization and later controlling attachment classification, and the two are often considered together. Unless otherwise specified, attachment has been assessed in relation to mothers.

We concentrate on psychopathology in childhood and rarely include research on adolescents, except when this might provide clues to fruitful future investigation. Given the heterogeneity of categories such as externalizing and internalizing, we also describe only a sampling of the studies that report these broad outcomes. Progress in the field will demand greater specificity to illuminate the processes and mechanisms that lead to particular behavioral outcomes, along with theoretical rationales outlining why particular attachment experiences or representations are expected to relate to specific outcomes.

With those caveats, what follows is our best assessment of what theory and research indicate about the associations between attachment and child psychopathology.

## Early Theory Linking Attachment and Disorder

From early on, theorists predicted differences in children's behavior in general and pathology in particular, based on the different forms of insecurity. Bowlby (1973) argued that the avoidantly attached child discovers that expressing anger in response to a caregiver's unresponsive or intrusive behavior will reduce the caregiver's proximity in stressful situations and so learns to redirect this anger toward the environment, perhaps resulting in hostile and aggressive behavior. In contrast, inconsistent or overprotective caregiving may engender vigilance and chronic anxiety in the ambivalently attached child, in response to fears that his or her needs will not be met. Bowlby traced depression to childhood experiences of separation from or loss of attachment figures, especially when hopelessness and helplessness ensue.

Rubin, Hymel, Mills, and Rose-Krasnor (1991) extended Bowlby's formulation to include child temperament, socioecological factors, and parental attitudes. They delineated a pathway in which an unresponsive, rejecting caregiver responds to an avoidant infant in an authoritarian, hostile manner, resulting in aggressive child behavior. Ambivalent infants are more likely to develop internalizing problems.

Sroufe (1983), on the other hand, suggested that both avoidant and ambivalent infants may develop externalizing problems, but the meaning and manifestations of these problems differ in predictable ways. Avoidant children might develop a hostile, antisocial pattern in response to rejecting, emotionally unavailable caregivers. The underlying anger, not directed at its source, might be manifested in lying, bullying, blaming, and insensitivity to others. Ambivalent children might be easily overstimulated and exhibit impulsivity, restlessness, short attention spans, and low frustration tolerance. Both kinds of children might be aggressive—but, Sroufe suggests, for different reasons.

These conceptualizations did not include the disorganized category, which has been demonstrated to occur at high rates in samples characterized by parent psychopathology, child abuse, and social or biological risk (see Hane & Fox, Chapter 11, this volume). Given its prevalence in children at risk for psychopathology, this pattern requires special attention. Main and Hesse (1990) have postulated that when a traumatized mother is unpredictably frightening, her child's response becomes disorganized. Egeland and Carlson (2004) argued that the child with a disorganized attachment is placed in an "unresolvable paradox," in that the putative source of safety (the caregiver) is simultaneously a source of fear. Unable either to regulate his or her arousal or to enlist the caregiver's assistance, the child may mentally isolate and fail to process disturbing stimuli, resulting in dissociation. Lyons-Ruth, Bronfman, and Atwood (1999) proposed that the child's fear may arise from sources other than the caregiver (e.g., abuse at the hands of others); if the parent responds to this fear with disruptive or contradictory affective communication, disorganization may result. This could explain some disorganization that develops postinfancy, following a child's exposure to maltreatment or trauma. Disorganization appears to be only weakly associated with maternal sensitivity and to have a more significant genetic component than other classifications (Rutter et al., 2009). Given its links with emotion regulation and cognitive processes, disorganized attachment has clear relevance to childhood psychopathology and must be part of any comprehensive theoretical model.

## Research Comparing Secure versus Insecure Attachment

Many early studies of the effects of attachment on development examined broad categories of secure versus insecure attachment. We reviewed this literature in the second volume of this handbook (DeKlyen & Greenberg, 2008) and only briefly summarize it here.

Initial work involved low-risk populations and asked whether insecure infant attachment was associated with behavior problems (e.g., Bates, Bayles, Bennett, Ridge, & Brown, 1991; Bates, Maslin, & Frankel, 1985; Fagot & Kavanaugh, 1990; Lewis, Feiring, McGuffog, & Jaskir, 1984). Main effects of insecure attachment on later problems were rarely found, and mediator or moderator effects were seldom tested. Studies of high-risk populations were generally more fruitful (e.g., El-Sheikh & Elmore-Staton, 2004; Lyons-

Ruth, Connell, Zoll, & Stahl, 1987; Munson, McMahon, & Spieker, 2001; Rodning, Beckwith, & Howard, 1991; Spieker & Booth, 1988; Sroufe et al., 2005; Vondra, Shaw, Swearingen, Cohen, & Owens, 2001).

The Minnesota Parent–Child Project was the most productive source of early results. A group of 174 infants of primarily young, single mothers was followed into early adulthood. Assessments during the preschool years (Erickson, Sroufe, & Egeland, 1985; Sroufe, 1983; Troy & Sroufe, 1987), the early elementary school period (Renken, Egeland, Marvinney, Mangelsdorf, & Sroufe, 1989; Sroufe, 1990; Sroufe, Egeland, & Kreutzer, 1990), preadolescence (Urban, Carlson, Egeland, & Sroufe, 1991), and adolescence (Carlson, 1998) consistently found that children in high-social-risk environments who exhibited early insecurity were more likely to have poor peer relations and symptoms of aggression, depression, and general maladjustment than children who had been secure. Later experiences that increased risk for secure infants or decreased risk for those who had been insecure also affected outcomes.

Other longitudinal investigations in high-risk populations confirmed the predictive value of early attachment (e.g., Cohn, 1990; Easterbrooks, Davidson, & Chazan, 1993; Goldberg, Gotowiec, & Simmons, 1995; Lyons-Ruth, Easterbrooks, & Cibelli, 1997; Lyons-Ruth, Easterbrooks, Davidson Cibelli, & Bronfman, 1995; Lyons-Ruth, Zoll, Connell, & Grunebaum, 1989; Turner, 1991).

Using sophisticated analyses to examine pathways linking attachment to subsequent antisocial outcomes, Kochanska and Kim (2012) assessed infant attachment (secure vs. insecure), child anger proneness, parent power assertion, and observed and parent-reported antisocial behavior in low-risk community samples. Although attachment security had no main effect on antisocial outcomes, it had an indirect effect, mediated by parents' power assertion and further modified by an interaction between child anger proneness and attachment. Insecure attachment in infancy appeared to create the context for coercive processes between a difficult toddler and his or her parent and for the emergence of antisocial behavior at age 6.5; this dynamic was not present in secure dyads.

Overall, these studies indicate that an insecure attachment in infancy may set a trajectory that increases risk for either externalizing or internalizing psychopathology, suggest that attachment serves as a general rather than a specific risk factor, and provide evidence of multifinality. In the remainder of this chapter we seek evidence of specificity for type of insecurity and for particular disorders.

## The Role of Specific Attachment Classifications in Disordered Behavior

### Externalizing Problems

Externalizing behaviors include a group of problems (e.g., oppositional defiant disorder (ODD), conduct disorder (CD), aggression, and antisocial behavior) that are often not clearly differentiated in research.

### THEORY

Several theories have been proposed concerning the role of attachment in the development of externalizing problems. Early theoretical arguments for expecting avoidantly attached children to be at increased risk for externalizing disorders have been reviewed above (e.g., Bowlby, 1973; Rubin et al., 1991; Sroufe, 1983).

Like Sroufe (1983), Mikulincer and Shaver (2011) suggest that antisocial behavior may result from either avoidant or ambivalent attachment models. The child with an avoidant stance might act out in order to maintain distance from or demonstrate a lack of concern for others. Ambivalently attached children, on the other hand, might do so to attract attention or to express anger or resentment.

Fonagy and colleagues (1997) present a model linking early insecure attachment, especially the avoidant classification, to later attachment and criminality. They hypothesize that as secure working models of attachment figures become more global, they facilitate bonding to social institutions and those who represent them (Hawkins et al., 1995). Children who lack this connection with institutions and have deviant peer relations are at increased risk for substance use and criminality. Secure attachments lead to greater awareness of the mental states of others, and this "mentalizing" inhibits malevolent acts and enhances relationship building. This theory raises a number of research questions that have only begun to be addressed (Dykas & Cassidy, 2011): How do "mentalizing" and related cognitive processes (e.g., joint attention, theory of mind) relate to attachment? Is this link relevant to depression and other disorders as well? And what might counterexamples (e.g., children with insecure working models who do bond to social institutions) tell us about the process?

Others theorists (e.g., Solomon, George, & DeJong, 1995) hypothesize that the absence of a coherent strategy (i.e., disorganization) rather than insecurity predisposes children to antisocial behavior; disorganization is also expected to increase vulnerability to internalizing disorders.

Consistent with the argument we presented earlier, several authors emphasize mediating and moderating processes that may link attachment and later problems. Fearon and colleagues (2010) posit several potential mediators, including self-confidence, social expectations, socialization of moral values, modeling of behavior, continuity of caregiving, and emotion regulation. Fearon and Belsky (2011) tested moderators (gender, social contextual risk, and age) and found that infant disorganization interacted with social risk in predicting school-age externalizing problems. Maternal sensitivity subsequent to the infant attachment assessment appeared especially influential for children who had been classified avoidant.

Kochanska and Kim (2012) describe two major sets of developmental goals served by attachment, one behavioral and focused on protection, the other fundamental to creating the context for socialization: The child who does not feel safe explores less and is less likely to develop adaptive emotion regulation strategies, and the insecure parent–child dyad's failure to establish reciprocity and responsiveness undermines positive socialization. Both mechanisms may contribute to antisocial behavior. The association between attachment and behavior problems is indirect and probabilistic, influenced by child characteristics and a cascade of later interactions and experiences.

## RESEARCH LINKING ATTACHMENT TO EXTERNALIZING PROBLEMS

A moderate association between attachment disorganization and externalizing problems was demonstrated in an early meta-analysis (Van IJzendoorn, Schuengel, & Bakermans-Kranenburg, 1999). More recently, Fearon and colleagues (2010) found that disorganization posed a higher risk than avoidant attachment, although both were associated with externalizing problems. Surprisingly, girls with disorganized attachments were significantly *less* likely than those with other classifications to be rated externalizing.

Following infants from the Minnesota Parent–Child Project, Aguilar, Sroufe, Egeland, and Carlson (2000) found that adolescents with early-onset antisocial behavior were more likely to have been avoidantly attached than adolescents with later-onset antisocial behavior or no disorder. However, they only compared avoidant with nonavoidant attachment, so no clear conclusions can be drawn regarding other classifications.

Avoidantly attached infants in the National Institute of Child Health and Human Development (NICHD) Study of Early Child Care had elevated externalizing scores in the first and second grades, but disorganized attachment predicted externalizing in grades 5 and 6 (Fearon & Belsky, 2011). For children with low contextual risk, there was no effect for any attachment classification, and few children had scores in the clinical range.

In high-risk samples, disorganized infant attachment predicted parent-rated externalizing problems when children were 5 years old (Shaw, Keenan, Vondra, Delliquadri, & Giovannelli, 1997) and teacher-rated externalizing in 7-year-olds (Lyons-Ruth et al., 1997). However, following children of teen mothers with high rates of depression, Keller and colleagues (2005) found that avoidant (but not disorganized) classification in infancy predicted an elevated trajectory for preschool disruptive behavior. The early-starting pattern, with escalating problems, was only prevalent when insecure attachment was combined with male gender and either high infant negativity or parenting risk, or when insecure attachment, parenting risk, and family ecological risk co-occurred. In the same sample, both avoidance and disorganization were associated with externalizing scores at 9 years of age (Munson et al., 2001).

Two low-risk samples in which attachment was assessed in early to middle childhood provide further evidence of the effect of the disorganized or controlling classification. In a French Canadian sample, children classified as controlling in a separation-reunion at ages 5–7 had the highest teacher-rated externalizing *and* internalizing problem scores concurrently and 2 years later (Moss, Cyr, & Dubois-Comtois, 2004; Moss et al., 2006). Both ambivalent and controlling children had elevated externalizing scores, using a composite of mother, teacher, and self-ratings. Controlling-punitive children had more externalizing problems, whereas controlling-caregiving children had more internalizing problems. Finally, using a story stem measure to assess attachment at 3–5 years of age, Roskam, Meunier, Stievenart, and Noel (2013) found that disorganization (but not security–insecurity) modestly predicted externalizing scores 2 years later.

We turn now to research focusing on specific types of externalizing behavior.

In a low-income sample, 60% of children classified disorganized at 12 months had clinically significant levels of aggression[1] on the Child Behavior Checklist at age 5, compared to 31% of avoidant, 28% of ambivalent, and 17% of secure infants (Shaw, Owens, Vondra, Keenan, & Winslow, 1996). Children with both disorganized attachment at 12 months and difficult temperament at age 2 had mean scores at the 99th percentile. Lyons-Ruth and colleagues (1995) reported that infant disorganization was associated with teacher-rated hostility; 55% of the children with disorganized classifications *and* mothers with psychosocial problems displayed hostile behavior in kindergarten, compared to 5% of those with neither risk factor.

Among low-risk children assessed at age 6, only those classified controlling were more likely to have conduct problems, as rated by parents, teachers, and peers (Solomon et al., 1995). Similarly, a study of high-risk first graders in which a story stem measure was used found that disorganization was related to higher teacher and parent ratings of conduct problems (Futh, O'Connor, Matias, Green, & Scott, 2008). However, Moss and colleagues (2004, 2006) reported that children classified either ambivalent or controlling at ages 5–7 were judged by mothers to be more aggressive (see Note 1) and to have more conduct problems 2 years later than were secure children.

Clinical samples provide a different perspective but may be limited by issues of selection or by the limited range of values. In the first two cohorts of our own research, described earlier, 80% of clinic-referred preschoolers meeting criteria for ODD were insecurely attached to their mothers, as opposed to 30% of typically developing children matched for age, socioeconomic status (SES), and family composition (Greenberg et al., 1991; Speltz et al., 1990). A disproportionate number received controlling classifications, and many were punitive or rejecting toward their mothers. In a third group of 80 clinically referred preschool boys and 80 carefully matched controls, 55% of those with ODD were insecure, with high rates of both avoidant and controlling categories (Speltz, DeKlyen, & Greenberg, 1999). This was one of the few studies to assess father–child attachment, and clinic-referred boys also had higher rates of insecurity with fathers (55 vs. 15%; DeKlyen, Speltz, & Greenberg, 1998). Boys insecurely attached to *both* parents were at greatest risk of being in the clinic group.

Note that a significant proportion of these clinically diagnosed boys exhibited secure attachments, indicating that a measure of insecure attachment does not merely assess oppositionality and is not a component of every pathway leading to ODD. Campbell (1990) similarly found that in some families of children with high rates of aggression and hyperactivity, the mother–child relationship appeared warm and trusting. Also, only the first cohort included girls, and the relation between attachment and clinic status held only for boys (there was little power to test this, but insecurity did not appear to characterize clinic girls; Speltz et al., 1990). Finally, in the second cohort, high concordance between child attachment and mothers' Adult Attachment Interview classification increased the probability that clinic boys were also insecure in infancy and that early attachment processes may have contributed to the development of disruptive problems (DeKlyen, 1996).

In another clinic sample of boys with ODD or CD diagnoses, Pasalich, Dadds, Hawes, and Brennan (2012) found that disorganized attachment was overrepresented (49%), but it was not associated with parent-reported severity of conduct problems. Boys with higher callous–unemotional (CU) ratings were more likely to have disorganized attachments, as predicted by the presumed inability of psychopaths to form intimate relationships. However, one-fourth of the children with high CU ratings were securely attached. Contrary to prediction, there was no relation to avoidant attachment (the authors suggest that their story stem measure underestimated avoidance).

Thus, there is evidence linking externalizing problems with all three insecure classifications, but the most consistent evidence implicates disorganization or controlling attachment, especially as children grow older. Many variables, including gender, social risk, and age at which problem behaviors were assessed, likely contribute to the varied findings, and the need for multirisk, transactional models in future research is clear.

### Internalizing Problems

As noted earlier, conceptual models have linked ambivalent attachment to internalizing problems because children with this pattern limit exploration, have poor emotion regulation, and are likely to feel fearful and helpless when faced with stressors (e.g., Cassidy & Berlin, 1994). Brumariu and Kerns (2010a) propose that three child characteristics link insecure attachment with internalizing symptoms: maladaptive and biased cognitions; impaired ability to identify, regulate, and cope with emotions; and self-concept/sense of worth. Each of these has been associated with anxiety and depression, and with early relations with caregivers; all except a diminished sense of self-worth are also linked with externalizing problems, which calls their specificity into question. Brumariu and Kerns suggest that excessive parental control may predict anxiety, whereas rejection may be more associated with depression. Disorganization is not discussed in their formulation. Some of the previously discussed research supports links between disorganization and internalizing outcomes; perhaps this is because disorganized children perceive themselves as helpless and vulnerable, and their attachment figures as unable to provide protection.

Two studies provide contrasting findings with respect to internalizing problems. In a longitudinal sample of high-risk families, avoidant but not disorganized infant attachment predicted teacher-reported internalizing symptoms at age 7; neither predicted clinically significant scores (Lyons-Ruth et al., 1997). On the other hand, Moss and her colleagues (2006) found that 5- to 7-year-old children with controlling classifications, and particularly the controlling-caregiving group, had the highest teacher-rated internalizing scores concurrently and 2 years later.

## ANXIETY DISORDERS

Given Bowlby's (1973) proposal that anxiety is fundamental to insecure attachment, it is surprising that little attention was initially paid to the relation between attachment and anxiety. Inadequate emotion regulation, manifested in intense fear or worry, is common to all anxiety disorders. Esbjorn, Bender, Reinholdt-Dunne, Munck, and Ollendick (2012) argue that children who experience an optimal balance of parent support and opportunities to establish self-regulation have the opportunity to develop flexible and effective strategies to regulate distress and reduce negative emotions. Both withdrawing and overly involved parents are more likely to have insecure children (avoidant or ambivalently attached, respectively) who either depend entirely on their own resources or have limited opportunities for self-regulation and rely primarily on others and are therefore at risk for anxiety disorders.

Carlson and Sroufe (1995) posit that ambivalent attachment is predictive of separation anxiety and school phobia given the child's worry about the attachment figure's availability (see also Manassis, 2001). Disorganization also might involve excessive concern about the caregiver's well-being, but we are unaware of specific theorizing about its association with anxiety. The link between avoidant attachment and restricted expression of negative emotions might predispose to somatic complaints or obsessive–compulsive symptoms.

A meta-analysis by Colonnesi and colleagues (2011) indicated a moderate association between ambivalent attachment and anxiety ($r = .37$); however, they compared only secure versus insecure and ambivalent versus nonambivalent categories. After surveying studies of attachment and anxiety, Esbjorn and colleagues (2012) also argued that insecure-ambivalent attachments increased children's vulnerability for anxiety, especially when combined with other risks. However, in their narrative review of the literature, Brumariu and Kerns (2010a) concluded that research attempting to link specific attachment classifications with childhood and adolescent anxiety has yielded mixed results and is limited because so few investigators have included measures of disorganization. A series of studies by their group used observational, story stem, and interview assessments of attachment, prospectively and concurrently, and found that disorganization, but not avoidance or ambivalence, was associated with anxiety in children age 10 years and older (Kerns & Brumariu, 2014). In contrast, in a multidomain study including concurrent attachment assessment at 4–5 years of age, insecurity had no direct effect and only a small indirect effect on anxiety symptoms (Hopkins, Lavigne, Gouze, LeBailly, & Bryant, 2013).

Studies including only three categories of attachment have generally found associations between ambivalent classification and anxiety. They have also often examined older children or adolescents. For example, in the Minnesota sample, adolescents with ambivalent infancy classifications were more likely to receive anxiety diagnoses; however, only nine children had an anxiety disorder and an ambivalent attachment in this follow-up sample (Warren, Huston, Egeland, & Sroufe, 1997). Only ambivalence predicted the number of anxiety disorder diagnoses; 28% of ambivalent infants had an anxiety disorder by age 17, compared with 16% of avoidant and 11% of secure infants. In a questionnaire-based study, ambivalent children had higher levels of anxiety than either avoidant or secure children at 12 years of age; assessment included only two insecure categories and was concurrent (Muris, Meesters, van Melick, & Zwambag, 2001). With an older sample (grades 6–10), Lee and Hankin (2009) found that self-reported ratings of both ambivalent and avoidant attachment were related to concurrent anxiety symptoms and changes in anxiety levels; again, disorganization was not assessed.

Shamir-Essakow, Ungerer, and Rapee (2005) used a four-category separation–reunion classification to assess high-risk Australian preschool children. Those with either disorganized or avoidant attachment had elevated levels of anxiety symptoms, after the researchers controlled for mothers' anxiety.

Overall, the evidence is inconclusive with respect to the association between particular attachment classifications and broad assessments of anxiety. We now consider research examining specific anxiety disorders.

## SEPARATION ANXIETY

Separation anxiety disorder is the most common anxiety diagnosis in prepubertal children, and both clinicians and researchers have theorized about the role played by parent–child relations (Klein, 1994; Manassis & Bradley, 1994; Thurber, 1996). Separation anxiety increases risk for a variety of adult psychiatric disorders, including depression, agoraphobia, and panic disorder; thus, research examining the association between attachment processes and separation anxiety could illuminate the pathways to these disorders as well.

Evidence linking infant attachment to separation anxiety is mixed. Dallaire and Weinraub (2005) found that children classified as ambivalent at 15 months reported higher levels of separation anxiety at 6 years than did secure (but not avoidant or disorganized) children, but the difference was marginal. Comparing only secure with ambivalent infant classifications, Bar-Haim, Dan, Eshel, and Sagi-Schwartz (2007) found that ambivalence was not associated with separation anxiety when children were 11 years of age. And comparing disorganization with organized patterns, MacDonald and colleagues (2008) reported no association between infant attachment and separation anxiety at 8 years.

In a study using a concurrent, four-category story stem measure, 10- to 12-year-old boys (but not girls) with ambivalent classifications were more likely to exhibit separation anxiety symptoms (Brumariu & Kerns, 2010b). However, the same investigators found no such association for children assessed with the Security Scale and Coping Strategies Questionnaire (Brumariu & Kerns, 2008).[2] Moss and colleagues (2006) reported that children classified controlling in a separation/reunion at ages 5–7 rated themselves higher on separation anxiety than did secure children.

Finally, in a unique clinical sample of 5- to 10-year-old children hospitalized for suicidal and/or assaultive behavior, Goodman, Stroh, and Valdez (2012) examined associations between attachment, based on the Attachment Story Completion Task, and separation anxiety, simple phobia, overanxious disorder, and posttraumatic stress disorder (PTSD). Their four-category measure was associated only with separation anxiety; the children with separation anxiety diagnoses were all classified either ambivalent or disorganized.

## OTHER ANXIETY DISORDERS

Using the Child Attachment Interview in a community sample, Borelli, David, Crowley, and Mayes (2010) reported that 8- to 12-year-old children with disorganized attachments had more social anxiety symptoms than organized children, and their problems were more likely to be clinically significant. With a four-category story stem measure, Brumariu and Kerns (2010b) also found that disorganization was associated with social anxiety, school phobia, and somatic symptoms in 10- to 12-year-olds, but a questionnaire assessment of attachment by the same researchers indicated that ambivalent attachment was the best predictor of social anxiety (Brumariu & Kerns, 2008). Neither a comparison of infant disorganized versus organized attachment (MacDonald et al., 2008) nor a contrast of controlling versus secure childhood attachment (Moss et al., 2006) predicted phobia or generalized anxiety.

## DEPRESSION

Bowlby and others have advanced theories for the role of attachment in the pathogenesis of depression (discussed earlier; also see Cicchetti & Cummings, 1990; Kobak et al., 1991). Egeland and Carlson (2004) postulate that ambivalence may lead to depression because the child is unable to satisfy the caregiver's demands and therefore perceives later difficulties or loss as yet another failure. Avoidant children may come to feel they are unlovable or inadequate and to see others as hostile; their alienation and sense of hopelessness may also lead to depression. And the child with a disorganized attachment is likely to feel overwhelmed by later difficulties and regard him- or herself as incapable, and therefore become depressed.

Morley and Moran (2011) suggest a pathway from early attachment involving negative representations of the self, leading to a helpless response to failure and vulnerability to depressed feelings; negative life events may then trigger depression. That is, attachment experiences result in cognitive biases that influence the child's interpretation of and response to negative events. This view is consistent with both cognitive and helplessness theories of depression (Abramson, Seligman & Teasdale, 1978; Beck, 1987). Morley and Moran argue that the inconsistent care that results in an ambivalent attachment undermines the stability and coherence of one's sense of self and self-worth, resulting in feelings of helplessness following failure. Individuals with avoidant attachments may ignore their deficiencies, attribute negative events to external causes, and therefore not be threatened by failure, but if they lack this sense of self-sufficiency and respond to failure—especially interpersonal failure—with a sense of helplessness, they may also be vulnerable to depression. Individuals with disorganized attachment may have tenuous coping strategies that break down under stress, leading to maladaptive responses and, again, vulnerability to depression. In short, any insecure attachment style may set the stage for depression.

Brumariu and Kerns (2010a) note that surprisingly few studies have investigated attachment and childhood depression. Adolescent research strongly suggests that insecurity is associated with depression, but a somewhat dated meta-analysis failed to find a link between disorganization and children's depression (Van IJzendoorn et al., 1999). Our review of the literature indicates that findings are mixed with respect to specific types of attachment (both ambivalence and disorganization have been implicated) and raises questions about causal direction in studies relying on concurrent self-reports of attachment and depression.

In a high-risk population, Bureau, Easterbrooks, and Lyons-Ruth (2009) reported that infant disorganization (vs. organized attachment) predicted depressive symptoms at 8 years, but insecurity did not. Every study we have reviewed that assessed disorganization or controlling attachment after infancy has found this category to be associated with depressive symptoms or diagnosis. For example, school-age children classified as controlling upon separation–reunion displayed more depressive symptoms than children with other classifications in a study by Graham and Easterbrooks (2000). Interestingly, low income predicted depressive symptoms for children with insecure attachments but not for securely attached children, suggesting that security might be protective against the effects of economic risk. Using the Child Attachment Interview to compare organized and disorganized 8- to 12-year-olds in a community sample, Borelli and colleagues (2010) found that disorganized children rated themselves as more depressed than children with organized patterns, but their parents did not. Disorganized children were also more likely to meet clinical criteria for depression. In the Moss and colleagues (2006) study, children classified as controlling at ages 5–7 rated themselves higher on depressive symptoms 2 years later than did secure children.

In Goodman and colleagues' (2012) sample of 5- to 10-year-old psychiatrically hospitalized children, assessed with a story completion task, disorganized children were more likely to meet criteria for a depressive disorder and reported more negative self-esteem than children with organized classifications. Although four-category attachment analyses were not significant, two-thirds of clinically depressed children, compared to one-fifth of those not clinically depressed, were classified as disorganized.

However, Lee and Hankin (2009), assessing only self-reported anxious and avoidant attachment, found that both were related to concurrent depression symptoms and to changes in depression levels of youth (grades 6–10). A middle childhood assessment using both three-category self-report attachment ratings and four-category scores from a story stem interview indicated that both self-reported avoidance and interview-based ambivalence and disorganization ratings were related to depressive symptoms (Kerns, Brumariu, & Seibert, 2011). These associations became insignificant after researchers controlled for demographics. The discrepancies between these results demonstrate the challenge of comparing findings based on three- versus four-category systems; how might the children rated as avoidant on the self-report questionnaire have been classified if disorganization were an option? Some researchers who have reported secondary organized classifications for disorganized children report that the majority of these appear avoidant (e.g., Borelli et al., 2010).

Starr, Hammen, Brennan, and Najman (2013) illustrate the role differential genetic susceptibility may play in links between attachment and childhood disorder. Participants ages 15–20, oversampled for maternal depression, were genotyped for polymorphisms in the serotonin transporter gene (*5-HTTLPR*) and assessed using the Bartholomew Relationship Questionnaire (Bartholomew & Horowitz, 1991), a self-rating of depressive symptoms, structured psychiatric interviews, and a life stress interview. For boys only, the short allele of *5-HTTLPR* predicted increased likelihood of depression among less secure boys and decreased likelihood among boys with higher security scores. The authors suggest that secure attachment serves as a buffer against the vulnerability associated with the short allele, which has been described as a marker for social reactivity: Boys who are genetically predisposed to be more reactive may suffer from negative parenting environments but thrive in more optimal situations. For girls but not for boys, security had a main effect, resulting in lower depression scores. However, gene × attachment classification interactions have often proven difficult to replicate, suggesting that this finding requires validation in other samples.

## Other Disorders

### ATTENTION-DEFICIT/HYPERACTIVITY DISORDER

We are unaware of theory linking specific attachment categories to attention-deficit/hyperactivity disorder (ADHD).

In Moss and colleagues' (2006) community sample (discussed earlier), children classified as controlling in a separation–reunion at ages 5–7 endorsed more ADHD symptoms 2 years later than did secure children. Using a child attachment interview, Borelli and colleagues (2010) found that disorganized children ages 8–12 had higher levels of parent-rated attention problems on the Child Behavior Checklist, and these problems were more likely to be clinically significant. Similarly, in a small Swedish cohort, disorganization, as assessed by a story stem measure at age 5, predicted ADHD symptoms at age 7 (Bohlin, Eninger, Brocki, & Thorell, 2012). Using the same sample, Thorell, Rydell, and Bohlin (2012) reported that children's representations of disorganized attachment at 8.5 years predicted ADHD

symptoms 1 year later. Finally, in a clinical sample of 4- to 9-year-old children with ODD or CD diagnoses, disorganization (vs. organization) was associated with a clinical diagnosis of ADHD (Green, Stanley, & Peters, 2007). Other types of insecurity were not analyzed in these studies, so comparisons between disorganized and avoidant or ambivalent attachments cannot be made.

Despite using a variety of measures and types of samples, this small set of studies is consistent in finding concurrent associations between disorganized or controlling attachment classifications and ADHD symptoms. Future research should differentiate between subsamples high in inattention and those characterized by hyperactive/impulsive symptoms.

### OBSESSIVE–COMPULSIVE DISORDER

Models of obsessive–compulsive disorder (OCD) have implicated insecurity in general. and avoidant and ambivalent attachment styles specifically. It has been suggested that compulsions result from the avoidant child's rigid self-reliance or the ambivalent child's difficulty learning from experience, given an early inflexible focus on caregivers (Ivarsson, Granqvist, Gillberg, & Broberg, 2010). In another formulation, Rezvan and colleagues (2012) note that the parents of children with OCD are more likely to be intrusive and interfering, resulting in avoidant attachment. Alternatively, children with frightening parents (i.e., disorganized or controlling children) may attempt through ritualized behaviors to ward off fear and control unavoidable dangers.

Few investigations have examined the relation between OCD and attachment, and only one has done so in childhood. Rezan and colleagues (2012) reported that insecurity (assessed with a self-report inventory) was associated with the number of obsessive–compulsive symptoms in a sample of 10- to 12-year-olds. In an adolescent study, 60% of those with OCD diagnoses were classified as dismissing (analogous to avoidant) on the Adult Attachment Interview (Ivarsson et al., 2010).

### POSTTRAUMATIC STRESS DISORDER

The correlates of disorganized attachment overlap with two of the three symptom clusters of PTSD diagnosis. The avoidance cluster includes dissociation (numbing), and the hyperarousal cluster includes irritability/angry outbursts; both are often exhibited by individuals who have been exposed to severe trauma. For this reason, it is reasonable to expect that disorganized attachment might be associated with PTSD.

Recoding the Minnesota data to include the disorganized/disoriented scale, Ogawa, Sroufe, Weinfield, Carlson, and Egeland (1997) and Carlson (1998) examined how infant attachment, developmental factors, and trauma experience were related to dissociation at ages 17 and 19. Both avoidance and disorganization in infancy predicted clinically significant dissociation in adolescence. These findings partially support Liotti's (1995) model linking early disorganization and trauma to later dissociative disorders.

More recently, MacDonald and colleagues (2008) followed a small group of infants, about half of whom were exposed to cocaine *in utero*, through their eighth birthday. Disorganization in infancy predicted number of PTSD symptoms and, in particular, symptoms in the avoidance and reexperiencing clusters, after researchers controlled for gender, cocaine exposure, and continuity of care. Significantly, children classified as disorganized were no more likely than controls to report having experienced trauma, although 64% indicated some traumatic exposure.

## AUTISM SPECTRUM DISORDER

Because the core criteria for autism spectrum disorder (ASD) involve impaired social interaction and communication, it was long assumed that children with these disorders might not form attachment relationships. They were also expected to exhibit some of the unusual behaviors associated with disorganized attachment.

Several studies have demonstrated that some children with ASD do form secure attachments (e.g., Dissnayake & Crossley, 1996; Rogers, Ozonoff, & Maslin-Cole, 1991), but insecure attachments occur more frequently than they do in nonclinical children. A meta-analysis of 16 studies concluded that although many children with autism exhibited secure attachments (53% in studies that assessed four categories), they were more likely than comparison children to be insecure (Rutgers, Bakermans-Kranenburg, Van IJzendoorn, & van Berckelaer-Onnes, 2004). However, this difference was evident only among children who were mentally delayed; studies with less delayed children showed no association with insecurity.

Studies examining multiple categories of attachment have provided mixed evidence, with some studies indicating an excess of disorganized attachments among children with ASD (e.g., Capps, Sigman, & Mundy, 1994) and others failing to do so. Notably, Capps and colleagues (1994) demonstrated that disorganization was overrrepresented even when unusual behaviors typical of ASD (e.g., stereotypies) were disregarded during coding. In a small study of toddlers with pervasive developmental disorder (PDD; a broader diagnostic category including autism), mental retardation, language delays, or typical development, Van IJzendoorn and colleagues (2007) found that children with PDD were more likely than those without this diagnosis to be classified as disorganized (vs. organized). However, 72% of the children with PDD also had mental retardation, which increased the risk of both insecure attachment and disorganization. This parallels earlier findings that only children with both PDD and mental retardation had elevated rates of disorganization (Rutgers et al., 2004; Willemsen-Swinkels, Bakermans-Kranenburg, Buitelaar, Van IJzendoorn, & van Engeland, 2000).

Naber and colleagues (2007) also reported that children with ASD were more likely than children without disorders to have disorganized attachment. However, children with ASD did not differ in rates of disorganization from other children with PDD, mental retardation, or language development disorders; mental developmental level, rather than severity of autistic symptoms, again appeared to account for disorganization. In a study by Bohlin and colleagues (2012), neither attachment insecurity nor disorganization (assessed with a story stem procedure at age 5) predicted autism symptoms at 7 years.

Given the consensus that autism is largely biologically determined, these findings may be more useful as aids in supporting children and families than for etiological understanding.

## GENDER DYSPHORIA

Few researchers have examined attachment processes in children with gender dysphoria (GD; formerly gender identity disorder). Goldberg (1997) reported a study in which boys with this disorder were more likely to be insecure than a community comparison group, and more likely to be ambivalent than a clinic comparison group. Secure, avoidant, and ambivalent classifications were approximately equally represented among the boys with GD, and disorganization was the least likely classification. Insecure attachment (based on the Separation Anxiety Test) was also overrepresented in another group of clinic-referred boys with this diagnosis (Birkenfeld-Adams, 2000). A related construct labeled "gender contentedness" was negatively associated with avoidant attachment for girls and boys and with preoccupied (ambivalent) attachment for boys in a fifth-grade sample (disorganization was not assessed; Cooper et al., 2013). Thus, although youth with GD appear to be at increased risk for insecure attachment, there is no consensus about what form this insecurity is likely to take.

## EATING DISORDERS

Although eating disorders are uncommon prior to adolescence, family relationships are frequently cited as a major etiological risk, so links with attachment are a promising target for research. Two studies are relevant. One involving Dutch preadolescents revealed that children reporting loss of control over eating rated their attachments with both parents as less secure (Goosens, Braet, Bosmans, & Decaluwe, 2011). In another, a unique investigation measuring prefrontal blood volume, Nagamisu and colleagues (2010) demonstrated that attachment-oriented images were particularly salient to young adolescent girls with anorexia nervosa. These youngsters responded with more prefrontal activation than comparison girls to images of mother–child interactions; surprisingly, no differences appeared in response to images of obese or slender bodies or of high-calorie food. The domain of eating disorders is one that requires further investigation.

# Disordered Attachment: Response to Extreme Caregiving Environments

## Diagnosing Disordered Attachment

So far we have focused on how attachment might serve as a risk or protective factor for specific disorders. What happens when a child has no specific caregiver to whom he or she can attach or when caregiving relationships are severely disrupted? Does this constitute disorder in itself, and if so, what might characterize this disorder?

These questions have informed studies of children raised in orphanages and others who have experienced maltreatment or the loss of caregivers, resulting in either the absence of a figure with whom to build a relationship or the traumatic disruption of a caregiving relationship. For many years clinicians have been aware of a small but seriously impaired group of children whose difficulties are believed to result from distorted or disrupted caregiving. Concerns about these children led to investigations of the effects of "maternal deprivation" after World War II (e.g., Bowlby, 1953; Goldfarb, 1955; Spitz, 1946). Children living in institutions, adopted after institutionalization, or removed from home because of maltreatment or neglect have been the subject of considerable recent research (e.g., Dozier, Albus, Stovall, & Bates, 2000; McCall, Van IJzendoorn, Juffer, Groark, & Groza, 2011; Rutter et al., 2010; O'Connor et al., 2003; St. Petersburg–USA Orphanage Research Team, 2008; Zeanah, Smyke, & Dumitrescu, 2002).

Official diagnostic systems first acknowledged that distorted attachment relationships might constitute a disorder when the third edition of the *Diagnostic and Statistical Manual of Mental Disorders* (DSM-III; American Psychiatric Association, 1980) included reactive attachment disorder (RAD). RAD was characterized as a pervasive disturbance across relationships, occurring before 10 months of age, with associated "failure to thrive" symptoms. The next revision (DSM-IV; American Psychiatric Association, 1994) and the *International Classification of Diseases* (ICD-10; World Health Organization, 1992) altered age of onset to 5 years or younger and dropped the failure to thrive criterion. Two types of the disorder were described: an inhibited form marked by hypervigilance, fear, withdrawal, and ambivalence, and a disinhibited subtype with indiscriminately friendly behavior and limited evidence of a specific attachment. DSM-IV also required documentation of pathogenic care.

These diagnoses recognized that disturbed attachment relationships may themselves represent disorder, but their formulation was inconsistent with attachment theory and research (Zeanah, 1996). Among other concerns, criteria focused on social behavior in general rather than relationships with primary caregivers, and the association between RAD and traditional attachment measures was problematic. Drawing from richly described case studies and their experiences with Romanian orphanages, Zeanah and Boris (2000) proposed alternative criteria, distinguishing "nonattachment," "disordered attachment," and "disruption of attachments." As in the DSM-IV and ICD-10 formulations, children in the first category (nonattachment), with no discriminated attachment figure, might either fail to differentiate among adults (indiscriminate sociability) or fail to seek or respond to caregivers in a developmentally typical manner. Zeanah and Boris did not require that these distortions occur in social situations beyond the caregiving context, and they specified that the child must have a mental age of at least 10 months, to distinguish attachment disorder from cognitive deficits or PDD. In the second category (disordered attachment), a selective attachment was thought to exist but to be disturbed, as evidenced by the child's self-endangerment, extreme inhibition, compulsive compliance, or role reversal. Finally, the third group (disruption of attachment) included children whose attachment to a primary caregiver had been disrupted; they might display grief reactions ranging from protest to despair to detachment. Initial studies suggested that these criteria, grounded in both attachment theory and clinical experience, permitted more reliable description of cases than the DSM-IV criteria (Boris, Fueyo, & Zeanah, 1997; Boris et al., 2004).

Zeanah and colleagues (2005) also developed a coding system to determine the extent to which a child displayed attachment behavior to a particular caregiver. Sroufe and colleagues (2005) and others have emphasized the importance of quality, not strength, of attachment, as all children in normal caregiving environments are expected to develop attachment bonds. However, in extreme circumstances such as institutional care, fostering, or adoption, it becomes critical to assess the degree to which any attachment relationship has developed. The Strange Situation was not designed to be sensitive to this, so the new coding system provides an important tool for understanding disorders involving atypical caregiving.

More recently, DSM-5 (American Psychiatric Association, 2013) separated the subtypes of the previous diagnostic category into two distinct disorders. RAD now refers to the emotional withdrawal/inhibited pattern and a new diagnostic category, disinhibited social engagement disorder (DSED), describes those children previously referred to as indiscriminately friendly. Research suggests that these two diagnoses can be reliably assigned and that each is cohesive and relatively stable, with distinct and predictable associations (Gleason et al., 2011).

Very limited information exists on the emotional withdrawal/inhibited form, but Gleason and colleagues (2011) report that in their small sample, it was modestly related to caregiving quality, and children who met criteria all received insecure-other attachment classifications. These children might be considered to have no selective attachment relationships.

More is known about disinhibited children. Aside from an initial experience of insufficient care, there is little evidence of a continuing association between caregiving quality and the disinhibited pattern, and there appears to be considerable stability over time even when children appear to have adapted well in adoptive families (Chisholm, Carter, Ames, & Morison, 1995; Gleason et al., 2011; Rutter et al., 2007). Although these children are often classified as insecure using traditional attachment measures, a substantial number receive organized and even secure classifications (Chisholm et al., 1995; O'Connor et al., 2003; Rutter et al., 2007; Zeanah et al., 2004). Multiple investigators have therefore concluded that this diagnosis does not reflect a disinhibited attachment with a specific caregiver but, instead, a general failure to inhibit social behavior and recognize boundaries (Bakermans-Kranenburg et al., 2011; Bruce, Tarullo, & Gunnar, 2009; Gleason & Zeanah, 2010). Disinhibition may be an example of a behavioral pattern that results from extremely deficient early caregiving but does not necessarily preclude a child's subsequent ability to form a secure attachment with caring adults.

Zeanah and colleagues found that children in standard orphanage care were more likely to exhibit indiscriminate behavior than either those in a special unit designed to provide more consistent care or a home-reared group (Smyke, Dumitrescu, & Zeanah, 2002; Zeanah et al., 2002). Interestingly, the pure withdrawn/inhibited pattern was relatively uncommon; most orphanage children displayed a mixture of inhibited and disinhibited behavior.

As noted, some children who have experienced extreme deprivation have been assigned organized and even secure attachment classifications, especially after receiving more adequate caregiving (Chisholm et al., 1995; O'Connor et al., 2003; Rutter et al., 2007; Zeanah et al., 2004), but it is not clear that their responses to traditional attachment protocols have the same meaning as those of other children (Bakermans-Kranenburg et al., 2011; Rutter et al., 2009). Also, most research has relied on the DSM-IV diagnosis, which combined the inhibited/withdrawn group with disinhibited cases. With those caveats, what do we know about the attachment relationships of children whose early caregiving was severely deficient and whom we therefore might expect to have disordered attachment?

Reviewing six studies of institutionally reared children, Van IJzendoorn and colleagues (1999) calculated that attachments with a favorite caregiver were secure in 17.1% of cases, avoidant in 5.5%, resistant in 4.6%, and disorganized in 72.8%. Marcovitch and colleagues (1997) assessed 3- to 5-year-old Romanian children adopted into Canadian families and also found higher than expected rates of insecurity. Not one adoptee was classified as avoidant; the authors argue that avoidance is particularly maladaptive for an adoptee, and that parents motivated to adopt are unlikely to exhibit parenting patterns related to avoidance during relationship formation. Subsequent studies using conventional measures of attachment have likewise found high rates of insecurity and, in particular, disorganization (Van den Dries, Juffer, Van IJzendoorn, & Bakermans-Kranenburg, 2009).

The focus so far has been on children who have spent significant periods of time (generally over 6 months) in institutions. What about the population that clinicians are more likely to encounter, children who have been maltreated? Using an interview developed for their work with Romanian orphans, Zeanah and colleagues (2004) demonstrated that RAD could be reliably diagnosed in toddlers in foster care, with a prevalence of 38–40%. A significant number displayed both withdrawn and indiscriminate social behavior, and clinician interviews indicated that some children who met criteria for indiscriminate/disinhibited RAD nonetheless had selective attachments to a caregiver, similar to institutionalized children. Boris and colleagues (2004) compared three groups of children (ages 18–48 months): one with a history of maltreatment, a second from a homeless shelter, and the last from HeadStart. Using Zeanah and Boris's (2000) alternative criteria, they found that maltreated children were the most likely to have an attachment disorder. Children with this diagnosis were less likely to be concurrently securely attached (to foster mothers, in the maltreated sample) and had lower security scores. However, children with an attachment disorder were no more likely than the others to be classified as disorganized. Finally, using ICD-10 criteria, Minnis and colleagues (2009) reported

that children with RAD diagnoses were far more likely (relative risk 2.4) than comparisons to be insecurely attached (27% disorganized), but 30% were rated secure on the Manchester Child Attachment Story Task.

## Other Disorders Associated with Severely Disrupted Attachment

Are there specific disorders that children with extremely deficient early caregiving or attachment disorders are particularly likely to exhibit? There is a good deal of evidence of impairment in this population, but less has been written about specific diagnoses. In a small sample, Hodges and Tizard (1989) reported that children adopted from an institution that provided adequate physical care but was deficient with respect to caregiver–child interaction had more problems with anxiety, antisocial behavior, and peer relationships than comparisons. In their sample of 3- to 5-year-old Romanian children adopted into Canadian families, Marcovitch and colleagues (1997) found that both length of institutionalization and insecure attachment to adoptive parents were associated with number of behavior problems. Comparing children in standard orphanage care with others receiving more consistent care and a home-reared group, Zeanah and colleagues reported that only those in the orphanage exhibited *severe* aggression, although many displayed no aggression at all (Smyke, Dumitrescu, & Zeanah, 2002; Zeanah et al., 2002). In contrast, home-reared children had relatively high rates of "moderate" aggression, so comparisons based on linear analyses were misleading. In a study by Gleason and colleagues (2011), children described as emotionally withdrawn/inhibited (similar to the new RAD category) had elevated depression symptoms. The indiscriminately social/disinhibited group was more likely to be characterized as impulsive and inattentive; 25% met criteria for ADHD. The disinhibited pattern has also been found by others to be associated with impaired attention regulation (Bakermans-Kranenburg et al., 2011; Bruce et al., 2009; Gleason & Zeanah, 2010). Examining a different population (high-risk home-reared infants) and using a new rating scale of infant–stranger engagement, Lyons-Ruth, Bureau, Riley, and Atlas-Corbett (2009) found that indiscriminate sociability, associated with early maltreatment or maternal psychiatric hospitalization, predicted aggressive and hyperactive behavior ratings at age 5.

## Summary

A lingering problem complicating interpretation of all of these findings is the absence of a widely accepted system that includes the entire spectrum of attachment experiences and successfully integrates these with a conceptualization of disordered attachment that is consistent with attachment theory and research. Most studies continue to rely on standard attachment classifications, although these do not adequately describe children who have experienced extremes of caregiving (Bakermans-Kranenburg et al., 2011). Despite considerable attention to the category of disorganized attachment over the past several years, exactly how it and its subtypes fit into this spectrum, and the mechanisms relating it to experience, to various outcomes, and to disorder, are still unclear.

The study of children deprived of an average, expectable caregiving environment both confirms the importance of these experiences to psychological health and illustrates the limitations of the conventional attachment measures on which we have long relied. Although many children with these disorders exhibit insecure or unclassifiable attachments, others appear secure in standard assessments. Regardless of attachment classification, they often display a variety of disordered behaviors that are clearly related to caregiving history. More research is needed, particularly with respect to children in the child protective system. Such investigations will help to inform the design of more effective interventions and are also likely to contribute to a deeper understanding of basic processes critical to both typical and pathological social and emotional development.

## Where Are We Now, and Where Should We Go from Here?

Since Mary Ainsworth first developed the Strange Situation, measurement has been central to our understanding of attachment and its relation with development. Measurement was a focal concern in our chapters in previous editions of this handbook (DeKlyen & Greenberg, 2008; Greenberg, 1999), and it remains a concern.

Significant progress has been made, for example, in creating tools to assess attachment in middle childhood, but we still know little about how measures from different developmental periods and using different methodologies relate to each other. Without such evidence, it is impos-

sible to determine whether outcomes are due to stable psychological structures established in early childhood, are dependent on the quality of ongoing relationships, or are perhaps caused by a third factor that influences both attachment and outcome. As Fearon and Belsky (2011) have argued, establishing causality will require well-validated measurement protocols that permit rigorous, cross-lagged longitudinal designs, and these are not yet available.

In 2008 we recommended a "return to the clinic." In recent years a significant body of research has described children who have suffered extremely deficient caregiving, providing a great deal of detail about the cognitive, behavioral, and physiological sequelae of severe neglect (see, e.g., monographs edited by McCall et al., 2011; Rutter et al., 2010). However, we still lack an integrated model that combines a taxonomy of disordered attachment with the classic attachment categories. Such a classification system should include and further describe subcategories of disorganized/disoriented attachment (e.g., controlling–punitive and controlling–caregiving), so that we can better understand why each develops, how each relates to specific disorders, and the environments and biology associated with each of these. Further development of measurements appropriate to children in extreme caregiving environments is needed for both theoretical and practical reasons. It would help us answer important clinical questions: How does a new attachment relationship form? How can disrupted attachments be repaired? What determines whether a secure attachment develops following maltreatment or trauma and whether disruptions are likely to leave lasting impairment? The lack of measures appropriate to the many clinical situations involving removal from home, the effects of foster care, and adaptation to later adoption is a major impediment to the practical application of attachment theory to these urgent social issues. Unfortunately, attachment concepts have too often been applied in a manner that is unsophisticated, inaccurate, or even dangerous (Mercer, Sarner, & Rosa, 2003).

Relatively few studies have examined disorders or behaviors that meet clinical criteria for concern. Diagnoses can provide a threshold of severity, as well as a degree of specificity that is missing in terms such as *externalizing* or *behavior problems*, although they do not ensure homogeneity of symptoms or etiology.[3] Some of the inconsistent findings reported in our review may be the result of poorly defined and heterogeneous constructs (e.g., externalizing, internalizing, behavior problems). Furthermore, when dimensional ratings are used, it is critical that authors provide information about the range of values represented in a given sample and their clinical significance. Also, low behavior ratings can be as much a cause for concern as elevated scores, so that interpreting scales solely by means of linear analyses may be problematic.

As already indicated, the field has been held back by lack of consistency in what researchers measure and how they report results. We have suggested that comparisons of secure versus insecure children are no longer very useful. Progress requires more specificity, and relatively few researchers have examined links between specific attachment classifications and specific disorders. Variability in how attachment is measured and reported (e.g., ambivalent vs. all other categories, three as opposed to four classifications) has further limited our ability to draw conclusions about specific attachment categories. Especially given the apparent significance of disorganization, we would encourage investigators always to assess and analyze all four attachment categories.

Researchers have begun to examine how differential susceptibility models, involving both environmental factors and gene × environment interactions, may relate to attachment (e.g., Kochanska, Philibert, & Barry, 2009; Spangler, Johann, Ronai, & Zimmermann, 2009; Starr et al., 2013). Epigenetic research has also provided new insights, for example, suggesting that trauma and stress influence health and well-being by changing the expression of genes (in this volume, see Bakermans-Kranenburg & Van IJzendoorn, Chapter 8; Hane & Fox, Chapter 11; and Ehrlich, Miller, Jones, & Cassidy, Chapter 9). These and other new approaches promise to provide fresh perspectives on the relation between attachment constructs and children's psychopathology. However, we must exercise caution before embracing these new methodologies too enthusiastically or abandoning old ones; exciting early findings do not always replicate (cf. Roisman, Booth-LaForce, Belsky, Burt, & Groh, 2013).

## Summary

In the *Handbook*'s first edition, this chapter posed the following question: Do specific attachment patterns lead to specific disorders? Greenberg (1999) concluded that attachment insecurity might be an important but nonspecific risk factor, increasing risk for several forms of psychopathology. It is not clear whether our inability to provide a more conclusive answer today is because the effect of attachment is indeed less specific than had been hypothesized, or because there has been insufficient research that reports on all attachment categories and clearly delineates outcomes to either confirm or dispute this assertion.

Although attachment processes show both predictive and concurrent associations with psychopathology in childhood, insecure attachment is rarely either a necessary or a sufficient cause of later disorder. Insecurity is not synonymous with disorder; secure children may be disordered and insecure children may function adequately. However, nonoptimal attachment experiences in infancy and beyond increase the risk for a variety of problems. With the intersection of multiple risk factors, maladaptation is increasingly probable. Further study of attachment as both mediator and moderator and the incorporation of concepts of differential susceptibility and gene × environment interaction are likely to be productive.

We have presented evidence that both avoidant and disorganized or controlling attachments are associated with externalizing problems, at least for boys. Disorganization may be a stronger predictor. The few relevant studies that exist suggest that ADHD is also often associated with disorganized attachment. The evidence for links between specific attachment styles and anxiety is less conclusive. A major roadblock is inconsistent reporting of attachment categories. Studies that assess three categories have often found ambivalent patterns predictive, while those that assess four categories more often implicate disorganization. Theoretical arguments have been advanced for links between each insecure category and depression, and empirical findings have been mixed, perhaps reflecting the disorder's heterogeneity. This may change with adolescence, when girls become far more likely than boys to be diagnosed with depression. Theory suggests that disorganization should be associated with PTSD, but little research has tested this in childhood. PTSD presents an especially interesting case, since the trauma involved often occurs after infancy, so internal working models may have undergone change. How important might early versus later attachment relationships be in this case? Contrary to expectations, many children in the autistic spectrum do form secure attachments, although they are less likely to do so than typically developing children. Disorganization is the most common form of insecurity in this group, but it appears to be more associated with cognitive delay than with the core symptoms of ASD.

Children in extremely compromised caregiving environments have been the subject of major studies in the last decade, and conceptualizations of RAD have undergone significant change. Youngsters meeting criteria for the new RAD diagnosis are likely to be classified as insecure, but many have likely failed to form a specific attachment. Children with disinhibited or indiscriminately friendly behavior are less associated with any one classification; some form secure attachments while maintaining indiscriminate social behavior. Standard attachment measures have proven inadequate to describe the relationships that many institutionalized, foster, adopted, or maltreated children have with caregivers, and we look for further development in this area.

The study of attachment and its relation to normality and psychopathology has advanced significantly in the past three decades. Yet further development and cross-validation of measures with older children and more comprehensive investigations that assess potential moderating and mediating processes and mechanisms are needed to illuminate the transactional relations linking attachment, other risks, and psychopathology. A continued emphasis on attachment-informed studies of children who have experienced extremes of caregiving will serve both to address urgent clinical and public health demands and to enrich our understanding of attachment. We look forward to more multifactorial, longitudinal studies of normative and high-risk populations and of samples with specific forms of psychopathology, utilizing complex models, to provide a fuller picture of the role of attachment in the development of childhood psychopathology.

## Notes

1. The items on the Child Behavior Checklist Aggression subscale include only a few descriptions of actual aggression along with many other behaviors (disobedience, temper, etc.) and in our opinion would more accurately be labeled "disruptive" or "oppositional behavior."

2. Kerns, Brumariu, and Seibert (2011) compared self-reported ratings of security, avoidance, and preoccupation with story stem interview ratings for security, avoidance, ambivalence, and disorganization. Security ratings assessed by the two methods were cor-

related ($r = .28$); neither avoidance nor ambivalence ratings were. Self-reported preoccupation (ambivalence) correlated with story stem disorganization ratings ($r = .24$).

3. The National Institute of Mental Health's Research Domain Criteria (RDoC) initiative is likely to further complicate future comparisons, but it may ultimately result in more clarity in reporting maladaptive outcomes (Cuthbert & Kozak, 2013).

## References

Abramson, L. Y., Seligman, M. E., & Teasdale, J. D. (1978). Learned helplessness in humans: Critique and reformulation. *Journal of Abnormal Psychology*, 87, 49–74.

Adam, K. S., Sheldon-Keller, A. E., & West, M. (1995). Attachment organization and vulnerability to loss, separation, and abuse in disturbed adolescents. In S. Goldberg, R. Muir, & J. Kerr (Eds.), *Attachment theory: Social, developmental, and clinical perspectives* (pp. 309–341). Hillsdale, NJ: Analytic Press.

Aguilar, B., Sroufe, L. A., Egeland, B., & Carlson, E. (2000). Distinguishing the early-onset/persistent and adolescence-onset antisocial behavior types: From birth to 16 years. *Development and Psychopathology*, 12, 109–132.

American Psychiatric Association. (1980). *Diagnostic and statistical manual of mental disorders* (3rd ed.). Washington, DC: Author.

American Psychiatric Association. (1994). *Diagnostic and statistical manual of mental disorders* (4th ed.). Washington, DC: Author.

American Psychiatric Association. (2013). *Diagnostic and statistical manual of mental disorders* (5th ed.). Arlington, VA: Author.

Bakermans-Kranenburg, M. J., Steele, H., Zeanah, C. H., Muhamedrahimov, R. J., Vorria, P., DubrovaKrol, N. A., et al. (2011). Attachment and emotional development in institutional care: Characteristics and catch-up. In R. B. McCall, M. H. Van IJzendoorn, F. Juffer, C. J. Groark, & V. K. Groza (Eds.), *Children without permanent parents: Research, practice and policy. Monographs of the Society for Research in Child Development*, 76, 62–91.

Bar-Haim, Y., Dan, O., Eshel, Y., & Sagi-Schwartz, A. (2007). Predicting children's anxiety from early attachment relationships. *Journal of Anxiety Disorders*, 21, 1061–1068.

Bartholomew, K., & Horowitz, L. M. (1991). Attachment styles among young adults: A test of a four–category model. *Journal of Personality and Social Psychology*, 61, 226–244.

Bates, J. E., Bayles, K., Bennett, D. S., Ridge, B., & Brown, M. M. (1991). Origins of externalizing behavior problems at eight years of age. In D. J. Pepler & K. H. Rubin (Eds.), *The development and treatment*

*development*. New York: International Universities Press.

Futh, A., O'Connor, T. G., Matias, C., Green, J., & Scott, S. (2008). Attachment narratives and behavioral and emotional symptoms in an ethnically diverse, at-risk sample. *Journal of the American Academy of Child and Adolescent Psychiatry, 47,* 709–718.

Galynker, I. I., Yaseen, Z. S., Katz, C., Zhang, X., Jennings-Donovan, G., Dashnaw, S., et al. (2012). Distinct but overlapping neural networks subserve depression and insecure attachment. *Social Cognitive and Affective Neuroscience, 7,* 896–908.

Gleason, M. M., Fox, N. A., Drury, S., Smyke, A., Egger, H. L., Nelson, C. A., et al. (2011). Validity of evidence-derived criteria for reactive attachment disorder: Indiscriminately social/disinhibited and emotionally withdrawn/inhibited types. *Journal of the American Academy of Child and Adolescent Psychiatry, 50,* 216–231.

Gleason, M. M., & Zeanah, C. H. (2010). *Reactive attachment disorder: A review for DSM-V.* Washington, DC: American Psychiatric Association.

Goldberg, S. (1997). Attachment and childhood behavior problems in normal, at-risk, and clinical samples. In L. Atkinson & K. Zucker (Eds.), *Attachment and psychopathology* (pp. 171–195). New York: Guilford Press.

Goldberg, S., Gotowiec, A., & Simmons, R. J. (1995). Infant–mother attachment and behavior problems in healthy and chronically ill preschoolers. *Development and Psychopathology, 7,* 267–282.

Goldfarb, W. (1955). Emotional and intellectual consequences of psychological deprivation in infancy: A reevaluation. In P. Hoch & D. Zubin (Eds.), *Psychopathology in childhood* (pp. 105–119). New York: Grune & Stratton.

Goodman, G., Stroh, M., & Valdez, A. (2012). Do attachment representations predict depression and anxiety in psychiatrically hospitalized prepubertal children? *Bulletin of the Menninger Clinic, 76,* 260–289.

Goossens, L., Braet, C., Bosmans, G., & Decaluwe, V. (2011). Loss of control over eating in pre-adolescent youth: The role of attachment and self-esteem. *Eating Behaviors, 12,* 289–295.

Graham, C. A., & Easterbrooks, M. A. (2000). School-aged children's vulnerability to depressive symptomatology: The role of attachment security, maternal depressive symptomatology, and economic risk. *Development and Psychopathology, 12,* 201–213.

Green, J., Stanley, C., & Peters, S. (2007). Disorganized attachment representation and atypical parenting in young school age children with externalizing disorder. *Attachment and Human Development, 9,* 207–222.

Greenberg, M. T. (1999). Attachment and psychopathology in childhood. In J. Cassidy & P. R. Shaver (Eds.), *Handbook of attachment* (pp. 469–496). New York: Guilford Press.

Greenberg, M. T., & Snell, J. (1997). The neurological basis of emotional development. In P. Salovey (Ed.), *Emotional development and emotional literacy* (pp. 93–119). New York: Basic Books.

Greenberg, M. T., Speltz, M. L., & DeKlyen, M. (1993). The role of attachment in the early development of disruptive behavior problems. *Development and Psychopathology, 5,* 191–213.

Greenberg, M. T., Speltz, M. L., DeKlyen, M., & Endriga, M. C. (1991). Attachment security in preschoolers with and without externalizing problems: A replication. *Development and Psychopathology, 3,* 413–430.

Greenberg, M. T., Speltz, M. L., DeKlyen, M., & Jones, K. (2001). Correlates of clinic referral for early conduct problems: Variable- and person-oriented approaches. *Development and Psychopathology, 13,* 255–276.

Greenspan, S. I. (1981). *Psychopathology and adaptation in infancy and early childhood: Principles of clinical diagnosis and preventive intervention.* New York: International Universities Press.

Groh, A. M., Roisman, G. I., Van IJzendoorn, M. H., Bakermans-Kranenburg, M. J., & Fearon, R. P. (2012). The significance of insecure and disorganized attachment for children's internalizing symptoms: A meta-analytic study. *Child Development, 83,* 591–610.

Gunnar, M. R. (2000). Early adversity and the development of stress reactivity and regulation. In C. A. Nelson (Ed.), *Minnesota Symposium on Child Psychology: Vol. 31. The effects of early adversity on neurobehavioral development* (pp. 163–200). Mahwah, NJ: Erlbaum.

Guttmann-Steinmetz, S., & Crowell, J. A. (2006). Attachment and externalizing disorders: A developmental psychopathology perspective. *Journal of the American Academy of Child and Adolescent Psychiatry, 45,* 440–450.

Hane, A. A., & Fox, N. A. (2006). Ordinary variations in maternal caregiving of human infants influence stress reactivity. *Psychological Science, 17,* 550–556.

Hawkins, J. D., Arthur, M. W., & Catalano, R. F. (1995). Preventing substance abuse. In M. Tonry & D. Farrington (Eds.), *Crime and justice: A review of research: Vol. 19. Building a safer society: Strategic approaches to crime prevention* (pp. 343–427). Chicago: University of Chicago Press.

Hertsgaard, L., Gunnar, M., Erickson, M. F., & Nachmias, M. (1995). Adrenocortical responses to the Strange Situation in infants with disorganized/disoriented attachment relationships. *Child Development, 66,* 1100–1106.

Hodges, J., & Tizard, B. (1989). IQ and behavioral adjustment in ex-institutional adolescents. *Journal of Child Psychology and Psychiatry, 30,* 53–75.

Hopkins, J., Lavigne, J. V., Gouze, K. R., LeBailly, S. A., & Bryant, F. B. (2013). Multi-domain models of risk factors for depression and anxiety symptoms in preschoolers: Evidence for common and specific factors. *Journal of Abnormal Child Psychology, 41,* 705–722.

Ivarsson, T., Granqvist, P., Gillberg, C., & Broberg, A. G. (2010). Attachment states of mind in adolescents with obsessive–compulsive disorder and/or depressive disorders: A controlled study. *European Child and Adolescent Psychiatry, 19*, 845–853.

Izard, C. E., Youngstrom, E. A., Fine, S. E., Mostow, A. J., & Trentacosta, C. J. (2006). Emotions and developmental psychopathology. In D. Cicchetti & D. J. Cohen (Eds.), *Developmental psychopathology: Vol. 1. Theory and method* (2nd ed., pp. 244–292). Hoboken, NJ: Wiley.

Keller, T. E., Spieker, S. J., & Gilchrist, L. (2005). Patterns of risk and trajectories of preschool problem behaviors: A person-oriented analysis of attachment in context. *Development and Psychopathology, 17*, 349–384.

Kerns, K. A., & Brumariu, L. E. (2014). Is insecure parent–child attachment a risk factor for the development of anxiety in childhood or adolescence? *Child Development Perspectives, 8*, 12–17.

Kerns, K. A., Brumariu, L. E., & Seibert, A. (2011). Multi-method assessment of mother–child attachment: Links to parenting and child depressive symptoms in middle childhood. *Attachment and Human Development, 13*, 315–333.

Klein, R. G. (1994). Anxiety disorders. In M. Rutter, E. Taylor, & L. Hersov (Eds.), *Child and adolescent psychiatry* (pp. 351–374). London: Blackwell.

Kobak, R., Cassidy, J., Lyons-Ruth, K., & Ziv, Y. (2006). Attachment, stress, and psychopathology: A developmental pathways model. In D. Cicchetti & D. J. Cohen (Eds.), *Developmental psychopathology: Vol. 1. Theory and method* (2nd ed., pp. 333–369). Hoboken, NJ: Wiley.

Kobak, R. R., Sudler, N., & Gamble, W. (1991). Attachment and depressive symptoms during adolescence: A developmental pathways analysis. *Development and Psychopathology, 3*, 461–474.

Kochanska, G., & Kim, S. (2012). Toward a new understanding of legacy of early attachments for future antisocial trajectories: Evidence from two longitudinal studies. *Development and Psychopathology, 24*, 783–806.

Kochanska, G., Philibert, R. A., & Barry, R. A. (2009). Interplay of genes and early mother–child relationship in the development of self-regulation from toddler to preschool age. *Journal of Child Psychology and Psychiatry, 50*, 1331–1338.

Kochanska, G., Woodard, J., Kim, S., Koenig, J. L., Yoon, J. E., & Barry, R. A. (2010). Positive socialization mechanisms in secure and insecure parent–child dyads: Two longitudinal studies. *Journal of Child Psychology and Psychiatry, 51*, 998–1009.

LeDoux, J. E. (1995). Emotion: Clues from the brain. *Annual Review of Psychology, 46*, 209–235.

Lee, A., & Hankin, B. L. (2009). Insecure attachment, dysfunctional attitudes, and low self-esteem predicting prospective symptoms of depression and anxiety during adolescence. *Journal of Clinical Child and Adolescent Psychology, 38*, 219–231.

Lewis, M., Feiring, C., McGuffog, C., & Jaskir, J. (1984). Predicting psychopathology in six-year-olds from early social relations. *Child Development, 55*, 123–136.

Lieberman, A. F., & Zeanah, C. H. (1995). Disorders of attachment in infancy. *Child and Adolescent Psychiatric Clinics of North America, 4*, 571–687.

Liotti, G. (1995). Disorganized/disoriented attachment in the psychotherapy of dissociative disorders. In S. Goldberg, R. Muir, & J. Kerr (Eds.), *Attachment theory: Social, developmental, and clinical perspectives* (pp. 343–366). Hillsdale, NJ: Analytic Press.

Lyons-Ruth, K., Bronfman, E., & Atwood, G. (1999). A relational diathesis model of hostile–helpless states of mind: Expressions in mother–infant interaction. In J. Solomon & C. George (Eds.), *Attachment disorganization* (pp. 33–69). New York: Guilford Press.

Lyons-Ruth, K., Bronfman, E., & Parsons, E. (1999). Maternal frightened, frightening or atypical behavior and disorganized infant attachment patterns. In J. I. Vondra & D. Barnett (Eds.), Atypical patterns of infant attachment: Theory, research, and current directions. *Monographs of the Society for Research in Child Development, 64*(3, Serial No. 258), 67–96.

Lyons-Ruth, K., Bureau, J.-F., Riley, C. D., & Atlas-Corbett, A. F. (2009). Socially indiscriminate attachment behavior in the strange situation: Convergent and discriminate validity in relation to caregiving risk, later behavior problems, and attachment security. *Development and Psychopathology, 21*, 355–372.

Lyons-Ruth, K., Connell, D., Zoll, D., & Stahl, J. (1987). Infants at social risk: Relationships among infant maltreatment, maternal behavior, and infant attachment behavior. *Developmental Psychology, 23*, 223–232.

Lyons-Ruth, K., Dutra, L., Schuder, M. R., & Bianchi, I. (2006). From infant attachment disorganization to adult dissociation: Relational adaptations or traumatic experiences? *Psychiatric Clinics of North America, 29*, 63–86.

Lyons-Ruth, K., Easterbrooks, M. A., & Cibelli, C. D. (1997). Infant attachment strategies, infant mental lag, and maternal depressive symptoms: Predictors of internalizing and externalizing problems at age 7. *Developmental Psychology, 33*, 681–692.

Lyons-Ruth, K., Easterbrooks, M. A., Davidson Cibelli, C. E., & Bronfman, E. (1995, April). *Predicting school-age externalizing symptoms from infancy: Contributions of disorganized attachment strategies and mild mental lag.* Paper presented at the biennial meeting of the Society for Research in Child Development, Indianapolis, IN.

Lyons-Ruth, K., Zoll, D., Connell, D., & Grunebaum, H. U. (1989). Family deviance and family disruption in childhood: Associations with maternal behavior and infant maltreatment during the first years of life. *Development and Psychopathology, 1*, 219–236.

Maccoby, E. E., & Martin, J. A. (1983). Socialization in the context of the family: Parent–child interaction. In P. H. Mussen (Series Ed.) & E. M. Hetherington (Vol. Ed.), *Handbook of child psychology: Vol. 4. Social-*

*ization, personality, and social development* (4th ed., pp. 469–546). New York: Wiley.

MacDonald, H. Z., Beeghly, M., Grant-Knight, W., Augustyn, M., Woods, R. W., Cabral, H., et al. (2008). Longitudinal association between infant disorganized attachment and childhood posttraumatic stress symptoms. *Development and Psychopathology, 20,* 493–508.

Mahler, M. S., Pine, F., & Bergman, A. (1975). *The psychological birth of the human infant.* New York: Basic Books.

Main, M., Cassidy, J., & Kaplan, N. (1985). Security in infancy, childhood and adulthood: A move to the level of representation. In I. Bretherton & E. Waters (Eds.), Growing points of attachment theory and research. *Monographs of the Society for Research in Child Development, 50*(1–2, Serial No. 209), 66–104.

Main, M., & Hesse, E. (1990). Parents' unresolved traumatic experiences are related to infant disorganized attachment status: Is frightened and/or frightening parental behavior the linking mechanism? In M. T. Greenberg, D. Cicchetti, & M. Cummings (Eds.), *Attachment in the preschool years: Theory, research, and intervention* (pp. 161–184). Chicago: University of Chicago Press.

Manassis, K. (2001). Child–parent relations: Attachment and anxiety disorders. In W. K. Silverman & P. D. A. Treffers (Eds.), *Anxiety disorders in children and adolescents: Research, assessment and intervention* (pp. 255–272). New York: Cambridge University Press.

Manassis, K., & Bradley, S. (1994). The development of childhood anxiety disorders: Toward an integrated model. *Journal of Applied Developmental Psychology, 15,* 345–366.

Marcovitch, S., Goldberg, S., Gold, A., Washington, J., Wasson, C., Krekewich, K., et al. (1997). Determinants of behavioral problems in Romanian children adopted in Ontario. *International Journal of Behavioral Development, 20,* 17–31.

Masten, A. S. (2001). Ordinary magic: Resilience processes in development. *American Psychologist, 56,* 227–238.

McCall, R. B., Van IJzendoorn, M. H., Juffer, F., Groark, C. J., & Groza, V. K. (2011). Children without permanent parents: Research, practice, and policy. *Monographs of the Society for Research in Child Development, 76.*

Mercer, J., Sarner, L., & Rosa, L. (2003). *Attachment therapy on trial: The torture and death of Candace Newmaker.* Westport, CT: Praeger.

Mikulincer, M., & Shaver, P. R. (2011). Attachment, anger, and aggression. In P. R. Shaver & M. Mikulincer (Eds.), *Human aggression and violence: Causes, Manifestations, and Consequences* (pp. 241–258). Washington, DC: American Psychological Association.

Minnis, H., Green, J., O'Connor, T. G., Liew, A., Glaser, D., Taylor, E., et al. (2009). An exploratory study of the association between reactive attachment disorder and attachment narratives in early school-age chil-dren. *Journal of Child Psychology and Psychiatry, 50,* 931–942.

Morisset, C. T., Barnard, K. E., Greenberg, M. T., Booth, C. L., & Spieker, S. J. (1990). Environmental influences on early language development: The context of social risk. *Development and Psychopathology, 2,* 127–149.

Morley, T. E., & Moran, G. (2011). The origins of cognitive vulnerability in early childhood: Mechanisms linking early attachment to later depression. *Clinical Psychology Review, 31,* 1071–1082.

Moss, E., Cyr, C., & Dubois-Comtois, K. (2004). Attachment at early school age and developmental risk: Examining family contexts and behavior problems of controlling–caregiving, controlling–punitive, and behaviorally disorganized children. *Developmental Psychology, 40,* 519–532.

Moss, E., Smolla, N., Cyr, C., Dubois-Comtois, K., Mazzarello, T., & Berthiaume, C. (2006). Attachment and behavior problems in middle childhood as reported by adult and child informants. *Development and Psychopathology, 18,* 425–444.

Munson, J. A., McMahon, R. J., & Spieker, S. J. (2001). Structure and variability in the developmental trajectory of children's externalizing problems: Impact of infant attachment, maternal depressive symptomatology, and child sex. *Development and Psychopathology, 13,* 277–296.

Muris, P., Meesters, C., van Melick, M., & Zwambag, L. (2001). Self-reported attachment style, attachment quality, and symptoms of anxiety and depression in young adolescents. *Personality and Individual Differences, 30,* 809–818.

Naber, F. B. A., Swinkels, S. H. N., Buitelaar, J. K., Bakermans-Kranenburg, M. J., Van IJzendoorn, M. H., Dietz, C., et al. (2007). Attachment in toddlers with autism and other developmental disorders. *Journal of Autism and Developmental Disorders, 37,* 1123–1138.

Nagamisu, S., Yamashita, F., Araki, Y., Iizuka, C., Ozono, S., Komatsu, H., et al. (2010). Characteristic prefrontal blood volume patterns when imaging body type, high-calorie food, and mother–child attachment in childhood anorexia nervosa: A near infrared spectroscopy study. *Brain and Development, 32,* 162–167.

O'Connor, T. G., Marvin, R. S., Rutter, M., Olrick, J. T., Britner, P. A., & the English and Romanian Adoptees Team. (2003). Child–parent attachment following early institutional deprivation. *Development and Psychopathology, 15,* 19–38.

Ogawa, J. R., Sroufe, L. A., Weinfield, N. S., Carlson, E. A., & Egeland, B. (1997). Development and the fragmented self: Longitudinal study of dissociative symptomatology in a nonclinical sample. *Development and Psychopathology, 9,* 855–879.

Olsavsky, A. K., Telzer, E. H., Shapiro, M., Humphreys, K. L., Flannery, J., Goff, B., et al. (2013). Indiscriminate amygdala response to mothers and strangers after early maternal deprivation. *Biological Psychiatry, 74,* 853–860.

Pasalich, D. S., Dadds, M. R., Hawes, D. J., & Brennan, J. (2012). Attachment and callous-emotional traits in children with early-onset conduct problems. *Journal of Child Psychology and Psychiatry, 53*, 838–845.

Patterson, G. R., DeBaryshe, B. D., & Ramsey, E. (1989). A developmental perspective on antisocial behavior. *American Psychologist, 44*, 329–335.

Patterson, G. R., Reid, J. B., & Dishion, T. J. (1992). *Antisocial boys*. Eugene, OR: Castalia.

Raikes, H. A., & Thompson, R. A. (2008). Attachment security and parenting quality predict children's problem-solving, attributions, and loneliness with peers. *Attachment and Human Development, 10*, 451–464.

Renken, B., Egeland, B., Marvinney, D., Mangelsdorf, S., & Sroufe, L. A. (1989). Early childhood antecedents of aggression and passive-withdrawal in early elementary school. *Journal of Personality, 57*, 257–281.

Rezvan, S., Rahrami, F., Abedi, M., MacLeod, C., Doost, H. T. N., & Ghasemi, V. (2012). Attachment insecurity as a predictor of obsessive-compulsive symptoms in female children. *Counseling Psychology Quarterly, 25*, 403–415.

Richters, J. E., & Waters, E. (1991). Attachment and socialization: The positive side of social influence. In M. Lewis & S. Feinman (Eds.), *Social influences and socialization in infancy* (pp. 185–213). New York: Plenum Press.

Rodning, C., Beckwith, L., & Howard, J. (1991). Quality of attachment and home environments in children prenatally exposed to PCP and cocaine. *Development and Psychopathology, 3*, 351–366.

Rogers, S. J., Ozonoff, S., & Maslin-Cole, C. (1991). A comparative study of attachment behavior in young children with autism or other psychiatric disorders. *Journal of the American Academy of Child and Adolescent Psychiatry, 30*, 483–488.

Roisman, G. I., Booth-LaForce, C., Belsky, J., Burt, K. B., & Groh, A. M. (2013). Molecular-genetic correlates of infant attachment: A cautionary tale. *Attachment and Human Development, 15*, 384–406.

Roskam, I., Meunier, J.-C., Stievenart, M., & Noel, M.-P. (2013). When there seem to be no predetermining factors: Early child and proximal family risk predicting externalizing behavior in young children incurring no distal family risk. *Research in Developmental Disabilities, 34*, 627–639.

Rubin, K. H., Hymel, S., Mills, S. L., & Rose-Krasnor, L. (1991). Conceptualizing different developmental pathways to and from social isolation in childhood. In D. Cicchetti & S. L. Toth (Eds.), *Rochester Symposium on Developmental Psychopathology: Vol. 2. Internalizing and externalizing expressions of dysfunction* (pp. 91–122). Hillsdale, NJ: Erlbaum.

Rutgers, A. H., Bakermans-Kranenburg, M. J., Van IJzendoorn, M. H., & Van Berckelaer-Onnes, I. A. (2004). Autism and attachment: A meta-analytic review. *Journal of Child Psychology and Psychiatry, 45*, 1123–1134.

Rutter, M. (1982). Prevention of children's psychoso-cial disorders: Myth and substance. *Pediatrics, 70*, 883–894.

Rutter, M., Colvert, E., Kreppner, J., Beckett, C., Castle, J., Groothuis, C., et al. (2007). Early adolescent outcomes for institutionally-deprived and non-deprived adoptees: I. Disinhibited attachment. *Journal of Child Psychology and Psychiatry, 48*, 17–30.

Rutter, M., Kreppner, J., & Sonuga-Barke, E. (2009). Emanuel Miller Lecture: Attachment insecurity, disinhibited attachment, and attachment disorders: Where do research findings leave the concepts? *Journal of Child Psychology and Psychiatry, 50*, 529–543.

Rutter, M., Sonuga-Barke, E. J., Beckett, C., Castle, J., Kreppner, J., et al. (2010). Deprivation-specific psychological patterns: Effects of institutional deprivation. *Monographs of the Society for Research in Child Development, 75*(1, Serial No. 295).

Schore, A. N. (2005). Attachment, affect regulation, and the developing right brain: Linking developmental neuroscience to pediatrics. *Pediatrics Review, 26*, 204–217.

Shamir-Essakow, G., Ungerer, J. A., & Rapee, R. M. (2005). Attachment, behavioral inhibition, and anxiety in preschool children. *Journal of Abnormal Child Psychology, 33*, 131–143.

Shaw, D. S., Keenan, K., Vondra, J. I., Delliquadri, E., & Giovannelli, J. (1997). Antecedents of preschool children's internalizing problems: A longitudinal study of low-income families. *Journal of the American Academy of Child and Adolescent Psychiatry, 36*, 1760–1767.

Shaw, D. S., Owens, E. B., Vondra, J. I., Keenan, K., & Winslow, E. B. (1996). Early risk factors and pathways in the development of early disruptive behavior problems. *Development and Psychopathology, 8*, 679–699.

Smyke, A. T., Dumitrescu, A., & Zeanah, C. H. (2002). Attachment disturbances in young children. I: The continuum of caretaking casualty. *Journal of the American Academy of Child and Adolescent Psychiatry, 41*, 972–982.

Solomon, J., George, C., & De Jong, A. (1995). Children classified as controlling at age 6: Evidence of disorganized representational strategies and aggression at home and at school. *Development and Psychopathology, 7*, 447–463.

Spangler, G., Johann, M., Ronai, Z., & Zimmermann, P. (2009). Genetic and environmental influence on attachment disorganization. *Journal of Child Psychology and Psychiatry, 50*, 952–961.

Spangler, G., & Schieche, M. (1998). Emotional and adrenocortical responses of infants to the Strange Situation: The differential function of emotional expression. *International Journal of Behavioral Development, 22*, 681–706.

Speltz, M. L., DeKlyen, M., & Greenberg, M. T. (1999). Attachment in boys with early onset conduct problems. *Development and Psychopathology, 11*, 269–286.

Speltz, M. L., Greenberg, M. T., & DeKlyen, M. (1990). Attachment in preschoolers with disruptive behavior: A comparison of clinic-referred and nonproblem children. *Development and Psychopathology, 2,* 31–46.

Spieker, S. J., & Booth, C. L. (1988). Maternal antecedents of attachment quality. In J. Belsky & T. Nezworski (Eds.), *Clinical implications of attachment* (pp. 95–135). Hillsdale, NJ: Erlbaum.

Spitz, R. (1946). Anaclitic depression: An inquiry into the genesis of psychiatric conditions in early childhood—II. *Psychoanalytic Study of the Child, 2,* 313–342.

Sroufe, L. A. (1983). Infant caregiver attachment and patterns of adaptation in preschool: The roots of maladaptation and competence. In M. Perlmutter (Ed.), *Minnesota Symposium on Child Psychology: Vol. 16. Development and policy concerning children with special needs* (pp. 41–81). Hillsdale, NJ: Erlbaum.

Sroufe, L. A. (1990). Pathways to adaptation and maladaptation: Psychopathology as developmental deviation. In D. Cicchetti (Ed.), *Rochester Symposium on Developmental Psychopathology: Vol. 1. The emergence of a discipline* (pp. 13–40). Hillsdale, NJ: Erlbaum.

Sroufe, L. A., Egeland, B., Carlson, E., & Collins, A. (2005). *The development of the person: The Minnesota Study of Risk and Adaptation from Birth to Adulthood.* New York: Guilford Press.

Sroufe, L. A., Egeland, B., & Kreutzer, T. (1990). The fate of early experience following developmental change: Longitudinal approaches to individual adaptation in childhood. *Child Development, 61,* 1363–1373.

Starr, L. R., Hammen, C., Brennan, P. A., & Najman, J. M. (2013). Relational security moderates the effect of serotonin transporter gene polymorphism (*5-HTTLPR*) on stress generation and depression among adolescents. *Journal of Abnormal Child Psychology, 41,* 379–388.

Stouthamer-Loeber, M., Loeber, R., Farrington, D. P., Zhang, Q., Van Kammen, W., & Maguin, E. (1993). The double edge of protective and risk factors for delinquency: Interrelations and developmental patterns. *Development and Psychopathology, 5,* 683–701.

St. Petersburg–USA Orphanage Research Team. (2008). The effects of early social-emotional and relationship experience on the development of young orphanage children. *Monographs of the Society for Research in Child Development, 73*(3),

Thorell, L. B., Rydell, A.-M., & Bohlin, G. (2012). Parent–child attachment and executive functioning in relation to ADHD symptoms in middle childhood. *Attachment and Human Development, 14,* 517–532.

Thurber, C. A. (1996). Separation anxiety disorder and the collapse of anxiety disorders of childhood and adolescence. *Anxiety Disorders Practice Journal, 2,* 115–135.

Troy, M., & Sroufe, L. A. (1987). Victimization among preschoolers: The role of attachment relationship history. *Journal of the American Academy of Child and Adolescent Psychiatry, 26,* 166–172.

Turner, P. (1991). Relations between attachment, gender, and behavior with peers in the preschool. *Child Development, 62,* 1475–1488.

Urban, J., Carlson, E., Egeland, B., & Sroufe, L. A. (1991). Patterns of individual adaptation across childhood. *Development and Psychopathology, 3,* 445–460.

van den Dries, L., Juffer, F., Van IJzendoorn, M. H., & Bakermans-Kranenburg, M. J. (2009). Fostering security?: A meta-analysis of attachment in adopted children. *Children and Youth Services Review, 31,* 410–421.

Van IJzendoorn, M. H., Rutgers, A. H., Bakermans-Kranenburg, M. J., Swinkels, S. H. N., van Daalen, E., Dietz, C., et al. (2007). Parental sensitivity and attachment in children with autism spectrum disorder: Comparison with children with mental retardation, with language delays, and with typical development. *Child Development, 78,* 597–608.

Van IJzendoorn, M. H., Schuengel, C., & Bakermans-Kranenburg, M. J. (1999). Disorganized attachment in early childhood: Meta-analysis of precursors, concomitants and sequelae. *Development and Psychopathology, 11,* 225–249.

Vondra, J. I., Shaw, D. S., Swearingen, L., Cohen, M., & Owens, E. B. (2001). Attachment stability and emotional and behavioral regulation from infancy to preschool age. *Development and Psychopathology, 13,* 13–33.

Warren, S. L., Huston, L., Egeland, B., & Sroufe, L. A. (1997). Child and adolescent anxiety disorders and early attachment. *Journal of the American Academy of Child and Adolescent Psychiatry, 36,* 637–644.

Waters, E., Kondo-Ikemura, K., Posada, G., & Richters, J. E. (1991). Learning to love: Mechanisms and milestones. In M. Gunnar & L. A. Sroufe (Eds.), *Minnesota Symposium on Child Psychology: Vol. 23. Self processes and development* (pp. 217–255). Hillsdale, NJ: Erlbaum.

Willemsen-Swinkels, S. H. N., Bakermans-Kranenburg, M. J., Buitelaar, J. K., Van IJzendoorn, M. H., & van Engeland, H. (2000). Insecure and disorganized attachment in children with a pervasive developmental disorder: Relationship with social interaction and heart rate. *Journal of Child Psychology and Psychiatry, 41,* 759–767.

Winnicott, D. W. (1965). *The maturational processes and the facilitating environment.* New York: International Universities Press.

World Health Organization. (1992). *The ICD-10 classification of mental and behavioural disorders: Clinical descriptions and diagnostic guidelines.* Geneva: Author.

Zaccagnino, M., Cussino, M., Callerame, C., Perinetti, B. A., Veglia, F., & Green, J. (2013). Attachment and social understanding in young school-age children: An investigation using the Manchester Child Attachment Story Task. *Minerva Psichiatrica, 54*(1), 59–69.

Zeanah, C. H. (1996). Beyond insecurity: A reconceptualization of attachment disorders in infancy. *Journal of Consulting and Clinical Psychology, 64,* 42–52.

Zeanah, C. H., & Boris, N. W. (2000). Disturbances and disorders of attachment in early childhood. In C. H. Zeanah (Ed.), *Handbook of infant mental health* (2nd ed., pp. 353–368). New York: Guilford Press.

Zeanah, C. H., Scheeringa, M., Boris, N. W., Heller, S. S., Smyke, A. T., & Trapani, J. (2004). Reactive attachment disorder in maltreated toddlers. *Child Abuse and Neglect, 28,* 877–888.

Zeanah, C. H., Smyke, A. T., & Dumitrescu, A. (2002). Attachment disturbances in young children: II. Indiscriminate behavior and institutional care. *Journal of the American Academy of Child and Adolescent Psychiatry, 41,* 983–989.

Zeanah, C. H., Smyke, A. T., Koga, S. F., Carlson, E., & the Bucharest Early Intervention Project Core Group (2005). Attachment in institutionalized and community children in Romania. *Child Development, 76,* 1015–1028.

shows other unusual signs of hesitation, confusion, apprehension, dysphoria, or conflict in relation to her. Disorganized-avoidant and disorganized-ambivalent infants often display unexpected combinations of distress, contact seeking, avoidance, resistance, or other apprehensive or conflict behaviors. Attachment disorganization, as a coding category, has been shown to be stable for periods ranging from 6 to 60 months ($r = .36$; $N = 515$) and has good interrater reliability (Van IJzendoorn et al., 1999).

## Prevalence of Disorganized Attachment Patterns

Meta-analyses indicate that 15% of infants are classified as disorganized in middle-class, nonclinical groups ($N = 1,882$) and 34% in low-income samples ($N = 493$) (Van IJzendoorn et al., 1999). Attachment disorganization (D) is accompanied by a secondary classification of ambivalent in 46% of cases, avoidant in 34%, and secure in 14%. However, these subtypes may be differentially distributed in low- and high-social-risk environments. In middle-income samples, more D infants are classified D-secure (50%, $N = 110$, Jacobvitz, Hazen, Zaccagnino, Messina, & Beverung, 2011; 62%, $N = 268$, Main & Solomon, 1990; 52%, $N = 1,131$, National Institute of Child Health and Human Development Early Child Care Research Network [NICHD ECCRN], 2001; K. McCartney, personal communication, October 12, 2005).

## Temperament, Genetics, and D Behavior

Given the contradictory nature of D behaviors, an important question is whether temperamental differences underlie them. Studies examining concordance in D classification across caregivers reveal that infants are unlikely to be classified as D with more than one caregiver (Fonagy et al., 1996; Main & Solomon, 1990). In addition, a meta-analysis showed a nonsignificant association between behavioral assessments of infant temperament and D ($r = .003$; Van IJzendoorn et al., 1999). Thus, the evidence does not indicate that infant temperament underlies D.

Only one study has examined temperamental variation *within* the D group. Padrón, Carlson, and Sroufe (2014) found that infants who were classified as D but did *not* display indices of fear during the Strange Situation were more likely than other D infants to have exhibited limited emotion regulation as newborns.

An important new area of study concerns possible genetic influences on D. Using *behavioral* genetic methods, Bokhorst and colleagues (2003) found that only nonshared environmental factors contributed to twin concordances in D. The authors speculated that nonshared factors such as trauma or differential parenting may be important in the etiology of D.

With the recent advent of *molecular* genetic techniques, it is easier to detect small effects of particular genes with modest sample sizes. The D4 dopamine receptor gene (*DRD4*) has been considered a candidate gene for infant attachment behavior because it is preferentially expressed in the mesocorticolimbic dopamine pathway that mediates reward related to social interaction, including mother–infant attachment (Insel, 2003). In a low-risk Hungarian sample, the risk for D increased fourfold among infants carrying the *DRD4*.7 polymorphism (Lakatos et al., 2000), and tenfold in the additional presence a *–521 C/T* single-nucleotide polymorphism (SNP) of the same *DRD4*.7 allele (Lakatos et al., 2002). Cicchetti, Rogosch, and Toth (2011), examining children with and without maltreatment, also found relations between the *DRD4*.7 allele and D. At age 2, *nonmaltreated children* with the *DRD4*.7 allele were more likely to be classified as D than children without the allele, replicating the Lakatos and colleagues (2000) finding. Also, 2-year-olds with the short allele of the serotonin transporter polymorphism (*5-HTTLPR*) were more often classified as D than children without that allele. These serotonin alleles have been associated with increased negative emotional response (Canli & Lesch, 2007). In contrast, for *maltreated children*, the *absence* of the *DRD4*.7 allele was associated with attachment disorganization but only at 1 year of age prior to the intervention. Following the intervention, no genetic differences were associated with disorganization. Cicchetti and colleagues (2011) speculated that genetic effects may be more evident in benign environments, while very adverse environments may override genetic contributions. However, a recent report using two large samples (the Generation R Study from the Netherlands [Gen R] and the NICHD SECCYD) failed to replicate the association between attachment disorganization and either the *DRD4* or *5-HTTLPR* polymorphisms (Luijk et al., 2011). (For further discussion, see Bakermans-Kranenburg & Van IJzendoorn, Chapter 8, this volume.)

## Disorganized Attachment and Gene–Environment Interaction

Studies have also examined *gene–environment interaction effects* in the formation of disorganized patterns of attachment. Gervai and colleagues (2007) reported that in the presence of the more prevalent *nonrisk DRD4.4* allele, infant disorganization was significantly related to disrupted mother–infant interaction, as expected on the basis of previous meta-analyses (e.g., Madigan et al., 2006). However, among infants with the *DRD4.7* risk allele, the expected relation between quality of caregiving and attachment disorganization did not hold. Luijk and colleagues (2011) found a similar interaction effect in the NICHD sample.

This interaction effect did not replicate in the Gen R study in the Netherlands (Luijk et al., 2011), possibly because the study did not adequately capture maternal behavior. Specifically, maternal sensitivity was not related to infant security of attachment, as would be expected (e.g., NICHD ECCRN, 1997; Van IJzendoorn et al., 1999). Thus, in the only two studies that have satisfied the prior expectation that maternal behavior would be related to infant attachment security, the *DRD4.7* allele conferred less sensitivity to maternal behavior.

In contrast, in relation to maternal unresolved (U) status on the AAI rather than maternal behavior, Van IJzendoorn and Bakermans-Kranenburg (2006) found that U predicted infant disorganization significantly *more often* if the infant also carried the *DRD4.7* allele. Thus, further work is needed to explore relations among dopamine function, maternal care, and infant attachment behavior. Also see Spangler, Johann, Ronai, and Zimmermann (2009) for a small-sample study of interaction between maternal insensitivity and children with two *5-HTT* short alleles. In summary, findings so far do not cohere in support of a strong genetic component. However, the *DRD4* polymorphism, in particular, warrants additional study. (See Bakermans-Kranenburg & Van IJzendoorn, Chapter 8, this volume, for further discussion of these issues.)

## Stress Hormone Levels, Neurobiology, and Disorganized Attachment Behaviors

In animal models, cortisol secretion is correlated with an animal's inability to mobilize an effective strategy to cope with a stressor (e.g., Levine, Wiener, & Coe, 1993). Consistent with Main and Solomon's (1990) view that D reflects the lack of an infant strategy for coping with stress, three studies report associations between D in infancy and infant reactivity to a stressor (Bernard & Dozier, 2010; Hertsgaard, Gunnar, Erickson, & Nachmias, 1995; Spangler & Grossmann, 1993).

In addition, infant D has been associated with atypical patterns of diurnal cortisol secretion. Whereas cortisol levels typically decrease over the course of the day, Luijk and colleagues (2010) reported that 2-year-olds previously classified as D at 14 months displayed a more flattened rate of change across the day than did those who were not D. In addition, differences in total daily cortisol were found *within the D group*, with D-secure infants secreting significantly more cortisol than either disorganized-avoidant or disorganized-resistant infants. Similar flattened rates of change in cortisol over the day have been observed among maltreated children in foster care (e.g., Dozier, et al., 2006), further suggesting that flattened slopes are markers for disturbed care.

Few studies have examined differences in brain structure or function among infants at risk for disorganization. Tharner and colleagues (2013) reported an increased risk for D among 14-month-olds with a smaller gangliothalamic ovoid at 6 months, assessed by ultrasound. The authors speculated that ovoid differences may contribute to difficulties in response selection and hence to the display of conflict behavior when distressed. Given current interest in how early relationships influence brain development, we can expect the literature on attachment and infant neurobiology to grow exponentially in the next decade.

## Developmental Timing: Prenatal Effects on D?

Animal studies provide clear evidence for the influence of prenatal experiences on brain structure and function (Del Cerro et al., 2010). A fetal programming hypothesis has been proposed to account for these effects (Barker, 1998). However, only a few human prenatal studies have included attachment assessments. In particular, maternal prenatal exposure to alcohol has been associated with D (Hay, Jacobson, Molteno, Viljoen, & Jacobson, 2004; O'Connor, Sigman, & Kasari, 1992; Rodning, Beckwith, & Howard, 1991), but only O'Connor and colleagues (1992) controlled for postnatal alcohol consumption. Bergman, Sarkar, Glover, and O'Connor (2008) also found that maternal prenatal stressful life events predicted infant disorganization. Other studies suggest that postnatal attachment experiences can attenuate the effects of prenatal stress on infant behavior (Bergman et al., 2008, 2010). However, specific effects of D were not explored in those studies.

## Is Indiscriminate Attachment Behavior Associated with D?

An important new area of study concerns how D may intersect with indiscriminate attachment behavior (IAB), now referred to as disinhibited social engagement disorder (DSED; American Psychiatric Association, 2013). DSED is a form of atypical attachment behavior first described among infants reared in orphanages with multiple caregivers, but it is also evident among some young children in high-risk home environments (Lyons-Ruth, Bureau, Riley, & Atlas-Corbett, 2009; O'Connor, Rutter, & English and Romanian Adoptees Study Team, 2000). DSED is characterized by non-normative engagement with strangers, including seeking close physical contact or going off readily with a stranger. DSED was first assessed by caregiver report, but direct observational assessments have now been validated (Gleason et al., 2014; Lyons-Ruth et al., 2009).

A few studies have examined how DSED is related to D. Zeanah, Smyke, Koga, Carlson, and the Bucharest Early Intervention Project Core Group (2005) found a high incidence of D (65%) and unclassifiable attachment behavior (13%) among 12- to 31-month-old institutionalized children in Romania (mean age 24 months). Only 3% showed a clearly recognizable pattern of organized attachment behavior toward the institutional caregiver. Consistent with normative samples, the quality of caregiver interaction was related to disorganized versus organized attachment. Surprisingly, institutional caregivers' reports of DSED were unrelated both to disorganized behavior and to quality of interaction with the institutional caregiver. However, at 54 months, Gleason and colleagues (2014) found that the only predictor of DSED was D with the institutional caregiver at study entry (mean age 22 months). At 54 months, DSED was assessed behaviorally rather than by institutional caregiver report, using the new Stranger at the Door procedure (see Gleason et al., 2014). No other measure at study entry predicted DSED, including quality of institutional care, time in institution, developmental quotient, or birthweight. These results are

particularly striking because half of the children had been placed in good-quality foster care at study entry. Thus, D predicted DSED over a 2½-year period regardless of quality of later care.

In the only other study to use a behavioral assessment of DSED, Lyons-Ruth and colleagues (2009) assessed home-reared socially at-risk infants and found that DSED was significantly more frequent among infants classified as D with the primary caregiver. In addition, DSED was associated with more severe caregiving risk and with more pervasive later behavior problems than was D behavior alone. Thus, in the only two studies that have assessed DSED in relation to infant attachment *with an early inadequate caregiver*, D behavior toward the inadequate caregiver was associated with DSED toward the stranger.

All other studies of the relations between attachment behavior in the Strange Situation and DSED toward a stranger have observed the child *with an adequate subsequent foster or adoptive parent*. Not surprisingly, those studies yield a very different picture, with DSED toward a stranger typically occurring in concert with organized, and often secure, behavior toward the new caregiver (see Lyons-Ruth et al., 2009, for review). Thus, it appears critical to distinguish between the quality of the original attachment relationship and the quality of later, more adequate attachment relationships in exploring the origins of DSED.

In the only randomized study of *change in D* among formerly institutionalized young children, Smyke, Zeanah, Fox, Nelson, and Guthrie (2010) found that after 19 months of foster care, children in foster care were significantly more likely than children in institutional care to exhibit organized rather than disorganized attachments. In addition, children in foster care displayed secure attachments at rates similar to those in the never-institutionalized comparison group. Yet, rates of DSED were not significantly different between children in foster placement and those who remained in institutional care, even after an average of 32 months in foster care. This converges with prior adoption studies, which also found that DSED can be shown long after placement into good care, at times in concert with apparently secure attachment behavior toward the new caregiver. Dozier and colleagues (2006) reported further that among maltreated children in foster care, these new secure-appearing behavioral organizations toward the foster mother may coexist with continued patterns of cortisol disregulation. Hence, it remains unclear to what extent new attachment organizations can compensate for the preceding periods of disorganization in the original attachment relationship in infancy. Primary prevention of DSED may depend on preventing D from forming in the *primary caregiving relationship*.

## Infant D and Family Risk Factors

### Maltreatment

A recent meta-analysis examined the effect of maltreatment (10 samples; $n$ = 456), as well as the effect of multiple socioeconomic risks, on the risk for D (Cyr, Euser, Bakermans-Kranenburg, & Van IJzendoorn, 2010). Large effect sizes were noted, with maltreated children more likely to be disorganized ($d$ = 2.19) than other socioeconomically at-risk children ($d$ = 0.48). However, children with five or more socioeconomic risks (eight studies; $d$ = 1.20) were also at elevated risk for disorganization. These results support Bernier and Meins's (2008) cumulative risk model proposing that multiple social risks will increase the incidence of D. Mechanisms underlying this association remain unclear but may include changes in parental behavior due to multiple economic stresses or more distal effects, such as multiple caregivers.

### Parental Psychopathology

Studies examining relations between maternal depression and D have yielded mixed results. A meta-analysis of 16 studies ($N$ = 1,053) found only a marginally significant relation between maternal depressive symptoms and infant D ($r$ = .06, $p$ = .06; Van IJzendoorn et al., 1999). However, a second meta-analysis revealed a significant effect of maternal depression when only serious depressive disorders requiring treatment were considered (Martins & Gaffan, 2000; see also Toth, Rogosh, Manly, & Cicchetti, 2006). More chronic and severe maternal depression resulting in significant clinical impairment may be necessary to produce an increase in infant D.

Maternal borderline personality disorder (BPD), characterized by intense and unstable relationships and impulsive, self-damaging behavior, including suicidality, has also been associated with elevated rates of D in infants. Compared to infants whose mothers did not have BPD, a higher proportion (80%) of 12-month-olds with mothers with BPD were classified as D (Hobson, Patrick, Crandell, García-Pérez, & Lee, 2005). Disorganization

was also more prevalent among children whose mothers were drug-addicted compared to other low-income mothers (Melnick, Finger, Hans, Patrick, & Lyons-Ruth, 2008). (Associations between prenatal maternal substance abuse and D were reported in an earlier section of this chapter, "Developmental Timing.")

### Parental Work Hours and Marital Conflict

In the Austin longitudinal study, Hazen, Allen, Umemura, Heaton, and Jacobvitz (2015) found an increased incidence of D if time in nonmaternal care exceeded 60 hours per week. A replication in the large NICHD sample confirmed that risk of D exponentially increased after 60 hours/week in nonmaternal care (Hazen et al., 2015). In the Austin sample, disorganization with fathers did not increase as a function of time spent in nonpaternal care, suggesting that D is not simply a function of lack of interaction. Conflict in the marriage is also related to infant D (Owen & Cox, 1997), but more research is needed to understand why this relation exists. It will be important to examine mechanisms underlying the relations between infant D and these family factors.

### Parental Unresolved States of Mind

According to attachment theory, children build expectations about future interactions with parents and others based on repeated patterns of interaction in close relationships. As these largely unconscious expectations become elaborated and organized, they form "internal working models" (Bowlby 1973) that guide children's interpretations and behaviors in new situations. Main, Kaplan, and Cassidy (1985) found that when parents' representations of their childhood attachment relationships were explored in an open-ended interview, the Adult Attachment Interview, four classifications of adults' states of mind regarding attachment could be reliably assigned. These four classifications, labeled autonomous, dismissing, preoccupied, and unresolved-disorganized (U), are analogous to the four infant attachment classifications—secure, avoidant, resistant, and disorganized.

The U classification is assigned to adults who show signs of disorientation and disorganization during discussions of potentially traumatic events (i.e., deaths, physical abuse, or sexual abuse). As detailed by Main, Goldwyn, and Hesse (2003), one sign of such lack of resolution is a lapse in the monitoring of discourse, whereby the speaker has "lost awareness of the discourse context." Examples include falling silent for 20 seconds mid-sentence, then completing the sentence or failing to finish the sentence. Another sign of unresolved loss or trauma is a lapse in the monitoring of reasoning. These lapses in the monitoring of reasoning are usually brief and should not be confused with "irrational" thinking across the transcript. Lapses include disbelief that the person is dead (e.g., discussing a parent in the present tense even though the parent died 20 years earlier) or beliefs that go against normal ideas about causality (e.g., "I killed him by saying one sentence"). Hesse (1996) suggested that lapses in the monitoring of reasoning or discourse involve "frightening and/or overwhelming experiences that may momentarily be controlling or altering discourse" (p. 8). Hesse and Main (2006) proposed that adults classified Unresolved are still overwhelmed either by the trauma itself, which is inherently frightening, or by "incompletely remembered loss experiences."

Similar to disorganized infants, adults classified as U are given a best-fitting alternate classification, identifying the pattern most closely corresponding to the overall organization of the interview (e.g., unresolved-autonomous). Main and colleagues (2003) also developed interview-wide criteria for designating an Adult Attachment Interview (AAI) item as "cannot classify." This may occur if both a dismissing and a preoccupied attachment strategy are evident in the same interview or if the participant exhibits low coherence across the interview.

Notably, Ainsworth and Eichberg (1991) did not find a significant association between being classified as U and either the mother's age when the loss occurred or her relationship to the deceased (attachment figure vs. someone else). Jacobvitz, Leon, and Hazen (2006) also found that the mother's age when the loss occurred was unrelated to her resolution of the loss. However, mothers who were classified as U were more likely to have lost a parent than to have lost a less important figure.

## Maternal Unresolved State of Mind and Infant D

Parental U state of mind is significantly related to infant D, with an effect size of 0.65 ($r = .31$, $N = 548$; Van IJzendoorn, 1995). This association has been confirmed in studies throughout North America, Western Europe, the Middle East, Africa, and Mexico, and occurs even when adults' attachment status is assessed prior to the child's birth (Van IJzendoorn et al., 1999). However, very few studies have examined correlates of U states among fathers.

One unique study examined the intergenerational transmission of U states from mother to *adult daughter* among Holocaust survivors and controls with no Holocaust background. Holocaust survivors were more often classified as U. However, the U state was not transmitted to the next generation (Sagi-Schwartz et al., 2003). The authors note that the traumatic events were not created by attachment figures but emerged from an outside destructive force (the Nazis), which may have allowed the survivors to establish organized attachment relationships with their own children. Living in Israel was also found to be a protective factor in a meta-analysis of 12,746 Holocaust survivors and controls (Barel, Van IJzendoorn, Sagi-Shwartz, & Bakermans-Kranenburg, 2010).

## U States of Mind and D Behavior in Adolescence

Obsuth, Hennighausen, Brumariu, and Lyons-Ruth (2014) examined the correlates of adolescent U states of mind in relation to observed adolescent–parent interaction in a conflict discussion paradigm at age 20 (details are provided in a later section). U states of mind were specifically related to patterns of interaction characterized by odd, out-of-context, or disoriented behaviors by both adolescent and parent but were not related to adolescent caregiving or punitive interaction with the parent.

## U States of Mind and Dissociative Symptoms

U states of mind have been associated with altered states of consciousness, such as trance-like states. For example, individuals classified as U showed elevated scores on the Tellegen Absorption Scale (TAS; Tellegen & Atkinson, 1974), which includes items such as "I sometimes 'step outside' my usual self and experience an entirely different state of mind" (Hesse & Van IJzendoorn, 1999). Two other studies have found an association between elevated dissociative symptoms and U states among both low- and high-risk mothers (Bailey,

Moran, & Pederson, 2007; Schuengel, Bakermans-Kranenburg, & Van IJzendoorn, 1999).

## Unresolved States of Mind and Other Psychiatric Symptoms

In a meta-analysis of the first 10,000AAIs, the distribution of classifications among North American nonclinical mothers indicated that 18% were U or cannot classify (U/CC) (Bakermans-Kranenburg & Van IJzendoorn, 2009). Distributions in European, Japanese and Israeli samples were similar. Gender was not associated with U/CC status. A lower than expected rate of U/CC was found among adolescent samples (11%), coupled with a higher than expected rate of dismissing classifications. The distribution in clinical samples was strikingly different, with U/CC strongly overrepresented (43% U/CC). U/CC was overrepresented among those with internalizing disorders (e.g., suicidality and borderline psychopathology) and externalizing disorders (e.g., antisocial personality disorder [APD]). Familial violence, extrafamilial violence, and violence against the self (e.g., childhood maltreatment, current posttraumatic stress disorder [PTSD]) were strongly associated with U/CC classification. Notably, however, depressed groups did not have a higher rate of U/CC classification, which echoes the lack of a clear association between parental depression and infant disorganization. U states were also more prevalent among veterans with PTSD than trauma-exposed veterans without PTSD (Harari et al., 2009). U states have also been related to substance abuse and parental separation/divorce, as well as suicidal ideation and emotional distress, in a nonclinical sample (Riggs & Jacobvitz, 2002). Though few relevant studies have been conducted, physical handicaps, including blindness and deafness, were not associated with attachment states of mind.

Elevated rates of cannot classify (CC) were found in adults diagnosed with BPD (Fonagy et al., 1996) and obsessive–compulsive disorder without depression (Ivarsson, Granqvist, Gillberg, Anders, & Broberg, 2010), and in criminal populations (Hesse, Hobson, Patrick, Maughan, & Main, 2011). Thus, higher rates of U/CC states were associated with many clinical presentations, pointing to the potential contribution of disturbed attachment relationships to a variety of clinical disorders.

## Unresolved States of Mind and Functional Brain Responses

Only two small studies have examined neurobiological correlates of U states of mind. In one study, Buchheim and colleagues (2006) administered the Adult Attachment Projective (AAP), a picture-based alternative for assessing U states of mind, to 11 healthy adult females while undergoing functional MRI, with five women classified as U. When responses to all pictures were included, there was no differential activation of brain regions evident for U versus non-U participants. However, as the traumatic imagery in the pictures increased, individuals classified as U increased activation in several emotion-related brain regions, including right inferior prefrontal cortex (PFC), left superior temporal gyrus, left caudate nucleus, and bilateral medial temporal regions, while others did not. In a second study of 11 patients with BPD and 17 controls (Buchheim et al., 2008), the only effects were related to patient status and not to U states of mind. Further work with larger samples is needed to assess the generalizability of these results.

## Unresolved Loss versus Unresolved Abuse

An individual can be classified as U in relation to loss or abuse, or both. Usually these are combined for analysis, but the few studies that have examined correlates of U-loss and U-abuse separately have found important differences. Vulliez-Cody, Obsuth, Torreiro-Casal, Ellertsdottir, and Lyons-Ruth (2013) found that U-loss was a correlate of maternal role confusion in relation to her child, whereas U-abuse was not. U-loss was accompanied by broad indicators of the parent's helplessness and need for the child's guidance, suggesting that mothers who experience U-loss may feel they need support from their child. In relation to this hypothesis, Moss, Cyr, and Dubois-Comtois (2004) found that maternal losses during the child's lifetime were related to the child's caregiving behavior toward the mother but not to punitive or disorganized behavior. Bailey and colleagues (2007) found that abuse was related to both U-loss and U-abuse in adolescent mothers, but Byun, Brumariu, and Lyons-Ruth (in press) found that only U-abuse, not U-loss, was related to the severity of the abuse in childhood. Thus, differential correlates of maternal U-loss and U-abuse deserve further exploration.

## A "Transmission Block" in the Assessment of Maternal U States of Mind?

The meta-analysis cited earlier revealed that only 53% of D infants had mothers with U states of mind (Van IJzendoorn, 1995). Although this is a robust effect, it also means that 47% of D infants did not have U mothers. One explanation is that U can only be assigned if the participant reports a specific loss or abuse experience. Therefore, discourse about loss or abuse per se may constitute a narrow window for capturing all anomalous attachment states of mind seen among adults with more difficult childhood experiences. Thus, investigators have also developed coding systems to capture more pervasive anomalies in the AAI that are not confined to discourse anomalies related to loss or abuse.

## CC States of Mind on the AAI

As noted earlier, one approach to coding transcriptwide anomalies is to code multiple states of mind in the same transcript, as noted earlier for the CC category (Hesse, 1996). However, to date, reliability and validity data on the CC classification has been limited, with Bakermans-Kranenburg and Van IJzendoorn (2009) noting that there were not enough reliably coded CC classifications in the first 10,000 AAIs to conduct a separate assessment.

## Hostile–Helpless States of Mind on the AAI

In another approach to coding transcriptwide anomalies, Lyons-Ruth, Yellin, Melnick, and Atwood (2005) developed a coding system for hostile–helpless (HH) states of mind on the AAI. This coding system focuses on indices of pervasively contradictory evaluations of the attachment relationship itself, rather than on lapses in monitoring during discussions of loss or trauma. Research reviewed below suggests that the HH coding system may be particularly relevant to understanding processes involved in the intergenerational transmission of maltreatment.

The central feature of an HH state of mind is the extent to which the individual has positively identified with the psychological stance of a childhood caregiver whom he or she also globally devalues elsewhere in the interview. HH interviews may combine "hot" but unelaborated devaluation,

a concise narrative, apparently frank discussion of both positive and negative aspects of childhood attachment relationships, and in some cases, an entertaining quality. This combination provides a poor fit with other existing AAI classifications and may erroneously lead to placement in the "earned secure" subgroup (see Lyons-Ruth, Yellin, et al., 2005). Both hostile and helpless subtypes may be seen. In the hostile subtype, one or more attachment figures are represented in globally devalued terms as hostile or malevolent, but there is also evidence of a competing positive representation and continued identification with the same attachment figure. For example, in different parts of the AAI interview, one speaker said, "We were friends, . . . we were enemies. . . . We're just alike but we fought all the time." Contradictory mental contents are seen in the juxtaposition of positive and globally devaluing evaluations of the same caregiver over the course of the interview. Theoretically, a hostile state of mind is viewed as a potential outcome of a controlling/punitive stance in childhood (see section on childhood attachment below).

In the helpless subtype, the participant globally devalues but also positively identifies with a helpless or parentally abdicating caregiver; for example, "We're best friends. . . . She's a basket case." Individuals with a helpless state of mind may describe having adopted a vigilant and protective caregiving role toward the parent in childhood. Anger is inhibited or expressed in assertions that are not integrated with the more predominant caregiving attitude. Theoretically, a helpless state of mind in adulthood is viewed as a potential outgrowth of a caregiving attachment stance in childhood. A "mixed" HH subtype is also commonly seen that includes aspects of both subtypes.

## HH States of Mind and Infant Disorganization

Parental HH states of mind have been significantly related to infant disorganization in two studies (Lyons-Ruth, Yellin, et al., 2005; Melnick et al., 2008), and in both, HH states of mind accounted for variance in infant disorganization not accounted for by U states of mind. In the Lyons-Ruth, Yellin, and colleagues (2005) study, U and HH states of mind were similarly good predictors of D-secure infant behavior, but HH was a stronger predictor than U for infants classified as D-insecure (i.e., disorganized-avoidant or disorganized-ambivalent). In the second study, 62 mothers receiving treatment for methadone dependence were compared to 87 women in a nonaddicted low-income control group, and again, HH better accounted for infants classified as D-insecure (Melnick et al., 2008).

## HH States of Mind and Maltreatment

Barone, Bramante, Lionettia, and Pastore (2014) evaluated factors that differentiated mothers who had murdered a child ($n = 23$) from mothers with mental illness ($n = 37$) and healthy controls ($n = 61$). Once variance associated with SES, traumatic events, and mental illness was accounted for, HH states of mind added to the prediction of child murder, but U states did not. Frigerio, Costantino, Ceppi, and Barone (2013) also found that HH states of mind were stronger in differentiating maltreating mothers from nonmaltreating mothers than were U states of mind. In addition, HH states of mind have been found to be prevalent among mothers followed by social services for documented neglect of a child (Milot et al., 2014), although U states were not examined in that study. Finally, among 104 young adults, HH state of mind mediated the relations between severity of childhood maltreatment and borderline and antisocial symptoms in young adulthood, whereas U state of mind was not a significant mediator (Finger, Byun, Melnick, & Lyons-Ruth, 2015). Thus, pervasively unintegrated evaluations of central attachment relationships may be particularly associated with experiencing, and possibly repeating, childhood maltreatment.

## HH States of Mind and Adolescent Attachment Behavior

Obsuth and colleagues (2014), studying adolescent–parent interaction among 104 dyads, found that adolescent HH states of mind were related to punitive interactions with parents at age 20, but not to caregiving or disoriented interaction patterns with parents. This contrasts with the earlier mentioned association between U states and disoriented forms of interaction in the same study. Thus, it appears that U and HH states of mind are associated with different forms of disorganization in interaction with a parent. It will be important to explore further these potentially distinct pathways encompassed within the broader framework of D relationships.

## HH States of Mind and Psychopathology

Other work has examined HH states of mind among adults with anxiety disorders and with borderline psychopathology. Young adults with anxiety disorders were rated higher on HH states of mind than were adolescents without Axis I diagnoses (Brumariu, Obsuth, & Lyons-Ruth, 2013). In relation to BPD, in a sample of 12 patients with BPD and 11 adult outpatients with dysthymia, significantly more women in the BPD group (100%) displayed an HH state of mind, compared to 55% of the dysthymic group. In addition, significantly more patients with BPD (75 vs. 27% in the dysthymic group) indicated in their responses on the AAI that in childhood they had engaged in punitive or caregiving forms of controlling behavior toward parents. These results indicate that in addition to U states of mind, patients with BPD exhibit a pervasive difficulty in integrating affective evaluations of attachment figures. Finally, as mentioned previously, Finger and colleagues (2015) found that HH states of mind mediate the relations between severity of childhood maltreatment and the extent of both borderline and antisocial features in young adulthood.

## Parental Frightened, Frightening, or Atypical Behavior

Why are parental U or HH states of mind related to infant D? Main and Hesse (1990) hypothesized that when the still-traumatized parent responds to memories or ideas related to loss or trauma, he or she may engage in inexplicably frightened or frightening behavior. A frightened or frightening attachment figure is thought to provoke conflict for an infant because the attachment figure is "at once the source of and the solution to its alarm" (p. 163). Unable to implement a coherent strategy of approaching or fleeing, the infant shows D behavior.

## Maternal Insensitivity

Ratings of maternal insensitivity, which have consistently distinguished secure from organized insecure infants (Van IJzendoorn, 1995), have not consistently distinguished infants displaying D (metaanalysis; Van IJzendoorn et al., 1999). Thus, the sensitivity scale may not be specific enough to capture the various forms of fear-related parental behavior related to infant D. Given this lack of prediction, both Main and Hesse (1992) and

Bronfman, Parsons, and Lyons-Ruth (1992) developed coding systems to capture the frightened, frightening, or other disrupted parental behaviors most strongly related to infant D. A number of subsequent studies have explored the hypothesis of "fright without solution" by examining whether frightening or disrupted parental behavior predicts infant D. A meta-analysis of studies using either of these two coding systems indicated that infants whose parents displayed frightened, frightening, or disrupted behavior were 3.7 times more likely to display D behavior ($r = .34$; $N = 851$; Madigan et al., 2006).

## Frightened or Frightening Maternal Behavior

Main and Hesse (1992, 1998) developed six scales to identify subtypes of frightening or frightened (FR) parental behavior:

1. *Threatening*—postures, facial expressions and movements that appear aggressive (e.g., sudden movements into the area surrounding the infant's face and eyes).
2. *Frightened*—behaviors indicating the mother is inexplicably frightened (e.g., a retreat sequence, as in pulling or backing away from the infant).
3. *Dissociative*—indications of possible entrance into an altered state of consciousness (e.g., stilling or freezing in trance-like postures or speaking in haunted voice tones).
4. *Timid or deferential*—behavior in which the parent appears submissive to the infant (e.g., very timid or deferential handling of the infant).
5. *Spousal or romantic*—excessive intimate or sexualized caressing of the baby.
6. *Disorganized*—parental behavior fitting Main and Solomon's (1990) description of infant disorganized/disoriented behaviors.

Several researchers have examined FR behavior in relation to parents' U states on the AAI. Jacobvitz and colleagues (2006) found that mothers classified as U displayed higher levels of FR behavior with their infants at 8 months but did not differ from other mothers on maternal insensitivity, interference, or rejection ($N = 125$). U was associated with FR regardless of the secondary secure or insecure subclassification. Moreover, U mothers who lost an attachment figure, or who were

younger than 16 at the time of the loss, were more likely to display FR behavior. Therefore, kinship and timing of the loss may contribute to whether the mother's U state impinges on her caregiving.

In contrast, Schuengel, Bakermans-Kranenburg, and Van IJzendoorn (1999) found a relation between maternal U states and maternal FR behavior toward an infant but only among the subgroup of mothers classified as U-insecure on the AAI (analogous to the D-insecure infant subgroup). Abrams, Rifkin, and Hesse (2006) found that U parents had significantly higher dissociative-FR scores than other parents, but U was not associated with any other FR subscales. In addition, in a study of village-dwelling mothers in Mali, True, Pasani, and Oumar (2001) found that infants whose mothers displayed *any* FR behavior were more often classified as D. Finally, both Jacobvitz and colleagues (2011) and Schuengel and colleagues (1999) found that mothers' FR behavior mediated the relation between maternal U states and infant D.

In the only study of high-risk participants to examine this issue, Lyons-Ruth, Bronfman, and Parsons (1999) also found that FR behavior was significantly related to infant D. However, when the two subgroups of D infants were examined, only mothers of D-insecure infants displayed more FR behavior. This finding resembled Schuengel and colleagues' (1999) finding that FR behavior was only elevated among mothers in the U-insecure subgroup of the AAI. By meta-analysis (Madigan et al., 2006), the effect size for the relation between U attachment and FR was $r = .28$ ($N = 242$), and the effect size for the relation between FR and infant D was $r = .32$ ($N = 325$). One of the few studies including fathers found that fathers' frightening-FR behavior ($N = 110$) predicted infant D with father, but only when fathers were both frightening *and* insensitive (Hazen, McFarland, Jacobvitz, & Boyd-Soisson, 2010). In addition, Abrams and colleagues (2006) examined the six FR subscales in both father–infant ($n = 25$) and mother–infant ($n = 50$) dyads. Both mothers and fathers of disorganized infants received significantly higher scores on the Threatening-FR and Dissociative-FR subscales. When all six FR subscales were considered simultaneously, only Dissociative-FR behavior uniquely predicted infant D. Given the importance of dissociative-type FR behavior, it is noteworthy that both Schuengel and colleagues (1999) and Lyons-Ruth, Hennighausen, and colleagues (2005) failed to find a relation between maternal scores on the Dissociative Experiences

Scale and infant D. Thus, *in vivo* interaction seems more important than symptom scores.

Jacobvitz and colleagues (2011) also created an assessment of FR maternal behavior with 24-month-olds. The infants' mothers were rated on four 9-point scales, including Frightening/Anomalous, Frightened by Child, Disoriented/Dissociated Behavior, and Boundary Diffusion (failing to keep appropriate boundaries with child). Maternal U states assessed prenatally, as well as FR behavior at 8 months and infant disorganization at 1 year, predicted mothers' FR behavior at 24 months. For related work on mother–toddler role confusion and infant D, see Macfie, Fitzpatrick, Rivas, and Cox (2008).

## Maternal Disrupted Communication

Lyons-Ruth, Bronfman, and Parsons (1999) expanded on Main and Hesse's (1990) construct of fright without solution to develop a broader coding system for disrupted communication between parent and infant (Atypical Maternal Behavior Instrument for Assessment and Classification, or AMBIANCE). Lyons-Ruth, Bronfman, and Atwood (1999) theorized that for all infants, fear arises from a variety of sources, in addition to parental behavior. For the infant to organize a consistent attachment strategy in the face of such fears, the parent must provide minimally adequate comfort and proximity, even if the parent him- or herself is not the source of infant fear. For example, a mother may engage in contradictory forms of affective communication with the infant around the need for comfort, such as moving away while asking tenderly, "What's the matter?" Or the parent may engage in role-confused behavior such as asking the infant for a kiss when the infant needs comfort. More dramatically, the parent may leave the infant to cry on the floor with no response. In this view, the parent's inability to provide a consistent response to the infant's need for comfort is extreme enough, or contradictory enough, that avoidant or ambivalent strategies cannot be organized in relation to the caregiver.

The AMBIANCE coding system (Bronfman et al., 1992; Bronfman, Madigan, & Lyons-Ruth, 2007) includes the items on the 1992 version of the Main and Hesse (1992) FR coding system. The system also includes aspects of caregiving behavior not included in the FR system that were observed among mothers at risk and are theoretically related to unmodulated infant fear and D. Five broad dimensions of disrupted parental affective communication with the infant are assessed:

1. *Negative-intrusive behavior*—behavior that is frightening, behavior that interferes with the infant's ongoing directions, or behavior that communicates a hostile attitude toward the infant (e.g., mocking or teasing the infant).
2. *Role confusion*—behavior that prioritizes the parent's needs over the infant's needs (e.g., asking for reassurance or affection from the infant when the infant is distressed).
3. *Disorientation*—behavior that appears frightened or affectively odd (e.g., unusual changes in pitch and intonation of voice or stiff and awkward body postures when interacting with infant).
4. *Affective communicative errors*—contradictory communications or failures to respond to clear infant cues for comfort (e.g., verbally inviting the infant to approach followed by physical distancing; leaving the infant to cry on the floor).
5. *Withdrawal*—behaviors that communicate reluctance to interact fully with the infant (e.g., walking around the infant, hesitating before responding, or interacting silently with infant).

Meta-analysis of studies using the AMBIANCE (Madigan et al., 2006) confirmed a significant relation between maternal disrupted communication and infant D attachment ($r = .35$; $N = 384$). Meta-analysis also revealed high test–retest stability of the AMBIANCE over 10 to 72 months ($r = .56$, $N = 203$).

In an initial study using both AMBIANCE and FR coding systems in a low-income sample (see the earlier section on FR), Lyons-Ruth, Bronfman, and Parsons (1999) found that, with all FR behaviors excluded, the frequency of disrupted communication still significantly predicted infant D. Only 17% of maternal behaviors coded on the AMBIANCE were FR behaviors. This suggests that FR behavior is occurring within a broader matrix of disturbed communication between mother and infant. In addition, when using the AMBIANCE to compare the two infant D subtypes, mothers of D-insecure infants showed significantly higher rates of negative intrusive behavior and role confusion, while mothers of D-secure infants exhibited higher levels of withdrawal (Lyons-Ruth, Bronfman, & Parsons, 1999). Finally, Forbes, Evans, Moran, and Pederson (2007) assessed mothers and infants at both 12 and 24 months. At both ages, disrupted communication was related to infant D, and change in maternal disrupted communication from 12 to 24 months predicted change in infant D.

Maternal behavior is not related to infant gender using either the FR system or the AMBIANCE (Lyons-Ruth, Bronfman, & Parsons, 1999). However, David and Lyons-Ruth (2005) found that gender differences in infant attachment behavior may emerge in the context of high levels of frightening maternal behavior. In the context of high levels of frightening behavior, males were more likely to show disorganized conflict behavior and avoidance than females, who often continued to approach their mothers. Thus, males' responses were more reliable indicators of the quality of parent–infant interaction.

Meta-analysis also confirmed a significant relation between maternal disrupted communication and U classification on the AAI ($r = .20$; $N = 311$; Madigan et al., 2006). Furthermore, among 45 adolescent mothers who were *not classified* as U on the AAI, Madigan, Moran, Schuengel, Pederson, and Otten (2007) found a robust relation between maternal disrupted communication and infant D. Therefore, the AMBIANCE may be helpful in identifying infants at risk of D whose mothers do not exhibit U states of mind on the AAI. Finally, Ballen, Bernier, Moss, Tarabulsy, and St-Laurent (2010) did not find an overall relation between U states of mind and disrupted communication among mothers interacting with a foster child. However, U-loss, in particular, was related to the Fearful/Disoriented subscale on the AMBIANCE, which captures more dissociative behaviors. Finally, in an innovative extension of work using the AMBIANCE, Crawford and Benoit (2009) developed criteria for coding the five dimensions of maternal disrupted communication at a representational rather than a behavioral level. Maternal disrupted communication coded on the Working Model of the Child Interview (WMCI) in the third trimester of pregnancy significantly predicted maternal U state, maternal disrupted communication, and infant D at 12 months.

As seen earlier, disrupted maternal communication can be patterned in many ways. Thus, it is also important to examine whether different patterns of disrupted behavior may predict different outcomes for the child. Lyons-Ruth, Bureau, Easterbrooks, Obsuth, and Hennighausen (2013) traced correlates of maternal withdrawal and maternal negative-intrusive behavior over the infancy, middle childhood, and adolescent periods, and found distinct correlates at each age. In infancy, maternal withdrawal was associated with continued attempts by the infant to approach and gain contact with the mother, despite concomitant disorganized behavior (D-secure subtype). In middle childhood, maternal withdrawal in infancy predicted child controlling–caregiving behavior toward mother, but not punitive behavior. In adolescence, maternal withdrawal in infancy predicted the mothers' role confusion and caregiving helplessness (George & Solomon, 1996). Maternal role confusion on interview was further related to caregiving/role confusion in observed adolescent–parent interaction (see the later section on adolescents). Thus, a strikingly coherent construct emerges relating maternal withdrawal to maternal role confusion and child caregiving. In contrast, maternal negative-intrusive behavior in infancy was unrelated to any of these above outcomes but predicted child externalizing problems in preschool and middle childhood (Lyons-Ruth, Alpern, & Repacholi, 1993; Lyons-Ruth, Easterbrooks, & Cibelli, 1997). Additional studies relating disrupted maternal communication to psychopathology in adulthood are reviewed below in the section "Prospective Prediction of Psychopathology in Adolescence/Young Adulthood."

### Disrupted Communication among Fathers

We do not know whether a father's disrupted communication has a similar relation to infant D. In the only study of fathers, Madigan and colleagues (2011) found no relation between fathers' disrupted communication and father–infant disorganization at 18 months, but only 6 infants among 31 father–infant dyads were classified D.

### Maternal Disrupted Communication and Maternal and Infant Cortisol

In one of the few studies examining maternal and infant cortisol, Crockett, Holmes, Granger, and Lyons-Ruth (2013) found that very disrupted maternal communication with a 4-month-old infant after a still-face procedure was associated with blunted maternal cortisol at study entry. Maternal cortisol, in turn, predicted infants' hyperreactive cortisol response to the still-face and recovery periods. Schechter and colleagues (2004) also assessed maternal cortisol levels in relation to disrupted maternal communication among violence-exposed mothers of preschoolers. Similar blunted levels of maternal cortisol were observed in mothers who exhibited disrupted, and, particularly, withdrawing behavior during reunion with their preschool child.

## Maternal Affective Communication Early in the First Year

Unfortunately, only a few studies have examined whether mother–infant interaction in the first 6 months of life forecasts later infant D. Tomlinson, Cooper, and Murray (2005) assessed maternal depression and caregiving behavior of 147 mothers with their infants at 2 months and 18 months, and found that both remote-disengaged and intrusive maternal behavior at 2 months uniquely predicted D at 18 months. Jaffe, Beebe, Feldstein, Crown, and Jasnow (2001) found that "hypervigilant" vocal rhythm tracking by both mother and baby forecast D. The authors proposed that hypervigilance stems from maternal stress or anxiety. Furthermore, Beebe and colleagues (2010) found that mothers of 4-month-old infants later classified as D displayed multiple disturbances in affective communication at 4 months. Their babies also showed more vocal distress and mirrored the mother's affective disturbances (e.g., smiling to mother's smile, while simultaneously whimpering from mother's rough handling). The authors suggested that D infants form working models characterized by emotional incoherence and expectations of emotional distress. More longitudinal studies over the first year are needed to explore how early parent–infant interaction and infant stress responses are related to the emergence of infant D.

## Maternal Disrupted Communication and Offspring Regional Brain Volumes

A promising new direction is examination of regional brain differences in relation to maternal disrupted communication and infant D. Lyons-Ruth, Pechtel, Yoon, Anderson, and Teicher (2014) examined regional brain volumes among 18 low-income young adults studied longitudinally from infancy. Examining multiple family risk factors over time, including maltreatment, only D and maternal disrupted communication at 18 months predicted left amygdala volume at 29 years. In addition, early attachment risk was further associated with dissociation and limbic irritability at age 29, and these relations were mediated by left amygdala volume. Thus, consistent with animal models, the quality of early care may have enduring influences on brain development. Other magnetic resonance imaging (MRI) and functional MRI (fMRI) studies to date have examined infant security and maternal sensitivity rather than D (for a review, see Pechtel, Murray, Brumariu, & Lyons-Ruth, 2013).

In the next decade we should see an explosion of studies examining how early care influences children's brain structure and function.

## Maternal Mind-Mindedness and Infant D

Meins and colleagues (2012) assessed mothers' mind-mindedness (MM) through maternal comments referring to infant mental states. They found that mothers of D infants did not differ from other mothers in attributing mental states to their infants. However, based on total comments, mothers of D infants made proportionally fewer *appropriate* mental state comments and proportionally more *nonattuned* mental state comments. Thus, mothers of D infants appear to think about their infants' mental states but in nonattuned ways.

## Randomized Interventions to Reduce D

The previous studies that relate parenting behavior to infant D are all correlational. Thus, they do not provide a strong basis for inferring causality. However, randomized controlled trials now provide strong evidence that D is amenable to change through interventions that focus on the mother–infant relationship (Bernard et al., 2012; Cicchetti, Rogosch, & Toth, 2006; Heinicke et al., 1999; Juffer, Bakermans-Kranenburg, & Van IJzendoorn, 2005; Moss, Bureau, St-Laurent, & Tarabulsy, 2011; Smyke et al., 2010; Tereno et al., 2014; Toth et al., 2006). These interventions have reduced the rate of D among dyads with a wide range of risk characteristics. However, despite the success of these programs, mechanisms contributing to change, such as changes in the caregiver's interactions with the child, have not been studied. Future randomized trials should address underlying mechanisms in order to advance our understanding of how parent-focused interventions prevent D.

# Disorganized/Controlling Attachment in Preschool and Middle Childhood

Main and Cassidy (1988), in a pioneering study of attachment beyond infancy, assessed 6-year-olds' behavioral and verbal responses to a reunion with the parent after an hour-long separation. They found that children could be classified into four categories that corresponded to the four infant attachment classifications, including secure-confident, insecure-avoidant, insecure-ambivalent, and insecure-controlling. Children were classified "insecure-controlling" if they "seem to actively attempt to control or direct the parent's attention and behavior and assume a role which is usually considered more appropriate for a parent with reference to a child" (p. 418).

## Age, Gender, and Stability of Disorganized/Controlling Attachment

Gender differences in the prevalence of D/controlling attachment were not found by meta-analysis (Van IJzendoorn et al., 1999; but see NICHD ECCRN, 2001). The effect size of the association between infant D and later D/controlling behavior has ranged from 20% (NICHD ECCRN, 2001) to 80% (Van IJzendoorn et al., 1999). However, the NICHD SECCYD assessed attachment behavior only up to age 3, so the lower stability in that study may reflect turbulence over the toddler period. Higher stability has been obtained when relating infant D to D/controlling behavior in the late preschool period. Finally, a sizable number of children who do not appear to have D in infancy begin to display controlling behaviors as preschoolers (Bureau, Easterbrooks, & Lyons-Ruth, 2009b; Main & Cassidy, 1988; NICHD ECCRN, 2001; Wartner, Grossmann, Fremmer-Bombik, & Suess, 1994).

Whether the child exhibits disorganized versus controlling forms of behavior also seems related to age. Moss, Cyr, Bureau, Tarabulsy, and Dubois-Comtois (2005) found that two-thirds of the young preschoolers classified as D/controlling displayed D behavior rather than controlling behavior. However, by age 6, two-thirds of the D/controlling group displayed controlling behavior. However, in high-risk samples, D behaviors continue to be observable through age 8 (Bureau et al., 2009b).

## D/Controlling Attachment and Cognitive Correlates

Bowlby (1969) posited that continued activation of the attachment system should inhibit exploration of the environment. Consistent with this formulation, Jacobsen, Edelstein, and Hofmann (1994) found that D/controlling children ($n$ = 6), assessed in middle childhood by the child's re-

sponses to a story task, differed significantly from other children in adolescence on tasks assessing syllogistic reasoning, even after they controlled for self-confidence, IQ, and attention problems. Moss and colleagues (1998; Moss & St-Laurent, 2001; Moss, St-Laurent, & Parent, 1999) found that despite the similarity in IQ between children with and without D, D/controlling children showed the poorest school performance in middle childhood. Moreover, D/controlling children demonstrated poorer math performance and difficulty becoming cognitively engaged in a problem-solving task. Finally, Stacks and Oshio (2009) found that preschoolers who produced disorganized narratives using George and Solomon's (2000) story completion task scored lower on assessments of school readiness than other children. This relation between D and less effective cognitive functioning has also been demonstrated in a Belgian cohort followed from ages 4 to 7 (Stievenart, Roskam, Meunier, & van de Moortele, 2011).

## D/Controlling Attachment and Parental Attachment Representations

Three studies have found an association between maternal U status on the AAI and D/controlling behavior in childhood (Behrens, Hesse, & Main, 2007; George & Solomon, 1996; Greenberg, Speltz, DeKlyen, & Endriga, 1991). In addition, George and Solomon (1996) developed a semistructured Experiences of Caregiving Interview that probes mothers' experiences of helplessness in the parenting role. A helpless stance could involve seeing the child in idealized terms as "larger than life" or could involve fear of the child and fear of one's own loss of control in relation to the child. Maternal helplessness was also associated with D/controlling behavior at age 6. Furthermore, Vulliez-Coady and colleagues (2013) found that maternal helplessness assessed in adolescence was associated with adolescent D/controlling behavior.

## D/Controlling Attachment and Children's Representations

D behavior is thought to occur because the infant experiences fear without solution. To evaluate this hypothesis, Main and colleagues (1985) examined children's depictions of self and caregiver on a doll-play story task, the Separation Anxiety Test. Children classified as D in infancy were more likely to give fearful and disorganized narratives (e.g., remaining silent, elaborating fearful or passive themes, or engaging in catastrophic fantasies). Solomon, George, and De Jong (1995) found that D/controlling kindergartners more often depicted themselves as helpless and their caregivers as frightening. Jacobsen and colleagues (1994) also found an association between D/controlling behavior and disorganized responses to cartoons depicting parent–child separation. Examining family drawings of 7-year-old, high-risk children, Madigan, Goldberg, Moran, and Pederson (2004) and Fihrer and McMahon (2009) did not replicate these findings. However, the high-risk nature of these samples may have affected the drawings of those who were *not* D. Thus, story stems may be more discriminating of D in low-risk samples.

## D/Controlling Attachment and Behavior Problems

### Externalizing Problems

A meta-analysis has indicated that children classified as D using infant, preschool, or school-age attachment assessments are more likely to display behavior problems ($N$ = 734; Van IJzendoorn et al., 1999). A more recent meta-analysis of 69 samples ($N$ = 5,947) confirmed those findings, indicating that children classified as D are at risk for externalizing problems ($d$ = 0.34), and this association is stronger than for other insecure classifications (avoidance: $d$ = 0.12; resistance: $d$ = 0.11; Fearon et al., 2010).

### Internalizing Problems and Dissociative Symptoms

Other meta-analyses have shown that attachment disorganization in infancy does not predict internalizing problems (Groh, Roisman, Van IJzendoorn, Bakermans-Kranenburg, & Fearon, 2012; Madigan, Atkinson, Laurin, & Benoit, 2013), with avoidant attachment more strongly related to internalizing symptoms. However, future studies are needed that differentiate between internalizing problems that are comorbid with externalizing problems and those that are not comorbid, as these likely occur in different groups. Comorbidity, in particular, has been associated with D/controlling behavior in preschool (Moss, Bureau, Cyr, Mongeau, & St-Laurent, 2004; Moss et al., 2004; O'Connor, Bureau, McCartney, &

Lyons-Ruth, 2011). In addition, Jacobvitz and colleagues (2011) found that maternal FR behavior at 8 months and/or FR/anomalous behavior at 24 months forecast depressive symptoms at age 7, as rated by teachers.

Dissociative symptoms in childhood, as reported by teachers, have also been investigated in relation to D. Carlson (1998) found that D in infancy predicted teacher reports of dissociation, internalizing behavior, and poorer overall emotional health in grades 1, 2, and 3. Smeekens, Riksen-Walraven, and van Bakel (2009) found that infants classified as D scored higher on teacher ratings of dissociation and externalizing behavior and lower on ego resiliency, peer social competence, and school adjustment at age 5. However, this relation between infant D and teacher-rated dissociation did not replicate in the large, low-risk NICHD sample (Haltigan & Roisman, 2014).

### Subtypes of D/Controlling Behavior in Relation to Behavior Problems

Meta-analyses have not yet evaluated whether there are differences in behavior problem profiles among the three D/controlling subgroups (*punitive, caregiving, behaviorally disorganized*). Moss and colleagues (2004), controlling for gender, IQ, and SES, found that controlling-punitive and behaviorally disorganized children, compared to secure children, were more likely to show externalizing behavior by age 8, whereas controlling-caregiving children were more likely to exhibit internalizing behavior. Parents of the three D/controlling subtypes also differed, with parents of caregiving children more likely to have experienced a loss, whereas parents of behaviorally disorganized children engaged in more marital conflicts (Moss et al., 2011). In the NICHD SECCYD data (O'Connor et al., 2011), behaviorally disorganized children at age 3 showed elevated rates of both internalizing and externalizing behavior, as well as poorer relationships with their teachers and peers, compared to other children. O'Connor and colleagues (2011) also found that mothers of behaviorally disorganized children had significantly worse partner relationships than did mothers of controlling-caregiving and controlling-punitive children. In addition, among 43 high-social-risk families, children higher in behavioral disorganization more often came from families who were referred for parenting help in infancy (Bureau et al., 2009b). Controlling-punitive behavior was associated with higher levels of maternal disrupted communication in infancy, whereas controlling-caregiving behavior was associated with greater maternal withdrawal in infancy.

## D/Controlling Attachment and the Development of Peer Relationships

Only a few studies have obtained ratings of friendship quality, either from trained observers or from peers. Wartner and colleagues (1994) found that 6-year-olds classified as D/controlling or avoidant were less competent in peer play and conflict resolution than were secure children. However, Cohn (1990) found that neither ratings of peer sociometric status nor peer nominations obtained from classmates differentiated D/controlling children from other children.

Jacobvitz and Hazen (1999), using case study data on 66 children ages 20–56 months, found that children classified as D in infancy more often engaged in fearful behavior and bizarre aggressive acts with peers, and more often acted very differently with different peers. They proposed that D children are more likely to carry unintegrated models of relationships into their interactions with others, so that they draw on different models with different peers. In two additional studies, D infants had poor peer relationships and greater difficulty adjusting to the stress induced by the school setting at age 5, as rated by teachers (Lyons-Ruth et al., 1997; Smeekens et al., 2009). Finally, McElwain, Booth-LaForce, and Wu (2011), using the SECCYD sample, found that children classified as D or avoidant in infancy experienced less maternal talk about mental states at age 2. Less mental state talk, in turn, mediated relations between D and poorer friendship quality at age 5. The authors suggested that restricted psychological discourse may hinder interactions with peers.

Very little is known about how D/controlling attachment relationships evolve from ages 8 to 18. An important agenda for future research will be to track the developmental pathways associated with these deviations in relation to the challenges associated with middle childhood and adolescence. In addition, we have very little understanding of the neurophysiological correlates of attachment strategies after infancy, even though the regulation of stressful arousal is at the heart of attachment theory. We need further studies of childhood attachment that incorporates biological markers.

In the final sections we review prediction of adolescent psychopathology from attachment in infancy and childhood, then conclude with studies of disorganized attachment in adolescence, assessed both with the AAI and with a new observational assessment of adolescent–parent attachment.

## Prospective Prediction of Psychopathology in Adolescence/Young Adulthood

### Dissociative Symptoms

Based on the lack of integration shared by D in infancy and dissociation in adulthood, Liotti (1992) proposed that D in infancy increases a child's vulnerability to later dissociative disorders. Several studies have now tested this hypothesis. In a longitudinal sample of 129 children, Ogawa, Sroufe, Weinfield, Carlson, and Egeland (1997; see also Carlson, 1998) found that mother's psychological unavailability and infant D in the first 2 years of life were the best predictors of scores on the Dissociative Experiences Scale (DES; Bernstein & Putnam, 1986) at age 19. Sexual or physical abuse did not predict dissociative symptoms on the DES after the quality of early caregiving was controlled. Only with regard to teacher-rated "dissociative" symptoms in elementary school did contemporaneous physical abuse explain additional unique variance. In a second longitudinal cohort (N = 56), Dutra, Bureau, Holmes, Lyubchik, and Lyons-Ruth (2009) also found that mother's disrupted communication, lack of positive involvement, and flatness of affect in infancy predicted dissociation on the DES at age 19, accounting for 50% of the variance in dissociation. Again, childhood abuse was a weaker predictor of dissociation than maternal behavior. Thus, in both prospective studies, quality of parent–infant interaction before age 2 was the strongest predictor of dissociative symptoms, stronger than either infant D or abuse experiences.

### Borderline Features and Suicidality

Two prospective studies have evaluated the contribution of early disorganized attachment relationships to features of BPD in adulthood (Carlson, Egeland, & Sroufe, 2009; Lyons-Ruth, Bureau, Holmes, Easterbrooks, & Brooks, 2013). Carlson and colleagues (2009) found that infant D predicted symptoms of BPD at age 28, but this relation was not significant when maternal hostility at 42 months and cumulative stress (3–42 months) were included in the model. However, the relation between infant D and BPD symptoms was mediated by children's self-representations at age 12. These self-representations were assessed by narratives designed to capture distortions in the organization of self–other relationships, such as feelings of guilt or fear, bizarre images related to the self, and/or references to violence related to the self.

Lyons-Ruth, Bureau, Holmes, and colleagues (2013) examined the interrelations between severity of childhood abuse and quality of attachment in predicting BPD features. Both abuse and attachment were significant predictors of BPD features at age 19, but maternal withdrawal on the AMBIANCE in infancy was the single most important predictor, accounting for unique variance in BPD features beyond the variance associated with abuse. D in infancy was not a predictor, but D/controlling attachment behavior in middle childhood also explained unique variance in BPD features. Taken together, the two studies suggest that mothers of 19-year-olds with elevated BPD symptoms may have been more withdrawn in infancy but became more hostile as the child moved into toddlerhood.

Lyons-Ruth, Bureau, Holmes, and colleagues (2013) also separately examined predictors of suicidality/self-injury at age 20. Maternal withdrawal in infancy again was the strongest predictor. In addition, suicidality was predicted by *D-secure* approach behavior toward mother in infancy. Neither *D-insecure* behavior in infancy nor D/controlling behavior in middle childhood predicted suicidality. Thus, suicidal young adults may have had a stronger propensity to seek proximity to the parent in infancy than did nonsuicidal young adults.

## APD and Substance Abuse

Shi, Bureau, Easterbrooks, Zhao, and Lyons-Ruth (2012) examined infancy and childhood predictors of APD among 56 low-income young adults. Childhood abuse, male gender, and maternal withdrawal in infancy all explained unique variance in APD features 20 years later. Infant D was not a predictor, but behavioral disorganization in middle childhood added to prediction of later antisocial features. Studies of antisocial behavior in the Minnesota Longitudinal Study did not include infant D in the models (Aguilar, Sroufe, Egeland, & Carlson, 2000; Siebenbruner, Englund, Egeland, & Hudson, 2006).

Pechtel, Woodman, and Lyons-Ruth (2012) examined predictors of substance abuse, which is often comorbid with both APD and BPD. Early maternal withdrawal forecast substance abuse in young adulthood, but only for those with a low nonverbal IQ in childhood.

## Depression and Anxiety

Two articles from the Minnesota Longitudinal Study have explored infancy, preschool, and school-age predictors of adolescent depressive or anxiety disorders but, again, D was not examined (Bosquet & Egeland, 2006; Duggal, Carlson, Sroufe, & Egeland, 2001). In the Harvard Longitudinal Study, mother's depressive symptoms in infancy, but not in childhood or young adulthood, were found to predict young adult depression (Bureau, Easterbrooks, & Lyons-Ruth, 2009a). Infant D did not add to the model.

In summary, the notable finding across all of the attachment–oriented prospective studies of maladaptation is that infant attachment behavior is an important predictor of some long-term outcomes, but more consistent and substantial prediction is obtained from maternal behavior (Belsky & Fearon, 2002; Dutra et al., 2009; Lyons-Ruth, Bureau, Holmes, et al., 2013; NICHD SECCYD, 2001; Shi et al., 2012; Sroufe, Egeland, Carlson, & Collins, 2005). This suggests that quality and consistency in parental care over time may account for continuities in children's development and underscores the need for additional focus on the deviations in parenting associated with a child's disorganization.

## Assessing D in Adolescence

### U States of Mind on the AAI in Adolescence

Assessment of attachment in infancy and childhood has primarily involved direct observation of parent–child interaction, but attachment assessments in adolescence and adulthood have relied mostly on the AAI. Also, the majority of adolescent AAI studies have examined organized patterns of attachment only (e.g., Kobak & Sceery, 1988; Waters, Merrick, Treboux, Crowell, & Albersheim, 2000). One exception is Allen, Hauser, and Borman-Spurrell's (1996) study of psychiatrically hospitalized adolescents and controls, studied from age 14. In that study, maternal behaviors promoting adolescent autonomy and relatedness at age 14 predicted coherence of transcript on the AAI 11 years later, but they did not predict AAI classifications, including U status.

Only two studies to date have examined continuity from infant disorganization to U/CC on the AAI in adolescence or adulthood (Main, Hesse, & Kaplan, 2005; Sroufe et al., 2005; Weinfield, Whaley, & Egeland, 2004). In a low-income sample, Weinfeld and colleagues found that D infants were more likely to be classified insecure at age 19 on the AAI but not as U/CC. In addition, at age 19, there was an atypical distribution of insecure AAI classifications, with 55% classified dismissing and only 15% as U despite the high-risk nature of the sample (Weinfield et al., 2004). By age 26, D infants were more likely to be classified as U (Sroufe et al., 2005). Main and colleagues (2005), in a low-risk sample, reported a trend-level relation between infant D and U classification at age 19, again with an unexpectedly high proportion of dismissing classifications.

## Observational Assessment of D in Adolescence

Given that adolescents who were disorganized in infancy may not be more likely to display U states on the AAI, the AAI may be limited as an index of disorganization in adolescence. This may occur because of coding constraints wherein individuals who do not report loss or abuse on the AAI cannot be judged U. One approach to this dilemma is to move away from a sole reliance on the AAI and include direct observational assessments of attachment in adolescence.

In the Minnesota Longitudinal Study, 175 mother–adolescent and 44 father–adolescent dyads were observed across a series of interaction and problem-solving tasks at age 13, but adolescent attachment scales/classifications were not specifically developed. Videotapes were rated on five scales: Engagement, Affect, Conflict, Conflict Resolution, Role/Boundary Maintenance, and Balance in the Relationship. Parent–child boundary dissolution at age 13 predicted change in behavior problems between grades 6 and 16 (Sroufe et al., 2005). Parental hostility at age 13 also discriminated heavy drinkers at age 16 (Englund, Hudson, & Egeland, 2003).

The Regensburg Longitudinal Study followed 96 families over time assessing adrenocortical responses during interactions between 12-year-olds and their mothers during a talk show task eliciting fear and a computer game eliciting anger. Increased cortisol levels were found only among adolescents classified as D in infancy, especially those adolescents showing fear (Spangler & Zimmermann, 2014).

In the Harvard Longitudinal Study, an important focus was to develop and validate an observational measure of attachment in adolescence. A secure base in adolescence has been conceptualized as a goal-corrected partnership, or sense of freedom to explore thoughts and feelings with a parent in a collaborative way (Allen et al., 1996; Kobak & Sceery, 1988). As with earlier attachment assessments, secure-base behavior during adolescence may become most salient during times of negotiation, conflict, and stress. Therefore, 104 low-income late adolescents (mean age 20 years) and their mothers were videotaped in a 5-minute unstructured reunion and a 10-minute discussion of an area of disagreement in their relationship. Videotapes were coded using the Goal-Corrected Partnership in Adolescence Coding System (GPACS; Lyons-Ruth, Hennighausen, et al., 2005), which includes 10 rating scales for organized and disorganized aspects of parent and adolescent behavior. A confirmatory factor analysis on the 10 scales yielded four dyadic factors: one factor for collaborative interaction and three factors for aspects of D/controlling behavior: disorientation, caregiving/role confusion, and punitive behavior (Obsuth et al., 2014). Structural models specifying only two factors (collaborative/disorganized) resulted in a significantly poorer fit to the data. Thus, the first important finding was that there were several empirically distinct dimensions underlying disorganized behavior in adolescence.

Each of the three disorganized factors was associated with distinct validating measures (Obsuth et al., 2014). As in infancy and childhood, disorientation in interaction was characterized by odd, out-of-context behavior (e.g., suddenly freezing with arms up during interaction with mother) and was significantly related to D behavior in infancy. For each 1-point increase in the factor score for adolescent disoriented interaction, the participant was 50% more likely to have been D in infancy in interaction with the same parent. In addition, disorientation was associated with U/CC classification but not HH classification on the adolescent's AAI. These findings provide construct validity for disorientation as a behavioral measure of D. Disorientation was also associated with poor quality romantic relationships, but not with partner abuse, suggesting a more distant relational stance. Finally, disorientation was robustly associated with concurrent dissociative symptoms. Notably, disorientation was not related to overall psychiatric morbidity, confirming that odd, out-of-context behavior with the parent is not simply the by-product of severe psychopathology.

Punitive and caregiving/role-confused interactions also had distinct correlates. Caregiving/role-confused adolescents reported providing more emotional and instrumental support to the parent, and mothers of caregiving adolescents were independently rated as more role confused on the Experiences of Caregiving Interview (ECI; Obsuth et al., 2014; Vulliez-Coady et al., 2013). Both punitive and caregiving/role-confused interactions were associated with maternal reports of helplessness on the Caregiving Helplessness Questionnaire (CHQ; George & Solomon, 2011) and with poor quality romantic relationships that included abuse to and from the partner. However, only punitive interactions were related to the adolescent's HH classification, but not U/CC classification, on the AAI.

Caregiving/role-confused interactions were not related to adolescent AAI classifications, so states of mind associated with caregiving behavior remain elusive. However, as noted earlier, *mothers* who were more role confused on the ECI interview were more likely to be classified U-loss on the AAI (Vulliez-Coady et al., 2013), suggesting that work exploring links between caregiving/role confusion, loss, and U-loss on the AAI would be fruitful.

A second validity study used GPACS attachment *classifications* rather than factor scores on a sample of 40 psychiatrically hospitalized and nonhospitalized adolescents and their families from the larger study of Allen and colleagues (1996). Significant four-way correspondence (73%, $\kappa$ = .51) was obtained between GPACS classifications at age 14 during a conflict discussion (facilitating, deflecting, entangled, and disorganized/controlling), and the corresponding AAI classifications at age 25 (autonomous, dismissing, preoccupied, and U/CC) (Hennighausen, Bureau, David, & Lyons-Ruth, 2011).

Finally, studies using the GPACS further underscore the importance of the quality of adolescent–parent interaction in pathways to disturbed functioning. All three aspects of disorganization in adolescence were associated with increased adolescent depressive and dissociative symptoms, and both punitive and caregiving/role-confused aspects were also associated with overall psychiatric morbidity on DSM-IV-R Axis I (Obsuth et al., 2014). Furthermore, Lyons-Ruth, Brumariu, Bureau, Hennighausen, and Holmes (2015) found that role confusion and disorientation in adolescent–parent interactions accounted for unique variance in both borderline features and recurrent suicidality/self-injury, beyond the contribution of childhood abuse. Brumariu and colleagues (2013) found that disorientation was also elevated among adolescents with anxiety disorders, which are often comorbid with BPD. Finally, studying 166 low-income adolescents, Kobak, Zajac, and Rosenthal (2014) found that caregiving/role-confused interactions at age 13 on the GPACS predicted increases in impulsive self-damaging behavior by age 15 among girls, including substance abuse and risky sexual behavior. In summary, the GPACS breaks new ground in differentiating disoriented and role-confused aspects of behavior in adolescence from the more typically studied hostile/punitive interactions and links all three disturbed interaction patterns to impairment in key developmental outcomes.

## Future Directions

We are now approaching the third decade of work on disorganized forms of attachment. The accumulated studies, including several meta-analyses of the literature, make clear that D relationships are associated with both current and future functional impairment, including impaired peer relations, poor adaptation to school, and child psychopathology. Thus, this work has several important implications for future research and policy.

First, our new understanding of epigenetics is creating a paradigm shift in the fields of genetics and development, which pushes work on D to the forefront of current science. Randomized rodent and primate studies have identified deviations in caregiving as one causal agent for change in the expression of numerous genes in early development (e.g., Meaney & Szyf, 2005; see Bakermans-Kranenburg & Van IJzendoorn, Chapter 8, this volume). Given these findings in other species, disturbed caregiving in humans may also contribute to changes in gene expression in the human infant.

It has become popular to frame neurobiological differences associated with psychopathology as the "underlying mechanisms" or potential root causes of behavioral disturbances. However, the "underlying" causal contributors may be hiding in plain sight in the form of repetitive patterns of child–caregiver interaction that shape the expression of genes and mold responses to stress and fearful arousal. There are relatively few bodies of work that identify tipping points for what constitutes disturbed care in human infancy. State-documented abuse or neglect or multiple changes of caregiver in institutional or foster settings are among the few widely substantiated indicators of disturbed care, but these are quite extreme deviations and rely on secondary indicators of quality of care. The extensive body of work on D is one of the few literatures to identify and validate the boundaries between adequate care and disturbances in caregiving based on direct observation of the quality of parent–child interaction.

Thus, in the next decade, the clinical applications of the body of work on D need to be more fully explored. As reviewed here, there is now an impressive array of evidence on the reliability of both infant and maternal disorganized/disrupted classifications, as well as on their construct and discriminant validity in relation to other measures of attachment quality, maltreatment, and dysregulation of the infant hypothalamic–pituitary–adrenal (HPA) axis. Most importantly, there is now overwhelming evidence of predictive validity in relation to later functional impairment and psychopathology. The empirical support for the morbidity associated with disorganized attachment is at least as strong, if not stronger, than the evidence base for many child psychiatric disorders now listed in DSM-5, especially those that are evident in infancy and early childhood. Thus, D is likely to be an important contributor to public health costs in the form of outpatient and inpatient mental health care, special education, delinquency, and emergency room treatment.

Second, current National Institutes of Health (NIH) research priorities call for a focus on the broad underlying processes or vulnerability factors that predispose to psychiatric morbidity and are likely to cut across diagnostic categories. We have long known that family factors contribute risk across the spectrum of psychiatric disturbance, including schizophrenia, bipolar disorder, and depression, as well as the pervasive personality disorders. As very recent work now indicates, gene variants that contribute to a variety of serious psychiatric diagnoses are also particularly open to epigenetic modifications by the environment (Cross-Disorder Group of the Psychiatric Genomics Consortium, 2013). Thus, if caregiving affects

gene expression in humans, as well as other species, it would not be surprising if the influence of the caregiving environment cuts across conventional diagnostic categories and affects a broad range of psychiatric morbidity.

Third, in accord with the NIH emphasis on examining broad underlying processes that are prominent in the pathways to a number of disorders, the next decade should focus on how caregiver–infant interaction shapes the maternal and infant neurobiology associated with these disorganized relationships. We know relatively little about the infant stress response system and how it is affected by serious deviations in care. The still sparse literature on HPA axis function in infancy focuses most strongly on infant responses in normative environments. There are a few additional studies on infants in extremely adverse environments, such as foster care, but a coherent picture of the environments that produce either HPA hyperresponsivity or HPA hyporesponsivity has yet to be fleshed out. In addition, we have virtually no literature on structural and functional neurobiological concomitants of these infant adaptations. Such data are critical to developing biological indicators that can facilitate early identification and intervention in these disturbed pathways. As we approach a more truly developmental understanding of pathways to adult, as well as childhood, disorders, we will need to incorporate an increasingly sophisticated view of how early stressors and inadequate environmental buffering may alter subsequent neurophysiology.

Finally, although the neurobiological data are of great importance, we do not need to wait for these data to develop and validate a clinically useful set of evidence-based indicators of disorganized/disordered attachment in infancy. Given the 15% incidence of D in normative samples, it will be important to narrow the current research criteria for D to include only the forms to be considered disordered. These criteria should be more selective than current research criteria, perhaps by focusing only on children who display the more extreme forms of disorganized behavior, as represented by the higher ratings on the 9-point scale for extent of disorganization. Different cutpoints and different types of disorganization need to be validated in relation to current environmental risk and to later functional impairment.

Importantly, the past three decades of work also underscore that D behavior is associated with deviations in care, and that indications for disorder should include parental, as well as child, behaviors. Indeed, there is a long-established historical precedent for including the caregiving environment in DSM and ICD criteria, as seen in the criteria for RAD and DSED, both of which specify a deviant caregiving environment as a criterion for diagnosis. The development of such criteria, combined with existing work on RAD and DSED, would give us an emerging scientific basis for early assessment and diagnosis of the spectrum of attachment disorders that present to clinical parent–infant services. Given the considerable childhood and young adult morbidity associated with D and disturbed parenting, it is now a priority to move this work into clinical application.

# References

Abrams, K., Rifkin, A., & Hesse, E. (2006). Examining the role of parental frightened/frightening subtypes in predicting disorganized attachment within a brief observational procedure. *Development and Psychopathology, 18,* 344–362.

Aguilar, B., Sroufe, L. A., Egeland, B., & Carlson, E. (2000). Distinguishing the early-onset/persistent and adolescent-onset antisocial behavior types: From birth to 16 years. *Development and Psychopathology, 12,* 109–132.

Ainsworth, M. D. S., Blehar, M., Waters, E., & Wall, S. (1978). *Patterns of attachment.* Hillsdale, NJ: Erlbaum.

Ainsworth, M. D. S., & Eichberg, C. G. (1991). Effects on infant–mother attachment of mother's unresolved loss of an attachment figure or other traumatic experience. In C. M. Parkes, J. Stevenson-Hinde, & P. Marris (Eds.), *Attachment across the life cycle* (pp. 160–183). London: Routledge.

Allen, J., Hauser, S., & Borman-Spurrell E. (1996). Attachment theory as a framework for understanding sequelae of severe adolescent psychopathology: An 11-year follow-up study. *Journal of Consulting and Clinical Psychology, 64,* 254–263.

American Psychiatric Association. (2013). *Diagnostic and statistical manual of mental disorders* (5th ed.). Arlington, VA: Author.

Bailey, H., Moran, G., & Pederson, D. (2007). Childhood maltreatment, complex trauma symptoms, and unresolved attachment in an at-risk sample of adolescent mothers. *Attachment and Human Development, 9,* 139–161.

Bakermans-Kranenburg, M., & Van IJzendoorn, M. (2009). The first 10,000 adult attachment interviews: Distributions of adult attachment representations in clinical and non-clinical groups. *Attachment and Human Development, 11*(3), 223–263.

Ballen, N., Bernier, A., Moss, E., Tarabulsy, G., & St-Laurent, D. (2010). Insecure attachment states of mind and atypical caregiving behavior among foster mothers. *Journal of Applied Developmental Psychology, 31,* 118–125.

Barel, E., Van IJzendoorn, M., Sagi-Schwartz, A., & Bakermans-Kranenburg, M. (2010). Surviving the Holocaust: A meta-analysis of the long-term sequelae of genocide. *Psychological Bulletin, 5,* 677–698.

Barker, D. (1998). *In utero* programming of chronic disease. *Clinical Science, 95,* 115–128.

Barone, L., Bramante, A., Lionettia, F., & Pastore, M. (2014). Mothers who murdered their child: An attachment-based study on filicide. *Child Abuse and Neglect, 38*(9), 1468–1477.

Beebe, B., Jaffe, J., Markese, S., Buck, K., Chen, H., Cohen, P., et al. (2010). The origins of 12-month attachment: A microanalysis of 4-month mother-infant interaction. *Attachment and Human Development, 12,* 3–141.

Behrens, K., Hesse, E., & Main, M. (2007). Mothers' attachment status as determined by the Adult Attachment Interview predicts their 6-year-olds' reunion responses: A study conducted in Japan. *Developmental Psychology, 43,* 1553–1567.

Belsky, J., & Fearon, R. (2002). Early attachment security, subsequent maternal sensitivity, and later child development: Does continuity in development depend upon continuity of caregiving? *Attachment and Human Development, 3,* 361–387.

Bergman, K., Sarkar, P., Glover, V., & O'Connor, T. (2008). Quality of child–parent attachment moderates the impact of antenatal stress on child fearfulness. *Journal of Child Psychology and Psychiatry, 49,* 1089–1098.

Bergman, K., Sarkar, P., Glover, V., & O'Connor, T. (2010). Maternal prenatal cortisol and infant cognitive development: moderation by infant–mother attachment. *Biological Psychiatry, 67,* 1026–1032.

Bernard, K., & Dozier, M. (2010). Examining infants' cortisol responses to laboratory tasks among children varying in attachment disorganization: Stress reactivity or return to baseline? *Developmental Psychology, 46,* 1771–1778.

Bernard, K., Dozier, M., Bick, J., Lewis-Morrarty, E., Lindhiem, O., & Carlson, E. (2012). Enhancing attachment organization among maltreated children: Results of a randomized clinical trial. *Child Development, 83,* 623–636.

Bernier, A., & Meins, E. (2008). A threshold approach to understanding the origins of attachment disorganization. *Developmental Psychology, 44,* 969–982.

Bernstein, E., & Putnam, F. (1986). Development, reliability, and validity of a dissociation scale. *Journal of Nervous and Mental Disease, 174,* 1769–1782.

Bokhorst, C., Bakermans-Kranenburg, M., Fearon, R., Van IJzendoorn, M., Fonagy, P., & Schuengel, C. (2003). The importance of shared environment in mother–infant attachment security: A behavioral genetic study. *Child Development, 74,* 1769–1782.

Bosquet, M., & Egeland, B. (2006). The development

and maintenance of anxiety symptoms from infancy through adolescence in a longitudinal sample. *Development and Psychopathology, 18*, 517–550.

Bowlby, J. (1969). *Attachment and loss: Vol. 1. Attachment.* New York: Basic Books.

Bowlby, J. (1973). *Attachment and loss: Vol. 2. Separation: Anxiety and anger.* New York: Basic Books.

Bronfman, E., Madigan, S., & Lyons-Ruth, K. (2007). *Atypical maternal behavior instrument for assessment and classification (AMBIANCE): Manual for coding disrupted affective communication: Version 2.0.* Unpublished manuscript, Harvard Medical School, Cambridge, MA.

Bronfman, E., Parsons, E., & Lyons-Ruth, K. (1992). *Atypical maternal behavior instrument for assessment and classification (AMBIANCE): Manual for coding disrupted affective communication: Version 1.0.* Unpublished manuscript, Harvard Medical School, Cambridge, MA.

Brumariu, L., Obsuth, I., & Lyons-Ruth, K. (2013). Quality of attachment relationships and peer relationship dysfunction among late adolescents with and without anxiety disorders. *Journal of Anxiety Disorders, 27*,116–124.

Buchheim, A., Erk, S., George, C., Kächele, H., Kirchele, H., Martius, P., et al. (2006). Neural correlates of attachment trauma in borderline personality disorder: a functional magnetic resonance imaging study. *Psychiatry Research, 163*(3), 223–235.

Buchheim, A., Erk, S., George, C., Kächele, H., Ruchsow, M., Spitzer, M., et al. (2008). Measuring attachment representation in an fMRI environment: A pilot study. *Psychopathology, 39*(3), 136–143.

Bureau, J.-F., Easterbrooks, M. A., & Lyons-Ruth, K. (2009a). Maternal depressive symptoms in infancy: Unique contribution to children's depressive symptoms in childhood and adolescence? *Development and Psychopathology, 21*, 519–537.

Bureau, J.-F., Easterbrooks, M. A., & Lyons-Ruth, K. (2009b). Attachment disorganization and role-reversal in middle childhood: Maternal and child precursors and correlates. *Attachment and Human Development, 11*, 265–284.

Byun, S., Brumariu, L., & Lyons-Ruth, K. (in press). Disorganized attachment in adolescence: Does it mediate the relation between severity of childhood abuse and dissociation? *Journal of Trauma and Dissociation.*

Canli, T., & Lesch, K. (2007). Long story short: Serotonin transporter in emotion regulation and social cognition. *Nature Neuroscience, 10*, 1103–1109.

Carlson, E. A. (1998). A prospective longitudinal study of attachment disorganization/disorientation. *Child Development, 69*, 1107–1128.

Carlson, E. A., Egeland, B., & Sroufe, L. A. (2009). A prospective investigation of the development of borderline personality symptoms. *Development and Psychopathology, 21*, 1311–1334.

Cicchetti, D., Rogosch, F., & Toth, S. (2006). Fostering secure attachment in infants in maltreating families through preventative interventions. *Development and Psychopathology, 18*, 623–649.

Cicchetti, D., Rogosch, F., & Toth, S. (2011). The effects of child maltreatment and polymorphisms of the serotonin transporter and dopamine D4 receptor genes on infant attachment and intervention efficacy. *Development and Psychopathology, 23*, 357–372.

Cohn, D. (1990). Child–mother attachment of six-year-olds and social competence at school. *Child Development, 61*,152–162.

Crawford, A., & Benoit, D. (2009). Caregivers' disrupted representations of the unborn child predict later infant–caregiver disorganized attachment and disrupted interactions. *Infant Mental Health Journal, 30*, 124–144.

Crockett, E., Holmes, B., Granger, D., & Lyons-Ruth, K. (2013). Maternal disrupted communication during face-to-face interaction at four months: Relation to maternal and infant cortisol among at-risk families. *Infancy, 18*, 1111–1134.

Cross-Disorder Group of the Psychiatric Genomics Consortium. (2013). Identification of risk loci with shared effects on five major psychiatric disorders: A genome-wide analysis. *Lancet, 381*, 1371–1379.

Cyr, C., Euser, E. M., Bakermans-Kranenburg, M., & Van IJzendoorn, M. (2010). Attachment security and disorganization in maltreating and high-risk families: A series of meta-analyses. *Development and Psychopathology, 22*(1), 87–108.

David, D., & Lyons-Ruth, K. (2005). Differential attachment responses of male and female infants to frightening maternal behavior: Tend or befriend versus fight or flight? *Infant Mental Health Journal, 26*, 1–18.

Del Cerro, M., Perez-Laso, C., Ortega, E., Martin, J., Gomez, F., Perez-Izquierdo, M., et al. (2010). Maternal care counteracts behavioral effects of prenatal environmental stress in female rats. *Behavioural Brain Research, 208*, 593–602.

Dozier, M., Manni, M., Gordon, M., Peloso, E., Gunnar, M., Stovall-McClough, K., et al. (2006). Foster children's diurnal production of cortisol: An exploratory study. *Child Maltreatment, 2*, 189–197.

Duggal, S., Carlson, E. A., Sroufe, L. A., & Egeland, B. (2001). Depressive symptomatology in childhood and adolescence. *Development and Psychopathology, 13*, 143–164.

Dutra, L., Bureau, J.-F., Holmes, B., Lyubchik, A., & Lyons-Ruth, K. (2009). Quality of early care and childhood trauma: A prospective study of developmental pathways to dissociation. *Journal of Nervous and Mental Disease, 197*, 383–390.

Englund, M., Hudson, K., & Egeland, B. (2003, April). *Common pathways to heavy alcohol use and abstinence in adolescence.* Paper presented at the annual meeting of the Society for Research in Child Development, Tampa, FL.

Fearon, R. M. P., Bakermans-Kranenburg, M. J., Van IJzendoorn, M. H., Lapsley, A., & Roisman, G. I.

(2010). The significance of insecure attachment and disorganization in the development of children's externalizing behavior: A meta-analytic study. *Child Development, 81*, 435–456.

Fihrer, I., & McMahon, C. (2009). Maternal state of mind regarding attachment, maternal depression and children's family drawings in the early school years. *Attachment and Human Development, 11*, 537–556.

Finger, B., Byun, S., Melnick, S., & Lyons-Ruth, K. (2015). Hostile–helpless states of mind mediate relations between childhood abuse severity and personality disorder features. *Translational Developmental Psychiatry, 3*, 28785.

Fonagy, P., Leigh, T., Steele, M., Steele, H., Kennedy, G., Mattoon, M., et al. (1996). The relation of attachment status, psychiatric classification, and response to psychotherapy. *Journal of Consulting and Clinical Psychology, 64*, 22–31.

Forbes, L. M., Evans, E. M., Moran, G., & Pederson, D. R. (2007). Change in atypical maternal behavior predicts change in attachment disorganization from 12 to 24 months in a high-risk sample. *Child Development 78*, 955–971.

Frigerio, A., Costantino, E., Ceppi, E., & Barone, L. (2013). Adult attachment interviews of women from low-risk, poverty, and maltreatment risk samples: Comparisons between the hostile/helpless and traditional AAI coding systems. *Attachment and Human Development, 4*, 424–442.

George, C., & Solomon, J. (1996). Representational models of relationships: Links between caregiving and attachment. *Infant Mental Health Journal, 17*, 198–216.

George, C., & Solomon, J. (2000). *Six-year attachment doll play classification system.* Unpublished classification manual, Mills College, Oakland, CA.

George, C., & Solomon, J. (2011). Caregiving helplessness: The development of a screening measure for disorganized maternal caregiving. In J. Solomon & C. George (Eds.), *Disorganized attachment and caregiving* (pp. 133–166). Guilford Press.

Gervai, J., Novak, A., Lakatos, K., Toth, I., Danis, I., Ronai, Z., et al. (2007). Infant genotype may moderate sensitivity to maternal affective communications: Attachment disorganization, quality of care, and the DRD4 polymorphism. *Social Neuroscience, 2*, 1–13.

Gleason, M. M., Fox, N. A., Drury, S. S., Smyke, A. T., Nelson, C. A., III, & Zeanah, C. H. (2014). Indiscriminate behaviors in previously institutionalized young children. *Pediatrics, 133*(3), 657–665.

Greenberg, M. T., Speltz, M. L., DeKlyen, M., & Endriga, M. C. (1991). Attachment security in preschoolers with and without externalizing behavior problems: A replication. *Development and Psychopathology, 3*, 413–430.

Groh, A. M., Roisman, G. I., Van IJzendoorn, M. H., Bakermans-Kranenburg, M. J., & Fearon, R. P. (2012). The significance of insecure and disorganized attachment for children's internalizing symptoms:

A meta-analytic study. *Child Development, 83*(2), 591–610.

Haltigan, J., & Roisman, G. (2014). *Infant attachment insecurity and dissociative symptomatology: Findings from the NICHD Study of Early Child Care and Youth Development.* Manuscript under review.

Harari, D., Bakermans-Kranenburg, M. J., de Kloet, C. S., Geuze, E., Vermetten, E., Westenberg, H. G. M., et al. (2009). Attachment representations in Dutch veterans with and without deployment-related PTSD. *Attachment and Human Development, 6*, 515–536.

Hay, A. M., Jacobson, S. W., Molteno, C. D., Viljoen, D., & Jacobson, J. L. (2004). Alcohol exposure and infant–mother attachment in a South-African community. *Alcoholism: Clinical and Experimental Research, 28*(Suppl. 5), 45A.

Hazen, N., Allen, S., Umemura, T., Heaton, C., & Jacobvitz, D. (2015). Very extensive non-maternal care predicts mother-infant attachment disorganization: Convergent evidence from two samples. *Development and Psychopathology, 27*(3), 649–661.

Hazen, N., McFarland, L. Jacobvitz, D., & Boyd-Soisson, E. (2010). Fathers' frightening behaviors and sensitivity with infants: Relations with fathers' attachment representations, father–infant attachment, and children's later outcomes. *Early Child Development and Care, 180*, 51–69.

Heinicke, C. M., Fineman, N. R., Ruth, G., Recchia, S. L., Guthrie, D., & Rodning, C. (1999). Relationship-based intervention with at-risk mothers: Outcome in the first year of life. *Infant Mental Health Journal, 20*, 349–374.

Hennighausen, K., Bureau, J.-F., David, D. H., & Lyons-Ruth, K. (2011). Disorganized attachment in adolescence: Validation in relation to Adult Attachment Interview classifications at age 25. In J. Solomon & C. George (Eds.), *Disorganized attachment and caregiving* (pp. 207–244). New York: Guilford Press.

Hertsgaard, L. Gunnar, M., Erickson, M. F., & Nachmias, M. (1995). Adrenocortical response to the Strange Situation in infants with disorganized/disoriented attachment relationships. *Child Development, 66*, 1100–1106.

Hesse, E. (1996). Discourse, memory, and the Adult Attachment Interview: A note with emphasis on the emerging cannot classify category. *Infant Mental Health Journal, 17*, 4–11.

Hesse, E., Hobson, P., Patrick, M., Maughan, B., & Main, M. (2011, March). *The AAI in a prison population: High scores for unresolved loss in psychopaths while derogation predicts murder and bodily harm.* Paper presented at the biennial meeting of the Society for Research in Child Development, Seattle, WA.

Hesse, E., & Main, M. (2006). Frightened, threatening, and dissociative parental behavior in low-risk samples: Description, discussion, and interpretations. *Development and Psychopathology, 18*, 309–343.

Hesse, E., & Van IJzendoorn, M. (1999). Propensities towards absorption are related to lapses in the monitoring of reasoning or discourse during the Adult Attachment Interview: A preliminary investigation. *Attachment and Human Development, 1*, 67–91.

Hobson, R. P., Patrick, M., Crandell, L., García-Pérez, R., & Lee, A. (2005). Personal relatedness and attachment in infants of mothers with borderline personality disorder. *Development and Psychopathology, 17*, 329–347.

Insel, T. (2003). Is social attachment an addictive disorder? *Physiology and Behavior, 79*, 351–357.

Ivarsson, T., Granqvist, P., Gillberg, C., Anders, G., & Broberg, A. (2010). Attachment states of mind in adolescents with obsessive–compulsive disorder and/or depressive disorders: A controlled study. *European Child and Adolescent Psychiatry, 19*, 845–853.

Jacobsen, T., Edelstein, W., & Hofmann, V. (1994). A longitudinal study of the relation between representations of attachment in childhood and cognitive functioning in childhood and adolescence. *Developmental Psychology, 30*, 112–124.

Jacobvitz, D., & Hazen, N. (1999). Developmental pathways from infant disorganization to childhood peer relationships. In J. Solomon & C. George (Eds.), *Attachment disorganization* (pp. 127–159). New York: Guilford Press.

Jacobvitz, D., Hazen, N., Zaccagnino, M., Messina, S., & Beverung, L. (2011). Frightening maternal behavior, infant disorganization, and risks for psychopathology. In D. Cicchetti & G. Roisman (Eds.), *The Minnesota Symposium on Child Psychology: The origins and organization of adaptation and maladaptation* (Vol. 36, pp. 283–322). New York: Wiley.

Jacobvitz, D., Leon, K., & Hazen, N. (2006). Does expectant mothers' unresolved trauma predict frightening/frightened maternal behavior?: Risk and protective factors. *Development and Psychopathology, 18*, 363–379.

Jaffe, J., Beebe, B., Feldstein, S., Crown, C., & Jasnow, M. (2001). Rhythms of dialogue in infancy: Coordinated timing in development. *Monographs of the Society for Research in Child Development, 66*, 1–149.

Juffer, F., Bakermans-Kranenburg, M., & Van IJzendoorn, M. (2005). The importance of parenting in the development of disorganized attachment: Evidence from a preventive intervention study in adoptive families. *Journal of Child Psychology and Psychiatry, 46*, 263–274.

Kobak, R. R., & Sceery, A. (1988). Attachment in late adolescence: Working models, affect regulation and representations of self and others. *Child Development, 59*, 135–146.

Kobak, R. R., Zajac, K., & Rosenthal, N. (2014). *Adolescent–caregiver attachment: Adaptation and risk in an economically disadvantaged sample.* Manuscript submitted for publication.

Lakatos, K., Nemoda, Z., Toth, I., Ronai, Z., Ney, K., Sasvari-Szekely, M., et al. (2002). Further evidence for the role of the dopamine D4 receptor gene (*DRD4*) in attachment disorganization: Interaction of the III exon 48 bp repeat and the –521 C/T promoter polymorphisms. *Molecular Psychiatry, 7*, 27–31.

Lakatos, K., Toth, I., Nemoda, Z., Ney, K., Sasvari-Szekely, M., & Gervai, J. (2000). Dopamine D4 receptor (*DRD4*) gene polymorphism is associated with attachment disorganization. *Molecular Psychiatry, 5*, 633–637.

Levine, S., Wiener, S., & Coe, C. L. (1993). Temporal and social factors influencing behavioral and hormonal responses to separation in mother and infant squirrel monkeys. *Psychoneuroendocrinology, 18*, 297–306.

Liotti, G. (1992). Disorganized/disoriented attachment in the etiology of the dissociative disorders. *Dissociation, 5*, 196–204.

Luijk, M., Roisman, G.,Haltigan, J., Tiemeier, H., Booth-LaForce, C., Van IJzendoorn, M., et al. (2011). Dopaminergic, serotonergic, and oxytonergic candidate genes associated with infant attachment security and disorganization?: In search of main and interaction effects. *Journal of Child Psychology and Psychiatry, 52*, 1295–1307.

Luijk, M. P., Saridjan, N., Tharner, A., Van IJzendoorn, M. H., Bakermans-Kranenburg, M. J., Jaddoe,V. W., et al. (2010). Attachment, depression, and cortisol: Deviant patterns in insecure-resistant and disorganized infants. *Developmental Psychobiology, 52*(5), 441–452.

Lyons-Ruth, K., Alpern, L., & Repacholi, B. (1993). Disorganized infant attachment classification and maternal psychosocial problems as predictors of hostile-aggressive behavior in the preschool classroom. *Child Development, 64*, 572–585.

Lyons-Ruth, K., Bronfman, E., & Atwood, G. (1999). A relational diathesis model of hostile-helpless states of mind: Expressions in mother–infant interaction. In J. Solomon & C. George (Eds.), *Attachment disorganization* (pp. 33–69). New York: Guilford Press.

Lyons-Ruth, K., Bronfman, E., & Parsons, E. (1999). Maternal disrupted affective communication, maternal frightened, frightening, or atypical behavior, and disorganized infant attachment strategies. In J. Vondra & D. Barnett (Eds.), Atypical patterns of infant attachment: Theory, research, and current directions. *Monographs of the Society for Research in Child Development, 64*, 67–96.

Lyons-Ruth, K., Brumariu, L., Bureau, J., Hennighausen, K., & Holmes, B. (2015). Role confusion and disorientation in young adult–parent interaction among individuals with borderline symptomatology. *Journal of Personality Disorders, 29*(5), 641–662.

Lyons-Ruth, K., Bureau, J.-F., Easterbrooks, A., Obsuth, I., & Hennighausen, K. (2013). Parsing the construct of maternal insensitivity: Distinct longitudinal pathways associated with early maternal withdrawal. *Attachment and Human Development, 15*, 562–582.

Lyons-Ruth, K., Bureau, J.-F., Holmes, B., Easterbrooks, A., & Brooks, N. (2013). Borderline symptoms and suicidality/self-injury in late adolescence: Prospectively observed relationship correlates in infancy and childhood. *Psychiatry Research, 206,* 273–281.

Lyons-Ruth, K., Bureau, J.-F., Riley, C., Atlas-Corbett, A. (2009). Socially indiscriminate attachment behavior in the Strange Situation: Convergent and discriminant validity in relation to caregiving risk, later behavior problems, and attachment insecurity. *Development and Psychopathology, 21,* 355–372.

Lyons-Ruth, K., Connell, D., Zoll, D., & Stahl, J. (1987). Infants at social risk: Relations among infant maltreatment, maternal behavior, and infant attachment behavior. *Developmental Psychology, 23,* 223–232.

Lyons-Ruth, K., Easterbrooks, M., & Cibelli, C. (1997) Disorganized attachment strategies and mental lag in infancy: Prediction of externalizing problems at age seven. *Developmental Psychology, 33,* 681–692.

Lyons-Ruth, K., Hennighausen, K., & Holmes, B. (2005). *Goal-corrected partnership in adolescence coding system (GPACS): Coding manual. Version 2.* Unpublished document. Department of Psychiatry, Harvard Medical School. Cambridge, MA.

Lyons-Ruth, K., Pechtel, P., Yoon, S., Anderson, C., & Teicher, M. (2014). *Infant disorganized attachment and maternal disrupted communication: Relations to left amygdala volume in adulthood.* Manuscript submitted for publication.

Lyons-Ruth, K., Yellin, C., Melnick, S., & Atwood, G. (2005). Expanding the concept of unresolved mental states: Hostile/helpless states of mind on the adult attachment interview are associated with atypical maternal behavior and infant disorganization. *Development and Psychopathology, 17,* 1–23.

Macfie, J., Fitzpatrick, K., Rivas, E., Cox, M. (2008). Independent influences upon mother–toddler role reversal: Infant–mother attachment disorganization and role reversal in mother's childhood. *Attachment and Human Development, 10,* 29–39.

Madigan, S., Atkinson, L., Laurin, K., & Benoit, D. (2013). Attachment and internalizing behavior in early childhood: A meta-analysis. *Developmental Psychology, 49,* 672–689.

Madigan, S., Bakermans-Kranenburg, M. J., Van IJzendoorn, M., Moran, G., Pederson, D., & Benoit, D. (2006). Unresolved states of mind, anomalous parental behavior, and disorganized attachment: A review and meta-analysis of a transmission gap. *Attachment and Human Development, 8,* 89–111.

Madigan, S., Benoit, D., & Boucher, C. (2011).Exploration of the links among fathers' unresolved states of mind with respect to attachment, atypical paternal behavior, and disorganized infant–father attachment. *Infant Mental Health Journal, 3,* 286–304.

Madigan, S., Goldberg, S., Moran, G., & Pederson, D. (2004). Naïve observers' perceptions of family drawings by 7-year-olds with disorganized attachment histories. *Attachment and Human Development, 6,* 223–239.

Madigan, S., Moran, G., Schuengel, C., Pederson, D., & Otten, R. (2007). Unresolved maternal attachment representations, disrupted maternal behavior and disorganized attachment in infancy: Links to toddler behavior problems. *Journal of Child Psychology and Psychiatry, 48,* 1042–1050.

Main, M., & Cassidy, J. (1988). Categories of response to reunion with the parent at age 6: Predicted from infant attachment classifications and stable over a 1-month period. *Developmental Psychology, 24,* 415–426.

Main, M., Goldwyn, R., & Hesse, E. (2003). *Adult attachment scoring and classification system.* Unpublished manuscript, University of California, Berkeley.

Main, M., & Hesse, E. (1990). Parents' unresolved traumatic experiences are related to infant disorganized attachment status: Is frightened and/or frightening parental behavior the linking mechanism? In M. T. Greenberg, D. Cicchetti, & E. M. Cummings (Eds.), *Attachment in the preschool years: Theory, research and intervention* (pp. 161–182). Chicago: University of Chicago Press.

Main, M., & Hesse, E. (1992). *Frightened, threatening, dissociative, timid-deferential, sexualized, and disorganized parental behavior: A coding system for frightened/frightening (FR) parent–infant interactions.* Unpublished manuscript, University of California at Berkeley.

Main, M., & Hesse, E. (1998). *Frightening, threatening, dissociative, timid-deferential, sexualized and disorganized parental behavior: A coding system for frightened/ frightening (FR) parent–infant interactions.* Unpublished manuscript, University of California, Berkeley.

Main, M., & Hesse, E. (2003). *Adult attachment scoring and classification system.* Unpublished manuscript, University of California, Berkeley.

Main, M., Hesse, E., & Kaplan, N. (2005). Predictability of attachment behavior and representational processes at 1, 6, and 18 years of age: The Berkeley Longitudinal Study. In K. E. Grossmann, K. Grossmann, & E. Waters (Eds.), *Attachment from infancy to adulthood* (pp. 245–304). New York: Guilford Press.

Main, M., Kaplan, N., & Cassidy, J. (1985). Security in infancy, childhood, and adulthood: A move to the level of representation. In I. Bretherton & E. Waters (Eds.), Growing points of attachment theory and research. *Monographs of the Society for Research in Child Development, 50* (1–2, Serial No. 209), 66–104.

Main, M., & Solomon, J. (1990). Procedures for identifying infants as disorganized/disoriented during the Ainsworth Strange Situation. In M. T. Greenberg, D. Cicchetti, & E. M. Cummings (Eds.), *Attachment in the preschool years: Theory, research, and intervention* (pp. 121–160). Chicago: University of Chicago Press.

Main, M., & Weston, D. (1981). The quality of the toddler's relationship to mother and to father: Related to conflict behavior and the readiness to establish new relationships. *Child Development, 52,* 932–940.

Martins, C., & Gaffan, E. (2000). Effects of early maternal depression on patterns of infant–mother attachment: A meta-analytic investigation. *Journal of Child Psychology and Psychiatry, 41,* 737–746.

McElwain, N. , Booth-LaForce, C., & Wu, X. (2011). Infant–mother attachment and children's friendship quality: Maternal mental-state talk as an intervening mechanism. *Developmental Psychology, 47,* 1295–1311.

Meaney, M., & Szyf, M. (2005). Environmental programming of stress responses through DNA methylation: Life at the interface between a dynamic environment and a fixed genome. *Dialogues Clinical Neuroscience, 7,*103–123.

Meins, E., Fernyhough, C., de Rosnay, M., Arnott, B., Leekam, S., & Turner, M. (2012). Mind-mindedness as a multidimensional construct: Appropriate and nonattuned mind-related comments independently predict infant–mother attachment in a socially diverse sample. *Infancy, 17,* 393-415.

Melnick, S., Finger, B., Hans, S., Patrick, M., Lyons-Ruth, K. (2008). Hostile–helpless states of mind in the AAI: A proposed additional AAI category with implications for identifying disorganized infant attachment in high-risk samples. In H. Steele & M. Steele (Eds.), *Clinical applications of the adult attachment interview* (pp. 399–423). NewYork: Guilford Press.

Milot, T., Lorent, A., St-Laurent, D., Bernier, A., Tarabulsy, G., Lemeline, J.-P., et al. (2014). Hostile-helpless state of mind as further evidence of adult disorganized states of mind in neglecting families. *Child Abuse and Neglect, 38,* 1351–1357.

Moss, E., Bureau, J.-F., Cyr, C., Mongeau, C., & St-Laurent, D. (2004). Correlates of attachment at age 3: Construct validity of the preschool attachment classification system. *Developmental Psychology, 40,* 323–334.

Moss, E., Bureau, J.-F., St-Laurent, D., & Tarabulsy, G. M. (2011). Understanding disorganized attachment at preschool and school age: Examining divergent pathways of disorganized and controlling children. In J. Solomon & C. George (Eds.), *Disorganized attachment and caregiving* (2nd ed., pp. 52–79). New York: Guilford Press.

Moss, E., Cyr, C., Bureau, J.-F., Tarabulsy, G., & Dubois-Comtois, K. (2005). Stability of attachment between preschool and early school-age and factors contributing to continuity/discontinuity. *Developmental Psychology, 41,* 773–783.

Moss, E., Cyr, C., & Dubois-Comtois, K. (2004). Attachment at early school age and developmental risk: Examining family contexts and behavior problems of controlling-caregiving, controlling-punitive, and behaviorally disorganized children. *Developmental Psychology, 40,* 519–532.

Moss, E., Rousseau, D., Parent, S., St-Laurent, D., & Saintong, J. (1998). Correlates of attachment at school age: Maternal reported stress, mother-child interaction, and behavior problems. *Child Development, 69,* 1390–1405.

Moss, E., & St-Laurent, D. (2001). Attachment at school age and academic performance. *Developmental Psychology, 37,* 863–874.

Moss, E., St-Laurent, D., & Parent, S. (1999). Disorganized attachment and developmental risk at school-

age. In J. Solomon & C. George (Eds.), *Attachment disorganization* (pp. 160–187). New York: Guilford Press.

National Institute of Child Health and Human Development (NICHD) Early Child Care Research Network (ECCRN). (1997). The effects of infant childcare on infant–mother attachment security: Results of the NICHD study of early childcare. *Child Development, 68,* 860–879.

National Institute of Child Health and Human Development (NICHD) Early Child Care Research Network (ECCRN). (2001). Child-care and family predictors of preschool attachment and stability from infancy. *Developmental Psychology, 37,* 847–862.

Obsuth, I., Hennighausen, K., Brumariu, L., & Lyons-Ruth, K. (2014). Disorganized behavior in adolescent–parent interaction: Relations to attachment state of mind, partner abuse, and psychopathology. *Child Development, 85,* 370–387.

O'Connor, E., Bureau, J.-F., McCartney, K., & Lyons-Ruth, K. (2011). Risks and outcomes associated with disorganized/controlling patterns of attachment at age three in the NICHD Study of Early Child Care and Youth Development. *Infant Mental Health Journal, 32,* 450–472.

O'Connor, M., Sigman, M., & Kasari, C. (1992). Attachment behavior of infants exposed to alcohol prenatally: Mediating effects of infant affect and mother–infant interaction. *Development and Psychopathology, 4,* 243–256.

O'Connor, T., Rutter, M., & the English and Romanian Adoptees Study Team. (2000). Attachment disorder behavior following early severe deprivation: Extension and longitudinal follow-up. *Journal of the American Academy of Child and Adolescent Psychiatry, 39,* 702–712.

Ogawa, J. R., Sroufe, L. A., Weinfield, N. S., Carlson, E. A., & Egeland, B. (1997). Development and the fragmented self: Longitudinal study of dissociative symptomatology in a nonclinical sample. *Development and Psychopathology, 9,* 855–879.

Owen, M. T., & Cox, M. J. (1997). Marital conflict and the development of infant–parent attachment relationships. *Journal of Family Psychology, 11,* 152–164.

Padrón, E., Carlson, E., & Sroufe, L. A. (2014). Frightened versus not frightened disorganized infant attachment: Newborn characteristics and maternal caregiving, *American Journal of Orthopsychiatry, 84,* 201–208.

Pechtel, P., Murray, L., Brumariu, L., & Lyons-Ruth, K. (2013). Reactivity, regulation, and reward responses to infant cues among mothers with and without psychopathology: An fMRI review. *Translational Developmental Psychiatry, 1,* 1–17.

Pechtel, P., Woodman, A., & Lyons-Ruth, K. (2012). Early maternal withdrawal and non-verbal childhood IQ as precursors for substance abuse diagnosis in young adulthood: Results of a 20-year prospective study. *International Journal of Cognitive Therapy, 5,* 316–329.

Riggs, S., & Jacobvitz, D. (2002). Expectant parents' representations of early attachment relationships: Associations with mental health and family history. *Journal of Consulting and Clinical Psychology, 70,* 195–204.

Rodning, C., Beckwith, L., & Howard, J. (1991). Quality of attachment and home environments in children prenatally exposed to PCP and cocaine. *Development and Psychopathology, 3,* 351–366.

Sagi-Schwartz, A., Van IJzendoorn, M., Grossmann, K. E., Joels, T., Grossmann, K., Scharf, M., et al. (2003). Attachment and traumatic stress in female holocaust child survivors and their daughters. *American Journal of Psychiatry, 160,* 1086–1092.

Schechter, D., Zeanah, C., Myers, M., Brunelli, S., Liebowitz, M., Marshal, R., et al. (2004). Psychobiological dysregulation in violence-exposed mothers: Salivary cortisol of mothers with very young children pre- and post-separation stress. *Bulletin of the Menninger Clinic, 68,* 313–336.

Schuengel, C., Bakermans-Kranenburg, M., & Van IJzendoorn, M. (1999). Frightening maternal behavior linking unresolved loss and disorganized infant attachment. *Journal of Consulting and Clinical Psychology, 67,* 54–63.

Shi, Z., Bureau, J.-F., Easterbrooks, M. A., Zhao, X., & Lyons-Ruth, K. (2012). Childhood maltreatment and prospectively observed quality of early care as predictors of antisocial personality disorder features. *Infant Mental Health Journal, 33,* 55–69.

Siebenbruner, J., Englund, M. M., Egeland, B., & Hudson, K. (2006). Developmental antecedents of late adolescence substance abuse patterns. *Development and Psychopathology, 18,* 551–571.

Smeekens, S., Riksen-Walraven, J., & van Bakel, H. (2009). The predictive value of different infant attachment measures for socioemotional development at age five. *Infant Mental Health Journal, 30,* 366–383.

Smyke, A., Zeanah, C., Fox, N., Nelson, C., & Guthrie, D. (2010). Placement in foster care enhances quality of attachment among young institutionalized children. *Child Development, 81,* 212–223.

Solomon, J., George, C., & De Jong, A. (1995). Children classified as controlling at age six: Evidence of disorganized representational strategies and aggression at home and at school. *Development and Psychopathology, 7,* 447–463.

Spangler, G., & Grossmann, K. E., (1993). Biobehavioral organization in securely and insecurely attached infants. *Child Development, 64,* 1439–1450.

Spangler, G., Johann, M., Ronai, Z., & Zimmermann, P. (2009). Genetic and environmental influence on attachment disorganization. *Journal of Child Psychology and Psychiatry, 50,* 952–996.

Spangler, G., & Zimmermann, P. (2014). Emotional and adrenocortical regulation in early adolescence: Prediction by attachment security and disorganization in infancy, *International Journal of Behavioral Development, 38,* 142–154.

Sroufe, L. A., Egeland, B., Carlson, E., & Collins, W. (2005). *The development of the person: The Minnesota study of risk and adaptation from birth to adulthood.* New York: Guilford Press.

Stacks, A., & Oshio, T. (2009). Disorganized attachment and social skills as indicators of Head Start children's school readiness skills, *Attachment and Human Development, 11,* 143–164.

Stievenart, M., Roskam, I., Meunier, J., & van De Moortele, G. (2011).The reciprocal relation between children's attachment representations and their cognitive ability. *International Journal of Behavioral Development, 35,* 58–66.

Tellegen, A., & Atkinson, G. (1974). Openness to absorbing and self-altering experiences ("absorption"), a trait related to hypnotic susceptibility. *Journal of Abnormal Psychology, 83,* 268–277.

Tereno, S., Guédeney, N., Wendland, J., Lyons- Ruth, K., Tubach, F., Lamas, C., et al. (2014). *Impact of a home-visiting program on maternal atypical behavior: The role of cumulative risk factors.* Manuscript submitted for publication.

Tharner, A., Dierckx, B., Luijk, M., Van IJzendoorn, M., Bakermans-Kranenburg, M., Ginkel, J. R., et al. (2013). Attachment disorganization moderates the effect of maternal postnatal depressive symptoms on infant autonomic functioning, *Psychophysiology, 50,* 195–203.

Tomlinson, M., Cooper, P., & Murray, L. (2005). The mother–infant relationship and infant attachment in a South African peri-urban settlement. *Child Development, 76,* 1044–1054.

Toth, S., Rogosch, F., Manly, J., & Cicchetti D. (2006). The efficacy of toddler–parent psychotherapy to reorganize attachment in the young offspring of mothers with major depressive disorder: A randomized preventive trial. *Journal of Consulting and Clinical Psychology, 74,* 1006–1016.

True, M., Pasani, L., & Oumar, F. (2001). Infant–mother interactions among the Dogon of Mali. *Child Development, 72,* 1451–1466.

Van IJzendoorn, M. (1995). Adult attachment representations, parental responsiveness, and infant attachment: A meta-analysis on the predictive validity of the Adult Attachment Interview. *Psychological Bulletin, 117,* 387–403.

Van IJzendoorn, M., & Bakermans-Kranenburg, M. (2006). DRD4.7-repeat polymorphism moderates the association between maternal unresolved loss or trauma and infant disorgnaization. *Attachment and Human Development, 8,* 291–307.

Van IJzendoorn, M., Schuengel, C., & Bakermans-Kranenburg, M. (1999). Disorganized attachment in early childhood: A meta-analysis of precursors, concomitants, and sequelae. *Development and Psychopathology, 11,* 225–249.

Vulliez-Coady, L., Obsuth, I., Torreiro-Casal, M., Ellertsdottir, L., & Lyons-Ruth, K (2013). Maternal role-confusion: Relations to maternal attachment and mother–child interaction from infancy to adolescence. *Infant Mental Health Journal, 34*, 117–131.

Wartner, U., Grossmann, K., Fremmer-Bombik, E., & Suess, G. (1994). Attachment patterns at age six in south Germany: Predictability from infancy and implications for preschool behavior. *Child Development, 65*, 1014–1027.

Waters, E., Merrick, S., Treboux, D., Crowell, J., & Albersheim, L. (2000). Attachment security in infancy and early adulthood: A twenty-year longitudinal study. *Child Development, 71*, 684–689.

Weinfield, N., Whaley, G., & Egeland, B. (2004). Continuity, discontinuity, and coherence in attachment from infancy to late adolescence: Sequelae of organization and disorganization. *Attachment & Human Development, 6*, 73–97.

Zeanah, C., Smyke, A., Koga, S., Carlson, E., & the Bucharest Early Intervention Project Core Group (2005). Attachment in institutionalized and community children in Romania. *Child Development, 76*, 1015–1028.

# Chapter 30

# Challenges to the Development of Attachment Relationships Faced by Young Children in Foster and Adoptive Care

Mary Dozier
Michael Rutter

Children are born biologically prepared to develop attachment relationships to primary caregivers. Parents are likewise biologically prepared to provide care for their young children (Numan & Insel, 2003). Foster care and adoption represent deviations from the more typical situation in which a child is raised continuously by birth parents. In some species, foster care and adoption do not occur, and in many other species, such care is rare (Maestripieri, 2005). The human caregiving system appears to be relatively flexible in this regard; nonetheless, there are challenges involved for both surrogate parents and children. Depending on the nature of the preplacement conditions, the postplacement conditions, and a child's vulnerabilities and strengths, different effects are seen across behavioral and biological systems.

In this chapter, we discuss young children in foster care, as well as those adopted both nationally and internationally. Although children in these groups experience different challenges, they are all raised by someone other than birth parents for at least part of their lives. Some of the challenges include institutional care, changes in caregivers, early experiences of maltreatment, and prenatal or genetic factors that confer vulnerability. We include a discussion of animal models of separation and neglect because they richly inform our understanding of the effects of infants' early experience.

## Changes Since Earler Editions

The first edition of the *Handbook* did not include a chapter on foster care and adoption, partly because the then-current research base was not sufficiently well developed to justify it. Earlier, Bowlby (1969/1982), Spitz (1945), and others had written about the deleterious effects of neglect and institutional care, and nonhuman researchers had documented the problematic effects of disruptions in care (e.g., Levine, Johnson, & Gonzalez, 1985). Nonetheless, research in more recent decades had been somewhat limited. The research base has grown in the last several decades, although we suggest that this is an emerging area with great potential for further growth.

Several pioneering longitudinal studies have been conducted in the last two decades that have documented both the severe consequences of early deprivation on children's functioning within institutional settings, and the impressive catch-up that often occurs when children are subsequently adopted or fostered (e.g., Bakermans-Kranenburg, Steele, et al., 2011; Nelson, Fox, & Zeanah, 2014; Rutter et al., 2007). Catch-up is seen across domains, with children showing dramatic physical, cognitive, and social growth upon placement in families (Bakermans-Kranenburg, Steele, et al., 2011; Nelson et al., 2014). Nonetheless, a minority of children continue to show deficits, most especially in domains of attention, indiscriminate sociability, and, although less frequently, quasi-autistic symptoms (Bakermans-Kranenburg, Steele, et al., 2011; Nelson et al., 2014).

These studies and others solidified the evidence that early deprivation has pervasive deleterious effects on children's biological and behavioral development, but that remediation is often possible when children subsequently have loving, supportive caregivers. The importance of subsequent care on children's ability to handle early adversity was not a new idea, but these studies are exemplary because some children showed dramatic recovery following such extreme neglect. Links between biological and behavioral functioning have been demonstrated in these and other studies in key ways (e.g., Nelson et al., 2014).

## Types of Surrogate Care

### Foster Care

About 400,000 children are in formal foster care in the United States, which represents a significant and linear decrease over the last several decades (U.S. Department of Health and Human Services [DHHS], 2013). Many children living in informal foster care arrangements (e.g., with relatives or neighbors) are not counted in this number. In the United States, about 6% of children entering foster care are less than 1 year old, and 26% are between 1 and 5 years of age. Thus, the associated disruptions in care and the forming of attachment relationships to new caregivers occur for many at a developmental point when forming and maintaining attachment relationships are key biologically programmed tasks. Children in foster care have a range of previous caregiving experiences, both prior to entering the foster care system and within it. With the exception of those placed into foster care at birth, most have been neglected by their birth parents, and some have experienced abuse, either by itself or in combination with neglect.

Although foster care is intended to be a temporary solution, children of all ages tend to stay in care for relatively long periods in the United States. Only 12% stay in foster care less than a month, with an additional 5% staying for less than a year. Twenty-seven percent stay in foster care between 1 and 2 years, and 28% remain more than 2 years. When children leave foster care, approximately 51% are reunited with birth parents and 22% are adopted, sometimes by their foster parents (DHHS, 2013). For those who reunify, about one-third return to foster care within 3 years.

### Adoption

The population of adopted children overlaps with the population of children who have been in foster care. The number of children adopted from the foster care system in the United States has been about 50,000 each year of the last decade (e.g., DHHS, 2013). About 8,700 children were adopted internationally during 2012 into the United States (U.S. Department of State, 2013). The number of children adopted internationally into the United States increased from 1990, when about 7,000 children were adopted, to 2005, when about 22,000 were adopted, but then decreased dramatically each year since 2005, to about 8,700 in 2012. Policies within various nations have partially driven these rates. Many of the children adopted internationally have been in institutional care for at least some period of time prior to adoption. The age of adoption has increased over the years, with about 50% adopted before age 1 in 1999, but few (10%) adopted before age 1 in 2012 (U.S. Department of State, 2013).

## Experiences Prior to Placement in Foster or Adoptive Care

Human young have a long period of immaturity and therefore remain dependent on caregivers for a number of years. Nonetheless, the period when the formation of initial selective attachments has the most biological significance is probably the first several years of life. During the second half of the first year of life, children typically develop attachment relationships to specific caregivers. From an evolutionary perspective, one of the functions of attachment behaviors is to keep children close to caregivers under potentially dangerous circumstances. Even before children develop selective attachment relationships, caregivers play critical roles in helping their infants begin to regulate physiological and behavioral states. For example, neonates are typically dependent upon their mothers for temperature regulation, and young infants are dependent on parents for physiological regulation. Thus, experiences of separation, maltreatment, and privation, even early in the first year of life, may have long-term developmental consequences.

Children experience a range of conditions prior to placement in foster care and adoptive care. At one end of a continuum are children who have lacked a caregiver altogether and experienced minimal stimulation. Although privation at this level is most often associated with institutional care, it is also sometimes seen among children reared with birth parents or foster parents. At the other end of the continuum are children who have been cared for by loving, committed caregivers who, for some reason (e.g., death, imprisonment), were not able to continue parenting. Many children who enter surrogate care fall between these two extremes; they have not been starkly deprived, but they also have not received consistently nurturing care. In the following sections, we consider experiences of institutional care, neglect, abuse, and separation from caregivers.

## Institutional Care

Historically, many children who did not have parents to care for them lived in group care or institutional care settings (Bowlby, 1951). Attention to the effects of these conditions in the 1940s and 1950s ended the widescale use of institutional care in the United States and the United Kingdom. Nonetheless, such institutional care continues to exist in some places within the United States, where it is often referred to as "group care" or "congregate care." About 15% of all children who are removed from their parents' care are placed in facilities that house more than 11 children (DHHS, 2013). Older children are especially likely to be placed in institutional care, although infants and young children are placed in such facilities as well. Reasons given for these placements include the shortage of foster parents, the desire to keep siblings together, and the high quality of the facilities. Even high-quality institutional care, however, has problematic effects (Kaufman et al., 2004). An international group of scholars (Dozier et al., 2014, p. 219) has recently issued a consensus statement that "group settings should not be used

as living arrangements, because of their inherently detrimental effects on the healthy development of children, regardless of age."

Compared to the United States and the United Kingdom, institutional care is seen more often in a number of other countries. The Children's Bureau (U.S. Department of Health and Human Services, 2015) defines congregate care as homes with 7–12 children, and institutional care as facilities with 12 or more children. Institutional care is common in Asia, Central and South American, Africa, and the Middle East, with the highest proportion of children in institutional care in Eastern Europe and central Asia (United Nations International Children's Emergency Fund [UNICEF], 2013).

In 1945, Spitz described the conditions of orphanages in the United States. In an attempt to reduce infection, and in response to low staff-to-child ratios, institutional environments had become increasingly sterile. Babies were handled as little as possible, kept in cribs from which they could not interact with each other or with staff members, and fed and changed in perfunctory fashion. Bowlby (1951) conducted a study of institutions in Europe for the WHO, describing similar conditions. Orphanages in Romania and St. Petersburg, Russia, were described in comparable ways over 50 years later (Groark, Muhamedrahimov, Palmov, Nikiforova, & McCall, 2005; Rutter, Kreppner, & O'Connor, 2001; St. Petersburg–USA Orphanage Research Team, 2008). For example, bottles were propped up so that babies could be fed without being held, and children were left lying in their cribs for extended periods.

### Effects of Institutional Care on Development

Starkly depriving conditions are associated with the most pervasive effects on child functioning. At the very basic level, death rates are high. Furthermore, these children are often delayed in physical growth. They show deficits in motor development, with many of them crawling and walking well behind schedule (Johnson et al., 1996). Extensive delays in cognitive functioning and language development are also seen (Carlson & Earls, 1997; Johnson et al., 1996; Nelson et al., 2014). In addition to developmental delays, institutionalized children show highly anomalous behaviors, including stereotypies such as rocking and self-stimulating behaviors. Social behaviors are odd and often include one of two extremes:

Some children are withdrawn and depressed in appearance, whereas others are indiscriminate in their attachment behaviors (Chisholm, 1998; Chisholm, Carter, Ames, & Morison, 1995; Nelson et al., 2014; O'Connor, Rutter, & the English and Romanian Adoptees Study Team, 2000; Tizard & Rees, 1975).

Nonhuman primates raised under isolated conditions show similar deficits in functioning (Suomi, Chapter 7, this volume). For example, rhesus infants reared without appropriate mother surrogates show highly anomalous behaviors that persist when the infants are placed back in their home cages. These monkeys show stereotypies, inappropriate social behaviors, and (when mating does occur) inadequate parenting. Reintegrating these isolates with other animals is difficult because their inappropriate behavior patterns often make them targets for abuse (Suomi & Harlow, 1972).

### Differences among Institutions

There are differences among institutions and even within institutions in the care provided (Groark et al., 2005; Gunnar, Bruce, & Grotevant, 2000). Key differences among institutions include different staff-to-child ratios and philosophies regarding staff interactions with children (Groark et al., 2005). There may be exceptions, and staff-to-child ratios and philosophies can be manipulated (Groark et al., 2005). Indeed, Groark and colleagues found that conditions in institutions can be substantially improved, resulting in changes in child behavioral outcomes. Reducing staff-to-child ratios, combined with altering expectations of child care workers, can result in profoundly altered interaction patterns.

Despite such results, even high-quality institutional care appears to have deleterious effects on young children's development (Kaufman et al., 2004). As a rule, children often miss the opportunity to develop selective attachment relationships to caregivers in institutions, and institutional care discourages caregivers from committing themselves to children. A number of forces operate to make caring for children in institutions perfunctory. Developing faster ways to feed and change children becomes important under such conditions. Institutional care seems to have specific adverse effects on children that other depriving conditions do not. In particular, the disinhibited attachment

seen among institutionalized children is rarely seen among children who have experienced other forms of deprivation, as we discuss later.

### Neglect

Neglect accounts for about three-fourths of all substantiated cases of child maltreatment (Institute of Medicine [IOM], 2013). *Neglect* is a caregiver's failure to provide for his or her child's basic safety or welfare. Examples include leaving young children home alone, failing to provide adequate food or shelter, and failing to protect children from dangerous conditions (e.g., exposure to violence). On the one hand, although this may seem similar to the description of institutional care, neglecting parents usually have relationships with their children, and their children typically form selective attachments to them or to other caregivers in the home. From an evolutionary perspective, it makes sense that the attachment system is adaptable to a range of caregiving conditions. We expect that the formation of a selective attachment protects neglected children from the long-term effects seen among some institutionalized children.

On the other hand, although neglect is less toxic than conditions of privation, it has pervasive, long-term effects (for a review, see Smith & Fong, 2004). Children who experience early neglect are at increased risk for a host of problematic outcomes. During school-age years, children who have experienced early neglect exhibit more internalizing and externalizing behavior problems and have greater difficulties in relationships with peers than do other children (Egeland, Sroufe, & Erickson, 1983). As adolescents and adults, these children continue to be at significantly increased risk for a range of problems, including depression, anxiety, eating disorders, substance abuse, posttraumatic stress disorder, suicide, and criminal activities (e.g., Spertus, Yehuda, Wong, Halligan, & Seremetis, 2003). There is some evidence that the consequences are most serious for children who experience neglect early in life (e.g., DHHS, 2013; IOM, 2013; Keiley, Howe, Dodge, Bates, & Pettit, 2001).

### Abuse

When abuse is documented, children are often removed from the home, at least for a period of time. As with children who experience neglect, abused children typically form selective attachment relationships with caregivers. In fact, Roth and Sullivan (2005) argued that abuse heightens the connectedness children feel with their caregivers. They found, studying rodent pups, that the pairing of pain with the mother's presence is associated with enhanced positive feelings for the mother (see also Polan & Hofer, Chapter 6, this volume). Rajecki, Lamb, and Obmascher (1978) reported similar findings with a broader range of animal species.

Nonetheless, children who experience abuse are involved in a "paradoxical situation," in the words of Hesse and Main (2006, p. 336). When children experience abuse at the hands of a caregiver, they are frightened of the person from whom they would normally seek support. Under more typical parenting conditions, young children are frightened by a variety of things, including the dark, being left alone, and a dog barking, but they can typically turn to a caregiver to protect and soothe them. For example, when children receive inoculations, they are likely to be both hurt and frightened; caregivers, however, can buffer the effects of the stress (Gunnar, Brodersen, Krueger, & Rigatuso, 1996). But when caregivers themselves are the source of the fear, they fail to protect their children effectively from danger. Children's "paradoxical situation" is seen in their behavior when reunited with abusive caregivers in the Strange Situation (Hesse & Main, 2006). Typical responses include freezing upon reunion or moving away from, rather than toward, the parent. The fear that children experience interferes with their approach to parents. Thus, such children have odd, inexplicable behaviors that are classified as disorganized or disoriented (see also Lyons-Ruth & Jacobvitz, Chapter 29, and George & Solomon, Chapter 18, this volume).

Repeated exposure to frightening conditions may result in children developing a sensitized neurobiology, whereby minor threats elicit strong behavioral and physiological reactions. Other effects of maltreatment include children's difficulty in developing a trusting relationship with a caregiver (Milan & Pinderhughes, 2000), differential processing of angry faces (Cicchetti & Curtis, 2005; Pollak & Tolley-Schell, 2003), lack of empathy for distressed peers (George & Main, 1979), negative attributional biases (Dodge, Pettit, Bates, & Valente, 1995; Gibb, 2001), and later dissociative and externalizing symptoms (Lyons-Ruth, Alpern, & Repacholi, 1993).

## Separations from Caregivers

Except when children are placed in foster or adoptive care at birth, placement involves separation from caregivers. Infants have a number of biological systems that maximize the likelihood of obtaining care from their biological mothers in particular. For example, at birth, an infant prefers the mother's smell to other smells, and this facilitates turning toward the nipple for breast feeding (Roth & Sullivan, 2005). Under benign conditions, the infant comes to anticipate certain rhythms of activity and responsiveness from the mother or caregiver (Beebe, Lachman, & Jaffe, 1997; Gianino & Tronick, 1988). Even prior to the development of a selective attachment, separations are likely to be experienced as dysregulating (see Polan & Hofer, Chapter 6, this volume).

Animal studies demonstrate how powerfully nonhuman primate and rodent young respond to separations from their mothers. Levine, Weiner, and Coe (1993) showed that infant squirrel monkeys never habituated to separations from their mothers. Even when infants had been separated many times, they continued to show neuroendocrine distress responses to the separations. A number of researchers (e.g., Levine et al., 1993; Sanchez, Ladd, & Plotsky, 2001) have found that these early separations have short-term and long-term effects on neuroendocrine regulation. For example, when rodent pups were separated from their mothers for periods of time longer than they would be separated in the wild, they developed a hyperreactive neuroendocrine system. Presumably, rodent pups' stress systems are not designed to deal with these long separations because there would be little chance of survival if their mothers did not return to the nest. Although these separations have been described as unnaturally long and therefore of limited usefulness in generalizing to the human condition, these longer separations may in fact be analogous to a human child's experience when placed in foster or adoptive care. Nonetheless, it is important to note that children often develop secure, organized attachments following transitions in care if placed in the home of nurturing parents (Dozier, Stovall, Albus, & Bates, 2001; Nelson et al., 2014).

Experiences of maltreatment and separation are often confounded for young children placed into foster and adoptive care, making it difficult to isolate effects. Animal studies may help point to which experiences are critical and which are not, although developing adequate models of abuse and separation remains complex, as does the generalization across species.

## Factors Affecting How Children Cope with Adversity

### Child Vulnerabilities

A number of prenatal and genetic factors affect how children cope with adversity. Some of these factors, such as prenatal exposure to alcohol and premature birth, may be overrepresented in the population of children that enter foster and adoptive care (e.g., Barth & Needell, 1996). There are also high rates of prior maternal substance abuse among children placed into foster care and domestic adoptive care in the United States. The rates of prenatal substance exposure are often highest among children placed at birth because detection of maternal use of illegal substances is often a cause for placement into foster care. This is important because there is often an inverse association between prenatal and postnatal risk factors for children placed in domestic foster and adoptive care. For example, children who are placed in foster or adoptive care at birth are likely to have higher levels of prenatal substance exposure, but lower levels of postnatal risk (e.g., abuse, neglect, separations), than children placed at later ages.

The incidence of maternal smoking and drinking, as well as maternal use of illegal substances (e.g., cocaine and amphetamines), is high for children placed into foster and adoptive care in the United States (Barth, 1991). Prenatal exposure to substances has been linked with a wide range of problems for children, including attentional problems (Savage, Brodsky, Malmud, Giannetta, & Hurt, 2005), substance abuse (Glantz & Chambers, 2006), and conduct disorder (Wakschlag & Hans, 2002).

The preponderance of evidence suggests that the effects of risk are generally additive, with each additional factor increasing the odds of problematic outcomes (Appleyard, Egeland, van Dulmen, & Sroufe, 2005; Sameroff, Bartko, Baldwin, Baldwin, & Seifer, 1998). Some investigators, in fact, have found that the effects of risk factors are multiplicative, with three or four risk factors showing a much stronger effect than fewer risk factors (e.g., Appleyard et al., 2005). There is growing evidence for gene–environment interactions. Genetic variants often have little or no main effect on maladaptive psychological outcomes but are nonethe-

less associated with an increased vulnerability to risks such as child abuse (Rutter, Moffitt, & Caspi, 2006). For example, Caspi and colleagues (2002, 2003) reported evidence for a gene–environment interaction involving the monoamine oxidase A (MAOA) gene that affects antisocial behavior and another gene (the short-allele variant of the serotonin transporter gene) that affects rates of depression (see also Kaufman et al., 2006). Suomi (2003) similarly found that the short-allele version of the serotonin transporter gene in rhesus monkeys was associated with maladaptive outcomes in peer-reared, but not mother-reared, monkeys. Bakermans-Kranenburg and Van IJzendoorn (2006, 2011; Bakermans-Kranenburg, Van IJzendoorn, Caspers, & Philibert, 2011) found a significant interaction between the 7-repeat variant of the dopamine D4 receptor (DRD4) gene and environment in predicting outcome. The same genetic variant has been found to moderate the effects of an intervention to promote sensitive parenting and positive discipline (Bakermans-Kranenburg, Van IJzendoorn, Mesman, Alink, & Juffer, 2008).

### Quality of Surrogate Caregiving Experiences

Among children in intact families and children who have been placed in foster or adoptive care, the later caregiving environment has proven to be important in affecting many outcomes (Ackerman, Kogos, Youngstrom, Schoff, & Izard, 1999; Duyme, Dumaret, & Tomkiewicz, 1999; Sinclair & Wilson, 2003). Children who are moved to privileged adoptive families after institutional care typically show a rapid catch-up in physical growth, followed by rapid cognitive development (Bakermans-Kranenburg, Steele, et al., 2011; Nelson et al., 2014). Nonetheless, some children continue to show deficits after being placed into stable foster or adoptive homes (Bakermans-Kranenburg et al., 2011; Nelson et al., 2014; Van IJzendoorn & Juffer, 2006). These issues are considered in more depth in a later section.

Sroufe and colleagues (Sroufe, Egeland, Carlson, & Collins, 2005; Weinfield, Sroufe, & Egeland, 2000) have suggested that when conditions in children's lives change, developmental outcomes follow rules of "lawful discontinuity." For the most part, the changes that have been studied have included parental death, divorce, and other similar life stressors. Although these changes are significant, they often pale in comparison with the changes in the lives of children who enter surrogate care. Such children typically change caregivers, sibling groups, neighborhoods, SES, and sometimes even nations, cultures, and languages spoken. We expect that for infants and young children, the caregivers' characteristics are most critical to children's adjustment.

Hinde and McGinnis (1977) found that rhesus infants adjusted much more quickly following separations if their mothers' returned to normal behavior rather than exhibiting distressed or aberrant behavior. This is similar to findings regarding a child's ability to adjust to such stressors as death and divorce. When the remaining caregiver is able to function as an effective support to the child, the child's adjustment is much better than if the caregiver cannot serve this role (Harris, Brown, & Bifulco, 1986).

### Adoptive, Foster, and Kinship Caregivers

In general, adoptive parents, traditional foster caregivers, and kinship caregivers represent somewhat different populations. Parents adopting across national boundaries are screened most extensively, and kinship caregivers are screened least extensively. Parents seeking to adopt internationally are typically screened to ensure that they do not present risks to any adopted child through their pattern of rearing. At the time of adoption, adopting parents have rates of psychopathology that are low by general population standards (Rutter, 2006). Accordingly, it might be expected that this population would mirror the general population with regard to attachment state of mind, or indeed might show high rates of autonomous states of mind.

### Screening Caregivers

Screening of foster parents is somewhat variable. Most child welfare agencies attempt to place children in foster homes within the same city or county system from which children were removed. Therefore, in areas where removal of children is high per capita (e.g., in high-poverty areas), the available pool of foster parents is often much smaller than the number needed. A smaller foster parent pool typically results in less screening. Qualifications for becoming kin caregivers depend on whether the caregiver is licensed as a foster parent or the arrangement is informal. Combined with the fact that kin caregivers are

often the parents of the child's parents (who were unable to care for the child), it is not surprising that these kin caregivers have fewer resources and experience more stressors than traditional foster parents do (Brooks & Barth, 1998; Cuddleback, 2004). To our knowledge, the distribution of kin caregivers' attachment state of mind has not been reported in the literature.

There have been adoptions by lesbian couples for quite some time, with findings from several studies that the children generally fare well (Goldberg, 2010). What is relatively new is the adoption by gay male couples, although the numbers involved have been growing (Brodzinsky & Pertman, 2011). Golombok and colleagues (2014) compared 41 two-parent gay father adoptive families, 40 two-parent lesbian adoptive families, and 40 two-parent heterosexual adoptive families. The inclusion criteria were that the target child would be between 4 and 8 years of age and have been placed with the adoptive family for at least 12 months. The main finding was that there were few differences among the groups with respect to the development of the children, although there was a tendency for those in gay father adoptive families to do somewhat better in some domains. A major strength of the study was the multimethod approach, which included interview, observation, and questionnaire data and multi-informants (involving parents, child, and teacher).

The authors considered the possible reasons for the somewhat better outcome for the children adopted by gay men, and noted that unlike both lesbian couples and heterosexual couples, scarcely any of the gay father couples had tried to have children before and had therefore not gone through all the stresses involved with infertility and failed fertility treatments. Also, there was no clash between the gay men as to who was the "mother" (as there was in some lesbian couples) because clearly neither was the biological mother. For obvious reasons, the sample was not an epidemiological one because in the current circumstances that was not possible. Nevertheless, as judged by the agencies that kept records, the participation rate of 71% was high. A further limitation is that the children are still relatively young, and it is not known how they will turn out when older. Of course, too, especially with the gay men, they cannot possibly be regarded as typical of most gay men because most gay men do not wish to adopt. However, the policy implications are clear-cut in indicating that gay adoptive families constitute a largely untapped pool of potential adoptive parents.

## Challenges for Children Forming Attachments to New Caregivers

To this point, we have considered the conditions associated with foster and adoptive care that are likely to affect children's adjustment. We now consider the challenges children face in developing attachments to new caregivers. The literature on attachment in relation to foster care and adoption falls into three general categories: foster placement, adoptive placement at birth or soon after, and adoptive care following institutional care. We consider each of these in turn.

### Attachments of Children in Foster Care

#### The Process of Forming New Attachment Relationships

When developing in typical mother–child dyads, children form selective attachments as a result of maturation and an extended history of interactions. In contrast, children who are placed into foster or adoptive care are often at a developmental stage in which selective attachment relationships would already have been formed with caregivers. Therefore, the process by which new selective attachments are formed is likely to move along a different trajectory, or to take a form different from the usual one.

To study this process, Stovall and Dozier (2000) developed a diary method for tracking children's attachment behaviors. They examined the formation of attachment relationships from as close to the first day of a child's placement in a new home as possible. Foster parents were asked to report on children's behaviors during incidents likely to elicit attachment behaviors. In particular, they recorded how children responded to being frightened, hurt, and separated from them. Foster parents also recorded their own reactions to their children's behaviors and children's subsequent responses. These behaviors were recorded on a checklist developed to be as complete as possible.

Stovall-McClough and Dozier used the attachment diary to study children's developing attachment relationships in a new foster home (Stovall & Dozier, 2000; Stovall-McClough & Dozier, 2004). For children placed into care before about 1 year of age, placements became stable quickly. Within 1–2 weeks, most infants and tod-

dlers developed a consistent pattern of responding to their caregivers (Stovall & Dozier, 2000). For children placed later than approximately 1 year of age, the process appeared to take longer than for younger children. Even after 2 months, these children often did not show stable patterns of attachment behavior. Furthermore, in this early period of attachment formation, diary data suggested that the children "led the dance" (Stern, 2002). That is, children's avoidant and resistant behaviors elicited complementary (i.e., rejecting) behaviors from caregivers, even for caregivers with an autonomous state of mind.

These findings regarding the formation of attachments to new caregivers are probably neither as encouraging as they seem for the younger infants, nor as discouraging as they seem for the older infants. First, the finding that children younger than about 1 year of age show secure behaviors quickly with an autonomous foster parent is promising in terms of children's ability to organize their behavior in relation to a new caregiver. A period of 1–2 weeks (i.e., the length of time it appears to take young infants to develop expectations concerning a new caregiver's availability) is probably a long time in the life of a young infant. Although infants adapt to the new caregivers by organizing attachment behaviors in relation to caregiver availability, disruptions may still have had dysregulating effects. Second, the findings suggest that children who are more than about 1 year of age at the time of placement have some difficulty trusting new caregivers and behaving in ways that elicit nurturing behaviors. Stovall and Dozier (2000) were concerned, based on these early findings, that the children's behaviors would be self-perpetuating—that children who behaved in avoidant or resistant ways would fail to elicit nurturance from caregivers, and would therefore not experience an environment that could positively challenge and change their expectations. As we discuss in the next section on consolidated attachment relationships, however, these children are eventually able to develop attachment relationships that reflect their caregivers' state of mind rather than the children's anticipation of a non-nurturing world.

### Consolidated Attachment Relationships among Foster Children

Dozier and colleagues (2001) studied the consolidated attachment relationships of children placed into foster care for at least 2 months. Infant attachment quality in this study was assessed in the Strange Situation, and foster mother state of mind with respect to attachment was assessed with the Adult Attachment Interview (George, Kaplan, & Main, 1984, 1985, 1996; see Hesse, Chapter 26, this volume). Foster mothers' states of mind were concordant with infant attachment 72% of the time (kappa = .43) in the Dozier and colleagues (2001) study, as compared with 76% (kappa = .49) in the meta-analysis.

When children are placed with autonomous foster parents, it seems that experiences of maltreatment and separation do not affect their ability to form organized attachment relationships. These results are surprising in one sense but are also consistent with the evidence that attachment formation is a relationship-specific construct for young children. For example, the quality of attachment relationships that children form with mothers, fathers, and preschool teachers have been found to be relatively independent (e.g., Goossens & Van IJzendoorn, 1990; Howes & Hamilton, 1992; see Howes & Spieker, Chapter 15, this volume, for a review).

Whereas the attachment outcomes for children placed with autonomous foster parents were quite positive, children placed with nonautonomous caregivers were disproportionately likely to develop disorganized attachment relationships. This disproportionate distribution resulted from foster children developing disorganized attachment relationships when parented by foster parents with either dismissive or unresolved states of mind. Among biologically intact dyads, disorganized infant attachment is predicted only by parental unresolved state of mind and not by a dismissive state of mind. Dozier and colleagues (2001) interpreted these results as suggesting that children who have experienced early adversity are especially in need of nurturing care. Without such care, they do not appear to be able to organize their attachment relationships.

## Attachment among Adopted Children

### Children Adopted Early in Infancy

A meta-analysis of unpublished data suggests that attachment security (as measured in the Strange Situation) is somewhat less frequent in adopted children than in nonclinical, nonadopted samples (47 vs. 67%; Van IJzendoorn & Juffer, 2006).

### Children Adopted Following Extended Institutional Care

Vorria and colleagues (2003, 2006) studied attachment among children in Greek orphanages, and with their parents at postadoption. There was a high rate of disorganized attachment (64 vs. 28%) while the children were in residential care, as found in other studies (Van IJzendoorn, Schuengel, & Bakermans-Kranenburg, 1999; Zeanah, Smyke, Koga, Carlson, & the Bucharest Early Intervention Project Core Group, 2005). At follow-up 2 years after adoption, attachment security, as measured with the Waters and Deane (1985) Attachment Q-Sort procedure (based on observer ratings), showed a lower level of security in the former Metera children than in a community comparison group, and less coherence and greater avoidance on the Bretherton (1985) Attachment Story Completion Task (ASCT). Thus, even after 2 years, there were continuing differences in attachment security associated with early institutional rearing. There was no effect of preadoption attachment security on the ASCT, and a negative effect on Q-sort-rated security. Disorganized attachment before adoption, as compared with security before adoption, was associated with more secure narratives after adoption. When studied at 13 years of age, these children showed generally positive attachment relationships with their adoptive parents, with only small differences between their functioning and that of a comparison group (Vorria, Ntouma, Vairami, & Rutter, 2015).

## Atypical Attachments

Sroufe and colleagues (2005) have emphasized that among intact dyads, strength of attachment is irrelevant. Except under very atypical circumstances, all infants in intact parent–child dyads are expected to become attached to their primary caregivers. Even when children have maltreating parents, they appear to develop specific attachment relationships with those parents (e.g., Crittenden, 1985; Egeland & Sroufe, 1981). It is quality of attachment that differentiates most children, rather than whether they have developed attachment relationships of a certain relative strength or intensity. Among children who have been placed into foster or adoptive care, however, it appears critical to consider the *extent* to which children develop attachment relationships to new caregivers. The

Strange Situation, the standard way of assessing attachment quality, does not assess whether the child is attached to the caregiver.

## Failure to Develop Specific Attachments

When children do not have an opportunity to develop early primary attachment relationships, they may fail to develop specific attachments to subsequent caregivers or may show odd behaviors with regard to those caregivers. Zeanah and colleagues (2005) have used a coding system developed by Carlson (2002) for assessing the extent to which a child shows attachment behaviors toward a particular figure in the Strange Situation. Ratings are made on the basis of the child's display of behaviors, ranging from typical behaviors shown by children from intact parent–child dyads (at the high end of the scale) to no display of attachment behaviors (at the low end of the scale). This system is important in considering differences among children who spent the early months of their lives in institutional care. In particular, Zeanah and colleagues found that early-institutionalized children displayed less discriminating attachment behaviors than never-institutionalized children. In fact, 100% of the never-institutionalized children showed clear attachment behavior patterns (coded as secure, avoidant, resistant, or disorganized), whereas only 3.2% of the institutionalized children showed clear attachment behaviors.

## Indiscriminate Friendliness and Disinhibited Attachment

Related to this failure to develop discriminating attachment relationships are disinhibited attachment and indiscriminate friendliness or indiscriminate sociability. Indiscriminate sociability was first described by Tizard and Hodges (1978); children who display it approach strangers as if they are attachment figures. Rutter and colleagues (2007) provided a multisource assessment of disinhibited attachment at age 11 years, after at least 7½ years in adoptive families. Among Romanian adoptees between 6 and 42 months of age, entering the United Kingdom after having experienced institutional rearing, 26% showed marked disinhibition as assessed by parental report, as compared with 9% of those who had not experienced institutional rearing or who had entered

the United Kingdom below 6 months of age, and 4% in domestic adoptees adopted under the age of 6 months. Investigator ratings showed that the features most strongly associated with disinhibited attachment were socially inappropriate physical contact, a lack of social reserve, an unusual relationship with the examiner, verbal and social violation of conventional boundaries, and a high rate of spontaneous comments. At age 6 years, disinhibited attachment had been associated with a high proportion of disorganized, insecure/other, and unclassifiable classifications, with 41% rated as secure. It was also noteworthy that the majority of the children with disinhibited attachment exhibited problems in several other domains of behavior.

Indiscriminate sociability and disinhibited attachment are seen relatively frequently among children who were previously institutionalized for longer than 6 months of the first 2 years of life (e.g., Chisholm, 1998; Zeanah & Smyke, 2005). Most of the existing evidence suggests that children who were in foster care do not show high rates of indiscriminate sociability

## The Meaning of Disinhibited Attachment

Several features of these findings stand out. First, disinhibited attachment constitutes a clinically significant problem that is remarkably persistent many years after adoption for children who were once in institutional care, and almost exclusively so for this population. In the Bucharest Early Intervention Project, Zeanah and Smyke (2005) reported that although inhibited attachment disorders were not disproportionately represented in frequency 18 months after the children were placed in foster families, disinhibited attachment disorders did not remit.

Second, disinhibited attachment is not a variant of attachment insecurity. Rather, it seems to represent an attachment *disorder* that involves a relative failure to develop normal attachment relationships.

Third, although the pattern was strongly associated with institutional deprivation, a substantial proportion of institutionally deprived children did *not* show this pattern. So far, the reasons for the individual differences in response remain obscure. Stevens, Sonuga-Barke, Asherson, Kreppner, and Rutter (2006) have suggested that genetic influences in susceptibility to environmental hazards may be implicated.

Fourth, it seems that the pattern rarely develops if the institutional deprivation does not persist beyond 6 months of age, but it is common with any persistence beyond 6 months. This suggests the possibility that some form of biological programming is involved in disinhibited attachment. The findings call for study of the biological processes that may be involved, but they also raise questions about possible sensitive periods in the development of selective attachment relationships.

## Caregiver Commitment

In biologically intact families, commitment is often assumed on the part of the children and parents. It is relatively rare to hear of parents who threaten their children with placement outside the family (e.g., in a juvenile delinquency center, with the gypsies, or on the street), or for underage children to think seriously about leaving home. For foster parents and foster children, however, these issues are often salient. Foster parents have the option of giving the children back to the agency for care. Furthermore, although adoption is intended as a permanent solution, nearly 8% of adoptions are disrupted annually, mostly because parents request the children's removal. Whereas young children form attachment relationships with their new caregivers, some children retain a sense of connection to other parents or to members of another family. These issues are considered in the sections below.

Under typical conditions, we would rarely expect to see a lack of commitment on a parent's part. Humans produce relatively few young and invest an enormous amount of resources in each. There are rare conditions when commitment appears low on the part of biological parents. When children are placed into foster care or with adoptive parents, however, parents' commitment can be variable.

Among some species, infants are adopted, but only under fairly limited conditions. For example, typically only lactating females and biologically related females appear to adopt orphaned or abandoned rhesus macaque infants (M. Gerald, personal communication, February 14, 2004). In general, humans are less under the control of hormonal influences than other species, perhaps partly because of a more highly developed prefrontal cortex. Nonetheless, it is important to remember that fostering and adopting occur without the usual biological preparedness that accompanies parenting under more typical conditions.

At one end of the continuum, some foster parents appear to think of their foster children as their own, investing emotionally in their children in ways not unlike parents with their birth children. At the other end of the continuum, some foster parents appear to think of themselves as temporary caregivers who should not invest emotionally in their children (Dozier & Lindhiem, 2006).

We have assessed commitment through an interview called the This Is My Baby Interview (Bates & Dozier, 1997) with foster parents. In the interview, a foster mother is asked to describe her child and to indicate how much she would miss the child if he or she were removed from her care, among other things. Differences in commitment are associated with how many children parents have fostered in the past, with the number of children fostered in the past being inversely related to commitment to current children (Dozier & Lindhiem, 2006). Foster parents who have fostered more children are less likely to commit to the children currently in their care than foster parents who have fostered fewer children. Also, commitment differs for children of different ages, with caregivers showing higher levels of commitment to children placed at younger ages.

Dozier and Lindhiem (2006) have suggested that having a committed caregiver is even more important to the child's sense of security than is the caregiver's responsiveness to the child's bids for reassurance. The two constructs of commitment and responsiveness to distress are largely orthogonal. For example, it is possible for a foster mother to be dismissing (and not responsive to child cues), yet highly committed to a child. From an evolutionary perspective, it is critical that the child have a caregiver who will be there to protect him or her under threatening conditions. Although it is optimal if the caregiver is also soothing and responsive, it may be less essential than the caregiver's commitment to the child. Parents who are more highly committed show more delight in their children than parents who are not as highly committed (Bernard & Dozier, 2011). Commitment is associated with whether the relationship endures or is disrupted, but there are probably subtle, as well as more obvious, ways of communicating commitment or its absence. Placements are more likely to be disrupted when caregivers are less committed than when caregivers are more committed (Dozier & Lindhiem, 2006).

## Open Adoption and Contact with the Biological Family

When foster children have visitation with birth parents, and/or move back and forth between birth parents' homes and foster homes, issues of "Whose child am I?" sometimes arise. For example, birth mothers may want children to think of them as their mothers, but children often refer to foster mothers as their mothers. The younger the child, the harder it is for the child to hold onto any notion of another parent at all (Piaget, 2000). As children become older, they may be raised by one set of parents while knowing about the existence of another set of parents. A similar set of circumstances faces children who are adopted.

These issues are salient in this era of open adoption, when there is the possibility for both biological parents and adopted children to search for each other. The research undertaken up to now regarding open adoption, although very useful in its own right, has not used attachment measures or assessed attachment issues. The move to open adoption was driven initially by the view that this would be beneficial for a child (Hale & Fortin, 2008). Nonetheless, open adoption has implications for all three groups of participants in what can be considered the *adoption triangle* (Triseliotis, Feast, & Kyle, 2005)—that is, the biological family, the adoptive family, and the adopted individual. What is the effect on the adoptive parents of having to share parenthood with another set of parents? What is the effect on the adopted child if continuing contact with the biological family is not possible in practice? What is the effect on attachment representations when, after an initially closed adoption, contact with the biological family is made after years of no contact? Attachment theory provides no clear guide to what is likely to happen or what should happen. What it does do, however, is highlight how contact or the impossibility of contact is likely to impinge on people's internal working models of themselves and of their relationships with other people.

Howe and Feast (2001) focused primarily on the adopted individual—comparing 394 individuals who had searched for their biological parents with 78 who had not, and who had been sought out and approached on behalf of a birth relative. Of those searchers who found a birth relative, few (7%) were rejected outright, and few (9%) had the contact terminated within a year after only one or two contacts, which was also experienced as a rejection. Most (71%) evaluated the reunion as emotionally satisfying, and nearly half claimed that it had improved their self-esteem. Few (11%) of the searchers and one-fourth of the nonsearchers felt that the reunion experience had been upsetting. Howe and Feast concluded that adopted individuals who did *not* search were on the whole well integrated into their adoptive families. Those placed transracially were less likely (56 vs. 71% in same-race placements) to report that they felt they "belonged" in their adoptive family.

Triseliotis and colleagues (2005) examined the outcome of contact with respect to all three members of the adoption triangle. Data were derived from a large-scale postal questionnaire, focusing only on adopted children included in the first study. A high participation rate (82%) was achieved. Approximately one-half of the birth mothers were under the age of 20 at the time of the adopted children's birth, and a minority (11%) were 16 or under. Most became pregnant during the 1950s and early 1960s, when social attitudes toward pregnancies outside marriage tended to be very censorious. Most of the girls' parents were initially shocked and upset, but eventually approximately one-third were supportive (despite usually keeping the pregnancies secret). Most women reported that they felt they had no choice about giving up their babies. Emotional support was usually lacking at the time of parting with their children, and most of the biological mothers came to feel lonely and abandoned. Nevertheless, many (70%) of the mothers said that as they looked back, they felt that adoption had been the right decision. Most did not think the experience had affected their capacity to make new relationships (although 14% said that it had). Similarly, some three-fifths did not think parting with their adopted children had affected the quality of their relationships with their other children, but two-fifths thought it had. These findings suggest that a more detailed study of social relationships, including a use of attachment concepts, would be worthwhile.

Regarding the contact with the adopted children many years later, mothers who were sought out were more likely than seekers to report that the contact felt comfortable. In two-thirds of cases, contact was stopped at the initiative of the adopted persons, especially in the case of seeker mothers. For most birth mothers, contact and reunion were happy and satisfying experiences, with about half feeling that their ability to relate to others had been improved by the reunion; however, some (1 in 10) were dissatisfied, and about the same proportion felt angrier since contact than before.

Most adopted people rated their relationships with their adoptive parents as close, but some (nearly 20%) described them as not close. Those who felt that their relationships were close were least likely to feel rejected by their biological parents. In cases in which there was a feeling of rejection, however, this tended to peak in adolescence. Some adopted persons reported a sense of loss. The experience of reunion with their biological mothers was reported by one-third of adopted persons as having enhanced their relationships with their adoptive families, but some (1 in 6) said that it had led to deterioration in these relationships. Eight years after the reunion, about three-fourths were still in contact with the biological relatives. Some (1 in 3) came to look upon their birth mothers as parents, but just over half viewed them as friends or friends/relatives. For the remaining subset (18%), the relationships were distant or their birth mothers felt like strangers. Many (80%) were pleased to have made contact, and where contact had been established, feelings of rejection or loss tended to diminish. Nevertheless, some (10–20%) of adopted people felt that adoption had adversely affected their marriage and social relationships.

Most (nearly 90%) adopting parents had disclosed the adoption when their children were 4 years of age or younger, and most felt that this had been the right time. Most adoptive parents talked (sometimes or often) with their children about the children's birth families, but a minority (1 in 5) felt that their children were reluctant to do this. Almost all adopting parents felt close to their adopted children and felt very happy about their relationship. Over three-fourths of adopters described their children's motivation to search as strong, and most were supportive of it. However, a few (1 in 6) felt frightened and worried. A prominent concern was that their children might be hurt by the contact, but some felt worried that reunion would mean that they would "lose" their children.

Most (70%) adopters reported that their relationships with their children were unchanged by the search and reunion, and for almost everyone else it had been enhanced. Nevertheless, some (1 in 8) said that, especially in the early stages of the search, their relationships were under strain. Overall, most (nearly 70%) reported that the contact experience had been positive, and very few (3%) reported it as clearly negative.

Viewed as a whole, the search and reunion were positive experiences. For an appreciable minority, the experience of parting with their children may have had an adverse effect on their social relationships. Similarly, for a minority of adopted individuals, there were concerns over some aspects of social relationships. A more detailed study of these variations would benefit from an attachment perspective, but it would be a mistake to ignore the broader social context, and the attachment features would need to be examined alongside other perspectives.

## Interventions to Enhance Attachment among Foster and Adopted Children

Harlow found that isolate-reared monkeys engaged in odd, aggressive, and self-destructive behaviors when placed back into their home cages following extended isolation. It turned out that younger monkeys best served as "therapist monkeys" for these isolate-reared monkeys; these younger monkeys allowed close contact while tolerating aberrant behavior without reprisal (Suomi & Harlow, 1972; Suomi, Harlow, & McKinney, 1972). The principle here might be that contact was needed, but in a context that would not result in injury. For children in institutional care, foster care and adoption represent interventions that often meet these two criteria. An interpersonally engaged but tolerant environment appears to result in excellent physical catch-up, as well as reasonable cognitive catch-up for children who had been institutionalized (Bakermans-Kranenburg, Steele, et al., 2011; Gunnar et al., 2000).

Even when provided with the company of "therapist monkeys," Harlow's isolate-reared monkeys continued to show odd behavior. Most did not mate as adults, and most that did mate showed very inappropriate parenting behaviors. Similarly, children adopted from orphanages continue to show anomalous behaviors, especially with regard to social behaviors and inhibitory control. Without nurturing parents, foster children may develop cognitively but have difficulty organizing attachment behaviors (Gunnar et al., 2000) The aspects of functioning that appear problematic, at least for some children, are regulation of neuroendocrine functioning, inhibitory control, and behavioral control (including risk for substance abuse and related problems), as well as disorganized attachment, nondiscriminating attachment relationships, and odd social behaviors (Gunnar et al., 2000). There has been relatively little research investigating how best to alter these behavioral trajectories. We suggest that interventions need to target the behaviors identified as specifically problematic. In some instances there will be overlap in intervention strategies for foster children, domestically adopted children, and internationally adopted children, and in other instances there will not be. The last two decades have seen an explosion of attachment-based interventions for young children (e.g., Hoffman, Marvin, Cooper, & Powell, 2006). A smaller number of interventions target the needs of children in foster or adoptive care (Dozier, Lindhiem, & Ackerman, 2005; Fisher & Chamberlain, 2000; Juffer, Hoksbergen, Riksen-Walraven, & Kohnstamm, 1997).

### Evidence-Based Interventions for Foster and Adopted Children

Several overlapping models of intervention that target attachment issues have been developed for foster and adopted children (Dozier et al., 2005; Lieberman, Ghosh Ippen, & Van Horn, 2006; Spieker, Oxford, Kelly, Nelson, & Fleming, 2012; Zeanah et al., 2001). Programs range from relatively brief interventions (Dozier et al., 2005, Spieker et al., 2012), to longer interventions (Lieberman et al., 2006), to comprehensive change in the nature of how foster care is provided (Zeanah et al., 2001). Some interventions target parent changes in sensitivity almost exclusively (Dozier et al., 2005), whereas others work to change parent reflective functioning (Lieberman et al., 2006; Spieker et al., 2012). These interventions developed explicitly for foster children overlap significantly with interventions for high-risk parents and infants (e.g., Powell, Cooper, Hoffman, & Marvin, 2013). Interventions for foster parents often target the challenges associated with caring for a child who has experienced early adversity (e.g., maltreatment, transitions in care) that affects his or her response to foster parents (e.g., Dozier et al., 2005; Spieker et al., 2012), in addition to more general intervention targets such as sensitivity. Dozier and colleagues (2014) have incorporated intervention components that target specific problems seen among children who experienced institutional care, including indiscriminate sociability and quasi-autistic behaviors.

Although several interventions have been developed that target these populations and are being tested through randomized clinical trials, the evidence base is relatively nascent. The evidence supporting intervention efficacy comes primarily from trials with high-risk birth parents rather than with foster or adoptive parents. Although preliminary, findings are promising at this point. Dozier and colleagues (2014) reported that foster children randomized to the Attachment and Biobehavioral Catch-Up (ABC) Intervention showed higher rates of security in the Preschool Strange Situation than children assigned to a control intervention. Lewis-Morrarty, Dozier, Bernard, Terracciano, and Moore (2012) found that infants assigned to the ABC condition showed stronger executive functioning in preschool years than children assigned to the control intervention. Spieker and colleagues (2012) saw improvements in sensitivity for parents at postintervention in their randomized clinical trial, although those effects were not sustained 6 months later.

Robust effects were seen in attachment and many other outcomes for children randomly assigned from institutional care to the model of foster care used in the Bucharest Early Intervention Project (Nelson et al., 2014). The model of intervention was comprehensive, including foster parents committing to the care of their children, receiving a stipend that supported intensive involvement with the children, and receiving visits that supported parents' sensitivity.

### Harmful Interventions for Foster and Adopted Children

In parallel with these positive developments in evidence-based interventions that target specific needs of foster and adopted children, there have been various coercive interventions claiming to be attachment-based but actually using concepts that are antithetical to attachment theory. These approaches, known as *attachment therapy* or *holding therapy*, lack empirical support and indeed have led to adverse effects, as suggested by Lillienfield (2007), Pignotti and Mercer (2007), and O'Connor and Zeanah (2003). Lillienfield includes holding therapy as one of the "potentially harmful therapies (PHTs)" (p. 53) in his *Psychological Science* review. Holding therapy is included as a Level 1 PHT, classified as "probably produc[ing] harm in some individuals" (p. 59). Several deaths have been associated with the use of this treatment (Pignotti & Mercer, 2007), and no randomized clinical trials that have been conducted support its efficacy (Lillienfield, 2007). Despite claims to the contrary, holding therapy does not provide a useful basis for further developments in the design of treatments for attachment disorders in adopted or nonadopted children. This treatment is unfortunately often referred to as attachment therapy. It seems critical to differentiate it from treatments derived from attachment theory.

## Conclusions

From an evolutionary perspective, it is advantageous that the human attachment system can adapt to a range of caregiving conditions. Children can form attachment relationships to new caregivers when a previous relationship has been disrupted or after the experience of adversity. When new caregivers are nurturing, children can organize their attachment behavior in relation to the new caregivers' availability. Nonetheless, when children experience conditions that are beyond those with which the attachment system is designed to deal, it seems that rigid means of coping (e.g., disinhibited attachment) or a neurobiology that predisposes to later disorder become more likely. Interventions need to target the specific issues with which children struggle most.

## References

Ackerman, B. P., Kogos, J., Youngstrom, E., Stroff, K., & Izard, C. (1999). Family instability and the problem behaviors of children from economically disadvantaged families. *Developmental Psychology, 35*, 258–268.

Appleyard, K., Egeland, B., van Dulmen, M. H. M., & Sroufe, L. A. (2005). When more is not better: The role of cumulative risk in child behavior outcomes. *Journal of Child Psychology and Psychiatry, 46*, 235–245.

Bakermans-Kranenburg, M. J., Steele, H., Zeanah, C. H., Muhamedrahimov, R. J., Vorria, P., Dobrova-Krol, N. A., et al. (2011). Attachment and emotional development in institutional care: Characteristics and catch up. *Monographs of the Society for Research in Child Development, 76*, 62–91.

Bakermans-Kranenburg, M. J., & Van IJzendoorn, M. H. (2006). Gene–environment interaction of the dopamine D4 receptor (*DRD4*) and observed maternal insensitivity predicting externalizing behavior in preschoolers. *Developmental Psychobiology, 48*, 406–409.

Bakermans-Kranenburg, M. J., & Van IJzendoorn, M. H. (2011). Differential susceptibility to rearing environment depending on dopamine-related genes: New

evidence and a meta-analysis. *Development and Psychopathology, 23*, 39–52.

Bakermans-Kranenburg, M. J., Van IJzendoorn, M. H., Caspers, K., & Philibert, R. (2011). *DRD4* genotype moderates the impact of parental problems on unresolved loss or trauma. *Attachment and Human Development, 13*, 253–269.

Bakermans-Kranenburg, M. J., Van IJzendoorn, M. H., Mesman, J., Alink, L. R., & Juffer, F. (2008). Effects of an attachment-based intervention on daily cortisol moderated by dopamine receptor D4: A randomized control trial on 1–3-year-olds screened for externalizing behavior. *Development and Psychopathology, 20*, 805–820.

Barth, R. P. (1991). Adoption of drug-exposed children. *Children and Youth Services Review, 13*, 323–342.

Barth, R. P., & Needell, B. (1996). Outcomes for drug-exposed children four years post-adoption. *Children and Youth Services Review, 18*, 37–56.

Bates, B., & Dozier, M. (1997). *This Is My Baby Interview*. Unpublished manuscript, University of Delaware.

Beebe, B., Lachmann, F., & Jaffe, J. (1997). Mother–infant interaction structures and presymbolic self- and object representations. *Psychoanalytic Dialogues, 7*, 133–182.

Bernard, K., & Dozier, M. (2011). This is my baby: Foster parents' feelings of commitment and displays of delight. *Infant Mental Health Journal. 32*, 251–262.

Bowlby, J. (1951). *Maternal care and mental health*. Geneva: World Health Organization.

Bowlby, J. (1982). *Attachment and loss: Vol. 1: Attachment*. New York: Basic Books. (Original work published 1969)

Bretherton, I. (1985). Attachment theory: Retrospect and prospect. In I. Bretherton & E. Waters (Eds.), Growing points of attachment theory and research. *Monographs of the Society for Research in Child Development, 50*(1–2, Serial No. 209), 3–35.

Brodzinsky, D., & & Pertman, A. (2011). *Adoption by lesbians and gay men: A new dimension in family diversity*. New York: Oxford University Press.

Brooks, D., & Barth, R. P. (1998). Characteristics and outcomes of drug-exposed and non-drug exposed children in kinship and non-relative foster care. *Children and Youth Services Review, 20*, 475–501.

Carlson, E. (2002). *Attachment formation scale*. Unpublished document, University of Minnesota.

Carlson, M., & Earls, F. (1997). Psychological and neuroendocrinological sequelae of early social deprivation in institutionalized children in Romania. *Annals of the New York Academy of Sciences, 807*, 419–428.

Caspi, A., McClay, J., Moffitt, T. E., Mill, J., Martin, J., Craig, I. W., et al. (2002). Role of genotype in the cycle of violence in maltreated children. *Science, 297*, 851–854.

Caspi, A., Sugden, K., Moffitt, T. E., Taylor, A., Craig, I. W., Harrington, H., et al. (2003). Influence of life stress on depression: Moderation by a polymorphism in the *5-HTT* gene. *Science, 301,* 386–389.

Chisholm, K. (1998). A three year follow-up of attachment and indiscriminate friendliness in children adopted from Romanian orphanages. *Child Development, 69,* 1092–1106.

Chisholm, K., Carter, M. C., Ames, E. W., & Morison, S. J. (1995). Attachment security and indiscriminately friendly behavior in children adopted from Romanian orphanages. *Development and Psychopathology, 7,* 283–294.

Cicchetti, D., & Curtis, W. J. (2005). An event-related potential study of the processing of affective facial expressions in young children who experienced maltreatment during the first year of life. *Development and Psychopathology, 17,* 641–677.

Crittenden, P. M. (1985). Maltreated infants: Vulnerability and resilience. *Journal of Child Psychology and Psychiatry, 26,* 85–96.

Cuddleback, G. S. (2004). Kinship family foster care: A methodological and substantive synthesis of research. *Children and Youth Services Review, 26,* 623–639.

Dodge, K. A., Pettit, G. S., Bates, J. E., & Valente, E. (1995). Social information-processing patterns partially mediate the effect of early physical abuse on later conduct problems. *Journal of Abnormal Psychology, 104,* 632–643.

Dozier, M., Kaufman, J., Kobak, R. R., O'Connor, T. G., Sagi-Schwartz, A., Scott, S., et al. (2014). Consensus statement on group care for children and adolescents. *American Journal of Orthopsychiatry, 84*(3), 219–225.

Dozier, M., & Lindhiem, O. (2006). This is my child: Differences among foster parents in commitment to their young children. *Child Maltreatment, 11,* 338–345.

Dozier, M., Lindhiem, O., & Ackerman, J. P. (2005). Attachment and Biobehavioral Catch-Up: An intervention targeting empirically identified needs of foster infants. In L. J. Berlin, Y. Ziv, L. Amaya-Jackson, & M. T. Greenberg (Eds.), *Enhancing early attachments: Theory, research, intervention, and policy* (pp. 178–194). New York: Guilford Press.

Dozier, M., Stovall, C., Albus, K., & Bates, B. (2001). Attachment for infants in foster care: The role of caregiver state of mind. *Child Development, 72,* 1467–1477.

Duyme, M., Dumaret, A.-C., & Tomkiewicz, S. (1999). How can we boost IQs of "dull children"?: A late adoption study. *Proceedings of the National Academy of Sciences USA, 96,* 8790–8794.

Egeland, B., & Sroufe, L. A. (1981). Attachment and early maltreatment. *Child Development, 52,* 44–52.

Egeland, B., Sroufe, L. A., & Erickson, M. (1983). The developmental consequence of different patterns of maltreatment. *Child Maltreatment, 7,* 459–469.

Fisher, P. A., & Chamberlain, P. (2000). Multidimensional Treatment Foster Care: A program for inten-

sive parent training, family support, and skill building. *Journal of Emotional and Behavioral Disorders, 8,* 155–164.

George, C., Kaplan, N., & Main, M. (1984). *Adult Attachment Interview protocol.* Unpublished manuscript, University of California at Berkeley.

George, C., Kaplan, N., & Main, M. (1985). *Adult Attachment Interview protocol* (2nd ed.). Unpublished manuscript, University of California at Berkeley.

George, C., Kaplan, N., & Main, M. (1996). *Adult Attachment Interview protocol* (3rd ed.). Unpublished manuscript, University of California at Berkeley.

George, C., & Main, M. (1979). Social interactions of young abused children: Approach, avoidance, and aggression. *Child Development, 50,* 306–318.

Gianino, A., & Tronick, E. Z. (1988). The mutual regulation model: The infant's self and interactive regulation coping and defensive capacities. In T. Field, P. McCabe, & N. Schneiderman (Eds.), *Stress and coping* (pp. 47–68). Hillsdale, NJ: Erlbaum.

Gibb, B. E. (2001). Childhood maltreatment and negative cognitive styles. *Clinical Psychology Review, 22,* 223–246.

Glantz, M. D., & Chambers, J. C. (2006). Prenatal drug exposure effects on subsequent vulnerability to drug abuse. *Development and Psychopathology, 18,* 893–922.

Goldberg, A. (2010). *Lesbian and gay parents and their children: Research on the family life cycle,* Washington, DC: American Psychological Association.

Golombok, S., Mellish, L., Jennings, S., Casey, P., Tasker, F., & Lamb, M. E. (2014). Adoptive gay father families: Parent–child relationships and children's psychological adjustment. *Child Development, 85*(2), 456–468.

Goossens, F., & Van IJzendoorn, M. H. (1990). Quality of infants' attachments to professional caregivers: Relation to infant–parent attachment and daycare characteristics. *Child Development, 61,* 832–837.

Groark, C. J., Muhamedrahimov, R. J., Palmov, O. I., Nikiforova, N. V., & McCall, R. B. (2005). Improvements in early care in Russian orphanages and their relationship to observed behaviors. *Infant Mental Health Journal, 26,* 96–109.

Gunnar, M. R., Brodersen, L., Krueger, K., & Rigatuso, J. (1996). Dampening of adrenocortical responses during infancy: Normative changes and individual differences. *Child Development, 67,* 877–888.

Gunnar, M. R., Bruce, J., & Grotevant, H. D. (2000). International adoption of institutionally reared children: Research and policy. *Development and Psychopathology, 12,* 677–693.

Hale, B., & Fortin, J. (2008). Legal issues in the care and treatment of children with mental health problems. In M. Rutter, D. Bishop, D. Pine, S. Scott, J. Stevenson, & E. Taylor (Eds.), *Rutter's child and adolescent psychiatry* (5th ed.). Oxford, UK: Blackwell.

Harris, T., Brown, G. W., & Bifulco, A. (1986). Loss of parent in childhood and adult psychiatric disorder:

The role of lack of adequate parental care. *Psychological Medicine, 16,* 641–659.

Hesse, E., & Main, M. (2006). Frightening, threatening, and dissociative behavior in low-risk parents: Description, discussion, and interpretations. *Development and Psychopathology, 18,* 309–343.

Hinde, R. A., & McGinnis, L. (1977). Some factors influencing the effects of temporary mother–infant separation: Some experiments with rhesus monkeys. *Psychological Medicine, 7,* 197–212.

Hoffman, K. T., Marvin, R. S., Cooper, G., & Powell, B. (2006). Changing toddlers' and preschoolers' attachment classifications: The Circle of Security intervention. *Journal of Consulting and Clinical Psychology, 74,* 1017–1026.

Howe, D., & Feast, J. (2001). The long-term outcome of reunions between adult adopted people and their birth mothers. *British Journal of Social Work, 31,* 351–368.

Howes, C., & Hamilton, C. E. (1992). Children's relationships with child care teachers: Stability and concordance with parental attachments. *Child Development, 63,* 867–878.

Institute of Medicine (IOM). (2013). *New directions in child abuse and neglect research.* Washington DC: National Academies Press.

Johnson, D., Albers, L., Iverson, S., Mathers, M., Dole, K., Georgieff, M., et al. (1996). Health status of U.S. adopted Eastern European (EE) orphans. *Pediatric Research, 39,* 134.

Juffer, F., Hoksbergen, R. A. C., Riksen-Walraven, J. M., & Kohnstamm, G. A. (1997). Early intervention in adoptive families: Supporting maternal sensitive responsiveness, infant–mother attachment, and infant competence. *Journal of Child Psychology and Psychiatry, 38,* 1039–1050.

Kaufman, J., Yang, B., Douglas-Palumberi, H., Grasso, D., Lipschitz, D., Houshyar, S., et al. (2006). Brain-derived neurotrophic factor–5-HHTLPR gene interactions and environmental modifiers of depression in children. *Biological Psychiatry, 59,* 673–680.

Kaufman, J., Yang, B., Douglas-Palumberi, H., Houshyar, S., Lipschitz, D., Krystal, J. H., et al. (2004). Social supports and serotonin transporter gene moderate depression in maltreated children. *Proceedings of the National Academy of Sciences USA, 101,* 17316–17321.

Keiley, M. K., Howe, T. R., Dodge, K. A., Bates, J. E., & Pettit, G. S. (2001). The timing of child physical maltreatment: A cross-domain growth analysis of impact on adolescent externalizing and internalizing problems. *Development and Psychopathology, 13,* 891–912.

Levine, S., Johnson, D. F., & Gonzalez, C. A. (1985). Behavioral and hormonal responses to separation in infant Rhesus monkeys and mothers. *Behavioral Neuroscience, 99,* 399–410.

Levine, S., Weiner, S. G., & Coe, C. L. (1993). Temporal and social factors influencing behavioral and hormonal responses to separation in mother and in-

fant squirrel monkeys. *Psychoneuroendocrinology, 4,* 297–306.

Lewis-Morrarty, E., Dozier, M., Bernard, K., Terracciano, S., & Moore, S. (2012). Cognitive flexibility and theory of mind outcomes among foster children: Preschool follow-up results of a randomized clinical trial. *Journal of Adolescent Health, 52,* S17–S22.

Lieberman, A. F., Ghosh Ippen, C., & Van Horn, P. (2006). Child–parent psychotherapy: 6-month follow-up of a randomized controlled trial. *Journal of the American Academy of Child and Adolescent Psychiatry, 45,* 913–918.

Lillienfeld, S. O. (2007). Psychological treatments that cause harm. *Psychological Science, 2,* 53–70.

Lyons-Ruth, K., Alpern, L., & Repacholi, B. (1993). Disorganized infant attachment classification and maternal psychosocial problems as predictors of hostile-aggressive behavior in the preschool classroom. *Child Development, 64,* 572–585.

Maestripieri, D. (2005). Early experience affects the intergenerational transmission of infant abuse in rhesus monkeys. *Proceedings of the National Academy of Sciences USA, 102,* 9726–9719.

Milan, S. E., & Pinderhughes, E. E. (2000). Factors influencing maltreated children's early adjustment in foster care. *Development and Psychopathology, 12,* 63–81.

Nelson, C. A., Fox, N. A., & Zeanah, C. H. (2014). *Romania's abandoned children: Deprivation, brain development and the struggle for recovery.* Cambridge, MA: Harvard University Press.

Numan, M. J., & Insel, T. R. (2003). *The neurobiology of parental behavior* (3rd ed.). New York: Springer.

O'Connor, T. G., Rutter, M., & the English and Romanian Adoptees Study Team. (2000). Attachment disorder behaviour following early severe deprivation: Extension and longitudinal follow-up. *Journal of the American Academy of Child and Adolescent Psychiatry, 39,* 703–712.

O'Connor, T. G., & Zeanah, C. (2003). Attachment disorders: Assessment strategies and treatment approaches. *Attachment and Human Development, 5,* 223–244.

Piaget, J. (2000). Childhood cognitive development: The essential readings. In K. Lee (Ed.), *Essential readings in cognitive development* (pp. 33–47). Oxford, UK: Blackwell.

Pignotti, M., & Mercer, J. (2007). Holding therapy and dyadic developmental psychotherapy are not supported and acceptable social work interventions: A systematic research synthesis revisited. *Research on Social Work Practice, 17,* 513–519.

Pollak, S. D., & Tolley-Schell, S. A. (2003). Selective attention to facial emotion in physically abused children. *Journal of Abnormal Psychology, 112,* 323–338.

Powell, B., Cooper, G., Hoffman, K., & Marvin, B. (2013). *The Circle of Security Intervention: Enhancing attachment in early parent–child relationships.* New York: Guilford Press.

Rajecki, D. W., Lamb, M. E., & Obmascher, P. (1978). Toward a general theory of infantile attachment: A comparative review of aspects of the social bond. *Behavioral and Brain Sciences, 3,* 417–464.

Roth, T. L., & Sullivan, R. M. (2005). Memory of early maltreatment: Neonatal behavioral and neuronal correlates of maternal maltreatment within the context of classical conditioning. *Biological Psychiatry, 57,* 823–831.

Rutter, M. (2006). *Genes and behavior: Nature–nurture interplay explained.* Oxford, UK: Blackwell.

Rutter, M., Colvert, E., Kreppner, J., Beckett, C., Castle, J., Groothues, C., et al. (2007). Early adolescent outcomes for institutionally-deprived and non-deprived adoptees: I. Disinhibited attachment. *Journal of Child Psychology and Psychiatry, 48,* 17–30.

Rutter, M., Kreppner, J. M., & O'Connor, T. G. (2001). Specificity and heterogeneity in children's responses to profound institutional privation. *British Journal of Psychiatry, 179,* 97–103.

Rutter, M., Moffitt, T. E., & Caspi, A. (2006). Gene–environment interplay and psychopathology: Multiple varieties by real effects. *Journal of Child Psychology and Psychiatry, 47,* 226–261.

Sameroff, A. J., Bartko, W. T., Baldwin, A., Baldwin, C., & Seifer, R. (1998). Family and social influences on the development of child competence. In M. Lewis & C. Feiring (Eds.), *Families, risk, and competence* (pp. 161–185). Mahwah, NJ: Erlbaum.

Sanchez, M. M., Ladd, C. O., & Plotsky, P. M. (2001). Early adverse experience as a developmental risk factor for later psychopathology: Evidence from rodent and primate models. *Development and Psychopathology, 13,* 419–449.

Savage, J., Brodsky, N. L., Malmud, E., Giannetta, J. M., & Hurt, H. (2005). Attentional functioning and impulse control in cocaine-exposed and control children at age ten years. *Journal of Developmental and Behavioral Pediatrics, 26,* 42–47.

Sinclair, I., & Wilson, K. (2003). Matches and mismatches: The contribution of carers and children to the success of foster placements. *British Journal of Social Work, 33,* 871–884.

Smith, M. G., & Fong, R. (2004). *The children of neglect: When no one cares.* New York: Brunner-Routledge.

Spertus, I. L., Yehuda, R., Wong, C. M., Halligan, S., & Seremetis, S. V. (2003). Childhood emotional abuse and neglect as predictors of psychological and physical symptoms in women presenting to a primary care practice. *Child Abuse and Neglect, 27,* 1247–1258.

Spieker, S. J., Oxford, M. L., Kelly, J. F., Nelson, E. M., & Fleming, C. B. (2012). Promoting First Relationships: Randomized trial of a relationship-based intervention for toddlers in child welfare. *Child Welfare, 17,* 271–286.

Spitz, R. (1945). Hospitalism: An inquiry into the genesis of psychiatric conditions in early childhood. *Psychoanalytic Study of the Child, 1,* 53–74.

Sroufe, L. A., Egeland, B., Carlson, E. A., & Collins, W. A. (2005). *The development of the person: The Minnesota Study of Risk and Adaptation from Birth to Adulthood.* New York: Guilford Press.

Stern, D. N. (2002). *The first relationship: Infant and mother.* Cambridge, MA: Harvard University Press.

Stevens, S., Sonuga-Barke, E., Asherson, P., Kreppner, J., & Rutter, M. (2006). A consideration of the potential role of genetic factors in individual differences in response to early institutional deprivation: The case of inattention/overactivity in the English and Romanian Adoptees Study. *ACAMH Occasional Papers: Genetics, 25,* 63–76.

Stovall, K. C., & Dozier, M. (2000). The development of attachment in new relationships: Single subject analyses for 10 foster infants. *Development and Psychopathology, 12,* 133–156.

Stovall-McClough, K. C., & Dozier, M. (2004). Forming attachments in foster care: Infant attachment behaviors during the first 2 months of placement. *Development and Psychopathology, 16,* 253–271.

St. Petersburg–USA Orphanage Research Team. (2008). The effects of early social emotional and relationship experience on the development of young orphanage children. *Monographs of the Society for Research in Child Development, 73,* 1–262.

Suomi, S. J. (2003). Gene–environment interactions and the neurobiology of social conflict. *Annals of the New York Academy of Sciences, 1008,* 132–139.

Suomi, S. J., & Harlow, H. F. (1972). Social rehabilitation of isolate-reared monkeys. *Developmental Psychology, 6,* 487–496.

Suomi, S. J., Harlow, H. F., & McKinney, W. T. (1972). Monkey psychiatrists. *American Journal of Psychiatry, 128,* 927–932.

Tizard, B., & Hodges, J. (1978). The effect of early institutional rearing on the development of eight year old children. *Journal of Child Psychology and Psychiatry, 19,* 99–118.

Tizard, B., & Rees, J. (1975). The effect of early institutional rearing on the behavioral problems and affectional relationships of four-year-old children. *Journal of Child Psychology and Psychiatry, 27,* 61–73.

Triseliotis, J., Feast, J., & Kyle, F. (2005). *The adoption triangle revisited: A study of adoption, search and reunion experiences.* London: British Association for Adoption and Fostering.

United Nations International Children's Emergency Fund (UNICEF). (2013). *End placing children under three years in institutions. A call to action.* Geneva: Author.

U.S. Department of Health and Human Services, Administration for Children and Families, Children's Bureau. (2015, May 15). *A national look at the use of congregate care in child welfare.* Available at http://www.acf.hhs.gov/sites/default/files/cb/cbcongregatecare_brief.pdf.

U.S. Department of Health and Human Services, Administration on Children, Youth and Families.

(2013). *Trends in foster care and adoption.* Washington, DC: U.S. Government Printing Office.

U.S. Department of State. (2013). International adoption. Retrieved from *http://adoption.state.gov/about_us/statistics.php.*

Van IJzendoorn, M. H., & Juffer, F. (2006). The Emanual Miller Memorial Lecture 2006: Adoption as intervention: Meta-analytic evidence for massive catch-up and plasticity in physical, socio-emotional and cognitive development. *Journal of Child Psychology and Psychiatry, 47,* 1228–1245.

Van IJzendoorn, M. H., Schuengel, C., & Bakermans-Kranenburg, M. J. (1999). Disorganized attachment in early childhood: Meta-analysis of precursors, concomitants, and sequelae. *Development and Psychopathology, 11,* 225–249.

Vorria, P., Ntouma, M., Vairami, M., & Rutter, M. (2015). Attachment relationships of adolescents who spent their infancy in residential group care: The Greek Metera study. *Attachment and Human Development, 17*(3), 257–271.

Vorria, P., Papaligoura, Z., Dunn, J., Van IJzendoorn, M. H., Steele, H., Kontopoulou, A., et al. (2003). Early experiences and attachment relationships of Greek infants raised in residential group care. *Journal of Child Psychology and Psychiatry, 44,* 1–13.

Vorria, P., Papaligoura, Z., Sarafidou, J., Kopakaki, M., Dunn, J., Van IJzendoorn, M. H., et al. (2006). The development of adopted children after institutional care: A follow-up study. *Journal of Child Psychology and Psychiatry, 47,* 1246–1253.

Wakschlag, L. S., & Hans, S. L. (2002). Maternal smoking during pregnancy and conduct problems in high-risk youth: A developmental framework. *Development and Psychopathology, 12,* 351–369.

Waters, E., & Deane, K. E. (1985). Defining and assessing individual differences in attachment relationships: Q-methodology and the organization of behavior in infancy and early childhood. In I. Bretherton & E. Waters (Eds.), Growing points of attachment theory and research. *Monographs of the Society for Research in Child Development, 50*(1–2, Serial No. 209), 41–65.

Weinfield, N. S., Sroufe, L. A., & Egeland, B. (2000). Attachment from infancy to early adulthood in a high-risk sample: Continuity, discontinuity, and their correlates. *Child Development, 71,* 695–702.

Zeanah, C. H., Larrieu, J. A., Heller, S. S., Valliere, J., Hinshaw-Fuselier, S., Aoki, Y, et al. (2001). Evaluation of a preventive intervention for maltreated infants and toddlers in foster care. *Journal of the American Academy of Child and Adolescent Psychiatry, 40,* 214–221.

Zeanah, C. H., & Smyke, A. T. (2005). Building attachment relationships following maltreatment and severe deprivation. In L. J. Berlin, Y. Ziv, L. Amaya-Jackson, & M. T. Greenberg (Eds.), *Enhancing early attachments: Theory, research, intervention, and policy* (pp. 195–216). New York: Guilford Press.

Zeanah, C. H., Smyke, A. T., Koga, S. F., Carlson, E., & the Bucharest Early Intervention Project Core Group. (2005). Attachment in institutionalized and community children in Romania. *Child Development, 76,* 1015–1028.

# Chapter 31

# Attachment States of Mind and Psychopathology in Adulthood

## K. Chase Stovall-McClough
## Mary Dozier

Bowlby (1969/1982, 1973, 1980) proposed a model of development with clearly articulated implications for psychopathology. According to this model, an infant's formation of an attachment to a caregiver is a key developmental task that not only influences the child's representations of self and other but also affects strategies for processing attachment-related thoughts and feelings. Attachment-related events, such as loss and abuse, lead to modifications in these internal representations and affect a child's strategies for processing thoughts and feelings. Bowlby (1973, 1980) suggested that when children develop negative representations of themselves or others, or when they adopt strategies for processing attachment-related thoughts and feelings that compromise realistic appraisals, they become more vulnerable to psychopathology. In this chapter, we consider how the quality of an infant's attachment to his or her caregiver, subsequent attachment-related experiences, and concurrently assessed states of mind with respect to attachment (Main, Goldwyn, & Hesse, 2003) may be related to risk for psychopathology or to psychological resilience in adulthood.

## Infant Attachment and Later Psychopathology

When infants' experiences lead to expectations that caregivers will be responsive to their needs,

they develop secure strategies for seeking out their caregivers when distressed or in need, with the expectation that their needs will be met. Insecure strategies vary primarily along the dimension of attempts to minimize or maximize the expression of attachment needs. When children use minimizing strategies, they defensively turn attention away from their distress and from issues of caregiver availability. They therefore have limited access to their own feelings and develop an unrealistic portrayal of parents' availability. When children use maximizing strategies, they defensively turn their attention to their own distress and to issues of caregiver availability. Because they are so "enmeshed" (Main et al., 2003) in issues of caregiver availability, they are unable to appraise accurately whether threats exist and whether caregivers are available. Either of these strategies may leave children at increased risk for psychopathology. Minimizing strategies may predispose a child to externalizing disorders because attention is turned away from the self, without the resolution of negative representations. Maximizing strategies may predispose a child to internalizing disorders because attention is riveted on caregiver availability and negative representations remain painfully alive.

Sroufe (e.g., 1997, 2005; Sroufe, Egeland, Carlson, & Collins, 2005b) have emphasized the importance of the organizational function of the attachment system in integrating affective, motivational, and behavioral components of experience. In this model, adaptations to early experiences set the stage for negotiating later experiences. Adult psychopathology is placed in a developmental context, with an emphasis on the interactions among prior experience, subsequent adaptation, and current contextual factors (Carlson, Egeland, & Sroufe, 2009). The quality of attachment in childhood can have both a direct impact on adult functioning and be modified by adaptations to caregiving experiences to predict typical or atypical development.

## Overview of the Chapter

A number of longitudinal studies have examined links between infant attachment and adult psychopathology (Dutra & Lyons-Ruth, 2005; Englund, Kuo, Puig, & Collins, 2011; Grossmann, Grossmann, & Waters, 2005; Lyons-Ruth, Bureau, Holmes, Easterbrooks, & Brooks, 2013; Shi, Bureau, Easterbrooks, Zhao, & Lyons-Ruth, 2012; Sroufe et al., 2005a, 2005b). In this chapter, we consider evidence from these longitudinal studies and cast our net more broadly to consider associations between attachment-relevant events in childhood (e.g., loss, trauma, and separation from parents) and later psychopathology. In addition, we examine the association between concurrently assessed attachment states of mind as assessed by the Adult Attachment Interview (AAI; George, Kaplan, & Main, 1985; Main et al., 2003) and psychopathology.

We consider specific disorders with regard to the importance of attachment as an etiological factor (with highly heritable disorders less influenced by attachment), and the extent to which disorders represent an internalizing versus an externalizing symptom picture. We start with mood disorders, followed by anxiety disorders. Both of these groups of disorders are heterogeneous with regard to heritability and symptomatology; therefore, it would be surprising if clear findings emerged with regard to attachment-related issues without further specification of parameters. We move from there to a discussion of dissociative disorders. The evidence linking attachment in infancy and attachment-related traumas to later dissociative symptoms and concurrent states of mind with dissociative symptoms converge to form a compelling picture. We consider eating disorders next; these disorders are often comorbid with personality disorders and mood disorders. We then turn our attention to

schizophrenia, a disorder that is highly heritable. From there, we move to a consideration of two of the most prevalent personality disorders: borderline personality disorder and antisocial personality disorder.

For each disorder or group of disorders considered, we begin with a general description of the disorder(s) and the latest evidence regarding genetic involvement. We then discuss attachment theory's contributions to an understanding of the disorder(s). From there we move to a consideration of the empirical evidence linking attachment phenomena to the disorder(s). We include the latest findings and consider them in light of our hypotheses outlined in earlier versions of the chapter in previous editions. Finally, we present the most recent data on links between infant attachment and adult psychopathology, and discuss changes in the state of the field.

## Mood Disorders

Unipolar and bipolar mood disorders differ considerably with respect to symptomatology, genetic involvement, course, and the probable role of attachment in their etiology. A large meta-analysis of twin studies found lifetime heritability of major depression to be 37% (Sullivan, Neale, & Kendler 2000). The heritability of major depressive disorder, however, is linearly related to severity, with more severe depression (defined by earlier onset and recurrence) more heritable than less severe depression (Bienvenu, Davydow, & Kendler, 2011). Bipolar disorders are highly heritable, with rates estimated to be as high as 85% (e.g., Bienvenu et al., 2011). There has been little attention paid to the developmental context of bipolar disorder. According to Parry (2010), no studies to date have examined the role of attachment, and few have considered the role of abuse and early trauma. Thus, we focus below on the role of attachment in later depression.

The heterogeneous nature of depression is important to consider in relation to attachment. First, severity seems to be an important dimension to consider (Brown & Harris, 1993), with some suggesting that a "disease-like endogenous" form of the disorder is more heritable than a "neurotic" form driven by environmental and personality vulnerabilities (Bienvenu et al., 2011). Second, the differential reliance on internalizing versus externalizing coping strategies is important, and is central to states of mind with respect to attachment. Some people with unipolar disorders show predominantly internalizing symptoms, with self-blame and self-deprecation primary. Others show a preponderance of externalizing symptoms, with interpersonal hostility primary. Preoccupied states of mind, which involve a preoccupation with one's own thoughts and feelings, are consistent with internalizing symptoms. On the other hand, dismissing states of mind, which involve a turning away from one's own distress, are consistent with externalizing symptoms.

## Attachment and Mood Disorder: Theoretical Links

Bowlby (1980) suggested that three major circumstances are most likely to be associated with the later development of depression. First, when a child's parent dies, and the child experiences little control over ensuing events, he or she is likely to develop a sense of hopelessness and despair in reaction to traumatic events. Second, when a child is unable to form stable and secure relationships with caregivers, he or she develops a model of the self as a failure. Any subsequent loss or disappointment is then likely to be perceived as reflecting that the child is a failure. Third, when a parent gives a child the message that he or she is incompetent or unlovable, the child develops complementary models of the self as unlovable and of others as unloving (Bretherton, 1985). Thus, the child and later the adult will expect hostility and rejection from others when he or she is in need. Cummings and Cicchetti (1990) have suggested that these experiences of having a psychologically unavailable parent are similar to the experience of actually losing a caregiver, in that the child experiences frequent or even chronic losses of the parent. Each of the sets of circumstances specified by Bowlby involves a sense of uncontrollability on the part of the child and is compatible with Seligman's learned helplessness theory of depression (Seligman, Abramson, Semmel, & von Baeyer, 1979).

## Children's Attachment-Related Experiences and Later Depression

The circumstances Bowlby proposed as central to the development of depression have received strong empirical support. Insecure attachment (both resistant and avoidant) predicts depression in adolescence (Duggal, Carlson, Sroufe, & Ege-

land, 2001), though to our knowledge those findings have not yet been extended to adulthood. Moreover, several studies provide converging evidence that the death of a parent in early childhood puts an individual at risk for later depression (e.g., Harris, Brown, & Bifulco, 1990; Kivela, Luukinin, Koski, Viramo, & Pahkala, 1998; Nickerson, Bryant, Aderka, Hinton, & Hofmann, 2013; Takeuchi et al., 2003). Harris and colleagues (1990) found that risk for later depression increased when the loss occurred before age 11 and involved the death of (vs. long-term separation from) a parent. Bowlby (1980) suggested that the death of a child's mother may well lead to a sense of total despair, whereas separation from the mother may lead to a belief that events are reversible.

Just as important as the loss itself are the child's subsequent experiences with caregivers (Harris, Brown, & Bifulco, 1986; Kendler, Sheth, Gardner, & Prescott, 2002; Nickerson et al., 2013; Oakley-Browne, Joyce, Wells, Bushnell, & Hornblow, 1995). Harris and colleagues (1986) found that inadequate care following the loss doubled the risk of depression in adulthood, particularly in cases of separation rather than death. More recently, Nickerson and colleagues (2013) found that adverse parenting following the early death of a parent was associated with increased risk for depression, as well as a multitude of other disorders in adulthood.

## Attachment States of Mind and Depression

Main and colleagues (2003) have proposed that different attachment states of mind are associated with different patterns of processing attachment-related thoughts, feelings, and memories. Secure *autonomous* transcripts are characterized by coherence; the speaker's representation of attachment experiences is straightforward, clear, and consistent with evidence presented. Insecure *nonautonomous* transcripts fall into several categories, including "dismissing," "preoccupied," "unresolved with respect to loss or trauma," and "cannot classify." A lack of recall, idealization of caregivers, and/or derogation of attachment experiences characterize dismissing transcripts. Preoccupied transcripts are characterized by current angry involvement with attachment figures or by passive speech, such as rambling discourse (Main et al., 2003). The category *unresolved* is used for transcripts in which the speaker experiences lapses in reasoning or lapses in monitoring of discourse regarding a loss or trauma. When an unresolved classification is given, a secondary classification (of autonomous, preoccupied, or dismissing) is also made.

The *cannot classify* category represents a mixture, or shifting, of information-processing strategies that are inconsistent with one another. For example, the individual may describe one parent in a highly dismissing way and relate incidents of distress concerning the other parent in an enmeshed way. The cannot classify category has been associated with high rates of psychopathology (e.g., Allen, Hauser, & Borman-Spurrell, 1996; Hesse, Hobson, Patrick, Maughan, & Main, 2011; Holtzworth-Munroe, Stuart, & Hutchinson, 1997; Riggs et al., 2007), but sample sizes are rarely large enough to examine associations between this category and specific forms of psychopathology. (See Hesse, Chapter 26, this volume, for a more detailed description of the AAI.)

In versions of this chapter in previous editions of this volume, we called attention to the inconsistent findings regarding the association between states of mind and depressive disorders, with some studies reporting depression associated with preoccupied states of mind (Cole-Detke & Kobak, 1996; Fonagy et al., 1996; Rosenstein & Horowitz, 1996), but others reporting depression associated more closely with dismissing states of mind (Patrick, Hobson, Castle, Howard, & Maughan, 1994). Such discrepant findings continue to appear in the literature. Borelli, Goshin, Joestl, Clark, and Byrne (2010) examined self-reported depressive symptoms and attachment state of mind in a sample of incarcerated women, and Ivarsson, Granqvist, Gillberg, and Broberg (2010) looked at attachment state of mind in a clinical sample of adolescents. Similar to Cole-Detke and Kobak (1996), Fonagy and colleagues (1996), and Rosenstein and Horowitz (1996), Borelli and colleagues found depressive symptomatology to be more highly associated with preoccupied states of mind than with secure or dismissing states of mind. On the other hand, Ivarsson and colleagues found that over half of the sample of outpatient depressed adolescents (64%) was classified as dismissing in a forced three-way distribution of secure, insecure/dismissing, and insecure/preoccupied.

Consistent with the point made by Sroufe and colleagues (2005a), we suggest that there may be systematic differences on the internalizing–externalizing dimension in the groups labeled as "depressed" in these studies, and that these may account for the discrepancies in findings. In the Rosenstein and Horowitz (1996) study, ado-

lescents who had been admitted to a psychiatric hospital were separated into three groups: a "pure affective disorder" group, which excluded those with comorbid conduct disorder, a conduct disorder group, and a comorbid group. Thus, adolescents in the pure affective disorder group excluded people who showed externalizing symptoms of conduct disorder but did not exclude those who were comorbid for a more internalizing disorder. They were classified as having preoccupied states of mind significantly more often than those in the comorbid or the conduct disorder group. More specifically, 69% of the pure affective disorder group was classified as preoccupied, whereas 25% of the comorbid group and 14% of the conduct disorder group were classified as preoccupied.

Cole-Detke and Kobak (1996) examined the states of mind of women who reported depressive symptoms, eating disorder symptoms, both types of symptoms, or neither type. The distribution of women who reported only depressed symptoms was relatively even across the three categories of attachment. Although depressed women were classified as preoccupied more often than were women with eating disorders, the majority fell into categories other than preoccupied. Again, the criteria for the depressed group excluded at least some with comorbid externalizing, but not internalizing, symptoms.

In Borelli and colleagues' (2010) study of incarcerated women residing with their infants, change in depression over the first year of incarceration was assessed. The sample as a whole was rated as primarily nonautonomous, with similar proportions of dismissing and preoccupied states of mind (28% dismissing, 32% preoccupied, and 40% unresolved in a four-way distribution). However, preoccupied states of mind were associated with increases in depression over the first year of incarceration. The sample excluded those incarcerated for violent offenses (and presumably those with externalizing behaviors).

Patrick and colleagues (1994) limited their depressed group to women inpatients without any borderline personality disorder symptomatology, thus excluding some with internalizing symptomatology. They assessed the states of mind of 24 female inpatients with diagnoses of either dysthymia or borderline personality disorder. Women were included in the dysthymic group only if they met none of the criteria for borderline personality disorder. The distribution of states of mind was significantly different for the two groups. All of the women in the borderline group were classified as preoccupied, as contrasted with 50% of those in the dysthymic group.

In Ivarsson and colleagues' (2010) study of outpatient adolescents with depression (*n* = 100), over half of the sample (64%) was classified as dismissing in a forced three-way distribution. With the five-way classification breakdown (secure, dismissing, preoccupied, unresolved, and cannot classify) 28% were classified as cannot classify and 40% were classified as unresolved. The sample included those with depression and comorbid obsessive–compulsive disorder (OCD), which may account for the high percentage of dismissing states of mind because OCD encompasses extreme efforts to avoid the internal experience of anxiety.

Given that the experience of loss is hypothesized to be a significant vulnerability factor for depression, it follows that people with unipolar mood disorders may be unresolved with respect to loss. In the several studies that have examined unresolved status among depressed people, the results have been inconsistent. In Fonagy and colleagues' (1996) large sample of inpatients, 72% of people with depression were classified as unresolved, compared with 18% in Rosenstein and Horowitz's (1996) adolescent inpatient sample and 16% of Patrick and colleagues' (1994) outpatient sample.

Fonagy and colleagues (1996) found that different subtypes of depression were differentially related to states of mind. Compared with dysthymia, major depression in this study was more often associated with autonomous states of mind. Fonagy and colleagues suggested that these findings could be attributable to the episodic nature of major depression. Major depression may not interfere with the maintenance of coherent states of mind as pervasively as chronic dysthymia does. Another possibility is that major depression is more heritable than dysthymia, so that it takes less unfavorable caregiving for the disorder to emerge.

These various findings point to the importance of diagnostic issues when one is considering linkages between attachment states of mind and mood disorders. Several distinctions among the unipolar mood disorders appear important. Compared with dysthymia, major depression is less frequently associated with autonomous states of mind. Within the categories of major depressive disorder and dysthymia, we suggest that differences in the extent to which disorders are self-blaming (internalizing) versus other-blaming (externalizing) are important in terms of states of mind. A related issue is comorbidity. Although a diagnosis of unipolar mood disorder may not provide evidence of the extent to which symptoms are internalizing or externalizing, other comorbid diagnoses (e.g.,borderline personality disorder, eating disorders, and particular anxiety disorders such as OCD) may provide such evidence. Several studies have highlighted how important it is to consider comorbid diagnoses in analyses.

## Anxiety Disorders

Similar to mood disorders, anxiety disorders are quite heterogeneous. Most, however, are characterized by a combination of anxiety and an effort to avoid the anxiety. When anxiety or fear predominates, the disorder typically involves internalizing symptoms, whereas when avoidance predominates, the disorder typically involves externalizing symptoms. As discussed previously, strategies that maximize the expression of attachment needs are expected to be associated with more internalizing disorders, and strategies that minimize the expression of attachment needs are expected to be associated with more externalizing disorders. The disorder in which fear most clearly predominates is generalized anxiety disorder (GAD). Individuals who have this disorder experience chronic ruminative anxiety regarding at least several life circumstances and there is little ability to stop or avoid the anxiety. Interestingly, however, newer models of GAD have reconceptualized the role of worry in the maintenance of the disorder, suggesting that worry itself serves as a method of *avoiding* conflict, social engagement, and negative internal states (Borkovec, Alcaine, & Behar, 2004; Mennin, Heimberg, Turk, & Fresco, 2002). Panic attacks are also characterized primarily by fear, but avoidance of triggers for panic is an important component of panic disorder. Similarly, phobic disorders (including specific phobia, social phobia, and agoraphobia) are characterized by fear when the individual does not successfully avoid the feared stimulus, but avoidance often predominates. In OCD, fear is experienced to the extent that the individual does not engage in self-prescribed compulsive behaviors. Posttraumatic stress disorder (PTSD) is characterized by vacillation between (1) emotional numbing and efforts to avoid reminders of the trauma, and (2) fear and anxiety associated with reexperiencing the trauma. Underlying this emotional instability is a generalized hypervigilance. It is the vacillation between avoidance and overwhelming fear that characterizes this disorder.

Comorbidity of anxiety disorders with other diagnoses is common; in particular, anxiety disorders and depressive disorders often co-occur (Hettema, Neale, & Kendler, 2001; Kendler, Heath, Martin, & Eaves, 1987). The estimates of heritability of anxiety disorders vary from study to study, but twin studies suggest between 20 and 40% heritability (Hettema et al., 2001; Hettema, Prescott, Myers, Neale, & Kendler, 2005). A meta-analysis by Hettema and colleagues (2001) found similar heritability across most mood disorders. Furthermore, there is no evidence that one anxiety disorder has a stronger genetic basis than another (Walter et al., 2013).

## Attachment and Anxiety Disorders: Theoretical Links

Bowlby (1973) proposed that all forms of anxiety disorders (with the exception of specific animal phobias) are best accounted for by early anxiety regarding the availability of the attachment figure. Several types of family environments were specified as most likely to create a real or perceived threat of parental loss. Included among these are family environments in which a child worries about a parent's survival in the child's absence or about being rejected or abandoned, when the child feels the need to remain home as a companion to a parent, and environments in which a parent has difficulty letting the child go because of overwhelming feelings that harm will come to the child.

## Infant Attachment and Later Anxiety Disorders

The Minnesota Study of Risk and Adaptation from Birth to Adulthood (Bosquet & Egeland, 2006; Warren, Huston, Egeland, & Sroufe, 1997) examined the association between attachment in infancy and later anxiety disorders. Anxiety disorders were diagnosed when children were 17½. Infants with resistant attachments were significantly more likely than infants with secure or avoidant attachments to be diagnosed with anxiety disorders as adolescents. Warren and colleagues also assessed whether this relation between resistant attachment and anxiety disorders was attributable to temperamental differences, as indicated by neonatal nurse ratings of reactivity (Terreira, 1960) as

well as the Neonatal Behavioral Assessment Scale (Brazelton, 1973). Even when researchers controlled for differences in temperament, resistant attachments emerged as significant predictors of later anxiety disorders.

In another longitudinal sample of low-risk children, infant attachment security was also found to be associated with anxiety symptoms at age 11. Bar-Haim, Dan, Eshel, and Sagi-Schwartz (2007) found that resistant attachment in particular predicted elevated levels of social phobia, as reported by parents and children, especially for boys. They noted, however, that the symptoms did not reach clinical significance.

## Children's Attachment-Related Experiences and Later Anxiety Disorder

Consistent with Bowlby's position, problematic family environments have been linked with anxiety disorders. Brown and Harris (1993) found an increased incidence of early loss of a caregiver and extremely inadequate caregiving in the histories of those with panic disorder compared to those without a psychiatric diagnosis. Faravelli, Webb, Ambonetti, Fonnesu, and Sessarego (1985) found agoraphobia to be associated with a higher incidence of early separation from mothers or parental divorce. In a larger meta-analysis, de Ruiter and Van IJzendoorn (1992) examined the association between early childhood separation anxiety and later agoraphobia. They found that adults with agoraphobia reported more childhood separation anxiety than controls, but were not more likely to suffer from separation anxiety disorder as children. Adults with agoraphobia were also more likely to rate their parents as low on affection and high on overprotection than controls. de Ruiter and Van IJzendoorn argued that this provided indirect support of Bowlby's hypothesized association between ambivalent (resistant) infant attachment and later agoraphobia.

Anxiety disorders in adulthood are also linked with retrospective accounts of negative views of caregiving experiences. Cassidy (1995) examined the cognitive processing characteristics of those with GAD and found they reported more rejection by their parents and role reversal than people without GAD. Similarly, Chambless, Gillis, Tran, and Steketee (1996) found that most people with anxiety disorders described their parents as unloving and controlling. Specific anxiety disorder diagnosis (OCD vs. panic disorder with agoraphobia) was not differentially associated with parental care (Chambless et al., 1996).

Bandelow and colleagues (2002) compared histories of patients with panic disorder ($n$ = 115) and normal controls ($n$ = 124). Based on retrospective report, the patients with panic disorder had experienced significantly more traumatic early life events, including parental death and separation, than adults without panic disorder. Such individuals also reported more parental restriction and less love than controls. In a study of adults with social anxiety disorder (social phobia), Bandelow and colleagues (2004) obtained similar results and concluded that, beyond a family history of mental illness, separation experiences in childhood were among the most important contributing factors to adult social anxiety. In these retrospective studies, it is not possible to disentangle the potential biasing effect of concurrent anxiety on recollection of caregiving experiences.

## Attachment States of Mind and Anxiety Disorders

In line with findings that resistant infant attachment is predictive of later anxiety symptoms, preoccupied states of mind have been found to be overrepresented in adults with anxiety disorders. Of adolescents with clinically elevated scores on the Anxiety scale of the Millon Multiaxial Personality Inventory (Millon, 1983), 65% had preoccupied states of mind (Rosenstein & Horowitz, 1996). Similarly, Fonagy and colleagues (1996) found that most adults with anxiety disorders were classified as preoccupied in the three-category system. Cassidy (1995) found that, contrasted with people without symptoms of GAD, those with GAD reported greater anger and vulnerability on the Perceptions of Adult Attachment Questionnaire (PAAQ; Lichtenstein & Cassidy, 1991). Feelings of anger and vulnerability are consistent with preoccupied states of mind.

In a few studies, unresolved loss and trauma has been overrepresented in those with anxiety disorders. In a small sample ($n$ = 18) of women diagnosed with a variety of anxiety disorders including panic, OCD, and GAD, Manassis, Bradley, Goldberg, Hood, and Swinson (1994) found that all were classified as nonautonomous, with 78% rated as unresolved. Because of the small sample size, it was not possible to analyze relations between specific anxiety disorders and attachment state of mind. Fonagy and colleagues (1996) found

that 86% of the sample of adults with mixed anxiety disorders was classified as unresolved. Brumariu, Obsuth, and Lyons-Ruth (2013) examined 109 adolescents with various DSM-IV Axis I disorders. Comparing those with anxiety disorders (including panic, phobias, PTSD, GAD, and OCD) to those without anxiety disorders (but diagnosed with other DSM IV Axis I disorders), adolescents were rated on a scale of incoherence from 1 to 3 based on AAI classifications. Those with anxiety disorders showed higher levels of overall disorganization or incoherence compared to adolescents without anxiety disorders.

Moving beyond studies that cut across the anxiety disorders, there is some support for the idea that specific anxiety disorders involving primarily avoidance of fear are most often associated with dismissing states of mind. Zeijlmans van Emmichoven, Van IJzendoorn, de Ruiter, and Brosschot (2003) examined attachment state of mind among 28 adults with anxiety disorders and 56 adult outpatients without such disorders. In the sample of outpatients, 39% were classified as dismissing, 29% as autonomous, 21% as preoccupied, and 11% as unresolved. Most (86%) of the adults with anxiety disorders were diagnosed with panic disorder and agoraphobia, supporting our contention that anxiety disorders involving mainly avoidance may be best characterized by dismissing states of mind. In a sample comparing adolescents without diagnosed disorders to adolescents with OCD and another group with depression, 80% of those with OCD were classified as dismissing compared to 64% of those with depression.

PTSD is diagnosed in those individuals who exhibit a number of intrusive, avoidant, and hypervigilant symptoms when confronted with either internal or external reminders of traumatic events. Its phenomenological similarity to unresolved trauma and loss, as measured in the AAI, has been noted by several researchers (Fearon & Mansell, 2001; Harari et al., 2009; Nye et al., 2008; Stovall-McClough & Cloitre, 2006). Growing support for the association between PTSD and unresolved loss/trauma supports this idea; however, we have identified only two studies that have examined PTSD and unresolved state of mind regarding the same traumatic event. Stovall-McClough and Cloitre (2006) examined attachment in a sample of 60 women with histories of childhood abuse, 30 of whom were diagnosed with PTSD related to child abuse. Sixty-three percent of those with PTSD were classified as unresolved regarding childhood trauma, compared to 27% of those without PTSD. Moreover, unresolved trauma on the AAI was associated specifically with PTSD avoidance symptoms, and not with reexperiencing or hypervigilant symptoms. Among Dutch veterans, Harari and colleagues (2009) found that 87% of the veterans with PTSD were unresolved with regard to combat trauma. Additionally, severity of the DSM-IV PTSD symptoms strongly correlated with lack of resolution scores derived from the AAI.

## Dissociative Disorders

*Dissociative disorders,* as the name suggests, are characterized by a dissociation of consciousness and even parts of the self that are usually integrated. Minor dissociative states are commonplace—for example, becoming so absorbed in a conversation while driving as to be unaware of the passing landscape. The dissociative disorders specified in DSM-5 (American Psychiatric Association, 2013) involve dissociation of one's identity (dissociative identity disorder and dissociative fugue), memory (dissociative amnesia), and consciousness (depersonalization/derealization disorder). Transient experiences of depersonalization are seen in about 40% of hospitalized patients (American Psychiatric Association, 2000) and appear to be experienced at some point by many people without elevated clinical symptoms as well. The more serious dissociative disorders have been diagnosed relatively rarely until recently, when there has been a sharp rise in such diagnoses (Johnson, Cohen, Kasen, & Brook, 2006). Waller and Ross (1997) found no evidence for genetic influences in dissociative disorders, but more recent studies suggest a potential link between genetic polymorphisms within the gene SCN9A (a gene associated with pain threshold) and dissociative symptoms (Savitz et al., 2008; Tadic et al., 2009).

### Attachment and Dissociation: Theoretical Links

Dissociation involves turning away, presumably not volitionally, from some aspect of the environment. Dissociation in the face of trauma clearly has an adaptive function, in that it allows a person to avoid being overwhelmed with the experience. Evolution has predisposed infants and children to experience dissociative states readily when threatened. The cost of experiencing dissociative states

frequently as a child, however, is a sensitized and compromised neurobiology (De Bellis, 2001). This is especially true because children pass through critical periods for the organization of brain systems. Once sensitization has occurred, less is required to evoke dissociative states (De Bellis, 2001). Thus, a child who repeatedly enters dissociative states will more readily enter such states under conditions of mild stress.

When a traumatic event (e.g., a natural disaster, loss, or abuse) is experienced, but the caregiver can provide sensitive care and a sense of protection, the child is not in a position of experiencing "fright without solution" (Main & Hesse, 1990). In these cases, a child can continue to rely on a caregiver for protection. If, however, the caregiver cannot protect the child under conditions that the child experiences as threatening, or if the parent is actually the source of the threat, the child may experience the threat as overwhelming and enter a dissociative state (Main & Morgan, 1996).

Such dissociative states can be seen among some infants in the Strange Situation who are classified as disorganized (see Lyons-Ruth & Jacobvitz, Chapter 29, this volume; Main & Morgan, 1996). For most children, the Strange Situation is distressing, but an organized attachment system orchestrates behaviors with the caregiver. Some infants, however, experience a breakdown of attachment strategies. Abused infants, as well as infants of caregivers who are unresolved with respect to trauma or loss, are likely to show this breakdown in strategies (Carlson, Cicchetti, Barnett, & Braunwald, 1989; Main & Morgan, 1996). Main and Hesse (1990) proposed that frightened or frightening parental behavior leaves these children "frightened without solution." According to Main and Hesse, as well as Liotti (2004), early experiences with a frightened or frightening caregiver cause a child to develop multiple, incompatible models of the self and the other. In interactions with the caregiver, the child experiences rapid shifts in which the caregiver is at first frightened, then no longer frightened, then caring for the child. With each shift, a different model of self (perpetrator of fright, rescuer, loved child) and of the caregiver (victim, rescued victim, competent caregiver) is operative. These multiple models of the self and other cannot be integrated by young children and are retained as multiple models (Liotti, 2004; Main & Hesse, 1990). These children have an unsolvable dilemma when distressed: They are neither able to go to their caregivers for nurturance nor able to turn away and distract themselves. Because they experience this continued threat without resolution, they are at risk for entering a minor dissociative state during the Strange Situation and under other threatening conditions.

Liotti (2004) pointed out that disorganized attachment behaviors are phenotypically similar to dissociative states in adulthood, suggesting a possible connection between early trance-like states and later dissociative disorders. Given evidence that the experience of dissociative states in childhood leads to a sensitized neurobiology that predisposes individuals to experiencing later dissociative states, disorganized attachment in infancy and childhood experiences of abuse without caregiver protection may predispose individuals to dissociative states in adulthood (Carlson, 1998).

### Infant Attachment and Dissociation in Adulthood

Carlson (1998) and Ogawa, Sroufe, Weinfield, Carlson, and Egeland (1997) examined the association between disorganized attachment in infancy and dissociative symptoms during childhood and adolescence in the Minnesota longitudinal study. Of the original sample, 35% of the infants were classified as disorganized/disoriented at 12 months, and 43% were classified as disorganized at 18 months. Infant disorganization was associated with higher teacher ratings of dissociative symptoms both in elementary and high school, and in adulthood (Carlson, 1998). Furthermore, disorganized/disoriented behavior in the Strange Situation predicted the self-report of more dissociative symptomatology at age 19 (Carlson, 1998) and into adulthood (Sroufe, Egeland, Carlson, & Collins, 2005a). Thus, two sets of raters converged in pointing to symptoms of dissociation for adolescents who were assessed as disorganized/disoriented in infancy, and the relations persisted over time. Ogawa and colleagues (1997) found that, combined with indices of maternal emotional availability, disorganized attachment accounted for 34% of the variance in later dissociative symptoms. In addition, no associations emerged between disorganized/disoriented attachment and any of the variables assessing endogenous vulnerability, such as prenatal difficulties, difficulties during childbirth, or maternal drug and alcohol use (Carlson, 1998; Ogawa et al., 1997).

Dutra and Lyons-Ruth (2005) obtained similar findings in their longitudinal study. Fifty-six late adolescents who had participated in the Strange Situation as infants were administered the Dissociative Experiences Scale. Measures of parent–infant affective communication, quality of care, parental psychopathology, and maltreatment history were also administered at several time periods. The strongest predictors of adolescent dissociative symptoms were disorganization of attachment during infancy, disrupted affective communication with the mother, and maternal neglect.

### Children's Attachment-Related Experiences and Later Dissociative Disorders

As noted earlier, Main and Hesse (1990) proposed that disorganized or disoriented behavior in the Strange Situation results from the caregiver behaving in a frightened or frightening manner toward the child. This caregiver, who is often unresolved with respect to attachment, is unable to protect the child adequately from later threats, or may even perpetrate threats. Thus, it seems that a child who is disorganized in infancy may be at increased risk for later abuse because of the caregiver's qualities. Children who have formed disorganized attachments to caregivers in infancy and are later repeatedly abused may be particularly susceptible to later dissociative disorders (Liotti, 2004). In fact, the incidence of abuse among people with dissociative disorders is extremely high, with figures as high as 97% reported in some studies (e.g., Putnam, 1991).

Main and Hesse (1990) proposed an intergenerational model of the transmission of dissociative symptoms. They suggested that unresolved loss and trauma are the underlying causes of parents behaving in frightening or frightened ways with their children. Indirect support for this idea is suggested by the finding that unresolved loss on the AAI is associated with levels of absorption as measured by Tellegen's Absorption Scale (Hesse & Van IJzendoorn, 1998). Losses require some time to resolve, according to Main and colleagues (2003). Very recent losses are not considered in the scoring of unresolved status in Main and colleagues' system because lack of resolution in such cases is normative. Even recent losses can have disorganizing effects on parental behavior, however. Therefore, it follows that a parent's experience of the death of someone close may make disorganized attachment and even later dissociative states in a child more likely. Indeed, Liotti (2004) found that 62% of adults diagnosed with dissociative disorders had mothers who had lost a close relative within 2 years of their children's birth. In a follow-up study, Pasquini, Liotti, Mazzotti, Fassone, and Picardi (2002) compared a sample of patients with dissociative disorders to clinical controls. Patients whose mothers had suffered a loss or other traumatic life event within 2 years of the patients' births had an increased risk of 2.6 for a dissociative disorder diagnosis.

## Attachment States of Mind and Dissociative Disorders

Several studies have examined unresolved attachment status and the presence of dissociative symptoms in patients and other high-risk samples. West, Adam, Spreng, and Rose (2001) found that adolescent inpatients with higher dissociation scores were classified as unresolved or cannot classify in the AAI more often than were adolescent inpatients with lower dissociation scores. In a study by Riggs and colleagues (2007), psychiatric inpatients with unresolved trauma showed more dissociative symptomatology than inpatients without unresolved trauma. And finally, in a sample of pregnant adolescents, Madigan, Vaillancourt, McKibbon, and Benoit (2012) found higher self-reported dissociative symptoms in adolescents with an unresolved attachment classification than in those without an unresolved classification.

Although, to our knowledge, there are no published studies documenting the distribution of attachment classifications among adults with dissociative disorders per se (rather than dissociative symptoms more generally), Steele (2003) reported that the AAI was routinely administered to patients at the Clinic for Dissociative Studies in London. When it was administered to people diagnosed with dissociative identity disorder, the transcripts were characterized by multiple organizational strategies. More specifically, separate identifiable personalities appear to be linked with their own personal histories and strategies for managing the affect and content elicited by AAI questions. Thomson and Jaque (2012) examined the association between unresolved trauma and loss and dissociation in a sample of artists. Among artists who reported pathological levels of dissociation as seen in dissociative disorders (e.g., dissociative amnesia and depersonalization/derealization), 53% were classified as unresolved on the AAI.

## Eating Disorders

Eating disorders include anorexia nervosa and bulimia nervosa. *Anorexia nervosa* is characterized by maintaining a body weight that is dangerously low, accompanied by distorted body image and fears of becoming fat. *Bulimia nervosa* is characterized by binge eating, accompanied by behaviors intended to compensate for the bingeing, such as purging and taking laxatives. Typically these disorders emerge in adolescence, particularly at stressful times, such as college entry. The vast majority (90%) of those diagnosed with eating disorders are women (American Psychiatric Association, 2000). Many women with eating disorders are also depressed, with rates of reported comorbidity as high as 75% (Mitchell & Pyle, 1985).

## Attachment and Eating Disorders: Theoretical Links

Bowlby (1973) suggested that a child feels inadequate and out of control if given the message that he or she will have difficulty functioning independently or is unlovable. As discussed previously, children who receive such messages may feel their own anxiety exquisitely—developing GAD or agoraphobia, for example. If these children have developed an avoidant strategy of turning their attention away from their own distress, however, they may be at increased risk for developing externalizing symptoms. Cole-Detke and Kobak (1996) suggested that young women who develop eating disorders might be attempting to control their world through eating behavior that directs attention away from their own feelings of distress.

## Children's Attachment-Related Experiences and Later Eating Disorders

Much of the evidence linking early attachment-related experiences to eating disorders relies on retrospective accounts of parenting availability. The findings that emerge are complicated but relatively consistent. First, women with anorexia nervosa typically describe both of their parents negatively (e.g., Palmer, Oppenheimer, & Marshall, 1988; Ratti, Humphrey, & Lyons, 1996; Rowa, Kerig, & Geller, 2001; Vidovic, Juresa, Begovac, Mahnik, & Tocilkj, 2005; Wade, Treloar, & Martin, 2001; Wallin & Hansson, 1999; Woodside et al., 2002).

Second, fathers are often described as emotionally unavailable and rejecting (Cole-Detke & Kobak, 1996; Rhodes & Kroger, 1992). Third, mothers are described as domineering, overprotective, and perfectionistic (Minuchin, Rosman, & Baker, 1980; Woodside et al., 2002). Finally, parents appear to act in ways that thwart efforts at independence (Ratti et al., 1996). Kenny and Hart (1992) found that women with eating disorders described their parents as generally unsupportive of their independence.

Thus, a picture generally emerges of an over-controlling, perfectionistic mother who communicates lack of support for her daughter's autonomy striving; an emotionally rejecting father; and a daughter who feels rejected, controlled, and inadequate. Although sexual abuse has been suggested as a causal factor for eating disorders, the preponderance of evidence suggests that such abuse is not strongly related to the development of either anorexia nervosa or bulimia nervosa (e.g., Carter, Bewell, Blackmore, & Woodside, 2006; Pope, Mangweth, Negrao, Hudson, & Cordas, 1994; Welch & Fairburn, 1994).

## Attachment States of Mind and Eating Disorders

Several studies have examined the association between AAI states of mind and eating disorders, with somewhat contradictory results. As reviewed previously, Cole-Detke and Kobak (1996) used the self-reports of a sample of college women for the assessment of eating disorders. The methodology yielded information about preoccupied, dismissing, and autonomous states of mind, but not about the unresolved or cannot classify categories. The breakdown of states of mind differed significantly for women reporting eating disorders, depression, a combination of the two, or neither. Women who reported eating disorders only were most frequently classified as dismissing. Women who reported a combination of eating disorders and depression were most frequently classified as preoccupied (similar to women who reported only depression). Similarly, Ward and colleagues (2001) found that the overwhelming majority (95%) of patients were classified as nonautonomous on the AAI, and that 79% were classified as dismissing. Barone and Guiducci (2009) found an overrepresentation of nonautonomous attachment states of mind (90%) among adults with eating disorders compared with adults without eating disorders. More specifically,

dismissing states of mind appeared to characterize those with eating disorders (47% for the eating disorders group vs. 20% for the comparison group). Unresolved states of mind also differentiated those with eating disorders, 27% of whom were classified as unresolved, compared to only 7% of the comparison group.

In contrast, Fonagy and colleagues (1996) found that 64% of people with eating disorders were classified as preoccupied. When the four-category system was used, 13 of the 14 individuals with eating disorders were classified as unresolved with respect to loss or trauma. Those with eating disorders did not differ significantly from those with other psychiatric disorders in the breakdown of state-of-mind classifications. In the Cole-Detke and Kobak (1996) study, over half (61%) of the women reporting eating disorders also reported depression, and were therefore not included in the "pure" eating disorder group. If a similar proportion of people in Fonagy and colleagues' study were comorbid for depression, the majority of the remaining "pure" eating disorder group might have been classified as dismissing, thus matching Cole-Detke and Kobak's results.

Consistent with the patterns of family interaction described earlier, Cole-Detke and Kobak (1996) and Ward and colleagues (2001) have argued that women with eating disorders are attempting to control their worlds through their eating behavior, and that the type of control exerted is externally oriented. This type of control is chosen because women with eating disorders do not have the ability to examine their own psychological states, and they cope instead by diverting their distress to focus on their own bodies. Cole-Detke and Kobak have therefore proposed that eating disorders allow the diversion of attention away from attachment-related concerns, and toward the more external and more "attainable" goal of body change.

Further differentiation between eating disorders may also be useful in considering the role of attachment states of mind. Primarily restrictive behavior, as seen in anorexia, may be associated with dismissing states of mind, whereas eating disorders characterized by primarily bingeing and purging may be associated with preoccupied states of mind. Dias, Soares, Klein, Cunha, and Roisman (2011) provide preliminary support for this hypothesis. In a sample of eating disordered patients, AAIs were rated using Kobak's continuous Q-sorting method (Kobak, 1993). The large majority of the clinical sample was classified as nonautonomous (70%), with hyperactivation of attachment differentiating the purging patients from the restrictive patients.

## Schizophrenia

The various types of schizophrenia are the disorders often associated with the greatest level of dysfunction. They are characterized most especially by *psychosis* (i.e., loss of touch with reality), as manifested often in delusions or hallucinations. The schizophrenias have high heritability (e.g., Thompson, Watson, Steinhauer, Goldstein, & Pogue-Geile, 2005). For example, the concordance for monozygotic twins is usually estimated at about 50%, as opposed to 15% for dizygotic twins (Gottesman, 1991). Even in adoption studies, when the influence of the environmental effects associated with biological parents is minimized, the influence of biological parents appears more predictive of the development of schizophrenia than the influence of adoptive parents (Gottesman, 1991). The mechanism for the transmission has not been clearly specified as a single-gene or single-chromosome locus. Many researchers are now exploring what seems the more likely explanation that multiple genes are involved, and that the involvement of specific genes will be variable across the schizophrenias (Baron, 2001; Gottesman, 1991).

### Children's Attachment-Related Experiences and Later Schizophrenia

The family environment variable that has been most widely suggested as causal in the etiology of schizophrenia is "expressed emotion" (Goldstein, 1985). High levels of expressed emotion are characterized by familial overinvolvement and/or criticality. Communication deviance and expressed emotion assessed in the families of adolescents with mild to moderate clinical disturbances predicted schizophrenia and schizophrenia spectrum disorders (schizoid, schizotypal, and paranoid personality disorders) 15 years later (Goldstein, 1985). Even though these results suggest that parental behavior is important in the onset of schizophrenia, it is also plausible that the parents' behaviors reflected sensitivity to different premorbid behaviors of their children who later developed schizophrenia. For example, Walker,

Grimes, Davis, and Smith (1993) found that in home videotapes taken years before the onset of schizophrenia, the children who later developed schizophrenia could be reliably differentiated from their siblings who did not develop schizophrenia.

### Attachment States of Mind and Schizophrenia

Only a handful of studies have examined the distribution of AAI classifications among individuals with schizophrenia or other psychoses. Dozier and colleagues have examined states of mind among individuals with schizophrenia (Dozier, Cue, & Barnett, 1994; Tyrrell, Dozier, Teague, & Fallot, 1999). Tyrrell and colleagues (1999) found that 89% of individuals with schizophrenia were classified as dismissing when unresolved status was not considered, but 44% were classified as unresolved when that category was included. (The insecure cannot classify category was not used in these studies.) MacBeth, Gumley, Schwannauer, and Fisher (2010) examined attachment states of mind in a sample of patients recovering from their first episode of psychosis. In this study, 26% of the patients were classified as autonomous and 62% were classified as dismissing (62%). The four-way classification breakdown revealed that 29% of the sample fell into the unresolved category.

We argue, however, that these results tell us little about factors predisposing individuals to schizophrenia. First, we suggest that findings of higher rates of unresolved status among people with schizophrenia should be interpreted with caution. Indeed, schizophrenia, characterized most especially by thought disorder, involves "lapses in monitoring of reasoning and discourse" (Main et al., 2003., p. 97)—the characteristics that define unresolved status. Thus, people with thought disorder may appear unresolved with respect to loss or abuse *because* of their thought disorder. Second, we suggest that the failure to find many autonomous transcripts among those with schizophrenia may reflect the deleterious effect of schizophrenia on the brain. The lack of coherence associated with formal thought disorder is inconsistent with a coherent transcript. Although we urge caution in thinking of states of mind as preceding psychopathology when measured concurrently, we suggest that differences in states of mind are important in how relationships are approached and how treatment is used. Indeed, in a review of studies examining attachment in those with psychotic disorders, an autonomous state of mind was related to better service engagement and follow-through than was a nonautonomous state of mind (Gumley, Taylor, Schwannauer, & MacBeth, 2014).

## Borderline Personality Disorder

People with borderline personality disorder have a notably unstable sense of self (American Psychiatric Association, 2000, 2013). Similarly, representations of others are undeveloped and unstable; that is, others are idealized at times and devalued at other times. A central issue is the fear of abandonment by an idealized other. Because the unstable sense of self is dependent on validation from the idealized other, the threat of abandonment is experienced as potentially devastating. This instability of internal representations is often associated with emotional volatility. In particular, strong feelings of anger and dysphoria can be readily precipitated by subtle suggestions of rejection. Thus, a number of contributing factors create conditions in which interpersonal relationships are likely to be intense and tumultuous. Such factors also point to probable attachment-relevant influences on the etiology of borderline personality disorder (Agrawal, Gunderson, Holmes, & Lyons-Ruth, 2004).

Although the prevalence of borderline personality disorder in the general population is about 6% (Torgersen, Kringlen & Cramer, 2001), the prevalence among people receiving treatment is much greater—about 15% among outpatients and 50% among outpatients diagnosed with personality disorders (Widiger, 1993). Thus, people with borderline personality disorder are relatively more likely than others to seek treatment; this is not surprising given that "crying out for help" is characteristic of the disorder.

Among personality disorders, studies investigating heritability among twins have found rates as low as 30% when personality traits are measured with standardized interview methods (Kendler et al., 2008) and as high as 70–80% when using self-report methods (Coolidge, Thede, & Jang, 2001). The heritability of borderline personality disorder specifically is also found to vary across self-report and interview-based measures. Torgersen and colleagues (2012) suggest that when the two methods of assessment are both taken into account in the same study, error variance between methods is eliminated, producing a more accurate estimate. In a large twin study using both self-report and in-

terview-based measures, Torgersen and colleagues (2000) established a heritability rate of 67% for borderline personality disorder among twins, suggesting a significant genetic influence. A predisposition toward emotional sensitivity, poor emotion regulation, and both internalizing and externalizing behavioral tendencies are likely the underlying traits (e.g., Crowell, Beauchaine, & Linehan, 2009; Torgersen et al., 2000).

There is growing evidence to support the diathesis-stress model of borderline personality disorder with early environmental factors interacting with genetic influences to increase the risk for the disorder. To test this model directly, Belsky and colleagues (2012) examined the interactions among a number of environmental and family history characteristics in a longitudinal study of over 1,000 pairs of same-sex twins followed from birth until age 12. The twin study estimated the heritability of borderline traits at age 12 to be about 66%, consistent with Torgersen and colleagues (2012). As predicted, both environmental adversity (harsh early parenting and maternal negative expressed emotion) and inherited risk (a family history of psychiatric illness) independently predicted borderline personality traits at age 12. The diathesis–stress model was also supported. Children with harsh early experiences were more likely to show borderline traits at age 12 if they also had a family history of psychiatric illness than were those children with harsh early experiences without a family psychiatric history. The authors concluded that both "acted as a more virulent risk factor in the presence of the other" (Belsky et al., 2012, p. 261).

### Attachment and Borderline Personality Disorder: Theoretical Links

Main and Hesse (1990) have suggested that the experience of trauma in the absence of a supportive caregiver predisposes individuals to develop either borderline or dissociative pathology. As described previously, Main and Hesse have proposed that a child cannot integrate the various qualities of a caregiver into single models of self and other when the caregiver behaves in a frightened or frightening way; thus, unintegrated models are maintained. This formulation is consistent with the organizational model of the developing self and borderline personality disorder suggested by Carlson and colleagues (2009). Early traumatic experiences overwhelm children's ability to regulate emotions and organize internal models of self and other, leading eventually to a breakdown in these capacities.

Borderline pathology is generally associated with exaggeration of symptomatology and negative affect, as well as a "preoccupation" with concerns about current and previous relationship difficulties. The readiness to report distress is consistent with maximizing the expression of attachment needs, seen in infants with resistant attachment and in adults who are preoccupied with respect to attachment. Internalized models of caregivers as incompetent or inconsistently available, and of the self as inconsistently valued, seem as central to a diagnosis of borderline personality disorder as to a classification of preoccupied attachment (Agrawal et al., 2004).

## Children's Attachment-Related Experiences and Later Borderline Personality Disorder

The evidence for problematic family conditions in the development of borderline personality disorder is compelling. Early abuse in particular is often seen in the histories of people diagnosed with borderline personality disorder (Brown & Anderson, 1991; Carlson et al., 2009; Herman, Perry, & van der Kolk, 1989; Ogata et al., 1990). Sanders and Giolas (1991) found evidence of higher rates of documented abuse histories in the hospital records of patients with this disorder than in the histories of other patients. Thus, these results do not appear to reflect a reporting bias only. In addition, people with borderline personality disorder report high rates of prolonged separations from caregivers during their childhoods (Zanarini, Gunderson, Marino, Schwartz, & Frankenburg, 1989), especially from their mothers (Soloff & Millward, 1983). They also report emotional neglect when their caregivers were physically present (Patrick et al., 1994; Zanarini et al., 1989). Liotti and Pasquini (2000) found a 2.5-fold increase in the risk for borderline personality disorder for individuals whose mothers had suffered a loss within 2 years of their birth, and a 5.3-fold increase for those with early maltreatment.

Since the previous Handbook was published, there is growing evidence pointing to a multidetermined model of borderline personality disorder that takes into account both genetic or endogenous characteristics and early environmental factors (including caregiving experiences) (Belsky et al., 2012; Carlson et al., 2009). With regard to infant attachment and its relationship with adult borderline personality disorder, the findings are mixed. To our knowledge, only two longitudinal studies have examined the association between infant attachment quality and later borderline symptoms. Lyons-Ruth, Yellin, Melnick, and Atwood (2005) reported on the development of borderline personality disorder features in a group of 56 high-risk infants in early adulthood. Early attachment status, including attachment disorganization, did not predict later borderline personality disorder symptoms, as measured by a psychiatric interview. Rather, early maltreatment and disrupted parent–infant communication were associated with a greater likelihood of developing borderline symptoms. In a study exploring the etiology of borderline personality disorder from a developmental psychopathology perspective, Carlson and colleagues (2009) examined the influence of early environmental variables, including infant attachment and early "endogenous" variables such as medical issues and representations of the self measured in middle childhood and early adolescence. Although infant disorganization, maternal hostility, abuse, family disruptions, and maternal stress predicted adulthood borderline personality disorder symptoms, only maternal hostility at age 3 continued to predict borderline symptoms after researchers controlled for the early endogenous variables. The influence of disorganized attachment on risk for borderline personality disorder was mediated by disturbances in self-representations measured at 12 years.

## Attachment States of Mind and Borderline Personality Disorder

A number of researchers have reported on the association between attachment state of mind, as measured by the AAI, and the incidence of diagnosed borderline personality disorder in clinical samples (Barone, 2003; Barone, Fossati, & Guiducci, 2011; Diamond, Stovall-McClough, Clarkin, & Levy, 2003; Fonagy et al., 1996; Patrick et al., 1994; Rosenstein & Horowitz, 1996; Stalker & Davies, 1995; Stovall-McClough & Cloitre, 2003). Using the three-way classification system, Fonagy and colleagues (1996) found that 75% of people with borderline personality disorder had preoccupied states of mind, and that half of those with preoccupied states of mind fell into the rarely used subgroup "fearfully preoccupied with respect to trauma" (E3). In Patrick and colleagues' (1994) study, all women with borderline personality disorder were classified as preoccupied, and 10 of the

12 were classified as E3. When the four-way classification system was used, 89 and 75% of people with borderline personality disorder were classified as unresolved in the Fonagy and colleagues and Patrick and colleagues studies, respectively. In a study of inpatient adolescents, Rosenstein and Horowitz (1996) found that the majority of those diagnosed with borderline personality disorder (64%) were also classified as preoccupied on the AAI. This study did not include the unresolved category. Barone (2003) examined attachment status in a sample of 80 subjects, 40 of whom were diagnosed with borderline personality disorder and 40 of whom were nonclinical controls. Using the four-way attachment classification system, he identified only 7% of those with borderline personality disorder as autonomous, whereas 23% were preoccupied, 20% were dismissing, and 50% were unresolved. This distribution was significantly different than that found in the control group, where 62% were identified as autonomous, 10% as preoccupied, and only 7% as unresolved.

Recent reviews suggest that, indeed, preoccupied and unresolved attachment states of mind appear to be the most commonly identified attachment classification in those with borderline personality disorder (Bakermans-Kranenburg & Van IJzendoorn, 2009; Barone et al., 2011). Looking more closely at subgroups within borderline personality disorder, Barone and colleagues (2011) divided a large sample of therapy-seeking participants who were diagnosed with borderline personality disorder into four subgroups based on their DSM-IV Axis I diagnoses: (1) mood disorders, (2) drug use/abuse disorders, (3) alcohol use/abuse disorders, and (4) eating disorders. Three-way analyses revealed that preoccupied states of mind distinguished those with mood disorders (52%) from the other three groups, whereas dismissing states of mind best characterized those with drug (57%) and alcohol use disorders (55%) as well as eating disorders (60%). Unresolved states of mind did not differentiate the four groups but was found in 28% of the sample.

## Antisocial Personality Disorder

Antisocial personality disorder is characterized by a consistent disregard for the rights and feelings of others and for the basic laws of society (American Psychiatric Association, 2000, 2013). Characteristics of antisocial personality disorder include deceitfulness, impulsivity, irresponsibility, irritability, and lack of remorse. The links between childhood and adolescent conduct disorder and later adult antisocial personality disorder have been noted in numerous studies (e.g., Blair, Peschardt, Budhani, Mitchell, & Pine, 2006). Indeed, one of the criteria for antisocial personality disorder is the presence of earlier conduct disorder.

### Attachment and Antisocial Personality Disorder: Theoretical Links

Bowlby (1973) proposed that when children experience separations from parents, and when parents threaten abandonment, children feel intense anger. Ordinary but stressful separations are often met with anger, which is functional in communicating to the parents the children's feelings about the separation. When prolonged separations are combined with frightening threats, however, Bowlby suggested that children are likely to feel a dysfunctional level of anger toward parents, often involving intense hatred. Initially, the anger may be directed toward the parents. Because that may prove dangerous in maintaining the relationship with the parents, however, the anger is often repressed and directed toward other targets (Bowlby, 1973).

### Children's Attachment-Related Experiences and Later Antisocial Personality Disorder

Prolonged separations from primary caregivers (as the result of divorce or separation rather than death), fathers' antisocial or deviant behavior, and mothers' unaffectionate, neglectful care are associated with antisocial personality disorder (McCord, 1979; Robins, 1966). Robins found that parental desertion, divorce, or separation was associated with the diagnosis of antisocial personality disorder. Zanarini and colleagues (1989) found that 89% of people with antisocial personality disorder had experienced prolonged separations from a caregiver at some point in childhood. Given that loss by death was not associated with later antisocial personality disorder, however, it does not seem to be simply the absence of a caregiver that is important (Robins, 1966). In a prospective longitudinal study, McCord (1979) found that antisocial personality disorder is a likely outcome only when mothers are also unaffectionate and do not provide adequate supervision, and when fathers are deviant.

## Attachment States of Mind and Antisocial Personality Disorder

Most of the empirical evidence suggests that antisocial personality disorder is associated with unresolved and dismissing states of mind (Allen et al., 1996; Frodi, Dernevik, Sepa, Philipson, & Brageslo, 2001; Levinson & Fonagy, 2004; Rosenstein & Horowitz, 1996). Allen and colleagues (1996) assessed states of mind in adolescent psychiatric inpatients and a control group of high school students. Criminality and use of "hard drugs" were then assessed approximately 10 years later. The most impressive finding was that ratings from the adolescents' attachment interviews predicted criminality 10 years later, even after researchers accounted for previous psychiatric hospitalization. In particular, derogation of attachment and lack of resolution of trauma predicted criminal behavior. In *derogation of attachment*, a rarely occurring feature of dismissing attachment, the person derogates attachment figures or attachment experiences. Among the sample of psychiatric inpatients in the Allen and colleagues study, 15% of the interviews were categorized as cannot classify because they met criteria for multiple, incompatible categories. This group of people reported the most criminal behavior, followed by people classified as dismissing and unresolved. Post hoc analyses revealed that the cannot-classify (termed *unclassifiable* at that time) group showed higher levels of criminal behavior than the autonomous and preoccupied groups, and that the dismissing group showed significantly higher levels than the autonomous group. Similarly, Hesse and colleagues (2011) examined the incidence of cannot classify and secondary dismissing (Ds2) classifications in a small sample of male prisoners (n = 19). Eleven of the men were classified as psychopaths based on the Psychopathy Checklist—Revised (PCL-R; Hare, Hart, & Harpur, 1991). All were classified as cannot classify regardless of the nature of their offense, but derogation of attachment did not appear to distinguish the psychopathic prisoners from those who were not classified as psychopaths. A secondary analysis, however, found that those incarcerated for crimes involving murder or violent bodily harm (n = 9) were more likely to fall in the rare Ds2 subcategory than were the men incarcerated for other offenses.

Rosenstein and Horowitz (1996) found that among adolescents with conduct disorder only, six of seven were classified as dismissing, and none was classified as unresolved. Among adolescents with comorbid conduct disorder and mood disorder, half were classified as dismissing, and nearly half were classified as unresolved with respect to loss or trauma. Fonagy and colleagues (1996) obtained very different results for a combined group of people with antisocial and paranoid personality disorders, however. When the three-category system was used, more were classified as preoccupied and autonomous than as dismissing. When the four-category system was used, most were classified as unresolved.

Findings have been relatively consistent when researchers have considered violence rather than antisocial personality disorder. In a study examining the association between attachment status and propensity toward domestic violence, Holtzworth-Munroe and colleagues (1997) administered the AAI to maritally distressed violent men (n = 30) and nonviolent men (n = 30). Men with histories of domestic violence were more likely than nonviolent men to be classified as nonautonomous, and 37% were rated as cannot classify. Babcock, Jacobson, Gottman, and Yerington (2000) conducted a study with a group of maritally distressed men with a history of domestic violence (n = 23) and those without such a history (n = 13). Similar to Holtzworth-Munroe and colleagues' (1997) findings, domestically violent men were more likely to be rated as nonautonomous. Moreover, the dismissing category was associated with higher scores on an antisocial scale than were other categories. Only 9% of the domestically violent men could not be classified on the AAI—a lower rate than that reported by Holtzworth-Munroe and colleagues, but higher than that seen in the general population.

## Summary: Current State of Theory and Research

### Attachment in Infancy: Links to Adult Psychopathology

Since we last visited these issues, it remains the case that the only clear connections between infant attachment and adult psychopathology are between disorganized attachment and dissociative symptoms in adolescence and early adulthood (Carlson, 1998; Sroufe et al., 2005a) and between resistant attachment and anxiety disorders in adolescence (Warren et al., 1997). These associations are compelling for a number of reasons. First, the "phenotypic similarity" of the phenomena is striking when one considers the link between disorganized attachment and dissociative symptoms (Liotti, 2004; Main & Morgan, 1996) and between resistant attachment and anxiety (Cassidy, 1995). Second, the caregiving experiences predictive of disorganized and resistant attachment are similar to the caregiving experiences predictive of dissociative symptoms and anxiety symptoms, respectively. More specifically, the occurrence of attachment-related trauma, especially abuse, is known to be associated with both disorganized attachment (Carlson et al., 1989) and dissociative disorders (e.g., Putnam, 1991). This connection between abuse and later dissociation may be accounted for partially by the development of a sensitized neurobiology when a child experiences frightening events from which escape is not possible. Similarly, unavailable or inconsistently available caregiving appears predictive of both resistant attachment and symptoms of anxiety (Cassidy, 1995). Carlson (1998) has suggested that a child who frequently becomes hyperaroused (rather than disorganized) when threatened with an unavailable caregiver develops a sensitized neurobiology that predisposes him or her to later anxiety.

Finally, the categories of adult attachment that parallel infant disorganized and resistant attachment are characterized by behaviors consistent with the predicted symptomatology (Sroufe et al., 2005a). Adults who are unresolved with respect to loss or trauma are characterized by a "lapse in reasoning or in the monitoring of discourse" when discussing loss or trauma (Main et al., 2003, p. 97). Similarly, the discourse of adults who are preoccupied with respect to attachment is affected by anxiety that may be either more diffuse (e.g., similar to the anxiety associated with GAD; Cassidy, 1995) or more focused (e.g., similar to the anxiety associated with a phobic disorder). Thus, the categories of adult attachment that parallel infant disorganized and resistant attachment are themselves characterized by some level of dissociation and anxiety, respectively.

## Attachment States of Mind: State of the Field

Following the publication of this volume in 2008, a meta-analysis was conducted to examine the distribution of AAI classifications among both clinical and nonclinical groups (Bakermans-Kranenberg & Van IJzendoorn, 2009). Drawing from studies published over the past 25 years, over 10,000 AAIs were included in the study.

Two robust findings emerged with regard to attachment states of mind and adult psychopathology. First, psychiatric disorders are nearly always associated with nonautonomous states of mind and/or unresolved status (Bakermans-Kranenberg & Van IJzendoorn, 2009). Cutting across all clinical samples, 76% (n = 1,956) of the AAI's were classified as nonautonomous, compared to 42% of nonclinical samples. A large percentage (43%) of the AAI's in the clinical samples were classified as unresolved or cannot classify, whereas only 18% of the interviews from the nonclinical group fell into these categories. What these findings mean in terms of the causal connection between attachment state of mind and psychiatric disorders remains unclear. Only the Allen and colleagues (1996) study provided evidence that ratings of derogation and lack of resolution of abuse can predict problematic behaviors (in particular, criminal behavior and hard drug use) in a high-risk sample. Some of the longitudinal studies now being conducted with high-risk samples will address the association between states of mind and the emergence of different psychiatric disorders more comprehensively.

The second finding highlighted by Bakermans-Kranenburg and Van IJzendoorn's (2009) meta-analysis is the connection between dismissing–preoccupied states of mind and externalizing–internalizing disorders. Meta-analytic results supported connections we had proposed in previous versions of this volume; namely, that externalizing disorders such as conduct disorder and antisocial personality disorder are associated with dismissing states of mind, and disorders characterized by internalizing symptoms, such as borderline personality disorder, are associated with preoccupied states of mind. Further support for this distinction was provided by the meta-analysis, which included studies of violent behavior separated into those studies involving violence against the family, the self, and society. Violence against the family was associated with preoccupied states of mind, whereas violence against society (criminal behaviors) and violence against the self (e.g., drug abuse and eating disorders) were associated with dismissing states of mind.

There are exceptions to this rule, however. Individuals with anxiety and depression tend to show a mixed picture with regard to attachment. At least one study including antisocial personality disorder appears to show a preponderance of preoccupied states of mind, contrary to our hypothesis (Fonagy et al., 1996). Bakermans-Kranenburg and Van IJzendoorn's (2009) meta-analysis, which included both adolescent and adult criminal samples, suggested that in addition to dismissing states of mind, preoccupied states of mind are also identified in externalizing/conduct disorder samples more often than autonomous states of mind. We suggest that the comorbidity of samples is critical to consider in such cases. Diversity of symptom pictures within a disorder may also contribute to inconsistent findings. For instance, both depression and anxiety are heterogeneous disorders, subsuming both those who are more self-focused (i.e., internalizing) and less self-focused (i.e., externalizing). Eating disorders, too, consist of both restricting symptoms requiring a tuning out of internal hunger/pain signals and purging behaviors resulting from an overreaction to internal feelings of satiation.

## The Metaphor of the Branching Railway Lines: New Directions

The research we have examined in this chapter provides growing support for Bowlby's (1973) model of the "branching railway lines." In this model there are no circumstances, including the quality of early caregiving or the experiences of loss or abuse, that fully constrain development. Nonetheless, certain developmental pathways become more or less likely with experience because there develops within a child an organized system for coping with his or her experiences (Sroufe et al., 2005a). Ways in which early attachment experiences may place children at risk for later psychopathology, however, still need to be tested. Large longitudinal studies are best suited to assessing how early attachment experiences place children at risk for later psychopathology, but such studies are expensive in terms of both time, money, and other resources. Indeed, such studies span full careers, and in the best-case scenarios are even then handed on to the next generation of researchers. Several longitudinal studies have focused on attachment experiences early, following participants throughout life. An example is the Minnesota Longitudinal Project, begun when Alan Sroufe and Byron Egeland were junior faculty members at University of Minnesota's Institute of Child Development and still being conducted by a second generation of faculty at the Institute. The Minnesota Longitudinal Project is extraordinary, most especially for the care with which the investigators set out to examine salient tasks at each point

in development. But, surely, these are challenging studies to undertake that require an impressive research infrastructure, ongoing support for the research, and a long-term commitment on the part of the research team.

Efforts to integrate theory and research findings from multiple disciplines including developmental psychology, clinical psychology, and cognitive neuroscience are on the rise; such research is certainly needed to more fully develop our understanding of "psychopathology as an outcome of development" (Sroufe, 1997, p. 251). Neuroscience in particular is a promising area for exploring the brain mechanisms involved in problematic adaptations to parental behavior and understanding why some children suffer adverse consequences while others demonstrate apparent resilience. Researchers have begun to uncover possible mechanisms by which environmental stress such as parental maltreatment may affect gene expression leading to later psychiatric symptoms and disorders. Also, study of gene × environment interactions have highlighted the potential role of the dopamine receptor gene (DRD4) and a particular allele (7-repeat allele) that appears to drive the dopaminergic networks of the brain. Children with the DRD4 7-repeat allele have been found to be particularly susceptible to both positive and negative parenting environments (Bakermans-Kranenburg, Van IJzendoorn, Caspers, & Philibert, 2011). The presence of these so called "risk genes" or "susceptibility genes" (Bakermans-Kranenburg et al., 2011) are involved in strong interaction effects enabling researchers to better understand why some children appear to be differentially vulnerable to their environments (see Bakermans-Kranenburg & Van IJzendoorn, Chapter 8, for further discussion of this topic). These represent examples of future research in the area.

Intervention studies will be important in the next generation of understanding the effects of attachment on later development. To the extent that attachment quality can be experimentally manipulated, claims of causal effects of caregiver availability and attachment quality on developmental outcomes can be made. In a number of randomized clinical trials, interventions targeting parental sensitivity have been shown to affect attachment quality (e.g., Bernard et al., 2012; Cicchetti, Rogosch, & Toth, 2006). If these experimental studies can be extended longitudinally, claims that early attachment affects later psychopathology can be made with greater confidence than has been allowed in the past.

## Acknowledgment

Support for this work was provided by National Institute of Mental Health Grant Nos. R01 52135, 84135, and 74374 to Mary Dozier.

## References

Agrawal, H. R., Gunderson, J., Holmes, B. M., & Lyons-Ruth, K. (2004). Attachment studies with borderline patients: A review. *Harvard Review of Psychiatry, 12,* 94–104.

Allen, J. P., Hauser, S. T., & Borman-Spurrell, E. (1996). Attachment theory as a framework for understanding sequelae of severe adolescent psychopathology: An 11-year follow-up study. *Journal of Consulting and Clinical Psychology, 64,* 254–263.

American Psychiatric Association. (2000). *Diagnostic and statistical manual of mental disorders* (4th ed., text rev.). Washington, DC: Author.

American Psychiatric Association. (2013). *Diagnostic and statistical manual of mental disorders* (5th ed.). Arlington, VA: Author.

Babcock, J. C., Jacobson, N. S., Gottman, J. M., & Yerington, T. P. (2000). Attachment, emotional regulation, and the function of marital violence: Differences between secure, preoccupied, and dismissing violent and nonviolent husbands. *Journal of Family Violence, 15,* 391–409.

Bakermans-Kranenburg, M. J., & Van IJzendoorn, M. H. (2009) The first 10,000 adult attachment interviews: Distributions of adult attachment representations in clinical and non-clinical groups. *Attachment and Human Development, 11*(3), 223–263.

Bakermans-Kranenburg, M. J., Van IJzendoorn, M. H., Caspers, K., & Philibert, R. (2011). DRD4 genotype moderates the impact of parental problems on unresolved loss or trauma, *Attachment and Human Development, 13*(3), 253–269.

Bandelow, B., Spath, C., Tichauer, G. A., Broocks, A., Hajak, G., & Ruther, E. (2002). Early traumatic life events, parental attitudes, family history, and birth risk factors in patients with panic disorder. *Comprehensive Psychiatry, 43,* 269–278.

Bandelow, B., Torrente, A. C., Wedekind, D., Broocks, A., Hajak, G., & Ruther, E. (2004). Early traumatic life events, parental rearing styles family history of mental disorders, and birth risk factors in patients with social anxiety disorder. *European Archives of Psychiatry and Clinical Neuroscience, 254,* 397–405.

Bar-Haim, Y, Dan, O., Eshel, Y., & Sagi-Schwartz, A. (2007). Predicting children's anxiety from early attachment relationships. *Journal of Anxiety Disorders, 21,* 1061–1068.

Baron, M. (2001). Genetics of schizophrenia and the new millennium: Progress and pitfalls. *American Journal of Human Genetics, 68,* 299–312.

Barone, L. (2003). Developmental protective and risk in borderline personality disorder: A study using the Adult Attachment Interview. *Attachment and Human Development, 5,* 64–77.

Barone, L., Fossati, A., & Guiducci, V. (2011). Attachment mental states and inferred pathways of development in borderline personality disorder: A study using the Adult Attachment Interview. *Attachment and Human Development, 13*(5), 451–469.

Barone, L., & Guiducci, V. (2009). Mental representations of attachment in eating disorders: A pilot study using the Adult Attachment Interview. *Attachment and Human Development, 11*(4), 405–417.

Belsky, D. W., Caspi, A., Arseneault, L., Bleidorn, W., Fonagy, P., Goodman, M., et al. (2012). Etiological features of borderline personality related characteristics in a birth cohort of 12-year-old children. *Development and Psychopathology, 24,* 251–265.

Bernard, K., Dozier, M., Bick, J., Lewis-Morrarty, E., Lindhiem, O., & Carlson, E. (2012). Enhancing attachment organization among maltreated infants: Results of a randomized clinical trial. *Child Development, 83,* 623–636.

Bienvenu, O. J., Davydow, D. S., & Kendler, K. S. (2011). Psychiatric "diseases" *versus* behavioral disorders and degree of genetic influence. *Psychological Medicine, 41,* 33–40.

Blair, R., Peschardt, K., Budhani, S., Mitchell, D., & Pine, D. (2006). The development of psychopathy. *Journal of Child Psychology and Psychiatry, 47,* 262–276.

Borelli, J. L., Goshin, L., Joestl, S., Clark, J., & Byrne, M. W. (2010). Attachment organization in a sample of incarcerated mothers: Distribution of classifications and associations with substance abuse history, depressive symptoms, perceptions of parenting competency, and social support. *Attachment and Human Development, 12*(4), 355–374.

Borkovec, T. D., Alcaine, O., & Behar, E. (2004). Avoidance theory of worry and generalized anxiety disorder. In R. G. Heimberg, C. L. Turk, & D. S. Mennin (Eds.), *Generalized anxiety disorder: Advances in research and practice* (pp. 77–108). New York: Guilford Press.

Bosquet, M., & Egeland, B. (2006). The development and maintenance of anxiety symptoms from infancy through adolescence in a longitudinal sample. *Development and Psychopathology, 18,* 517–550.

Bowlby, J. (1973). *Attachment and loss: Vol. 2. Separation: Anxiety and anger.* New York: Basic Books.

Bowlby, J. (1980). *Attachment and loss: Vol. 3. Loss: Sadness and depression.* New York: Basic Books.

Bowlby, J. (1982). *Attachment and loss: Vol. 1. Attachment.* New York: Basic Books. (Original work published 1969)

Brazelton, T. B. (1973). *Neonatal Behavioral Assessment Scale.* Philadelphia: Lippincott.

Bretherton, I. (1985). Attachment theory: Retrospect and prospect. In I. Bretherton & E. Waters (Eds.), *Growing points of attachment theory and research.*

*Monographs of the Society for Research in Child Development, 50*(1–2, Serial No. 209), 3–35.

Brown, G. R., & Anderson, B. (1991). Psychiatric morbidity in adult inpatients with childhood histories of sexual and physical abuse. *American Journal of Psychiatry, 148*, 55–61.

Brown, G. W., Birley, J. L. T., & Wing, J. K. (1972). Influence of family life on the course of schizophrenic disorders: A replication. *British Journal of Psychiatry, 121*, 241–258.

Brown, G. W., & Harris, T. O. (1993). Aetiology of anxiety and depressive disorders in an inner city population: 1. Early adversity. *Psychological Medicine, 23*, 143–154.

Brumariu, L., Obsuth, I., & Lyons-Ruth, K. (2013). Quality of attachment relationships and peer relationship dysfunction among late adolescents with and without anxiety disorders. *Journal of Anxiety Disorders, 27*, 116–124.

Carlson, E. A. (1998). A prospective longitudinal study of disorganized/disoriented attachment. *Child Development, 69*, 1107–1128.

Carlson, E. A., Egeland, B., & Sroufe, A. (2009) A prospective investigation of the development of borderline personality symptoms, *Development and Psychopathology, 21*, 1311–1334.

Carlson, V., Cicchetti, D., Barnett, D., & Braunwald, K. (1989). Disorganized/disoriented attachment relationships in maltreated infants. *Developmental Psychology, 25*, 525–531.

Carter, J. C., Bewell, C., Blackmore, E., & Woodside, D. B. (2006). The impact of childhood sexual abuse in anorexia nervosa. *Child Abuse and Neglect, 30*, 257–269.

Cassidy, J. (1995). Attachment and generalized anxiety disorder. In D. Cicchetti & S. Toth (Eds.), *Rochester Symposium on Developmental Psychopathology: Vol. 6. Emotion, cognition, and representation* (pp. 343–370). Rochester: University of Rochester Press.

Chambless, D. L., Gillis, M. M., Tran, G. Q., & Steketee, G. S. (1996). Parental bonding reports of clients with obsessive compulsive disorder and agoraphobia. *Clinical Psychology and Psychotherapy, 3*, 77–85.

Cicchetti, D. Rogosch, F. A., & Toth, S. L. (2006). Fostering secure attachments in infants in maltreating families through preventive interventions. *Development and Psychopathology, 18*(1), 623–649.

Cole-Detke, H., & Kobak, R. (1996). Attachment processes in eating disorder and depression. *Journal of Consulting and Clinical Psychology, 64*, 282–290.

Coolidge, F. L., Thede, L. L., & Jang, K. L. (2001). Heritability of childhood personality disorders: A preliminary study. *Journal of Personality Disorders, 15*, 33–40.

Crowell, S. E., Beauchaine, T. P., Linehan, M. M. (2009). A biosocial developmental model of borderline personality: An elaboration and extension of Linehan's biosocial theory. *Psychological Bulletin, 135*, 495–510.

Cummings, E. M., & Cicchetti, D. (1990). Toward a transactional model of relations between attachment and depression. In M. T. Greenberg, D. Cicchetti, & E. M. Cummings (Eds.), *Attachment in the preschool years* (pp. 339–372). Chicago: University of Chicago Press.

De Bellis, M. D. (2001). Developmental traumatology: The psychobiological development of maltreated children and its implications for research, treatment, and policy. *Development and Psychopathology, 13*, 539–564.

de Ruiter, C., & Van IJzendoorn, M. H. (1992). Agoraphobia and anxious-ambivalent attachment: An integrative review. *Journal of Anxiety Disorders, 6*, 365–381.

Diamond, D., Stovall-McClough, K. C., Clarkin, J. F., & Levy, K. N. (2003). Patient–therapist attachment in the treatment of borderline personality disorder. *Bulletin of the Menninger Clinic, 67*, 227–259.

Dias, P., Soares, I., Klein, J., Cunha, J. P. S., & Roisman, G. I., (2011). Autonomic correlates of attachment insecurity in a sample of women with eating disorders. *Attachment and Human Development, 13*(2), 155–167.

Dozier, M., Cue, K., & Barnett, L. (1994). Clinicians as caregivers: Role of attachment organization in treatment. *Journal of Consulting and Clinical Psychology, 62*, 793–800.

Duggal, S., Carlson, E. A., Sroufe, L. A., & Egeland, B. (2001). Depressive symptomatology in childhood and adolescence. *Development and Psychopathology, 13*, 143–164.

Dutra, L., & Lyons-Ruth, K. (2005, April). *Maltreatment, maternal and child psychopathology, and quality of early care as predictors of adolescent dissociation.* Paper presented at the biennial meeting of the Society for Research in Child Development, Atlanta, GA.

Englund, M., Kuo, S. I., Puig, J., Collins, W. A. (2011). Early roots of adult competence: The significance of close relationships from infancy to early adulthood. *International Journal of Behavioral Development, 35*, 490–496.

Faravelli, C., Webb, T., Ambonetti, A., Fonnesu, F., & Sessarego, A. (1985). Prevalence of traumatic early life events in 31 agoraphobic patients with panic attacks. *American Journal of Psychiatry, 142*, 1493–1494.

Fearon, R. M., & Mansell, W. (2001). Cognitive perspectives on unresolved loss: Insights from the study of PTSD. *Bulletin of the Menninger Clinic, 65*, 380–396.

Fonagy, P., Leigh, T., Steele, M., Steele, H., Kennedy, R., Mattoon, G., et al. (1996). The relation of attachment status, psychiatric classification, and response to psychotherapy. *Journal of Consulting and Clinical Psychology, 64*, 22–31.

Frodi, A., Dernevik, M., Sepa, A., Philipson, J., & Bragesjo, M. (2001). Current attachment representations of incarcerated offenders varying in degree of psychopathy. *Attachment and Human Development, 3*, 269–283.

George, C, Kaplan, N., & Main, M. (1985). *Adult Attachment Interview.* Unpublished manuscript, University of California at Berkeley.

Goldstein, M. J. (1985). Family factors that antedate the onset of schizophrenia and related disorders: The results of a fifteen year prospective study. *Acta Psychiatrica Scandinavica, 71*, 7–18.

Gottesman, I. I. (1991). *Schizophrenia genesis.* New York: Freeman.

Grossmann, K. E., Grossmann, K., & Waters, E. (Eds.). (2005). *Attachment from infancy to adulthood: The major longitudinal studies.* New York: Guilford Press.

Gumley, A. I., Taylor, H. E. F., Schwannauer, M., & MacBeth, A. (2014). A systematic review of attachment psychosis: measurement, construct validity and outcomes. *Acta Psychiatrica Scandinavica, 129*(4), 257–274.

Harari, D., Bakermans-Kranenburg, M. J, de Kloet, C., S., Geuze, E., Vermetten, E., Westenberg, H. G. M., et al. (2009) Attachment representations in Dutch veterans with and without deployment-related PTSD, *Attachment and Human Development, 11*(6), 515–536.

Hare, R., Hart, S., & Harpur, T. (1991). Psychopathy and the DSM-IV criteria for antisocial personality disorder. *Journal of Abnormal Psychology, 100*(3), 391–398.

Harris, T. O., Brown, G. W., & Bifulco, A. T. (1986). Loss of parent in childhood and adult psychiatric disorder: The Walthamstow Study. 1. The role of lack of adequate parental care. *Psychological Medicine, 16*, 641–659.

Harris, T. O., Brown, G. W., & Bifulco, A. T. (1990). Depression and situational helplessness/mastery in a sample selected to study childhood parental loss. *Journal of Affective Disorders, 20*, 27–41.

Herman, J. L., Perry, J. C., & van der Kolk, B. A. (1989). Childhood trauma in borderline personality disorder. *American Journal of Psychiatry, 146*, 490–495.

Hesse, E., Hobson, P., Patrick, M., Maughan, B., & Main, M. (2011, March). *The AAI in a prison population: High scores for unresolved loss in psychopaths, while derogation predicts murder and bodily harm.* Poster presented at the biennial meeting of the Society for Research in Child Development, Montreal, Canada.

Hesse, E., & Van IJzendoorn, M. H. (1998). Parental loss of close family members and propensities towards absorption in offspring. *Developmental Science, 1*, 299–305.

Hettema, J. M., Neale, M. C., & Kendler, K. S. (2001). A review and meta-analysis of the genetic epidemiology of anxiety disorders. *American Journal of Psychiatry, 158*, 1568–1578.

Hettema, J. M., Prescott, C. A., Myers, J. M., Neale, M. C., & Kendler, K. S. (2005). The structure of genetic and environmental risk factors for anxiety disorders in men and women. *Archives of General Psychiatry, 62*, 182–189.

Holtzworth-Munroe, A., Stuart, G. L., & Hutchinson, G. (1997). Violent versus nonviolent husbands: Differences in attachment patterns, dependency, and jealousy. *Journal of Family Psychology, 11*, 314–331.

Ivarsson, T., Granqvist, P., Gillberg, C., & Broberg, A. G. (2010). Attachment states of mind in adolescents with obsessive compulsive disorder and/or depressive disorders: A controlled study. *European Child and Adolescent Psychiatry, 19*, 845–853.

Johnson, J. G., Cohen, P., Kasen, S., & Brook, J. S. (2006). Dissociative disorders among adults in the community, impaired functioning, and Axis I and II comorbidity. *Journal of Psychiatric Research, 40*, 131–140.

Kendler, K., Aggen, S., Czajkowski, N., Roysamb, E., Tambs, K., Torgersen, S., et al. (2008). The structure of genetic and environmental risk factors for DSM-IV personality disorders: A multivariate twin study. *Archives of General Psychiatry, 65*(12), 1438–1446.

Kendler, K. S., Sheth, K., Gardner, C. O., & Prescott, C. A. (2002). Childhood parental loss and risk for first-onset of major depression and alcohol dependence: The time-decay of risk and sex differences. *Psychological Medicine, 323*, 1187–1194.

Kendler, K. S., Heath, A. C., Martin, N. G., & Eaves, L. J. (1987). Symptoms of anxiety and symptoms of depression. *Archives of General Psychiatry, 44*, 451–457.

Kenny, M. E., & Hart, K. (1992). Relationship between parental attachment and eating disorders in an inpatient and a college sample. *Journal of Counseling Psychology, 39*, 521–526.

Kivela, S., Luukinin, H., Koski, K., Viramo, P., & Pahkala, K. (1998). Early loss of mother or father predicts depression in old age. *International Journal of Geriatric Psychiatry, 13*, 527–530.

Kobak, R. (1993). *The Adult Attachment Interview Q-set.* Unpublished manuscript, University of Delaware.

Levinson, A., & Fonagy, P. (2004). Offending and attachment: The relationship between interpersonal awareness and offending in a prison population with psychiatric disorder. *Canadian Journal of Psychoanalysis, 12*, 225–251.

Lichtenstein, J., & Cassidy, J. (1991, April). *The Inventory of Adult Attachment: Validation of a new measure.* Paper presented at the biennial meeting of the Society for Research in Child Development, Seattle, WA.

Liotti, G. (2004). Trauma, dissociation, and disorganized attachment: Three strands of a single braid. *Psychotherapy: Theory, Research, Practice, Training, 41*, 472–486.

Liotti, G., & Pasquini, P. (2000). Predictive factors for borderline personality disorder: Patients' early traumatic experiences and losses suffered by the attachment figure. *Acta Psychiatrica Scandinavica, 102*, 282–289.

Lyons-Ruth, K., Bureau, J., Holmes, B., Easterbrooks, A., Brooks, N. H. (2013). Borderline symptoms and suicidality/self-injury in late adolescence: Prospectively observed relationship correlates in infancy and childhood. *Psychiatry Research, 206*, 273–281.

Lyons-Ruth, K., Yellin, C., Melnick, S., & Atwood, G. (2005). Expanding the concept of unresolved mental states: Hostile/helpless states of mind on the Adult

Attachment Interview are associated with disrupted mother–infant communication and infant disorganization. *Development and Psychopathology, 17*, 1–23.

MacBeth, A., Gumley, A., Schwannauer, M., & Fisher, R. (2010). Attachment states of mind, mentalization, and their correlates in a first-episode psychosis sample. *Psychology and Psychotherapy: Theory, Research and Practice, 84*, 42–57.

Madigan, S., Vaillancourt, K., McKibbon, A., & Benoit, D. (2012) The reporting of maltreatment experiences during the Adult Attachment Interview in a sample of pregnant adolescents. *Attachment and Human Development, 14*(2), 119–143.

Main, M., Goldwyn, R., & Hesse, E. (2003). *Adult attachment scoring and classification system.* Unpublished manuscript, University of California at Berkeley.

Main, M., & Hesse, E. (1990). Parents' unresolved traumatic experiences are related to infant disorganized attachment status: Is frightened and/or frightening parental behavior the linking mechanism? In M. T. Greenberg, D. Cicchetti, & E. M. Cummings (Eds.), *Attachment in the preschool years* (pp. 161–182). Chicago: University of Chicago Press.

Main, M., & Morgan, H. (1996). Disorganization and disorientation in infant Strange Situation behavior. In L. K. Michelson & W. J. Ray (Eds.), *Handbook of dissociation: Theoretical, empirical, and clinical perspectives* (pp. 107–138). New York: Plenum.

Manassis, K., Bradley, S., Goldberg, S., Hood, J., & Swinson, R. P. (1994). Attachment in mothers with anxiety disorders and their children. *Journal of the American Academy of Child and Adolescent Psychiatry, 33*, 1106–1113.

McCord, J. (1979). Some child-rearing antecedents of criminal behavior in adult men. *Journal of Personality and Social Psychology, 37*, 1477–1486.

Mennin, D. S., Heimberg, R. G., Turk, C. L., & Fresco, D. M. (2002). Applying an emotion regulation framework to integrative approaches to generalized anxiety disorder. *Clinical Psychology: Science and Practice, 9*, 85–90.

Millon, T. (1983). *The Millon Clinical Multiaxial Inventory manual* (3rd ed.). Minneapolis, MN: National Computer Systems.

Minuchin, S., Rosman, B. L., & Baker, L. (1980). *Psychosomatic families: Anorexia nervosa in context.* Cambridge, MA: Harvard University Press.

Mitchell, J. E., & Pyle, R. L. (1985). Characteristics of bulimia. In J. E. Mitchell (Ed.), *Anorexia nervosa and bulimia: Diagnosis and treatment* (pp. 29–47). Minneapolis: University of Minnesota Press.

Nickerson, A., Bryant, R. A., Aderka, I. M., Hinton, D. E., & Hofmann, St. G. (2013). The impacts of parental loss and adverse parenting on mental health: Findings from the national comorbidity survey-replication. *Psychological Trauma: Theory, Research, Practice,Policy, 5*, 119–127.

Nye, E. C., Katzman, J., Bell, J. B., Kilpatrick, J., Brainard, M., & Haaland, K. Y. (2008). Attachment organization in Vietnam combat veterans with posttraumatic stress disorder. *Attachment and Human Development, 10*, 41–57.

Oakley-Browne, M. A., Joyce, P. R., Wells, J. E., Bushnell, J. A., & Hornblow, A. R. (1995). Adverse parenting and other childhood experiences as risk factors for depression in women aged 18–44 years. *Journal of Affective Disorders, 34*, 13–23.

Ogata, S. N., Silk, K. R., Goodrich, S., Lohr, N. E., Westen, D., & Hill, E. M. (1990). Childhood sexual and physical abuse in adult patients with borderline personality disorder. *American Journal of Psychiatry, 147*, 1008–1013.

Ogawa, J., Sroufe, L. A., Weinfield, N. S., Carlson, E. A., & Egeland, B. (1997). Development and the fragmented self: A longitudinal study of dissociative symptomatology in a non-clinical sample. *Development and Psychopathology, 9*, 855–879.

Palmer, R. L., Oppenheimer, R., & Marshall, P. D. (1988). Eating disordered patients remember their parents: A study using the Parental Bonding Instrument. *International Journal of Eating Disorders, 7*, 101–106.

Parry, P. (2010). Paediatric bipolar disorder: Are attachment and trauma factors considered? In J. Barnhill (Ed.), *Bipolar disorder: A portrait of a complex mood disorder* (pp. 165–190). Rijeka, Croatia: InTech.

Pasquini, P., Liotti, G., Mazzotti, E., Fassone, G., & Picardi, A. (2002). Risk factors in the early family life of patients suffering from dissociative disorders. *Acta Psychiatrica Scandinavica, 105*, 110–116.

Patrick, M., Hobson, R. P., Castle, D., Howard, R., & Maughan, B. (1994). Personality disorder and the mental representation of early social experience. *Development and Psychopathology, 6*, 375–388.

Pope, H. G., Mangweth, B., Negrao, A. B., Hudson, J. I., & Cordas, T. A. (1994). Childhood sexual abuse and bulimia nervosa: A comparison of American, Austrian, and Brazilian women. *American Journal of Psychiatry, 151*, 732–737.

Putnam, F. W. (1991). Recent research on multiple personality disorder. *Psychiatric Clinics of North America, 14*, 489–502.

Ratti, L. A., Humphrey, L. L., & Lyons, J. S. (1996). Structural analysis of families with a polydrug-dependent, bulimic, or normal adolescent daughter. *Journal of Consulting and Clinical Psychology, 64*, 1255–1262.

Rhodes, B., & Kroger, J. (1992). Parental bonding and separation–individuation difficulties among late adolescent eating disordered women. *Child Psychiatry and Human Development, 22*, 249–263.

Riggs, S. A., Paulson, A., Tunnell, E., Sahl, G., Atkison, H., & Ross, C. A. (2007). Attachment, personality, and psychopathology among adult inpatients: Self-reported romantic attachment style versus Adult Attachment Interview states of mind. *Development and Psychopathology, 19*, 263–291.

Robins, L. (1966). *Deviant children grown up.* Baltimore: Williams & Wilkins.

Rosenstein, D. S., & Horowitz, H. A. (1996). Adolescent attachment and psychopathology. *Journal of Consulting and Clinical Psychology, 64,* 244–253.

Rowa, K., Kerig, P. K., & Geller, J. (2001). The family and anorexia nervosa: Examining parent–child boundary problems. *European Eating Disorders Review, 9,* 97–114.

Sanders, B., & Giolas, M. H. (1991). Dissociation and childhood trauma in psychologically disturbed adolescents. *American Journal of Psychiatry, 148,* 50–54.

Savitz, J. B., van der Merwe, L., Newman, T. K., Solms, M., Stein, D. J., & Ramesar, R. S. (2008). The relationship between childhood abuse and dissociation: Is it influenced by catechol-O-methyltransferase (COMT) activity? *International Journal of Neuropsychopharmacology, 11*(2), 149–161.

Seligman, M. E. P., Abramson, L. Y., Semmel, A., & von Baeyer, C. (1979). Depressive attributional style. *Journal of Abnormal Psychology, 88,* 242–247.

Shi, Z., Bureau, J., Easterbrooks, M.A., Zhao, X., & Lyons-Ruth, K. (2012). Childhood maltreatment and prospectively observed quality of early care as predictors of antisocial personality disorder features. *Infant Mental Health Journal, 33,* 55–69.

Soloff, H. P., & Millward, J. W. (1983). Developmental histories of borderline patients. *Comprehensive Psychiatry, 24,* 574–588.

Sroufe, L. A. (1997). Psychopathology as development. *Development and Psychopathology, 9,* 251–268.

Sroufe, L. A. (2005). Attachment and development: A prospective, longitudinal study from birth to adulthood. *Attachment and Human Development, 7,* 349–367.

Sroufe, L. A., Egeland, B., Carlson, E., & Collins, W. A. (2005a). *The development of the person: The Minnesota Study of Risk and Adaptation from Birth to Adulthood.* New York: Guilford Press.

Sroufe, L. A., Egeland, B., Carlson, E., & Collins, W. A. (2005b). Placing early attachment experiences in developmental context: The Minnesota longitudinal study. In K. E. Grossmann, K. Grossmann, & E. Waters (Eds.), *Attachment from infancy to adulthood: The major longitudinal studies* (pp. 48–70). New York: Guilford Press.

Stalker, C. A., & Davies, F. (1995). Attachment organization and adaptation in sexually-abused women. *Canadian Journal of Psychiatry, 40,* 234–240.

Steele, H. (2003). Unrelenting catastrophic trauma within the family: When every secure base is abusive. *Attachment and Human Development, 5,* 353–366.

Stovall-McClough, K. C., & Cloitre, M. (2003). Reorganization of unresolved childhood traumatic memories following exposure therapy. *Annals of the New York Academy of Sciences, 1008,* 297–299.

Stovall-McClough, K. C., & Cloitre, M. (2006). Unresolved attachment, PTSD, and dissociation in women with childhood abuse histories. *Journal of Consulting and Clinical Psychology, 74,* 219–228.

Sullivan, P. F., Neale, M. C., & Kendler, K. S. (2000). Genetic epidemiology of major depression: Review and meta-analysis. *American Journal of Psychiatry, 157,* 1552–1562.

Tadic, A., Victor, A., Başkaya, O., von Cube, R., Hoch, J., Kouti, I., et al. (2009). Interaction between gene variants of the serotonin transporter promoter region (5-HTTLPR) and catechol O-methyltransferase (COMT) in borderline personality disorder. *American Journal of Medical Genetics, Part B, Neuropsychiatric Genetics, 150B*(4), 487–495.

Takeuchi, H., Hiroe, T., Kanai, T., Morinobu, S., Kitamura, T., Takahashi, K., et al. (2003). Childhood parental separation experiences and depressive symptomatology in acute major depression. *Psychiatry and Clinical Neurosciences, 57*(2), 215–219.

Terreira, A. (1960). The pregnant woman's attitude and its reflection on the newborn. *American Journal of Orthopsychiatry, 30,* 553–561.

Thompson, J. L., Watson, J. R., Steinhauer, S. R., Goldstein, G., & Pogue-Geile, M. F. (2005). Indicators of genetic liability to schizophrenia: A sibling study of neuropsychological performance. *Schizophrenia Bulletin, 31,* 85–96.

Thomson, P., & Jaque, V. (2012). Dissociation and the Adult Attachment Interview in artists and performing artists. *Attachment and Human Development, 14,* 145–160.

Torgersen, S., Kringlen, E., & Cramer, V. (2001). The prevalence of personality disorders in a community sample. *Archives of General Psychiatry, 58,* 590–596.

Torgersen, S., Lygren, S., Oeien, P. A., Skre, I., Onstad, S., Edvardsen, J., et al. (2000). A twin study of personality disorders. *Comprehensive Psychiatry, 41,* 416–425.

Torgersen, S., Myers, J., Reichborn-Kjennerud, T., Roysamb, E., Kubarych, T. S., & Kendler, K. S. (2012) The heritability of cluster B personality disorders assessed both by personal interview and questionnaire. *Journal of Personality Disorders, 26,* 848–866.

Tyrrell, C. L., Dozier, M., Teague, G. B., & Fallot, R. D. (1999). Effective treatment relationships for persons with serious psychiatric disorders: The importance of attachment states of mind. *Journal of Clinical Psychology, 67*(5), 725–733.

Vidovic, V., Juresa, V., Begovac, I., Mahnik, M., & Tocilkj, G. (2005). Perceived family cohesion, adaptability and communication in eating disorders. *European Eating Disorders Review, 13,* 19–28.

Wade, T. D., Treloar, S. A., & Martin, N. G. (2001). A comparison of family functioning, temperament, and childhood conditions in monozygotic twin pairs discordant for lifetime bulimia nervosa. *American Journal of Psychiatry, 158,* 1155–1157.

Walker, E. F., Grimes, K. E., Davis, D. M., & Smith, A. J. (1993). Childhood precursors of schizophrenia: Facial expressions of emotion. *American Journal of Psychiatry, 150,* 1654–1660.

Waller, N. G., & Ross, C. (1997). The prevalence and biometric structure of pathological dissociation in the general population: Taxonomic and behavior genetic findings. *Journal of Abnormal Psychology, 106,* 499–510.

Wallin, U., & Hansson, K. (1999). Anorexia nervosa in teenagers: Patterns of family function. *Nordic Journal of Psychiatry, 53,* 29–35.

Walter, S., Glymour, M. M., Koenen, K., Liang, L., Tchetgen, E. J. T., Cornelis, M., et al. (2013). Performance of polygenic scores for predicting phobic anxiety. *PLoS ONE, 8*(11), e80326.

Ward, A., Ramsay, R., Turnbull, S., Steele, M., Steele, H., & Treasure, J. (2001). Attachment in anorexia nervosa: A transgenerational perspective. *British Journal of Medical Psychology, 74,* 497–505.

Warren, S. L., Huston, L., Egeland, B., & Sroufe, L. A. (1997). Child and adolescent anxiety disorders and early attachment. *Journal of the American Academy of Child and Adolescent Psychiatry, 36,* 637–644.

Welch, S. L., & Fairburn, C. G. (1994). Sexual abuse and bulimia nervosa: Three integrated case control comparisons. *American Journal of Psychiatry, 15,* 402–407.

West, M., Adam, K., Spreng, S., & Rose, S. (2001). Attachment disorganization and dissociative symptoms in clinically treated adolescents. *Canadian Journal of Psychiatry, 46,* 627–631.

Widiger, T. A. (1993). The DSM-III-R categorical personality diagnoses: A critique and an alternative. *Psychological Inquiry, 4,* 75–90.

Woodside, D. B., Bulik, C. M., Halmi, K. A., Fichter, M. M., Kaplan, A., Berrettini, W. H., et al. (2002). Personality, perfectionism, and attitudes toward eating in parents of individuals with eating disorders. *International Journal of Eating Disorders, 31,* 290–299.

Zanarini, M. C., Gunderson, J. G., Marino, M. F., Schwartz, E. O., & Frankenberg, F. R. (1989). Childhood experiences of borderline patients. *Comprehensive Psychiatry, 30,* 18–25.

Zeijlmans van Emmichoven, I. A., Van IJzendoorn, M. H., de Ruiter, C., & Brosschot, J. F. (2003). Selective processing of threatening information: Effects of attachment representation and anxiety disorder on attention and memory. *Development and Psychopathology, 15,* 219–237.

# Chapter 32

# Prevention and Intervention Programs to Support Early Attachment Security

## A Move to the Level of the Community

Lisa J. Berlin
Charles H. Zeanah
Alicia F. Lieberman

The opportunity to revisit the topic of attachment-based interventions for this third edition of the *Handbook of Attachment* comes at a particularly exciting time for several reasons. First, supporting early child development is a prominent goal among practitioners and policymakers. Galvanized by large studies linking early adversity to diverse negative outcomes (e.g., Edwards, Holden, Anda, & Felitti, 2003), concerns about young children's exposure to "toxic stress" are being widely voiced (e.g., Bornstein, 2013; Shonkoff, 2010). Simultaneously, and informed in large part by attachment theory and research, supportive parenting is increasingly recognized as a crucial buffer to toxic stressors (Shonkoff; 2010; Tough, 2012). President Barack Obama's 2014 State of the Union address called for the expansion of services that support early child development and early parenting.

Another reason to be especially enthusiastic about attachment-based interventions concerns the depth of the evidence base. Rigorous evaluations are increasingly demonstrating lasting and diverse positive effects of several attachment intervention programs. Moreover, attachment interventions are increasingly moving from university-based trials to community-based implementation, creating the possibility for attachment-based programs to play a sustained role in the broader provision of social services to children and families.

We begin by reviewing the implications of attachment theory and research for attachment-based intervention. We then review the four attachment-based intervention programs with the strongest evidence base: Child–Parent Psychotherapy, the Attachment and Biobehavioral Catch-up program, the Video-Feedback Intervention to Promote Positive Parenting program, and the Circle of Security program. We next describe several efforts to translate attachment interventions from university research-driven endeavors to community-based programs. We conclude with a set of recommendations for sustaining the "real-world" implementation of attachment-based interventions. Throughout, we highlight progress in attachment-based interventions since our previous version of this *Handbook* chapter (Berlin, Zeanah, & Lieberman, 2008) and offer suggestions for the continued development of the field.

## Implications of Attachment Theory and Research for Attachment-Based Intervention

### The Attachment "Transmission Gap" and Infants' Differential Susceptibility

As we have previously discussed at length (Berlin et al., 2008), attachment theory and research have direct implications for intervention. Van IJzendoorn's (1995) "transmission model" and his identification of a "transmission gap" concisely summarize this theory and research. According to the transmission model, a parent's internal working models of attachment drive parenting behaviors, which in turn shape the quality of the child's attachment to that parent. Parents' internal working models influence parenting behaviors by guiding the parent's responsiveness to the child's needs (Main, 1990). The parent's sensitive responsiveness fosters emotional security, whereas less supportive parenting is characterized by partial or inconsistent responsiveness.

Through two meta-analyses, Van IJzendoorn (1995; deWolff & Van IJzendoorn, 1997) provided strong support for direct links between (1) parents' internal working models and their sensitive parenting behaviors, (2) parents' internal working models and their child's attachment to them, and (3) sensitive parenting behaviors and child attachment. Sensitive parenting behaviors, however, accounted for a relatively small proportion of the association between parental internal working models and child attachment (Van IJzendoorn, 1995). Thus, sensitive parenting did not appear to be the principal mediator of the effects of parental working models on child attachment. This "transmission gap" was subsequently replicated in several other investigations (for reviews, see Atkinson et al., 2000, 2005; Madigan et al., 2006) and is still not well understood.

We (2008) previously discussed several emerging areas of research helping to clarify the transmission gap and its implications for intervention. Of these, Belsky's differential susceptibility framework (Belsky & Pleuss, 2009) has been especially valuable. According to this framework, individuals are differentially susceptible to rearing influences. Moreover, individuals are differentially susceptible "for better *and* for worse," meaning that some highly sensitive and often temperamentally irritable infants both suffer more in response to early adversity and also benefit more from early

support (Bakermans-Kranenburg & Van IJzendoorn, 2007; Belsky, Bakermans-Kranenburg, & Van IJzendoorn, 2007).

Differential susceptibility may be due, in part, to genes that regulate dopamine in the brain, as illustrated by a recent meta-analysis (Bakermans-Kranenburg & Van IJzendoorn, 2011). For example, a 2006 study found that infants with a dopamine receptor polymorphism (*D4DR* 7-repeat allele) whose mothers had unresolved losses or traumas were at increased risk for attachment disorganization (Van IJzendoorn & Bakermans-Kranenburg, 2006). Moreover, infants with this 7-repeat allele whose mothers did not have unresolved losses or traumas exhibited significantly less disorganization than infants without the 7-repeat allele, regardless of whether these less susceptible infants had mothers who were resolved or unresolved with respect to loss or trauma. Another inquiry illustrated that children with the *D4DR* 7-repeat allele whose mothers treated them less sensitively at 10 months were reported to have more externalizing behavior problems at age 3 than children without the 7-repeat allele, regardless of their mothers' sensitivity (Bakermans-Kranenburg & Van IJzendoorn, 2006). Furthermore, children with the 7-repeat allele whose mothers treated them more sensitively during infancy had the lowest externalizing behavior problem scores. Other research examining gene–environment interactions as predictors of attachment-related phenomena has pointed to polymorphisms of serotonin transporter genes (e.g., Cicchetti, Rogosch, & Toth, 2011; Drury et al., 2012; Spangler, Johann, Ronai, & Zimmermann, 2009). For further discussion of attachment, genetics, and differential susceptibility, see Bakermans-Kranenburg and Van IJzendoorn (Chapter 8, this volume).

Taken as a whole, the growing evidence of gene–environment interactions as predictors of attachment-related phenomena implies that one reason for the transmission gap may be that the transmission model is more relevant to some (more susceptible) children than to others. By extension, the implications of the transmission model for attachment programs may also need to be considered in the context of the differential susceptibility approach (Bakermans-Kranenburg & Van IJzendoorn, 2015). Much about the transmission gap and about differential susceptibility remains to be specified. Understanding of both will likely draw on attachment intervention work guided by the transmission model.

## Implications of the Attachment "Transmission Model" for Attachment-Based Intervention

As we have previously described (Berlin et al., 2008), the attachment transmission model suggests two points of intervention: the parent's internal working models and parenting behavior(s). In keeping with Bowlby's (1980, 1988) proposal that new attachments are one of the factors most likely to alter internal working models, we have emphasized the importance of the intervener serving as a secure base for the parent. As we describe further later in this chapter, the relationship between the intervener and the parent plays at least some role in all the attachment-based interventions we review.

## Prevention and Intervention Programs to Support Early Attachment Security: The Evidence Base

In this section we review the four attachment-based intervention programs that have amassed the strongest evidence bases: Child–Parent Psychotherapy, the Attachment and Biobehavioral Catch-up program, the Video-Feedback Intervention to Promote Positive Parenting program, and the Circle of Security program. In so doing, we describe key intervention targets and processes, as well as the latest evaluation findings. We also revisit three questions identified in our earlier work as requiring clarification. The first question stems from evidence that different services fit some families better than others: *What works for whom?* The second question refers to mechanisms of therapeutic change: *What drives program success?* The third question concerns the criteria for positive outcomes: *What is program success?*

## Child–Parent Psychotherapy

Child–Parent Psychotherapy (CPP) is a dyadic intervention based on infant–parent psychotherapy, a psychoanalytic treatment for infants under age 3 and their parents. In this intervention, the metaphor of "ghosts in the nursery" is used to describe the intergenerational transmission of unresolved childhood conflicts from the parent to the infant (Fraiberg, 1980). The principal goals are to help the parent (1) reconnect with the pain, fear, anger,

and helplessness evoked by frightening childhood experiences and (2) understand his or her current negative feelings toward his or her infant as a reenactment of unresolved conflicts about his or her own parents or other important childhood figures resulting from these frightening experiences. The therapist's empathic guidance is considered the essential ingredient for helping the parents explore their past, practice new parenting behaviors, and free their child from engulfment in the parents' conflicted childhood experiences.

Lieberman and Van Horn (2005, 2008) expanded this model to CPP, a manualized, 12-month intervention for children between birth and 5 years of age. CPP incorporates Bowlby's emphasis on the importance of external reality as a source of traumatic stressors and other adverse influences that may have a dual impact on the child and on parental perceptions and behaviors toward the child. It does this while also retaining an appreciation for the role of the parents' unresolved childhood experiences in shaping their working models of attachment and their relationship with the child (Lieberman & Van Horn, 2008). CPP simultaneously targets the parent's pathogenic perceptions and behaviors, and the child's mental health symptoms, and aims to support attachment security primarily as a mechanism for promoting the child's mental health.

The initial CPP assessment of the dyad includes a structured questionnaire about child and parent exposure to traumatic experiences, an evaluation of safety concerns and concrete needs, and an exploration of the parents' culturally based caregiving values and practices. The assessment ends with a feedback session in which the parent is engaged in co-creating a treatment plan that includes psychoeducation about the impact of trauma and adverse experiences on the child and the parent.

CPP sessions are conducted jointly with the parent(s) and the child. The CPP therapist uses play and unstructured interactions as vehicles to promote a goal-corrected partnership, translate the motivations and feelings of the child and the parent toward each other, address trauma reminders, and reframe mutual negative attributions. When this therapeutic focus on the present is not sufficient to promote improvement, the CPP therapist guides the parent into an exploration of her or his childhood experiences that are being reenacted in relation to the child. CPP therapists also provide case management and connect the family to relevant community services when concrete problems of living interfere with the parent's ability to create a safe family environment.

CPP efficacy is supported by five randomized trials. Lieberman, Weston, and Pawl (1991) randomly assigned 59 newly immigrated, impoverished, and highly stressed Latina mothers and their insecurely attached 1-year-olds to 1 year of weekly, 90-minute, home-based CPP or to a control group. When the children were 2 years old, the CPP group had higher scores on observed maternal empathy and dyadic goal-corrected partnership, and lower levels of children's avoidance, resistance, and anger toward their mothers. The Attachment Q-Sort did not show group differences, a finding attributed by the authors to insufficient training of the assessors in using this measure. Within the CPP group, a measure of "level of therapeutic process" predicted attachment security, maternal empathy, initiation of interaction and involvement, dyadic goal-corrected partnership, and lower child avoidance.

CPP was also found to foster attachment security in infants and preschoolers from maltreating families (Cicchetti, Rogosch, & Toth, 2006; Toth, Maughan, Manly, Spagnola, & Cicchetti, 2002). In a randomized trial with 137 infants, those receiving CPP between ages 12 months and 24 months were significantly more likely to be securely attached at 26 months than control infants receiving services as usual. A 1-year follow-up study found higher rates of attachment security (according to Schneider-Rosen, Braunwald, Carlson, & Cicchetti's [1985] coding scheme) among CPP 3-year-olds compared to controls (Stronach, Toth, Rogosch, & Cicchetti, 2013). A subsequent follow-up study revealed that by age 3, the CPP children were showing increasingly higher (normal) production of morning cortisol, a hormonal index of stress regulation that often shows atypical patterns in traumatized children (Cicchetti, Rogosch, Toth, & Sturge-Apple, 2011).The control infants' morning cortisol production declined over time to atypically low levels. Thus, in this case, CPP appeared to prevent hormonal dysregulation. There were not significant group differences in maternal sensitivity when children were 26 months old or in mother-reported behavior problems at age 3. There was also no evidence of any genetic moderators of the efficacy of the intervention (Cicchetti, Rogosch, & Toth, 2011).

Interestingly, immediately postintervention, there were no group differences in attachment between the CPP group and a group receiving a home-based psychoeducational parenting intervention (Cicchetti et al., 2006). At follow-up, however, CPP 3-year-olds were more likely to be securely attached than children in the comparison group (Stronach et al., 2013). Similar findings emerged from a randomized trial of 87 maltreated preschoolers (Toth et al., 2002).

CPP also fostered attachment security in toddlers of depressed mothers (Cicchetti, Toth, & Rogosch, 1999; Toth, Rogosch, Manly, & Cicchetti, 2006). At age 3, the CPP group had higher IQ scores than the control group (Cicchetti, Rogosch, & Toth, 2000). No CPP effects were found on maternal depression, and maternal depression did not moderate intervention effects.

A final randomized trial included 75 preschoolers exposed to marital violence and other traumatic stressors (Lieberman, Van Horn, & Ghosh Ippen, 2005). Compared to case management plus community treatment as usual, those who received weekly CPP for 1 year showed fewer mother-reported behavior problems and traumatic stress symptoms and were less likely to meet criteria for traumatic stress disorder. Mothers reported significantly fewer symptoms of posttraumatic stress disorder (PTSD)-related avoidance (Lieberman et al., 2005). A 6-month follow-up study reexamining 50 of these dyads showed that children in the CPP group maintained their lower behavior problems relative to the control group, and their mother reported significantly fewer psychiatric symptoms (Lieberman, Ghosh Ippen, & Van Horn, 2006). A data reanalysis comparing children with four or more traumatic events and children with fewer than four traumatic events showed that CPP effects were stronger for children and mothers who had experienced more risk (Ghosh Ippen, Harris, Van Horn, & Lieberman, 2011).

In summary, in keeping with its overarching concerns with children's mental health, CPP has demonstrated largely positive effects on both attachment-specific and broader mental health outcomes. Three of four randomized trials with high-risk families tested and found effects of CPP on attachment security in infants, toddlers, or preschoolers. In the one study in which there were no program effects on attachment security, there were positive effects on relevant maternal and child behaviors such as maternal empathy and child avoidance (Lieberman et al., 1991). In some, but not all, subsequent studies demonstrating effects on attachment security, there were also effects on maternal sensitivity (e.g., Cicchetti et al., 2006). In some, but not all, studies CPP demonstrated positive effects on child behavior problems. CPP has shown sustained effects on attachment security, maternal mental health, and child behavior problems (Lieberman et al., 2006; Stronach et al., 2013). Finally, CPP has shown positive effects on hormonal (cortisol) regulation (Cicchetti, Rogosch, Toth, & Sturge-Apple, 2011). This body of findings is important because CPP is attachment-informed rather than attachment-derived and addresses the child–parent relationship broadly, rather than focusing more narrowly on attachment behaviors. The fact that CPP's effects on attachment security are as powerful as they are speaks to the centrality of attachment in child–parent relationships.

As we discuss later in this chapter, CPP has been broadly disseminated worldwide, and it is increasingly being implemented in community settings. Given its duration and intensity, CPP requires extensive resources. Current and future efforts for program development center on mechanisms for ensuring fidelity and long-term sustainability, often within the context of broad-based social service systems (e.g., Van Horn et al., 2012).

### Attachment and Biobehavioral Catch-up

Developed by Dozier and her colleagues to promote attachment security and biological regulation in children who have experienced early adversity, the manualized Attachment and Biobehavioral Catch-up (ABC) program consists of 10 home-based sessions delivered by a trained parent coach (Dozier, Lindheim, & Ackerman, 2005). Each session includes mother and child together and addresses a specific topic. Each session also includes a review of video-recorded mother–infant interactions, starting with stock Strange Situation clips and moving to video feedback specific to the dyad, both to reinforce supportive parenting behaviors and to facilitate gentle suggestions for alternatives.

The ABC program has undergone continual refinement during the past several years. It now emphasizes explicit parent coaching in reference to three behavioral targets: (1) nurturance; (2) following the child's lead; and (3) reducing frightening caregiving behavior. Two sessions are devoted to the topic of "overriding" one's own parenting history and/or non-nurturing instincts. In addition, parent coaches provide frequent "in-the-moment" comments in response to opportunities that they observe for the parent to provide nurturance or to follow the child's lead. The parent coach explicitly connects the parent's ongoing behaviors to these behavioral targets and to the infant's responses and/or longer-term developmental benefits. Comments are deliberately disproportionately positive. For example, if the parent coach notices the mother hugging her distressed toddler, the parent coach will immediately praise the mother for providing nurturance and note how helpful it is for her child (e.g., "Great job cuddling him after he fell down. . . . See how he is calming down so quickly in your arms. . . . You are teaching him that you are there for him . . ."). An ABC parent coach is expected to make at least one comment per minute during every session. The quantity and content of a parent coach's in-the-moment commenting has become the focal point of ABC training, supervision, and monitoring.

Two large randomized trials have provided strong evidence of program efficacy. Both have compared the ABC program to a 10-session, home-based control intervention that targets cognitive and language development. The first randomized trial included 96 foster infants and their foster mothers. Following intervention, the ABC foster mothers showed greater pre- to postintervention improvements in sensitive parenting behaviors than control foster mothers (Bick & Dozier, 2013). The ABC foster infants demonstrated more secure attachment behaviors and less avoidance than the control foster infants, according to the Parent Attachment Diaries (Dozier et al., 2009). Within ABC recipients, foster mothers who began the ABC program with autonomous (secure) states of mind with respect to attachment according to the Adult Attachment Interview also received higher coder-rated score for understanding of intervention concepts and "reflective functioning" (insight and self-awareness) than foster mothers who began ABC with nonautonomous states of mind (Bick, Dozier, & Moore, 2012).

A follow-up analysis of cortisol production revealed that, compared to the control group, children in the ABC group exhibited more normal patterns of cortisol production and that this pattern did not differ significantly from the pattern observed in a comparison group of 104 children who had never been in foster care (Dozier et al., 2006; Dozier, Peloso, Lewis, Laurenceau, & Levine, 2008). Moreover, ABC foster mothers of toddlers reported fewer behavior problems than control foster mothers (Dozier et al., 2006). Another follow-up study examined 37 of the original participants' cognitive flexibility and theory of mind (perspective-taking) skills between the ages of 4 and 6 (Lewis-Morrarty, Dozier, Bernard, Terracciano, & Moore, 2012). Findings again favored the ABC children, who demonstrated stronger cognitive flexibility and theory-of-mind skills than control children, and cognitive flexibility and theory-of-mind skills equal to those of 24 never-fostered comparison children.

A second randomized trial targeted 212 custodial biological mothers and their infants or toddlers (age two or younger) receiving child protective services after being identified as being at risk for child neglect (Bernard et al., 2012). Analysis of postintervention Strange Situations for 120 infants and toddlers (mean age 19 months) revealed that ABC children were significantly less likely to be disorganized and more likely to be securely attached than controls (Bernard et al., 2012). Observation of 117 toddlers' problem-solving abilities during a challenging tool task with their mothers indicated that ABC toddlers displayed less sadness and anger than controls (Lind, Bernard, Ross, & Dozier, 2014).

In keeping with its original goals, the ABC program has demonstrated positive effects on both biological and behavioral outcomes. Specifically, a postintervention study including 101 participants found that children in the ABC group exhibited higher morning levels of cortisol and more normal diurnal patterns of cortisol production (i.e., higher morning levels followed by lower evening levels), whereas control children showed a flatter pattern across the day (Bernard, Dozier, Bick, & Gordon, 2014). A follow-up study including 125 preschoolers revealed strikingly similar findings, with the ABC preschoolers again exhibiting higher morning levels of cortisol and more normal diurnal patterns of cortisol production approximately 3 years after the end of the ABC intervention (Bernard, Hostinar, & Dozier, 2015).

Finally, analysis of parent coaches' in-the-moment comments is beginning to illuminate the mechanisms underlying ABC program effects. Two different, relatively recent studies indicated that coders' ratings of the frequency and content of parent coaches' in-the-moment comments predicted positive changes in observed parenting behaviors (Meade & Dozier, 2012; Meade, Dozier, Weston-Lee, & Neely, 2014).

In summary, the ABC program has demonstrated consistently positive short-term effects on attachment-specific outcomes, including child security and caregivers' sensitive behaviors, long-term effects on child behaviors such as cognitive flexibility, and short- and longer-term effects on

hormonal (cortisol) regulation. The program's combined features of manualization, a short duration, and substantive intensity make it an especially appealing candidate for community-based implementation outside of controlled evaluation studies. As we discuss later in this chapter, increasingly ABC is in fact being broadly disseminated and folded into child- and family-serving systems such as child welfare services. It is important to note that parent coaching according to ABC requires considerable skill. Parent coaches work relatively independently, must address session-specific intervention topics with caregivers while simultaneously observing and commenting on ongoing caregiving behaviors, and must be dexterous users of video recordings. As will be discussed further, the process of ABC adoption by community-based providers requires attending carefully to all of these demands.

With respect to the evaluation and thorough "unpacking" of the mechanisms underlying both attachment-based interventions and attachment relationships, we (2008) previously noted that there are no attachment-based intervention studies with both pre- and postintervention assessments of maternal state of mind with respect to attachment, parenting behaviors, and child attachment security. This is still the case, though with the exception of preintervention measure of child attachment security and postintervention measures of maternal states of mind (Adult Attachment Interviews), Dozier's ABC database contains all of the other components noted and therefore is currently the most comprehensive attachment intervention database.

### Video-Feedback Intervention to Promote Positive Parenting

Juffer, Bakermans-Kranenburg, and Van IJzendoorn (2008) have developed and evaluated several versions of the Video-Feedback Intervention to Promote Positive Parenting (VIPP), which is a home-based program that includes four to six sessions of approximately 90 minutes each. Trained interveners focus on promoting parental sensitivity through interveners' presentation of written materials and review of in-home, videotaped infant–parent interactions. Using an approach called "speaking for the child," interveners aim to help the parent notice the infant's signals, interpret them accurately, and respond promptly and appropriately. Video reviews highlight "sensitivity chains" in which the parent's sensitive responsivity is met with a positive reaction from the infant (Juffer, Bakermans-Kranenburg, & Van IJzendoorn, 2014).

Multiple randomized trials support program efficacy. VIPP has typically been contrasted with a light control "intervention," such as weekly phone check-ins with the parent. Positive effects of the program have been concentrated in improvements in sensitive caregiving behaviors. For example, one randomized trial targeted 81 first-time mothers preliminarily classified as having insecure states of mind with respect to attachment (Klein Velderman, Bakermans-Kranenburg, Juffer, & Van IJzendoorn, 2006a). VIPP mothers received home visits between their infants' seventh and 10th months. When their infants were 11 and 13 months old, VIPP mothers were rated as significantly more sensitive than no-treatment control mothers. Interestingly, the intervention had stronger effects on increasing maternal sensitivity for mothers of temperamentally "highly reactive" infants. There were no significant intervention effects on infant–mother attachment at 13 months. Among the highly reactive infants who received VIPP, there was a significant association between pre- to posttest change in maternal sensitivity and infant attachment security. This association was not significant among the less reactive infants who received VIPP. Together these findings lend support to Belsky's differential susceptibility framework by illustrating stronger intervention effects for the highly reactive and presumably more sensitive and susceptible infants, as well as greater susceptibility among these infants to their mothers' evolving parenting behaviors.

In a follow-up study conducted when these children were of preschool age, children who had received VIPP during infancy were less likely to meet clinical criteria for externalizing behavior problems (Klein Velderman et al., 2006b). These effects were not mediated by earlier maternal sensitivity. In addition, there were no program effects on maternal sensitivity or on Attachment Q-Sort scores at this time, nor any evidence of moderation of program effects by infant reactivity.

Another randomized trial with approximately 130 adoptive parents found some positive effects on attachment security of an enhanced version of VIPP (VIPP-R), in which the duration of the home visits was expanded to 3 hours in order to include discussion of parents' childhood attachment experiences (Juffer, Hoksbergen, Riksen-Walraven, & Kohnstamm, 1997; Juffer, Rosenboom, Hoksbergen, Riksen-Walraven, & Kohnstamm,

1997). Among adoptive families without—but not with—birth children, those who had participated in VIPP-R evinced a higher proportion of securely attached infants compared to the control group. Follow-up analyses of both types of adoptive families indicated positive effects of VIPP-R (but not VIPP) on attachment organization (i.e., fewer infants classified disorganized; Juffer, Bakermans-Kranenburg, & Van IJzendoorn, 2005) and on children's behavior problems at age 7 (Stams, Juffer, Van IJzendoorn, & Hoksbergen, 2001).

Another version of the program, Video-Feedback Intervention to Promote Positive Parenting and Sensitive Discipline (VIPP-SD), emphasizes both parental sensitivity and positive disciplinary practices for children showing early signs of externalizing problems (Mesman et al., 2007). In a randomized trial of 237 families selected on the basis of their 1- to 3-year-old child's high scores for externalizing behaviors, 1 year after completing treatment, program mothers exhibited significantly more sensitive disciplinary attitudes and behaviors than control mothers (van Zeijl et al., 2006).

Two follow-ups of this study have examined the dopamine receptor polymorphism (*D4DR* 7-repeat allele) as a moderator of the effects of VIPP-SD. The first examined the *D4DR* 7-repeat allele as a moderator of program effects on 157 children's externalizing behavior problems, as reported by their mothers, an outcome for which there was not a main effect in the original study with all 237 families (Bakermans-Kranenburg, Van IJzendoorn, Pijlman, et al., 2008). As expected, the children with the *D4DR* 7-repeat allele were differentially susceptible to the intervention such that VIPP-SD reduced behavior problems only for these children (VIPP-SD did not have an effect for children without the *D4DR* 7-repeat allele). This effect was especially pronounced in VIPP-SD families whose mothers showed more improvement in their use of sensitive discipline. A second follow-up study investigated the *D4DR* 7-repeat allele as a moderator of program effects on 130 children's daily cortisol production (Bakermans-Kranenburg, Van IJzendoorn, Mesman, Alink, & Juffer, 2008). Again, the children with the *D4DR* 7-repeat allele were differentially susceptible to the intervention, such that VIPP-SD reduced daily—and particularly morning—production of cortisol for these children only.

The VIPP program continues to undergo development and expansion. For example, VIPP has been implemented for mothers with eating disorders (Stein et al., 2006) and with children with autism spectrum disorders (Poslawsky et al., 2015). A randomized trial of VIPP-SD in Portugal including 42 poor, high-risk families with toddlers found positive effects on observed mother–child interactions, harsh discipline, and mother-reported family environment (Negrão, Pereira, Soares, & Mesman, 2014; Pereira, Negrão, Soares, & Mesman, 2014). Another randomized trial of VIPP-SD targeting 76 Turkish minority families in the Netherlands revealed positive effects on maternal sensitivity and (reduced) intrusiveness (Yagmur, Mesman, Malda, Bakermans-Kranenburg, & Ekmekci, 2014). Finally, an initial randomized trial with 120 home-based child care providers has demonstrated positive effects on care quality of the newly developed Video-Feedback Intervention to Promote Positive Parenting and Child Care (VIPP-CC; Groenveld; Vermeer, Van IJzendoorn, & Linting, 2011).

In summary, VIPP is the briefest attachment-based intervention considered here. It has typically been provided to lower-risk families than those targeted by CPP, ABC, or the Circle of Security, and it emphasizes preventing or reducing children's behavior problems. Although brief, the program is precisely targeted, and it has shown positive effects on sensitive caregiving behaviors and child outcomes, especially externalizing behavior problems. VIPP's effects have been more pronounced for more temperamentally reactive infants (Klein Velderman et al., 2006a) and for those carrying the *D4DR* dopamine receptor polymorphism (e.g., for cortisol production; Bakermans-Kranenburg, Van IJzendoorn, Mesman, et al., 2008). It is also important to note that with the exception of an earlier, more intensive version of the program (VIPP-R) delivered to adoptive families, program effects on infant–mother attachment security have not been obtained. VIPP has been multiply adapted not only to focus on sensitive discipline but also for child care providers and special needs children. As we later discuss, VIPP is also being implemented in multiple community-based settings.

### Circle of Security

The Circle of Security (COS) program is an attachment-based intervention that has undergone tremendous development in the past several years (see Powell, Cooper, Hoffman, & Marvin, 2014). Whereas the evidence base for this program is more limited than that supporting the other three attachment programs, several versions of the program have been evaluated and have demonstrated positive effects. All versions of the program implement core components of the COS approach that include a trained intervener in either a group or individual meeting who teaches the parent(s) attachment theory and research, and helps them to reflect on their own histories and parenting behaviors. The centerpiece of the program content is the COS graphic, a remarkably simple yet comprehensive pictorial depiction of attachment theory's key constructs about (1) children's needs for both intimate connection and autonomy, and (2) parenting behaviors that support these needs. The COS also focuses on children's cues, emphasizing that children sometimes "miscue" their parents about their true needs.

To guide the intervener's approach to parenting behaviors, COS includes consideration of parents' "core sensitivities" regarding separation, esteem, and safety. In addition, the COS program uses the innovative concept of "shark music" to help parents think about why specific child behaviors that are not actually dangerous might *feel* threatening to parents and elicit negative responses (i.e., activate a parent's "shark music"). All versions of the COS program emphasize video review with parents. The Circle of Security Interview (COSI) taps parents' working models of attachment and can be used to guide the intervener's understanding of the parent's core sensitivities and parenting challenges.

Three separate evaluations attest to the promise of the COS program. The first evaluation used a pre- and posttreatment design to evaluate 65 dyads in a 20-week, group-based version of the program (Hoffman, Marvin, Cooper, & Powell, 2006). Trained group leaders delivered the intervention in 75-minute weekly sessions to groups of six to eight parents of Head Start or Early Head Start toddlers or preschoolers. Preintervention Strange Situations and COSI's were administered for research purposes and to help individualize program foci. Comparisons of pre- and postintervention Strange Situations revealed significant decreases in both insecure and disorganized classifications. At baseline, 80% of the children were classified as insecure and 60% were disorganized. Postintervention, 46% of the children were classified as insecure, and 25% were disorganized.

The second evaluation consisted of a randomized trial including 220 low-income mothers with firstborn, temperamentally irritable infants (Cassidy, Woodhouse, Sherman, Stupica, & Lejuez, 2011). Dyads were randomly assigned to a four-session, home-based version of the COS program or to a psychoeducational control intervention. Interestingly, although there were no main effects of the intervention, infants subclassified as "highly irritable" in the COS group were more likely to be securely attached than highly irritable controls. Mothers' self-reported attachment styles also moderated the intervention's effects. For highly irritable infants only, when mothers were more secure, there was an effect of COS participation on (increased likelihood of) infant attachment security at age 1, whereas when mothers were less secure, there was no COS effect. For highly irritable infants with more dismissing mothers, there was a positive effect of COS on attachment security, whereas when mothers were less dismissing (and more preoccupied), there was no effect. Moreover, within the control group, highly irritable infants with more dismissing mothers were significantly less likely to be secure than moderately irritable infants with more dismissing mothers. As Cassidy and her colleagues noted, these findings are consistent with Belsky's differential susceptibility framework. They illustrate not only a targeted benefit of the intervention for the highly irritable and presumably more sensitive and susceptible infants, but also increased challenge (i.e., attachment insecurity) for these same infants under less beneficial conditions (i.e., in the absence of the intervention and when their mothers also reported more dismissing attachment styles).

The third evaluation of the COS program consisted of an evaluation of COS groups provided as a supplemental treatment to mothers and their infants in a jail-diversion program (Cassidy et al., 2010). This study is discussed in greater detail in the following section addressing the wider dissemination of attachment-based interventions.

In summary, COS is the newest attachment-based intervention considered here. It derives most directly from attachment theory and in fact teaches parents and caregivers attachment theory in the course of the intervention. It is the only attachment-based intervention considered here that does not include the child or allow for opportunities to practice new parenting behaviors during the intervention sessions. Initial studies of the COS program indicate positive effects on infant or toddler attachment security. The program requires further evaluation, however, especially in the context of rigorous randomized trials. The one existing randomized trial demonstrated positive effects on infant attachment security, although these effects were limited to highly irritable infants. Interestingly, at the same time, effects were also moderated by maternal attachment style, such that when high infant irritability and maternal attachment style combined to increase infants' risk for developing attachment insecurity, the program significantly reduced that risk. As we discuss further, dissemination of COS has vastly outpaced program evaluation. The next steps for this program center on the development of the most recent, unified, and highly scalable version of the program and, concurrently, on strengthening its evidence base.

## Summary

Each of the four programs just reviewed is directly informed by attachment theory and research. CPP has the longest history and the most intensive approach, with the program typically lasting at least 1 year and targeting parents' internal working models and parenting behaviors. Moreover, CPP also invests heavily in the relationship between the intervener (therapist) and parent; the "level of therapeutic process" developed in this relationship has been found to magnify program outcomes (Lieberman et al., 1991).

The other three programs provide between four and 20 individual or group sessions. Although significantly shorter and more narrowly focused than CPP, these three programs also aim to promote parental reflection and to help parents make explicit connections between their own histories and what parenting behaviors they do and do not want to replicate. The three newer programs all incorporate video review to enhance parental reflection. Moreover, like CPP, the ABC, VIPP, and COS program approaches all consider the intimate and often delicate nature of attachment intervention work. All attend carefully to the nature of the interaction between the intervener and the parent, and to the model of relating that the intervener provides. For example, in the ABC program, more challenging in-the-moment comments are not provided during earlier sessions but rather are reserved for later sessions, after a supportive foundation has been laid. Similarly, the early sessions of both the VIPP and COS programs emphasize building the relationship between the intervener and the mother.

The evaluations of these four interventions demonstrate that attachment-based interventions can indeed support the development of attachment security and can reduce the risk of developing or maintaining attachment insecurity. Positive effects have emerged from multiple rigorous randomized trials conducted with participants with varying levels of risk, both within and outside the United States. Especially—but not exclusively—with respect to attachment-specific outcomes, attachment-based interventions have consistently outperformed not only light or no-treatment control conditions but also more didactic and/or cognitively focused interventions of equal duration and intensity. As detailed in our review, increasingly attachment-based interventions are demonstrating long-term effects on attachment security (e.g., Stronach et al., 2013) and other socio-emotional outcomes such as behavior problems (e.g., Klein Velderman et al., 2006b).

Attachment-based interventions are also increasingly demonstrating effects on biological outcomes. Four studies have reported intervention effects on children's cortisol production (Bakermans-Kranenburg, Van IJzendoorn, Mesman, et al., 2008; Bernard et al., 2014; Cicchetti, Rogosch, Toth, & Sturge-Apple, 2011; Dozier et al., 2006). These effects are somewhat inconsistent, however. For example, Bakermans-Kranenburg, Van IJzendoorn, Mesman, and colleagues (2008) found that VIPP-SD reduced morning production of cortisol for the intervention children with the D4DR 7-repeat allele. Both Cicchetti, Rogosch, Toth, and Sturge-Apple (2011) and Bernard and colleagues (2014) found that attachment-based intervention *raised* the production of morning cortisol. These inconsistencies may well reflect variation in these studies' samples—especially with regard to prior risk exposure—and/or to variation in intervention approach. Regardless, one task for future research is to help clarify such apparent discrepancies. Analyzing biological outcomes elucidates not only the mechanisms underlying the associations between increased maternal sensitivity and young children's self-regulation but also the connections between biological and behavioral processes writ large.

## Key Questions

In 2008, we highlighted three questions within the field of attachment-based intervention: (1) What works for whom? (2) What drives program success? And (3) What *is* program success? Recent progress in the field has helped to address these questions. With regard to what works for whom, there is evidence of stronger effects for dyads with more secure mothers and/or with children at higher risk, especially those who are more temperamentally and/or genetically sensitive (susceptible). For example, Bick and her colleagues

(2012) found that foster mothers with autonomous states of mind demonstrated better understanding of intervention concepts and more reflective functioning during intervention sessions. Cassidy and her colleagues (2011) found that highly irritable infants with more secure mothers (compared to those with less secure mothers) derived positive effects from COS. Furthermore, Ghosh Ippen and her colleagues (2011) discerned stronger effects of CPP for children who had experienced more traumatic events, and both Cassidy and colleagues' study and several evaluations of the VIPP program (Bakermans-Kranenburg, Van IJzendoorn, Mesman, et al., 2008; Bakermans-Kranenburg, Van IJzendoorn, Pijlman, et al., 2008; Klein Velderman et al., 2006a) found stronger intervention effects for "highly irritable," "highly reactive," and/or genetically more vulnerable children (with the D4DR 7-repeat allele). More vulnerable infants with less secure mothers also experienced greater benefits in some cases (Cassidy et al., 2011; Klein Velderman et al., 2006a). Taken together, these findings help to illuminate what works for whom and may also inform the tailoring of intervention approaches. Infants who are more temperamentally and/or genetically sensitive might be prioritized for attachment-based interventions, for example. Program providers might also consider the *fit* between a parent's attachment security and his or her child's emotional reactivity.

With respect to what drives program success, Dozier and her colleagues have made important strides by specifying the components of the intervener's behavior toward the mother (i.e., more frequent and more targeted in-the-moment comments) that increase the mother's sensitive parenting behaviors (Meade & Dozier, 2012; Meade et al., 2014). The in-the-moment comments are designed to provide explicit feedback to parents as they practice ABC target behaviors in their typical parenting environments. Notably, the ABC program approach is consistent with the findings of a 2008 meta-analysis of "parent training" programs indicating that one of the intervention components associated with larger program effects was the requirement for parents to practice new skills with their children during training sessions (Kaminski, Vale, Filene, & Boyle, 2008).

At the same time, much remains to be understood more generally about how attachment-based interventions with as few as four sessions can induce such important changes in human development. Bakermans-Kranenburg, Van IJzendoorn,

Mesman, and colleagues (2008) have discussed the merits of briefer attachment–based interventions, including (1) precise, short-term goals, and (2) relative ease of adherence to program requirements for typical interveners. The use of video feedback, which is an important component of ABC, VIPP, and COS, also deserves mention. Video review may be especially conducive for attachment-based intervention because it concretely facilitates the observation of parent–child interaction, which in turn may stimulate parental reflection (Juffer & Steele, 2014). Moreover, the coviewing of video between the intervener and parent may increase their therapeutic alliance and galvanize the action of "putting feelings into words . . . [that] has often been described as fundamental to the therapeutic process" (Steele et al., 2014, p. 409).

We further suggest the importance of considering how rewarding it is for both parent and child to be harmoniously in step with one another. For example, it was notable to us that CPP reduced psychiatric symptoms among mothers (Lieberman et al., 2006) because CPP does not focus on maternal mental health per se. CPP's focus on the mother–child relationship may have improved maternal mental health through the mothers' increased satisfaction with their relationships with their children and/or through mothers' own increased reflective capacities. In addition, to the extent that attachment-based interventions increase children's biological and behavioral self-regulation, they often make parenting easier and more enjoyable. Last, more harmonious parent–child interactions may be so rewarding that they quickly perpetuate themselves. As Bakermans-Kranenburg, Van IJzendoorn, and Pijlman (2008, pp. 816–817) note, "the children's reinforcement of their parents' successful interactive behaviors may partly explain the long-term effects of relatively brief interventions. . . . The process of feedback may continue after the intervener leaves the home."

Finally, with respect to defining program success, Shonkoff (2010) has urged those concerned with supporting early childhood development to articulate common short- and long-term goals. Attachment-based interventions are in many ways more specific than other early interventions in identifying sensitive parenting behaviors and/or child attachment security as the key outcomes to target. As attachment-based interventions move from more tightly controlled research endeavors to more widely and often more loosely implemented

initiatives, considering the criteria for intervention success remains an important task.

## Community Implementation of Attachment-Based Interventions

The impressive evidence supporting attachment interventions has helped to galvanize policy initiatives for early child development. It has also increased demand from practitioners in many spheres for services to support early attachment security. Increasingly, community-based agencies are seeking to integrate attachment-focused protocol into ongoing, broad-based social services. This trend bodes well for the long-term sustainability of attachment-based programs. As Greenberg (2005) argued a decade ago, transforming new evidence-based interventions into widespread practice requires integrating the interventions into existing systems. In this section we describe several different examples of recent or ongoing community implementation initiatives.

### Community Implementation of CPP

Facilitated in part by the National Child Traumatic Stress Network, CPP has now been implemented in 30 states in the United States and in Israel and Sweden (Substance Abuse and Mental Health Services Administration, n.d.). One interesting example is provided by the Florida Infant Mental Health Pilot Program, funded by the Florida state legislature (Osofsky et al., 2007). Participants were 57 mothers with infants or young children who had been investigated or substantiated for child maltreatment. The principal treatment was CPP. Notably, during and immediately after 25 CPP sessions, there were no further maltreatment reports for participants. There were also some positive changes in observed maternal and child behaviors. Building on these findings, the national advocacy organization Zero to Three established the Safe Babies Court Teams Project, which provides similar court teams in five other states (Zero to Three, 2014). One study has indicated that children served by the Court Teams achieved a permanent placement sooner than comparison children, and that Court Team children were more likely to reach permanency with a member of their biological family (McCombs-Thornton & Foster, 2012).

Another example of community-based implementation of CPP is a 2009 initiative in which

CPP was one of three interventions integrated into a wraparound foster care program for a diverse population of 216 three- to 18-year-olds (Weiner, Schneider, & Lyons, 2009). CPP was provided to children 6 years old and younger who had experienced a moderate or severe trauma and who had a caregiver willing to participate in the program. Pre- to posttreatment analyses revealed positive effects on ongoing clinical assessments of children's traumatic stress symptoms and "behavioral and emotional needs" for African American, Hispanic, and biracial (but not white) children.

A final example is provided by the Building Healthy Children program, an ongoing multipronged initiative for high-risk families that includes CPP as one component (Paradis, Sandler, Manly, & Valentine, 2013; Toth & Gravener, 2012). The program is being provided collaboratively by the Mt. Hope Family Center and the Departments of Social Work and Pediatrics at the University of Rochester. Services are integrated into children's medical homes, and funding is provided by the county Department of Human Services and the United Way. The program focuses on low-income young mothers (age 20 or younger) with two or fewer children under the age of 3. Eligible families are enrolled into a randomized trial in which CPP is one of three home-based interventions provided to families depending on a baseline needs assessment. Control families receive community services as usual. The program includes active, culturally sensitive outreach and careful coordination across multiple service sectors. In 2013, the program had enrolled approximately 500 (program and control) families, provided CPP to 56 (11%) of the dyads, and retained 85% of all families by the target child's third birthday. Initial findings from health and developmental assessments included greater compliance with well-child visits and avoidance of child welfare services in the program group (Paradis et al., 2013). Upcoming outcome assessments will include observer-sorted Q-Sets assessing infant–parent attachment and maternal behavior in the home.

## Community Implementation of the ABC Program

The ABC program has been implemented in several locations in the United States and abroad, including Germany and Australia. One recent pilot randomized trial tested the feasibility and efficacy of supplementing services as usual for new mothers in residential substance abuse treatment with ABC (Berlin, Shanahan, & Appleyard Carmody, 2014). Findings were promising: Mothers who were randomly assigned to receive supplemental ABC home visits scored higher than control mothers on observational ratings of sensitive parenting behaviors.

An ongoing project located in Hawaii is examining ABC as one component of community-based child welfare services (Meade et al., 2014). Initial analyses have examined 78 families with infants or toddlers referred to child protective services. Families received ABC from one of nine trained child welfare staff members. Initial findings have indicated pre- to posttreatment increases in observed maternal sensitivity and positive regard, as well as decreases in observed intrusive parenting behaviors.

Finally, in another ongoing project, Berlin, Jones Harden, and their colleagues are conducting a randomized trial to examine home-based Early Head Start services for low-income families with and without ABC. Initial findings have indicated strong feasibility and acceptance of this model by both mothers and Early Head Start staff. Qualitative maternal interviews have highlighted the unique benefits of receiving ABC in addition to Early Head Start home visits (Denmark, Aparicio, Berlin, & Jones Harden, 2014). Outcome assessments will include observed maternal sensitivity and measures of both mothers' and children's cortisol production.

## Community Implementation of VIPP

Since 2000, VIPP has been offered to all adoptive parents in the Netherlands. It is also used on a regular basis by several Dutch organizations providing clinical services to youth. In Flemish Belgium, VIPP is being implemented with foster parents countywide (M. J. van IJzendoorn, personal communication, January 14, 2015). These initiatives have not been formally evaluated.

## Community Implementation of the COS Program

The COS program has been has been implemented in multiple locations in the United States and abroad, including Canada, Australia, New Zealand, Africa, Asia, Europe, and South America. Moreover, several U.S. states are incorporating COS into their service systems. For example, in New Mexico, COS is provided to families receiving child protective services. In Nebraska, one region has set a goal of 80% of the parents of birth-to 3-year-old children receiving COS by 2017. The Minnesota Department of Human Services is providing COS training to adult mental health service providers. New York City's Department of Health has launched COS services throughout the city's five boroughs. In Norway, COS is being implemented with foster and adoptive parents nationwide. In Australia, COS is widely used and underpins a cross-agency collaborative for children between birth and age 8 (G. Cooper & K. Hoffman, personal communication, January 28, 2015).

Whereas COS dissemination has far outpaced evaluation, one evaluation of a jail-diversion program for pregnant women and new mothers with a history of substance abuse who were involved in the criminal justice system yielded positive findings (Cassidy et al., 2010). A prenatal–early infancy version of COS was created for this program and provided by doctoral-level therapists in 20 weekly group sessions as a supplement to the program's other services (e.g., substance abuse treatment, trauma treatment, job training). Analysis of postintervention Strange Situations for twenty 12-month-old infants illustrated rates of attachment security (70%) and disorganization (20%) characteristic of low-risk samples.

Most recently, a new version of COS was developed deliberately for purposes of program scalability (Circle of Security International, n.d.). The Circle of Security Parenting (COS-P) consists of eight sessions led by a trained group leader. COS-P can also be provided on an individual basis. This version of the program uses standard video clips to teach basic tenets of attachment theory and research and to promote parental reflection. As of 2015, COS-P had been translated into nine languages, over 6,000 providers had been trained in this model, and randomized trials were under way to test it.

## Community Implementation of Attachment-Based Interventions for Maltreated Children

The Tulane Infant Team and Family Resource Center in New Orleans, Louisiana, draws on multiple attachment-based interventions to serve children and families involved with child protective services within a six-parish (county) region. The program is supported through contracts with the state and private foundations. The Family Resource Center provides basic interventions to 200

children and their parents per year, and the Infant Team provides targeted interventions to children younger than 5 years old and their parents. This work involves collaboration with legal, child welfare, educational, health, and mental health systems to provide attachment theory- and research-based assessments and treatments to young children. The Infant Team sometimes provides simultaneous intervention to the child and foster parent, who must co-construct a new attachment relationship, and to the child and birth parents, with whom the child has disrupted and usually disturbed relationships. Treatment plans are individualized and may include CPP, ABC, and COS.

Following their placement in foster care, approximately half of the children treated by the Infant Team are returned to their parents or relatives, and about half are freed for adoption following voluntary or involuntary termination of parental rights (Zeanah et al., 2001). Although randomized assignment to the program is not possible, Zeanah and his colleagues (2001) have studied outcomes for maltreated children in the 4 years following the intervention to the 4 years that immediately preceded the intervention. They found that the intervention led to a 68% reduction in recidivism for the same child. In addition, they found a 75% reduction in maltreatment recidivism for children born subsequently to the same mother. Ten years later, both child and maternal recidivism rates were essentially unchanged from the original evaluation (Larrieu, 2014). In addition, a 5-year follow-up of graduates of the intervention demonstrated few differences between maltreated children who had received the intervention and age- and gender-matched peers who had never been maltreated (Robinson et al., 2012). Taken as a whole, these findings illustrate the value of translating attachment based interventions to community-based services for maltreated young children and their caregivers.

## Summary

Multiple attachment-based programs with increasing evidence of efficacy are increasingly being implemented in community settings, explicitly outside of controlled research trials and with an eye toward integrating attachment-based intervention protocol into comprehensive social service systems. Results so far are promising, both in terms of broadening the reach of attachment theory- and research-based interventions and in terms of demonstrated positive effects. At the same time, it is important to bear in mind that evaluations of these community-based efforts are often not as rigorous as the randomized trials that initially demonstrated program efficacy. For example, as Toth and Gravener (2012, p. 134) noted, "it is unclear what impact CPP has on the attachment relationship when applied in a community setting." The attachment outcomes from the ongoing Building Healthy Children initiative should clarify this question, however. In another example, Berlin and her colleagues (2014) not only implemented a rigorous (pilot) randomized trial but also provided expert ABC parent coaches to the agency with whom they partnered. Sustaining the integration of ABC into residential substance abuse treatment will require agency staff becoming ABC parent coaches, as is being done in the ongoing ABC project with child welfare staff in Hawaii. Thus, going forward, an important task will be rigorous evaluations of attachment-based interventions *as they are being implemented in the community*. Finally, we note that evaluating attachment interventions within broader service agencies provides a unique opportunity to examine program effects on nonattachment outcomes. For example, the COS/ jail-diversion program demonstrated preliminary success in terms of infant attachment outcomes. Program successes in terms of maternal substance use and criminal recidivism can also be examined, as can the interplay among direct and indirect program impacts.

## Implementing and Sustaining Attachment-Based Programs in Community Settings

In light of the increasing community implementation of attachment-based interventions and in the interest of supporting their long-term sustainability, here we discuss three sets of issues: (1) *fidelity and quality control*; (2) *family culture and belief systems*; and (3) *community collaboration*. First, the replication of positive intervention effects requires careful attention to fidelity and quality control. Both CPP and ABC have been implemented in community settings through the learning collaborative model, which focuses on high-quality implementation at the community level. Developed by Ebert and her colleagues at the National Center for Child Traumatic Stress, the learning collaborative model is based on previous work conducted

by the Institute for Healthcare Improvement. The model also incorporates Fixsen and Blase's (2008) concepts of "implementation drivers" to promote fidelity and sustainable practice. *Implementation drivers* refer to the key components of the infrastructure required to support practice, organizational, and systems change (see also Blome, Bennett, & Page, 2010, for a related discussion of organizational dynamics). Moreover, sustainability planning is incorporated into the initial stages of program implementation.

The learning collaborative model involves the development of multiple partnerships and takes a data-driven approach. The model includes the assessment of organizational readiness for change, involvement of senior administrative staff, and careful attention to fidelity. Intervention developers and expert consultants help to initiate the collaboration. Multilevel teams including intervention trainers, trainees, supervisors, and agency administrators work together for a specifically defined time punctuated by frequent meetings and incremental process evaluations. Initial studies of learning collaboratives point to positive outcomes including community-based practitioners' sustained use of high-fidelity practices and increased organizational capacity for implementing and sustaining such practices (Ebert, Amaya-Jackson, Markiewicz, Kisiel, & Fairbank, 2012).

The learning collaborative approach has guided numerous community implementations of CPP, including implementation of CPP within wraparound foster care and within the Safe Babies Court Teams Project (i.e., Weiner et al., 2009; Zero to Three, 2014). The CPP development team also recently released a package of fidelity instruments designed to measure fidelity to process and content. Specific procedures are prescribed for the assessment and engagement phase of treatment, with the later phase of treatments tailored to the needs of the dyad (Ghosh Ippen, Van Horn, & Lieberman, 2012).

The learning collaborative approach has also guided community implementations of the ABC program with multiple child-serving agencies in North Carolina (Appleyard Carmody, Dozier, Amaya-Jackson, Murphy, & Alvord, 2013). The ABC manual prescribes specific content for particular sessions, and there are specific fidelity requirements. These requirements center on both the frequency and foci of the parent coach's in-the-moment commenting (e.g., one comment per minute, focusing on the program's target parenting behaviors). These concrete fidelity markers inform not only training and supervision practices but also parent coach selection processes. For example, Dozier and her colleagues have used a screening instrument that includes asking prospective parent coaches to make in-the-moment comments in response to video clips of mother–child interaction. A study of 16 prospective parent coaches found that the quality of their in-the-moment comments during screening predicted the quality of their commenting during actual ABC sessions (Meade, Blackwell, Roben, & Dozier, 2013).

With regard to *family culture and belief systems*, the developers of CPP have long emphasized the importance of attending to the role of culture in defining nuclear and extended family dynamics, acceptable help-seeking behaviors, and family–community relationships, all factors that inevitably influence the alignment of an attachment intervention's aims and any family's uptake of that intervention (e.g., Lieberman & Van Horn, 2008). Initial qualitative findings from Berlin and her colleagues' ongoing randomized trial of Early Head Start plus ABC support this point (Denmark et al., 2014). Because over 80% of study participants are Latinas who were not born in the United States, mothers were queried specifically about the fit between their culture(s) and ABC program objectives. Mothers highlighted the value of having Latina parent coaches, especially when addressing the program's behavioral target of following the child's lead, which, while appealing, ran counter to many mothers' own upbringings.

With regard to *community collaboration*, we emphasize here the importance of communication and support among multiple stakeholders for strong implementation and sustainability of attachment-based programs in the community. Stakeholders often include multiple parties from different disciplinary backgrounds and professional cultures, and with differing agendas and constraints (e.g., university-based researchers, community practitioners, agency administrators, local funders). A lengthy trust-building period is often required, as is a demonstrated willingness to compromise. One example of an area in which to compromise is the selection of outcome measures. In our experience, whereas university-based researchers pursue numerous and often nuanced program outcomes, community agency personnel and local funders are most interested in basic public health and child welfare indicators, such as rate of children in foster placements, or rates of children referred for special needs services, both of which have large financial implications for local and state governments. An early-stage discussion of outcome measures could incorporate plans for both types of data. In short, as Toth and Gravener noted (2012, p. 135), both implementation and sustainability require "commitment across systems and the ability to recognize and build on the strengths of diverse organizations." We encourage both researchers and practitioners interested in the community implementation of attachment-based interventions to attend carefully to such commitments.

## Conclusion

Our revisiting of the topic of attachment-based interventions for this third edition of the *Handbook of Attachment* has both illustrated significant progress and led to a number of suggestions for the continued development of the field. Whereas virtually all attachment interventions are based on the transmission model, Belsky's differential susceptibility framework has been especially valuable for improving understanding of mechanisms of influence in early attachments and variation in intervention effects. Four attachment-based intervention programs have amassed a strong evidence base: CPP, the ABC program, the VIPP program, and the COS program. The evidence indisputably demonstrates the effects of attachment interventions on both promoting the development of attachment security and preventing or altering attachment insecurity, in addition to other outcomes. Three of these four programs are being implemented in community settings, often in the context of broad-based social service systems. The learning collaborative approach, enacted to date with the CPP and ABC programs, offers one promising avenue toward ensuring and sustaining high-fidelity, community-based program implementation. The impressive evidence supporting attachment interventions has helped to galvanize policy initiatives for early child development. Maintaining a "place at the table" among such initiatives for attachment-based interventions will require continued careful attention to fidelity, family culture and belief systems, and community collaboration. At the same time, rigorous research must continue to elucidate the role of early attachments in human development and how best to support them.

# References

Appleyard Carmody, K., Dozier, M., Amaya-Jackson, L., Murphy, R. A., & Alvord, A. (2013). Best practices for disseminating early childhood maltreatment evidence-based care: The LAUNCHing ABC in NC Project. *Section on Child Maltreatment Newsletter: American Psychological Association, Division 37, 18*(1), 6–10. Retrieved from: *www.apadivisions.org/division-37/publications/newsletters/maltreatment/2013/01/issue.pdf*.

Atkinson, L., Goldberg, S., Raval, V., Pederson, D. R., Benoit, D., Moran, G., et al. (2005). On the relation between maternal state of mind and sensitivity in the prediction of infant attachment security. *Developmental Psychology, 41*(1), 42–53.

Atkinson, L., Niccols, A., Paglia, A., Coolbear, J., Parker, K. C. H., Poulton, L., et al. (2000). A meta-analysis of time between maternal sensitivity and attachment assessments: Implications for internal working models of infancy/toddlerhood. *Journal of Social and Personal Relationships, 17*(6), 791–810.

Bakermans-Kranenburg, M. J., & Van IJzendoorn, M. H. (2006). Gene–environment interaction of the dopamine D4 receptor (*DRD4*) and observed maternal insensitivity predicting externalizing behavior in preschoolers. *Developmental Psychobiology, 48*(5), 406–409.

Bakermans-Kranenburg, M. J., & Van IJzendoorn, M. H. (2007). Research review: Genetic vulnerability or differential susceptibility in child development: The case of attachment. *Journal of Child Psychology and Psychiatry, 48*(12), 1160–1173.

Bakermans-Kranenburg, M. J., & Van IJzendoorn, M. H. (2011). Differential susceptibility to rearing environment depending on dopamine-related genes: New evidence and a meta-analysis. *Development and Psychopathology, 23*(1), 39–52.

Bakermans-Kranenburg, M. J., & Van IJzendoorn, M. H. (2015). The hidden efficacy of interventions: Gene × environment experiments from a differential susceptibility perspective. *Annual Review of Psychology, 66*, 1–29.

Bakermans-Kranenburg, M. J., Van IJzendoorn, M. H., Mesman, J., Alink, L., & Juffer, F. (2008). Effects of an attachment-based intervention on daily cortisol moderated by dopamine receptor D4: A randomized control trial on 1- to 3-year-olds screened for externalizing behavior. *Development and Psychopathology, 20*(3), 805–820.

Bakermans-Kranenburg, M. J., Van IJzendoorn, M. H., Pijlman, F. A., Mesman, J., & Juffer, F. (2008). Experimental evidence for differential susceptibility: Dopamine D4 receptor polymorphism (*DRD4 VNTR*) moderates intervention effects on toddlers' externalizing behavior in a randomized controlled trial. *Developmental Psychology, 44*(1), 293–300.

Belsky, J., Bakermans-Kranenburg, M. J., & Van IJzendoorn, M. H. (2007). For better and for worse: Differential susceptibility to environmental influences. *Current Directions in Psychological Science, 16*(6), 300–304.

Belsky, J., & Pluess, M. (2009). Beyond diathesis stress: Differential susceptibility to environmental influences. *Psychological Bulletin, 135*(6), 885–908.

Berlin, L. J., Jones Harden, B., Raymond, M., & Denmark, N. (2012, June). *Buffering children from toxic stress through attachment-based intervention: An Early Head Start–University Partnership.* Poster presented at the Head Start National Research Conference, Washington, DC.

Berlin, L. J., Shanahan, M., & Appleyard Carmody, K. A. (2014). Promoting supportive parenting in new mothers with substance use problems: A pilot randomized trial. *Infant Mental Health Journal, 35*(1), 81–85.

Berlin, L. J., Zeanah, C. H., & Lieberman, A. F. (2008). Prevention and intervention programs for supporting early attachment security. In J. Cassidy & P. R. Shaver (Eds.), *Handbook of Attachment* (2nd ed., pp. 745–761). New York: Guilford Press.

Bernard, K., Dozier, M., Bick, J., & Gordon, M. K. (2014). Normalizing blunted diurnal cortisol rhythms among children at risk for neglect: The effects of an early intervention. *Development and Psychopathology, 8*, 1–13.

Bernard, K., Dozier, M., Bick, J., Lewis-Morrarty, E., Lindhiem, O., & Carlson, E. (2012). Enhancing attachment organization among maltreated children: Results of a randomized clinical trial. *Child Development, 83*(2), 623–636.

Bernard, K., Hostinar, C., & Dozier, M. (2015). Intervention effects on diurnal cortisol rhythms of CPS-referred infants persist into early childhood: Preschool follow-up results of a randomized clinical trial. *JAMA Pediatrics, 69*(2), 112–119.

Bick, J., & Dozier, M. (2013). The effectiveness of an attachment-based intervention in promoting foster mothers' sensitivity toward foster infants. *Infant Mental Health Journal, 34*(2), 95–103.

Bick, J., Dozier, M., & Moore, S. (2012). Predictors of treatment use among foster mothers in an attachment-based intervention program. *Attachment and Human Development, 14*(5), 439–452.

Blome, W., Bennett, S., & Page, T. F. (2010). Organizational challenges to implementing attachment-based practices in public child welfare agencies: An example using the Circle of Security® model. *Journal of Public Child Welfare, 4*(4), 427–449.

Bornstein, D. (2013, November 3). Protecting children from toxic stress. *The New York Times.* p. SR4.

Bowlby, J. (1980). *Attachment and Loss, Vol. 3: Loss.* New York: Basic Books.

Bowlby, J. (1988). *A secure base.* New York: Basic Books.

Cassidy, J., Woodhouse, S. S., Sherman, L. J., Stupica, B., & Lejuez, C. W. (2011). Enhancing infant attachment security: An examination of treatment efficacy and differential susceptibility. *Development and Psychopathology, 23*(1) 131–148.

Cassidy, J., Ziv, Y., Stupica, B., Sherman, L. J., Butler, H., Karfgin, A., et al. (2010). Enhancing attachment security in the infants of women in a jail-diversion program. *Attachment and Human Development, 12*(4), 333–353.

Cicchetti, D., Rogosch, F. A., & Toth, S. L. (2000). The efficacy of toddler–parent psychotherapy for fostering cognitive development in offspring of depressed mothers. *Journal of Abnormal Child Psychology, 28*(2), 135–148.

Cicchetti, D., Rogosch, F. A., & Toth, S. L. (2006). Fostering secure attachment in infants in maltreating families through preventive interventions. *Development and Psychopathology, 18*(3), 623–649.

Cicchetti, D., Rogosch, F. A., & Toth, S. L. (2011). The effects of child maltreatment and polymorphisms of the serotonin transporter and dopamine D4 receptor genes on infant attachment and intervention efficacy. *Development and Psychopathology, 23*(2), 357–372.

Cicchetti, D., Rogosch, F. A., Toth, S. L., & Sturge-Apple, M. (2011). Normalizing the development of cortisol regulation in maltreated infants through preventive interventions. *Development and Psychopathology, 23*(3), 789–800.

Cicchetti, D., Toth, S. L., & Rogosch, F. A. (1999). The efficacy of toddler–parent psychotherapy to increase attachment security in offspring of depressed mothers. *Attachment and Human Development, 1*(1), 34–66.

Circle of Security International (n.d.). *Brief history of the research and development of COS interventions.* Retrieved July 14, 2014, from *http://circleofsecurity.org/about-us/history.*

Denmark, N., Aparicio, E., Berlin, L. J., & Jones Harden, B. (2014, April). *Latina mothers' experiences of a supplemental parenting program within an Early Head Start–University partnership.* Poster presented at the Society for Research in Child Development Special Topic Meeting, "Strengthening Connections among Child and Family Research, Policy, and Practice," Alexandria, VA.

de Wolff, M. S., & Van IJzendoorn, M. H. (1997). Sensitivity and attachment: A meta-analysis on parental antecedents of infant attachment. *Child Development, 68*(4), 571–591.

Dozier, M., Lindheim, O., & Ackerman, J. P. (2005). Attachment and biobehavioral catch-up. In L. J. Berlin, Y. Ziv, L. Amaya-Jackson, & M. T. Greenberg (Eds.), *Enhancing early attachments: Theory, research, intervention and policy* (pp. 178–194). New York: Guilford Press.

Dozier, M., Lindheim, O., Lewis, E., Bick, J., Bernard, K., & Peloso, E. (2009). Effects of a foster parent training program on young children's attachment behaviors: Preliminary evidence from a randomized clinical trial. *Child and Adolescent Social Work Journal, 26*(4), 321–332.

Dozier, M., Peloso, E., Lewis, E., Laurenceau, J., & Levine, S. (2008). Effects of an attachment-based intervention of the cortisol production of infants and toddlers in foster care. *Development and Psychopathology, 20*(3), 845–859.

Dozier, M., Peloso, E., Lindheim, O., Gordon, M. K., Manni, M., Sepulveda, S., et al. (2006). Developing evidence-based interventions for foster children: An example of a randomized clinical trial with infants and toddlers. *Journal of Social Issues, 62*(4), 767–785.

Drury, S. S., Gleason, M. M., Theall, K. P., Smyke, A. T., Nelson, C. A., Fox, N. A., Zeanah, C.H. (2012). Genetic sensitivity to the caregiving context: The influence of *5HTTLPR* and *BDNF* val66met on indiscriminate social behavior. *Physiology and Behavior, 106*, 728–735.

Ebert, L., Amaya-Jackson, L., Markiewicz, J., & Fairbank, J. (2012). Development and application of the NCCTS Learning Collaborative Model for the implementation of evidence-based child trauma treatment. In R. K. McHugh & D. H. Barlow (Eds.), *Dissemination and implementation of evidence-based psychological interventions* (pp. 97–123). New York: Oxford University Press.

Ebert, L., Amaya-Jackson, L., Markiewicz, J., Kisiel, C., & Fairbank, J. (2012). Use of the Breakthrough Series Collaborative to support broad and sustained use of evidence-based trauma treatment for children in community practice settings. *Administration and Policy in Mental Health and Mental Health Services Research, 39*(3), 187–199.

Edwards, V. J., Holden, G. W., Anda, R. F., & Felitti, V. J. (2003). Experiencing multiple forms of childhood maltreatment and adult mental health: Results from the Adverse Childhood Experiences (ACE) study. *American Journal of Psychiatry, 160*(8), 1453–1460.

Fixsen, D. L., & Blase, K. A. (2008). *Drivers framework.* Chapel Hill: National Implementation Research Network, Frank Porter Graham Child Development Institute, University of North Carolina.

Fraiberg, S. (1980). *Clinical studies in infant mental health: The first year of life.* New York: Basic Books.

Ghosh Ippen, C., Harris, W. W., Van Horn, P., & Lieberman, A. F. (2011). Traumatic and stressful events in early childhood: Can treatment help those at highest risk? *Child Abuse and Neglect, 35*(7), 504–513.

Ghosh Ippen, C., Van Horn, P., & Lieberman, A. F. (2012). *Child–parent psychotherapy fidelity measures protocol.* Unpublished manuscript, Child Trauma Research Program, University of California.

Greenberg, M. T. (2005). Enhancing early attachments: Synthesis and recommendations for research, practice, and policy. In L. J. Berlin, Y. Ziv, L. Amaya-Jackson, & M. T. Greenberg (Eds.), *Enhancing early attachments: Theory, research, intervention, and policy* (pp. 327–343). New York: Guilford Press.

Groeneveld, M. G., Vermeer, H. J., Van IJzendoorn, M. H., & Linting, M. (2011). Enhancing home-based child care quality through video-feedback intervention: A randomized controlled trial. *Journal of Family Psychology, 25*(1), 86–96.

Hoffman, K. T., Marvin, R. S., Cooper, G., & Powell, B. (2006). Changing toddlers' and preschoolers' attachment classifications: The Circle of Security intervention. *Journal of Consulting and Clinical Psychology*, 74(6), 1017–1026.

Juffer, F., Bakermans-Kranenburg, M. J., & Van IJzendoorn, M. H. (2005). The importance of parenting in the development of disorganized attachment: Evidence from a preventive intervention study in adoptive families. *Journal of Child Psychology and Psychiatry*, 46(3), 263–274.

Juffer, F., Bakermans-Kranenburg, M. J., & Van IJzendoorn, M. H. (2008). *Promoting positive parenting: An attachment-based intervention.* Mahwah, NJ: Erlbaum.

Juffer, F., Bakermans-Kranenburg, M. J., & Van IJzendoorn, M. H. (2014). Attachment-based interventions: Sensitive parenting is the key to positive parent–child relationships. In P. Holmes & S. Farnfield (Eds.) *Attachment: The guidebook to attachment theory and interventions.* New York: Routledge.

Juffer, F., Hoksbergen, R. A. C., Riksen-Walraven, J. M., & Kohnstamm, G. A. (1997). Early intervention in adoptive families: Supporting maternal sensitive responsiveness, infant–mother attachment, and infant competence. *Journal of Child Psychology and Psychiatry*, 38, 1039–1050.

Juffer, F., Rosenboom, L. G., Hoksbergen, R. A. C., Riksen-Walraven, J. M. A., & Kohnstamm, G. A. (1997). Attachment and intervention in adoptive families with and without biological children. In W. Koops, J. B. Hoeksma, & D. C. van den Boom (Eds.), *Development of interaction and attachment: Traditional and non-traditional approaches* (pp. 93–108). Amsterdam: North-Holland.

Juffer, F., & Steele, M. (2014). What words cannot say: The telling story of video in in attachment-based interventions. *Attachment and Human Development*, 16, 307–314.

Kaminski, J. W., Vale, L. Z., Filene, J. H., & Boyle, C. L. (2008). A meta-analytic review of components associated with parent training program effectiveness. *Journal of Abnormal Child Psychology*, 36(4) 567–589.

Klein Velderman, M., Bakermans-Kranenburg, M. J., Juffer, F., & Van IJzendoorn, M. H. (2006a). Effects of attachment-based interventions on maternal sensitivity and infant attachment: Differential susceptibility of highly reactive infants. *Journal of Family Psychology*, 20(2), 266–274.

Klein Velderman, M., Bakermans-Kranenburg, M. J., Juffer, F., Van IJzendoorn, M. H., Mangelsdorf, S. C., et al. (2006b). Preventing preschool externalizing behavior problems through video-feedback intervention in infancy. *Infant Mental Health Journal*, 27(5), 466–493.

Larrieu, J. (June, 2014). *A model for intervening with maltreated infants translated across three countries: The Tulane Infant Team Intervention for maltreated infants and their families.* Paper presented at the 14th World Association for Infant Mental Health Congress, Edinburgh,UK.

Lewis-Morrarty, E., Dozier, M., Bernard, K., Terracciano, S. M., & Moore, S. V. (2012). Cognitive flexibility and theory of mind outcomes among foster children: Preschool follow-up results of a randomized clinical trial. *Journal of Adolescent Health*, 51(2), S17–S22.

Lieberman, A. F., Ghosh Ippen, C., & Van Horn, P. (2006). Child–parent psychotherapy: 6-month follow-up of a randomized controlled trial. *Journal of the American Academy of Child and Adolescent Psychiatry*, 45(8), 913–917.

Lieberman, A. F., Padrón, E., Van Horn, P., & Harris, W. W. (2005). Angels in the nursery: The intergenerational transmission of benevolent parental influences. *Infant Mental Health Journal*, 26(6), 504–520.

Lieberman, A. F., & Van Horn, P. (2005). *Don't hit my mommy: A manual for child–parent psychotherapy with young witnesses of family violence.* Washington, DC: Zero to Three Press.

Lieberman, A. F., & Van Horn, P. (2008). *Psychotherapy with infants and young children: Repairing the effects of stress and trauma on early attachment.* New York: Guilford Press.

Lieberman, A. F., Van Horn, P., & Ghosh Ippen, C. (2005). Toward evidence-based treatment: Child-parent psychotherapy with preschoolers exposed to marital violence. *Journal of the American Academy of Child and Adolescent Psychiatry*, 44(12), 1241–1248.

Lieberman, A. F., Weston, D. R., & Pawl, J. H. (1991). Preventive intervention and outcome with anxiously attached dyads. *Child Development*, 62(1), 199–209.

Lind, T., Bernard, K., Ross, E., & Dozier, M. (2014). Intervention effects on negative affect of CPS-referred children: Results from a randomized clinical trial. *Child Abuse and Neglect*, 38(9), 1459–1467.

Madigan, S., Bakermans-Kranenburg, M. J., Van IJzendoorn, M. H., Moran, G., Pederson, D. R., & Benoit, D. (2006). Unresolved states of mind, anomalous parental behavior, and disorganized attachment: A review and meta-analysis of a transmission gap. *Attachment and Human Development*, 8(2), 89–111.

Main, M. (1990). Cross-cultural studies of attachment organization: Recent studies, changing methodologies, and the concept of conditional strategies. *Human Development*, 33(1), 48–61.

McCombs-Thornton, K. L., & Foster, E. M. (2012). The effect of the ZERO TO THREE Court Teams initiative on types of exits from the foster care system—a competing risks analysis. *Children and Youth Services Review*, 34, 169–178.

Meade, E., Blackwell, M., Roben, C., & Dozier, M. (2013, April). *Using screening interviews to predict parent coach performance in the Attachment and Biobehavioral Catch-Up intervention.* Poster presentation at the biennial meeting of Society for Research in Child Development, Seattle, WA.

Meade, E., & Dozier, M. (2012). "In the moment" commenting: A fidelity measurement and active ingredient in *a parent training program.* Unpublished manuscript, University of Delaware.

Meade, E., Dozier, M., Weston-Lee, P., & Neely, E. (2014, May). *Implementation of Attachment and Biobehavioral Catch-Up: Preliminary findings of effectiveness and predictors of change.* Poster presentation at the annual meeting of the Society for Prevention Research, Washington, DC.

Mesman, J., Stolk, M N., Van Zeijl, J., Alink, L. R. A., Juffer, F., Bakermans-Kranenburg, M. J., et al. (2007). Extending the video-feedback intervention to sensitive discipline: The early prevention of antisocial behavior. In F. Juffer, M. J. Bakermans-Kranenburg, & M. H. Van IJzendoorn (Eds.), *Promoting positive parenting: An attachment-based intervention* (pp. 171–192). Mahwah, NJ: Erlbaum.

Negrão, M., Pereira, M., Soares, I., & Mesman, J. (2014). Enhancing positive parent–child interactions and family functioning in a poverty sample: A randomized control trial. *Attachment and Human Development, 16,* 315–328.

Osofsky, J. D., Kronenberg, M., Hammer, J. H., Lederman, C., Katz, L., Adams, S., et al. (2007). The development and evaluation of the intervention model for the Florida Infant Mental Health Pilot Program. *Infant Mental Health Journal, 28,* 259–280.

Paradis, H., Sandler, M., Manly, J., & Valentine, L. (2013). Building healthy children: Evidence-based home visitation integrated with pediatric medical homes. *Pediatrics, 132,* S174–S179.

Pereira, M., Negrão, M., Soares, I., & Mesman, J. (2014). Decreasing harsh discipline in mothers at risk for maltreatment: A randomized control trial. *Infant Mental Health Journal, 35*(6), 604–613.

Poslawsky, I. E., Naber, F. B. A., Bakermans-Kranenburg, M. J., van Daalen, E., van England, H., & Van IJzendoorn, M. H. (2015). Video-Feedback Intervention to Promote Positive Parenting Adapted to Autism (VIPP-AUTI): A randomized controlled trial. *Autism, 19,* 588–603.

Powell, B., Cooper, G., Hoffman, K., & Marvin, B. (2014). *The Circle of Security intervention: Enhancing attachment in early parent–child relationships.* New York: Guilford Press.

Robinson, L., Boris, N., Heller, S., Rice, J., Zeanah, C., Clark, C., et al. (2012). The good enough home?: Home environment and outcomes of young maltreated children. *Child and Youth Care Forum, 41*(1), 73–88.

Schneider-Rosen, K., Braunwald, K. G., Carlson, V., & Cicchetti, D. (1985). Current perspectives in attachment theory: Illustrations from the study of maltreated infants. *Monographs of the Society for Research in Child Development, 50*(1/2), 194–210.

Shonkoff, J. (2010). Building a new biodevelopmental framework to guide the future of early childhood policy. *Child Development, 81*(1), 357–367.

Spangler, G., Johann, M., Ronai, Z., & Zimmermann, P. (2009). Genetic and environmental influence on attachment disorganization. *Journal of Child Psychology and Psychiatry, 50*(8), 952–961.

Stams, G. J. J. M., Juffer, F., Van IJzendoorn, M. H., & Hoksbergen, R. A. C. (2001). Attachment-based intervention in adoptive families in infancy and children's development at age seven: two follow-up studies. *British Journal of Developmental Psychology, 19*(2), 159–180.

Steele, M., Steele, H., Bate, J., Knafo, H., Kinsey, M., Bonuck, K., et al. (2014). Looking from the outside in: The use of video in attachment-based interventions. *Attachment and Human Development, 16,* 402–415.

Stein, A., Woolley, H., Senior, R., Hertzmann, L., Lovel, M., Lee, J., et al. (2006). Treating disturbances in the relationship between mothers with bulimic eating disorders and their infants: A randomized, controlled trial of video feedback. *American Journal of Psychiatry, 16,* 899–906.

Stronach, E. P., Toth, S. L., & Rogosch, F. A., Cicchetti, D. (2013). Preventative interventions and sustained attachment security in maltreated children. *Development and Psychopathology, 25,* 919–930.

Substance Abuse and Mental Health Services Administration. (n.d.). National Registry of Evidence-Based Practices. Intervention summary: Child–parent psychotherapy. Retrieved July 14, 2014, from *www.nrepp.samhsa.gov/viewintervention.aspx?id=194.*

Toth, S. L., & Gravener, J. (2012). Review: Bridging research and practice: Relational interventions for maltreated children. *Child and Adolescent Mental Health, 17*(3), 131–138.

Toth, S. L., Maughan, A., Manly, J. T., Spagnola, M., & Cicchetti, D. (2002). The relative efficacy of two interventions in altering maltreated preschool children's representational models: Implications for attachment theory. *Development and Psychopathology, 14*(4), 877–908.

Toth, S. L., Rogosch, F. A., Manly, J. T., & Cicchetti, D. (2006). The efficacy of toddler–parent psychotherapy to reorganize attachment in the young offspring of mothers with major depressive disorder: A randomized preventive trial. *Journal of Consulting and Clinical Psychology, 74*(6), 1006–1016.

Tough, P. (2012). *How children succeed: Grit, curiosity, and the hidden power of character.* Boston: Houghton Mifflin/Harcourt.

Van Horn, P., Osofsky, J. D., Henderson, D., Korfmacher, J., Thomas, K., & Lieberman, A. F. (2012). Replication of child–parent psychotherapy in community settings: Models for training. *Zero to Three, 33*(2), 48–54.

Van IJzendoorn, M. H. (1995). Adult attachment representations, parental responsiveness, and infant attachment: A meta-analysis on the predictive validity of the adult attachment interview. *Psychological Bulletin, 117*(3), 387–403.

Van IJzendoorn, M. H., & Bakermans-Kranenburg, M. J. (2006). DRD4 7-repeat polymorphism moderates the association between maternal unresolved loss or trauma and infant disorganization. *Attachment and Human Development, 8*(4), 291–307.

Van Zeijl, J., Mesman, J., Van IJzendoorn, M. H., Bakermans-Kranenburg, M. J., Juffer, F., Stolk, M. N., et al. (2006). Attachment-based intervention for enhancing sensitive discipline in mothers of 1- to 3-year-old children at risk for externalizing behavior problems: A randomized controlled trial. *Journal of Consulting and Clinical Psychology, 74*(6), 994–1005.

Yagmur, S., Mesman, J., Malda, M., Bakermans-Kranenburg, M. J., & Ekmekci, H. (2014). Video-feedback intervention increases sensitive parenting in ethnic minority mothers: A randomized control trial. *Attachment and Human Development, 16,* 371–386.

Weiner, D. A., Schneider, A. A., & Lyons, J. S. (2009). Evidence-based treatments for trauma among culturally diverse foster care youth: Treatment retention and outcomes. *Children and Youth Services Review, 31*(11), 1199–1205.

Zeanah, C. H., Larrieu, J. A., Heller, S. S., Valliere, J., Hinshaw-Fuselier, S., Aoki, Y., et al. (2001). Evaluation of a preventive intervention for maltreated infants and toddlers in foster care. *Journal of the American Academy of Child and Adolescent Psychiatry, 40,* 214–221.

Zero to Three. (2014). The Safe Babies Court Team approach: Championing children, encouraging parents, engaging communities. Retrieved from: *www.zerotothree.org/maltreatment/safe-babies-court-team.*

# Chapter 33

# Attachment and Adult Psychotherapy
## Theory, Research, and Practice

### Arietta Slade

Attachment theory evolved from John Bowlby's (1969/1982, 1973, 1980, 1988) elegant and parsimonious conceptualization of the nature and function of human attachment. His influence on the field of developmental psychology became apparent in the 1960s, largely as a result of the work of his colleague and friend Mary Ainsworth (Ainsworth, Blehar, Waters, & Wall, 1978; for reviews, see Karen, 1998; Slade & Holmes, 2013). However, despite the fact that Bowlby was a psychoanalyst and psychotherapist, his work was largely ignored by clinicians and clinical researchers for decades. Writing in 1988, Bowlby expressed his dismay at this state of affairs:

> It is a little unexpected that, whereas attachment theory was formulated by a clinician for use in the diagnosis and treatment of emotionally disturbed patients and families, its usage hitherto has been mainly to promote research in developmental psychology. Whilst I welcome the findings of this research as enormously extending our understanding of personality development and psychopathology, and thus as of the greatest clinical relevance, it has none the less been disappointing that clinicians have been so slow to test the theory's uses. (pp. ix–x)

The reasons behind what Bowlby rightly described as the failure of clinicians to embrace his work are complex (see Holmes, 1993, 1995), and to a large extent this situation has changed considerably over the past 25 years. Beginning in the early 1990s, but particularly in the last 15 years, researchers and clinicians working from a variety of perspectives have (to paraphrase Bowlby) *tested the theory's uses* in a number of ways. Thus, whereas there was hardly any research on attachment and psychotherapy in 1990 (save Mary Dozier's groundbreaking study, published that year), there is today a considerable research literature in this area. Likewise, whereas in 1990 it would have been fair to say that most clinicians were largely unaware of attachment theory, and even less aware of its relevance to their work, it is equally fair to say that the situation is largely reversed today. And yet, as I hope to make clear in this chapter, there is still a great deal of work to be done to truly realize Bowlby's vision.

When I set out to prepare this chapter, my goal was primarily to update the one I had written for the 2008 *Handbook of Attachment*. However, perhaps because I had reviewed a number of classic articles in attachment theory, research, and clinical practice for a collection compiled with Jeremy Holmes (Slade & Holmes, 2013), I now read the literature through a different lens. What I began to see was that many tests of attachment theory's use in psychotherapeutic research and practice over the last 25 years have been limited in significant ways.

On the *research* side, this has been—until very recently—reflected in the relative absence of outcome measures sensitive to the dynamically meaningful and theoretically predictable differences among secure, avoidant, preoccupied, and unresolved/disorganized patients[1] in their patterns of relating and of regulating affect (for reviews, see Daniel, 2006; Mikulincer, Shaver, & Berant, 2013; Steele, Steele, & Murphy, 2009), particularly within the often emotionally arousing context of psychotherapy. These differences are of utmost importance clinically because the course and outcome of treatment, as well as the technical demands for treating secure, avoidant, preoccupied, and unresolved/disorganized patients, are quite distinct (Holmes, 2001; Slade, 2000; Wallin, 2007). However, these differences are evident only as trends in the research literature, the net result being that the only clear and unsurprising conclusion is that insecure attachment (both the patient's and the therapist's) makes for a more problematic course in psychotherapy. Fortunately, as I describe below, Sarah Daniel, Alessandro Talia, and their colleagues (Daniel, 2006, 2009, 2011, 2014; Talia et al., 2014) have begun to publish work that transcends these trends in crucial ways, moving the study of attachment and psychotherapy research to what they refer to as "the level of the relation" (Talia et al., 2014). As I outline below, this refers to the impact of attachment organization on the dynamic relationship between patient and therapist, specifically the ways the patient's discourse elicits, maintains, or disrupts emotional proximity with the therapist.

On the *clinical* side, these limitations have been manifest in a surprising lack of depth in the way attachment constructs are applied to the clinical enterprise. On the face of it, attachment is a dominant construct in the theory and practice of psychotherapy today (there were 4.3 million results of a Google search of "attachment and psychotherapy"). This would include not only dynamic psychotherapy, but also more behaviorally oriented therapies (e.g., attachment is an important concept in Linehan's [1993] dialectical behavior therapy, or DBT). But what many clinicians mean by the term *attachment* and what Bowlby and his followers mean by it are quite different. The vast majority of clinicians use the term *attachment* as a way of talking about the early mother–child relationship. Although this is to a certain extent

accurate, using the term in this way robs it of the evolutionary, motivational contexts that were so central to Bowlby's thinking. For Bowlby, the term *attachment* referred to a dynamic relational system that is activated by threat, shaped by interaction with the caregiving environment, and powered by the instinct to survive, on multiple levels (Slade, 2014). Thus, the assumption that *attachment* is shorthand for *relationship* is both incorrect and incomplete. There are other clinicians who do in fact describe patients in terms of their purported attachment organizations, but often these simply become another form of diagnosis uncoupled from a discussion of more dynamic processes and outcomes. I would think of these as *flirtations* with attachment rather than the love affair that would be implied by over 4 million Google hits.

At the same time, there is a core group of writers who eschew the generic use of the term *attachment*, and who write about psychotherapy and about their adult patients in ways that are deeply *attachment informed*. This work began to take shape in the 1980s, when Mary Main's work (Main, Kaplan, & Cassidy, 1985) captured the imagination of the psychoanalytic establishment, and "attachment" returned to its original home after years of exile. In 1987, Larry Aber and I gave a talk to a predominantly psychoanalytic audience on the clinical implications of attachment theory (Slade & Aber, 1992). The large auditorium was packed, with more than a few psychoanalytic luminaries in the audience. Nevertheless, the questions at the end of the day suggested that curiosity and acceptance were still very far apart. "How could a 30-minute procedure tell us anything about the complexity of a child's internal life?" (This from clinicians who were fully prepared to accept the validity of another, relatively brief, procedure, the Rorschach.) "What about the drives?" "What about the unconscious?" And most memorably, "What does Mary Main think about sex?" Over the next decade, however, this resistance, which was initially focused on the nondynamic nature of classification, began to give way, and attachment theory slowly began to take hold of the imaginations of clinicians working from a psychodynamic perspective.

The most prolific and influential of these is certainly Jeremy Holmes (1997, 1998, 2001, 2004, 2009, 2014), who—as Bowlby's biographer—has been studying attachment since he began his psychiatry training in the 1960s. Others in this group include Sarah Daniel (2009, 2014), Morris Eagle (2013), Peter Fonagy and his colleagues Mary

Target and Anthony Bateman (2001; Bateman & Fonagy, 2009; Fonagy & Target, 1996), Karlen Lyons-Ruth (Lyons-Ruth, 1999, Lyons-Ruth, Dutra, Schuder, & Bianchi, 2006), Pat Sable (2000), Howard and Miriam Steele (2008), David Wallin (2007), and myself (1999, 2004a, 2004b, 2014). Sue Johnson's work (2008) on attachment processes in couple therapy also belongs in this group (see Brassard & Johnson, Chapter 35, this volume). A number of important additional contributions to the literature on attachment-informed psychotherapy practice have been compiled in three volumes published in the last decade: Oppenheim and Goldsmith (2007); Steele and Steele (2008), and Obegi and Berant (2009).

It is important to note that none of these clinicians see attachment classifications as *defining* patients. From a clinical perspective, classifications are less relevant than the dynamics that underlie them and the defenses that these evoke; that is, thinking about attachment "*informs* rather than *defines* intervention and clinical thinking, and offers a broad and far-reaching view of human functioning that has the potential to change the way clinicians think about and respond to their patients, and the way they understand the dynamics of the therapeutic relationship" (Slade, 2008, p. 763, emphasis added).

This review and critique is organized around the questions that have dominated the research and clinical literatures, albeit in different ways. The first question is whether a *patient's* attachment organization or style affects the process and outcome of treatment. That is, does the patient's attachment affect the nature of the therapeutic alliance, the transference, the capacity to engage in the process of psychotherapy, or symptom remission? The second question is whether the *therapist's* attachment organization or style affects the process and outcome of treatment, and the third is whether treatment should be tailored to a patient's attachment organization. The final question is whether attachment organization or style can be changed by psychotherapy. Here, attachment is the *target* of change (rather than the predictor of change).

Each of these questions is based on a single key assumption: Psychodynamic psychotherapy—by virtue of its emphasis on the therapeutic relationship and on discovering or recovering memories and affects from the past and in the present—inherently activates an individual's attachment system. It requires that the patient form a relationship with the "stronger and wiser" therapist (which will have multiple levels of meaning and functions), that the patient remember elements of his or her early experiences with parents or caregivers, and that the patient confront intense and presumably negative feelings in relation to both past and present experiences with significant others. Each of these circumstances would be expected to trigger attachment-related patterns of defense and affect regulation in the patient (and, as we shall see, the therapist), even if (as in some behavioral therapies) transforming these is not an explicit goal of treatment.

I write this chapter not only as an attachment theorist and researcher, trained in both the Strange Situation (Ainsworth et al., 1978) and the Adult Attachment Interview (AAI; George, Kaplan, & Main, 1996), but also as a dynamically oriented psychotherapist with 40 years' experience working with a broad array of patients, teaching assessment and psychotherapy, and supervising clinicians at all levels of experience. Although I am reasonably acquainted with other forms of therapy, and—like most experienced therapists—do at times incorporate various adjunctive methods in my work, my lens is (primarily) long-term work with patients that assumes a link between past experience and present psychological organization.

I begin with a background section laying out the historical contexts for the study of attachment and psychotherapy. This will be followed by an exploration of research and clinical "answers" to each of the four questions posed earlier. Because of the complex nature of both the research and clinical literatures in this area, I focus here primarily on research. In the concluding sections, I suggest directions for future integrative research and practice.[2]

## Attachment Theory: Dynamics and Classifications

Bowlby introduced attachment theory over the course of 30 years, beginning with his paper on juvenile thieves in 1944. By 1980, when the final volume of his trilogy was published, attachment theory had evolved as a complex motivational and dynamic theory of development and personality (Bowlby 1969/1982, 1973; see Cassidy, Chapter 1, this volume). Attachment theory was from the start deeply grounded in evolutionary theory and, as such, Bowlby viewed much of human development in light of the individual's instinct to survive. He described a number of key biological systems designed to ensure this. Of these, he saw the attachment–behavioral system as primary, in that it establishes the social relationships essential both to immediate survival in infancy and to the proper functioning of other key biological systems—the exploratory system, the affiliative system, the sexual/reproductive system, and the caregiving system. Bowlby described these systems as *inherently dynamic*, each being in a state of "activation" or relative "deactivation." Thus, for example, when a child needs care (either because of external threats, illness, or exhaustion), the attachment–behavioral system will be activated, and the child will signal a "stronger and wiser" caregiver, and (in whatever way development to that point allows) seek proximity. When the child feels safe, or the immediate needs are met, the attachment system will be relatively "deactivated," and the child will feel free to explore the environment, again in whatever way is developmentally possible. At the same time, it is important to note that—for critical evolutionary reasons—the attachment system itself is never fully deactivated; rather, attachment *behavior* is deactivated (Bowlby, 1969/1982).

Equally crucial in Bowlby's thinking was another dynamic construct, that of adaptation. He believed that an individual will *adapt* in whatever way is necessary to ensure safety, and to maintain the relationships that are key to emotional and physical survival. Thus, if a mother cannot tolerate her infant's needs, the infant will learn to express them in ways that she can tolerate. Finally, Bowlby saw the relationship between caregiver and infant as *dynamic*, in that the infant's response shapes that of the mother, who in turn shapes that of the child, and so on. This dynamic interaction is ultimately *internalized* by the child, and forms what Bowlby called "internal working models of attachment." Mary Main and her colleagues (1985) aptly link internal working models to the dynamic "attempts and outcomes" (p. 75) of the child's search for safety. Thus, *relational* patterns, including both sides of the relationship (Sroufe & Fleeson, 1986) are internalized.

These ideas, grounded in dynamic systems theory and ethology, gave rise to the idea of attachment *patterns*. Over time, Bowlby suggested that individuals—as a function of their lived experience in their primary relationships—are likely to develop *characteristic* ways of responding to their internal experience, and *characteristic* ways of seeking care and closeness from important others. These are typical *ways of being in relation to*

significant others, and of ensuring that vital relationships can be maintained and one's relative safety is ensured. In this way, attachment patterns serve *particular interpersonal functions* with respect to attachment: to maintain closeness and allow for autonomy (security); to maintain distance (avoidance); to ensure negative proximity (preoccupation); or to preserve safety in the face of interpersonal danger (unresolved/disorganized). Insecure organizations also serve defensive functions, in that they protect the individual from feelings or thoughts that might threaten the attachment relationship (Bowlby, 1969/1982).

Bowlby's work laid the foundation for the tripartite classification system formalized by Mary Ainsworth's study of mother–infant attachment (Ainsworth et al., 1978) and Mary Main's study of adult attachment (Main et al., 1985), both of which outlined three major "organized" patterns: secure, avoidant/dismissing, and resistant/preoccupied. Some years later, disorganized infant and unresolved adult patterns were introduced (Main & Hesse, 1990; Main & Solomon, 1990).[3]

The study of classifications led to a subtle shift away from Bowlby's original dynamic model. Whereas dynamic and interpersonal functions are clearly *implied* in each of the organized and disorganized patterns (indeed, Main calls them "*states of mind*"), researchers and even clinicians often refer to attachment classifications or styles as if these are static attributes of an individual. This tendency persists despite the fact that both the Ainsworth and Main classification systems are based on evaluation of a range of dynamic and interrelated processes that are triggered by the activation of the attachment system. For example, in the Strange Situation, it is not proximity seeking per se that is crucial for classification, but when, how, and why it occurs. It is the *pattern* of proximity seeking relative to other behaviors that is relevant to classification. Likewise, in the AAI, incoherence occurs in particular ways and in response to particular questions; these distinctions are key to scoring. It is the *pattern* and type of incoherence that reveal meaningful differences among insecure organizations. Each pattern serves distinct, interpersonal, and defensive functions that are triggered when the attachment system is activated. Thus, it is crucial to remember that attachment classifications and styles refer to dynamic interpersonal processes, and not static internal (trait-like) characteristics. *It is the dynamic nature of attachment orientations that offers the promise of change through psychotherapy.*

## Attachment and Psychotherapy: A Look from Both Sides

### *Issues of Method*

There are two distinct strands of research in studies of attachment and psychotherapy: one relies on paper-and-pencil assessments of attachment style or orientation, while the other relies on in-depth assessment of attachment organization using the AAI. While these two methods are in some sense complementary, they are not one and the same. This makes it more difficult to compare findings across studies and adds another layer of complexity to an already multifaceted field.

The bulk of research on attachment and psychotherapy process and/or outcome assesses adult attachment using one or more of a set of related instruments to measure "global" attachment style: the Relationship Styles Questionnaire (RSQ; Griffin & Bartholomew, 1994) and the Experiences in Close Relationships scale (ECR; Brennan, Clark, and Shaver, 1998). The RSQ gave rise to the ECR, and both are brief, self-report questionnaires that can be administered in under 20 minutes, yielding a score on two dimensions: anxiety and avoidance. An individual's "attachment *style*" refers to the degree to which attachment-related anxiety or avoidance is a prominent feature of expectations regarding close relationships. Although both dimensions can be analyzed continuously, both can also be scored categorically. Individuals who score high on avoidance and low on anxiety are considered "avoidant"; those who score high on anxiety and low on avoidance are considered "anxious"; and individuals high on both dimensions are described as "fearful avoidant." The key difference between the anxiety and avoidance dimensions concerns the strategies subjects report using to manage a variety of attachment-related threats. Whereas the psychotherapy research literature includes studies based on other questionnaire or Q-sort assessments of attachment style, the RSQ and ECR are by far the most prevalent instruments in this area.

These instruments, and the picture they yield, are distinct from the assessment of "attachment *organization*" using the AAI (George et al., 1996). This is an hour-long, 16-question, in-depth interview that leads to a verbatim transcript for scoring. It takes an experienced coder an average of 2 hours to score each AAI. The AAI yields attachment classifications of secure-autonomous; insecure-dismissing; insecure-preoccupied; and a fourth classification, insecure-unresolved. This fourth classification can either be scored as a second classification in a forced three-way solution (i.e., secure, dismissing, or preoccupied individuals can also be unresolved in relation to loss or trauma, with "U" scored as a secondary classification), or as a classification in its own right in a four-way solution. While this is an enormously rich instrument that has tremendous face validity for clinicians, it is important to note that the AAI is used almost exclusively to yield attachment categories, and therefore does not distinguish among *degrees* of avoidance, preoccupation, or disorganization. Although severity is to some extent reflected in subclassifications, these have never been used in psychotherapy research. The absence of an assessment of degree is unfortunate because if we think of attachment classifications as manifestations of different ways of managing intense, attachment-related affects, and of defending against those that might threaten vital relations, the flexibility and or rigidity of any defense is crucial. There are the "wounded well" who use organized insecure defenses in reasonably successful ways, in contrast to the deeply disturbed, who rely on them in rigid and primitive ways.

Although it might seem that measures of attachment style and organization assess similar aspects of "attachment," and that results would appear be comparable across studies, the results of a recent meta-analysis (Roisman et al., 2007) indicate that, in fact, these measures converge only slightly, suggesting that they are measuring distinct phenomena and should not be conflated. Psychotherapy researchers working with large samples have understandably tended to use the RSQ and ECR because of their ease of administration and scoring, and the analytic flexibility that is afforded by a continuous rather than categorical measure. These instruments also permit the evaluation of dynamic change. Yet these instruments lack the potential for deeper examination of attachment-related psychological processes that is provided by the AAI. The fact that the increasingly complex research literature on attachment and psychotherapy is based on two quite different measures, with much conceptual but little methodological overlap, complicates the interpretation of many findings and makes the translation of research for clinicians even more difficult.

A related issue of method is that studies of patients in very diverse settings and with dramatically different levels of functioning and psychopathology (college counseling centers, inpatient units, residential treatment centers) are often lumped together for the purpose of meta-analysis. Not only are these groups quite different from one another, but also it is likely that attachment orientations *or* organizations manifest themselves in different ways depending on overall level of functioning. In this context, the degree of avoidance, preoccupation, or disorganization becomes especially crucial. Going forward, more nuanced thinking about both levels of psychopathology, as well as the interrelationship between psychopathology and attachment processes, is necessary.

I now turn to an examination of the four questions outlined earlier. I ground these questions in the 2001 report of the American Psychological Association Division 29 Task Force on Empirically Supported Treatments (Ackerman et al., 2001). These American Psychological Association guidelines are directly relevant both to general questions of contemporary psychotherapy research and practice, and to the particular importance of attachment processes in psychotherapy.

### Does a patient's attachment organization or style affect the process and outcome of treatment?

In 2001, the American Psychological Association Division 29 Task Force on Empirically Supported Treatments concluded that "the therapy relationship makes substantial and consistent contributions to psychotherapy outcome independent of specific type of treatment" (Ackerman et al., 2001, p. 495). This is entirely consistent with the belief held by most experienced therapists that the *therapeutic* relationship with a patient is essential to successful outcomes, and that the corrective emotional experience provided by the therapist is itself a potent agent for change.

Attachment theory would, of course, predict that the capacity to form a trusting relationship with a therapist will be determined, at least in part, by the patient's attachment organization. Attachment theory would also predict—particularly for insecure individuals—that the vulnerability and therefore the threat inherent in forming a therapeutic relationship is likely to activate the attachment system in a variety of ways, revealing distinct patterns of defense and interpersonal relatedness.[4] Indeed, activation of the attachment system within the confines of good psychotherapy

is a *sine qua non* of a successful treatment because it offers the possibility for change, adaptation, and thus transformation.

Mary Dozier's 1990 study was one of the first to examine the impact of attachment on psychotherapy. She assessed the attachment organization of 40 individuals with schizophrenic or bipolar mood disorders using Kobak's Q-set methodology for scoring the AAI (Kobak, Cole, Ferenz-Gillies, & Fleming, 1993), which yields ratings of deactivation–activation, as well as security–anxiety (and in this sense is conceptually similar to the RSQ and ECR). She then collected clinician ratings of patient compliance, help seeking, self-disclosure, and general treatment use. She found that clinician ratings of treatment compliance were associated with the secure dimension of attachment, whereas patients who were more avoidant were less likely to seek help from their therapists, less likely to comply with treatment, and less likely to make productive use of treatment. More preoccupied patients were more likely to self-disclose than those scoring high on the avoidance dimension. This pioneering study confirmed attachment theory's assumptions about the value of a secure orientation in promoting a helping relationship. Also, because many of the outcomes were designed to detect theoretically meaningful differences in the behavior and attitudes of avoidant and preoccupied patients, the study also offered the first hints as to how these two insecure organizations might differentially affect process and outcome in psychotherapy.

### Patient Attachment and the Working Alliance

Psychotherapy researchers have long used measures of what is termed the *working* or *therapeutic* alliance to assess the strength of the patient–therapist relationship. Following Dozier (1990), the first wave of research on attachment and psychotherapy focused on the relation between an individual's global orientation to attachment and the strength of the working alliance, using a range of attachment assessments, including the AAI and ECR (and its variants), as well as other questionnaire-based measures of attachment style. A recent meta-analysis of 17 of these studies (Diener & Monroe, 2011) indicates that a patient's attachment style (only one study used the AAI) predicts the quality of the alliance. Patients with secure attachment styles are more likely to have stronger alliances, whereas those with insecure attachment styles are likely to have weaker alliances. Neither attachment anxiety nor attachment-related avoidance (as variously measured) differentially predicted the weakness of the alliance. None of the moderation analyses were significant, including those assessing the effects of treatment type, alliance measure, attachment measure, or treatment length. The one difference that did emerge is that patient ratings of the alliance were more strongly correlated with patient attachment style than were therapist ratings of alliance; this presumably reflects the fact that patients are likely influenced by their attachment style in rating their connection to and relationship with the therapist. The effect size of the relation between attachment and working alliance was small to medium ($r = .17$) (Diener, Hilsenroth, & Weinberger, 2009; Diener & Monroe, 2011).

These results confirm the notion that a sense of security allows for closeness in relationships and promotes exploration, curiosity, and reflection, and that insecurity, by contrast, inhibits the development of a healing partnership. But is this anything but a confirmation of what most clinicians and psychotherapy researchers already know—that healthier, more flexible patients do better in treatment, no matter what kind of treatment they receive? And that more rigid, defended, chaotic, or disorganized patients are more difficult to connect with and help? A measure that assesses alliance in a linear way (e.g., all poor alliances are grouped together) at a single point in time is unlikely to reveal anything about the nature of these poor alliances and how therapists might tailor their work to the *particular* weaknesses associated with *particular* forms of attachment insecurity. Given that the bulk of patients in clinical samples are insecure (Van IJzendoorn & Bakermans-Kranenburg, 2009), the need for more nuanced answers is great.

Of the many investigations of attachment and therapeutic alliance conducted over the past 20 years, only two involved investigation of differences between avoidant and preoccupied patients in *patterns* of alliance. Eames and Roth (2000) studied the link between attachment organization and patterns of treatment rupture, and found that preoccupied patients reported more frequent ruptures, whereas dismissing patients reported lower rates of rupture. These patterns are consistent with theoretical predictions that preoccupied patients would be likely to engage with their therapists in more intense and volatile ways, and that dismissing patients would be more

affectively constrained and perhaps less engaged (again in line with their defensive strategies for regulating interpersonal relationships). Parenthetically, this study used a rupture-and-repair methodology that—despite being widely used in psychotherapy research (Safran & Muran, 2003)—has rarely been used in research on attachment and psychotherapy. Because this method permits the identification of specific moments of emotional arousal and defense, its rarity in the attachment literature is unfortunate.

Kanninen, Salo, and Punamaki (2000) examined changes in alliance over time and found that whereas secure patients reported few shifts in therapeutic alliance over the course of treatment, there was a steep drop in therapeutic alliance ratings for preoccupied patients in the middle of therapy, with a steep rise at the end of therapy. Dismissing patients, by contrast, showed a drop in alliance ratings at the end of therapy. Thus, patterns of change in the alliance distinguished avoidant and preoccupied patients.

By focusing on the dynamics of the alliance—of rupture or of change—these two studies allowed researchers to track differences between avoidant and preoccupied patients in their response to the emotional context of treatment and the therapeutic relationship in distinct, theoretically predictable, and clinically significant ways. Preoccupied patients in particular—in a way that is entirely consistent with Ainsworth's observations of insecure/resistant infants (Ainsworth et al., 1978)—appear to be intensely engaged with the therapist but then resist this closeness over the course of treatment.

## Patient Attachment and Psychotherapy Outcomes

Several studies have examined whether attachment organization or styles differentially predict outcomes, as measured by reduction in symptoms. In a recent meta-analysis, Levy, Ellison, Scott, and Bernecker (2011) compared results across 14 studies, all of which assessed symptom remission in light of attachment style at the start of treatment; of these, nine studies used the RSQ or ECR, and the rest used a variety of other paper-and-pencil attachment assessments. The results of this meta-analysis indicated that patients scoring high in attachment anxiety showed least remission in symptoms, whereas patients rated as high in attachment security had the most positive outcomes.

Attachment avoidance appeared to be minimally related to treatment outcome. The findings of this meta-analysis again reflect a trend that recurs throughout the research literature, which is quite consistent with theory, namely, that avoidant individuals tend to look less affected by therapy and the therapeutic relationship on a number of fronts, whereas preoccupied individuals tend to have more stormy and intense courses of therapy, and do less well overall.

A small number of studies do suggest that shifts in attachment avoidance may sometimes occur. In one of the studies included in the meta-analysis, Muller and Rosenkranz (2009) studied outcomes of an 8-week group treatment for PTSD, and described treatment outcome as moderated by change in attachment orientation, such that the lessening of both attachment anxiety *and* attachment-related avoidance over the course of treatment were associated with decreases in overall symptomatology. Thus, if a treatment is successful in lowering avoidance, symptoms may lessen. Fonagy and colleagues (1996) used the AAI to measure the relation between attachment and outcome in a sample of psychiatric inpatients receiving psychoanalytic psychotherapy ($N = 85$). These researchers found that dismissing patients were more likely to show changes in the Global Assessment of Functioning Scale on the DSM-IV than were those who were preoccupied or unresolved/disorganized. In another study that *was* included in the meta-analysis, McBride, Atkinson, Quilty, and Bagby (2006) likewise found that depressed patients who scored high on avoidant attachment did better than their anxiously attached (i.e., more preoccupied) peers.

Although these results are hardly conclusive, they do align with the view that individuals with preoccupied attachments have the worst outcomes in therapy, whereas the picture is more mixed and ambiguous for those who are avoidant in their attachments. This general trend, indicating a bumpier course in treatment (more ruptures, shifting alliances) and likely poorer outcomes for patients who are preoccupied and unresolved/disorganized is consistent with the finding that these classifications are often linked with borderline personality disorder (BPD) and other severe personality disorders (see Westen, Nakash, Thomas, & Bradley, 2007, for a review), and require treatment that is targeted specifically to their diagnosis (Bateman & Fonagy, 2009; Levy et al., 2006; Linehan, 1993).

## *The Patient's Attachment to the Therapist*

In 1995, research on attachment and psychotherapy took a new turn when Brent Mallinckrodt and his colleagues introduced a method for assessing the quality of the patient's *attachment to the therapist* (Mallinckrodt, Gantt, & Coble, 1995), as distinct from the patient's more general or global attachment organization or style (as measured by the AAI or ECR). The Client Attachment to Therapist Scale (CATS) is a 36-item self-report measure that distinguishes among secure, avoidant-fearful, and preoccupied-merged attachment to the therapist. It is important to note that this three-category model collapses the ECR avoidant and fearful dimensions into a single category, complicating comparison with other measures. In later research, Mallinckrodt and colleagues (2005) documented the specific contribution that the patient's attachment to the therapist makes to the working alliance, over and above global attachment style. In general, this measure is only modestly correlated with global attachment style or organization (Mikulincer et al., 2013), suggesting that global insecurity does not necessarily preclude forming a secure attachment to the therapist, presumably because the therapist defies the patient's expectations of relationships.

## ATTACHMENT TO THE THERAPIST AND THE WORKING ALLIANCE

In their initial research, Mallinckrodt and his colleagues (1995) found that secure attachment to the therapist on the CATS predicted a strong working alliance; this finding has been replicated in a number of subsequent studies (see Mikulincer et al., 2013). In related work, Gelso and his colleagues (Fuertes et al., 2007; Marmarosh et al., 2009) found that patients' positive feelings about the real relationship with the therapist were correlated with secure attachment to the therapist and a stronger working alliance. Once again, these results shed little light on the differential impact of avoidant and preoccupied attachment to the therapist on the clinical process.

Several of the findings in Mallinckrodt and his colleagues' (1995) original study do, however, point to important differences in these two insecure groups. Consistent with prior research, they found that avoidant attachment to the therapist was associated with a poor alliance. Interestingly, they also found that patients whose attachment to the therapist was judged to be preoccupied rated their alliance with the therapist as strong, as did those with secure attachments. This finding raises a crucial question: Are these apparently equally "strong" attachments the same?

Research by Woodhouse, Schlosser, Crook, Ligiero, and Gelso (2003) raised a similar set of questions. These researchers examined the relation between a patient's attachment to his or her therapist and therapist ratings of the patient's negative and positive transference, namely, the patient's tendency to project his or her own interpersonal expectations and childhood fantasies onto the therapist. Avoidant/fearful attachment to the therapist was unrelated to any aspect of transference. And, contrary to their predictions, there was no connection between a patient's secure attachment to the therapist and the positive transference. Rather, secure attachment was related to both the negative transference and the overall amount of transference. In other words, secure attachment to the therapist allowed room for a powerful and even negative transference to emerge. Most important, however, and consistent with the findings of Mallinckrodt and colleagues (1995), preoccupied/merged attachment to the therapist was *also* strongly correlated with negative transference and amount of transference.

In both studies, secure and preoccupied attachment patterns look superficially alike; both types of patients feel connected to the therapist and have powerful feelings about him or her. But to return again to the question of dynamics, although we would expect patients with both secure and preoccupied attachments to the therapist to have intense feelings during the treatment, particularly negative ones, *the meaning and interpersonal function of these feelings would be entirely different.* The securely attached patient would feel free to express negative feelings about the therapist without fear of retribution, and would expect appropriate coregulation. The preoccupied patient would know of no other way to experience closeness than through heightened negative affect (Cassidy, 1994) and efforts to control these feelings through resistance. Thus, the outcomes are different for the two groups, despite some apparent similarities in their experience of the transference. In other words, it is quite likely that the *fate* of both negative transference and overall transference would differ for secure and preoccupied patients; also, we would expect the patients' capacity to reflect on the meaning of the transference to differ considerably, as would the flexibility and/or intractability of transference feelings.

## ATTACHMENT TO THE THERAPIST AND THE DEPTH OF ENGAGEMENT

Two studies (Romano, Fitzpatrick, & Janzen, 2009; Saypol & Farber, 2010) have linked secure attachment to the therapist to the capacity to explore significant issues in psychotherapy, whereas avoidant attachment to the therapist was linked to less self-disclosure and meaningful exploration. Related to this work is a recent study by Janzen, Fitzpatrick, and Drapeau (2008), in which reports of emotionally charged moments, even after a short period in therapy, were linked to increases in avoidant patients' experience of security in relation to the therapist, and appeared to enhance their feeling that the therapy was helpful. Avoidant patients appear to be more likely to engage when their concerns about closeness are somehow addressed. Thus, as in the Eames and Roth (2000) and Kanninen and colleagues (2000) studies described earlier, these researchers attempted to focus on transformational moments within the therapy and to link these in a meaningful way to attachment. For clinicians, these shifts are where attachment issues reveal themselves dramatically and where change is most likely to occur.

As I hope I have made clear, despite the fact that a number of researchers have examined the relation between a patient's attachment orientation and the process and outcome of psychotherapy, the only clear outcome to emerge thus far is that secure patients do better in psychotherapy and insecure patients do more poorly. The small number of studies that *have* detected meaningful differences among secure, avoidant, and preoccupied patients—in their patterns of response to the therapist and to the therapeutic process—have typically relied on more novel methodologies that allow for the assessment of change in the alliance over time, patterns of rupture, the study of critical incidents, and so forth. These kinds of methodologies allow researchers to examine *dynamic relational processes* in the treatment, namely, what happens when the attachment system is activated (via ruptures, critical incidents, etc.), either over the course of a single session or over the course of a treatment. It is in these contexts that we are most likely to see attachment defenses triggered and change is most likely to occur. When does change happen and in what context? Can these changes be understood in light of attachment? One-time assessments using linear outcome measures (e.g., the working alliance, self-disclosure) make it difficult to detect the patterns that reveal the "coherence of individual development" (Sroufe, 1979). Unless outcomes are considered in relation to each other (i.e., as patterns), it is very difficult to detect differences between avoidant and preoccupied strategies.

### The Clinical Perspective

In rather sharp contrast to the relative ambiguity of the research literature regarding the differential effects of avoidant and preoccupied ways of relating and being, there is a small body of writing about the clinical utility of attachment theory and classification in thinking about and organizing psychotherapeutic material. In myriad ways, attachment processes are seen as providing vital clues to understanding shifts in alliance, degrees of engagement, the evolving attachment to the therapist, and an individual's capacity to change. Although few clinicians routinely administer the AAI (but see Steele & Steele, 2008) or are indeed trained in either the AAI or the Strange Situation procedure, the distinctions among avoidant, preoccupied, and unresolved/disorganized patterns have enormous face validity for clinicians. As I have described elsewhere (1999, 2000, 2007, 2014), thinking about and listening for attachment dynamics and themes helps me find metaphors and language that are experience-near for patients, encompass the nature of both defenses and treatment ruptures, make sense of relational patterns, and provide an imaginative picture of early experiences of seeking and receiving care. The differences among the narratives of avoidant, preoccupied, and unresolved/disorganized adults are striking (also see Daniel, 2009, 2014; Holmes, 1997, 1998, 2004, 2009), and alert the clinician in powerful ways to moments when the attachment system is activated or deactivated. These moments also tell us a great deal about an individual's vulnerability to threat and defense (Slade, 2014), and as such offer significant opportunities for change and reorganization.

Although rarely the focus of research, the unresolved/disorganized category has been particularly meaningful to clinicians and provides a useful entrée into thinking about the long-term sequelae of unresolved fear and trauma. Giovanni Liotti (2004) has been making important contributions in this area for over 20 years. His suggestion that disorganized attachment in infancy might well lead to dissociative processes in adults inspired Main and Hesse (1990) to study the link between maternal frightened and frightening behavior and infant disorganization. Karlen Lyons-Ruth has also been a major contributor in this area, tracking the long-term sequelae of atypical maternal behavior, and in particular the multiple clinical and developmental consequences of the "hostile–helpless" diathesis in setting the stage for severe pathology in later life (see Holmes, 2004; Lyons-Ruth & Jacobvitz, Chapter 29, this volume; Slade, 2007; ). Of particular note is Lyons-Ruth and colleagues' astute observation regarding the complexities of working with patients who are unresolved/disorganized in relation to attachment:

> The resolution of discrete traumatic events in treatment may come about more quickly than the resolution of long-standing patterns of role-reversal, disorientation, and disrupted forms of affect communication in the transference. Among dissociative young adults, current research suggests that disrupted communication patterns with attachment figures tend to be a subtle and implicit part of dyadic interaction from a very early age, and therefore, may be extremely difficult for the patient to articulate until forms of a healthier and more genuine implicit and explicit dialog around heightened affective experiences are worked out in the therapeutic relationship. (p. 82)

This observation makes it clear why these difficulties, which are challenging to track in clinical work, present major challenges for researchers.

### Does the therapist's attachment organization affect the process and outcome of treatment?

The second conclusion of the American Psychological Association Division 29 Task Force is as follows: "Practice and treatment guidelines should explicitly address therapist behaviors and qualities that promote a facilitative therapy relationship" (Ackerman et al., p. 495). Thus, the task force not only placed particular importance on the therapy relationship, but it also placed the responsibility for the formation and maintenance of this relationship squarely on the shoulders of the therapist. As is clear from the previous sections, we know that the bulk of patients will be insecure, making it likely that they will struggle in some way or other to form a solid alliance and working relationship. This makes the therapist's capacity to build relationships despite the challenges of a patient's insecurity all the more important. From an attachment perspective, not only is the patient's attachment organization relevant to outcome, *so is the therapist's*. Therapists who are able to provide a secure and safe base for their patients, to remain emotionally present and compassionate while managing complex and potentially intense affects within a therapy session, are likely to be those who best facilitate their patients' development.

Again, it was Mary Dozier who opened the door to studying how therapists' attachment organization affects outcomes (Dozier, Cue, & Barnett, 1994). Dozier assessed the attachment organization of the 18 case managers who had provided treatment to the patients described in her 1990 study. She coded the clinician AAIs using Kobak and colleagues' (1993) Q-set; the patients' AAIs had also been classified using this method. Dozier found that a therapist's security predicted her ability to "respond therapeutically to the individual needs of her clients" (Dozier et al., 1994, p. 798). A number of studies have since confirmed that security in the therapist is correlated with the strength of the working alliance and patients' experience of being helped by the therapy (for reviews, see Daniel, 2006; Mikulincer et al., 2013).

But Dozier's research took the issue of therapist attachment one crucial step further: She examined how therapist attachment style *interacts* with that of the patient (here, again, we see her dynamic and deeply attachment-informed perspective). What she found was that secure therapists are able to work flexibly with patients, regardless of their attachment style, whereas insecure therapists are more inclined to get sidetracked by the patient's defenses and respond to them in nontherapeutic ways. In particular, whereas insecure therapists responded to what was *apparent or manifest* in patient communications, secure therapists were able to recognize and respond to *underlying* (and presumably more disruptive) feelings and needs. Thus, secure therapists responded to dependency needs in dismissing patients, and were more autonomy promoting with preoccupied patients. Insecure therapists, by contrast, were much more likely to "perceive greater dependency needs and intervene more intensively with clients who are preoccupied than they are with those who are dismissing" (Dozier et al., 1994, p. 798). In other words, insecure therapists are likely to heighten and magnify patient defenses rather than explore the needs that are *provoking* attachment-related defenses, presumably because of the ways the patient activates their own defenses and anxieties. Dozier and colleagues' (1994) findings have been replicated and expanded in studies published over

the past 15 years (Petrowski, Nowacki, Pokorny, & Buchheim, 2011; Romano, Janzen, & Fitzpatrick, 2009; Tyrrell, Dozier, Teague, & Fallot, 1999). As we shall see, study of the interaction between patient and therapist attachment has important implications for the question of how therapists should respond to signs of avoidance and anxiety in their patients.

Unlike the literature on attachment and both therapy process and outcome, this literature quite explicitly outlines the differences between the ways avoidant and preoccupied patients defend themselves against their needs for closeness and autonomy within the activating context of psychotherapy. These differences are found to have differential effects on therapists, who, like their patients, defend against affect and relatedness within the activating context of psychotherapy in theoretically predictable ways. Thus, the literature on the therapist's attachment classification is inherently a much more dynamic research literature, with much clearer implications for clinical training, supervision, and practice.

### The Clinical Perspective

With the exception of Holmes (1998, 2001) and Wallin (2010), clinical writers have had surprisingly little to say about how a therapist's attachment organization or style affects the process and outcome of psychotherapy. This omission is particularly striking given that the notion of countertransference has its roots in classical psychoanalytic theory. The importance of countertransference is implicit in the directive to young clinicians to pursue both personal treatment and supervision, yet explicit consideration in case studies of the impact of the therapist's own defenses and anxiety has been notably absent from the clinical literature (even relational psychoanalysis, with its intersubjective focus, seems to skirt these issues). Given the highly robust research finding that the therapist's attachment style has an effect on both process and outcome, and provides explicit evidence for the *relational nature* of attachment processes, this omission is particularly unfortunate.

### Should psychotherapy be tailored to the patient's attachment organization?

For reasons that should by now not be surprising, the American Psychological Aassociation Division 29 Task Force on Empirically Supported

Psychotherapy concluded in 2001 that "current research on [attachment] is insufficient for a clear judgment to be made on whether customizing the therapy relationship to these [attachment] characteristics improves treatment outcomes" (Ackerman et al., 2001, p. 496). However, evidence gathered since then suggests that there may well be value—once the therapeutic relationship has been established—in tailoring the treatment process to the patient's predominant attachment style or organization. In particular, research suggests that there is value in responding "against" the patient's attachment style, and that the ability to do so is likely a reflection of the therapist's own attachment organization. Much of this research is attachment-informed in the sense that it is based on the assumption that avoidant and preoccupied patients have "typical" ways of defending against and regulating affect and relationships, and that these patterns or styles of relating have distinct implications for practice.

Researchers originally suggested that therapists are inclined to respond with more cognitive interventions (interpretations and suggestions) with dismissing/deactivating patients, and with more affective interventions (reflection of feelings, empathy) to more preoccupied/hyperactivating patients (Rubino, Barker, Roth, & Fearon, 2000). However, these linear trends do not obtain when the therapist's attachment organization is taken into account. As described earlier, Dozier and colleagues (1994) reported that secure case managers are less likely than insecure case managers to become enmeshed with hyperactivating patients or to shut down in concert with their deactivating patients. Secure therapists are inclined to adopt styles that are noncomplementary to those of their patients. In a later study of patient–therapist interaction, Tyrrell and colleagues (1999) reported similar findings. Even though therapists in this sample were all classified as secure, those who were *less* dismissing/deactivating were able to form stronger alliances with patients who were *more* dismissing/deactivating. These same researchers also reported that more dismissing patients did better with more preoccupied/hyperactivating clinicians. Petrowski and colleagues (2011) likewise reported that patients scoring high on attachment anxiety found therapists with higher attachment avoidance more helpful, suggesting that the containment provided by a more avoidant therapist was therapeutic, as compared with the hyperactivating strategies that might be used by a therapist whose attachment style was anxious.

One of the conclusions that can be drawn from this work is that secure therapists are more able than their insecure peers to respond in a noncomplementary way to a patient's defenses, presumably because they are themselves less likely to respond defensively with patients and less likely to be dysregulated by the content of sessions. Gentle challenges to the patient's attachment organization have the effect of softening rather than provoking characteristic defensive styles, thereby enhancing flexibility and change (see Daniel, 2006). In a fascinating article supporting this research, Daly and Mallinckrodt (2009) presented data (based on detailed interviews with experienced therapists) to support the notion that more experienced clinicians (regardless of their orientation) are able to move "in" and "out" of attachment style with a patient over the course of treatment. Noting that most studies of attachment and psychotherapy are carried out with inexperienced therapists in training clinics, Daly and Mallinckrodt suggested that in the early stages of therapy, when the relationship and alliance are just getting established, experienced clinicians are likely to respond "in style" to patient defenses. This makes patients feel more understood and mirrored. As therapy progresses, however, and the relationship is more secure, experienced therapists move toward responding in ways that are "out of style," pushing more dismissing patients to express intolerable emotions and become more engaged in relation to the therapist, and pushing more preoccupied patients to contain powerful emotions, function more autonomously, and deintensify transference manifestations and expectations. Although Daly and Mallinckrodt did not study these patterns in relation to therapist attachment style, it seems likely that therapists become more flexible and sensitive to both manifest defenses and latent affect as they become more experienced. It may be that experience—at least to some extent—will override therapists' own attachment-related anxiety and defenses, such that they are able to respond more therapeutically to a range of patients and clinical situations. This kind of flexibility is much more difficult for inexperienced therapists, who, unfortunately, most often serve as the therapists in psychotherapy research.

### The Clinical Perspective

Most, if not all, dynamically oriented clinicians adjust what they do in treatment on the basis of the patient's defenses, psychic organization, and interpersonal functioning. Again, the clinical attachment literature documents this in many ways; in work with avoidant patients, therapists must find ways to engage them emotionally, and "break" their rigid stories (Holmes, 1998). The therapists of preoccupied patients must help them contain and regulate intense emotions by creating meaningful narratives and (following Talia et al., 2014) derive comfort from the contact they seek. The "strategies" for doing this are not unique to an attachment perspective; the softening of defenses and the containment of pain is the essential work of psychotherapy. But when the question is framed in terms of whether to respond "in" or "out" of style (see Holmes, 1998; Slade, 1999), it is, in effect, framing therapeutic action in attachment terms. Here, I think it is clear that challenging the patient's defenses is likely what will be most useful, and that either the "secure" and/or experienced therapist (and experience, of course, makes most professionals feel safe) is in the best position to do this.

## Can psychotherapy change attachment orientations?

The literature reviewed up to this point addressed the impact of attachment organization on therapy process and outcomes. A small number of studies have come at this question in a different way, examining whether attachment status itself can be changed by psychotherapy: Rather than assess the impact of attachment on psychotherapy, they assess the impact of psychotherapy on attachment. Change in attachment status itself becomes the target of treatment.

In their study of 35 nonpsychotic inpatients, Fonagy and colleagues (1995) gave the AAI to patients upon admission for intensive inpatient treatment and on follow-up, 1 year postdischarge. The authors reported that whereas all patients were insecure at the start of treatment, 40% were secure upon discharge. Unfortunately, the distribution of classifications before and after treatment is not reported, so it is difficult to assess who changed and in what way. Clearer evidence for the utility of the AAI as an outcome measure emerged in a large-sample randomized clinical trial conducted by Levy and his colleagues (2006). This group compared the effectiveness of transference-focused psychotherapy (TFP) with that of DBT and modified psychodynamic supportive psychotherapy in treating individuals with BPD. They re-

ported that in a sample of 60 outpatients following 1 year of treatment, TFP (but not DBT or supportive psychotherapy) led to a significant increase in the number of individuals classified as secure in relation to attachment. These results suggest that a treatment that works directly on the patient's feelings about the therapist may be particularly suited to changing attachment organization. However, Diamond, Stovall-McClough, Clarkin, and Levy (2003) reporting on a subsample of Levy and colleagues' (2006) larger sample, examined changes in attachment status in 10 patients receiving TFP. Here the shifts described in the Levy and colleagues study did not obtain. Only two of the nine subjects who were insecure on intake shifted to secure. The rest either stayed the same or shifted to other insecure categories.

In third study, reported by Stovall-McClough and Cloitre (2003), 18 women with posttraumatic stress disorder (PTSD) diagnoses were treated using either exposure therapy or skills training. At intake, 72% were classified as unresolved/disorganized with regard to trauma, and only 11% of the sample was judged secure. Over half of patients who were unresolved/disorganized (62%; n = 8) shifted from the unresolved/disorganized status following treatment, and 50% of the total sample was secure at termination.

To date, these appear to be the only studies that have examined change in AAI status as a function of treatment. As a whole, especially given the relatively small sample sizes, they provide at best only modest support for the idea that AAI status can change in psychotherapy, and even less evidence that therapy can bring about shifts from insecure to secure status. Thus the question remains whether it is reasonable to assess treatment outcome or establish the empirical basis for one treatment over another using change in AAI classification as a criterion measure. Attachment classifications are overt manifestations of deep structures that take time to change, even in the most successful of treatments. As Everett Waters and his colleagues pointed out (Waters, Hamilton, & Weinfeld, 2000), stability in attachment classifications is the rule rather than the exception, with negative life events being most clearly associated with instability. Thus, to return to one of the themes of this chapter, it is probably much more useful to assess change in a more dynamic and nuanced way.

One way to do this would be to assess change in attachment dimensions, but even here the results are modest and mixed. Two studies have examined the impact of psychotherapy on attachment style, which is potentially a way to study change in a more dynamic way. Travis, Bliwise, Binder, and Horne-Meyer (2001) reported findings similar to those of Diamond and colleagues (2003), namely, that while a significant proportion of patients shifted attachment styles, the number who shifted to a secure style was not significant. In a more recent study, Muller and Rosenkranz (2009) examined changes in attachment style over the course of an 8-week intensive group psychotherapy treatment for PTSD. They reported that the treatment group (as opposed to the waiting-list controls) was more likely to move from an insecure to secure style of attachment. Attachment anxiety decreased from admission to discharge to follow-up, whereas changes in attachment avoidance were more difficult to detect.

### The Clinical Perspective

Most clinical writers suggest that when treatment is going well, anxiety diminishes, avoidance softens, and psychological organization improves. And, indeed, the clinical attachment literature, which includes many case studies, routinely documents shifts in attachment processes and dynamics over the course of treatment, with many patients moving from insecure-unresolved/disorganized to insecure-organized to secure modes of regulating affect and being "in relation" to significant others. These changes are typically observed rather than measured, but from a clinical perspective, these are meaningful and observable transformations.

### New Directions: Narrative Processes, and a "Move to the Level of the Relation"

As mentioned early in this chapter, I view recent work by Sarah Daniel, Alessandro Talia, and their colleagues as leading the way toward a paradigm shift in attachment-informed research and clinical practice (Daniel, 2009, 2014; Talia et al., 2014). Recall that from Bowlby's perspective, attachment classifications and styles refer to dynamic relational processes, and not static internal (trait-like) characteristics. These processes are the explicit focus of Daniel and Talia's research, which uses novel methods and approaches to measure both dynamic patterns of attachment activation and their relational functions within a treatment context.

In 2006, Daniel published a remarkably detailed, comprehensive, and integrated review of the literature on adult attachment patterns and individual psychotherapy. Several years later, she published an exploratory study examining the relation between adult attachment insecurity and narrative processes in psychotherapy. As Mary Main's work makes so explicit, assessing the *quality* of narrative processes is at the heart of attachment classification. And, as Holmes and I have both pointed out elsewhere (Holmes, 1998, 2001; Slade 1999, 2014), narrative patterns within the context of a single psychotherapy session provide crucial information about defensive structures and other features of attachment organization, as well as crucial opportunities for intervention and transformation. In her 2011 study, Daniel coded three key elements of narrative processes in psychotherapy: verbal productivity, narrative initiative, and topic segments. These were subdivided on the basis of semantic content into those focusing on external, internal, or reflexive processes. The participants, who were evaluated within the context of a randomized clinical trial of cognitive-behavioral and psychoanalytic treatments for bulimia, were assessed on the AAI prior to treatment. Later, their in-session discourse was coded along the dimensions described earlier. Daniel reported significant differences between dismissing and preoccupied patients in their verbal productivity during psychotherapy sessions, with preoccupied patients talking more and taking more speech turns per session than their dismissing counterparts, who were more likely to pause during sessions. Likewise, preoccupied patients were more likely to initiate narratives in therapy. Type of treatment, cognitive-behavioral therapy (CBT) or psychoanalytic psychotherapy (PPT), had no apparent effect on these patterns. Differences in content were less clear, and interacted with treatment type, leading Daniel to suggest the need for more "fine-grained" analysis of discourse patterns, and for the inclusion of secure and unresolved/disorganized patients in future research.

Several features distinguished Daniel's early work from other research on attachment and psychotherapy, and indeed from other adult attachment research. Main and her colleagues (1985) have from the start emphasized the importance of assessing narrative *coherence* in determining an individual's attachment organization. Moments of incoherence are critical indicators of both the activation of the attachment system and as typical defenses against such activations. In line with this, a secure narrative must meet all four of Grice's

(1989) maxims for narrative coherence: quantity, quality, relevance, and manner. But because it is a linear scale, the coherence scale does not capture these variations, nor does it capture the *kinds of incoherence* that distinguish subtypes of insecurity. Main has always emphasized how differently avoidant, preoccupied, and unresolved/disorganized individuals are incoherent. Daniel's work on discourse patterns takes two important steps toward developing ways of detecting these differences: She directly evaluated quantity by measuring rate of verbal production (which, as anyone who has coded AAIs knows, usually does in fact distinguish avoidant and preoccupied adults), and she evaluates manner by tracking narrative initiative. Finally, Daniel also evaluated the *content* of psychotherapy sessions. To my knowledge, no one working in this area has considered the question of content or theme. Given that *what* patients talk about can often be quite significant, this seems like a crucial oversight. Although Daniel's sample was small and her findings with respect to thematic content ambiguous, her inclusion of these variables signals another important shift in the work. In particular, it would seem crucial going forward to examine shifts in attachment dynamics within a session (through analyzing shifts in coherence and/or discursive behavior) in light of session content.

Recently, Talia and colleagues (2014) reported another set of groundbreaking developments in the study of attachment and psychotherapy. In their study, the in-session speech of patients classified as secure, dismissing, or preoccupied on the AAI was analyzed in light of the ways that their discourse *elicited and maintained emotional proximity* with the therapist. Transcripts of therapist–patient discourse were analyzed using the Patient Attachment Coding System (PACS), developed by Talia and Miller-Bottome (2014). The PACS is made up of three main scales, which derive directly from the core principles of attachment theory: the Contact Seeking scale, which rates discursive behaviors that "tend to increase emotional proximity and the likelihood of receiving support from the therapist" (p. 7); the Avoidance scale, which rates discursive behaviors that decrease emotional closeness between patient and therapist; and the Resistance scale, which rates discursive behaviors that "tend to thwart the therapist's attempts to support patients and to make sense of their experience" (p. 7).

In a combined sample of 56 patients in different types of psychotherapy, the AAI was administered prior to treatment, and AAI classifica-

tions were shown to predict distinctive in-session discursive patterns, as rated with the PACS by external observers. Patients judged secure on the AAI had significantly higher scores on the Contact Seeking scale than either preoccupied and dismissing patients (although preoccupied patients were significantly more likely to seek contact than dismissing patients), and tended to express distress openly, ask for help, and show gratitude. Avoidant patients were characterized by higher scores on the Avoidance scale than the other two groups, and tended to minimize any disclosure, convey self-sufficiency, and downplay their distress. Preoccupied patients were characterized by higher scores than the others on the Resistance scale, and tended to obstruct the therapist's attempts to intervene, failed to enlist the therapists' own points of view, and conveyed their experience in a vague or confusing way. Particularly fascinating is the discovery that preoccupied patients not only seek contact but also *resist* it. This is, of course, completely in line with Ainsworth's observation of ambivalence in resistant infants' behavior (Ainsworth et al., 1978), and it very much clarifies what it is that can be both so challenging and irritating about working with preoccupied patients.

As Talia and his colleagues (2014) noted, by providing a more precise understanding of the interpersonal functions of particular narrative patterns, this research takes the study of attachment narratives from "the level of representation" and moves it to "the level of the relation" (p. 205). As a result of this study, and a second validation study (Talia, Miller-Bottome, & Daniel, 2015), we not only know that insecurity makes it difficult to engage in treatment at a variety of levels but also how these difficulties are manifest in form and interpersonal function across categories of attachment. These findings are entirely in line with the dynamic and *relational* aspects of Bowlby's theory, aspects that, as I mentioned earlier, are so often lost in research. And, by detecting the interpersonal aims of discourse and meaningfully linking these to attachment classification, Talia and colleagues were able to track explicitly what were simply trends or hints in previous studies. This demonstrates how crucial it is for research and its methods to be meaningfully grounded in theory.

It is important to underscore the fact that this study grew out of a collaboration across a number of sites. This collaboration allowed the researchers to combine samples in which both AAI data and session transcripts were available. Thus, rather than rely on a series of paper-and-pencil measures, this study was able to examine in-session processes in a meaningful way across a large number of subjects. Obviously, this is time-intensive, expensive work. But the yields are potentially very significant.

From a clinical perspective, I view these methodologies as allowing researchers and clinicians to track minute-by-minute change in both the therapist's and the patient's discursive *relational* behavior. Presumably, these changes can tell us when a patient's attachment system is activated during the course of a session, and when an intervention (a question, an observation, an interpretation, or even a silence) has helped overcome avoidance or resistance in the patient, or heightened it. Likewise, they can help identify points of activation and defense in the therapist as well, and help track opportunities for repair and therapeutic progress. These are the moments of true change in psychotherapy.

## Future Directions

### The Integration of Theory, Research, and Practice

If Bowlby were alive today, he would surely be happy to discover that the once vilified term *attachment* has now become a part of the lexicon of psychotherapy researchers and psychotherapists alike. But I believe that he would also encourage us to keep pushing further, to deepen our understanding of attachment processes, and to build bridges across disciplines still in so many respects far apart. In the spirit of such forward momentum, and in light of the work reviewed in this chapter, I close with a list of potential ways to use attachment theory and research to deepen our understanding of our patients and their relational dynamics, to identify what is helpful to whom, and to address aspects of how therapists bring their own difficulties and challenges into the work.

1. *Deepen the way attachment is written about and taught.*

There is today a vast and complex literature on attachment processes (see, e.g., Mikulincer & Shaver, 2007; Slade & Holmes, 2013). Yet, as I hope I have made clear in this chapter, researchers and clinicians alike have often lost sight of the dynamic and relational elements of this theory,

elements that have great implications for clinical research and practice. These were at the heart of Bowlby's writings and shaped the evolution of the theory and its methods. Only recently have these returned to the forefront in research and practice. When we write about attachment, or teach it to our students (whether they are research or clinical students), it is important not to limit our discussions to classifications or styles, but to fully explore and set in context what these classifications *mean* on a number of critical levels.

2. *Expose clinicians to the methods of attachment theory, so that they become better observers of these processes.*

The best way to learn about attachment processes is to *observe* them *in situ*. Yet, except for those lucky clinicians who have really studied the Strange Situation procedure, the AAI, or any other attachment measure, there are few opportunities really to learn about attachment from the inside out. One of the most compelling and attachment-informed interventions in the field today, the Circle of Security intervention (Powell, Cooper, Hoffman, & Marvin, 2013) grew out of the years Glen Cooper, Kent Hoffman, and Bert Powell spent studying attachment with Jude Cassidy, watching Strange Situation procedures together, reading AAI transcripts, and deeply immersing themselves in the theory and research. Likewise, my training on the AAI with Mary Main and Mary Ainsworth was one of the most valuable forms of clinical supervision I ever had. Currently there are few hands-on ways for clinicians to learn really deeply about attachment processes in all their complexity (see Steele & Steele, 2008). For this reason, those of us in the field with this knowledge must become more involved in the training of clinicians if our goal is to ensure that their work is truly attachment-informed.

3. *Explore new methodologies in attachment psychotherapy research.*

As I detailed earlier, I believe that much of the research on psychotherapy and attachment has relied on outcome measures unlikely to distinguish the differential impact of avoidant and preoccupied modes of defense on the process and outcome of psychotherapy. The methods introduced by Daniel and Talia, as well as the rupture and repair methodologies described by Safran and Muran (2003) and the "critical incident" methodologies (e.g., Janzen et al., 2008), are most likely not only to pick up meaningful differences in the course and outcome of therapy but also to help identify what works best for whom at moments when the attachment system is activated in psychotherapy.

4. *Pay more attention to clinicians' own psychological health.*

It is fascinating to me to realize how little attention has been given in any of the literatures I have reviewed to the importance of a clinician's "security." Obviously, it would be Draconian and in fact absurd to suggest that only secure individuals be allowed to work as clinicians. For one (and I say this with my tongue only slightly in my cheek), such a requirement would significantly decrease the number of practitioners in the field. And the familiarity and comfort with emotional pain, with the loss, separation, trauma, and other hardships that often come out of painful attachment experiences, give many clinicians a special ear and heart for the work. But it is evident from the research (and this has certainly been my experience as a supervisor) that while painful attachment experiences can enrich a therapist's perspective, unmetabolized and unintegrated affect in a therapist has a profound and negative impact on the work. Thus, an individual's relative attachment security should be a relevant to the determination of whether he or she will make a good therapist. In the clinical psychology doctoral program in which I taught for over 30 years (at the City College of New York), in-depth clinical interviews aimed at evaluating some of these characteristics were a key step in the admission process and allowed at least some assessment of important personal characteristics. Even more important, professional development should from the very beginning include individual supervision, with an emphasis on understanding clinical process, transference and countertransference, as well as separate personal psychotherapy. Both are key to clinicians' separating their own struggles from those of their patients, and to having a secure base from which they can think about and regulate their experiences in this activating, challenging work.

In conclusion, I reiterate that the study of the clinical implications of attachment is fascinating, challenging, and complicated. I tip my hat to the generations of researchers and clinicians who struggled with these complexities over the last quarter century, and look forward to joining with future generations as they expand upon these rich foundations.

## Acknowledgments

I would like to thank Jeremy Holmes—colleague, friend, and keen reader—for his hugely helpful edits on an early draft. As always, his comments helped me polish the chapter stylistically and conceptually. Thanks, too, to Sarah Daniel, who graciously shared her work (including prepublication drafts) during the writing process, and—together with Alessandro Talia—reviewed and sharpened my descriptions of their research.

## Notes

1. In an effort to use terms that are the most descriptive and least confusing, I refer to secure adults as *secure*; avoidant or dismissing adults as *avoidant*; and preoccupied or anxious adults as *preoccupied*. Although not an ideal solution, it seems the clearest, simplest, and least controversial one. Likewise, I refer to adults who are unresolved in relation to loss or trauma as *unresolved/disorganized*, as many clinicians use the term *disorganized* to refer to both children and adults.

2. I regret that space limitations preclude my discussing the literature on mentalization and mentalization-based interventions (e.g., Allen, 2013; Bateman & Fonagy, 2009), both of which are deeply attachment informed. Some of this work is discussed by Fonagy, Luyten, Allison, and Campbell, Chapter 34, this volume.

3. In 1996, Erik Hesse described a fourth insecure adult attachment classification, "cannot classify." This classification has rarely been included either in either research or clinical studies of psychotherapy.

4. Interestingly, Bateman and Fonagy (2009) caution against activating the attachment system of patients with borderline personality disorder by talking about the past, until they have developed the reflective capacities necessary to tolerate such threats.

## References

Ackerman, S. J., Benjamin, L. S., Beutler, L. E., Gelso, C. J., Goldfried, M. R., Hill, C., et al. (2001). Empirically supported therapy relationships: Conclusions and recommendations of the Division 29 Task Force. *Psychotherapy, 38*, 495–497.

Ainsworth, M. D. S., Blehar, M. C., Waters, E., & Wall, S. (1978). *Patterns of attachment: A psychological study of the Strange Situation*. Hillsdale, NJ: Erlbaum.

Allen, J. G. (2013). *Mentalizing in the development and treatment of attachment trauma*. London: Karnac.

Bateman, A., & Fonagy, P. (2009). Randomized controlled trial of outpatient mentalization-based treatment versus structured clinical management for borderline personality disorder. *American Journal of Psychiatry, 166,* 1355–1364.

Bowlby, J. (1944). Forty-four juvenile thieves: Their characters and home life. *International Journal of Psychoanalysis, 25,* 19–52, 107–127.

Bowlby, J. (1973). *Attachment and loss: Vol. 2. Separation.* New York: Basic Books.

Bowlby, J. (1980). *Attachment and loss: Vol. 3. Loss.* New York: Basic Books.

Bowlby, J. (1982). *Attachment and loss: Vol. 1. Attachment.* New York: Basic Books. (Original work published 1969)

Bowlby, J. (1988). *A secure base: Parent–child attachment and healthy human development.* New York: Basic Books.

Brennan, K. A., Clark, C. L., & Shaver, P. R. (1998). Self-report measurement of adult attachment: An integrative overview. In J. A. Simpson & W. S. Rholes (Eds.), *Attachment theory and close relationships* (pp. 46–76). New York: Guilford Press.

Cassidy, J. (1994). Emotion regulation: Influences of attachment relationships. *Monographs of the Society for Research in Child Development, 59,* 228–249.

Daly, K., & Mallinckrodt, B. (2009). A grounded-theory model of experts' approach to psychotherapy for clients with attachment avoidance or attachment anxiety. *Journal of Counseling Psychology, 56,* 549–563.

Daniel, S. I. F. (2006). Adult attachment patterns and individual psychotherapy: A review. *Clinical Psychology Review, 26,* 968–984.

Daniel, S. I. F. (2009). The developmental roots of narrative expression in therapy: Contributions from attachment theory and research. *Psychotherapy: Theory, Research, Practice, Training, 46*(3), 301–316.

Daniel, S. I. F. (2011). Adult attachment insecurity and narrative processes in psychotherapy: An exploratory study. *Clinical Psychology and Psychotherapy, 18,* 498–511.

Daniel, S. I. F. (2014). *Adult attachment patterns in a treatment context: Relationship and narrative.* London: Routledge.

Diamond, D., Stovall-McClough, C., Clarkin, J., & Levy, K. N. (2003). Patient–therapist attachment in the treatment of borderline personality disorder. *Bulletin of the Menninger Clinic, 67,* 227–259.

Diener, M. J., Hilsenroth, M. J., & Weinberger, J. (2009). A primer on meta-analysis of correlation coefficients: The relationship between patient-reported therapeutic alliance and adult attachment style as an illustration. *Psychotherapy Research, 19,* 519–526.

Diener, M. J., & Monroe, J. M. (2011). The relationship between adult attachment style and therapeutic alliance in individual psychotherapy: A meta-analytic review. *Psychotherapy, 48*(3), 237–248.

Dozier, M. (1990). Attachment organization and treatment use for adults with serious psychopathological disorders. *Development and Psychopathology, 2,* 47–60.

Dozier, M., Cue, K., & Barnett, L. (1994). Clinicians as caregivers: Role of attachment organization in treatment. *Journal of Consulting and Clinical Psychology, 62,* 793–800.

Eagle, M. N. (2013). *Attachment and psychoanalysis: Theory, research, and clinical implications.* New York: Guilford Press.

Eames, V., & Roth, A. (2000). Patient attachment orientation and the early working alliance: A study of patient and therapist reports of alliance quality and ruptures. *Psychotherapy Research, 10,* 421–434.

Fonagy, P. (2001). *Attachment theory and psychoanalysis.* New York: Other Press.

Fonagy, P., Leigh, T., Steele, M., Steele, H., Kennedy, R., Mattoon, G., et al. (1996). The relation of attachment status, psychiatric classification and response to psychotherapy. *Journal of Consulting and Clinical Psychology, 64,* 22–31.

Fonagy, P., Steele, M., Steele, H., Leigh, T., Kennedy, R., Mattoon, G., et al. (1995).Attachment, the reflective self, and borderline states: The predictive specificity of the Adult Attachment Interview and pathological emotional development. In S. Goldberg, R. Muir, & J. Kerr (Eds.), *Attachment theory: Social, developmental, and clinical perspectives* (pp. 233–279). Hillsdale, NJ: Analytic Press.

Fonagy, P., & Target, M. (1996). Playing with reality: I. Theory of mind and the normal development of psychic reality. *International Journal of Psycho-Analysis, 77,* 217–233.

Fuertes, J. N., Mislowack, A., Brown, S., Gur-Arie, S., Wilkinson, S., & Gelso, C. J. (2007). Correlates of the real relationship in psychotherapy: A study of dyads. *Psychotherapy Research, 17*(4), 423–430.

George, C., Kaplan, N., & Main, M. (1996). *Adult Attachment Interview* (3rd ed.). Unpublished manuscript, University of California at Berkeley.

Grice, H. P. (1989). *Studies in the way of words.* Cambridge, MA: Harvard University Press.

Griffin, D. W., & Bartholomew, K. (1994) Models of the self and other: Fundamental dimensions underlying measures of adult attachment. *Journal of Personality and Social Psychology, 3,* 430–445.

Hesse, E. (1996). Discourse, memory, and the Adult Attachment Interview: A note with emphasis on the emerging cannot classify category. *Infant Mental Health Journal, 17,* 4–11.

Holmes, J. A. (1993). *John Bowlby and attachment theory.* London: Routledge.

Holmes, J. A. (1995). *Something there is that doesn't love a wall: John Bowlby, attachment theory, and psychoanalysis.* In S. Goldberg, R. Muir, & J. Kerr (Eds.), *Attachment theory: Social, developmental, and clinical perspectives* (pp. 19–43). Hillsdale, NJ: Analytic Press.

Holmes, J. A. (1997). *Attachment, intimacy, and autonomy: Using attachment theory in adult psychotherapy.* Northvale, NJ: Aronson.

Holmes, J. A. (1998). Defensive and creative uses of narrative in psychotherapy: An attachment perspective. In G. Roberts & J. Holmes (Eds.), *Narrative in psychotherapy and psychiatry* (pp. 49–68). Oxford, UK: Oxford University Press.

Holmes, J. A. (2001). *The search for the secure base: Attachment theory and psychotherapy.* London: Routledge.

Holmes, J. A. (2004). Disorganized attachment and borderline personality disorder: A clinical perspective. *Attachment and Human Development, 6(2),* 181–190.

Holmes, J. A. (2009). *Exploring in security: Toward an attachment-informed psychoanalytic psychotherapy.* London: Routledge.

Holmes, J. A. (2014). *Attachments: Psychiatry, psychotherapy, psychoanalysis.* London: Routledge.

Janzen, J., Fitzpatrick, M., & Drapeau, M. (2008). Processes involved in client-nominated relationship building incidents: Client attachment, attachment to therapist, and session impact. *Psychotherapy: Theory, Research, Practice, Training, 45,* 377–390.

Johnson, S. (2008). Couple and family therapy: An attachment perspective. In J. Cassidy & P. R. Shaver (Eds.), *Handbook of attachment: Theory, research, and clinical applications* (2nd ed., pp. 811–829). New York: Guilford Press.

Kanninen, K., Salo, J., & Punamaki, R. L. (2000). Attachment patterns and working alliance in trauma therapy for victims of political violence. *Psychotherapy Research, 10,* 435–449.

Karen, R. (1998). *Becoming attached: First relationships and how they impact our capacity to love.* New York: Oxford University Press.

Kobak, R. R., Cole, H. E., Ferenz-Gillies, R., & Fleming, W. S. (1993). Attachment and emotion regulation during mother–teen problem solving: A control theory analysis. *Child Development, 64,* 231–245.

Levy, K. N., Ellison, W. D., Scott, L. N., & Bernecker, S. L. (2011). Attachment style. *Journal of Clinical Psychology, 67(2),* 193–203.

Levy, K. N., Meehan, K., Kelly, K. M., Reynoso, J., Weber, M., Clarkin, J., et al. (2006). Changes in attachment patterns and reflective function in a randomized control trial of transference-focused psychotherapy for borderline personality disorder. *Journal of Consulting and Clinical Psychology, 74,* 1027–1040.

Linehan, M. M. (1993). *Cognitive-behavioral treatment of borderline personality disorder.* New York: Guilford Press.

Liotti, G. (2004). Trauma, dissociation, and disorganized attachment: Three strands of a single braid. *Psychotherapy: Theory, Research, Practice, Training, 41,* 472–486.

Lyons-Ruth, K. (1999). The two-person unconscious: Intersubjective dialogue, enactive relational representation and the emergence of new forms of relational organization. *Psychoanalytic Inquiry, 19,* 576–617.

Lyons-Ruth, K., Dutra, L., Schuder, M., & Bianchi, I. (2006). From infant attachment disorganization to adult dissociation: Relational adaptations of traumat-

ic experiences. In R. Chevetz (Ed.), Dissociative disorders. *Psychiatric Clinics of North America, 29,* 63–86.

Main, M., & Hesse, E. (1990). Parents' unresolved traumatic experiences are related to infant disorganized attachment status: Is frightened and/or frightening parental behavior the linking mechanism? In M. T. Greenberg, D. Cicchetti, & E. M. Cummings (Eds.), *Attachment in the preschool years: Theory, research, and intervention* (pp. 161–182). Chicago: University of Chicago Press.

Main, M., Kaplan, N., & Cassidy, J. (1985). Security in infancy, childhood, and adulthood: A move to the level of representation. In I. Bretherton & E. Waters (Eds.), Growing points of attachment theory and research. *Monographs of the Society for Research in Child Development, 50(1–2,* Serial No. 209), 66–107.

Main, M., & Solomon, J. (1990). Procedures for identifying infants as disorganized/disoriented during the Ainsworth Strange Situation. In M. T. Greenberg, D. Cicchetti, & E. M. Cummings (Eds.), *Attachment in the preschool years: Theory, research, and intervention* (pp. 95–124). Chicago: University of Chicago Press.

Mallinckrodt, B., Gantt, D. L., & Coble, H. M. (1995). Attachment patterns in the psychotherapy relationship: Development of the client attachment to therapist scale. *Journal of Counseling Psychology, 42,* 307–317.

Mallinckrodt, B., Porter, M. J., & Kivlighan, D. M., Jr. (2005). Client attachment to therapist, depth of in-session exploration, and object relations in brief psychotherapy. *Psychotherapy: Theory, Research, Practice, Training, 42,* 85–100.

Marmarosh, C. L., Gelso, C. J., Markin, R. D., Majors, R., Mallery, C., & Choi, J. (2009). The real relationship in psychotherapy: Relationships to adult attachments, working alliance, transference, and therapy outcome. *Journal of Counseling Psychology, 56,* 337–350.

McBride, C., Atkinson, L., Quilty, L. C., & Bagby, R. M. (2006). Attachment as moderator of treatment outcome in major depression: A randomized control trial of interpersonal psychotherapy vs. cognitive behaviour therapy. *Journal of Consulting and Clinical Psychology, 74,* 1041–1054.

Mikulincer, M., & Shaver, P. R. (2007). *Attachment in adulthood: Structure, dynamics, and change.* New York: Guilford Press.

Mikulincer, M., Shaver, P. R., & Berant, E. (2013). An attachment perspective on therapeutic processes and outcomes. *Journal of Personality, 81,*606–616.

Muller, R. T., & Rosenkranz, S. E. (2009). Attachment and treatment response among adults in inpatient treatment for posttraumatic stress disorder. *Psychotherapy: Theory, Research, Practice, Training, 46(1),* 82–96.

Obegi, J. H., & Berant, E. (Eds.). (2009). *Attachment theory and research in clinical work with adults.* New York: Guilford Press.

Oppenheim, D., & Goldsmith, D. F. (2007). *Attachment*

theory in clinical work with children: Bridging the gap between research and practice. New York: Guilford Press.

Petrowski, K., Nowacki, K., Pokorny, D., & Buchheim, A. (2011). Matching the patient to the therapist: The roles of the attachment status and the helping alliance. *Journal of Nervous and Mental Disease, 199,* 839–844.

Powell, B., Cooper, G., Hoffman, K., & Marvin, R. (2013). *The Circle of Security intervention: Enhancing attachment in early parent–child relationships.* New York: Guilford Press.

Roisman, G. I., Holland, A., Fortuna, K., Fraley, R. C., Clausell, E., & Clarke, A. (2007). The adult attachment interview and self-reports of attachment style: An empirical rapprochement. *Journal of Personality and Social Psychology, 92,* 678–697.

Romano, V., Fitzpatrick, M., & Janzen, J. (2008). The secure-base hypothesis: Global attachment, attachment to counsellor, and session exploration in psychotherapy. *Journal of Counselling Psychology, 55,* 495–504.

Romano, V., Janzen, J. I., & Fitzpatrick, M. R. (2009). Volunteer client attachment moderates the relationship between trainee therapist attachment and therapist interventions. *Psychotherapy Research, 19,* 666–676.

Rubino, G., Barker, C., Roth, T., & Fearon, P. (2000). Therapist empathy and depth of interpretation in response to potential alliance ruptures: The role of therapist and patient attachment styles. *Psychotherapy Research, 10,* 408–420.

Sable, P. (2000). *Attachment and adult psychotherapy.* New York: Aronson.

Safran, J. D., & Muran, J. C. (2003). *Negotiating the therapeutic alliance: A relational treatment guide.* New York: Guilford Press.

Saypol, E., & Farber, B. A. (2010). Attachment style and patient disclosure in psychotherapy. *Psychotherapy Research, 20*(4), 462–471.

Slade, A. (1999) Attachment theory and research: Implications for the theory and practice of individual psychotherapy with adults. In J. Cassidy & P. R. Shaver (Eds.), *Handbook of attachment: Theory, research, and clinical applications* (pp. 575–594). New York: Guilford Press.

Slade, A. (2000). The development and organization of attachment: Implications for psychoanalysis. *Journal of the American Psychoanalytic Association, 48,* 1147–1174.

Slade, A. (2004a). Two therapies: Attachment organization and the clinical process. In L. Atkinson & S. Goldberg (Eds.), *Attachment issues in psychopathology and intervention* (pp. 181–206). Hillsdale, NJ: Erlbaum.

Slade, A. (2004b). The move from categories to phenomena: Attachment processes and clinical evaluation. *Infant Mental Health Journal, 25,* 1–15.

Slade, A. (2007). Disorganized mother, disorganized child: The mentalization of affective dysregulation and therapeutic change. In D. Oppenheim & D. F. Goldsmith (Eds.), *Attachment theory in clinical work with children: Bridging the gap between research and practice* (pp. 226–250). New York: Guilford Press.

Slade, A. (2008). The implications of attachment theory and research for adult psychotherapy: Research and clinical perspectives. In J. Cassidy & P. R. Shaver (Eds.), *Handbook of attachment: Theory, research, and clinical applications* (2nd ed., pp. 762–782). New York: Guilford Press.

Slade, A. (2014). Imagining fear: Attachment, threat, and psychic experience. *Psychoanalytic Dialogues, 24,* 254–266.

Slade, A., & Aber, J. L. (1992). Attachments, drives and development: Conflicts and convergences in theory. In J. Barron, M. Eagle, & D. Wolitzky (Eds.) *Interface of psychoanalysis and psychology* (pp. 154–186). Washington, DC: American Psychiatric Association Press.

Slade, A., & Holmes, J. A. (2013). *Attachment theory.* London: Sage.

Sroufe, L. A. (1979). The coherence of individual development: Early care, attachment, and subsequent developmental issues. *American Psychologist, 34,* 834–841.

Sroufe, L. A., & Fleeson, J. (1986). Attachment and the construction of relationships. In W. W. Hartup & Z. Rubin (Eds.), *Relationships and development* (pp. 51–71). Hillsdale, NJ: Erlbaum.

Steele, H., & Steele, M. (Eds.). (2008). *Clinical applications of the Adult Attachment Interview.* New York: Guilford Press.

Steele, H., Steele, M., & Murphy, A. (2009). Use of the adult attachment interview to measure process and change in psychotherapy. *Psychotherapy Research, 19,* 633–643.

Stovall-McClough, C., & Cloitre, M. (2003). Reorganization of traumatic childhood memories following exposure therapy. *Annals of the New York Academy of Science, 1008,* 297–299.

Talia, A., Daniel, S. I. F., Miller-Bottome, M., Brambilla, A., Miccoli, D., Safran, J. D., et al. (2014). AAI predicts patients' in-session interpersonal behavior and discourse: A "move to the level of the relation" for attachment-informed psychotherapy research. *Attachment and Human Development, 16*(2), 192–209.

Talia, A., & Miller-Bottome, M. (2014). *Patient Attachment Coding System.* Unpublished manuscript, University of Copenhagen.

Talia, A., Miller-Bottome, M., & Daniel, S. I. F. (2015). Assessing attachment in psychotherapy: Validation of the Patient Attachment Coding System (PACS). *Clinical Psychology and Psychotherapy.* DOI: 10.1002/cpp.1990.

Travis, L. A., Bliwise, N. G., Binder, J. L., & Horne-Meyer, H. L. (2001). Changes in clients' attachment styles over the course of time-limited dynamic psychotherapy. *Psychotherapy: Theory, Research, Practice, and Training, 38,* 149–159.

Tyrrell, C. L., Dozier, M., Teague, G. B., & Fallot, R. D. (1999). Effective treatment relationships for persons with serious psychiatric disorders: The importance of attachment states of mind. *Journal of Consulting and Clinical Psychology, 67*, 725–733.

Van IJzendoorn, M. H., & Bakermans-Kranenburg, M. J. (2009). The first 10,000 Adult Attachment Interviews: Distributions of adult attachment representations in clinical and non-clinical groups. *Attachment and Human Development, 11*, 223–263.

Wallin, D. J. (2007). *Attachment and psychotherapy.* New York: Guilford Press.

Wallin, D. J. (2010). From the inside out: The therapist's attachment patterns as sources of insight and impasse. In M. Kerman (Ed.) *Clinical pearls of wisdom* (pp. 245–256). New York: Norton.

Waters, E., Hamilton, C. E., & Weinfield, N. S. (2000). The stability of attachment from infancy to adolescence and early adulthood: General introduction. *Child Development, 71*, 678–683.

Westen, D., Nakash, O., Thomas, C., & Bradley, R. (2007). Clinical assessment of attachment patterns and personality disorder in adolescents and adults. *Journal of Consulting and Clinical Psychology, 74*, 1065–1085.

Woodhouse, S. S., Schlosser, L. Z., Crook, R. E., Ligiero, D. P., & Gelso, C. J. (2003). Client attachment to therapist: Relations to transference and client recollections of parental caregiving. *Journal of Counseling Psychology, 50*, 395–408.

# Chapter 34

# Reconciling Psychoanalytic Ideas with Attachment Theory

Peter Fonagy
Patrick Luyten
Elizabeth Allison
Chloe Campbell

The relationship between attachment theory and psychoanalysis, historically, has not been an easy one (Eagle, 2013; Fonagy, 2001; Fonagy, Gergely, & Target, 2008). But in recent years, developments in both fields have led to a growing rapprochement (Eagle, 2013; Holmes, 2009). Changes in psychoanalytic thinking have made it more accommodating of attachment thinking; conversely, aspects of the development of attachment findings, applications, and theory have made it more pertinent to psychoanalysis.

In this chapter we examine the disagreements between psychoanalysis and attachment theory, and point to some of the two disciplines' common foundations. We then describe an approach to the role of attachment in human development that considers it in relation to the capacity to *mentalize*, that is, to understand ourselves and others in terms of intentional mental states, and places both attachment and mentalizing in the context of the development of *epistemic trust*—the capacity to trust others as a source of knowledge about the world. This approach builds on some of Bowlby's assumptions drawn from evolutionary biology, placing some of the better founded psychoanalytic criticisms of attachment theory in a different perspective. We suggest that this context allows the

ongoing significance of Bowlby and Ainsworth's thinking for the psychoanalytic project to be appreciated.

## I. Traditional Psychoanalytic Developmental Theory and Attachment Theory: More Different Than Alike?

In his biography of Bowlby, Holmes (1993) identified four points of disagreement with psychoanalysis: (1) the psychoanalytic emphasis on the patient's *internal phantasies* (unconscious imaginative activity) at the expense of environmental influences and the patient's real, lived experiences; (2) what Bowlby perceived as the spirit of *rigid dogmatism* within the psychoanalytic world, which was at odds with intellectual creativity and scientific inquiry; (3) psychoanalytic metapsychology, which Bowlby considered to be a speculative approach to understanding the human mind, which is not open to empirical verification; and (4) the lack of empirical observation to underpin psychoanalytic theories.

Through his focus on the measurable and on the child's environment, Bowlby demanded causal clarity and an epistemological refinement of psychoanalytic thinking. The adoption of an empirical approach to clarifying and examining the validity of psychoanalytic ideas is still controversial within the clinical psychoanalytic tradition (Aron, 2012; Hoffman, 2009; Stern, 2013), although certain strands within psychoanalysis have taken a more positive approach to empirical research (Luyten, Blatt, & Corveleyn, 2006; Luyten, Blatt, Van Houdenhove, & Corveleyn, 2006).

Bowlby's ethological approach raised considerable challenges for the psychoanalytic position. Attachment was depicted by Bowlby as a form of behavior that the infant adapts according to environmental stimuli. The reflexive, flatly uniform quality that derived from an evolutionary and ethological perspective on attachment seemed starkly opposed to the humanism of the psychoanalytic impulse to recognize and engage with the complexity of individual subjectivity (Chused, 2012; Quinodoz, 1996).

Attachment was also at odds with traditional drive-oriented psychoanalytic theory, which posited that the first few weeks and months of an infant's life are almost solely characterized by drive discharge. Hence, drives were seen as primary; *objects* (i.e., attachment figures) were seen as secondary (Greenberg & Mitchell, 1983). Objects entered the scene only because of the failure of pure primary process functioning, when hallucinatory wish-fulfilments (e.g., imagining the mother's breast) failed to yield real gratification, which secondarily generated social awareness and engagement (Freud, 1915/1957). This view could not be reconciled with Bowlby's insistence on the primacy of attachment relationships, their evolutionary functions and, by implication, the fact that infants were fundamentally and from the beginning of life positively oriented toward others.

Finally, attachment theory was accused of neglecting the developmental role of sexuality and aggression, which are seen as the central human urges in traditional psychoanalysis, responsible for continuous internal conflict and justifying defensive operations (Meissner, 2009). In contrast to the psychoanalytic understanding of human nature and relationships in terms of conflict and compromise (Geyskens, 2003), attachment theory appeared to reduce human relationships to a smooth, evolutionary, prewired unfolding process. Thus, particularly in Neo-Freudian and Lacanian circles, adopting attachment theory would mean a betrayal of fundamental hard-fought insights

into the nature of human development (Symons, 2008; Widlocher & Fairfield, 2004; Zamanian, 2011).

## 2. The Response of Major Psychoanalytic Thinkers

Predictably, given the major differences in assumptions about the fundamentals of development, attachment theory met with fierce resistance from the psychoanalytic community.

Bowlby's focus on the impact of the lived reality of the child's early emotional experiences, normally in relation to the mother, has distinct parallels with Winnicott's (1965) recognition of the significance of the early caring environment. However, Winnicott, one of the best-known psychoanalytic developmentalists, was unhappy with Bowlby's use of ethology and the statistical approach at the expense of the clinical case study, and was concerned about the loss of the complexity of individual subjectivity (Abram, 2008). Thus, although in retrospect we might locate Bowlby's work within the object relations school of psychoanalytic thinking, with both Bowlby and Winnicott emphasizing the significance of the relationship between infant and caregiver, this was not straightforwardly perceived as a shared intellectual project (Keller, 2011).

Anna Freud, one of the great psychoanalysts of Bowlby's era, was also one of the first psychoanalysts to adopt a coherent developmental perspective on psychopathology. She argued that psychological disorder is most effectively studied in its developmental evolution, asserting that it is the profile or pattern among different *developmental lines* that best captures the nature of the risk faced by the individual child. This view foreshadowed and laid part of the foundation of contemporary developmental psychopathology (Cicchetti, 2013). Anna Freud's developmental lines included, for instance, the line from dependency to self-reliance to adult object relations, so central in attachment theory. But her theory was broader and also included the line from irresponsibility to responsibility in body management, the line from egocentrism to social partnership, and so forth. Unevenness of development was considered a risk factor, and treatment in certain cases adopted the modified aim of restoring the child to the path of normal development (developmental help) (Midgley, 2012).

Despite their shared emphasis on development, Anna Freud was deeply unsympathetic to attachment theory. And, despite her own observations to the contrary, in her theoretical writings Anna Freud based the child's early relationship with the mother on sexual instinctual needs, in line with traditional drive theory. Although she was well aware of unevenness in ego development, she rarely saw this as caused by relationship disturbance. While her clinical focus and interventions were to a marked extent focused on optimizing the social context of the child, her theoretical writings appeared to be constrained by an adherence to classical psychoanalytical ideas (Young-Bruehl, 2011).

Melanie Klein (1936/1964) was the third great thinker who shaped the psychoanalytic milieu within and against which Bowlby worked. Klein's disagreements with Anna Freud have been well documented (Gabbard & Scarfone, 2002); their shared suspicion of attachment theory was perhaps one of the few things that united them. Klein was one of the founders of the object relations school, which, with its conception that subjective experience shapes one's behavior and relationships, considerably narrowed the gap between attachment theory and psychoanalysis (Mikulincer & Shaver, 2007). The relationship between Klein's and Bowlby's thinking was both intimate and highly adversarial, and the points of contact are worth examining because of the great influence of Kleinian thinking on contemporary psychoanalysis (e.g., Brown, 2011).

Klein saw mental structures as arising out of a variety of internal objects (phantasies about people in the infant's life), which change in character as the child develops from infancy. The infant's phantasies are modified by actual experiences of interaction with the environment. Bowlby was deeply influenced by Kleinian thought, and traces of his training and experience in the British Psychoanalytic Society, which was predominantly Kleinian, can be readily identified in his writings. For example, his focus on the first year of life as a crucial determinant of later developmental outcomes is highly compatible with the Kleinian approach. Perhaps most important is the intimate connection that both bodies of work envision between emotional experiences and the cognitive apparatus underpinning thought. This is expressed most clearly in the last volume of Bowlby's trilogy (1980) and in Bion's (1997) elaboration of Klein's ideas. Even in opposition, many of Bowlby's ideas were reactions against the Kleinian influence on him.

One of Bowlby's central objections to Kleinian psychoanalytic theory was its neglect of actual experience and the assumption that a child's anxieties arise predominantly from constitutional tendencies, such as innate (i.e., drive-related) aggression (Klein, 1936/1964). However, recent post-Kleinian psychoanalysts have been quite successful at integrating environmental accounts with Klein's ideas (e.g., Ferro, 2006). The child's capacity to cope with the pain and anxiety of the depressive position, seeing him- or herself as destructive and envious, is now generally attributed in more contemporary Kleinian views to external as well as constitutional factors (Vermote, 2011).

## 3. Areas of Integration between Psychoanalysis and Attachment Theory

Several trends within psychoanalysis have paved the way for a rapprochement with attachment theory. For a start, psychoanalysis has become more pluralistic and accepting of differences (Holmes, 2009). The emergence of a relational and relationship-focused emphasis in modern psychoanalysis has also led to increasing interest in the formative nature of the child's social environment, and object relations theory has played a pivotal role in this context (Aron & Leichich, 2011; Brown, 2010; Epstein, 2010). In this section we consider more closely some of the most important areas of integration between psychoanalysis and attachment theory.

### a. The Internal Working Model

Bowlby's attachment theory, like classical psychoanalysis, has a biological focus (see especially Bowlby, 1969). Bowlby's critical contribution was his unwavering focus on the infant's need for an unbroken (secure) early attachment to the mother. He emphasized the survival value of attachment in enhancing safety through proximity to the caregiver in addition to feeding, learning about the environment and social interaction, and protection from predators.

Perhaps not surprisingly, psychoanalysts were horrified by this apparently simplistic approach, which bore the hallmarks of the worst excesses of behaviorist reductionism. However, in the second volume of *Attachment and Loss*, Bowlby established the set-goal of the attachment system as maintaining *the caregiver's accessibility and responsiveness*, which he covered with a single term: *availability* (Bowlby, 1973, p. 202). This availability translates into the confident expectation, gained from "tolerably accurately" (p. 202) represented experience, over a significant time period, that the attachment figure will be available. The attachment behavioral system thus came to be underpinned by a set of representational models or, following the pioneering psychologist Craik (1943), internal working models (IWMs; see Bretherton & Munholland, Chapter 4, this volume).

The positing of a representational system underpinning attachment permitted a far more sophisticated consideration of individual differences (Bowlby, 1973, 1980). Given the power of the biological forces driving the human attachment system, Bowlby assumed that almost all human beings will become attached. The concept of the disorganization of the attachment system was not yet available (Main & Solomon, 1986); for Bowlby, attachment could be only secure or insecure. Secure attachment implied a representational system in which the attachment figure was seen as accessible and responsive when needed. Anxious attachment implied a somewhat dysfunctional system in which the caregiver's responsiveness was not assumed and the child adopted strategies for circumventing his or her perceived unresponsiveness (Ainsworth, Blehar, Waters, & Wall, 1978).

Thus, the central feature of the IWM concerned the infant's encoding of interactions in terms of what they implied about the expected availability of the attachment figure. Bowlby also envisioned a complementary working model of the self. The key feature of this was how acceptable or unacceptable the child felt in the eyes of the attachment figure. A child whose IWM of the caregiver focused on rejection was expected to evolve a complementary working model of the self as unlovable, unworthy, and flawed. Although not explicitly stated by Bowlby, these models of the attachment figure and the self were somewhat transactional, interactive models representing self–other relationships. The explanatory power of Bowlby's model rested in his proposal that these encoded expectations were capable of providing prototypes for all later close relationships.

Bowlby's original concept has been elaborated by some of the greatest minds in the attachment field (see Bretherton & Munholland, 2008). Through the working model, Bowlby created a wider theory about the construction of the psyche, which is sometimes underrepresented in the more schematic portrayals of attachment theory. In *Loss*, for instance, Bowlby (1980) described how an individual defensively excludes stimuli that are incompatible with the IWM, leading to an inability to accommodate external reality, often in relation to other people's emotional states or attachment needs. This led to a new take by Bowlby on repression and dissociative phenomena (the kind of territory more normally associated with psychoanalytic thinking), which are often the result of deactivation of the attachment system (Dykas & Cassidy, 2011)—most notably in a disorganized individual dealing with grief or bereavement (Bretherton & Munholland, 1999).

The concept of the IWM was key to the rapprochement with psychoanalytic object relations theory and psychoanalysis more generally (e.g., Blatt, Auerbach, & Levy, 1997; Wachtel, 2009, 2010). This so-called "move to the level of representation" elaborated by Main, Kaplan, and Cassidy (1985) has had enormous influence, particularly via the Adult Attachment Interview (AAI). Main and colleagues' work (Main, Hesse, & Hesse, 2011; Main et al., 1985) reconceptualized individual differences in attachment organization as individual differences in the mental representation of the self in relation to attachment; it enabled the examination of attachment in older children and adults.

## b. Object Relations

The notion of IWMs is consistent with psychoanalytic object relations theory's emphasis on the central role of self and object representations in development (Blatt et al., 1997; Greenberg & Mitchell, 1983; Kernberg & Caligor, 2005). In both perspectives, representations of self and others are seen as the fundamental building blocks of normal and disrupted development, with representations of self and others becoming increasingly integrated, differentiated, and positive in normal development. Fairbairn's (1952, 1963) simple insight that people are fundamentally driven by relationships and their need for them, and that the pursuit of relationships is not a secondary by-product of the primary drives for gratification described by Freud, is in essence highly congruent with Bowlby's insight in relation to the biological priority of the "secure base." For both attachment theory and object relations theory, it is axiomatic that the infant's psyche, his or her relationship representational structure, is shaped by early relationship experiences. As the object relations model replaced ego psychology as a dominant international psychoanalytic paradigm, attachment theory's emphasis on the innate need for a relationship came to be embraced by a majority within the field.

Psychopathology, from these perspectives, is seen as reflecting impairments in the structure and content of mental representations of self and others (e.g., Blatt, 1974; Westen, 1991). This led to a burgeoning research literature (Huprich & Greenberg, 2003; Mikulincer & Shaver, 2007) that uses concepts denoting very similar constructs, but often with somewhat different names, ranging from object representations (Brinich, 1980) to cognitive–affective schemas of self and others (self–object–affect triads) (Kernberg, 2014), role responsiveness (Sandler & Sandler, 1998), representations of interactions that have been generalized (Stern, 1985), and IWMs (Blatt et al., 1997). The strong psychometric contributions of attachment research were recognized and further developed by psychoanalytic researchers. In particular, the links between the adult attachment construct and object relations patterns of self–other representation have been carefully studied (Blatt et al., 1997; Loeffler-Stastka & Blueml, 2010; Luyten & Blatt, 2013; Priel & Besser, 2001).

Attachment theory's emphasis on an autonomous need for a relationship has not gone completely unchallenged within psychoanalysis (e.g., Geyskens, 2003; Green, 2005; Widlocher & Fairfield, 2004). However, the embarrassment caused by the apparently endemic neglect of childhood maltreatment (Masson, 1984; Simon, 1992) has been followed by an embrace of the trauma concept and the role of early relationships more broadly (e.g., Levine, 2014; Person & Klar, 1994). More generally, the emergence and dominance of object relations theory in the 1980s and 1990s contributed to increasing psychoanalytic recognition of the formative nature of the child's external, social environment. Engaging with the psychological consequences of childrearing patterns characteristic of families with serious social disadvantages has forced psychoanalysts to rethink the concept of trauma (e.g., Bohleber, 2007), bringing their conceptualization closer to attachment formulations (Allen, Fonagy, & Bateman, 2008).

Yet, as noted, not everyone agrees, and it is striking that with the growing popularity of attachment and object relations theory, interest in sexuality in psychoanalysis has declined significantly (Fonagy, 2008). This has happened despite the fact that sexuality, along with aggression, remains one of the most problematic human experiences, as evidenced by the role of sexuality and aggression in a variety of psychological problems and disorders (Fonagy & Luyten, 2016; Zamanian, 2011). With some exceptions (e.g., Kernberg, 2012), the integration of attachment theory with a comprehensive theory of human sexuality and aggression remains to be developed (see Birnbaum, Chapter 22, this volume).

### c. Relational and Relationship-Focused Psychoanalysis

The 1980s saw the beginning of an integration of relational approaches augmented and modified by the intersubjectivist vision of philosophically oriented psychoanalysts such as Stolorow (1997) and infant researchers such as Emde (Emde, Kubicek, & Oppenheim, 1997). This interpersonal relationship-focused perspective is perhaps best exemplified by the so-called "relational school," partly rooted in the work of Sullivan (1953; Benjamin, 1998; Bromberg, 1998; Mitchell & Aron, 1999). The theory is more of an orientation than a coherent body of ideas, and many theoreticians and clinicians who emphasize relational issues do not necessarily identify themselves as "relational psychoanalysts." Yet relational psychoanalysis combines the concerns of modern psychoanalysis with the traditional concerns of attachment theory. It emerged as psychoanalysis moved toward the developmental framework established within attachment theory and other dynamic psychological approaches rooted in observing early development. Psychodynamic therapists who wish to embrace the relational approach often move toward an attachment model, albeit unwittingly (Cortina, 2001).

The relational model assumes that subjectivity is interpersonal: that is, the intersubjective replaces the intrapsychic (Mitchell, 1988). This renders the individual human mind a contradiction in terms, since subjectivity is invariably rooted in an intersubjective matrix of relational bonds within which personal meanings are embedded (Mitchell, 2000) rather than in biological drives. Unlike most other psychoanalytic theories, the relational model lacks a specific explanation of how relationality and intersubjectivity develop. For this reason, attachment theory and conclusions drawn from the observation of attachment relationships may be helpful.

Bowlby's focus on child–caregiver interaction as the primary driver of social development makes him a quintessential relational theorist. Among others he influenced, Bowlby clearly influenced Trevarthen (e.g., Trevarthen & Aitken, 2001), who argues that infants are innately predisposed to social relationships and that primary intersubjectivity characterizes the mental experience of infants during infant–caregiver interactions (Trevarthen, 1993; Trevarthen, Aitken, Vandekerckhove, Delafield-Butt, & Nagy, 2006). In addition to a predisposition to relate, attachment theory posits and describes other adaptations—including defensive processes—that develop in the context of specifically elaborated relational processes, which themselves occur at the interface between infant distress and caregiver response. That is, attachment theory, like relational theory, is a two-person theory of conflict and defense, which sees defenses as arising from the conflict between the infant's needs and the caregiver's responses (Lyons-Ruth, 1999, 2003).

The hypothesis of procedural representations of implicit relational knowing raises the theory of internal object relations to a more general "systems" conception. The implicit relational knowing of two partners or of a patient and an analyst will be altered by moments of meeting—by the enactment of a new potential that will come to be represented as a future possibility. The best-documented forms of procedural implicit relational knowing are displayed during the first 2 years of life, when interactions are registered in representations of interpersonal events in a nonsymbolic form. The unique configuration of adaptive strategies that emerges from the attachment relationship constitutes the initial organization of the child's domain of implicit relational knowing (IWMs, protonarrative envelopes, themes of organization, relational scripts).

In general, both attachment theorists and interpersonalists are reluctant to privilege fantasy over actuality. Interpersonal and intrapsychic factors are seen as equally important. Sullivan's break from traditional psychoanalysis mirrors Bowlby's conflict with the British psychoanalytic community: Bowlby shared an emphasis on dyadic relationships with interpersonalists, but he also shared with Sullivan (1964) an interest in observable behavior. Neither Bowlby nor Sullivan could specifically be labeled "behaviorist," but they shared a systematic interest in what happens between people. For Sullivan, this entailed a detailed inquiry into who said what to whom, whereas Bowlby's focus was on what happened in the past to explain the present.

Current relational thinking often uses psychopathological accounts of trauma to highlight the relational aspects of actual experience (e.g., Davies, 1996). "What really happened" is combined with attention to the patient's subjective experience, not in order to separate veridical events from distortions associated with unconscious fantasy, but rather to elaborate the overwhelming nature of the experience itself—especially because the context of trauma is assumed to preclude awareness of its meanings (Pizer, 2003). It is the inherent paradox of attachment trauma that a stance of "not knowing what one knows" (Bowlby, 1988, p. 99) may be adopted to keep the crucial relationship intact. Relational psychoanalytic (Stern, 1997) and attachment-inspired (Hesse & Main, 2006) clinical descriptions provide similar formulations of dissociation linked with traumatic experience.

### d. The Self Psychology Tradition

The emergence of self psychology from the work of Heinz Kohut (1971) has, like attachment theory, contributed to focusing psychoanalytic interest on the earliest phases of development. Self psychology grew out of the increasing dominance of object relations theory, but because its origins were in North America, it was less affected by the Kleinian focus on aggression and destructiveness. The work of Kohut revolutionized North American psychoanalysis in the last decades of the 20th century. Kohut broke the iron grip of ego psychology by forcing psychoanalysts to think in less mechanistic terms—in terms of selfhood rather than psychological function and *selfobjects* rather than the drive gratification provided by the object.

Self psychology holds empathy to be central in both development and therapy (Ornstein, 2008); without it we would not have access to the world of the other. *Empathy* is a process that emerges between two or more people when their interaction creates the possibility of a world of meanings based on mutual understanding, and empathy generates a sense of connection through dialogue (Orange, 2009). The seminal contribution of Kohut (1971, 1977; Kohut & Wolf, 1978), at least in the context of this chapter, lies in his innovative suggestion that the development of *narcissism* (originally self-love or self-esteem) has its own developmental path, and that caregiving individuals (objects) serve special functions along this line of development, as selfobjects that evoke the experience of selfhood. Empathic responses from the selfobject facilitate the unfolding of infantile grandiosity and encourage feelings of omnipotence, which enable the building of an idealized image of the parent, with whom the child wishes to merge. This "transmuting internalization of the mirroring function" gradually leads to a consolidation of a nuclear self (Kohut & Wolf, 1978, pp. 414–416). The idealization of the selfobject leads to the development of ideals. At the opposite pole of this "bipolar self" is a representation of natural talents gained through the mirroring function. Selfobjects continue to be needed throughout life, to some degree, to sustain self-cohesion (Kohut, 1984). Kohut's self psychology relies on the notion of attachment as a central motivation for the establishment and maintenance of self-cohesiveness (Shane, Shane, & Gales, 1997). Like Bowlby, Kohut replaced the dual drives of classical analysis with a relational construct. Like Winnicott, he linked self-development with mirroring or maternal sensitivity. And like attachment theorists, he reversed the relationship of drives and self-structure, regarding the self as superordinate and drive conflicts as indications of "an enfeebled self" (Kohut, 1977).

Unlike attachment theorists, however, self psychologists view the cohesion of the self as the primary motivation guiding human behavior rather than as a biologically predefined relationship pattern. Kohut separated anxiety about object loss from anxiety about disintegration of the self. For self psychology, the root of anxiety is the self's experience of a defect, a lack of cohesiveness and continuity (Cohler & Weiner, 2011). This subtle but important shift of emphasis relegates the attachment figure to second place.

It is also difficult to identify within attachment theory a concept analogous to grandiosity or omnipotence as naturally occurring in infant development. The notion of infantile omnipotence is certainly challenged by findings indicating that on the majority of occasions the infant is not able to elicit synchronous (mirroring) behavior from the mother (Tronick, 2007). Although infants undoubtedly enjoy experiences of mastery (Rochat, 2009), there is no evidence that this leads to a sense of omnipotence. It seems far more likely that we are once more encountering the problematic tendency of psychoanalytic thinkers to describe infant behavior in terms of adultomorphic constructs. This is the very problem Bowlby's entire theoretical effort aimed to address.

## e. Developmental Research and Attachment

The work of Daniel Stern (1985) bridged the gulf between infant researchers and psychoanalysts in a highly successful and productive way. His primary concern was with the development of self-structure. He distinguished four stages of early formation of the self: (1) the sense of emergent self (0–2 months) involves the process of the self's coming into being and forming initial connections; (2) the sense of core self and the domain of core relatedness (2–6 months) are based on the single organizing subjective perspective and a coherent physical self; (3) the sense of subjective self and the domain of intersubjective relatedness (7–15 months) emerge with the discovery of subjective mental states beyond physical events; and (4) the sense of verbal self forms after 15 months.

Stern (1985, 1994) described three types of relationships of self-with-other: (1) self–other complementing, (2) state sharing, and (3) state transforming. Although these relationships can be characterized by the degree of attachment or separateness they imply, Stern was interested in their contribution to structuring the self through the schematization of experience. Stern's most important point of contact with attachment theory is probably in the elaboration of the IWM. His starting point is the "emerging moment," which is the subjective integration of all aspects of lived experience. The "moment" takes its input from emotions, behaviors, sensations, and all other aspects of the internal and external world from schematic representations of various types (e.g., event representations, semantic representations or conceptual schemas, perceptual schemas, and sensorimotor representations). He adds two further modes of representations: "feeling shapes" and "protonarrative envelopes." These schemas form a network, which he terms "the schema of a-way-of-being-with." The schema of a-way-of-being-with is conceptualized by Stern (1998) from the assumed subjective perspective of the infant in interaction with the caregiver.

The infant organizes his or her experience around a motive and a goal. The goals are not only biological, but include object relatedness (Fairbairn), affect states (Kernberg), states of self-esteem (Kohut), and safety (Sandler), as well as the gratification of physical needs, whether hunger, thirst, sexuality, or aggression. Stern's theory elaborates that of Winnicott (1971): attunement satisfies the infant's need for omnipotence, while the caregiver's capacity to accept protest without retaliation or anxiety allows the child to have confidence in the caregiver as resilient to the infant's attacks.

Stern's framework has much to offer attachment theory, particularly in terms of the careful integration of infant observation studies with concepts concerning interpersonal development. Nevertheless, it lacks two critical dimensions essential to attachment theory. First, it lacks a genuine longitudinal observational perspective. A great strength of attachment theory is its almost unique empirical handle on longitudinal and cross-generational predictions. Although Stern's observations are well operationalized in terms of mother–infant interaction and infant development, they lack operationalization in the context of adult behavior; therefore, longitudinal studies based on Stern's framework have rarely been attempted. Second, while Stern (1998) probably appropriately claims that schemas of ways-of-being-with are the building blocks of IWMs, close links between the two systems have not yet been demonstrated. However, important pioneering work by Beatrice Beebe and her group (Beebe, Lachmann, & Jaffe, 1997) has drawn on this ambition. In the tradition of pioneers such as Stern and Emde (e.g., Emde & Spicer, 2000), this work has sought to demonstrate the significance of the growth of scientific understanding of early development for clinical and theoretical psychoanalysis. It has led to the gradual modification of the image of the "psychoanalytic infant" from a hypothetical creature based on speculative reconstruction from adult narratives, to a picture that is constrained and moderated by actual systematic observations of children.

The Beebe and Lachmann (2014) microanalytic studies of mother–infant interactions, from as young as 4 months of age, provide a robust way to apply attachment thinking to psychodynamic psychotherapy. Video microanalysis allows for the capture of rapid and often very subtle communicative events that can help us to tease out the origins of communication disturbances in infancy. The detailed empiricism of Beebe's observations is reminiscent of the complex and meticulous observational work originally undertaken by Mary Ainsworth (Beebe & Lachmann, 2014).

Tronick (2003) has also deepened our understanding of the uniqueness of attachment relationships and proposed an important model for how these relationships increasingly differentiate themselves. This work has taken us beyond attachment theory's early, reductive views on proximity, and

has helped us to conceptualize the nuances of the mother–infant relationship and the mechanisms through which attachment is achieved and maintained. In particular, by pointing to the uniqueness of each attachment bond, Tronick's (2008) contribution has challenged the view that the child's relationship with the mother is paradigmatic for later relationships. At the same time, however, the model radically revised our understanding of how relationships do influence one another (Tronick, 2005, 2007).

Tronick's (1989, 2007) mutual regulation model (MRM) of infant–adult interaction focuses on the subtle, nonverbal, microregulatory and socioemotional processes that unfold in mother–infant interactions. The MRM postulates that infants have "self-organizing neurobehavioral capacities" and "biopsychological processes" that allow them to "organize behavioral states" and make "sense of themselves and their place in the world" (Tronick, 2007, pp. 8–9). At the same time, Tronick pointed to the limits of these capacities and stated that they need to be supplemented by a "larger dyadic regulatory system" in which the infant participates with the caregiver (Tronick, 2007, p. 9). In this way Tronick brings together the notion of sensitivity with the overriding construct of meaning making.

Successful mutual regulation is achieved when an infant and caregiver together generate, communicate, and integrate meaningful elements of consciousness. This creates a synchrony in implicit relational knowing, allowing each to anticipate and "know" the moves of the other. This "knowing" is initially of a pattern of physiological responses or activations rather than of intentional states, although clearly it can be the platform for knowing of intention given developmental time. The parent–infant collaboration results in a singular, organized dyadic state that is believed to be more than the sum of its parts. This leads to what Tronick terms a state of "co-creativity" in which infant and caregiver shape their relationship through a process of mutual regulation (Tronick, 2003, p. 476).

The focus of both Beebe and colleagues' (1997) interactive regulation model and Tronick's (1989, 2007) MRM includes the "messiness" of interpersonal communications, as well as the greater cohesion allowed through reparation and co-creativity. These models allow us to operationalize such psychoanalytic concepts as the *holding environment* (Winnicott, 1965) and *background of safety* (Sandler, 1960), and take us toward a genuinely relational model of change in psychoanalytic treatment. Furthermore, studies of the contingency between the mother's and infant's vocalizations can help us to predict secure attachment relationships (Jaffe, Beebe, Feldstein, Crown, & Jasnow, 2001).

Work by Mayes (e.g., Mayes & Leckman, 2007) has taken some of the ideas first plotted in psychoanalytic terms and powerfully worked them through an empirical, child-development perspective. Mayes has been particularly notable in her use of Winnicott's (1958) clinical and theoretical insights. His idea of maternal primary preoccupation and his thoughts on maternal care and its role in child development have, for example, been explored by Mayes in her study of the course of and fluctuations in early primary preoccupation (Leckman & Mayes, 1999). The study found that parents' perceptions of the maternal care they received during childhood predicted postpartum fluctuations in mood. Mayes and colleagues suggest that parents whose representations of early parenting are colored by perceptions and experiences of unavailable or inadequate care are less able to sustain the intense, adaptive preoccupied focus on their new infant without also experiencing dysphoria. In this model, early parenting experiences may determine the extent to which new parents might be vulnerable in the peripartum period (Mayes & Leckman, 2007; for clinical applications, see Berlin, Zeanah, & Lieberman, Chapter 32, this volume).

## 4. Mentalizing Theory and Attachment

The mentalizing model is a recent psychoanalytic extension of attachment theory and research that claims a synergistic relationship between attachment processes and the growth of a child's capacity to understand interpersonal behavior in terms of mental states (Fonagy, Gergely, Jurist, & Target, 2002). This capacity is referred to as *mentalizing* or *reflective functioning*. Recent elaborations of this theory have pointed to the key role of attachment relationships in the development of the capacity for epistemic trust (which we discuss later). Both evolutionary considerations and experimental developmental research suggest that epistemic trust plays a key role in the intergenerational transmission of knowledge and in learning that is specific to human beings (Fonagy, Luyten, & Allison,

2015). These new theoretical and empirical developments, which have emerged out of a new dialogue among attachment theory, the mentalizing approach, and evolutionary theory, also shed new light on the nature and emergence of personality disorders (PDs), as outlined below, and attest to the ongoing productivity of the interface between psychoanalytic ideas and attachment theory.

Mentalizing is often simplistically understood, but research findings clearly demonstrate that it involves a spectrum of capacities. It is underpinned by four dimensions involving relatively distinct neural circuits: (1) automatic versus controlled, (2) based on external features (e.g., facial expression, posture) versus internal indicators, (3) regarding the self and others, and (4) cognitive versus affective (Bateman & Fonagy, 2012). Effective mentalizing requires the individual to maintain a balance across these four dimensions.

Over the past 25 years, a systematic program of research has demonstrated that the capacity to mentalize emerges in the context of early attachment relationships and is a key determinant of self-organization and affect regulation. Specifically, studies examining different ways in which caregiver mentalizing is operationalized—including prenatal reflective function (Fonagy, Steele, Steele, Moran, & Higgitt, 1991), child-specific reflective function (Slade, Grienenberger, Bernbach, Levy, & Locker, 2005), mind-related comments (Meins, Fernyhough, Fradley, & Tuckey, 2001; Meins et al., 2002), and a diverse range of other measures (Aber, Slade, Berger, Bresgi, & Kaplan, 1985; Koren-Karie, Oppenheim, Dolev, Sher, & Etzion-Carasso, 2002; Oppenheim, Koren-Karie, & Sagi, 2001; Solomon & George, 1999)—indicate that each of these aspects of mentalizing capacity predicts attachment security in the child. Furthermore, the caregiver's capacity to mentalize can offer protection from risk factors in the caregiver that are associated with generating attachment insecurity, such as maternal trauma and disruptive maternal behaviors. We also now know that the benefits of caregiver mentalizing extend beyond attachment outcomes: it is associated with children's better performance in social cognition tasks (Laranjo, Bernier, Meins, & Carlson, 2010; Meins et al., 2002), as well as general social-cognitive development (Meins et al., 2003). By contrast, social environments characterized by adversity in child development (e.g., neglect, abuse) impair the development of cognition (Ayoub et al., 2009; Fernald, Weber, Galasso, & Ratsifandrihamanana, 2011; Goodman, Quas,

& Ogle, 2010; Rieder & Cicchetti, 1989). The mentalizing approach proposes that problems in affect regulation, attentional control, and self-control stemming from dysfunctional attachment relationships (Agrawal, Gunderson, Holmes, & Lyons-Ruth, 2004; Lyons-Ruth, Yellin, Melnick, & Atwood, 2005; Sroufe, Egeland, Carlson, & Collins, 2005), as manifested perhaps most clearly in severe personality problems such as borderline personality disorder (BPD), are mediated through a failure to develop a robust mentalizing capacity (Bateman & Fonagy, 2010).

While the mentalization-focused model of development places strong emphasis on the relationship between attachment and mentalizing, this relationship is situated within a broader developmental approach that also emphasizes the role of gene–environment interplay (for a fuller discussion of this point, see Fonagy & Luyten, 2016). Although the capacity to mentalize is not a constitutional given, it does seem to be a capacity that is partly prewired (Kovacs, Teglas, & Endress, 2010). Thus, this is not a naive environmentalist model: the interaction between genetic predisposition and early and later influences on the development of the capacity to mentalize is thought to be crucially important.

In this section we outline the mentalizing model and show how certain observed associations between attachment and psychopathology can be understood in terms of the vicissitudes of the development of the capacity to mentalize, taking BPD as a paradigmatic example.

### a. Disordered Attachment in BPD

Studies using both self-report and interview-based measures of attachment have shown that BPD is associated with increased levels of attachment insecurity (Agrawal et al., 2004). Cross-sectional investigations show that individuals with borderline features have preoccupied, disorganized, and unresolved patterns of attachment (Levy, Beeney, & Temes, 2011). A cross-sectional study examining the attachment styles of patients with mood disorder and those with BPD found that although both groups showed greater preoccupation and fearfulness than controls, only patients with BPD simultaneously showed preoccupation *and* fearfulness. This study therefore confirms the suggestion from a number of attachment theorists that the key marker of BPD may be a lack of any functional regulation strategy to reduce attachment distress (Fonagy & Bateman, 2008; Main, 2000).

To understand these associations, we must consider the nature of early attachments. Our model hypothesizes that suboptimal early attachment experiences are robust predictors of BPD in later life, not so much because of the attachment experiences themselves, but because it is in the context of attachment relationships that the infant learns to understand his or her own emotional states, acquires the capacity for affect regulation, and discovers him- or herself as a psychological entity through marked mirroring interactions (Fonagy et al., 2002; Fonagy, Gergely, & Target, 2007). In line with this hypothesis, Carlson, Egeland, and Sroufe (2009) reported significant, although weak, correlations between borderline symptoms at 28 years of age and indicators of a suboptimal early environment (maltreatment, maternal hostility, attachment disorganization, and family stress in the first 3–4 years of life). These culminated in a range of social-cognitive anomalies—attentional disturbance, emotional instability, and relational disturbance—that were evident by 12 years of age. A path-analytic approach offered strong evidence that disturbances in self-representation in early adolescence mediated the link between disorganization of early attachment relationships and PD.

### b. BPD and Childhood Adversity

The role of developmental trauma in BPD in general has been a significant focus of research. Among individuals with PDs, rates of childhood trauma are very high (Ball & Links, 2009). Compared with nonclinical adults, patients with PDs are four times as likely to have suffered early trauma (Johnson, Cohen, Brown, Smailes, & Bernstein, 1999), and BPD is more consistently associated with childhood maltreatment than any other PD diagnosis (e.g., Baird, Veague, & Rabbitt, 2005; Battle et al., 2004; Buchheim et al., 2008).

A particularly impressive study following up several hundred abused and neglected children and matched controls into adulthood reported a 2.5-fold increase in the prevalence of BPD associated with abuse and neglect (Widom, Czaja, & Paris, 2009). In this prospective investigation of children who were identified as maltreated by child protection services, early neglect appeared to be the most potent risk factor for both genders, whereas physical abuse represented a risk only for males. A systematic review of the literature on BPD and trauma by Crombie (2013) found that generally high-quality studies across a range of designs and measurement methodologies converge in showing, both prospectively and retrospectively, that emotional neglect and abuse predict BPD symptoms and diagnosis in line with or in excess of the impact that can be observed to be associated with physical and sexual abuse. This observation supports our expectation that even in the absence of dramatic maltreatment, the individual's competence to represent mental states may be undermined by the absence of contingent responses to their subjective experience, resulting in increased vulnerability for BPD. Subsequent brutality in an attachment context may then further disrupt mentalizing as part of an adaptive adjustment to adversity (Fonagy, Steele, Steele, Higgitt, & Target, 1994; Stein, Fonagy, Ferguson, & Wisman, 2000). Hence, early emotional neglect in particular, rather than physical or sexual abuse as such, may predispose individuals to the development of BPD by limiting their opportunity to acquire the capacity to mentalize and leaving them vulnerable to disruptions in mentalizing under the influence of later stress.

### c. Disruptions of the Caregiving Environment and the Development of Mentalizing

Consistent with these claims, studies show that insecurely attached children do not perform as well as secure children in mentalizing tasks (e.g., de Rosnay & Harris, 2002). The London Parent–Child Project (Fonagy, Steele, Steele, & Holder, 1997), for instance, found that 82% of children who were secure with their mother in the Strange Situation passed Harris's Belief–Desire–Reasoning Task at 5.5 years, compared with 50% of those who were avoidant and 33% of the small number who were preoccupied. The mentalizing approach has emphasized the importance of secure attachment in providing a context in which the child is allowed to develop the ability to mentalize and regulate his or her own emotions. But even more importantly, in an environment that is invalidating and emotionally abusive, an insecure and disorganized attachment pattern is likely to develop, and this is likely to seriously hinder development of the capacity for mentalizing (Fonagy, 2000; Fonagy & Luyten, 2009).

Again, the broader context seems to be key here. Significantly, Widom and colleagues (2009) found that the impact of child abuse and neglect became nonsignificant in a regression model pre-

dicting BPD features when other family and lifestyle characteristics were included (e.g., parental substance use, employment, education level, and Axis I disorders). These authors concluded that maltreatment may represent a marker for family dysfunction, and that family dysfunction may actually be more significant in leading to a greater risk of BPD. This is congruent with the notion that abuse and neglect are typically part of a broader context characteristic of "risky families and environments" (Repetti, Taylor, & Seeman, 2002) or "pathogenic relational environments" (Cicchetti & Toth, 2005). A number of family-related factors—all likely to undermine the acquisition of mentalizing—have been reported to be significant predictors of BPD, including parental psychopathology, witnessing domestic violence in childhood, and parental imprisonment and suicide attempts (Afifi et al., 2011; Helgeland & Torgersen, 2004; Widom et al., 2009; Zanarini, Frankenburg, Hennen, Reich, & Silk, 2006). More detailed prospective studies of caregiver–child interactions are needed to investigate these assumptions further, but we may expect growing up in an environment of insecure and unpredictable attachment relationships to disrupt the acquisition of robust mentalizing. In this context, a recent comprehensive systematic review (Macintosh, 2013) identified five studies (Bouchard et al., 2008; Fonagy & Bateman, 2006; Fossati et al., 2009; Fossati, Feeney, Maffei, & Borroni, 2011; Stein & Allen, 2007) supporting the assumption that impairments in mentalizing mediated the relationship between insecure attachment and/or adversity and adult functioning. However, more research is clearly needed in this area.

Considered in relation to attachment, mentalizing deficits associated with childhood maltreatment may be a form of decoupling, inhibition, or even a phobic reaction to mentalizing. Various studies indeed suggest that (1) adversity may undermine cognitive development in general (Cicchetti, Rogosch, & Toth, 2000; Crandell & Hobson, 1999; Stacks, Beeghly, Partridge, & Dexter, 2011), (2) mentalizing problems as a result of maltreatment may reflect arousal problems associated with exposure to chronic stress (see Cicchetti & Walker, 2001), and (3) the child may avoid mentalizing to avoid perceiving the abuser's hostile and malevolent thoughts and feelings about him or her (e.g., Fonagy, 1991; Goodman et al., 2010).

Regardless of the precise nature of the impact of early adversity on mentalizing, these findings imply that the foundations of subjective selfhood will be less robustly established in those who have experienced early neglect. However, whereas some readers might interpret this approach as a deficit theory, our emphasis is on adaptation. The specific configuration of mentalizing capacities characterizing individuals with BPD (and other types of psychopathology associated with impairments in mentalizing) may be conceived of as optimizing the child's adaptation to the challenges of his or her social context (Blair & Raver, 2012; Frankenhuis & Panchanathan, 2011; Frankenhuis, Panchanathan, & Clark Barrett, 2013). Our speculation that in circumstances of neglect and/or abuse, it may be preferable to forgo reflective considerations—particularly of the cognitions of others (Fonagy, 1991)—is consistent with an evolutionary–developmental view that suggests we have to study the likely impact for survival and the costs and benefits (to children) of developing particular mental capacities in particular social contexts (Belsky, 2012; Ellis et al., 2012). While the impairments in mentalizing that we have noted may bring benefit to the child under some social conditions, in normal adult contexts, they render the individual more vulnerable—even in the face of social adversity in adulthood. The precise nature of these impairments, research suggests, largely depends on individuals' dominant secondary attachment strategies for dealing with experiences, which become increasingly generalized. In the next section, we review these strategies and their influence on mentalizing in more detail.

### d. Neurobiology of Stress, Attachment, and Mentalizing

Beyond the general impact of attachment disruptions on mentalizing, secondary attachment strategies (deactivation or hyperactivation of the attachment system in an effort to cope with threats; Cassidy & Kobak, 1987) have a more specific influence on mentalizing and may explain individual differences in mentalizing profiles.

Following the model outlined by Arnsten and colleagues (1998, 1999) and Mayes (2000, 2006), we suggest that with increased arousal a switch occurs from cortical to subcortical systems, from controlled to automatic mentalizing, and, subsequently, to nonmentalizing modes. Two points are critical for understanding impairments in mentalizing in this context. First, owing to the neurochemical switch associated with escalating emotional stress, patterns of brain functioning can shift from flexibility to automatic functioning: that is,

from relatively slow executive functions mediated by the prefrontal cortex (PFC) to faster habitual behaviors mediated by posterior cortical (e.g., parietal) and subcortical (e.g., amygdala, hippocampus, and striatum) structures. At the same time, mentalizing seems to disappear as self-protective physical reactions (i.e., fight–flight–freeze) begin to dominate behavior. This has the presumed evolutionary value of promoting immediate adaptive responses to danger. However, in situations of interpersonal stress, where complex cognitive–emotional functioning (i.e., mentalizing) may be helpful, the switch from executive (mentalizing) to automatic (fight–flight–freeze) responses may be counterproductive, to say the least. We also assume, following Arnsten and colleagues and Mayes (2000), that exposure to early stress and trauma can lower the threshold for switching, an assumption that has received considerable empirical support in the meantime. Second, both situational and more stable within-person variations play a role in the switch from more controlled to automatic mentalizing (for detailed discussion, see Fonagy & Luyten, 2009; Luyten, Fonagy, Lowyck, & Vermote, 2012).

In individuals with *secure attachment*, activation of the attachment system predictably involves a relaxation of normal strategies of interpersonal caution. There is good evidence that intense activation of the neurobehavioral system underpinning attachment is associated with deactivation of the arousal and affect-regulation systems (Fonagy & Luyten, 2009; Luyten et al., 2012), as well as the deactivation of neurocognitive systems likely to generate interpersonal suspicion, that is, those systems and brain regions involved in social cognition or mentalizing, including the lateral PFC, medial PFC (mPFC), lateral parietal cortex, medial parietal cortex, medial temporal lobe, and rostral anterior cingulate cortex (Bartels & Zeki, 2000, 2004; Lieberman, 2007; Satpute & Lieberman, 2006; Van Overwalle, 2009). For example, with increased intimacy, regions of the brain associated with reflective mentalizing will be deactivated—which perhaps explains the many linguistic and cultural variations of the popular sentiment that love is blind.

Moreover, as noted, the neuropeptides oxytocin and vasopressin play key roles in two aspects of creating attachment relationships: (1) by activating the reward/attachment system, and (2) by deactivating neurobehavioral systems that are involved in mediating social avoidance (Bartels & Zeki, 2004). For instance, oxytocin and vasopressin have been shown to inhibit aversion of both female and male rodents to infant pups, and to promote a number of affiliative behaviors, including caregiving behavior (Heinrichs, von Dawans, & Domes, 2009; Insel & Young, 2001). Oxytocin also reduces behavioral and neuroendocrine responses to social stress and seems to enable animals to overcome their natural avoidance of proximity and to inhibit defensive behavior, thereby facilitating approach behavior (Simeon et al., 2011). Vasopressin has primarily been implicated in male-typical social behaviors, including aggression and pair-bond formation, and mediates anxiogenic effects (Heinrichs & Domes, 2008). Thus, in the context of secure attachment, activation of the attachment system will generate not only increased experience of reward, increased sensitivity to social cues, and decreased social avoidance, but also the potential for the reward to override lack of trust. This complex set of associations with social behavior may help to account for the puzzling combination of facilitative and inhibitory associations between attachment history and social cognition. For instance, in two separate imaging studies, Bartels and Zeki (2000, 2004) reported that the activation of areas mediating maternal and/or romantic attachments appeared simultaneously to suppress brain activity in several regions mediating different aspects of cognitive control, including those associated with making social judgments and mentalizing. The second set of brain areas observed to be deactivated by the activation of attachment concerns included the temporal poles, temporoparietal junction, amygdala, and mPFC—areas consistently linked to explicit and internally focused mentalizing, including judgments of social trustworthiness, moral judgments, theory of mind tasks, and attention to one's own emotions.

In contrast, studies suggest that *anxious-preoccupied attachment strategies* are associated with simultaneously lowered thresholds for attachment system activation and deactivation of controlled mentalizing. In these individuals, more automatic, subcortical systems, including the amygdala, have a lower threshold for responding to stress.

*Attachment deactivating strategies* have in turn been shown to be associated with the capacity to keep systems involved in controlled mentalizing online for longer, including systems involved in judging the trustworthiness of other individuals (i.e., the "pull" mechanism associated with attachment; Vrticka, Andersson, Grandjean, Sander, & Vuilleumier, 2008). Yet whereas securely attached individuals are able to keep the controlled men-

talizing system online even when stress increases, which means that the attachment system is less likely to be triggered, the deactivating strategy of dismissive individuals is likely to fail in these circumstances. If securely attached individuals are those who are able to retain a relatively high activation of prefrontal areas in the presence of activation of the dopaminergic mesolimbic pathways (the attachment and reward system), then differences in mentalizing between securely attached individuals and those individuals who primarily rely on attachment deactivating strategies may become apparent only under increasing stress; this seems consistent with the findings of experimental studies (Mikulincer & Shaver, 2007).

This model allows us to explain why, for instance, mentalizing deficits in BPD are more likely to be observed in experimental settings that trigger the attachment system, such as in studies collecting AAI narratives (e.g., Fonagy et al., 1996; Levinson & Fonagy, 2004), and also why patients with BPD who mix deactivating and hyperactivating strategies, as is characteristic of *disorganized attachment*, show tendencies for both hypermentalizing and mentalizing failure. On the one hand, because attachment deactivating strategies are typically associated with minimizing and avoiding affective content, patients with BPD often have a tendency for hypermentalizing; that is, continuing attempts to mentalize, but without integrating cognition and affect. On the other hand, because the use of hyperactivating strategies is associated with a decoupling of controlled mentalizing, this leads to failure of mentalizing as a result of overreliance on modes of social cognition that antedate full mentalizing (Bateman & Fonagy, 2006).

We see BPD as being in some ways at the opposite end of the spectrum from *interpersonal resilience* (Gunderson & Lyons-Ruth, 2008; Higgitt & Fonagy, 1992). Studies suggest that the ability to continue to mentalize even under considerable stress leads to so-called "broaden and build" (Fredrickson, 2001) cycles of attachment security, which reinforce feelings of secure attachment, personal agency, and affect regulation ("build") and lead one to be pulled into different and more adaptive environments ("broaden") (Mikulincer & Shaver, 2007). Congruent with these assumptions, studies on resilience have shown that positive attachment experiences are related to resilience in part through relationship recruiting, that is, the capacity of resilient individuals to become attached to caring others (Hauser, Allen, & Golden, 2006). Hence, high levels of mentalizing and the associated use of security-based attachment strategies when faced with stress are good candidates to explain the effect of relationship recruiting and resilience in the face of stress. In contrast, attachment hyperactivation and deactivation have been shown to limit the ability to broaden and build in the face of stress. Moreover, they have also been shown to inhibit other behavioral systems that are involved in resilience, such as exploration, affiliation, and caregiving (Insel & Young, 2001; Mikulincer & Shaver, 2007; Neumann, 2008). This may also partially explain these individuals' difficulties in entering lasting relationships (including relationships with mental health care professionals) and the intergenerational transmission of borderline pathology.

To summarize, we may envision three types of association between aspects of mentalizing and attachment. These are created by (1) attachment relationships based on intense romantic or maternal love, (2) attachment relationships based on threat/fear, and (3) secure and predictable attachment relationships. Although any given attachment relationship may have features of each of these three types, they are important to distinguish because the relationship between attachment activation and mentalizing may differ considerably depending on which feature is activated within an attachment relationship: (1) mediated by dopaminergic structures of the reward system in the presence of oxytocin and vasopressin, the love-related activation of the attachment system can inhibit the neural systems that underpin the generation of negative affect; (2) threat-related activation of the attachment system (e.g., triggered by perceived threat, loss, or harm) may also evoke intense arousal and overwhelming negative affect, bringing about an activation of posterior cortical and subcortical areas and switching off frontal cortical activity, including mentalizing (Arnsten, 1998; Arnsten et al., 1999; Mayes, 2000); (3) meanwhile, a secure and predictable attachment relationship may be most effective in *preempting* threat, which possibly reduces the need for frequent activation of the attachment system.

## e. Attachment, Mentalizing, and Epistemic Trust

Recent elaborations of thinking about mentalizing have pointed to a further important function of attachment relationships: the development of epistemic trust, enabling social learning in a constantly changing environment (Fonagy & Luyten, 2016; Fonagy et al., 2015).

As we have seen, there is now considerable evidence that the caregiver's capacity to mentalize predicts secure attachment in the child. This raises the related question: how does the child learn from their caregiver's behavior? This question has powerful ramifications for our understanding of human social development. We have argued elsewhere (Fonagy et al., 2015), based on both evolutionary findings and theory (Sperber et al., 2010; Wilson & Sperber, 2012), as well as experimental developmental research (e.g., Corriveau et al., 2009), that secure attachment experiences pave the way for not only the acquisition of mentalizing but also, potentially more generally, the formation of epistemic trust, that is, an individual's willingness to consider another person's communication of new knowledge as trustworthy, generalizable, and relevant to the self. As noted, these theoretical developments promise to lead to major changes in our views concerning the importance of attachment relationships in human development.

The theory of natural pedagogy (ToNP; Csibra & Gergely, 2009) has offered a compelling empirically based model to explain how attachment history can create distinct types of epistemic states. ToNP is based on research suggesting a human-specific, cue-driven social-cognitive adaptation of mutual design dedicated to ensuring the most effective and efficient transfer of culturally relevant knowledge. This fast route for transmission of knowledge is needed in humans because most of our knowledge about the world is cognitively opaque. Csibra and Gergely (2009) used an idea first discussed by Bertrand Russell (1940), but extensively used by Sperber and Wilson (1995), suggesting that certain signals (*ostensive cues*) are employed by an agent to indicate his or her intent to communicate to the addressee. These cues may also serve to counteract natural *epistemic vigilance* (an adaptive self-protection against potentially damaging, deceptive, or inaccurate information). The ToNP model claims that ostensive cues generate a particular attentional state in which natural disbelief is temporarily suspended and the addressee feels that the communication contains information specifically relevant to him or her, which should be remembered and encoded as knowledge that is generally relevant to social situations. The information can be laid down and used as part of procedural and semantic memory, not uniquely or primarily episodic memory.

Research in this context suggests that a securely attached child is more likely to feel that the caregiver is a reliable source of knowledge because the predictors of secure attachment relationships are in essence also ostensive communication cues. A sensitive caregiver's consistent emotional responses to the child are communicated via the caregiver's ostensive cues, which include eye contact, turn taking, contingent reactivity, and the use of a special tone of voice, all of which appear to trigger a special mode of learning in the infant. The caregiver's marked mirroring of the infant's emotional expression that underpins the development of emotion understanding can be seen as ostensive in nature, signaling the relevance of the caregiver's display to the infant's accumulating knowledge base about his or her own subjective experience (Fonagy et al., 2007).

In brief, ostensive cues trigger epistemic trust and simultaneously engender secure parent–child attachment (Fonagy et al., 2007). They set aside the biological protection provided by epistemic vigilance. They open a channel of information exchange about the social and personally relevant world (an "epistemic superhighway") that allows us to acquire new knowledge rapidly. The knowledge transmitted is generalized beyond the specific experience in which it is acquired, remembered, and encoded with the authority but not the person of the communicator. Epistemic trust is necessary to allow us to change our position safely in the light of new experiences.

Several fascinating developmental experiments summarized by Csibra and Gergely (2009) offer compelling evidence from infancy for the power of this dialogic learning process. In one simple demonstration, 6-month-old infants were shown to follow an agent's gaze-shift selectively to an object only if it had been preceded either by eye contact with the infant or by infant-directed speech (Senju & Csibra, 2008). Shared attention with an agent is triggered by the infant experiencing the agent's interest. The interest triggers the infant's expectation (epistemic trust) that there may be something relevant for the infant to learn.

A second study employing an automated eye-tracker used an infant-induced contingent reactivity paradigm (Deligianni, Senju, Gergely, & Csibra, 2011). During the familiarization phase, 8-month-old infants observed a display of five unfamiliar animated objects (looking more like jugs or kettles than anything else). Four of these, in the four corners of the display, moved unpredictably. The object at the center acted differently in two conditions. In the interactive condition, whenever the infant's gaze wandered toward the object, it would apparently respond to the infant's gaze with movements and sound. In the control condition, the central object would move a comparable amount, but this would be independent of the infant's gaze. In the test phase, only three objects were present. The central object in this phase turned toward either the left or the right object. It should be noted that although none of the five jug-like objects had eyes, they had a clear, unequivocal front signaled by a pointed "hat" and an elongated "nose" (somewhat reminiscent of a kettle with an upturned beak). The 8-month-olds in the interactive condition detected the contingent activity of the central object and looked at the object it turned toward (i.e., followed its "gaze") far more. In the noncontingent control condition, the infants did not look longer, more frequently, or more promptly at the object toward which the central object turned. It seems that the contingent reactivity of this nonhuman and somewhat bizarre object was sufficient to influence the infant's orientation. The study is important in showing that it is the experience of response-induced contingencies that creates epistemic trust and elicits a "joint attention response."

As noted, studies in this context emphasize the key importance of attachment history. For example, in a longitudinal study of attachment, 147 children assessed for attachment in infancy were tested twice for epistemic trust at the ages of 50 and 61 months (Corriveau et al., 2009). In this study, the child's mother and a stranger made conflicting claims to a child concerning (1) the name of a novel object, (2) the name of a hybrid animal made up of 50% of each of two animals (e.g., an image made up of 50% rabbit and 50% squirrel; the mother might call it a squirrel, while the stranger says it is a rabbit), and (3) the name of a hybrid animal made up of 75% of one animal and 25% of another. In the third case it was always the mother who made the improbable claim (e.g., that a picture made up of 75% bird and 25% fish was a fish), while the stranger gave the more likely answer (in this example, "bird"). The nature of a child's attachment relationship powerfully conditioned the child's trust in the information imparted by the attachment figure (mother) and others (strangers) as informants. Children who were securely attached in infancy displayed a flexible strategy, showing a preference toward accepting claims made by their mother when appropriate. Insecure-avoidant children withheld trust in their mother, preferring to attend to information from the stranger, while insecure-resistant children withheld trust in the stranger even when their mother made improbable claims. Children with insecure-disorganized histories evidenced what we may call *epistemic hypervigilance*; they appeared to regard both sources of information with suspicion.

Hence, security of attachment, rooted in a history of feeling recognized, appears to increase the likelihood of trust in the source of communication when it is reasonably credible. Yet a secure attachment history also generates confidence in one's own experience and belief, and empowers one's (i.e., the child's) judgment. A history of attachment avoidance may generate epistemic mistrust, while anxious attachment creates epistemic uncertainty through overreliance on the views of the attachment figure. Disorganized attachment, rooted in a history of chronic misattunement, unsurprisingly can create mistrust of both the attachment figure and strangers as a source of information. It is the unresolvable question of "Whom can I trust?" that might contribute to epistemic hypervigilance in a child with a history of disorganized attachment.

Here, attachment researchers are faced with a conundrum. While these studies suggest that attachment may be a key mechanism for the mediation of epistemic trust, the theoretical formulations reviewed suggest that it may be secondary to an underlying biological process preserved by evolution. We have seen that stimuli such as the bizarre kettle-shaped object in the study described earlier are capable of at least momentarily triggering the same category of response as human beings. In other words, secure attachment is not likely to be a necessary condition for generating epistemic trust, but it may be sufficient, and perhaps the most pervasive in early childhood because it is a highly evolutionarily effective indicator of trustworthiness.

Looked at from a distance, microanalytic (e.g., Beebe et al., 2010) and more global (e.g., DeWolf & Van IJzendoorn, 1997; Isabella, Belsky, & von Eye, 1989; Kiser, Bates, Maslin, & Bayles, 1986; Mills-Koonce et al., 2007) ratings of sensitive caregiving can be seen as in essence recognizing the child's agentive self. It is this recognition that we believe offers the cognitive advantage to secure attachment, which has been fairly consistently noted, although not, to our knowledge, commonly studied (e.g., Crandell & Hobson, 1999; Jacobsen & Hofmann, 1997; Moss, Rousseau, Parent, St-Laurent, & Saintong, 1998) and contributes to the cognitive disadvantage of developmental adversity (Ayoub et al., 2009; Fernald et al., 2011; Goodman et al., 2010; Rieder

& Cicchetti, 1989). We believe that through the down-regulation of affect triggered by proximity seeking in the distressed infant, attachment not only establishes a lasting bond but also opens a channel for information to be used for the transfer of knowledge between the generations.

Attachment insecurity is likely to be associated with a greater likelihood of cognitive closure, a lower tolerance for ambiguity, and a more pronounced tendency for dogmatic thinking (Mikulincer, 1997). Saving intellectual effort and adopting stereotypes is also more likely in individuals whose attachment is insecure (Mikulincer, 1997). The same predisposition to knowledge inflexibility is revealed by the tendency of insecure individuals to make judgments on the basis of early information and to pay insufficient heed to subsequent data even if it is incompatible with the configuration first created (Green-Hennessy & Reis, 1998; Mikulincer, 1997). Insecure individuals, who fear the loss of attachment figures, also anxiously hold on to their initial constructions. Kruglanski (1989; Kruglanski & Webster, 1996; Pierro & Kruglanski, 2008) proposed the concept of *epistemic freezing*, characterized by a tendency to defend existing knowledge structures, even when they are incorrect or misleading (see also Fiske & Taylor, 1991).

Returning to the earlier theme of seeing adversity as leading not to deficit but rather to a superior adaptation to challenging environments (Frankenhuis et al., 2013), we may see such a defensive strategy as adaptive if an individual's self-esteem is vulnerable. Cognitive closure, dogmatism, and conservatism may simply be strategies to create a bulwark to safeguard an inadequately individuated self (Bowlby, 1980). By contrast, the greater confidence of secure individuals that they will be able to recover from dysregulation also enables them to be less defensive and more able to open their minds to information that may challenge their assumptions.

Mikulincer (1997) suggested that insecure individuals are more readily threatened by information that challenges their knowledge structures because of the vulnerability of their sense of self, and their vulnerability in particular to being emotionally overwhelmed. If emotional dysregulation is experienced as a real and imminent threat, they may opt for knowledge stability, as it temporarily serves to down-regulate arousal. Such individuals are less likely to revise their knowledge in the face of information that challenges their assumptions (Green & Campbell, 2000; Green-Hennessy & Reis, 1998; Mikulincer, 1997; Mikulincer & Arad,

1999) as if they not only have less confidence in the robustness of their bond to their attachment figure but also fear the loss of epistemic trust. In summary, we assume that the epistemic superhighway provided to us by evolution in order to learn from experience is partially closed to those whose attachment to their caregiver is insecure.

Anomalies of early parent–infant communication that predict attachment disorganization and later personality pathology (e.g., Lyons-Ruth, Bureau, Holmes, Easterbrooks, & Brooks, 2013) may be, from this perspective, understood as cases of *misuse of ostensive cueing*, by which we mean using cues to lead the infant to anticipate personally relevant, generalizable knowledge through a kind of pseudosensitivity followed by the transmission of disruptive and even destructive knowledge. From the perspective of epistemic trust as the mediator of culture, and its key underlying engine for progression, we see the destruction of trust in social knowledge as a key mechanism in pathological personality development. Developmental adversity, perhaps most deeply attachment trauma (Allen, 2012, 2013), may trigger a profound destruction of trust. The absence of epistemic trust generates an apparent rigidity in the eyes of the communicator, who, in accordance with the principles of theoretical rationality, expects the recipient to modify his or her behavior on the basis of the information received and apparently understood. But in the absence of trust, the capacity for change is absent. The information presented is not used to update the individual's social understanding. In terms of the ToNP (Csibra & Gergely, 2009) the person has (temporarily) lost the capacity for learning. From a therapist's standpoint, he or she has become "hard to reach" and interpersonally inaccessible.

According to the evolutionary perspective we are advancing, a particular attachment style should be seen less as a measure of the extent to which the caregiver succeeded in generating infant attachment security and, more broadly, as the child learning of the most appropriate method for his or her social survival in a complex interpersonal world (Belsky, 2006; Ein-Dor, Mikulincer, & Shaver, 2011; Mikulincer & Shaver, 2007; Simpson & Belsky, 2008). An avoidant-dismissive model of attachment might be more protective in certain environments than a secure one. Similarly, the anxious-preoccupied style may be an effective means of ensuring a child learns to effectively harness interpersonal attention and resources in a context of resource uncertainty. Even serious PDs

such as BPD, while conspicuously dysfunctional in our normative social setting, may have adaptive benefits for individuals living in an emergency milieu characterized by high levels of interpersonal violence, where there is a need for extreme vigilance on issues of self-protection and significant benefit in being able to form intense emotional relationships, which might elicit critical protection or resource supply, very quickly. The mentalizing strengths that have been noted in many individuals with BPD—a tendency to be able to make quick inferences of other people's mental states on the basis of their visual and emotional cues, hypersensitivity to facial expressions, hyperreactivity to positive and emotional stimuli—are all suggestive of a mentalizing profile that may be an adaptation to functioning in a threatening or high-risk environment.

## 5. The Future of Attachment Theory and Psychoanalysis

Despite the limitations of attachment theory, it is clear that the attachment relationship provides the context in which we learn to make sense of ourselves and others, or, to use the language of psychoanalysis, in which we create our internal world. Yet we contend that the future of attachment theory lies in developing our understanding of the relationship of attachment and mentalizing.

The mentalizing construct bridges the gap between psychodynamic and attachment models by focusing on the relationship of attachment processes and the growth of the child's sense of self and his or her capacity to comprehend the mental states of others. The future clinical importance of attachment lies in understanding how mentalizing difficulties, impairments, and imbalances are generated and how they can be alleviated. Mentalizing also provides a broader developmental model within which we can reconsider and accommodate the developmental challenges and themes traditionally emphasized within psychoanalytic thinking: the ways in which individuals differently respond to the developmental, environmental, and instinctual challenges posed by sexuality and aggression, and cope with these challenges in a complex social world. Any genuinely convincing developmental understanding of the ways in which the emotional environment may affect the mind in infancy and childhood must accommodate the reality of evolutionarily driven adaptiveness. We postulate that mentalizing provides the missing link in understanding the evolutionary mechanism at work in the transmission of attachment. This broader evolutionary perspective, rather than creating a reflexive, flatly Pavlovian model for human development, allows us to appreciate the richness of human subjectivity through a theory that accommodates the complex mix of factors that makes us who we are: that is, the early emotional environment, genes, and the barrage of wider social pressures that each individual learns to interpret and respond to in particular ways depending on his or her epistemic history and mentalizing capacities.

At one level, our views on the relationship among attachment, mentalizing, and epistemic trust may appear to downplay the clinical significance of attachment. However, we would argue that attachment thinking remains fundamental to understanding the mechanism through which mentalizing and epistemic trust are made possible. From the outset, the most effective way an infant is first mentalized and first able to develop epistemic trust is in the context of a secure attachment relationship. Similarly, it is only in the context of stable attachment relationships, and then within the wider social environment, that mentalizing can be developed and epistemic hypervigilance can safely be relaxed. According to this thinking, as humans evolved greater social complexity, the attachment relationship became coaxial with the transmission of other, more species-specific social-cognitive processes, such as mentalizing and the promotion of natural pedagogy.

This latest elaboration of thinking in relation to attachment takes us back to one of Bowlby's original intentions in the formulation of attachment theory: making sense of emotional development and psychopathology in an evolutionary context. Psychoanalytic thinking, and psychology more broadly, has been criticized for failing to take into account the impact of the socioeconomic environment on the individual psyche (Fonagy, Target, & Gergely, 2006). We can no longer neglect this influence. For instance, there is accumulating evidence that increasing levels of social inequality are connected with an increased prevalence of BPD (Grant et al., 2008; Wilkinson & Pickett, 2009). If we consider that the evolutionary drive behind mentalizing was to enable our survival in increasingly complex social situations involving matters of hierarchy, cooperation, exclusion, and inclusion, it makes eminent sense that representations of ourselves and those around us should calibrate the extent to which we are experiencing social isolation, alienation, or inferiority. Psychological resilience enables the individual to resist these pressures to some degree; individuals with BPD are often conspicuously reactive to such pressures—to be wholly impervious to their effects suggests mentalizing impairments of a different nature altogether. Both extremes, however, derive from an inability to absorb information from the social environment in a way that is compatible with the construction of a normatively coherent sense of self.

## References

Aber, J., Slade, A., Berger, B., Bresgi, I., & Kaplan, M. (1985). *The Parent Development Interview*. Unpublished manuscript, Barnard College, Columbia University, New York, NY.

Abram, J. (2008). Donald Woods Winnicott (1896–1971): A brief introduction. *International Journal of Psychoanalysis, 89*, 1189–1217.

Afifi, T. O., Mather, A., Boman, J., Fleisher, W., Enns, M. W., Macmillan, H., et al. (2011). Childhood adversity and personality disorders: Results from a nationally representative population-based study. *Journal of Psychiatric Research, 45*, 814–822.

Agrawal, H. R., Gunderson, J., Holmes, B. M., & Lyons-Ruth, K. (2004). Attachment studies with borderline patients: A review. *Harvard Review of Psychiatry, 12*, 94–104.

Ainsworth, M. D. S., Blehar, M. C., Waters, E., & Wall, S. (1978). *Patterns of attachment: A psychological study of the Strange Situation*. Hillsdale, NJ: Erlbaum.

Allen, J. G. (2012). *Restoring mentalizing in attachment relationships: Treating trauma with plain old therapy*. Washington, DC: American Psychiatric Press.

Allen, J. G. (2013). *Mentalizing in the development and treatment of attachment trauma*. London: Karnac Books.

Allen, J. G., Fonagy, P., & Bateman, A. W. (2008). *Mentalizing in clinical practice*. Washington, DC: American Psychiatric Press.

Arnsten, A. F., Mathew, R., Ubriani, R., Taylor, J. R., & Li, B. M. (1999). Alpha-1 noradrenergic receptor stimulation impairs prefrontal cortical cognitive function. *Biological Psychiatry, 45*, 26–31.

Arnsten, A. F. T. (1998). The biology of being frazzled. *Science, 280*, 1711–1712.

Aron, L. (2012). Rethinking "doublethinking": Psychoanalysis and scientific research—an introduction to a series. *Psychoanalytic Dialogues, 22*, 704–709.

Aron, L., & Leichich, M. (2011). Relational psychoanalysis. In G. Gabbard, B. Litowitz, & P. Williams (Eds.), *Textbook of psychoanalysis* (pp. 211–224). Arlington, VA: American Psychiatric Press.

Ayoub, C., O'Connor, E., Rappolt-Schlictmann, G.,

Vallotton, C., Raikes, H., & Chazan-Cohen, R. (2009). Cognitive skill performance among young children living in poverty: Risk, change, and the promotive effects of Early Head Start. *Early Child Research Quarterly, 24*, 289–305.

Baird, A. A., Veague, H. B., & Rabbitt, C. E. (2005). Developmental precipitants of borderline personality disorder. *Development and Psychopathology, 17*, 1031–1049.

Ball, J. S., & Links, P. S. (2009). Borderline personality disorder and childhood trauma: Evidence for a causal relationship. *Current Psychiatry Reports, 11*, 63–68.

Bartels, A., & Zeki, S. (2000). The neural basis of romantic love. *NeuroReport, 11*, 3829–3834.

Bartels, A., & Zeki, S. (2004). The neural correlates of maternal and romantic love. *NeuroImage, 21*, 1155–1166.

Bateman, A. W., & Fonagy, P. (2006). *Mentalization based treatment for borderline personality disorder: A practical guide*. Oxford, UK: Oxford University Press.

Bateman, A. [W.], & Fonagy, P. (2010). Mentalization based treatment for borderline personality disorder. *World Psychiatry, 9*, 11–15.

Bateman, A. W., & Fonagy, P. (Eds.). (2012). *Handbook of mentalizing in mental health practice*. Washington, DC: American Psychiatric Publishing.

Battle, C. L., Shea, M. T., Johnson, D. M., Yen, S., Zlotnick, C., Zanarini, M. C., et al. (2004). Childhood maltreatment associated with adult personality disorders: Findings from the Collaborative Longitudinal Personality Disorders Study. *Journal of Personality Disorders, 18*, 193–211.

Beebe, B., Jaffe, J., Markese, S., Buck, K., Chen, H., Cohen, P., et al. (2010). The origins of 12-month attachment: A microanalysis of 4-month mother-infant interaction. *Attachment and Human Development, 12*, 3–141.

Beebe, B., Lachmann, F., & Jaffe, J. (1997). Mother–infant interaction structures and presymbolic self and object representations. *Psychoanalytic Dialogues, 7*, 113–182.

Beebe, B., & Lachmann, F. M. (2014). *The origins of attachment: Infant research and adult treatment*. New York: Routledge.

Belsky, J. (2006). The developmental and evolutionary psychology of intergenerational transmission of attachment. In C. S. Carter, L. Ahnert, K. E. Grossmann, S. B. Hrdy, M. E. Lamb, S. W. Porges, et al. (Eds.), *Attachment and bonding: A new synthesis* (pp. 169–198). Cambridge, MA: MIT Press.

Belsky, J. (2012). The development of human reproductive strategies: Progress and prospects. *Current Directions in Psychological Science, 21*, 310–316.

Benjamin, J. (1998). *The shadow of the other: Intersubjectivity and gender in psychoanalysis*. New York: Routledge.

Bion, W. (1997). *Taming wild thoughts*. London: Karnac Books.

Blair, C., & Raver, C. C. (2012). Child development

in the context of adversity: Experiential canalization of brain and behavior. *American Psychologist, 67*, 309–318.

Blatt, S. J. (1974). Levels of object representation in anaclitic and introjective depression. *Psychoanalytic Study of the Child, 29*, 107–157.

Blatt, S. J., Auerbach, J. S., & Levy, K. N. (1997). Mental representations in personality development, psychopathology, and the therapeutic process. *Review of General Psychology, 1*, 351–374.

Bohleber, W. (2007). Remembrance, trauma and collective memory: The battle for memory in psychoanalysis. *International Journal of Psychoanalysis, 88*, 329–352.

Bouchard, M. A., Target, M., Lecours, S., Fonagy, P., Tremblay, L. M., Schachter, A., et al. (2008). Mentalization in adult attachment narratives: Reflective functioning, mental states, and affect elaboration compared. *Psychoanalytic Psychology, 25*, 47–66.

Bowlby, J. (1969). *Attachment and loss: Vol. 1. Attachment*. London: Hogarth Press and Institute of Psycho-Analysis.

Bowlby, J. (1973). *Attachment and loss: Vol. 2. Separation: Anxiety and anger*. London: Hogarth Press and Institute of Psycho-Analysis.

Bowlby, J. (1980). *Attachment and loss: Vol. 3. Loss: Sadness and depression*. London: Hogarth Press and Institute of Psycho-Analysis.

Bowlby, J. (1988). *A secure base: Clinical applications of attachment theory*. London: Routledge.

Bretherton, K., & Munholland, K. A. (1999). Internal working models in attachment relationships: A construct revisited. In J. Cassidy & P. R. Shaver (Eds.), *Handbook of attachment: Theory, research, and clinical applications* (pp. 89–114). New York: Guilford Press.

Bretherton, K., & Munholland, K. A. (2008). Internal working models in attachment relationships: Elaborating a central construct in attachment theory. In J. Cassidy & P. R. Shaver (Eds.), *Handbook of attachment: Theory, research, and clinical applications* (2nd ed., pp. 102–127). New York: Guilford Press.

Brinich, P. M. (1980). Some potential effects of adoption on self and object representations. *Psychoanalytic Study of the Child, 35*, 107–133.

Bromberg, P. M. (1998). *Standing in the spaces*. Hillsdale, NJ: Analytic Press.

Brown, L. J. (2010). Klein, Bion, and intersubjectivity: Becoming, transforming, and dreaming *Psychoanalytic Dialogues, 20*, 669–682.

Brown, L. J. (2011). *Intersubjective processes and the unconscious: An integration of Freudian, Kleinian, and Bionian perspectives*. New York: Routledge.

Buchheim, A., Erk, S., George, C., Kachele, H., Kircher, T., Martius, P., et al. (2008). Neural correlates of attachment trauma in borderline personality disorder: A functional magnetic resonance imaging study. *Psychiatry Research, 163*, 223–235.

Carlson, E. A., Egeland, B., & Sroufe, L. A. (2009). A prospective investigation of the development of borderline personality symptoms. *Development and Psychopathology, 21,* 1311–1334.

Cassidy, J., & Kobak, R. (1987). Avoidance and its relation to other defensive processes. In J. Belsky & T. Nezworski (Eds.), *Clinical implications of attachment* (pp. 300–323). Hillsdale, NJ: Erlbaum.

Chused, J. F. (2012). The analyst's narcissism. *Journal of the American Psychoanalytic Association, 60,* 899–915.

Cicchetti, D. (2013). Annual research review: Resilient functioning in maltreated children—past, present, and future perspectives. *Journal of Child Psychology and Psychiatry, 54,* 402–422.

Cicchetti, D., Rogosch, F. A., & Toth, S. L. (2000). The efficacy of toddler–parent psychotherapy for fostering cognitive development in offspring of depressed mothers. *Journal of Abnormal Child Psychology, 28,* 135–148.

Cicchetti, D., & Toth, S. L. (2005). Child maltreatment. *Annual Review of Clinical Psychology, 1,* 409–438.

Cicchetti, D., & Walker, E. F. (2001). Editorial: Stress and development: Biological and psychological consequences. *Development and Psychopathology, 13,* 413–418.

Cohler, B. J., & Weiner, T. (2011). The inner fortress: Symptom and meaning in Asperger's syndrome *Psychoanalytic Inquiry, 31,* 208–221.

Corriveau, K. H., Harris, P. L., Meins, E., Fernyhough, C., Arnott, B., Elliott, L., et al. (2009). Young children's trust in their mother's claims: Longitudinal links with attachment security in infancy. *Child Development, 80,* 750–761.

Cortina, M. (2001). Sullivan's contributions to understanding personality development in light of attachment theory and contemporary models of the mind. *Contemporary Psychoanalysis, 37,* 193–238.

Craik, K. (1943). *The nature of explanation.* Cambridge, UK: Cambridge University Press.

Crandell, L. E., & Hobson, R. P. (1999). Individual differences in young children's IQ: A social-developmental perspective. *Journal of Child Psychology and Psychiatry, 40,* 455–464.

Crombie, T. (2013). *Stability over time and the role of attachment in emerging personality disorder in adolescence: A two year longitudinal study. Part 1: Literature review. A systematic literature review into the relationship between childhood emotional abuse and emotional neglect and borderline personality disorder.* Unpublished doctoral thesis, University College London .

Csibra, G., & Gergely, G. (2009). Natural pedagogy. *Trends in Cognitive Sciences, 13,* 148–153.

Davies, J. M. (1996). Linking the "pre-analytic" with the postclassical: Integration, dissociation, and the multiplicity of unconscious processes. *Contemporary Psychoanalysis, 32,* 553–576.

Deligianni, F., Senju, A., Gergely, G., & Csibra, G. (2011). Automated gaze-contingent objects elicit orientation following in 8-month-old infants. *Developmental Psychology, 47,* 1499–1503.

de Rosnay, M., & Harris, P. L. (2002). Individual differences in children's understanding of emotion: The roles of attachment and language. *Attachment and Human Development, 4,* 39–54.

DeWolf, M. S., & Van IJzendoorn, M. H. (1997). Sensitivity and attachment: A meta-analysis on parental antecedents of infant attachment. *Journal of Marriage and the Family, 68,* 571–591.

Dykas, M. J., & Cassidy, J. (2011). Attachment and the processing of social information across the life span: Theory and evidence. *Psychological Bulletin, 137,* 19–46.

Eagle, M. N. (2013). *Attachment and psychoanalysis: Theory, research, and clinical implications* New York: Guilford Press.

Ein-Dor, T., Mikulincer, M., & Shaver, P. R. (2011). Attachment insecurities and the processing of threat-related information: Studying the schemas involved in insecure people's coping strategies. *Journal of Personality and Social Psychology, 101,* 78–93.

Ellis, B. J., Del Giudice, M., Dishion, T. J., Figueredo, A. J., Gray, P., Griskevicius, V., et al. (2012). The evolutionary basis of risky adolescent behavior: Implications for science, policy, and practice. *Developmental Psychology, 48,* 598–623.

Emde, R., Kubicek, L., & Oppenheim, D. (1997). Imaginative reality observed during early language development. *International Journal of Psychoanalysis, 78,* 115–133.

Emde, R. N., & Spicer, P. (2000). Experience in the midst of variation: New horizons for development and psychopathology. *Development and Psychopathology, 12,* 313–332.

Epstein, O. B. (2010). And what about the "bad breast"? An attachment viewpoint on Klein's theory. *Attachment: New Directions in Relational Psychoanalysis and Psychotherapy, 4,* ix–xiv.

Fairbairn, W. R. D. (1952). *An object-relations theory of the personality.* New York: Basic Books.

Fairbairn, W. R. D. (1963). Synopsis of an object-relations theory of the personality. *International Journal of Psychoanalysis, 44,* 224–225.

Fernald, L. C., Weber, A., Galasso, E., & Ratsifandrihamanana, L. (2011). Socioeconomic gradients and child development in a very low income population: Evidence from Madagascar. *Developmental Science, 14,* 832–847.

Ferro, A. (2006). Clinical implications of Bion's thought. *International Journal of Psychoanalysis, 87,* 989–1003.

Fiske, S. T., & Taylor, S. E. (1991). *Social cognition* (2nd ed.). New York: McGraw-Hill.

Fonagy, P. (1991). Thinking about thinking: Some clinical and theoretical considerations in the treatment of a borderline patient. *International Journal of Psychoanalysis, 72,* 639–656.

Fonagy, P. (2000). Attachment and borderline personality disorder. *Journal of the American Psychoanalytic Association, 48,* 1129–1146.

Fonagy, P. (2001). *Attachment theory and psychoanalysis.* New York: Other Press.

Fonagy, P. (2008). A genuinely developmental theory of sexual enjoyment and its implications for psychoanalytic technique. *Journal of the American Psychoanalytic Association*, 56, 11–36.

Fonagy, P., & Bateman, A. W. (2006). Mechanisms of change in mentalization-based treatment of BPD. *Journal of Clinical Psychology*, 62, 411–430.

Fonagy, P., & Bateman, A. W. (2008). The development of borderline personality disorder: A mentalizing model. *Journal of Personality Disorders*, 22, 4–21.

Fonagy, P., Gergely, G., Jurist, E., & Target, M. (2002). *Affect regulation, mentalization, and the development of the self*. New York: Other Press.

Fonagy, P., Gergely, G., & Target, M. (2007). The parent–infant dyad and the construction of the subjective self. *Journal of Child Psychology and Psychiatry*, 48, 288–328.

Fonagy, P., Gergely, G., & Target, M. (2008). Psychoanalytic constructs and attachment theory and research. In J. Cassidy & P. R. Shaver (Eds.), *Handbook of attachment* (2nd ed., pp. 783–810). New York: Guilford Press.

Fonagy, P., Leigh, T., Steele, M., Steele, H., Kennedy, R., Mattoon, G., et al. (1996). The relation of attachment status, psychiatric classification, and response to psychotherapy. *Journal of Consulting and Clinical Psychology*, 64, 22–31.

Fonagy, P., & Luyten, P. (2009). A developmental, mentalization-based approach to the understanding and treatment of borderline personality disorder. *Development and Psychopathology*, 21, 1355–1381.

Fonagy, P., & Luyten, P. (2016). A multilevel perspective on the development of borderline personality disorder. In D. Cicchetti (Ed.), *Developmental psychopathology: Vol. 3. Risk, disorder, and adaptation* (3rd ed., pp. 726–742). New York: Wiley.

Fonagy, P., Luyten, P., & Allison, E. (2015). Epistemic petrification and the restoration of epistemic trust: A new conceptualization of borderline personality disorder and its psychosocial treatment. *Journal of Personality Disorders*, 29, 575–609.

Fonagy, P., Steele, H., Steele, M., & Holder, J. (1997). Attachment and theory of mind: Overlapping constructs? *Association for Child Psychology and Psychiatry Occasional Papers*, 14, 31–40.

Fonagy, P., Steele, M., Steele, H., Higgitt, A., & Target, M. (1994). The Emanuel Miller Memorial Lecture 1992. The theory and practice of resilience. *Journal of Child Psychology and Psychiatry*, 35, 231–257.

Fonagy, P., Steele, M., Steele, H., Moran, G. S., & Higgitt, A. C. (1991). The capacity for understanding mental states: The reflective self in parent and child and its significance for security of attachment. *Infant Mental Health Journal*, 12, 201–218.

Fonagy, P., Target, M., & Gergely, G. (2006). Psychoanalytic perspectives on developmental psychopathology. In D. Cicchetti & D. J. Cohen (Eds.), *Developmental psychopathology: Vol. 1. Theory and method* (2nd ed., pp. 701–749). Hoboken, NJ: Wiley.

Fossati, A., Acquarini, E., Feeney, J. A., Borroni, S., Grazioli, F., Giarolli, L. E., et al. (2009). Alexithymia and attachment insecurities in impulsive aggression. *Attachment and Human Development*, 11, 165–182.

Fossati, A., Feeney, J., Maffei, C., & Borroni, S. (2011). Does mindfulness mediate the association between attachment dimensions and borderline personality disorder features?: A study of Italian non-clinical adolescents. *Attachment and Human Development*, 13, 563–578.

Frankenhuis, W. E., & Panchanathan, K. (2011). Balancing sampling and specialization: An adaptationist model of incremental development. *Proceedings of the Royal Society of London B: Biological Sciences*, 278, 3558–3565.

Frankenhuis, W. E., Panchanathan, K., & Clark Barrett, H. (2013). Bridging developmental systems theory and evolutionary psychology using dynamic optimization. *Developmental Science*, 16, 584–598.

Fredrickson, B. L. (2001). The role of positive emotions in positive psychology. The broaden-and-build theory of positive emotions. *American Psychologist*, 56, 218–226.

Freud, S. (1957). Instincts and their vicissitudes. In J. Strachey (Ed.), *The standard edition of the complete psychological works of Sigmund Freud* (Vol. 14, pp. 109–140). London: Hogarth Press. (Original work published 1915)

Gabbard, G. O., & Scarfone, D. (2002). "Controversial discussions." The issue of differences in method. *International Journal of Psychoanalysis*, 83, 453–456.

Geyskens, T. (2003). Imre Hermann's Freudian theory of attachment. *International Journal of Psychoanalysis*, 84, 1517–1529.

Goodman, G. S., Quas, J. A., & Ogle, C. M. (2010). Child maltreatment and memory. *Annual Review of Psychology*, 61, 325–351.

Grant, B. F., Chou, S. P., Goldstein, R. B., Huang, B., Stinson, F. S., Saha, T. D., et al. (2008). Prevalence, correlates, disability, and comorbidity of DSM-IV borderline personality disorder: Results from the Wave 2 National Epidemiologic Survey on Alcohol and Related Conditions. *Journal of Clinical Psychiatry*, 69, 533–545.

Green, A. (2005). The illusion of common ground and mythical pluralism. *International Journal of Psychoanalysis*, 86, 627–632.

Green, J. D., & Campbell, W. K. (2000). Attachment and exploration in adults: Chronic and contextual accessibility. *Personality and Social Psychology Bulletin*, 26, 452–461.

Greenberg, J. R., & Mitchell, S. A. (1983). *Object relations in psychoanalytic theory*. Cambridge, MA: Harvard University Press.

Green-Hennessy, S., & Reis, H. T. (1998). Openness in processing social information among attachment types. *Personal Relationships*, 5, 449–466.

Gunderson, J. G., & Lyons-Ruth, K. (2008). BPD's interpersonal hypersensitivity phenotype: A gene-environment-developmental model. *Journal of Personality Disorders*, 22, 22–41.

Hauser, S. T., Allen, J. P., & Golden, E. (2006). *Out of the woods. Tales of resilient teens.* Cambridge, MA: Harvard University Press.

Heinrichs, M., & Domes, G. (2008). Neuropeptides and social behaviour: Effects of oxytocin and vasopressin in humans. *Progress in Brain Research, 170,* 337–350.

Heinrichs, M., von Dawans, B., & Domes, G. (2009). Oxytocin, vasopressin, and human social behavior. *Frontiers in Neuroendocrinology, 30,* 548–557.

Helgeland, M. I., & Torgersen, S. (2004). Developmental antecedents of borderline personality disorder. *Comprehensive Psychiatry, 45,* 138–147.

Hesse, E., & Main, M. (2006). Frightened, threatening, and dissociative parental behavior in low-risk samples: Description, discussion, and interpretations. *Development and Psychopathology, 18,* 309–343.

Higgitt, A., & Fonagy, P. (1992). Psychotherapy in borderline and narcissistic personality disorder. *British Journal of Psychiatry, 161,* 23–43.

Hoffman, I. Z. (2009). Doublethinking our way to "scientific" legitimacy: The dessication of human experience. *Journal of the American Psychoanalytic Association, 57,* 1043–1069.

Holmes, J. (1993). *John Bowlby and attachment theory.* London: Routledge.

Holmes, J. (2009). *Exploring in security: Towards an attachment-informed psychoanalytic psychotherapy.* London: Routledge.

Huprich, S. K., & Greenberg, R. P. (2003). Advances in the assessment of object relations in the 1990s. *Clinical Psychology Review, 23,* 665–698.

Insel, T. R., & Young, L. J. (2001). The neurobiology of attachment. *Nature Reviews Neuroscience, 2,* 129–136.

Isabella, R. A., Belsky, J., & von Eye, A. (1989). Origins of infant–mother attachment: An examination of interactional synchrony during the infant's first year. *Developmental Psychology, 25,* 12–21.

Jacobsen, T., & Hofmann, V. (1997). Children's attachment representations: Longitudinal relations to school behavior and academic competency in middle childhood and adolescence. *Developmental Psychology, 33,* 703–710.

Jaffe, J., Beebe, B., Feldstein, S., Crown, C. L., & Jasnow, M. D. (2001). Rhythms of dialogue in infancy: Coordinated timing in development. *Monographs of the Society for Research in Child Development, 66,* i–viii, 1–132.

Johnson, J. G., Cohen, P., Brown, J., Smailes, E. M., & Bernstein, D. P. (1999). Childhood maltreatment increases risk for personality disorders during early adulthood. *Archives of General Psychiatry, 56,* 600–605.

Keller, L. E. (2011). Repairing links: Building attachments in the preschool classroom. *Journal of the American Psychoanalytic Association, 59,* 737–763.

Kernberg, O. F. (2012). *The inseparable nature of love and aggression: Clinical and theoretical perpsectives.* Arlington, VA: American Psychiatric Publishing.

Kernberg, O. F. (2014). Some comments about Ronald Fairbairn's impact today. In G. S. Clarke & D. E. Scharff (Eds.), *Fairbairn and the object relations tradition* (pp. 115–126). London: Karnac Books.

Kernberg, O. F., & Caligor, E. (2005). A psychoanalytic theory of personality disorders. In M. F. Lenzenweger & J. F. Clarkin (Eds.), *Major theories of personality disorder* (2nd ed., pp. 114–156). New York: Guilford Press.

Kiser, L. J., Bates, J. E., Maslin, C. A., & Bayles, K. (1986). Mother–infant play at six months as a predictor of attachment security of thirteen months. *Journal of the American Academy of Child Psychiatry, 25,* 68–75.

Klein, M. (1964). The psychotherapy of the psychoses. In *Contributions to psychoanalysis, 1921–1945.* New York: McGraw-Hill. (Original work published 1936)

Kohut, H. (1971). *The analysis of the self.* New York: International Universities Press.

Kohut, H. (1977). *The restoration of the self.* New York: International Universities Press.

Kohut, H. (1984). *How does analysis cure?* Chicago: University of Chicago Press.

Kohut, H., & Wolf, E. S. (1978). The disorders of the self and their treatment: An outline. *International Journal of Psychoanalysis, 59,* 413–426.

Koren-Karie, N., Oppenheim, D., Dolev, S., Sher, E., & Etzion-Carasso, A. (2002). Mothers' insightfulness regarding their infants' internal experience: Relations with maternal sensitivity and infant attachment. *Developmental Psychology, 38,* 534–542.

Kovacs, A. M., Teglas, E., & Endress, A. D. (2010). The social sense: Susceptibility to others' beliefs in human infants and adults. *Science, 330,* 1830–1834.

Kruglanski, A. W. (1989). *Lay epistemics and human knowledge: Cognitive and motivational bases.* New York: Plenum Press.

Kruglanski, A. W., & Webster, D. M. (1996). Motivated closing of the mind: "Seizing" and "freezing." *Psychological Review, 103,* 263–283.

Laranjo, J., Bernier, A., Meins, E., & Carlson, S. M. (2010). Early manifestations of children's theory of mind: The roles of maternal mind-mindedness and infant security of attachment. *Infancy, 15,* 300–323.

Leckman, J. F., & Mayes, L. C. (1999). Preoccupations and behaviors associated with romantic and parental love. Perspectives on the origin of obsessive–compulsive disorder. *Child and Adolescent Psychiatric Clinics of North America, 8,* 635–665.

Levine, H. B. (2014). Psychoanalysis and trauma. *Psychoanalytic Inquiry, 34,* 214–224.

Levinson, A., & Fonagy, P. (2004). Offending and attachment: The relationship between interpersonal awareness and offending in a prison population with psychiatric disorder. *Canadian Journal of Psychoanalysis, 12,* 225–251.

Levy, K. N., Beeney, J. E., & Temes, C. M. (2011). Attachment and its vicissitudes in borderline personality disorder. *Current Psychiatry Reports, 13,* 50–59.

Lieberman, M. D. (2007). Social cognitive neuroscience: A review of core processes. *Annual Review of Psychology, 58*, 259–289.

Loeffler-Stastka, H., & Blueml, V. (2010). Assessment tools for affect regulation and quality of object relations in personality disorders: The predictive impact on initial treatment engagement. *Bulletin of the Menninger Clinic, 74*, 29–44.

Luyten, P., & Blatt, S. J. (2013). Interpersonal relatedness and self-definition in normal and disrupted personality development: Retrospect and prospect. *American Psychologist, 68*, 172–183.

Luyten, P., Blatt, S. J., & Corveleyn, J. (2006). Minding the gap between positivism and hermeneutics in psychoanalytic research. *Journal of the American Psychoanalytic Association, 54*, 571–610.

Luyten, P., Blatt, S. J., Van Houdenhove, B., & Corveleyn, J. (2006). Depression research and treatment: Are we skating to where the puck is going to be? *Clinical Psychology Review, 26*, 985–999.

Luyten, P., Fonagy, P., Lowyck, B., & Vermote, R. (2012). Assessment of mentalization. In A. W. Bateman & P. Fonagy (Eds.), *Handbook of mentalizing in mental health practice* (pp. 43–65). Washington, DC: American Psychiatric Publishing.

Lyons-Ruth, K. (1999). The two person unconscious: Intersubjective dialogue, enactive relational representation and the emergence of new forms of relational organisation. *Psychoanalytic Inquiry, 19*, 576–617.

Lyons-Ruth, K. (2003). Dissociation and the parent-infant dialogue: A longitudinal perspective from attachment research. *Journal of the American Psychoanalytic Association, 51*, 883–911.

Lyons-Ruth, K., Bureau, J. F., Holmes, B., Easterbrooks, A., & Brooks, N. H. (2013). Borderline symptoms and suicidality/self-injury in late adolescence: Prospectively observed relationship correlates in infancy and childhood. *Psychiatry Research, 206*, 273–281.

Lyons-Ruth, K., Yellin, C., Melnick, S., & Atwood, G. (2005). Expanding the concept of unresolved mental states: Hostile/helpless states of mind on the Adult Attachment Interview are associated with disrupted mother–infant communication and infant disorganization. *Development and Psychopathology, 17*, 1–23.

Macintosh, H. (2013). Mentalizing and its role as a mediator in the relationship between childhood experiences and adult functioning: Exploring the empirical evidence. *Psihologija, 46*, 193–212.

Main, M. (2000). The organized categories of infant, child, and adult attachment: Flexible vs. inflexible attention under attachment-related stress. *Journal of the American Psychoanalytic Association, 48*, 1055–1096.

Main, M., Hesse, E., & Hesse, S. (2011). Attachment theory and research: Overview with suggested applications to child custody. *Family Court Review, 49*, 426–463.

Main, M., Kaplan, N., & Cassidy, J. (1985). Security in infancy, childhood, and adulthood: A move to the level of representation. *Monographs of the Society for Research in Child Development, 50*, 66–104.

Main, M., & Solomon, J. (1986). Discovery of an insecure-disorganized/disoriented attachment pattern. In T. B. Brazelton & M. W. Yogman (Eds.), *Affective development in infancy* (pp. 95–124). Norwood, NJ: Ablex.

Masson, J. (1984). *The assault on truth: Freud's suppression of the Seduction Theory.* New York: Farrar, Straus & Giroux.

Mayes, L. C. (2000). A developmental perspective on the regulation of arousal states. *Seminars in Perinatology, 24*, 267–279.

Mayes, L. C. (2006). Arousal regulation, emotional flexibility, medial amygdala function, and the impact of early experience: Comments on the paper of Lewis et al. *Annals of the New York Academy of Sciences, 1094*, 178–192.

Mayes, L. C., & Leckman, J. F. (2007). Parental representations and subclinical changes in postpartum mood. *Infant Mental Health Journal, 28*, 281–295.

Meins, E., Fernyhough, C., Fradley, E., & Tuckey, M. (2001). Rethinking maternal sensitivity: Mothers' comments on infants' mental processes predict security of attachment at 12 months. *Journal of Child Psychology and Psychiatry, 42*, 637–648.

Meins, E., Fernyhough, C., Wainwright, R., Clark-Carter, D., Das Gupta, M., Fradley, E., et al. (2003). Pathways to understanding mind: Construct validity and predictive validity of maternal mind-mindedness. *Child Development Perspectives, 74*, 1194–1211.

Meins, E., Fernyhough, C., Wainwright, R., Das Gupta, M., Fradley, E., & Tuckey, M. (2002). Maternal mind-mindedness and attachment security as predictors of theory of mind understanding. *Child Development, 73*, 1715–1726.

Meissner, W. W. (2009). The question of drive vs. motive in psychoanalysis: A modest proposal. *Journal of the American Psychoanalytic Association, 57*, 807–845.

Midgley, N. (2012). *Reading Anna Freud.* London: Routledge.

Mikulincer, M. (1997). Adult attachment style and information processing: Individual differences in curiosity and cognitive closure. *Journal of Personality and Social Psychology, 72*, 1217–1230.

Mikulincer, M., & Arad, D. (1999). Attachment working models and cognitive openness in close relationships: A test of chronic and temporary accessibility effects. *Journal of Personality and Social Psychology, 77*, 710–725.

Mikulincer, M., & Shaver, P. R. (2007). *Attachment in adulthood: Structure, dynamics, and change.* New York: Guilford Press.

Mills-Koonce, W. R., Gariepy, J. L., Propper, C., Sutton, K., Calkins, S., Moore, G., et al. (2007). Infant and parent factors associated with early maternal sensitivity: A caregiver-attachment systems approach. *Infant Behavior and Development, 30*, 114–126.

Mitchell, S. A. (1988). *Relational concepts in psychoanaly-*

sis: An integration. Cambridge, MA: Harvard University Press.

Mitchell, S. A. (2000). Relationality: From attachment to intersubjectivity. Hillsdale, NJ: Analytic Press.

Mitchell, S. A., & Aron, L. (Eds.). (1999). Relational psychoanalysis: The emergence of a tradition. Hillsdale, NJ: Analytic Press.

Moss, E., Rousseau, D., Parent, S., St-Laurent, D., & Saintong, J. (1998). Correlates of attachment at school-age: Maternal reported stress, mother–child interaction and behavior problems. Child Development, 69, 1390–1405.

Neumann, I. D. (2008). Brain oxytocin: A key regulator of emotional and social behaviours in both females and males. Journal of Neuroendocrinology, 20, 858–865.

Oppenheim, D., Koren-Karie, N., & Sagi, A. (2001). Mothers' empathic understanding of their preschoolers' internal experience: Relations with early attachment. International Journal of Behavioral Development, 25, 16–26.

Orange, D. M. (2009). Kohut Memorial Lecture: Attitudes, values and intersubjective vulnerability International Journal of Psychoanalytic Self Psychology, 4, 235–253.

Ornstein, P. H. (2008). Heinz Kohut's self psychology—and ours: Transformations of psychoanalysis. International Journal of Psychoanalytic Self Psychology, 3, 195–214.

Person, E., & Klar, H. (1994). Establishing trauma: The difficulty distinguishing between memories and fantasies. Journal of the American Psychoanalytic Association, 42, 1055–1081.

Pierro, A., & Kruglanski, A. W. (2008). "Seizing and freezing" on a significant-person schema: Need for closure and the transference effect in social judgment. Personality and Social Psychology Bulletin, 34, 1492–1503.

Pizer, B. (2003). When the crunch is a (k)not: A crimp in relational dialogue. Psychoanalytic Dialogues, 13, 171–192.

Priel, B., & Besser, A. (2001). Bridging the gap between attachment and object relations theories: A study of the transition to motherhood. British Journal of Medical Psychology, 74, 85–100.

Quinodoz, J. M. (1996). The sense of solitude in the psychoanalytic encounter. International Journal of Psychoanalysis, 77, 481–496.

Repetti, R. L., Taylor, S. E., & Seeman, T. E. (2002). Risky families: Family social environments and the mental and physical health of offspring. Psychological Bulletin, 128, 330–366.

Rieder, C., & Cicchetti, D. (1989). Organizational perspective on cognitive control functioning and cognitive–affective balance in maltreated children. Developmental Psychology, 25, 382–393.

Rochat, P. (2009). Others in mind: Fear of rejection and the social origin of self-consciousness. Cambridge, UK: Cambridge University Press.

Russell, B. (1940). An inquiry into meaning and truth. London: Allen & Unwin.

Sandler, J. (1960). The background of safety. International Journal of Psychoanalysis, 41, 191–198.

Sandler, J., & Sandler, A.-M. (1998). Object relations theory and role responsiveness. London: Karnac Books.

Satpute, A. B., & Lieberman, M. D. (2006). Integrating automatic and controlled processes into neurocognitive models of social cognition. Brain Research, 1079, 86–97.

Senju, A., & Csibra, G. (2008). Gaze following in human infants depends on communicative signals. Current Biology, 18, 668–671.

Shane, M., Shane, E., & Gales, M. (1997). Intimate attachments: Toward a new self psychology. New York: Guilford Press.

Simeon, D., Bartz, J., Hamilton, H., Crystal, S., Braun, A., Ketay, S., & Hollander, E. (2011). Oxytocin administration attenuates stress reactivity in borderline personality disorder: A pilot study. Psychoneuroendocrinology, 36, 1418–1421.

Simon, B. (1992). "Incest—see under Oedipus complex": The history of an error in psychoanalysis. Journal of the American Psychoanalytic Association, 40, 955–988.

Simpson, J. A., & Belsky, J. (2008). Attachment theory within a modern evolutionary framework. In J. Cassidy & P. R. Shaver (Eds.), Handbook of attachment: Theory, research, and clinical applications (2nd ed., pp. 131–157). New York: Guilford Press.

Slade, A., Grienenberger, J., Bernbach, E., Levy, D., & Locker, A. (2005). Maternal reflective functioning, attachment, and the transmission gap: A preliminary study. Attachment and Human Development, 7, 283–298.

Solomon, J., & George, C. (1999). The caregiving system in mothers of infants: A comparison of divorcing and married mothers. Attachment and Human Development, 1, 171–190.

Sperber, D., Clement, F., Heintz, C., Mascaro, O., Mercier, H., Origgi, G., et al. (2010). Epistemic vigilance. Mind and Language, 25, 359–393.

Sperber, D., & Wilson, D. (1995). Relevance: Communication and cognition (2nd ed.). Malden, MA: Blackwell.

Sroufe, L. A., Egeland, B., Carlson, E. A., & Collins, W. A. (2005). The development of the person: The Minnesota Study of Risk and Adaptation from Birth to Adulthood. New York: Guilford Press.

Stacks, A. M., Beeghly, M., Partridge, T., & Dexter, C. (2011). Effects of placement type on the language developmental trajectories of maltreated children from infancy to early childhood. Child Maltreatment, 16, 287–299.

Stein, H., & Allen, J. G. (2007). Mentalizing as a framework for integrating therapeutic exposure and relationship repair in the treatment of a patient with complex posttraumatic psychopathology. Bulletin of the Menninger Clinic, 71, 273–290.

Stein, H., Fonagy, P., Ferguson, K. S., & Wisman, M. (2000). Lives through time: An ideographic approach to the study of resilience. *Bulletin of the Menninger Clinic, 64*, 281–305.

Stern, D. B. (1997). *Unformulated experience: From dissociation to imagination in psychoanalysis.* Hillsdale, NJ: Analytic Press.

Stern, D. B. (2013). Psychotherapy is an emergent process: In favor of acknowledging hermeneutics and against the privileging of systematic empirical research. *Psychoanalytic Dialogues, 23*, 102–115.

Stern, D. N. (1985). *The interpersonal world of the infant: A view from psychoanalysis and developmental psychology.* New York: Basic Books.

Stern, D. N. (1994). One way to build a clinically relevant baby. *Infant Mental Health Journal, 15*, 9–25.

Stern, D. N. (1998). The process of therapeutic change involving implicit knowledge: Some implications of developmental observations for adult psychotherapy. *Infant Mental Health Journal, 19*, 300–308.

Stolorow, R. D. (1997). Review of "A dynamic systems approach to the development of cognition and action." *International Journal of Psychoanalysis, 78*, 620–623.

Sullivan, H. S. (1953). *The interpersonal theory of psychiatry.* New York: Norton.

Sullivan, H. S. (1964). *The fusion of psychiatry and social science.* New York: Norton.

Symons, S. (2008). Lacan's concept of desire and its vicissitudes. *American Journal of Psychoanalysis, 68*, 379–398.

Trevarthen, C. (1993). The self born in intersubjectivity: an infant communicating. In U. Neisser (Ed.), *The perceived self: Ecological and interpersonal knowledge of the self* (pp. 121–173). Cambridge, UK: Cambridge University Press.

Trevarthen, C., & Aitken, K. J. (2001). Infant intersubjectivity: research, theory, and clinical applications. *Journal of Child Psychology and Psychiatry, 42*, 3–48.

Trevarthen, C., Aitken, K. J., Vandekerckhove, M., Delafield-Butt, J., & Nagy, E. (2006). Collaborative regulations of vitality in early childhood: Stress in intimate relationships and postnatal psychopathology. In D. Cicchetti & D. J. Cohen (Eds.), *Developmental psychopathology. Vol. 2: Developmental neuroscience* (2nd ed., pp. 65–126). New York: Wiley.

Tronick, E. (1989). Emotions and emotional communication in infants. *American Psychologist, 44*, 112–119.

Tronick, E. (2005). Why is connection with others so critical?: The formation of dyadic states of consciousness and the expansion of individuals' states of consciousness: Coherence governed selection and the cocreation of meaning out of messy meaning making. In J. Nadel & D. Muir (Eds.), *Emotional development* (pp. 293–315). Oxford, UK: Oxford University Press.

Tronick, E. (2007). *The neurobehavioral and social–emotional development of infants and children.* New York: Norton.

Tronick, E. (2008, March). *Meaning making and the dyadic expansion of consciousness model.* Paper presented at the Festschrift in Honor of Arnold Modell at the Boston Psychoanalytic Society and Institute, Boston.

Tronick, E. Z. (2003). "Of course all relationships are unique": How co-creative processes generate unique mother–infant and patient–therapist relationships and change other relationships. *Psychoanalytic Inquiry, 23*, 473–491.

Van Overwalle, F. (2009). Social cognition and the brain: A meta-analysis. *Human Brain Mapping, 30*, 829–858.

Vermote, R. (2011). On the value of "late Bion" to analytic theory and practice. *International Journal of Psychoanalysis, 92*, 1089–1098.

Vrticka, P., Andersson, F., Grandjean, D., Sander, D., & Vuilleumier, P. (2008). Individual attachment style modulates human amygdala and striatum activation during social appraisal. *PLoS ONE, 3*, e2868.

Wachtel, P. L. (2009). Knowing oneself from the inside out, knowing oneself from the outside in: The "inner" and "outer" worlds and their link through action. *Psychoanalytic Psychology, 26*, 158–170.

Wachtel, P. L. (2010). One-person and two-person conceptions of attachment and their implications for psychoanalytic thought. *International Journal of Psychoanalysis, 91*, 561–581.

Westen, D. (1991). Social cognition and object relations. *Psychological Bulletin, 109*, 429–455.

Widlocher, D., & Fairfield, S. (Eds.). (2004). *Infantile sexuality and attachment* (2nd ed.). London: Karnac Books.

Widom, C. S., Czaja, S. J., & Paris, J. (2009). A prospective investigation of borderline personality disorder in abused and neglected children followed up into adulthood. *Journal of Personality Disorders, 23*, 433–446.

Wilkinson, R., & Pickett, K. (2009). *The spirit level: Why equality is better for everyone.* London: Penguin Books.

Wilson, D., & Sperber, D. (2012). *Meaning and relevance.* Cambridge, UK: Cambridge University Press.

Winnicott, D. W. (1958). Primary maternal preoccupation. In D. W. Winnicott (Ed.), *Collected papers: Through paediatrics to psycho-analysis* (pp. 300–305). London: Tavistock.

Winnicott, D. W. (1965). *The maturational processes and the facilitating environment.* London: Hogarth Press.

Winnicott, D. W. (1971). *Playing and reality.* London: Routledge.

Young-Bruehl, E. (2011). *Childism: Confronting prejudice against children.* New Haven, CT: Yale University Press.

Zamanian, K. (2011). Attachment theory as defense: What happened to infantile sexuality? *Psychoanalytic Psychology, 28*, 33–47.

Zanarini, M. C., Frankenburg, F. R., Hennen, J., Reich, D. B., & Silk, K. R. (2006). Prediction of the 10-year course of borderline personality disorder. *American Journal of Psychiatry, 163*, 827–832.

# Chapter 35

# Couple and Family Therapy

## *An Attachment Perspective*

Audrey Brassard
Susan M. Johnson

Attachment theory, as a well-researched perspective on close relationships, can guide a therapist to the heart of a couple's difficulties, elucidating the task of restructuring key interactions, cognitions, and emotional responses. Attachment theory highlights the need for secure emotional connections with specific loved ones, and the regulation of emotions such as fear of loss and disconnection, as the implicit organizing elements in the interactions observed during couple and family therapy (C&FT). Bowlby (1973, p. 180) spoke of the relation between an individual and his or her environment (most essentially, loved ones) as the "outer ring" of a system, proposing that this outer ring is complementary to the "inner ring" that maintains an emotional "homeostasis" within each person's body and mind. Attachment is systemically oriented, in the traditional sense used in family therapy, and it also adds this "inner ring" to our understanding of relationships. Key concepts of child and adult attachment have been progressively integrated into existing models, such as behavioral couple therapy (Davila, 2003; Mondor et al., 2013) and multidimensional family therapy (Liddle, 1999). Attachment-centered C&FT interventions have also been adapted to specific difficulties and tested in a variety of settings. These include attachment-based family therapy (ABFT; Diamond, Siqueland, & Diamond, 2003), emotionally focused therapy (EFT) for couples, and emotionally focused family therapy (EFFT) (Johnson, 2004).

Attachment theory and research are crucial parts of an emerging relationship science (Johnson, 2013) that has begun to address the core mysteries of human relationships. In this emerging field of science, many different kinds of research, relationship concepts, and clinical findings are coming together to form a coherent whole, for example, data on the dyadic interplay of attachment, conflict, and support in determining satisfaction in couple partnerships (Brassard, Lussier, & Shaver, 2009: Kane et al., 2007), research on the nature of love as outlined by attachment theory and research (Johnson, 2003), and understandings of emotion and the "panic" triggered by disconnection (Panksepp, 1998). This research suggests that emotional responsiveness between adult partners predicts stability and satisfaction in relationships, and that positive cycles of interactions in which each partner responds to the other's attachment vulnerabilities are key to relationship repair and to the regulation of the primal panic that arises in negative interactions. Attachment theory and relationship science offer a perspective that integrates physiology, emotion, and interactional patterns, allowing a therapist to home in on, bring into focus, and restructure the organizing elements of close relationships.

In this chapter, we outline the unique contributions of attachment theory to C&FT and explain how these contributions are significant departures from the traditions of the field of C&FT. We then present prominent clinical models of C&FT based on attachment theory, along with recent outcome research. Finally, we outline future promising directions for attachment-oriented interventions in C&FT.

## Attachment: A Unique Perspective on Couple and Family Systems

### What Attachment Theory Offers to C&FT

On a general level, attachment theory offers couple and family therapists a broad, integrated theory of close relationships and normal growth within such relationships, including a clear outline of basic human needs and emotional processes from the cradle to the grave. For a therapist, this is invaluable. The theory is specific enough to guide the formulation of individual couples' or families' problems, then to shape interventions enacted in therapy sessions. The process of change includes helping partners to recognize and "own" their attachment needs and to guide partners to ask for these needs to be met in a clear, cogent way that fosters partner responsiveness.

Attachment theory also provides a compass in the intrapsychic and interpersonal maelstrom of couple and family distress. The goal of therapy is the creation of new, positive interaction cycles of emotional responsiveness that redefine the relationship as a whole. By providing a picture of relationship health, attachment theory offers an answer to the long-standing clinical question: What constitutes necessary and sufficient change? Attachment theory is arguably the only relational theory that offers a large body of research detailing the key interactions in healthy relationships and documenting the specific results of these interactions. Attachment theory and research inform a therapist about the nature of the pivotal processes and watershed events that define close relationships, and they offer guidance about how

to restructure these events in therapy. In all of the attachment-oriented models of C&FT described in this chapter, key change events and specific interventions are explained.

Finally, primary relationships have great healing power. Attachments to key people provide our "primary protection against feelings of helplessness and meaninglessness" (McFarlane & van der Kolk, 1996, p. 24). Attachment theory empowers a therapist to link self and system, and to create interactions that not only change a relationship but also address individual problems within that relationship. Attachment-oriented interventions have been used successfully to address a variety of clinical issues, including depression in adults and adolescents (Denton, Wittenborn, & Golden, 2012; Diamond et al., 2010), traumatic stress in adults (Dalton, Greenman, Classen, & Johnson, 2013), and negative, defiant behaviors in adolescents (Moretti & Holland, 2003).

The remainder of this section provides a closer examination of how the main tenets of attachment theory are relevant for couple and family therapists. These may be summarized in terms of how attachment theory addresses the following key issues: Attachment theory depathologizes dependency, emphasizes the power of emotion in organizing interactions, has clear implications for the therapeutic alliance and the role of the therapist in C&FT, offers a therapist a map to individual differences in relationship style, adds a cognitive component of working models to the focus on emotional response and interaction patterns, helps to explain how behaviors are passed on and perpetuated in families, and fosters engagement in therapy in that it is highly relevant to the lived realities clients bring to therapy (Johnson & Talitman, 1996).

### Depathologizing Dependency

The dominant discourse in the field of C&FT has long been one that promotes autonomy and is critical of dependency (Fishbane, 2005). In contrast, the central tenet of attachment theory is that seeking and maintaining contact with significant others is an innate, primary motivating force in human beings at all phases of the lifespan. Dependency is an innate part of being human, not a sign of enmeshed relationships or of lack of differentiation from others (Bowlby, 1988). Rejection and emotional isolation are inherently traumatizing. A sense of connection with loved ones can be maintained more readily on the cognitive, representational (working model) level as we mature, but contact is still a primary need. This need is universal across cultures (Mesman, Van IJzendoorn, & Sagi-Schwartz, Chapter 37, this volume), although it may be expressed somewhat differently in different contexts. The attachment perspective focuses the therapy on issues of connection and disconnection, and allows for the active validation of needs and fears concerning attachment. It offers the therapist a language for the "emotional starvation" (Levy, 1937) that characterizes an insecure relationship.

This perspective suggests that members grow and differentiate *with* each other rather than *from* each other. A felt sense of secure connection is seen as the best route to confident autonomy—a state that is often a key goal in family therapy, especially with adolescents. The *secure base* provided by a loving attachment figure encourages a cognitive openness to new information (Mikulincer, 1997). It promotes the confidence necessary to risk, learn, and continually update models of self and others, so that adjustment to new contexts is facilitated. It also strengthens the ability to stand back and reflect on oneself, including one's behavior and mental states (Fonagy, Luyten, Allison, & Campbell, Chapter 34, this volume). An increase in emotional accessibility and responsiveness is therefore a key goal in attachment-oriented C&FT, rather than focusing only on setting boundaries and developing assertiveness skills.

### The Pivotal Role of Emotion

Emotion is central to attachment, and attachment theory provides a guide for understanding and normalizing many of the extreme emotions that accompany distressed relationships. *Separation distress*, indicated by powerful emotions of anger, panic, and abandonment and sadness, results from the perception that an attachment figure is inaccessible or does not care. It is in attachment relationships that our strongest emotions arise and seem to have the most impact. When an individual is threatened—either by traumatic events or by a sense of disconnection in an attachment relationship—powerful affect arises, attachment needs for comfort and connection become particularly compelling, and attachment behaviors are activated.

A positive sense of connection with a loved one is a primary emotion regulation device (Mikulincer & Shaver, Chapter 24, this volume). The attachment view of family members as "hidden regulators" of each other's physiological and emotional worlds is supported by empirical studies (Coan, Schaefer, & Davidson, 2006; Johnson et al., 2013)

Attachment theory focuses the therapist on emotional experience and elucidates the logic and meaning of emotional responses. The valuing and active recognition of emotion has not, until recently, been a primary focus in C&FT. Emotion was considered to be either part of the problem or epiphenomenal to changes in family systems or individual behavior. In contrast, the models mentioned in this chapter are used to explore and reprocess key emotions, use emotion as a key change mechanism, and focus on barriers to emotional responsiveness.

### The Nature of the Therapeutic Alliance

The tenet of attachment theory that outlines the need for a safe haven and a secure base suggests that the creation of safe emotional engagement with a therapist is central to the clinical change process (Bowlby, 1988). Although C&FT has long espoused therapeutic alliances of a collaborative nature, the explicit validation and careful creation of a secure base in the therapies presented in this chapter, as well as the level of emotional engagement fostered between therapist and clients, reflects the attachment perspective. An attachment-oriented therapist acts as a surrogate attachment figure by actively helping clients regulate emotion, particularly the attachment-related anxiety or panic (Panksepp, 1998) that triggers negative emotional flooding or requires strongly avoidant suppression in insecure relationships.

Emotion is also more differentiated in the attachment perspective and so can be addressed and regulated in a more specific fashion by an emotionally present and attuned therapist. Therapists who understand the process of separation distress can tune in to a client's emotional perspective, look beyond disruptive responses such as hostile criticism or stonewalling, and place them in the context of legitimate attachment needs and fears, translating what might appear to be characterological deficits or lack of social skills into context-specific responses to loss of connection—responses that can be validated and restructured.

Bowlby (1988) noted that human beings are "strongly inclined towards self-healing" (p. 152). The therapist's job is to provide the context—namely, a secure base—that allows this natural healing process to occur. This is a very different theoretical frame from the one that casts the therapist as a magician or creator of miraculous reversals of negativity, which has been sometimes seen in the C&FT field.

## Understanding and Addressing Individual Differences

Attachment theory also offers the couple and family therapist a way to understand and address individual differences in affect regulation and engagement with partners. There has been an increasing emphasis in this field on respecting individual differences and moving away from a one-size-fits-all set of interventions. There are only so many ways of coping with disconnection—that is, with a negative response to the question, "Can I depend on you when I need you?" Attachment strategies in both parent–child and adult relationships can be described in terms of two main dimensions, anxiety and avoidance (Ainsworth, Blehar, Waters, & Wall, 1978; Brennan, Clark, & Shaver, 1998; see also Crowell, Fraley, & Roisman, Chapter 27, this volume).

When the connection with an irreplaceable other is threatened, the attachment system may become hyperactivated. Attachment behaviors become heightened and intense as anxious clinging, pursuit, and even aggressive attempts to obtain a response from the loved one escalate. The second strategy for dealing with the lack of safe emotional engagement, especially when hope for responsiveness has been lost, is to deactivate the attachment system and suppress attachment needs. This is done by focusing on other issues, such as work, and avoiding distressing attempts to engage emotionally with attachment figures (Mikulincer & Shaver, Chapter 24, this volume). These two strategies, anxious clinging and detached avoidance, can develop into habitual styles of engagement with intimate others.

A third insecure pattern has been identified—a combination of yearning for closeness, then fearfully avoiding reliance on a relationship partner because of potential emotional pain. This pattern is referred to as *fearfully avoidant* in the adult social-psychological literature (Bartholomew & Horowitz, 1991). In infants, a failure to establish a coherent, organized strategy is associated with chaotic or traumatic attachment experiences with frightening or abusive attachment figures (Main & Hesse, 1990).

All of these insecure patterns, which begin as accommodations to the ways in which key attach-

ment figures fail to provide a secure base/safe haven, can be rigidly and inappropriately applied in subsequent relationships, thereby generating ongoing negative cycles of interaction and lack of connection with loved ones. These adaptations become "self-maintaining patterns of social interaction and emotion regulation" (Shaver & Clark, 1994, p. 119). For example, when a partner anxiously demands contact, then withdraws when it is offered, a therapist sees a pattern of fearful avoidance and understands the dilemma of the client who not only longs for closeness but also turns it down, unable to regulate the associated fear and pain.

Attachment research has shown that these habitual forms of engagement can be modified by new or changed relationships (Simpson, Collins, Tran, & Haydon, 2007), which suggests that new interaction patterns created in therapy can have a significant impact on individuals and their relationships. In distressed relationships, attachment-related styles of perceiving and responding to others often operate outside awareness and are so habitual that they cannot easily be modified by the skills-building and cognitive reframing interventions so often used in C&FT. In the attachment-oriented models, the focus is expanded to include new attachment-related emotional experiences; a clearer way to address attachment needs; and the potential alteration of working models of self, partner, and relationship.

## Working Models: The Self in the System

Secure attachment is theoretically characterized by a working model of self as worthy of love and care and as competent. Research has strongly supported this aspect of the theory by showing that measured attachment security is associated with greater self-efficacy and a more coherent, articulated, and positive view of self (e.g., Mikulincer, 1995). Secure individuals, who have experienced their attachment figures as responsive and supportive when needed, also tend to have working models of others as dependable and trustworthy. These models of self and others are based on thousands of social interactions. They are carried forward into new interactions and new relationships not as one-dimensional cognitive schemas, but as emotionally charged procedural scripts for how to create relatedness under particular conditions. A person may have multiple and conflicting models, but most often one is dominant in a given context.

Working models are formed, elaborated, maintained, and—most importantly for the couple and family therapist—*changed* through emotional communication. The therapist can point out the pitfalls of specific perceptions that arise from negative working models, showing how they prohibit openness toward loved ones, block relationship change, and ultimately keep a person stuck with self-damaging perceptions and behaviors. At the end of therapy, for example, a 13-year-old boy might be able to say to his stepfather, "When I was little, with my first dad, I decided I was a bad kid. That was why he was so mad at me. Now I assume you think I'm bad, and when you get upset with me, I just tell you I don't care. I'll never please you anyway. I just give up." His stepfather can now tell him, "I don't want you to feel like you're a bad kid. You are my kid now—my special son. I don't want you to give up with me. And I want to learn to be a kinder dad."

### A Relevant Focus for Intervention

Bowlby began his career as a health care professional by studying the effects of maternal deprivation and separation on children. Attachment theory describes and explains the trauma of deprivation, loss, rejection, and abandonment by those we need most. Couple and family therapists know about the stress of deprivation and separation. They can see, for example, what Bowlby described in his 1944 article, "Forty-Four Juvenile Thieves"—that "behind the mask of indifference [of avoidant children] is bottomless misery and behind apparent callousness, despair" (p. 39). Bowlby saw his young charges as frozen in the attitude "I will never be hurt again" and paralyzed by their isolation and rage. Attachment theory encourages a therapist to reach, with empathic questions, reflections, and conjectures, behind partners and family members' masks and unpack separation distress, anger about rejections and hurts, and the attachment longings that color emotional reactions. Attachment theory has supreme relevance to the lived experience and dilemmas of couple and family members in distressed relationships.

### Attachment-Oriented Models of Intervention in Family Therapy

Although there are some emerging and potentially promising attachment-based family interventions with adolescents (Mackey, 2003; Moretti & Holland, 2003) and younger children (Hughes, 2011), there are only two family therapy models that have received empirical validation of their effectiveness and that systematically use an attachment framework to assess and address problems in families. These are ABFT (Diamond, 2005; Diamond et al., 2003) and EFFT (Johnson & Lee, 2000; Johnson, Maddeaux, & Blouin, 1998). These approaches assume that adolescents who enter therapy need to reconnect with parents in order to move toward more confident autonomy, and that a new level of emotional communication is necessary for this to occur. They address a wide range of symptoms, both internalizing (e.g., depression) and externalizing (e.g., conduct disorder). Both assume that attachment issues such as rejection, neglect, and abandonment are often obscured by conflicts related to behavioral problems (e.g., neglecting chores or homework), and that therapy must foster empathic, attuned conversations about relationship ruptures and attachment injuries.

### Attachment-Based Family Therapy

For adolescents, secure attachment nurtures healthy development, whereas insecure attachment is associated with depression and other problems in adaptation (Allen, Porter, McFarland, McElhaney, & Marsh, 2007; Herring & Kaslow, 2002). Practitioners of ABFT—an approach whose clinical procedures draw from many systems approaches, including EFT (Diamond et al., 2003)—have specialized in working with depressed and/or suicidal adolescents, who benefit from more direct communication with parents. Secure attachment is characterized by this kind of communication, which fosters perspective taking and effective, collaborative problem solving (Allen & Tan, Chapter 19, this volume; Kobak & Duemmler, 1994). ABFT aims to improve the family's capacity for problem solving, affect regulation, and organization. This strengthens family cohesion, which can buffer against suicidal thinking, depression, and risk behaviors.

Diamond and colleagues (2003) note that depressed adolescents usually talk in the first therapy session about feeling hopeless, alone, and angry at their parents. The parents speak of frustration about their own perceived failure to help their children. The parents' lack of availability at critical moments has often become a source of injury and alienation for the adolescents. ABFT is an attempt to help parents and adolescents address these "relational ruptures," address core attachment concerns (including increasing the adolescents' sense of entitlement to care), and develop a coherent understanding of attachment events. All of this increases the adolescents' sense of felt security and helps them to revise negative working models of self and other. A major challenge in this approach, and in all attachment-based family interventions, is to build the parents' capacity for providing a sense of security in their children. Diamond and colleagues point out that an adolescent's ability to express vulnerability and attachment needs often rekindles the desire for a parent's care, and the parent can then be helped by the therapist to connect with the child. This approach targets parental criticism and ineffective parenting, and the adolescent's withdrawal/hopelessness, inability to regulate emotions, and negative self-concept. The first session involves the family unit; the second is with the adolescent alone; and the third is with the parent(s) alone. The remaining sessions involve combinations of one or both parents and the adolescent, the adolescent alone, or a parent alone.

Treatment focuses on five specific tasks:

1. The *relational reframe task*, which aims at reducing hostility and criticism by reframing the problem in terms of negative interaction cycles (e.g., parental reaching out, adolescent rejection of help, parental criticism, and adolescent withdrawal).

2. The *alliance-building task with the adolescent*, in which the therapist connects with the adolescent, validating any sense of abandonment, acknowledging the burden of being "parentified" (i.e., having to take care of a parent), and empathizing with the pain of being triangulated in conflicts between the parents, as well as helping the adolescent to identify his or her concerns and goals.

3. The *alliance-building task with the parents*, in which the therapist prepares the parents to listen to and respond to the adolescent's concerns, reducing the parents' distress, which promotes their motivation to provide attachment security to their children and their willingness to learn emotion-focused parenting skills.

4. The *reattachment task*, in which the therapist sets up a conversation addressing core relationship failures, encouraging parents to respond to the adolescent's grievances with empathy, so that a new kind of family encounter can occur.

Parents at least acknowledging, when not apologizing, for past attachment failures promotes forgiveness and renewed mutual trust, thus revising the adolescent's expectancy and desire for parents protection and support.

5. The *competency promoting task*, in which the therapist promotes the adolescent's self-esteem and competency by encouraging parents to challenge and support the adolescent, and urging the adolescent to take more responsibility for his or her behavior.

### Emotionally Focused Family Therapy

The goals of EFFT are to modify the distressing cycles of interaction that amplify conflict and undermine the potentially secure connection between parents and children, and to shape positive cycles of accessibility and responsiveness that offer the developing adolescent a safe haven and secure base (Johnson, 2004). Therapy takes place in three stages: deescalation of negative cycles, restructuring of attachment interactions, and consolidation, across 10–20 sessions. The first two of these include the entire family. Once the network of alliances has been mapped out, the family members' views of the problem have been grasped, and the adolescent's problematic behavior has been placed in the context of family attachment patterns, sessions may be conducted with the adolescent alone or with any combination of family members. The therapist focuses on two tasks: the elucidation and reprocessing of key attachment-related emotions and emotional responses (the "music" of the relational "dance") and the gradual revision of key patterns of interaction to create a more secure attachment. The therapist focuses on emotion as the organizing element in interactions and acts as less of a coach than the therapist does in ABFT, relying instead on the power of new emotional signals to evoke new behaviors and revise expectations, perceptions, and models of relationships in both parents and children. The recognition, validation, and expression of attachment needs is a key part of EFFT, as is addressing the adolescent's frustration and despair over disconnection.

In the first stage of EFFT, the therapist focuses on the presenting problem and assesses dynamics with relevant family members, while validating each family member's perception of the presenting problem, and identifying and reflecting the family's negative interaction pattern. The therapist explores the impact of the negative family patterns on different family subsystems (e.g., the parental or sibling subsystem, mother and adolescent). The therapist then reframes the family problem as one arising out of an attachment crisis, thus normalizing family difficulties without blaming anyone (Palmer & Efron, 2007). At the end of the first stage, the therapist reframes dysfunctional or secondary emotional responses as part of a broader negative interactional pattern fueled by underlying primary emotions (e.g., fear, hurt, sadness, feelings of failure or unlovability) and attachment needs. Accessing the primary emotions creates empathy and responsiveness among family members, and helps the family deescalate (Johnson et al., 2005).

In the second stage of EFFT, the goal is to facilitate the restructuring of the family negative interactional pattern identified in the first stage. The therapist focuses on accessing and highlighting the unmet attachment needs of children and adolescents, while promoting parental accessibility and responsiveness to children's underlying emotions and needs. The change event in this stage occurs when the therapist facilitates the enactment of children reaching out to their parents with these underlying needs, followed by the parents' responsiveness to the child's vulnerability and bids for care, connection, and comfort. The therapist needs to support both parents and children in working through the fears associated with the vulnerability experienced in distressed family relationships and reengaging in new patterns of availability and responsiveness (Johnson, 2004).

In the final stage of EFFT, the therapist focuses on consolidating the changes family members have made in the second stage. At the end of this stage, the family is able to integrate the new ways of engaging in discussions, which are characterized by openness, responsiveness, and engagement among family members. The family new sense of connection can then translate into everyday cooperation and problem solving.

There are some similarities between both EFFT and ABFT and the work of John Gottman on emotional communication between parents and children. However, Gottman's model is more focused on teaching parents how to coach their children directly about emotions and emotion regulation (e.g., Gottman, Katz, & Hooven, 1997). Both EFFT and ABFT promote a particular way of being emotionally present with and attuning to family members. Trevarthen and Aitken's (2001) concept of *primary intersubjectivity* within an attachment framework, which explains how children's view of themselves emerges from their experience of what their parents tune in to and respond to in them, would also appear to be relevant here. In both EFFT and ABFT, there is more recognition of emotion than has been customary in the majority of family therapies; even so, ABFT appears to be somewhat more cognitive than EFFT and to use heightened emotion less when creating new kinds of parent–child interactions. All attachment-oriented models and interventions referred to in this chapter focus on helping parents and children repair attachment rifts and injuries, and elucidate interaction patterns and responses in a way that makes "the attachment needs that underlie problem behaviors visible" (Moretti & Holland, 2003, p. 245).

### Dyadic Developmental Psychotherapy

Dyadic developmental psychotherapy (DDP) was originally developed by Dan Hughes to treat children in foster or adoptive homes who have suffered abuse and neglect, and who manifest severe psychological difficulties associated with complex trauma and difficulties with attachment (Hughes, 2004, 2006). DDP has as its core the maintenance of a contingent, collaborative, sensitive, reflective, and affectively attuned relationship between therapist and child, between caregiver and child, and between therapist and caregiver. DDP focuses on and relies on the intersubjective sharing and joint development and organization of emotional experience. Hughes (2011) gradually expanded DDP into a comprehensive model of family therapy, also referred to as attachment-focused family therapy. The therapy model focuses on the attachment bond as a way to navigate complex emotions and behaviors in parent–child relationships, and understands problematic child behaviors in the context of past attachment traumas or injuries, as well as current stresses on the attachment relationship.

DDP is very similar to EFFT in terms of clinical process given their joint focus on emotion and bonding interactions, and removing the blocks to those interactions. In DDP, children are assisted in regulating and expressing their emotions and communicating emotional messages in ways that foster secure connection with a parent who is supported and responds with an attitude characterized by playfulness, acceptance, curiosity, and empathy. DDP is different from EFFT in that it is used not only with adolescents but also with children (as young as age 4 or 5) and their parents.

## Empirical Support for Attachment-Based Family Interventions

Two important randomized controlled trials of ABFT (12 sessions) have been conducted in the United States. In the first, Diamond, Reis, Diamond, Siqueland, and Isaacs (2002) randomly assigned 32 adolescents suffering from major depressive disorder (and their parents) to either ABFT or a 6-week waiting list. Results showed the efficacy of ABFT in reducing depressive symptoms posttreatment and at a 6-month follow-up. Treatment also significantly decreased adolescent levels of anxiety symptoms and family conflict. According to Diamond (2005), when parents were shown videotapes of sessions and asked to discuss changes that had occurred, the key factor seemed to be that the parents had come to understand how ruptures in their relationships with their adolescents contributed to the depression, and that their adolescents desired and needed their love. In ABFT, an adolescent first discloses anger about relationship failures. A parent is supported to remain nondefensive, apologize, and explain his or her own inability to make better choices. The parent and adolescent then share more vulnerable feelings and needs, and come to a better appreciation of each other's struggles. In a more recent randomized controlled trial, Diamond and colleagues (2010) showed that ABFT is more efficacious than enhanced usual care (EUC) in reducing suicidal ideation posttreatment and at 6-month follow-up in a sample of 66 adolescents. ABFT was more effective than EUC, regardless of whether adolescents had a sexual trauma history (Diamond, Creed, Gillham, Gallop, & Hamilton, 2012).

Examining the mechanisms of change, Shpigel, Diamond, and Diamond (2012) found that increases in maternal autonomy led to increases in adolescents' perceived parental care (during treatment) and decreases in attachment-related anxiety and avoidance (at follow-up) but were not related to change in depression or suicidal ideation. In terms of recent developments, Kissil (2011) proposed an application of ABFT to adolescent self-injury and presented a case study supporting the use of ABFT in this population. ABFT may be especially relevant to this problem, considering that self-harm is often conceptualized as an affect regulation strategy, a way to self-soothe that is more likely to be used by insecurely attached adolescents. According to De Silva and colleagues

(2013), ABFT is a "promising" empirically supported practice for the treatment of suicidal ideation and self-harm.

There has been less empirical support for the effectiveness of EFFT. In a preliminary study, the effectiveness of EFFT was supported in a study of 13 young women diagnosed with bulimia nervosa at an outpatient hospital clinic (Johnson et al., 1998). Most also met criteria for clinical depression, and several had attempted suicide. All subjects except one rated themselves as having either an anxious or a fearfully avoidant attachment, as assessed with the Relationship Questionnaire (Bartholomew & Horowitz, 1991). A cognitive-behavioral educational group ($n = 4$) was compared with an EFFT group ($n = 9$). Both treatments (10 sessions) were supervised by experts in these interventions, and implementation checks were conducted. Both were found to result in decreased severity of bulimic symptoms, lower scores on the Beck Depression Inventory, and reduced general psychiatric symptomatology. Remission rates for bingeing and vomiting were better than those reported for individual therapy. More recently, Robinson, Dolhanty, and Greenberg (2015) revisited EFFT as a promising model of therapy for families dealing with eating disorders (EDs) in children and adolescents, and case studies have provided some support to the efficacy of EFFT as a therapeutic intervention with families in which adolescents are struggling with symptomatic behaviors (Bloch & Guillory, 2011; Palmer & Efron, 2007), including nonsuicidal self-injury (Schade, 2013), or interventions with stepfamilies facing adjustment issues (Furrow & Palmer, 2007).

Although DDP does not meet criteria as an evidence-based treatment, the theoretical validity for DDP and what might be considered an initial pilot study are summarized by Becker-Weidman and Hughes (2008). Further study of DDP and its efficacy using larger samples, randomization, and restricted age range of the participants is warranted.

## Attachment-Oriented Couple Therapy

The couple therapy field appears to be moving toward greater recognition of adult attachment needs and the desirability of promoting emotional connection and nurturance in couples. A few commentators (e.g., Davila, 2003) have suggested ways in which the attachment perspective could be used to enhance behavioral couple therapy. In a recent study, Mondor and colleagues (2013) showed that attachment anxiety predicts early termination in cognitive-behavioral couple therapy. They suggested that because attachment insecurities might interfere with treatment continuation, therapists should assess and address attachment orientations in couple therapy, regardless of their therapeutic model.

Attachment theory suggests that many relationship problems are essentially due to the insecurity of the bond between partners and to the struggle to define the relationship as a potential safe haven and a secure base (Bowlby, 1969/1982, 1988). The key issue in distressed relationships is the negative cycles that maintain disconnection and limited responsiveness to emotional signals and attachment cues. As a distressed woman remarked to her husband, "It's not the fights that really matter. I could handle disagreements if I felt like you were there for me. But I can never find you when I need you. I feel alone in this relationship."

There is now an impressive body of research on the relevance of attachment theory to adult relationships (reviewed, e.g., by Mikulincer & Shaver, 2007, Chapter 24, this volume; J. A. Feeney, Chapter 21, this volume) both in clinical and nonclinical samples. Secure attachment, whether measured by questionnaires or interviews (see Crowell, Fraley, & Roisman, Chapter 27, this volume, for a review of measures), has been found to predict such positive aspects of relationship functioning as greater interdependence, commitment, trust, and satisfaction in couples (e.g., Mondor, McDuff, Lussier, & Wright, 2011); higher levels of seeking and providing support (e.g., Davila & Kashy, 2009; Kane et al., 2007); greater empathy and less withdrawal and verbal aggression (e.g., Fournier, Brassard, & Shaver, 2011; Péloquin, Lafontaine, & Brassard, 2011); more sensitive and appropriate caregiving behavior (B. C. Feeney, 2004, 2007; Millings & Walsh, 2009); and more satisfying sexual interactions (e.g., Brassard, Péloquin, Dupuy, Wright, & Shaver, 2012; Dewitte, 2012). Recent studies have also documented the interplay among the attachment, caregiving, and sexual systems (Péloquin, Brassard, Delisle, & Bédard, 2013; Péloquin, Brassard, Lafontaine, & Shaver, 2014). This research parallels other findings that indicate the pivotal importance of soothing and supportive responses in high-functioning relationships and the absolute requirement for safe emotional engagement (e.g., Gottman, 1994; Pasch & Bradbury, 1998).

EFT uses systemic and experiential interventions to promote change in couple relationships but places these in the context of an attachment–theoretical understanding of adult love relationships. As a couple therapy based on attachment theory, EFT is characterized by the following:

1. A focus on and validation of attachment needs and fears, and the promotion of safe emotional engagement, comfort, and support.
2. A privileging of emotional responses and communication, and directly addressing attachment vulnerabilities and fears to foster emotional attunement and responsiveness.
3. The creation of a respectful collaborative alliance, so that the therapy setting itself is a safe haven and a secure base.
4. An explicit shaping of responsiveness and accessibility (withdrawn partners are to be reengaged, and blaming partners are guided to ask that their attachment needs be met in a positive manner, so that bonding events can occur and serve as an antidote to negative cycles and insecurity).
5. A focus on self-definitions that can be redefined through emotional communication with partners (attachment figures).
6. An explicit shaping of pivotal attachment responses that redefine a relationship (as each person asks that attachment needs be met, and the other partner responds to ensure that positive bonding interactions occur).
7. Addressing and healing specific attachment injuries, including betrayals (e.g., infidelity) and abandonment at key moments of need (e.g., at the time of a miscarriage).

This approach has received extensive empirical validation in terms of both relationship outcomes and defined change processes. A meta-analysis of the most rigorous studies of EFT found that 70–73% of couples recovered from relationship distress after 10–12 sessions (with therapists who were receiving clinical supervision), and that 86% rated their relationship as significantly improved (Johnson, Hunsley, Greenberg, & Schindler, 1999). This meta-analysis also revealed a mean effect size of 1.3 across studies reviewed, which is considerable in psychotherapy research. The effectiveness of EFT does not appear to be as heavily influenced as other approaches by initial relationship distress levels. Specifically, initial distress was found to account for only 4% of the variance in satisfaction at follow-up, compared to an estimated 46% in the behavioral approaches tested (Whisman & Jacobson, 1990).

The attachment framework offers both clinicians and scientists a way of understanding how to create lasting changes and avoid relapse, even in brief therapy. There is evidence that results are stable, even in very stressed, high-risk relationships in which relapse might be expected (Clothier, Manion, Gordon-Walker, & Johnson, 2002; Halchuk, Makinen, & Johnson, 2010). If interventions reach to the heart of the matter (attachment injuries), they are more likely to create lasting change.

The nine steps in EFT are well documented in the couple therapy literature (Johnson, 2004; Johnson et al., 2005). The process of change moves from outlining negative interaction patterns and their attachment consequences to deepening the awareness of the core attachment-related emotions underlying these interaction patterns. A silent, withdrawn partner (typically a man) is able to attune to and express his helplessness and hopelessness when he sees the anger in his partner, and he can link this anger to his tendency to remain silent. He also begins to understand that his silence creates panic in his partner, which then fuels her critical complaining. In Stage 1 of EFT, *deescalation*, both partners begin to express newly accessed and formulated emotions, and to frame the negative cycle and disconnection as a mutual enemy. Once this cycle is deescalated, partners are guided in Stage 2 of EFT, *restructuring the bond*, to engage authentically with their emotions and to express the fear, sadness, or shame that keeps them blaming or distancing. Longings for connection and comfort can then emerge and be used to create more explicit and coherent bids for responsiveness from each other. This process is crystallized into key change events in Stage 2, in which the focus is on restructuring attachment responses and building positive cycles of connection. Here, more withdrawn, avoidant partners can assert their needs for validation and safety, and more anxiously attached, blaming partners can ask that their needs for comfort and connection be met. Stage 2 of EFT ends with a new kind of safe emotional engagement for both partners. These changes are then consolidated in Stage 3, *consolidation*: A new narrative or story about of how the relationship was threatened and repaired is created; new attachment behaviors are highlighted; and it becomes easier to solve pragmatic problems from a position of safety.

In the key change events of Stage 2, change occurs on multiple levels. As a blaming partner (typically a woman) finds herself asking that her attachment needs be met, she moves to a new level of affect regulation in which vulnerable emotions can be encountered, ordered, and expressed congruently, so that her attachment needs are made clear. She also moves away from her attributions of weakness and accepts her "softer side" as legitimate, integrating attachment fears and needs into her sense of self. As her partner responds favorably, her image of others as untrustworthy is challenged. As new, more secure interactions occur, a new pattern of attuned responsiveness is created that expands the couple's behavioral repertoire and model of relatedness.

In a typical session, attachment not only provides an overall perspective on a couple's problems but also elicits specific interventions. Empathic reflection of emotional responses and interaction processes, validation, and empathic questioning are used to create a sense of safety and focus the process on attachment needs. Here is an example:

"Peter, you said you try not to react so as to stop the fights. You also said, 'I put up a wall, and that is kind of sad.' The word *sad* really struck me. It *is* sad. It's a loss to you when you wall out someone you love. Yes? I wonder what it feels like behind that wall—the wall that Mary then rails against and 'hurls' herself toward with more and more fury. Do you ever talk to *her* about that sadness?"

The therapist then distills inner emotions and outer moves with the client, and clarifies attachment-oriented messages to the other while promoting new, more attachment-friendly interactions through enactments (i.e., directing one partner to talk to the other as the therapist intervenes in the evolving, moment-to-moment processes; see Tilley & Palmer, 2013):

"So you say that Mary sees this 'cool' guy, but inside you feel small and sad and lonely. You just don't know what to do when she tells you she isn't happy. You're scared of making a mistake, so you freeze up. You freeze not because she is unimportant, as she believes, but because she has such an impact on you. Can you tell her, please, 'When I feel small and scared, I do shut you out, and I see now how that upsets and frustrates you. I am so unsure of how to please you, I shut down before I can even think.'"

The therapist then turns to Mary and helps her respond to this new kind of interaction. Attachment theory has great breadth, but it is also specific enough to focus on the agreed-upon priority for most clinicians (Beutler, Williams, & Wakefield, 1993)—that is, to specify the therapist and client behaviors that create important moments of change.

A major development in EFT—the focus on the forgiveness of attachment injuries that block the creation of new levels of trust—speaks to the fact that a powerful theoretical map elucidates the nature of impasses in the therapeutic process and suggests how to deal with these impasses. Attachment theorists have pointed out that incidents in which one partner responds or fails to respond at times of urgent need seem to influence the quality of an attachment relationship disproportionately (Simpson & Rholes, 1994). Attachment injuries have been described as a perceived abandonment, betrayal, or breach of trust in a critical moment of need for support expected of attachment figures (Johnson, Makinen, & Millikin, 2001). Such incidents either shatter or confirm one partner's assumptions about attachment relationships and the dependability of the other partner, causing seemingly irreparable damage to close relationships. Many partners enter therapy not only in general distress, but also with the goal of bringing closure to such events and thereby restoring lost intimacy and trust. During therapy, these events often reemerge in an alive and intensely emotional manner and overwhelm the injured partner, creating an impasse and hindering the process of change. These incidents usually occur in the context of life transitions, loss, physical danger, or uncertainty (e.g., after a medical diagnosis or miscarriage), when attachment needs are most salient and compelling; as such, they can be considered relationship traumas. Attachment theory offers an explanation of why certain painful events, such as specific abandonments, become pivotal in a relationship, as well as an understanding of what the key features of such events will be, how they will affect a particular couple's relationship, and how such events can be optimally resolved. Such events are taken into account throughout therapy but are focused on and worked through in Stage 2 of EFT.

Makinen and Johnson (2006) conducted a study to test the effectiveness of the formulation of the EFT attachment injury resolution model (AIRM). The injured party is encouraged to clarify his or her pain associated with the event and to frame it in attachment terms. The other partner is then guided to respond with empathy and regret in a congruent and engaged manner. The injured party is supported to face his or her fears of becoming vulnerable again, and is able to ask that the attachment needs aroused by the incident be addressed. The other partner can now respond empathically, creating a positive reenactment of the original injuring event. This process is then integrated into the couple's story of the injury and their new ability to repair it. In Makinen and Johnson's study, all distressed couples with a single attachment injury recovered from relationship distress, reduced the pain caused by the injury, and reached positive levels of forgiveness. These results were maintained over a 3-year period (Halchuk et al., 2010). Couples with more than one attachment injury and very low initial levels of trust did experience reduced pain but had less positive results in the domains of forgiveness and relationship satisfaction. Dealing with these more seriously damaged kinds of relationships may be difficult or require more sessions than the limited number offered in this study. The steps of the AIRM were further validated in a recent psychotherapy process study (Zuccarini, Johnson, Dalgleish, & Makinen, 2013). Greenberg, Warwar, and Malcolm (2010) examined the impact of a similar EFT approach in 20 couples who experienced what they called "emotional interpersonal injury" and found that most individuals rated themselves at the end of treatment as forgiving their partners. They showed a significant improvement in dyadic satisfaction, trust, and forgiveness, as well as improvement on symptom and target complaint measures. These couples were able to maintain their gains at 3-month follow-up. Meneses and Greenberg (2014) identified three processes that predicted change in couple satisfaction and forgiveness among 33 couples: the "injurer's expression of shame," the "injured partner's accepting response to the shame," and "the injured partner's in-session expression of forgiveness."

## Recent Empirical Support for EFT for Couples

Based on an extensive review of research, EFT is considered to be an evidence-based treatment for couple distress (Snyder, Castellani, & Whisman, 2006), and it has been successfully adapted to clinical populations in which relational distress was either comorbid with or exacerbated by other stressful couple or family concerns, including parenting chronically ill children (Walker, Johnson, Manion, & Cloutier, 1996), facing postpartum depression (Whiffen & Johnson, 1998), or dealing with posttraumatic stress disorder (PTSD) (Johnson, 2002). Here we review recent evidence relevant to empirical validation of EFT for couples as a treatment for comorbid depression, chronic illness, and trauma/PTSD.

## Depression

Dessaulles, Johnson, and Denton (2003) initially randomly assigned 12 couples in which the female partner was clinically depressed to either EFT alone or antidepressant pharmacotherapy. They found no significant differences between the two conditions, but their results showed that levels of depression decreased from pre- to posttreatment in both groups. Moreover, only women from the EFT group continued to decrease their depressive symptoms from posttreatment to the 6-month follow-up. More recently, Denton and colleagues (2012) conducted the first study to compare antidepressant medication alone to antidepressant medication augmented with EFT for women with comorbid major depressive disorder and relationship discord. Although both treatments contributed to a diminution in depressive symptoms, women who received medication plus EFT reported more improvement in relationship satisfaction than did women who received medication alone. Replication of these results with larger samples is needed.

## Chronic Illness

EFT has also been viewed as a promising treatment option for couples experiencing psychological and relational distress following the diagnosis and treatment of chronic illness (see Tie & Poulsen, 2013, for a review). In early studies, McLean and Nissim (2007) provided two case studies of couples facing advanced cancer (colon, ovaries) and treated with EFT; in both cases, couples were able to switch from unresponsive or compulsive caregiving to reciprocal caregiving. Couture-Lalande, Greenman, Naaman, and Johnson (2007) studied two patients diagnosed

with breast cancer and their spouses; these couples received 16 sessions of EFT. Qualitative results suggest that the therapeutic process experienced by couples facing breast cancer is similar to that experienced by couples with partners in normal physical health. Significant improvement in symptoms of depression and couple satisfaction among patients diagnosed with advanced cancer and partners were also found in a study of 16 couples receiving EFT (McLean et al., 2008). More recently, a randomized controlled trial (McLean, Walton, Rodin, Esplen, & Jones, 2013) supported the efficacy of EFT in the treatment of relationship distress in end-stage cancer patients and their partners (but not their depressive symptoms) as compared to a standard care approach. Chawla and Kafescioglu (2012) presented case examples of the application of EFT to couples coping with traumatic brain injury and couples coping with cardiovascular disease. Their case studies suggest that EFT can produce deep couple/family attachment experiences in therapy and contribute to positive relationship outcomes.

## Trauma/PTSD

A preliminary qualitative study by MacIntosh and Johnson (2008) revealed that affect regulation is the most significant area of challenge for sexual abuse survivors in EFT. Shame, anger, hypervigilance, and an inability to trust and take risks were significant challenges for the studied couples. This type of extreme relational trauma and the relationship problems that it causes normally require a minimum of 30 couple therapy sessions (Johnson & Courtois, 2009). In a pilot study of seven couples in which one partner was a war veteran suffering from PTSD, there were statistically significant decreases in veterans' PTSD symptoms after participation in an average of 30 sessions of EFT (Weissman et al., 2011). Greenman and Johnson (2012) presented a case example to support the relevance of EFT in the treatment of couples in which one partner was diagnosed with PTSD. They suggested that EFT is suited to numerous aspects of the clinical presentation of PTSD, including difficulties with affect regulation, isolation, flashbacks, and dissociation. More recently, Dalton and colleagues (2013) published the first randomized controlled trial on the efficacy of EFT for relationship distress in which the female partner was a victim of severe childhood abuse. It showed significant increases in relationship satisfaction among the EFT treatment group at posttest, providing evidence of the effectiveness of a couple-based treatment for women with comorbid relationship distress and a history of childhood abuse.

## Process-of-Change Studies

Couple therapists need a detailed guide for their interventions to make significant differences in the lives of the couples with whom they work because they are managing two individuals whose thoughts, behaviors, and emotions are in constant interaction. This is problematic in light of repeated findings over the past 30 years suggesting that between 25 and 30% of couples who receive therapy do not demonstrate significant improvement, and that there are substantial rates of relapse (close to 40%) among those who do show improvement (Halford & Snyder, 2012; Halford et al., 2012). Despite claims of the relevance of process research for the day-to-day practice of couple therapy (e.g., Gurman, 2011) and calls for more practice-focused research with an emphasis on "specific mechanisms of change" (Sexton et al., 2011, p. 379), there has been scant research linking the process of therapy (i.e., what therapists actually do in session and how their clients respond to their interventions) to successful outcomes.

In a recent review of EFT process studies, Greenman and Johnson (2013) concluded that research conducted to date has allowed the validation of certain key assumptions of EFT. A growing number of studies has indicated that deep emotional experiencing in both partners is related to positive outcomes such as greater relationship satisfaction and a preponderance of empathic interactions (e.g., Couture-Lalande et al., 2007; Zuccarini et al., 2013). McRae, Dalgleish, Johnson, Burgess Moser, and Killian (2014) recently showed that EFT is successful in helping to increase partners' levels of emotional experiencing throughout therapy. Studies have also supported the assumption that critical change events, such as "blamer softening" when a previously hostile/critical partner asks, from a position of vulnerability and within a high level of experiencing, for reassurance, comfort, or for an attachment need to be met, are essential components of relationship improvement (Bradley & Furrow, 2004; Furrow, Edwards, Choi, & Bradley, 2012). Most such studies have relied on a task analysis of proximal outcomes to assess the process of change (Heatherington, Friedlander, & Greenberg, 2005).

## Attachment and C&FT: Where Do We Go from Here?

The attachment perspective is changing the field of C&FT. It is giving rise to systematic, empirically validated interventions and as part of the new science of relationships (Johnson 2013), it is also offering the field an explanatory framework for relationship problems, a detailed, research-based model of health, and a map for intervention. There have been important developments during the last decade, yet there are many additional questions to answer.

There is now preliminary functional magnetic resonance imaging (fMRI) research showing that a couple's participation in EFT is related to modification of neural responses to threat (Johnson et al., 2013). In a recent study of 24 couples, insecure female partners in distressed relationships at pretest did not benefit from holding hands with their partner to counter their fearful response to anticipated electric shocks or to dampen their perception of pain. At posttest, upon completion of EFT for couples, they were less sensitive to threat cues when they held their husbands' hands, compared to handholding with a stranger or being alone. This study supports the theoretical claim that, in addition to improving relationship satisfaction, EFT can affect couple members' ability to soothe each other's difficult emotions by strengthening their attachment bond and modifying the way in which the brain responds to threats in the presence of a romantic partner.

Another important development is the recent finding that EFT can change couples' levels of attachment insecurity, as assessed with both observational coding of attachment behaviors and a self-report measure of attachment anxiety and avoidance (Burgess Moser et al., 2015). More specifically, 32 moderately distressed and insecurely attached couples attended an average of 21 sessions of EFT. Couples significantly increased their secure base use and secure base provision from pre- to posttherapy, as assessed with the Secure Base Scoring System (SBSS; Crowell et al., 2002). Attachment-related avoidance significantly decreased over the course of EFT, whereas results were less consistent for attachment anxiety. Significant decreases in attachment anxiety occurred only for the subset of partners (16 of 32) who were able to engage in a key change event in EFT, the blamer-softening event, wherein a partner is able to ask for his or her needs to be met from a position of soft vulnerability (Burgess Moser, Dalgleish, Johnson, Wiebe, & Tasca, 2015).

A third development worth mentioning is that couple therapists using EFT, as well as behavioral clinical approaches, are now recognizing the importance of attachment insecurity as a predictor of change in marital satisfaction (Dalgleish et al., 2015), as a risk factor for early therapy termination (Mondor et al., 2013), or as an outcome of couple therapy (Benson, Sevier, & Christensen, 2013).

In the coming decade, attachment theory and research could contribute to our understanding of and ability to address pivotal transitions in close relationships. The transition to parenthood—a time when many relationships begin to unravel, and many women succumb to depression—is being examined through the lens of attachment (Rholes et al., 2011). The emotional support offered by the new father appears to affect the number of women who become more anxiously attached at this time (Simpson, Rholes, Campbell, Tran, & Wilson, 2003). If we understand these transitions in attachment terms rather than simply in terms of factors such as role change or general stress, we can more effectively help struggling couples and reduce the likelihood of clinical problems such as postpartum depression (Whiffen, 2003). Other transitions such as remarriage also warrant clinical and empirical research, as it may involve several attachment challenges such as attachment loss, loyalty struggles, unrealistic expectations, or competing attachment needs (Furrow & Palmer, 2011; see B. C. Feeney & Woodhouse, Chapter 36, this volume).

Another potential development is that attachment theory and research, paired with recent clinical evidence, can refine our understanding of sexual difficulties within a relationship (Johnson & Zuccarini, 2010, 2011). In a clinical sample of 242 couples seeking therapy, 60% of women and 64% of men were dissatisfied with their sex lives even though they were not necessarily seeking therapy for sexual difficulties (Brassard et al., 2012). This study also showed that attachment insecurity (anxiety, avoidance) was related not only to individuals' own sexual well-being but also their partners' sexual satisfaction (see Birnbaum, Chapter 22, for discussion of attachment and sex). Johnson and Zuccarini (2010, 2011) have proposed that EFT be adapted to deal with a number of sexual issues experienced by couples seeking EFT treatment (e.g., low sexual desire, erectile dysfunction). By reframing the sexual issues and

patterns as part of the dysfunctional interactional dynamic, it is possible to restructure them into a more functional and secure dynamic in which "emotional responsiveness, tender touch, and erotic playfulness can all come together" (Johnson & Zuccarini, 2010, p. 436). Empirical studies are needed to support the efficacy of EFT with couples facing sexual difficulties.

As research continues, it should contribute to the refinement and validation of C&FT interventions in couples where relationship distress is complicated by comorbid symptomatology, such as depression, PTSD, and other anxiety disorders. In addition to the recent evidence presented in this chapter, Priest (2013) has suggested the adaptation of EFT to the treatment of generalized anxiety disorder (GAD), a syndrome often associated with marital distress (e.g., Whisman, 2007) and insecure attachment orientations (Eng & Heimberg, 2006). Soltani, Shairi, Roshan, and Rahimi (2014) have also provided early support for EFT in reducing stress, depression, and anxiety symptoms in couples facing infertility. Attachment theory gives us a way of seeing the coherence in the web of symptoms and interpersonal difficulties that our clients present; it therefore helps us identify the most effective targets for change.

Recent work by EFT therapists has also provided descriptions of the application of EFT for same-sex couples (Hardtke, Armstrong, & Johnson, 2010; Zuccarini & Karos, 2011) and culturally diverse couples (Liu & Wittenborn, 2011). To our knowledge, only one study (Diamond et al., 2013) has obtained preliminary data on the feasibility and efficacy of the adapted ABFT treatment with suicidal lesbian, gay, and bisexual (LGB) adolescents.

Many studies have supported the associations between attachment insecurity and intimate partner violence (IPV) in couples from the community (e.g., Lafontaine & Lussier, 2005; Péloquin et al., 2011) and among clinical samples of men seeking treatment (e.g., Brassard et al., 2014; Fournier et al., 2011). They have identified mechanisms by which more insecure individuals behave aggressively toward their partners: poor anger regulation and empathy, low relationship satisfaction, and the presence of a demand–withdraw pattern of communication. Because EFT requires a secure environment in which deeper and more vulnerable emotions can be addressed, IPV has been used as an exclusion criterion for couples seeking therapy. Research could examine the possibility of carefully using EFT when minor aggressive behaviors are perpetrated by partners in the context of a dysfunctional interactional dynamic.

The promise of attachment research is that with the conceptual map provided by this perspective, interventions can both systematize relationship repair and thereby stabilize families and also open the door to all the benefits associated with more secure attachment, such as resilience and increased empathy for others. Einstein asked how the sciences could ever hope to explain so important a biological phenomenon as love. The science of attachment is in fact continuing to expand our understanding of the bonds of love between family members and adult partners, and this understanding allows us to provide better therapeutic interventions. We believe that relationship-oriented, attachment-informed interventions are among the most exciting developments in the field of psychotherapy and psychology more generally.

## References

Ainsworth, M. D. S., Blehar, M. C., Waters, E., & Wall, S. (1978). *Patterns of attachment: A psychological study of the Strange Situation*. Hillsdale, NJ: Erlbaum.

Allen, J. P., Porter, M. R., McFarland, F. C., McElhaney, K. B., & Marsh, P. A. (2007). The relation of attachment security to adolescents' paternal and peer relationships, depression, and externalizing behavior. *Child Development, 78*, 1222–1239.

Bartholomew, K., & Horowitz, L. (1991). Attachment styles among young adults. *Journal of Personality and Social Psychology, 61*, 226–244.

Becker-Weidman, A., & Hughes, D. (2008). Dyadic developmental psychotherapy: An evidence-based treatment for children with complex trauma and disorders of attachment. *Child and Family Social Work, 13*, 329–337.

Benson, L. A., Sevier, M., & Christensen, A. (2013). The impact of behavioral couple therapy on attachment in distressed couples. *Journal of Marital and Family Therapy, 39*, 407–430.

Beutler, L. E., Williams, R. E., & Wakefield, P. J. (1993). Obstacles to disseminating applied psychological science. *Applied and Preventive Psychology, 2*, 53–58.

Bloch, L., & Guillory, P. T. (2011). The attachment frame is the thing: Emotion-focused family therapy in adolescence. *Journal of Couple and Relationship Therapy, 10*, 229–245.

Bowlby, J. (1944). Forty-four juvenile thieves: Their characters and home life. *International Journal of Psycho-Analysis, 25*, 19–52.

Bowlby, J. (1973). *Attachment and loss: Vol. 2. Separation: Anxiety and anger*. New York: Basic Books.

Bowlby, J. (1982). *Attachment and loss: Vol. 1. Attach-

ment*. New York: Basic Books. (Original work published 1969)

Bowlby, J. (1988). *A secure base: Clinical applications of attachment theory*. London: Routledge.

Bradley, B., & Furrow, J. (2004). Toward a mini-theory of blamer softening. *Journal of Marital and Family Therapy, 30*, 233–246.

Brassard, A., Darveau, V., Péloquin, K., Lussier, Y., & Shaver, P. R (2014). Childhood sexual abuse and intimate partner violence in a clinical sample of men: The mediating roles of adult attachment and anger management. *Journal of Aggression, Maltreatment and Trauma, 23*, 683–704.

Brassard, A., Lussier, Y., & Shaver, P. R. (2009). Attachment, conflict, and couple satisfaction: Test of a mediational dyadic model. *Family Relations, 58*, 634–646.

Brassard, A., Péloquin, K., Dupuy, E., Wright, J., & Shaver, P. R., (2012). Romantic attachment insecurity predicts sexual dissatisfaction in couples seeking marital therapy. *Journal of Sex and Marital Therapy, 38*, 245–262.

Brennan, K. A., Clark, C. L., & Shaver, P. R. (1998). Self-report measurement of adult romantic attachment: An integrative overview. In J. A. Simpson & W. S. Rholes (Eds.), *Attachment theory and close relationships* (pp. 46–76). New York: Guilford Press.

Burgess Moser, M., Dalgleish, T. L., Johnson, S. M., Lafontaine, M. F., Wiebe, S., & Tasca, G. A. (in press). Changes in relationship-specific romantic attachment in emotionally focused couple therapy. *Journal of Marital and Family Therapy*.

Burgess Moser, M., Dalgleish, T. L., Johnson, S. M., Wiebe, S., & Tasca, G. (2015). The impact of blamer softening on romantic attachment in emotionally focused therapy. Manuscript in preparation.

Chawla, N., & Kafescioglu, N. (2012). Evidence-based couple therapy for chronic illnesses: Enriching the emotional quality of relationships with emotionally focused therapy. *Journal of Family Psychotherapy, 23*, 42–53.

Clothier, P., Manion, I., Gordon-Walker, J., & Johnson, S. M. (2002). Emotionally focused interventions for couples with chronically ill children: A two year follow-up. *Journal of Marital and Family Therapy, 28*, 391–399.

Coan, J., Schaefer, H., & Davidson, R. (2006). Lending a hand. *Psychological Science, 17*, 1–8.

Couture-Lalande, M. E., Greenman, P. S., Naaman, S. S., & Johnson, S. M. (2007) [La thérapie de couple axée sur l'émotion (EFT) pour traiter les couples dont la femme a le cancer du sein: Une étude exploratoire [Emotion-focused therapy (EFT) to treat couples in which the women suffers from breast cancer: An exploratory study]. *Psycho-Oncology, 1*, 257–264.

Crowell, J. A., Treboux, D., Gao, Y., Fyffe, C., Pan, H., & Waters, E. (2002). Assessing secure base behavior in adulthood: Development of a measure, links to adult attachment representations, and relations to couples' communication and reports of relationships. *Developmental Psychology, 38,* 679–693.

Dalgleish, T. L., Johnson, S. M., Burgess Moser, M., Lafontaine, M. F., Wiebe, S. A., & Tasca, G. A. (2015). Predicting change in marital satisfaction throughout emotionally focused couples therapy. *Journal of Marital and Family Therapy, 41,* 276–291.

Dalton, E., Greenman, P. S., Classen, C. C., & Johnson, S. M. (2013). Nurturing connections in the aftermath of childhood trauma: A randomized controlled trial of emotionally focused couple therapy for female survivors of childhood abuse. *Couple and Family Psychology: Research and Practice, 2,* 209–221.

Davila, J. (2003). Attachment processes in couple therapy: Informing behavioral models. In S. M. Johnson & V. E. Whiffen (Eds.), *Attachment processes in couple and family therapy* (pp. 124–143). New York: Guilford Press.

Davila, J., & Kashy, D. A. (2009). Secure base processes in couples: Daily associations between support experiences and attachment security. *Journal of Family Psychology, 23,* 76–88.

Davis, P. T., & Cummings, M. E. (1994). Marital conflict and child adjustment: An emotional security hypothesis. *Psychological Bulletin, 116,* 387–411.

Denton, W. H., Wittenborn, A. K., & Golden, R. N. (2012). Augmenting antidepressant medication treatment of depressed women with emotionally focused therapy for couples: A randomized pilot study. *Journal of Marital and Family Therapy, 38,* 23–38.

De Silva, S., Parker, A., Purcell, R., Callahan, P., Liu, P., & Hetrick, S. (2013). Mapping the evidence of prevention and intervention studies for suicidal and self-harming behaviors in young people. *Crisis, 34,* 223–232.

Dessaulles, A., Johnson, S. M., & Denton, W. H. (2003). Emotion-focused therapy for couples in the treatment of depression: A pilot study. *American Journal of Family Therapy, 31,* 345–353.

Dewitte, M. (2012). Different perspectives on the sex–attachment link: Towards an emotion-motivational account. *Journal of Sex Research, 49,* 105–124.

Diamond, G. (2005). Attachment–based family therapy for depressed and anxious adolescents. In J. Lebow (Ed.), *Handbook of clinical family therapy* (pp. 17–41). Hoboken, NJ: Wiley.

Diamond, G., Siqueland, L., & Diamond, G. M. (2003). Attachment-based family therapy for depressed adolescents: Programmatic treatment development. *Clinical Child and Family Psychology Review, 6,* 107–128.

Diamond, G. M., Diamond, G. S., Levy, S., Closs, C., Ladipo, T., & Siqueland, L. (2013). Attachment-based family therapy for suicidal lesbian, gay, and bisexual adolescents: A treatment development study and open trial with preliminary findings. *Psychology of Sexual Orientation and Gender Diversity, 1,* 91–100.

Diamond, G. S., Creed, T. A., Gillham, J., Gallop, R., & Hamilton, J. L. (2012). Sexual trauma history does not moderate treatment outcome in attachment-based family therapy (ABFT) for adolescents with suicide ideation. *Journal of Family Psychology, 26,* 595–605.

Diamond, G. S., Reis, B. F., Diamond, G. M., Siqueland, L., & Isaacs, L. (2002). Attachment-based family therapy for depressed adolescents: A treatment development study. *Journal of the American Academy of Child and Adolescent Psychiatry, 41,* 1190–1196.

Diamond, G. S., Wintersteen, M. B., Brown, G. K., Diamond, G. M., Gallop, R., Shelef, K., et al. (2010). Attachment-based family therapy for suicidal adolescents: A randomized controlled trial. *Journal of the American Academy of Child and Adolescent Psychiatry, 49,* 122–131.

Eng, W., & Heimberg, R. G. (2006). Interpersonal correlates of generalized anxiety disorder: Self versus other perception. *Anxiety Disorders, 20,* 380–387.

Feeney, B. C. (2004). A secure base: Responsive support of goal strivings and exploration in adult intimate relationships. *Journal of Personality and Social Psychology, 87,* 631–648.

Feeney, B. C. (2007). The dependency paradox in close relationships: Accepting dependence promotes independence. *Journal of Personality and Social Psychology, 92,* 268–285.

Fishbane, M. (2005). Differentiation and dialogue in intergenerational relationships. In J. Lebow (Ed.), *Handbook of clinical family therapy* (pp. 543–568). Hoboken, NJ: Wiley.

Fournier, B., Brassard, A., & Shaver, P. R. (2011). Attachment and intimate partner violence: The demand-withdraw communication pattern and relationship satisfaction as mediators. *Journal of Interpersonal Violence, 26,* 1982–2003.

Furrow, J. L., Edwards, S. A., Choi, Y., & Bradley, B. (2012). Therapist presence in emotionally focused couple therapy blamer softening events: Promoting change through emotional experience. *Journal of Marital and Family Therapy, 38,* 39–49.

Furrow, J. L., & Palmer, G. (2007). EFFT and blended families: Building bonds from the inside out. *Journal of Systemic Therapies, 26,* 44–58.

Furrow, J. L., & Palmer, G. (2011). Emotionally focused therapy for remarried couples: Making new connections and facing competing attachments. In J. L. Furrow, S. M. Johnson, & B. A. Bradley (Eds.), *The emotionally focused casebook: New directions in treating couples* (pp. 271–294). New York: Routledge.

Gottman, J. M. (1994). *What predicts divorce?* Hillsdale, NJ: Erlbaum.

Gottman, J. M., Katz, L. F., & Hooven, C. (1997). *Meta-emotion: How families communicate emotionally.* Hillsdale, NJ: Erlbaum.

Greenberg, L., Warwar, S., & Malcolm, W. (2010). Emotion-focused couples therapy and the facilitation of forgiveness. *Journal of Marital and Family Therapy, 36,* 28–42.

Greenman, P. S., & Johnson, S. M. (2012). United we

stand: Emotionally focused therapy for couples in the treatment of posttraumatic stress disorder. *Journal of Clinical Psychology: In Session, 68,* 561–569.

Greenman, P. S., & Johnson, S. M. (2013). Process research on emotionally focused therapy (EFT) for couples: Linking theory to practice. *Family Process, 52,* 46–61.

Gurman, A. S. (2011). Couple therapy research and the practice of couple therapy: Can we talk? *Family Process, 50,* 280–292.

Halchuk, R. E., Makinen, J. A., & Johnson, S. M. (2010). Resolving attachment injuries in couples using emotionally focused therapy: A three-year follow-up. *Journal of Couple and Relationship Therapy, 9,* 31–47.

Halford, W. K., Hayes, S., Christensen, A., Lambert, M. J., Baucom, D. H., & Atkins, D. C. (2012). Toward making progress feedback an effective common factor in couple therapy. *Behavior Therapy, 43,* 49–60.

Halford, W. K., & Snyder, D. K. (2012). Universal processes and common factors in couple therapy and relationship education. *Behavior Therapy, 43,* 1–12.

Hardtke, K. K., Armstrong, M. S., & Johnson, S. (2010). Emotionally focused couple therapy: A full-treatment model well-suited to the specific needs of lesbian couples. *Journal of Couple and Relationship Therapy, 9,* 312–326.

Heatherington, L., Friedlander, M. L., & Greenberg, L. S. (2005). Change process research in couples and family therapy: Methodological challenges and opportunities. *Journal of Family Psychology, 19,* 18–27.

Herring, M., & Kaslow, N. J. (2002). Depression and attachment in families: A child-focused perspective. *Family Process, 41,* 494–506.

Hughes, D. (2004). An attachment-based treatment of maltreated children and young people. *Attachment and Human Development, 6,* 263–278.

Hughes, D. (2006). *Building the bonds of attachment* (2nd ed.). New York: Aronson.

Hughes, D. (2011). *Attachment-focused family therapy workbook.* New York: Norton.

Johnson, S. M. (2002). *Emotionally focused couple therapy with trauma survivors: Strengthening attachment bonds.* New York: Guilford Press.

Johnson, S. M. (2003). Attachment theory: A guide for couple therapy. In S. M. Johnson & V. E. Whiffen (Eds.), *Attachment processes in couple and family therapy* (pp. 103–123). New York: Guilford Press.

Johnson, S. M. (2004). *The practice of emotionally focused couple therapy: Creating connection* (2nd ed.). New York: Brunner-Routledge.

Johnson, S. M. (2013). *Love sense: The revolutionary new science of romantic relationships.* New York: Little, Brown.

Johnson, S. M., Bradley, B., Furrow, J., Lee, A., Palmer, G., Tilley, D., et al. (2005). *Becoming an emotionally focused couple therapist: The workbook.* New York: Brunner-Routledge.

Johnson, S. M., Burgess Moser, M., Beckes, L., Smith, A., Dalgleish, T., Halchuk, R., et al. (2013). Soothing the threatened brain: Leveraging contact comfort with emotionally focused therapy, *PLoS ONE, 8*(11), 1–10.

Johnson, S. M., & Courtois, C. A. (2009). Couple therapy. In C. A. Courtois & J. D. Ford (Eds.), *Treating complex traumatic stress disorders: An evidence-based guide* (pp. 371–390). New York: Guilford Press.

Johnson, S. M., Hunsley, J., Greenberg, L., & Schlindler, D. (1999). Emotionally focused couples therapy: Status and challenges. *Clinical Psychology: Science and Practice, 6,* 67–79.

Johnson, S. M., & Lee, A. (2000). Emotionally focused family therapy: Restructuring attachment. In C. E. Bailey (Ed.), *Children in therapy: Using the family as a resource* (pp. 112–136). New York: Norton.

Johnson, S. M., Maddeaux, C., & Blouin, J. (1998). Emotionally focused family therapy for bulimia: Changing attachment patterns. *Psychotherapy, 35,* 238–247.

Johnson, S. M., Makinen, J., & Millikin, J. (2001). Attachment injuries in couple relationships: A new perspective on impasses in couples therapy. *Journal of Marital and Family Therapy, 27,* 145–155.

Johnson, S. M., & Talitman, E. (1996). Predictors of success in emotionally focused marital therapy. *Journal of Marital and Family Therapy, 23,* 135–152.

Johnson, S. M., & Zuccarini, D. (2010). Integrating sex and attachment in emotionally focused couple therapy. *Journal of Marital and Family Therapy, 36,* 431–445.

Johnson, S. M., & Zuccarini, D. (2011). EFT for sexual issues: An integrated model of couple and sex therapy. In J. L. Furrow, S. M. Johnson, & B. A. Bradley (Eds.), *The emotionally focused casebook: New directions in treating couples* (pp. 219–246). New York: Routledge.

Kane, H. S., Jaremka, L. M., Guichard, A. C., Ford, M. B., Collins, N. L., & Feeney, B. C. (2007). Feeling supported and feeling satisfied: How one partner's attachment style predicts the other partner's relationship experiences. *Journal of Social and Personal Relationships, 24,* 535–555.

Kissil, K. (2011). Attachment-based family therapy for adolescent self-injury. *Journal of Family Psychotherapy, 22,* 313–327.

Kobak, R., & Duemmler, S. (1994). Attachment and conversation: Toward a discourse analysis of adolescent security. In K. Bartholomew & D. Perlman (Eds.), *Advances in personal relationships: Vol. 5. Attachment processes in adulthood* (pp. 121–149). London: Jessica Kingsley.

Lafontaine, M. F., & Lussier, Y. (2005). Does anger towards the partner mediate and moderate the link between romantic attachment and intimate violence? *Journal of Family Violence, 20,* 349–361.

Levy, D. (1937). Primary affect hunger. *American Journal of Psychiatry, 94,* 643–652.

Liddle, H. A. (1999). Theory development in a family-based therapy for adolescent drug abuse. *Journal of Clinical Child Psychology, 28,* 521–532.

Liu, T., & Wittenborn, A. (2011). Emotionally focused therapy with culturally diverse couples. In J. L. Furrow, S. M. Johnson, & B. A. Bradley (Eds.), *The emotionally focused casebook: New directions in treating couples* (pp. 295–316). New York: Routledge.

MacIntosh, H. B., & Johnson, S. (2008).Emotionally focused therapy for couples and childhood sexual abuse survivors. *Journal of Marital and Family Therapy, 34,* 298–315.

Mackey, S. K. (2003). Adolescence and attachment: From theory to treatment implications. In P. Erdman & T. Caffery (Eds.), *Attachment and family systems: Conceptual, empirical, and therapeutic relatedness* (pp. 79–113). New York: Brunner-Routledge.

Main, M., & Hesse, E. (1990). Parents' unresolved traumatic experiences are related to infant disorganized attachment status: Is frightened and/or frightening parental behavior the linking mechanism? In M. T. Greenberg, D. Cicchetti, & E. M. Cummings (Eds.), *Attachment in the preschool years: Theory, research, and intervention* (pp. 161–182). Chicago: University of Chicago Press.

Makinen, J. A., & Johnson, S. M. (2006). Resolving attachment injuries in couples using emotionally focused therapy: Steps toward forgiveness and reconciliation. *Journal of Consulting and Clinical Psychology, 74,* 1055–1064.

McFarlane, A. C., & van der Kolk, B. A. (1996). Trauma and its challenge to society. In B. A. van der Kolk, A. C. McFarlane, & L. Weisaeth (Eds.), *Traumatic stress: The effects of overwhelming experience on mind, body, and society* (pp. 24–46). New York: Guilford Press.

McLean, L. M., Jones, J. M., Rydall, A. C., Walsh, A., Esplen, M. J., Zimmermann, C., et al. (2008). A couples intervention for patients facing advanced cancer and their spouse caregivers: Outcomes of a pilot study. *Psycho-Oncology, 17,* 1152–1156.

McLean, L. M., & Nissim, R. (2007). Marital therapy for couples facing advanced cancer: Case review. *Palliative and Supportive Care, 5,* 303–313.

McLean, L. M., Walton, T., Rodin, G., Esplen, M., & Jones, J. M. (2013). A couple-based intervention for patients and caregivers facing end-stage cancer: Outcomes of a randomized controlled trial. *Psycho-Oncology, 22,* 28–38.

McRae, T. R., Dalgleish, T. L., Johnson, S. M., Burgess Moser, M., & Killian, K. D. (2014). Emotion regulation and key change events in Emotionally Focused Couple Therapy. *Journal of Couple and Relationship Therapy, 13,* 1–24.

Meneses, C. W., & Greenberg, L. S. (2011). The construction of a model of the process of couples' forgiveness in emotion-focused therapy for couples. *Journal of Marital and Family Therapy, 37,* 491–502.

Meneses, C. W., & Greenberg, L. S. (2014). Interpersonal forgiveness in emotion-focused couples' therapy: Relating process to outcome. *Journal of Marital and Family Therapy, 40,* 49–67.

Mikulincer, M. (1995). Attachment style and the mental representation of self. *Journal of Personality and Social Psychology, 69,* 1203–1215.

Mikulincer, M. (1997). Adult attachment style and information processing. *Journal of Personality and Social Psychology, 72,* 1217–1230.

Mikulincer, M., & Shaver, P. R. (2007). *Attachment in adulthood: Structure, dynamics, and change.* New York: Guilford Press.

Millings, A., & Walsh, J. (2009). A dyadic exploration of attachment and caregiving in long-term couples. *Personal Relationships, 16,* 437-453.

Mondor, J., McDuff, P., Lussier, Y., & Wright, J. (2011). Couples in therapy: Actor–partner analyses of the relationships between adult romantic attachment and marital satisfaction. *American Journal of Family Therapy, 39,* 112–123.

Mondor, J., Sabourin, S., Wright, J., Poitras-Wright, H., McDuff, & Lussier, Y. (2013). Early termination from couple therapy in a naturalistic setting: The role of therapeutic mandates and romantic attachment. *Contemporary Family Therapy, 35,* 59–73.

Moretti, M. M., & Holland, R. (2003). The journey of adolescence: Transitions in self in the context of attachment relationships. In S. M. Johnson & V. E. Whiffen (Eds.), *Attachment processes in couple and family therapy* (pp. 234–257). New York: Guilford Press.

Palmer, G., & Efron, D. (2007). Emotionally focused family therapy: Developing the model. *Journal of Systemic Therapies, 26,* 17–24.

Panksepp, J. (1998). *Affective neuroscience: The foundations of human and animal emotions.* New York: Oxford University Press.

Pasch, L. A., & Bradbury, T. N. (1998). Social support, conflict, and the development of marital dysfunction. *Journal of Consulting and Clinical Psychology, 66,* 219–230.

Péloquin, K., Brassard, A., Delisle, G., & Bédard, M. M. (2013). Integrating the attachment, caregiving and sexual systems into the understanding of sexual satisfaction. *Canadian Journal of Behavioural Science, 45,* 185–195.

Péloquin, K., Brassard, A., Lafontaine, M. F., & Shaver, P. R. (2014). Sexuality examined through the lens of attachment theory: Attachment, caregiving, and sexual satisfaction. *Journal of Sex Research, 51,* 561–576.

Péloquin, K., Lafontaine, M. F., & Brassard, A. (2011). Romantic attachment, dyadic empathy, and intimate partner violence: Examination of the direct relationships and underlying mechanism. *Journal of Social and Personal Relationships, 28,* 915–942.

Priest, J. B. (2013). Emotionally focused therapy as treatment for couples with generalized anxiety disorder and relationship distress. *Journal of Couple and Relationship Therapy, 12,* 22–37.

Rholes, W. S., Simpson, J. A., Kohn, J. L., Wilson, C. L., McLeish Martin, A., Tran, S., et al. (2011). Attachment orientations and depression: A longitudinal study of new parents. *Journal of Personality and Social Psychology, 100,* 567–586.

Robinson, A. L., Dolhanty, J., & Greenberg, L. (2015). Emotion-focused family therapy for eating disorders in children and adolescents. *Clinical Psychology and Psychotherapy, 22*(1), 75–82.

Schade, L. C. (2013). Non-suicidal self-injury (NSSI): A case for using emotionally focused family therapy. *Contemporary Family Therapy, 35,* 568–582.

Sexton, T., Gordon, K. C., Gurman, A., Lebow, J., Holtzworth-Munroe, A., & Johnson, S. (2011). Guidelines for classifying evidence-based treatments in couple and family therapy. *Family Process, 50,* 377–392.

Shaver, P. R., & Clark, C. L. (1994). The psychodynamics of adult romantic attachment. In J. M. Masling & R. F. Bornstein (Eds.), *Empirical perspectives on object relations theories* (pp. 105–156). Washington, DC: American Psychological Association.

Shpigel, M. S., Diamond, G. M., & Diamond, G. S. (2012). Changes in parenting behaviors, attachment, depressive symptoms, and suicidal ideation in attachment-based family therapy for depressive and suicidal adolescents. *Journal of Marital and Family Therapy, 38,* 271–283.

Simpson, J. A., Collins, W. A., Tran, S., & Haydon, K. C. (2007). Attachment and the experience and expression of emotions in romantic relationships: A developmental perspective. *Journal of Personality and Social Psychology, 92,* 355–367.

Simpson, J. A., & Rholes, W. S. (1994). Stress and secure base relationships in adulthood. In K. Bartholomew & D. Perlman (Eds.), *Advances in personal relationships: Vol. 5. Attachment processes in adulthood* (pp. 181–204). London: Jessica Kingsley.

Simpson, J. A., Rholes, W. S., Campbell, L., Tran, S., & Wilson, C. L. (2003). Adult attachment, the transition to parenthood, and depressive symptoms. *Journal of Personality and Social Psychology, 84,* 1172–1187.

Snyder, D. K., Castellani, A. M., & Whisman, M. A. (2006). Current status and future directions in couple therapy. In S. T. Fiske, A. E. Kazdin, & D. L. Schacter (Eds.), *Annual review of psychology* (Vol. 57, pp. 317–344). Palo Alto, CA: Annual Reviews.

Soltani, M., Shairi, M. R., Roshan, R., & Rahimi, C. R. (2014). The impact of emotionally focused therapy on emotional distress in infertile couples. *International Journal of Fertility and Sterility, 7,* 337–344.

Tie, S., & Poulsen, S. (2013). Emotionally focused couple therapy with couples facing terminal illness. *Contemporary Family Therapy, 35,* 557–567.

Tilley, D., & Palmer, G. (2013). Enactments in emotionally focused couple therapy: Shaping moments of contact and change. *Journal of Marital and Family Therapy, 39,* 299–313.

Trevarthen, C., & Aitken, K. J. (2001). Infant intersubjectivity: Research, theory, and clinical applications. *Journal of Child Psychology and Psychiatry, 42,* 3–48.

Walker, J. G., Johnson, S., Manion, I., & Cloutier, P. (1996). Emotionally focused marital intervention for couples with chronically ill children. *Journal of Consulting and Clinical Psychology, 64,* 1029–1036.

Weissman, N., Batten, S. V., Dixon, L., Pasillas, R. M., Potts, W., Decker, M., et al. (2011, August). *The effectiveness of emotionally focused couples therapy (EFT) with veterans with PTSD.* Poster presented at the Veterans Affairs National Annual Conference: Improving Veterans Mental Health Care for the 21st Century, Baltimore.

Whiffen, V. E. (2003). Adult attachment and child bearing depression. In S. M. Johnson & V. E. Whiffen (Eds.), *Attachment processes in couple and family therapy* (pp. 321–341). New York: Guilford Press.

Whiffen, V. E., & Johnson, S. M. (1998). An attachment theory framework for the treatment of childbearing depression. *Clinical Psychology: Science and Practice, 5,* 478–493.

Whisman, M. A. (2007). Marital distress and DSM-IV psychiatric disorders in a population-based national survey. *Journal of Family Psychology, 116,* 638–643.

Whisman, M. A., & Jacobson, N. S. (1990). Power, marital satisfaction, and response to marital therapy. *Journal of Family Psychology, 4,* 202–212.

Zuccarini, D., Johnson, S. M., Dalgleish, T., & Makinen, J. (2013). Forgiveness and reconciliation in emotionally focused therapy for couples: The client change process and therapist interventions. *Journal of Marital and Family Therapy, 39,* 148–162.

Zuccarini, D., & Karos, L. (2011). Emotionally focused therapy for gay and lesbian couples: Strong identities, strong bonds. In J. L. Furrow, S. M. Johnson, & B. A. Bradley (Eds.), *The emotionally focused casebook: New directions in treating couples* (pp. 317–342). New York: Routledge.

# PART VI

## SYSTEMS, CULTURE, AND CONTEXT

# Chapter 36

# Caregiving

Brooke C. Feeney
Susan S. Woodhouse

Attachment theory provides an ideal framework for understanding caregiving because it stipulates that the need for security is one of the most fundamental of all basic needs (for individuals of all ages), and it provides a basis for understanding the complex interpersonal dynamics involved in three important and interrelated components of human nature: attachment, exploration, and caregiving (Bowlby, 1969/1982, 1973, 1980, 1988). All three systems are presumed to have survival value; thus, the urge to engage in each form of behavior is likely to be preprogrammed to some degree. The three systems are briefly described below as a backdrop for our discussion of caregiving processes.

First, drawing on ethological principles, *attachment theory* regards the propensity to form strong emotional bonds with particular individuals (attachment) as an innate human characteristic, present in infancy and continuing through adulthood and old age. According to the theory (Bowlby, 1973, 1969/1982), individuals come into the world equipped with an attachment system that functions to maintain their safety and security through contact with nurturing caregivers (also referred to as *attachment figures*). The attachment system becomes activated most strongly in adversity, so that when distressed (e.g., alarmed, anxious, frightened, tired, or ill), the individual feels an urge to seek protection, comfort, and support from

a primary caregiver (Bowlby, 1973, 1969/1982; Bretherton, 1987; Gillath et al., 2006). Attachment theory emphasizes that the desire for comfort and support in adversity should not be regarded as childish or immature dependence; instead, it should be respected as an intrinsic part of human nature that contributes to health and well-being.

Second, attachment theory states that another basic component of human nature is the urge *to explore the environment*—to work, play, discover, pursue goals, and take part in activities with peers (Bowlby, 1988). However, true or unencumbered exploration is expected to occur only when attachment needs have been satisfied (when the attachment system is deactivated). In this sense, exploration can be antithetical to attachment behavior, and vice versa (Bowlby, 1988); that is, when an individual of any age is feeling safe and secure, he or she is able to explore away from the attachment figure (or caregiver) and pursue autonomous activities. However, when feeling distressed in any way, he or she feels an urge to increase proximity. According to the theory, when individuals are confident that an attachment figure (e.g., a parent in childhood, a spouse in adulthood) is available when needed and will be responsive when called upon, they typically feel secure enough to explore the environment, take on challenges, engage in independent activities, and make discoveries. Exploration is also presumed to contribute to optimal health and well-being.

A third major component of human nature, according to attachment theory, is *caregiving* (Bowlby, 1969/1982, 1988). Caregiving includes a broad array of behaviors that complement (and support) a relationship partner's attachment *and* exploration behavior (Bowlby, 1969/1982, 1988; Kunce & Shaver, 1994). Thus, caregiving is viewed as serving two major functions: (1) providing a *safe haven* for the attached person by supporting his or her attachment behaviors, and (2) providing a *secure base* for the attached person by supporting his or her exploration of the environment. A major postulate of attachment theory is that individuals who thrive emotionally and socially, and who make the most of their opportunities, are those who have at least one caregiver (e.g., a parent in childhood or a spouse in adulthood) who is encouraging of the individual's autonomy yet responsive to needs when called upon.

We begin this chapter by elaborating on each caregiving function. We then review research on attachment and caregiving in parent–child relationships, followed by a review of research on attachment and caregiving in adult relationships. Following each of these reviews, we discuss directions for future research.

## Safe Haven

To remain within easy access of a familiar individual known to be ready and willing to come to our aid in an emergency is clearly a good insurance policy—whatever our age.
                              —JOHN BOWLBY (1988, p. 27)

A safe haven functions to support behavior that involves "coming in" to the relationship for comfort, reassurance, and assistance in times of stress (Bowlby, 1988; Collins & Feeney, 2000). From an attachment perspective, good caregivers are those who are able to effectively restore their partner's felt security when needed—by providing emotional comfort and facilitating problem resolution. Being *sensitive* and *responsive* to an attached partner's needs and distress cues as they arise is crucial to the maintenance of felt security (Ainsworth, Blehar, Waters, & Wall, 1978; Feeney & Collins, 2014). This involves the provision of the type and amount of support that is dictated by the situation and by the partner's needs—flexibly responding to attachment needs by taking into ac-

count the other's point of view, feelings, and intentions; by encouraging expression of feelings; and by adjusting one's own behavior in response to the contingencies of the situation. A sensitive and responsive caregiver is one who regulates his or her behavior so that it meshes with that of the person who is being cared for, takes his or her cues from and allows his or her interventions to be paced by the recipient, is attuned to the recipient's nonverbal signals, attends to the details of the recipient's behavior, interprets the recipient's signals and behaviors correctly, discovers what response is most appropriate for the individual recipient, responds promptly and appropriately, and monitors the effects of his or her behavior on the recipient and modifies it accordingly (Bowlby, 1988). In response, the care-receiver behaves in ways that take account of the caregiver's interventions. Thus, in a well-functioning partnership, each person is adapting to the other.

In contrast, an insensitive and unresponsive caregiver may not notice the recipient's attachment behaviors or signals, may misinterpret or ignore them when they are noticed, may interfere in an arbitrary way or behave in a rejecting manner, and/or respond late, inappropriately, or not at all to a need for support (Bowlby, 1969/1982, 1988). Thus, these caregivers may be neglectful, overinvolved, or out of sync with their partner's needs (Collins, Ford, Guichard, Kane, & Feeney, 2010; Kunce & Shaver, 1994). Thus, there are many ways that caregivers may be insensitive and unresponsive in times of need because being sensitive and responsive is not always easy, and even well-intended caregiving efforts may have unintended negative consequences. For example, caregivers may offer support in a way that makes the recipient feel weak, needy, or inadequate; that induces guilt or indebtedness; that makes the recipient feel like a burden; that minimizes or discounts the recipient's problem; or that blames or criticizes the recipient for his or her misfortune.

In his writings regarding responses to attachment system activation, Bowlby (1988) emphasized that adequate time and a relaxed atmosphere are necessary conditions for caregivers to behave in a sensitive manner. He also suggested that there is a strong tendency to treat others the same way that we ourselves have been treated; that is, although caregiving behavior is thought to be preprogrammed to some degree (meaning that it is ready to develop along certain lines when certain conditions elicit it), all the detail is learned. Thus, individuals are likely to learn either healthy or unhealthy caregiving patterns from the significant people who have previously been responsible for their care.

## Secure Base

*All of us, from the cradle to the grave, are happiest when life is organized as a series of excursions, long or short, from the secure base provided by our attachment figure(s).*
—JOHN BOWLBY (1988, p. 62)

A secure base functions to support behavior that involves "going out" from the relationship for autonomous exploration in the environment (Bowlby, 1988; Feeney, 2004; see also Crowell et al., 2002; Waters & Cummings, 2000). Good caregivers must know how to not only respond appropriately to attachment behavior and signals of distress but also support their partner's autonomous exploration (e.g., goal strivings, personal growth; Bowlby, 1988). This involves providing a base from which an attached person can make excursions into the outside world (to play, work, learn, discover, create, make new friends), knowing that he or she can return for comfort, reassurance, and/or assistance should he or she encounter difficulties along the way. Bowlby (1988) describes the concept of a secure base as one in which caregivers create the conditions that enable their relationship partners to explore the world in a confident way:

> In essence this role is one of being available, ready to respond when called upon to encourage and perhaps assist, but to intervene actively only when clearly necessary. In these respects it is a role similar to that of the officer commanding a military base from which an expeditionary force sets out and to which it can retreat, should it meet with a setback. Much of the time the role of the base is a waiting one but it is none the less vital for that. For it is only when the officer commanding the expeditionary force is confident his base is secure that he dare press forward and take risks. (p. 11)

Based on this description, three important characteristics of a secure base have been extrapolated (Feeney & Thrush, 2010). First, a secure base supports exploration by being *available* in the event that the base is needed (e.g., to assist in removing obstacles). Second, a secure base supports exploration by *not unnecessarily interfering* with it. According to attachment theory, intrusive/interfering behavior is antithetical to sensitive/responsive caregiving, and it is a major inhibi-

tor of exploration. This behavior likely inhibits exploration because it communicates a variety of negative messages to the recipient (e.g., that he or she is not capable of engaging in independent exploration, that autonomous exploration is threatening to close others). Third, a secure base supports exploration by being *encouraging and accepting* of it (Feeney & Thrush, 2010). Encouragement is expected to facilitate exploration because it conveys an excitement/enthusiasm regarding exploration, as well as confidence in the explorer's abilities.

Insensitive caregivers who do not provide an adequate, secure base are likely to take little notice of the partner's goals and goal-related feelings, to intrude in the partner's explorations, to fail to respect the person's desire for autonomy by discouraging or impeding exploration, to discourage bids for support and encouragement, or to respond in an ill-timed and unhelpful manner. Nonetheless, the importance of a secure base is evident for individuals of all ages. Just as children can be seen using their parents as a secure base for exploration by keeping track of the parents' whereabouts, exchanging glances, and from time to time returning to the parents to share in mutually enjoyable contact, adults can be seen engaging in similar types of behaviors. For example, an adult is likely to maintain phone contact when exploring away from a spouse for an extended period of time and share details of his or her explorations with the spouse. Bowlby (1988) suggested that individuals who are confident that their base is secure and ready to respond if called upon are likely to take it for granted. Yet should the base suddenly become unavailable or inaccessible, the importance of the base to the emotional equilibrium of the individual is immediately apparent.

## Research on Attachment and Caregiving in Parent–Child Relationships

Over 40 years ago, Mary Ainsworth and her colleagues (see Ainsworth, Bell, & Stayton, 1971; Ainsworth et al., 1978) were the first to report evidence that sensitive maternal caregiving (in response to both attachment and exploration needs, in both safe haven and secure base contexts) is linked to later infant attachment. Ainsworth and colleagues (1978) defined *sensitivity* as a caregiver's ability to perceive and accurately interpret infant cues, then respond promptly and appropriately to those infant cues. Their view of sensitivity included prompt and appropriate caregiver responses to both attachment and exploration needs. This seminal work inspired many other researchers to examine the role of parental caregiving (primarily mothers', but also fathers' caregiving, as discussed below) in attachment. A meta-analysis by De Wolff and Van IJzendoorn (1997) established that that there is a significant link between maternal sensitivity and later child attachment security, with a moderately strong effect size of $r = .24$. In fact, according to a meta-analysis of intervention studies, interventions that improved parental sensitivity were more effective than other interventions in terms of attachment outcomes (Bakermans-Kranenburg, Van IJzendoorn, & Juffer, 2003). This meta-analysis was influential because it provided empirical support for a causal link between caregiving quality and child attachment.

Moreover, the data suggest that sensitivity is important in predicting not only infant–mother attachment but also infant–father attachment. A meta-analysis of 16 studies conducted over a 30-year period showed a significant link between fathers' sensitivity and infant attachment, with a small effect size of $r = .12$ (Lucassen et al., 2011). It is not clear why the effect size was small. It has been theorized that there may be other factors uniquely important in paternal caregiving, such as stimulating play (Grossmann, Grossmann, Kindler, & Zimmermann, 2008), that should be considered in assessing fathers' sensitivity. The meta-analysis, however, showed that sensitivity in combination with stimulating play did not predict attachment outcomes better than paternal sensitivity alone (Lucassen et al., 2011). Thus, despite evidence that some but not all cultures have differing expectations of mothers and fathers (Lewis & Lamb, 2003), it appears that the sensitivity construct is relevant for understanding both maternal and paternal caregiving.

We now know that sensitivity is linked not only to later child attachment but also to a number of other important child outcomes. For example, low sensitivity early in life has been empirically linked to both later internalizing problems (e.g., Mount, Crockenberg, Jó, & Wagar, 2010) and externalizing problems (e.g., Shaw, Lacourse, & Nagin, 2005). Cassidy (1994) proposed that emotion regulation is a mechanism through which the link between attachment and later psychopathology occurs, and that children adapt their own behavioral and regulatory strategies to the caregiving environment in which they find themselves.

Sensitive responding to infant distress is linked to decreases in infant distress (e.g., Jahromi, Putnam, & Stifter, 2004), suggesting that sensitive caregiving plays a role in regulating the infant at a time when it is developing the capacity to self-regulate. In fact, research shows that maternal sensitivity in infancy is associated with child emotion regulation both in infancy (Glöggler & Pauli-Pott, 2008) and later in childhood (Lecuyer & Houck, 2006). There is also empirical evidence that parental caregiving is linked to physiological regulation, as indexed by vagal tone, an indicator of parasympathetic nervous system activation (e.g., Moore & Calkins, 2004), and that patterns of vagal regulation vary depending on maternal sensitivity (Moore et al., 2009). Likewise, maternal sensitivity is linked to infant adrenocortical function (i.e., infant cortisol reactivity and recovery; Atkinson et al., 2013).

## Parental Caregiving and the Intergenerational Transmission of Attachment: The Transmission Gap

Much of the research on parental caregiving has focused on the intergenerational transmission of attachment from parent to child. Parental caregiving is theorized to be rooted in parents' representations of their own attachment experiences. Secure representations of attachment allow the caregivers to remain nondefensively open to a child's needs and to respond in a way that provides the child with a secure base from which he or she can explore, and a safe haven to which the child can return in times of distress (Ainsworth et al., 1978; Bowlby, 1988). In short, we would expect caregivers' attachment representations to be linked directly to infant attachment, with caregiver sensitivity as the mediating mechanism for this intergenerational transmission. A series of meta-analyses have addressed each of these links and have shown that (1) there is a robust link ($d = 1.09$, a large effect size) between adult attachment representations and infant attachment, with a 75% concordance between the two at the level of secure–insecure (Van IJzendoorn, 1995); (2) there is a significant link between adult attachment representations and sensitivity, with a moderate effect size of 0.72 ($r = .34$); and (3) the link between sensitivity and infant attachment is significant with a moderate effect size ($r = .24$). Yet this final link is, statistically speaking, the weakest link in the meditational model, and it is significantly weaker in low-income families (De Wolff & Van IJzendoorn, 1997). A meta-analytic test of the full model showed that parenting behavior accounted for a smaller-than-expected proportion of the association between parental attachment representations and child attachment, which Van IJzendoorn (1995) termed the *transmission gap*. This transmission gap remains one of the most vexing puzzles in attachment research. We are left with a question: How are we to understand the role of caregiving in the development of attachment? Clearly, sensitivity matters, but what else is important?

One possibility is that researchers may rely too heavily on brief observations of sensitivity in standardized laboratory interactions. A meta-analysis, however, showed that the results were no different for studies with longer observation periods (De Wolff & Van IJzendoorn, 1997) or for those that assessed sensitivity via more ecologically valid home observations (e.g., Tarabulsy et al., 2005). The effect size (corrected $r = .85$) found by Ainsworth and colleagues (1978) was far larger than subsequent ones, yet De Wolff and Van IJzendoorn (1997) noted that had their meta-analysis been limited to those studies that used the Ainsworth (1969) scale, there would have been no increase in the effect size. Van IJzendoorn (1995) raised the question of whether genetics (instead of caregiving) may explain the intergenerational transmission of attachment. However, a number of studies examining this question indicated that the link between parent attachment representations and child attachment cannot be explained genetically (e.g., Fearon et al., 2006; Mesquita et al., 2013; Roisman, Booth-LaForce, Belsky, Burt, & Groh, 2013; Roisman & Fraley, 2008).

Belsky and Fearon (2008) argued that the transmission gap may be due to unidentified moderators, such as child characteristics. Indeed, a large body of research on temperament × environment interactions supports the idea that not all children are equally affected by their caregiving environments (Rothbart & Bates, 2006). Two new hypotheses suggest that children may vary in their neurobiological sensitivity to environmental influence, whether for the worse or for the better: (1) the differential susceptibility hypothesis (Belsky & Pluess, 2009) and (2) the hypothesis of biological sensitivity to context (Boyce & Ellis, 2005). Both approaches suggest that infant negativity should not be considered a risk factor, but rather an endophenotypic marker of susceptibility to the environment. In fact, studies provide some support for the idea that more negatively reactive/irritable infants may benefit more than other infants from caregiving interventions (e.g., Cassidy, Woodhouse, Sherman, Stupica, & Lejuez, 2011).

Another possibility in trying to understand the relatively weak link between parental sensitivity and child attachment is that researchers have been conceptualizing and/or measuring sensitivity incorrectly—or perhaps not measuring all important facets of what it means to provide a sensitive and responsive safe haven and secure base. Bowlby (1969/1982) theorized that attachment is based on real experiences with important caregivers. The question then becomes, *which* experiences are important? The answer has important implications for not only the science of attachment but also clinical intervention. Effective intervention relies on knowing which parenting behaviors to target. Different researchers have focused on different aspects of parental caregiving in assessing sensitivity.

Mesman and Emmen (2013) reviewed the eight most commonly used observational measures of parental sensitivity, out of the 50 or so existing observational systems. They pointed out that the scales were quite different from one another in terms of how they defined and operationalized sensitivity. Some of the scales differed from Ainsworth's definition of sensitivity by including positive affect and/or warmth as one of the indicators of sensitivity. Only one scale, the National Institute of Child Health and Human Development Studies of Early Child Care and Youth Development (NICHD SECCYD; Owen, 1992), like Ainsworth's, did not include warmth or positive maternal affect at all in its definition of sensitivity. Ainsworth (1967) believed that warmth was not necessary for attachment security because in her work with mothers and infants in Uganda, she had seen that the mothers tended to be sensitive and responsive, yet were not typically affectionate; nevertheless, the majority of the infants were securely attached. MacDonald (1992) suggested that warmth and sensitivity might belong to different motivational systems and presented data indicating that they were independent. MacDonald argued that warmth may serve as a reward but is not related to protection in the context of fear or distress. More recently, Davidov and Grusec (2006) found that sensitivity was associated with child regulation of negative affect and empathy toward others who were in distress, but that warmth was linked to child regulation of positive affect.

Some researchers (e.g., Raval et al., 2001) have emphasized the importance of examining context in trying to better understand the link between parental caregiving and child attachment, arguing that unmeasured aspects of the larger context may influence child attachment security above and beyond the effects of parental caregiving. Tarabulsy and colleagues (2005) found that the meditational role of maternal sensitivity in the link between maternal and child attachment emerged more clearly if contextual variables (i.e., maternal education, maternal depression, paternal support, infant maternal grandmother support) were accounted for in the model. More research is needed to confirm such ecological effects and understand the mechanisms through which they function.

Much of the research on parental sensitivity toward children has not distinguished between sensitivity to distress (safe haven) and sensitivity during exploration (secure base). Rather, parental sensitivity has been conceptualized in terms of parental capacity to respond flexibly to child cues *across contexts* in ways that match those cues (i.e., responding appropriately to cues for either safe haven or secure base). Thus, sensitivity has been conceptualized as flexible and appropriate responding to children's cues in what Ainsworth and colleagues (1971) termed the *attachment–exploration balance*. Given that infants and children move rapidly between exploration and attachment needs, an ability to move flexibly between different types of caregiving (i.e., both secure base and safe haven) may be important. In theory and research on attachment in childhood, the term *secure base* has often appeared as a shorthand for secure base and safe haven together (Dykas, Woodhouse, Cassidy, & Waters, 2006; Sroufe & Waters, 1977; Steele et al., 2014; Waters & Cummings, 2000; Woodhouse, Dykas, & Cassidy, 2009). Such usage is likely rooted in early writings on attachment. Ainsworth and colleagues (1978) and Bowlby (1988) theorized that a secure base is impossible without availability of the caregiver to provide a safe haven when needed. Nevertheless, research has begun to differentiate between sensitivity to infant distress (safe haven) and sensitivity to nondistress (secure base).

A number of studies have found that caregiver sensitivity in the context of infant distress predicts infant attachment and other key child outcomes (e.g., social competence, adjustment, affect regulation) better than concurrently assessed caregiver sensitivity in response to infant nondistress (e.g., Davidov & Grusec, 2006; Leerkes, 2011; Leerkes, Blankson, & O'Brien, 2009). Leerkes, Weaver, and O'Brien (2012) argued that these findings are consistent with Bowlby's (1969/1982) focus on the evolutionary importance of infant crying as a compelling social cue signaling to the caregiver that the infant needs safety, protection, and comfort. This suggests that differentiating between caregiving for attachment needs in times of stress (safe-haven caregiving) and caregiving for exploration (secure-base caregiving) could be important in understanding the links between caregiving and later child outcomes.

It is important to note, however, that classifying infant or child distress as always signaling a need for a safe haven may be too simplistic (Cassidy, Jones, & Shaver, 2013). Upon reunion, an infant who has been left alone in the Strange Situation may cry with arms lifted up toward the mother as a signal of wanting to be picked up. This would be an example of infant distress in a situation that is clearly related to the child's need for a safe haven. Alternatively, an infant may cry when a toy it was actively exploring is taken away (e.g., when limits need to be set for safety or other reasons). In this case, the distress is not related to a need for a safe haven. In fact, the distress may be terminated immediately if the toy is returned and the child is able to return to exploration. If the parent attempts to soothe a child who is crying due to frustration of exploration, the child's distress may increase because the exploration needs are not being met. Thus, it is possible for distress to occur in secure-base contexts. Such distress may best be dealt with through the provision of secure-base caregiving, with parental attention to helping the child explore. Likewise, there may be times when a child is expressing a need for safe haven without exhibiting any distress. Cassidy and colleagues (2013) give an example of an infant who has been playing contentedly for 20 minutes while her mother sits with a toddler in her lap and braids the toddler's hair. After the toddler leaves the mother's lap, the infant goes to the mother's lap and snuggles with her. This proximity seeking signals attachment needs because the infant's exploration ceased until she was able to experience the comforting assurance of the mother's presence and closeness. The movement toward the mother is linked to the mother as a safe haven of reassurance, safety, and emotional refueling.

Thus, the distinction between distress and nondistress contexts may not precisely indicate a need for a safe haven or a secure base. Instead, it may be better to examine the caregiving context (exploratory/secure-base context vs. safe-haven context) *in conjunction with* distress (distress vs. nondistress) to best understand parental caregiving and its links to later child attachment. Cassidy and colleagues (2013) proposed that such a two-dimensional approach may allow for stronger links to emerge between specific types of parental caregiving and later child attachment, as well as other important child outcomes.

Another conceptualization of caregiving has been proposed as a potential solution to the transmission gap (Cassidy et al., 2005). In an effort to understand whether there may be a way to conceptualize and measure caregiving that could help to bridge the transmission gap and address the fact that the sensitivity–attachment link is significantly weaker in low-income mother–infant dyads (De Wolff & Van IJzendoorn, 1997), Cassidy and colleagues (2005) conducted a qualitative study that focused on a sample of racially and ethnically diverse, low-income mothers. The researchers observed mother–infant interactions including structured tasks in the laboratory when the infant was 4.5 months old and three 30-minute, naturalistic, videotaped home visits that occurred on three separate days when the infant was between 4.5 and 9 months old. Surprisingly, the majority of the mothers were not even minimally sensitive to infant cues when the infant was 4.5 to 9 months old. Nevertheless, approximately half of the infants were securely attached at 12 months. It appeared that infants could tolerate an unexpectedly high level of maternal insensitivity, as long as two conditions were met. First, certain negative behaviors could not be present (e.g., frightening behavior, extremely cold or hostile behavior, or consistent intrusive efforts to keep the infant's attention on the mother). Any mother who exhibited these negative behaviors had an insecure infant. Second, the mother needed to communicate that both sides of the attachment–exploration balance were acceptable to her by ultimately meeting exploration and attachment needs, even if she was insensitive along the way. Cassidy and colleagues observed that most of the insensitive behavior observed during exploration at 4.5 to 9 months had little association with attachment at 12 months. For example, mothers could be quite intrusive during infant play by introducing too many toys at too rapid a pace, pulling away toys in which the baby was interested, and following the mothers' rather than the infants' interests. Despite high levels of intrusion, infants were secure at 12 months as long as mothers were not intrusive in ways that activated the child's attachment system. As long as

mothers were *comfortable enough* with exploration that they did not terminate it, the child developed a secure attachment. Likewise, mothers of both insecure and secure infants might ignore infant crying or too quickly turn a crying baby away from her. Mothers of infants who would later be secure finally relented and "got the job done" of soothing the baby to calm in a chest-to-chest position. Cassidy and colleagues referred to this conceptualization of caregiving as *secure-base provision* and defined it in terms of doing a "good-enough" job of supporting both attachment (safe haven) and exploration (secure base) needs.

Based on this work, Woodhouse, Beeney, Doub, and Cassidy (2015) developed a quantitative measure of secure-base provision and found that it predicted 12-month infant attachment in a racially and ethnically diverse, low-socioeconomic status (SES) sample, whereas sensitivity did not. The findings of Brody and Flor (1998) are relevant to the way in which Woodhouse and her colleagues interpreted their findings. Brody and Flor suggested that parents living in dangerous or stressful conditions may adopt parenting strategies such as more stringent child management techniques, more authoritarian parenting, and more parent-centered (rather than child-centered) parenting in an effort to support child adaptation to those stressful conditions. What they termed *nononsense parenting* is meant to promote children's self-regulation and independence, to protect children from danger, and to help children avoid involvement with antisocial activities and its potential consequences. Brody and Flor's data provided no evidence that such no-nonsense parenting practices were linked to later insecure attachment. Woodhouse and her colleagues argued that use of the secure-base provision approach in assessing caregiving avoids emphasizing certain culturally bound parenting practices found in white, middle-class samples (e.g., sweet tone of voice, affectionate verbal comments).

Other researchers have found evidence that sensitivity during nondistress may also be important in predicting attachment in older infants. Bernier, Matte-Gagné, Belanger, and Whipple (2014) found that both sensitivity (at 12 months) and autonomy support (at 15 months) fully accounted for the relation between maternal attachment representations (assessed at 7 months) and child attachment at 24 months. They argued that researchers have not attended enough to parental support for exploration in the relation between maternal and child attachment. These results raise the question of whether particular aspects of caregiving matter at different stages of child development. It could be that the balance of attachment and exploration looks different depending on the child's stage of development. It may be that in the first year of life, the regulation of distress is the predominant role of caregivers, whereas by 15 months, support for exploration becomes equally important.

Interestingly, there is not a strong empirical link between parental sensitivity and child disorganization (e.g., NICHD Early Child Care Research Network, 1997). Empirical evidence suggests that it is atypical or anomalous parenting that is linked to disorganized attachment (e.g., Lyons-Ruth, Bronfman, & Parsons, 1999), such as parents' frightened or frightening behavior (Main & Hesse, 1990). Lyons-Ruth and colleagues (1999) proposed that infants may become disorganized when caregiving is disrupted in other ways, such as parents presenting irresolvable caregiving strategies to the child (e.g., heightening arousal of the infant's attachment system while simultaneously rejecting attachment cues). Longitudinal work has highlighted maternal withdrawal in infancy (e.g., distanced interactions and a lack of initiative in greeting or comforting) as a key predictor of a variety of types of psychopathology in the transition to young adulthood (e.g., Lyons-Ruth, Bureau, Holmes, Easterbrooks, & Brooks, 2013; Shi, Bureau, Easterbrooks, Zhao, & Lyons-Ruth, 2012). See Lyons-Ruth and Jacobvitz (Chapter 29, this volume) for further discussion of caregiving and disorganized attachment.

### Research on Factors that Predict Caregiving Quality

Adult attachment representations as assessed by the Adult Attachment Interview (AAI; George, Kaplan, & Main, 1984, 1985, 1996), as discussed earlier, are a robust predictor of parenting quality based on meta-analytic findings (Van IJzendoorn, 1995). Yet, as Jones, Cassidy, and Shaver (2015) noted in a review of the 64 relevant studies that appeared between 1994 and 2013, parents' adult attachment styles, as assessed by self-report measures of attachment emerging from social psychology, such as the Experiences in Close Relationships Scale (ECR; Brennan, Clark, & Shaver, 1998), are also empirically linked to parental caregiving. The fact that both adult attachment representations and attachment styles are linked to parenting is intriguing given that the two approaches

to assessing adult attachment are only modestly linked with one another (Roisman et al., 2007). Taxonomic work on measures of adult attachment style has shown that adult style can best be conceptualized in terms of two dimensions: attachment anxiety and avoidance (Fraley & Waller, 1998). Avoidance reflects the degree to which an individual tends to deactivate the attachment system, and to avoid interpersonal closeness or disclosure of emotions within relationships. Attachment anxiety, in contrast, reflects a tendency toward hyperactivating the attachment system, preoccupation with abandonment or rejection in relationships, and a desire to be unusually close in interpersonal relationships that can be unsettling to relational partners. Jones and colleagues (2015) found that across multiple studies, avoidance was linked to less sensitive and responsive caregiving. In contrast, results for attachment anxiety were more mixed. Nevertheless, the review showed that attachment styles were linked in theoretically expected ways with parenting behaviors, emotions related to parenting, and parent cognitions.

Researchers have considered parental mental states (e.g., the capacity " . . . to see things from the [child's] point of view"; Ainsworth, 1969, "Scale 1: Sensitivity vs. Insensitivity to the Baby's Signals," para. 3) as predictors of caregiving quality. First, a body of research has linked maternal reflective functioning to parental caregiving (e.g., Rosenblum, McDonough, Sameroff, & Muzik, 2008; Stacks et al., 2014), and improvements in reflective functioning have been linked to improvements in parenting (Suchman, DeCoste, Leigh, & Borelli, 2010). *Reflective functioning* is defined as parents' ability to keep their children's (and their own) mental states (e.g., feelings, thoughts, intentions, and desires) in mind and to link this understanding to their own and their children's behavior (Fonagy, Gergely, Jurist, & Target, 2002). Second, research has shown consistent links between mind-mindedness and sensitivity (e.g., Demers, Bernier, Tarabulsy, & Provost, 2010; Laranjo, Bernier, & Meins, 2008; Meins et al., 2012). *Mind-mindedness* is defined as "the mother's proclivity to treat her infant as an individual with a mind, rather than merely as a creature with needs that must be satisfied" (Meins, Fernyhough, Fradley, & Tuckey, 2001, p. 638). Third, Dix (1991, 1992) theorized that parents with child-oriented parenting goals (that focus on the child's perspective) would be more sensitive. Consistent with this idea, Leerkes (2010) showed that mothers with more infant-oriented goals responded to infant distress more sensitively than did mothers with self-oriented goals.

Attachment theory suggests that parental emotions that are self-focused (e.g., anger, anxiety) rather than infant-focused (i.e., empathic) interfere with sensitive caregiving because they may lead mothers to avoid the distress, withdraw from the child, or respond intrusively (Cassidy, 1994; Dix, 1991). This idea has been empirically supported (Dix, Gershoff, Meunier, & Miller, 2004; Leerkes, 2010; Leerkes, Parade, & Gudmundson, 2011).

There has been little research on links between maternal physiological regulation and maternal caregiving, despite evidence from research on animals that maternal physiological regulation is important in organizing parenting behavior (e.g., Insel, 2000). A notable exception is a study showing that sensitivity to distress was linked to vagal withdrawal (a physiological sign of attending to a challenge) for mothers of 6-month-old infants who would later be insecure-avoidant, suggesting that these mothers experience sensitivity to distress as challenging (Mills-Koonce et al., 2007). Another study showed that mothers of secure 12-month-old infants showed greater vagal withdrawal during the final reunion of the Strange Situation than did mothers of avoidant infants, suggesting that mothers of secure infants were attending more to their children than were mothers of insecure-avoidant infants (Hill-Soderlund et al., 2008). Similarly, Leerkes and colleagues (2015) found that less adaptive physiological regulation prenatally was associated with lower maternal sensitivity to infant distress at 6 months. This link was mediated by mothers' self-focused and negative processing of infant cues.

## Parental Caregiving and Attachment across Cultures

Ainsworth (1967) began her research on maternal caregiving in Uganda. Thus, from the beginning, her thinking about caregiving was rooted in repeated naturalistic observations in a cross-cultural context. Bowlby's (1969/1982) theory of attachment was based in an ethological perspective in which caregiving and attachment are thought to be how the human species evolved to promote survival. Thus, theory would suggest that although there may be cultural differences in parenting beliefs, goals, and behaviors, there should be underlying similarities as well. Much of the research on caregiving and attachment, however, has tended to neglect cultural/contextual differences and has instead focused on middle-class families in Western industrialized societies. Van IJzendoorn and Sagi-Schwartz (2008; see also Mesman, Van IJzendoorn, & Sagi-Schwartz, Chapter 37, this volume) made a case that more research is needed to better understand attachment across cultures. There is some evidence suggesting that sensitivity is important across cultures. For example, Posada (2013) summarized a series of studies assessing the link between parental sensitivity and child attachment in different cultural and SES groups in Colombia and the United States, and found the expected associations between sensitivity and attachment in all groups.

Similarly, True, Pisani, and Oumar (2001) examined the link between maternal sensitivity and infant attachment in a sample of mothers and their infants from the Dogon ethnic group of Mali, West Africa. Despite culturally based parenting practices that differed from typical Western parenting practices and differences in infant behaviors, the associations between parent sensitivity and infant attachment approached significance in this small sample ($n = 27$), and frightened/frightening behaviors significantly predicted insecurity (typically disorganized attachment). Maternal sensitivity and frightened/frightening behaviors explained 19% of the variance in infant attachment. Nevertheless, there are likely cultural/contextual issues that should be considered in connection with caregiving (see Yovsi, Kärtner, Keller, & Lohaus, 2009, for a discussion of this issue).

A systematic review of the literature on observational studies of parental sensitivity in racial/ethnic minority groups showed that parental sensitivity tends to be lower in these parents than in racial/ethnic majority groups (Mesman, Van IJzendoorn, & Bakermans-Kranenburg, 2012). This difference, however, appeared to be associated with the confounding effects of low SES, which was linked to minority status. SES is typically more strongly related to sensitivity than is ethnicity or race (e.g., Chaudhuri, Easterbrooks, & Davis, 2009). Moreover, SES is linked to within-group differences in sensitivity in the United States (e.g., Barnett, Shanahan, Deng, Haskett, & Cox, 2010) and the Netherlands (e.g., Bocknek, Brophy-Herb, & Banerjee, 2009). These results are consistent with a family stress model (e.g., Yaman, Mesman, Van IJzendoorn, Bakermans-Kranenburg, & Linting, 2010) in which economic difficulties diminish parents' ability to parent sensitively (Conger & Donnellan, 2007).

## Directions for Future Research on Parent–Child Caregiving

Despite the fact that research on caregiving has been vigorously pursued since the seminal work by Ainsworth and her colleagues (1978) on the link between parental caregiving and child attachment, there is still much to learn. Research demonstrates that caregiving matters for later attachment and other important outcomes. However, we need to know more about the dimensions of caregiving that matter and empirically map how important aspects of caregiving may change during a child's development. For example, it may be that emotion regulation (support for attachment needs) is the key function of caregiving in infancy, but that as the child grows, support for active, autonomous exploration and limit setting (to create a sense of safety as children engage in more autonomous exploration) may become important aspects of caregiving.

## Research on Attachment and Caregiving in Adulthood

While research on parent–child caregiving has typically viewed the safe-haven and secure-base functions jointly (as part of the same sensitivity construct), research in the adult literature has more commonly viewed the provision of a safe haven (support for attachment needs) and secure base (support for exploration) as two different caregiving functions that occur in two different life contexts. Also, in adult relationships, the caregiving and care-seeking roles are bidirectional, with each partner at times providing care and at other times receiving care. In well-functioning adult attachment relationships, "taking care" of a partner involves supporting that person's need for comfort/assistance when the attachment system is activated, and supporting his or her explorations (personal growth, goal strivings) when the attachment system is not activated.

## Safe-Haven Processes: Support of Attachment Needs

An assumption of attachment theory is that across the lifespan, when individuals are distressed (attachment system activation), they feel an urge toward proximity to attachment figures (who may include romantic partners, close friends, parents,

or other family members in adulthood), and that attachment behavior will be activated with greater intensity as the degree of perceived threat increases. Consistent with these assumptions, observational and daily diary studies have shown that care-seeking behavior in adulthood increases in response to stressful or threatening events (Collins & Feeney, 2000, 2005; Collins, Kane, Guichard, & Ford, 2008), and that secure individuals have a higher threshold for attachment system activation than do insecure individuals (Bartholomew, Cobb, & Poole, 1997; Mikulincer & Florian; 1995; Ognibene & Collins, 1998; Simpson & Rholes, 1994) and show a greater willingness/ability to seek/mobilize support (e.g., Collins & Feeney, 2000; Feeney, Cassidy, & Ramos-Marcuse, 2008; Florian, Mikulincer, & Bucholtz, 1995; Mikulincer & Florian, 1995; Mikulincer, Florian, & Weller, 1993; Ognibene & Collins, 1998; Rholes, Simpson, & Orina, 1999; Simpson, Rholes, & Nelligan, 1992).

## Links between Care-Seeking and Caregiving Behaviors

Normatively, signs of distress in a close other should activate the attachment figure's caregiving system. Because care-seeking and caregiving behaviors are directed toward the same goal (i.e., reducing distress and restoring felt security) in well-functioning partnerships, they should be linked in complementary ways. Research in support of this idea has shown that specific care-seeking behaviors were associated with specific caregiving behaviors enacted during discussions of stressful life events (Collins & Feeney, 2000; Feeney et al., 2008). For example, clear and direct expressions of need were associated with helpful forms of support, whereas indirect expressions of need were associated with unhelpful forms of support, and the type of help offered (e.g., instrumental or emotional support) was matched to the type of help sought (Collins & Feeney, 2000). Similarly, in a daily diary study of couples, participants received more support on days when they expressed greater need (Collins & Feeney, 2005). Also, in an experimental study in which expressions of distress (a form of care seeking) was experimentally manipulated, caregivers wrote more supportive messages to their partner when they believed the partner was more distressed (Feeney & Collins, 2001). Thus, the evidence suggests that safe-haven care-seeking and caregiving behaviors are coordinated in complementary ways.

## Individual Differences in Safe-Haven Caregiving

Theoretically, and consistent with evidence for parental caregiving, secure individuals should find it easier to perceive and respond to others' distress than do insecure individuals. This is because sensitive and compassionate reactions to the needs of others are products of a well-functioning caregiving behavioral system, which cannot function effectively when one's own needs for security have not been met (Collins et al., 2010; Mikulincer & Shaver, 2005). Secure individuals are also more likely to possess the skills, resources, and adaptive caregiving motives that are necessary for being responsive to the needs of others (Feeney & Collins, 2001, 2003, 2014).

Corroborating this, a series of self-report studies reveal that secure attachment (low anxiety and avoidance) is associated with more effective caregiving in intimate relationships (Carnelley, Pietromonaco, & Jaffe, 1996; B. C. Feeney & Collins, 2001; J. A. Feeney, 1996; Kane et al., 2007; Kunce & Shaver, 1994). Overall, secure adults are sensitive to their partner's cues and willing to provide physical comfort when needed; they are more cooperative than controlling in their caregiving style, and they are less likely to be overinvolved in their caregiving efforts. In contrast, insecure attachment (high anxiety and/or avoidance) is associated with less effective caregiving behavior, but the particular pattern of ineffective care depends on the particular type of insecurity. Avoidant individuals are relatively neglectful and controlling, whereas anxious individuals are relatively intrusive, overinvolved, and controlling.

Observational studies provide converging evidence for attachment differences in patterns of caregiving. In a series of studies, Simpson, Rholes, and colleagues (Rholes et al., 1999; Simpson, Rholes, Orina, & Grich, 2002; Simpson et al., 1992) showed that avoidant attachment is associated with less effective caregiving behavior. For example, when men were placed in the caregiving role (Simpson et al., 1992), those who were high in avoidance provided less reassurance and support as their partner's level of distress increased; they also expressed more anger toward their partners during the stress period, and interacted more negatively with them during the recovery period (after the stressor was removed), especially when their partners sought more support (Rholes et al., 1999). These findings suggest that avoidant men found their partner's expressions of need to be aversive,

and that they responded by distancing themselves from their partners. In these studies, anxious attachment was unrelated to observed caregiving behavior. However, an observational study that examined individual differences in caregiving behavior while one member of the couple described a personal stressor to his or her partner (Collins & Feeney, 2000) revealed that attachment anxiety is associated with less effective support behavior. Anxious individuals provided less instrumental support, were less responsive, and exhibited more negative support behavior, especially when their partner's needs were less clear—indicating that attachment anxiety (as well as avoidance) limits one's ability to be a good caregiver.

A study designed to examine attachment differences in responsiveness to attachment needs experimentally manipulated the caregiver's belief that his or her partner was either extremely distressed about an upcoming speech task (high need for support) or not at all distressed (low need for support; Feeney & Collins, 2001). From an attachment perspective, responsive caregiving should be appropriately contingent on the partner's needs; thus, support providers should show increased support effort in response to greater need. However, results revealed that avoidant individuals showed no evidence of responsiveness; they provided relatively low levels of emotional support regardless of their partner's level of need, and they provided more instrumental support in the low-need condition (when their partner had little need for it) than in the high-need condition (when their partner needed it most). Anxious individuals showed some evidence of responsiveness, but they were not always in sync with their partner's needs; they provided more instrumental support in the high-need condition than the low-need condition (a pattern of responsiveness), but they provided the same relatively high level of emotional support regardless of their partner's level of need (a pattern of overinvolvement).

Westmaas and Silver (2001) also showed that insecure attachment impeded effective caregiving when women interacted with a peer whom they were led to believe had just been diagnosed with cancer. Avoidant women were rated by observers as less supportive and as making less eye contact during the interaction. Attachment anxiety was unrelated to behavioral support but was associated with reports of feeling uneasy during the interaction and self-critical thoughts (occupied with thoughts about their own interpersonal performance).

Taken together, observational studies provide clear evidence that secure individuals are more sensitive to the needs of others and better able to modulate their cognitive, emotional, and behavioral resources in ways that are contingent on their partner's expression of distress. In contrast, insecure adults have substantial deficits in their ability to support and care for others, but the specific nature of the deficit differs for avoidant and anxious individuals. One limitation of these studies is our inability to draw causal inferences concerning the effect of secure attachment on caregiving behavior. However, recent experimental studies (in which attachment security was manipulated using priming techniques) have shown that experimentally induced attachment security increases empathy, the endorsement of prosocial values, and prosocial behavior (Mikulincer et al., 2001, 2003; Mikulincer & Shaver, 2001; Mikulincer, Shaver, Gillath, & Nitzberg, 2005). These investigations provide evidence for a causal link between feeling secure and compassionate responses to others in need.

## Mechanisms That Explain Individual Differences in Caregiving

In taking an attachment–theoretical approach to understanding caregiving, it is important to go beyond the mere documentation of attachment differences to identify the mechanisms that explain these patterns. Research and theorizing in this area have suggested that effective caregiving (sensitively responding to needs as they arise) requires a constellation of skills, resources, and motivations that individuals possess to varying degrees (Feeney & Collins, 2003, 2014). One study using observational, survey, and experimental methods (Feeney & Collins, 2001) showed that unique patterns of motives (e.g., egoistic vs. altruistic motives for helping one's partner), skills (e.g., knowledge about how to support others), and resources (e.g., self-focus) can explain why people with different attachment characteristics differ in their caregiving. Avoidant adults are unresponsive because they lack knowledge about how to support others, lack a prosocial orientation toward others, and fail to develop the deep sense of relationship closeness, commitment, and trust that appear to be critical for motivating effective caregiving behavior. Anxious adults are overinvolved caregivers because although they feel close and committed to their partners, they simultaneously distrust their partners and are selfishly motivated in their caregiving attempts.

Other research examining specific motives that underlie the provision of responsive or unresponsive caregiving (Feeney & Collins, 2003) has revealed that avoidant individuals help their partners for relatively egoistic reasons (e.g., they feel obligated to help, want to avoid sanctions for not helping, or expect to get something in return), whereas anxious individuals help for both egoistic and altruistic reasons (e.g., they not only feel concern for their partner's welfare but they also want to gain their partner's love or make their partner dependent upon them). These motives, in turn, predicted the quality of support provided in the relationship. Altruistic motives were linked with a responsive caregiving style, whereas egoistic motives were linked with an unresponsive or overinvolved caregiving style (see also Feeney, Collins, Van Vleet, & Tomlinson, 2013).

With regard to emotional mechanisms, researchers have examined caregivers' emotional reactions to their partners' expressions of anxiety in times of stress (Monin, Feeney, & Schultz, 2012). Caregivers who are unable to regulate their own emotions or who are uncomfortable with others' emotion expression may have negative emotional reactions to witnessing a significant other's distress, which should impede effective caregiving. This was supported in an observational study in which one member of married/dating couples was exposed to a stressor, and in an experimental study in which participants watched standardized videos of clear versus ambiguous emotion expression. Results indicated that insecure-avoidant individuals felt angry in response to their partners' expression of distress, whereas insecure-anxious individuals felt anxious/nervous. These results are consistent with research showing that avoidant (and sometimes anxious) individuals display anger when their partners are distressed or seek support from them (Rholes et al., 1999).

## Safe-Haven Caregiving as a Predictor of Important Outcomes for Recipients

An individual who receives safe-haven caregiving should experience immediate outcomes, including problem resolution, reduced stress/physiological arousal, better coping capacity, enhanced feelings of security, and enhanced relationship satisfaction. Consistent with these ideas, research has shown that small acts of caring from a partner can have immediate effects on well-being and relationship quality. For example, in a daily diary study, both men and women felt more loved/valued and happier in their relationship on days when their partner provided more caring support, and these positive effects lingered the following day (Collins & Feeney, 2005). Likewise, an observational study of couples in which one partner disclosed a personal worry to the other showed that care-recipients experienced immediate improvements in emotional well-being when their partner provided more responsive support (Collins & Feeney, 2000). Similarly, Simpson and colleagues (1992) found that participants who were waiting to begin a stressful procedure were more calmed when their romantic partners made more supportive remarks, and they were less calmed when their partners avoided or downplayed their concerns (see also Cutrona, 1986; Winstead & Derlega, 1985). There is also evidence that the receipt of safe-haven support facilitates problem resolution; studies have shown that supportive behavior provided by companions (e.g., talking about a problem-solving task) is a strong predictor of subsequent problem-solving performance (e.g., Lakey & Heller, 1988; Winstead, Derlega, Lewis, Sanchez-Hucles, & Clarke, 1992).

Experimental research also shows that caring support from a partner can have immediate effects on emotional well-being and relationship functioning. In one study, immersive virtual environment technology was used to create a frightening task for one member of each couple and to experimentally manipulate their romantic partner's attentiveness and emotional support in the virtual world (Kane, McCall, Collins, & Blascovich, 2012). Relative to those with an inattentive/neglectful partner in the virtual world, those with an attentive/responsive partner reported lower anxiety, more positive self-evaluations, and increased relationship satisfaction following the frightening task. Also, individuals who had been exposed to an inattentive/neglectful partner kept greater physical distance between themselves and their partner during a subsequent, unrelated task.

These findings suggest that responsive caregiving can reduce stress and foster relationship quality, and that unresponsive behaviors can erode both physical and emotional closeness between partners. The findings also indicate a causal link between receipt of caring support and immediate improvements in personal and relational well-being. This is consistent with research with both

dating and married adults indicating that the extent to which individuals are satisfied and adjusted in their relationship depends in part on whether their partner is a good caregiver who can provide a safe haven of comfort, support, and security (Carnelley et al., 1996; J. A. Feeney, 1996).

In addition, researchers have shown that the provision and receipt of responsive care within a close relationship, particularly emotional/esteem support, is one of the best predictors of satisfaction in those relationships (Buhrmester, Furman, Wittenberg, & Reis, 1988; Katz, Beach, & Anderson, 1996; Kotler, 1985). In fact, Barbee and Yankeelov (1992; cited in Barbee & Cunningham, 1995) found that the lack of an attempt to support a partner and the use of dismissing behaviors (e.g., minimizing the importance of the problem) during a support interaction were significant predictors of later romantic relationship dissolution. And other research has shown that caregiving patterns observed in the laboratory (and reported by both couple members) predict the quality, functioning, and stability of relationships concurrently (Collins & Feeney, 2000) and over time (Feeney & Collins, 2001).

Additional evidence for the importance of responsive caregiving in adult relationships comes from studies showing that cardiovascular reactivity is buffered in individuals who experience a stressor in the presence of a close, nonevaluative support provider relative to individuals who experience the stressor alone, with a stranger, or with an evaluative other (e.g., Allen, Blascovich, Tomaka, & Kelsey, 1991; Edens, Larkin, & Abel, 1992; Kamarck, Manuck, & Jennings, 1990; Snydersmith & Cacioppo, 1992). Negative and unsupportive interactions, however, predict slower recovery (Fritz, Nagurney, & Helgeson, 2003). In addition, soothing touch or close physical contact (with a close relationship partner) during a stressful task has been found to decrease heart rate and blood pressure (e.g., Ditzen et al., 2007; Fishman, Turkheimer, & DeGood, 1995; Grewen, Anderson, Girdler, & Light, 2003; Lynch, Thomas, Pasketwitz, Katchar, & Weir, 1977; Whitcher & Fisher, 1979) and to attenuate neural activation in brain regions associated with emotional and behavioral responses to threat (Coan, Schaefer, & Davidson, 2006; see also Coan, Chapter 12, this volume).

Finally, a large literature that is beyond the scope of this chapter indicates that social support in times of stress is associated with better mental and physical health outcomes (e.g., Cohen,

1988, 2004; Cohen & Syme, 1985; Cohen & Wills, 1985; Kawachi & Berkman, 2001; Sarason, Sarason, & Gurung, 1997; Uchino, Cacioppo, & Kiecolt-Glaser, 1996). This literature generally indicates that people with satisfying levels of social support are healthier (both psychologically and physically); they recover from illness more quickly (have better immune functioning) and are better adjusted (both personally and socially). It is important to note that in these studies, "social support" is typically conceptualized and assessed via reports of general perceptions of available support, social network size, and support received within a certain period of time. Very few of these studies have included observations of caregiving behaviors (and related interpersonal processes) as they unfold during actual support interactions with close relationship partners, nor have they followed people over time to assess the extent to which specific caregiving dynamics predict health outcomes.

### Individual Differences in Outcomes of Safe-Haven Caregiving

Some research has considered individual differences in outcomes of safe-haven caregiving. Two studies examined attachment differences in the extent to which the presence of a supportive other buffers autonomic reactivity to stress (Carpenter & Kirkpatrick, 1996; Feeney & Kirkpatrick, 1996). One study indicated that separation from a partner during a stressful situation had adverse effects on insecure individuals' cardiovascular reactivity (Feeney & Kirkpatrick, 1996), and the other indicated that for insecure (avoidant and anxious) participants, physiological reactivity in response to a stressor was greater when the partner was present than when absent (Carpenter & Kirkpatrick, 1996). For both types of insecure individuals, the partner's presence resulted in a negative immediate outcome—perhaps because these individuals were dealing with not only the stressful laboratory task but also the prospect of being rejected by their partners while trying to cope with this threat. In contrast, partner proximity had no discernible effect on secure individuals' autonomic responses to stress—perhaps because the psychological availability of the partner transcends physical separation in secure relationships because secure individuals may be confident of their ability to cope with stress, or because they have a higher threshold for attachment system activation.

Other research that considers the moderating effects of attachment on caregiving outcomes during a stressful situation demonstrated that avoidant women were more calmed than secure women by the supportive comments of their male partners, despite the fact that they were less likely to mention the stressful impending event to their partners (Simpson et al., 1992). The researchers suggested that supportive behaviors may have a stronger and more positive impact on avoidant than on secure individuals because they do not typically expect to receive support. These findings are noteworthy because they indicate that avoidant individuals do benefit from receiving support, even though they are unlikely to seek it out.

Another study examining individual differences in the effects of experimentally provided social support showed similar effects (Sarason & Sarason, 1986). Participants who scored high and low in general perceptions of available support were either provided with support or given no special intervention before working on a difficult task. Interestingly, individuals who were low in perceived support (characteristic of insecure individuals) performed significantly better when support was experimentally offered to them. However, individuals who were high in perceived support (characteristic of secure individuals) performed similarly regardless of the experimental support manipulation. These results point to a facilitative effect of manipulated caregiving for individuals low in perceived support.

More research is needed to specify outcomes of safe-haven caregiving for individuals with different attachment characteristics. In particular, it will be important to identify the conditions under which insecure adults are able to derive comfort/security from their partners. Most research on this topic has been conducted with children and has shown that attachment security predicts the ability to be soothed by caregivers: Secure children seek support when distressed and are easily comforted; avoidant children fail to seek proximity to caregivers and do not derive comfort; and although anxious/ambivalent children seek proximity to caregivers, they are difficult to soothe (Ainsworth et al., 1978). Similarly, research has shown that when highly anxious adults discuss relationship conflicts with their partners, they are more distressed relative to less anxious people, and remain more distressed even when their partners are rated as behaving positively toward them (Simpson, Campbell, & Weisberg, 2006). Likewise, research with adolescents has shown that anxious individuals exhibit heightened heart rate and blood pressure during interactions with peers, whereas avoidant adolescents experience fewer overall interactions with peers and heightened heart rate and blood pressure during experiences of conflict (Gallo & Matthews, 2006). However, much remains to be discovered about the ability of adults with different attachment characteristics to derive comfort from relationship partners. Individuals with different attachment characteristics may require different forms of responsive care in order to feel soothed. For example, Simpson, Winterheld, Rholes, and Orina (2007) found that secure individuals are more calmed when their partners provide emotional care, whereas insecure (dismissive) individuals react more favorably to instrumental support.

## Research on Secure Base Support Processes: Support of Exploration

Although adults routinely assign credit for their accomplishments to the support of the significant people in their lives (people who have encouraged them to grow as individuals and strive to reach their full potential), empirical investigations of this caregiving function represent a newer and less developed aspect of the adult caregiving literature.

### Links between Exploration Behaviors and Secure-Base Caregiving

As described earlier, three important characteristics of a secure base include supporting exploration by (1) being available in the event that the base is needed, (2) not unnecessarily interfering with exploration, and (3) being encouraging and accepting of exploration. In an initial test of the idea that these three components predict exploration behavior in adulthood, Feeney and Thrush (2010) created a laboratory situation to permit the observation of one couple member's exploration behavior as a function of the other couple member's secure-base behavior (by giving the "explorer" a novel exploration activity to try out in the presence of his or her spouse). Results indicated that spouse availability was associated with greater persistence at the exploration task, whereas spouse interference predicted less persistence, poorer performance, and less enthusiasm in the process of the task. Spouse encouragement predicted better performance and greater expressed enthusiasm for the task. Taken together, these results indicate

that availability and encouragement facilitate exploration, whereas interference is an inhibitor of exploration (Feeney & Thrush, 2010).

Results of this investigation also revealed an ambivalent behavioral pattern for explorers with interfering spouses. Specifically, although explorers with interfering spouses expressed greater concern about the spouse watching their explorations, they also sought task assistance from them. In addition, explorers with interfering spouses were receptive to both solicited and unsolicited task assistance, and they were simultaneously rejecting of both solicited and unsolicited task assistance. This seems to reflect a fundamental tension that individuals with interfering spouses experience in exploration contexts: People with interfering caregivers may come to believe that they are incapable of successful independent exploration, and these self-doubts may make them receptive to task assistance. However, they may be simultaneously rejecting of this assistance because the negative messages conveyed by spouse interference are likely to feel demeaning, and because spouse interference impedes one's own goals/efforts.

Another study examined links between secure-base behavior and exploration behavior in the context of discussing personal goals (Feeney, 2004). Caregivers who were coded by observers as being supportive of and comfortable with their partners' autonomous goals had partners who discussed their goals openly, confidently explored avenues for achieving their goals, and were receptive to support attempts. In contrast, caregivers who were coded by observers as avoiding discussion of their partner's goals had partners who did not discuss their goals openly, did not confidently explore avenues for achieving their goals, were not receptive to support attempts (when they occurred), and avoided discussion of the goals themselves. Interestingly, caregivers who were intrusive and controlling during the discussion had partners who modified and minimized the importance of their original goals.

### Individual Differences in Secure-Base Caregiving

To date, not much research has considered individual differences in secure-base caregiving within adult relationships. One study has shown that avoidant spouses are less available to their partners during exploration, whereas anxious spouses are more interfering with, and less encouraging of, exploration (Feeney & Thrush, 2010). These findings are consistent with the infant literature indicating that insecure parents tend to interfere with their baby's exploratory activity (Cassidy & Berlin, 1994; Grossmann, Grossmann, & Zimmermann, 1999). With regard to who is more or less likely to receive secure-base support from their partners, results indicated that both types of insecure individuals (avoidant and anxious) had spouses who were less available to them during exploration, and attachment avoidance was specifically linked with the receipt of less encouragement for exploration. Thus, the characteristics of both interaction partners matter in predicting the provision and receipt of secure-base support.

### Secure-Base Caregiving as a Predictor of Important Outcomes for Recipients

Given that research on secure-base caregiving in adult relationships is in its infancy, the research that has been conducted thus far primarily has considered immediate outcomes of receiving (or failing to receive) this important type of care. Initial studies have focused on state self-esteem and mood as important immediate outcomes. One study revealed that when recipients felt that their goals were supported by their partners (during a discussion of personal goals), they experienced increases in self-esteem and positive mood after the discussion (Feeney, 2004). Similarly, spouses' secure-base behavior during an exploration activity, in which "explorers" worked on a novel and challenging task, predicted changes in the explorer's mood and state self-esteem from before to after the activity (Feeney & Thrush, 2010). Specifically, spouse encouragement predicted increases in positive mood, decreases in concerned mood, and decreases in frustrated mood from before to after the activity. Although spouse availability also predicted decreases in concerned mood, spouse encouragement was the component of secure base support that was most strongly predictive of emotionality. This suggests that encouragement may serve an important emotional and motivational function that the other components of secure-base caregiving (availability and nonintrusiveness) do not serve. With regard to self-esteem, spouse interference during exploration predicted significant decreases in self-esteem, whereas spouse encouragement predicted increases in self-esteem. Finally, experimental evidence for the detrimental effect of intrusive support on self-esteem and positive affect was obtained in a study that manipulated intrusive support during a computer exploration activity

(Feeney, 2004). Individuals who received intrusive support, and who perceived their partners' support as being intrusive and insensitive, experienced decreases in state self-esteem and positive mood from before to after the activity.

Another immediate outcome of intrusive support is poor performance on exploration tasks (Feeney, 2004; Feeney & Thrush, 2010). This may reflect the fact that explorers with interfering partners are interrupted frequently and less able to concentrate on performing well. Also, because explorers with interfering partners perform poorly even when given the answers to challenging tasks (Feeney, 2004), they may be rejecting their partners' intrusive assistance. Although these speculations await future investigation, it is noteworthy that these results with adults are consistent with research showing that parental interference in children's exploratory activities is associated with a variety of negative outcomes for children, including disrupted concentration, less persistence and enthusiasm in exploration, more passivity, more negative emotion, less competence, and less curiosity (e.g., Ainsworth, Bell, & Stayton, 1974; Cassidy & Berlin, 1994; Egeland & Farber, 1984; Main, 1983; Matas, Arend, & Sroufe, 1978).

Perceptions of exploration, and of one's ability to explore successfully, are additional immediate outcomes of receiving secure-base support. In one study, spouse encouragement during exploration predicted subsequent perceptions that exploration is enjoyable and that one is smart and competent to engage in it, whereas spouse interference had the opposite effect (Feeney & Thrush, 2010). Another study showed that when recipients felt that their goals were supported by their partners (during a discussion of personal goals), they rated their likelihood of achieving their goals to be greater after the discussion than before the discussion (Feeney, 2004).

With regard to longer-term outcomes, in one observational/longitudinal study, individuals whose partners exhibited availability to them (during goal discussions) at one point in time were more likely to have accomplished their goals 6 months later, and they showed greater evidence of increases in independent functioning over this period of time (Feeney, 2007). Corroborating these findings using self-report methods, Brunstein, Dangelmayer, and Schultheiss (1996) found that reports of the amount of goal support received from romantic partners predicted the enactment of both relationship and individual goals over a 4 week period of time. A longitudinal investigation of newlyweds showed that a spouses' secure-base support during the first year of marriage predicts increases in personal growth and relationship quality, as well as reports of better psychological and physical health 1 year later (Van Vleet & Feeney, 2011).

There are also some studies indicating that the successful pursuit of personally meaningful goals is related to indicators of well-being including elated rather than depressed mood and satisfaction with life (Brunstein, 1993; Brunstein, Schultheiss, & Grassman, 1998; Emmons, 1986; Emmons & King, 1988; Omodei & Wearing, 1990; Palys & Little, 1983; Ruehlman & Wolchik, 1988; Yetim, 1993; Zaleski, 1987). As a whole, these studies have shown that individuals with high well-being, in contrast to those with low well-being, pursue goals that are important, fulfilling, challenging, fueled by optimistic expectations, and assisted by others. This is consistent with attachment theory's notion that it is the interpersonal dynamics surrounding the *assistance by others* that is responsible for driving the effects of goal strivings on personal well-being. In longitudinal studies that support this idea, Brunstein and colleagues (1996) found that perceptions of goal attainability and social support for personal goals were predictive of changes in subjective well-being over time, and Brunstein (1993) showed that favorable conditions to attain personal goals led to more progress in goal achievement that translated into enhanced well-being. In fact, of all the personal goal variables assessed in their study, support of personal goals by significant others was the most powerful predictor of subjective well-being (Brunstein, 1993).

Studies have shown that support for personal goals by intimate partners accounts for how satisfied people feel with their relationship (Brunstein et al., 1996; Kaplan & Maddux, 2002). The idea is that perceiving high goal support from a partner should facilitate the enactment of personal goals, thereby enhancing the individual's relationship satisfaction. In contrast, perceiving a partner as undermining the pursuit of personal goals should impair relationship satisfaction by posing a threat to the accomplishment of highly valued goal states. Consistent with attachment–theoretical propositions regarding the importance of the secure-base caregiving function, this research showed that reports of goal support received from dating partners predicted increases in relationship satisfaction over a period of 4 weeks, and that both receiving and giving personal goal support were

systematically linked to spouses' marital satisfaction. These findings suggest that personal goal attainment and relationship outcomes are linked in important ways (Gore & Cross, 2006).

Overall, this work provides important evidence for attachment–theoretical propositions regarding the importance of secure-base caregiving in adulthood. However, more research is needed to assess a variety of potential long-term outcomes of secure-base caregiving, including effects on learning/knowledge/discovery, global self-esteem, achievements, approach to challenges, and changes in exploration behavior over time.

## Individual Differences in Outcomes of Secure-Base Caregiving

Although all individuals are expected to benefit from secure-base caregiving, it is possible that the care receiver's attachment characteristics will moderate this link and influence the degree to which he or she benefits. For example, the exploration behavior of avoidant individuals may be less tied to the support they receive (given that they have learned not to depend on it). Moreover, even if anxious individuals receive secure-base caregiving, their fear of failure and chronic attachment system activation may inhibit their ability to fully embrace the value of exploration. These possibilities await future investigation.

## Directions for Future Research on Caregiving in Adult Relationships

In addition to future research directions we have already discussed, there is a need for theoretical elaboration and research that considers the interrelations among the attachment, caregiving, and exploration systems as they play out in dyadic interactions. For example, researchers must consider ways in which caregiving processes might change when the attachment and caregiving systems are simultaneously activated in the same individual (e.g., when relationship partners are simultaneously distressed). It is also noteworthy that our discussion of secure-base caregiving processes emphasizes explorations of the external world that are likely to have important implications for the inner self in terms of self-esteem, perceptions of self-competency, and so on. However, effective secure-base caregiving should include not only the support of a relationship partner's exploration of the physical world but also the exploration of his or her inner psychological world (e.g., exploration of thoughts, feelings, and emotions related to self-understanding and self-discovery). In fact, Main and her colleagues have described the uninhibited exploration of attachment-related events, thoughts, and emotions as a hallmark of secure attachment (Main, 1995; Main, Kaplan, & Cassidy, 1985). Thus, the support of this type of exploration, in particular, may have important implications for the development of secure attachment orientations in adulthood (e.g., Byng-Hall, 1999). Finally, it will be important to consider the ways in which the attachment, caregiving, and exploration systems function together in the context of everyday interactions between relationship partners. Attachment theory predicts that a delicate balance of encouraging autonomy (secure-base caregiving) yet accepting dependence when needed (safe-haven caregiving) is vital for healthy personal and relationship functioning. Thus, studies that simultaneously consider both caregiving functions will be important in advancing this research area.

## Concluding Statement

Our goal in this chapter has been to consider caregiving from an attachment–theoretical perspective by reviewing theory and research on caregiving in both parent–child and adult relationships. Safe-haven and secure-base caregiving represent two complementary caregiving functions, and they are connected in the sense that attachment figures will be unable to effectively provide a secure base (and support exploration behavior) unless they understand and respect that attachment behavior is a part of human nature (even in adulthood), and is not a negative sign of dependency that should be outgrown (Bowlby, 1969/1982, 1988; Feeney, 2007). Good caregivers must have a genuine understanding and respect for not only individuals' need to grow, learn, discover, and accomplish personal goals but also the the ingrained need of all individuals for affection, intimacy, and comfort in times of stress. Although it requires effort to provide a sensitive and responsive safe haven and secure base (and to balance these caregiving responsibilities), attachment theory highlights that the rewards of such care are likely to be great: Recipients of such care are likely to be happy and trusting, confident that others will be helpful when needed, confident in their own abili-

ties and capabilities, self-reliant and bold in their explorations of the world, cooperative with others, effective citizens who are unlikely to break down in adversity, active contributors to society, sympathetic/helpful to others in distress, and capable of maintaining healthy/stable relationships.

## References

Ainsworth, M. (1969). *Maternal care scales*. Retrieved from *www.psychology.sunysb.edu/attachment/measures/content/ainsworth_scales.html*.

Ainsworth, M. D. S. (1967). *Infancy in Uganda: Infant care and the growth of love*. Baltimore: Johns Hopkins Press.

Ainsworth, M. D. S., Bell, S. M., & Stayton, D. (1971). Individual differences in strange situation behavior of one-year-olds. In H. R. Schaffer (Ed.), *The origins of human social relations* (pp. 17–57). London: Academic Press.

Ainsworth, M. D. S., Bell, S. M., & Stayton, D. (1974). Infant–mother attachment and social development. In M. P. Richards (Ed.), *The introduction of the child into a social world* (pp. 99–135). London: Cambridge University Press.

Ainsworth, M. D. S., Blehar, M. C., Waters, E., & Wall, S. (1978). *Patterns of attachment: Psychological study of the strange situation*. Hillsdale, NJ: Erlbaum.

Allen, K. M., Blascovich, J., Tomaka, J., & Kelsey, R. M. (1991). Presence of human friends and pet dogs as moderators of autonomic responses to stress in women. *Journal of Personality and Social Psychology, 61*, 582–589.

Atkinson, L., Gonzalez, A., Kashy, D. A., Basile, V. S., Masellis, M., Pereira, J., et al. (2013). Maternal sensitivity and infant and mother adrenocortical function across challenges. *Psychoneuroendocrinology, 38*, 2943–2951.

Bakermans-Kranenburg, M., Van IJzendoorn, M., & Juffer, F. (2003). Less is more: Meta-analyses of sensitivity and attachment interventions in early childhood. *Psychological Bulletin, 129*, 195–215.

Barbee, A. P., & Cunningham, M. R. (1995). An experimental approach to social support communications: Interactive coping in close relationships. *Communication Yearbook, 18*, 381–413.

Barnett, M. A., Shanahan, L., Deng, M., Haskett, M. E., & Cox, M. J. (2010). Independent and interactive contributions of parenting behaviors and beliefs in the prediction of early childhood behavior problems. *Parenting: Science and Practice, 10*, 43–59.

Bartholomew, K., Cobb, R. J., & Poole, J. (1997). Adult attachment patterns and social support processes. In G. R. Pierce, B. Lakey, I. G. Sarason, & B. R. Sarason (Eds.), *Sourcebook of social support and personality*. New York: Plenum Press.

Belsky, J., & Fearon, R. M. P. (2008). Precursors of attachment security. In J. Cassidy & P. R. Shaver (Eds.), *Handbook of attachment: Theory, research, and clinical applications* (2nd ed., pp. 295–316). New York: Guilford Press.

Belsky, J., & Pluess, M. (2009). Beyond diathesis stress: Differential susceptibility to environmental influences. *Psychological Bulletin, 135,* 885–908.

Bernier, A., Matte-Gagné, C., Bélanger, M. È., & Whipple, N. (2014). Taking stock of two decades of attachment transmission gap: Broadening the assessment of maternal behavior. *Child Development, 85,* 1852–1865.

Bocknek, E. L., Brophy-Herb, H. E., & Banerjee, M. (2009). Effects of parental supportiveness on toddlers' emotion regulation over the first three years of life in a low-income African American sample. *Infant Mental Health Journal, 30,* 452–476.

Bowlby, J. (1973). *Attachment and loss: Separation, anxiety and anger.* New York: Basic Books.

Bowlby, J. (1980). *Attachment and loss: Sadness and depression.* New York: Basic Books.

Bowlby, J. (1982). *Attachment and loss: Vol. 1. Attachment.* New York: Basic Books. (Original work published 1969)

Bowlby, J. (1988). *A secure base.* New York: Basic Books.

Boyce, W. T., & Ellis, B. J. (2005). Biological sensitivity to context: I. An evolutionary–developmental theory of the origins and functions of stress reactivity. *Development and Psychopathology, 17,* 271–301.

Brennan, K. A., Clark, C. L., & Shaver, P. R. (1998). Self-report measurement of adult attachment: An integrative overview. In J. A. Simpson & W. S. Rholes (Eds.), *Attachment theory and close relationships* (pp. 46–76). New York: Guilford Press.

Bretherton, I. (1987). New perspectives on attachment relations: Security, communication, and internal working models. In J. D. Osofsky (Ed.), *Handbook of infant development* (2nd ed., pp. 1061–1100). New York: Wiley.

Brody, G. H., & Flor, D. L. (1998). Maternal resources, parenting practices, and child competence in rural, single-parent African American families. *Child Development, 69*(3), 803–816.

Brunstein, J. C. (1993). Personal goals and subjective well-being: A longitudinal study. *Journal of Personality and Social Psychology, 65,* 1061–1070.

Brunstein, J. C., Dangelmayer, G., & Schultheiss, O. C. (1996). Personal goals and social support in close relationships: Effects on relationship mood and marital satisfaction. *Journal of Personality and Social Psychology, 71,* 1006–1019.

Brunstein, J. C., Schultheiss, O. C., & Grassman, R. (1998). Personal goals and emotional well-being: The moderating role of motive dispositions. *Journal of Personality and Social Psychology, 75,* 494–508.

Buhrmester, D., Furman, W., Wittenberg, M. T., & Reis, H. T. (1988). Five domains of interpersonal competence in peer relationships. *Journal of Personality and Social Psychology, 55,* 991–1008.

Byng-Hall, J. (1999). Family and couple therapy: Toward greater security. In J. Cassidy, & P. R. Shaver (Eds.), *Handbook of attachment: Theory, research, and clinical applications* (pp. 625–645). New York: Guilford Press.

Carnelley, K. B., Pietromonaco, P. R., & Jaffe, K. (1996). Attachment, caregiving, and relationship functioning in couples: Effects of self and partner. *Personal Relationships, 3,* 257–278.

Carpenter, E. M., & Kirkpatrick, L. A. (1996). Attachment style and presence of a romantic partner as moderators of psychophysiological responses to a stressful laboratory situation. *Personal Relationships, 3,* 351–367.

Cassidy, J. (1994). Emotion regulation: Influences of attachment relationships. *Monographs of the Society for Research in Child Development, 59,* 228–249.

Cassidy, J., & Berlin, L. J. (1994). The insecure/ambivalent pattern of attachment: Theory and research. *Child Development, 65,* 971–991.

Cassidy, J., Jones, J. D., & Shaver, P. R. (2013). Contributions of attachment theory and research: A framework for future research, translation, and policy. *Development and Psychopathology, 25,* 1415–1434.

Cassidy, J., Woodhouse, S. S., Cooper, G., Hoffman, K., Powell, B., & Rodenberg, M. (2005). Examination of the precursors of infant attachment security: Implications for early intervention and intervention research. In L. J. Berlin, Y. Ziv, L. Amaya-Jackson, & M. T. Greenberg (Eds.), *Enhancing early attachments: Theory, research, intervention, and policy* (pp. 34–60). New York: Guilford Press.

Cassidy, J., Woodhouse, S. S., Sherman, L. J., Stupica, B., & Lejuez, C. W. (2011). Enhancing infant attachment security: An examination of treatment efficacy and differential susceptibility. *Development and Psychopathology, 23,* 131–148.

Chaudhuri, J. H., Easterbrooks, M. A., & Davis, C. R. (2009). The relation between emotional availability and parenting style: Cultural and economic factors in a diverse sample of young mothers. *Parenting: Science and Practice, 9,* 277–299.

Coan, J., Schaefer, H. S., & Davidson, R. J. (2006). Lending a hand: Social regulation of the neural response to threat. *Psychological Science, 17,* 1032–1039.

Cohen, S. (1988). Psychosocial models of the role of social support in the etiology of physical disease. *Health Psychology, 7,* 269–297.

Cohen, S. (2004). Social relationships and health. *American Psychologist, 59,* 676–684.

Cohen, S., & Syme, S. L. (1985). *Social support and health.* San Diego, CA: Academic Press.

Cohen, S., & Wills, T. A. (1985). Stress, social support, and the buffering hypothesis. *Psychological Bulletin, 98,* 310–357.

Collins, N. L., & Feeney, B. C. (2000). A safe haven: An attachment theory perspective on support-seeking and caregiving in adult romantic relationships. *Journal of Personality and Social Psychology, 78,* 1053–1073.

Collins, N. L., & Feeney, B. C. (2005, May). *Attachment*

*processes in intimate relationships: Support-seeking and caregiving behavior in daily interaction.* Paper presented at the annual meeting of the American Psychological Society, Los Angeles.

Collins, N. L., Ford, M. B., Guichard, A. C., Kane, H. S., & Feeney, B. C. (2010). Responding to need in intimate relationships: Social support and caregiving processes in couples. In M. Mikulincer & P. R. Shaver (Eds.), *Prosocial motives, emotions, and behavior: The better angels of our nature* (pp. 367–389). Washington, DC: American Psychological Association.

Collins, N, L., Kane, H. S., Guichard, A. C., & Ford, M. B. (2008). *Will you be there when I need you?: Perceived partner responsiveness shapes support-seeking behavior and motivations.* Unpublished manuscript, University of California, Santa Barbara.

Conger, R. D., & Donnellan, M. B. (2007). An interactionist perspective on the socioeconomic context of human development. *Annual Review of Psychology, 58,* 175–199.

Crowell, J., Treboux, D., Gao, Y., Fyffe, C., Pan, H., & Waters, E. (2002). Assessing secure base behavior in adulthood: Development of a measure, links to adult attachment representations and relations to couples' communication and reports of relationships. *Developmental Psychology, 38,* 679–693.

Cutrona, C. E. (1986). Behavioral manifestations of social support: A microanalytic investigation. *Journal of Personality and Social Psychology, 51,* 201–208.

Davidov, M., & Grusec, J. E. (2006). Untangling the links of parental responsiveness to distress and warmth to child outcomes. *Child Development, 77,* 44–58.

Demers, I., Bernier, A., Tarabulsy, G. M., & Provost, M. A. (2010). Mind-mindedness in adult and adolescent mothers: Relations to maternal sensitivity and infant attachment. *International Journal of Behavioral Development, 34,* 529–537.

De Wolff, M., & Van Ijzendoorn, M. (1997). Sensitivity and attachment: A meta-analysis on parental antecedents of infant attachment. *Child Development, 68,* 571–591.

Ditzen, B., Neumann, I. D., Bodenmann, G., von Dawans., B., Turner, R. A., Ehler, U., et al. (2007). Effects of different kinds of couple interaction on cortisol and heart rate responses to stress in women. *Psychoneuroendocrinology, 32,* 565-574.

Dix, T. (1991). The affective organization of parenting: Adaptive and maladaptative processes. *Psychological Bulletin, 110,* 3–25.

Dix, T. (1992). Parenting on behalf of the child: Empathic goals in the regulation of responsive parenting. In I. E. Sigel, A. V. McGillicuddy-DeLisi, & J. J. Goodnow (Eds.), *Parental belief systems: The psychological consequences for children* (2nd ed., pp. 319–346). Hillsdale, NJ: Erlbaum.

Dix, T., Gershoff, E. T., Meunier, L. N., & Miller, P. C. (2004). The affective structure of supportive parenting: Depressive symptoms, immediate emotions, and child-oriented motivation. *Developmental Psychology, 40,* 1212–1227.

Dykas, M. J., Woodhouse, S. S., Cassidy, J., & Waters, H. S. (2006). Narrative assessment of attachment representations: Links between secure base scripts and adolescent attachment. *Attachment and Human Development, 8,* 221–240.

Edens, J. L., Larkin, K. T., & Abel, J. L. (1992). The effect of social support and physical touch on cardiovascular reactions to mental stress. *Journal of Psychosomatic Research, 36,* 371–382.

Egeland, B., & Farber, E. (1984). Infant–mother attachment: Factors related to its development and changes over time. *Child Development, 55,* 753–771.

Emmons, R. A. (1986). Personal strivings: An approach to personality and subjective well-being. *Journal of Personality and Social Psychology, 51,* 1058–1068.

Emmons, R. A., & King, L. A. (1988). Conflict among personal strivings: Immediate and long-term implications for psychological and physical well-being. *Journal of Personality and Social Psychology, 54,* 1040–1048.

Fearon, R., Van IJzendoorn, M., Fonagy, P., Bakermans-Kranenburg, M., Schuengel, C., & Bokhorst, C. (2006). In search of shared and nonshared environmental factors in security of attachment: A behavior-genetic study of the association between sensitivity and attachment security. *Developmental Psychology, 42,* 1026–1040.

Feeney, B. C. (2004). A secure base: Responsive support of goal strivings and exploration in adult intimate relationships. *Journal of Personality and Social Psychology, 87,* 631–648.

Feeney, B. C. (2007). The dependency paradox in close relationships: Accepting dependence promotes independence. *Journal of Personality and Social Psychology, 92,* 268–285.

Feeney, B. C., Cassidy, J., & Ramos-Marcuse, F. (2008). The generalization of attachment representations to new social situations: Predicting behavior during initial interactions with strangers. *Journal of Personality and Social Psychology, 95,* 1481–1498.

Feeney, B. C., & Collins, N. L. (2001). Predictors of caregiving in adult intimate relationships: An attachment theoretical perspective. *Journal of Personality and Social Psychology, 80,* 972–994.

Feeney, B. C., & Collins, N. L. (2003). Motivations for caregiving in adult intimate relationships: Influences on caregiving behavior and relationship functioning. *Personality and Social Psychology Bulletin, 29,* 950–968.

Feeney, B. C., & Collins, N. L. (2014). A new look at social support: A theoretical perspective on thriving through relationships. *Personality and Social Psychology Review.* [Epub ahead of print]

Feeney, B. C., Collins, N. L., Van Vleet, M., & Tomlinson, J. M. (2013). Motivations for providing a secure base: Links with attachment orientation and secure base support behavior. *Attachment and Human Development, 15,* 261–280.

Feeney, B. C., & Kirkpatrick, L. A. (1996). The effects

of adult attachment and presence of romantic partners on physiological responses to stress. *Journal of Personality and Social Psychology, 70,* 255–270.

Feeney, B. C., & Thrush, R. L. (2010). Relationship influences on exploration in adulthood: The characteristics and function of a secure base. *Journal of Personality and Social Psychology, 98,* 57–76.

Feeney, J. A. (1996). Attachment, caregiving, and marital satisfaction. *Personal Relationships, 3,* 401–416.

Fishman, E., Turkheimer, E., & DeGood, D. (1995). Touch relieves stress and pain. *Journal of Behavioral Medicine, 18,* 69–79.

Florian, V., Mikulincer, M., & Bucholtz, I. (1995). Effects of adult attachment style on the perception and search for social support. *Journal of Psychology, 129,* 665–676.

Fonagy, P., Gergely, G., Jurist, E. L., & Target, M. (2002). *Affect regulation, mentalization, and the development of the self.* New York: Other Press.

Fraley, R., & Waller, N. G. (1998). Adult attachment patterns: A test of the typological model. In J. A. Simpson & W. S. Rholes (Eds.), *Attachment theory and close relationships* (pp. 77–114). New York: Guilford Press.

Fritz, H. L., Nagurney, A. J., Helgeson, V. S. (2003). Social interactions and cardiovascular reactivity during problem disclosure among friends. *Personality and Social Personality Bulletin, 29,* 713–725.

Gallo, L. C., & Matthews, K. A. (2006). Adolescents' attachment orientation influences ambulatory blood pressure responses to everyday social interactions. *Psychosomatic Medicine, 68,* 253–261.

George, C., Kaplan, N., & Main, M. (1984). *Adult Attachment Interview protocol.* Unpublished manuscript, University of California, Berkeley.

George, C., Kaplan, N., & Main, M. (1985). *Adult Attachment Interview protocol* (2nd ed.). Unpublished manuscript, University of California, Berkeley.

George, C., Kaplan, N., & Main, M. (1996). *Adult Attachment Interview protocol* (3rd ed.). Unpublished manuscript, University of California, Berkeley.

Gillath, O., Mikulincer, M., Fitzsimons, G. M., Shaver, P. R., Schachner, D. A., & Bargh, J. A. (2006). Automatic activation of attachment-related goals. *Personality and Social Psychology Bulletin, 32,* 1375–1388.

Glöggler, B., & Pauli-Pott, U. (2008). Different fear-regulation behaviors in toddlerhood: Relations to preceding infant negative emotionality, maternal depression, and sensitivity. *Merrill–Palmer Quarterly, 54,* 86–101.

Gore, J. S., & Cross, S. E. (2006). Pursuing goals for us: Relationally autonomous reasons in long-term goal pursuit. *Journal of Personality and Social Psychology, 90,* 848–861.

Grewen, K., Anderson, B., Girdler, S., & Light, K. C. (2003). Warm partner contact is related to lower cardiovascular reactivity. *Behavioral Medicine, 29,* 123–130.

Grossmann, K., Grossmann, K. E., Kindler, H., & Zimmermann, P. (2008). A wider view of attachment and exploration: The influence of mothers and fathers on the development of psychological security from infancy to young adulthood. In J. Cassidy & P. R. Shaver (Ed.), *Handbook of attachment: Theory, research, and clinical applications* (2nd ed., pp. 857–879). New York: Guilford Press.

Grossmann, K. E., Grossmann, K., & Zimmermann, P. (1999). A wider view of attachment and exploration. In J. Cassidy & P. R. Shaver (Eds.), *Handbook of attachment theory and research: Theory, research, and clinical applications* (pp. 760–786). New York: Guilford Press.

Hill-Soderlund, A. L., Mills-Koonce, W. R., Propper, C., Calkins, S. D., Granger, D. A., Moore, G. A., et al. (2008). Parasympathetic and sympathetic responses to the strange situation in infants and mothers from avoidant and securely attached dyads. *Developmental Psychobiology, 50,* 361–376.

Insel, T. R. (2000). Toward a neurobiology of attachment. *Review of General Psychology, 4,* 176–185.

Jahromi, L. B., Putnam, S. P., & Stifter, C. A. (2004). Maternal regulation of infant reactivity from 2 to 6 months. *Developmental Psychology, 40,* 477–487.

Jones, J. D., Cassidy, J., & Shaver, P. R. (2015). Parents' self-reported attachment styles: A review of links with parenting behaviors, emotions, and cognitions. *Personality and Social Psychology Review, 19,* 44–76.

Kamarck, T. W., Manuck, S. B., & Jennings, J. R. (1990). Social support reduces cardiovascular reactivity to psychological challenge: A laboratory model. *Psychosomatic Medicine, 52,* 42–58.

Kane, H. S., Jaremka, L. M., Guichard, A. C., Ford, M. B., Collins, N. L., & Feeney, B. C. (2007). Feeling supported and feeling satisfied: How one partner's attachment style predicts the other partner's relationship experiences. *Journal of Social and Personal Relationships, 24,* 535–555.

Kane, H. S., McCall, C., Collins, N. L., & Blascovich, J. A. (2012). Mere presence is not enough: Responsive support in a virtual world. *Journal of Experimental Social Psychology, 48,* 37–44.

Kaplan, M., & Maddux, J. E. (2002). Goals and marital satisfaction: Perceived support for personal goals and collective efficacy for collective goals. *Journal of Social and Clinical Psychology, 21,* 157–164.

Katz, J., Beach, S. R. H., & Anderson, P. (1996). Self-enhancement versus self-verification: Does spousal support always help? *Cognitive Therapy and Research, 20,* 345–360.

Kawachi, I., & Berkman, L. F. (2001). Social ties and mental health. *Journal of Urban Health, 78,* 458–467.

Kotler, T. (1985). Security and autonomy within marriage. *Human Relations, 38,* 299–321.

Kunce, L. J., & Shaver, P. R. (1994). An attachment-theoretical approach to caregiving in romantic relationships. In K. Bartholomew & D. Perlman (Eds.), *Advances in personal relationships* (Vol. 5, pp. 205–237). London: Jessica Kingsley.

Lakey, B., & Heller, K. (1988). Social support from a friend, perceived support, and social problem solving. *American Journal of Community Psychology, 16*, 811–824.

Laranjo, J., Bernier, A., & Meins, E. (2008). Associations between maternal mind-mindedness and infant attachment security: Investigating the mediating role of maternal sensitivity. *Infant Behavior and Development, 31*, 688–695.

Lecuyer, E., & Houck, G. M. (2006). Maternal limit-setting in toddlerhood: Socialization strategies for the development of self-regulation. *Infant Mental Health Journal, 27*, 344–370.

Leerkes, E. M. (2010). Predictors of maternal sensitivity to infant distress. *Parenting: Science and Practice, 10*, 219–239.

Leerkes, E. M. (2011). Maternal sensitivity during distressing tasks: A unique predictor of attachment security. *Infant Behavior and Development, 34*, 443–446.

Leerkes, E. M., Blankson, A. N., & O'Brien, M. (2009). Differential effects of maternal sensitivity to infant distress and nondistress on socioemotional functioning. *Child Development, 80*, 762–775.

Leerkes, E. M., Parade, S. H., & Gudmundson, J. A. (2011). Mothers' emotional reactions to crying pose risk for subsequent attachment insecurity. *Journal of Family Psychology, 25*, 635–643.

Leerkes, E. M., Supple, A. J., O'Brien, M., Calkins, S. D., Haltigan, J. D., Wong, M. S., et al. (2015). Antecedents of maternal sensitivity during distressing tasks: Integrating attachment, social information processing, and psychobiological perspectives. *Child Development, 86*(1), 94–111.

Leerkes, E. M., Weaver, J. M., & O'Brien, M. (2012). Differentiating maternal sensitivity to infant distress and non-distress. *Parenting: Science and Practice, 12*, 175–184.

Lewis, C., & Lamb, M. E. (2003). Fathers' influences on children's development: The evidence from two-parent families. *European Journal of Psychology of Education, 18*, 211–228.

Lucassen, N., Tharner, A., Van IJzendoorn, M. H., Bakermans-Kranenburg, M. J., Volling, B. L., Verhulst, F. C., et al. (2011). The association between paternal sensitivity and infant–father attachment security: A meta-analysis of three decades of research. *Journal of Family Psychology, 25*, 986–992.

Lynch, J. J., Thomas, S. A., Paskewitz, D. A., Katcher, A. H., & Weir, L. O. (1977). Human contact and cardiac arrhythmia in a coronary care unit. *Psychosomatic Medicine, 39*, 188–192.

Lyons-Ruth, K., Bronfman, E., & Parsons, E. (1999). Maternal frightened, frightening, or atypical behavior and disorganized infant attachment patterns. *Monographs of the Society for Research in Child Development, 64*, 67–96.

Lyons-Ruth, K., Bureau, J.-F., Holmes, B., Easterbrooks, A., & Brooks, N. H. (2013). Borderline symptoms and suicidality/self-injury in late adolescence: Prospectively observed relationship correlates in infancy and childhood. *Psychiatry Research, 206*, 273–281.

MacDonald, K. (1992). Warmth as a developmental construct: An evolutionary analysis. *Child Development, 63*, 753–773.

Main, M. (1983). Exploration, play, and cognitive functioning related to infant–mother attachment. *Infant Behavior and Development, 6*, 167–174.

Main, M. (1995). Attachment: Overview, with implications for clinical work. In S. Goldberg, R. Muir, & J. Kerr (Eds.), *Attachment theory: Social, developmental, and clinical perspectives* (pp. 407–474). Hillsdale, NJ: Analytic Press.

Main, M., & Hesse, E. (1990). Parents' unresolved traumatic experiences are related to infant disorganized attachment status: Is frightened and/or frightening parental behavior the linking mechanism? In M. T. Greenberg, D. Cicchetti, & E. M. Cummings (Eds.), *Attachment in the preschool years: Theory, research, and intervention* (pp. 161–182). Chicago: University of Chicago Press.

Main, M., Kaplan, N., & Cassidy, J. (1985). Security in infancy, childhood, and adulthood: A move to the level of representation. In I. Bretherton & E. Waters (Eds.), Growing points in attachment theory and research. *Monographs of the Society for Research in Child Development, 50*, 66–104.

Matas, L., Arend, R., & Sroufe, L. A. (1978). Continuity of adaptation in the second year: The relationship between quality of attachment and later competence. *Child Development, 49*, 547–556.

Meins, E., Fernyhough, C., de Rosnay, M., Arnott, B., Leekam, S. R., & Turner, M. (2012). Mind-mindedness as a multidimensional construct: Appropriate and nonattuned mind-related comments independently predict infant–mother attachment in a socially diverse sample. *Infancy, 17*, 393–415.

Meins, E., Fernyhough, C., Fradley, E., & Tuckey, M. (2001). Rethinking maternal sensitivity: Mothers' comments on infants' mental processes predict security of attachment at 12 months. *Journal of Child Psychology and Psychiatry, 42*, 637–648.

Mesman, J., & Emmen, R. A. G. (2013). Mary Ainsworth's legacy: A systematic review of observational instruments measuring parental sensitivity. *Attachment & Human Development, 15*, 485–506.

Mesman, J., Van IJzendoorn, M. H., & Bakermans-Kranenburg, M. J. (2012). Unequal in opportunity, equal in process: Parental sensitivity promotes positive child development in ethnic minority families. *Child Development Perspectives, 6*, 239–250.

Mesquita, A. R., Soares, I., Roisman, G. I., Van IJzendoorn, M., Bakermans-Kranenburg, M., Luijk, M., et al. (2013). Predicting children's attachment behaviors from the interaction between oxytocin and glucocorticoid receptors polymorphisms. *Psychiatry Research, 210*, 1322–1323.

Mikulincer, M., & Florian, V. (1995). Appraisal of and

coping with a real-life stressful situation: The contribution of attachment styles. *Personality and Social Psychology Bulletin, 21,* 406–414.

Mikulincer, M., Florian, V., & Weller, A. (1993). Attachment styles, coping strategies, and posttraumatic psychological distress: The impact of the Gulf War in Israel. *Journal of Personality and Social Psychology, 64,* 817–826.

Mikulincer, M., Gillath, O., Halevy, V., Avihou, N., Avidan, S., & Eshkoli, N. (2001). Attachment theory and reactions to others' needs: Evidence that activation of the sense of attachment security promotes empathic responses. *Journal of Personality and Social Psychology, 81,* 1205–1224.

Mikulincer, M., Gillath, O., Sapir-Lavid, Y., Yaakobi, E., Arias, K., Tal-Aloni, L., et al. (2003). Attachment theory and concern for others' welfare: Evidence that activation of the sense of secure base promotes endorsement of self-transcendence values. *Basic and Applied Social Psychology, 25,* 299–312.

Mikulincer, M., & Shaver, P. R. (2001). Attachment theory and intergroup bias: Evidence that priming the secure base schema attenuates negative reactions to out-groups. *Journal of Personality and Social Psychology, 81,* 97–115.

Mikulincer, M., & Shaver, P. R. (2005). Attachment security, compassion, and altruism. *Current Directions in Psychological Science, 14,* 34–38.

Mikulincer, M., Shaver, P. R., Gillath, O., & Nitzberg, R. A. (2005). Attachment, caregiving, and altruism: Boosting attachment security increases compassion and helping. *Journal of Personality and Social Psychology, 89,* 817–839.

Mills-Koonce, W. R., Gariepy, J.-L., Propper, C., Sutton, K., Calkins, S., Moore, G., et al. (2007). Infant and parent factors associated with early maternal sensitivity: A caregiver-attachment systems approach. *Infant Behavior and Development, 30,* 114–126.

Monin, J. K., Feeney, B. C., & Schulz, R. (2012). Attachment orientation and reactions to anxiety expression in close relationships. *Personal Relationships, 19,* 535–550.

Moore, G. A., & Calkins, S. D. (2004). Infants' vagal regulation in the still-face paradigm is related to dyadic coordination of mother-infant interaction. *Developmental Psychology, 40,* 1063–1080.

Moore, G. A., Hill-Soderlund, A. L., Propper, C. B., Calkins, S. D., Mills-Koonce, W. R., & Cox, M. J. (2009). Mother–infant vagal regulation in the face-to-face still-face paradigm is moderated by maternal sensitivity. *Child Development, 80,* 209–223.

Mount, K. S., Crockenberg, S. C., Jó, P. S., & Wagar, J.-L. (2010). Maternal and child correlates of anxiety in 2½-year-old children. *Infant Behavior and Development, 33,* 567–578.

National Institute of Child Health and Human Development (NICHD) Early Child Care Research Network. (1997). The effects of infant child care on infant–mother attachment security: Results of the NICHD study of early child care. *Child Development, 68,* 860–879.

Ognibene, T. C., & Collins, N. L. (1998). Adult attachment styles, perceived social support, and coping strategies. *Journal of Social and Personal Relationships, 15,* 323–345.

Omodei, M. M., & Wearing, A. J. (1990). Need satisfaction and involvement in personal projects: Toward an integrative model of subjective well-being. *Journal of Personality and Social Psychology, 59,* 762–769.

Owen, M. T. (1992). *The NICHD study of Early Child Care Mother–Infant Interaction Scales.* Unpublished manuscript, Timberlawn Psychiatric Research Foundation, Dallas, TX.

Palys, T. S., & Little, B. R. (1983). Perceived life satisfaction and the organization of personal project systems. *Journal of Personality and Social Psychology, 44,* 1221–1230.

Posada, G. (2013). Piecing together the sensitivity construct: Ethology and cross-cultural research. *Attachment and Human Development, 15,* 637–656.

Raval, V., Goldberg, S., Atkinson, L., Benoit, D., Myhal, N., Poulton, L., et al. (2001). Maternal attachment, maternal responsiveness and infant attachment. *Infant Behavior and Development, 24,* 281–304.

Rholes, W. S., Simpson, J. A., & Orina, M. M. (1999). Attachment and anger in an anxiety-provoking situation. *Journal of Personality and Social Psychology, 76,* 940–957.

Roisman, G. I., Booth-LaForce, C., Belsky, J., Burt, K. B., & Groh, A. M. (2013). Molecular-genetic correlates of infant attachment: A cautionary tale. *Attachment and Human Development, 15,* 384–406.

Roisman, G. I., & Fraley, R. C. (2008). A behavior-genetic study of parenting quality, infant attachment security, and their covariation in a nationally representative sample. *Developmental Psychology, 44,* 831–839.

Roisman, G. I., Holland, A., Fortuna, K., Fraley, R., Clausell, E., & Clarke, A. (2007). The Adult Attachment Interview and self-reports of attachment style: An empirical rapprochement. *Journal of Personality and Social Psychology, 92,* 678–697.

Rosenblum, K. L., McDonough, S. C., Sameroff, A. J., & Muzik, M. (2008). Reflection in thought and action: Maternal parenting reflectivity predicts mind-minded comments and interactive behavior. *Infant Mental Health Journal, 29,* 362–376.

Rothbart, M. K., & Bates, J. E. (2006). Temperament. In N. Eisenberg, W. Damon, & R. M. Lerner (Eds.), *Handbook of child psychology: Vol. 3. Social, emotional, and personality development* (6th ed., pp. 99–166). Hoboken, NJ: Wiley.

Ruehlman, L. S., & Wolchik, S. A. (1988). Personal goals and interpersonal support and hindrance as factors in psychological distress and well-being. *Journal of Personality and Social Psychology, 55,* 293–301.

Sarason, B. R., Sarason, I. G., & Gurung, R. A. R. (1997). Close personal relationships and health outcomes: A key to the role of social support. In S.

Duck (Ed.), *Handbook of personal relationships* (pp. 547–573). New York: Plenum Press.

Sarason, I. G., & Sarason, B. R. (1986). Experimentally provided social support. *Journal of Personality and Social Psychology, 50,* 1222–1225.

Shaw, D. S., Lacourse, E., & Nagin, D. S. (2005). Developmental trajectories of conduct problems and hyperactivity from ages 2 to 10. *Journal of Child Psychology and Psychiatry, 46,* 931–942.

Shi, Z., Bureau, J.-F., Easterbrooks, M. A., Zhao, X., & Lyons-Ruth, K. (2012). Childhood maltreatment and prospectively observed quality of early care as predictors of antisocial personality disorder features. *Infant Mental Health Journal, 33,* 55–69.

Simpson, J. A., Campbell, L., & Weisberg, Y. J. (2006). Daily perceptions of conflict and support in romantic relationships: The ups and downs of anxiously attached individuals. In M. Mikulincer & G. S. Goodman (Eds.), *Dynamics of romantic love: Attachment, caregiving, and sex* (pp. 216–239). New York: Guilford Press.

Simpson, J. [A.], & Rholes, W. S. (1994). Stress and secure base relationships in adulthood. In K. Bartholomew & D. Perlman (Eds.), *Advances in personal relationships* (Vol. 5, pp. 181–204). London: Jessica Kingsley.

Simpson, J. A., Rholes, W. S., & Nelligan, J. S. (1992). Support seeking and support giving within couples in an anxiety-provoking situation: The role of attachment styles. *Journal of Personality and Social Psychology, 62,* 434–446.

Simpson, J. A., Rholes, W. S., Orina, M. M., & Grich, J. (2002). Working models of attachment, support giving, and support seeking in a stressful situation. *Personality and Social Psychology Bulletin, 28,* 598–608.

Simpson, J. A., Winterheld, H. A., Rholes, W. S., & Orina, M. M. (2007). Working models of attachment and reactions to different forms of caregiving from romantic partners. *Journal of Personality and Social Psychology, 93,* 466–477.

Snydersmith, M. A., & Cacioppo, J. T. (1992). Parsing complex social factors to determine component effects: I. Autonomic activity and reactivity as a function of human association. *Journal of Social and Clinical Psychology, 11,* 263-278.

Sroufe, L. A., & Waters, E. (1977). Attachment as an organizational construct. *Child Development, 48,* 1184–1199.

Stacks, A. M., Muzik, M., Wong, K., Beeghly, M., Huth-Bocks, A., Irwin, J. L., et al. (2014). Maternal reflective functioning among mothers with childhood maltreatment histories: Links to sensitive parenting and infant attachment security. *Attachment and Human Development, 16,* 515–533.

Steele, R. D., Waters, T. E. A., Bost, K. K., Vaughn, B. E., Truitt, W., Waters, H. S., et al. (2014). Caregiving antecedents of secure base script knowledge: A comparative analysis of young adult attachment representations. *Developmental Psychology, 50,* 2526–2538.

Suchman, N. E., DeCoste, C., Leigh, D., & Borelli, J. (2010). Reflective functioning in mothers with drug use disorders: Implications for dyadic interactions with infants and toddlers. *Attachment and Human Development, 12,* 567–585.

Tarabulsy, G. M., Bernier, A., Provost, M. A., Maranda, J., Larose, S., Moss, E., et al. (2005). Another look inside the gap: Ecological contributions to the transmission of attachment in a sample of adolescent mother–infant dyads. *Developmental Psychology, 41,* 212–224.

True, M. M., Pisani, L., & Oumar, F. (2001). Infant–mother attachment among the Dogon of Mali. *Child Development, 72,* 1451–1466.

Uchino, B. N., Cacioppo, J. T., & Kiecolt-Glaser, J. K. (1996). The relationship between social support and physiological processes: A review with emphasis on underlying mechanisms and implications for health. *Psychological Bulletin, 119,* 488–531.

Van IJzendoorn, M. (1995). Adult attachment representations, parental responsiveness, and infant attachment: A meta-analysis on the predictive validity of the Adult Attachment Interview. *Psychological Bulletin, 117,* 387–403.

Van IJzendoorn, M. H., & Sagi-Schwartz, A. (2008). Cross-cultural patterns of attachment: Universal and contextual dimensions. In J. Cassidy & P. R. Shaver (Eds.), *Handbook of attachment: Theory, research, and clinical applications* (2nd ed., pp. 880–905). New York: Guilford Press.

Van Vleet, M., & Feeney, B. C. (2011). *A longitudinal investigation of the consequences of secure base support in close relationships.* Unpublished manuscript, Carnegie Mellon University.

Waters, E., & Cummings, E. (2000). A secure base from which to explore close relationships. *Child Development, 71,* 164–172.

Westmaas, J. L., & Silver, R. C. (2001). The role of attachment in responses to victims of life crises. *Journal of Personality and Social Psychology, 80,* 425–438.

Whitcher, S. J., & Fisher, J. D., (1979). Multidimensional reaction to therapeutic touch in a hospital setting. Journal of Personality and Social Psychology, 37, 87-96.

Winstead, B. A., & Derlega, V. J. (1985). Benefits of same-sex friendships in a stressful situation. *Journal of Social and Clinical Psychology, 3,* 378–384.

Winstead, B. A., Derlega, V. J., Lewis, R. J., Sanchez-Hucles, J., & Clarke, E. (1992). Friendship, social interaction, and coping with stress. *Communication Research, 19,* 193–211.

Woodhouse, S. S., Dykas, M. J., & Cassidy, J. (2009). Perceptions of secure base provision within the family. *Attachment and Human Development, 11,* 47–67.

Woodhouse, S. S., Beeney, J. R. S., Doub, A. E., & Cassidy, J. (2015). *Secure base provision: A new approach to links between maternal caregiving and attachment.* Manuscript in preparation.

Yaman, A., Mesman, J., Van IJzendoorn, M. H., Bakermans-Kranenburg, M. J., & Linting, M. (2010). Parenting in an individualistic culture with a collectivistic cultural background: The case of Turkish immigrant families with toddlers in the Netherlands. *Journal of Child and Family Studies, 19,* 617–628.

Yetim, U. (1993). Life satisfaction: A study based on the organization of personal projects. *Social Indicators Research, 29,* 277–289.

Yovsi, R. D., Kärtner, J., Keller, H., & Lohaus, A. (2009). Maternal interactional quality in two cultural environments: German middle class and Cameroonian rural mothers. *Journal of Cross-Cultural Psychology, 40,* 701–707.

Zaleski, Z. (1987). Behavioral effects of self-set goals for different time ranges. *International Journal of Psychology, 22,* 17–38.

# Chapter 37

# Cross-Cultural Patterns of Attachment
## Universal and Contextual Dimensions

Judi Mesman
Marinus H. van IJzendoorn
Abraham Sagi-Schwartz

It was in Uganda, a former British protectorate in East Africa, that Mary Ainsworth (1967) began to create the famous tripartite classification system of infant–mother attachment relationships. In her short-term longitudinal field study, carried out in 1954–1955, she found three patterns of attachment behavior in a small sample of 28 infants. The "securely attached group" of 16 infants cried infrequently, seemed especially content when they were with their mothers, and used their mothers as a secure base from which to explore the environment. The "insecurely attached group" of seven infants cried frequently, not only when left alone by their mothers but also in the mothers' presence; they cried to be picked up, cried when they were put down, and wanted continuous physical contact with their mothers, mingled with ambivalence about their mothers' presence. A "nonattached" group of five infants responded similarly to their mothers and to other adults, were not upset about being left alone by their mothers, and avoided interaction with the mothers upon their return. From Ainsworth's detailed case studies of these infants, it can be inferred that in the Strange Situation procedure (Ainsworth, Blehar, Waters, & Wall, 1978) they would have been classified as "avoidant."

The Uganda study laid the foundation for not only the notion of attachment classification but also the development of the sensitivity construct that would later be captured in the still widely used Sensitivity–Insensitivity to Infant Signals and Communications Observational Scale (Ainsworth, Bell, & Stayton, 1971, 1974). Ainsworth described how it was not warmth that seemed to distinguish between the different attachment classifications because almost all of the observed mothers in the Uganda sample showed warmth in interaction with their babies, but rather the amount of caregiving for the baby, and the mother's excellence as an informant about the baby. From Ainsworth's descriptions it becomes clear that these two factors amount to a pattern of proximity and availability, interest in the baby, perceptiveness about the baby's needs, and prompt responsiveness to the baby's signals. Ainsworth's work in a context with multiple caregivers in the non-Western setting of Uganda was the starting point from which she initiated a replication study in a Western setting, as described in her Baltimore study (Ainsworth & Wittig, 1969). Thus, the Uganda study provided all the main ingredients for decades of research and theorizing about attachment and the role of parental sensitivity

852

in predicting differences in the quality of attachment.

Bowlby (1969/1982) suggested that the formation of an attachment relationship between infants and their protective caregivers is the outcome of evolution; "inclusive fitness" (Trivers, 1974) was deemed to be facilitated by an ethologically based innate bias to become attached to a conspecific (see Simpson & Belsky, Chapter 5, this volume). Therefore, a core element of attachment theory is the universality of this bias in infants to become attached, regardless of their specific cultural niche. Furthermore, secure attachment is expected to be normative within contexts that are not inherently threatening to human health, survival, and successful reproduction. In circumstances not too strongly deviating from the "environment of evolutionary adaptedness" (Bowlby, 1969/1982), it is assumed to be most adaptive to develop an attachment pattern that allows for exploration of the environment from the security of a safe haven in case of distress. However, if a cultural niche is harsh and socioeconomic circumstances are extremely stressful for parents, infants may be prepared by their parents to develop, for example, an avoidant attachment pattern to cope with the socioeconomic stresses. In such a niche, the avoidant attachment pattern may well be normative in that it promotes inclusive fitness by stimulating a quantitative strategy of procreation with lower investment in more offspring at an earlier age (Simpson & Belsky, Chapter 5, this volume). Similarly, a resistant attachment pattern may be more common in environments that induce stress associated with intractable wars (Belsky, 2008). Evolution may not have equipped human beings with rigid behavioral strategies that would have made it difficult to adapt to changing (natural and social) environments (Hinde, 1982; Simpson & Belsky, Chapter 5, this volume). According to Hinde's (1982) position on conditional strategies, both mothers and babies are equipped to elicit not one set of interactions but a wide range of potential relationships compatible with specific environmental requirements. Nevertheless, one may wonder whether the secure attachment pattern is the primary strategy for adapting to a social environment that is basically supportive of the infant, and whether the insecure strategies should be considered as secondary, in that they constitute deviating but adaptive patterns provoked by less supportive contexts (Main, 1990). Although insecure attachments may emerge to the benefit of inclusive fitness, the long-term costs for

the individual's psychological and physical well-being might be considerable.

Regarding the antecedents of attachment, consistent responsive care is expected to foster a secure attachment bond, converging with observational studies of both human and nonhuman primates (e.g., Harlow, 1958; Nelson, Fox, & Zeanah, 2014; Van IJzendoorn, Bard, Bakermans-Kranenburg, & Ivan, 2009). Even in rodents it is found that early-life stress is provoked by fragmentation and unpredictability of parental care and signaling, and such stress leads to persistent emotional dysfunction in offspring (Baram et al., 2012; Meaney, 2010). Indeed, the role of parental sensitivity is to provide a secure base from which the child can explore in the secure knowledge that the caregiver will be physically and emotionally available in case of distress, and will alleviate this distress (Ainsworth et al., 1974, 1978). Genetics seems to play only a minor role in forming variations in attachment patterns (Bakermans-Kranenburg & Van IJzendoorn, Chapter 8, this volume).

It can be argued that when the broader child-rearing context allows for consistent responsive care, the formation of a secure attachment to this responsive caregiver is most likely to result in adaptive development and inclusive fitness. Similarly, in environments not deviating strongly from the environment of evolutionary adaptedness (Bowlby, 1969/1982), secure attachment is expected to lead to positive child outcomes across domains given that attachment security has been found to predict more optimal basic human prerequisites for adaptive functioning such as stress regulation (Lupien, McEwen, Gunnar, & Heim, 2009), nutritional status (Black & Aboud, 2011), and immune system functioning (Ehrlich, Miller, Jones, & Cassidy, Chapter 9, this volume; Miller, Chen, & Parker, 2011; see also Thompson, Chapter 16, this volume).

These universality assumptions have been widely tested and confirmed in North American and European samples, but the question is: What has nearly half a century of cross-cultural attachment research yielded regarding these issues? In this chapter, we describe and evaluate the cross-cultural attachment studies that have followed Ainsworth's Uganda example. We limit our discussion to cultures other than the Anglo-Saxon and European cultures because these are amply represented in other chapters in this volume (e.g., Fearon & Belsky, Chapter 14; Thompson, Chapter 16; Lyons-Ruth & Jacobvitz, Chapter

29; DeKlyen & Greenberg, Chapter 28; Chase-Stovall & Dozier, Chapter 31). We discuss the following hypotheses (originally suggested by Van IJzendoorn, 1990):

1. The *universality hypothesis*: When given an opportunity, all infants without severe neurophysiological impairments will become attached to one or more specific caregivers.
2. The *normativity hypothesis*: The majority of infants are securely attached in contexts that are not inherently threatening to human health and survival.
3. The *sensitivity hypothesis*: Attachment security is dependent on childrearing antecedents, particularly sensitive and prompt responses to infant attachment signals.
4. The *competence hypothesis*: Secure attachment leads to positive child outcomes in a variety of developmental domains.

## Attachment and Sensitivity in Africa: A Network of Caregivers

In her Uganda study, Ainsworth (1967, 1977) described the development of attachment in a multiple-caregiver context. Since then, it has also been established that in a Western context, infants' attachment to their mothers does not impede attachment relationships with other caregivers, such as fathers and professional caregivers in day care (Ahnert, Pinquart & Lamb, 2006; Goossens & Van IJzendoorn, 1990; Lucassen et al., 2011; Sagi et al., 1995). Thus, even in a childrearing environment in which mothers share their caregiving responsibilities with several other adults (and in Uganda also with older children), infants nevertheless become attached to their mothers and use them as a secure base to explore the world. The Uganda study, however, was rather small and exploratory, and certainly not representative of the various African cultures, each with its own patterns of multiple caregiving. In this section we discuss studies of attachment in Africa conducted in the years following Ainsworth's (1967) research. We place special emphasis on child development in a network of (child and adult) caregivers, in order to examine whether a multiple-caregiver environment is compatible with a unique attachment relationship between child and parent. Attachment in a network of multiple caregivers (or *alloparents*) is of crucial im-

portance because cross-cultural evidence indicates that in most societies, nonparental caretaking is either the norm or a common form (Hewlett & Winn, 2014; Hrdy, 2009), although this view has been contested (Bogin, Bragg, & Kuzawa, 2014), and paternal grandparents in a patrilineal society are likely to compete for the same resources as the child, challenging the often hypothesized benefits of alloparenting (Strassman, 2011). In this section we discuss ethnographic studies and studies using standardized instruments addressing attachment in the African context, which often involves multiple caregivers.

### Ethnographic Studies of Attachment and Sensitivity in Africa

We start by describing five studies of multiple caregiving in African societies that provide ethnographic descriptions of secure-base behavior and discriminative attachment to one or more caregivers, and patterns of sensitive responsive care. Four of these studies concern hunter–gatherer societies, characterized by small seminomadic groups with a fluid group structure, absence of strict social rules, and flexible subsistence strategies (Lee & Daly, 1999). Bowlby (1969/1982) developed his evolutionary theory of attachment on the basis of speculations about child development and childrearing in the original environment in which the human species spent about 99% of its historical time as hunters and gatherers. In this "environment of evolutionary adaptedness" an infant would be protected against predators and other dangers by staying in close proximity to a protective adult. The four societies resembling this original way of living are described here.

Konner (1977, 2005) studied the !Kung San or Bushmen of northwestern Botswana, and described the general rules of childrearing in the !Kung society as reflecting indulgence, stimulation, and nonrestriction (Konner, 1977). The !Kung infants were fed whenever they cried and reached for the breast. At night they slept in close proximity to their mothers and were also fed on demand—even without the mothers' awakening. An infant was carried around in a sling, giving the infant constant access to the mother's breast and to decorative objects hanging around her neck. The infant could look around freely and experience extensive physical and cognitive stimulation. The 2- and 3-year-old children studied by Konner were involved in multiage peer groups, spending more time there than with their mothers, and readily establishing new bonds. Nevertheless, !Kung mothers were most comforting in response to infant crying, even when excluding breast feeding, always responding to crying bouts lasting longer than 30 seconds (Konner, 2005). The !Kung study showed that there is room for both multiple attachment relationships and a preferred primary bond with the mother. It further highlights that sensitive responsiveness is an integral part of infant care within a multiple-caregiver context.

Morelli and Tronick (1991) studied the Efé of the Ituri forest in northeastern Zambia, a group that employs a system of multiple caregivers throughout the first few years of life, with newborns allowed to suckle other adult females even when their mothers are present (Tronick, Morelli, & Winn, 1987). Even the physical care is shared with other caregivers. Morelli and Tronick reported that the number of caregivers in the first 18 weeks amounted to 14.2 on average. This extremely dense social network led to prompt responses to any sign of infant distress. During the second half of the first year, the infants began to show preference for the care of their own mothers, were more likely to protest against their mothers leaving, and wanted to be carried by their mothers on trips outside the camp. Morelli and Tronick pointed to the 1-year-olds' interference with adults' work activities, which prevented nonmaternal caregivers from taking on caregiving responsibility during work. They also noted that at night, only the mothers cared for their infants, and sleep was regularly interrupted by episodes of playful interaction exclusively between infants and their mothers (Morelli & Tronick, 1991), which may have facilitated the emergence of a special infant–mother bond. From the perspective of attachment theory, the night may be an especially stressful time, during which infants need a protective caregiver the most (see description of Israeli communal kibbutzim, below). The Efé study supports the universality hypothesis, also suggesting that sensitive responsiveness at night fosters attachment relationships.

The child care pattern among the Hadza of Tanzania also consists of multiple caregivers, with close, indulgent, and affectionate physical caregiver–infant proximity and responsiveness in the first years of life (Marlowe, 2005). Hadza women usually forage in groups containing only women and children, taking young infants with them and leaving toddlers at the camp. Marlowe (2005) found that mothers held infants more often than

all other caregivers combined, also showing how despite mothers' willingness to hand their children over to other available caregivers, the child was not always equally willing, signifying a preference for mothers as primary attachment figures. When a child started crying when handed over to another caregiver, the mother usually took the child back, which is consistent with the notions of secure-base behavior and maternal sensitive responsiveness. In addition, Marlowe noted how all caregivers seemed to be equally sensitive to fussing and crying, but that mothers, compared with other caregivers, were generally much more effective at soothing and calming their child. Thus, descriptions of Hadza child care are consistent with the universality and sensitivity hypotheses.

For part of the year, the Bofi live in settlements near farming villages in the southwest region of the Central African Republic, and live in camps in the forest for the other part of the year. In their study of 22 Bofi children who also experienced multiple careving, Fouts and Lamb (2005) reported that the average length of bouts of crying and/or fussing was substantially longer when the mother was absent than when she was present. The difference was not statistically significant, but given the small sample size, this is not surprising. Calculating the effect size reveals a large one ($d = 0.70$), suggesting that in maternal absence, children try to elicit the mother's presence and care, which is consistent with other descriptions of attachment behavior. Furthermore, crying children were more likely to be responded to when the mother was present than when she was absent, and context- and caregiver-specific patterns of sensitive responsiveness appeared to explain individual differences in crying frequency. These findings confirm the universality hypothesis concerning a preferential attachment bond with the mother within a multiple-caregiving context, and they also support the sensitivity hypothesis, in that patterns of responsive caregiving, albeit specific to the ecology of each child's family circumstances, were predictive of less crying.

In contrast to these four societies, the Hausa in Nigeria represent a polymatric culture that practices mostly agriculture. An average of four caregivers share the tasks of social, verbal, and playful interactions with children, but the biological mothers take almost complete responsibility for physical care activities, such as feeding and bathing (Marvin, VanDevender, Iwanaga, LeVine, & LeVine, 1977). In their ethnographic study of 18 infants, Marvin and colleagues found that

Hausa infants were almost always in close physical contact with or close proximity to available adult caregivers, while not allowed to explore the wider environment alone because of the dangers involved. The high social density of the Hausa compound led to prompt adult or older sibling responses to any infant attachment signals, such as crying. The Hausa caregivers therefore appeared to be indulgent and sensitive, and at the same time restrictive toward their infants. The restriction of locomotion also led to a different use of adult caregivers as a secure base: Hausa infants explored their immediate environment in visual and manipulative ways, but only in close proximity to an attachment figure, and they ceased to explore as soon as the caregiver left. Nevertheless, Hausa infants clearly used adult caregivers as safe bases from which to explore, and they differentiated between attachment figures and strangers. Furthermore, all infants displayed attachment behavior toward an average of three to four different figures. Although being raised in an attachment relationships network, most Hausa infants were principally attached to one adult (generally the one holding the baby and interacting with him or her most often, whether or not this was the mother) to whom they addressed their attachment behavior most frequently (Marvin et al., 1977). This study provides evidence for the universality hypothesis and suggests that sensitive responsiveness is part of routine care for infants.

## Standardized Observations of Attachment and Sensitivity in Africa

Only a few studies in multiple-caregiver African societies have used standardized procedures such as the Strange Situation procedure (Ainsworth et al., 1978) or the Attachment Q-Sort (AQS; Vaughn & Waters, 1990) to classify infants formally as securely or insecurely attached. This is, of course, due to the substantial practical barriers to conducting standardized procedures in contexts lacking laboratory facilities. The four studies that successfully did so are therefore very important and are discussed further here.

Childrearing among the Gusii of Kenya is characterized by alloparenting, but the division of tasks between mothers and other caregivers is rather strict. Mothers provide most of the physical care and are responsible for their children's health, whereas the activities of child caregivers are limited to social and playful interactions

(Kermoian & Leiderman, 1986). In their study, Kermoian and Leiderman (1986) included 26 infant–caretaker dyads. Outside each mother's hut, a modified Strange Situation procedure was implemented, with two separation–reunion episodes for mother, caregiver, and stranger each. The extra separations were meant to compensate for the lack of a Strange Situation laboratory environment. Gusii infants are used to being greeted with a handshake by their mothers and caretakers, and during the reunions, the Gusii infants anticipated the handshake in the same way as North American or European infants anticipate a hug. The secure Gusii infants would reach out to an adult with one arm, to receive the handshake enthusiastically, whereas the insecure infants would avoid the adult or reach and then pull away after the adult approached. The distribution of patterns of attachment was comparable with Western findings: Secure attachment was found in 61 and 54% of infants to mothers and to nonmaternal caregivers, respectively. The authors concluded that the development of differential or person-specific attachment behaviors for "polymatric" infants is similar to that observed in "monomatric" Western societies; that is, infants do become uniquely attached to a protective adult caregiver, regardless of the presence of one or more mother figures (Reed & Leiderman, 1981). This study also provides evidence for the universality and normativity hypotheses. Interestingly, positive nutritional or health status of the infants was related to the security of the infant–mother bond, whereas the infants' cognitive development was related to the security of attachment to the nonmaternal caregiver. These findings might be expected given the clear task division between mothers (physical care, focus on health) and other caregivers (social and playful interactions), and provide evidence also for the competence hypothesis.

Attachment classifications based on the traditional Strange Situation procedure were available in a study of 26 mothers and their 1-year-old infants among the Dogon subsistence farmers in Mali, among whom maternal care is flexibly supplemented with care from siblings and other family members (True, 1994; True, Pisani, & Oumar, 2001). The Dogon mothers breast-fed their infants on demand very frequently and kept them in close proximity almost all the time. The percentage of secure infant–mother dyads was high (69%), whereas the avoidant classification appeared to be absent, and few resistant infant–mother dyads were found (8%). The percentage of disorganized infants was high (23%) compared to percentages in normal Western samples (15–20%). The study supports the universality hypothesis in showing how the Strange Situation procedure is classifiable with the ABCD (anxious-avoidant, secure, anxious-resistant, disorganized) coding system in an African culture, and supports the normativity hypothesis, because the majority of infants were securely attached (True et al., 2001). To explain the lack of avoidant attachments, True (1994) hypothesized that the Strange Situation procedure in the Dogon society may have been experienced as highly stressful instead of mildly stressful, forcing avoidant infants to seek proximity, and may also have increased the number of disorganized infants. Finally, True also found that infant attachment security was related to caregiving patterns characterized by sensitivity, a lack of frightening/frightened behaviors, and fewer violations of communication coherence and cooperativeness. This seminal study among the Dogon therefore provides evidence for the universality hypothesis, the normativity hypothesis, and the sensitivity hypothesis. Importantly, it also shows that contrary to some claims (e.g., Otto [2014], who calls the procedure "cruel"), it is possible to find creative and culture-sensitive ways of administering the Strange Situation procedure that are not overly stressful for the infants.

There is some evidence that the extensive shared infant care in forager communities might influence infant behavior in separation–reunion situations. In a study among the Aka foragers of the Central African Republic, sensitive responsiveness by nonmaternal caregivers negatively predicted infant's distress during mother's absence (Meehan & Hawks, 2013), and positively predicted infant engagement of mother upon her return (Meehan & Hawks, 2015), suggesting that infant behavior toward mothers in separation–reunion situations needs to be interpreted with consideration for the caregiving context.

In South Africa, Tomlinson, Cooper, and Murray (2005) studied attachment in a black sample of 98 mother–infant dyads, and assessed them at 2, 6, and 18 months postpartum. Families were living in Khayelitsha, an impoverished black settlement close to Cape Town. Only 5% lived in brick houses, and 49% of the houses were without modern plumbing, 58% of the families had no regular income, and 51% of the pregnancies were unplanned. The researchers undertook the challenging job of conducting the Strange Situation, observing the quality of the home environment

and maternal sensitive responsiveness. Despite the poor living circumstances, the majority of infants were securely attached to their mothers (62%), although a rather large number of infants did develop a disorganized attachment (26%). Only 4% were avoidantly attached, and the remaining 8% were resistantly attached (Tomlinson et al., 2005). Furthermore, a remarkably high incidence of postpartum depression was found in the mothers (35% when infants were 2 months old), compared to similar samples in Western countries (with about 10% of mothers experiencing postpartum depression). The presence of postpartum depression was strongly associated with attachment insecurity and disorganization, and sensitivity at 2 months, as well as at 18 months, predicted attachment security significantly and independently of depression. The study therefore provides support for the universality hypothesis, the normativity hypothesis, and the sensitivity hypothesis.

In another South African study by Minde, Minde, and Vogel (2006), 46 mother–child dyads (children ages 18-40 months) living in an impoverished black township of Johannesburg were observed using the AQS. The results showed a roughly equal distribution of secure attachment (47%) and insecure attachment (53%), although we should mention that the AQS was not designed to yield attachment classifications. The relatively low rate of secure attachment is likely to be due to the extremely disadvantaged nature of the sample. Not only did all mothers report financial problems but also almost half of them reported a history of abuse, and about one-third had been placed away from home for prolonged periods before they were 5 years old (Minde et al., 2006). Furthermore, the sample's depression and anxiety levels were just under the 90th percentile of the norm distribution, and similar to findings in Western countries, both the severity of financial problems and the experience of abuse were related to lower rates of attachment security (Minde et al., 2006). The AQS was successfully applied in this South African sample, providing evidence in support of the universality hypothesis. The normativity hypothesis was not properly tested because the AQS was not designed to yield classifications. The sensitivity hypothesis was indirectly confirmed, as higher rates of problems known to adversely affect maternal sensitivity (financial problems and a history of abuse) were related to insecure attachment.

Family life in Africa has changed drastically in the past decades, due to the HIV/AIDS pandemic; many infants of infected mothers are born with

HIV. Peterson, Drotar, Olness, Guay, and Kiziri-Mayengo (2001) investigated a Ugandan sample of 35 HIV-positive mothers with or without AIDS, and 25 HIV-negative mothers, all with infants in their first year of life, 10 of whom were HIV-infected themselves. The researchers used the AQS to rate the attachment security of the infants during a 4-hour home visit. The average AQS score reflecting infants' secure-base behavior in the subsample of 50 infants who were not infected with HIV (.35) was very similar to those found in other countries in different parts of the world (average of 34 samples = .31; Van IJzendoorn, Vereijken, Bakermans-Kranenburg, & Riksen-Walraven, 2004). Peterson and colleagues also found that 32% of the variance of AQS attachment security in the Ugandan sample was predicted by maternal affect, which consisted of ratings of expressivity and affective involvement, stimulation and activity, and responsivity and sensitivity. Thus, almost half a century after the original Uganda study, the new Ugandan findings support Ainsworth's (1967) observations of attachment bonds within a multiple-caregiver context (universality hypothesis) and her suggestion that sensitive parenting fosters a secure attachment relationship (the sensitivity hypothesis). Furthermore, the normativity hypothesis was supported by showing that security scores were similar to those found elsewhere.

## Attachment and Sensitivity in East Asia

Countries in East Asia have been described as favoring the cultural model of *interdependence* (Kagitcibasi, 2007) and have been labeled as having a *collectivistic culture* (Oyserman, Coon, & Kemmelmeier, 2002). Both terms refer to a cultural context in which the importance of the group and social harmony are emphasized more than the needs of the individual, and in which adherence to group norms, filial piety, and self-sacrifice are expected (Hofstede, 1984). The label *autonomous-relatedness* has been coined to describe cultural groups that allow room for a focus on autonomy within an interdependent context, which generally characterizes urbanized or migrated groups that originally came from collectivistic cultural backgrounds but now reside in a more individualistic context (Kagitcibasi, 2007). Indeed, the rapid urbanization, globalization, and increased wealth in

several regions of East Asia may have moved the social and psychological identities of its (urban) inhabitants closer to those of Western countries (e.g., Naftali, 2010). Consistent with this idea, a recent meta-analysis showed that urban Chinese parents display lower levels of authoritative parenting (i.e., warmth and support for autonomy) than parents from North American countries, but not necessarily higher authoritarian parenting in terms of a focus on unquestioning obedience (Wang & Mesman, 2015).

Multiple caregivers are also common in most East Asian cultures, although nonparental care is mostly restricted to care by grandparents, who often coreside with the nuclear family and tend to provide extensive care for their grandchildren when both parents are working (e.g., Nauck & Suckow, 2006), and may in those situations be the primary attachment figures for the children. Grandparental coresidence is also fostered by housing shortages in urban areas and the absence of professional child care facilities for families in which both parents work outside the home (Goh & Kuczynski, 2010). Sibling care is very uncommon given the one-child policy in China and the very low fertility rates in Japan and South Korea. However, we note that demographic and cultural differences within the East Asian region are substantial. For instance, in a country such as Indonesia, fertility rates are higher than elsewhere in the region (although declining fast), and the relatively recent colonial past of this country and its current predominant Muslim identity also sets it apart from countries such as China and Japan. A total of 18 studies using standardized observational instruments focusing on attachment are available from Papua New Guinea, China, Taiwan, Japan, South Korea, and Indonesia. We discuss these in some detail below.

### Attachment among the Trobriander

In a unique study among 20 mother–toddler dyads living in the horticulturalist village of Tauwema on the Trobriand Islands (part of Papua New Guinea), written ethnographic records were collected, as well as standardized observations in the Strange Situation procedure (Grossmann, Grossmann, & Keppler, 2005). All observed toddlers showed attachment behavior and used their mothers as safe havens in times of distress in both field observations and the standardized Strange Situation, supporting the universality hypothesis.

In addition, all toddlers showed separation distress when involuntarily separated from their mothers (Grossmann et al., 2005). Secure attachment was normative, with 16 of the 20 infants falling into this category, supporting the normativity hypothesis. Maternal sensitivity was not systematically observed, but the ethnographic records suggest that mothers of insecure infants were less accessible to their toddlers, and slower and harsher in their responses (Grossmann et al., 2005), which indicates tentative support for the sensitivity hypothesis.

### Attachment in China and Taiwan

Nine studies of attachment have been conducted in normative urban samples in China, but only three were published in English, and only one obtained attachment classifications by coders officially trained by experts (Archer et al., 2009). In that study, 62 infants and toddlers were examined in the Strange Situation procedure, yielding a distribution of 57% secure, 13% avoidant, 16% resistant, and 13% disorganized (with forced classification: B = 62%, A = 15%, C = 23%). The other two studies found a rate of 68% of securely attached infants (Ding, Xu, Wang, Li, & Wang, 2012; Hu & Meng, 1996), which is very similar to results from studies conducted in other parts of the world (Van IJzendoorn & Kroonenberg, 1988). The pattern within the insecure category was somewhat different, with Hu and Meng (1996) reporting 16% avoidant and 16% resistant (disorganized was not coded), whereas Ding and colleagues (2012) reported 7.5% avoidant and 21.8% resistant (and 2.5% disorganized). The six studies published in Chinese yielded the following distributions: B = 65%, A = 17%, C = 13% , D = 4% (Li et al., 2004); B = 73%, A = 11%, C = 7%, D = 9% (Liang, Chen, & Chen, 2000); B = 53%, A = 13%, C = 27%, D = 7% (Hu & Meng, 2003); B = 72%, A = 10%, C = 10%, D = 8% (Yue, Zhang, Chen, Liang, & Zhang, 2010); B = 68%, A = 6%, C = 26%, D = 0% (Ding et al., 2008); and B = 67%, A = 6%, C = 23%, D = 4% (Gu et al., 1997). As can be readily noticed, all studies conducted in China confirm both the universality hypothesis (by successfully classifying all children into one of the attachment categories) and the normativity hypothesis (by showing that the majority of children are securely attached).

What is also notable is the relatively low prevalence of avoidant attachment in the majority of these studies compared to the rates of avoid-ance reported in Western studies (Van IJzendoorn & Kroonenberg, 1988; Van IJzendoorn, Sagi, & Lambermon, 1992). Hu and Meng (1996) expressed doubts about the validity of the avoidant category, noting that the avoidant infants did not show stranger anxiety, and expressed indifference toward their mothers at reunion. The Chinese mothers' stress on early independence in their infants, as well as their reliance on nonparental caregivers, may have been responsible for this pattern. In some cases, grandparents may have served as the primary attachment figures. An alternative interpretation, however, might be based on the subtle avoidant behaviors that are difficult for even well-trained coders to observe in infants. However, as we see later, the lower prevalence of the avoidant category is in line with findings of other studies in non-Western cultures and may reflect the cultural context of parenting.

In view of the (until recently) strict birth control policy in China and the traditional preference for a male child, it is important to note that the distributions of attachment classifications for male and female infants were virtually the same in the two studies that reported gender (Ding et al., 2012; Hu & Meng, 1996). It has been suggested that firstborn daughters who "survive" parental choices regarding gender-driven abortion or postnatal abandonment are apparently welcome (Short, Fengying, Siyuan, & Mingliang, 2001) and have indeed been shown to have been treated better than those with a male sibling (Fong, 2002). Regarding the role of grandparents, all but one family in the Hu and Meng study (1996) coresided with one or more grandparents. The rate of grandparental coresidence was not reported in the Ding and colleagues study (2012), but they did report that infants with an insecure attachment to their mothers were also more likely to sleep with nonmaternal caregivers at night. In both studies, the possibility that a grandparent was the primary caregiver of the infants in those samples was suggested as a potential explanation for the results, namely, the high rate of avoidance and what appeared to be infant indifference toward the mothers (Hu & Meng, 1996), and the lower rate of security in infants with more caregivers during the day and at night (Ding et al., 2012). The issue of sleeping arrangements is also discussed in the section on the Israeli kibbutz below.

Of the nine studies conducted in China, none examined the sensitivity hypothesis using observational studies. However, three studies examined the competence hypothesis and reported evidence to support this assumption. In one study, securely attached 2-year-old children exhibited fewer internalizing and externalizing problems than nonsecurely attached children both concurrently and at ages 4 and 7 years (Yue et al., 2010). In the second study, securely attached infants possessed more advanced cognitive skills than insecurely attached infants, but there were no differences in physical development (Ding, Wang, Li, Chi, & Xu, 2008), and the final study to examine outcomes of attachment found that secure toddlers had fewer behavior problems and displayed better self-regulation (Gu et al., 1997).

Posada and colleagues (2013) conducted a cross-cultural study involving nine countries, including a sample of 68 mothers and their 4-year-old children in Taiwan, which we discuss under the same heading as the studies from mainland China because of geographical and cultural proximity. Importantly, Taiwan does not have a one-child policy, but its fertility rate is also very low. In the Posada and colleagues study, 3-hour home observations were conducted, and the AQS was used to rate the child's secure-base behavior. The results showed that the average security scores for the Taiwanese sample (.32) were similar to scores found in other studies (.31; see Van IJzendoorn et al., 2004).

## The Japanese Case: Amae, Dependence, and Attachment

One of the most severe critiques of attachment theory has come in the form of an accusation of "cultural blindness" among attachment researchers to alternative conceptions of relatedness (Rothbaum, Weisz, Pott, Miyake, & Morelli, 2000). This "cultural blindness" accusation of a Western bias in attachment theory was based specifically on the Japanese case (rebutted in Van IJzendoorn & Sagi, 2001). The Japanese case can indeed be considered a real challenge to attachment theory's universality, normativity, and sensitivity hypotheses, and we address these challenges below.

It has been argued that the concept of attachment may not be relevant to the Japanese culture, in which the idea of amae (Doi, 1973, 1992) seems to play a more prominent and effective role in describing family relationships and their societal implications (Emde, 1992). (Amae refers to relational dependence, including aspects such as the desire for interpersonal closeness, the presence of

indulgence, and relying on the other person [Behrens, 2004].) Furthermore, it has been argued that "Amae has an advantage over attachment because it implies a psychological dependence" (Doi, 1989, p. 350). Vereijken (1996) asked eight native Japanese behavioral scientists to describe the concepts of amae, attachment, and dependence with the help of the AQS. The descriptions of amae and dependence were very similar, whereas the descriptions of attachment security and amae were not associated (Vereijken, 1996). Furthermore, when the descriptions of the ideal child according to Japanese mothers were compared with the Japanese experts' definitions, only attachment security (and not amae) appeared to be desirable (cf. Posada et al., 1995). Furthermore, an observational study of Japanese sojourners in the united states by Mizuta, Zahn-Waxler, Cole, and Hiruma (1996; see also Nakagawa, Teti, & Lamb, 1992) confirmed Vereijken's (1996) conclusion that amae and attachment are orthogonal dimensions that can be reliably distinguished. Furthermore, Behrens (2004), a psychologist of Japanese origin, analyzed the use of the term and related terminology in natural Japanese discourse. she concluded that for many native Japanese speakers, amae has a negative connotation involving social enforcement of obligations, and that amae lacks the biological roots of the attachment concept, is not associated with the regulation of stress, but can occur any time there is a desire or a motive on the part of the amae provider (Behrens, 2004; Behrens, Main, & Hesse, 2007). Because of the fundamental conceptual, linguistic, and biological differences between the two constructs, attachment research in japan cannot be considered a challenge to the concept of amae, and amae cannot be considered a refutation of the concept of attachment.

### Studies Using the Strange Situation Procedure in Japan

We now turn to observational studies of attachment in Japan. Three studies using the Strange Situation procedure to assess attachment security in Japan have been reported in the international literature. The first was conducted by Durrett, Otaki, and Richards (1984), who studied a middle-class sample of 39 intact families with their 12-month-old firstborns in Tokyo. This study showed a pattern of avoidant, secure, and resistant infant–mother attachments, consistent with the global distribution, with 13% A, 61% B, 18%

C, and 8% unclassifiable cases. The Tokyo study confirms the universality and normativity hypotheses because the authors did not report difficulties in applying the attachment coding system to this population, and because the normative "modal" category was secure. The unclassifiable cases could be a sign of culture-specific problems in applying the tripartite model but could also be due to the fact that the disorganized (D) classification was not yet available (notably, the D category was particularly instrumental in solving unclassifiable cases; Main & Solomon, 1990; see also Lyons-Ruth & Jacobvitz, Chapter 29, and Solomon & George, Chapter 18, in this volume). Furthermore, the mothers of securely attached infants indicated that they felt more supported by their husbands than did the mothers of avoidantly attached infants, but they did not differ in this regard from the mothers of resistantly attached infants (Durrett et al., 1984). This finding provides indirect support for the sensitivity hypothesis because partner support has been found to foster maternal sensitivity (e.g., Van Bakel & Riksen-Walraven, 2002).

The second Japanese study, conducted in Sapporo (Miyake, Chen, & Campos, 1985; Nakagawa, Lamb, & Miyake, 1992; Takahashi, 1986), was unfortunately weakened by some methodological flaws and unclear reporting (see Van IJzendoorn & Sagi-Schwartz, 2008, for a full discussion of this study) and is therefore not discussed further in this section. The third Japanese study was also conducted in Sapporo with 43 mother–child dyads (Behrens, Hesse, & Main, 2007). Attachment distributions were based on Main and Cassidy's sixth-year reunion assessment procedure (see Solomon & George, Chapter 18, this volume). In contrast to the previous Sapporo study, children's three-way or forced "organized" attachment classification distribution did not differ from the global distribution: 68% secure, 22% avoidant, 10% resistant (three children remained unclassified). The ABCD distribution was 49% B, 2% A, 0%C, and 49% D. The high proportion of D could be due to the fact that the non-Japanese coders had to judge maternal talk from translated transcripts and may have missed important cues from the tone of voice (Behrens et al., 2007). Furthermore, maternal attachment representations as measured with the Adult Attachment Interview (AAI; see Hesse, Chapter 26, this volume) predicted child reunion classification (Behrens et al., 2007), with proportions very similar to matches reported worldwide. This is indirect support for the sensitivity hypothesis because adult attachment representations have been found to predict maternal sensitivity (also in Asian samples, see, e.g., Liang et al., 2015), which in turn is known to predict infant attachment security (De Wolff & Van IJzendoorn, 1997). Thus, maternal sensitivity is likely to have (partially) mediated the relation between maternal attachment representations and infant attachment security. Notably, mothers' unresolved attachment status strongly predicted child D status ($r = .65$).

## Studies Using the Attachment Q-Sort in Japan

Three studies using the AQS have been conducted in Japan. Vereijken (1996) studied a Tokyo sample of 48 families with 14-month-old infants. More sensitive mothers had more secure children, and the association between sensitivity and attachment was impressively strong (all correlations—based on reports from independent coders—were .59 or higher). In a follow-up study 10 months later, the association between sensitivity and attachment was replicated (Vereijken, 1996). In another study, 50 Japanese mothers and their preschool children were observed (Kazui, Endo, Tanaka, Sakagami, & Suganuma, 2000). The results showed that the children of secure mothers (as assessed with the AAI) had the highest security scores on the AQS, whereas children of unresolved mothers had the lowest AQS scores. The children of the dismissing and preoccupied mothers scored in between. The majority of the mothers were classified as secure (66%). Knowing that secure mothers generally have more sensitive interactions with their children than do insecure mothers, this outcome represents another indirect confirmation of attachment theory's sensitivity hypothesis. The last Japanese study was conducted in the context of a larger cross-cultural context (Posada et al., 2013). In a sample of 45 infants, the average security score was the lowest (.19) of those reported for nine countries in total, but the majority of scores were positive, indicating a predominance of secure-base behavior. The low average score appeared to be predominantly due to lower scores on the Smooth Interactions with Mother and the Interactions with Other Adults scales (and not the scales reflecting physical proximity and contact with the mother). These findings may reflect the potential discomfort that Japanese mothers convey when observed in the home (Nakagawa, Lamb, et al., 1992).

## Attachment and Sensitivity in South Korea

In the first and only study to use the Strange Situation procedure in South Korea, Jin, Jacobvitz, Hazen, and Jung (2012) observed 87 mother–infant dyads. The results showed that 70% of the infants were classified as securely attached, 1% as avoidant, 17% as resistant, and 9% as disorganized. Jin and colleagues noted that in the reunion episodes of the Strange Situation, the mothers were more likely to approach their infants immediately and sit beside them than was the case in Ainsworth's Baltimore sample, even when the infants were no longer distressed. The authors also discussed the low prevalence of avoidant attachment in their sample by pointing to the generally lower percentage of infants in the avoidant category in other studies of East Asian samples, such as those from Indonesia (Zevalkink, Riksen-Walraven, & Van Lieshout, 1999) and China (e.g., Archer et al., 2015; Ding et al., 2012). Jin and colleagues (2012) speculated that a caregiving context in which mother–infant relationships are generally characterized by physical closeness, indulgence, and the discouragement of mother–infant separation is very unlikely to produce avoidant children. As they put it, "Instead, when insecure attachment occurs, it is more likely to be resistant, since mothers are more likely to err on the side of being overly enmeshed, overprotective, or overinvolved, rather than rejecting" (p. 41). As we see later in this chapter, this may be relevant even for other non-Western cultures outside of East Asia. Finally, observations of maternal sensitivity during free play in this study revealed that infants of more sensitive mothers were more likely to be securely attached than infants of less sensitive mothers. Thus, this unique study in South Korea confirmed the universality hypothesis, the normativity hypothesis, and the sensitivity hypothesis.

## Muslim Families in Indonesia

Indonesia is the fourth most populous country in the world and has the largest Islamic population of any country in the world. Zevalkink (1997) conducted the first attachment study on Islamic families of Sundanese Indonesian origin in West Java. Sundanese Indonesian children generally experience relatively extensive periods of close physical proximity to their mothers because they are carried in a carrying cloth, or *slendang*, during the first year. They are breast-fed on demand until 2 or 3 years of age and sleep in the same beds as their mothers during the first 4 years of life. When an infant is fussy or cries, the mother promptly responds with soothing or feeding. Sundanese Indonesian women, however, marry at a very young age, and their divorce rate is high. A stable income and permanent job are rare, which adds to the instability of family life. Poverty and health problems lead to rather high infant mortality (Zevalkink et al., 1999). Zevalkink and colleagues (1999) reported Strange Situation assessments of 46 children, ages 12–30 months. They also conducted extensive home observations on maternal sensitivity and observed maternal support in structured play sessions. The distribution of attachment classifications was as follows: 52% secure, 7% avoidant, 20% resistant, and 22% disorganized (Zevalkink et al., 1999). More maternal support in structured play sessions was associated with attachment security; disorganized children received low maternal support. In addition, a higher-quality home caregiving environment was related to higher rates of secure attachment (Zevalkink, Riksen-Walraven, & Bradley, 2008). Thus, in these Muslim families, the universality hypothesis was confirmed because all children could be classified based on the Strange Situation procedure. Furthermore, a majority of children were securely attached (supporting the normativity hypothesis), and secure attachment was associated with the quality of caregiving in the predicted way (supporting the sensitivity hypothesis).

## Attachment and Sensitivity in Latin America

In this section, we examine the four hypotheses of attachment theory within the Latin American cultural context, mostly reflecting urban parenting, but also in one case of rural parenting. We found seven studies using standardized methods to assess attachment conducted in Latin American countries, including studies from Chile, Colombia, Peru, and Mexico. Each is discussed below.

### Chile: A Study on Malnourished Infants

The first study using the strange situation procedure in a Latin American context was conducted in Chile by Valenzuela (1997) among 84 mother–infant dyads living in poverty, with half of the infants classified as chronically underweight. For the total sample, only 27% of infants were categorized as securely attached, 26% as avoidant, 25% as resistant, and 21% as A/C (probably classifiable now as D). However, when distinguishing two groups based on infant nutritional status, the results revealed that the attachment distribution was much closer to the global distribution in the adequately nourished infants: 50% secure, 23% avoidant, 22% resistant, and 2% A/C (Valenzuela, 1997). Indeed, consistent with findings in the Gusii study (Kermoian & Leiderman, 1986), attachment security was significantly related to infant nutritional status. Finally, in the Chilean study, observations of maternal sensitivity were also significantly related to attachment security in the expected direction (Valenzuela, 1997). This set of findings is consistent with studies showing that responsive feeding (which basically refers to sensitivity during feeding) is related to children's more optimal weight status (Black & Aboud, 2011). In fact, both the World Health Organization and United Nations International Children's Emergency Fund (Who/UNICEF; 2003) have incorporated responsive feeding into their guidelines for promoting healthy child development. In summary, the study provides evidence for all four key hypotheses formulated to represent the key tenets of attachment theory.

### Studies from Colombia and Peru

The AQS was used to assess child secure-base behavior in four studies from urban Colombia (the first three with partially overlapping samples), each of which revealed high average security scores (comparing to the average of .31 across 34 samples in Van IJzendoorn et al., 2004). First, an average security score of .43 was found by Posada and colleagues (2002) in a sample of 61 infants, and observed maternal sensitivity was positively related to attachment security in this study. Second, an average AQS score of .46 was found in a sample of 30 infants (Posada, Carbonell, Alzate, & Plata, 2004). Third, Vaughn and colleagues (2007) reported an average score of .48 for a sample of 25 Colombian infants; they found that maternal secure-base narratives were related to attachment security in the expected direction. Finally, Posada and colleagues (2013) report an average score of .32 in a group of 83 toddlers. In one of these four studies, ethnographic descriptions of maternal care were analyzed to examine the appropriateness of attachment theory's con-

ceptualization of early care (Posada et al., 2004). The authors concluded that "most of the domains of maternal behavior found in this study matched well those identified by Ainsworth; our characterization of maternal early care displays a direct relation to that of attachment theory (e.g., Ainsworth et al., 1978)" (p. 516). Within the cross-cultural study by Posada and colleagues (2013), an urban sample of 30 mothers and preschoolers from Peru was also included, showing an average AQS security scores of .30, similar to that found for the Colombian sample reported in the same article. Given the positive and moderate-to-high security scores found in the five studies described here, support is provided for the universality and normativity hypotheses. Furthermore, the results of two studies directly support the sensitivity hypothesis, and another provides indirect support by showing that maternal secure-base narratives (conceptually relevant to sensitive parenting) relate positively to infant secure attachment.

### Attachment and Sensitivity in Urban and Rural Mexico

In a study by Gojman and colleagues (2012), intergenerational relations of attachment and caregiving quality were investigated in a sample of 35 urban, upper-middle-class Mestizo families, and a sample of 31 rural poor Indian families in Mexico. For the urban middle-class families, the Strange Situation procedure revealed a rate of 77% secure attachment, 3% avoidant, 3% resistant, and 14% disorganized (Gojman et al., 2012). In the poor rural sample, rates of security (32%) were clearly lower, and disorganization (35%) was more prevalent than in the upper-middle-class urban sample. The finding that attachment security is less common in poor rural samples than in more affluent urban samples is consistent with the family stress model, which describes how financial strains lead to parental stress, which in turn compromises family functioning in general and parenting quality in particular, leading to unfavorable child outcomes (Conger & Donnellan, 2007). This indirect evidence for the sensitivity hypothesis was corroborated by results showing a partial mediation model, with maternal autonomous attachment representations, as measured with the AAI, predicting observed maternal sensitivity, which in turn predicted infant attachment security (Gojman et al., 2012). As noted by the authors, these results clearly support the cross-cultural robustness of core features of attachment theory.

## Attachment in Israel

For the purpose of this chapter, we include Israel within the Anglo-Saxon and European cultures, and therefore do not review urban-normative samples that have been studied with similar outcomes as those found in many Western countries (e.g., Sagi, Koren-Karie, Gini, Ziv, & Joels, 2002). We focus on two unique samples in Israel: infants raised in kibbutzim and the Arab minority.

### Attachment and Collective Sleeping Practices

Following a visit to Israeli kibbutzim in the early 1950s, Bowlby (1951) noted the rich opportunities for research provided by kibbutz upbringing and predicted that this childrearing context, though clearly different from institutional care, might produce higher rates of attachment insecurity. The communal bedrooms in the children's house were shared by three or four children, who each had private corners in which they kept their personal things, and which were decorated according to each child's preference. When collective sleeping was still in effect (starting a few months after birth), family time was in the afternoon and evening, and children were returned to the children's house for the night by their parents, who put them to bed. A caregiver or a parent then remained with them until the night watchwomen took over (Aviezer, Van IJzendoorn, Sagi, & Schuengel, 1994). Whereas most institutionalized childrearing in Western cultures involves multiproblem populations, the collective sleeping arrangements in the kibbutzim were designed for middle-class, well-functioning families. Although the system of multiple caregiving in the kibbutz was in many ways similar to multiple-caregiver contexts elsewhere (Rabin & Beit-Hallahmi, 1982), a worldwide sample of 183 societies showed that in none of them did infants sleep away from their parents (Barry & Paxton, 1971).

In support of the universality hypothesis, several studies of the attachments of communally sleeping kibbutz children to their parents and caregivers revealed that they do form attachment bonds with their caregivers, and most often with their mothers (Aviezer & Sagi-Schwartz, 2008). The first communal kibbutz study conducted with the ABC system found 57% of securely attached infants (Sagi, Lamb, Lewkowicz, Shoham, Dvir, & Estes, 1985). Using the ABCD system in a more recent sample, a rate of 26% secure infant–mother attachment was found (Sagi, Van IJzendoorn, Aviezer, Donnell, & Mayseless, 1994). In the ABC classification system D/B cases could have been classified as secure, hence inflating the rate of security. The rate of security in the communal sleep kibbutz was lower than that found in Israeli nonkibbutz samples (e.g., 66% in Koren-Karie, Oppenheim, Dolev, Sher, & Etzion-Carasso, 2002; 70% in Sagi, et al., 2002), and lower than that in a kibbutz sample with family-based sleeping (60% in Sagi et al., 1994). To rule out alternative explanations for the effect of communal sleeping arrangements, assessments were also made of the ecology of the children's house during the day, maternal separation anxiety, infants' temperaments, and mother–infant play interactions. The two groups (i.e., family-based and communal sleepers) were found to be comparable on all of these variables. Thus, it was concluded that collective sleeping, experienced by infants as a time when mothers were largely unavailable and inaccessible, was responsible for the greater insecurity found in this group.

Interestingly, resistant attachment was found to be overrepresented in the communal-sleeping kibbutz samples (Sagi et al., 1985, 2002). Inconsistent responsiveness was inherent in the reality of these infants, given that sensitive responding by a mother or caregiver during the day contrasted sharply with the presence of an unfamiliar person at night. This supports the sensitivity hypothesis because inconsistent responsiveness has been described as an important antecedent of resistant attachment (Ainsworth et al., 1978; Cassidy & Berlin, 1994). The rate of disorganized infants was also rather high for the second communal-sleeping kibbutz sample (44%), which could be attributed to the unpredictable circumstances that these children experienced, especially during the nights. It should also be noted that in several Israeli studies (Jewish sample: Koren-Karie et al., 2002; Sagi et al., 1985, 1994, 1997, 2002; Sagi-Schwartz, Van IJzendoorn, & Bakermans-Kranenburg, 2008; Arab sample: Zreik, 2014; see details below), the resistant classification appeared to be overrepresented and the avoidant classification to be underrepresented compared to the global distribution (Van IJzendoorn & Kroonenberg, 1988). We speculate that the resistant attachment strategy may be elicited in the context of continual threats to national and personal security more readily than the avoidant strategy—the threat is external to the family. Parental preoccupation with these daily stresses may lead to exaggerated overprotective-ness and impaired sensitivity to children's attachment signals (see Belsky, 2008, for an evolutionary perspective).

## Networks of Attachment Relationships

The kibbutz context has also made a unique contribution to the evaluation of the competence hypothesis. In a follow-up of most of the subjects in the Sagi and colleagues' (1985) sample when they were 5 years old, Oppenheim, Sagi, and Lamb (1990) found that secure attachment to a nonparental caregiver (the *metapelet*) during infancy was the strongest predictor of a child's being empathic, dominant, independent, achievement-oriented, and behaviorally purposive in kindergarten. No significant associations were found between these socioemotional developments and the quality of children's attachment to their parents, suggesting that the influence of attachment relationships may be domain-specific (see also the Gusii study described earlier). Because the infants' relations with caregivers had been formed in the context of the infant house, those relationships were the best predictor of children's socioemotional behavior in similar contexts. Furthermore, the extended network of infants' attachments to the three types of caregivers (i.e., mothers, fathers, and *metapelet*) was a better predictor of later functioning than attachments in the family network only (attachments to mothers and fathers) and the attachment to mothers only (Sagi & Van IJzendoorn, 1996; Van IJzendoorn et al., 1992), which is consistent with findings in other samples (Howes, Rodning, Galluzzo, & Myers, 1988; Tavecchio & Van IJzendoorn, 1987). This outcome may be interpreted as support for the integration model, which assumes that in a network of multiple-attachment relationships, secure attachments may compensate for insecure attachments in a linear way (Van IJzendoorn et al., 1992). Beyond kindergarten, however, networks of infant attachment relations did not contribute as much to the explanation of later behavior (Sagi-Schwartz & Aviezer, 2005). Instead, the data were more supportive of the hierarchy model (Van IJzendoorn et al., 1992), suggesting that early relations with mother as the primary caregiver contributed most to later adaptive functioning at all ages (except in kindergarten), even in the kibbutz environment (Aviezer, Resnick, Sagi, & Gini, 2002).

## Ecological Constraints on Intergenerational Transmission of Attachment

*Intergenerational transmission of attachment* refers to the process through which parents' mental representations of their past attachment experiences influence their parenting behavior and the quality of their children's attachment to them (Bowlby, 1969/1982; see Hesse, Chapter 26, this volume). In several studies of Western cultures, a concordance rate of about 75% has been found between the security of the parents' mental representation of attachment and the security of the child–parent attachment (for a review, see Van IJzendoorn, 1995). In an Israeli study, Sagi and colleagues (1997) administered the AAI to 20 mothers from kibbutzim maintaining collective sleeping arrangements and to 25 mothers from home-sleeping kibbutzim. Parent–child concordance in attachment classifications was low for the communally sleeping group (40%), whereas it was rather high for the home-sleeping group (76%). Thus, contextual factors such as communal sleeping may override the influence of parents' attachment representation and their sensitive responsiveness. This finding indicates the limits of a context-free, universal model of transmission.

## Attachment in the Arab Minority Residing in Israel

In a unique study on attachment in Arab families, infant–mother attachment relationships among Arabs living in Israel were assessed (Zreik, 2014; Zreik, Oppenheim, & Sagi-Schwartz, 2015). The sample included 85 Arab mother-infant dyads, and attachment was assessed using the Strange Situation Procedure. Maternal sensitivity was assessed using the Emotional Availability Scales (Biringen, Robinson, & Emde, 2000) and the Maternal Behavior Q-Sort (Pederson & Moran, 1995). Secure attachment was found to be the modal classification, with a rate of 67%, which supports the universality and normativity hypotheses. Moreover, similar to the studies involving Jewish infants in Israel, the ambivalent classification (13%) also appeared to be overrepresented in this Arab sample, with an underrepresentation of the avoidant classification (4%). Perhaps the fact that both groups live in a similar stressful geopolitical ecology contributed to this finding. Sixteen percent of the sample was classified as disorganized. The expected association between sensitivity and attachment security is not clear-cut when religion, maternal education, and measurement of sensitivity are taken into consideration, thus only partially supporting the sensitivity hypothesis (see Zreik, 2014, for details).

## Universal and Contextual Dimensions of Attachment

Figures 37.1 and 37.2 provide overviews of the results presented in each of the earlier sections. In this section, we review the findings of cross-cultural attachment research in relation to the four core hypotheses of attachment theory, discussing both their universal and their contextual aspects.

### The Universality Hypothesis

The universality hypothesis appears to be supported most strongly. In every study on attachment(-related) caregiving patterns in non-Anglo-Saxon and European countries, children were observed to show attachment behavior in stressful circumstances and to have a preferential bond with one or more caregivers, based on both ethnographic descriptions and standardized assessments. The cross-cultural studies included here support Bowlby's (1969/1982) idea that attachment is indeed a universal phenomenon, and an evolutionary explanation seems to be warranted. Although in many cultures children grow up with a network of attachment figures, the parent or caregiver who takes responsibility for the care of a child during part of the day or the night becomes the favorite target of infant attachment behaviors. Not only the attachment phenomenon itself, but also the different types of attachment, appear to be present in various Western and non-Western cultures. Avoidant, secure, and resistant attachments have been observed in the African, East Asian, and Latin American studies, in samples ranging from hunter–gatherer societies characterized by high levels of alloparenting to affluent and deprived urban contexts. Even in the extremely diverging childrearing context of the Israeli kibbutzim with communal sleep at night, the differentiation between secure and insecure attachment could be made.

These results do not, however, preclude culture-specific patterns. Several studies have noted the attachment to multiple caregivers, and the identity of those caregivers depends on the specific caregiving arrangements that are common in a given cultural context. For instance, infant secure attachment was found in relation to not only the infant's mother but also nonmaternal caregivers (Goossens & Van IJzendoorn, 1990; Kermoian & Leiderman, 1986; Sagi et al., 1995). In addition, infants' ways of expressing attachment and exploration behaviors have been found to vary depending on cultural norms and customs. Hausa infants are generally physically restricted in their locomotion by their caregivers and are thus less free to explore the environment by themselves (Marvin et al., 1977). Instead, these infants explored their immediate environment in visual and manipulative ways, but only in close proximity to an attachment figure, and they ceased to explore as soon as the caregiver left. Nevertheless, the Hausa infants clearly used adult caregivers as secure bases from which to explore, and they differentiated between attachment figures and strangers (Marvin et al., 1977). Among the Gusii, culture-specific modes of attachment behavior were described, in that infants are accustomed to greeting their caregivers with a handshake, which was differentially observed depending on attachment classifications (Kermoian & Leiderman, 1986), showing how local cultural customs can be taken into account in attachment research using standardized assessments.

### The Normativity Hypothesis

The cross-cultural evidence for the normativity hypothesis is rather strong as well. In almost all cross-cultural studies included here, the majority of infants were classified as securely attached. Figure 37.2 summarizes the attachment classification distributions found in the studies discussed earlier. When these are combined with AQS findings about the cross-cultural preference among experts, as well as mothers, for securely attached children, we may be confident that secure attachment is not just a North American invention or a Western ideal, but instead is a rather widespread and preferred phenomenon. As we described early on in this chapter, the category of secure attachments emerged from Ainsworth's Uganda study, not from her Baltimore study (as is often suggested). In further support of the normativity hypothesis, Posada and colleagues (1995, 2013) showed that maternal beliefs about ideal child behavior overlapped considerably with attachment theory's notion of the secure-base phenomenon, and that the secure-base phenomenon is clearly present in maternal

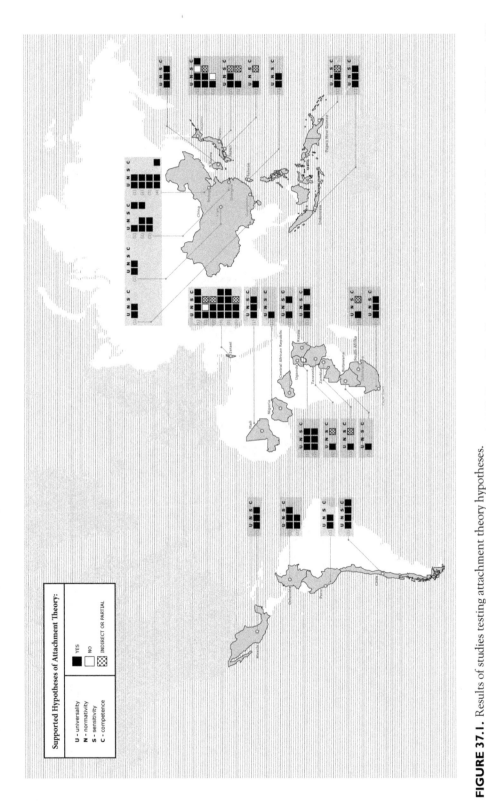

**FIGURE 37.1.** Results of studies testing attachment theory hypotheses.

**Africa:** Botswana–1 (!Kung San; Konner, 1977); Central African Republic–1 (Bofi; Fouts & Lamb, 2005); Kenya–1 (Gusii; Kermoian & Leiderman, 1986); Mali–1 (Dogon; True et al., 2001); Nigeria–1 (Hausa; Marvin et al., 1977); South Africa, Cape Town–1 (Tomlinson et al., 2005); South Africa, Johannesburg–1 (Minde et al., 2006); Tanzania–1 (Hadza; Marlowe, 2005); Uganda–1 (Ganda; Ainsworth & Wittig, 1969); Uganda–2 (Peterson et al., 2001); Zambia–1 (Efé; Morelli & Tronick, 1991).

**East Asia:** China, Beijing–1 (Hu & Meng, 1996); China–Beijing–2 (Liang et al., 2000); China–Beijing–3 (Hu & Meng, 2003); China, Beijing–4 (Yue et al., 2010); China, Guangzhou–1 (Li et al., 2004); China, Shanghai–1 (Gu et al., 1997); China, Shanghai–2 (Ding et al., 2008); China, Shanghai–3 (Ding et al., 2012); China, Xi'an (Archer et al., 2009); Indonesia–1 (Zevalkink et al., 1999); Japan, Tokyo–1 (Durrett et al., 1984); Japan, Tokyo–2 (Kazui et al., 2000); Papua New Guinea–1 (Trobriand Islands, Grossmann et al., 2005); Japan, Sapporo–1 (Takahashi, 1986; Nakagawa et al., 1992); Japan, Sapporo–2 (Behrens et al., 2007); Japan, Sapporo–3 (Posada et al., 2013); South Korea–1 (Jin et al., 2012); Taiwan–1 (Posada et al., 2013).

**Latin America:** Chile–1 (Valenzuela, 1997); Colombia–1 (Posada et al., 2002, 2004; Vaughn et al., 2007); Colombia–2 (Posada et al., 2013); Mexico–1 (Gojman et al., 2012); Peru–1 (Posada et al., 2013).

**Israel:** Israel–1 (first kibbutz cohort communal sleeping; Sagi et al., 1985); Israel–2 (second kibbutz cohort communal sleeping; Sagi et al., 1994); Israel–3 (second kibbutz cohort family sleeping; Sagi et al., 1994); Israel–4 (first urban cohort; Sagi et al., 2002); Israel–5 (second urban cohort; Koren–Karie et al., 2002); Israel–6 (Arabs; Zreik, 2014).

867

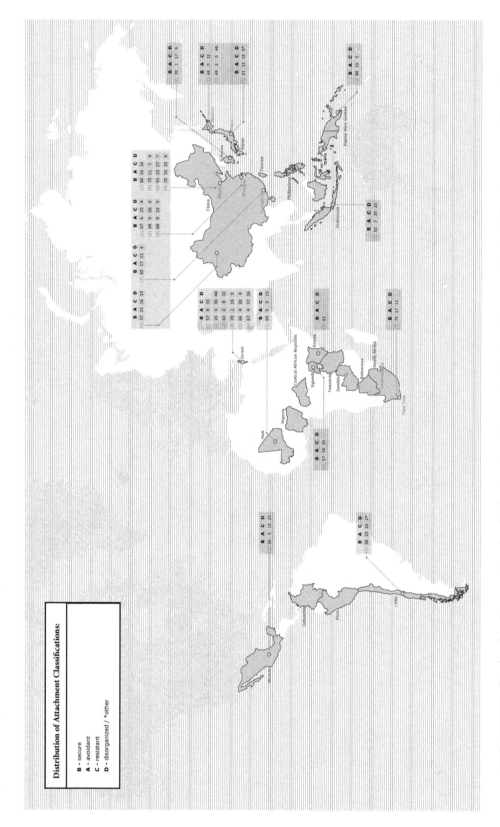

**FIGURE 37.2.** Results of studies examining the distribution of attachment classifications. See paragraphs that follow the caption in Figure 37.1.

descriptions of the behaviors of their own children across different cultural contexts (Posada et al., 1995).

Even though secure attachment appears to be the norm across cultures, there are variations in the rates of secure attachment reported in the studies in non-Anglo-Saxon and European contexts. For instance, rates of security were particularly low in the rural poor Mexican sample (32%; Gojman et al., 2012) and in the undernourished Chilean sample (7%; Valenzuela, 1997). These findings emphasize the importance of socioeconomic circumstances in shaping family life and parenting patterns. This is consistent with the family stress model, which describes how adverse economic circumstances interfere with optimal parenting through their influence on parental stress, ultimately leading to negative effects on child development (Conger & Donnellan, 2007; see also McLoyd, 1998). Not having the economic resources to reliably provide basic care for children in terms of nutrition, health care, safe housing, and clothing is likely to be universally stressful for parents. We suggest investing in studies on the relation between economic stress and attachment-related processes across cultures to evaluate the family stress model. In many studies comparing parent–child relations in different cultural groups, cultural and socioeconomic variables are confounded (e.g., Bakermans-Kranenburg, Van IJzendoorn, & Kroonenberg, 2004). Therefore, as also shown by the Mexican and Chilean studies, it is pivotal for future cross-cultural studies of attachment to examine different socioeconomic groups within cultures.

The normativity hypothesis does not address the distribution of classifications within the insecure category. However, interesting patterns of the prevalence rates of avoidant versus resistant attachment emerge from the studies discussed in this chapter (see Figure 37.2). Whereas results from Anglo-Saxon and European samples generally show a higher rate of A than C classifications, with A mostly (well) above 20% (Van IJzendoorn et al., 1992; Van IJzendoorn & Kroonenberg, 1988), the range of avoidant attachment classifications in the studies discussed in this chapter lies between 0 and 23%, with only two studies reporting a rate higher than 20% (Behrens et al., 2007; Valenzuela, 1997), and half of the studies reporting a rate lower than 10% in a variety of non-Western countries. Because avoidant attachment is generally associated with consistently unresponsive parenting, we hypothesize that in countries empha-

sizing relatedness, customs of highly proximal and indulgent parenting may be responsible for the low rates of avoidance. As Jin and colleagues (2012) noted, insensitive care in these cultures may be more likely to be intrusive rather than unavailable (and therefore potentially inconsistently sensitive as well), which is generally found to foster resistant attachment rather than avoidance.

## The Sensitivity Hypothesis

The sensitivity hypothesis was not tested in most of the studies, but when examined, the data almost invariably supported it (except for the procedurally flawed first Sapporo study). Indirect support for the sensitivity hypothesis comes from studies reporting that secure attachment was related to factors known to be associated with maternal sensitivity. Furthermore, several ethnographic studies provide accounts of sensitive parenting as apparently normative in hunter–gatherer societies. It is also interesting to note that in a sample of no less than 1,150 Asian families living in the United States, 87% of whom were born in Asia, observations of maternal sensitivity were significantly related to observations of infant attachment security (Huang, Lewin, Mitchell, & Zhang, 2012). Further support for the cross-cultural relevance of the sensitivity construct was provided by Mesman and colleagues (2015), who reported strong convergence between maternal beliefs about the ideal mother and attachment theory's description of the sensitive mother across 26 cultural groups from 15 countries (see also Emmen et al., 2012).

The potentially universal role of sensitive caregiving in fostering attachment security is consistent with the idea that when the socioeconomic context allows for sensitive care, the formation of a secure attachment to a sensitive caregiver is most likely to result in adaptive functioning and inclusive fitness. Notably, the function and outcome of the parental behaviors are more important than their specific manifestation, which is consistent with the form–function distinction drawn by Bornstein, Cote, Haynes, Suwalsky, and Bakeman (2012), which states that different parental behaviors can have the same function in different cultural contexts. As such, the sensitivity construct reflects an organizational approach to the attachment relationship in that neither parent nor child behaviors can be captured by a predefined and exhaustive set of concrete behaviors (Sroufe & Waters, 1977), but reflect a history of patterns of interaction rather than individual behaviors (Weinfield, Sroufe, Egeland, & Carlson, 2008). Indeed, there is evidence that whereas the rates of contingent responding are very similar across very different cultures, the modalities through which responsiveness is channeled are culture-dependent (e.g., Kärtner, Keller, & Yovsi, 2010). In some cultures, appropriate responding to infant vocalization may consist of touching or stroking the infant, whereas in other cultures it may be to imitate the sound that the infant made or to smile at the infant (Kärtner, Keller, & Yovsi, 2010; Keller, Borke, Yovsi, Lohaus, & Jensen, 2005; Keller et al., 2009). Similarly, infant distress may be dealt with appropriately in many different ways. For instance, soothing through nursing/feeding is much more common in non-Western than in Western cultures (e.g., Ainsworth, 1967; True et al., 2001). Many more concrete aspects of responsiveness may be examined to fine-tune our understanding of what it means to be sensitive in different cultures both in infancy and beyond, to paint a comprehensive picture of the similarities and differences in the concrete behavioral characteristics of sensitive responsiveness across cultures and their particular role in fostering secure attachment.

### The Competence Hypothesis

The competence hypothesis has been tested only sporadically in cross-cultural research; this concurs with the relative lack of Western studies on the association between attachment and (later) competence (Groh et al., 2014; Sroufe, Egeland, Carlson, & Collins, 2005; Van IJzendoorn, Dijkstra, & Bus, 1995). In the Gusii study (Kermoian & Leiderman, 1986), the nutritional status of the secure infants was better than that of the insecure infants. This outcome has been replicated by Valenzuela (1997) in her Chilean study of undernourished infants. Although the relation between attachment and health status is truly remarkable, it is still not clear whether attachment security serves only as the cause and nutritional status only as the effect. It may be that more healthy infants evoke more care in general and more sensitive care in particular, especially in situations of economic deprivation when parents are forced to be selective in their investment of time and energy (Finerman, 1994; Scheper-Hughes, 1993). A more intricate causal pattern cannot be completely excluded on the basis of the correlational evidence

that Kermoian and Leiderman (1986) and Valenzuela (1997) have provided. The Dogon study (True, 1994; True et al., 2001) does not allow for differentiation between cause and effect, either. Only the Israeli studies on children raised in a kibbutz and city children showed some longitudinal relations between secure attachment and future adaptive functioning (Aviezer, Sagi, & Van IJzendoorn, 2002; Gini, Oppenheim, & Sagi-Schwartz, 2007; Oppenheim, Koren-Karie, & Sagi-Schwartz, 2007; Sagi- Schwartz & Aviezer, 2005). We should therefore conclude that the cross-cultural support for the competence hypothesis is still insufficient. Given the convincing support for the other three key hypotheses postulated by attachment theory, it seems more than feasible to extend attachment research in non-Western countries to children's developmental outcomes. Furthermore, the concept of attachment networks may be fruitfully applied in studies of the competence hypothesis in societies where multiple caregivers are the norm.

### Conclusions

Our analysis and integration of cross-cultural attachment research suggest a balance between universal trends and contextual determinants. Attachment theory without contextual components is as difficult to conceive of as attachment theory without a universalistic perspective. If all infants across cultures used the same fixed strategies to deal with attachment challenges, it would leave no room for adaptation to dynamic changes in the environment (Hinde & Stevenson-Hinde, 1990) and to the constraints imposed by different developmental niches (DeVries, 1984; Harkness & Super, 1992, 1996; LeVine & Miller, 1990; see Simpson & Belsky, Chapter 5, this volume). Without variation, selection of optimal behavioral strategies would become obsolete (Darwin, 1859/1985; see Van IJzendoorn, Bakermans-Kranenburg, & Sagi-Schwartz, 2006, for an evolutionary attachment model integrating universal and contextual dimensions of attachment).

The studies reviewed in this chapter emphasize the importance of investigating attachment within the wider social networks in which children grow and develop. In Western as well as non-Western cultures, most children communicate with several attachment figures, including siblings. Examining the competence hypothesis only on the basis of infant–mother attachment may decrease predictive power substantially, and more conceptual and empirical work is needed to determine how experiences with different attachment figures become organized to form a coherent internal working model (Sagi-Schwartz & Aviezer, 2005). Furthermore, several studies reviewed here emphasize the importance of including variations in the socioeconomic context within countries, so that attachment patterns can be elucidated from both a cultural and a resource perspective.

Last, the current cross-cultural database is almost absurdly small compared to the domain that should be covered. Data on attachment in a populous country such as India and most Islamic countries are still lacking, and large parts of Africa, Asia, and Latin America are uncharted territories with respect to the development of attachment. Although the studies including samples from these parts of the world represent admirable contributions to the attachment literature, they cannot be considered to be representative of their respective continents. This lack of studies outside of North America and Europe, of course, is partly due to the difficulties of conducting standardized research in countries where facilities and resources are lacking. And even if researchers manage to, for instance, conduct the Strange Situation procedure, in many cases the coding is done by researchers who have not been formally trained by experts, which makes the quality of the classifications unclear. It is also the task of Western attachment researchers to provide adequate and affordable training opportunities to those researchers in other parts of the world who want to study attachment.

In our chapter of this third edition, which includes attachment data from five new countries or cultures compared to the previous edition (Van IJzendoorn & Sagi-Schwartz, 2008), we pay special attention to cross-cultural beliefs about attachment and sensitivity, and we provide more details on attachment and sensitivity in Latin America and with Arabs living in Israel. What has not changed since 2008 is that the available cross-cultural studies have not refuted the bold conjectures of attachment theory about the universality of attachment, the normativity of secure attachment, the link between sensitive caregiving and attachment security, and the competent child outcomes of secure attachment. In fact, taken as a whole, the studies are remarkably consistent with the theory. Until further notice, attachment theory may therefore claim cross-cultural validity.

## Acknowledgments

Support for the preparation of this chapter was provided by the Spinoza Prize of the Netherlands Foundation for Scientific Research (NWO) to Marinus H. van IJzendoorn, and by NORFACE (New Opportunities for Research Funding Agency Cooperation in Europe, Grant No. 292) to Judi Mesman.

## References

Ahnert, L., Pinquart, M., & Lamb, M. E. (2006). Security of children's relationships with nonparental care providers: A meta-analysis. *Child Development, 74,* 664–679.

Ainsworth, M. D. S. (1967). *Infancy in Uganda: Infant care and the growth of love.* Baltimore: Johns Hopkins University Press.

Ainsworth, M. D. S. (1977). Infant development and mother–infant interaction among Ganda and American families. In P. H. Leiderman, S. R. Tulkin, & A. H. Rosenfeld (Eds.), *Culture and infancy* (pp. 119–150). New York: Academic Press.

Ainsworth, M. D. S., Bell, S. M., & Stayton, D. J. (1971). Individual differences in Strange Situation behavior of one year olds. In H. R. Schaffer (Ed.), *The origins of human social relations* (pp. 17–58). New York: Academic Press.

Ainsworth, M. D. S., Bell, S. M., & Stayton, D. J. (1974). Infant–mother attachment and social development: Socialisation as a product of reciprocal responsiveness to signals. In M. P. M. Richards (Ed.), *The introduction of the child into a social world* (pp. 9–135). London: Cambridge University Press.

Ainsworth, M. D. S., Blehar, M. C., Waters, E., & Wall, S. (1978). *Patterns of attachment.* Hillsdale, NJ: Erlbaum.

Ainsworth, M. D. S., & Wittig, B. A. (1969). Attachment and exploratory behavior of one year olds in a strange situation. In B. M. Foss (Ed.), *Determinants of infant behavior* (Vol. 4, pp. 113–136). London: Methuen.

Archer, M., Steele, H., Steele, M., Jin, X., Herreros, F., & Lan, J. (2009, April). *Infant–mother attachment in a Chinese community sample.* Poster presented at the biennial meeting of the Society for Research in Child Development, Denver, CO.

Archer, M., Steele, M., Lan, J., Jin, X., Herreros, F., & Steele, H. (2015). Attachment between infants and mothers in China: Strange Situation procedure findings to date and a new sample. *International Journal of Behavioral Development* [Epub ahead of print].

Aviezer, O., Resnick, G., Sagi, A., & Gini, M. (2002). School competence in young adolescence: Links to early attachment relationships beyond concurrent self-perceived competence and representations of relationships. *International Journal of Behavioral Development, 26,* 397–409.

Aviezer, O., Sagi, A. & Van IJzendoorn, M.H. (2002). Collective sleeping for kibbutz children: An experiment in nature predestined to fail. *Family Process, 41,* 435–454.

Aviezer, O., & Sagi-Schwartz, A. (2008). Attachment and non-maternal care: Towards contextualizing the quantity versus quality debate. *Attachment and Human Development, 10,* 275–285.

Aviezer, O., Van IJzendoorn, M. H., Sagi, A., & Schuengel, C. (1994). "Children of the dream" revisited: 70 years of collective early child care in Israeli kibbutzim. *Psychological Bulletin, 116,* 99–116.

Bakermans-Kranenburg, M. J., Van IJzendoorn, M. H., & Kroonenberg, P. M. (2004). Differences in attachment security between African-American and white children: Ethnicity or socio-economic status? *Infant Behavior and Development, 27,* 417–433.

Baram, T. Z., David, E. P., Obenaus, A., Sandman, C. A., Small, S. L., Solodkin, A., et al. (2012). Fragmentation and unpredictability of early-life experience in mental disorders. *American Journal of Psychiatry, 169*(9), 907–915.

Barry, H. I., & Paxton, L. M. (1971). Infancy and early childhood: Cross-cultural codes 2. *Ethnology, 10,* 466–508.

Behrens, K. (2004). A multifaceted view of the concept of *amae:* Reconsidering the indigenous Japanese concept of relatedness. *Human Development, 47,* 1–27.

Behrens, K. Y., Hesse, E., & Main, M. (2007). Mothers' attachment status as determined by the Adult Attachment Interview predicts their 6-year-olds' reunion responses: A study conducted in Japan. *Developmental Psychology, 43,* 1553–1567. [Verified online]

Belsky, J. (2008). War, trauma and children's development: Observations from a modern evolutionary perspective. *International Journal of Behavioral Development, 32,* 260–271.

Biringen, Z., Robinson, J. L., & Emde, R. N. (2000). Appendix B: The Emotional Availability Scales (3rd ed.; an abridged infancy/early childhood version). *Attachment and Human Development, 2,* 256–270.

Black, M. M., & Aboud, F. E. (2011). Responsive feeding is embedded in a theoretical framework of responsive parenting. *Journal of Nutrition, 141,* 490–494.

Bogin, B., Bragg, J., & Kuzawa, C. (2014). Humans are not cooperative breeders but practice biocultural reproduction. *Annals of Human Biology, 41,* 368–380.

Bornstein, M. H., Cote, L. R., Haynes, O. M., Suwalsky, J. T. D., & Bakeman, R. (2012). Modalities of infant–mother interaction in Japanese, Japanese American immigrant, and European American dyads. *Child Development, 83,* 2073–2088.

Bowlby, J. (1951). *Maternal care and mental health.* Geneva: World Health Organization.

Bowlby, J. (1982). *Attachment and loss: Vol. 1. Attachment.* New York: Basic Books. (Original work published 1969)

Cassidy, J., & Berlin, L. J. (1994). The insecure/ambivalent pattern of attachment: Theory and research. *Child Development, 65,* 971–991.

Conger, R. D., & Donnellan, M. B. (2007). An interactionist perspective on the socioeconomic context of human development. *Annual Review of Psychology, 58,* 175–199.

Darwin, C. (1985). *On the origin of species by means of natural selection, or the preservation of favoured races in the struggle for life.* Harmondsworth, UK: Penguin. (Original work published 1859)

De Wolff, M., & Van IJzendoorn, M. H. (1997). Sensitivity and attachment. A meta-analysis on parental antecedents of infant attachment. *Child Development, 68,* 571–591.

DeVries, M. W. (1984). Temperament and infant mortality among the Masai of East Africa. *American Journal of Psychiatry, 141,* 1189–1194.

Ding, Y. H., Wang, Z. Y., Li, H. R., Chi, Z. Y., & Xu, H. (2008). Study of 62 infants' attachment in Shanghai and their relationship with infants' temperament and cognitive development. *Chinese Child Healthcare Journal, 16,* 163–165.

Ding, Y. H., Xu, X., Wang, Z., Li, H., & Wang, W. (2012). Study of mother–infant attachment patterns and influence factors in Shanghai. *Early Human Development, 88,* 295–300.

Doi, T. (1973). *The anatomy of dependence.* New York: Kodansha.

Doi, T. (1989). The concept of *amae* and its psychoanalytic implications. *International Review of Psychoanalysis, 16,* 349–354.

Doi, T. (1992). On the concept of *amae. Infant Mental Health Journal, 13,* 7–11.

Durrett, M. E., Otaki, M., & Richards, P. (1984). Attachment and the mother's perception of support from the father. *International Journal of Behavioral Development, 7,* 167–176.

Emde, R. N. (1992). *Amae,* intimacy, and the early moral self. *Infant Mental Health Journal, 13,* 34–42.

Emmen, R. A. G., Malda, M., Mesman, J., Ekmekci, H., & Van IJzendoorn, M. H. (2012). Sensitive parenting as a cross-cultural ideal: Sensitivity beliefs of Dutch, Moroccan, and Turkish mothers in the Netherlands. *Attachment and Human Development, 14,* 601–619.

Finerman, R. (1994). "Parental incompetence" and "selective neglect": Blaming the victim in child survival. *Social Science and Medicine, 40,* 5–15.

Fong, V. L. (2002). China's one-child policy and the empowerment of urban daughters. *American Anthropologist, 104,* 1098–1109.

Fouts, H. N., & Lamb, M. E. (2005). Weaning emotional patterns among the Bofi foragers of Central Africa: The role of maternal availability and sensitivity. In M. E. Lamb & B. S. Hewlett (Eds.), *Hunter–gatherer childhoods: Evolutionary, developmental, and cultural perspectives* (pp. 19–64). New Brunswick, NJ: Transaction.

Gini, M., Oppenheim, D., & Sagi-Schwartz, A. (2007).

Negotiation styles in mother–child narrative co-construction in middle childhood: Associations with early attachment. *International Journal of Behavioral Development, 31,* 149–160.

Goh, E. C. L., & Kuczynski, L. (2010). "Only children" and their coalition of parents: Considering grandparents and parents as joint caregivers in urban Xiamen, China. *Asian Journa of Social Psychology, 13,* 221–231.

Gojman, S., Millán, S., Carlson, E., Sánchez, G., Rodarte, A., González, P., et al. (2012). Intergenerational relations of attachment: A research synthesis of urban/rural Mexican samples. *Attachment and Human Development, 14,* 553–566.

Goossens, F. A., & Van IJzendoorn, M. H. (1990). Quality of infants' attachments to professional caregivers: Relation to infant–parent attachment and day-care characteristics. *Child Development, 61,* 832–837.

Groh, A. M., Fearon, R. P., Bakermans-Kranenburg, M. J., Van IJzendoorn, M. H., Steele, R. D., & Roisman, G. I. (2014). The significance of attachment security for children's social competence with peers: A meta-analytic study. *Attachment and Human Development, 16,* 103–136.

Grossmann, K. E., Grossmann, K., & Keppler, A. (2005). Universal and culture-specific aspects of human behavior: The case of attachment. In W. Friedlmeier, P. Chakkarath, & B. Schwarz (Eds.), *Culture and human development: The importance of cross-cultural research for the social sciences* (pp. 71–91). New York: Psychology Press.

Gu, H., Cen, G., Li, D., Gao, X., Li, Z., & Chen, X. (1997). Two-year-old children's social behaviour development and related family factors. *Psychological Science, 20,* 519–524.

Harkness, S., & Super, C. M. (1992). Shared child care in East Africa: Sociocultural origins and developmental consequences. In M. E. Lamb, K. J. Sternberg, C. P. Hwang, & A. G. Broberg (Eds.), *Child care in context: Cross-cultural perspectives* (pp. 441–459). Hillsdale, NJ: Erlbaum.

Harkness, S., & Super, C. M. (Eds.). (1996). *Parents' cultural belief systems: Their origins, expressions, and consequences.* New York: Guilford Press.

Harlow, H. (1958). The nature of love. *American Psychologist, 13,* 673–685.

Hewlett, B. S., & Winn, S. (2014). Allomaternal nursing in humans. *Current Anthropology, 55,* 200–229.

Hinde, R. A. (1982). Attachment: Some conceptual and biological issues. In C. Parkes, & J. Stevenson-Hinde (Eds.), *The place of attachment in human behavior* (pp. 60–76). New York: Basic Books.

Hinde, R. A., & Stevenson-Hinde, J. (1990). Attachment: Biological, cultural, and individual desiderata. *Human Development, 33,* 62–72.

Hofstede, G. (1984). *Culture's consequences: International differences in work-related values.* Newbury Park, CA: Sage.

Howes, C., Rodning, C., Galluzzo, D. C., & Myers, L. (1988). Attachment and child care: Relationships with mother and caregiver. *Early Childhood Research Quarterly, 3,* 403–416.

Hrdy, S. B. (2009). *Mothers and others: The evolutionary origins of mutual understanding.* Cambridge, MA: Harvard University Press.

Hu, P., & Meng, Z. (1996). *An examination of infant–mother attachment in China.* Poster presented at the 14th meeting of the International Society for the Study of Behavioral Development, Quebec City, Canada.

Hu, P., & Meng, Z. (2003). Research on discrimination of mother-infant attachment type. *Acta Psychologica Sinica, 35,* 201–208.

Huang, Z. J., Lewin, A., Mitchell, S. J., & Zhang, J. (2012). Variations in the relationship between maternal depression, maternal sensitivity, and child attachment by race/ethnicity and nativity: Findings from a nationally representative cohort study. *Maternal and Child Health Journal, 16,* 40–50.

Jin, M. K., Jacobvitz, D., Hazen, N., & Jung, S. H. (2012). Maternal sensitivity and infant attachment security in Korea: Cross-cultural validation of the Strange Situation. *Attachment and Human Development, 14,* 33–44.

Kagitcibasi, C. (2007). *Family, self, and human development across cultures: Theory and applications* (2nd ed.). Mahwah, NJ: Erlbaum.

Kärtner, J., Keller, H., & Yovsi, R. D. (2010). Mother-infant interaction during the first 3 months: The emergence of culture-specific contingency patterns. *Child Development, 81,* 540–554.

Kazui, M., Endo, T., Tanaka, A., Sakagami, H., & Suganuma, M. (2000). Intergenerational transmission of attachment: Japanese mother–child dyads. *Japanese Journal of Educational Psychology, 48,* 323–332.

Keller, H., Borke, J., Staufenbiel, T., Yovsi, R. D., Abels, M., Papaligoura, Z., et al. (2009). Distal and proximal parenting as alternative parenting strategies during infants' early months of life: A cross-cultural study. *International Journal of Behavioral Development, 33,* 412–420.

Keller, H., Borke, J., Yovsi, R., Lohaus, A., & Jensen, H. (2005). Cultural orientations and historical changes as predictors of parenting behaviour. *International Journal of Behavioral Development, 29,* 229–237.

Kermoian, R., & Leiderman, P. H. (1986). Infant attachment to mother and child caretaker in an East African community. *International Journal of Behavioral Development, 9,* 455–469.

Konner, M. (1977). Infancy among the Kalahari Desert San. In P. H. Leiderman, S. R. Tulkin, & A. Rosenfeld (Eds.), *Culture and infancy: Variations in the human experience* (pp. 287–328). New York: Academic Press.

Konner, M. (2005). Hunter–gatherer infancy and childhood: The !Kung and others. In M. E. Lamb & B. S. Hewlett (Eds.), *Hunter–gatherer childhoods: Evolutionary, developmental, and cultural perspectives* (pp. 19–64). New Brunswick, NJ: Transaction.

Koren-Karie, N., Oppenheim, D., Dolev, S., Sher, E., &

Etzion-Carasso, A. (2002). Mothers' insightfulness regarding their infants' internal experience: Relations with maternal sensitivity and infant attachment. *Developmental Psychology, 38,* 534–542.

Lee, R. B., & Daly, R. (1999). *The Cambridge encyclopedia of hunters and gatherers.* Cambridge, UK: Cambridge University Press.

LeVine, R. A., & Miller, P. M. (1990). Commentary. *Human Development, 33,* 73–80.

Li, X., Jing, J., Yang, D., Cai, X., Chen, X., & Su, X. (2004). Characters of 75 infants' attachment towards their mothers. *Chinese Mental Health Journal, 18,* 291–293.

Liang, L., Chen, H., & Chen, X. (2000). Pattern of toddler–mother attachment. *Psychological Science, 23*(3), 324–328.

Liang, X., Wang, Z.-Y., Liu, H.-Y., Lin, Q., Wang, Z., & Liu, Y. (2015). Adult attachment status predicts the developmental trajectory of maternal sensitivity in new motherhood among Chinese mothers. *Midwifery, 31*(1), 68–73.

Lucassen, N., Tharner, A., Van IJzendoorn, M. H., Bakermans-Kranenburg, M. J., Volling, B. L., Verhulst, F. C., et al. (2011). The association between paternal sensitivity and infant–father attachment security: A meta-analysis of three decades of research. *Journal of Family Psychology, 25,* 986–992.

Lupien, S. J., McEwen, B. S., Gunnar, M. R., & Heim, C. (2009). Effects of stress throughout the lifespan on the brain, behavior and cognition. *Nature Reviews Neuroscience, 10,* 434–445.

Main, M. (1990). Cross-cultural studies of attachment organization: Recent studies, changing methodologies, and the concept of conditional strategies. *Human Development, 33,* 48–61.

Main, M., & Solomon, J. (1990). Procedures for identifying infants as disorganized/disoriented during the Ainsworth Strange Situation. In M. T. Greenberg, D. Cicchetti, & E. M. Cummings (Eds.), *Attachment in the preschool years: Theory, research, and intervention* (pp. 121–160). Chicago: University of Chicago Press.

Marlowe, F. W. (2005). Who tends Hadza children? In M. E. Lamb & B. S. Hewlett (Eds.), *Hunter–gatherer childhoods: Evolutionary, developmental, and cultural perspectives* (pp. 19–64). New Brunswick, NJ: Transaction.

Marvin, R. S., VanDevender, T. L., Iwanaga, M. I., LeVine, S., & LeVine, R. A. (1977). Infant–caregiver attachment among the Hausa of Nigeria. In H. McGurk (Ed.), *Ecological factors in human development* (pp. 247–259). Amsterdam: North-Holland.

McLoyd, V. C. (1998). Socioeconomic disadvantage and child development. *American Psychologist, 53,* 185–204.

Meaney, M. J. (2010). Epigenetics and the biological definition of gene × environment interactions. *Child Development, 1,* 41–79.

Meehan, C. L., & Hawks, S. (2013). Cooperative breeding and attachment among the Aka foragers. In N.

Quinn & J. M. Mageo (Eds.), *Attachment reconsidered: Cultural perspectives on a Western theory* (pp. 85–113). New York: Palgrave Macmillan.

Meehan, C. L., & Hawks, S. (2015). Multiple attachments: Allomothering, stranger anxiety, and intimacy. In H. Otto & H. Keller (Eds.), *Different faces of attachment: Cultural variations on a universal human need* (pp. 113–140). Cambridge, UK: Cambridge University Press.

Mesman, J., Van IJzendoorn, M., Behrens, K., Carbonell, O. A., Cárcamo, R., Cohen-Paraira, I., et al. (2015). Is the ideal mother a sensitive mother? Beliefs about early childhood parenting in mothers across the globe. [Epub ahead of print]

Miller, G. E., Chen, E., & Parker, K. J. (2011). Psychological stress in childhood and susceptibility to the chronic diseases of aging: Moving toward a model of behavioral and biological mechanisms. *Psychological Bulletin, 137,* 959–997.

Minde, K., Minde, R., & Vogel, W. (2006). Culturally sensitive assessment of attachment in children aged 18–40 months in a South African township. *Infant Mental Health Journal, 27,* 544–558.

Miyake, K., Chen, S. J., & Campos, J. J. (1985). Infant temperament, mother's mode of interaction, and attachment in Japan: An interim report. *Monographs of the Society for Research in Child Development, 50*(1-2), 276–297.

Mizuta, I., Zahn-Waxler, C., Cole, P. M., & Hiruma, N. (1996). A cross cultural study of preschoolers' attachment: Security and sensitivity in Japanese and U.S. dyads. *International Journal of Behavioral Development, 19,* 141–159.

Morelli, G. A., & Tronick, E. Z. (1991). Efé multiple caretaking and attachment. In J. L. Gewirtz & W. M. Kurtines (Eds.), *Intersections with attachment* (pp. 41–52). Hillsdale, NJ: Erlbaum.

Naftali, O. (2010). Recovering childhood: Play, pedagogy, and the rise of psychological knowledge in contemporary urban China. *Modern China, 36,* 589–616.

Nakagawa, M., Lamb, M. E., & Miyake, K. (1992). Antecedents and correlates of the Strange Situation behavior of Japanese infants. *Journal of Cross-Cultural Psychology, 23,* 300–310.

Nakagawa, M., Teti, D. M., & Lamb, M. E. (1992). An ecological study of child–mother attachments among Japanese sojourners in the United States. *Developmental Psychology, 28,* 584–592.

Nauck, B., & Suckow, J. (2006). Intergenerational relationships in cross-cultural comparison: How social networks frame intergenerational relations between mothers and grandmothers in Japan, Korea, China, Indonesia, Israel, Germany, and Turkey. *Journal of Family Issues, 27,* 1159–1185.

Nelson, C. A., Fox, N. A., & Zeanah, C. H. (2014). *Romania's abandoned children: Deprivation, brain development, and the struggle for recovery.* Cambridge, MA: Harvard University Press.

Oppenheim, D., Koren-Karie, N., & Sagi-Schwartz, A. (2007). Emotional dialogues between mothers and children at 4.5 and 7.5 years: Relations with children's attachment at 1 year. *Child Development, 78,* 38–52.

Oppenheim, D., Sagi, A., & Lamb, M. E. (1990). Infant–adult attachments on the kibbutz and their relation to socioemotional development four years later. In S. Chess & M. E. Hertzig (Eds.), *Annual progress in child psychiatry and child development* (pp. 92–106). New York: Brunner/Mazel.

Otto, H. (2014). Don't show your emotions!: Emotion regulation and attachment in the Cameroonian Nso. In H. Otto & H. Keller (Eds.), *Different faces of attachment: Cultural variations on a universal human need* (pp. 215–229). Cambridge, UK: Cambridge University Press.

Oyserman, D., Coon, H. M., & Kemmelmeier, M. (2002). Rethinking individualism and collectivism: Evaluation of theoretical assumptions and meta-analyses. *Psychological Bulletin, 128,* 3–72.

Pederson, D. R., & Moran, G. (1995). A categorical description of infant–mother relationships in the home and its relation to Q-sort measures of infant–mother interaction. *Monographs of the Society for Research in Child Development, 60* (2-3), 111–132.

Peterson, N. J., Drotar, D., Olness, K., Guay, L., & Kiziri-Mayengo, R. (2001). The relationship of maternal and child HIV infection to security of attachment among Ugandan infants. *Child Psychiatry and Human Development, 32,* 3–17.

Posada, G., Carbonell, O. A., Alzate, G., & Plata, S. J. (2004). Through Colombian lenses: Ethnographic and conventional analyses of maternal care and their associations with secure base behavior. *Developmental Psychology, 40,* 508–518.

Posada, G., Gao, Y., Wu, F., Posado, R., Tascon, M., Schoelmerich, A., et al. (1995). The secure-base phenomenon across cultures: Children's behavior, mothers' preferences, and experts' concepts. In E. Waters, B. E. Vaughn, G. Posada, & K. Kondo-Ikemura (Eds.), Caregiving, cultural, and cognitive perspectives on secure-base behavior and working models: New growing points of attachment theory and research. *Monographs of the Society for Research in Child Development, 60* (2–3, Serial No. 244), 27–48.

Posada, G., Jacobs, A., Richmond, M., Carbonell, O. A., Alzate, G., Bustamante, M. R., et al. (2002). Maternal caregiving and infant security in two cultures. *Developmental Psychology, 38,* 67–78.

Posada, G., Lu, T., Trumbell, J., Kaloustian, G., Trudel, M., Plata, S. J., et al. (2013). Is the secure-base phenomenon evident here, there, and anywhere?: A cross-cultural study of child behavior and experts' definitions. *Child Development, 84,* 1896–1905.

Rabin, A. I., & Beit-Hallahmi, B. (1982). *Twenty years later.* New York: Springer.

Reed, G., & Leiderman, P. H. (1981). Age-related changes in attachment behavior in polymatrically reared infants: The Kenyan Gusii. In T. M. Field, A. M. Sostek, P. Vietze, & P. H. Leiderman (Eds.), *Culture and early interactions* (pp. 215–236). Hillsdale, NJ: Erlbaum.

Rothbaum, F., Weisz, J., Pott, M., Miyake, K., & Morelli, G. (2000). Attachment and culture: Security in the United States and Japan. *American Psychologist, 55,* 1093–1104.

Sagi, A., Koren-Karie, N., Gini, M., Ziv, Y., & Joels, T. (2002). Shedding further light on the effects of various types and quality of early child care on infant–mother attachment relationship: The Haifa study of early child care. *Child Development, 73,* 1166–1186.

Sagi, A., Lamb, M. E., Lewkowicz, K. S., Shoham, R., Dvir, R., & Estes, D. (1985). Security of infant–mother, –father, and –metapelet attachments among kibbutz-reared Israeli children. In I. Bretherton & E. Waters (Eds.), Growing points of attachment theory and research. *Monographs of the Society for Research in Child Development, 50* (1–2, Serial No. 209), 257–275.

Sagi, A., & Van IJzendoorn, M. H. (1996). Multiple caregiving environments: The kibbutz experience. In S. Harel & J. P. Shonkoff (Eds.), *Early childhood intervention and family support programs: Accomplishments and challenges* (pp. 143–162). Jerusalem: JDC–Brookale Institute.

Sagi, A., Van IJzendoorn, M. H., Aviezer, O., Donnell, F., Koren-Karie, N., Joels, T, et al. (1995). Attachments in a multiple-caregiver and multiple-infant environment: The case of the Israeli kibbutzim. In E. Waters, B. E. Vaughn, G. Posada, & K. Kondo-Ikemura (Eds.), Caregiving, cultural, and cognitive perspectives on secure-base behavior and working models: New growing points of attachment theory and research (Special issue). *Monographs of the Society for Research on Child Development, 60*(Serial No. 244, No. 2–3), 71–91.

Sagi, A., Van IJzendoorn, M. H., Aviezer, O., Donnell, F., & Mayseless, O. (1994). Sleeping out of home in a kibbutz communal arrangement: It makes a difference for infant–mother attachment. *Child Development, 65,* 992–1004.

Sagi, A., Van IJzendoorn, M. H., Scharf, M., Joels, T., Koren-Karie, N., Mayseless, O., et al. (1997). Ecological constraints for intergenerational transmission of attachment. *International Journal of Behavioral Development, 20,* 287–299.

Sagi-Schwartz, A., & Aviezer, O. (2005). Correlates of attachment to multiple caregivers in kibbutz children from birth to emerging adulthood: The Haifa longitudinal study. In K. E. Grossmann, K. Grossmann, & E. Waters (Eds.), *Attachment from infancy to adulthood* (pp. 165–197). New York: Guilford Press.

Sagi-Schwartz, A., Van IJzendoorn, M. H., Bakermans-Kranenburg, M. J. (2008). Does intergenerational transmission of trauma skip a generation?: No meta-analytic evidence for tertiary traumatization with third generation of Holocaust survivors. *Attachment and Human Development, 10,* 105–121.

Scheper-Hughes, N. (1993). *Death without weeping: The violence of everyday life in Brazil.* Berkeley: University of California Press.

Short, S. E., Fengying, Z., Siyuan, X., & Mingliang, Y. (2001). China's one-child policy and the care of children: An analysis of qualitative and quantitative data. *Social Forces, 79,* 913–943.

Sroufe, L. A., Egeland, B., Carlson, E., & Collins, W. A. (2005). *The development of the person: The Minnesota Study of Risk and Adaptation from Birth to Adulthood.* New York: Guilford Press.

Sroufe, L. A., & Waters, E. (1977). Attachment as an organizational construct. *Child Development, 48,* 1184–1199.

Strassman, B. I. (2011). Cooperation and competition in a cliff-dwelling people. *PNAS, 108,* 10894-10901.

Takahashi, K. (1986). Examining the Strange Situation procedure with Japanese mothers and 12-month-old infants. *Developmental Psychology, 22,* 265–270.

Takahashi, K. (1990). Are the key assumptions of the "Strange Situation" procedure universal?: A view from Japanese research. *Human Development, 33,* 23–30.

Tavecchio, L. W. C., & Van IJzendoorn, M. H. (1987). *Attachment in social networks: Contributions to the Bowlby–Ainsworth attachment theory.* Amsterdam: North-Holland.

Tomlinson, M., Cooper, P., & Murray, L. (2005). The mother–infant relationship and infant attachment in a South-African peri-urban settlement. *Child Development, 76,* 1044–1054.

Trivers, R. L. (1974). Parent–offspring conflict. *American Zoologist, 14,* 249–264.

Tronick, E. Z., Morelli, G. A., & Winn, S. (1987). Multiple caretaking of Efé (Pygmy) infants. *American Anthropologist, 89,* 96–106.

True, M. M. (1994). *Mother–infant attachment and communication among the Dogon of Mali.* Unpublished doctoral dissertation, University of California, Berkeley.

True, M. M., Pisani, L., & Oumar, F. (2001). Infant–mother attachment among the Dogon of Mali. *Child Development, 72,* 1451–1466.

Valenzuela, M. (1997). Maternal sensitivity in a developing society: The context of urban poverty and infant chronic undernutrition. *Developmental Psychology,* 845–855.

Van Bakel, H. J. A., & Riksen-Walraven, J. M. A. (2002). Parenting and development of one-year-olds: Links with parental, contextual, and child characteristics. *Child Development, 73,* 256–273.

Van IJzendoorn, M. H. (1990). Developments in cross-cultural research on attachment: Some methodological notes. *Human Development, 33,* 3–9.

Van IJzendoorn, M. H. (1995). Adult attachment representations, parental responsiveness, and infant attachment: A meta-analysis on the predictive validity of the Adult Attachment Interview. *Psychological Bulletin, 117,* 387–403.

Van IJzendoorn, M. H., Bakermans-Kranenburg, M. J., & Sagi-Schwartz, A. (2006). Attachment across diverse sociocultural contexts. The limits of universality. In K. Rubin & O. B. Chung (Eds.), *Parenting beliefs, behaviors, and parent–child relations: A cross-cultural perspective* (pp. 107–142). New York: Psychology Press.

Van IJzendoorn, M. H., Bard, K. A., Bakermans-Kranenburg, M. J., & Ivan, K. (2009). Cognitive development of young nursery-reared chimpanzees in responsive versus standard care. *Developmental Psychobiology, 51,* 173–185.

Van IJzendoorn, M. H., Dijkstra, J., & Bus, A. G. (1995). Attachment, intelligence, and language. *Social Development, 4,* 115–128.

Van IJzendoorn, M. H., & Kroonenberg, P. M. (1988). Cross-cultural patterns of attachment: A meta-analysis of the Strange Situation. *Child Development, 59,* 147–156.

Van IJzendoorn, M. H., & Sagi, A. (2001). Cultural blindness or selective inattention? *American Psychologist, 56,* 824–825.

Van IJzendoorn, M. H., Sagi, A., & Lambermon, M. W. E. (1992). The multiple caretaker paradox: Data from Holland and Israel. *New Directions for Child Development, 57,* 5–24.

Van IJzendoorn, M. H., & Sagi-Schwartz, A. (2008). Cross-cultural patterns of attachment: Universal and contextual dimensions. In J. Cassidy & P. R. Shaver (Eds.), *Handbook of attachment: Theory, research, and clinical applications* (2nd ed., pp. 880–905). New York: Guilford Press.

Van IJzendoorn, M. H., Vereijken, C. M. J. L., Bakermans-Kranenburg, M. J., & Riksen-Walraven, J. M. (2004). Assessing attachment security with the Attachment Q-Sort: Meta-analytic evidence for the validity of the observer AQS. *Child Development, 75,* 1188–1213.

Vaughn, B. E., Coppola, G., Verissimo, M., Monteiro, L., José Santos, A., Posada, G., et al. (2007). The quality of maternal secure-base scripts predicts children's secure-base behavior at home in three sociocultural groups. *International Journal of Behavioral Development, 31,* 65–76.

Vaughn, B. E., & Waters, E. (1990). Attachment behavior at home and in the laboratory: Q-sort observations and Strange Situation classifications of one-year-olds. *Child Development, 61,* 1965–1973.

Vereijken, C. M. J. L. (1996). *The mother–infant relationship in Japan: Attachment, dependency, and amae.* Unpublished doctoral dissertation, Catholic University of Nijmegen, The Netherlands.

Vereijken, C. M. J. L., Riksen-Walraven, M., & Kondo-Ikemura, K. (1997). Maternal sensitivity and infant attachment security in Japan: A longitudinal study. *International Journal of Behavioral Development, 21,* 35–49.

Wang, L., & Mesman, J. (2015). *Parenting and child development in China: A narrative and meta-analytic review of the cross-cultural literature.* Manuscript submitted for publication.

Weinfield, N. S., Sroufe, L. A., Egeland, B., & Carlson, E. (2008). Individual differences in infant-caregiver attachment: Conceptual and empirical aspects of security. In J. Cassidy & P. R. Shaver (Eds.), *Handbook of attachment: Theory, research, and clinical applications* (2nd ed., pp. 78–101). New York: Guilford Press.

WHO/UNICEF (2003). *Global strategy for infant and young child feeding.* Geneva: WHO.

Yue, Y., Zhang, G., Chen, H., Liang, Z., & Zhang, P. (2010). The relations between children's attachment and problem behaviour. *Psychological Science, 33,* 318–320.

Zevalkink, J. (1997). *Attachment in Indonesia: The mother–child relationship in context.* Ridderkerk, The Netherlands: Ridderprint.

Zevalkink, J., Riksen-Walraven, J. M., & Van Lieshout, C. F. M. (1999). Attachment in the Indonesian caregiving context. *Social Development, 8,* 21–40.

Zevalkink, J., Riksen-Walraven, M., & Bradley, R. H. (2008). The quality of children's home environment and attachment security in Indonesia. *Journal of Genetic Psychology: Research and Theory on Human Development, 169,* 72–91.

Zreik, G (2014). *Attachment in a cross-cultural perspective: The case of Arab infants and mothers in Israel.* Unpublished doctoral thesis, University of Haifa, Department of Psychology, Faculty of Social Sciences, Ramat-Gan, Israel.

Zreik, G., Oppenheim, D., Sagi-Schwartz, A. (2015, March). *Attachment in a cross-cultural perspective: The case of Arab infants and mothers in Israel.* Poster presented at the biennial meeting of the Society for Research in Child Development Philadelphia .

# Chapter 38

# A Lifespan Perspective on Attachment and Care for Others

## Empathy, Altruism, and Prosocial Behavior

Phillip R. Shaver
Mario Mikulincer
Jacquelyn T. Gross
Jessica A. Stern
Jude Cassidy

Attachment theory (Bowlby, 1969/1982, 1973, 1980) is, at its core, a theory of prosocial behavior. It explains how, in early childhood, interactions with mindful, caring, and supportive parental figures ("attachment figures") create and solidify children's positive mental representations of others (as competent, dependable, and well intentioned), their pervasive sense of safety and security, and their ability to recognize, acknowledge, and regulate emotions. The theory has been supported by decades of developmental research, summarized in this volume, which implies the existence of an intergenerational transmission of security (or insecurity) that potentially creates a continuing cross-generational stream of prosocial behavior—or its absence. The extension of the theory to some of the topics encountered in the broader psychological literature on prosocial behavior—empathy, compassion, generosity, forgiveness, and altruism (Mikulincer & Shaver, 2010, 2012) —is quite natural, and in recent years it has been accomplished in studies of the prosocial behavior of children, adolescents, and adults.

Our purpose in this chapter is to highlight attachment-related research on prosocial behavior in different phases of the lifespan. We begin with a brief explanation of how the theory's basic concepts relate to prosocial attitudes, motives, emotions, and behavior. This explanation is summarized in a conceptual model of the association between parental sensitive responsiveness on one hand, and a child's empathy and prosocial behavior on the other, mediated by the child's attachment security, internal working models (IWMs), and effective emotion regulation. We follow the theoretical introduction with two major sections on prosocial emotions and behavior in childhood and in adulthood. We conclude the chapter with suggestions for future research involving children and adults.

## Basic Concepts of Attachment Theory in Relation to Prosociality

As explained more fully in other chapters of this volume, attachment theory is organized in terms of several basic concepts: the attachment behavioral system, the caregiving behavioral system, the felt sense of security, working models of self and others, and emotion regulation (see, in this volume, Cassidy, Chapter 1; Bretherton & Munholland, Chapter 4; B. C. Feeney & Woodhouse, Chapter 36; and Mikulincer & Shaver, Chapter 24). The attachment behavioral system was postulated by Bowlby (1969/1982) to explain the observable tendency of primate infants to maintain proximity to their mother, especially in novel or unpredictable environments, and to cling to her when threats arise (often, in the natural environment, as she moves into and through trees to avoid predators). In the human case, although we are born with a grasping reflex that allowed our primate ancestors to cling to a mother's fur, the attachment system emerges slowly during the first months of life, but it gradually matures sufficiently to orient a baby to its familiar caregivers, to move the baby closer to them in response to threats and fears, and to regulate the baby's sense of safety in response to a caregiver's protection, support, and soothing.

Bowlby (1969/1982) also postulated the existence of a caregiving behavioral system to explain humans' seemingly natural capacity for empathy, compassion, and care—features evident in the behavior of parents who respond sensitively to their children's signs of vulnerability and need. These features are not limited to parental behavior but also are evident in the observable tendency of children and adults to become concerned when they encounter other people who are suffering or in need and, often, to be motivated to relieve this suffering or respond to others' needs. Within a person's developmental history, parameters of the universally present attachment behavioral system are modified in response to caregivers' behavior, and the same experiences affect the caregiving behavioral system, causing a complex web of connections between the person's attachment and caregiving cognitions, emotions, and behavior.

According to Bowlby (1969/1982), the caregiving system is designed to provide protection and support to others who are either chronically dependent or temporarily in need. It is inherently altruistic in nature, being aimed at the alleviation of others' distress, although the system itself presumably evolved because it increased inclusive fitness by making it more likely that children and tribe members with whom the individual shared genes would survive and reproduce (Batson, 2010; de Waal, 2008; Hamilton, 1964; MacLean, 1985). Within attachment theory, the caregiving system

provides an entrée to the study of compassion and altruism; moreover, understanding this system provides a foundation for devising ways to increase people's compassion and effective altruism.

The caregiving system is focused on the welfare of others and therefore directs attention to others' distress rather than to one's own needs. In its prototypical form—that is, in the parent–child relationship—the goal of the child's attachment system (proximity that fosters protection, reduces distress, increases safety, and establishes a secure base) is also the goal of the parent's caregiving system. Extending this conceptualization to the broader realm of compassion and altruism, we view the caregiving system as activated by the presence of a distressed person, even a stranger in need, its aim being to alter the needy person's condition until signs of increased safety, well-being, and security appear. This system's functioning can be undermined by anxiety and self-concern on the part of the potential care provider, which is why attachment insecurity often undermines or interferes with effective care. In contrast, a sense of attachment security allows a person to attend less to his or her own concerns and shift attention to providing care.

Theoretically, being secure implies that one has witnessed, experienced, and benefited from generous attachment figures' sensitive and effective care, which provides a model to follow when one encounters a vulnerable or needy other. Secure individuals also feel more comfortable than insecure ones with intimacy and interdependence, so they can more readily accept other people's needs for closeness, sympathy, and support. The positive mental representations (working models) of others that are associated with attachment security (see Bretherton & Munholland, Chapter 4, this volume) make it easier to construe others as deserving of sympathy and support, hence compelling one to care for them. Moreover, secure individuals' positive model of self (Bartholomew & Horowitz, 1991; Bowlby, 1969/1982) allows them to feel more confident about their ability to handle another person's needs while effectively regulating their own emotions (e.g., Batson, 2010).

In contrast, an insecure person is likely to have vulnerable, defended self-esteem, if not an outright negative model of self. He or she is likely to be wary of others' potential for neglect, harsh criticism, rejection, or abuse. Stated this baldly, it is clear why security might be conducive to empathy and prosocial behavior, whereas insecurity might be conducive to self-concern, self-protection, defensive rejection of others' needs, and mistimed or misguided efforts to understand and help others.

As explained in other chapters in this volume (e.g., Solomon & George, Chapter 18), Ainsworth, Blehar, Waters, and Wall (1978) established methods for identifying and categorizing different patterns of attachment (secure, anxious/ambivalent or resistant, and avoidant) that emerge during the first two years of life as a result of caregivers' behavior. In their book, Ainsworth and colleagues (1978) also demonstrated that two main dimensions, anxiety and avoidance, underlie the three patterns of attachment. Subsequent research on adult attachment established similar categorization schemes for adults, using either interviews (e.g., the Adult Attachment Interview [AAI]; Hesse, Chapter 26, this volume) or adult self-report measures of attachment anxiety and avoidance (e.g., the Experiences in Close Relationships scale [ECR]; Brennan, Clark, & Shaver, 1998; see Crowell, Fraley, & Roisman, Chapter 27, this volume). In the following section, we explore attachment-related childhood roots of care for others.

## Childhood Roots of Care for Others

The capacity to care for others' well-being is rooted in early development. Children as young as 8 months of age display concern for others' suffering and in some contexts will act to relieve their pain (Roth-Hanania, Davidov, & Zahn-Waxler, 2011; Zahn-Waxler, Radke-Yarrow, Wagner, & Chapman, 1992). Among the multiple factors that comprise care for others, two of the most important are empathy and prosocial behavior. *Empathy* is an experience of affective resonance with another's emotions, along with a sense of concern for his or her welfare; it may also include cognitive apprehension of another's condition or needs (Decety & Meyer, 2008; Eisenberg, 2000; Hoffman, 1984, 2001). *Prosocial behavior* is voluntary behavior intended to benefit others (Grusec, Hastings, & Almas, 2011); like empathy, prosocial behavior may occur in response to distress, but it may also arise in response to other cues such as instrumental or material need (Dunfield & Kuhlmeier, 2013). In addition to these dimensions, *compassion* refers to the feeling of care for others' suffering, as well as the intention to relieve their suffering (Dalai Lama, 2001; Gillath, Shaver, & Mikulincer, 2005; Halifax, 2012; Siegel & Germer, 2012). Compassion is similar in many respects to empathy, but it involves a sense of acceptance, tenderness, and motivation to act to relieve suffering, and it tends to result in more positive affect than does empathy (Klimecki, Leiberg, Richard, & Singer, 2014). Despite its clear connection to concern for others, virtually no research has specifically examined the development of compassion in children, although some classroom interventions cite compassion as a desired outcome (Greenberg & Harris, 2012).

Together, empathy and prosocial behavior have been the foci of most of the empirical and theoretical work on children's capacity to care. Because this chapter is concerned with care for others, we focus on empathy and prosocial behavior in this section, emphasizing children's comforting of others in response to distress and/or global measures of prosociality, and omit discussion of specific noncaring social capacities such as compliance, cooperation, social competence, affection, and moral reasoning (but see Thompson, Chapter 16, this volume).

Although concern for others' welfare is part of normative development, clear individual differences in empathy and prosocial behavior are evident across childhood, with some children responding to a peer's distress with immediate and overt concern and helpful overtures, and others responding with wariness, hostility, indifference, or distress of their own. These differences are linked to important developmental outcomes, such as peer acceptance, friendship quality, school performance, loneliness, and aggression (Asher & McDonald, 2009; Cassidy & Asher, 1992; Clark & Ladd, 2000; Findlay, Girardi, & Coplan, 2006; Ladd, Birch, & Buhs, 1999; Wentzel, 2003). Given the theoretical basis for expecting a link between attachment and care for others described in the previous section, a key question becomes: Are individual differences in children's empathy and prosocial behavior related to attachment?

We begin by exploring theoretical considerations regarding the link between attachment security and children's emerging capacity to care for others, first by exploring potential mediators of this link, then by discussing the role of parental sensitivity in supporting the development of both security and care for others. We then discuss definitions and operationalizations of empathy and prosocial behavior. Next, we review empirical investigations of the attachment–care link from infancy through adolescence.

## Theoretical Considerations

### Mediators

As mentioned earlier, Bowlby (1973) proposed that security provides a foundation for the development of children's emotional functioning, particularly the capacity to regulate emotions. Ainsworth's (1969) observations suggested that individual differences in children's attachment representations guide specific patterns of behavior, and that a secure IWM provides the blueprint for mutually responsive social interaction. Both of these concepts—emotion regulation and the secure IWM—are relevant to empathy and prosocial behavior, and provide potential mediating mechanisms in the link between attachment and care for others.

With regard to children's emotional functioning, researchers studying empathy and prosocial behavior in children have long recognized that multiple emotional competencies underlie the capacity to care for others, including emotion recognition and understanding, intersubjectivity, affective resonance, distinction between self and other, perspective taking, and effortful control (Batson, 1991; Davis, 1996; Decety & Jackson, 2004; Ickes, 2003; Kochanska, 1993; Laible, 2004). Attachment has been empirically linked to many of these, with securely attached children consistently showing, for example, better emotion understanding (Denham, Blair, Schmidt, & De-Mulder, 2002; Laible & Thompson, 1998; Raikes & Thompson, 2006; see also Thompson, Chapter 16, this volume) and better effortful control compared to their insecure peers (Viddal et al., 2015).

One of the most important and well researched of these competencies is *emotion regulation* (e.g., Eisenberg & Fabes, 1992; Trommsdorff, Friedlmeier, & Mayer, 2007), which allows children to perceive and respond to others' distress without becoming overly distressed themselves. Research has shown that behavioral and physiological indicators of self-regulation are related to children's empathy and prosocial behavior, whereas personal distress (i.e., self-focused, dysregulated negative emotion) is inversely related to or unassociated with empathy and prosocial behavior (Eisenberg, 2000; Eisenberg & Fabes, 1990, 1991, 1995; Fabes, Eisenberg, & Eisenbud, 1993).

The extent to which emotion regulation capacities are linked to individual differences in attachment is striking. Attachment theory holds that emotion regulation arises from repeated experiences of caregivers' sensitive coregulation of children's distress, and views this capacity as a major mediating mechanism explaining how early experience affects later functioning (Bowlby, 1973, 1980, 1988; Calkins & Leerkes, 2011; Cassidy, 1994; Hofer, 1994; Mikulincer, Shaver, & Pereg, 2003; Schore, 2000; Sroufe, 1996, 2000; Thompson, 1994; see Mikulincer & Shaver, Chapter 24, this volume). Considerable research has demonstrated that securely attached infants, children, and adolescents are better able to regulate emotional arousal (Contreras, Kerns, Weimer, Gentzler, & Tomich, 2000; Kerns, Abraham, Schlegelmilch, & Morgan, 2007; Kobak, Cole, Ferenz-Gillies, Fleming, & Gamble, 1993; Kopp, 1989; Leerkes & Wong, 2012; Nachmias, Gunnar, Mangelsdorf, Parritz, & Buss, 1996; Sroufe, 1983, 2005; see Thompson, Chapter 16, this volume). Thus, based on theory and empirical evidence, we join others who have proposed a model in which emotion regulation mediates the link between attachment security and care for others (e.g., Panfile & Laible, 2012).

With regard to cognition, a second pathway by which attachment may be linked to care for others is via the IWM. Through repeated experiences with a responsive caregiver, secure attachment provides children with a mental representation of the self as worthy of and effective in eliciting care, of others as available and responsive to distress, and of the world as a generally safe and caring place. One line of evidence for this part of the model comes from visual habituation studies of infants' responses to geometric representations of a caregiver and child: a large oval and a small oval (Johnson, Dweck, & Chen, 2007; Johnson et al., 2010). In these studies, securely attached infants looked longer at visual displays in which the "caregiver" oval was unresponsive to the "child" oval's distress upon separation, whereas insecure infants looked longer at displays in which the "caregiver" oval was responsive. In each case, infants attended longer to visual displays that were presumed to violate their expectations—that is, their mental representations—that distress would be met with responsive care (in the case of secure infants) or unresponsive care (in the case of insecure infants) (Johnson et al., 2007, 2010). These findings provide evidence for the existence of attachment-based expectations about how social actors respond to others' distress. Specifically, the secure child develops a representation of others as caring, attuned, and responsive (in addition to a representation of the self as likely to receive empathic care from others; Bowlby, 1973; Bretherton, Ridgeway,

& Cassidy, 1990). (For discussions of topics related to the concept of the IWM, see Lyons-Ruth et al., 1998, for the idea of *implicit relational knowing*, and Waters & Waters, 2006, for the idea of *secure-base scripts*.)

The precise mechanism by which the secure model of others as caring becomes integrated into a model of the self as caring for others remains unclear; however, Sroufe and Fleeson (1986) proposed that care leading to secure attachment shows children both sides of a responsive relationship, and that children can draw upon both representations when responding to the needs of others. Empirically, securely attached children tend to have more positive, reciprocal friendships in childhood (Elicker, Englund, & Sroufe, 1992; Shulman, Elicker, & Sroufe, 1994) and more secure IWMs of romantic relationships in adolescence (Furman & Wehner, 1997), suggesting that implicit knowledge of what it means both to give and to receive responsive care is conserved as children enter into close relationships with peers. It is also possible that children incorporate behavioral routines for care in the same way they model other kinds of behavior, such as eating with a spoon, brushing teeth, dancing, or throwing a ball.

### Parental Sensitivity

Beyond the roles of emotion regulation and a secure IWM as mediators of the link between attachment and care for others (see solid lines in Figure 38.1), there are other conceptual models that may further illuminate this link. One model

to consider is one in which security and care for others share common developmental antecedents (see dashed lines in Figure 38.1). A wealth of research demonstrates that caregivers' emotionally attuned, consistent responsiveness predicts attachment security in young children (Ainsworth, 1969; Ainsworth et al., 1978; Egeland & Farber, 1984; Isabella, 1993; van den Boom, 1994), and theories of empathic development posit that sensitive parental behavior also contributes to the development of children's care for others (Hoffman, 1977; for evidence, see Eisenberg, Fabes, & Murphy, 1996; Eisenberg et al., 1992, 1993; Garner, 2006; Hastings, Utendale, & Sullivan, 2007; Taylor, Eisenberg, Spinrad, Eggum, & Sulik, 2013).

In addition to being influenced by parental sensitivity, children's care for others appears to be guided by *rules* for responding to distress. According to recent empirical work, even young children (age 3 years) appear to decide which emotional displays are "appropriate" or "inappropriate" and show greater empathy and willingness to help an adult experimenter whose distress is perceived as appropriate to the harm that caused it (Hepach, Vaish, & Tomasello, 2013b). Thus, children assess the appropriateness of emotions and use this assessment to guide their empathy and prosocial responses. It is reasonable to suspect that children learn these decision rules for what constitutes "appropriate" distress through experiences of how their own distress was responded to, which is a key contributor to secure child attachment (e.g., Beckes & Coan, 2015; Leerkes, 2011).

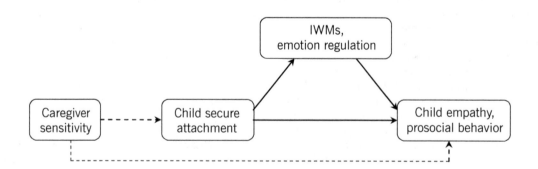

**FIGURE 38.1.** Model of the link between secure attachment and care for others (i.e., empathy and prosocial behavior) in childhood. Solid lines represent the principal model presented in this chapter, in which the link between secure attachment and care for others are mediated by (1) secure internal working models (IWMs) of self and other, and (2) emotion regulation. Dashed lines represent an additional model, in which caregiver sensitivity provides a common developmental antecedent for both security and care for others.

The perspective of attachment theory on the role of parenting in the development of concern for others differs from that of other conceptual models. Traditional theories of socialization, social learning, and conditioning tend to rest on a top-down, behaviorally oriented approach in which parents' instruction, modeling, reinforcement, and punishment shape children's desired social behavior and the internalization of parental values (Maccoby, 1992). In fact, historically, much of the research on parents' role in the development of concern for others has focused on socialization practices such as discipline and modeling of prosocial action (Hoffman, 1970). In support of these theories, considerable evidence indicates that adults' gentle discipline, inductive reasoning, emotion-focused dialogue, prosocial modeling, and authoritative, noncontrolling parenting style promote children's empathy and prosocial behavior (e.g., Grusec, 1972; Krevans & Gibbs, 1996; Perry, Bussey, & Frieberg, 1981; Rushton, 1975; also see Hastings, Utendale, & Sullivan, 2007). More recently, these models have included the child's role in socialization, with a focus on how children's temperament and view of their parents influence their receptivity to the socialization efforts (e.g., Grusec & Goodnow, 1994; Kochanska, 1997; Maccoby, 1992).

According to Ainsworth, Bell, and Stayton (1974), attachment theory offers a different view. Rather than requiring parents' active socialization efforts, children are thought to be inherently social, biologically predisposed to respond to the social signals of members of their species, and intrinsically motivated to comply with maternal requests, especially within the context of a sensitive, trusting relationship. For instance, Ainsworth and colleagues proposed that the greater compliance with maternal requests that is characteristic of securely attached infants reflects the mutual responsivity inherent to their IWMs of relationships. (In other words, secure children represent relationships as contexts within which recognition of and responsiveness to the needs of other people are the norm.) The central thesis of this argument is that "socialization results from reciprocal mother–infant responsiveness. When the mother is less sensitive and less responsive to her infant than is expected in the social environment of evolutionary adaptedness, the infant more than likely will be less responsive and hence less compliant to the signals of his mother and other social companions" (pp. 118–119). Extending this view to care for others, we can speculate that empathy and prosocial behavior need not be explicitly taught, but

instead develop naturally in the context of a mutually responsive relationship. Such a relationship provides the repeated firsthand, felt experience of having a secure base and safe haven in times of distress, which may then allow secure individuals to extend such care to distressed others. For recent similar viewpoints about a biologically based predisposition toward caring for others, see Bartal, Decety, and Mason (2011), de Waal (2008), and Warneken and Tomasello (2006).

To point out these distinctions between the attachment and socialization perspectives is not to discount the unique contributions of each to the development of care for others in children. Kochanska (2002) suggested that attachment and socialization work in concert in fostering children's conscience, with security representing a "mutually responsive orientation" that renders children more willing to accept and integrate parents' socialization influence. In support of this view, she observed that the effects of positive parenting on children's conscience held only for securely attached children (Kochanska, Aksan, Knaack, & Rhines, 2004). Similarly, Zahn-Waxler, Radke-Yarrow, and King (1979) posited that children must not only witness parents' prosocial modeling and be exposed to prosocial values but must also *experience parents' empathy and prosocial actions themselves* in order to develop these capacities. Thus, socialization may be important, but it does not provide a full picture of parents' role in the development of children's care for others; crucially, the lived experience of having a secure base and safe haven in times of distress provides the foundation for children's ability to regulate emotion and care for others, upon which socialization influences can build.

In summary, multiple theoretical pathways link attachment security to a child's capacity to care for others. Here we focus on how security may contribute to the development of empathy and prosocial behavior, particularly in response to others' distress.

### Definitions and Operationalization

In childhood, the definition and operationalization of care for others is particularly complex. As described earlier, *empathy* is the felt, emotional dimension of concern for others' welfare, whereas *prosocial behavior* is the active, behavioral manifestation of that emotion, which encompasses actions intended to benefit others. A critical distinction is that the former refers to an internal state, the latter to expressed behavior. Thus, a key issue for researchers is how to measure each construct with sensitivity and specificity in young children, before self-reports of internal experience are possible.

Relatedly, some prosocial behavior may be motivated by empathy, but not in every case (Hastings et al., 2007). For example, a child may share a toy with a sad peer out of compliance with a teacher's expectations, or out of deference to the peer's social dominance, rather than out of genuine concern for the peer's well-being (see Hepach, Vaish, & Tomasello, 2013a, for consideration of empirical methods for examining children's underlying motivations for prosocial behavior). Furthermore, children's internal experiences of empathy may not always manifest in prosocial behavior, particularly when the situation is complex or when prosocial intervention would be especially difficult. Therefore, one can neither measure children's prosocial behavior and infer that it reflects empathy, nor measure empathy and assume that prosocial behavior will follow.

Researchers mindful of this distinction have developed separate criteria to measure each dimension (e.g., Zahn-Waxler, Radke-Yarrow, et al., 1992): Empathy is reflected in young children's looks of concern ("concerned attention") or expressions of sadness in response to a sad peer, adult, or parent; prosocial behavior takes the form of helping, sharing, or comforting (among other behaviors), but may or may not be a response to others' distress (Dunfield & Kuhlmeier, 2013). Understanding the link between attachment and children's capacity to care for others requires specificity in measurement and attention to the unique contributions of both empathy and prosocial behavior. With this in mind, we review empirical work on the links between attachment and both empathy and prosocial behavior in childhood.

## Empirical Work

Several studies have examined attachment-related differences in care for others from infancy through adolescence. In this section, we divide these studies by developmental period (based on the age of the children when care for others was assessed), and further by the measurement of care (i.e., empathy, prosocial behavior, or a composite). For each developmental period, we begin with a brief summary of age-related changes in attachment relationships, care for others, or both. Then, after reviewing studies of the link between attachment

and care for others within each age group, we discuss evidence for the purported mediational role of child emotion regulation.

### Infancy and Toddlerhood

Children's initial attachment relationships develop during their first year of life (Bowlby, 1969/1982; see Marvin, Britner, & Russell, Chapter 13, this volume). Early precursors of empathy are evident during this time as well, such as affect mirroring and "empathic distress" (Hoffman, 2001), as are early indications of empathy (e.g., Roth-Hanania et al., 2011, who noted modest levels of affective and cognitive empathy as early as 8 months). Prosocial behaviors are rare in the first year of life (Roth-Hanania et al., 2011) but become increasingly common between ages 1 and 2 (Zahn-Waxler, Radke-Yarrow, et al., 1992). By their second birthday, almost all infants readily provide instrumental help (Warneken & Tomasello, 2006, reported that 92% of 18-month-old infants provided help in at least one simple situation), and some show concerned attention or provide comfort in response to the distress of peers, siblings, strangers, or their mother (Eisenberg, Fabes, & Spinrad, 2006). In addition, even young infants are able to make social evaluations of others based on their prosocial and antisocial behaviors. For example, 6- and 10-month-old infants show a preference for actors (represented by colored shapes) who helped compared to those who hindered another actor's attempt to attain a goal, an evaluation that may serve as the foundation for later moral action (Hamlin, Wynn, & Bloom, 2007).

Surprisingly, only a handful of studies have investigated attachment-related differences in empathy and/or prosocial behavior among infants and toddlers. In one study, 36-month-olds' attachment security (assessed with mothers' ratings using the Attachment Q-Set [AQS; Waters & Deane, 1985]) was linked to mother-rated empathy, yet was linked only indirectly to observed prosocial behavior through empathy (Panfile & Laible, 2012). In another study, mothers' reports of neither their 1-year-old infants' empathy nor prosocial behavior were associated with infant behavior in the Strange Situation (Carter, Little, Briggs-Gowan, & Kogan, 1999).

Two additional studies used composite measures containing elements of both empathy and prosocial behavior. One longitudinal study of 22- to 23-month-olds recorded empathic responses toward an experimenter who was simulating distress

(Bischof-Köhler, 2000). Toddlers who had been classified as securely attached in the Strange Situation as infants were more likely to show concern and provide help than those who had been classified as insecurely attached. Additional longitudinal evidence came from a study measuring infants' attachment and observed care for others at both 16 and 22 months, toward both the mother and an experimenter simulating distress. Only one of the eight potential associations (two behaviors, two care recipients, two time points) was significant: Infants' security in the Strange Situation at 22 months was positively related to their concurrent empathic concern for the experimenter (van der Mark, Van IJzendoorn, & Bakermans-Kranenburg, 2002). We also mention a third study that, although it lacks a measure of attachment security, seems relevant to the links considered here. Main and George (1985) observed children in a day care setting and reported that abused toddlers (who typically are insecurely attached; Cyr, Euser, Bakermans-Kranenburg, & Van IJzendoorn, 2010) never reacted to a peer's distress with concern, but instead often reacted with physical attacks, fear, or anger.

In contrast to the mixed evidence concerning infants' and toddlers' *behaviors* and *emotions*, studies of their *expectations* about the concern that will be shown in response to the distress of others reveal more consistent attachment-based differences. In a series of studies using a visual habituation paradigm (briefly described earlier), Johnson and colleagues (2007, 2010) demonstrated that securely attached infants expected others (i.e., a large oval) to help someone in distress (i.e., a small oval simulating distress), whereas insecure-avoidant and insecure-resistant infants expected others to withhold comfort. These studies suggest that infants' attachment patterns influence their representations of the ways in which people treat each other, including whether caring and comforting are typical responses to distress.

Earlier, we described a mediation model (Figure 38.1) in which attachment security supports the development of effective emotion regulation, which in turn underlies children's ability to show concern for others without becoming overly aroused with personal distress. The evidence for each of these pathways in infancy and toddlerhood (from attachment to emotion regulation, and from emotion regulation to empathy and prosocial behavior) supports the possibility that such a mediating pathway exists during this developmental period. As noted earlier, several investigators have

argued that the quality of infants' developing attachments contributes to individual differences in emotion regulation (e.g., Cassidy, 1994), and several studies provide empirical evidence (e.g., Hill-Soderlund et al., 2008; Kim, Stifter, Philbrook, & Teti, 2014; Sherman, Stupica, Dykas, Ramos-Marcuse, & Cassidy, 2013). Infants' greater regulatory skills, in turn, have been associated with prosocial behaviors and empathy (e.g., Carter et al., 1999), as well as the ability to maintain an optimal level of arousal in the face of others' distress (Geangu, Benga, Stahl, & Striano, 2011), a crucial part of empathic concern (Davidov, Zahn-Waxler, Roth-Hanania, & Knafo, 2013). A recent test of this mediation model revealed that toddlers' emotion regulation mediated the association between attachment security and empathy (all mother-reported variables), such that more secure toddlers were better able to regulate their emotions, which then predicted greater empathy (Panfile & Laible, 2012). Furthermore, greater empathy in this study predicted more prosocial behavior toward an experimenter seeking a pacifier to soothe the (recorded) cries of a nearby baby.

In summary, few studies have examined the link between attachment and caring for others during the infancy/toddler period. The mixed evidence that emerges from these studies suggests that other factors may relate to empathy and prosocial behavior more than attachment during this period. Such factors may include genetics (Zahn-Waxler, Robinson, & Emde, 1992, reported modest evidence for heritability of empathy and prosocial behavior at 14 and 20 months) and temperament (van der Mark et al., 2002, found that temperamental fearfulness in 16-month-old girls predicted less empathic concern for a distressed stranger at 22 months). The possibility that infants and toddlers are too young to experience complex social feelings such as empathy in the ways that become more evident by the preschool years may also influence the consistency of the link between attachment and caring for others during this period.

## Preschool

The preschool period ushers in developmental changes that affect both children's attachment relationships, such as the emergence of a goal-corrected partnership (see Marvin et al., Chapter 13, this volume), and factors underlying care for others, such as maturing emotion regulation and enhanced executive functioning (Eisenberg & Sulik, 2012; Rothbart, Sheese, Rueda, & Posner,

2011). Opportunities to care for peers in the classroom or for younger siblings in the home increase as preschoolers spend more time in the company of other children.

Evidence for attachment-related differences in care for others during this developmental period emerges from some studies and not from others. Two longitudinal studies of attachment found links with later empathy. In one of these, 1-year-old infants who were classified as secure in the Strange Situation were later rated by their mothers as more sympathetic to their peers' distress at age 3 compared to children who were insecure as infants (Waters, Wippman, & Sroufe, 1979). In the other study, secure attachment (mother-reported with the AQS) and care for others were measured at both 42 and 48 months. Although neither concurrent link was significant, attachment security at 42 months predicted concerned facial expressions during a baby-cry procedure at 48 months, even after researchers controlled for earlier empathy (Murphy & Laible, 2013). In contrast, in a third longitudinal study, attachment quality in the Strange Situation at age 2 did not predict children's reports of their affective responses to emotional photographs at age 5 (Iannotti, Cummings, Pierrehumbert, Milano, & Zahn-Waxler, 1992).

Studies of prosocial behavior are also somewhat mixed. For example, when children (ages 2–7) were left alone in an unfamiliar room with their younger (toddler) sibling, children rated as more secure by their mothers on the AQS were more likely to respond to the sibling's distress with comfort (Teti & Ablard, 1989); however, Volling (2001) found no differences in sibling comforting between 4-year-olds previously classified as secure or insecure in the Strange Situation (with both mother and father) at 12 months. Additionally, in two studies of preschool children, child attachment (mother-reported AQS) was related to concurrent mother-reported prosocial behavior directly (Laible, 2006) and, in a separate sample, indirectly via child effortful control (Laible, 2004).

When peers are the targets of children's prosocial behavior, evidence is similarly mixed, although the inconsistencies may be due to differences in the measurement of attachment. For example, security in the Strange Situation at age 2 predicted observed prosocial behavior toward a peer 3 years later (Iannotti et al., 1992). In contrast, security assessed with an observer-rated AQS did not relate to naturalistic observations of preschoolers' prosociality in the classroom (Mitchell-Copeland, Denham, & DeMulder, 1997), nor did

mother- and father-reported AQS relate to teacher-reported prosociality (Lafrenière, Provost, & Dubeau, 1992). There is also some evidence that secure children are more prosocial with peers than are avoidant, but not resistant, children, a finding that is only possible using a measure of attachment that differentiates the two insecure subtypes (e.g., the Strange Situation). Children who had been secure in the Strange Situation at 12 and 18 months were observed to be more prosocial and empathic in the classroom as preschoolers than those who had been avoidant, but not more than those who had been resistant (Kestenbaum, Farber, & Sroufe, 1989). In the same sample, Sroufe (1983) found that teacher reports of empathic responding were "characteristic" of children who had been secure infants and "uncharacteristic" of children who had been avoidant. The children who had been classified as resistant were between these other two groups.

Turning again to the model wherein the link between attachment and children's care for others is mediated by emotion regulation, we note that emotion regulation continues to develop throughout preschool and remains an important contributor to social interactions. Preschoolers vary widely in their ability to self-regulate, with individual differences in this ability relating to differences in empathy (e.g., Eisenberg & Fabes, 1995). Well-regulated preschoolers can focus on the distress of others in need and respond with empathy because they are better able to control their own emotional arousal (Eisenberg et al., 1990). A recent longitudinal study provides some additional evidence for preschoolers' emotion regulatory capacities predicting concern for others using physiological measures of respiratory sinus arrythmia (RSA), an indicator of heart rate variability thought to underlie individual differences in emotion regulation and arousal (Taylor, Eisenberg, & Spinrad, 2015). In this study, baseline RSA (for girls and boys) and RSA suppression (for boys only) at 42 months were positively correlated with concurrent mother-reported sympathy. Moreover, a marginally significant indirect path was evident from baseline RSA, at 42 months, to greater mother- and teacher-reported sympathy, at 72 and 84 months, through effortful control at 52 months.

In summary, the majority of studies support a link between secure attachment and care for others among preschoolers, although some inconsistent findings highlight the need for further research. It is worth noting that longitudinal studies provide more consistent evidence than concurrent studies when care for others is measured during the preschool period and attachment is measured during infancy/toddlerhood, particularly when peers are the targets of care. This pattern could be due to chance, methodological constraints (e.g., perhaps prosocial behavior and empathy are more easily measured in preschoolers), or developmental realities (e.g., early attachment may play a larger role than current attachment in preschoolers' care for others, particularly their peers in the classroom); future research could help tease apart these possibilities. We also note that some studies using the Strange Situation as the measure of attachment quality provide evidence for differential relations between the insecure subtypes, with secure children showing more care for others than avoidant, but not resistant, children.

### Early and Middle Childhood

By early and middle childhood, peers begin to play a greater role in children's social development, and demonstration of empathy and prosocial behavior toward peers contributes to friendship formation and popularity (Eisenberg et al., 2006). Developmental advances in theory of mind (i.e., understanding that other people have minds), emotion regulation, and cognitive flexibility allow for enhanced understanding of others' needs (e.g., Devine & Hughes, 2013; Murphy, Eisenberg, Fabes, Shepard, & Guthrie, 1999; Piekny & Maehler, 2013). The attachment behavioral system makes significant developmental advances as well: Its goal shifts from caregiver *proximity* to caregiver *accessibility*, as children are able to handle longer separations with the knowledge that attachment figures will be available if needed (see Kerns & Brumariu, Chapter 17, this volume).

Studies examining attachment-related differences in care for others during early and middle childhood generally assess only behavior (e.g., volunteering to help others, kindness to younger children), rather than empathic internal states. In fact, all but one study assessed care for others using parent or teacher reports of prosocial behavior. The single exception contained observations of 6-year-olds' unsolicited prosocial interactions with their younger siblings in the home and found no behavioral differences between children with secure and insecure attachment histories (assessed at 12 months with the Strange Situation; Volling & Belsky, 1992).

Among the studies using parent and teacher reports of prosocial behavior, the evidence favors

a positive link between security of attachment and prosocial behavior. Two longitudinal studies provide evidence that children who were securely attached earlier in life are more prosocial than children who had been avoidant, but not more than children who had been resistant. In one of these studies, 8- and 9-year-old children who had been secure in the Strange Situation at 15 months were rated as more prosocial (based on a composite of parent and teacher reports) than those who had been avoidant, but not those who had been resistant (Bohlin, Hagekull, & Rydell, 2000). A concurrent link between attachment and prosocial behavior was absent in this study, however, when childhood attachment was assessed with the Separation Anxiety Test (SAT; Slough & Greenberg, 1990; adapted from Klagsbrun & Bowlby, 1976), a measure that does not differentiate insecure subgroups. In the other study, 5-year-olds responding to a modified version of the Attachment Story Completion Task (ASCT; Bretherton & Ridgeway, 1990), with themes indicative of secure attachment representations to parents were rated as more prosocial by their teachers 1 year later than children who had responded with avoidant (but not resistant) themes (Rydell, Bohlin, & Thorell, 2005). An additional longitudinal study suggests that children with secure attachment histories are more prosocial than those with disorganized, but not avoidant or resistant, attachment histories (Seibert & Kerns, 2015). In this study, third- and fifth-grade children who had been classified disorganized at 36 months in the Strange Situation were rated as less prosocial by their mothers than children who had been secure; ratings of previously avoidant and resistant children did not differ from those of any other group. Teacher ratings in this study followed a similar trend, with secure children given the highest ratings and disorganized children given the lowest; however, although omnibus analyses revealed significant differences in prosocial behavior among the four classifications, post hoc tests to clarify the nature of these differences were not significant. In contrast to these three studies, a fourth longitudinal study reported no concurrent or longitudinal associations between attachment (measured at 6 years with observed separation and reunion behavior; Main & Cassidy, 1988, and at 8 years with a modified version of the ASCT) and teacher reports of prosocial behavior at 6 and 8 years (Bureau & Moss, 2010).

Two studies with concurrent measures of attachment and care for others offer mixed findings. First, in a sample of low-income, ethnically diverse families, 5-year-olds' attachment-related narra-tives in a story stem task were related to teacher reports—but not mother reports—of the children's prosocial behavior controlling for verbal IQ and sociodemographic risk (Futh, O'Connor, Matias, Green, & Scott, 2008). Second, late elementary school children's perceived attachments to both mother and father (assessed with the self-report Security Scale; Kerns, Klepac, & Cole, 1996) were associated with prosocial behavior (a composite of mother, father, and teacher reports), but only in an overall model that also included "positive parental affection," and only for girls (Michiels, Grietens, Onghena, & Kuppens, 2010). When child-report-ed attachment was tested as a unique predictor, the association disappeared.

In considering which factors may explain these attachment-based differences in care for oth-ers, we once again turn to the example of the emo-tion regulation mediation model (Figure 1). The evidence supporting this model in early and mid-dle childhood comes from several studies showing that children's ability to regulate emotional arous-al predicts greater empathy and prosocial behavior, whereas their dysregulated emotions in response to others' distress (i.e., personal distress) relate nega-tively to their concern for others (e.g., Eisenberg, Fabes, et al., 1996; Eisenberg et al., 1995, 1998; Fabes, Eisenberg, Karbon, Troyer, & Switzer, 1994; Rothbart, Ahadi, & Hershey, 1994). Additionally, a few studies can be viewed as providing evidence relevant to the full mediational model because they indicate that sensitive parenting (which is consistently linked to attachment security) pre-dicts emotion regulation during early and middle childhood, which in turn predicts child prosocial behavior during this developmental period (see, e.g., Chan, 2011; Davidov & Grusec, 2006).

In conclusion, studies of attachment and care for others in early and middle childhood, as is the case in other developmental periods, are few. In fact, studies of attachment-related differences in empathy during early and middle childhood do not, to our knowledge, exist. The research on prosocial behavior, however, supports a modest as-sociation. As with the preschool period, some evi-dence points to diminished care for others among insecure-avoidant but not insecure-resistant chil-dren. We also note another pattern similar to that evident in the preschool period: Longitudinal as-sociations between early-life attachment security and care for others in early and middle childhood are more likely to be present than links between attachment and prosocial behavior when mea-

sured concurrently. Once again, more research is needed, particularly studies using more diverse measures of children's care for others, beyond par-ent or teacher reports of behavior.

## Adolescence

As children enter adolescence, close, intimate friendships and romantic relationships begin to form, opening the possibility of attachment to peers, as well as the potential for practicing the provision of care within these new relational con-texts. Significant advances in cognitive and brain development (Paus, 2009; Piaget, 1972), provide adolescents with a more complex understanding of others' emotions and needs, and sophisticated meta-awareness allows adolescents to report more accurately on their own empathy and prosocial behavior. Moreover, adolescents' representations of specific previous and current attachment re-lationships are gradually joined to form a more global, integrated attachment organization (see Allen & Tan, Chapter 19, this volume). Adoles-cent attachment is typically examined through self-report measures of attachment to parents (e.g., the Inventory of Parent and Peer Attach-ment [IPPA]; Armsden & Greenberg, 1987), self-report measures of attachment style more broadly (e.g., the ECR (Brennan et al., 1998), or an in-terview-based measure of "state of mind with re-spect to attachment" (the AAI; George, Kaplan, & Main, 1985).

Given the similar methods used for assess-ing attachment and care for others in adults and adolescents, and the multitude of studies on at-tachment-based differences in care for others in adulthood (reviewed in the next section), it is sur-prising that few studies have examined this link during adolescence. The existing studies, however, consistently find that secure adolescents are more empathic and prosocial than insecure adoles-cents, which provides a point of continuity with the adult literature. Using the IPPA (Armsden & Greenberg, 1987) and the Interpersonal Reactiv-ity Index (IRI; Davis, 1980), Laible, Carlo, and Raffaelli (2000) found that 16-year-olds reporting higher secure attachment to peers (but not to par-ents) also reported being more empathic, and a combination of high attachment security scores in relation to both peers and parents predicted the highest levels of empathy (although see Andretta et al., 2015, for evidence with African American adolescents involved in the juvenile criminal jus-tice system indicating that, using the same measures, secure adolescents were not more empathic than their insecure peers; they were, however, substantially more prosocial on the self-reported Adolescent Prosocial Behavior Scale [APBS; Andretta, Woodland, & Worrell, 2014]). In a similar study, Thompson and Gullone (2008) found that 12- to 18-year-old adolescents reporting higher scores on a measure of secure attachment to parents (the parent scale of the revised IPPA; Gullone & Robinson, 2005) also reported being more empathic (using the Index of Empathy for Children and Adolescents; Bryant, 1982) and prosocial (using the Strengths and Difficulties Questionnaire; SDQ; Goodman, 2001). In that study (Thompson & Gullone, 2008), empathy partially mediated the link between attachment and prosocial behavior. In a study with 11- to 16-year-old British students using the same measures of attachment (revised IPPA) and prosocial behavior (SDQ), higher attachment security scores were associated with more prosocial behavior (Oldfield, Humphrey, & Hebron, 2015; see also Chan et al., 2013, for similar results in an ethnically and racially diverse sample using a different self-report measure of prosocial behavior). Another study using the IPPA found evidence for a model wherein attachment to mother and/or peers affects bullying behavior in seventh, eighth, and ninth graders indirectly via their self-reported empathy on the Basic Empathy Scale (BES; Jolliffe & Farrington, 2006). For boys, *cognitive* empathy mediated the indirect effects of attachment to both mother and peers on bullying behavior, whereas for girls, *affective* empathy mediated the effect of attachment to peers on bullying (You, Lee, Lee, & Kim, 2015). Consistent with these studies using the IPPA, studies with other measures of attachment demonstrate positive links as well. One such study found that the level of self-reported secure attachment to the mother and to a friend (using the Relationship Questionnaire; Bartholomew & Horowitz, 1991), but not to father, related to self-reported prosocial behavior among youth in middle and early high school (Markiewicz, Doyle, & Brendgen, 2001; see also Keskin & Çam, 2010, for similar evidence among Turkish youth).

Notably, the two studies from this developmental period with measures of attachment that differentiate the insecure subtypes—the observer-rated Attachment Behavior Classification Procedure (ABCP; Cobb, 1996; Hilburn-Cobb, 1998) and the interview-based AAI—found that only dismissing, and not preoccupied, adolescents reported lower empathy/prosocial behavior, mirroring some of the findings from studies of preschoolers and grade school children demonstrating lower empathy/prosocial behavior among avoidant, but not resistant, children. In one of these studies, using the ABCP, both secure and preoccupied adolescents (ages 11–18) reported greater empathy on the IRI than avoidant adolescents (Hilburn-Cobb, 2004). In the other study, using the AAI, 11th-grade students with a secure/autonomous state of mind were more likely than students with an insecure/dismissing state of mind to be nominated by their peers as being prosocial (Dykas, Ziv, & Cassidy, 2008).

We again consider the emotion regulation mediation model described in relation to previous developmental periods. Adolescence is an important period for the development of brain regions involved in emotion regulation and executive functioning, such as the prefrontal cortex and anterior cingulate cortex; it is not until late adolescence that these regions reach full maturity (Decety & Meyer, 2008). In support of our mediation model, evidence suggests that teens who are more effective at regulating their emotions are also more prosocial (Cui et al., 2015; Kanacri, Pastorelli, Eisenberg, Zuffianò, & Caprara, 2013) and empathic (MacDermott, Gullone, Allen, King, & Tonge, 2010), whereas teens who struggle with self-regulation, such as those with conduct disorder, are less empathic than their peers (Cohen & Strayer, 1996). Moreover, considerable research indicates that secure adolescents are more effective at regulating their emotions than insecure adolescents, and use more adaptive forms of emotion regulation (e.g., Cooper, Shaver, & Collins, 1998; Kobak & Sceery, 1988; Zimmermann, Maier, Winter, & Grossmann, 2001).

In summary, the evidence suggests that securely attached adolescents are more empathic and prosocial than their insecurely attached counterparts, mirroring evidence from the adult literature (reviewed in the next section). More studies of this developmental period are needed, especially ones using non-self-report measures, to provide a more fully developed understanding of the role of secure attachment in adolescents' care for others.

## Empirical Studies of Children and Adolescents: Discussion

Research to date provides moderate evidence for a link between attachment security and care for others in childhood. The majority of the empirical work has focused on preschool-age children, utilizing both adult report and observational measures in naturalistic and laboratory settings, with the weight of the evidence in favor of the hypothesized link. In early and middle childhood, studies have employed a wider variety of methods for assessing attachment and care for others and have yielded less conclusive findings. By the time children enter adolescence, however, the use of self-report measures provides a more direct, standardized methodology for tapping children's empathic and prosocial capacities. Accordingly, although studies with adolescents are few, they provide the most consistent support for an association between attachment security and concern for others before adulthood, and these studies offer a point of continuity with findings from the adult literature (Mikulincer & Shaver, 2005).

The inconsistent findings in the research on children merit exploration. Methodological differences across studies, sometimes as a result of child age, may account for some of the inconsistencies. Before the use of self-report measures becomes possible in adolescence, questionnaire measures of care for others alternately tap parents' and teachers' perceptions of children's apparent concern for peer distress, tendency to share with others spontaneously, helpfulness toward adults, or a combination of these. These reports are likely shaped in part by normative levels of care for others in the child's culture or social group, as well as reporter biases, such as teachers' esteem for more compliant children or parents' social desirability tendencies and the degree to which the parents hold prosocial values themselves. When observational measures are used, children's care for others may be influenced by contextual factors such as a child's relationship to the person in distress (e.g., sibling, peer, mother, teacher, experimenter), the presence of other individuals, the salience of emotional cues, and the setting in which observation occurs (e.g., classroom, playground, home, laboratory), which also may influence the degree of *felt* security the child experiences in the moment he or she witnesses others' distress. Both the variety of measures employed and the multiplicity of factors influencing children's emotions and behavior at any one moment are likely to give rise to variability in the data.

Beyond the diversity of measures used, a more fundamental distinction can be made between measures of care for others in the presence–absence of an emotional display (i.e., whether children are responding to distress or to a non-

emotional need, such as a bid for instrumental help). This is an important distinction to make when considering the role played by secure attachment in emotional development. Specifically, security fosters the development of cognitive and regulatory skills that support children's ability to respond to others' distress, such as emotion regulation and emotion understanding (e.g., Panfile & Laible, 2012), which may not play as large a role in children's prosocial response to nondistressed others. Whereas measures of empathy almost always exclusively involve response to emotion, several of the studies of prosocial behavior reviewed here, particularly studies using mother- and teacher-reports, simultaneously assessed children's ability to comfort or demonstrate compassion in response to distress, along with children's responses to instrumental or material needs (e.g., "helps clean up," "shares toys") in the absence of emotional stimuli. Given recent evidence that prosocial behavior is a multifaceted construct, and that comforting, sharing, and instrumental helping behaviors show unique developmental trajectories (Dunfield & Kuhlmeier, 2013), unique neural and parenting correlates (Brownell, Svetlova, Anderson, Nichols, & Drummond, 2013; Paulus, Kühn-Popp, Licata, Sodian, & Meinhardt, 2013), and few intercorrelations among types of prosocial behavior (e.g., Richman, Berry, Bittle, & Himan, 1988), these disparate forms of behavior may have differential relations with attachment. Perhaps, for example, comforting, which typically occurs within an emotional context, relates to secure attachment, whereas other forms of prosocial behavior do not.

An additional explanation for the inconsistent findings in studies of children concerns the possible nonlinear relation between attachment and care for others. Investigators of this topic have observed that children with secure attachment histories score neither extremely high nor extremely low on measures of care for others, and propose that middle scores may be optimal for young children (van der Mark et al., 2002). This may help to account for findings from some studies that the highest frequencies of empathic behavior were from children of severely depressed mothers or from single mothers who depended on their children as a source of comfort (Radke-Yarrow & Zahn-Waxler, 1984; Rehberg & Richman, 1989; Richman et al., 1988). Indeed, young children of depressed mothers are more likely to develop disorganized attachments, characterized by caregiving toward the mother and parent–child role reversal (Teti, Gelfand, Messinger, & Isabella, 1995; Van IJzendoorn, Schuengel, & Bakermans-Kranenburg, 1999). Relatedly, Eisenberg and colleagues (1995) have argued that maintenance of a moderate, but nonaversive, level of emotional arousal is important for feeling sympathy in the absence of debilitating personal distress; it may be that attachment security helps maintain an optimal level of arousal, such that secure children neither avoid responding to others' distress nor engage in "compulsive caregiving" out of personal distress. Consideration of "compulsive caregiving" may also help to explain why insecure-resistant children sometimes do not show reduced prosocial behavior; for these children, providing care for others may serve as an adaptive strategy for maintaining closeness with others, even if the care is motivated by personal distress rather than genuine, attuned concern for others' welfare (for discussion of compulsive care and adult anxious attachment, see Bowlby, 1980; Feeney & Collins, 2001; Kunce & Shaver, 1994).

Another possibility is that the inconsistent findings are in part due to moderating factors such as parent socialization. As previously mentioned, although attachment and socialization are constructs from distinct theoretical frameworks and have unique pathways to care for others in childhood, there is some evidence that attachment and socialization interact to predict moral development (Kochanska et al., 2004). Security may provide a foundation upon which socialization can build a stronger ethic of care across development. When measured within the same study, the unique effects of attachment and socialization practices (e.g., elaborative discourse, response to distress, gentle discipline) may reveal a more complete and nuanced picture of the roots of care for others in childhood.

Finally, we cannot rule out the possibility that attachment does not, in fact, play a role in children's care for others, and that the links observed thus far are explained by other factors, such as parent socialization, genetics, child temperament, cultural or contextual influences, or interactions with teachers and peers. It may be that parents who use sensitive, warm discipline and reinforce prosocial behavior also use sensitive parenting more broadly, contributing to children's care for others and to secure attachment via independent pathways. Alternatively, there is some evidence that more empathic parents tend to have securely attached children (Oppenheim, Koren-Karie, & Sagi, 2001; Stern, Borelli, & Smiley, 2015), so it

may be that secure children learn to empathize simply by observing empathic adult models, or that empathy is transmitted from parent to child via genetic mechanisms (Knafo, Zahn-Waxler, Van Hulle, Robinson, & Rhee, 2008). It is also possible that children with high negative emotionality (i.e., a fearful temperament) elicit insensitive parental behavior and are more prone to personal distress, limiting their capacity to care for others. These and other pathways merit exploration as we consider new directions for research on the development of children's concern for others.

## Caring for Others in Adulthood

Adult attachment researchers in the fields of personality and social psychology have tended to consider prosocial motives, emotions, and behaviors as related to the caregiving behavioral system proposed by Bowlby (1969/1982) in his effort to explain why parents (and also older children, as well as adults other than the parents) respond to an infant's, and indeed to any person's, needs for help, protection, or support (e.g., Mikulincer, Shaver, & Gillath, 2008; Shaver, Mikulincer, & Shemesh-Iron, 2010). Although this reliance on the caregiving system construct is not essential for studying links between attachment orientations and prosocial emotions and behavior (and was not emphasized in the previous section of this chapter), it has proved to be a useful way to conceptualize adults' responses to people in need. That is, caregiving is not only a primary ingredient of parental behavior but also a major part of romantic and marital relationships, and a key to all forms of prosocial behavior in adulthood.

An adult's caregiving behavior is related to his or her attachment orientation because the parameters of the attachment and caregiving systems are shaped by some of the same forces (most notably, parenting), and because attachment insecurity involves a degree of self-focus and self-protection that interferes with attention to others' needs (just as attachment insecurity interferes with curiosity and exploration in infancy, according to Ainsworth et al., 1978). The two major kinds of attachment insecurity, anxiety and avoidance, are therefore expected to have somewhat different implications for providing care and support to a person in need. Anxiety is associated with feelings of vulnerability and a focus on one's own negative feelings (in particular, what empathy researcher

Daniel Batson [1991, 2010] called "personal distress," as distinct from empathy). Avoidance is associated with not feeling comfortable getting close to other people and attempting to avoid situations that interfere with personal independence (Mikulincer et al., 2008).

Theoretically, the goal of the caregiving system is to reduce other people's suffering, to protect them from harm, and to foster their growth and development—in other words, to provide a safe haven and secure base for them (Collins, Ford, Guichard, Kane, & Feeney, 2010; B. C. Feeney & Woodhouse, Chapter 36, this volume; Mikulincer et al., 2008). According to Collins and colleagues (2010), the caregiving system is activated in two kinds of situations: (1) when another person has to cope with danger, stress, or discomfort and is either openly seeking help or would clearly benefit from it, and (2) when another person has an opportunity for exploration, learning, or mastery and either needs help in taking advantage of the opportunity or seems eager to talk about it or to be validated for having aspirations or achieving desired goals. In either case, once a person's caregiving system is activated (whether appropriately or not), he or she calls on a repertoire of behaviors aimed at restoring or advancing another person's welfare. This repertoire includes showing interest in the other person's problems or goals; providing an open, accepting space in which the other person's needs are heard; affirming the other's competence and ability to cope with the situation; expressing love and affection; providing advice and instrumental aid as needed, without interfering with the person's own problem-solving efforts or exploratory activities; and admiring and applauding the person's successes.

Optimal functioning of the caregiving system requires psychological assets associated with attachment security, as explained throughout the earlier sections of this chapter—assets such as emotion regulation strategies that allow caregivers to deal effectively with the discomfort entailed by witnessing another person's distress. Deficient emotion regulation can cause a caregiver to feel overwhelmed by personal distress, to slip into the role of another needy person rather than occupying the role of caregiver, or to maintain distance from the needy other as a way of reducing his or her own negative emotions. Optimal caregiving also requires effective self-regulation strategies beyond emotion regulation. Addressing another person's problems often requires temporary suspension of one's own goals and plans. Moreover,

one has to diagnose the other person's problem, develop a plan for assisting the person sensitively and effectively, and suppress motives that interfere with effective helping. According to Collins, Guichard, Ford, and Feeney (2006), caregiving can be disrupted by social skills deficits, depletion of psychological resources, lack of a desire to help, and egoistic motives that interfere with empathic sensitivity.

### Attachment Orientations and Patterns of Care

Bowlby (1969/1982) noticed that activation of the attachment system can interfere with the operation of the caregiving system because potential caregivers may feel that obtaining safety and care for themselves is more urgent than providing a safe haven or secure base for others. At such times, adults are likely to be so focused on their own vulnerability that they lack the mental resources necessary to attend sensitively to others' needs. Only when a sense of security is restored can a potential caregiver perceive others as not only potential sources of security and support but also as worthy human beings who themselves need and deserve sympathy and support.

Reasoning along these lines, adult attachment researchers (e.g., Collins et al., 2010; Mikulincer et al., 2008) hypothesized that attachment security is an important foundation for optimal caregiving. Moreover, being *secure* implies (given the theory and the research reviewed in earlier sections of this chapter) that a secure person has witnessed, experienced, and benefited from his or her attachment figures' effective care (with those figures being either parents or other important care providers), which provides a model to follow when the person comes to occupy the caregiving role. Because secure individuals are more comfortable with intimacy and interdependence (Hazan & Shaver, 1987), they can allow other people to approach them for help and express feelings of vulnerability and need (Lehman, Ellard, & Wortman, 1986). Secure individuals' confidence about other people's goodwill makes it easier for them to construe others as deserving sympathy and support, and their positive model of self allows them to feel more confident about their ability to handle another person's needs while effectively regulating their own emotions and helping behavior.

Adults who are insecure with respect to attachment (i.e., are either anxious or avoidant, or both) are likely to find it difficult to provide effective care. Although those who suffer from attachment anxiety may have some of the qualities necessary for effective caregiving (e.g., willingness to experience and express emotions, and comfort with psychological intimacy and physical closeness), their deficits in self-regulation make them vulnerable to personal distress, which interferes with sensitive and responsive care. Their tendency to become sidetracked by self-focused worries, misplaced projections, and blurred interpersonal boundaries can interfere with focusing accurately on other people's pain and suffering. Moreover, attachment-anxious adults' lack of confidence can make it difficult for them to adopt the role of "stronger and wiser" pillar of support. In addition, their strong desire for closeness and approval may cause them to become intrusive or overinvolved, blurring the distinction between another person's welfare and their own.

Attachment-anxious individuals may use caregiving as a means of satisfying their own unmet needs for closeness, acceptance, and inclusion. According to Collins and colleagues (2010), these self-centered motives result in intrusive caregiving that is insensitive to a needy person's signals. Anxious people may try to get too close or too involved when an interaction partner does not want help, and this can generate resentment, anger, and conflict, which in turn leave the anxious person feeling unappreciated or falsely accused.

Avoidant adults' lack of comfort with closeness and negative working models of others may also interfere with optimal caregiving. Their discomfort with expressions of need and dependence may cause them to back away rather than get involved with someone whose needs are strongly expressed. As a result, avoidant individuals may attempt to detach themselves emotionally and physically from needy others, may feel superior to those who are vulnerable or distressed, or may experience disdainful pity rather than empathic concern (Mikulincer et al., 2008). In some cases, avoidant people's cynical or hostile attitudes and negative models of others may replace sympathy or compassion with *schadenfreude*, or gloating.

## Providing Care in Parent–Child and Romantic Relationships

B. C. Feeney and Woodhouse (Chapter 36, this volume) reviewed studies of caregiving in parent–child relationships, demonstrating that parents' attachment orientations systematically affect their caregiving-related mental representations and be-

haviors (see also Jones, Cassidy, & Shaver, 2015a, 2015b). Secure parents find it easier to perceive their children's needs accurately and to respond sensitively and appropriately. Anxious parents tend to be anxious themselves, and their self-preoccupation and biased perceptions can cause them to miss or misread their children's needs and calls for help. Avoidant parents tend not to be comfortable with children's expressions of need, and they act in ways that lead their children to become more emotionally inhibited and self-reliant. Viewed in terms of empathy or kindness, these insecure parents' attitudes and behaviors are problematic.

In the romantic and marital domains, research and common sense both indicate that a person's ability and willingness to respond sensitively to a relationship partner's needs are major determinants of relationship quality (e.g., Collins & Feeney, 2000). Adult romantic love involves not only the attachment system, which helps maintain proximity to a relationship partner, but also the caregiving system, which motivates one partner to attend and respond to the other's needs (Shaver & Hazan, 1988). As a result, romantic and marital relationships provide good opportunities to discover how attachment patterns shape caregiving orientations. Many of the relevant studies are reviewed by B. C. Feeney and Woodhouse (Chapter 36, this volume); others are discussed in detail by Mikulincer and Shaver (2007a). These studies indicate that attachment insecurity interferes with compassion, empathy, and loving-kindness in couple relationships. A few examples are provided here.

For example, attachment security is associated with care provision by adult spouses of cancer victims—people who are clearly in need. Kim and Carver (2007) found that greater attachment security (assessed with self-report scales) was associated with more frequent provision of emotional support to a spouse with cancer. Attachment security was also associated with favorable motives for providing care, such as accepting the need for caregiving, feeling loving, and respecting the care recipient (Kim, Carver, Deci, & Kasser, 2008). As expected, attachment anxiety was associated with more self-focused motives for caregiving (e.g., providing care in order to be appraised as a good person). In another study, Braun and colleagues (2012) found that avoidant attachment was associated with less responsive and less sensitive care for a spouse with cancer, whereas anxious attachment was associated with more compulsive caregiving (insisting on care, being intrusive, failing to be sensitive to the spouse's actual needs). This harks back to an early study by Kunce and Shaver (1994) in which anxious adults and their mates both agreed that the anxious adults' caregiving efforts tended to be unempathic, self-focused, and intrusive.

In two laboratory experiments, B. Feeney and Collins (2001) and Collins and colleagues (2010) provided a detailed analysis of avoidant and anxious adults' caregiving deficits. Dating couples were brought to a laboratory, and one member of the couple (the "care seeker") was informed that he or she would perform a stressful task—preparing and delivering a videotaped speech. The other couple member (the "caregiver") was led to believe that his or her partner was either extremely nervous (high-need condition) or not at all nervous (low-need condition) about the speech task, and was given the opportunity to write a private note to the partner. In both studies, the note was coded in terms of the degree of support it conveyed. In addition, the caregiver's attentiveness to the partner's needs was assessed by counting the number of times the caregiver checked a computer monitor for messages from the partner while the caregiver was working on a series of puzzles (in a separate room). To assess the caregiver's state of mind, Collins and colleagues added measures of empathic feelings toward the partner, rumination about the partner's feelings, willingness to switch tasks with the partner, partner-focused attention, and causal attributions regarding the partner's feelings. More avoidant participants wrote less emotionally supportive notes in both high- and low-need conditions, and provided less instrumental support in the high- than in the low-need condition, when the partner most needed support. Moreover, avoidant participants reported less empathy for their partner, were less willing to switch tasks with the partner, and were less distracted by thoughts about the partner while doing puzzles. More anxious participants were easily distracted by thoughts about their partner and reported relatively high levels of empathy and rumination, but failed to write more supportive notes as their partner's needs increased.

Because most such studies of attachment and caregiving in parent–child and adult couple relationships have been correlational rather than experimental, making it impossible to determine causality, Mikulincer, Shaver, Sahdra, and Bar-On (2013) conducted a study, in both the United States and Israel, to see whether *experimentally augmented security* ("security priming"; in this case, subliminal presentation of attachment figures' names) would improve care provision to a roman-

tic partner who was asked to discuss a personal problem. A second goal of the study was to see whether security priming could overcome barriers to responsive caregiving caused by mental depletion or fatigue. Couples came to a laboratory and were informed that they would be video-recorded during an interaction in which one of them (the care seeker) disclosed a personal problem to the other (the caregiver). Caregivers were taken to another room, where they performed a task that induced (or did not induce) mental fatigue, while also being subliminally exposed to either the names of security providers or the names of unfamiliar people. Following these manipulations, couple members were videotaped while talking about the care seeker's problem, and the recording was later coded to assess the caregiver's supportive or unsupportive behavior. As predicted, attachment security (security priming) was associated with greater sensitivity and responsiveness to the disclosing partner, and the priming overcame the detrimental effects of mental depletion on sensitive responsiveness.

## Providing Care and Expressing Social Virtues in the Wider Social World

### Empathy, Compassion, and Altruism

The discovery of connections between attachment orientation and caregiving in both the parent–child and romantic/marital domains led researchers to explore the possibility that attachment insecurity interferes with compassion toward suffering others, even if the sufferers do not belong to the caregiver's family. If all forms of lovingkindness draw from the same caregiving well, then contamination of that well by attachment-related worries and defenses is likely.

In fact, studies of adult attachment and prosocial attitudes and behavior do show that avoidant people score lower on diverse measures of prosocial reactions to other people's needs. For example, more avoidant adults report less empathic concern (e.g., B. Feeney & Collins, 2001; Joireman, Needham, & Cummings, 2002; Lopez, 2001; Wayment, 2006), less inclination to take the perspective of a distressed person (Corcoran, & Mallinckrodt, 2000; Joireman et al., 2002), less ability to share another person's feelings (Trusty, Ng, & Watts, 2005), less sense of communion with others, and less willingness to take responsibility for others' welfare (Collins & Read, 1990; Shaver et al., 1996; Zuroff, Moskowitz, & Cote, 1999). Avoidant adults are also less likely to be cooperative and other-oriented (DeDreu, 2012; Hawley, Shorey, & Alderman, 2009; Van Lange, DeBruin, Otten, & Joireman, 1997), to write comforting messages to a distressed person (Weger & Polcar, 2002), to offer help to needy others in hypothetical scenarios (Bailey, McWilliams, & Dick, 2012; Drach-Zahavy, 2004), or to be sensitive to moral transgressions that can damage other people (Albert & Horowitz, 2009). Sommerfeld (2009) also found that more avoidant people (assessed with the ECR) were more likely to feel a sense of burden when acting generously.

With regard to attachment anxiety, research once again suggests a pattern of overinvolvement and intrusiveness during encounters with people in distress. In particular, although Lopez (2001) found a positive association between attachment anxiety and a measure of emotional empathy, people who score relatively high on measures of attachment anxiety also report higher levels of personal distress while witnessing others' suffering (Britton & Fuendeling, 2005; Joireman et al., 2002; Monin, Schulz, Feeney, & Clark, 2010; Vilchinsky, Findler, & Werner, 2010). Moreover, anxious adults score higher on a measure of unmitigated communion, which taps a compulsive need to help others even when they are not asking for assistance, and even when the help comes at the expense of one's own health and legitimate needs (Fritz & Helgeson, 1998; Shaver et al., 1996).

In an observational laboratory study, Westmaas and Silver (2001) videotaped people while they interacted with a confederate of the experimenter who, they thought, had recently been diagnosed with cancer. The authors found that both kinds of attachment insecurity created specific impediments to effective caregiving. As expected, avoidant participants were rated by observers as less verbally and nonverbally supportive and as making less eye contact during the interaction. Attachment anxiety was not associated with supportiveness, but more anxious participants reported greater discomfort while interacting with the confederate and were more likely to report self-critical thoughts after the interaction. These are signs of emotional overinvolvement and self-related worries, which can sometimes interfere with caregiving.

It is worth mentioning, however, that Ein-Dor and Orgad (2012) found that attachment-anxious people acted prosocially when a real danger threatened them and their group. In their study, participants were led to believe that they accidentally activated a computer virus that erased an experimenter's computer. They were then asked to alert the department's computer technicians to the incident. On their way, they were presented with four decision points at which they could choose either to delay their warning or continue directly to the technicians' office. More anxious individuals (assessed with the ECR) were less willing to be delayed on their way to deliver a warning message. This finding fits with the "sentinel" mental script characteristic of attachment-anxious individuals (Ein-Dor, Mikulincer, & Shaver, 2011), which might automatically cause them to act prosocially in a dangerous situation by rapidly communicating the threat to others. Kogut and Kogut (2013) also found that attachment-anxious people tend to help others when they can identify with the help receiver or feel similar to or specially connected with him or her, probably thereby satisfying unmet needs for merger and love.

There is also evidence that the link between avoidant attachment and unhelpfulness can be mitigated in specific relational contexts. For example, Richman, DeWall, and Wolff (2015) found that when highly avoidant participants were convinced that helping would not increase closeness to the receiver of help or would not change their own emotions, they tended to help others as much as less avoidant participants; that is, by reducing the psychological linkage between helping and emotional closeness, Richman and colleagues reduced avoidant people's fears of becoming more intimate with the needy other, allowing them to act more prosocially toward him or her. This finding fits with our belief that avoidant people's reluctance to help others is in part due to attachment system deactivation and a preference for emotional distance rather than intimacy.

In an influential study of adolescents that spurred similar research with adults, McKinney (2002) found that those who were insecurely attached to their parents were less involved than more securely attached adolescents in voluntary altruistic activities, such as caring for older adults or donating blood. Gillath, Shaver, Mikulincer, Nitzburg, and colleagues (2005) extended this line of research by assessing young adults' motives for volunteering in their communities. Avoidant attachment was associated with engaging in fewer volunteer activities; among those who did volunteer, avoidance was associated with being involved for less altruistic reasons. Attachment anxiety was not directly related to engaging in volunteer activities per se, but it was associated with more egoistic reasons for volunteering (e.g., hoping to be socially accepted and receive approval), another indication of anxious people's self-focus. These findings were replicated in a subsequent study with Dutch students (Erez, Mikulincer, Van IJzendoorn, & Kroonenberg, 2008). In all of these studies, more avoidant adults were less likely to volunteer.

Insecure people's relative lack of a prosocial orientation is also manifested in career choice. Using the AAI to measure adult attachment, Horppu and Ikonen-Varila (2004) found that insecure students at a college for kindergarten teachers endorsed less altruistic, less prosocial motives for becoming teachers, compared with more secure students. Similarly, Roney, Meredith, and Strong (2004) found that less secure occupational therapy students (identified with self-report scales) were less likely to say they chose a therapeutic career because they wanted to help people. In a sample of medical students, Ciechanowski, Russo, Katon, and Walker (2004) found that less secure students (based on self-report scales) were more likely not to choose primary care specialties because primary care demands intense patient–physician relationships that can cause patients to become emotionally attached to their physician.

Recently, a number of investigators have examined the effects of security priming on feelings and attitudes toward needy people. For example, Bartz and Lydon (2004) primed attachment-related mental representations by asking people to think about a close relationship in which they felt either secure, anxious, or avoidant, then assessed the implicit and explicit activation of communion-related thoughts (thoughts about devoting oneself to others and maintaining supportive and warm interactions with them). Implicit activation was assessed in a word fragment completion task (which identified the number of word fragments completed with a communion-related word); explicit activation was assessed with the Communion scale of the Extended Personality Attributes Questionnaire. Contextual priming of representations of avoidant attachment led to lower levels of implicit and explicit communion-related thoughts than did contextual priming of secure attachment.

Along the same lines, Mikulincer and colleagues (2001, Study 1) performed an experiment assessing compassionate responses to others' suffering. Dispositional attachment anxiety and avoidance were assessed with the ECR scales, and a sense of attachment security was activated in one condition by having participants read a story about

support provided by a loving attachment figure. This condition was compared with the activation of neutral or positive affect. Following the priming procedure, all participants read a brief story about a student whose parents had been killed in an automobile accident and rated how much they experienced compassion and personal distress when thinking about the distressed student. As expected, dispositional attachment anxiety and avoidance were inversely related to compassion, and attachment anxiety (but not avoidance) was positively associated with personal distress. In addition, enhancement of attachment security, but not enhancement of positive affect, strengthened compassion and inhibited personal distress in reaction to others' distress. These findings were replicated in four additional studies (Mikulincer et al., 2001, Studies 2–5).

In another set of three experiments, Mikulincer, Gillath, and colleagues (2003) found theoretically predictable attachment-related differences in value orientations. Avoidant attachment, assessed with the ECR, was inversely associated with endorsement of two self-transcendent values, benevolence (concern for close others) and universalism (concern for all humanity), supporting our notion that avoidant strategies interfere with concern for others' needs. In addition, experimental priming of mental representations of attachment figure availability, as compared with enhancing positive affect or exposing participants to a neutral priming condition, strengthened endorsement of these two prosocial values. The findings fit well with Van IJzendoorn and Zwart-Woudstra's (1995) discovery that secure attachment (assessed with the AAI) is associated with more humanistic moral reasoning. The conclusion is further supported by Clark and colleagues' (2011) findings that contextual priming of attachment security reduced the endorsement of materialistic values and decreased the importance people assigned to material objects.

Mikulincer, Shaver, Gillath, and Nitzberg (2005) examined the effects of security priming on the actual decision to help or not to help a person in distress. In the first two experiments, participants watched a confederate (an actress) while she performed a series of increasingly aversive tasks. As the study progressed, the confederate became increasingly distressed by the aversive tasks, and the actual participant (who was merely an observer) was given an opportunity to take the distressed person's place, thereby self-sacrificing for the benefit of the distressed confederate. Shortly before the scenario just described, participants had been exposed to a series of security or neutral primes subliminally (rapid presentation of the name of an attachment figure or a neutral control person) or supraliminally (vividly recalling an interaction with a supportive person), or in the control condition (recalling a neutral person). At the point of making a decision about replacing the distressed confederate, participants completed brief measures of compassion and personal distress. In both studies, dispositional avoidance was related to lower reported compassion and lower willingness to help the distressed confederate. Dispositional attachment anxiety was related to self-reported personal distress but not to either compassion or willingness to help. In addition, subliminal or supraliminal priming of representations of a security-providing figure decreased personal distress and increased participants' compassion and willingness to take the place of the distressed confederate.

In two additional studies, Mikulincer and colleagues (2005, Studies 3–4) examined whether the contextual bolstering of attachment security overrides egoistic motives for helping, such as mood enhancement (Schaller & Cialdini, 1988) or empathic joy (Smith, Keating, & Stotland, 1989), and results in genuinely altruistic (unselfish) helping. Participants were divided into two conditions (security priming, neutral priming), read a true newspaper article about a woman in dire personal and financial distress, and rated their emotional reactions to the article (compassion and personal distress). In one study, half of the participants anticipated mood enhancement by means other than helping (e.g., expecting to watch a comedy film). In the other study, half of the participants were told that the needy woman was chronically depressed and her mood might be beyond their ability to repair (no empathic joy condition). Schaller and Cialdini (1988) and Smith and colleagues (1989) had found that these two conditions, expecting to improve one's mood by other means or anticipating no sharing of joy with the needy person, reduced egoistic motives for helping because a potential helper would gain no mood-related benefit from helping. However, these conditions failed to inhibit altruistic motives for helping when helping was augmented by security priming. The security-supported increased willingness to help seemed to be genuinely unselfish. These findings support our theoretical view that a sense of attachment security reduces selfishness (defensive self-protection) and allows a person to activate his or her caregiving behavioral system, direct attention to others' distress, take the perspective of a distressed other, and engage in altruistic behavior with the primary goal of benefiting the other person.

## Generosity

Generous actions are among the building blocks of positive and stable social relations. However, although extensive theoretical and empirical work has been devoted to the study of empathy, compassion, and altruistic helping in adults, there is little systematic research on acts of generosity, the subjective experiences of people when they act generously, or the associations of these experiences with attachment orientations. One preliminary exploration (Sommerfeld, 2009) involved the development of the Experience of Generosity Questionnaire, a measure of the extent to which adults are prosocially oriented when acting generously or feel a sense of burden, self-criticism/guilt, or self-congratulation when being "generous." Sommerfeld (2009) examined associations between these experiential aspects of generosity and ECR attachment insecurity scores (anxiety and avoidance). She found that attachment anxiety was associated with greater feelings of personal burden and self-criticism/guilt, whereas avoidance was associated with a less prosocial orientation, in addition to feelings of personal burden. Much more research is needed on attachment and generosity.

## Gratitude

Gratitude has been portrayed in the psychological literature in diverse ways: as a positive emotion, as a personality trait, as a positive attitude toward others, as a moral virtue, and as a constructive approach to interpersonal relations (Emmons & McCullough, 2003; Weiner, 1985). Emmons and McCullough (2003) proposed that gratitude be conceptualized in terms of three propositions. First, the object of gratitude is always an "other," whether a human being, a nonhuman natural being (e.g., an animal, the weather), or a supernatural being (e.g., God). Second, gratitude is a response to a perceived personal benefit (e.g., a material, emotional, or spiritual gain) resulting from another's actions—a benefit that has not necessarily been earned or deserved. Third, gratitude stems from appraising the benefactor's actions as intentionally designed to benefit the recipient, even if the intention is metaphorical, as in the case of good weather ("Thank you for not raining on my parade"). According to Lazarus and Lazarus (1994), gratitude results from recognizing another's goodwill and appreciating the other's generous action as an altruistic gift. Agreeing with this conception, Tsang (2006) defined *gratitude* as "a positive emotional reaction to the receipt of a benefit that is perceived to have resulted from the good intentions of another" (p. 139).

In Peterson and Seligman's (2004) taxonomy of human strengths and virtues, the capacity for gratitude is viewed as a core strength that improves people's well-being and mental health (Snyder & McCullough, 2000). Similarly, Emmons and McCullough (2003) portrayed gratitude as a remedy for many of life's hardships and as a way to achieve peace of mind, happiness, and satisfying interpersonal relationships. In line with this view, Watkins, Woodward, Stone, and Kolts (2003) found that grateful people tend to experience greater "abundance" in their lives, feel more thankful to other people for contributions to their personal well-being, and are more likely than other people to appreciate even the small pleasures in life. Moreover, the expression of gratitude to a generous relationship partner has been found to have beneficial effects on relationship satisfaction, emotional and physical closeness, and positive appraisals of the partner (e.g., Algoe, Gable, & Maisel, 2010; Algoe & Haidt, 2009; Lambert, Clark, Durtschi, Fincham, & Graham, 2010).

From an attachment perspective, the experience of gratitude can be expected to be associated with feelings of being protected, accepted, and valued by others. Warm, comforting interactions with a sensitive, responsive, and supportive caregiver during childhood foster not only positive mental representations (working models) of others but also a feeling that one has received a gift that "keeps on giving" (as advertisers sometimes boast). This feeling makes it easier, in later phases of life, to feel grateful for other people's kindness and generosity. In other words, attachment security can be expected to correlate with dispositional gratitude. In contrast, attachment-related avoidance may constrict feelings of gratitude in response to others' generous behavior because avoidant people tend to doubt other people's good intentions. Moreover, expressions of gratitude toward a relationship partner can be interpreted as a sign of closeness or dependence, which is inconsistent with avoidant people's preference for emotional distance.

Attachment anxiety may lead to ambivalent reactions to others' generous behavior. People who score high on attachment anxiety tend not to believe they deserve others' kindness and worry that they will not be able to reciprocate adequately or meet a generous person's needs and expectations (Mikulincer & Shaver, 2007a). This, in turn, may taint gratitude with anxiety. In addition, for attachment-anxious people, positive interpersonal experiences may be reminiscent of previous experiences that began well but ended poorly. Once attuned to negative memories, the anxious mind suffers from a spread of negative affect (Mikulincer & Orbach, 1995), which is likely to interfere with genuine gratitude.

In two studies, Mikulincer, Shaver, and Slav (2006) explored links between attachment scores and feelings of gratitude toward a generous relationship partner. The first study was cross-sectional and correlational; it indicated that secure participants scored higher on a dispositional measure of gratitude than avoidant participants and reported more feelings of security, happiness, love, and generosity—and fewer feelings of narcissistic threat and distrust—when feeling grateful. Attachment anxiety was not significantly associated with dispositional gratitude, but it was associated with a more ambivalent experience of gratitude. People who scored higher on attachment anxiety recalled experiencing security-related feelings (e.g., "I felt there was someone who cared for me"), happiness, and love, together with narcissistic threats and inferiority feelings (e.g., "I felt weak and needy"), which seemed to mar the otherwise positive experience of gratitude.

In a second study (Mikulincer et al., 2006), newlywed couples (both husbands and wives) completed a daily questionnaire each evening for 21 days. In it, they listed positive and negative behaviors exhibited by their partner on a given day and rated the extent to which they felt grateful toward the partner that day. For both husbands and wives, attachment security predicted higher levels of daily gratitude across the 21-day period. Moreover, more secure husbands reported greater gratitude on days when they perceived more positive spousal behavior, whereas more avoidant husbands reported relatively low levels of gratitude even on days when they noticed their wife's positive behavior.

Attachment insecurities also seem to interfere with the positive effects that gratitude normally has on prosocial behavior. Mikulincer and Shaver (2009) randomly assigned undergraduates to a gratitude condition ("Think about the many things in life for which you might feel grateful") or a control condition ("Think about your typical day"). They then measured the extent to which participants helped an experimenter's confederate, who asked them to complete a cognitively taxing problem-solving survey. The major dependent variable was the time spent working on the survey. The results indicated that participants in the gratitude condition spent more time helping with the survey than did participants in the control condition, and more anxious and/or avoidant participants spent less time helping. However, these effects were qualified by significant interactions between gratitude and attachment insecurity scores: The gratitude exercise led to more helping behavior than the control condition mainly when participants scored relatively low on anxiety and/or avoidance. The prosocial effect of gratitude was lower when attachment anxiety or avoidance was relatively high.

Overall, research findings reported thus far suggest that gratitude and its links with prosocial behavior are complex and moderated by attachment orientations. It seems relatively easy for a secure person to feel grateful, especially after being rewarded by someone else. It is difficult for an insecure person to be unambivalent about receiving a benefit from another person, and to pass the benefit along to someone else. To an important extent, gratitude depends on feeling loved, valued, supported, and cared for, both in the moment and over the years.

## Forgiveness

Forgiveness is often key to maintaining relational harmony and affectional bonds following conflicts, offenses, and transgressions in relationships (e.g., Fincham & Beach, 2010; Gordon, Hughes, Tomcik, Dixon, & Litzinger, 2009; Karremans & Van Lange, 2004). In addition, forgiveness contributes to positive emotions toward an offending other, to intimacy and emotional closeness, and to relationship satisfaction and stability (e.g., Finkel, Rusbult, Kumashiro, & Hannon, 2002). Moreover, the ability to forgive is related to psychological and even to physical well-being (e.g., Karremans, Van Lange, Ouwerkerk, & Kluwer, 2003). However, forgiveness is not an automatic response to another person's offenses and transgressions. It often requires a transformation (or what Rusbult, Verette, Whitney, Slovik, & Lipkus, 1991, called "accommodation") of interpersonal motives—containment of angry feelings and regulation of the impulse to act destructively,

while finding a constructive way to overcome an impasse created by another person's hurtful behavior (e.g., McCullough, 2000). According to McCullough, Worthington, and Rachal (1997), forgiveness requires "a set of motivational changes, whereby one becomes decreasingly motivated to retaliate against and maintain estrangement from an offending relationship partner and increasingly motivated by conciliation and goodwill for the offender, despite the offender's hurtful actions" (pp. 321–322).

From an attachment perspective, the motivational transformation involved in forgiving an offending other is likely to be facilitated by attachment security. Secure people are confident of others' availability and love, view others as generally trustworthy and dependable, and believe in others' goodwill (Shaver & Hazan, 1993). In addition, secure people have been found to provide more benign explanations for others' hurtful actions and attribute them to less intentional and less stable causes. Therefore, they are more inclined to forgive. In contrast, avoidant individuals are likely to be less forgiving because they possess negative working models of others and tend to attribute others' objectionable behavior to bad intentions.

In the case of individuals who score high on attachment anxiety, reactions to others' offending behavior are likely to be influenced by two conflicting forces. On the one hand, their inclination to intensify negative emotions and ruminate about threats should fuel intense and prolonged bouts of anger toward an offending other, thereby interfering with forgiveness. On the other hand, such people's fears of rejection and separation may cause them to suppress or hide resentment and anger and incline them toward self-protective forgiveness. This kind of forgiveness might be accompanied by recurrent intrusive thoughts about the transgression and heightened doubts about others' availability and dependability. In other words, although attachment anxiety may not preclude forgiveness, it may engender ambivalence about forgiveness and therefore reduce its relational and personal benefits.

Correlational evidence indicates that attachment anxiety and avoidance are in fact associated with lower scores on measures of dispositional forgiveness (e.g., Burnette, Taylor, Worthington, & Forsyth, 2007; Kachadourian, Fincham, & Davila, 2004; Lawler-Row, Younger, Piferi, & Jones, 2006; Mikulincer et al., 2006; Yárnoz-Yaben, 2009). Moreover, Mikulincer and colleagues (2006) found that less secure people were more inclined to report intense feelings of vulnerability or humiliation and a strong sense of relationship deterioration when forgiving a partner. In other words, attachment insecurities were associated with a less constructive experience of forgiveness. Burnette, Davis, Green, Worthington, and Bradfield (2009) provided evidence concerning the potential mediators of such effects: Whereas the link between attachment anxiety and reduced forgiveness was mediated by excessive rumination on relational injuries, the link between avoidance and reduced forgiveness was mediated by lack of prosocial attitudes.

In a diary study of daily fluctuations in the tendency to forgive a spouse, Mikulincer and colleagues (2006) found that attachment insecurities predicted lower levels of forgiveness across 21 consecutive days. Moreover, whereas secure people were more inclined to forgive their spouse on days when they perceived more positive spousal behavior, less secure people reported little forgiveness even on days when they perceived their spouse to be available, attentive, and supportive. In other words, attachment insecurities not only prevented forgiveness but they also interfered with the ability of a partner's positive behavior to restore understanding and empathy.

Beyond these associations between dispositional measures of attachment and forgiveness, there is increasing evidence that state-like senses of security or insecurity can alter the tendency to forgive a hurtful partner. For example, Finkel, Burnette, and Scissors (2007) experimentally enhanced attachment anxiety or measured its natural weekly fluctuations for 6 months and found that heightened attachment anxiety reduced forgiveness for a partner's offenses. In addition, Hannon, Rusbult, Finkel, and Kumashiro (2010) found that a betraying partner's provision of security to the injured partner (by genuinely expressing interest in being responsive to the victim's needs) promoted forgiveness and restoration of relational harmony. Karremans and Aarts (2007) found that security priming (with the name of a loving other) elicited more automatic forgiving responses to interpersonal offenses than neutral priming.

In a series of experimental and longitudinal studies, Luchies, Finkel, McNulty, and Kumashiro (2010) showed that situational *felt security* (the extent to which a partner is perceived to be responsive and able to provide a sense of security and stability) is a prerequisite for the beneficial effects of forgiveness. For example, they found that the association between marital forgiveness and

heightened self-respect over the first 5 years of marriage depended on the extent to which spouses appraised their partners as safe and responsive. Moreover, the positive effects of forgiveness on self-respect and self-concept clarity following an experimentally induced hurtful relational episode depended on the perpetrator's expression of genuine interest in being responsive to the victim's needs. Overall, these findings imply that, under insecurity-heightening circumstances, forgiveness negatively affects feelings about oneself, which may help to explain why dispositionally insecure people are often reluctant to forgive an offending partner.

### Empirical Studies of Adults: Discussion

Based on only the relatively small sample of studies of adult attachment and caregiving reviewed here (for a fuller treatment, see Mikulincer & Shaver, 2007a), a clear and quite general pattern emerges. Adults who score high on self-report measures of attachment anxiety have difficulty caring for another person without becoming personally distressed in an unproductive manner, often because they are more focused on their own needs and sense of vulnerability than on the needs of a person who needs their help. They are lacking not in empathy but in what Buddhists call *effective compassion*, which goes beyond empathy to include "skillful" action. Attachment-anxious adults' ineffective compassion is evident in parent–child relationships, romantic/marital relationships, and interactions with peers and strangers. Their failure to take effective action is also affected by their somewhat negative models of self, which includes a sense of poor self-efficacy. It is worth mentioning, however, that although anxious adults' heightened sensitivity to threats (to self) often results in poorly timed or poorly considered efforts to help others, their heightened vigilance can sometimes benefit members of the groups to which they belong because their ability to detect threats can sometimes save their own and other people's lives (Ein-Dor, Mikulincer, Doron, & Shaver, 2010; Ein-Dor et al., 2011).

Adults who score high on self-report measures of attachment-related avoidance are quite different. They are generally less empathic, less compassionate, and less willing to help others. They are often uncomfortable with other people's reliance on them, especially if it requires close physical or emotional contact or prolonged assistance. At the group level, however, their self-preoccupation, and what Bowlby (1969/1982) called their "compulsive self-reliance," can sometimes make them quick to figure out, in a threatening situation, how to escape or save themselves, and this can provide a useful model for other members of their group to escape danger (Ein-Dor et al., 2010, 2011).

Both anxious and avoidant adults are capable of feeling and being generous, grateful, and forgiving, but their versions of these feelings are often colored by qualifications, such as feeling depleted, "ripped off," or overly obligated. Underlying such complicated forms of what would otherwise be positive feelings is a sense of insecurity, doubts about one's own value to others, and fear of vulnerability.

To date, an advantage of the literature on adult care is the relative ease of conducting experimental studies involving various kinds of security priming: guided imagery or recall of being treated well by attachment figures; pictures of attachment figures' faces; subliminal stimulation with attachment figures' names or words such as *being loved, hug, support,* or *affection* (Mikulincer & Shaver, 2007a, 2007b). This adds considerably to the huge volume of correlational research, which indicates that self-reported individual differences in security, anxiety, and avoidance are associated strongly with many questionnaire and behavioral measures of empathy, compassion, gratitude, and forgiveness. Activating an adult's network of mental associations related to security (associations that are both cognitive and affective) increases prosocial feelings and motivates prosocial behavior. Fewer studies have been conducted with "insecurity primes," but those studies show that being reminded of insecurity (e.g., memories of past rejections and hurt feelings) reduces empathy and prosocial behavior. Taken in combination with the developmental studies of children and adolescents reviewed earlier in this chapter, the adult studies offer convincing evidence that attachment security and insecurity influence a wide range of prosocial motives, feelings, and behaviors.

## Future Directions

Despite the impressive size of the literature reviewed in this chapter, indicating that attachment orientations are related to various aspects of concern for others, there are still many needs and possibilities for future research. Because our large sections on attachment and care in childhood and attachment and care in adulthood are somewhat different in focus and methods (because of the different developmental levels of the research participants, requiring different verbal and nonverbal measures, and the different social contexts in which they live; with parents, in university communities, in homes with their spouses, etc.), we consider future directions separately for the two large research domains.

### Future Directions for Research on Attachment and Prosocial Phenomena in Childhood

Existing research and its limitations indicate that the field is ripe for further investigation of the link between attachment security and the development of care for others in childhood, when these capacities are first coming online and there is the greatest opportunity to influence their development in the next generation. To do this, a first priority is to improve the sensitivity and specificity of measures used to assess care for others at different developmental stages. When operationalizing constructs, researchers should delineate clear boundaries around empathy and prosocial behavior, so that the unique developmental antecedents and consequences of each can be identified. Further insights may be gained by measuring specific dimensions of both constructs. For example, it may be important to assess both cognitive aspects of empathy (e.g., emotion recognition and understanding, perspective taking) and its affective aspects (e.g., emotional resonance, compassion, concern). Similarly, future research should consider specific dimensions of prosocial behavior such as sharing, helping, and comforting behaviors, verbal versus nonverbal responses, the relative success or effectiveness of prosocial overtures, and whether they occur in the presence or absence of emotional stimuli.

Central to the pursuit of valid measures of care for others is observational research in the home, neighborhood, and school, as well as in laboratory settings. Research has shown that responses to hypothetical situations (e.g., to imagine donating to someone in need) do not always map onto actual behavior (e.g., Ajzen, Brown, & Carvajal, 2004). For example, although children may know that they should share a prized teddy bear with a child who has no toys, they may not do so when faced with the immediate conflict between their own desires and another's needs. Observational measures used to study the normative development of children's empathy and prosocial behavior provide creative and ecologically valid tools that can be extended to the study of attachment-related individual differences. These include home-based observations of children's reactions to naturalistic and simulated distress (e.g., Zahn-Waxler, Radke-Yarrow, et al., 1992); laboratory situations in which an adult experimenter displays needs that differentially call for helping, sharing, and comforting (e.g., Dunfield & Kuhlmeier, 2013); and tasks that isolate specific motives (e.g., sympathy vs. seeking social rewards) underlying prosocial behavior (e.g., Hepach et al., 2013a). In addition, observational paradigms used with adults, such as donating behavior and willingness to help a distressed confederate (e.g., Mikulincer & Shaver, 2005), have been used successfully with children (e.g., Benenson, Pascoe, & Radmore, 2007) and provide other valid approaches to the study of attachment-related individual differences in care for others in childhood.

Exploring potential interactions of empathy with other mental capacities such as emotion regulation, theory of mind, and social information processing may illuminate connections that help to explain the development of care for others. Moving beyond cross-sectional, correlational studies toward intervention and longitudinal designs may shed light on questions of continuity and change, sensitive periods, and the temporal sequence of this link. For example, research examining the effects of attachment interventions such as the Circle of Security (Hoffman, Marvin, Cooper, & Powell, 2006) on children's empathy and prosocial behavior may illuminate whether enhancing security might support the development of greater capacities for extending care to others beyond the parent–child relationship.

Furthermore, priming studies of the kinds developed by researchers studying adult attachment provide a promising paradigm for investigating causal pathways in the short term. It is reasonable to hypothesize that experimental priming of attachment security in children will enhance their empathy and prosocial behavior given evidence of this link in the adult literature. Indeed, one study by Over and Carpenter (2009) demonstrated that subliminal priming of affiliation (i.e., a picture of two dolls facing each other) significantly enhanced 18-month-old children's spontaneous helping toward an experimenter who had dropped her pencils. In adult samples, however, attachment priming has been shown to have specific effects beyond those of affiliation in enhancing empathy and willingness to help a distressed other (Mikulincer et al., 2005). It remains to be seen whether attachment priming has similarly unique effects beyond affiliation in children.

Alongside developmental questions regarding individual differences, future research may be informed by the recent upsurge of creative methods used to examine the normative development of human altruism, which have shed light on contextual, motivational, and evolutionary factors influencing children's care for others (e.g., Warneken & Tomasello, 2009). For example, evidence suggests that toddlers sympathize with and are motivated to help victims of harm, even when the victims show no emotion, suggesting that children's early perspective taking and understanding of harm support their care for others, even in the absence of distress cues (Vaish, Carpenter, & Tomasello, 2009). It may be that the link between attachment and children's care for others is moderated by whether harm occurs in the presence or absence of emotional distress. A study of 5-year-olds demonstrated that children show the bystander effect made famous by social psychologists (Darley & Latane, 1968), helping at high levels when alone but less often when others are available to help (Plötner, Over, Carpenter, & Tomasello, 2015). Attachment security may moderate children's susceptibility to the bystander effect. Other research has shown that children are more prosocial following reciprocal (vs. simply friendly) social interactions with an adult (Barragan & Dweck, 2014) and following synchronous music making (Kirschner & Tomasello, 2010), suggesting that responsive, coordinated social interactions experimentally boost children's care for others. On one level, attachment security involves similar experiences of responsivity and mutual coordination; however, questions remain regarding how specific the role of caregiver–child interactions may be in promoting children's concern for others. Future investigations may benefit from drawing on the novel methods and context-specific paradigms in the emerging literature on child altruism to illuminate the nature of attachment-related individual differences.

In addition, it will be important to continue the search for further mechanisms underlying the link between security and care for others. For example, it may be that security reduces attention to threat to oneself, which allows children to shift mental resources away from the self and toward others in need (as described in this chapter in relation to adults). Examining the parameters of the automatic nature of some prosocial behavior should also prove useful. Alternatively, security may foster openness to emotional pain and vulnerability (Cassidy, Shaver, Mikulincer, & Lavy, 2009), such that others' suffering need not be defensively excluded. One particularly interesting avenue to explore is the biological basis of the ways in which attachment gets "under the skin" (in this volume, see Polan & Hofer, Chapter 6, and Ehrlich, Miller, Jones, & Cassidy, Chapter 9), and how, in turn, this may influence the capacity to care for others who are suffering. A viable starting point may be to examine the role of oxytocin in the development of children's concern for others, as it has been implicated in attachment and pair bonding (Carter, 1998; Feldman, Weller, Zagoory-Sharon, & Levine, 2007; Young & Wang, 2004), parenting (Bakermans-Kranenburg & Van IJzendoorn, 2008; Feldman et al., 2012; Galbally, Lewis, Van IJzendoorn, & Permezel, 2011), empathy (Bartz et al., 2010; Hurlemann et al., 2010), and altruistic behavior (De Dreu et al., 2010; Zak, Stanton, & Ahmadi, 2007). (See also Hane & Fox, Chapter 11, this volume.) These mechanisms likely interact with emotion regulation in linking security and concern for others.

Pursuing further research along these lines has broader implications for attachment theory. Specifically, a better understanding of attachment-related differences in children's care for others may prove useful in illuminating key processes involved in the intergenerational transmission of attachment. In parents, self-reported attachment security has been linked to their own enhanced emotion regulation capacities, which in turn are associated with parents' more empathic responses to their children's distress (Jones, Brett, Ehrlich, Lejuez, & Cassidy, 2014). A similar model may apply to children, whereby attachment security in childhood supports the development of both emotion regulation capacities and the capacity to care for others, so that, in adulthood, secure individuals are able to extend such care to their own children in the form of sensitive, empathic parenting. Indeed, evidence suggests that empathy and prosocial behavior early in development are carried forward into adulthood (Eisenberg et al., 2002), that adults' empathic concern is positively related to retrospective accounts of their parents' sensitive responses to their distress in childhood (Kanat-Maymon & Assor, 2009), and that parental empathy mediates the link between parent and child attachment security (Stern et al., 2015). Assembling the pieces of the intergenerational puzzle

calls for future longitudinal work on attachment and concern for others across the lifespan.

More broadly, there is a need for a positive psychology of children—encompassing virtues such as compassion, gratitude, mindfulness, and forgiveness (e.g., Froh et al., 2011; Greenberg & Harris, 2012)—that includes the potential influence of attachment. The extensive and exciting findings reported in the adult literature provide an avenue for similar exploration in childhood, with the creative adaptation of existing measures, as well as the development of new paradigms and methods for enhancing concern for others in the short and long term. We echo Greenberg and Turksma's (2015) call for leveraging the unique insights from developmental research to foster kindness and empathy in homes, neighborhoods, and schools, and add that these efforts likely need to be rooted in secure human relationships if they are to be effective, sustainable, and transmitted to the next generation. Understanding the developmental roots of care for others in childhood is central not only to attachment research but also to the broader goal of cultivating a kinder, more compassionate society.

## Future Directions for Research on Attachment and Prosocial Phenomena in Adulthood

As demonstrated in this chapter, there is extensive evidence linking attachment security and two major forms of insecurity (attachment anxiety and avoidance) with prosocial motives, emotions, and behavior. The connections between attachment and prosociality have been demonstrated in the laboratory and in the community, using both correlational and experimental designs. It is now important to branch out in new directions.

One rich source for new studies would be a search for both mediating and moderating factors. In particular, future studies should examine times and situations in which secure attachment fails to promote prosocial behavior as well as the conditions that may favor prosocial behavior among insecure people. The priming studies conducted thus far clearly indicate that security can be heightened temporarily by priming. It has been assumed that longer-term priming (1) would produce stronger and more lasting effects on mental and behavioral processes, and (2) might be similar to what happens naturally in security-enhancing close relationships with friends, romantic partners, mentors, leaders, or therapists. But more work is needed to explore the process of security enhancement in real-world relationships and to determine whether that kind of natural security enhancement results in increased empathy and care for other people. If it does have this bonus benefit, it will be important to learn how the effects are mediated (e.g., through changes in working models of self, such as increased self-esteem and self-efficacy, or changes in working models of others, such as formerly avoidant individuals changing their critical, skeptical working models of others).

In addition, research should examine how cultural settings and variables moderate the link between attachment and prosocial behavior given that physical and cultural settings can shape cognitive representations of people and relationships. For example, although there is evidence to suggest that security priming attenuates hostile attitudes toward outgroup members, even among groups engaged in years of intractable conflict (Mikulincer & Shaver, 2001, 2007c), one pilot study found that more secure Palestinians living in the territories occupied by Israeli soldiers were more, rather than less, hostile toward Israeli Jews and more accepting of violence against them (Mikulincer & Shaver, 2007c). Thus, although the pursuit of the possible benefits of psychological security enhancement is promising, the assumption that security and pacifism are synonymous would be faulty. Achieving a world at peace requires humane ethics, a more tolerant cultural and educational climate, and good judgment and effective political will on the part of leaders, not just securely attached individual citizens.

Because of the growing emphasis in adult attachment research on physiological and neurological underpinnings (in this volume, see Coan, Chapter 12, and Hane & Fox, Chapter 11), it will be important to explore further how the brain and various hormones underlie the link between attachment orientations and prosocial behavior. There are already numerous studies showing that self-reported anxiety and avoidance are related to various neurophysiological processes (e.g., reactions to social rejection; DeWall et al., 2012; Gillath, Bunge, Shaver, Wendelken, & Mikulincer, 2005). The next step would be to extend these studies into the realm of prosocial emotions and behavior.

Bowlby (1969/1982) viewed attachment and caregiving as two innate behavioral systems, both of which evolved because they increased the likelihood that primate (including human) infants would survive in a world of full of danger,

despite these infants' immaturity at birth. The attachment and caregiving behavioral systems presumably develop throughout life as a function of experiences in important relationships, and by the time adults enter psychological studies, their dispositional attachment and caregiving orientations, although not identical or totally unified, are clearly intertwined. In adult attachment research, prosocial emotions and behavior have generally been viewed as aspects of the caregiving system, but in the child attachment literature, less attention has been given to the concept of a developing caregiving system. Ideally, future research would involve measurement of both the attachment and the caregiving systems and then would determine, using longitudinal designs, how the two influence each other over time, and how each is influenced, separately or simultaneously, by social experiences of various kinds, with parents, other caregivers, teachers, coaches, and so on.

There might be other kinds of influences worth assessing, such as books, films, television series, and religious practices. Granqvist, Mikulincer, and Shaver (2010; see also Granqvist & Kirkpatrick, Chapter 39, this volume), for example, have reviewed literature showing that religious figures, such as Jesus or the Virgin Mary, can serve as symbolic attachment figures, and many religions encourage their adherents to pray to such figures for help in times of distress or crisis. In Buddhism, there have long been meditation practices that involve imagining being loved by a family member (e.g., one's mother) or a religious figure (e.g., the Buddha), then turning that feeling of love, in one's mind, toward other people, including "difficult" ones, which might make it easier to engage in constructive (prosocial) relationships with such people in real life (e.g., Hoffman, 2015b; Mipham, 2013; Nhat Hanh, 2014). Empirically, these loving-kindness practices have been shown in turn to strengthen feelings of social connectedness (Hutcherson, Seppala, & Gross, 2008) and boost prosocial behavior (Block-Lerner, Adair, Plumb, Rhatigan, & Orsillo, 2007; Kemeny et al., 2012; Leiberg, Klimecki, & Singer, 2011).

The role of the attachment system in prayer and Buddhist loving-kindness meditation is indicated by prayers that stress such factors as being protected in times of danger, and being "nearer" to God. A common Buddhist prayer is "I take *refuge* in the Buddha, the Dharma (the Buddha's teachings and Buddhist practices), and the Sangha (the community of fellow practitioners)." Many of these religious practices are being recast in a more secular form as Buddhist practices such as mind-fulness meditation and self-compassion medita-tion make their way into Western psychology and psychiatry (e.g., Hoffman, 2015a, 2015b; Miller, 2009, 2015). In the same way that mindfulness meditation is being studied by psychologists and neuroscientists, it should be possible to assess the effects of other forms of meditation—focusing on self-compassion, compassion for others, and lov-ing-kindness—on the brain, and on people's pro-social emotions and behavior.

## Concluding Comments

It is interesting that ideas stemming at first from close scrutiny of the parent–child relationship have proven to apply not only to other close relation-ships but also to all kinds of social relationships in which concern for others' welfare arises. It seems that all forms of sensitive, responsive, and compas-sionate care across the lifespan (e.g., caregiving in parent–child relationships, in adult romantic re-lationships, in relationships between middle-aged adults and their infirm older adult parents) and in different contexts (e.g., in close relationships and in the wider social world, where thousands of strangers need help and support) have a common basis and resemble each other. This implies that the research literatures on parenting, romantic caregiving, social support, helping, empathy, and counseling and psychotherapy—and even social justice/human rights and peace-building—are fun-damentally related, and that further theoretical and empirical efforts should be made to create an overarching perspective on them.

Generous caregivers—human, nonhuman, spiritual, and symbolic—can contribute to a per-son's sense of security and to his or her caregiving propensities; they can also provide models of com-passion and loving-kindness that can be copied. Thus, if we wish to create a kinder and more peace-ful world, we need to foster better parenting, more nurturing romantic relationships, better mentor-ing, and more positive and prosocial spiritual mod-els. Simply championing virtues in the abstract or using socialization practices alone to encourage virtue, without providing a sense of love and se-curity, is unlikely to be very helpful because, as we have shown here, insecure individuals do not ex-perience opportunities for kindness and virtue in simple, unadulterated ways. They tend not to have confidence in the possibility of goodness.

## References

Ainsworth, M. D. S. (1969). Individual differences in strange-situational behaviour of one-year-olds. In H. R. Schaffer (Ed.), *The origins of human social relations.* London: Academic Press.

Ainsworth, M. D. S., Bell, S. M., & Stayton, D. J. (1974). Infant–mother attachment and social development: "Socialisation" as a product of reciprocal responsive-ness to signals. In M. P. M. Richards (Ed.), *The inte-gration of a child into a social world* (pp. 99–135). New York: Cambridge University Press.

Ainsworth, M. D. S., Blehar, M. C., Waters, E., & Wall, S. (1978). *Patterns of attachment: A psychological study of the strange situation.* Hillsdale, NJ: Erlbaum.

Ajzen, I., Brown, T. C., & Carvajal, F. (2004). Explain-ing the discrepancy between intentions and actions: The case of hypothetical bias in contingent valua-tion. *Personality and Social Psychology Bulletin, 30*(9), 1108–1121.

Albert, L. S., & Horowitz, L. M. (2009). Attachment styles and ethical behavior: Their relationship and significance in the marketplace. *Journal of Business Ethics, 87,* 299–316.

Algoe, S. B., Gable, S. L., & Maisel, N. C. (2010). It's the little things: Everyday gratitude as a booster shot for romantic relationships. *Personal Relationships, 17,* 217–233.

Algoe, S. B., & Haidt, J. (2009). Witnessing excellence in action: The "other-praising" emotions of elevation, gratitude, and admiration. *Journal of Positive Psychol-ogy, 4,* 105–127.

Andretta, J. R., Ramirez, A. M., Barnes, M. E., Odom, T., Roberson-Adams, S., & Woodland, M. H. (2015). Perceived parental security profiles in African Amer-ican adolescents involved in the juvenile justice system. *Journal of Family Psychology.* [Epub ahead of print]

Andretta, J. R., Woodland, M., & Worrell, F. C. (2014). *Adolescent Prosocial Behavior Scale.* Wash-ington, DC: Child Guidance Clinic, Court Social Services Division, Superior Court of the District of Columbia.

Armsden, G. C., & Greenberg, M. T. (1987). The In-ventory of Parent and Peer Attachment: Individual differences and their relationship to psychological well-being in adolescence. *Journal of Youth and Ado-lescence, 16*(5), 427–454.

Asher, S. R., & McDonald, K. L. (2009). The behav-ioral basis of acceptance, rejection, and perceived popularity. In K. H. Rubin, W. M. Bukowski, & B. Laursen (Eds.), *The handbook of peer interactions, relationships, and groups* (pp. 232–248). New York: Guilford Press.

Bailey, S. J., McWilliams, L. A., & Dick, B. D. (2012). Expanding the social communication model of pain: Are adult attachment characteristics associated with observers' pain-related evaluations? *Rehabilitation Psy-chology, 57,* 27–34.

Bakermans-Kranenburg, M. J., & Van IJzendoorn, M. H. (2008). Oxytocin receptor (*OXTR*) and serotonin transporter (*5-HTT*) genes associated with observed parenting. *Social Cognitive and Affective Neuroscience, 3*, 128–134.

Barragan, R. C., & Dweck, C. S. (2014). Rethinking natural altruism: Simple reciprocal interactions trigger children's benevolence. *Proceedings of the National Academy of Sciences, 111*(48), 17071–17074.

Bartal, I. B. A., Decety, J., & Mason, P. (2011). Empathy and pro-social behavior in rats. *Science, 334*(6061), 1427–1430.

Bartholomew, K., & Horowitz, L. M. (1991). Attachment styles among young adults: A test of a four-category model. *Journal of Personality and Social Psychology, 61*(2), 226–244.

Bartz, J. A., & Lydon, J. E. (2004). Close relationships and the working self-concept: Implicit and explicit effects of priming attachment on agency and communion. *Personality and Social Psychology Bulletin, 30,* 1389–1401.

Bartz, J. A., Zaki, J., Bolger, N., Hollander, E., Ludwig, N. N., Kolevzon, A., et al. (2010). Oxytocin selectively improves empathic accuracy. *Psychological Science, 21*(10), 1426–1428.

Batson, C. D. (1991). *The altruism question: Toward a social-psychological answer.* Hillsdale, NJ: Erlbaum.

Batson, C. D. (2010). Empathy-induced altruistic motivation. In M. Mikulincer & P. R. Shaver (Eds.), *Prosocial motives, emotions, and behavior: The better angels of our nature* (pp. 15–34). Washington, DC: American Psychological Association.

Beckes, L., & Coan, J. A. (2015). The distress-relief dynamic in attachment bonding. In V. Zayas & C. Hazan (Eds.), *Bases of adult attachment* (pp. 11–33). New York: Springer.

Benenson, J. F., Pascoe, J., & Radmore, N. (2007). Children's altruistic behavior in the dictator game. *Evolution and Human Behavior, 28*(3), 168–175.

Bischof-Köhler, D. (2000). Empathie, prosoziales Verhalten und Bindungsqualität bei Zweijährigen [Empathy, prosocial behavior and security of attachment in two-year-olds]. *Psychologie in Erziehung und Unterricht, 47*(2), 142–158.

Block-Lerner, J., Adair, C., Plumb, J. C., Rhatigan, D. L., & Orsillo, S. M. (2007). The case for mindfulness-based approaches in the cultivation of empathy: Does nonjudgmental, present-moment awareness increase capacity for perspective-taking and empathic concern? *Journal of Marital and Family Therapy, 33*(4), 501–516.

Bohlin, G., Hagekull, B., & Rydell, A. M. (2000). Attachment and social functioning: A longitudinal study from infancy to middle childhood. *Social Development, 9*(1), 24–39.

Bowlby, J. (1973). *Attachment and loss: Vol. 2. Separation.* New York: Basic Books.

Bowlby, J. (1980). *Attachment and loss: Vol. 3. Loss, sadness and depression.* New York: Basic Books.

Bowlby, J. (1982). *Attachment and loss: Vol. 1. Attachment.* New York: Basic Books. (Original work published 1969)

Bowlby, J. (1988). *A secure base: Parent–child attachment and healthy human development.* London: Routledge.

Braun, M., Hales, S., Gilad, L., Mikulincer, M., Rydall, A., & Rodin, G. (2012). Caregiving styles and attachment orientations in couples facing advanced cancer. *Psycho-Oncology, 21,* 935–943.

Brennan, K. A., Clark, C. L., & Shaver, P. R. (1998). Self-report measurement of adult attachment: An integrative overview. In J. A. Simpson & W. S. Rholes (Eds.), *Attachment theory and close relationships* (pp. 46–76). New York: Guilford Press.

Bretherton, I., & Ridgeway, D. (1990). Story completion task to assess children's internal working models of child and parent in the attachment relationship. In M. T. Greenberg, D. Cicchetti, & E. M. Cummings (Eds.), *Attachment in the preschool years: Theory, research, and intervention* (pp. 300–305). Chicago: University of Chicago Press.

Bretherton, I., Ridgeway, D., & Cassidy, J. (1990). Assessing internal working models of the attachment relationship: An attachment story completion task for three-year-olds. In M. T. Greenberg, D. Cicchetti, & E. M. Cummings (Eds.), *Attachment in the preschool years: Theory, research, and intervention* (pp. 273–308). Chicago: University of Chicago Press.

Britton, P. C., & Fuendeling, J. M. (2005). The relations among varieties of adult attachment and the components of empathy. *Journal of Social Psychology, 145,* 519–530.

Brownell, C. A., Svetlova, M., Anderson, R., Nichols, S. R., & Drummond, J. (2013). Socialization of early prosocial behavior: Parents' talk about emotions is associated with sharing and helping in toddlers. *Infancy, 18*(1), 91–119.

Bryant, B. K. (1982). An index of empathy for children and adolescents. *Child Development, 53*(2), 413–425.

Bureau, J. F., & Moss, E. (2010). Behavioural precursors of attachment representations in middle childhood and links with child social adaptation. *British Journal of Developmental Psychology, 28*(3), 657–677.

Burnette, J. L., Davis, D. E., Green, J. D., Worthington, E. L., & Bradfield, E., Jr. (2009). Insecure attachment and depressive symptoms: The mediating role of rumination, empathy, and forgiveness. *Personality and Individual Differences, 46,* 276–280.

Burnette, J. L., Taylor, K., Worthington, E. L., Jr., & Forsyth, D. R. (2007). Attachment working models and trait forgivingness: The mediating role of angry rumination. *Personality and Individual Differences, 42,* 1585–1596.

Calkins, S. D., & Leerkes, E. M. (2011). Early attachment processes and the development of emotional self-regulation. In K. D. Vohs & R. F. Baumeister (Eds.), *Handbook of self-regulation: Research, theory, and applications* (2nd ed., pp. 355–373). New York: Guilford Press.

Carter, A. S., Little, C., Briggs-Gowan, M. J., & Kogan, N. (1999). The Infant–Toddler Social and Emotional Assessment (ITSEA): Comparing parent ratings to laboratory observations of task mastery, emotion regulation, coping behaviors and attachment status. *Infant Mental Health Journal, 20*(4), 375–392.

Carter, C. S. (1998). Neuroendocrine perspectives on social attachment and love. *Psychoneuroendocrinology, 23*(8), 779–818.

Cassidy, J. (1994). Emotion regulation: Influences of attachment relationships. *Monographs of the Society for Research in Child Development, 59*(2-3), 228–283.

Cassidy, J., & Asher, S. R. (1992). Loneliness and peer relations in young children. *Child Development, 63*(2), 350–365.

Cassidy, J., Shaver, P. R., Mikulincer, M., & Lavy, S. (2009). Experimentally induced security influences responses to psychological pain. *Journal of Social and Clinical Psychology, 28,* 463–478.

Chan, C. S., Rhodes, J. E., Howard, W. J., Lowe, S. R., Schwartz, S. E., & Herrera, C. (2013). Pathways of influence in school-based mentoring: The mediating role of parent and teacher relationships. *Journal of School Psychology, 51*(1), 129–142.

Chan, S. M. (2011). Social competence of elementary-school children: Relationships to maternal authoritativeness, supportive maternal responses and children's coping strategies. *Child: Care, Health and Development, 37*(4), 524–532.

Ciechanowski, P. S., Russo, J. E., Katon, W. J., & Walker, E. A. (2004). Attachment theory in health care: The influence of relationship style on medical students' specialty choice. *Medical Education, 38,* 262–270.

Clark, K. E., & Ladd, G. W. (2000). Connectedness and autonomy support in parent–child relationships: Links to children's socioemotional orientation and peer relationships. *Developmental Psychology, 36*(4), 485–498.

Clark, M. S., Greenberg, A., Hill, E., Lemay, E. P., Clark-Polner, E., & Roosth, D. (2011). Heightened interpersonal security diminishes the monetary value of possessions. *Journal of Experimental Social Psychology, 47,* 359–364.

Cobb, C. H. (1996). Adolescent–parent attachments and family problem-solving styles. *Family Process, 35*(1), 57–82.

Cohen, D., & Strayer, J. (1996). Empathy in conduct-disordered and comparison youth. *Developmental Psychology, 32*(6), 988–998.

Collins, N. L., & Feeney, B. C. (2000). A safe haven: An attachment theory perspective on support seeking and caregiving in intimate relationships. *Journal of Personality and Social Psychology, 78,* 1053–1073.

Collins, N. L., Ford, M. B., Guichard, A. C., Kane, H. S., & Feeney, B. C. (2010). Responding to need in intimate relationships: Social support and caregiving processes in couples. In M. Mikulincer & P. R. Shaver (Eds.), *Prosocial motives, emotions, and behavior: The better angels of our nature* (pp. 367–389). Washington, DC: American Psychological Association.

Collins, N. L., Guichard, A. C., Ford, M. B., & Feeney, B. C. (2006). Responding to need in intimate relationships: Normative processes and individual differences. In M. Mikulincer & G. S. Goodman (Eds.), *Dynamics of romantic love: Attachment, caregiving, and sex* (pp. 149–189). New York: Guilford Press.

Collins, N. L., & Read, S. J. (1990). Adult attachment, working models, and relationship quality in dating couples. *Journal of Personality and Social Psychology, 58,* 644–663.

Contreras, J. M., Kerns, K. A., Weimer, B. L., Gentzler, A. L., & Tomich, P. L. (2000). Emotion regulation as a mediator of associations between mother–child attachment and peer relationships in middle childhood. *Journal of Family Psychology, 14*(1), 111–124.

Cooper, M. L., Shaver, P. R., & Collins, N. L. (1998). Attachment styles, emotion regulation, and adjustment in adolescence. *Journal of Personality and Social Psychology, 74*(5), 1380–1397.

Corcoran, K. O., & Mallinckrodt, B. (2000). Adult attachment, self-efficacy, perspective taking, and conflict resolution. *Journal of Counseling and Development, 78,* 473–483.

Cui, L., Morris, A. S., Harrist, A. W., Larzelere, R. E., Criss, M. M., & Houltberg, B. J. (2015). Adolescent RSA responses during an anger discussion task: Relations to emotion regulation and adjustment. *Emotion, 15*(3), 360–372.

Cyr, C., Euser, E. M., Bakermans-Kranenburg, M. J., & Van Ijzendoorn, M. H. (2010). Attachment security and disorganization in maltreating and high-risk families: A series of meta-analyses. *Development and Psychopathology, 22*(1), 87–108.

Dalai Lama. (2001). *An open heart: Practicing compassion in everyday life* (N. Vreeland, Ed.). New York: Little, Brown.

Darley, J., & Latane, B. (1968). Bystander intervention in emergencies: Diffusion of responsibility. *Journal of Personality and Social Psychology, 8,* 377–383.

Davidov, M., & Grusec, J. E. (2006). Untangling the links of parental responsiveness to distress and warmth to child outcomes. *Child Development, 77*(1), 44–58.

Davidov, M., Zahn-Waxler, C., Roth-Hanania, R. & Knafo, A. (2013). Concern for others in the first year of life: Theory, evidence, and avenues for research. *Child Development Perspectives, 7*(2), 126–131.

Davis, M. H. (1980). A multidimensional approach to individual differences in empathy. *JSAS Catalog of Selected Documents in Psychology, 10,* 85.

Davis, M. H. (1996). *Empathy: A social psychological approach.* Boulder, CO: Westview.

Decety, J., & Jackson, P. L. (2004). The functional architecture of human empathy. *Behavioral and Cognitive Neuroscience Reviews, 3*(2), 71–100.

Decety, J., & Meyer, M. (2008). From emotion resonance to empathic understanding: A social developmental neuroscience account. *Development and Psychopathology, 20*(4), 1053–1080.

De Dreu, C. K. W. (2012). Oxytocin modulates the link between adult attachment and cooperation through reduced betrayal aversion. *Psychoneuroendocrinology*, *37*, 871–880.

De Dreu, C. K. W., Greer, L. L., Handgraaf, M. J., Shalvi, S., Van Kleef, G. A., Baas, M., et al. (2010). The neuropeptide oxytocin regulates parochial altruism in intergroup conflict among humans. *Science*, *328*, 1408–1411.

Denham, S. A., Blair, K., Schmidt, M., & DeMulder, E. (2002). Compromised emotional competence: Seeds of violence sown early? *American Journal of Orthopsychiatry*, *72*(1), 70–82.

Devine, R. T., & Hughes, C. (2013). Silent films and strange stories: Theory of mind, gender, and social experiences in middle childhood. *Child Development*, *84*(3), 989–1003.

de Waal, F. B. (2008). Putting the altruism back into altruism: The evolution of empathy. *Annual Review of Psychology*, *59*, 279–300.

DeWall, C. N., Masten, C. L., Powell, C., Combs, D., Schurtz, D. R., & Eisenberger, N. I. (2012). Do neural responses to rejection depend on attachment style?: An fMRI study. *Social Cognitive and Affective Neuroscience*, *7*, 184–192.

Drach-Zahavy, A. (2004). Toward a multidimensional construct of social support: Implications of provider's self-reliance and request characteristics. *Journal of Applied Social Psychology*, *34*, 1395–1420.

Dunfield, K. A., & Kuhlmeier, V. A. (2013). Classifying prosocial behavior: Children's responses to instrumental need, emotional distress, and material desire. *Child Development*, *84*(5), 1766–1776.

Dykas, M. J., Ziv, Y., & Cassidy, J. (2008). Attachment and peer relations in adolescence. *Attachment and Human Development*, *10*, 123–141.

Egeland, B., & Farber, E. A. (1984). Infant-mother attachment: Factors related to its development and changes over time. *Child Development*, *55* (3), 753–771.

Ein-Dor, T., Mikulincer, M., Doron, G., & Shaver, P. R. (2010). The attachment paradox: How can so many of us (the insecure ones) have no adaptive advantages? *Perspectives on Psychological Science*, *5*, 123–141.

Ein-Dor, T., Mikulincer, M., & Shaver, P. R. (2011). Attachment insecurities and the processing of threat-related information: Studying schemas involved in insecure people's coping strategies. *Journal of Personality and Social Psychology*, *101*, 78–93.

Ein-Dor, T., & Orgad, T. (2012). Scared saviors: Evidence that people high in attachment anxiety are more effective in alerting others to threat. *European Journal of Social Psychology*, *42*, 667–671.

Eisenberg, N. (2000). Emotion, regulation, and moral development. *Annual Review of Psychology*, *51*(1), 665–697.

Eisenberg, N., & Fabes, R. A. (1990). Empathy: Conceptualization, measurement, and relation to prosocial behavior. *Motivation and Emotion*, *14*(2), 131–149.

Eisenberg, N., & Fabes, R. A. (1991). Prosocial behavior and empathy: A multimethod, developmental perspective. In M. S. Clark (Ed.), *Prosocial behavior: Review of personality and social psychology* (Vol. 12, pp. 34–61). Newbury Park, CA: Sage.

Eisenberg, N., & Fabes, R. A. (1992). Emotion, regulation, and the development of social competence. In M. S. Clark (Ed.), *Emotion and social behavior: Review of personality and social psychology* (Vol. 14, pp. 119–150). Thousand Oaks, CA: Sage.

Eisenberg, N., & Fabes, R. A. (1995). The relation of young children's vicarious emotional responding to social competence, regulation, and emotionality. *Cognition and Emotion*, *9*(2–3), 203–228.

Eisenberg, N., Fabes, R. A., Carlo, G., Speer, A. L., Switzer, G., Karbon, M., et al. (1993). The relations of empathy-related emotions and maternal practices to children's comforting behavior. *Journal of Experimental Child Psychology*, *55*(2), 131–150.

Eisenberg, N., Fabes, R. A., Carlo, G., Troyer, D., Speer, A. L., Karbon, M., et al. (1992). The relations of maternal practices and characteristics to children's vicarious emotional responsiveness. *Child Development*, *63*(3), 583–602.

Eisenberg, N., Fabes, R. A., Miller, P. A., Shell, R., Shea, C., & May-Plumee, T. (1990). Preschoolers' vicarious emotional responding and their situational and dispositional prosocial behavior. *Merrill–Palmer Quarterly*, *36*(4), 507–529.

Eisenberg, N., Fabes, R. A., & Murphy, B. C. (1996). Parents' reactions to children's negative emotions: Relations to children's social competence and comforting behavior. *Child Development*, *67*(5), 2227–2247.

Eisenberg, N., Fabes, R. A., Murphy, B. [C.], Karbon, M., Smith, M., & Maszk, P. (1996). The relations of children's dispositional empathy-related responding to their emotionality, regulation, and social functioning. *Developmental Psychology*, *32*(2), 195–209.

Eisenberg, N., Fabes, R. A., Murphy, B. [C.], Maszk, P., Smith, M., & Karbon, M. (1995). The role of emotionality and regulation in children's social functioning: A longitudinal study. *Child Development*, *66*(5), 1360–1384.

Eisenberg, N., Fabes, R. A., Shepard, S. A., Murphy, B. C., Jones, S., & Guthrie, I. K. (1998). Contemporaneous and longitudinal prediction of children's sympathy from dispositional regulation and emotionality. *Developmental Psychology*, *34*(5), 910–924.

Eisenberg, N., Fabes, R. A., & Spinrad, T. L. (2006). Prosocial development. In N. Eisenberg, W. Damon, R. M. Lerner, & N. Eisenberg (Eds.), *Handbook of child psychology: Vol. 3. Social, emotional, and personality development* (6th ed., pp. 646–718). Hoboken, NJ: Wiley.

Eisenberg, N., Guthrie, I. K., Cumberland, A., Murphy, B. C., Shepard, S. A., Zhou, Q., et al. (2002). Prosocial development in early adulthood: A longitudinal study. *Journal of Personality and Social Psychology*, *82*(6), 993–1006.

Eisenberg, N., & Sulik, M. J. (2012). Emotion-related self-regulation in children. *Teaching of Psychology*, *39*(1), 77–83.

Elicker, J., Englund, M., & Sroufe, L. A. (1992). *Family–peer relationships: Modes of linkages.* Hillsdale, NJ: Erlbaum.

Emmons, R. A., & McCullough, M. E. (2003). Counting blessings versus burdens: An experimental investigation of gratitude and subjective well-being in daily life. *Journal of Personality and Social Psychology*, *84*(2), 377–389.

Erez, A., Mikulincer, M., Van IJzendoorn, M. H., & Kroonenberg, P. M. (2008). Attachment, personality, and volunteering: Placing volunteerism in an attachment–theoretical framework. *Personality and Individual Differences*, *44*, 64–74.

Fabes, R. A., Eisenberg, N., & Eisenbud, L. (1993). Behavioral and physiological correlates of children's reactions to others in distress. *Developmental Psychology*, *29*(4), 655–663.

Fabes, R. A., Eisenberg, N., Karbon, M., Troyer, D., & Switzer, G. (1994). The relations of children's emotion regulation to their vicarious emotional responses and comforting behaviors. *Child Development*, *65*(6), 1678–1693.

Feeney, B. C., & Collins, N. L. (2001). Predictors of caregiving in adult intimate relationships: An attachment theoretical perspective. *Journal of Personality and Social Psychology*, *80*(6), 972–994.

Feldman, R., Weller, A., Zagoory-Sharon, O., & Levine, A. (2007). Evidence for a neuroendocrinological foundation of human affiliation plasma oxytocin levels across pregnancy and the postpartum period predict mother–infant bonding. *Psychological Science*, *18*(11), 965–970.

Feldman, R., Zagoory-Sharon, O., Weisman, O., Schneiderman, I., Gordon, I., Maoz, R., et al. (2012). Sensitive parenting is associated with plasma oxytocin and polymorphisms in the *OXTR* and *CD38* genes. *Biological Psychiatry*, *72*(3), 175–181.

Fincham, F. D., & Beach, S. R. (2010). Marriage in the new millennium: A decade in review. *Journal of Marriage and Family*, *72*, 630–649.

Findlay, L. C., Girardi, A., & Coplan, R. J. (2006). Links between empathy, social behavior, and social understanding in early childhood. *Early Childhood Research Quarterly*, *21*(3), 347–359.

Finkel, E. J., Burnette, J. L., & Scissors, L. E. (2007). Vengefully ever after: Destiny beliefs, state attachment anxiety, and forgiveness. *Journal of Personality and Social Psychology*, *92*, 871–886.

Finkel, E. J., Rusbult, C. E., Kumashiro, M., & Hannon, P. A. (2002). Dealing with betrayal in close relationships: Does commitment promote forgiveness? *Journal of Personality and Social Psychology*, *82*, 956–974.

Fritz, H., & Helgeson, V. S. (1998). Distinctions of unmitigated communion from communion: Self-neglect and over-involvement with others. *Journal of Personality and Social Psychology*, *75*, 121–140.

Froh, J. J., Fan, J., Emmons, R. A., Bono, G., Huebner, E. S., & Watkins, P. (2011). Measuring gratitude in youth: Assessing the psychometric properties of adult gratitude scales in children and adolescents. *Psychological Assessment*, *23*(2), 311–324.

Furman, W., & Wehner, E. A. (1997). Adolescent romantic relationships: A developmental perspective. *New Directions for Child and Adolescent Development*, *78*, 21–36.

Futh, A., O'Connor, T. G., Matias, C., Green, J., & Scott, S. (2008). Attachment narratives and behavioral and emotional symptoms in an ethnically diverse, at-risk sample. *Journal of the American Academy of Child and Adolescent Psychiatry*, *47*(6), 709–718.

Galbally, M., Lewis, A. J., Van IJzendoorn, M., & Permezel, M. (2011). The role of oxytocin in mother–infant relations: A systematic review of human studies. *Harvard Review of Psychiatry*, *19*(1), 1–14.

Garner, P. W. (2006). Prediction of prosocial and emotional competence from maternal behavior in African American preschoolers. *Cultural Diversity and Ethnic Minority Psychology*, *12*(2), 179–198.

Geangu, E., Benga, O., Stahl, D., & Striano, T. (2011). Individual differences in infants' emotional resonance to a peer in distress: Self–other awareness and emotion regulation. *Social Development*, *20*(3), 450–470.

George, C., Kaplan, N., & Main, M. (1985). *Adult Attachment Interview.* Unpublished manuscript, Department of Psychology, University of California, Berkeley.

Gillath, O., Bunge, S. A., Shaver, P. R., Wendelken, C., & Mikulincer, M. (2005). Attachment-style differences and ability to suppress negative thoughts: Exploring the neural correlates. *NeuroImage*, *28*, 835–847.

Gillath, O., Shaver, P. R., & Mikulincer, M. (2005). An attachment–theoretical approach to compassion and altruism. In P. Gilbert (Ed.), *Compassion: Conceptualizations, research and use in psychotherapy* (pp. 121–147). New York: Routledge.

Gillath, O., Shaver, P. R., Mikulincer, M., Nitzberg, R. E., Erez, A., & Van IJzendoorn, M. H. (2005). Attachment, caregiving, and volunteering: Placing volunteerism in an attachment-theoretical framework. *Personal Relationships*, *12*, 425–446.

Goodman, R. (2001). Psychometric properties of the Strengths and Difficulties Questionnaire. *Journal of the American Academy of Child and Adolescent Psychiatry*, *40*(11), 1337–1345.

Gordon, K. C., Hughes, F. M., Tomcik, N. D., Dixon, L. J., & Litzinger, S. C. (2009). Widening spheres of impact: The role of forgiveness in marital and family functioning. *Journal of Family Psychology*, *23*, 1–13.

Granqvist, P., Mikulincer, M., & Shaver, P. R. (2010). Religion as attachment: Normative processes and individual differences (Special issue). *Personality and Social Psychology Review*, *14*, 49–59.

Greenberg, M. T., & Harris, A. R. (2012). Nurturing mindfulness in children and youth: Current state of research. *Child Development Perspectives*, 6(2), 161–166.

Greenberg, M. T., & Turksma, C. (2015). Understanding and watering the seeds of compassion. *Research in Human Development*, 12(3–4), 280–287.

Grusec, J. E. (1972). Demand characteristics of the modeling experiment: Altruism as a function of age and aggression. *Journal of Personality and Social Psychology*, 22(2), 139–148.

Grusec, J. E., & Goodnow, J. J. (1994). Impact of parental discipline methods on the child's internalization of values: A reconceptualization of current points of view. *Developmental Psychology*, 30(1), 4–19.

Grusec, J. E., Hastings, P. D., & Almas, A. (2011). Helping and prosocial behavior. In C. Hart & P. Smith (Eds.), *Handbook of child social development* (2nd ed., pp. 549–566). Malden, MA: Wiley-Blackwell.

Gullone, E., & Robinson, K. (2005). The Inventory of Parent and Peer Attachment—Revised (IPPA-R) for children: A psychometric investigation. *Clinical Psychology and Psychotherapy*, 12(1), 67–79.

Halifax, J. (2012). A heuristic model of active compassion. *Current Opinion in Supportive and Palliative Care*, 6, 228–235.

Hamilton, W. D. (1964). The genetical evolution of social behaviour I and II. *Journal of Theoretical Biology*, 7, 1–16, 17–52.

Hamlin, J. K., Wynn, K., & Bloom, P. (2007). Social evaluation in preverbal infants. *Nature*, 450(7169), 557–559.

Hannon, P. A., Rusbult, C. E., Finkel, E. J., & Kumashiro, M. A. (2010). In the wake of betrayal: Perpetrator amends, victim forgiveness, and the resolution of betrayal incidents. *Personal Relationships*, 17, 253–278.

Hastings, P. D., Utendale, W. T., & Sullivan, C. (2007). The socialization of prosocial development. In J. E. Grusec & P. D. Hastings (Eds.), *Handbook of socialization: Theory and research* (pp. 638–664). New York: Guilford Press.

Hawley, P. H., Shorey, H. S., & Alderman, P. M. (2009). Attachment correlates of resource-control strategies: Possible origins of social dominance and interpersonal power differentials. *Journal of Social and Personal Relationships*, 26, 1097–1118.

Hazan, C., & Shaver, P. R. (1987). Romantic love conceptualized as an attachment process. *Journal of Personality and Social Psychology*, 52, 511–524.

Hepach, R., Vaish, A., & Tomasello, M. (2013a). A new look at children's prosocial motivation. *Infancy*, 18(1), 67–90.

Hepach, R., Vaish, A., & Tomasello, M. (2013b). Young children sympathize less in response to unjustified emotional distress. *Developmental Psychology*, 49(6), 1132–1138.

Hilburn-Cobb, C. (1998). *Coding manual and scoring directions for adolescent attachment behavior, 5th revision*. Unpublished manuscript, University of Toronto.

Hilburn-Cobb, C. (2004). Adolescent psychopathology in terms of multiple behavioral systems: The role of attachment and controlling strategies and frankly disorganized behavior. In L. Atkinson & S. Goldberg, (Eds.), *Attachment issues in psychopathology and intervention* (pp. 95–135). Mahwah, NJ: Erlbaum.

Hill-Soderlund, A. L., Mills-Koonce, W. R., Propper, C., Calkins, S. D., Granger, D. A., Moore, G. A., et al. (2008). Parasympathetic and sympathetic responses to the Strange Situation in infants and mothers from avoidant and securely attached dyads. *Developmental Psychobiology*, 50(4), 361–376.

Hofer, M. A. (1994). Early relationships as regulators of infant physiology and behavior. *Acta Paediatrica Supplement*, 397, 9–18.

Hoffman, K. T. (2015a). Eighty-seven minutes: What we were never told about why we suffer and how to live with tenderness. Retrieved from *www.eightysevenminutes.com*.

Hoffman, K. T. (2015b). Taking refuge in the family of things: Exploring the nature of attachment. *The Arrow: A Journal of Wakeful Society, Culture, and Politics*, 2, 1–30.

Hoffman, K. T., Marvin, R. S., Cooper, G., & Powell, B. (2006). Changing toddlers' and preschoolers' attachment classifications: The Circle of Security intervention. *Journal of Consulting and Clinical Psychology*, 74(6), 1017–1026.

Hoffman, M. L. (1970). Conscience, personality, and socialization techniques. *Human Development*, 13(2), 90–126.

Hoffman, M. L. (1977). Empathy, its development and prosocial implications. *Nebraska Symposium on Motivation*, 25, 169–218.

Hoffman, M. L. (1984). Interaction of affect and cognition in empathy. In C. E. Izard, J. Kagan, & R. B. Zajonc (Eds.), *Emotions, cognition, and behavior* (pp. 103–131), Cambridge, UK: Cambridge University Press.

Hoffman, M. L. (2001). *Empathy and moral development: Implications for caring and justice*. Cambridge, UK: Cambridge University Press.

Horppu, R., & Ikonen-Varila, M. (2004). Mental models of attachment as a part of kindergarten student teachers' practical knowledge about caregiving. *International Journal of Early Years Education*, 12, 231–243.

Hurlemann, R., Patin, A., Onur, O. A., Cohen, M. X., Baumgartner, T., Metzler, S., et al. (2010). Oxytocin enhances amygdala-dependent, socially reinforced learning and emotional empathy in humans. *Journal of Neuroscience*, 30(14), 4999–5007.

Hutcherson, C. A., Seppala, E. M., & Gross, J. J. (2008). Loving-kindness meditation increases social connectedness. *Emotion*, 8(5), 720–724.

Iannotti, R. J., Cummings, E. M., Pierrehumbert, B., Milano, M. J., & Zahn-Waxler, C. (1992). Parental influences on prosocial behavior and empathy in early childhood. In J. Janssens & J. Gerris (Eds.), *Child rearing: Influences on prosocial and moral development* (pp. 77–100). Amsterdam: Swets & Zeitlinger.

Ickes, W. (2003). *Everyday mind reading: Understanding*

*what other people think and feel.* Amherst: Prometheus Books.

Isabella, R. A. (1993). Origins of attachment: Maternal interactive behavior across the first year. *Child Development, 64*(2), 605–621.

Johnson, S. C., Dweck, C. S., & Chen, F. S. (2007). Evidence for infants' internal working models of attachment. *Psychological Science, 18*(6), 501–502.

Johnson, S. C., Dweck, C. S., Chen, F. S., Stern, H. L., Ok, S. J., & Barth, M. (2010). At the intersection of social and cognitive development: Internal working models of attachment in infancy. *Cognitive Science, 34*(5), 807–825.

Joireman, J. A., Needham, T. L., & Cummings, A. L. (2002). Relationships between dimensions of attachment and empathy. *North American Journal of Psychology, 4*, 63–80.

Jolliffe, D., & Farrington, D. P. (2006). Development and validation of the Basic Empathy Scale. *Journal of Adolescence, 29*(4), 589–611.

Jones, J. D., Brett, B. E., Ehrlich, K. B., Lejuez, C. W., & Cassidy, J. (2014). Maternal attachment style and responses to adolescents' negative emotions: The mediating role of maternal emotion regulation. *Parenting, 14*(3–4), 235–257.

Jones, J. D., Cassidy, J., & Shaver, P. R. (2015a). Adult attachment style and parenting. In J. A. Simpson & W. S. Rholes (Eds.), *Attachment theory and research: New directions and emerging themes* (pp. 234–260). New York: Guilford Press.

Jones, J. D., Cassidy, J., & Shaver, P. R. (2015b). Parents' self-reported attachment styles: A review of links with parenting behaviors, emotions, and cognitions. *Personality and Social Psychology Review, 19*, 14–76.

Kachadourian, L. K., Fincham, F., & Davila, J. (2004). The tendency to forgive in dating and married couples: The role of attachment and relationship satisfaction. *Personal Relationships, 11*, 373–393.

Kanacri, B. L., Pastorelli, C., Eisenberg, N., Zuffianò, A., & Caprara, G. V. (2013). The development of prosociality from adolescence to early adulthood: The role of effortful control. *Journal of Personality, 81*(3), 302–312.

Kanat-Maymon, M., & Assor, A. (2010). Perceived maternal control and responsiveness to distress as predictors of young adults' empathic responses. *Personality and Social Psychology Bulletin, 36*(1), 33–46.

Karremans, J. C., & Aarts, H. (2007). The role of automaticity in the inclination to forgive close others. *Journal of Experimental Social Psychology, 43*, 902–917.

Karremans, J. C., & Van Lange, P. A. M. (2004). Back to caring after being hurt: The role of forgiveness. *European Journal of Social Psychology, 34*, 207–227.

Karremans, J. C., Van Lange, P. A. M., Ouwerkerk, J. W., & Kluwer, E. S. (2003). When forgiveness enhances psychological well-being: The influence of interpersonal commitment. *Journal of Personality and Social Psychology, 84*, 1011–1026.

Kemeny, M. E., Foltz, C., Cavanagh, J. F., Cullen, M.,

Giese-Davis, J., Jennings, P., et al. (2012). Contemplative/emotion training reduces negative emotional behavior and promotes prosocial responses. *Emotion, 12*(2), 338–350.

Kerns, K. A., Abraham, M. M., Schlegelmilch, A., & Morgan, T. A. (2007). Mother–child attachment in later middle childhood: Assessment approaches and associations with mood and emotion regulation. *Attachment and Human Development, 9*(1), 33–53.

Kerns, K. A., Klepac, L., & Cole, A. (1996). Peer relationships and preadolescents' perceptions of security in the child–mother relationship. *Developmental Psychology, 32*(3), 457–466.

Keskin, G., & Çam, O. (2010). Adolescents' strengths and difficulties: Approach to attachment styles. *Journal of Psychiatric and Mental Health Nursing, 17*(5), 433–441.

Kestenbaum, R., Farber, E. A., & Sroufe, L. A. (1989). Individual differences in empathy among preschoolers: Relation to attachment history. *New Directions for Child and Adolescent Development, 44*, 51–64.

Kim, B., Stifter, C. A., Philbrook, L. E., & Teti, D. M. (2014). Infant emotion regulation: Relations to bedtime emotional availability, attachment security, and temperament. *Infant Behavior and Development, 37*(4), 480–490.

Kim, Y., & Carver, C. S. (2007). Frequency and difficulty in caregiving among spouses of individuals with cancer: Effects of adult attachment and gender. *Psycho-Oncology, 16*, 714–728.

Kim, Y., Carver, C. S., Deci, E. L., & Kasser, T. (2008). Adult attachment and psychological well-being in cancer caregivers: The meditational role of spouses motives for caregiving. *Health Psychology, 27*, S144–S154.

Kirschner, S., & Tomasello, M. (2010). Joint music making promotes prosocial behavior in 4-year-old children. *Evolution and Human Behavior, 31*(5), 354–364.

Klagsbrun, M., & Bowlby, J. (1976). Responses to separation from the parents: A clinical test for young children. *British Journal of Projective Psychology and Personality Study, 21*, 7–27.

Klimecki, O., Leiberg, S., Richard, M., & Singer, T. (2014). Differential pattern of functional brain plasticity after compassion and empathy training. *Social Cognitive and Affective Neuroscience, 9*, 873–879.

Knafo, A., Zahn-Waxler, C., Van Hulle, C., Robinson, J. L., & Rhee, S. H. (2008). The developmental origins of a disposition toward empathy: Genetic and environmental contributions. *Emotion, 8*(6), 737–752.

Kobak, R. R., Cole, H. E., Ferenz-Gillies, R., Fleming, W. S., & Gamble, W. (1993). Attachment and emotion regulation during mother-teen problem solving: A control theory analysis. *Child Development, 64*(1), 231–245.

Kobak, R. R., & Sceery, A. (1988). Attachment in late adolescence: Working models, affect regulation, and representations of self and others. *Child Development, 59*(1), 135–146.

Kochanska, G. (1993). Toward a synthesis of parental socialization and child temperament in early development of conscience. *Child Development, 64*(2), 325–347.

Kochanska, G. (1997). Mutually responsive orientation between mothers and their young children: Implications for early socialization. *Child Development, 68*(1), 94–112.

Kochanska, G. (2002). Mutually responsive orientation between mothers and their young children: A context for the early development of conscience. *Current Directions in Psychological Science, 11*(6), 191–195.

Kochanska, G., Aksan, N., Knaack, A., & Rhines, H. M. (2004). Maternal parenting and children's conscience: Early security as moderator. *Child Development, 75*(4), 1229–1242.

Kogut, T., & Kogut, E. (2013). Exploring the relationship between adult attachment style and the identifiable victim effect in helping behavior. *Journal of Experimental Social Psychology, 49*, 651–660.

Kopp, C. B. (1989). Regulation of distress and negative emotions: A developmental view. *Developmental Psychology, 25*(3), 343–354.

Krevans, J., & Gibbs, J. C. (1996). Parents' use of inductive discipline: Relations to children's empathy and prosocial behavior. *Child Development, 67*(6), 3263–3277.

Kunce, L. J., & Shaver, P. R. (1994). An attachment-theoretical approach to caregiving in romantic relationships. In K. Bartholomew & D. Perlman (Eds.), *Attachment processes in adulthood: Advances in personal relationships* (Vol. 5, pp. 205–237). London: Jessica Kingsley.

Ladd, G. W., Birch, S. H., & Buhs, E. S. (1999). Children's social and scholastic lives in kindergarten: Related spheres of influence? *Child Development, 70*(6), 1373–1400.

Lafrenière, P. J., Provost, M. A., & Dubeau, D. (1992). From an insecure base: Parent–child relations and internalizing behaviour in the pre-school. *Early Development and Parenting, 1*(3), 137–148.

Laible, D. (2004). Mother–child discourse in two contexts: Links with child temperament, attachment security, and socioemotional competence. *Developmental Psychology, 40*(6), 979–992.

Laible, D. (2006). Maternal emotional expressiveness and attachment security: Links to representations of relationships and social behavior. *Merrill–Palmer Quarterly, 52*(4), 645–670.

Laible, D. J., Carlo, G., & Raffaelli, M. (2000). The differential relations of parent and peer attachment to adolescent adjustment. *Journal of Youth and Adolescence, 29*(1), 45–59.

Laible, D. J., & Thompson, R. A. (1998). Attachment and emotional understanding in preschool children. *Developmental Psychology, 34*(5), 1038–1045.

Lambert, N. M., Clark, M. S., Durtschi, J., Fincham, F. D., & Graham, S. M. (2010). Benefits of expressing gratitude: Expressing gratitude to a partner changes one's view of the relationship. *Psychological Science, 21*, 574–580.

Lawler-Row, K. A., Younger, J. W., Piferi, R. L., & Jones, W. H. (2006). The role of adult attachment style in forgiveness following an interpersonal offense. *Journal of Counseling and Development, 84*, 493–502.

Lazarus, R. S., & Lazarus, B. N. (1994). *Passion and reason: Making sense of our emotions.* New York: Oxford University Press.

Leerkes, E. M. (2011). Maternal sensitivity during distressing tasks: A unique predictor of attachment security. *Infant Behavior and Development, 34*(3), 443–446.

Leerkes, E. M., & Wong, M. S. (2012). Infant distress and regulatory behaviors vary as a function of attachment security regardless of emotion context and maternal involvement. *Infancy, 17*(5), 455–478.

Lehman, D. R., Ellard, J. H., & Wortman, C. B. (1986). Social support for the bereaved: Recipients' and providers' perspectives of what is helpful. *Journal of Consulting and Clinical Psychology, 54*, 438–446.

Leiberg, S., Klimecki, O., & Singer, T. (2011). Short-term compassion training increases prosocial behavior in a newly developed prosocial game. *PLoS One, 6*, e17798.

Lopez, F. G. (2001). Adult attachment orientations, self–other boundary regulation, and splitting tendencies in a college sample. *Journal of Counseling Psychology, 48*, 440–446.

Luchies, L. B., Finkel, E. J., McNulty, J. K., & Kumashiro, M. (2010). The doormat effect: When forgiving erodes self-respect and self-concept clarity. *Journal of Personality and Social Psychology, 98*, 734–749.

Lyons-Ruth, K., Bruschweiler-Stern, N., Harrison, A. M., Morgan, A. C., Nahum, J. P., Sander, L., et al. (1998). Implicit relational knowing: Its role in development and psychoanalytic treatment. *Infant Mental Health Journal, 19*, 282–289.

Maccoby, E. E. (1992). The role of parents in the socialization of children: An historical overview. *Developmental Psychology, 28*(6), 1006–1017.

MacDermott, S. T., Gullone, E., Allen, J. S., King, N. J., & Tonge, B. (2010). The Emotion Regulation Index for Children and Adolescents (ERICA): A psychometric investigation. *Journal of Psychopathology and Behavioral Assessment, 32*(3), 301–314.

MacLean, P. D. (1985). Brain evolution relating to family, play, and the separation call. *Archives of General Psychiatry, 42*, 405–417.

Main, M., & Cassidy, J. (1988). Categories of response to reunion with the parent at age 6: Predictable from infant attachment classifications and stable over a 1-month period. *Developmental Psychology, 24*(3), 415–426.

Main, M., & George, C. (1985). Responses of abused and disadvantaged toddlers to distress in agemates: A study in the day care setting. *Developmental Psychology, 21*(3), 407–412.

Markiewicz, D., Doyle, A. B., & Brendgen, M. (2001). The quality of adolescents' friendships: Associations with mothers' interpersonal relationships, attachments to parents and friends, and prosocial behaviors. *Journal of Adolescence, 24*(4), 429–445.

McCullough, M. E. (2000). Forgiveness as human strength: Theory, measurement, and links to wellbeing. *Journal of Social and Clinical Psychology, 19*, 43–55.

McCullough, M. E., Worthington, E. L., & Rachal, K. C. (1997). Interpersonal forgiving in close relationships. *Journal of Personality and Social Psychology, 73*, 321–336.

McKinney, K. G. (2002). Engagement in community service among college students: Is it affected by significant attachment relationships? *Journal of Adolescence, 25*, 139–154.

Michiels, D., Grietens, H., Onghena, P., & Kuppens, S. (2010). Perceptions of maternal and paternal attachment security in middle childhood: Links with positive parental affection and psychosocial adjustment. *Early Child Development and Care, 180*(1–2), 211–225.

Mikulincer, M., Gillath, O., Halevy, V., Avihou, N., Avidan, S., & Eshkoli, N. (2001). Attachment theory and reactions to others' needs: Evidence that activation of the sense of attachment security promotes empathic responses. *Journal of Personality and Social Psychology, 81*, 1205–1224.

Mikulincer, M., Gillath, O., Sapir-Lavid, Y., Yaakobi, E., Arias, K., Tal-Aloni, L., et al. (2003). Attachment theory and concern for others' welfare: Evidence that activation of the sense of secure base promotes endorsement of self-transcendence values. *Basic and Applied Social Psychology, 25*, 299–312.

Mikulincer, M., & Orbach, I. (1995). Attachment styles and repressive defensiveness: The accessibility and architecture of affective memories. *Journal of Personality and Social Psychology, 68*, 917–925.

Mikulincer, M., & Shaver, P. R. (2001). Attachment theory and intergroup bias: Evidence that priming the secure base schema attenuates negative reactions to out-groups. *Journal of Personality and Social Psychology, 81*(1), 97–115.

Mikulincer, M., & Shaver, P. R. (2005). Attachment security, compassion, and altruism. *Current Directions in Psychological Science, 14*(1), 34–38.

Mikulincer, M., & Shaver, P. R. (2007a). *Attachment in adulthood: Structure, dynamics, and change.* New York: Guilford Press.

Mikulincer, M., & Shaver, P. R. (2007b). Boosting attachment security to promote mental health, prosocial values, and inter-group tolerance. *Psychological Inquiry, 18*(3), 139–156.

Mikulincer, M., & Shaver, P. R. (2007c). Reflections on security dynamics: Core constructs, psychological mechanisms, relational contexts, and the need for an integrative theory. *Psychological Inquiry, 18*, 197–209.

Mikulincer, M., & Shaver, P. R. (2009). An attachment and behavioral systems perspective on social support (Special issue). *Journal of Social and Personal Relationships, 26*, 7–19.

Mikulincer, M., & Shaver, P. R. (Eds.). (2010). *Prosocial motives, emotions, and behavior: The better angels of our nature.* Washington, DC: American Psychological Association.

Mikulincer, M., & Shaver, P. R. (Eds.). (2012). *The social psychology of morality: Exploring the causes of good and evil.* Washington, DC: American Psychological Association.

Mikulincer, M., Shaver, P. R., & Gillath, O. (2008). A behavioral systems perspective on compassionate love. In B. Fehr, S. Sprecher, & L. G. Underwood (Eds.), *The science of compassionate love: Theory, research, and applications* (pp. 225–256). Malden, MA: Wiley-Blackwell.

Mikulincer, M., Shaver, P. R., Gillath, O., & Nitzberg, R. E. (2005). Attachment, caregiving, and altruism: Boosting attachment security increases compassion and helping. *Journal of Personality and Social Psychology, 89*, 817–839.

Mikulincer, M., Shaver, P. R., & Pereg, D. (2003). Attachment theory and affect regulation: The dynamics, development, and cognitive consequences of attachment-related strategies. *Motivation and Emotion, 27*(2), 77–102.

Mikulincer, M., Shaver, P. R., Sahdra, B. K., & Bar-On, N. (2013). Can security-enhancing interventions overcome psychological barriers to responsiveness in couple relationships? *Attachment and Human Development, 15*, 246–260.

Mikulincer, M., Shaver, P. R., & Slav, K. (2006). Attachment, mental representations of others, and gratitude and forgiveness in romantic relationships. In M. Mikulincer & G. S. Goodman (Eds.), *Dynamics of romantic love: Attachment, caregiving, and sex* (pp. 190–215). New York: Guilford Press.

Miller, W. (2009). *Everyday dharma.* Wheaton: Quest Books.

Miller, W. (2015, June). *Devotion as a doorway to existential trust: Rethinking devotion in light of attachment theory.* Invited lecture at the Mind and Life Summer Research Institute, Garrison, NY.

Mipham, S. (2013). *The Shambhala principle: Discovering humanity's hidden treasure.* New York: Harmony Books.

Mitchell-Copeland, J., Denham, S. A., & DeMulder, E. K. (1997). Q-sort assessment of child–teacher attachment relationships and social competence in the preschool. *Early Education and Development, 8*(1), 27–39.

Monin, J. K., Schulz, R., Feeney, B. C., & Clark, T. B. (2010). Attachment insecurity and perceived partner suffering as predictors of caregiver distress. *Journal of Experimental Social Psychology, 46*, 1143–1147.

Murphy, B. C., Eisenberg, N., Fabes, R. A., Shepard, S., & Guthrie, I. K. (1999). Consistency and change in children's emotionality and regulation: A longitudinal study. *Merrill–Palmer Quarterly, 45*(3), 413–444.

Murphy, T. P., & Laible, D. J. (2013). The influence of attachment security on preschool children's empathic concern. *International Journal of Behavioral Development*, *37*(5), 436–440.

Nachmias, M., Gunnar, M., Mangelsdorf, S., Parritz, R. H., & Buss, K. (1996). Behavioral inhibition and stress reactivity: The moderating role of attachment security. *Child Development, 67*(2), 508–522.

Nhat Hanh, T. (2014). *No mud, no lotus: The art of transforming suffering.* Berkeley, CA: Parallel Press.

Oldfield, J., Humphrey, N., & Hebron, J. (2015). The role of parental and peer attachment relationships and school connectedness in predicting adolescent mental health outcomes. *Child and Adolescent Mental Health.* [Epub ahead of print]

Oppenheim, D., Koren-Karie, N., & Sagi, A. (2001). Mother's empathic understanding of their preschoolers' internal experience: Relations with early attachment. *International Journal of Behavioral Development, 25*, 16–26.

Over, H., & Carpenter, M. (2009). Eighteen-month-old infants show increased helping following priming with affiliation. *Psychological Science, 20*(10), 1189–1193.

Panfile, T. M., & Laible, D. J. (2012). Attachment security and child's empathy: The mediating role of emotion regulation. *Merrill–Palmer Quarterly, 58*(1), 1–21.

Paulus, M., Kühn-Popp, N., Licata, M., Sodian, B., & Meinhardt, J. (2013). Neural correlates of prosocial behavior in infancy: Different neurophysiological mechanisms support the emergence of helping and comforting. *NeuroImage, 66*, 522–530.

Paus, T. (2009). Brain development. In R. M. Lerner & L. Steinberg (Eds.), *Handbook of adolescent psychology: Vol. 1. Individual bases of adolescent development* (3rd ed., pp. 95–115). Hoboken, NJ: Wiley.

Perry, D. G., Bussey, K., & Freiberg, K. (1981). Impact of adults' appeals for sharing on the development of altruistic dispositions in children. *Journal of Experimental Child Psychology, 32*(1), 127–138.

Peterson, C., & Seligman, M. E. P. (2004). *Character strengths and virtues: A handbook and classification.* New York: Oxford University Press.

Piaget, J. (1972). Intellectual evolution from adolescence to adulthood. *Human Development, 15*(1), 1–12.

Piekny, J., & Maehler, C. (2013). Scientific reasoning in early and middle childhood: The development of domain-general evidence evaluation, experimentation, and hypothesis generation skills. *British Journal of Developmental Psychology, 31*(2), 153–179.

Plötner, M., Over, H., Carpenter, M., & Tomasello, M. (2015). Young children show the bystander effect in helping situations. *Psychological Science, 26*(4), 499–506.

Radke-Yarrow, M., & Zahn-Waxler, C. (1984). Roots, motives, and patterns in children's prosocial behavior. In E. Staub, D. Bar-Tal, J. Karylowski, & J. Reykowski (Eds.), *Development and maintenance of prosocial behavior: International perspectives on positive behavior* (pp. 81–99). New York: Plenum Press.

Raikes, H. A., & Thompson, R. A. (2006). Family emotional climate, attachment security and young children's emotion knowledge in a high risk sample. *British Journal of Developmental Psychology, 24*(1), 89–104.

Rehberg, H. R., & Richman, C. L. (1989). Prosocial behaviour in preschool children: A look at the interaction of race, gender, and family composition. *International Journal of Behavioral Development, 12*(3), 385–401.

Richman, C. L., Berry, C., Bittle, M., & Himan, K. (1988). Factors related to helping behavior in preschool-age children. *Journal of Applied Developmental Psychology, 9*(2), 151–165.

Richman, S. B., DeWall, C. N., & Wolff, M. N. (2015). Avoiding affection, avoiding altruism: Why is avoidant attachment related to less helping?. *Personality and Individual Differences, 76*, 193–197.

Roney, A., Meredith, P., & Strong, J. (2004). Attachment styles and factors affecting career choice of occupational therapy students. *British Journal of Occupational Therapy, 67*, 133–141.

Rothbart, M. K., Ahadi, S. A., & Hershey, K. L. (1994). Temperament and social behavior in childhood. *Merrill–Palmer Quarterly, 40*(1), 21–39.

Rothbart, M. K., Sheese, B. E., Rueda, M. R., & Posner, M. I. (2011). Developing mechanisms of self-regulation in early life. *Emotion Review, 3*(2), 207–213.

Roth-Hanania, R., Davidov, M., & Zahn-Waxler, C. (2011). Empathy development from 8 to 16 months: Early signs of concern for others. *Infant Behavior and Development, 34*(3), 447–458.

Rusbult, C. E., Verette, J., Whitney, G. A., Slovik, L. F., & Lipkus, I. (1991). Accommodation processes in close relationships: Theory and preliminary empirical evidence. *Journal of Personality and Social Psychology, 60*, 53–78.

Rushton, J. P. (1975). Generosity in children: Immediate and long-term effects of modeling, preaching, and moral judgment. *Journal of Personality and Social Psychology, 31*(3), 459–466.

Rydell, A. M., Bohlin, G., & Thorell, L. B. (2005). Representations of attachment to parents and shyness as predictors of children's relationships with teachers and peer competence in preschool. *Attachment and Human Development, 7*(2), 187–204.

Schaller, M., & Cialdini, R. B. (1988). The economics of empathic helping: Support for a mood management motive. *Journal of Experimental Social Psychology, 24*, 163–181.

Schore, A. N. (2000). Attachment and the regulation of the right brain. *Attachment and Human Development, 2*(1), 23–47.

Seibert, A., & Kerns, K. (2015). Early mother–child attachment: Longitudinal prediction to the quality of peer relationships in middle childhood. *International Journal of Behavioral Development, 39*(2), 130–138.

Shaver, P. R., & Hazan, C. (1988). A biased overview of the study of love. *Journal of Social and Personal Relationships, 5*, 473–501.

Shaver, P. R., & Hazan, C. (1993). Adult romantic attachment: Theory and evidence. In D. Perlman & W. Jones (Eds.), *Advances in personal relationships* (Vol. 4, pp. 29–70). London, England: Jessica Kingsley.

Shaver, P. R., Mikulincer, M., & Shemesh-Iron, M. (2010). A behavioral systems perspective on prosocial behavior. In M. Mikulincer & P. R. Shaver (Eds.), *Prosocial motives, emotions, and behavior: The better angels of our nature* (pp. 73–91). Washington, DC: American Psychological Association.

Shaver, P. R., Papalia, D., Clark, C. L., Koski, L. R., Tidwell, M., & Nalbone, D. (1996). Androgyny and attachment security: Two related models of optimal personality. *Personality and Social Psychology Bulletin, 22,* 582–597.

Sherman, L. J., Stupica, B., Dykas, M. J., Ramos-Marcuse, F., & Cassidy, J. (2013). The development of negative reactivity in irritable newborns as a function of attachment. *Infant Behavior and Development, 36*(1), 139–146.

Shulman, S., Elicker, J., & Sroufe, L. A. (1994). Stages of friendship growth in preadolescence as related to attachment history. *Journal of Social and Personal Relationships, 11*(3), 341–361.

Siegel, R., & Germer, C. (2012). Wisdom and compassion: Two wings of a bird. In C. K. Germer & R. D. Siegel (Eds.), *Wisdom and compassion in psychotherapy* (pp. 7–35). New York: Guilford Press.

Slough, N. M., & Greenberg, M. T. (1990). Five-year-olds' representations of separation from parents: Responses from the perspective of self and other. *New Directions for Child Development, 48,* 67–84.

Smith, K. D., Keating, J. P., & Stotland, E. (1989). Altruism revisited: The effect of denying feedback on a victim's status to an empathic witness. *Journal of Personality and Social Psychology, 57,* 641–650.

Snyder, C. R., & McCullough, M. E. (2000). A positive psychology field of dreams: "If you build it, they will come. . . . " *Journal of Social and Clinical Psychology, 19,* 151–160.

Sommerfeld, E. (2009). The subjective experience of generosity. In M. Mikulincer & P. R. Shaver (Eds.), *Prosocial motives, emotions, and behavior: The better angels of our nature* (pp. 303–323). Washington, DC: American Psychological Association.

Sroufe, L. A. (1983). Infant–caregiver attachment and patterns of adaptation in preschool: The roots of maladaptation and competence. In M. Perlmutter (Ed.), *Development and policy concerning children with special needs: The Minnesota Symposia on Child Psychology* (Vol. 16, pp. 41–79). Hillsdale, NJ: Erlbaum.

Sroufe, L. A. (1996). *Emotional development: The organization of emotional development in the early years.* New York: Cambridge University Press.

Sroufe, L. A. (2000). Early relationships and the development of children. *Infant Mental Health Journal, 21*(1–2), 67–74.

Sroufe, L. A. (2005). Attachment and development: A prospective, longitudinal study from birth to adulthood. *Attachment and Human Development, 7*(4), 349–367.

Sroufe, L. A., & Fleeson, J. (1986). Attachment and the construction of relationships. In W. Hartup & Z. Rubin (Eds.), *Relationships and development* (pp. 51–71). Hillsdale, NJ: Erlbaum.

Stern, J. A., Borelli, J. L., & Smiley, P. A. (2015). Assessing parental empathy: A role for empathy in child attachment. *Attachment and Human Development, 17*(1), 1–22.

Taylor, Z. E., Eisenberg, N., & Spinrad, T. L. (2015). Respiratory sinus arrhythmia, effortful control, and parenting as predictors of children's sympathy across early childhood. *Developmental Psychology, 51*(1), 17–25.

Taylor, Z. E., Eisenberg, N., Spinrad, T. L., Eggum, N. D., & Sulik, M. J. (2013). The relations of ego-resiliency and emotion socialization to the development of empathy and prosocial behavior across early childhood. *Emotion, 13*(5), 822–831.

Teti, D. M., & Ablard, K. E. (1989). Security of attachment and infant–sibling relationships: A laboratory study. *Child Development, 60*(6), 1519–1528.

Teti, D. M., Gelfand, D. M., Messinger, D. S., & Isabella, R. (1995). Maternal depression and the quality of early attachment: an examination of infants, preschoolers, and their mothers. *Developmental Psychology, 31*(3), 364–376.

Thompson, K. L., & Gullone, E. (2008). Prosocial and antisocial behaviors in adolescents: An investigation into associations with attachment and empathy. *Anthrozoös, 21*(2), 123–137.

Thompson, R. A. (1994). Emotion regulation: A theme in search of definition. *Monographs of the Society for Research in Child Development, 59*(2–3), 25–52.

Trommsdorff, G., Friedlmeier, W., & Mayer, B. (2007). Sympathy, distress, and prosocial behavior of preschool children in four cultures. *International Journal of Behavioral Development, 31*(3), 284–293.

Trusty, J., Ng, K. M., & Watts, R. E. (2005). Model of effects of adult attachment on emotional empathy of counseling students. *Journal of Counseling and Development, 83,* 66–77.

Tsang, J. (2006). Gratitude and prosocial behavior: An experimental test of gratitude. *Cognition and Emotion, 20,* 138–148.

Vaish, A., Carpenter, M., & Tomasello, M. (2009). Sympathy through affective perspective taking and its relation to prosocial behavior in toddlers. *Developmental Psychology, 45*(2), 534–543.

van den Boom, D. C. (1994). The influence of temperament and mothering on attachment and exploration: an experimental manipulation of sensitive responsiveness among lower-class mothers with irritable infants. *Child Development, 65,* 1457–1477.

van der Mark, I. L., Van IJzendoorn, M. H., & Bakermans-Kranenburg, M. J. (2002). Development of empathy in girls during the second year of life: Associations with parenting, attachment, and temperament. *Social Development, 11*(4), 451–468.

Van IJzendoorn, M. H., Schuengel, C., & Bakermans–Kranenburg, M. J. (1999). Disorganized attachment in early childhood: Meta-analysis of precursors, concomitants, and sequelae. *Development and Psychopathology, 11*(02), 225–250.

Van IJzendoorn, M. H., & Zwart-Woudstra, H. A. (1995). Adolescents' attachment representations and moral reasoning. *Journal of Genetic Psychology, 156*, 359–372.

Van Lange, P. A. M., DeBruin, E. M. N., Otten, W., & Joireman, J. A. (1997). Development of prosocial, individualistic, and competitive orientations: Theory and preliminary evidence. *Journal of Personality and Social Psychology, 73*, 733–746.

Viddal, K. R., Berg-Nielsen, T. S., Wan, M. W., Green, J., Hygen, B. W., & Wichstrøm, L. (2015). Secure attachment promotes the development of effortful control in boys. *Attachment and Human Development, 17*(3), 319–335.

Vilchinsky, N., Findler, L., & Werner, S. (2010). Attitudes toward people with disabilities: The perspective of attachment theory. *Rehabilitation Psychology, 55*, 298–306.

Volling, B. L. (2001). Early attachment relationships as predictors of preschool children's emotion regulation with a distressed sibling. *Early Education and Development, 12*(2), 185–207.

Volling, B. L., & Belsky, J. (1992). The contribution of mother–child and father–child relationships to the quality of sibling interaction: A longitudinal study. *Child Development, 63*(5), 1209–1222.

Warneken, F., & Tomasello, M. (2006). Altruistic helping in human infants and young chimpanzees. *Science, 311*, 1301–1303.

Warneken, F., & Tomasello, M. (2009). The roots of human altruism. *British Journal of Psychology, 100*(3), 455–471.

Waters, E., & Deane, K. E. (1985). Defining and assessing individual differences in attachment relationships: Q-methodology and the organization of behavior in infancy and early childhood. *Monographs of the Society for Research in Child Development, 50*(1–2), 41–65.

Waters, E., Wippman, J., & Sroufe, L. A. (1979). Attachment, positive affect, and competence in the peer group: Two studies in construct validation. *Child Development, 50*(3), 821–829.

Waters, H. S., & Waters, E. (2006). The attachment working models concept: Among other things, we build script-like representations of secure base experiences. *Attachment and Human Development, 8*(3), 185–197.

Watkins, P. C., Woodward, K., Stone, T., & Kolts, R. L. (2003). Gratitude and happiness: Development of a measure of gratitude, and relationships with subjective well-being. *Social Behavior and Personality, 31*, 431–452.

Wayment, H. A. (2006). Attachment style, empathy, and helping following a collective loss: Evidence from the September 11 terrorist attack. *Attachment and Human Development, 8*(1), 1–9.

Weger, H., Jr., & Polcar, L. E. (2002). Attachment style and person-centered comforting. *Western Journal of Communication, 66*, 84–103.

Weiner, B. (1985). An attributional theory of achievement motivation and emotion. *Psychological Review, 92*, 548–573.

Wentzel, K. R. (2003). Sociometric status and adjustment in middle school: A longitudinal study. *Journal of Early Adolescence, 23*(1), 5–28.

Westmaas, J., & Silver, R. C. (2001). The role of attachment in responses to victims of life crises. *Journal of Personality and Social Psychology, 80*, 425–438.

Yárnoz-Yaben, S. (2009). Forgiveness, attachment, and divorce. *Journal of Divorce and Remarriage, 50*, 282–294.

You, S., Lee, J., Lee, Y., & Kim, A. Y. (2015). Bullying among Korean adolescents: The role of empathy and attachment. *Psychology in the Schools, 52*(6), 594–606.

Young, L. J., & Wang, Z. (2004). The neurobiology of pair bonding. *Nature Neuroscience, 7*(10), 1048–1054.

Zahn-Waxler, C., Radke-Yarrow, M., & King, R. A. (1979). Child rearing and children's prosocial initiations toward victims of distress. *Child Development, 50*(2), 319–330.

Zahn-Waxler, C., Radke-Yarrow, M., Wagner, E., & Chapman, M. (1992). Development of concern for others. *Developmental Psychology, 28*(1), 126–136.

Zahn-Waxler, C., Robinson, J. L., & Emde, R. N. (1992). The development of empathy in twins. *Developmental Psychology, 28*(6), 1038–1047.

Zak, P. J., & Stanton, A. A., & Ahmadi, S. (2007). Oxytocin increases generosity in humans. *PLoS One, 2*(11), e1128.

Zimmermann, P., Maier, M. A., Winter, M., & Grossmann, K. E. (2001). Attachment and adolescents' emotion regulation during a joint problem-solving task with a friend. *International Journal of Behavioral Development, 25*(4), 331–343.

Zuroff, D. C., Moskowitz, D. S., & Cote, S. (1999). Dependency, self-criticism, interpersonal behavior and affect: Evolutionary perspectives. *British Journal of Clinical Psychology, 38*, 231–250.

# Chapter 39

# Attachment and Religious Representations and Behavior

Pehr Granqvist
Lee A. Kirkpatrick

In my hour of darkness, in my time of need,
Oh, Lord grant me vision.
Oh, Lord grant me speed.
—Gram Parsons, "In My Hour of Darkness,"
*Grievous Angel* (1974)

Although Bowlby's theorizing about attachment focused largely on the evolutionary origins of the attachment system and its manifestation in infant–mother relationships, he clearly believed from the beginning that the processes and dynamics of attachment have broad implications for social development and psychological functioning across the lifespan. In this chapter we argue that with increased cognitive maturation, people can and do develop attachments to unseen figures (e.g., God). More specifically, we argue that some core aspects of religious beliefs and behavior are interpretable in terms of attachment dynamics.

Serious attachment scholars are well aware of the dangers inherent in extending the theory beyond its valid limits. Bowlby's choice of the term *attachment* was in one sense unfortunate because of the word's much broader meaning in everyday language: People speak of feeling *attached* to many things in their lives, from important possessions (cars, smartphones), to locations (home), to social groups, to sports teams, to rock stars. In our view, such phenomena can typically not be understood properly in terms of attachment, as defined by Bowlby. Nevertheless, we argue that some core as-

pects of religious belief and behavior represent real manifestations of attachment processes that may, in fact, provide a unique window into attachment processes in adulthood.[1]

This chapter is divided into five major sections. In the first, we argue that people's perceived relationships with God meet the defining criteria of attachment relationships reasonably well, and hence function psychologically much as other attachments do. We examine in the second section lifespan maturational issues involved in the development of attachment and religion. These first two sections deal with normative/typical aspects of the attachment–religion connection. In the third section, we review empirical connections between religion and individual differences in attachment. This section is subdivided into two subsections—the first focusing on a "compensation" pathway and the second describing a "correspondence" pathway to religion. We address in the fourth major section research findings and implications of the religion-as-attachment model with respect to psychological outcomes. In the final major section, which is new to this edition, we address the current state of theory and research on the attachment–religion connection.

## Believers' Perceived Relationships with God in Relation to the Criteria for an Attachment Relationship

The obvious starting point for the application of attachment theory to religion is the observation that central to monotheistic religions, particularly Christianity, is the belief in a personal God with whom believers maintain a personal, interactive relationship. The word *religion* stems from the Latin *religare* or *relegere*, which means "being bound" (see Ferm, 1945). This relationship connotation has a clear counterpart in how people evaluate their own faith. For example, when asked, "Which of the following four statements comes closest to your own view of 'faith': a set of beliefs, membership in a church or synagogue, finding meaning in life, or a relationship with God?," a majority of people in a national (U.S.) Gallup sample chose "a relationship with God" (compared to notably lower proportions for the other alternatives; Gallup & Jones, 1989).

It is also important to note that other supernatural figures may fill this relationship role in addition to or instead of "God." In many Christian traditions, it is Jesus with whom one maintains an active day-to-day relationship, while "God the Father" remains a more distant background figure. In Roman Catholicism, Mary typically represents the "maternal functions" related to attachment (Wenegrat, 1989). Outside Christianity, the worlds of different groups of believers are populated by a variety of gods and other deities, some (but by no means all) of whom function as attachment figures. Even in countries dominated by Eastern religions such as Hinduism and Buddhism, which Westerners may think of as godless philosophies, believers often focus on the more theistic components of the belief system and on personal gods imported from ancient folk religions (e.g., Kirkpatrick, 1994). In this chapter, we refer to "God" as an attachment figure, but it should be understood that in many cases another supernatural figure may fill this role.

A second point of departure for discussing an attachment–religion connection is the centrality of the emotion of love in people's perceived relationships with God and in religious belief systems more generally. The powerful emotional experiences associated with religion are often expressed "in the language of human love," particularly in the writing of mystics (Thouless, 1923, p. 132). Similarly, the process of religious conversion has been likened frequently, by both scholars and religious writers, to falling in love (James, 1902; Thouless, 1923; Ullman, 1982).

The "love" experienced by a worshipper in the context of a relationship with God is, of course, qualitatively different from that experienced in adult romantic relationships; the latter typically includes sexuality, whereas the former usually does not. The form of "love" experienced in the context of a relationship with God resembles more closely the prototypical attachment of a child to his or her mother. In Greeley's (1990, p. 252) words, "The Mary Myth's powerful appeal is to be found . . . in the marvelous possibility that God loves us the way a mother loves her baby."

The idea that God is experienced psychologically as a kind of parental figure is, of course, hardly new. The most familiar version of this idea is Freud's (e.g., 1927/1961) characterization of God as an "exalted father figure" (but see Granqvist, 2006). Wenegrat (1989), however, observed that the deities of the oldest known religions were largely maternal figures. Whether images of God more closely resemble maternal or paternal images has been a topic of much empirical research in the psychology of religion, with decidedly mixed results (e.g., Hood, Hill, & Spilka, 2009). The most reasonable conclusion from this research seems to be that images of God combine elements of both stereotypically maternal and paternal qualities (Vergote & Tamayo, 1981): God is neither an exalted father nor a mother figure but rather an "exalted attachment figure."

There is considerable evidence to support the notion that believers view God as a kind of exalted attachment figure (AF). One line of suggestive evidence comes from religious writings and songs, perhaps most notably in the Psalms (Wenegrat, 1989). God seems clearly to capture the essence of the protective other that a parent represents to a child. As summarized by the theologian Kaufman (1981, p. 67), "The idea of God is the idea of an absolutely adequate attachment-figure. . . . God is thought of as a protective and caring parent who is always reliable and always available to its children when they are in need."

Similarly, factor-analytic studies of God images consistently find a large first factor laden with attachment-related descriptors (see Hood et al., 2009). For example, Gorsuch's (1968) first factor (labeled "benevolent deity") included descriptors such as "comforting," "loving," and "protective," and the reverse of "distant" and "inaccessible."

In summary, there are several notable parallels between religious belief and experience on the one hand, and attachment relationships on the other. Below, we argue, using Ainsworth's (1985) and Bowlby's (1969/1982) criteria for distinguishing attachments from other types of relationships, that these resemblances are more than interesting analogies and in fact reflect genuine attachment processes.

## Seeking and Maintaining Proximity to God

The biological function of the attachment system, as described by Bowlby (1969/1982), is the maintenance of proximity between an infant and a protective AF. To obtain physical proximity, infants engage in behaviors such as crying, raising arms, and clinging (however, see below for maturational considerations).

Religions provide various ways of enhancing perceptions about the proximity of God. A crucial tenet of most theistic religions is that God is omnipresent; one is always in "proximity" to God. God is frequently described in religious literature as always being by one's side, holding one's hand, or watching over one. Nevertheless, other, more concrete cues may be valuable in enhancing perceptions of proximity to God. For example, virtually all religions provide places of worship where one can go to be closer to God. In addition, a diverse array of idols and symbols (e.g., graven images, crosses on necklaces, paintings) seem designed to remind the believer continually of God's presence.

The most important form of proximity-maintaining behavior directed toward God is prayer (Reed, 1978), which is not coincidentally also "the most often practiced form of religiosity" (Trier & Shupe, 1991, p. 354). Among the major forms of prayer reviewed in the comprehensive psychology-of-religion text by Hood, Spilka, Hunsberger, and Gorsuch (1996, pp. 394ff.), two seem clearly related to proximity maintenance: "contemplative" prayer ("an attempt to relate deeply to one's God") and "meditational" prayer ("concern with one's relationship to God"). Prayer seems analogous to social referencing (Campos & Stenberg, 1981; cf. secure base behaviors) in children; an intermittent checking back to make sure the AF is accessible.

## God as a Safe Haven

A second defining aspect of attachment is that an AF serves as a safe haven in times of potential danger, which fulfills the evolutionary function of protecting otherwise defenseless infants from danger.

Bowlby (1969/1982) discussed three sets of natural clues to danger that activate the attachment system and elicit attachment behavior: (1) frightening/alarming environmental events; (2) illness, injury, fatigue; and (3) separation (or threat thereof) from AFs.

As Freud (1927/1961) and many others have long speculated, religion does appear to be rooted at least partly in needs for protection and felt security. Although to be taken with a grain of salt (see Granqvist & Moström, 2014), as the adage goes, there are no atheists in foxholes. Hood and colleagues (1996, pp. 386–387) concluded that people are most likely to "turn to their gods in times of trouble and crisis," listing three general classes of potential triggers: "illness, disability, and other negative life events that cause both mental and physical distress; the anticipated or actual death of friends and relatives; and dealing with an adverse life situation." This list bears a striking resemblance to Bowlby's (1969/1982) discussion of factors postulated to activate the attachment system.

Considerable evidence supports the view that people turn to religion particularly in times of distress and crisis, and it is important to note that they primarily turn at such times to prayer—a form of religious attachment behavior—rather than to church (Argyle & Beit-Hallahmi, 1975). Pargament (1997) has outlined various religious coping strategies that people have employed in stressful situations, including attachment-like responses such as "experienced God's love and care" and "took control over what I could and gave up the rest to God." Furthermore, research undertaken within a coping framework has documented that religious individuals are inclined to turn to God particularly when faced with threats (e.g., danger) and loss (e.g., death of a loved one; e.g., Bjorck & Cohen, 1993).

### Frightening or Alarming Events

With respect to environmental stressors, empirical research suggests that there are indeed few atheists in some foxholes: Combat soldiers do pray frequently (Stouffer, 1949). From his interviews with combat veterans, Allport (1950, p. 57) concluded: "The individual in distress craves affection and security. Sometimes a human bond will suffice, more often it will not." As one combat veteran reported to Allport, "There were atheists in foxholes, but most of them were in love" (p. 56).

Although warfare provides an extreme example, other kinds of severe stressors can lead to emotional crises in which other AFs may be perceived as inadequate. A century of research supports the claim that sudden religious conversions are most likely during times of severe emotional distress and crisis (e.g., Galanter, 1979; James, 1902; Starbuck, 1899; Ullman, 1982). According to James (1902), the climax of the crisis-driven conversion process comes when one surrenders oneself to God and places one's problems in God's hands. Hence, even individuals who did not experience a relationship with God prior to a crisis may come to do so if sufficiently distressed. It is also noteworthy that the source of the distress precipitating religious conversions is often relationship-related; in our own studies, relationship problems with parents and romantic partners have been frequently cited (Granqvist, 1998; Kirkpatrick & Shaver, 1990).

Moreover, experimental studies suggest that appraisal of threat does not require conscious processing to result in increased God-related cognitions (Birgegard & Granqvist, 2004; Granqvist, Mikulincer, Gewirtz, & Shaver, 2012). For example, in a recent study explicitly set up to test the religion-as-attachment model in a Jewish sample of Israeli college students, participants showed a greater psychological accessibility of God (or the concept of God) following subliminal exposure to threats (i.e., failure and death) compared to neutral material (Granqvist, Mikulincer, et al., 2012).

### Illness, Injury, and Fatigue

Several studies show prayer to be an especially common method of coping with serious physical illnesses of various types (e.g., for reviews, see Koenig, King, & Carson, 2012; Pargament, 1997). For example, O'Brien (1982) observed in his interviews with patients experiencing renal failure that many of them saw God as providing comfort, nurturance, and a source of personal strength for getting through this difficult time. Other studies have shown religion to be particularly helpful to people in coping with *chronic* illness (Mattlin, Wethington, & Kessler, 1990).

### Separation and Loss

Research also suggests that religiousness and prayer tend to increase following the death of or (threat of) separation from loved ones, and that religious beliefs are correlated positively with successful coping at these times (e.g., Loveland, 1968; Parkes, 1972). Relevant research has focused

mostly on effects of spousal separation/bereavement (i.e., the ending of the principal attachment relationship in adulthood). Loss of a principal AF is a particularly powerful stressor: Not only is it a stressful event in itself but it also eliminates the availability of the person to whom one would otherwise turn for support in a stressful situation.

We (Granqvist, 1998; Kirkpatrick & Shaver, 1990) have observed that the crises reported retrospectively by religious converts often involved relationship-focused difficulties including loss of or separation from AFs, particularly through relationship breakups and divorce. Similarly, in a prospective study using a population-based sample of older adults—some of whom were destined to suffer bereavement during the course of the study and others who were not—Brown, Nesse, House, and Utz (2004) found a prospective increase in the importance of the religious beliefs for the bereaved compared to the nonbereaved, and specifically as a function of the bereavement. This study also showed that grief over the loss decreased specifically as a function of the increased significance of the bereaved individual's religious beliefs, indicating that the attachment component of the individual's religiousness may be what is activated in such situations and contributes to a more favorable outcome.

In a controlled attachment experiment, theistic believers who were primed with a subliminal separation threat ("Mother is gone") targeting their relationship with their mothers (i.e., typically the principal AF in childhood) showed an increase in their wish to be close to God compared with participants in an attachment-neutral control condition (Birgegard & Granqvist, 2004). We suggest that the effects of loss and separation are due to two factors: (1) Loss of a loved one activates the attachment system, thus giving rise to religious attachment behaviors such as prayer; and (2) bereaved/separated persons may find in God a surrogate AF to replace the absent AF.

### God as a Secure Base

Another defining characteristic of an attachment is that it provides a sense of felt security and a secure base for exploration of the environment. As noted, religious literature is replete with references to God's being "by my side" and "watching over me." Perhaps the best-known example is the 23rd Psalm: "Yea, though I walk through the valley of the shadow of death, I will fear no evil: for thou art with me; thy rod and thy staff they comfort me."[2]

It is easy to imagine how an AF who is simultaneously omnipresent, omniscient, and omnipotent can provide the most secure of secure bases. This is precisely what led Kaufman (1981) to his previously quoted conclusion that God represents an "absolutely adequate attachment-figure." It also led Johnson (1945, p. 191), a psychologist of religion, to conclude: "The emotional quality of faith is indicated in a basic confidence and security that gives one assurance. In this sense faith is the opposite of fear, anxiety, and uncertainty." This description of faith bears a striking resemblance to Bowlby's (1973, p. 202) own later descriptions of the secure base and its psychological effects: "When an individual is confident that an AF will be available to him whenever he desires it, that person will be much less prone to either intense or chronic fear than will an individual who for any reason has no such confidence."

Researchers have paid less attention to the question of how religious beliefs affect behavior and cognition in the absence of stressors. Thus, there is considerably less direct evidence for a secure-base function of religion than for a safe-haven function. Nevertheless, there is both direct and indirect support for such a function. Some of the research that is supportive of indirect effects is reviewed when we examine psychological outcomes associated with "attachment to God." Regarding direct effects, Granqvist, Mikulincer, and colleagues (2012) found in their experiments with theistic Jews in Israel that subliminal priming with the word God heightened participants' cognitive access to secure-base-related concepts (e.g., "loving," "accepting") in a lexical decision task and that priming with a religious symbol (a Torah scroll) caused neutral material (Chinese ideographs) to be better liked.

## Responses to Separation and Loss

We have noted in a previous section that certain aspects of religiousness often become more salient in response to bereavement and (threatened or actual) separations from loved ones. However, the fourth and fifth defining aspects of attachment, as outlined by Ainsworth (1985), concern responses to separation from, or loss of, the AF per se: The threat of separation causes anxiety in the attached person, and loss of the AF causes grief.

Determining whether God meets these criteria is difficult; God does not die, sail off to fight wars, or file for divorce. The potential for true separation

from God is usually seen by believers to come only in the hereafter, at which time one either spends eternity with God or is separated from God. It is noteworthy, however, that in most Christian belief systems, separation from God is the essence of hell.

Also, there are instances in religious life when believers are unable to experience a previously felt communion with God, which may also occur in situations in which the urge to feel such a communion is experienced as acute. In religious and mystical literature, such states are often referred to as a "wilderness experience" or a "dark night of the soul" (St. John of the Cross, 1990). Perhaps the best-known example is when Christ himself, nailed on the cross, cried out: "My God, my God, why hast thou forsaken me?" (Matthew 27:46). In an experimental paraphrase of this situation, Birgegard and Granqvist (2004) subliminally exposed theistic (mostly Christian) believers to either a separation prime targeting their God relationship ("God has abandoned me") or attachment-neutral control primes ("People are walking," "God has many names"), and examined whether the wish to be close to God would increase as expected from pre- to postexposure as a result of the separation-from-God priming. In other words, this was an attempt to create a conceptually analogous situation for adult believers to the separation situation in which infants studied in the Ainsworth Strange Situation find themselves (Ainsworth, Blehar, Waters, & Wall, 1978). Although modest support was obtained for the prediction, the effects were strongly moderated by individual differences, analogous to those observed in the Strange Situation (which we discuss in detail later in this chapter).

## Perceiving God as Stronger and Wiser

To highlight the inherently asymmetrical nature of attachment, Bowlby (1969/1982) used the term attachment relationship to denote the relationship that a weaker, less competent individual has with another individual perceived as stronger and wiser—prototypically, the mammalian offspring with its adult caregiver(s). Concerning believers' perceived relation with God, believers undoubtedly do perceive God as very much stronger and wiser than themselves. In fact, God is supposedly omnipotent and omniscient—attributes that are difficult for any earthly caregiver to compete with, as sensitive as he or she may be.

## Maturational Aspects in the Development of Attachment and Religion

So far, we have mostly considered adult expressions of religious experience in relation to attachment processes. The story of attachment starts in early childhood, however, as does the story of how a perceived relationship with God develops. We argue here that the relationship with God develops in temporal conjunction with the maturation of attachment, and especially with the cognitive developments thought to be intertwined with this maturation (Bowlby, 1973). Furthermore, we demonstrate that situational experiences associated with heightened attachment activation are already associated in childhood with increased significance of the individual's relationship with God (for reviews, see Granqvist, 2014b; Richert & Granqvist, 2013).

As noted, the biological function of the attachment system is to maintain proximity between an infant and a protective AF. With increasing cognitive abilities, older children are often satisfied by visual or verbal contact, or eventually by mere knowledge of an AF's whereabouts (Bretherton, 1987). This observation led Sroufe and Waters (1977) to suggest that "felt security" is the set-goal of the attachment system. Likewise, the consideration of cognitive abilities was an important part of the "move to the level of representation" (Main, Kaplan, & Cassidy, 1985) that was undertaken in attachment research 30 years ago. This move also opened the door, we argue, to the possibility of representing noncorporeal figures (e.g., gods, imaginary figures) as AFs, although physical contact with such a figure is not possible.

Far from being able to grasp symbolic thought or master mentalizing abilities, the human infant's behavioral repertoire initially consists of a series of fixed action patterns (cf. reflexive behaviors) that are necessary to obtain the biological set-goals of nourishment and proximity to a protective caregiver. However, in preschool, attachment to primary caregivers increasingly moves toward goal-corrected partnerships. This is presumably because of an emerging capacity for symbolic thought and mentalizing abilities (Bowlby, 1969/1982), which enable the child to represent the AF symbolically and to imagine the intentions and goals underlying the AF's behaviors. As a consequence, children become increasingly able to tolerate longer separations as they get older.

It is easy to see how symbolic thought and mentalizing abilities may similarly pave the way for an emerging understanding of God. As children experience themselves thinking and planning, and imagine the intentions of their social interaction partners, they may also apply their increasingly sophisticated mentalizing abilities to abstract, symbolic others. Naturally, related cognitive inclinations, such as a propensity for anthropomorphic thinking, naive physics, naive biology, and agency attributions, contribute further to making God an intuitively sensible ontology to the young child's mind (e.g., Barrett, 2004). As a case in point, young children (even from atheistic contexts) intuitively invent creationist ideas to explain origins but are hard pressed to entertain evolutionary explanations (Evans, 2001). Of course, the child's cognitive elaborations with God-related ideas are particularly likely to become consolidated and endure when adults provide consonant information (Evans, 2001; Granqvist, 2014b).

Although children's God concepts can be viewed as abstractions, they tend to be comparatively concrete and anthropomorphic by adult standards. A preschooler may, for example, explain the rain as a result of God's need to pee. For another example, God is typically described and drawn as a person (Heller, 1986). Common themes observed by Heller in his extensive study of children's images of God included many characteristics reminiscent of a secure attachment figure, such as nurturance, intimacy, and omnipresence. Interestingly, two other themes observed by Heller seem to parallel insecure attachment patterns, *inconsistent God* and *God, the distant thing in the sky*.

Once the requisite cognitive development has occurred, if a child's attachment system is highly activated (e.g., during a separation) the child may draw on God as an abstract yet anthropomorphized attachment surrogate. In a related discussion, Rizzuto (1979) suggested that at roughly age 5–6 years, children develop a "living" God representation, with God being an alternative, affectively charged safe haven rather than a purely cognitive representation in the child's mind.

In middle childhood, as children enter school and move even farther from their parents' immediate care, their God concepts become somewhat less anthropomorphic, although, at the same time, God is typically viewed as personally closer than in early childhood (Eshleman, Dickie, Merasco, Shepard, & Johnson, 1999; Tamminen, 1994). From early childhood on, empirical data indicate that God is indeed perceived as an available safe haven in times of stress. For example, Tamminen found that a high proportion of Finnish 7- to 12-year-olds reported that they felt close to God, particularly during emergencies and periods of loneliness. In addition, Eshleman and colleagues (1999) found that American preschoolers and elementary schoolchildren placed a God symbol closer to a fictional child when the fictional child was in attachment-activating situations (e.g., sick and in the hospital) than when the fictional child was in situations that contained less clear-cut attachment activators (e.g., the child had stolen an apple).

These findings have now been conceptually replicated in at least three studies, conducted in Sweden, the United States, and Italy, with children from 5 to 8 years of age (Cassibba, Granqvist, & Costantini, 2013; Dickie, Charland, & Poll, 2005; Granqvist, Ljungdahl, & Dickie, 2007). The results of these studies were based on a clearer distinction between attachment-activating and non-attachment-activating situations. Even then, children placed the God symbol closer to the fictional child in the attachment-activating situations. Interestingly, so did children raised by nonreligious parents (Granqvist, Ljungdahl, et al., 2007).

Adolescence and early adulthood have long been known to be periods of major religious transformations (e.g., Granqvist, 2012; James, 1902). These are the life periods most intimately associated with sudden religious conversions and other significant changes in one's relationship with God. Argyle and Beit-Hallahmi (1975, p. 59) referred to adolescence as "the age of religious awakening," although it is notably also the age of apostasy (Roof & McKinney, 1987). It is well known that cult recruiters make teenagers and young adults primary targets of their proselytizing and recruitment activities. Because adolescence is a unique and complex developmental period, it is not surprising that a wide range of explanations has been offered for the prevalence of conversion at this time. These include postulated links to puberty and sexual instincts (e.g., Thouless, 1923); the increased need for meaning, purpose, and sense of identity (Starbuck, 1899); and self-realization (Hood et al., 1996). From an attachment perspective, it is notable that adolescence represents a period of transition between principal AFs—usually from parents to peers (Zeifman & Hazan, 1997). According to Weiss (1982, p. 178), relinquishing one's parents as AFs has a number of predictable consequences, including vulnerability to emotional loneliness, which he defines as "the absence from one's in-

ternal world of an attachment figure." At such a time, adolescents may turn to God (or perhaps a charismatic religious leader) as a substitute AF (for a review, see Granqvist, 2012). As noted, sudden religious conversions and other major religious changes are also typically precipitated by significant emotional turmoil, which is likely to keep the attachment system hyperactivated in this sensitive period of attachment transition.

Compared to the preceding age periods, middle adulthood is typically less associated with attachment transitions and religious drama, and more associated with religious and other forms of "habit . . . the enormous fly-wheel of society, its most precious conservative agent" (James, 1890/1950, p. 121). However, there are notable exceptions, the most pronounced being marital separations and divorce. In old age, a person's relationship with God often regains importance, particularly when the person loses close friends or a spouse to death. As noted, such attachment transitions have been found to be associated with increased emphasis on one's relationship with God (e.g., Brown et al., 2004; Cicirelli, 2004; Granqvist & Hagekull, 2000; Kirkpatrick, 2005).

## Religion and Individual Differences in Attachment

An important characteristic of attachment theory is its integration of a normative model featuring a control system dynamic on the one hand, and a model of individual differences in the functioning of that system on the other. To be complete, a theory of religion-as-attachment must do the same. In the preceding sections, we have sketched a normative model within which many aspects of religious belief and behavior, and particularly perceived relationships with God, function psychologically as attachment processes. We turn in this section to the topic of relations between religion and individual differences in attachment. As it turns out, just as individual differences in attachment security modulate the behavioral and linguistic output of the attachment system in general, so do they modulate the effects of attachment activation in the context of believers' perceived God relations.

From the outset, Kirkpatrick (1994; Kirkpatrick & Shaver, 1990) noted that two somewhat opposing hypotheses could be derived from attachment theory concerning relations between religion and attachment security or insecurity, referred to as the *compensation* and *correspondence* hypotheses. These hypotheses may be seen as delineating two distinct developmental pathways to religion: one (compensation) following experiences with insensitive caregivers, and the other (correspondence) via experiences with sensitive, typically religious caregivers (Granqvist, Ivarsson, Broberg, & Hagekull, 2007; Kirkpatrick, 2005). It is in this developmental-pathway sense that the two hypotheses are conceptualized in the following sections. We describe findings from studies employing both self-reports (e.g., of romantic attachment) and more indirect, implicit assessments of attachment, such as the Adult Attachment Interview (AAI; Main, Goldwyn, & Hesse, 2003).[3] Moreover, we argue that essentially the same conclusions can be drawn from studies that have used different kinds of methods.

### The Compensation Pathway

According to Bowlby's control system model of attachment, the attachment system continually monitors internal states and external circumstances in relation to the question, "Is the attachment figure sufficiently near, attentive, responsive, approving, etc.?" (Hazan & Shaver, 1994, p. 3). The set point of the system is variable, depending on expectancies (i.e., components of internal working models, or IWMs) concerning the AF and perceived cues of environmental dangers. A negative answer to the question, according to the theory, activates a suite of potential attachment behaviors designed to restore an adequate degree of proximity. Under certain conditions, however, the individual may anticipate (based on prior experience and/or current circumstances) that efforts to achieve adequate proximity and comfort from the primary AF are unlikely to be successful. If so, a search for an alternative and more adequate AF may be initiated, which in some cases will lead to God. In the sections dealing with normative aspects of attachment and religion, we have noted a number of such situations. In this section, we are concerned with whether individual differences in attachment history and attachment security are associated with the use of God and religion in times of distress.

Both Ainsworth (1985) and Bowlby (1969/1982) expected a history of unsatisfactory attachments to predispose a person to search for substitute AFs. Ainsworth argued that children who fail to establish secure attachments to parents are likely to seek surrogates, including teachers,

older siblings, other relatives, or any stronger and wiser other who reliably proves to be accessible and responsive. Subsequent students of attachment largely neglected to pursue further the use of attachment surrogates in their research. However, it should be recalled that insecure (i.e., avoidant and resistant/ambivalent) attachment is believed to reflect a developmentally secondary (or conditional) attachment strategy stemming from defensive processes (e.g., exclusion of attachment-related information and diversion of attention) in the face of a failed primary strategy of obtaining sufficiently sensitive care from the AF (Main, 1991). The use of surrogate attachments may provide a unique opportunity to observe the presumed remnants of such a primary (or secure) attachment strategy. Although Ainsworth did not include God in her list of potential surrogates, it seems reasonable to assume that God may fill this role for many people with insecure attachment histories. In a word, God may provide a kind of attachment relationship one never had with one's parents or other primary AFs. We hypothesize that regulation of distress is at the core of this surrogate use of God and religion. Besides conditional strategies, people who have experienced abuse, frightening, or other aberrant forms of caregiving behavior from AFs (i.e., those with disorganized attachment) are predisposed to enter dissociative states of consciousness, which may also be expressed in the religious and spiritual realm, and consequently be analyzed as a form of compensation.

### Compensation and Theistic Religion

Some of the findings reported and arguments advanced in the normative attachment-and-religion sections of this chapter have been found to hold in particular for individuals who were likely to have experienced parental insensitivity while growing up, whether their estimated attachment-related experiences were based on self-reports (e.g., Granqvist, 1998, 2002; Granqvist & Hagekull, 1999, 2003; Halama, Gasparikova, & Sabo, 2013; Kirkpatrick & Shaver, 1990; Pirutinsky, 2009; Schnitker, Porter, Emmons, & Barrett, 2012) or assessed with the AAI (Granqvist, Ivarsson, et al., 2007). For example, sudden religious conversions, the most pronounced examples of religious drama, are associated with estimates of parental insensitivity. This connection was reported in the first study of attachment and religion (Kirkpatrick & Shaver, 1990). Since then, these findings have been strongly supported by a meta-analysis of all studies conducted before 2004, including almost 1,500 participants (Granqvist & Kirkpatrick, 2004), and later by additional studies (e.g., Halama et al., 2013; Schnitker et al., 2012).

In addition, confirmative evidence has accrued in relation to the "probable experience of parenting scales" used to score the AAI. For example, in an AAI study, participants whose parents were estimated by an independent coder to have been relatively less loving/sensitive self-reported more sudden and intense increases in religiousness (Granqvist, Ivarsson, et al., 2007). Notably, although all studies cited earlier were conducted on largely Christian samples, a later study of converts to Orthodox Judaism provided much needed cross-religion evidence for the association between attachment insecurity and sudden conversion (Pirutinsky, 2009).

In the meta-analysis (Granqvist & Kirkpatrick, 2004), sudden converts outscored both nonconverts and gradual converts on attachment insecurity with parents. Also, as would be expected given the distress-regulating aspect of sudden conversions, we found in the meta-analysis that sudden converts scored higher on a scale created to tap distress-regulating aspects of believers' perceived relations with God—focusing explicitly on attachment aspects of the relationship (e.g., God being viewed as a safe haven and secure base).

Moreover, several studies have shown that the increases in religiousness reported by individuals whose parents were judged to be low in sensitivity were typically precipitated by significant emotional turmoil ("themes of compensation") that was typically relationship-related (e.g., Granqvist & Hagekull, 1999; Granqvist, Ivarsson, et al., 2007; Halama et al., 2013). These studies assessed religious changes retrospectively, but Granqvist and Hagekull (2003) showed that the association could also be obtained prospectively; that is, reports of parental insensitivity prospectively predicted increased religiousness—particularly an increased importance of the perceived relationship with God, following the breakup of a romantic relationship.

Similarly, insecure romantic attachment has reliably predicted essentially the same kinds of religious changes. For example, Kirkpatrick (1997) found that over a 4-year period, women with insecure (particularly anxious) attachments established a new relationship with God and reported religious experiences, such as being "born again" and speaking in tongues, to a larger extent than did securely attached women. Findings of pro-

spectively predicted increases in the religiousness of adults reporting insecure romantic attachment were replicated in a second study by Kirkpatrick (1998), this time over a 5-month period, and in both males and females. Unlike the 1997 study, which used Hazan and Shaver's (1987) three-category measure of attachment orientations, this study utilized Bartholomew and Horowitz's (1991) four-category model, based on two dimensions: positive versus negative model of self, and positive versus negative model of other. Again, increases in the image of a loving God and in a perceived personal relationship with God were predicted by not only ambivalent/preoccupied romantic attachment but also by fearful-avoidant attachment, both of which are characterized by a negative model of self. Although the magnitude of the effects was modest in these two studies, when the contextual condition of romantic relationship breakup—possibly indicating an increased need to regulate distress via attachment—was considered in yet another sample, insecure romantic attachment prospectively predicted increases in aspects of religiousness somewhat more strongly (Granqvist & Hagekull, 2003).

One interpretation of the findings from these studies is that for people who view themselves as unworthy of love and care, turning to God may be possible because of God's unique characteristics as compared with other relationship partners. First, turning to God is comparatively risk free because a noncorporeal figure's responsiveness can always be imagined and need never be experienced as disconfirmed. Also, in most religious belief systems, God's love is either unconditional—so one need not be "worthy" of love to receive it—or available through particular courses of action (e.g., good deeds, prayer) that allow an otherwise "unworthy" person to "earn" God's love and forgiveness.

Although these studies might seem to suggest that individuals with insecure attachment patterns become increasingly religious over time, it should be recalled that this is expected primarily in the context of a need to regulate distress. Accordingly, religiousness may also decrease for such individuals (Granqvist, 2002). As expected, this happens under conditions in which the need to regulate distress through attachment surrogates is comparatively low, such as after establishing a new intimate human relationship (Granqvist & Hagekull, 2003).

In summary, the developmental pathway to religion in the case of parental insensitivity and insecure attachment is one marked by attachment system (hyper)activation, under conditions where a perceived relationship with God helps to regulate a believer's distress when no other adequate AFs are available. This conclusion corresponds well with the general speculations about the use of attachment surrogates offered by Bowlby (1969/1982) and Ainsworth (1985). As we have noted elsewhere (Granqvist, 2003; Granqvist & Hagekull, 1999; Kirkpatrick, 2005), this religious profile bears a striking resemblance to William James's (1902) more than century-old characterization of the "religion of the sick-souled."

However, whereas the AAI judges' estimates of parental insensitivity during interviewees' childhoods did predict the interviewees' history of using religion to regulate distress, classifications of the interviewees' *current* attachment organization were generally unrelated to such compensatory use of religion (Granqvist, Ivarsson, et al., 2007). Similarly, self-reported romantic attachment (particularly a negative self-model or a high degree of attachment anxiety) has been linked to increasing religiousness over time (longitudinal compensation), whereas self-reported secure attachment has been linked to higher religiousness at a given time (contemporaneous correspondence; see Kirkpatrick, 2005). An intriguing possibility is that this discrepancy results from the possibility that some individuals who suffered attachment-related difficulties (e.g., rejection, role reversal) in the past may have "earned" a certain degree of attachment security from their surrogate relationship with God. This interpretation is admittedly speculative, but if supported, it would indicate that religion as compensation may sometimes be psychologically reparative and conducive of growth, not just defensively reactive.

## Compensation and Altered Spiritual States (Mystical Experiences and New Age Spirituality)

Religion is doctrinal and communal, but all world religions also have an undercurrent of personal spiritual experiences that are not necessarily interpreted doctrinally by the persons having the experiences (e.g., Hood et al., 2009). Experiences known as "mystical" are probably the best example. Mystical experiences represent markedly altered states of consciousness, more specifically, a dissolution of one's usual, integrated sense of self (Stace, 1960). From his extensive studies of religious mystics, Stace noted that mystical experiences usually take the form of a pure, content-free

consciousness, where perceptual objects "disappear," resulting in an experience of "nothingness" (i.e., introvertive states), or a sense of all objects being unified into a perception of totality or oneness with all things (i.e., extrovertive states). The unity experience of extrovertive states may or may not be described as "God"; other examples are "Nature" and "Cosmos."

In much of the contemporary, pluralistic Western world, religious doctrines and communities have lost their privileged position as sources of legitimacy for peoples' spiritual experiences. Religions now coexist with one another and lead a largely marginalized life on the side of the many "nonreligious" movements in the mainstream, which are often individually rather than communally oriented, but some of which still have their say on experiences understood as spiritual. In this "spiritual revolution," the spirit has been taken out of religion/God and moved into the self (Heelas, Woodhead, Seel, & Szerszynski, 2005). The New Age movement is probably the best example. The term *New Age* refers not to a formalized movement but to a wide range of beliefs and activities that typically combine esotericism/occultism, astrology, parapsychology, alternative medicine, outgrowths of humanist psychology, and Eastern thinking in a Western context, and in which the individual is free to pick any ingredient suitable to the self from the diverse spiritual smorgasbord that characterizes the New Age (Farias & Granqvist, 2007). Notably, altered states of consciousness, such as out-of-body experiences, trance states (e.g., in conjunction with "drum trips"), and responses to hypnotic suggestions (e.g., past-life regression), are both prevalent and subjected to affirmative metaphysical interpretations within the New Age movement (Farias & Granqvist, 2007).

Thus, both mysticism and New Age spirituality should be associated with altered states of consciousness. As noted earlier, disorganized (D) attachment (as well as its adult counterpart, unresolved loss/abuse) is believed to be an important developmental precursor to the proclivity to enter altered states (e.g., Main & Morgan, 1996). Indeed, D behaviors such as freezing and stilling have been suggested to represent (proto-)dissociative states, already evident in infancy, and provoked by the approach–avoidance conflict thought to characterize D attachment (Hesse & Main, 2006; Main & Morgan, 1996). In other words, when the infant's attachment system is activated, instead of approaching the AF—who is simultaneously the source of threat *and* of potential comfort—the infant "spaces out" or dissociates. If this becomes a habitual mode of responding when faced with stress, D attachment should make the individual prone to later experiences of dissociative mental states (e.g., experiences of depersonalization, out-of-body experiences). Confirmatory evidence for this idea comes from studies linking infant D status to later dissociative states throughout childhood and adolescence, and unresolved loss/abuse to a more general propensity to experience altered states ("absorption"; for a review, see Granqvist, Reijman, & Cardeña, 2011).

Putting these pieces together, one of us (Granqvist, Ivarsson, et al., 2007) has proposed a mediational model in which D attachment (including unresolved loss/abuse) is hypothesized to predict altered spiritual states, via dissociation (e.g., absorption) as a mediating variable. This mediational model has now been supported in a prospective follow-up of the Swedish AAI study referenced earlier (Granqvist, Ivarsson, et al., 2007), both with mystical experiences (Granqvist, Hagekull, & Ivarsson, 2012) and New Age spirituality (Granqvist, Fransson, & Hagekull, 2009) as outcomes, and as predicted by unresolved loss/abuse. Moreover, support for this model has recently been independently replicated and extended in a study using unresolved loss as predictor, "supernatural beliefs" (i.e., paranormal beliefs plus mystical experiences) as outcome, and psychopathology-related forms of dissociation as mediator (Thomson & Jaque, 2014). Supporting the discriminant validity of the mediational model, more conventional forms of religiousness, such as theistic beliefs and strength of religious commitment, were unrelated both to unresolved loss/abuse and absorption in the former study (Granqvist, Hagekull, et al., 2012). The findings from these studies are particularly noteworthy when considering that AAI classifications are often unrelated to self-reports of external phenomena (see Hesse, Chapter 26, this volume).

Given that New Age spirituality typically does not revolve around God as an AF, it is reasonable to question whether the attachment model in general and the compensation hypothesis in particular are at all conceptually applicable (see Kirkpatrick, 2005). We speculate that the adoption of New Age practices and beliefs may be driven by motivation similar to that underlying religion as compensation, but that the generalization of IWMs of others (e.g., as frightening) restrict New Agers' use of God as an attachment surrogate. Note also that although the idea of a single, the-

istic God is usually absent from New Age beliefs, the world of New Agers is often inhabited by imagined angels and spirits, as well as human spiritual advisors and gurus who may fill some attachment-surrogate functions. Of course, the appeal of the New Age for disorganized individuals may also be due, in part, to its provision of metaphysical affirmations of these individuals' psychological states and experiences (e.g., of telepathy, contact with the dead, possession by abusive perpetrators). Prior to the individuals' introduction to the New Age, such states and experiences may well have been regarded, by self and others alike, as worrisome signs of poor reality contact.

Finally, we note that this mediational model might seem to "pathologize" New Age spirituality and mystical experiences. This is because virtually all *other* theorizing and research efforts on D attachment portray it as a risk factor in development. However, appearances should always be treated with caution. We have in fact argued that there is a major gap in the literature on potential nonpathological sequelae of D attachment, and that altered spiritual states represent a rare example that helps to fill that gap (Granqvist, Ivarsson, et al., 2012); mystical experiences, in particular, are not linked to psychopathology, although they are often preceded by stress and turmoil (e.g., Hood et al., 2009). Unusual forms of creativity might represent another example.

## The Correspondence Pathway

According to Bowlby's model, continuity of attachment patterns across time and transmission of attachment patterns across generations are traced to IWMs (Bowlby, 1973; see also Bretherton & Munholland, Chapter 4, this volume; Main et al., 1985). As a consequence of repeated experiences in interactions with their AFs, children develop beliefs and expectations (IWMs) about the availability and responsiveness of caregivers, and these models guide future behavioral, emotional, and cognitive responses in other social interactions. Moreover, the models of interaction partners are linked to models of the self—beliefs about the degree to which one sees oneself as worthy of love, care, and protection.

Although the level at which IWMs operate is a matter of debate, it seems likely that people maintain both (1) mental models of AFs in general and (2) mental models specific to particular relationships. Bretherton and Munholland (Chapter 4, this volume) suggest that such models are hierarchically arranged: The top level comprises a highly general model of self and others; a second level comprises models of parent–child relationships as distinct from peer relationships; and so on. We suggest that for many individuals, IWMs of God (or perceived relationships with God) hold an important place somewhere in this hierarchy.

Whether or not various levels of attachment-relevant mental representations are arranged in this precise hierarchical structure, consideration of the interrelatedness of IWMs leads to a straightforward set of predictions, which we refer to as IWM *correspondence*: Individual differences in religious beliefs and experience should correspond with individual differences in IWMs of self and other. Individuals who possess positive or "secure" generalized IWMs of themselves and their AFs may be expected to represent God and other deities in similar terms. Likewise, an "avoidant" attachment may be expected to manifest itself in the religious realm as agnosticism or atheism, or in a representation of God as remote and inaccessible. In addition, an "anxious" or "ambivalent" attachment may find expression in a deeply emotional, all-consuming, and "clingy" relationship to God. Finally, a disorganized (or fearful) attachment may relate to a representation of God as frightening and ominous.

Besides IWM correspondence, the developmental attachment literature has suggested that caregiver sensitivity and offspring attachment security facilitate the offspring's internalization of parental standards in general (e.g., Ainsworth, Bell, & Stayton, 1974; Kochanska, Aksan, Knaack, & Rhines, 2004; Richters & Waters, 1991). This conclusion converges with the literature on imitation (or social learning), in which a model's nurturance has been shown to facilitate children's imitation of the model's behaviors (e.g., Hetherington & Frankie, 1967), as well as with previous findings in the psychology of religion, which have repeatedly shown warm, high-quality caregiving to be linked to high parent–offspring similarity in religiousness (see Hood et al., 2009). Thus, a socially based aspect of religion (and religious membership) can be added to the IWM aspect of the correspondence hypothesis (Granqvist, 2002; Granqvist & Hagekull, 1999); that is, the religious beliefs and behaviors of people who are securely attached can be expected in part to reflect their sensitive AF's (say, a loving parent's) religious standards. In contrast, insecure offspring can be expected to be less likely to adopt their relatively insensitive or unresponsive AF's religious standards. This aspect of the correspondence

hypothesis is referred to as *social correspondence* (Granqvist, 2002, 2010). Through this addition, securely attached individuals are expected to become actively religious insofar as their caregivers were (i.e., social correspondence). If so, their perceived relations with God are expected to exhibit attributes of security (i.e., IWM correspondence).[4]

### A Review of Social Correspondence Findings

In line with the idea of social correspondence, individuals reporting experiences of being sensitively cared for by parents have been shown to score higher in religiousness than those reporting experiences of being less sensitively cared for, but only insofar as their parents also displayed high levels of religiosity (Granqvist, 1998, 2002; Granqvist & Hagekull, 1999; Kirkpatrick & Shaver, 1990). In addition, such people score higher on a scale created to assess religiosity as socially rooted in the parental relationship (Granqvist, 2002; Granqvist & Hagekull, 1999). Moreover, both sets of findings were supported in the Swedish AAI study, when coded estimates of parental sensitivity rather than direct self-reports were used (Granqvist, Ivarsson, et al., 2007). Similarly, in the case of romantic attachment, secure attachment is associated with scores on the scale measuring religiosity as socially based in the parental relationship (Granqvist, 2002).

Notably, the idea of social correspondence has now been supported in not only Christian populations but also a Jewish Israeli sample (Pirutinsky, 2009), and not only in samples drawn from the normal population but also from a maltreatment sample (Reinert & Edwards, 2009). Social correspondence has also been supported in prospective studies. In a study of adolescents about to undergo a Young Life Evangelical summer camp (Schnitker et al., 2012), secure attachment with parents prospectively predicted an at-camp reaffirmation of the faith one had been brought up with (cf. Halama et al., 2013; Wright, 2008).

We note that parental religiousness has often been portrayed in the psychology of religion as the single strongest predictor of offspring religiousness, especially by scholars who approach the topic from a social learning perspective (e.g., Batson, Schoenrade, & Ventis, 1993; Spilka, Hood, Hunsberger, & Gorsuch, 2003). However, the "effect" of parental religiousness is importantly moderated by the estimated quality of the offspring–parent attachment relationship. In fact, whereas parent–offspring correlations for retrospectively defined secure dyads have been large ($r \approx .50$), they have usually been nonsignificant and close to zero for insecure dyads (e.g., Granqvist, 1998; Kirkpatrick & Shaver, 1990). An implication of these findings for religious parents who wish their children to embrace their own religion is that religious preaching/teaching is not enough; in fact, it may fall on entirely deaf ears unless combined with placing a high priority on sensitive caregiving that meets the children's needs for protection and security. It is even possible that sensitive caregiving—in the absence of explicit religious training—suffices as long as a child has an opportunity to observe a caregiver engage in religious speech and behavior.

### A Review of IWM Correspondence Findings

Evidence for IWM correspondence between the interpersonal attachment and religious domains has also accrued in relation to attachment history as estimated through the AAI. The AAI study described earlier revealed that coded estimates of probable experiences with loving/sensitive parents were associated with participants' reports of a loving, as opposed to a distant, God image (Granqvist, Ivarsson, et al., 2007). Conversely, inferred experiences with rejecting and role-reversing parents were associated positively with a distant God image and negatively with a loving image of God.

Similar findings have been reported in an Italian AAI study (Cassibba, Granqvist, Costantini, & Gatto, 2008) that contained two subsamples: a highly religious group (Catholic nuns, priests, and seminarians) and a comparison group of lay Catholic believers, matched for sex. The highly religious group was coded significantly higher on not only loving experiences with mothers but also a continuous dimension of current security/coherence of discourse, and this group contained a higher proportion of secure-autonomous classifications than the worldwide nonclinical meta-analytic distribution (Bakermans-Kranenburg & Van IJzendoorn, 2009). Finally—regardless of subsample—secure-autonomous participants reported a more loving God image than insecure-nonautonomous participants.

Although religious transformations are less frequent for individuals who have experienced sensitive caregiving, they sometimes do occur. When they do, the life context and the constituents of the change are very different from those reported in the sections on the compensation pathway. For example, prospectively predicted increases in religiousness occurred *not* following romantic relationship dissolution, but rather after the establishment of a new intimate relationship, for participants who reported sensitive parenting (Granqvist & Hagekull, 2003). Also, religious changes tend to be gradual rather than sudden and to occur at a comparatively young age for these individuals (Granqvist & Hagekull, 1999; Granqvist, Ivarsson, et al., 2007; Halama et al., 2013; Schnitker et al., 2012).

Regarding romantic attachment, IWM correspondence has typically been supported in contemporaneous relations between religious variables and romantic attachment security. For example, Kirkpatrick and Shaver (1992) found that people with a secure romantic attachment displayed a higher personal belief in and relationship with God, as well as perceptions of God as loving, whereas people reporting avoidant romantic attachment were agnostic or atheist to a larger extent. These findings have since been conceptually replicated in a number of studies (e.g., Byrd & Boe, 2000; Granqvist & Hagekull, 2000, 2003; Kirkpatrick, 1998; TenElshof & Furrow, 2000). For example, Byrd and Boe (2000) found that participants reporting secure romantic attachments engaged more in prayer that served to maintain closeness to God. Moreover, even in prospective analyses, IWM correspondence between romantic attachment security and religious change has been supported in expected contexts—for example, following the formation of a romantic relationship in between assessments of religiosity (Granqvist & Hagekull, 2003).

Besides the correlational studies just reviewed, four sets of attachment and religion experiments (or quasi-experiments) involving subtle attempts to activate attachment have been performed (Birgegard & Granqvist, 2004; Cassibba et al., 2013; Granqvist, Ljungdahl, et al., 2007; Granqvist, Mikulincer, et al., 2012). The normative/main effects of attachment activation observed in these studies have already been described. However, in all four sets of studies, the main effects were qualified, or moderated, by perceived attachment history or current attachment security in a manner that supports the notion of IWM correspondence.

As we have seen, individuals who have experienced insensitive care are more likely to regulate intense distress through their perceived relationship with God than are those who have experienced sensitive care (i.e., a compensation effect). However, across the three experiments conducted by Birgegard and Granqvist (2004), an increase in the use of God to regulate distress was observed following subliminal separation primes among adult believers who had reported sensitive experiences with parents, thus supporting IWM correspondence instead. Because indirect assessments of religiosity (i.e., regression residuals from pre- to postpriming) were used in the context of *subliminal* priming, participants were unaware of attachment activation. Birgegard and Granqvist speculated that these conditions might have undermined the possibility of a compensatory use of religion in individuals who had experienced parental insensitivity, resulting in their withdrawal from God or (put differently) their defensive shift of attention away from attachment (e.g., Main et al., 1985). Conversely, presumably via automatic activation of IWMs, individuals with more sensitive experiences with caregivers could draw upon God in this situation, or turn their attention to attachment.[5]

In line with these speculations, the heightened psychological accessibility of God concepts following subliminal threat exposures (i.e., God as an implicit safe haven), observed by Granqvist, Mikulincer, and colleagues (2012), was particularly notable in participants with a relatively secure (nonavoidant) romantic attachment orientation. This experiment therefore conceptually replicated and extended those of Birgegard and Granqvist (2004). Similarly, concerning implicit access to God as a secure base, participants with a relatively secure romantic attachment style had particularly heightened cognitive access to secure base-related concepts following subliminal priming with the word *God* (Study 3) and implicitly reacted with more positive affect following subliminal exposure to a religion-related picture (Study 4) (Granqvist, Mikulincer et al., 2012). Hence, not only was attention to God more heightened for individuals reporting relatively secure romantic attachment than for those reporting insecure attachment when faced with unconscious threat, but the former individuals were also more likely to implicitly associate God with secure-base-related constructs and to benefit more implicitly from being unconsciously exposed to God-related material.

In addition, in the Swedish "felt board" study of 5- to 7-year-old children who were asked to place a God symbol at a chosen distance from a fictional child who was in attachment-activating or attachment-neutral situations (Granqvist, Ljungdahl, et al., 2007), secure children placed the God symbol closer to the fictional child when the fictional child was in attachment-activating situations. However, the pattern was reversed when the fictional child was in attachment-neutral situations (i.e., insecure children placed God closer).

Overall, the discrepancy in God symbol proximity between the two types of situations was much larger in secure than in insecure children. Our interpretation of this interaction is that secure children's attention shifted to God following attachment activation, whereas insecure children's attention to God did not shift as a function of attachment activation. Importantly, this study used the adapted Separation Anxiety Test (SAT; Kaplan, 1987), an indirect (semiprojective) method, to measure security, and the God symbol placement procedure was similarly semiprojective (i.e., the fictional child, not the study participant, was in different situations that were more or less likely to activate a child's attachment system). As in the adult experiments using subliminal priming techniques, this semiprojective procedure may have undermined a compensatory use of religion in insecure children, and instead yielded automatic activation of IWMs, thus supporting the correspondence hypothesis.

Cassibba and colleagues (2013) extended these findings in an Italian sample, showing that just as attachment security tends to be transmitted across generations from mother to child (Van IJzendoorn, 1995), *maternal* security on the AAI strongly predicted a higher degree of proximity in *their children's* God symbol placements relative to the fictional child. These findings are theoretically important in illustrating, perhaps for the first time, that mothers' IWMs generalize to the next generation's perceptions of the availability of another AF besides the mother.

In summary, substantial empirical support has been obtained for the idea that the developmental pathway to religion for individuals with secure attachments runs through extensive experience with sensitive, often religious caregivers and leads to the development of a security-enhancing representation of God. Moreover, in such cases, God, like other good AFs (Mikulincer & Shaver, 2004), is implicitly seen as available in times of need, although secure individuals are unlikely to need to use the perceived relationship with God specifically to regulate distress.

## Attachment to God and Psychological Outcomes

To the extent that having a safe haven and secure base prevents or reduces fear and anxiety, as argued by Bowlby (1969/1982) and others, a representation of God as a safe haven and secure base should confer certain psychological benefits. The connections between religion and mental health/well-being, which are both very complex, multifaceted constructs, are immensely complex: It seems clear that religious belief and commitment can have highly positive, highly negative, or neutral effects on mental health as variously defined (see Paloutzian & Kirkpatrick, 1995, for examples). In other words, the connection between religion and mental health is heavily influenced by moderators. A thorough review of this largely atheoretical and fragmented literature is beyond the scope of this chapter, but in this section, we argue that attachment–theoretical considerations may provide insight into why certain moderators underlie the links observed between religion and mental health. In order to facilitate a more systematic understanding of these links, we suggest three sets of moderators (for a more detailed discussion, see Granqvist, 2014a).

First, *contextual factors* associated with heightened attachment activation (e.g., stress, unavailability of one's secular AFs, low social welfare) increase the strength of the links observed between religion and mental health. For example, the positive effects of religious variables, such as those of "positive" religious coping (e.g., designed to increase the experience of spiritual support; Pargament, 1997) and "intrinsic" religiousness (i.e., religion as an end to itself, a master motive in life), on mental health outcomes are typically moderated by levels of stress, such that religion confers its most beneficial effects in times of real trouble. A meta-analysis of studies of religion and depression offers more specific evidence: Aspects of religion were negatively linked to depression, especially under conditions of high stress, whereas the main effect of religion on depression was relatively modest (Smith, McCullough, & Poll, 2003). Conversion research provides further evidence. Not only are intense/sudden conversion experiences likely to occur during times of stress, but such experiences are associated with marked attenuation of distress and at least short-term increases in well-being (Hood et al., 2009; Pargament, 1997).

Besides stress, research suggests that religion may be especially helpful in contexts in which other AFs are unavailable or insufficient as security providers. For example, in an early study by Kirkpatrick and Shaver (1992), the "effects" of attachment to God on psychological outcomes were moderated by perceived attachment history with

the mother. Respondents who remembered their mothers as relatively insensitive but perceived themselves as having a secure attachment to God (i.e., viewing God as responsive, loving, and caring) appeared to benefit the most from their perceived relationship with God.

The broader societal and cultural context should also be borne in mind. In particular, demographic data indicate that the one specific parameter that explains most (roughly 50%) of the statistical international variance in population estimates of religiosity (including seeking comfort, or a safe haven, in religion) is governmental welfare spending (i.e., proportion of gross national product [GNP] spent on schools, health care, health insurances, etc.). The conclusion from this literature is very clear: People are much less religious in welfare states. Parts of Europe (especially Scandinavia) are the very best cases in point, and this strong association seems to withstand control for every conceivable covariate (Gill & Lundsgaarde, 2004; Scheve & Stasavage, 2006). In these countries, state agencies and other functions of the welfare system appear to have replaced many of the functions historically served by religion. From an attachment–theoretical viewpoint, it may be that the successful implementation of welfare politics normally helps to keep people relatively safe and secure from alarm; they need not be shaken to their bones by misfortune because there is usually a safety net on which to fall back. As a corollary, religion may be especially likely to be conducive to mental health in societies marked by lower social welfare, that is, in contexts in which religion is typically both "needed" and culturally normative.

Second, *aspects of mental health* that are most notably affected by having a safe haven to turn to and a secure base to depart from are particularly reliably linked to religion. The psychological desideratum of a safe haven is the sense of having someone perceived as a protective, stronger, and wiser other to turn to when alarmed and distressed, which should be accompanied by attenuated worry and fear. The psychological desideratum of a secure base is that it promotes a sense of personal competence and control, which enables calm and confident exploration. Not coincidentally, in their review of research on associations between aspects of mental health and religious orientations, Batson and colleagues (1993) concluded that the most consistent positive links were obtained between freedom from worry and fear, and personal competence and control on the one hand, and intrinsic religiousness on the other.

As noted, another attachment-related aspect of mental health that religion appears to promote is the attenuation of grief (e.g., Brown et al., 2004; Cicirelli, 2004). Relatedly, it is also possible that religion may aid in reparation of maladaptive IWMs, for example, following loss of and/or experiences of having been insensitively cared for by other AFs. The possibility of the latter "earned security" form of reparation was discussed earlier in the section on compensation. Concerning loss, Bowlby (1980) noted that to proceed favorably in terms of promoting adaptation to a life without the loved one physically available, the mourning process requires that bereaved individuals ultimately accommodate information regarding the permanence of the loved one's death into their representational world, or else they are at risk of remaining unresolved/disorganized with respect to the loss (e.g., may display continued searching behaviors; Main et al., 2003). Available evidence indicates that the proportion of unresolved loss is somewhat lower in religious samples (3–17%; Cassibba et al., 2008, 2013; Granqvist, Ivarsson, et al., 2007) than in the nonclinical meta-analytic sample (16%; Bakermans-Kranenburg & Van IJzendoorn, 2009). Religion may promote mental resolution of loss by offering the bereaved both (1) the prospect of reunion with the deceased in the hereafter (Cassibba et al., 2008) and (2) the perfect surrogate AF (i.e., God) for dealing with the grief.

Finally, *aspects of religion* that are most consistently linked to mental health are partially those that express attachment components, including belief in a personal, loving God with whom one experiences a close and secure relationship. In fact, based on comprehensive research reviews, leading scholars on the religion–mental health connection have even suggested that "belief in/attachment to God" is the very source of religion/spirituality that makes people engage in other, more specific health-enhancing religious behaviors (e.g., rituals, commitment, coping) (Koenig et al., 2012, p. 587). Similarly, Pargament (2002) has concluded that mental health and well-being are predicted, positively and uniquely, by a secure relationship with God and perceived closeness to God (cf. secure attachment to God), whereas a tenuous (cf. insecure) relationship with God has an unfavorable effect on mental health and well-being.

Unfortunately, however, the empirical evidence for the vital role of attachment to God is far from conclusive. Interpretation of the data collected so far is limited by several methodological problems (Granqvist, 2014a). As one example, the causal direction of cross-sectional correlations between religion and various outcomes remains open to question. For another example, the (self-report) mode of measuring attachment to God and well-being in the studies conducted to date (e.g., Beck & McDonald, 2004; Kirkpatrick & Shaver, 1992; Rowatt & Kirkpatrick, 2002; Sim & Loh, 2003; Zahl & Gibson, 2012) leaves us unable to exclude the possibility that (any combination of) self-deception, impression management, shared method variance, semantic overlap, and so on, may be at least partly responsible for the associations obtained. Therefore, it is imperative to use less explicit methods for evaluating individual differences in believers' perceived relationship with God. Based on a longitudinal follow-up of our AAI study sample (Granqvist, Ivarsson, et al., 2007), we currently address this issue by using an interview about believers' representations of God in relation to the self (Granqvist & Main, 2003), which was adapted from the AAI protocol. One aim in developing this interview is to be able to undermine some of the potential validity threats to the self-reports of attachment to God. This method may ultimately prove to be useful also for shedding light on the attachment foundation of the religion–mental health connection, and particularly on the important question of whether earned security is sometimes derived from one's attachment to God.

## Current State of Theory and Research on the Attachment–Religion Connection

Since the previous edition of this volume in 2008, religion-as-attachment research has continued to mature. In fact, this field has been singled out in an authoritative handbook as the last decade's most promising "midlevel" theoretical contribution to the psychology of religion as a whole (Paloutzian & Park, 2013). This continuing maturation is remarkable considering that the religion-as-attachment model has been around for approximately a quarter of a century. We believe that there are two broad sets of reasons for the progress that has been made, one relating to increasing methodological rigor, and the other to conceptual expansions (Granqvist, 2010).

Regarding increasing methodological rigor, past attachment–religion research was predominantly correlational, whereas experimental and quasi-experimental designs have been increasingly added to the database in more recent years (e.g.,

Cassibba et al., 2013; Granqvist, Mikulincer, et al., 2012). Also, whereas past studies predominantly used samples of convenience, which were often drawn from student populations, recent studies have increasingly used more careful sample recruitment strategies and well-defined study populations (e.g., Cassibba et al., 2008; Reinert & Edwards, 2009; Schnitker et al., 2012). In addition, although past research was almost exclusively based on Christian samples in the Western world, recent studies have also used non-Christian samples from other parts of the world (e.g., Granqvist, Mikulincer, et al., 2012; Pirutinsky, 2009). Finally, whereas most past studies used explicit self-report assessments of both religion and attachment constructs, indirect, implicit assessments have been increasingly added to the research in recent years (e.g., Cassibba et al., 2008, 2013; Granqvist et al., 2009; Granqvist, Mikulincer, et al., 2012; see also Zahl & Gibson, 2012). Consequently, we are now better able to make causal inferences, to understand what populations—drawn from which religions—our inferences apply to, and to rule out self-report biases as an alternative explanation of some of the key findings.

Regarding conceptual expansions, several are noteworthy. First, as a complement to the many single-generation studies conducted, Cassibba and colleagues (2013) conducted a two-generation study focusing on intergenerational links between mothers' states of mind regarding attachment and their children's sense of God's closeness. As noted, this study is noteworthy in documenting that a mother's attachment organization is linked not only to her child's attachment to the mother herself (reviewed by Van IJzendoorn, 1995) but also to the child's sense of the availability of another AF besides the mother (i.e., God). Future research might show that similar generalizing effects extend to other attachment-related targets as well. Second, whereas the safe-haven function of religion has been supported and is particularly strongly emphasized in prior religion-as-attachment research, two recent experiments have provided equally compelling support for the secure-base function of religion (Granqvist, Mikulincer, et al., 2012). Third, most prior research focused on links between organized attachment patterns and theistic forms of religion, but recent research has also focused on other aspects of spirituality, such as in religious syncretism (Granqvist, Broberg, & Hagekull, 2014), in the context of Buddhism (Granqvist, Mikulincer, & Shaver, 2010), and in links between unresolved loss/abuse and altered spiritual states (Granqvist et al., 2009; Granqvist, Hagekull, et al., 2012;

Thomson & Jaque, 2014). Finally, although the attachment–religion connection was placed in the context of a broader evolutionary psychology perspective on religion several years ago (e.g., Kirkpatrick, 2005), more specific conceptual connections have recently been suggested between attachment and central parameters of cognitive science in explaining an individual's development of religious beliefs and representations (Granqvist, 2014b; Richert & Granqvist, 2013). In this context, special attention has been given to cultural and environmental factors (e.g., religious models) that presumably serve to calibrate human psychological mechanisms, such as the attachment system, to make religious "output" highly likely to occur and also to remain stable and important in people's lives (Granqvist, 2014b).

Much of the progress made in religion-as-attachment research in recent years builds coherently on the heuristic potential of attachment theory and on associated research in other areas of mainstream psychology. However, the database on the attachment–religion connection is still evolving relatively slowly, at least as far as high-quality empirical contributions are concerned, and as compared to some other branches of psychological science. Thus, there is ample room for continued progress. We believe that the most important factor holding back the speed of progress is that the psychology of religion is not institutionally anchored in the psychological mainstream. Although the psychology of religion is quickly becoming less marginalized (e.g., Paloutzian & Park, 2013), it is still in many ways a fringe field, garnering almost no academic positions and funding opportunities compared to other psychological subfields. This state of affairs reflects psychology's undisputed bias against religion, including the psychological study of it (e.g., American Psychological Association Council of Representatives, 2007). This bias is likely to make most psychologists deaf and blind to the fascinating and socially relevant aspects of religion. We hope that this chapter removes some of the barriers to accepting the psychology of religion into mainstream psychology.

## Conclusions and Future Directions

In this chapter, we have marshaled evidence from various sources pertinent to the hypothesis that many aspects of religious belief and experience, particularly those related to perceived relationships with God or other supernatural figures, reflect (at least in part) the operation of attachment processes. From a normative perspective, although God is a noncorporeal figure, God evinces all of the defining characteristics of an AF to whom people turn for a safe haven and secure base. We have also attempted to demonstrate that the attachment components of believers' perceived relations with God are far from surface aspects of religion but are instead central components of it. Moreover, we have argued that people's perceived relationships with God develop in tandem with the maturation of the attachment system and associated aspects of cognitive development (e.g., IWMs). From an individual-differences perspective, we have described two attachment-related pathways relevant to the development of religion. One of these runs through experiences with insensitive caregivers and the resulting attachment insecurity, in which case a relationship with God is sometimes a surrogate attachment that is useful in regulating distress (the compensation pathway). The other path runs through experiences with sensitive, often religious caregivers and attachment security, in which case religion is socially rooted in the parental relationship and reflects a generalization of IWMs of the self as worthy of care, and of others (including God) as willing and able to provide it (the correspondence pathway). We have also addressed attachment-related individual differences, in particular disorganized attachment and unresolved loss/abuse, associated with spiritually relevant altered states, as present in mystical experiences and New Age spirituality. We have discussed ways in which attachment-related individual differences are linked to implicit versus more explicit uses of religion. Finally, we have discussed evidence suggesting that the representation of attachment to a God perceived as a reliable safe haven and secure base may confer the kinds of psychological benefits associated with secure interpersonal attachments, especially in times of personal trouble, when other AFs are insufficient or unavailable.

As we have seen, for some individuals, religious beliefs seem to reflect responses to insecure interpersonal attachments; for others, religious beliefs are established early in life, during childhoods characterized by secure attachment, in which cases they remain fairly constant across the lifespan. This distinction raises a host of interesting empirical questions. For example, do the religious beliefs emerging from these alternative processes differ qualitatively with respect to their effects on psychological outcomes? The prospective longitudinal findings from Brown and colleagues (2004), along with other lines of evidence, suggest that individuals who either are currently insecure or have suffered attachment-related difficulties in the past are particularly well served by religion. However, additional prospective longitudinal research is needed before a firm conclusion can be drawn. Such research should also aim to clarify whether—and if so, when and how—religion may be both a salutary factor and a risk factor for psychological outcomes in the context of insecure attachment and past attachment difficulties.

A related set of questions concerns the interaction of correspondence and compensation processes within individuals across time. For example, in cases in which religious change is motivated by insecure interpersonal attachment, does one's orientation toward interpersonal attachments change concomitantly? We have noted the possibility of "earned security" effects from religion for some individuals, but much remains to be done methodologically to secure such an interpretation, to predict for whom and under what conditions earned security might develop, and to pinpoint more precisely the psychological processes involved. Increased knowledge in this area might provide a useful basis for the development of therapeutic strategies for dealing with relationship-related difficulties, particularly in religious populations.

An additional aspect of correspondence and compensation processes that warrants future research is the distinction between implicit- and explicit-level uses of religion. Our expectation, based on the conclusions drawn from the studies reviewed here, is that when activation of the attachment system causes high levels of subjective distress (e.g., in the context of overwhelming anxiety and personal crises), individuals with insecure attachment experiences with insensitive caregivers will be more inclined to regulate distress specifically by turning to God. This is because the insecure "conditional" strategies (i.e., minimization/avoidance and maximization/preoccupation; Main, 1991) are likely to prove insufficient during intense stress. If the insecure individual cannot bear the high levels of suffering experienced sufficiently well by employing his or her usual strategy for managing stress, God may be sought in a final attempt to find a security-providing AF. This could be conceived of as a way of retrying the failed "primary" attachment strategy of seeking closeness and security (Main, 1991), albeit in relation to a different and less psychologically threatening target than one's usual AFs.

In contrast, when attachment activation is unconscious or subtle, and God is the only AF available in the situation, automatic activation of

IWMs and associated neural networks may lead individuals with secure attachment experiences with sensitive caregivers to experience God as psychologically accessible, due to a generalized coherent/singular representation (Bowlby, 1973; Main, 1991) of God. Thus, the IWM aspect of correspondence may apply particularly at an implicit level. Notably, insecure individuals with insensitive caregivers would instead shy away in such situations, due to a generalized incoherent/multiple representation (Main, 1991).

Regarding limitations in the foci of attachment and religion studies to date, two are particularly important. First, there are still no long-term longitudinal studies that have followed participants from early childhood, when their first attachments developed, to later in development, when their God relationship and other attachment relationships unfold. Second, few attachment–religion studies have been conducted outside the Western world, and, to the best of our knowledge, none outside the major monotheistic traditions other than the New Age beliefs discussed previously.

Concerning general theoretical issues, we have found in discussions with colleagues that a common misconception of the religion-as-attachment model is that it would be built on, or even require, an adaptationist understanding of religion (i.e., an assumption that religion itself promoted inclusive fitness in our environments of evolutionary adaptation, or EEAs). In contrast, our view has consistently been that religion is more likely to be an evolutionary by-product than a direct adaptation (or set of adaptations); that is, whereas the attachment system has a clear and very important biological function within its usual sphere of operation (promoting inclusive fitness through caregivers' protection and support of offspring), it is unlikely that a relationship with (an imagined) God increased inclusive fitness by systematically protecting individuals who had such a relationship from danger in our EEAs. Although some theorists would suggest that the God relationship promoted inclusive fitness in some other ways, such as through sexual selection or group selection mechanisms, we believe that there are a number of good arguments against an adaptationist view of religion (for extensive discussion, see Kirkpatrick, 1999, 2005, 2006). Nevertheless, once a mechanism has established itself within the gene pool of a species, it may well continue to operate within individuals and in contexts that are not associated with its original biological function. Therefore, the question of religion's biological functional-ity is more or less orthogonal to the question of whether the relationship between a believer and God involves the attachment system and is a kind of attachment relationship.

Another general issue is the conceptual limit of attachment theory in the psychology of religion. We have deliberately restricted most of our discussion to aspects of religion that we believe to be psychologically grounded in the attachment system per se. Many other applications of attachment constructs to religion are tempting: "attachment" to human religious leaders (pastors, cult leaders, shamans); "attachment" to religious groups (congregations, cults, denominations); and the concept of "nonattachment" in Buddhism—to name just a few. Although these and other religious phenomena may seem analogous to attachment in certain ways, we suspect that many reflect the operation of psychological processes and systems other than attachment (Kirkpatrick, 1999, 2005, 2006). In short, we make no claim that attachment theory constitutes a comprehensive psychology of religion. What we do claim, however, is that attachment is a central component underlying individuals' beliefs about, ways of relating to, and representations of God, particularly, but by no means exclusively, in Christianity.

Notwithstanding many unanswered questions, we submit that no model of adult interpersonal relationships in general, or attachment relationships in particular, will be complete without explicit acknowledgment of the role of God and other imaginary figures in people's relationship networks. Incorporating religious beliefs into research on adult relationships may be useful in addressing vexing questions in the attachment literature concerning issues such as the content, structure, and generality of IWMs, and the dynamic processes underlying change in attachment patterns and IWMs over time. Thus, application of attachment theory to religion has not only held promise for the psychology of religion, but it may also have much to offer the study of attachment processes and individual differences across the lifespan.

## Notes

1. God is obviously different from human AFs by being unobservable. Therefore, it is not possible to have a physical, face-to-face relationship with God. Notably, attachments typically develop based on a joint interaction history between the attached person and the AF. Without getting into the realm of metaphys-

ics, we cannot determine that a believer's perceived relationship with God is based on such an interaction history (i.e., an expression of theism), but neither can we determine that it is not (i.e., an expression of atheism). However, our primary concern is whether, despite this difference from other attachments, a believer's perceived relationship with God can *function* psychologically like an attachment relationship. For the sake of readability and simplicity, throughout this chapter we speak of God "as" an attachment figure and of a believer's relationship with God "as" an attachment relationship, recognizing that some readers might prefer to characterize these phenomena as merely "attachment-like" or as "symbolic attachments."

2. All Biblical quotes are from the King James Version.

3. All attachment data reported in this chapter that required coding were coded by evaluators who were unaware of participants' religiousness and spirituality.

4. Although IWM correspondence and social correspondence are independent in principle, they are not so in practice. For example, insofar as a caregiver has an overtly expressed God image, a secure offspring is expected to adopt his or her caregiver's God image to a larger extent than an insecure offspring, even if the image is of, for example, a distant God (social correspondence). On the other hand, the secure offspring is anticipated to have a less distant God image, due to the operation of a generalized, positive set of IWMs (IWM correspondence). In practice, this is not a serious problem because a reliably sensitive caregiver's God image is unlikely to be distant. Hence social and IWM correspondence will usually operate in concert rather than in opposition.

5. In the social cognition literature, these distinctions are paralleled by distinctions between *contrast* (cf. compensation) and *assimilation* (cf. correspondence) effects (e.g., Wheeler & Petty, 2001). Contrast effects tend to occur when conditions or response modes require explicit processing (e.g., guided imagery, self-reports), whereas assimilation effects tend to occur when only implicit processes are operating (e.g., subliminal priming, lexical decision tasks).

## References

Ainsworth, M. D. S. (1985). Attachments across the life span. *Bulletin of the New York Academy of Medicine, 61,* 792–812.

Ainsworth, M. D. S., Bell, S. M., & Stayton, D. J. (1974). Infant–mother attachment and social development: "Socialization" as a product of reciprocal responsiveness to signals. In M. P. M. Richards (Ed.), *The integration of a child into a social world* (pp. 99–137). Cambridge, UK: Cambridge University Press.

Ainsworth, M. D. S., Blehar, M. C., Waters, E., & Wall, S. (1978). *Patterns of attachment: A psychological study of the Strange Situation.* Hillsdale, NJ: Erlbaum.

Allport, G. W. (1950). *The individual and his religion.* New York: Macmillan.

American Psychological Association Council of Representatives. (2007). *Resolution on religious, religion-based and/or religion-derived prejudice.* Washington, DC: American Psychological Association.

Argyle, M., & Beit-Hallahmi, B. (1975). *The social psychology of religion.* London: Routledge & Kegan Paul.

Bakermans-Kranenburg, M. J., & Van IJzendoorn, M. H. (2009). The first 10.000 Adult Attachment Interviews: Distributions of attachment representations in clinical and non-clinical groups. *Attachment and Human Development, 11,* 223–263.

Barrett, J. L. (2004). *Why would anyone believe in God?* Lanham, MD: AltaMira Press.

Bartholomew, K., & Horowitz, L. M. (1991). Attachment styles in young adults: A test of a four-category model. *Journal of Personality and Social Psychology, 61,* 226–244.

Batson, C. D., Schoenrade, P., & Ventis, W. L. (1993). *Religion and the individual: A social psychological perspective.* New York: Oxford University Press.

Beck, R., & McDonald, A. (2004). Attachment to God: The Attachment to God Inventory, tests of working model correspondence, and an exploration of faith group differences. *Journal of Psychology and Theology, 32,* 92–103.

Birgegard, A., & Granqvist, P. (2004). The correspondence between attachment to parents and God: Three experiments using subliminal separation cues. *Personality and Social Psychology Bulletin, 30,* 1122–1135.

Bjorck, J. P., & Cohen, L. H. (1993). Coping with threats, losses, and challenges. *Journal of Social and Clinical Psychology, 12,* 56–72.

Bowlby, J. (1973). *Attachment and loss: Vol. 2. Separation: Anxiety and anger.* New York: Basic Books.

Bowlby, J. (1980). *Attachment and loss. Vol. 3. Loss.* New York: Basic Books.

Bowlby, J. (1982). *Attachment and loss: Vol. 1. Attachment.* New York: Basic Books. (Original work published 1969)

Bretherton, I. (1987). New perspectives on attachment relations: Security, communication, and internal working models. In J. D. Osofsky (Ed.), *Handbook of infant development* (2nd ed., pp. 1061–1100). New York: Wiley.

Brown, S. L., Nesse, R. M., House, J. S., & Utz, R. L. (2004). Religion and emotional compensation: Results from a prospective study of widowhood. *Personality and Social Psychology Bulletin, 30,* 1165–1174.

Byrd, K. R., & Boe, A. D. (2000). The correspondence between attachment dimensions and prayer in college students. *International Journal for the Psychology of Religion, 11,* 9–24.

Campos, J. J., & Stenberg, C. (1981). Perception, appraisal, and emotion: The onset of social referencing. In M. E. Lamb & L. R. Sherrod (Eds.), *Infant social cognition: Empirical and theoretical considerations* (pp. 273–314). Hillsdale, NJ: Erlbaum.

Cassibba, R., & Granqvist, P., & Costantini, A. (2013). Mothers' attachment security predicts their children's sense of God's closeness. *Attachment and Human Development, 15*, 51–64.

Cassibba, R., & Granqvist, P., Costantini, A., & Gatto, S. (2008). Attachment and God representations among lay Catholics, priests, and religious: A matched comparison study based on the Adult Attachment Interview. *Developmental Psychology, 44*, 1753–1763.

Cicirelli, V. G. (2004). God as the ultimate AF for older adults. *Attachment and Human Development, 6*, 371–388.

Dickie, J. R., Charland, K., & Poll, E. (2005). *Attachment and children's concepts of God*. Unpublished manuscript, Hope College, Hope, MI.

Eshleman, A. K., Dickie, J. R., Merasco, D. M., Shepard, A., & Johnson, M. (1999). Mother God, father God: Children's perceptions of God's distance. *International Journal for the Psychology of Religion, 9*, 139–146.

Evans, E. M. (2001). Cognitive and contextual factors in the emergence of diverse belief systems: Creation versus evolution. *Cognitive Psychology, 42*, 217–266.

Farias, M., & Granqvist, P. (2007). The psychology of the New Age. In D. Kemp (Ed.), *Handbook of New Age* (pp. 123–150). Leiden, The Netherlands: Brill.

Ferm, V. (1945). *The encyclopedia of religion*. Secaucus, NJ: Poplar.

Freud, S. (1961). *The future of an illusion* (J. Strachey, Trans.). New York: Norton. (Original work published 1927)

Galanter, M. (1979). The "Moonies": A psychological study of conversion and membership in a contemporary religious sect. *American Journal of Psychiatry, 136*, 165–170.

Gallup, G., Jr., & Jones, S. (1989). *One hundred questions and answers: Religion in America*. Princeton, NJ: Princeton Religious Research Center.

Gill, A., & Lundsgaarde, E. (2004). State welfare spending and religiosity: A cross-national analysis. *Rationality and Society, 16*, 399–436.

Gorsuch, R. L. (1968). The conceptualization of God as seen in adjective ratings. *Journal for the Scientific Study of Religion, 7*, 56–64.

Granqvist, P. (1998). Religiousness and perceived childhood attachment: On the question of compensation or correspondence. *Journal for the Scientific Study of Religion, 37*, 350–367.

Granqvist, P. (2002). Attachment and religiosity in adolescence: Cross-sectional and longitudinal evaluations. *Personality and Social Psychology Bulletin, 28*, 260–270.

Granqvist, P. (2003). Attachment theory and religious conversions: A review and a resolution of the classic and contemporary paradigm chasm. *Review of Religious Research, 45*, 172–187.

Granqvist, P. (2006). On the relation between secular and divine relationships: An emerging attachment perspective and a critique of the depth approaches. *International Journal for the Psychology of Religion, 16*, 1–18.

Granqvist, P. (2010). Religion as attachment: The Godin award lecture. *Archive for the Psychology of Religion, 32*, 5–24.

Granqvist, P. (2012). Attachment and religious development in adolescence: The implications of culture. In G. Trommsdorff & X. Chen (Eds.), *Values, religion, and culture in adolescent development* (pp. 315–340). New York: Cambridge University Press.

Granqvist, P. (2014a). Mental health and religion from an attachment viewpoint: Overview with implications for future research. *Mental Health, Religion and Culture, 17*(8), 777–793.

Granqvist, P. (2014b). Religion and cognitive, emotional, and social development. In V. Saroglou (Ed.), *Religion, personality, and social psychology* (pp. 283–312). New York: Psychology Press.

Granqvist, P., Broberg, A. G., & Hagekull, B. (2014). Attachment, religiousness, and distress among the religious and spiritual: Links between religious syncretism and compensation. *Mental Health, Religion and Culture, 17*, 726–740.

Granqvist, P., Fransson, M., & Hagekull, B. (2009). Disorganized attachment, absorption, and New Age spirituality – A mediational model. *Attachment and Human Development, 11*, 385–403.

Granqvist, P., & Hagekull, B. (1999). Religiousness and perceived childhood attachment: Profiling socialized correspondence and emotional compensation. *Journal for the Scientific Study of Religion, 38*, 254–273.

Granqvist, P., & Hagekull, B. (2000). Religiosity, adult attachment, and why "singles" are more religious. *International Journal for the Psychology of Religion, 10*, 111–123

Granqvist, P., & Hagekull, B. (2003). Longitudinal predictions of religious change in adolescence: Contributions from the interaction of attachment and relationship status. *Journal of Social and Personal Relationships, 20*, 793–817.

Granqvist, P., Hagekull, B., & Ivarsson, T. (2012). Disorganized attachment promotes mystical experiences via a propensity for alterations in consciousness (Absorption). *International Journal for the Psychology of Religion, 22*, 180–197.

Granqvist, P., Ivarsson, T., Broberg, A. G., & Hagekull, B. (2007). Examining relations between attachment, religiosity, and New Age spirituality using the Adult Attachment Interview. *Developmental Psychology, 43*, 590–601.

Granqvist, P., & Kirkpatrick, L. A. (2004). Religious conversion and perceived childhood attachment: A meta-analysis. *International Journal for the Psychology of Religion, 14*, 223–250.

Granqvist, P., Ljungdahl, C., & Dickie, J. R. (2007). God is nowhere, God is now here: Attachment activation, security of attachment, and perceived closeness to God among 5–7 year-old children from religious and non-religious homes. *Attachment and Human Development, 9,* 55–71.

Granqvist, P., & Main, M. (2003). *The Representation of God in Relation to Self Interview (RGSI).* Unpublished manuscript, Uppsala University, Uppsala, Sweden.

Granqvist, P., Mikulincer, M., Gewirtz, V., & Shaver, P. R. (2012). Experimental findings on God as an AF: Normative processes and moderating effects of internal working models. *Journal of Personality and Social Psychology, 103,* 804–818.

Granqvist, P., Mikulincer, M., & Shaver, P. R. (2010). Religion as attachment: Normative processes and individual differences. *Personality and Social Psychology Review, 14,* 49–59.

Granqvist, P., & Moström, J. (2014). There are plenty of atheists in foxholes—in Sweden. *Archive for the Psychology of Religion,36*(2), 199–213.

Granqvist, P., Reijman, S., & Cardeña, E. (2011). Altered consciousness and human development. In E. Cardeña & M Winkelman (Eds.), *Altering consciousness: A multidisciplinary perspective* (pp. 211–234). New York: Praeger.

Greeley, A. (1990). *The Catholic myth: The behavior and beliefs of American Catholics.* New York: Scribner.

Halama, P, Gasparikova, M., & Sabo, M. (2013). Relationship between attachment styles and dimensions of the religious conversion process. *Studia Psychologica, 55,* 195–207.

Hazan, C., & Shaver, P. (1987). Romantic love conceptualized as an attachment process. *Journal of Personality and Social Psychology, 52,* 511–524.

Hazan, C., & Shaver, P. (1994). Attachment as an organizational framework for research on close relationships. *Psychological Inquiry, 5,* 1–22.

Heelas, P, Woodhead, L., Seel, B., & Szerszynski, B. (2005). *The spiritual revolution: Why religion is giving way to spirituality.* Oxford, UK: Blackwell.

Heller, D. (1986). *The children's God.* Chicago: University of Chicago Press.

Hesse, E., & Main, M. (2006). Frightened, threatening, and dissociative (FR) parental behavior as related to infant D attachment in low-risk samples: Description, discussion, and interpretations. *Development and Psychopathology, 18,* 309–343.

Hetherington, E., & Frankie, G. (1967). Effects of parental dominance, warmth, and conflict on imitation in children. *Journal of Personality and Social Psychology, 6,* 119–125.

Hood, R. W., Jr., Hill, P. C., & Spilka, B. (2009). *The psychology of religion: An empirical approach* (4th ed.). New York: Guilford Press.

Hood, R. W., Jr., Spilka, B., Hunsberger, B., & Gorsuch, R. (1996). *The psychology of religion: An empirical approach* (2nd ed.). New York: Guilford Press.

James, W. (1890). *The principles of psychology* (2 vols.). New York: Dover. (Original work published 1890)

James, W. (1902). *The varieties of religious experience.* New York: Longmans, Green.

Johnson, P. E. (1945). *Psychology of religion.* New York: Abingdon-Cokesbury.

Kaplan, N. (1987). *Individual differences in 6-years olds' thoughts about separation: Predicted from attachment to mother at age 1.* Unpublished doctoral dissertation, University of California, Berkeley.

Kaufman, G. D. (1981). *The theological imagination: Constructing the concept of God.* Philadelphia: Westminster.

Kirkpatrick, L. A. (1994). The role of attachment in religious belief and behavior. In K. Bartholomew & D. Perlman (Eds.), *Advances in personal relationships: Vol. 5. Attachment processes in adulthood* (pp. 239–265). London: Jessica Kingsley.

Kirkpatrick, L. A. (1997). A longitudinal study of changes in religious belief and behavior as a function of individual differences in adult attachment style. *Journal for the Scientific Study of Religion, 36,* 207–217.

Kirkpatrick, L. A. (1998). God as a substitute AF: A longitudinal study of adult attachment style and religious change in college students. *Personality and Social Psychology Bulletin, 24,* 961–973.

Kirkpatrick, L. A. (1999). Toward an evolutionary psychology of religion. *Journal of Personality, 67,* 921–952.

Kirkpatrick, L. A. (2005). *Attachment, evolution, and the psychology of religion.* New York: Guilford Press.

Kirkpatrick, L. A. (2006). Religion is not an adaptation. In P. McNamara (Ed.), *Where God and science meet: How brain and evolutionary studies alter our understanding of religion* (Vol. 1, pp. 159–179). Westport, CT: Praeger.

Kirkpatrick, L. A., & Shaver, P. R. (1990). Attachment theory and religion: Childhood attachments, religious beliefs, and conversion. *Journal for the Scientific Study of Religion, 29,* 315–334.

Kirkpatrick, L. A., & Shaver, P. R. (1992). An attachment theoretical approach to romantic love and religious belief. *Personality and Social Psychology Bulletin, 18,* 266–275.

Kochanska, G., Aksan, N., Knaack, A., & Rhines, H. M. (2004). Maternal parenting and children's conscience: Early security as moderator. *Child Development, 75,* 1229–1242.

Koenig, H. G., King, D. E., & Carson, V. B. (2012). *Handbook of religion and health* (2nd ed.). New York: Oxford University Press.

Loveland, G. G. (1968). The effects of bereavement on certain religious attitudes. *Sociological Symposium, 1,* 17–27.

Main, M. (1991). Metacognitive knowledge, metacognitive monitoring, and singular (coherent) vs. multiple (incoherent) models of attachment: Findings and directions for future research. In C. M. Parkes, J. Stevenson-Hinde, & P. Marris (Eds.), *Attachment across the life cycle* (pp. 127–159). London: Tavistock/Routledge.

Main, M., Goldwyn, R., & Hesse, E. (2003). *Adult attachment scoring and classification system*. Unpublished manuscript, University of California, Berkeley.

Main, M., Kaplan, N., & Cassidy, J. (1985). Security in infancy, childhood, and adulthood: A move to the level of representation. In I. Bretherton & E. Waters (Eds.), Growing points of attachment theory and research. *Monographs of the Society for Research in Child Development, 50*(1–2, Serial No. 209), 66–104.

Main, M., & Morgan, H. (1996). Disorganization and disorientation in infant Strange Situation behavior: Phenotypic resemblance to dissociative states. In L. Michelson & W. Ray (Eds.), *Handbook of dissociation: Theoretical, empirical, and clinical perspectives* (pp. 107–138). New York: Plenum Press.

Mattlin, J. A., Wethington, E., & Kessler, R. C. (1990). Situational determinants of coping and coping effectiveness. *Journal of Health and Social Behavior, 31*, 103–122.

Mikulincer, M., & Shaver, P. R. (2004). Security-based self-representations in adulthood: Contents and processes. In W. S. Rholes & J. A. Simpson (Eds.), *Adult attachment: Theory, research, and clinical implications* (pp. 159–195). New York: Guilford Press.

O'Brien, M. E. (1982). Religious faith and adjustment to long-term hemodialysis. *Journal of Religion and Health, 21*, 68–80.

Paloutzian, R. F., & Kirkpatrick, L. A. (Eds.). (1995). Religious influences on personal and societal well-being [Special issue]. *Journal of Social Issues, 51*(2).

Paloutzian, R. F., & Park, C. (Eds.). (2013). *Handbook of the psychology of religion and spirituality* (2nd ed., pp. 165–182). New York: Guilford Press

Pargament, K. (1997). *The psychology of religion and coping*. New York: Guilford Press.

Pargament, K. (2002). The bitter and the sweet: An evaluation of the costs and benefits of religiousness. *Psychological Inquiry, 13*, 168–181.

Parkes, C. M. (1972). *Bereavement: Studies of grief in adult life*. New York: International Universities Press.

Pirutinsky, S. (2009). Conversion and attachment insecurity among Orthodox Jews. *International Journal for the Psychology of Religion, 19*, 200–206.

Reed, B. (1978). *The dynamics of religion: Process and movement in Christian churches*. London: Darton, Longman & Todd.

Reinert, D. F., & Edwards, C. E. (2009). Attachment theory, childhood mistreatment, and religiosity. *Psychology of Religion and Spirituality, 1*, 25–34.

Richert, R., & Granqvist, P. (2013). Religious and spiritual development in childhood. In R. F. Paloutzian & C. Park (Eds.), *Handbook of the psychology of religion and spirituality* (2nd ed., pp. 165–182). New York: Guilford Press.

Richters, J. E., & Waters, E. (1991). Attachment and socialization: The positive side of social influence. In M. Lewis & S. Feinman (Eds.), *Genesis of behavior: Vol. 6. Social influences and socialization in infancy* (pp. 185–213). New York: Plenum Press.

Rizzuto, A. M. (1979). *The birth of the living God: A psychoanalytical study*. Chicago: University of Chicago Press.

Roof, W. C., & McKinney, W. (1987). *American mainline religion: Its changing shape and future*. New Brunswick, NJ: Rutgers University Press.

Rowatt, W. C., & Kirkpatrick, L. A. (2002). Two dimensions of attachment to God and their relation to affect, religiosity, and personality constructs. *Journal for the Scientific Study of Religion, 41*, 637–651.

Scheve, K. & Stasavage, D. (2006). Religion and preferences for social insurance. *Quarterly Journal of Political Science, 1*, 255–286.

Schnitker, S. A., Porter, T. J., Emmons, R. A., & Barrett, J. L. (2012). Attachment predicts adolescent conversions at Young Life religious summer camps. *International Journal for the Psychology of Religion, 22*, 216–230.

Sim, T. N., & Loh, B. S. M. (2003). Attachment to God: Measurement and dynamics. *Journal of Social and Personal Relationships, 20*, 373–389.

Smith, T. B., McCullough, M. E., & Poll, J. (2003). Religiousness and depression: Evidence for a main-effect and the moderating influence of stressful life-events. *Psychological Bulletin, 129*, 614–636.

Spilka, B., Hood, R. W., Jr., Hunsberger, B., & Gorsuch, R. (2003). *The psychology of religion: An empirical approach* (3rd ed.). New York: Guilford Press.

Sroufe, L. A., & Waters, E. (1977). Attachment as an organizational construct. *Child Development, 48*, 1184–1199.

Stace, W. T. (1960). *Mysticism and philosophy*. Philadelphia: Lippincott.

Starbuck, E. D. (1899). *The psychology of religion*. New York: Scribner.

Stouffer, S. A. (1949). *The American soldier: Vol. 2. Combat and its aftermath*. Princeton, NJ: Princeton University Press.

St. John of the Cross. (1990). *Dark night of the soul*. New York: Doubleday.

Tamminen, K. (1994). Religious experiences in childhood and adolescence: A viewpoint of religious development between the ages of 7 and 20. *International Journal for the Psychology of Religion, 4*, 61–85.

TenElshof, J. K., & Furrow, J. L. (2000). The role of secure attachment in predicting spiritual maturity of students at a conservative seminary. *Journal of Psychology and Theology, 28*, 99–108.

Thomson, P., & Jaque, V. (2014). Unresolved mourning, supernatural beliefs, and dissociation: A mediation analysis. *Attachment and Human Development, 16*(5), 499–514.

Thouless, R. H. (1923). *An introduction to the psychology of religion*. New York: Macmillan.

Trier, K. K., & Shupe, A. (1991). Prayer, religiosity, and healing in the heartland, USA: A research note. *Review of Religious Research, 32*, 351–358.

Ullman, C. (1982). Change of mind, change of heart: Some cognitive and emotional antecedents of religious conversion. *Journal of Personality and Social Psychology, 42,* 183–192.

Van IJzendoorn, M. H. (1995). Adult attachment representations, parental responsiveness, and infant attachment: A meta-analysis on the predictive validity of the Adult Attachment Interview. *Psychological Bulletin, 117,* 387–403.

Vergote, A., & Tamayo, A. (Eds.). (1981). *The parental figures and the representation of God.* The Hague: Mouton.

Weiss, R. S. (1982). Attachment in adult life. In C. M. Parkes & J. Stevenson-Hinde (Eds.), *The place of attachment in human behavior* (pp. 171–184). New York: Basic Books.

Wenegrat, B. (1989). *The divine archetype: The socio-biology and psychology of religion.* Lexington, MA: Lexington Books.

Wheeler, S. C., & Petty, R. E. (2001). The effects of stereotype activation on behavior: A review of possible mechanisms. *Psychological Bulletin, 127,* 797–826.

Wright, P. J. (2008). Predicting reaction to a message of ministry: An audience analysis. *Journal for the Scientific Study of Religion, 47,* 63–81.

Zahl, B. P., & Gibson, N. J. (2012). God representations, attachment to God, and satisfaction with life: A comparison of doctrinal and experiential representations of God in Christian young adults. *International Journal for the Psychology of Religion, 22,* 216–230.

Zeifman, D., & Hazan, C. (1997). A process model of adult attachment formation. In S. Duck (Ed.), *Handbook of personal relationships* (pp. 179–195). Chichester, UK: Wiley.

# Chapter 40

# Divorce through the Lens
# of Attachment Theory

Brooke C. Feeney
Joan K. Monin

The only thing more unthinkable than leaving was staying; the only thing more impossible than staying was leaving.

—Elizabeth Gilbert, *Eat, Pray, Love*

Divorce is a significant life event because it involves the termination of one of the strongest affectional bonds formed by adults. In this chapter, we consider divorce and its aftermath from an attachment–theoretical perspective. We consider the process of divorce, the effects of divorce on the couple members' postdivorce adjustment, and the effects of divorce on children. In doing so, we review the literature and consider how individual differences in attachment orientation may affect the process and outcome of divorce. We conclude by discussing important next steps for research.

## The Relevance of Attachment
## Theory to the Study of Divorce

First, it is important to emphasize that one of the most common attachment bonds formed in adulthood is the one formed with a romantic/marriage partner. According to attachment theory, neither love nor grief nor other forms of strong emotion are felt for just any person; instead, they are felt for particular individuals with whom one has estab-

lished an attachment bond (Bowlby, 1969/1982, 1979). *Attachment bonds* are strong, persistent ties that cause each member of a dyad to maintain proximity to the other and to engage in proximity-seeking behavior when greater protection or support is needed. The biological function of attachment bonds is protection, and the capacity to make and maintain bonds appropriate to each phase of life is as important for species survival as are nutrition and reproduction (Bowlby 1969/1982, 1979). Once formed, an attachment bond tends to endure, and its disruption is strongly resisted. To the extent that dissolving a marriage requires the dissolution or reorganization of an attachment bond, divorce is a very significant life transition.

Although attachment theory does not specifically delineate the factors that contribute to divorce, it provides an important foundation for understanding the mechanisms underlying this prevalent form of social disruption in adulthood. The theory stipulates two important criteria for healthy human functioning: First, every individual (throughout the lifespan) requires the presence and availability of a trustworthy figure who is willing and able to provide a *safe haven* (where a person can retreat for comfort and support in times of need) and a *secure base* (from which to engage in exploration of the world and one's own capacities). Second, everyone must be able both to recognize when another person is a trustworthy attachment figure and to collaborate with him or her to maintain a mutually rewarding relationship (Bowlby, 1979). The absence of one or both of these important features of a marriage—for one or both partners—sets the stage for dysfunctional relations and eventual separation and divorce.

## What Happens When a Spouse Fails to Function as a Trustworthy Attachment Figure?

Human beings of all ages are happiest and able to deploy their talents to best advantage when they are confident that, standing behind them, there are one or more trusted persons who will come to their aid should difficulties arise.
—JOHN BOWLBY (1979, p. 103)

This proposition from attachment theory is important to the stability and dissolution of marriages because "trusted persons" in adulthood often include a person's spouse. Attachment theory specifies the characteristics of a trustworthy figure—one who enhances a person's safety and security by providing (1) a safe haven to which he or she can retreat in times of need and (2) a secure base from which to explore (to learn, discover, work, play, engage in challenging activities, develop relationships with peers, and grow as an individual). Attachment figures who foster security recognize and respect their partner's needs/desire for a safe haven and secure base, and they act accordingly. Such attachment figures understand, accept, and respect both attachment behavior (proximity seeking in times of need) and exploratory behavior, and recognize that one of the most common causes of negative emotion is frustration of one's desires for love and care. Emotions such as anxiety and anger often stem from uncertainty about whether attachment figures will be available and responsive to one's needs (Bowlby, 1979).

Of course, spousal provision of a safe haven and a secure base can vary considerably, and a person's ability to fulfill the role of reliable caregiver to a romantic/marital partner is often influenced by one's previous attachment history. As Bowlby (1979) said, "Each of us is apt to do unto others as we have been done by" (p. 141). Attachment theory and research suggests that when spouses provide favorable conditions for each other (as

just described), each is likely to feel secure and self-reliant, trusting, cooperative, and helpful in dealing with the other, and with their children. When favorable conditions are not provided, spouses are likely to be insecure in their relationship and plagued by feelings of anxiety, hurt, anger, mistrust, resistance to cooperation, and frustrated personal growth (Bowlby, 1979, 1988).

Spouses may encourage each other's attachment anxiety (worry about rejection or abandonment) or avoidance (discomfort with intimacy) by being unresponsive to signals of need for care, behaving in a rejecting/disparaging manner, threatening the partner or family as a means of controlling the partner, and not being consistently available (Bowlby, 1969/1982, 1979, 1988). Such experiences may cause the partner to live in constant anxiety, have a low threshold for activation of attachment behavior, and be overly solicitous/dependent. Alternatively, the partner may react to inadequate spousal care by inhibiting attachment feelings/behavior, being distrustful of the spouse, and insisting on extreme self-reliance.

According to attachment theory, all kinds of poor care are likely simultaneously to arouse anger toward one's attachment figure and to inhibit its expression (Bowlby, 1969/1982, 1979, 1988). The result is often underlying resentment that contributes to dysfunctional relations because everyone, even people who have learned to be what Bowlby (1969/1982) called "compulsively self-reliant," needs love, care, and support. Moreover, when a person's attachment needs go unmet, he or she is more vulnerable to stress and less capable of dealing with it. In fact, unmet attachment needs may be expressed in aberrant forms of care-eliciting behavior (substance use, sexual infidelity) that are likely to take a great toll on marriage and family relations (Bowlby, 1979).

## What Causes a Person to be Unable to Recognize a Trustworthy Attachment Figure and Collaborate in a Mutually Rewarding Relationship?

There is a strong causal relationship between an individual's experiences with his parents and his later capacity to make affectional bonds.
—JOHN BOWLBY (1979, p. 135)

According to attachment theory, a healthy person is able to trust and rely on others, and to know who can be relied upon (Bowlby, 1969/1982,

1988). A healthy adult is also capable of exchanging roles when the situation calls for it, at one time providing a secure base and safe haven from which a partner can operate, and at other times being able to rely on the partner to provide a secure base and safe haven in return. Each partner must have the capacity to adopt either role as circumstances require. Each must be able to express a desire for help/support in a direct and effective way, and each, in turn, must be able to give to the other—and to their children (Bowlby, 1979, 1988).

The theory also stipulates that impairment of the ability to collaborate in a mutually rewarding relationship can take many forms. For example, a person who has difficulty trusting his or her spouse may either be unable to express a desire for support when needed or do so in a demanding, aggressive way. Both kinds of behavior reflect lack of confidence that support will be forthcoming and dissatisfaction with what is given when provided. Marriage partners with these impairments may exhibit anxious clinging and make excessive demands or be aloof, unavailable emotionally, and defiantly independent (Bowlby, 1979, 1988). They may exhibit either an inability to give spontaneously to others or a compulsively overinvolved caregiving style in order to meet attachment needs. According to attachment theory, these impairments may stem from inadequate care from previous attachment figures, most often one's parents.

A major claim of the theory is that mental and behavioral patterns learned in prior attachment relationships tend to persist because people construct representational models of self and attachment figures during childhood and adolescence, and new partners get assimilated to these models, often despite extensive evidence that the model is no longer appropriate. These biased perceptions result in misconceptions of others, false expectations about the way people behave, and inappropriate actions intended to forestall expected negative experiences. For example, Bowlby (1979, p. 142) said,

A man who during childhood was frequently threatened with abandonment can easily attribute such intentions to his wife. He will then misinterpret things she says or does in terms of such intent, and then take whatever action he thinks would best meet the situation he believes to exist. Misunderstanding and conflict must follow. In all this he is as unaware he is being biased by his past experience as he is that his present beliefs and expectations are mistaken.

Bowlby (1979) further stated that inappropriate but persistent representational models often coexist with more appropriate ones: "A husband may oscillate between believing his wife to be loyal to him and suspecting her of plans to desert" (p. 142). Bowlby contended that the stronger the emotions aroused in a relationship, the more likely are the earlier, less conscious models to become dominant and guide perception and behavior. Thus, in order to collaborate in a mutually rewarding relationship with a spouse, an adult must consider how his or her prior experiences may influence needs, worries, expectations, and relational behavior. A major premise of attachment theory is that representational models, and patterns of behavior based on them, can be so entrenched that they continue unchecked, even when they are dysfunctional.

For example, people who have learned a pattern of fault finding, punishment, revenge, guilt induction, or evasion tend to carry those patterns into their marriages, where they are likely to contribute to a destructive downward spiral that is difficult to break. Breaking such a negative interaction cycle may require (1) discovering the specific situations (current or past) that may underlie the negative interaction patterns and recognizing that negative interaction patterns are either responses to those situations or side effects of trying not to respond to them; (2) identifying the representational models of self and attachment figures that govern one's perceptions, predictions, and actions, often without conscious awareness or clarity; and (3) reevaluating relationships, modifying representational models in light of more recent experiences, and making deliberate changes in ways of treating others (Bowlby, 1979). Such changes are typically slow and patchy; they require a great deal of motivation and effort, and insecurity often hinders this process (Bowlby, 1979). This may explain why many marriages end despite couples having sought marital counseling.

### Relevant Empirical Work

Empirical work specifically linking attachment history and attachment orientation to the prediction of divorce is scarce. However, attachment theory offers a useful framework for explaining and integrating the processes that have been shown to predict marital dissolution. Personal characteristics and marital interaction patterns that predict divorce are indicative of either having a spouse who is not a trustworthy attachment figure and/or being unable to recognize, benefit from, and maintain a mutually rewarding relationship with a trustworthy figure.

As we explained earlier, attachment theory stipulates that every individual builds experience-based representational models of self and others that affect how he or she perceives events, forecasts the future, constructs plans, and selects strategies for interacting with others (Bowlby, 1969/1982, 1973, 1980). These models are thought to underlie individual differences in attachment orientation that have proven strongly predictive of relationship dynamics, including conflict behaviors (Brassard, Lussier, & Shaver, 2009; Saavedra, Chapman, & Rogge, 2010; Simpson, Rholes, & Phillips, 1996), caregiving behaviors (Feeney & Collins, 2001; Feeney & Thrush, 2010; Kunce & Shaver, 1994), motivations (Feeney, Collins, Van Vleet, & Tomlinson, 2013), biased information processing (Collins & Feeney, 2004; Ein-Dor, Mikulincer, & Shaver, 2011; Feeney & Cassidy, 2003), coping strategies (Mikulincer & Florian, 1998; Schmidt, Blank, Bellizzi, & Park, 2012), physiological responses to stress (Jaremka et al., 2013; Pietromonaco & Powers, 2015; Roisman, 2007), emotion regulation/expression (Monin, Feeney, & Schulz, 2012; Simpson, Collins, Tran, & Haydon, 2007), trust (Mikulincer, 1998), defensiveness (Fraley, Garner, & Shaver, 2000; Kohn, Rholes, & Schmeichel, 2012; Mikulincer & Orbach, 1995), and forgiveness (Liao & Wei, 2015; Mikulincer, Shaver, & Slav, 2006). Specifically within the context of marriage, attachment insecurity has been linked with relationship dissatisfaction, poor communication, poor emotion regulation, poor problem solving, and poor support behavior (Davila, Karney, & Bradbury, 1999; J. A. Feeney, Noller, & Callan, 1994; Kohn, Rholes, & Schmeichel, 2012).

In happy, well-functioning relationships, the attachment system works, so that both partners feel secure and protected, each is able to depend on the other, and each is unafraid of the other's dependence or both partners' interdependence (Fisher & Crandell, 1997). In a securely attached couple this reciprocity is achieved, but in insecure couples, there is rigidity (Reibstein, 1998). In insecure couples, protecting oneself is the primary objective, and it often overrides one's ability to respond empathically to one's partner. Insecure couples include ones in which (1) both partners defensively avoid dependency, each fleeing or withdrawing in times of distress; (2) one partner feels deprived of responsive support, while the other feels overwhelmed by what seem to be the other's insatiable needs; and (3) one partner always occupies the dependent role, while the other is defensively accusatory and dismissive, which

may appear as one partner continuously giving and sacrificing, while the receiving partner is continuously dissatisfied, controlling, unappreciative, and demanding (Fisher & Crandell, 1997). In all such cases, the attachment relationship, which ideally is supportive and rewarding, has become painful, conflictual, and unsatisfying, and the defensive processes that ensue—the very ones delineated so well and extensively by Gottman and colleagues (Gottman, 1994; Gottman & Levenson, 1992, 2000)—are likely to result in marital dissolution.

Attachment theory and research provide additional insight into the mechanisms underlying stability or instability of marriages. In a 4-year longitudinal study of newlyweds, Davila and Bradbury (2001) found that, compared with spouses in happy marriages and divorced spouses, spouses in stable but unhappy marriages showed the highest levels of attachment insecurity both initially and over time. It seems that insecurity causes spouses to be dissatisfied with their marriages yet simultaneously keeps them tied to the marriage. Although dissatisfaction is a proximal predictor of divorce (Karney & Bradbury, 1995), many couples do remain together despite dissatisfaction. Anxious/preoccupied individuals, who are chronically concerned about abandonment and love-worthiness, may attempt to maintain their relationships at any cost (Kirkpatrick & Davis, 1994), whereas avoidant individuals may view divorce as a suitable way to avoid intimacy. Consistent with this idea, research has shown that avoidant attachment is a risk factor for multiple marriages (Ceglian & Gardner, 1999).

## Effects of Divorce on Couple Members

Attachment theory describes the propensity of human beings to form strong emotional bonds with particular others and explains the many forms of emotional distress and personality disturbance (including anxiety, anger, depression, and emotional detachment) to which unwilling separation and loss can give rise (Bowlby, 1973, 1979). Because attachment is an instinctive process that is elicited particularly during times of threat and stress, the loss of an attachment figure may intensify feelings of distress and have an adverse effect on a person's health and well-being if the attachment bond is not broken for both couple members.

## Psychological and Physical Health

Studies of divorce have focused primarily on adjustment to divorce and the effects of divorce on physical and psychological well-being. Most such studies have examined the link between marital status and various indicators of individual well-being, and have found consistently that separated and divorced individuals have higher rates of physical and mental health disturbance than married individuals, and often higher rates even than widowed individuals (Blumenthal, 1967; Mirowsky & Ross, 2003). Specifically, separated and divorced individuals experience increased rates of acute (infectious diseases, respiratory illnesses) and chronic (diabetes, heart disease) physical illnesses, physical limitations, psychopathology, depression, suicide, homicide, violence, substance abuse (alcoholism), accidents and injuries, and disease-caused mortality (Aseltine & Kessler, 1993; Bloom, Asher, & White, 1978; Booth & Amato, 1991; Burman & Margolin, 1992; Chatav & Whisman, 2007; Hu & Goldman, 1990; Kiecolt-Glaser et al., 1987; Lorenz, Wickrama, Conger, & Elder, 2006; Overbeek et al., 2006; Perrig-Chiello, Hutchison, & Morselli, 2014; Sbarra, 2015; Sbarra, Hasselmo, & Nojopranoto, 2012; Stack & Scourfield, 2015; Williams & Umberson, 2004). Divorced individuals also report lower levels of happiness, life satisfaction, self-esteem, self-confidence, and competence (Amato, 2000; Glenn & Weaver, 1988; Gustavson, Røysamb, von Soest, Helland, & Mathiesen, 2012; Kurdek, 1991; Lucas, 2005; Spanier & Casto, 1979).

It is important to note that although divorced individuals are worse off than married people in general, if divorced people are compared with people in the most unhappy marriages, the divorced have higher morale, fewer physical problems, fewer depressive symptoms, and greater life satisfaction, self-esteem, and overall health (Hawkins & Booth, 2005; Overbeek et al., 2006). Thus, the more unhappiness and distress experienced in a marriage, the greater the relief and potential benefit that may follow divorce (see also Gustavson, Nilsen, Orstavik, & Røysamb, 2014; Gustavson et al., 2012; Spanier & Thompson, 1984). Also consistent with the idea that divorce is not uniformly harmful, research has shown that following a period of both emotional and physical upheaval, most adults cope successfully with divorce (Amato, 2000; Aseltine & Kessler, 1993; Booth & Amato, 1991; Hetherington & Kelly, 2002; Perrig-Chiello et al., 2014; Sbarra & Emery, 2005), and some re-port opportunities for growth, increased independence, and increased life satisfaction (Huddleston & Hawkings, 1991; Maatta, 2011; Marks, 1996; Symoens, Colman, & Bracke, 2014).

Nonetheless, a great deal of research indicates that divorce is generally very taxing and distressing. Although some studies have suggested that marital dissolution affects men more than women (Hu & Goldman, 1990; Symoens, Van de Velde, Colman, & Bracke, 2014), and others have suggested the reverse (Aseltine & Kessler, 1993; Gottman & Levenson, 1992; Kiecolt-Glaser et al., 1987), the effects of separation and divorce on psychological and physical health have been extensively documented for both sexes. It appears, however, that the processes responsible for the link between divorce and particular health outcomes may be different for women and men. For example, the health effects of marital loss have been attributed to the economic hardships and material conditions suffered by women when marriages dissolve (Lillard & Waite, 1995) and to the loss of social networks and social control that encourages healthy living for men (Gove & Shin, 1989; Umberson, 1987; see Dupre & Meadows, 2007, for a review). Also, Gottman (1994) found that the health of women is directly affected by marital distress, whereas for men it is mediated through loneliness.

It is important to note, however, that most of the studies in this area provide little information about why or how marital status is related to health or well-being (Mirowsky & Ross, 2003). Most researchers explain their results in terms of the protective effects of marriage, which include a healthier lifestyle, higher socioeconomic status, more financial resources, and a stable social network. Other explanations include (1) a social selectivity or preexisting pathology model, according to which people who divorce are less physically or psychologically fit for marriage, and (2) a crisis model, according to which divorce is a traumatic event that induces psychological distress and health problems that lessen as a person adjusts to a changed social situation (Bloom et al., 1978; Kitson, 1982; Lucas, 2005; Solomon & Jackson, 2014). The crisis model identifies divorce-related stressors likely to affect health and well-being, such as the emotional strain of marital breakdown, continuing conflict with the ex-spouse, fewer material and economic resources, more risky behaviors (drinking, driving recklessly), less stringent health monitoring, loss of supportive social networks, loss of social status, social isolation, hardships of single parenthood, time constraints, role strain, and the need to rebuild one's life. Attachment theory provides an integrative account of both perspectives by postulating that although separation anxiety and distress are normative responses to loss, some people are predisposed by previous experiences to react more strongly to losses (Kitson, 1982; Simos, 1979; Weiss, 1975).

### Individual Differences in Adjustment

Because attachment theory predicts differential experiences of relationships, appraisals of threats, emotion regulation, and coping strategies, depending on attachment styles (Mikulincer & Florian, 1998; Shaver & Mikulincer, 2007; Mikulincer & Shaver, Chapter 24, this volume), there are likely to be systematic individual differences in adjustment to divorce. In fact, individual differences should be especially evident in the context of divorce because divorce raises a core attachment issue (loss of an attachment figure), and the stresses/challenges associated with divorce are likely to heighten activation of the attachment system. According to attachment theory, stressful life events such as divorce should be particularly taxing for individuals with troubled attachment histories (insecure attachment orientations) (Bowlby, 1979). Insecure individuals are particularly likely to break down after loss or separation because the separation confirms their worst fears and expectations. The divorce is likely to reactivate earlier unresolved separations from attachment figures, and because insecure individuals lack the inner resources and coping strategies needed for adjusting to divorce, they are likely to have difficulty dealing with the loss (Mikulincer & Florian, 1996).

When discussing bereavement in adult life, Bowlby (1979) noted that adults generally respond to separation and loss in a series of stages, including numbness, yearning and searching, disorganization and despair, then reorganization. He also identified characteristics of loss situations that interfere with healthy adjustment. These include (1) having been in a relationship that provided considerable self-esteem and role identity, which are less sustainable without the lost partner; (2) having no close relationship with another person to whom the individual can transfer some of the feelings that were bound up with the lost spouse; and (3) a marriage that was conflicted or ambivalent. Bowlby emphasized that in order for mourning to result in a favorable outcome, the bereaved person must be able to express his or her feelings

(yearning, anger, sadness, fear of loneliness) and may need the support of another trusted person.

Attachment theory makes predictions regarding individual differences in adjustment to divorce. The divorce-related distress experienced by secure individuals is likely to be buffered by social and personal resources that facilitate coping (e.g., the ability to seek and elicit support from others; Vareschi & Bursik, 2005). In contrast, insecure individuals view stressors as more threatening. Those high in attachment anxiety view themselves as less capable of coping and report greater distress (Davis, Shaver, & Vernon, 2003); those high in avoidant tendencies use distancing to cope, do not turn to others for support, and report greater hostility (Mikulincer & Florian, 1998; Ognibene & Collins, 1998).

A few studies have specifically examined divorcing adults' adjustment as a function of attachment orientation. Birnbaum, Orr, Mikulincer, and Florian (1997) found that dispositional attachment anxiety and avoidance are associated with greater divorce-related distress and poorer coping (see also Cohen & Finzi-Dottan, 2012). Lee, Sbarra, Mason, and Law (2011) found that separated adults high in attachment anxiety showed higher levels of hyperactivating coping strategies and the highest levels of blood pressure during a divorce-specific task. Fraley and Bonanno (2004) studied a group of bereaved (not divorced) adults and found differences between two kinds of avoidance: Whereas some avoidant individuals (those who are also high in anxiety, called *fearful avoidants*) have difficulty adapting to the loss of a loved one, those who are *dismissing avoidants* seem resilient in adapting to loss, perhaps because they were not as invested in their relationship before the loss. In extremely threatening situations in which it is impossible to maintain a defensively dismissive stance, both anxious and avoidant attachment are associated with symptoms (Mikulincer, Horesh, Eilati, & Kotler, 1999; Mikulincer & Shaver, 2007). Corroborating these findings, Yamoz-Yaben (2010) found poor adjustment to divorce particularly among preoccupied and fearful (high anxiety) individuals. In another study, among avoidant individuals, those who were able to self-regulate (as indexed by heart rate variability during a divorce-related mental activation task) showed improvements in their self-concept over 3 months, whereas those who were less able to self-regulate showed either no improvement or worsening of their self-concept over the subsequent 3 months (Sbarra & Borelli, 2013), which suggests that some people (perhaps dismissing avoidants) are better able to deactivate attachment-related thoughts and feelings than others. It will be important to conduct more in-depth studies of the links between attachment security and adjustment to divorce, as well as the mechanisms underlying these links, one of which may be the ability to self-regulate.

## Continuing Attachment and Postdivorce Contact between Ex-Spouses

Although there are many problems and stressors with which divorced individuals must cope (economic problems, legal issues, property settlements, social network changes, concerns regarding children and coparenting, formation of new relationships; see Bohannon, 1970; Spanier & Casto, 1979), the loss of the marital relationship itself, combined with continuing contact and involvement with the ex-spouse, has been viewed as the most stressful part of the divorce experience (Bohannon, 1970; Hetherington, Cox, & Cox, 1982; Weiss, 1975, 1976). Separation from a spouse elicits conflicting emotions in both partners, including anger, contempt, regret, resentment, longing, affection, wish for reconciliation, guilt, anxiety, panic, sadness, and loneliness—regardless of what led to the divorce (Weiss, 1976). This mixture of positive and negative emotions can be confusing and is attributed to the persistence of the attachment bond when intimate relationships are disrupted (Berman, 1988a, 1988b; Weiss, 1975).

Studies have shown that many men and women going through divorce continue to have feelings of attachment toward their ex-spouses (Berman, 1988b; Brown, Felton, Whiteman, & Manela, 1980; Kitson, 1982; Spanier & Casto, 1979; Weiss, 1975). Although feelings of attachment are greatest when the divorce is recent and the spouse was the one who initiated it, attachment does not seem to be influenced by the length of marriage, suggesting that attachment bonds may be established fairly quickly but are broken slowly (Brown et al., 1980; Brown & Reimer, 1984; Kitson, 1982) and that the loss of an attachment bond is as difficult for those married a few years as for those married many years (Weiss, 1975). Once partners have significantly bonded, attachment often persists and resists dissolution—even in the face of anger, hurt, and knowledge that the relationship should be terminated (Aydintug,

1995; Davis et al., 2003; Mazor, Batiste-Harel, & Gampel, 1998).

These continued feelings of attachment for an ex-spouse have been considered to be a primary cause of the emotional and adjustment problems that follow separation (Berman, 1988a, 1988b; Brown et al., 1980; Kitson, 1982; Weiss, 1976). Although not consistently shown (Masheter, 1991; Spanier & Casto, 1979), continuing attachment to an ex-spouse has been linked with a variety of symptoms, including depression, anxiety, distress, loneliness, anger, lowered self-efficacy, lack of social self-confidence, less autonomy, less life satisfaction, and poor self-rated adjustment (Brown & Reimer, 1984; Emery, 1994; Madden-Derdich & Arditti, 1999; Masheter, 1997).

Continuing attachment to an ex-spouse may be accounted for by the biological predisposition to use attachment figures as a safe haven and a secure base. Losing an attachment figure eliminates these protective functions and creates both separation anxiety and attachment system activation. The many challenges associated with divorce are stressors that are likely to intensify activation of the attachment system and create a desire for proximity to one's attachment figure (which may have been the spouse prior to the divorce). The process of detachment and reorganization (Bowlby, 1980) is likely to be more difficult than either spouse anticipates because attachment bonds are likely to be partly unconscious and sometimes masked by feelings of dissatisfaction with the spouse (Weiss, 1975, 1976). This idea is consistent with research indicating that partners are often unaware of their emotional investment in their relationship until the relationship ends (Berscheid, 1983). This may explain why 42% of couples headed for divorce separate and then reconcile at least once before ending the relationship (Kitson & Raschke, 1981), why some ex-spouses end up having sex when they were intending only to transfer their children from one parent to the other (Davis et al., 2003), and why only a few years after their divorce, a majority of remarried men say they regret having divorced their former wives (Reibstein & Bamber, 1997).

Because of the difficulty of detaching, Reibstein (1998) notes that divorced individuals often experience a deep vulnerability to their former spouse, which they feel they must guard against with defensive strategies to prevent the pain of reevoked attachment feelings. Regardless of who initiated the divorce, both couple members are likely to be vulnerable, and the process of detachment is likely to be slow and painful for both. In fact, Bowlby (1973) noted that before detachment occurs, the attachment bond may be reactivated if the attachment figure reappears and invites renewed attachment. Attachment feelings and behaviors can be easily reactivated by drawing the former spouse back into old behavior patterns (Reibstein, 1998). Mikulincer and Florian (1996) proposed that adaptation to loss of an attachment figure involves a dialectical interplay of two opposing forces: the desire to maintain proximity to the lost person and the simultaneous desire to detach from the person to form new relationships.

Despite a large empirical literature on other aspects of the divorce experience, little is known about postdivorce relationships between ex-spouses. This is surprising given that postdivorce relations are likely to have important effects on the entire family system (Cole & Cole, 1999). It was once assumed that all postdivorce relations reflect separation distress and should be avoided (Kressel, Lopez-Morillas, Weinglass, & Deutsch, 1978). Clinical and empirical reports have shown that continued relations with a former spouse are often problematic (Aydintug, 1995; Kitson & Morgan, 1990) and that postdivorce harmony is rare, particularly when children are involved (Ambert, 1988; Buunk & Mutsaers, 1999). For example, research has shown that one-half of divorced women and one-third of divorced men continue to be intensely angry at their former spouses, even 10 years after the breakup (Wallerstein & Blakeslee, 1989). Moreover, a study of remarried individuals found little continued friendship between former spouses (Buunk & Mutsaers, 1999). Few relationships offer as many opportunities for anger, blame, hatred, retaliation, desires for revenge, and violence as the ones between former spouses (Guisinger, Cowan, Schuldberg, 1989), particularly given that ex-spouses know each other's vulnerabilities. Remarriages may also contribute to poor postdivorce relations because a close relationship with a former spouse may be threatening to a new spouse and create conflict in the new marriage (Buunk & Mutsaers, 1999).

Attachment theory provides a basis for explaining some of the negative ways in which former spouses behave toward each other. Bowlby (1969/1982) knew that behavior of an aggressive sort (protest, anger) often plays a role in maintaining affectional bonds. Anger can be functional when separation is perceived to be temporary because it may hasten reunion and make it less likely that another separation will occur. This may explain why high levels of disagreement and conflict typically occur during the first year of marital separation (Toews, McKenry, & Catlett, 2003), why many women continue to suffer physical and verbal abuse after separation and divorce, typically by men who do not want the relationship to end (Arendell, 1995; Jasinski & Williams, 1998), and why many relationships without a history of violence often become violent at the time of separation (Ellis & DeKeseredy, 1989; Toews, McKenry, & Catlett, 2003).

Although research has indicated the downside of continuing attachment to one's ex-spouse, it is important to note that a majority of divorced individuals report at least occasional contact with their ex-spouses, and that continuing attachment (presumably relatively secure attachment) might be associated with healthy development as well (Masheter, 1991). For example, research on children's continued contact with both parents has acknowledged the benefits of postdivorce relationships between ex-spouses (Ahrons & Rodgers, 1987; Ahrons & Wallisch, 1986; Dozier, Sollie, Stack, & Smith, 1993). Cooperative postdivorce parenting can reduce role strain for custodial parents and the sense of estrangement and loss for noncustodial parents (Hetherington & Camara, 1984; Masheter, 1991). In fact, it has been argued that for couples who share custody of children, detachment can be only limited (Reibstein, 1998) and some degree of attachment, if transferred effectively into constructive behavior, might be beneficial (Furstenberg & Cherlin, 1991; Madden-Derdich & Arditti, 1999; Masheter, 1991).

Reibstein (1998) argued that, given the strength of the attachment bond, divorced couples need protection from each other during and after divorce in the form of limited and rule-bound contact (agreed-upon rules of engagement and civility to set limits on dysfunctional behavior). Just as children need clarity, predictability, and consistency in the divorce context, so do the divorcing adults. The challenge for divorced couples is to redefine their relationship in a way that is mutually supportive, while minimizing behaviors that adversely affect adjustment (Madden-Derdich & Arditti, 1999). Because the relationship between former spouses often determines the emotional climate in which families function after a divorce (Ahrons & Rodgers, 1987; Hetherington et al., 1982), this redefinition process has significant implications for the functioning of the family in its new form.

Thus, both theoretical and empirical work on the redefinition process is needed. In some ways this process may be like the reorganization of attachment representations following bereavement. At first, Bowlby (1969/1982) viewed this as a case of "detachment," but in his later years (Bowlby, 1988), he viewed it as a matter of reorganization of attachment representations (Fraley & Shaver, 2008). Perhaps as postdivorce attachments can be reorganized so that some of the earlier positive feelings and a new commitment to cooperative interdependence (in parenting) can be beneficial, whereas the disappointment/animosity engendered by the failed marital relationship can fade into the background of memory. This redefinition process may involve a process of transition from an attachment bond to an affiliative bond, which, according to attachment theory, relies on a separate behavioral system. This redefinition process also involves the coordination and maintenance of joint caregiving responsibilities toward the children, while recognizing that other aspects of the prior marital relationship (attachment, sexuality, and caregiving toward the spouse) no longer apply. Positive relations between ex-spouses serve the interests of both spouses' caregiving systems, enhancing the children's well-being and the divorced parents' reproductive fitness.

Divorcing parents with secure attachment orientations are at an advantage because qualities associated with secure attachment (good communication skills, constructive coping strategies, ability to regulate emotions, and the ability to solve conflicts cooperatively) should enable them to share parenting while keeping their children's best interests in mind (Cohen & Finzi-Dottan, 2005; Roberson, Sabo, & Wickel, 2011; Shimkowski & Schrodt, 2012). Interventions may assist in this redefinition process. For example, Vareschi and Bursik (2005) found that parenting workshops increase positive and decrease negative parental interactions for insecure participants, suggesting that interventions can provide insecure individuals with previously unused or unfamiliar tools/strategies for diffusing conflict and facilitating cohesion in shared parenting (for an intervention to increase attachment security, see Bowers, Ogolsky, Hughes, & Kanter, 2014; Yamoz, Plazaola, & Etxeberria, 2008).

## Effects of Divorce on Children

Not only does divorce present attachment-related challenges for children, but the divorce-related stressors experienced by parents frequently interfere with their ability to respond sensitively, responsively, and consistently to their children's needs for safety and security (Page & Bretherton, 2001). Next we describe theory and research regarding the effects of divorce on children's attachment security, psychological and physical health, and future relationship functioning.

### Attachment Security

Again, a major proposition of attachment theory is that, based on experiences with caregivers, people build representational models of themselves and others, and these models are the essence of attachment security and insecurity (Bowlby, 1969/1982, 1973, 1980). To the extent that divorce reduces a child's confidence in who and where his or her attachment figures are; in his or her perceived acceptability in the eyes of attachment figures; and in the availability, accessibility, and sensitive responsiveness of attachment figures (all core aspects of working models), divorce is likely to affect children's attachment security. The mere fact that parents are living apart may undermine a child's feelings of security because parental accessibility becomes more tenuous (Maccoby, Buchanan, Mnookin, & Dornbusch, 1993; Page & Bretherton, 2001). In fact, Bowlby (1980) noted that some children who have experienced loss of or separation from one parent may fear the loss of or separation from the other.

### Infants and Children

Few studies have investigated the effects of divorce on infants' and young children's attachment patterns, and the few that exist have yielded mixed results. Nair and Murray (2005) found that 3- to 6-year-old children from divorced families had lower security scores on the Attachment Q-Set. Clarke-Stewart, Vandell, McCartney, Owen, and Booth (2000) also found that children from divorced families were less secure, as measured by the Strange Situation at 15 months, the Attachment Q-Set at 24 months, and a modified Strange Situation at 36 months. Similarly, Solomon, George, and Wallerstein (1995; cited in Nair & Murray, 2005) found that infants from divorced families were more likely than infants from intact families to be classified as insecure in the Strange Situation. However, Kier and Lewis (1997) found no differences between infants from divorced versus intact families using the Strange Situation. Also, Vaughan, Gove, and Egeland (1980) found only a trend for infants from nonintact families to be more anxiously attached to their mothers than children from intact families.

Investigators have identified several factors that moderate the association between divorce and attachment security in young children and are likely to explain the inconsistent links. First, as predicted by attachment theory, quality of parenting moderates the link. For example, mothers from intact families are more likely than divorced mothers to use positive/authoritative parenting styles (involving sensitivity and responsiveness), which directly affects attachment security (Hetherington et al., 1982; Nair & Murray, 2005). One study indicated that maternal emotional availability (the ability to read and respond appropriately to a child's emotional cues) contributed to the child's secure attachment above and beyond age of onset of overnight stays and interparental conflict (Altenhofen, Sutherland, & Biringen, 2010).

Second, father visitation patterns influence mother–infant attachment. For example, repeated overnight separation from a primary caregiver, usually the mother, is associated with disruption in mother–infant attachment when the conditions of visitation are poor (e.g., when parents do not provide adequate psychological support to the child) (Hodges, Landis, Day, & Oderberg, 1991; Solomon & George, 1999). However, mothers who function as a secure base for their children promote attachment security despite separations due to overnight visits with fathers. Furthermore, mothers who provide psychological protection to their children in the context of father visitation (by being sensitively responsive to the child during the visitation) also promote secure attachment to the father (Solomon & George, 1999). Interestingly, attachment transmission from fathers to children occurs only when fathers function as the primary caregivers (when divorced fathers have full custody; Bernier & Miljkovitch, 2009).

Third, maternal education and family income reduce the effects of divorce on attachment security (Clarke-Stewart et al., 2000) and psychological well-being (Mandemakers & Kalmijn, 2014), perhaps because better education and finances facilitate the kind of parenting that fosters attachment security. Finally, a child's cognitive ability (associated with age) has been identified as a protective factor. Kier and Lewis (1997) tested two contradicting predictions about the effects of parental separation on infants' attachment to

mother: Whereas the "early adversity" hypothesis predicts that infants will be adversely affected by negative life events and therefore develop an anxious attachment to mother, the "protective" hypothesis predicts that infants are resistant to stressors because of their limited cognitive ability. Results supported the protective hypothesis, suggesting that cognitive ability associated with age and incomplete attachment formation to the father protected young children against the ill effects of divorce.

Overall, research supports a context-sensitive view in which separation effects are moderated by the conditions of separation and reunion (Solomon & George, 1999). Observations of young children undergoing separations under varying circumstances (Heinicke & Westheimer, 1965; Robertson & Robertson, 1971) show, consistent with attachment theory, that a familiar and sensitive caretaking environment during separation can mitigate or even prevent infant distress and detachment (Solomon & George, 1999). According to this view, separation is a risk factor for attachment insecurity that may be potentiated by adverse conditions or prevented by conditions known to promote security.

## Adolescents and Young Adults

A larger number of studies have investigated the impact of divorce on children's attachment later in life. With some exceptions (e.g., Bernstein, Keltner, & Laurent, 2012; Washington & Hans, 2013), the consensus is that adolescents and young adults from divorced families are more likely to be insecurely attached than those from intact families, with most evidence pointing toward a greater likelihood of becoming fearful or preoccupied (more anxious) as an adult (Brennan & Shaver, 1998; Kilman, Carranza, & Vendemia, 2006; Ozen, 2003). For example, Beckwith, Cohen, and Hamilton (1999) found that adverse life events through age 12, particularly parental divorce, reduced the likelihood of secure attachment and increased the likelihood of preoccupied representations at 18 years of age. Similarly, other longitudinal investigations have shown that divorce is predictive of an insecure attachment status at 18 years (Crowell, Treboux, & Brockmeyer, 2009; Lewis, Feiring, & Rosenthal, 2000), and that stressful life events, which included divorce in some cases, were significantly related to the likelihood of an infant classified as secure in the Strange Situation becoming insecure by early adulthood (Waters, Merrick, Treboux, Crowell, & Albersheim, 2000; see also Ruschena, Prior, Sanson, & Smart, 2005). Riggs and Jacobvitz (2002) also found that adults classified as preoccupied and unresolved on the Adult Attachment Interview (AAI) were more likely than others to report a history of divorce or parental separation during childhood. And Mickelson, Kessler, and Shaver (1997) found parental divorce or separation to be negatively associated with secure attachment and positively related to anxious attachment in a nationally representative sample (see also McCabe, 1997; Shaver & Mikulincer, 2004; Summers, Forehand, Armistead, & Tannenbaum, 1998). Thus, it appears that parental separation or divorce is linked with attachment anxiety, which underlies both fearful and preoccupied attachment orientations.

The studies that do not support this conclusion found no relation between parental divorce and offsprings' later attachment style (Brennan & Shaver, 1993; J. A. Feeney & Noller, 1990; Hazan & Shaver, 1987; Hazelton, Lancee, & O'Neil, 1998). Fraley and Heffernan's (2013) research, using two Internet surveys of adults between ages 18 and 65, suggests that parental divorce has selective rather than broad implications for insecure attachment. This study showed that parental divorce was more strongly related to insecure relationships with parents in adulthood than insecure relationships with romantic partners or friends. Also, insecurity was more pronounced when parental divorce took place in early childhood, suggesting that there may be sensitive periods in attachment development.

Although the majority of empirical evidence suggests that divorce has a negative impact on adolescents' and young adults' attachment security, many factors have been shown to moderate this association. First, Brennan and Shaver (1993) found that parents' postdivorce marital status was related to their offsprings' attachment style. It seems that having either a mother or both parents remarry is associated with the best attachment outcome for young adults. Second, researchers have shown that individuals who come from divorced families do not differ from those who come from unhappy/intact families in their attachment security, indicating that the quality of the parents' relationship is important (Sprecher, Cate, & Levin, 1998). Third, perceptions of the reasons for divorce are important (Walker & Ehrenberg, 1998). For example, young people who felt that they were not involved in their parents' decision to divorce scored higher

on measures of attachment security, whereas those who felt they were involved were more likely to be preoccupied or fearful. Fourth, among adult children of divorce, exposure to parental alienation strategies (one parent speaking negatively about the other parent) is related to young adults' insecure attachment (Baker & Ben-Ami, 2011a). Fifth, gender of the child has sometimes been a moderator, such that women from divorced families are less likely to be securely attached and are more sensitive to the divorce experience than men from divorced families (Barber, 1998; Crowell et al., 2009; Evans & Bloom, 1996).

Finally, the quality of parent–child relationships is a key mediator between parental divorce and children's later adjustment (Amato, 2000; Amato & Sobolewski, 2001). Because divorce entails significant changes in family structure, it has the potential to influence the sensitive responsiveness and accessibility (both physical and psychological) of attachment figures, and thus affect the safe haven and secure base functions that parents normally provide. Parents may fail to provide these functions following divorce by inverting the parent–child relationship such that the child becomes a major attachment figure for the parent, or by becoming psychologically and/or physically unavailable to the child (Bowlby, 1969/1982, 1979). Not surprisingly, the influence of divorce on parent–child relationships has been an important topic in the literature (Bretherton & Page, 2004; Bulduc, Caron, & Logue, 2007; Cohen & Finzi-Dottan, 2005; Fabricius & Leucken, 2007; Hetherington, 1999; Hetherington, Cox, & Cox, 1978). Recent longitudinal studies have shown that divorce negatively impacts the mother–child relationship due to marital conflict and a collapse in parenting (Wallerstein, Lewis, & Packer Rosenthal, 2013; Yu, Pettit, Lansford, Dodge, & Bates, 2010), and that maternal sensitivity is lower in mother–child dyads in divorced families compared to intact married families (Sutherland, Altenhofen, & Biringen, 2012). Also, studies indicate that attachment to the father is particularly affected by divorce (Hannum & Dvorak, 2004; Tayler, Parker, & Roy, 1995), and that boys are more distressed than girls by separation from their fathers because of their strong identification with the same-sex parent (Hetherington et al., 1978). However, girls are most likely to feel a burden or responsibility for the father's well-being when the parents engage in conflict (Bretherton & Page, 2004; Bretherton, Ridgeway, & Cassidy, 1990; Page & Bretherton, 2001).

## Psychological and Physical Health

Children of divorce may experience the effects of separation and loss to an even greater extent than the divorcing adults because children typically have no control over the decision, and it often seems to them to occur suddenly and without warning. For children, the disruption of important attachment bonds occurs not only with regard to one or both parents, but often also with regard to friends and extended family members. The cumulative toll of these separations and losses, coupled with other divorce-related stressors (economic hardship, moving, changing schools, and parental remarriage), may complicate the child's psychological development and influence adjustment (Amato, 2000).

Thus, an enormous amount of research has focused on the effects of divorce on children's psychological health. There are some studies showing that divorce may have a positive effect on children's adjustment (Bernstein et al., 2012; Crosnoe & Elder, 2004; Hagerty, Williams, & Oe, 2002), and that children may benefit if stress decreases or resources increase following divorce (Amato, 1993). However, the majority of studies indicate that children from divorced families score lower on a wide range of outcome measures associated with well-being, including academic achievement, psychological adjustment, self-esteem, conduct, and social competence, and that they are at increased risk for developmental delays, psychopathology, anxiety, depression, phobia, and problematic behavior such as aggression (Amato, 2000, 2010; Bray & Hetherington, 1993; Brennan & Shaver; 1998; Chase-Lansdale, Cherlin, & Kiernan, 1995; Clarke-Stewart et al., 2000; Kilman et al., 2006; Sirvanli-Ozen, 2005; Strohschein, 2012; Uphold-Carrier & Utz, 2012; Wallerstein & Blakeslee, 1989). Longitudinal studies suggest that the effects for some children may be quite large and enduring (Gilman, Kawachi, Fitzmaurice, & Buka, 2003; Laumann-Billings & Emery, 2000; Wallerstein & Lewis, 2004).

Researchers have also found that physical health problems are associated with exposure to distressing parental divorce processes (Bloch, Peleg, Koren, Aner, & Klein, 2007; Fabricius & Luecken, 2007; Luecken & Fabricius, 2003; Mechanic & Hansell, 1989). For example, Troxel and Matthews (2004) highlighted five studies that demonstrated a link between parental divorce and increased physical health problems (Dawson, 1991; DeGoede & Spruijt, 1996; Guidubaldi & Clemen-

shaw, 1985; Maier & Lachman, 2000). Overall, research indicates that parental divorce in childhood is associated with increased risk for unintentional injuries, illness, hospitalization, somatic symptoms, premature mortality, and suicide (Aro & Palosaari, 1992; De Jong, 1992; D'Onofrio et al., 2006; Schwartz et al., 1995; Tucker et al., 1997). Parental divorce has also been linked with health-related behaviors, including irregular eating and sleeping patterns (Sirvanli-Ozen, 2005) and risky health behaviors such as substance abuse (Amato & Keith, 1991; Bray & Hetherington, 1993), alcohol use (Hope, Power, & Rodgers, 1998; Sartor, Lynskey, Heath, Jacob, & True, 2007), smoking (Isohanni, Moilanen, & Rantakallio, 1991), marijuana use (Hoffman, 1995), early sexual activity (Amato & Keith, 1991; Barber, 1998), and teen pregnancy (Aseltine & Doucet, 2003).

Of course, important moderating variables have been identified and are consistent with attachment theory's predictions that disruptions in important attachment bonds adversely affect individual functioning (Rogers, 2004). First, the increased risk for children from divorced homes stems from discordant, conflictual relationships that precede or follow the losses associated with divorce (Cherlin et al., 1991; Rutter, 1994), and not from the divorce itself. In fact, children experience better outcomes when parents in high-conflict marriages divorce rather than remain together (Amato & Booth, 2000; Amato & Keith, 1991; Booth & Amato, 2002; Emery, 1982; Hetherington, 1999). The quality of marital and familial relations is more predictive than marital status of health outcomes, including physical symptoms (Mechanic & Hansell, 1989; Sweeting & West, 1995), cancer (Duszynski, Shaffer, & Thomas, 1981; Shaffer, Duszynski, & Thomas, 1982), and mortality (Lundberg, 1993). Thus, the overall toxicity of the home environment is a central factor in explaining the link between divorce and adverse outcomes. Corroborating this, research examining biomarkers shows that divorce has significant and sustained effects on children's hypothalamic–pituitary–adrenal (HPA) axis only in the context of traumatic separation (stress at home and disrupted parental bonding; Bloch et al., 2007). Similarly, in undergraduates whose parents divorced before age 16, Fabricius and Luecken (2007) found that exposure to parental conflict was related to poorer physical health status and more distress, and other research has shown that regardless of family type, children whose parents had a hostile interparental relationship had poorer emotional well-being than children whose parents had a nonhostile relationship (Baxter, Weston, & Qu, 2011).

Second, high levels of warmth, affection and availability in the custodial mother-child relationship are negatively associated with post-divorce adjustment problems (Bretherton et al., 2013; Brown, Wolchik, Tein, & Sandler, 2007; Simons, Lin, Gordon, Conger, & Lorenz, 1999; Wolchik, Wilcox, Tein, & Sandler, 2000). Negative aspects of the mother–child relationship that contribute to adjustment problems include maternal depressive mood, which has been directly related to child/adolescent functioning (Forehand, McCombs, & Brody, 1987), and fear of abandonment, which mediates the link between mother–child relationship quality and internalizing–externalizing problems (Wolchik, Tein, Sandler, & Doyle, 2002). In fact, recent preventive interventions with the goal of enhancing relations between mothers and children going through divorce show positive effects on children's postdivorce adjustment (Velez, Wolchik, Tein, & Sandler, 2011; Wolchik et al., 2013). This makes theoretical sense given that a hallmark of secure attachment is open and relaxed communication between parent and child (Bowlby, 1969/1982).

Third, a strong social support network moderates the effects of divorce on children's well-being. Divorce mediation for the parents and extended family support (Emery, 1999) protect against maladjustment, particularly if the parent is psychologically unable to provide quality parenting following a divorce. For adolescents, peer support also moderates the effect of low parental support after divorce on internalizing symptoms (Rodgers & Rose, 2002). However, in a 3-year longitudinal investigation of divorcing families, Maccoby and colleagues (1993) found that the factors most powerfully associated with good adolescent adjustment were having a close relationship with a residential parent who monitored the child and remained involved in decisions concerning his or her life, and not feeling caught in the middle of parental conflict. Noncustodial parent involvement (Furstenberg, Morgan, & Allison, 1987 Sirvanli-Ozen, 2005), strong father–child or noncustodial parent–child relations (Fabricius & Luecken, 2007; Sandler, Wheeler, & Braver, 2013), and attachment to the family home (Stirtzinger & Cholvat, 1991) have also been identified as potentially protective factors. These network supports may reduce negative feelings about parental divorce, which has been linked with hostility, somatic complaints, and illness reports, indicating that it

is the negativity of experiences associated with divorce (and not the divorce itself) that increases vulnerability (Leucken & Fabricius, 2003).

Consistent with this research and with attachment theoretical predictions, Troxel and Matthews (2004) proposed that many health effects of divorce are mediated through disrupted parenting, specifically diminished warmth/sensitivity and reduced physical and psychological availability (see also Ross & Wynne, 2010). Inadequate parenting or physical absence of the parent, in turn, is hypothesized to cause children's emotional insecurity regarding their parents' love and ability to care for them (Davies & Cummings, 1994; Wolchik et al., 2002). Emotional insecurity is hypothesized to disrupt emotion regulation processes and render children susceptible to stress-related health problems. Consistent with this idea, maltreatment (most often in the form of denying emotional responsiveness) has been reported by adults whose parents divorced when they were 15 years of age or younger, and was positively associated with reports of physical and sexual abuse, and negatively associated with attachment security, self-sufficiency, and self-esteem (Baker & Ben-Ami, 2011b). Researchers have identified biopsychosocial pathways from the parental marital system to childhood health that require future study (Krantz & McCeney, 2002; Troxel & Matthews, 2004).

There is a large literature on custody issues and a fierce, two-sided debate about whether it is detrimental or beneficial for young children to have a consistent home for sleeping versus ensuring adequate sleeping time at both parent's houses—with each side interpreting attachment theory differently. One side emphasizes that secure attachment is fostered by stability with one parent and emphasizes the risk engendered by frequent/lengthy absences from a primary caregiver in disrupting attachment organization with that parent (Main, Hesse, & Hesse, 2011; McIntosh, Smyth, & Kelaher, 2013; Sroufe & McIntosh, 2011), whereas the other side argues for ensuring that children develop secure attachment with both parents and posit that the necessary mechanism for doing so is spending equal time with both parents (Kelly & Lamb, 2000; Lamb & Kelly, 2001). Existing empirical work on this issue is mixed and suggests that outcomes may depend on factors such as age of the child, parental conflict, strained relationships with parents, and whether parents have new partners (McIntosh et al., 2013; Tornello et al., 2013; Vanassche, Sodermans, Matthijs, & Swicegood, 2013). It remains for future research to establish the ideal means by which emotional security and optimal outcomes are attained for children of differing ages with regard to living arrangements with divorced parents.

## Future Romantic Relations

Attachment theory stipulates that working models of attachment and forecasts derived from them, once developed, guide behavior, feelings, and the processing of information in future relationships (Bowlby, 1980). Because the construction of these working models is thought to be influenced by experiences of separation and loss, attachment theory predicts that (particularly unresolved) experiences of separation/loss should be linked to the quality of one's future romantic relationships.

Although some investigators have found that young adults from divorced versus intact families do not differ on measures of intimacy (Nelson, Hughes, Handal, Katz, & Searight, 1993; Sinclair & Nelson, 1998), dating behavior (Greenberg & Nay, 1982), or quality of attachment to adult intimates (Olivas & Stoltenberg, 1997; Tayler et al., 1995), a majority of studies do find differences in later romantic relationship functioning between those who grew up in intact versus postdivorce families (see Amato, 1999). First, young adults from divorced families are likely to hold less positive attitudes toward marriage/relationships (Sirvanli-Ozen, 2005), show less trust (Southworth & Schwartz, 1987; Sprague & Kinney, 1997), have problems with dependency and control (Bolgar, Zweig-Frank, & Paris, 1995), be less optimistic (Sprecher et al., 1998), and believe that disagreement is destructive (Sinclair & Nelson, 1998; but see Coleman & Ganong, 1984, for an exception). Second, parental divorce increases the risk of marital instability and dissolution in offspring (Amato & DeBoer, 2001; Glenn & Kramer, 1987; Wolfinger, 2000) and of conflict in romantic relationships (Chen et al., 2006). Both divorce and marital conflict in the family of origin contribute to couple instability in offspring (Hetherington, 2003). Third, a history of parental conflict and divorce predicts lower intimacy in romantic relationships (Ensign, Scherman, & Clark, 1998; Sprecher et al., 1998), avoidance of short-term relationships (Knox, Zusman, & DeCuzzi, 2004), and perpetration of teen dating violence (Banyard, Cross, & Modecki, 2006). Corroborating these findings, Cui and Fincham (2010) showed that parental divorce and marital conflict were independently associated

with young adult children's romantic relationships, but through different mechanisms: Parental divorce was associated with young adults' low level of relationship quality through a negative attitude toward marriage (positive attitude toward divorce) and lack of commitment to their own current relationships, whereas parental marital conflict was associated with young adults' low level of relationship quality through their conflict behavior with their partner (see also Cui, Fincham, & Durtschi, 2011). In addition, adults who experienced multiple parental divorces are more likely (than adults with a single parental divorce) to claim that they are hard on their romantic partners (South, 2013), and one study suggests that parental remarriage quality has more influence on adults' current relational outcomes than the quality of their parents' first marriage (Yu & Adler-Baeder, 2007).

It is important to consider, however, that not all children from divorced families have the same risks for troubled romantic relationships in adulthood, and not every child from a divorced family experiences later relationships in the same way. Closeness to parents and positive appraisals of parental divorce have been identified as protective factors (Coleman & Ganong, 1984; Haaz, Kneavel, & Browning, 2014; Shulman, Scharf, Lumer, & Maurer, 2001), whereas parental conflict associated with divorce has a particularly negative effect on children's later relationships. The significant differences between those from intact and postdivorce families are often due to dysfunctional family dynamics and not to the divorce per se (Sprecher et al., 1998). In support of this conclusion, Hayashi and Strickland (1998) found that college students who experienced protracted interparental conflict, parental rejection, or overprotective parents were more likely to report jealousy and fears of abandonment in their love relationships, regardless of whether their parents divorced. Also, in a study of couples assessed 3 months prior to their weddings and 6 years later, those who were classified as secure (compared to those classified as insecure) were less likely to divorce in the early years of marriage (Crowell et al., 2009), indicating that attachment security is a protective factor.

Although several explanations have been offered for the intergenerational transmission of relationship instability (Amato & DeBoer, 2001; Glenn & Kramer, 1987; Hetherington & Kelly, 2002; McGue & Lykken, 1992), attachment theory offers a particularly comprehensive explanation for why some children from divorced families grow up to have more problems with relationships than do children from intact families (Brennan & Shaver, 1993). Because the process of divorce is taxing on the separating parents (who are the primary, and perhaps the only, attachment figures for their children), it is likely to have a large influence on their caregiving capacity. The separation anxiety and attachment system activation that is often experienced by separating adults is likely to interfere with their caregiving system. In fact, in the absence of personal and social resources for coping, simultaneous activation of the attachment and caregiving systems is likely to result in caregiving that is more self-focused than other-focused (Kunce & Shaver, 1994). These caregiving dynamics, coupled with parental modeling of poor marital communication, are likely to play an important role in shaping the child's attachment orientation and experiences in romantic relationships (Brennan & Shaver, 1993).

## The State of the Research since the Previous Edition of the *Handbook*

Additional research has been conducted on adults' adjustment to divorce and potential mechanisms that may account for positive or negative adjustment, and a few additional studies have focused specifically on attachment differences in adjustment. There is still a scarcity of research overall that considers the process of divorce from an attachment perspective, particularly research regarding postdivorce relations between ex-spouses.

Recent research continues to suggest that parental divorce can increase risk for negative mental and physical health outcomes in children, but this is often through parental conflict or traumatic separation. Research has continued to examine moderators of the association between divorce and well-being, identifying factors that are protective. New studies have examined mechanisms through which young children's attachment is influenced by divorce, and researchers are more often considering fathers in attachment transmission. Studies continue to show that parental divorce is associated with adult children's insecure attachment; however, new research suggests that divorce may have relationship-specific rather than broad implications for young adults' attachment. Recent longitudinal studies corroborate past research showing that divorce can negatively affect

parent–child relationships due to a breakdown in parenting, and studies continue to show effects of parental divorce on adult children's romantic relationships and attitudes toward marriage. Recent preventive interventions for families going through divorce show positive effects. A debate regarding custody issues and optimal distribution of time with divorced parents for young children will require additional empirical work.

## Conclusions

Our purpose in this chapter has been to explore the relevance of attachment theory for understanding the divorce process. Although divorce has received a great deal of attention, the research on divorce lacks theoretical motivation and integration, and many aspects of divorce have not been thoroughly investigated. More work is needed to (1) specify the combinations of intrapersonal and interpersonal processes (both distal and proximal) that lead to divorce; (2) establish the mechanisms responsible for the links between divorce and health for both adults and children; (3) determine the benefits and costs of various forms of postdivorce contact between ex-spouses, particularly where children are involved; and (4) specify the connections between parental divorce and future romantic relationship functioning, particularly with regard to the intergenerational transmission of the tendency to divorce. Attachment theory provides an integrative framework for such a research program because it suggests that divorce is a *process* of disrupted attachment that has far-reaching roots in previous relationships and profound implications for future relationships.

In taking an attachment–theoretical approach to divorce, it will be necessary to elaborate and test more detailed hypotheses concerning the normative processes involved in detaching from or reorganizing attachment bonds. Although Bowlby discussed separation and loss extensively, most of his insights came from observations of children who were separated from their attachment figures, and there was much less attention given to separation in adult relationships, except in the case of bereavement. Because divorce often requires a continuing and evolving relationship with a living person, the issue of negotiated reorganization becomes important (e.g., the possibility of transforming a primary attachment with sexual components into an affiliative relationship).

Surprisingly little research or theorizing has focused on individual differences in attachment orientations that affect the divorce process. Clinicians have provided some theoretical elaboration regarding the ways that attachment patterns may affect the divorce process (Cohen, Finzi, & Avi-Yonah, 1999; Finzi, Cohen, & Ram, 2000; Johnson, 2003; Todorski, 1995). They propose that individuals with different attachment orientations deal differently with divorce, experience separation differently, have different coping capacities/strategies, and interact differently with ex-spouses as coparents, and they offer guidelines for clinical intervention. These ideas require empirical testing. Given the significance of divorce for adult and children, theory-guided investigations of divorce processes are important for revealing approaches that separating couples can take to ensure the health and well-being of all family members.

## References

Ahrons, C. R., & Rodgers, R. H. (1987). *Divorced families: A multidisciplinary development view*. New York: Norton.

Ahrons, C. R., & Wallisch, L. S. (1986). The relationship between former spouses. In S. Duck & D. Perlman (Eds.), *Close relationships: Development, dynamics, and deterioration* (pp. 269–296). Beverly Hills, CA: Sage.

Altenhofen, S., Sutherland, K., & Biringen, Z. (2010). Families experiencing divorce: Age at onset of overnight stays, conflict, and emotional availability as predictors of child attachment. *Journal of Divorce and Remarriage, 51*, 141–156.

Amato, P. R. (1993). Children's adjustment to divorce: Theories, hypotheses, and empirical support. *Journal of Marriage and the Family, 55*, 23–38.

Amato, P. R. (1999). Children of divorced parents as young adults. In E. M. Hetherington (Ed.), *Coping with divorce, single parenting, and remarriage: A risk and resiliency perspective* (pp. 147–163). Mahwah, NJ: Erlbaum.

Amato, P. R. (2000). The consequences of divorce for adults and children. *Journal of Marriage and the Family, 62*, 1269–1287.

Amato, P. R. (2010). Research on divorce: Continuing trends and new developments. *Journal of Marriage and Family, 72*, 650–666.

Amato, P. R., & Booth, A. (2000). *A generational risk: Growing up in an era of family upheaval*. Cambridge, MA: Harvard University Press.

Amato, P. R., & DeBoer, D. D. (2001). The transmission of marital instability across generations: Relationship skills or commitment to marriage? *Journal of Marriage and the Family, 63*, 1038–1051.

Amato, P. R., & Keith, B. (1991). Parental divorce and the well-being of children: A meta-analysis. *Psychological Bulletin, 110*, 26–46.

Amato, P. R., & Sobolewski, J. M. (2001). The effects of divorce and marital discord on adult children's psychological well-being. *American Sociological Review, 66*, 900–921.

Ambert, A. (1988). Relationships between ex-spouses: Individual and dynamic perspectives. *Journal of Social and Personal Relationships, 5*, 327–346.

Arendell, T. (1995). *Fathers and divorce*. Thousand Oaks, CA: Sage.

Aro, H. M., & Palosaari, U. K. (1992). Parental divorce, adolescence, and transition to young adulthood: A follow-up study. *American Journal of Orthopsychiatry, 62*, 421–429.

Aseltine, R. H., Jr., & Doucet, J. (2003). The impact of parental divorce on premarital pregnancy. *Adolescent and Family Health, 3*, 122–129.

Aseltine, R. H., Jr., & Kessler, R. C. (1993). Marital disruption and depression in a community sample. *Journal of Health and Social Behavior, 34*, 237–251.

Aydintug, C. D. (1995). Former spouse interaction: Normative guidelines and actual behavior. *Journal of Divorce and Remarriage, 22*, 147–161.

Baker, A. J., & Ben-Ami, N. (2011a). To turn a child against a parent is to turn a child against himself: The direct and indirect effects of exposure to parental alienation strategies on self-esteem and well-being. *Journal of Divorce and Remarriage, 52*, 472–489.

Baker, A. J., & Ben-Ami, N. (2011b). Adult recall of childhood psychological maltreatment in "adult children of divorce": Prevalence and associations with concurrent measures of well-being, *Journal of Divorce and Remarriage, 52*, 203–219.

Banyard, V. L., Cross, C., & Modecki, K. L. (2006). Interpersonal violence in adolescence: Ecological correlates of self-reported perpetration. *Journal of Interpersonal Violence, 21*, 1314–1332.

Barber, N. (1998). Sex differences in dispositions towards kin, security of adult attachment, and sociosexuality as a function of parental divorce. *Evolution and Human Behavior, 19*, 125–132.

Baxter, J., Weston, R., & Qu, L. (2011). Family structure, co-parental relationship quality, post-separation paternal involvement and children's emotional well-being. *Journal of Family Studies, 17*, 86–109.

Beckwith, L., Cohen, S. E., & Hamilton, C. E. (1999). Maternal sensitivity during infancy and subsequent life events relate to attachment representation at early adulthood. *Developmental Psychology, 35*, 693–700.

Berman, W. H. (1988a). The relationship of ex-spouse attachment to adjustment following divorce. *Journal of Family Psychology, 1*, 312–328.

Berman, W. H. (1988b). The role of attachment in the post-divorce experience. *Journal of Personality and Social Psychology, 54*, 496–503.

Bernier, A., & Miljkovitch, R. (2009). Intergenerational transmission of attachment in father–child dyads: The case of single parenthood. *Journal of Genetic Psychology, 170,* 31–52.

Bernstein, R., Keltner, D., & Laurent, H. (2012). Parental divorce and romantic attachment in young adulthood: Important role of problematic beliefs. *Marriage and Family Review, 48,* 711–731.

Berscheid, E. (1983). Emotions in close relationships. In H. H. Kelly, E. Berscheid, A. Christensen, J. Harvey, T. Huston, G. Levinger, et al. (Eds.), *The psychology of close relationships* (pp. 110–168). New York: Freeman.

Birnbaum, G. E., Orr, I., Mikulincer, M., & Florian, V. (1997). When marriage breaks up: Does attachment style contribute to coping and mental health? *Journal of Social and Personal Relationships, 14,* 643–654.

Bloch, M., Peleg, I., Koren, D., Aner, H., & Klein, E. (2007). Long-term effects of early parental loss due to divorce on the HPA axis. *Hormones and Behavior, 51,* 516–523.

Bloom, B. L., Asher, S. J., & White, S. W. (1978). Marital disruption as a stressor: A review and analysis. *Psychological Bulletin, 85,* 867–894.

Blumenthal, M. D. (1967). Mental health among the divorced: A field study of divorced and never divorced persons. *Archives of General Psychiatry, 16,* 603–608.

Bohannan, P. (1970). *Divorce and after.* New York: Doubleday.

Bolgar, R., Zweig-Frank, H., & Paris, J. (1995). Childhood antecedents of interpersonal problems in young adult children of divorce. *Journal of the American Academy of Child and Adolescent Psychiatry, 34,* 143–150.

Booth, A., & Amato, P. (1991). Divorce and psychological stress. *Journal of Health and Social Behavior, 32,* 396–407.

Bowers, J. R., Ogolsky, B. G., Hughes, R., & Kanter, J. B. (2014). Coparenting through divorce or separation: A review of an online program. *Journal of Divorce and Remarriage, 55,* 464–484.

Bowlby, J. (1973). *Attachment and loss: Separation, anxiety, and anger.* New York: Basic Books.

Bowlby, J. (1979). *The making and breaking of affectional bonds.* London: Tavistock.

Bowlby, J. (1980). *Attachment and loss: Sadness and depression.* New York: Basic Books.

Bowlby, J. (1982). *Attachment and loss: Attachment* (2nd ed.). New York: Basic Books. (Original work published 1969)

Bowlby, J. (1988). *A secure base.* New York: Basic Books.

Brassard, A., Lussier, Y., & Shaver, P. R. (2009). Attachment, perceived conflict, and couple satisfaction: Test of a mediational dyadic model. *Family Relations, 58,* 634–646.

Bray, J. H., & Hetherington, E. M. (1993). Families in transition: Introduction and overview. *Journal of Family Psychology, 7,* 3–8.

Brennan, K. A., & Shaver, P. R. (1993). Attachment styles and parental divorce. *Journal of Divorce and Remarriage, 21,* 161–175.

Brennan, K. A., & Shaver, P. R. (1998). Attachment styles and personality disorders: Their connections to each other and to parental divorce, parental death, and perceptions of parental caregiving. *Journal of Personality, 66,* 835–878.

Bretherton, I., Gullón-Rivera, Á. L., Page, T. F., Oettel, B. J., Corey, J. M., & Golby, B. J. (2013). Children's attachment-related self-worth: a multi-method investigation of postdivorce preschoolers' relationships with their mothers and peers. *Attachment and Human Development, 15,* 25–49.

Bretherton, I., & Page, T. (2004). Shared or conflicting working models?: Relationships in postdivorce families seen through the eyes of mothers and their preschool children. *Development and Psychopathology, 16,* 551–575.

Bretherton, I., Ridgeway, D., & Cassidy, J. (1990). Assessing internal working models of the attachment relationship: An attachment story completion task for 3-year-olds. In M. T. Greenberg, D. Cicchetti, & M. E. Cummings (Eds.), *Attachment in the preschool years: Theory, research, and intervention* (pp. 273–308). Chicago: University of Chicago Press.

Brown, A. C., Wolchik, S. A., Tein, J. Y., & Sandler, I. N. (2007). Maternal acceptance as a moderator of the relation between threat to self appraisals and mental health problems in adolescents from divorced families. *Journal of Youth and Adolescence, 36,* 927–938.

Brown, P., Felton, B. J., Whiteman, V., & Manela, R. (1980). Attachment and distress following marital separation. *Journal of Divorce, 3,* 303–317.

Brown, S. D., & Reimer, D. A. (1984). Assessing attachment following divorce: Development and psychometric evaluation of the Divorced Reaction Inventory. *Journal of Counseling Psychology, 31,* 520–531.

Bulduc, J. L., Caron, S. L., & Logue, M. E. (2007). The effects of parental divorce on college students. *Journal of Divorce and Remarriage, 46,* 83–104.

Burman, B., & Margolin, G. (1992). Analysis of the association between marital relationships and health problems: An interactional perspective. *Psychological Bulletin, 112,* 39–63.

Buunk, B. P., & Mutsaers, W. (1999). The nature of the relationship between remarried individuals and former spouses and its impact on marital satisfaction. *Journal of Family Psychology, 13,* 165–174.

Ceglian, C. P., & Gardner, S. (1999). Attachment style: A risk for multiple marriages? *Journal of Divorce and Remarriage, 31,* 125–139.

Chase-Lansdale, P. L., Cherlin, A. J., & Kiernan, K. K. (1995). The long-term effects of parental divorce on the mental health of young adults: A developmental perspective. *Child Development, 66,* 1614–1634.

Chatav, Y., & Whisman, M. A. (2007). Marital dissolution and psychiatric disorders: An investigation of risk factors. *Journal of Divorce and Remarriage, 47,* 1–13.

Chen, H., Cohen, P., Kasen, S., Johnson, J. G., Ehrensaft, M., & Gordon, K. (2006). Predicting conflict within romantic relationships during the transition to adulthood. *Personal Relationships, 13,* 411–427.

Cherlin, A. J., Furstenberg, F. F., Chase-Lansdale, P. L., Kiernan, K. E., Robins, P. K., Morrison, D. R., et al. (1991). Longitudinal studies of effect of divorce on children in Great Britain and the United States. *Science, 252,* 1386–1389.

Clarke-Stewart, K. A., Vandell, D. L., McCartney, K., Owen, M. T., & Booth, C. (2000). Effects of parental separation and divorce on very young children. *Journal of Family Psychology, 14,* 304–326.

Cohen, O., Finzi, R., & Avi-Yonah, O. K. (1999). An attachment-based typology of divorced couples. *Family Therapy, 26,* 167–190.

Cohen, O., & Finzi-Dottan, R. (2005). Parent–child relationships during the divorce process: From attachment theory and intergenerational perspective. *Contemporary Family Therapy, 27,* 81–99.

Cohen, O., & Finzi-Dottan, R. (2012). Reasons for divorce and mental health following the breakup. *Journal of Divorce and Remarriage, 53,* 581–601.

Cole, C. L., & Cole, A. L. (1999). Boundary ambiguities that bind former spouses together after the children leave home in post-divorce families. *Family Relations, 48,* 271–272.

Coleman, M., & Ganong, L. H. (1984). Effects of family structure on family attitudes and expectations. *Family Relations, 33,* 425–432.

Collins, N. L., Feeney, B. C. (2004). Working models of attachment shape perceptions of social support: Evidence from experimental and observational studies. *Journal of Personality and Social Psychology, 87*(3), 363–383.

Crosnoe, R., & Elder, G. H., Jr. (2004). Family dynamics, supportive relationships, and educational resilience during adolescence. *Journal of Family Issues, 25,* 571–602.

Crowell, J. A., Treboux, D., & Brockmeyer, S. (2009). Parental divorce and adult children's attachment representations and marital status. *Attachment and Human Development, 11,* 87–101.

Cui, M., & Fincham, F. D. (2010). The differential effects of parental divorce and marital conflict on young adult romantic relationships. *Personal Relationships, 17,* 331–343.

Cui, M., Fincham, F. D., & Durtschi, J. A. (2011). The effect of parental divorce on young adults' romantic relationship dissolution: What makes a difference? *Personal Relationships, 18,* 410–426.

Davies, P. T., & Cummings, E. M. (1994). Marital conflict and child adjustment: An emotional security hypothesis. *Psychological Bulletin, 116,* 387–411.

Davila, J., & Bradbury, T. N. (2001). Attachment insecurity and the distinction between unhappy spouses who do and do not divorce. *Journal of Family Psychology, 15,* 371–393.

Davila, J., Karney, B. R., & Bradbury, T. N. (1999). Attachment change processes in the early years of marriage. *Journal of Personality and Social Psychology, 76,* 783–802.

Davis, D., Shaver, P. R., & Vernon, M. L. (2003). Physical, emotional, and behavioral reactions to breaking up: The roles of gender, age, emotional involvement, and attachment style. *Personality and Social Psychology Bulletin, 29,* 871–884.

Dawson, D. A. (1991). Family structure and children's health and well-being: Data from the 1988 National Survey of Child Health. *Journal of Marriage and the Family, 53,* 573–584.

DeGoede, M., & Spruijt, E. (1996). Effects of parental divorce and youth unemployment on adolescent health. *Patient Education and Counseling, 29,* 269–276.

De Jong, M. J. (1992). Attachment, individuation, and risk of suicide in late adolescence. *Journal of Youth and Adolescence, 21,* 357–373.

D'Onofrio, B. M., Turkheimer, E., Emery, R. E., Slutske, W. S., Heath, A. C., & Madden, P. A. (2006). A genetically informed study of the processes underlying the association between parental marital instability and offspring adjustment. *Developmental Psychology, 42,* 486–499.

Dozier, B. S., Sollie, D. L., Stack, S. J., & Smith, T. A. (1993). The effects of postdivorce attachment on coparenting relationships. *Journal of Divorce and Remarriage, 19,* 109–123.

Dupre, M. E., & Meadows, S. O. (2007). Disaggregating the effects of marital trajectories on health. *Journal of Family Issues, 28,* 623–652.

Duszynski, K. R., Shaffer, J. W., & Thomas, C. B. (1981). Neoplasm and traumatic events in childhood: Are they related? *Archives of General Psychiatry, 38,* 327–331.

Ein-Dor, T., Mikulincer, M., & Shaver, P. R. (2011). Attachment insecurities and the processing of threat-related information: Studying the schemas involved in insecure people's coping strategies. *Journal of Personality and Social Psychology, 101,* 78–93.

Ellis, D., & DeKeseredy, W. D. (1989). Marital status and woman abuse: The DAD model. *International Journal of Sociology of the Family, 19,* 67–87.

Emery, R. E. (1982). Interparental conflict and the children of discord and divorce. *Psychological Bulletin, 92,* 310–330.

Emery, R. E. (1994). *Renegotiating family relationships: Divorce, child custody, and mediation.* New York: Guilford Press.

Emery, R. E. (1999). Postdivorce family life for children: An overview of research and some implications for policy. In R. A. Thompson & P. R. Amato (Eds.), *The postdivorce family: Children, parenting, and society* (pp. 3–27). Thousand Oaks, CA: Sage.

Ensign, J., Scherman, A., & Clark, J. J. (1998). The relationship of family structure and conflict to levels of intimacy and parental attachment in college students. *Adolescence, 33*, 575– 582.

Evans, J. J., & Bloom, B. L. (1996). Effects of parental divorce among college undergraduates. *Journal of Divorce and Remarriage, 26*, 69–91.

Fabricius, W. V., & Luecken, L. J. (2007). Postdivorce living arrangements, parental conflict, and long-term physical health correlates for children of divorce. *Journal of Family Psychology, 21*, 195–205.

Feeney, B. C., & Cassidy, J. (2003). Reconstructive memory related to adolescent–parent conflict interactions: The influence of attachment-related representations on immediate perceptions and changes in perceptions over time. *Journal of Personality and Social Psychology, 85*, 945–955.

Feeney, B. C., & Collins, N. L. (2001). Predictors of caregiving in adult intimate relationships: An attachment theoretical perspective. *Journal of Personality and Social Psychology, 80*, 972–994.

Feeney, B. C., Collins, N. L., Van Vleet, M., & Tomlinson, J. M. (2013). Motivations for providing a secure base: Links with attachment orientation and secure base support behavior. *Attachment and Human Development, 15*, 261–280.

Feeney, B. C., & Thrush, R. L. (2010). Relationship influences on exploration in adulthood: The characteristics and function of a secure base. *Journal of Personality and Social Psychology, 98*, 57–76.

Feeney, J. A., & Noller, P. (1990). Attachment style as a predictor of adult romantic relationships. *Journal of Personality and Social Psychology, 58*, 281–291.

Feeney, J. A., Noller, P., & Callan, V. J. (1994). Attachment style, communication and satisfaction in the early years of marriage. In K. Bartholomew & D. Perlman (Eds.), *Attachment processes in adulthood* (pp. 269–308). London: Jessica Kingsley.

Finzi, R., Cohen, O., & Ram, A. (2000). Attachment and divorce. *Journal of Family Psychotherapy, 11*, 1–20.

Fisher, J. V., & Crandell, L. E. (1997). Complex attachment: Patterns of relating in the couple. *Sexual and Marital Therapy, 12*, 211–223.

Forehand, R., McCombs, A., & Brody, G. H. (1987). The relationship between parental depressive mood states and child functioning. *Advances in Behaviour Research and Therapy, 9*, 1–20.

Fraley, R. C., & Bonanno, G. A. (2004). Attachment loss: A test of three competing models on the association between attachment-related avoidance and adaptation to bereavement. *Personality and Social Psychology Bulletin, 30*, 878–890.

Fraley, R. C., Garner, J. P., & Shaver, P. R. (2000). Adult attachment and the defensive regulation of attention and memory: Examining the role of perspective and postemptive defensive processes. *Journal of Personality and Social Psychology, 79*, 816–826.

Fraley, R. C., & Heffernan, M. E. (2013). Attachment and parental divorce: A test of the diffusion and sensitive period hypotheses. *Personality and Social Psychology Bulletin, 39*, 1199–1213.

Fraley, R. C., & Shaver, P. R. (2008). Attachment theory and its place in contemporarypersonality theory and research. In O. P. John, R. W. Robins, & L. A. Pervin (Eds.), *Handbook of personality: Theory and research* (3rd ed., pp. 518–541). New York: Guilford Press.

Furstenberg, F. F., Jr., & Cherlin, A. J. (1991). *Divided families: What happens to children when parents part.* Cambridge, MA: Harvard University Press.

Furstenberg, F. F., Morgan, S. P., & Alison, P. D. (1987). Paternal participation and children's well-being after marital dissolution. *American Sociological Review, 52*, 695–701.

Gilman, S. E., Kawachi, I., Fitzmaurice, G. M., & Buka, S. L. (2003). Family disruption in childhood and risk of adult depression. *American Journal of Psychiatry, 160*, 939–946.

Glenn, N. D., & Kramer, K. B. (1987). The marriages and divorces of the children of divorce. *Journal of Marriage and the Family, 49*, 811–825.

Glenn, N. D., & Weaver, C. N. (1988). The changing relationship of marital status to reported happiness. *Journal of Marriage and the Family, 50*, 317–324.

Gottman, J. M. (1994). *What predicts divorce?: The relationship between marital processes and marital outcome.* Hillsdale, NJ: Erlbaum.

Gottman, J. M., & Levenson, R. W. (1992). Marital processes predictive of later dissolution: Behavior, physiology, and health. *Journal of Personality and Social Psychology, 63*, 221–233.

Gottman, J. M., & Levenson, R. W. (2000). The timing of divorce: Predicting when a couple will divorce over a 14-year period. *Journal of Marriage and the Family, 62*, 737–745.

Gove, W. R., & Shin, H. (1989). The psychological well-being of divorced and widowed men and women: An empirical analysis. *Journal of Family Issues, 10*, 122–144.

Greenberg, E. F., & Nay, W. R. (1982). The intergenerational transmission of marital instability reconsidered. *Journal of Marriage and the Family, 44*, 335–347.

Guidubaldi, J., & Cleminshaw, H. K. (1985). Divorce, family health, and child adjustment. *Family Relations, 34*, 35–41.

Guisinger, S., Cowan, P. A., & Schuldberg, D. (1989). Changing parent and spouse relations in the first years of remarriage of divorced fathers. *Journal of Marriage and the Family, 51*, 445–456.

Gustavson, K., Nilsen, W., Orstaik, R., & Røysamb, E. (2014). Relationship quality, divorce, and well-being: Findings from a three-year longitudinal study. *Journal of Positive Psychology, 9*, 163–174.

Gustavson, K., Røysamb, E., von Soest, T., Helland, M. J., & Mathiesen, K. S. (2012). Longitudinal associations between relationship problems, divorce, and life satisfaction: Findings from a 15-year population-based study. *Journal of Positive Psychology, 7*, 188–197.

Haaz, D. H., Kneavel, M., & Browning, S. W. (2014). The father–daughter relationship and intimacy in the marriages of daughters of divorce. *Journal of Divorce and Remarriage, 55,* 164–177.

Hagerty, B. M., Williams, R. A., & Oe, H. (2002). Childhood antecedents of adult sense of belonging. *Journal of Clinical Psychology, 58,* 793–801.

Hannum, J. W., & Dvorak, D. M. (2004). Effects of family conflict, divorce, and attachment patterns on the psychological distress and social adjustment of college freshmen. *Journal of College Student Development, 45,* 27–42.

Hawkins, D. N., & Booth, A. (2005). Unhappily ever after: Effects of long-term, low-quality marriages on well-being. *Social Forces, 84,* 451–471.

Hayashi, G. M., & Strickland, B. R. (1998). Long-term effects of parental divorce on love relationships: Divorce as attachment disruption. *Journal of Social and Personal Relationships, 15,* 23–38.

Hazan, C., & Shaver, P. R. (1987). Romantic love conceptualized as an attachment process. *Journal of Personality and Social Psychology, 52,* 511–524.

Hazelton, R., Lancee, W., & O'Neil, M. K. (1998). The controversial long term effects of parental divorce: The role of early attachment. *Journal of Divorce and Remarriage, 29,* 1–17.

Heinicke, C. M., & Westheimer, I. (1965). *Brief separation.* New York: International Universities Press.

Hetherington, E. M. (1999). Should we stay together for the sake of the children. In E. M.

Hetherington, E. M. (Ed.). *Coping with divorce, single parenting, and remarriage: A risk and resiliency perspective* (pp. 93–116). New York: Psychology Press.

Hetherington, E. M. (2003). Intimate pathways: Changing patterns in close personal relationships across time. *Family Relations, 52,* 318–331.

Hetherington, E. M., & Camara, K. A. (1984). Families in transition: The process of dissolution and reconstitution. In R. D. Parke (Ed.), *Review of child development: Vol. 7. The family* (pp. 398–440). Chicago: University of Chicago Press.

Hetherington, E. M., Cox, M., & Cox, R. (1978). The aftermath of divorce. In J. H. Stevens, Jr. & M. Matthews (Eds.), *Mother–child, father–child relationships* (pp. 149–176). Washington, DC: National Association for the Education of Young Children.

Hetherington, E. M., Cox, M., & Cox, R. (1982). The effects of divorce on parents and children. In M. Lamb (Ed.), *Nontraditional families* (pp. 233–288). Hillsdale, NJ: Erlbaum.

Hetherington, E. M., & Kelly, J. (2002). *For better or for worse: Divorce reconsidered.* New York: Norton.

Hodges, W. F., Landis, T., Day, E., & Oderberg, N. (1991). Infant and toddlers and post divorce parental access: An initial exploration. *Journal of Divorce and Remarriage, 16,* 239–252.

Hoffman, J. P. (1995). The effects of family structure and family relations on marijuana use. *International Journal of the Addictions, 30,* 1207–1241.

Hope, S., Power C., & Rodgers, B. (1998). The relationships between parental separation in childhood and problem drinking in adulthood. *Addiction, 93,* 505–514.

Hu, Y. R., & Goldman, N. (1990). Mortality differentials by marital-status: An international comparison. *Demography, 27,* 233–250.

Huddleston, R. J., & Hawkings, L. D. (1991). A comparison of physical and emotional health after divorce in a Canadian and United States sample. *Journal of Divorce and Remarriage, 15,* 193–207.

Isohanni, M., Moilanen, I., & Rantakallio, P. (1991). Determinants of teenage smoking with special reference to non-standard family background. *British Journal of Addiction, 86,* 391–398.

Jaremka, L. M., Glaser, R., Loving, T. J., Malarkey, W. B., Stowell, J. R., Kiecolt-Glaser, J. K. (2013). Attachment anxiety is linked to alterations in cortisol production and cellular immunity. *Psychological Science, 24,* 272–279.

Jasinski, J. L., & Williams, L. M. (Eds.). (1998). *Partner violence: A comprehensive review of 20 years of research.* Thousand Oaks, CA: Sage.

Johnson, S. M. (2003). Attachment theory: A guide for couple therapy. In S. M. Johnson & V. E. Whiffen (Eds.), *Attachment processes in couple and family therapy* (pp. 103–123). New York: Guilford Press

Karney, B. R., & Bradbury, T. N. (1995). The longitudinal course of marital quality and stability: A review of theory, methods, and research. *Psychological Bulletin, 118,* 3–34.

Kelly, J. B., & Lamb, M. E. (2000). Special issue child custody evaluations: Using child development research to make appropriate custody and access decisions for young children. *Family and Conciliation Courts Review, 38,* 297–514.

Kiecolt-Glaser, J. K., Fisher, L. D., Ogrocki, P., Stout, J. C., Speicher, C. E., & Glaser, R. (1987). Marital quality, marital disruption, and immune function. *Psychosomatic Medicine, 49,* 13–34.

Kier, C., & Lewis, C. (1997). Infant–mother attachment in separated and married families. *Journal of Divorce and Remarriage, 26,* 185–194.

Kilman, P. R., Carranza, L. V., & Vendemia, J. M. C. (2006). Recollections of parent characteristics and attachment patterns for college women of intact vs. non-intact families. *Journal of Adolescence, 29,* 89–102.

Kirkpatrick, L. A., & Davis, K. E. (1994). Attachment style, gender, and relationship stability: A longitudinal analysis. *Journal of Personality and Social Psychology, 66,* 502–512.

Kitson, G. C. (1982). Attachment to the spouse in divorce: A scale and its application. *Journal of Marriage and the Family, 44,* 379–393.

Kitson, G. C., & Morgan, L. A. (1990). The multiple consequences of divorce: A decade review. *Journal of Marriage and the Family, 52,* 913–924.

Kitson, G. C., & Raschke, H. J. (1981). Divorce research: What we know, what we need to know. *Journal of Divorce, 4*, 1–37.

Knox, D., Zusman, M., & DeCuzzi, A. (2004). The effect of parental divorce on relationships with parents and romantic partners of college students. *College Student Journal, 38*, 597.

Kohn, J. L., Rholes, W. S., & Schmeichel, B. J. (2012). Self-regulatory depletion and attachment avoidance: Increasing the accessibility of negative attachment-related memories. *Journal of Experimental Social Psychology, 48*, 375–378.

Kohn, J. L., Rholes, W. S., Simpson, J. A., Martin, A. M., Tran, S., & Wilson, C. L. (2012). Changes in marital satisfaction across the transition to parenthood: The role of adult attachment orientations. *Personality and Social Psychology Bulletin, 38*, 1506–1522.

Krantz, D. S., & McCeney, M. K. (2002). Effects of psychological and social factors on organic disease: A critical assessment of research on coronary heart disease. *Annual Review of Psychology, 53*, 341–369.

Kressel, K., Lopez-Morillas, M., Weinglass, J., & Deutsch, M. (1978). Professional intervention in divorce: A summary of views of lawyers, psychotherapists, and clergy. *Journal of Divorce, 2*, 119–155.

Kunce, L. J., & Shaver, P. R. (1994). An attachment theoretical approach to caregiving in romantic relationships. In R. Bartholomew & D. Perlman (Eds.), *Advances in personal relationships* (Vol. 5, pp. 205–237). London: Jessica Kingsley.

Kurdek, L. A. (1991). The relations between reported well-being and divorce history, availability of a proximate adult, and gender. *Journal of Marriage and the Family, 53*, 71–78.

Lamb, M. E., & Kelly, J. B. (2001). Using the empirical literature to guide the development of parenting plans for young children. *Family Court Review, 39*, 365–371.

Laumann-Billings, L., & Emery, R. E. (2000). Distress among young adults from divorced families. *Journal of Family Psychology, 14*, 671–687.

Lee, L. A., Sbarra, D. A., Mason, A. E., & Law, R. W. (2011). Attachment anxiety, verbal immediacy, and blood pressure: Results from a laboratory analog study following marital separation. *Personal Relationships, 18*, 285–301.

Lewis, M., Feiring, C., & Rosenthal, S. (2000). Attachment over time. *Child Development, 71*, 707–720.

Liao, K. Y., & Wei, M. (2015). Insecure attachment and depressive symptoms: Forgiveness of self and others as moderators. *Personal Relationships, 22*(2), 216–229.

Lillard, L. A., & Waite, L. J. (1995). 'Til death do us part: Marital disruption and mortality. *American Journal of Sociology, 100*, 1131–1156.

Lorenz, F. O., Wickrama, K. A. S., Conger, R. D., & Elder, G. H., Jr. (2006). The short-term and decade-long effects of divorce on women's midlife health. *Journal of Health and Social Behavior, 47*, 111–125.

Lucas, R. E. (2005). Time does not heal all wounds: A longitudinal study of reaction and adaptation to divorce. *Psychological Science, 16*, 946–950.

Luecken, L. J., & Fabricius, W. V. (2003). Physical health vulnerability in adult children from divorced and intact families. *Journal of Psychosomatic Research, 55*, 221–228.

Lundberg, O. (1993). The impact of childhood living conditions on illness and mortality in adulthood. *Social Science and Medicine, 36*, 1047–1052.

Maatta, K. (2011). The throes and relief of divorce. *Journal of Divorce and Remarriage, 52*, 415–434.

Maccoby, E. E., Buchanan, C. M., Mnookin, R. H., & Dornbusch, S. M. (1993). Postdivorce roles of mothers and fathers in the lives of their children. *Journal of Family Psychology, 7*, 24–38.

Madden-Derdich, D. A., & Arditti, J. A. (1999). The ties that bind: Attachment between former spouses. *Family Relations, 48*, 243–249.

Maier, E. H., & Lachman, M. E. (2000). Consequences of early parental loss and separation for health and well-being in midlife. *International Journal of Behavioral Development, 24*, 83–189.

Main, M., Hesse, E., & Hesse, S. (2011). Attachment theory and research: Overview with suggested applications to child custody. *Family Court Review, 49*, 426–463.

Mandemakers, J. J., & Kalmijn, M. (2014). Do mother's and father's education condition the impact of parental divorce on child well-being? *Social Science Research, 44*, 187–199.

Marks, N. F. (1996). Flying solo at midlife: Gender, marital status, and psychological well-being. *Journal of Family Issues, 58*, 917–932.

Masheter, C. (1991). Postdivorce relationships between ex-spouses: The roles of attachment and interpersonal conflict. *Journal of Marriage and the Family, 53*, 103–110.

Masheter, C. (1997). Healthy and unhealthy friendship and hostility between ex-spouses. *Journal of Marriage and the Family, 59*, 463–475.

Mazor, A., Batiste-Harel, P., & Gampel, Y. (1998). Divorcing spouses' coping patterns, attachment bonding and forgiveness processes in the post-divorce experience. *Journal of Divorce and Remarriage, 29*, 65–81.

McCabe, K. (1997). Sex differences in the long term effects of divorce on children depression and heterosexual relationship difficulties in the young adult years. *Journal of Divorce and Remarriage, 27*, 123–135.

McGue, M., & Lykken, D. T. (1992). Genetic influence on risk of divorce. *Psychological Science, 3*, 368–373.

McIntosh, J. E., Smyth, B. M., & Kelaher, M. (2013). Overnight care patterns following parental separation: Associations with emotion regulation in infants and young children. *Journal of Family Studies, 19*, 224–239.

Mechanic, D., & Hansell, S. (1989). Divorce, conflict, and adolescents' well-being. *Journal of Health and Social Behavior, 30*, 105–116.

Mickelson, K. D., Kessler, R. C., & Shaver, P. R. (1997).

Adult attachment in a nationally representative sample. *Journal of Personality & Social Psychology, 73,* 1092-1106.

Mikulincer, M. (1998). Attachment working models and the sense of trust: An exploration of interaction goals and affect regulation. *Journal of Personality and Social Psychology, 74,* 1209–1224.

Mikulincer, M., & Florian, V. (1996). Emotional reactions to interpersonal losses over the life span: An attachment theoretical perspective. In C. Magai & S. H. McFadden (Eds.), *Handbook of emotions, adult development, and aging* (pp. 269–285). San Diego, CA: Academic Press.

Mikulincer, M., & Florian, V. (1998). The relationship between adult attachment styles and emotional and cognitive reactions to stressful events. In J. A. Simpson & W. S. Rholes (Eds.), *Attachment theory and close relationships* (pp. 143–165). New York: Guilford Press.

Mikulincer, M., Horesh, N., Eilati, I., & Kotler, M. (1999). The association between adult attachment style and mental health in extreme life-endangering conditions. *Personality and Individual Differences, 27,* 831–842.

Mikulincer, M., & Orbach, I. (1995). Attachment styles and repressive defensiveness: The accessibility and architecture of affective memories. *Journal of Personality and Social Psychology, 68,* 917.

Mikulincer, M., & Shaver P. R. (2007). Attachment, group-related processes, and psychotherapy. *International Journal of Group Psychology, 57,* 233–245.

Mikulincer, M., Shaver, P. R., & Slav, K. (2006). Attachment, mental representations of others, and gratitude and forgiveness in romantic relationships. In M. Mikulincer & G. S. Goodman (Eds.), *Dynamics of romantic love: Attachment, caregiving, and sex* (pp. 190–215). New York: Guilford Press.

Mirowsky, J., & Ross, C. E. (2003). *Education, social status, and health.* Hawthorne, NY: Aldine de Gruyter.

Monin, J. K., Feeney, B. C., & Schulz, R. (2012), Attachment orientation and reactions to anxiety expression in close relationships. *Personal Relationships, 19,* 535–550.

Nair, H., & Murray, A. D. (2005). Predictors of attachment security in preschool children from intact and divorced families. *Journal of Genetic Psychology, 166,* 245–263.

Nelson, W. L., Hughes, H. M., Handal, P., Katz, B., & Searight, H. R. (1993). The relationship of family structure and family conflict to adjustment in young adult college students. *Adolescence, 28,* 29–40.

Ognibene, T. C., & Collins, N. L. (1998). Adult attachment styles, perceived social support and coping strategies. *Journal of Social and Personal Relationships, 15,* 323–345.

Olivas, S. T., & Stoltenberg, C. D. (1997). Post-divorce father custody: Are mothers the true predictors of adult relationship satisfaction? *Journal of Divorce and Remarriage, 28,* 119–137.

Overbeek, G., Vollebergh, W., de Graaf, R., Scholte, R, de Kemp, R., & Engels, R. (2006). Longitudinal associations of marital quality and marital dissolution with the incidence of DSM-III-R disorders. *Journal of Family Psychology, 20,* 284–291.

Ozen, D. S. (2003). The impact of interparental divorce on adult attachment styles and perceived parenting styles of adolescents: Study in Turkey. *Journal of Divorce and Remarriage, 40,* 129–149.

Page, T., & Bretherton, I. (2001). Mother– and father–child attachment themes in the story completions of pre-schoolers from post-divorce families: Do they predict relationships with peers and teachers? *Attachment and Human Development, 3,* 1–29.

Perrig-Chiello, P., Hutchison, S., & Morselli, D. (2014). Patterns of psychological adaptation to divorce after a long-term marriage. *Journal of Social and Personal Relationships.* [Epub ahead of print]

Pietromonaco, P. R., & Powers, S. I. (2015). Attachment and health-related physiological stress processes. *Current Opinion in Psychology, 1,* 34–39.

Reibstein, J. (1998). Attachment, pain, and detachment for the adults in divorce. *Sexual and Marital Therapy, 13,* 351–360.

Reibstein, J., & Bamber, R. (1997). *The family through divorce: How you can limit the damage.* London: Thorsons.

Riggs, S. A., & Jacobvitz, D. (2002). Expectant parents' representations of early attachment relationships: Associations with mental health and family history. *Journal of Consulting and Clinical Psychology, 70,* 195–204.

Roberson, P. N. E., Sabo, M., & Wickel, K. (2011). Internal working models of attachment and postdivorce coparent relationships. *Journal of Divorce and Remarriage, 52,* 187–201.

Robertson, J., & Robertson, J. (1971). Young children in brief separation: A fresh look. *The Psychoanalytic Study of the Child, 26,* 264-315.

Rodgers, K. B., & Rose, H. A. (2002). Risk and resiliency factors among adolescents who experience marital transitions. *Journal of Marriage and Family, 64,* 1024–1037.

Rogers, K. N. (2004). A theoretical review of risk and protective factors related to post divorce adjustment in young children. *Journal of Divorce and Remarriage, 40* (3/4), 135–147.

Roisman, G. I. (2007). The psychophysiology of adult attachment relationships: Autonomic reactivity in marital and premarital interactions. *Developmental Psychology, 43,* 39–53.

Ross, L. T., & Wynne, S. (2010). Parental depression and divorce and adult children's well-being: the role of family unpredictability. *Journal of Child and Family Studies, 19,* 757–761.

Ruschena, E., Prior, M., Sanson, A., & Smart, D. (2005). A longitudinal study of adolescent adjustment following family transitions. *Journal of Child Psychology and Psychiatry, 46,* 353–363.

Rutter, M. (1994). Family discord and conduct disorder: Cause, consequence, or correlate? *Journal of Family Psychology, 8,* 170–186.

Saavedra, M. C., Chapman, K. E., & Rogge, R. D. (2010). Clarifying links between attachment and relationship quality: Hostile conflict and mindfulness as moderators. *Journal of Family Psychology, 24,* 380–390.

Sandler, I. N., Wheeler, L. A., & Braver, S. L. (2013). Relations of parenting quality, interparental conflict, and overnights with mental health problems of children in divorcing families with high legal conflict. *Journal of Family Psychology, 27,* 915–924.

Sartor, C. E., Lynskey, M. T., Heath, A. C., Jacob, T., & True, W. (2007). The role of childhood risk factors in initiation of alcohol use and progression to alcohol dependence. *Addiction, 102,* 216–225.

Sbarra, D. A. (2015). Divorce and health: Current trends and future directions. *Psychosomatic Medicine, 77*(3), 227–236.

Sbarra, D. A., & Borelli, J. L. (2013). Heart rate variability moderates the association between avoidance and self-concept reorganization following marital separation. *International Journal of Psychophysiology, 88,* 253-260.

Sbarra, D. A., & Emery, R. E. (2005). Comparing conflict, nonacceptance, and depression among divorced adults: Results from a 12-year follow-up study of child custody mediation using multiple imputations. *American Journal of Orthopsychiatry, 75,* 63–75.

Sbarra, D. A., Hasselmo, K. & Nojopranoto, W. (2012). Divorce and death: A case study for health psychology. *Social and Personality Psychology Compass, 6,* 905–919.

Schmidt, S. D., Blank, T. O., Bellizzi, K, M., & Park, C. L. (2012). The relationship of coping strategies, social support, and attachment style with posttraumatic growth in cancer survivors, *Journal of Health Psychology, 17,* 1033–1040.

Schwartz, J. E., Friedman, H. S., Tucker, J. S., Tomlinson-Keasey, C., Wingard, D. L., & Criqui, M. H. (1995). Sociodemographic and psychosocial factors in childhood as predictors of adult mortality. *American Journal of Public Health, 85,* 1237–1245.

Shaffer, J. W., Duszynski, K. R., & Thomas, C. B. (1982). Family attitudes in youth as a possible precursor of cancer among physicians: A search for explanatory mechanisms. *Journal of Behavioral Medicine, 5,* 143–163.

Shaver, P. R., & Mikulincer, M. (2004). What do self-report attachment measures assess? In W. S. Rholes & J. A. Simpson (Eds.), *Adult attachment: Theory, research, and clinical implications* (pp. 17–54). New York: Guilford Press.

Shaver, P. R., & Mikulincer, M. (2007). Adult attachment strategies and the regulation of emotions. In J. J. Gross (Ed.), *Handbook of emotion regulation* (pp. 446–465). New York: Guilford Press.

Shimkowski, J. R., & Schrodt, P. (2012). Coparental communication as a mediator of interparental conflict and young adult children's mental well-being. *Communication Monographs, 79,* 48–71.

Shulman, S., Scharf, M., Lumer, D., & Maurer, O. (2001). How young adults perceive parental divorce: The role of their relationships with their fathers and mothers. *Journal of Divorce and Remarriage, 34,* 3–17.

Simons, E. L., Lin, K.-H., Gordon, L. C., Conger, R. D., & Lorenz, F. O. (1999). Explaining the higher incidence of adjustment problems among children of divorce compared with those in two-parent families. *Journal of Marriage and the Family, 61,* 1020–1033.

Simos, B. G. (1979). *A time to grieve: Loss as a universal human experience.* New York: Family Services Association of America.

Simpson, J. A., Collins, W. A., Tran, S., & Haydon, K. C. (2007). Attachment and the experience and expression of emotions in romantic relationships: A developmental perspective. *Journal of Personality and Social Psychology, 92,* 355–367.

Simpson, J. A., Rholes, W. S., & Phillips, D. (1996). Conflict in close relationships: An attachment perspective. *Journal of Personality and Social Psychology, 71,* 899–914.

Sinclair, S. L., & Nelson, E. S. (1998). The impact of parental divorce on college students' intimate relationships and relationship beliefs. *Journal of Divorce and Remarriage, 29,* 103–129.

Sirvanli-Ozen, D. (2005). Impacts of divorce on the behavior and adjustment problems, parenting styles, and attachment styles of children: Literature review including Turkish studies. *Journal of Divorce and Remarriage, 42,* 127–151.

Solomon, B. C., & Jackson, J. J. (2014). Why do personality traits predict divorce? Multiple pathways through satisfaction. *Journal of Personality and Social Psychology, 106,* 978–996.

Solomon, J., & George, C. (1999). The development of attachment in separated and divorced families: The effects of overnight visitation, parent and couple variables. *Attachment and Human Development, 1,* 2–33.

South, A. L. (2013). Perceptions of romantic relationships in adult children of divorce. *Journal of Divorce & Remarriage, 54,* 126–141.

Southworth, S., & Schwartz, J. C. (1987). Post-divorce contact, relationship with father, and heterosexual trust in female college students. *American Journal of Orthopsychiatry, 57,* 371–382.

Spanier, G. B., & Casto, R. F. (1979). Adjustment to separation and divorce: An analysis of 50 case studies. *Journal of Divorce, 2,* 241-253.

Spanier, G. B., & Thompson, L. (1984). *Parting.* Beverly Hills, CA: Sage.

Sprague, H. E., & Kinney, J. M. (1997). The effects of interparental divorce and conflict on college students' romantic relationships. *Journal of Divorce and Remarriage, 27,* 85–104.

Sprecher, S., Cate, R., & Levin, L. (1998). Parental divorce and young adults' beliefs about love. *Journal of Divorce and Remarriage, 28,* 107–120.

Sroufe, A., & McIntosh, J. (2011). Divorce and attachment relationships: The longitudinal journey. *Family Court Review, 49,* 464–473.

Stack, S., & Scourfield, J. (2015). Recency of divorce, depression, and suicide risk. *Journal of Family Issues, 36,* 695–715.

Stirtzinger, R., & Cholvat, L. (1991). The family home as attachment object for preschool age children after divorce. *Journal of Divorce and Remarriage, 15,* 105–124.

Strohschein, L. (2012). Parental divorce and child mental health: accounting for predisruption differences. *Journal of Divorce and Remarriage, 53,* 489–502.

Summers, P., Forehand, R., Armistead, L., & Tannenbaum, L. (1998). Parental divorce during early adolescence in Caucasian families: The role of family process variables in predicting the long-term consequences for early adult psychosocial adjustment. *Journal of Consulting and Clinical Psychology, 66,* 327–336.

Sutherland, K. E., Altenhofen, S., & Biringen, Z. (2012). Emotional availability during mother–child interactions in divorcing and intact married families. *Journal of Divorce and Remarriage, 53,* 126–141.

Sweeting, H., & West, P. (1995). Family life and health in adolescence: A role for culture in the health inequalities debate? *Social Science and Medicine, 40,* 163–175.

Symoens, S., Colman, E., & Bracke, P. (2014). Divorce, conflict, and mental health: How the quality of intimate relationships is linked to post-divorce well-being. *Journal of Applied Social Psychology, 44,* 220–233.

Symoens, S., Van de Velde, S., Colman, E., & Bracke, P. (2014). Divorce and the multidimensionality of men and women's mental health: The role of social-relational and socio-economic conditions. *Applied Research in Quality of Life, 9,* 197–214.

Tayler, L., Parker, G., & Roy, K. (1995). Parental divorce and its effects on the quality of intimate relationships in adulthood. *Journal of Divorce and Remarriage, 24,* 181–202.

Todorski, J. (1995). Attachment and divorce: A therapeutic view. *Journal of Divorce and Remarriage, 22,* 189–204.

Toews, M. L., McKenry, P. C., & Catlett, B. S. (2003). Male-initiated partner abuse during marital separation prior to divorce. *Violence and Victims, 18,* 387–402.

Tornello, S. L., Emery, R., Rowen, J., Potter, D., Ocker, B., & Xu, Y. (2013). Overnight custody arrangements, attachment, and adjustment among very young children. *Journal of Marriage and Family, 75,* 871–885.

Troxel, W. M., & Matthews, K. A. (2004). What are the costs of marital conflict and dissolution to children's physical health? *Clinical Child and Family Psychological Review, 7,* 29–57.

Tucker, J. S., Friedman, H. S., Schwartz, J. E., Criqui, M. H., Tomlinson-Keasey, C., & Wingard, D. L., et al. (1997). Parental divorce: Effects on individual behavior and longevity. *Journal of Personality and Social Psychology, 73,* 381–391.

Umberson, D. (1987). Family status and health behaviors: Social control as a dimension of social integration. *Journal of Health and Social Behavior, 28,* 306–319.

Uphold-Carrier, H., & Utz, R. (2012). Parental divorce among young and adult children: A long-term quantitative analysis of mental health and family solidarity. *Journal of Divorce and Remarriage, 53,* 247–266.

Vanassche, S., Sodermans, A. K., Matthijs, K., & Swicegood, G. (2013). Commuting between two parental households: The association between joint physical custody and adolescent wellbeing following divorce. *Journal of Family Studies, 19,* 139–158.

Vareschi, C. G., & Bursik, K. (2005). Attachment style differences in the parental interactions and adaptation patterns of divorcing parents. *Journal of Divorce and Remarriage, 42,* 15–32.

Vaughn, B. E., Gove, F. L., & Egeland, B. (1980). The relationship between out-of-home care and the quality of infant–mother attachment in an economically disadvantaged population. *Child Development, 51,* 1203–1214.

Velez, C. E., Wolchik, S. A., Tein, J., & Sandler, I. (2011). Protecting children from the consequences of divorce: A longitudinal study of the effects of parenting on children's coping processes. *Child Development, 82,* 244–257.

Walker, T. R., & Ehrenberg, M. F. (1998). An exploratory study of young persons' attachment styles and perceived reasons for parental divorce. *Journal of Adolescent Research, 13,* 320–342.

Wallerstein, J. S., & Blakeslee, S. (1989). *Second chances: Men, women, and children a decade after divorce.* New York: Ticknor & Fields.

Wallerstein, J. [S.], Lewis, J., & Packer Rosenthal, S. (2013). Mothers and their children after divorce: Report from a 25-year longitudinal study. *Psychoanalytic Psychology, 30,* 167–184.

Wallerstein, J. S., & Lewis, J. M. (2004). The unexpected legacy of divorce: Report of a 25-year study. *Psychoanalytic Psychology, 21,* 353–370.

Washington, K. N., & Hans, J. D. (2013). Romantic attachment among young adults: The effects of parental divorce and residential instability. *Journal of Divorce and Remarriage, 54,* 95–111.

Waters, E., Merrick, S., Treboux, D., Crowell, J., & Albersheim, L. (2000). Attachment security in infancy and early adulthood: A twenty-year longitudinal study. *Child Development, 71,* 684–689.

Weiss, R. S. (1975). *Marital separation.* New York: Basic Books.

Weiss, R. S. (1976). The emotional impact of marital separation. *Journal of Social Issues, 32,* 135–145.

Williams, K., & Umberson, D. (2004). Marital status, marital transitions, and health: A gendered life course perspective. *Journal of Health and Social Behavior, 45,* 81–98.

Wolchik, S. A., Sandler, I. N., Tein, J. Y., Mahrer, N. E., Millsap, R. E., Winslow, E., et al. (2013). Fifteen-year follow-up of a randomized trial of a preventive intervention for divorced families: Effects on mental health and substance use outcomes in young adulthood. Journal of Consulting and Clinical Psychology, 81, 660–673.

Wolchik, S. A., Tein, J. Y., Sandler, I. N., & Doyle, K. W. (2002). Fear of abandonment as a mediator of the relations between divorce stressors and mother–child relationship quality and children's adjustment problems. *Journal of Abnormal Child Psychology*, 30, 401–418.

Wolchik, S. A., Wilcox, K. L., Tein, J.-Y., & Sandler, I. N. (2000). An experimental evaluation of theory-based mother and mother–child programs for children of divorce. *Journal of Consulting and Clinical Psychology*, 68, 843–856.

Wolfinger, N. H. (2000). Beyond the intergenerational transition of divorce: Do people replicate the patterns of marital instability they grew up with? *Journal of Family Issues, 21*, 1061–1086.

Yamoz, S., Plazaola, M., & Etxeberria, J. (2008). Adaptation to divorce: An attachment-based intervention with long-term divorced parents. *Journal of Divorce and Remarriage, 49*, 291–307.

Yamoz-Yaben, S. (2010). Attachment style and adjustment to divorce. *Spanish Journal of Psychology, 13*, 210–219.

Yu, T., & Adler-Baeder, F. (2007). The intergenerational transmission of relationship quality: The effects of parental remarriage quality on young adults' relationships. *Journal of Divorce & Remarriage, 47*, 87–102.

Yu, T., Pettit, G. S., Lansford, J. E., Dodge, K. A., & Bates, J. E. (2010). The interactive effects of marital conflict and divorce on parent–adult children's relationships. *Journal of Marriage and Family, 72*, 282–292.

# Chapter 41

# Attachment and School Readiness

Amanda P. Williford
Lauren M. Carter
Robert C. Pianta

Research in the fields of education and psychology demonstrate the critical importance of a child possessing a diverse toolbox of school readiness skills upon kindergarten entry (e.g., Duncan et al., 2007). This toolbox includes skills related to academics, such as preliteracy and premathematics skills, as well as those related to socioemotional competence, including cooperation, frustration tolerance, and social problem-solving skills (Bierman et al., 2008; Snow, 2006; Webster-Stratton, Reid, & Stoolmiller, 2008). School readiness skills have been examined in both the education and developmental literatures, and are most often defined as the skills that a child acquires through his or her experiences in the home and early childhood education environments prior to entering formal schooling—usually kindergarten. The interactions that occur between a young child and the important adults in his or life are considered to be one of the key ongoing experiences from which children develop school readiness skills (e.g., Ainsworth, Blehar, Waters, & Wall, 1978; Mashburn et al., 2008). Early research in this topic area focused on the role that parents play in a child's cognitive, social, and emotional development during the first several years of life, but more recent research has examined the interactions and relationships between a young child and his or her teacher as a significant contributor to the development of school readiness skills.

Attachment theory provides a useful framework to further our understanding and thinking about the predictors of a child's academic, socioemotional, and behavioral development within the early education setting. This chapter synthesizes the research literature linking the quality of children's interactions with their parents and their teachers to the development of school readiness skills. We begin by examining research on the links between child–parent attachment and school readiness skills. However, the links between child–parent attachment and children's development are described in more detail in other chapters in this handbook. Thus, although we provide a brief review of the literature linking child–adult attachment to the development of children's readiness skills, our focus is on the quality of teacher–child interactions and relationships as contributors to the development of children's school readiness skills. We end the chapter by providing implications for both practice and future research.

## Conceptual Frameworks and Definitions

In the next section, we provide an overview of several key conceptual frameworks and definitions that have informed how researchers and practitioners understand the field of teacher–child relationships and how it relates to the development of school readiness skills. The following are included: school readiness, attachment theory, developmental systems theory, and the concept that relationships comprise daily interactions. Each of these frameworks is directly applicable to understanding the implications that attachment theory has for teacher–child relationships and the promotion of school readiness skills.

## School Readiness

Our focus in this chapter is the links between a child's attachment to adults (particularly teachers) and the development of school readiness skills. The term *school readiness* has become increasingly popular as more attention has turned to early childhood education and preparing children for kindergarten entry. School readiness has been defined as a set of skills that children possess when they enter school that prepares them for later school success. These skills can be classified into several key domains: language and literacy development; cognition and general knowledge; approaches to learning; physical health (including well-being and motor development); and social and emotional development (Bierman et al., 2008; U.S. Department of Health and Human Services, 2010; Snow, 2006; Webster-Stratton et al., 2008). We specifically stress the importance of both academic (e.g., language, literacy, mathematics) and traditionally socioemotional (e.g., emotional competence, self-regulation, executive functioning) school readiness skills for a child to be successful in kindergarten and later schooling.

Current conceptualizations of school readiness strongly emphasize the role of context, seeing a child's skills as situated within and dependent on the environment (Downer, Driscoll, & Pianta, 2006; Ramey & Ramey, 1998). This conceptualization of school readiness highlights how a child's learning and development are shaped by interactions with others. As the majority of young children now spend a significant portion of their time within a child care/preschool setting outside the home before entering into formal schooling (American Community Survey, 2005–2007), it is important to describe how the quality of the teacher–child relationship in addition to the parent–child relationship contributes to early success in school.

## Attachment Theory

Attachment theory is built on the belief that the quality of a child's relationships with one or more caregivers serves a critical role in the child's de-

velopment (e.g., Ainsworth et al., 1978; Sroufe, 1983). In a secure attachment relationship, the adult serves as (1) a secure base from which the child can explore new environments and (2) a safe haven for a child to return to when he or she needs to feel safe, comforted, or delighted in (Ainsworth et al., 1978). Broad constructs from attachment theory have informed the conceptualization of high-quality teacher–child relationships (Pianta, Hamre, & Stuhlman, 2003). For example, the *quality of emotional support* can be defined as the warmth, sensitivity, and support for individuality that a teacher provides to children in his or her classroom; this parallels the attachment concept of a secure base. Additionally, when children enter preschool at the age of 3 or 4 years, they carry with them the ongoing influence of the bond developed with one or both parents. The level of security achieved through the child–parent bond is theorized to influence directly the child's ability to successfully interact in and navigate this new environment.

To further extend attachment theory, one may view the daily relational interactions between a teacher and child as contributing to the creation of the child's internal working model, or schema, of the relationship that creates expectations and may guide subsequent perceptions by both the teacher and the child (Pianta, 1999). The quality of information conveyed (e.g., tone of voice, posture and proximity, timing) is just as important as the content of what is said or done within the dyad. When the quality of teacher–child interactions is high, it promotes a child's feeling of attachment and security toward the teacher. This, in turn, allows a child to engage more fully in learning activities, which supports his or her school adjustment. When teachers are able to establish an emotional connection and match levels of support to a child's abilities, they are more effective in addressing a child's problems and concerns. This responsiveness is thought to optimize the child's ability to use the classroom environment to its maximum potential in order to learn, develop, and grow.

## Developmental Systems Theory

An additional theory that influences the way we think about the connections between child–adult attachments and the development of children's school readiness skills is developmental systems theory (DST). This ecologically oriented theory portrays a child as embedded within layers of systems that are both organized and dynamic (Bronfenbrenner & Morris, 1998; Good & Weinstein, 1986; Pianta, 1999). Systems may be either proximal, such as the child's family or classroom, or distal, such as the government or a parent's place of employment. DST informs how we view a child's relationships with both teacher(s) and parent(s). This theory emphasizes that a child (and subsequently, his or her relationships) exists within a multilevel system, where each level (community, classroom, family, and individual) has a dynamic bidirectional influence on relational processes (Bronfenbrenner & Morris, 1998; Sameroff, 1995). Thus, a shift in any of these levels has the potential to influence the child in either a direct or indirect manner (depending on the level of proximity of the change). For example, if, at a distal level, a child's caregiver's employer requires him or her to begin to work more hours, this will affect, among other things, the caregiver's level of stress and the amount of time available to devote to the child, which may lead to consequences for the child. At a more proximal level, a change in classroom dynamics (e.g., a new teacher or new peers) may influence the child's immediate environment and the ways in which he or she interacts in the classroom.

## Relationships Comprised of Interactions

The development of school readiness skills, including academic and socioemotional skills, has been repeatedly linked to the quality of relationships that children form with their teachers (e.g., Hamre & Pianta, 2001; Mashburn et al., 2008; Pianta et al., 2003). High-quality teacher–child relationships often include high levels of warmth, sensitivity, and emotional connection, and low levels of dependency, negativity, and conflict (Pianta, 1999; Spilt, Koomen, Thijs, & Van der Leij, 2012). The quality of the teacher–child relationship is built, in part, through the daily interactions that occur between the child and teacher; these reciprocal exchanges continuously provide information to each participant and help to establish and maintain the quality of the relationship. For example, a teacher may notice that a child and a peer are struggling to work together in a learning center. The teacher acknowledges this challenge (e.g., "You two are working hard to figure this out") and provides a scaffold (e.g., "I'm here if you need me to help"). This provides the support the child needs to resolve a conflict with a peer. Additionally, this interaction provides evidence to the child that the teacher is an adult who notices his or her struggles and is available for help, if necessary.

The quality of teacher–child relationships can be measured at the global level, with a measure such as the Student–Teacher Relationship Scale (STRS; Pianta & Hamre, 2001), or at the discrete level, with an individualized child–teacher observational measure, such as the Individualized Classroom Assessment Scoring System (inCLASS; Downer, Booren, Lima, Luckner, & Pianta, 2010). Patterns of interactions are created that are based on the daily teacher–child interactions, which form the basis of the teacher–child relationship. The temporal interactions and subsequent relationships are the primary mechanisms through which children develop and learn.

This framework dovetails with attachment theory, in that the manner in which a child engages in daily interactions with a primary attachment figure, such as a parent, may form an internal model of relationships. These mental representations formed with early caregivers subsequently guide the interpretation and behavior of other relational patterns (e.g., with teachers; Buyse, Verschueren, Verachtert, & Van Damme, 2009; Rydell, Bohlin, Thorell, 2005; Zajac & Kobak, 2006). For example, the quality of the child's interactions with his or her caregiver may influence the quality of his or her interactions with a teacher or at least the expectations the child has for adults and their ability to provide emotional support. In a similar vein, interactions with a sensitive and warm teacher may help shape (or reshape) a child's interactional models that influence how he or she responds to future teachers during progression through school (Sabol & Pianta, 2012).

## Empirical Support

In the next section, we describe seminal and recent research that supports the links among child–parent attachment, child–teacher attachment, and a child's school readiness skills (see Figure 41.1).

### Children's School Readiness and Child–Parent Attachment

The quality of a child's attachment to a parent has been repeatedly associated with the development of school readiness skills across a wide

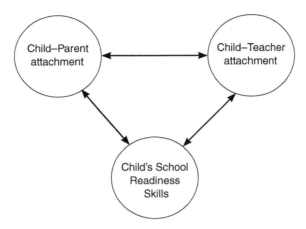

**FIGURE 41.1.** Empirical connections between child–parent attachment, child–teacher attachment, and a child's school readiness skills.

range of early learning domains (e.g., Bus, Belsky, Van IJzendoorn, & Crnic, 1997; Cassidy, Jones, & Shaver, 2013; Sroufe, 1983). With regard to academic skills, preschool children who display a secure parent attachment develop better reading and prereading skills compared to children who display an insecure attachment (Bus et al., 1997; Bus & Van IJzendoorn, 1997). Granot and Mayseless (2001) confirmed this link between attachment and preliteracy skills and extended it to prematematics skills. In their study, children with an insecure attachment tended to display lower verbal and math skills, lower reading comprehension skills, and lower overall academic achievement compared to children evidencing a secure parent attachment. Thus, children who do not experience a secure child–parent attachment are more likely to enter kindergarten displaying lower academic skills compared to securely attached peers. Furthermore, children with a secure child–mother attachment at 24 or 36 months of age demonstrated higher cognitive abilities in later years of childhood (West, Matthews, & Kerns, 2013). For some children, particularly children experiencing multiple risk factors such as poverty or a poor school environment (Akiba, LeTendre, & Scribner, 2007; Burchinal et al., 2011), this initial achievement gap initiates a trajectory of lower school achievement that tends to widen over time and consequently leads to future academic difficulties (Martoccio, Brophy-Herb, & Onaga, 2014).

Although academic skills are an important component of school readiness, findings from Rimm-Kaufman, Pianta, and Cox (2000) suggest

that socioemotional skills, such as a child's behavioral or emotional control, problem solving, or working memory, are even more important to teachers at kindergarten entry. Sroufe (1983) conducted one of the first studies to establish the association between child–parent attachment quality and socioemotional school readiness skills. In this seminal study, child–parent attachment was evaluated at 12 months and again at 18 months of age. Several years later, children with an insecure attachment to their mother were rated by their preschool teachers and were found to demonstrate lower curiosity, empathy, compliance, and social competence. Additionally, children who were insecurely attached had lower self-esteem and displayed greater dependence on their teacher (Sroufe, 1983). Granot and Mayseless (2001) confirmed and extended the link between insecure attachment and lower levels of socioemotional skills in a more recent study. In this study, over 100 fourth- and fifth-grade students were assessed to determine their level of maternal attachment security. Based on teacher report and sociometric data, secure children experienced better school adjustment and had a higher social status with peers. This is important in the classroom context because children with higher socioemotional skills may be more likely to take a risk in learning or to access available experiences more fully at school.

Children's attention skills, often considered an aspect of executive functioning, are another kind of key school readiness skill because they heavily influence a child's ability to focus on and process information being presented within the classroom. Research demonstrates that young children who evidence insecure attachments to their mother have shorter attention spans and tend to perform worse on cognitive functioning tasks than do those with secure attachments (e.g., Frankel & Bates, 1990; Main, 1983; Moss & St-Laurent, 2001). This may keep these children from fully accessing instruction in the classroom setting.

The quality of a child's attachment to a caregiver has also been linked repeatedly to child behavioral outcomes; children who do not display secure child–parent attachments are at higher risk for displaying externalizing and antisocial behavior (e.g., Fearon & Belsky, 2011; Kobak, Cassidy, Lyons-Ruth, & Ziv, 2006). Disruptive behavior in early childhood predicts multiple maladaptive outcomes, including the development of negative relationships with adults (Howes, 2000; Ladd & Burgess, 2001), unsuccessful kindergarten entry (Rimm-Kaufman et al., 2000), school failure, and long-term social adjustment problems (Conyers, Reynolds, & Ou, 2003). Kochanska and Kim (2012) provide support for the theory that the quality of child–parent attachment early in life moderates the impact of future socialization strategies, such as parenting practices, on children's outcomes. They found that only within the context of a prior insecure child–parent attachment relationship was there evidence of a causal pathway between child anger proneness, power assertive parenting practices in preschool, and children's later antisocial behavior problems. For children who experienced a secure child–parent attachment, anger proneness was not related to power assertive parenting practices, and power assertive parenting practices were not related to children's later antisocial behaviors.

As outlined earlier, educational and psychological research provide strong evidence that the quality of a child's attachment to a primary caregiver (with most research examining the relationship between child and mother) is linked to school readiness skills across a wide range of academic and socioemotional early learning domains. This provides a framework within which to understand the relationships that develop between the child and additional important adults; our focus in this chapter is on preschool/child care teachers. When a child enters school, he or she spends on average 30 hours per week with this adult (Blau & Currie, 2006). Thus, it is important to understand how the attachment quality that a child has developed with his or her parent(s) extends into the school environment and the attachment the child develops with his or her teacher.

## Connections between Child–Parent and Child–Teacher Attachment Quality

A child engages across multiple ecological systems, including those that are more proximal (e.g., home and school), as well as those that are more distal (e.g., community and government) (Bronfenbrenner & Morris, 1998). Evidence suggests that the attachment quality a child develops with an adult who plays a significant role in that child's experiences within one of these ecological systems, such as the home, may transfer to another system, such as the school, leading to an association between a child's attachment to a caregiver and the quality of attachment to a teacher. There are multiple reasons this may occur. The child elicits interactions from others across settings, which influence attachment (e.g., characteristics of the child or his or her behavior may lead adults to interact with him or her in similar ways; Belsky, 2005). In addition, the child forms an attachment with an adult in one setting, which is theorized to inform the creation of an internal working schema of how relationships with adults are expected to be. Thus, the child's attachment experience with his or her parent can be expected to apply to a subsequent relationship the child forms with a teacher. It is important to note that in early childhood, a teacher's role with a child often has many parallels with a parent's role; for example, a teacher may help a child develop important adaptive and self-care skills, such as solving problems independently or managing basic hygiene skills. Teachers also provide support and give evaluative feedback as children navigate the classroom environment (Hamre & Pianta, 2001; Myers & Pianta, 2008; O'Connor & McCartney, 2007). Hence, we would expect that the quality of a child's relationship with his or her early childhood teacher would prove important for the quality of later relationships. This is demonstrated in research indicating that a child's level of closeness with a teacher (as reported by the teacher) is stable across different teachers in the early school years (O'Connor & McCartney, 2007).

Booth, Kelly, Spieker, and Zuckerman (2003) studied the association between child–mother and child–teacher attachment quality in 24-month-old children. They found a significant correlation ($r = .31$, $p < .05$) between the observer-reported secure-base composite score of the mother–child and teacher–child attachment using the Attachment Q-Set (AQS) instrument. Booth and colleagues noted an additional reason this may occur—selection bias (i.e., sensitive mothers choose sensitive caregivers). This link between the quality of the child–parent and child–teacher attachment continues into the preschool years, although at a modest level (Ahnert, Pinquart, & Lamb, 2006; Sroufe, 1983). Ahnert and colleagues (2006) conducted a meta-analysis that examined the extent to which observed security with teachers matches the observed security with parents. Findings suggested that, overall, children's security with parents was significantly, albeit modestly, correlated with children's security with teachers ($r = .14$, $p < .001$).

These findings support the idea that children's early attachments to their parents guide the formation of internal models of relationships, which may influence the manner in which a child interprets the behavior of subsequent relational partners (Buyse, Verschueren, Verachtert, & Van Damme, 2009; Rydell et al., 2005). By integrating the theories of attachment and developmental systems, theorists postulate that teacher/caregiver characteristics, such as sensitivity, may change the internal working models that the child previously developed through their attachment experiences with their parents. This would subsequently revise the child's previous mental representation of adult relationships (for better or worse), which may then shift subsequent relationships with new important adults.

## Children's School Readiness and Child–Teacher Attachment

A positive relationship with a teacher, particularly in early childhood, increases the likelihood that a child will have higher academic performance, lower levels of externalizing behaviors, and better social skills (Crosnoe, Johnson, & Elder, 2004; Ladd & Burgess, 2001; Mashburn et al., 2008; Pianta & Stuhlman, 2004; Shields et al., 2001). The attachment framework can easily be applied to the teacher–child relationship. In the school context, the quality of this relationship may serve as a secure base from which the child explores the classroom environment, learns new skills, and to which he or she returns to for help, comfort, and support.

Howes and Ritchie (1999) described four primary types of child–teacher attachment that mirror child–parent attachment styles—secure, near secure, avoidant, and resistant. Additionally, a child–teacher attachment may not fit into any of the categories and is therefore labeled as inse-

cure/unclassifiable or may demonstrate an avoidant/resistant pattern. Below are brief descriptions of each type (for a more detailed description, see Howes & Ritchie, 1999):

- *Secure:* A secure child–teacher attachment relationship looks similar to a secure parent–child relationship. A child views the teacher as a secure base, accepting comfort and going to the teacher for help and with new discoveries.
- *Near-secure:* In a near secure child–teacher attachment pattern, the child responds somewhat positively to the teacher, if the *teacher* initiates contact, but does not tend to initiate contact independently. The child has a tendency to avoid interactions with the teacher and is more interested in classroom materials/activities.
- *Avoidant:* An avoidant style characterizes a child who is more interested in the classroom materials, does not approach the teacher for help, and ignores the teacher if he or she approaches.
- *Resistant:* In a resistant child–teacher attachment, the child tends to be upset and irritable, and cries frequently. The child often resists classroom rules and routines, and may engage in physical or verbal aggression with the teacher (i.e., kicking, crying for attention, being angry).

Howes and Ritchie (1999) validated these categories with a sample of 3,062 preschool children and their primary teacher; the sample was drawn from five studies of children enrolled in center-based child care and intervention programs. The majority of child–teacher attachments (35.4%) fit into the near-secure classification. The remaining children fit into categories labeled secure (29%), avoidant (20%), insecure/unclassifiable (10%), resistant (4%), and avoidant/resistant (0.4%). Children with a secure attachment to their teacher engaged in more complex play with peers compared to children categorized into one of the other attachment classifications; in contrast, those with an unclassifiable, resistant, or avoidant classification had a higher level of conflict with peers.

More recently, Commodari (2013) conducted a study of 152 Italian children between the ages 4 and 5. Results from this study suggest that the quality of a child's attachment to a preschool teacher is significantly correlated with multiple school readiness skills, including linguistic developmental level (linguistic and phonological skills), psychomotor skills, attention and metacognitive skills, and specific cognitive abilities (those involved in the prerequisites of mathematics, reading, and writing). These results may have important implications for how schools provide intervention services for children who are behind in school readiness skills. Commodari suggests that the early identification of children who demonstrate insecure teacher attachment and subsequent intervention to improve school adjustment may be critical pieces of a strategy to prevent future academic difficulties.

Williford, Maier, Downer, Pianta, and Howes (2013) conducted another study that examined teacher–child interactions at both the classroom level and the individual-child level. Results suggest that the quality of teacher–child interactions at the classroom level were predictive of gains across all school readiness skills, including language, literacy, and self-regulation. The effect of an individual child's level of engagement in the classroom was moderated by the quality of the teacher–child interactions at the classroom level; that is, in classrooms with high-quality teacher–child interactions, the gap in the development of school readiness skills between children with typical engagement and those with high levels of engagement was reduced (Williford, Maier, et al., 2013).

As discussed in the previous sections, existing empirical evidence provides support for connections among child–parent attachment, child–teacher attachment, and a child's readiness skills. However, much of the research linking the quality of the relationship between a child and teacher to a child's school readiness skills does not take into account a child's prior attachment experiences with his or her parent. Therefore, we currently cannot answer the question of whether the quality of children's early relationships with their parents moderates the associations between the child–teacher relationship and children's development of school readiness skills. However, there is evidence that the links between the quality of the teacher–child relationship and children's school readiness development is stronger for certain children. Children's positive relationships with teachers have been found to protect against poor academic and social outcomes for children classified as being at risk due a range of factors, including an unsupportive home environment, minority ethnicity, authoritarian parenting practices, or low academic achievement (Baker, 2006; Burchinal, Peisner-Feinberg, Pianta, & Howes, 2002; Ladd & Burgess, 2001). The evidence connecting the

quality of teacher–child relationships and social interactions with children's school readiness skills is summarized below.

Children who struggle academically often have reduced levels of behavioral and socioemotional outcomes, and for these children, a strong teacher–child relationship is particularly important (Eisenhower, Baker, & Blacher, 2007). Children who display lower academic skills also tend to experience less close and more conflictual relationships with teachers. However, research evidence suggests that when these children develop a warm and responsive relationship with their teacher, they tend to demonstrate more adaptive behavioral outcomes and lower levels of delinquency and socioemotional problems (Al-Yagon & Milulincer, 2004; Murray & Greenberg, 2001).

The quality of the teacher–child relationship has been found to link directly to children's socioemotional outcomes (behavior, social skills, self-regulation, executive functioning), as well as to moderate the relation between children's disruptive behavior and their later school outcomes. For children who display externalizing or disruptive behavior (i.e., aggression, hyperactivity, impulsivity), the teacher–child relationship tends to be negative and conflictual (Doumen et al., 2008; Howes, 2000; Ladd & Burgess, 2001; Spilt & Koomen, 2009). The reciprocal (and often negative) interactions that occur as a result of this may get worse over time and lead to poorer attachment quality with the current, as well as with future teachers. For example, there is growing empirical evidence suggesting that the quality of the teacher–child relationship longitudinally predicts children's behavior (e.g., Baker, Grant, & Morlock, 2008; Hamre & Pianta, 2001; Meehan, Hughes, & Cavell, 2003; Pianta & Stuhlman, 2004). Researchers found that after controlling for children's initial problem behaviors, teacher–child relationship quality significantly predicted children's later socioemotional adjustment, especially when there were concurrent ratings of relational quality (Pianta, Nimetz, & Bennett, 1997; Pianta & Stuhlman, 2004). In contrast, when teacher–child relations are negative and conflictual, children are at risk for increased problem behaviors, decreased academic and social skills, and increased school disengagement (e.g., Birch & Ladd, 1998; Graziano, Reavis, Keane, & Calkins, 2007; Henricsson & Rydell, 2004; Mantzicopoulos, 2005; Stipek & Miles, 2008).

However, a close and supportive teacher–child relationship has been found to be protective for children who display early disruptive behaviors. When children who display impulsivity and aggression are paired with teachers who are able to establish a positive emotional bond with them and meet their behavioral and regulatory needs in the classroom with low frustration and negativity, these children are more likely to evidence declines in aggression and exhibit greater socioemotional development, including acceptance by peers (e.g., Baker et al., 2008; Decker, Dona, & Christenson, 2007; Meehan et al., 2003).

Self-regulation is a school readiness skill within the socioemotional domain that can be defined as a child's ability to focus attention, manage emotions appropriately, and cope with environmental demands and stimuli (Baumeister & Vohs, 2004; Blair & Razza, 2007; Calkins & Williford, 2009; Rimm-Kaufman, Curby, Grimm, Nathanson, & Brock, 2009). During the early childhood period, children develop substantially in this skill domain and are increasingly expected to demonstrate self-regulation in order to be successful in the classroom environment (Williford, Whittaker, Vitiello, & Downer, 2013). Williford, Whittaker, and colleagues (2013) found that children's positive engagement with their teacher was related to the development of behavioral compliance and executive functioning skills during the preschool year. Results from this study also indicate that children who engage in a positive manner with their teacher or peers are more likely to show gains in their active task engagement and decreases in their emotion dysregulation during preschool.

## Improving the Teacher–Child Relationship to Support Children's School Readiness

The empirical evidence that supports the importance of a child's attachment to an early childhood teacher for his or her early learning has multiple implications for how we can support teachers in their efforts to develop accepting, sensitive, and responsive relationships with the young children in their classroom that facilitate children's early learning and later success in school. In this section, we describe recent experimental and quasi-experimental research that provides support for the hypothesis that improving the quality of teacher–child interactions and relationships leads to children's improved school readiness skills.

Multiple professional development/early intervention programs have been developed that target the improvement of teachers' skills in initiating and maintaining high-quality affective relationships with children in their classroom. Many of these interventions have been created using attachment theory as a foundation. Until the past decade, few experimental studies examined the extent to which targeted relational professional development systems improve the teacher–child relationship. These studies have assessed the more proximal observed teacher–child interactions as a proxy for measuring the more global construct of teacher–child relationship quality (e.g., Arnett Caregiver Interaction Scale [CIS; Arnett, 1989], inCLASS [Downer et al., 2010]), whereas other research has used teacher report of the teacher–child relationship quality, such as the STRS [Pianta & Hamre, 2001]). In aggregate, this research provides good evidence that improving teacher interaction behaviors through a relational lens can improve children's outcomes (e.g., Murray & Malmgren, 2005; Webster-Stratton, Reid, & Hammond, 2004).

Research suggests that targeting the teacher–child relationship holds particular promise as a strategy to prevent negative outcomes for children at higher risk. Early intervention may deflect children from poor school adjustment, particularly children who are socially and academically at risk. This section describes interventions/professional developments that focus on improving the teacher–child relationships or teacher–child interactions as a mechanism for improving children's academic and/or socioemotional outcomes.

## Incredible Years Training Programs—Teacher Classroom Management Program

The Incredible Years intervention (Webster-Stratton, Reid, & Hammond, 2001) is an evidence-based, multicomponent intervention that targets children ages 4-8 years old. The components of this program include a parent-training program, a child-training program, a teacher-training program, and a socioemotional curriculum ("Dinosaur School"), which can be used as a package or independently. For the purposes of this chapter, we describe the teacher-training program designed to improve teachers' classroom management skills by using five techniques: building positive relationships, using encouragement and praise, providing behavioral incentives, preventing negative behaviors, and addressing inappropriate behaviors. The teacher-training program is extensive and can take as long as 36 hours total (Webster-Stratton et al., 2004). In this training, teachers learn classroom management strategies as a group, then discuss videos of teacher–child interactions (Webster-Stratton et al., 2001).

The first element of the teacher program focuses on the importance of the teacher–child relationship (Webster-Stratton et al., 2004). The beginning sessions help teachers understand that high-quality relationships lead to increased motivation and cooperation on the part of children, as well as greater engagement in learning activities in the classroom. Additionally, emphasis is placed on the importance of becoming familiar with students by asking about their interests outside of school. Teachers are also encouraged to spend individual time with children. Other strategies include sending home "happy grams," having children celebrate each other's accomplishments, and encouraging a safe climate. Teachers are encouraged to model their own thoughts and to share feelings with the use of positive self-talk. In addition, teachers use behavior-based techniques (e.g., labeled praise, selective attention) to increase children's positive behaviors.

The effectiveness of the Incredible Years curriculum and training to improve both teacher practice and children's outcomes, particularly behavioral outcomes, can be found in multiple studies (e.g., Webster-Stratton et al., 2001, 2004). Webster-Stratton and colleagues (2001) demonstrated the effectiveness of both the parent and teacher training components in a randomized controlled trial (RCT). Results suggest that the program improved teachers' management techniques, children's social competence, and children's observed school behavior, while reducing conduct problems. A follow-up RCT conducted by Webster-Stratton and colleagues (2004) provided evidence for the importance of including individual child therapy in the model. More recently, the Incredible Years teacher-training program and the Dinosaur School curriculum were implemented, and together, they improved school readiness skills (including socioemotional skills) and child behavior (reduced conduct problems) (Reinke, Stormont, Webster-Stratton, Newcomer, & Herman, 2012; Webster-Stratton, Reid, & Stoolmiller, 2008). These results suggest that the suite of Incredible Years programs can reduce negative child behavior and improve children's school readiness skills, specifically their socioemotional skills.

## Chicago School Readiness Program

In 2008 and 2009, Raver and colleagues adapted the Incredible Years teacher-training program for use within an early childhood, multicomponent teacher consultation model. Results indicate that this adaptation may improve teacher practices and children's socioemotional and behavioral school readiness skills. The Chicago School Readiness Program (CSRP) is an example of an evidence-based, multicomponent treatment that delivers a combination of programs largely through mental health consultation in the schools (Raver et al., 2009). The project targeted children attending Head Start (a federally funded preschool program for children living in poverty; National Head Start Association, 1974). The primary purpose of the CSRP was to improve emotional and behavioral outcomes of young children living in poverty and at increased risk for negative school-based outcomes. The intervention contains four distinct phases: (1) teacher training, (2) coaching focused on strategy implementation, (3) mental health consultation for teacher stress reduction, and (4) mental health consultation for challenging children.

The first part of the intervention occurs at the beginning of the year and consists of 30 hours of teacher training over 5 weeks (based on the Incredible Years program [Webster-Stratton et al., 2004]), targeting teacher management strategies. Then, teachers work with trained mental health consultants to implement the learned strategies using a collaborative consultation process. After winter break, the third part of the intervention is implemented, which focuses on teacher stress reduction and strategies for coping with difficult situations. The final component of the intervention, child mental health consultation, occurs during the final 10 weeks, during which consultants provide direct services to children with high levels of behavior problems (individual and group therapy).

Results suggest increased positive teacher practices and reduced children's behavior problems (Raver et al., 2008). Teachers in the intervention condition demonstrated increased attachment-related caregiving behaviors (e.g., teacher sensitivity) and were more likely to demonstrate improved behavior management skills relative to controls (Raver et al., 2008). The intervention also improved child behaviors, with significant reductions in behavior problems (Raver et al., 2009). These results demonstrate an improvement in classroom dynamics and child behavioral outcomes. Furthermore, results cannot be attributed to an extra adult in the classroom because control classrooms were staffed with a teacher aide. CSRP has subsequently been replicated in two larger trials (now known as the Foundations of Learning Project [FLP]), and each of these trials also showed improvements in child outcomes, including improved academic and socioemotional school readiness skills (Morris, Millenky, Raver, & Jones, 2013). Collectively, the results from the CSRP suggest that targeting teacher skills with an attachment lens has the potential to improve children's ability to manage their own behavior. Unfortunately, there is a limited ability to disentangle the various components that may have produced change due to the multicomponent nature of the intervention.

## My Teaching Partner

My Teaching Partner (MTP) is an individualized coaching model focused on improving teacher–child interactions (Pianta, Mashburn, Downer, Hamre, & Justice, 2008). It is based on the hypothesis that the quality of teacher–child interactions directly contributes to children's achievement by increasing engagement, motivation, and on-task behavior (Hamre & Pianta, 2005). The program uses the Classroom Assessment Scoring System (CLASS; Pianta, La Paro, & Hamre, 2008) as a foundation for observing and analyzing video and giving feedback on teacher practice. The CLASS organizes teacher–child interactions into three broad domains—emotional support, classroom organization, and instructional support. MTP coaching provides several key opportunities for teachers. Teachers are given the chance to (1) observe videotaped high-quality teacher–child interactions, (2) identify effective responses to children's cues, and (3) receive ongoing individualized feedback concerning their own teacher–child interactions. The MTP coach and teacher go through five steps together: (1) The teacher videotapes interactions with children in the classroom (e.g., a math lesson, circle time, or small-group instruction); (2) the coach edits the video and prepares written prompts that focus on particular dimensions of the CLASS (e.g., support for child autonomy) to facilitate the teacher's self-analysis skills; (3) the teacher views the video and responds; (4) the teacher and coach conference by phone; and (5) the two collaborate to construct an action plan for the teacher to change his or her interactions. Each MTP coaching cycle takes about 2 weeks to complete and repeats continually throughout the school year (–12

cycles. Teachers and coaches interface through an online portal that includes a video library of over 200 effective teacher–child video clips. The intervention and coaching focuses on helping teachers become better observers of their own practice in order to improve their interactions with children, which subsequently encourage positive child behavior and engagement in the classroom.

The impact of MTP within preschool classrooms has been examined in two large trials. In the first preschool trial, MTP coaching was combined with implementation of a language and literacy and socioemotional curriculum (Pianta et al., 2008). Results demonstrated that teachers in the intervention condition improved their teacher–child interactions as measured with CLASS scores. These effects were more substantial for those whose classroom composition included a higher proportion of at-risk children (Pianta et al., 2008). With regard to children, those whose teachers were engaged in MTP demonstrated improved school readiness skills, including literacy, receptive vocabulary, task orientation, and assertiveness (Hamre et al., 2012; Mashburn, Downer, Hamre, Justice, & Pianta, 2010). Downer and colleagues (2015) conducted a study that suggested that MTP specifically increases a preschool teacher's instructional support. Additionally, children in the intervention condition of this study displayed improved positive engagement with their teachers as measured through classroom observations (Downer et al., 2015). Although there were no main treatment effects on children's readiness indicators during the coaching year, in the postintervention year, children with teachers who had participated in MTP had, on average, higher levels of inhibitory control (Pianta et al., 2015). Together, these results suggest that improving teacher–child interactions at the classroom level by using targeted professional development and consultation have the potential to improve children's academic and socioemotional school readiness skills.

## Banking Time

Banking Time is an attachment-based, dyadic intervention intended to improve a teacher's relationship with a specific child with whom he or she has had trouble connecting (Driscoll & Pianta, 2010; Pianta & Hamre, 2001). The difficulty may be due to the child's disruptive behavior or lack of social skills. It may also be due to the teacher, for any number of reasons (e.g., too many children), not engaging individually with a particular child.

The name of the intervention, Banking Time, comes from the idea that when a teacher invests in his or her relationship with a child, the relationship can become a resource in the classroom for both the child and the teacher during times of challenge (e.g., when the teacher is asking the child to complete a task). The hypothesized mechanism for change is strengthening the bond between the child and teacher, which in turn helps the child develop important socioemotional skills (e.g., better communication, more effective help-seeking behavior, and better self-management skills). These skills can be used in the classroom with adults and peers to improve school success in both socioemotional and academic areas.

In each session, a teacher and child engage in brief, 10- to 15-minute, one-on-one interactions in which the teacher conveys messages of support to the child, specifically in the areas of exploration, sensitivity, predictability, and encouragement. These sessions occur when the teacher is available to provide individualized attention and are not contingent on the child's behavior. The child leads each Banking Time session by choosing materials and guiding the interactions and play. The teacher is instructed not to ask questions, give commands, or teach a lesson, but rather to observe and describe the child's actions, label the child's positive and negative emotions, and emphasize positive relational themes. Teachers describe what the child is doing through narration or imitation; this shows that the adult is attending to the child and validates the child's action. Teachers label the child's positive and negative emotions in order to emphasize acceptance. Finally, the teacher chooses a specific theme that conveys a message to the child about the importance of the teacher's relationship with the child. For example, if the child tends not to seek help from the teacher, the theme may be "I'm here for help if you need me." These techniques are intended to enhance the teacher's and child's relationship with one another, which in turn recasts the teacher as a secure base for the child to use in the general classroom setting.

The effectiveness of Banking Time on teacher and child outcomes has been examined in several samples. Two studies show that the implementation of Banking Time increases a teacher's perceptions of closeness with children. In a quasi-experimental study, information about Banking Time was made available to teachers who were participating in a Web-based teacher professional development intervention (Driscoll, Wang, Mashburn, & Pianta, 2011). Teachers could implement the techniques in order to improve teacher–child relationships if they chose. Results from this study indicated that over the course of the year, teachers who chose to implement these techniques reported closer relationships. It is important to note that this study did not use random assignment of children to the intervention, but the trial does provide preliminary support for the effectiveness of Banking Time. In a second study that was an RCT, researchers found that teachers participating in Banking Time reported increased child–teacher closeness (Driscoll & Pianta, 2010). Furthermore, teacher reports of classroom behavior revealed that children participating in the intervention demonstrated improved behavioral outcomes. These trials suggest that Banking Time is a promising intervention for improving teacher perceptions of their relationships with disruptive preschool children. Importantly, because a warm teacher–child relationship is related to positive child outcomes, changing this relationship may be helpful in improving children's school readiness and decreasing levels of disruptive behavior (Driscoll & Pianta, 2010).

A large, federally funded RCT of Banking Time is currently under way. This study examined whether teachers' implementation of Banking Time with 3- and 4- year-old children at risk for a disruptive behavior disorder can improve children's behavioral and emotional outcomes. This study used classroom observations, direct assessment, and informant report (teachers', parents' and children's) to assess the teacher–child interactions and children's behavioral outcomes. Results indicated that use of Banking Time was effective in decreasing children's behavior problems and improving the observed quality of teacher–child interactions (Williford et al., 2015).

### Playing-2-gether

Playing-2-gether is a school or center-based intervention designed for teachers and their preschool children with moderate to high levels of disruptive behavior (e.g., impulsivity, hyperactivity, aggression). The mechanism for changing a child's disruptive behavior that is targeted by the intervention is the interactions between the teacher and child. Playing-2-gether consists of two components: the Relationship-Game and the Rule-Game. For each component, the teacher and child meet for approximately 15 minutes, at least twice weekly for 6 weeks. During the first component, the teacher and child meet for sessions that are consistent with the guidelines of Banking Time sessions: child-led, teacher as observer, and the teacher conveying understanding and sensitivity toward the child. This first component is heavily rooted in attachment theory. In the second session, the Rule-Game, the teacher leads the activity and uses skills to encourage appropriate behavior, such as clear commands, rules for good behavior, praising the child for following good behavior, and so forth. The second component draws on principles from learning theory and effective behavior management.

Vancraeyveldt and colleagues (2015) conducted a three-wave, randomized study of a sample of 175 teacher–child dyads. All children were identified as having elevated levels of externalizing behavior. Teachers were randomly assigned to the intervention or a business-as-usual condition. After intervention implementation, the teachers and children in the intervention group had made significant gains with regard to the teacher–child relationship and child behavior. Within this group, teachers rated their relationships as having significantly less conflict, and children were identified as having decreased conduct and behavioral problems (e.g., hyperactivity, impulsivity). Interestingly, the positive effects of the two-part intervention all occurred after the first component of the intervention—the attachment-based, relationship-focused component. These positive effects remained but did not strengthen during the second component. Additionally, teachers in the intervention group rated their relationships with children as closer after the first component, but this effect disappeared after the second component. This study supports the effectiveness of engaging in Banking Time sessions with children who display disruptive behavior.

In summary, results from recent experimental research provide evidence that early intervention/professional development programs that focus on improving the quality of teacher–child interactions can help children develop school-readiness skills with most of the interventions targeting children's behavior. However, with the exception of Banking Time, all of these programs consist of multiple components based on multiple theories of how to affect children's development and learning. In the next section, we conclude our chapter by describing how future research can extend our understanding of how the quality of children's attachment to their parents and their teachers contributes to their development of school readiness skills.

## Future Research Directions

Recent research has made significant gains in describing the nature of teacher–child relationships and understanding the association between the quality of teacher–child relationships and interactions, and children's development of school readiness skills. Attachment theory has been used heavily to conceptualize the key characteristics that should comprise high-quality teacher–child relationships and interactions, and to explain why relationships characterized by interactions that are consistent, responsive, and warm allow children to take full advantage of learning opportunities, engage maximally in the classroom, and develop the skills needed to be successful in kindergarten. The review of empirical work in this chapter demonstrates the complexity of examining teacher–child relationships, particularly when researchers expand beyond describing the nature of the child–teacher dyad in order to investigate multiple ecological levels of influence (e.g., the association between parent–child and teacher–child relationships), and how these levels of influence independently and jointly contribute to children's school readiness skills. Significant gains in research methodology, as well as greater integration across disciplines, pave the way for future research into the complexities of understanding the impact of teacher–child and parent–child relationships on children's school readiness skills.

Statistical techniques, such as multilevel modeling, allow researchers to expand beyond the child–teacher dyad paradigm and examine the effects of multiple levels within the child's developmental system. Developing a better understanding of home-, school-, classroom-, and community-level factors associated with close teacher–child relationships will help schools and teachers to create environments and experiences that support children's success in school across academic, behavioral, emotional, and social domains.

Another area of potential research is a deeper exploration of how the quality of teacher–child attachment may serve as a moderator for children at risk due to an insecure child–parent attachment. Additional studies examining children's school readiness skills with tighter controls and research designs must be conducted in order to examine the extent to which the quality of the teacher–child relationship during early childhood may moderate the relation between the quality of the parent–child relationship and children's development of school readiness skills. There are few studies that have included *both* the quality of parent–child and teacher–child relationships when examining how early child–adult relationships predict children's school readiness skills.

The majority of the research on teacher–child relationship quality has used teacher report of the teacher–child relationship or naturalistic observations of the quality of a teacher's interactions across all children in the classroom. New measures that examine the quality of a teacher's interactions with an individual child may help us understand how a teacher differentiates his or her level of sensitivity and support to individual children in the classroom (Williford et al., 2013). Additionally, current classroom-based measures examine teacher's interactions as they occur naturally in the classroom during an allocated block of time. Conducting observations in natural settings is important for ecologically valid measurement. However, the lack of standardization across activities limits our ability to understand whether the quality of interactions is due to characteristics of the child, the teacher, or the demands of the activity. The development of a standardized task, similar to laboratory-based research examining the quality of child–mother interactions, may help us understand the factors that influence the quality of teacher–child relationships and has implications for early intervention efforts to improve the affective quality of teacher–child interactions.

With regard to future experimental work, except for studies examining Banking Time, the intervention programs described in this chapter focus on improving the quality of teacher–child interactions as one component of a more comprehensive program. Therefore, we do not know whether the enhanced teacher–child relationship, another aspect of the program, or the combination of components is responsible for improvements in the quality of teachers' interactions with children or children's improved outcomes. Research is needed that "unpacks" these comprehensive intervention programs to determine whether particular components are critical for improving the quality of the teacher–child relationship and whether this improvement is responsible for improved child outcomes.

## Conclusion

The increase in the number of multidisciplinary studies allows researchers to examine ideas with a new lens. By applying the attachment framework

from the field of child development to the field of early childhood education, we are better able to understand how the teacher serves as a resource for children, helping them to engage maximally with activities in the classroom and acquire skills needed to be successful in school. Empirical evidence supports links between a child's attachment to a parent, to a teacher, and to the development of essential academic and socioemotional school readiness skills. The creation of interventions based on these findings has already begun; there are several evidence-based interventions that increase the quality of the child–teacher attachment and, consequently, the child's school readiness skills. Future work devoted to understanding the mechanisms explaining how the teacher–child relationship serves as a protective factor for children at risk may enhance current and future interventions, so that they more effectively and efficiently promote a young child's school readiness skills.

## Acknowledgments

We would like to thank Sarah Brooks for helping us to complete this chapter. This work was supported in part by a grant awarded to Amanda P. Williford by the Institute of Education Sciences, U.S. Department of Education, through Grant No. R324A100215 to the University of Virginia. The opinions expressed are those of the authors and do not represent views of the U.S. Department of Education.

## References

Ahnert, L., Pinquart, M., & Lamb, M. E. (2006). Security of children's relationships with nonparental care providers: A meta-analysis. *Child Development, 77*(3), 664–679.

Ainsworth, M. D. S., & Blehar, M., Waters, E., & Wall, S. (1978). *Patterns of attachment: A psychological study of the strange situation.* Mahwah, NJ: Erlbaum.

Akiba, M., LeTendre, G., & Scribner, J. (2007). Teacher quality, opportunity gap, and national achievement in 46 countries. *Educational Researcher, 36*(7), 369–387.

Al-Yagon, M., & Mikulincer, M. (2004). Socioemotional and academic adjustment among children with learning disorders: The mediational role of attachment-based factors. *Journal of Special Education, 38*(2), 111–123

American Community Survey. (2005–2007). *Three-year summary file.* Washington, DC: U.S. Census Bureau.

Arnett, J. (1989). Caregivers in day-care centers: Does training matter? *Journal of Applied Developmental Psychology, 10*(4), 541–552.

Baker, J. A. (2006). Contributions of teacher–child relationships to positive school adjustment during elementary school. *Journal of School Psychology, 44,* 211–229.

Baker, J. A., Grant, S., & Morlock, L. (2008). The teacher–student relationship as a developmental context for children with internalizing or externalizing behavior problems. *School Psychology Quarterly, 23*(1) 3–15.

Baumeister, R. F., & Vohs, K. D. (Eds.). (2004). *Handbook of self-regulation: Research, theory, and applications.* New York: Guilford Press.

Belsky, J. (2005). Differential susceptibility to rearing influence: An evolutionary hypothesis and some evidence. In B. Ellis & D. Bjorklund (Eds.), *Origins of the social mind: Evolutionary psychology and child development* (pp. 139–163). New York: Guilford Press.

Bierman, K., Domitrovich, C., Nix, R., Gest, S., Welsh, J., Greenberg, M., et al. (2008). Promoting academic and socioemotional school readiness: The Head Start REDI Program. *Child Development, 79*(6), 1802–1817.

Birch, S. H., & Ladd, G. W. (1998). Children's interpersonal behaviors and the teacher–child relationship. *Developmental Psychology, 34*(5), 934–946.

Blair, C., & Razza, R. P. (2007). Relating effortful control, executive function, and false belief understanding to emerging math and literacy ability in kindergarten. *Child Development, 78*(2), 647–663.

Blau, D., & Currie, J. (2006). Pre-school, day care, and after-school care: Who's minding the kids? *Handbook of the Economics of Education, 2,* 1163–1278.

Booth, C., Kelly, J., Spieker, S., & Zuckerman, T. G. (2003). Toddlers' attachment security to child-care providers: The Safe and Secure Scale. *Early Education and Development, 14*(1), 83–100.

Bronfenbrenner, U., & Morris, P. (1998). The ecology of developmental processes. *Handbook of Child Psychology, 1,* 993–1028.

Burchinal, M., McCartney, K., Steinberg, L., Crosnoe, R., Friedman, S., McLoyd, V., et al. (2011). Examining the black–white achievement gap among low-income children using the NICHD study of early child care and youth development. *Child Development, 82*(5), 1404–1420.

Burchinal, M. R., Peisner-Feinberg, E., Pianta, R., & Howes, C. (2002). Development of academic skills from preschool through second grade: Family and classroom predictors of developmental trajectories. *Journal of School Psychology, 40*(5), 415–436.

Bus, A., & Belsky, J., Van IJzendoorn, M., & Crnic, K. (1997). Attachment and bookreading patterns: A study of mothers, fathers, and their toddlers. *Early Childhood Research Quarterly, 12*(1), 81–98.

Bus, A., & Van IJzendoorn., M. (1997). Affective dimension of mother–infant picturebook reading. *Journal of School Psychology, 35*(1), 47–60.

Buyse, E., Verschueren, K., Verachtert, P., & Van Damme, J. (2009). Predicting school adjustment in early elementary school: Impact of teacher–child relationship quality and relational classroom climate. *Elementary School Journal, 110*(2), 119–141.

Calkins, S., & Williford, A. (2009). Taming the terrible twos: Self-regulation and school readiness. In O. A. Barbarin & B. H. Wasik (Eds.), *Handbook of child development and early education: Research to practice* (pp. 172–198). New York: Guilford Press.

Cassidy, J., Jones, J. D., & Shaver, P. R. (2013). Contributions of attachment theory and research: A framework for future research, translation, and policy. *Development and Psychopathology, 25*(4, Pt 2), 1415–1434.

Commodari, E. (2013). Preschool teacher attachment, school readiness and risk of learning difficulties. *Early Childhood Research Quarterly, 28*(1), 123–133.

Conyers, L., Reynolds, A., & Ou, S. (2003). The effect of early childhood intervention and subsequent special education services: Findings from the Chicago child–parent centers. *Educational Evaluation and Policy Analysis, 25*(1), 75–95.

Crosnoe, R., Johnson, M. K., & Elder, G. H. (2004). Intergenerational bonding in school: The behavioral and contextual correlates of student-teacher relationships. *Sociology of Education, 77*(1), 60–81.

Decker, D. M., Dona, D. P., & Christenson, S. L. (2007). Behaviorally at-risk African American students: The importance of student–teacher relationships for student outcomes. *Journal of School Psychology, 45*(1), 83–109.

Doumen, S., Verschueren, K., Buyse, E., Germeijs, V., Luyckx, K., & Soenens, B. (2008). Reciprocal relations between teacher–child conflict and aggressive behavior in kindergarten: A three-wave longitudinal study. *Journal of Clinical Child and Adolescent Psychology, 37*(3), 588–599.

Downer, J., Booren, L., Lima, O., Luckner, A., & Pianta, R. (2010). The Individualized Classroom Assessment Scoring System (inCLASS): Preliminary reliability and validity of a system for observing preschoolers' competence in classroom interactions. *Early Childhood Research Quarterly, 25*(1), 1–16.

Downer, J. T., Driscoll, K., & Pianta, R. C. (2006). *The transition from kindergarten to first grade: A developmental, ecological approach.* Washington, DC: National Association for the Education of Young Children.

Downer, J. T., Pianta, R., Burchinal, M., Field, S., Hamre, B., Locasale-Crouch, J. L., et al. (2015). *Coaching and coursework focused on teacher-child interactions during language/literacy instruction: Effects on teacher outcomes and children's classroom engagement.* Manuscript under review.

Driscoll, K., & Pianta, R. (2010). Banking Time in Head Start: Early efficacy of an intervention designed to promote supportive teacher–child relationships. *Early Education and Development, 21*(1), 38–64.

Driscoll, K., Wang, L., Mashburn, A., & Pianta, R. (2011). Fostering supportive teacher–child relationships: Intervention implementation in a state-funded preschool program. *Early Education and Development, 22*(4), 593–619.

Duncan, G., Dowsett, C., Claessens, A., Magnuson, K., Huston, A., Klebanov, P., et al. (2007). School readiness and later achievement. *Developmental Psychology*, *43*(6), 1428–1446.

Eisenhower, A., Baker, B., & Blacher, J. (2007). Early student–teacher relationships of children with and without intellectual disability: Contributions of behavioral, social, and self-regulatory competence. *Journal of School Psychology*, *45*(4), 363–383.

Fearon, R. M. P., & Belsky, J. (2011). Infant–mother attachment and the growth of externalizing problems across the primary-school years. *Journal of Child Psychology and Psychiatry*, *52*, 782–791.

Frankel, K. A., & Bates, J. E. (1990). Mother–toddler problem solving: Antecedents in attachment, home behavior, and temperament. *Child Development*, *61*(3), 810–819.

Good, T., & Weinstein, R. (1986). Schools make a difference: Evidence, criticism, and new directions. *American Psychologist*, *41*(10), 1090–1097.

Granot, D., & Mayseless, O. (2001). Attachment security and adjustment to school in middle childhood. *International Journal of Behavioral Development*, *25*(6), 530–541.

Graziano, P., Reavis, R., Keane, S., & Calkins, S. (2007). The role of emotion regulation in children's early academic success. *Journal of School Psychology*, *45*(1), 3–19.

Hamre, B. [K.], & Pianta, R. (2001). Early teacher–child relationships and the trajectory of children's school outcomes through eighth grade. *Child Development*, *72*(2), 625–638.

Hamre, B. K., & Pianta, R. C. (2005). Can instructional and emotional support in the first-grade classroom make a difference for children at risk of school failure? *Child Development*, *76*(5), 949–967.

Hamre, B. [K.], Pianta, R. [C.], Burchinal, M., Field, S., LoCasale-Crouch, J., Downer, J., et al. (2012). A course on effective teacher–child interactions effects on teacher beliefs, knowledge, and observed practice. *American Educational Research Journal*, *49*(1), 88–123.

Henricsson, L., & Rydell, A. (2004). Elementary school children with behavior problems: Teacher–child relations and self-perception. A prospective study. *Merrill–Palmer Quarterly-Journal of Developmental Psychology*, *50*(2), 111–138.

Howes, C. (2000). Socioemotional classroom climate in child care, teacher–child relationships and children's second grade peer relations. *Social Development*, *9*(2), 191–204.

Howes, C., & Ritchie, S. (1999). Attachment organizations in children with difficult life circumstances. *Development and Psychopathology*, *11*(2), 251–268.

Kobak, R., Cassidy, J., Lyons-Ruth, K., & Ziv, Y. (2006). Attachment, stress, and psychopathology: A developmental pathways model. In D. Cicchetti & D. J. Cohen (Eds.), *Developmental psychopathology: Vol. 1. Theory and method* (2nd ed., pp. 333–369). Hoboken, NJ: Wiley.

Kochanska, G., & Kim, S. (2012). Toward a new understanding of legacy of early attachments for future antisocial trajectories: Evidence from two longitudinal studies. *Development and Psychopathology*, *24*(3), 783–806.

Ladd, G., & Burgess, K. (2001). Do relational risks and protective factors moderate the linkages between childhood aggression and early psychological and school adjustment? *Child Development*, *72*(5), 1579–1601.

Main, M. (1983). Exploration, play, and cognitive functioning related to infant-mother attachment. *Infant Behavior and Development*, *6*(2), 167–174.

Mantzicopoulos, P. (2005). Conflictual relationships between kindergarten children and their teachers: Associations with child and classroom context variables. *Journal of School Psychology*, *43*(5), 425–442.

Martoccio, T. L., Brophy-Herb, H. E., & Onaga, E. E. (2014). Road to readiness: Pathways from low-income children's early interactions to school readiness skills. *Infants and Young Children*, *27*(3), 193–206.

Mashburn, A. J., Downer, J. T., Hamre, B. K., Justice, L. M., & Pianta, R. C. (2010). Consultation for teachers and children's language and literacy development during pre-kindergarten. *Applied Developmental Science*, *14*(4), 179–196.

Mashburn, A. [J.], Pianta, R., Hamre, B., Downer, J., Barbarin, O., Bryant, D., et al. (2008). Measures of classroom quality in prekindergarten and children's development of academic, language, and social skills. *Child Development*, *79*(3), 732–749.

Meehan, B., Hughes, J., & Cavell, A. (2003). Teacher–student relationships as compensatory resources for aggressive children. *Child Development*, *74*, 1145–1157.

Morris, P., Millenky, M., Raver, C., & Jones, S. (2013). Does a preschool social and emotional learning intervention pay off for classroom instruction and children's behavior and academic skills?: Evidence from the foundations of learning project. *Early Education and Development*, *24*(7), 1020–1042.

Moss, E., & St-Laurent, D. (2001). Attachment at school age and academic performance. *Developmental Psychology*, *37*(6), 863–874.

Murray, C., & Greenberg, M. (2001). Relationships with teachers and bonds with school: Social emotional adjustment correlates for children with and without disabilities. *Psychology in Schools*, *38*(1), 25–41.

Murray, C., & Malmgren, K. (2005). Implementing a teacher–student relationship program in a high-poverty urban school: Effects on social, emotional, and academic adjustment and lessons learned. *Journal of School Psychology*, *43*(2), 137–152.

Myers, S., & Pianta, R. (2008). Developmental commentary: Individual and contextual influences on student–teacher relationships and children's early problem behaviors. *Journal of Clinical Child and Adolescent Psychology*, *37*(3), 600–608.

National Head Start Association. (1974). Head Start. Retrieved from *www.nhsa.org*.

O'Connor, E., & McCartney, K. (2007). Examining teacher–child relationships and achievement as part of an ecological model of development. *American Educational Research Journal, 44*(2), 340–369.

Pianta, R. C. (1999). *Enhancing relationships between children and teachers.* Washington, DC: American Psychological Association.

Pianta, R. C., Burchinal, M., Hamre, B. K., Downer, J. T., LoCasale-Crouch, J., Cabell, S. Q., et al. (2015). *Early childhood professional development: Coaching and coursework effect on indicators of children's school readiness.* Manuscript submitted for publication.

Pianta, R. C., & Hamre, B. (2001). *Students, Teachers, And Relationship Support (STARS).* Odessa, FL: Psychological Assessment Resources.

Pianta, R. C., Hamre, B., & Stuhlman, M. (2003). Relationships between teachers and children. In I. Weiner, D. Freedheim, J. Schinka, & W. Velicer (Eds.), *Handbook of psychology* (pp. 199–234). New York: Wiley.

Pianta, R. C., La Paro, K., & Hamre, B. (2008). *The Classroom Assessment Scoring System Pre-K manual.* Baltimore: Brookes.

Pianta, R. C., Mashburn, A., Downer, J., Hamre, B., & Justice, L. (2008). Effects of web-mediated professional development resources on teacher–child interactions in pre-kindergarten classrooms. *Early Childhood Research Quarterly, 23*(4), 431–451.

Pianta, R. C., Nimetz, S., & Bennett, E. (1997). Mother–child relationships, teacher–child relationships, and school outcomes in preschool and kindergarten. *Early Childhood Research Quarterly, 12,* 263–280.

Pianta, R. C., & Stuhlman, M. (2004). Teacher–child relationships and children's success in the first years of school. *School Psychology Review, 33*(3), 444–458.

Ramey, C. T., & Ramey, S. L. (1998). Prevention of intellectual disabilities: Early interventions to improve cognitive development. *Preventive Medicine, 27*(2), 224–232.

Raver, C., Jones, S., Li-Grining, C., Metzger, M., Champion, K., & Sardine, L. (2008). Improving preschool classroom processes: Preliminary findings from a randomized trial implemented in head start settings. *Early Childhood Research Quarterly, 23*(1), 10–26.

Raver, C., Jones, S., Li-Grining, C., Metzger, M., Champion, K., & Sardine, L. (2009). Targeting children's behavior problems in preschool classrooms: A cluster-randomized controlled trial. *Journal of Consulting and Clinical Psychology, 77*(2), 302–316.

Reinke, W., Stormont, M., Webster-Stratton, C., Newcomer, L., & Herman, K. (2012). The incredible years teacher classroom management program: Using coaching to support generalization to real-world classroom settings. *Psychology in the Schools, 49*(5), 416–428.

Rimm-Kaufman, S., Curby, T., Grimm, K., Nathanson, L., & Brock, L. L. (2009). The contribution of children's self-regulation and classroom quality to children's adaptive behaviors in the kindergarten classroom. *Developmental Psychology, 45,* 958–972.

Rimm-Kaufman, S., Pianta, R., Cox, M. (2000). Teachers' judgments of problems in the transition to kindergarten. *Early Childhood Research Quarterly, 14*(2), 147–166.

Rydell, A., Bohlin, G., & Thorell, L. B. (2005). Representations of attachment to parents and shyness as predictors of children's relationships with teachers and peer competence in preschool. *Attachment and Human Development, 7*(2), 187–204.

Sabol, T., & Pianta, R. (2012). Recent trends in research on teacher–child relationships. *Attachment and Human Development, 14*(3), 213–231.

Sameroff, A. (1995). General systems theories and developmental psychopathology. In D. Cichetti & D. Cohen (Eds.), *Developmental psychopathology: Theory and methods* (pp. 659–695). Oxford, UK: Wiley.

Shields, A., Dickstein, Seifer, R., Giusti, I., Magee, K., & Spritz B. (2001). Emotional competence and early school adjustment: A study of preschoolers at risk. *Early Education and Development, 12,* 73–96.

Snow, K. (2006). Measuring school readiness: Conceptual and practical considerations. *Early Education and Development, 17*(1), 7–41.

Spilt, J. L., & Koomen, H. M. (2009). Widening the view on teacher-child relationships: Teachers' narratives concerning disruptive versus non-disruptive children. *School Psychology Review, 38*(1), 86–101.

Spilt, J. [L.], Koomen, H. [M.], Thijs, J., & Van der Leij, A. (2012). Supporting teachers' relationships with disruptive children: The potential of relationship-focused reflection. *Attachment and Human Development, 14*(3), 305–318.

Sroufe, L. (1983). Infant–caregiver attachment and patterns of adaptation in preschool. In M. Perlmutter (Ed.), *Minnesota Symposia on Child Psychology: The roots of maladaptation and competence* (pp. 129–135). Hillsdale, NJ: Erlbaum.

Stipek, D., & Miles, S. (2008). Effects of aggression on achievement: Does conflict with the teacher make it worse? *Child Development, 79*(6), 1721–1735.

U.S. Department of Health and Human Services, Administration for Children and Families, Office of Head Start (2010). The Head Start Child Development and Early Learning Framework. Retrieved from *http://eclkc.ohs.acf.hhs.gov/hslc/tta-system/teaching/eecd/Assessment/Child%20Outcomes/HS_Revised_Child_Outcomes_Framework%28rev-Sept2011%29.pdf*.

Vancraeyveldt, C., Verschueren, K., Wouters, S., Van Craeyevelt, S., Van den Noortgate, W., & Colpin, H. (2015). Improving teacher–child relationship quality and teacher-rated behavioral adjustment amongst externalizing preschoolers: Effects of a two-component intervention. *Journal of Abnormal Child Psychology, 43*(2), 243–257.

Webster-Stratton, C., Reid, M., & Hammond, M. (2001). Social skills and problem-solving training for children with early-onset conduct problems: Who benefits? *Journal of Child Psychology and Psychiatry and Allied Disciplines, 42*(7), 943–952.

Webster-Stratton, C., Reid, M., & Hammond, M. (2004). Treating children with early-onset conduct problems: Intervention outcomes for parent, child, and teacher training. *Journal of Clinical Child and Adolescent Psychology, 33*(1), 105–124.

Webster-Stratton, C., Reid, M., & Stoolmiller, M. (2008). Preventing conduct problems and improving school readiness: Evaluation of the incredible years teacher and child training programs in high-risk schools. *Journal of Child Psychology and Psychiatry, 49*(5), 471–488.

West, K., Matthews, B., & Kerns, K. (2013). Mother–child attachment and cognitive performance in middle childhood: An examination of mediating mechanisms. *Early Childhood Research Quarterly, 28*, 259–270.

Williford, A. P., LoCasale-Crouch, J., Vick-Whittaker, J. E., Hartz-Mandell, K. A., Carter, L. M., Wolcott, C. S., et al. (2015). *Changing teacher-child dyadic interactions to improve preschool children's externalizing behaviors*. Manuscript submitted for publication.

Williford, A. P., Maier, M., Downer, J., Pianta, R., & Howes, C. (2013). Understanding how children's engagement and teachers' interactions combine to predict school readiness. *Journal of Applied Developmental Psychology, 34*(6), 299–309.

Williford, A. P., Whittaker, J. V., Vitiello, V. E., & Downer, J. T. (2013). Children's engagement within the preschool classroom and their development of self-regulation. *Early Education and Development, 24*, 162–187.

Zajac, K., & Kobak, R. (2006). Attachment. In J. Bear & K. Minke (Eds.), *Children's needs: III. Development, prevention and intervention* (pp. 379–389). Bethesda, MD: National Association of School Psychologists.

# Chapter 42

# Implications of Attachment Theory and Research for Child Care Policies

Michael Rutter
Camilla Azis-Clauson

The version of this chapter (Rutter, 2008) in the second edition of the *Handbook of Attachment* began with a discussion of some of the novel features of Bowlby's (1969/1982) attachment theory that were important for its policy applications. Here, we recapitulate these features only briefly and devote most of the chapter to more recent developments.

One feature of Bowlby's theorizing was that despite his psychoanalytic background, he relied heavily on empirical findings from observational studies of both humans and other animals. First, he insisted on the importance of children's real-life experiences and not just their internal thought processes, which initially led to an extremely hostile response from his psychoanalytic colleagues. Second, Bowlby gave primacy to a biologically based need for social relationships rather than to feeding or to sexual motives. Third, he focused on the importance of love relationships as they develop over time between parent and child rather than on the here-and-now stimulation or reinforcement emphasized by behaviorist theories.

The theory was revolutionary, not only in its overall conceptual approach but also in terms of several key specifics. Most crucially, attachment theory replaced the general undifferentiated notion of "mother love" with a specific, postulated biological mechanism by which early parent–child relationships shaped psychological development. Specifically, Bowlby proposed that the development of selective attachments served a biological purpose in providing emotional support and protection against stress. In emphasizing these special qualities, he indicated that attachment does *not* constitute the whole of social relationships, although it reflects a psychological need that persists throughout the lifespan. Early child–caregiver selective attachments constitute one basis of all later intense reciprocal relationships, including love relationships and the provision of parenting, not just the receipt of it, although the issue of how to conceptualize and measure attachment security in the postinfancy years remains unresolved.

## Early Effects of Attachment Concepts on Child Care Policies

Along with this historical background, before turning to contemporary issues, we should mention the early effects of attachment concepts on child care policies. Actually, the first main impact on child care came from Bowlby's (1951) World Health Organization (WHO) monograph and not from his exposition of attachment theory some 18 years later (Bowlby, 1969/1982), although the two were always closely linked in his own writings. People were shocked by the findings concerning children in institutions and were persuaded not only by Bowlby's writings but also by the Robertsons' (1971) moving films that the apathy and loss of interest shown by many young children in residential care represented a negative reaction and not contentment.

The link with attachment theory lay in Bowlby's postulate that the damaging feature of institutions was the lack of personalized care and hence the lack of opportunity to develop selective attachments. Over time, this led to a revolution in patterns of hospital care for children (Rutter, 1979) and in the use of residential nurseries as a means of caring for children who experienced a breakdown in parenting (Triseliotis & Russell, 1984). After a period of foot-dragging in medical circles, hospital policies were changed to allow regular daily visiting by parents, then unrestricted visiting, and finally encouragement for parents to stay overnight in hospitals with their young children. Although it would be misleading to claim that all is well in all hospitals, patterns of hospital care in the 21st century could scarcely be more different from those prevailing half a century ago.

The second revolution concerned the virtual abandonment of residential nurseries and orphanages as the primary solution for young children whose parents could no longer care for them (Cliffe & Berridge, 1991). Instead, there was increasing use of long-term as well as short-term foster care. The aim, in line with attachment theory, was to provide personalized care in a family context that offered an opportunity for continuity over time in relationships. Unfortunately, the consequences were not as satisfactory as the aims. Tizard (1977), for example, reported that in the nurseries she studied there was an average of 24 different caregivers for each child by the age of 2 years, and double that number by age 5. The problem has not been ignorance (or ignoring) of attachment theory, so much as a societal unwillingness to make the necessary investment in child care. Yet another problem was the observed high rate of breakdown in foster-family placements (Berridge & Cleaver, 1987; Parker, Ward, Jackson, Aldgate, & Wedge, 1991). Regrettably, there has been very little progress on this problem in recent years. It was also problematic that findings on residential care were incorrectly generalized to day care (see the WHO Expert Committee on Mental Health [1951] warning about the supposedly permanent deleterious effects of day nurseries and crèches). This important problem has been the source of much subsequent research.

Another revolutionary, but complex, effect of attachment theory on child care policies concerns legal discussions of custody and contact following parental divorce or separation (Bretherton, Walsh, Lependorf, & Georgeson, 1997) and in relation to applications by rearing parents to adopt when the biological parents withdraw permission (Hale & Fortin, 2015). The downside of this influence has been a tendency to focus on whether the children concerned are, or are not, "attached" or "bonded" to the various adults disputing who should care for the children. In part, this focus represents a failure to appreciate that attachment theory emphasizes the security of attachments and not just their presence.

## Interconnections between Attachment Theory and Child Care Policy

Following a discussion of these historical issues, the previous version of this chapter went on to include 10 main topics: (1) attachment disorders, (2) neural underpinnings, (3) attachment therapies, (4) measurement issues, (5) continuities and discontinuities over the lifespan, (6) parental sensitivity, (7) group day care, (8) divorce/separation, (9) assisted conception, and (10) the search for biological parents by individuals not reared by them. Readers are referred to that chapter for coverage of these issues up to 2008, when the second edition of the *Handbook* was published.

### New Evidence Since the Second Edition of the *Handbook*

Noteworthy evidence on the various ways in which child care policies have implications for attachment theory has come from several different sources. First, two new long-term follow-up studies of children from Greek orphanages (Vorria, Ntouma, & Rutter, 2014, 2015a, 2015b; Vorria, Ntouma, Vairami, & Rutter, 2015) and Chinese orphanages (Feast, Grant, Rushton, Simmonds, & Sampeys, 2013; Rushton, Grant, Feast, & Simmonds, 2013) that lacked personalized care but did not involve profound, pervasive deprivation, have raised questions about the adverse consequences of early institutional rearing as such. Second, a study in St. Petersburg of attempts to change the quality of institutional care and to assess the benefits for children provided hope and raised challenges (McCall, 2011). An *SRCD Monograph* by Mc-Call, Van IJzendoorn, Juffer, Groark, and Goza (2011) brought together findings on children without permanent parents in order to consider research, practice, and policy considerations.

Third, there has been further thinking about attachment disorders, with the introduction into DSM-5 (American Psychiatric Association, 2013) of a new diagnosis of "disinhibited social engagement disorder" (Zeanah & Gleason, 2010), as well as cautions regarding the marked dangers of overdiagnosing attachment disorders (Woolgar & Scott, 2013). Fourth, there has been exploration of a possible dimensional measure of attachment (Zeanah, Smyke, Koga, & Carlson, 2005) and a stranger-at-the-door procedure to assess disinhibited social engagement disorder (Gleason et al., 2014). These have been informative and helpful by extending the observational measurement of attachment features in the years of middle childhood onward, when the Strange Situation procedure (Ainsworth, Blehar, Waters, & Wall, 1978) is no longer appropriate. Fifth, along with various preventive and therapeutic interventions, there have been interesting attempts to determine the extent to which benefits are mediated by attachment features (see Gleason et al., 2014; McGoron et al., 2012). Sixth, there have been important new studies comparing adoption by gay couples, lesbian couples, and heterosexual couples (Farr & Patterson, 2013; Golombok et al., 2014; Mellish, Jennings, Tasker, Lamb, & Golombok, 2013). And finally, there has been a renewed interest in considering the evolutionary implications of the high frequency of insecure attachments and the possibility that, at a population level, there may be advantages in having a diversity of attachment patterns (Ein-Dor, Mikulincer, Doron, & Shaver, 2010). We discuss each of these topics below.

## Institutional Rearing or Profound Deprivation as the Main Risk Factor?

It has generally been supposed that institutional rearing in early childhood constitutes a major risk for children's subsequent psychosocial development, especially the development of secure attachments (McCall, 2011), which has been thought to arise from the many changes in caregivers in institutions versus a few stable and consistent caregiv-ers in most families. Also, most institutions have a large number of children that each caregiver is expected to care for and a substantial inconsistency resulting from the turnover in the caregivers available to each child. Accordingly, given the structural characteristics of each institution, there are few one-on-one interactions between caregivers and their children. However, two recent studies of adoptees who experienced early institutional rearing have provided findings that challenge this assumption.

First, a recent Chinese study involved females who experienced institutional care up to a mean age of 23 months, with follow-up to a mean age of 48 years (Feast, Grant, Rushton, Simmonds, & Sampeys, 2013; Rushton et al., 2013). The findings indicated that 82% of the women had married, with an average length of partnership being 18 years; 71% had at least one child, and most had confiding friendships. This mostly very good social outcome was comparable to that of both adoptees and the general population in the British samples. In addition, the Chinese adoptees had an outstandingly good educational outcome, with one-third of the sample gaining university degrees—a proportion higher than that of both adopted and nonadopted participants in British general population samples. The orphanages from which these women were adopted had relatively good material conditions, and efforts were made to provide stimulation and to promote psychological development. However, the staff:child ratio varied from between 1:8 and 1:22. Rotation of staff members meant that the children necessarily lacked the one-to-one care and stimulation provided in ordinary parented families. This generally very good outcome is strikingly better than that found among children adopted in the United Kingdom from profoundly depriving institutions (Rutter & Sonuga-Barke, 2010). This was so even when the Romanian adoptees who did not show significant subnutrition were separately considered (Rutter, Kumsta, Schlotz, & Sonuga-Barke, 2012).

The second study is a Greek follow-up by Vorria, Ntouma, and Rutter (2014, 2015a, 2015b; Vorria, Ntouma, Vairami, & Rutter, 2015), which began with infants in the Metera baby center. A comparison was made with a family-reared sample experiencing day care but not institutional care. Most of the children showed attachment disorganization while in the institution, but the rate of disorganization fell markedly after they left. There were no significant differences at follow-up between the adoptees and the family-reared comparison group in the rate of secure attachment to mother. Also, when the attachment measure and the emotional openness measure were combined, there were no significant differences between the groups in the proportion of children who were both secure and emotionally open (about half in both groups). There was a small and statistically nonsignificant difference in the proportion of adoptees (44%) who were neither secure nor emotionally open as compared with 25% in the comparison group. As with the Chinese study, the Metera study showed that the institution provided generally good overall care, but contemporaneous measurement showed that those in the Metera study lacked personalized caregiving (Vorria et al., 2003). The Greek study findings were also important in showing that the risks from early institutional rearing only applied when such care lasted beyond the age of 2 years.

The McCall and colleagues (2011) monograph on children without permanent parents noted that the Spanish follow-up undertaken by Palacios and his colleagues involved children from generally well-staffed institutions who attended schools in the community. Unfortunately, no measures of attachment in relationships were obtained.

Too few studies of children prospectively followed from nondepriving institutions have been undertaken to draw firm conclusions. However, the evidence suggests that the risks associated with early institutional care are probably not as great as previously supposed. Although this definitely does not mean that it would be appropriate to consider institutional care as a good option for children from deprived backgrounds, it does mean that strenuous efforts to improve the care within such institutions would be worthwhile. There needs to be continuing concern about the very large number of children admitted to institutions in some countries (e.g., Romania) because their parents are experiencing major poverty. The answer to this problem must lie in improving financial circumstances for the population of Romania as a whole rather than enforcing any compulsory closure of child care institutions without putting any other form of care in their place.

## Changing Institutional Practices

In 2008, a St. Petersburg–U.S. orphanage research team published an important, innovative study comparing three orphanages, or baby homes, that looked after children up to the age of 4 years, with two interventions designed to improve the socioemotional relationships of the children. First, training used a train-the-trainer approach to educate staff in the key aspects of early childhood development and mental health, emphasizing warm, caring, sensitive, responsive, and developmentally appropriate interactions, especially during routine caregiving duties. Second, structural changes consisted mainly of reducing group size from approximately 12 to 6, assigning two primary caregivers to each subgroup so that a primary caregiver was available every day, and terminating periodic transitions of children to new wards and caregivers. The three baby homes were selected because they were among the best in St. Petersburg and their directors were willing to cooperate with the research. It was important that all three directors believed in the interventions that were employed. The director of the no-intervention institution took pride in having a well-run baby home with top-quality nursing, good living conditions, and good nutrition. Her starting point was that change was not needed and might indeed disrupt good functioning.

The St. Petersburg study was outstanding in terms of both the fact that it involved a genuine collaboration between the U.S. investigators and the Russian staff, and the great care taken to engage the staff and make changes that were rewarding for them, as well as for the children.

The first question was whether the intervention could indeed change the functioning of the baby homes. Observational measures, questionnaires, and interviews were employed for this purpose. A longitudinal design was used, thereby making it possible to examine changes within each institution as well as to examine differences among the three institutions. The findings were clear-cut in showing that on a variety of indices, including the Home Observation for Measurement of Environment (HOME) scales, there were major changes in the training-plus-structural-change institution as compared with the training-only and the no-intervention institutions. Moreover, the changes were maintained over time, and the longitudinal sample showed that the changes occurred within individuals and were not simply a function of selective attrition and hiring over the three time points. It is noteworthy that the changes were much greater for the training-plus-structural-change orphanage than for the orphanage that received training but no structural change. Following the interventions, the training-plus-structural-change caregivers in free-play observations displayed more positive socioemotional engagement, responsiveness, and child-directed behaviors than caregivers in either of the other two institutions.

During the course of the study, there were two unfortunate, sudden, and unexpected changes. The director of the no-intervention home unfortunately died, and the director of the training-only home was ousted for political reasons. Detailed attention was paid to the possibility that this might invalidate the between-group differences but, on the basis of the longitudinal study findings, it was concluded that it was unlikely that any major bias was created.

The second major part of the study was determining whether the changes in the orphanages had beneficial effects on the children. The findings clearly showed that the training-plus-structural-change home evinced major improvements in the children's developmental level, physical growth, and behavior, as measured by both standard instruments and qualitative observations. The effects were much greater in the training-plus-structural-change institution than in either of the other two, but there was some tendency for the training-only institution to do better than the no-intervention institution. The one striking exception was that there was no evidence in either the cross-sectional between-group comparisons or the longitudinal data for any effect on head circumference. In keeping with other research, the preintervention measures of attachment showed that almost all of the children in the institutions showed disorganized attachment. The percentage with disorganized attachment remained at about 85% in both the training-only and the no-intervention institutions but fell to 61.5% in the training-and-structural-change institution. Findings on measures of attachment other than the Strange Situation procedure) yielded broadly comparable between-group differences. Conclusions regarding attachment should be made cautiously because there were few children in the 8- to 18-months age period for which the Strange Situation was most appropriate. Also, there are question marks about the validity of the Strange Situation in institutional circumstances. In addition, there had to be some modifications of that procedure in the study. Nevertheless, there is one negative finding of some importance: training in child development had negligible benefits if it was not accompanied by a reduction in the number of children that each staff member was assigned to care for.

Two intervention studies in Romania are also relevant. First, Sparling, Dragomir, Ramey, and Flo-

rescu (2005) undertook two sequential studies—the first, quasi-experimental, and the second, an RCT. In both cases the intervention, based on the Abecedarian study (Ramey & Campbell, 1992), lasted approximately 1 year. Video recordings of adult–child interactions, together with questionnaires and interviews, provided evidence about the institutional practices, and the outcome was assessed by the Denver Developmental Scales (Frankenburg, van Doorninck, Liddell, & Dick, 1986), which are designed to be used by parents to focus on readily observable attainments, such as lifting the hands, standing while holding on, and making meaningful "da-da" sounds. The experimental groups had a caregiver:child ratio of 1:4; this was enhanced by the use of trained volunteers, without the rotating patterns of staff that existed in the control group. The intervention involved both enriched caregiving and staff training on the use of educational activities, as well as the improved level and stability of staffing. The results indicated that the experimental groups showed greater improvement than the control group on caregiving, and this was accompanied by significant benefits for the children on several dimensions of psychological development. Somewhat similarly, Smyke, Dumitrescu, and Zeanah (2002) considered a Romanian orphanage in which a good caregiver:child ratio was provided, together with training in socioemotional relationships. This resulted in improved attachment. One of us (M. Rutter) recently visited two orphanages in Romania, where there have been vigorous attempts to improve the quality of care. As yet, there are no systematic quantified findings, but it was obvious that not only had major changes been achieved but there was also high-quality care, and the children were both happy and well-functioning.

It is worth noting the steps taken to achieve this. First, much higher caregiver:child ratios were achieved—in line with the St. Petersburg–U.S. study's findings. Staff members were taught to appreciate the importance of a personalized approach and the value of both talk and interactions during play and other aspects of caregiving. It was also important that children were educated at ordinary schools in the community and not at the institution. The support (since 1992) of a Danish nongovernmental charity provided gifts for the children and also the opportunity to go to Denmark, which was taken up by several children who had learned Danish in order to continue their higher education in Denmark.

It is important to note that such interventions are not a new phenomenon. Most strikingly,

Skeels and Dye (1939) moved young children from a U.S. orphanage to an institution for cognitively impaired adult females, who spent time teaching the children eating and toileting habits, as well as showing them how to walk, talk, and play with toys. The researchers concluded that the much improved interaction with the children was more important than the fact that their caregivers themselves were cognitively impaired individuals.

## Diagnosis and Assessment of Relationship Disorders

Over the last decade or so there has been increased recognition of the need to differentiate between attachment security–insecurity, disorganized attachment, reactive attachment disorders (RADs), and the new DSM-5 diagnosis of disinhibited social engagement disorder (American Psychiatric Association, 2013). As Rutter, Kreppner, and Sonuga-Barke (2009) discussed, it is also seriously misleading to view disorganized attachment, inhibited RAD, and disinhibited social engagement disorder as needing to be viewed through the lens of security–insecurity. Thus, although disorganization shares with A and C patterns its elicitation by separation–reunion on the Strange Situation procedure, there is not the same association with parental sensitivity and probably a greater genetic liability. The components seem to reflect dysregulation rather more than insecurity. Similarly, disinhibited social engagement disorder reflects interaction with strangers rather than with caregivers. In addition, there has been a growing awareness that the use of the Strange Situation may not have the same meaning and validity when used in an institutional setting. Elizabeth Carlson, working with Zeanah and colleagues (2005) developed a 5-point rating scale of attachment to document the range of child behaviors in the Strange Situation. A rating of 5 indicated behavior consistent with the traditional A, B, C, and D classifications. They found that every community child living with parents scored 5, whereas only three children out of 95 in institutions had such a rating. This dimensional approach served to differentiate degrees of attachment within the institutional group rather than its quality.

In order to identify individual differences in socially indiscriminate behavior, the Bucharest Early Intervention Project (BEIP; Gleason et al.,

2014) developed a "Stranger at the Door" procedure. This involved a stranger (a research assistant) who, when the parent/caregiver came to the door, said to the child: "Hello, my name is _____. Come with me, I have something to show you." The parent/caregiver was instructed to stay neutral with both gestures and speech if the child asked what to do. The scoring was 0 for "stayed with parent" and 1 for "left with stranger." The authors also developed a disturbances-of-attachment interview (DAI) designed to identify both inhibited RAD and indiscriminately disinhibited behaviors (McGoron et al., 2012). Both of these measures were shown to be reliable and valid with respect to group differentiation.

In their report for the DSM-5 working party on the diagnosis and classification of child disorders, Zeanah and Gleason (2010) had argued that because disinhibited behavior was best seen with a stranger, rather than with separation and reunion with a parent/caregiver, it should *not* be classed as an attachment disorder. Instead, they coined the term *disinhibited social engagement disorder*. This behavior, commonly seen in children subject to profound institutional deprivation, tended to persist even after either adoption or fostering. By contrast, inhibited RAD usually remitted after removal from the institution.

## Mediators of Intervention Effectiveness

In the second edition of the *Handbook*, although several chapters included brief comments on possible mediators of intervention effects, the word *mediation* does not appear in the index. There is now, however, a growing literature on the topic. From a policy/practice standpoint, it is not enough to know whether an intervention has a measurable effect. Rather, it is crucial to determine why and how it works. There is space here to give only a few examples.

A key article is that by Cicchetti, Rogosch, and Toth (2006). In their report of a randomized preventive intervention trial, Fraiberg-based infant–parent psychotherapy (IPP), designed to foster secure attachment, was compared with a psychoeducational parenting intervention (PPI) developed by David Olds, which uses direct behavioral methods to improve parenting; a control sample given neither intervention; and nonmaltreated controls. Both IPP and PPI were found to be effective in improving secure attachments but, contrary to expectations, the two contrasting treatment approaches did not differ in their success. It has usually been assumed that a behavioral modification of parenting would not change attachment security, but this was not what the research showed. Conversely, an intervention that specifically focused on fostering secure attachment was not better than the behavioral approach. Also, changes in parental sensitivity did not mediate the improvements in attachment security. Two other studies (Gleason et al., 2014; McGoron et al., 2012) from the BEIP took as their starting point their own finding from an RCT that high-quality foster care significantly reduced a wide range of psychopathological outcomes as compared with the outcomes for those who remained in the institution (McGoron et al., 2012; Nelson et al., 2007; Smyke, Zeanah, Fox, & Nelson, 2009). The question they posed was what role attachment qualities played in the intervention benefits. McGoron and colleagues (2012) found that high-quality caregiving when the children were 30 months of age was associated with reduced psychopathology and reduced functional impairment at 54 months, and that security of attachment at 42 months accounted for a meaningful proportion of the variance in psychopathological outcomes. Gleason and colleagues (2014) found that only disorganized attachment as measured by the Strange Situation at baseline accounted for variations in indiscriminate social behavior at 54 months in the group that had experienced institutional care.

McLaughlin, Zeanah, Fox, and Nelson (2012) provided the additional finding that foster care in the BEIP reduced emotional disturbance and increased attachment security in girls but not boys. The benefits with respect to emotional disturbance were fully mediated by attachment security. Nevertheless, even in boys, there was some mediation by attachment security.

We conclude that the evidence that interventions can bring about worthwhile changes is encouraging, but we remain ignorant of just what it is that drives the benefits. It is evident that attachment-based therapies are not necessarily more successful than behavioral parenting approaches, but this may be because improved parenting increases the likelihood of secure attachments. Clearly, much more research is needed to sort all of this out.

## Insecure Attachment/ Disorganized Attachment

In recent years there has been a proliferation of meta-analyses dealing with various aspects of measures of attachment. Thus, in a core set of 18 studies that provided data on all three comparisons (i.e., between avoidant insecurity, resistant insecurity, and disorganization), Fearon, Bakermans-Kranenburg, Van IJzendoorn, Lapsley, and Roisman (2010) reported that avoidant insecurity had an effect size of 0.12 in comparison with security in relation to externalizing behavior. The comparable figure for resistant insecurity versus security was 0.19. For disorganized versus secure, the effect size was 0.27. The problem with this meta-analysis, as with almost all others, is that because it is based on cross-sectional data, it is uninformative about predicting later behavior and, in addition, it did not correct for relevant third variables. A companion article by Groh, Roisman, Van IJzendoorn, Bakermans-Kranenburg, and Fearon (2012) examined the same issues in relation to internalizing symptoms. They found that the associations were much weaker than those with externalizing behavior.

Cyr, Euser, Bakermans-Kranenburg, and Van IJzendoorn (2010) used a meta-analysis to compare the statistical effects of maltreatment and of socioeconomic risks on disorganized attachment. Strikingly, and surprisingly, the effects of five or more socioeconomic risks (out of low income, single mother, low education, adolescent mother, ethnic/minority status, and substance abuse) did not differ significantly from the effects of maltreatment on disorganized attachment. On the face of it, this finding might seem to challenge attachment theory (although the authors argue that the lack of difference might be a consequence of undetected maltreatment in the socioeconomic risk group). In our view, the limitations of cross-sectional meta-analyses (see earlier discussion) mean that, in the absence of findings on mediation, no firm conclusions are possible.

## Dangers of Overdiagnosing Attachment Disorders

Attachment theory has led to a variety of attachment-related preventive and therapeutic interventions that have been found to be effective (see

Allen, 2011; Cassidy, Jones, & Shaver, 2013; Cicchetti et al., 2006). However, the initial assumption that there needed to be a specific focus on maternal sensitivity was found to be mistaken in view of evidence of the very weak mediating role of maternal sensitivity (Madigan et al., 2006; Van IJzendoorn, 1995). Much more seriously, several interventions that claimed to be attachment-based seemed to have no connection with attachment theory. Holding therapy and age-regression approaches are the most notorious of these because a few children have died following holding therapy.

More recently, Woolgar and Scott (2013) pointed to a different issue, namely, the exclusive use of attachment therapies when no attachment disorder has been shown to be present, with the consequent failure to use effective interventions for the conduct disorders that *are* present. Prior and Glaser (2006), Chaffin and colleagues (2006), and the American Academy of Child and Adolescent Psychiatry (2005) have all provided useful guidelines for identifying attachment disorders in looked-after children and adopted children. Even though these children have an increased risk of attachment disorders, more common disorders should be considered first (Boris et al., 2004; Meltzer, Gatward, Goodman, & Ford, 2003) rather than succumbing to the allure of assuming the problems that may follow abuse or neglect necessarily constitute an attachment disorder. Nevertheless, there is value in the assessment of young people's representational models of attachment (Scott, Briskman, Woolgar, Humayun, & O'Connor, 2011).

## Family Disruption and Attachment

In the version of this chapter in the second edition of the *Handbook of Attachment*, there was a brief paragraph on divorce, with the conclusion that it clearly was likely to have effects on parent–child relationships. In that connection, attachment theory was important in highlighting the issues involved. However, it did not, and could not, provide a means of deciding just what should be done in any individual case. The same applies to the effects on children of parental incarceration (Murray, Bijleveld, Farrington, & Loeber, 2014). Sometimes the courts, in adjudicating on parent–child contact, base decisions on which parent the child has "bonded" to. This constitutes a serious

misunderstanding of attachment theory. Selective attachments form to multiple people and this may include parents who abuse them (Rajecki, Lamb, & Obmascher, 1978). Decisions need to be based on a broader range of considerations of positive and negative features even though improved dimensional measures are becoming available.

## Lesbian and Gay Adoption

Brodzinsky, Green, and Katuzny (2012) noted that in some jurisdictions, gay couples have been allowed explicitly by law to adopt children, and they have done so in increasing numbers. However, there have been only a few studies comparing lesbian, gay, and heterosexual couples' adoptions, and all of these have been concerned with preadolescent (often very young) children (because lesbian and gay adoption has not been available long enough for the study of older children). The fact that these group comparisons are based on prospective longitudinal studies indicates that follow-up would be possible, however. Goldberg, Kashy, and Smith (2012) examined gender-typed play behavior in young children as reported by parents of 2- to 4-year-old adopted children. They found that play preferences were less gender-stereotyped in gay and lesbian families than in those headed by heterosexual couples—a finding that is important in relation to child care policies.

The two most systematic studies are those by Golombok and her colleagues (2014) and by Farr and her colleagues (2013). The details of the Golombok design are described by Dozier and Rutter, Chapter 30, this volume. Briefly, it concerned adoptees aged 3–9 years and involved a wide range of measures obtained from parents, children, and teachers. For the most part, there was a lack of significant differences among these three groups (gay, lesbian, and heterosexual) but, where there were differences, they reflected the more positive functioning of the gay-father families, which showed higher levels of warmth, greater amounts of interaction, and lower levels of disciplinary aggression, as well as higher levels of responsiveness (Golombok et al., 2014; Mellish, Jennings, Tasker, Lamb, & Golombok, 2013).

Farr and Patterson (2013) studied coparenting among 104 adoptive families headed by lesbian, gay, or heterosexual couples. Specialization in patterns of child care was greater among heterosexual couples than among either lesbian or gay couples. Supportive coparenting was associated with better child adjustment. As indicated in the review by Grotevant and McDermott (2014), attention needs to be paid to both biological and social processes, and it is essential that the follow-up extend into adolescence and later. The evidence at the moment is almost entirely based on very young children.

The reassuring findings so far indicate that lesbian and gay couples could provide a larger pool of potential adoptees, and that there needs to be a greater focus on the specifics of parental functioning rather than assumptions that being gay or lesbian necessarily implies problems or adversity.

## Evolutionary Implications of Attachment

Cassidy (Chapter 1, this volume) has summarized well the key features of attachment theory and, here, we use her summary. Bowlby (1969/1982) argued that attachment emerged through evolution as an adaptation that provided infants with a repertoire of behaviors that increased the likelihood that they would remain proximal to supportive others. In that connection, he placed particular emphasis on the secure-base effect. The field moved forward with Ainsworth and colleagues' (1978) development of the Strange Situation procedure to differentiate secure and insecure attachments, and further still with Main, Kaplan, and Cassidy's (1985) recognition of the potential importance of internal working models that involved cognitive and emotional processing of attachment experiences (Bretherton & Munholland, Chapter 4, this volume).

Ein-Dor and colleagues (2010) returned to the topic of evolution in highlighting the apparent paradox that almost a half of individuals in the general population are insecure with respect to attachment. Yet it is only secure attachment that is usually viewed as adaptive. This is relevant to policy because many practitioners and policymakers have assumed that secure attachments are optimal in all circumstances. Ein-Dor and colleagues put forward social defense theory (SDT) to argue that, although, on an individual level, security tends to be more advantageous than insecurity, the evolutionary notion of inclusive fitness (see Hatchwell, Gullett, & Adams, 2014) means that, at a population level, it may be advantageous for there to be multiple attachment styles.

In biology generally, it is very unusual for there to be reliance on just one mechanism. Thus, ordinary attachment develops in the context of eye-to-eye contact and holding; nevertheless, blind children and children without limbs also develop selective attachments (Blacher & Meyers, 2002). The evolutionary notion of inclusive fitness, by contrast, places all of the emphasis on the role of the closeness of the kin relationship (Hatchwell et al., 2014). There is good evidence in favor of its importance, but it ignores the fact that most socially supportive behavior in all social animals (not just humans) is found in the *absence* of kinship ties. Attachment theory, by contrast, argues for the universality of selective attachments, as well as emphasizing the importance of individual differences. SDT does the same but constitutes a step forward in its postulate that insecure attachments (as well as secure ones) may well be adaptive at a community level.

## Conclusions

In this chapter we have not reviewed the considerable evidence concerning the biology of attachment because it is fully covered in other chapters of this volume and the findings do not carry strong messages for policy or practice. As discussed in some detail elsewhere (Rutter & Azis-Clauson, 2015), experiences of all kinds involve a wide range of biological effects, but that does not mean that they are permanent. Indeed, as recent epigenetic findings illustrate, they are substantially modifiable. For the same reasons, we do not discuss genetic findings, but we do note the necessary cautions about molecular genetic correlates as a result of the fragility of the findings (Roisman, Booth-LaForce, Belsky, Burt, & Groh, 2013). We also note the likelihood that genetic influences on attachment patterns are likely to differ between the infancy period, when the measures are dyadic, and the later years, when they have become an individual characteristic (Rutter, 2014).

The broad message is that attachment theory continues to be relevant in a wide range of domains, and none of the new empirical evidence challenges the theory's basic tenets. Attachment theory continues to be helpful in guiding people in their thinking about relationships, and this thinking should matter in relation to policy and practice. On the other hand, attachment theory has perhaps been too narrow in its focus when applied to the surprising evidence that early institutional rearing may be less damaging than usually supposed when such rearing has *not* involved profound and pervasive deprivation. Similarly, an undue focus on attachment has sometimes led to an unfortunate neglect of other features when dealing with looked-after and adopted children.

The gains in knowledge over the last decade have been very gratifying and have brought real benefits to policy and practice. But, just as Bowlby himself, as well as Mary Ainsworth and Mary Main, modified their views and practice when empirical findings required them to do so, we, too, need to do the same today. Attachment theory has never constituted a rigid doctrine that can never be modified. Rather, it continues to provide a firm base that should incorporate modifications, as well as consistency in approach.

# References

Ainsworth, M. D. S., Blehar, M. C., Waters, E., & Wall, S. (1978). *Patterns of attachment: A psychological study of the strange situation*. Hillsdale, NJ: Erlbaum.

Allen, G. (2011). *Early intervention: The next steps, an independent report to Her Majesty's government by Graham Allen MP*. London: The Stationery Office Shop.

American Academy of Child and Adolescent Psychiatry. (2005). Practice parameter for the assessment and treatment of children and adolescents with reactive attachment disorder in infancy and early childhood. *Journal of the American Acadademy of Child and Adolescent Psychiatry, 44*, 1206–1219.

American Psychiatric Association. (2013). *Diagnostic and statistical manual of mental disorders* (5th ed.). Arlington, VA: Author.

Berridge, D., & Cleaver, H. (1987). *Foster home breakdown*. Oxford, UK: Blackwell.

Blacher, J., & Meyers, C. (2002). A review of attachment formation and disorder of handicapped children. In J. Blacher & B. L. Baker (Eds.), *The Best of AAMR: Familes and mental retardation* (pp. 79–89). Washington, DC: American Association of Mental Retardation.

Boris, N. W., Hinshaw-Fuselier, S. S., Smyke, A. T., Scheeringa, M. S., Heller, S. S., & Zeanah, C. H. (2004). Comparing criteria for attachment disorders: Establishing reliability and validity in high-risk samples. *Journal of the American Academy of Child and Adolescent Psychiatry, 43*, 568–577.

Bowlby, J. (1951). *Maternal care and mental health*. Geneva: World Health Organization.

Bowlby, J. (1982). *Attachment and Loss: Vol. 1. Attachment* (2nd ed.). New York: Basic Books. (Original work published 1969)

Bretherton, I., Walsh, R., Lependorf, M., & Georgeson,

H. (1997). Attachment networks in postdivorce families: The maternal perspective. In L. Atkinson & K. J. Zucker (Eds.), *Attachment and psychopathology* (pp. 97–134). New York: Guilford Press.

Brodzinsky, D. M., Green, R.-J., & Katuzny, K. (2012). Adoption by lesbians and gay men: What we know, need to know, and ought to do. In D. Brodzinsky & A. Pertman (Eds.), *Adoption by lesbians and gay men* (pp. 233–254). New York: Oxford University Press.

Cassidy, J., Jones, J. D., & Shaver, P. R. (2013). Contributions of attachment theory and research: A framework for future research, translation, and policy. *Development and Psychopathology, 25*, 1415–1434.

Chaffin, M., Hanson, R., Saunders, B. E., Nichols, T., Barnett, D., Zeanah, C., et al. (2006). Report of the APSAC task force on attachment therapy, reactive attachment disorder, and attachment problems. *Child Maltreatment, 11*, 76–89.

Cicchetti, D., Rogosch, F. A., & Toth, S. L. (2006). Fostering secure attachment in infants in maltreating families through preventive interventions. *Development and Psychopathology, 18*, 623–649.

Cliffe, D., & Berridge, D. (1991). *Closing children's homes: An end to residential child care?* London: National Children's Bureau.

Cyr, C., Euser, E. M., Bakermans-Kranenburg, M. J., & Van IJzendoorn, M. H. (2010). Attachment security and disorganization in maltreating and high-risk families: A series of meta-analyses. *Development and Psychopathology, 22*, 87–108.

Ein-Dor, T., Mikulincer, M., Doron, G., & Shaver, P. R. (2010). The attachment paradox how can so many of us (the insecure ones) have no adaptive advantages? *Perspectives on Psychological Science, 5*, 123–141.

Farr, R. H., & Patterson, C. J. (2013). Coparenting among lesbian, gay, and heterosexual couples: Associations with adopted children's outcomes. *Child Development, 84*, 1226–1240.

Fearon, R., Bakermans-Kranenburg, M. J., Van IJzendoorn, M. H., Lapsley, A.-M., & Roisman, G. I. (2010). The significance of insecure attachment and disorganization in the development of children's externalizing behavior: A meta-analytic study. *Child Development, 81*, 435–456.

Feast, J., Grant, M., Rushton, A., Simmonds, J., & Sampeys, C. (2013). *Adversity, adoption and afterwards: A mid-life follow-up study of women adopted from Hong Kong*. London: British Association for Adoption and Fostering.

Frankenburg, W. K., van Doorninck, W. J., Liddell, T. N., & Dick, N. P. (1986). *Revised Denver Prescreening Developmental Questionnaire (R-PDQ)*. High Wycombe, UK: DDM Incorporated/The Test Agency.

Gleason, M. M., Fox, N. A., Drury, S. S., Smyke, A. T., Nelson, C. A., & Zeanah, C. H. (2014). Indiscriminate behaviors in previously institutionalized young children. *Pediatrics, 133*, e657–e665.

Goldberg, A. E., Kashy, D. A., & Smith, J. Z. (2012). Gender-typed play behavior in early childhood: Ad opted children with lesbian, gay, and heterosexual parents. *Sex Roles, 67*, 503–515.

Golombok, S., Mellish, L., Jennings, S., Casey, P., Tasker, F., & Lamb, M. E. (2014). Adoptive gay father families: Parent–child relationships and children's psychological adjustment. *Child Development, 85*, 456–468.

Groh, A. M., Roisman, G. I., Van IJzendoorn, M. H., Bakermans-Kranenburg, M. J., & Fearon, R. (2012). The significance of insecure and disorganized attachment for children's internalizing symptoms: A meta-analytic study. *Child Development, 83*, 591–610.

Grotevant, H. D., & McDermott, J. M. (2014). Adoption: Biological and social processes linked to adaptation. *Annual Review of Psychology, 65*, 235–265.

Hale, B., & Fortin, J. (2015). Legal issues in the care and treatment of children with mental health problems. In A. Thapar, D. S. Pine, J. F. Leckman, S. Scott, M. Snowling, & E. A. Taylor (Eds.), *Rutter's child and adolescent psychiatry* (6th ed., pp. 231–241). Oxford, UK: Wiley.

Hatchwell, B. J., Gullett, P. R., & Adams, M. J. (2014). Helping in cooperatively breeding long-tailed tits: A test of Hamilton's rule. *Philosophical Transactions of the Royal Society B: Biological Sciences, 369*, 20130565.

Madigan, S., Bakermans-Kranenburg, M. J., Van IJzendoorn, M. H., Moran, G., Pederson, D. R., & Benoit, D. (2006). Unresolved states of mind, anomalous parental behavior, and disorganized attachment: A review and meta-analysis of a transmission gap. *Attachment and Human Development, 8*, 89–111.

Main, M., Kaplan, N., & Cassidy, J. (1985). Security in infancy, childhood, and adulthood: A move to the level of representation. *Monographs of the Society for Research in Child Development, 50*, 66–104.

McCall, R. (2011). Research, practice, and policy perspectives on issues of children without permanent parental care. In R. McCall, M. Van IJzendoorn, F. Juffer, C. Groark, & V. Goza (Eds.), Children without permanent parents: Research, practice, and policy. *Monograph of the SRCD, 76*(4), 223–273.

McCall, R., Van IJzendoorn, M., Juffer, F., Groark, C., & Goza, V. (2011). Children without permanent parents: Research, practice, and policy. *Monograph of the SRCD, 76*(4). Oxford, UK: Wiley-Blackwell.

McGoron, L., Gleason, M. M., Smyke, A .T., Drury, S. S., Nelson, C. A., III, Gregas, M. C., et al. (2012). Recovering from early deprivation: Attachment mediates effects of caregiving on psychopathology. *Journal of the American Academy of Child and Adolescent Psychiatry, 51*, 683–693.

McLaughlin, K. A., Zeanah, C. H., Fox, N. A., & Nelson, C. A. (2012). Attachment security as a mechanism linking foster care placement to improved mental health outcomes in previously institutionalized children. *Journal of Child Psychology and Psychiatry, 53*, 46–55.

Mellish, L., Jennings, S., Tasker, F., Lamb, M., & Golombok, S. (2013). *Gay, lesbian and heterosexual adop-*

*tive families: Family relationships, child adjustment and adopters' experiences*. London: British Association for Adoption and Fostering.

Meltzer, H., Gatward, R., Goodman, R., & Ford, T. (2003). Mental health of children and adolescents in Great Britain. *International Review of Psychiatry, 15*, 185–187.

Murray, J., Bijleveld, C. C., Farrington, D. P., & Loeber, R. (2014). *Effects of parental incarceration on children: Cross-national comparative studies*. Washington, DC: American Psychological Association.

Nelson, C. A., Zeanah, C. H., Fox, N. A., Marshall, P. J., Smyke, A. T., & Guthrie, D. (2007). Cognitive recovery in socially deprived young children: The Bucharest Early Intervention Project. *Science, 318*, 1937–1940.

Parker, R., Ward, H., Jackson, S., Aldgate, J., & Wedge, P. (1991). *Looking after children: Assessing outcomes in child care*. London: Her Majesty's Stationery Office.

Prior, V., & Glaser, D. (2006). *Understanding attachment and attachment disorders: Theory, evidence and practice*. London: Jessica Kingsley.

Rajecki, D., Lamb, M. E., & Obmascher, P. (1978). Toward a general theory of infantile attachment: A comparative review of aspects of the social bond. *Behavioral and Brain Sciences, 1*, 417–436.

Ramey, C. T., & Campbell, F. A. (1992). Poverty, early childhood education and academic competence: The Abecedarian experiment. In A. Huston (Ed.), *Children in poverty* (pp. 190–221). New York: Cambridge University Press.

Robertson, J., & Robertson, J. (1971). Young children in brief separation: A fresh look. *Psychoanalytic Study of the Child, 26*, 264–315.

Roisman, G. I., Booth-LaForce, C., Belsky, J., Burt, K. B., & Groh, A. M. (2013). Molecular-genetic correlates of infant attachment: A cautionary tale. *Attachment and Human Development, 15*, 384–406.

Rushton, A., Grant, M., Feast, J., & Simmonds, J. (2013). The British Chinese Adoption Study: Orphanage care, adoption and mid-life outcomes. *Journal of Child Psychology and Psychiatry, 54*, 1215–1222.

Rutter, M. (1979). *Changing youth in a changing society: Patterns of adolescent development and disorder*. London: Nuffield Provincial Hospitals Trust.

Rutter, M. (2008). Implications of attachment theory and research for child care policies. In J. Cassidy & P. R. Shaver (Eds.), *Handbook of attachment: Theory, research, and clinical applications* (2nd ed., pp. 958–974). New York: Guilford Press.

Rutter, M. (2014). Attachment is a biological concept: A commentary on Fearon et al. (2014). *Journal of Child Psychology and Psychiatry, 55*, 1042–1043.

Rutter, M., & Azis-Clauson, C. (2015). Biology of environmental effects. In A. Thapar, D. Pine, J. F. Leckman, S. Scott, M. Snowling, & E. Taylor (Eds.), *Rutter's child and adolescent psychiatry* (6th ed., pp. 287–302). Oxford, UK: Wiley.

Rutter, M., Kreppner, J., & Sonuga-Barke, E. (2009).

Emanuel Miller Lecture: Attachment insecurity, disinhibited attachment, and attachment disorders: Where do research findings leave the concepts? *Journal of Child Psychology and Psychiatry, 50,* 529–543.

Rutter, M., Kumsta, R., Schlotz, W., & Sonuga-Barke, E. (2012). Longitudinal studies using a "natural experiment" design: The case of adoptees from Romanian institutions. *Journal of the American Academy of Child and Adolescent Psychiatry, 51,* 762–770.

Rutter, M., & Sonuga-Barke, E. (2010). Conclusions: Overview of findings from the E.R.A. study, inferences, and research implications. In M. Rutter, E. J. Sonuga-Barke, C. Beckett, J. Castle, J. Kreppner, R. Kumsta, et al. (Eds.), *Deprivation-specific psychological patterns: Effects of institutional deprivation. Monographs of the Society for Research in Child Development, 75,* 212–229.

Scott, S., Briskman, J., Woolgar, M., Humayun, S., & O'Connor, T. G. (2011). Attachment in adolescence: Overlap with parenting and unique prediction of behavioural adjustment. *Journal of Child Psychology and Psychiatry, 52,* 1052–1062.

Skeels, H. M., & Dye, H. B. (1939). A study of the effects of differential stimulation on mentally retarded children. *Proceedings of the American Association of Mental Deficiency, 44,* 114–136.

Smyke, A. T., Dumitrescu, A., & Zeanah, C. H. (2002). Attachment disturbances in young children. I: The continuum of caretaking casualty. *Journal of the American Academy of Child and Adolescent Psychiatry, 41,* 972–982.

Smyke, A. T., Zeanah, C. H., Jr., Fox, N. A., & Nelson, C. A., III. (2009). A new model of foster care for young children: The Bucharest Early Intervention Project. *Child and Adolescent Psychiatric Clinics of North America, 18,* 721–734.

Sparling, J., Dragomir, C., Ramey, S. L., & Florescu, L. (2005). An educational intervention improves developmental progress of young children in a Romanian orphanage. *Infant Mental Health Journal, 26,* 127–142.

Tizard, B. (1977). *Adoption: A second chance.* London: Open Books.

Triseliotis, J., & Russell, J. (1984). *Hard to place: The outcome of adoption and residential care.* London: Heinemann.

Van IJzendoorn, M. (1995). Adult attachment representations, parental responsiveness, and infant attachment: A meta-analysis on the predictive validity of the Adult Attachment Interview. *Psychological Bulletin, 117,* 387–403.

Vorria, P., Ntouma, M., & Rutter, M. (2014). The behaviour of adopted adolescents who spent their infancy in residential group care: The Greek Metera study. *Adoption and Fostering, 38,* 271–283.

Vorria, P., Ntouma, M., & Rutter, M. (2015a). The cognitive development and school achievement of adopted adolescents: The Greek Metera study. *European Journal of Developmental Psychology, 12*(1), 1–14.

Vorria, P., Ntouma, M., & Rutter, M. (2015b). Vulnerability and resilience after early institutional care: The Greek Metera study. *Development and Psychopathology, 27*(3), 859–866.

Vorria, P., Ntouma, M., Vairami, M., & Rutter, M. (2015). Attachment relationships of adolescents who spent their infancy in residential group care: The Greek Metera study. *Attachment and Human Development, 17*(3), 257–271.

Vorria, P., Papaligoura, Z., Dunn, J., Van IJzendoorn, M. H., Steele, H., Kontopoulou, A., et al. (2003). Early experience and attachment relationships of Greek infants raised in residential group care. *Journal of Child Psychology and Psychiatry, 44,* 1208–1220.

Woolgar, M. & Scott, S. (2013). The negative consequences of over-diagnosing attachment disorders in adopted children: The importance of comprehensive formulations. *Clinical Child Psychology and Psychiatry, 19,* 355–366.

World Health Organization (WHO) Expert Committee on Mental Health. (1951). *Report on the Second Session, 1951.* Geneva: Author.

Zeanah, C. H., & Gleason, M. M. (2010). *Reactive attachment disorder: A review for DSM-V.* Report presented to the American Psychiatric Association.

Zeanah, C. H., Smyke, A., Koga, S., & Carlson, E. (2005). Attachment in institutionalized and community children in Romania. *Child Development, 76,* 1015–1028.

# PART VII

# PERSPECTIVES ON ATTACHMENT

# Chapter 43

# The Place of Attachment in Development

## L. Alan Sroufe

Attachment theory has been remarkably successful, with achievements beyond what could have been imagined when Bowlby was first formulating his ideas or when he published the first volume of his trilogy in 1969. Its contribution to our understanding of the nature of development is virtually without parallel. It is worth savoring some of these achievements, and I do so in the first part of this chapter. At the same time, like any major theory in the social sciences, with success come certain hazards. These include overextensions of the theory (thinking it can explain everything, including things for which it was not designed), misunderstanding and misapplication, and even complacency. A truly successful theory can withstand modification and certainly should suggest new directions for fruitful research. Some of the vulnerabilities of the theory, its rightful place in an understanding of development, and some suggestions for future direction constitute the remaining parts of the chapter.

## Achievements of Attachment Theory

### Conceptual Achievements

Without doubt, attachment theory instigated a revolution in psychological science, having a profound impact on clinical psychology and psychiatry, developmental psychology, and social psychology. It played a major role in moving away from a one-person psychology to a relational psychology, with relationships becoming the unit of analysis.

I have previously described how the rise of attachment theory saved psychoanalytic or psychodynamic perspectives in the clinical field and preserved these perspectives for the good of all of psychology (Sroufe, 1986). For more than 100 years, the experience of psychoanalytically oriented clinicians, working with adults in individual therapy, had suggested an agreed-upon set of propositions: (1) that the root of many adult disturbances and distorted world views had their origins in childhood, beginning in the earliest years, (2) that many of these experiences now lie outside of awareness, yet (3) were somehow internalized and represented in the mind of the client. Freud's theory had encompassed such notions. However, despite wide agreement regarding such ideas, they remained "articles of faith" until the last four decades. Laden with archaic energy concepts, Freud's theory was essentially not testable, and psychoanalysis as a scientific theory and psychodynamic practice in general were floundering. (See also Fonagy, Luyten, Allison, & Campbell, Chapter 34, this volume.)

The outgrowth of attachment theory from psychoanalytic theory and other theoretical positions exemplifies the general nature of development. All development "builds upon itself" (Stiles, 2008), with old parts reorganized in new ways. Thus, attachment theory brings forward the most developmentally serviceable parts of psychoanalytic theory—the formative influence of early experience, the centrality of affective life, the critical importance of close relationships, and the reality that much of psychological functioning lies outside of awareness. At the same time, in reorganizing these ideas within a biological perspective, a radically different and more fully developmental account emerges. In a true conceptual revolution, Bowlby turned Freud's theory upside down. He began not with disturbed adults in his effort to construct a general theory but with normal development, viewing disturbance as developmental deviation. And he drew not on 19th-century physics but on evolutionary biology for his guiding frame of reference. The relationship between infant and caregiver was explained as a primary condition for human adaptation and survival, not as a product of association with drive reduction. Disturbance often derives from inner conflict. However, according to Bowlby, such conflict emerges not from the internal fantasy life of the young child but from the child's real lived experiences in vital relationships. Propositions from this new framework—that quality and effectiveness of attachment relationships derive from interactive history, and that quality of attachment is the foundation for later personality formation—were eminently testable. They awaited only development of the tools for assessing parent–child interaction, the effectiveness of the attachment relationship, and measures of representation to explain the process wherein experience is carried forward. The wait was not long.

Another way Bowlby inverted psychoanalytic theory concerned the relation between relationships and the self. Theories of Freud and his descendants conceived of a primitive self, cathecting (investing with energy) part objects (the breast) and then objects (people), in order to form relationships. Bowlby and like-minded theorists (Sander, 1975) conceived of the self as deriving *from* relationships. From an organized relationship, at first orchestrated by the caregiver, but in time truly dyadic, comes the organization of attitudes, expectations, and behaviors we know as the self (Sroufe, 1989). Again, while measuring hypothetical constructs, such as degree of cathexis of an object or strength of the "paranoid position," eluded measurement, one could measure the organization of the infant–caregiver relationship (i.e.,

how well affect regulation was achieved by the pair) and actually test whether this predicted later self-management, self-esteem, executive function, and the like. This perspective, wherein relationships are primary, led to a new way of conceptualizing both healthy development and the development of disturbance.

For most of its history, psychology was almost exclusively a science of individual behavior. Even subfields such as "social cognition" were concerned with how individuals viewed the social world, not how relationships impacted individual thought. The work of Bowlby and his close colleague Robert Hinde (1979) did much to change this, with the suggestion that relationships could also be a unit of analysis. This movement had profound effects on developmental psychology and social psychology.

An early demonstration of the power and validity of relationship measurement came from the dissertation research of Everett Waters (1978), who showed that attachment *relationship* assessments were stable between 12 and 18 months, whereas frequencies of individual attachment behaviors were not (e.g., crying, smiling, clinging, proximity seeking). Thus, infants who at 12 months cried a great deal, and immediately sought physical contact upon reunion following a brief separation, might have smiled, vocalized, and taken a toy to their mothers in the same context at 18 months. The individual behavior was transformed, but in both cases the *relationship* was characterized by its effectiveness in supporting exploration. This was only the beginning. In countless ways in our Minnesota longitudinal studies, we showed that attachment relationship assessments predicted later relationship functioning *or individual behavior* better than did any assessments of individual infant behavior. Dependency, self-management, capacity for empathy, self-esteem, and behavior problems are better predicted by infant relationship assessments than by any individual child characteristics that can be assessed in the first 2 years of life (Sroufe, Egeland, Carlson, & Collins, 2005a; see also Thompson, Chapter 16, this volume).

Some of the most powerful achievements of a relationship perspective derive from the study of peer relationships (see Groh et al., 2014, for a recent summary). Understanding peer relationships as relationships—in terms of their symmetry and age changes—opened the way for an intensive study of the role of peers in individual development (Hartup, 1999). Some of the strongest findings in the attachment field concern the links between early attachment and later functioning with peers. Social competence is strongly related to attachment history (e.g., Sroufe, Egeland, & Carlson, 1999), but beyond this, so too are measures of the quality of specific peer relationships. Both frequency of close friendships and closeness of friendships are related to attachment history (e.g., Elicker, Englund, & Sroufe, 1992; Shulman, Elicker, & Sroufe, 1994). One final example here concerns bullying relationships (Troy & Sroufe, 1987). Again, no measure of individual behavior in the first years has been shown to predict later bullying. Within an attachment perspective, prediction became possible. Moreover, this study showed that the most powerful predictions came from consideration of the attachment histories of *both* partners. Those with secure histories neither bullied nor were the victims of bullies in our extensive play pair assessments. Those with insecure/resistant histories were bullied by those with insecure/avoidant histories but nurtured by those with secure histories.

In adult social psychology as well, the power of studying relationship quality, as opposed to simply individual characteristics or perceptions, has become manifest (e.g., Mikulincer & Shaver, 2007; Simpson & Rholes, 2012). In addition to studying the quality of adult attachment relationships, investigators are probing the details about how adult relationships work, both poorly and well. Thus, for example, studies have concerned mutual regulation between partners and how partners are or are not able to resolve conflict (which itself is predicted by relationship history measures; Salvatore, Kuo, Steele, Simpson, & Collins, 2011; Simpson & Overall, 2014).

Another conceptual advance came from the methodology developed by Ainsworth (e.g., Ainsworth, Blehar, Waters, & Wall 1978). Direct observation is a key to rigorous psychological science, yet observational work is fraught with challenges. For years it seemed that there were only two choices, neither of which was adequate. On the one hand, one could record frequencies of very reliable discrete behaviors (how often a baby cries or smiles, or a mother vocalizes or picks up the infant). Numerous problems plagued this approach. First, much observation was required for such measures to be stable. Second, the same behavior could mean many different things depending on context. (Did the mother pick up the baby when it wanted to be picked up or did her behavior in fact interfere with an infant goal?). Finally, even apparently clear behaviors were ambiguous (was

the verbalization too loud?). Attempts were made to solve some of these problems with complex contingency analyses of behavioral chains, but this proved unwieldy. The second option relied on judgments of observers who typically would watch entire episodes of behavior, then make ratings based on their impressions. Although this had the virtue of attempting to capture the meaning of behavior, such judgments were notably unreliable across raters.

Ainsworth provided a third option, both for her scales of maternal behavior and her attachment rating scales (Ainsworth et al., 1978). She retained the goal of capturing meaning, but she also utilized specific behavioral referents. For illustration, consider the following three vignettes: immediately upon reunion following a brief separation, a baby (1) begins approaching the caregiver, then halfway to her turns off to the side; (2) starts to approach the mother, then halfway to her stops and shows her a toy, smiling broadly; (3) starts to approach, then turns away to a toy, picks it up and, smiling, shows it to the mother. Only the first of these would receive a score for avoidance, and that score would be higher or lower depending on what happened next (e.g., higher, if the infant subsequently ignored the mother's efforts to gain his or her attention). Ainsworth and colleagues (1978) provided multiple possible scenarios for each scale point. While she could, of course, not describe every possible scenario, the varied scenarios allow the rater to engage in template matching, with quite adequate reliability. We used this same approach in many of our behavioral observations across the Minnesota longitudinal study (Sroufe et al., 2005a).

Attachment theory also played a crucial role in solving conceptual problems that were of great importance in the soon-to-emerge field of developmental psychopathology (e.g., Sroufe & Rutter, 1984). These included the problems of explaining continuity and change, understanding the particular role of early experience, and explicating pathology as a developmental outcome. The concept of "developmental pathways," adapted by Bowlby from the work of Waddington (1957), was central to each of these problems.

The pathways model dissolved the question of whether development was characterized by continuity or change by suggesting that there would be increasing probability of following a pathway the longer it had been followed, and that continuity would not be in terms of identical behavior; rather, it would be characterized by transformation and a branching family of outcomes related in terms of meaning. Change was possible at any point of development, but change was constrained by previous adaptation. As Bowlby (1973, p. 412) put it: "Development turns on each and every stage of the journey on an interaction between the organism as it has developed up to that moment and the environment in which it then finds itself." Early experience has a special place in this model because of the cumulative nature of development, always building on what was there before. It certainly does not preordain all outcomes, but neither is it without significance or "erased" (Kagan, 1984) by later experience. Finally, psychopathology is viewed as a product of the cumulative adaptations of the individual as he or she faces the series of developmental issues and challenges. Predictably, problems tend to become more stable with development, and pathway is a more powerful predictor of outcome than are manifest symptoms at a given age (e.g., Moffitt, 1993).

The heterogeneity of all childhood disorders and the ubiquitous comorbidity among them becomes understandable within this framework (Sroufe, 1997). Most important, this approach leads to a new research agenda. The first objectives become to identify early variations in patterns of adaptation that mark initiation of pathways and identify the complex of factors that initiate such patterns. Attachment experiences—that is, parental responsiveness and secure-base provision—are only a part of this picture, but an important part. Other objectives are to trace continuity and change in adaptations in the face of subsequent developmental issues and determine factors that maintain individuals or deflect them from the pathway previously "chosen." In time, this approach would potentially lead to a new system for classifying later problems. In addition, it provokes new attention to prevention and early intervention efforts (see Berlin, Zeanah, & Lieberman, Chapter 32, this volume).

## Empirical Achievements

Empirical achievements of attachment theory, both in adult social psychology and in developmental psychology, are found throughout this volume. Therefore, here I feature only a few, drawing primarily from the Minnesota Longitudinal Study of Risk and Adaptation (e.g., Sroufe et al., 2005a). I group achievements in terms of core hypotheses from attachment theory. These include the fol-

lowing: that variations in infant attachment are rooted in the quality of early parent–infant interaction, that these attachment variations are the foundation for personality formation, and that "internal working models" or representations of the interactive history are the means by which lived experience is carried forward. Work on continuity, change, and "resilience" is highlighted.

### Predicting Attachment Variations from Parent–Infant Interactive History

Based on her extensive observation (72 hours per case), Ainsworth showed that, indeed, caregivers' sensitive responsiveness predicted later attachment security (e.g., Ainsworth et al., 1978). Others using less extensive but still substantial observation replicated these results, with a correlation of about .50 (Pederson, Gleason, Moran, & Bento, 1998; Posada et al., 1999). Correlations are more modest with less observation but are still consistently found (see De Wolff & Van IJzendoorn, 1997, for a meta-analysis). Moreover, studies that included measures of infant temperament find that only caregiver sensitivity, not temperament, predicts attachment outcomes (e.g., National Institute of Child Health and Human Development Early Child Care Research Network [NICHD ECCRN], 1997; Sroufe et al., 2005a). (See also Fearon & Belsky, Chapter 14, and Vaughn & Bost, Chapter 10, this volume.)

### Predictability of Later Behavior from the Early Years

In the 1960s and early 1970s, before attachment theory had taken hold, developmental psychology was in a strange place. It was being put forward that there was little to no continuity in development, especially from the early years of life (Kagan & Moss, 1962). Moreover, it was claimed that constructs such as attachment (Masters & Wellman, 1974) and even personality (Mischel, 1968) were of little use because behavior of individuals was so unstable across time and contexts. Thus, it has been of great importance to the entire field to establish that such cross-time and even cross-context linkages can be established. As discussed earlier, this was done by moving to the level of the organization of behavior and showing that individual patterns of organization in early life forecast patterns of adaptation with regard to the salient issues of subsequent developmental periods. Behavior is expected to change across contexts; for example, the well-adapted infant explores actively in the caregiver's presence but effectively seeks contact when distressed, and the well-adapted preschooler plays with exuberance in the play yard but sits quietly during story time (Block & Block, 1980). And behavior must change with development. Children who are ineffective in using the caregiver for comforting, including those who show avoidance, later are more dependent, whereas those who are effectively dependent infants later are more autonomous (Sroufe, Fox, & Pancake, 1983). No one expects loyal friendships among infants, but they are a hallmark of successful adaptation in middle childhood. Using such an understanding, clear evidence of continuity (coherence of adaptation) from infancy to adulthood has been demonstrated (Sroufe et al., 2005a). Links are especially strong to measures of self-management, dependency, and peer relationships. With adequate outcome data, which we were able to obtain in our extensive preschool and summer camp studies, correlations in the .40s and .50s were common. Nothing in the early years predicted better than attachment history, likely because it summarizes so much of what is going on in the development of the infant.

A more recent body of work provided dramatic evidence of intergenerational continuity. Every step in a cyclical chain beginning with disorganized attachment has been established. Disorganized attachment in one generation predicts disorganized attachment in the next (Main, Hesse, & Kaplan, 2005; Raby, Steele, Carlson, & Sroufe, 2015). More important are the links in the chain. Disorganized attachment predicts the tendency to dissociate throughout childhood and into adulthood (Carlson, 1998). As reviewed by Lyons-Ruth and Jacobvitz (Chapter 29, this volume), disorganized attachment and dissociation predict lack of resolution of loss or trauma in the Adult Attachment Interview (AAI), and lack of resolution in the AAI predicts frightening parental behavior. Furthermore, frightening parental behavior predicts, as theoretically specified, disorganized attachment in the infant of the next generation, so the cycle is complete (Jacobvitz, Hazen, & Riggs, 1997; Schuengel, Bakermans-Kranenburg, Van IJzendoorn, & Blom, 1999).

For many reasons it is not surprising that early attachment experiences forecast later development (Sroufe, Egeland, Carlson, & Collins, 2005b). First, having experienced responsive care, those with secure histories tend to experience a basic sense of connection with others and a be-

lief that relationships are valuable. Second, such individuals also begin life with positive expectations about themselves and their ability to elicit support from others. Having had a secure base for exploration, they bring to the social world a curiosity, a zest for discovery, a positive problem-solving attitude, and a set of instrumental skills that make them attractive social partners. Having experienced effective dyadic affect regulation during infancy, children with secure histories have a solid foundation for emotion regulation and self-management in later years. They believe that self-regulation in the face of challenge and recovery from periods of dysregulation are possible, and they have brain excitatory and inhibitory systems that are properly tuned for achieving both. Finally, as part of an empathic, reciprocating relational system, they now have an understanding of how effective relationships work and a capacity for empathic responsiveness to others. (See also Thompson, Chapter 16, this volume.)

None of this is to say that attachment experiences by themselves determine later development, or that early secure attachments are a guarantee of later healthy adjustment, or that anxious early attachments cannot be overcome. Change, as well as continuity, is central to the theory.

## Continuity, Change, and Studies of Representation

Although demonstrating continuity from the early years forward was an important achievement, the predictability and coherence of change also followed from Bowlby's theory. Indeed, in the Minnesota Longitudinal Study of Risk and Adaptation, we were able to account for change, age by age (Sroufe et al., 2005a). During the infancy period, when family stress decreased or social support increased, change from anxious to secure attachment was more likely. At later ages also, as family stress and support changed, or as maternal depression waxed and waned, so too did child behavior problems. Moreover, we were able to show that representations of experience played a key role in continuity and change (Carlson, Sroufe, & Egeland, 2004). First, assessments of representation—through stories, drawings, projective techniques, and narrative interviews—were predictable throughout childhood and adolescence into adulthood from infant attachment variations. Second, there was interplay between representation and experience as predicted by theory. At any given age, measures of representation predicted adaptation at the next age, with earlier behavior held constant. At the same time, measures of behavior predicted representation at the later age, with prior representation controlled. This is the same thing as saying that representation predicted change in behavior, while, reciprocally, experience predicted change in representation, age by age. (For discussion of representational processes, see Bretherton & Munholland, Chapter 4, this volume.)

### The Fate of Early Experience Following Change: Resilience

According to Bowlby's pathways model, one's entire developmental history is always part of the array of influences acting on the person. This suggests that, even following change, early experience is not erased. The Minnesota longitudinal study provided data for examining this hypothesis (Sroufe et al., 2005a; Sroufe, Egeland, & Kreutzer, 1990). We began by defining what we viewed as two groups of preschool-age children. They had in common a consistently high level of behavior problems across three assessment periods. (Indeed, based on a position that change erases early experience, there is only one group.) What distinguished them was that some had a history of secure attachment, whereas others had an insecure history. When we conducted follow-up research when children were in third grade, children with secure histories had significantly fewer behavior problems than those with insecure histories. We repeated such a demonstration at subsequent ages. Similarly, those with insecure attachment histories, who for a time do well, are more vulnerable to subsequent problems. Early experience is not erased.

These findings shed light on the phenomenon of *resilience* as a developmental process. Had our study only begun, for example, in the preschool years, we still would have found that some children bounced back from their period of difficulty and by this criterion could be said to be resilient. However, it would have been fallacious to consider this capacity simply an inherent characteristic of some children. It is simply a label for the phenomenon of recovery. More of an explanation derives from knowing the history that provides the foundation for recovery. When history and current supports are taken into account, very little mystery remains in this kind of resilience.

A more classic definition of *resilience* is the capacity to do well in the face of adversity (Masten, 2001). For example, high family stress is as-

sociated with child behavior problems. But not all children facing high stress show such problems, and it would be possible to "explain" this by saying they are resilient. Once again, our data show that those with histories of secure attachment are significantly less likely to manifest problems in the face of stress (Pianta, Egeland, & Sroufe, 1990). A secure attachment history provides a foundation for coping with adversity, likely both because of internal resources and the capacity to draw on external social support. The capacities to rebound, to cope with adversity, and to take advantage of turning points for growth all are predicted by attachment history (Sroufe et al., 2005a).

## Vulnerabilities of Attachment Theory

All theories have vulnerabilities—incoherence in propositions, illogical deductions, predictions that are not distinctive, and the like. But a very successful theory faces two particular and related hazards. These are overreaching, or trying to explain everything, and the belief that the theory is the total explanation for any phenomenon. These are certainly risks for attachment theory. With such expansionism, the theory risks losing its core, losing sight of what it was specifically designed to explain and explain well. As Sandra Scarr (personal communication, September 1978) once asked, "Is attachment theory simply a theory that all good things go together?" Were this so, it would not be much of a theory.

Over the years almost everything has been suggested at one time or another to be related to attachment variations, from grammatical language acquisition to map reading to IQ. One actual finding from our study is that infant attachment security predicted math achievement scores in high school. Although one can come up with a rationale to explain this finding (and possibly even posit post hoc some common underlying brain mechanisms), we resisted the idea of publishing this finding that we believed to be misleading. It is not likely that attachment evolved to prepare individual brains for understanding math. In fact, the most likely explanation of this correlation is that math achievement is highly related to school attendance, and for a variety of reasons (including getting along with peers and teachers, and having parents who support schooling), those with secure histories have better attendance. In support of this, attachment history does not predict reading achievement, which is not as dependent on attendance as is math achievement.

Attachment theory makes very specific predictions—to positive expectations concerning self, other, and relationships; to a basic sense of security; to the capacity to draw support from, and offer support to, others; to emotion regulation; and to a well functioning personality. It should not and does not predict to everything, including many aspects of cognitive functioning.

Likewise, attachment history is not the only thing that predicts important outcomes, even in the social arena. There are many critical influences on development, including other relationships both inside and outside of the family, as well as the broader contextual situation surrounding the developing child. Siblings, peers, schools, neighborhoods, and socioeconomic status all are known to have important influences. As pointed out in the earlier discussion of resilience, attachment history was important; but intervening changes in social support and life stress being experienced by the family also played a role. To account fully for resilience, all of these factors needed to be considered.

Attachment is not even all there is to parenting. Parents do much more than provide a haven of safety and a secure base for exploration, important as these provisions are. Parents provide limits and boundaries, socialize the expression of emotion, instill values through their example, promote or inhibit exchanges with the broader social environment, select and encourage a range of experiences to which the child is exposed, among many other things (see Table 43.1). Assimilating all of this to attachment will curtail our knowledge of parental influence and even interfere with the task of understanding attachment because it disallows the possibility of studying how attachment experiences work in concert with other experiences.

We developed strong measures of several key aspects of early parenting that we viewed as outside the purview of attachment. These included measures of limit setting, parent–child boundary dissolution (a form of overstimulation), and parental scaffolding of problem solving. In addition, we also assessed parental intrusiveness (Ainsworth's Cooperation–Interference Scale in infancy), the quality and stability of the home environment, and promotion of autonomy in early adolescence (Sroufe et al., 2005b). Although each of these show some correlation with attachment security, they certainly are not identical to attachment, and they play distinctive roles in development.

A first example concerns school outcomes. Attachment history does correlate with a range of school outcomes, mostly tapping relationships with school personnel and commitment to school. For example, it predicts dropping out of school. But parental scaffolding for problem solving, which we measured at age 3½ years in our laboratory, was a far stronger predictor. This measure tapped how well the parent structured four problems for the child, provided relevant help, and properly sequenced this help, moving neither too fast nor too slow, helping but not taking over (Englund, Luckner, Whaley, & Egeland, 2004; Sroufe et al., 2005a). This single measure predicted a host of educational outcomes, everything we measured, from years of school completed to returning for a general equivalency degree (GED) for those who dropped out.

Prediction of attention-deficit/hyperactivity disorder (ADHD) symptoms provides another example. Although insecure attachment is probabilistically related to behavior problems in general

**TABLE 43.1. The Tasks of Parenting**

- Regulation of arousal
- Appropriately modulated stimulation
- Provision of secure base and safe haven
- Appropriate guidance, limits, and structure
- Maintenance of parent–child boundaries
- Socialization of emotional expression and containment
- Scaffolding for problem solving
- Supporting mastery and achievement
- Supporting contacts with the broader social world
- Accepting the child's growing independence

and certain forms of specific problems, it is not at all well related to ADHD symptoms in particular (Sroufe et al., 2005a). In contrast, certain other aspects of parenting, as well as other features of the developmental landscape, are clearly predictive of ADHD, both as a category and as symptom scores. Ainsworth's Intrusiveness measure at 6 months and parent–child boundary problems at 24 and 42 months are all related to ADHD. The 42-month measure, taken from the problem-solving task described earlier, was the single best predictor at multiple follow-up ages (Carlson, Jacobvitz, & Sroufe, 1995). This measure taps a particular issue with dysregulation. A high score results when the parent provokes, cajoles, teases, flirts with, or otherwise increases the child's level of stimulation precisely at those times when the child is already becoming overtaxed by the problems and is beginning to lose control. Thus, as the child approaches the edge of overarousal and loss of control, the parental behavior pushes the child over the edge, undermining the child's belief in his or her ability to modulate arousal, as well as the actual capacity for self-control. Parents receiving low scores maintain a calm, reassuring presence at these times and increase their support, helping the child achieve both the sense of and capacity for self-regulation. This is a critically important parental role. In addition to this parenting measure, we found that measures of family life stress and stability or chaos in the home environment also predicted ADHD symptoms. When the measures of overstimulating parenting were combined with these measures of the surrounding environment, predictions to ADHD symptoms became quite strong, dwarfing endogenous measures of neurological status or temperament. But security of attachment played a minor role in this picture.

Even when we focus on an outcome with clear theoretical links to attachment, such as quality of later social relationships, other aspects of parenting proved to be important as well. For example, in our summer camp studies, we were able to develop a measure of "friendship competence" (forming and maintaining a reciprocal, loyal friendship; Elicker et al., 1992). This was indeed related to attachment history, while accounting for 13% of the variance. However, when attachment was combined with the other measures of supportive parenting described earlier, the variance accounted for doubled, with a multiple $r$ of .52. Time after time, with a range of outcome measures, the broader measure of parenting was almost always more powerful than attachment alone.

Peer experiences also are an important influence on development, without doubt. The question of whether they are more important than attachment or other parenting variables misses the mark (Harris, 1998). The most important developmental question concerns how the two influences work together. We miss this question entirely when we try to explain everything in terms of attachment.

As reported earlier, infant attachment security is a clear predictor of peer competence, at every age. It provides an important motivational foundation for close relationships and exploratory and regulation capacities that make one attractive to peers. Still, what one gains from peer experiences also contributes to later social competence. We see social competence as constructed step by step, with each phase based on the foundation that was laid down before. Thus, with preschool peers, one learns a great deal about sustaining and chaining interactions in the face of difficulties, about selecting preferred partners, and about participating in groups per se. These experiences are unique because peers are equals (as the word signifies): One does not hold authority over the other. All of these experiences prepare the child for the loyal friendships and adherence to peer group norms that are the hallmark of middle childhood. These latter experiences then support the more intimate relationships of adolescence and negotiating the complexities of the adolescent social world, with same- and cross-gender friendships and same- and mixed-gender group functioning. It is no surprise that peer functioning at each age predicts social competence measures at the next. Moreover, when peer experiences are combined with attachment history and other aspects of parenting history, predictions increase over what either parenting or peer experiences alone can predict. In the case of the middle childhood friendship competence measure I discussed earlier, adding preschool teacher peer competence ratings to the equation raises the resulting multiple $r$ to .62 ($r^2 = .38$), now triple the variance accounted for by attachment history alone.

Early attachment history and later family experiences or later peer experiences can combine in a variety of complex ways depending on the particular outcome (Sroufe et al., 2005b). Sometimes the joint influence is simply additive, as I have just described. Another example of this concerns the prediction of observed hostility in adult couple interaction. Such hostility is predicted by insecure attachment in infancy. But it is also predicted by teacher rankings of peer competence in grades 1–3. These are independent predictors, with neither mediating the other.

Sometimes the impact of early attachment is partially mediated by another influence. We obtained observation-based measures of parental support for the 13-year-old child's emerging autonomy. Some of the variance of attachment history in predicting hostility in adult relationships was mediated by this later parenting measure. Still, early attachment remained a significant predictor. But with another adult outcome—conflict resolution, infant attachment history fell to nonsignificance once the age-13 measure was included. Depending on outcome, a variety of results were obtained, and this was also true when peer relationship measures at various ages were combined with attachment history. Sometimes only attachment history predicted, and sometimes only the peer measure predicted. But much more often, consideration of both was critical, with joint effects, including mediation, being the rule (Sroufe et al., 2005b). None of this trivializes the importance of attachment history. In fact, infant attachment gains importance as a construct when it is considered within a broader developmental framework.

Another potential hazard in attachment research is assuming the existence of a causal link when infant attachment is related to some later outcome. First, it is important to show that a third factor, such as IQ, life stress, or other experiential variables, is not a primary player. Second, as I just discussed, it is important to explore whether the link is mediated by some third variable. It is perhaps even more hazardous to conclude causal developmental linkages in the case of correlates of adult attachment measures. Not only must there be controls for relevant third variables, in addition, one must be cautious regarding assuming developmental antecedents. One example here will suffice.

Individuals with borderline personality disorder (BPD) features have been reported to be both "unresolved" and "preoccupied" in the AAI. This is a replicable finding (Dozier, Stovall-McClough, & Albus, 2008; Macfie, Swan, Fitzpatrick, Watkins, & Rivas, 2014; Stovall-McClough & Dozier, Chapter 31, this volume). Given the prevalence of trauma in the history of these problems, it is almost statistically guaranteed that they will more likely be unresolved regarding trauma. (One cannot be unresolved with regard to trauma if there was no history of trauma.) It is also plausible given the emotional volatility of such persons

that nonmodulated anger would characterize the transcripts of these individuals when describing their parental relationships. So these results make sense. But the conclusion that these interview responses and BPD itself are the result of resistant attachment in infancy is not a logical deduction and cannot be justified by the adult correlation itself. This can only be determined with prospective, longitudinal data. Although such data confirm that disorganized attachment in infancy and a history of trauma predict borderline symptoms (Carlson, Egeland, & Sroufe, 2009), anxious/resistant attachment in infancy does not predict borderline symptoms. In fact, with the exception of anxiety, and to a lesser extent depression, we did not find resistant attachment to be a risk factor for severe psychopathology. In our high-quality data set, in which infant attachment was assessed twice and efforts were made to distinguish resistant from disorganized attachment, resistance does not even predict conduct problems (Sroufe et al., 2005a). This is in contrast to avoidant attachment. This does not make the correlation between preoccupied AAI status and borderline symptoms meaningless. It has the importance of any other marker of a disturbed process. But it is an overreach to speak of preoccupied status as a cause of borderline symptoms.

## The Place of Attachment in Development

Our understanding that attachment experiences work in concert with other developmental influences raises larger questions about how to conceptualize the place of attachment in the organic *process* of development. I suggested earlier that attachment provides a foundation for entrée into the peer group, but then peer experiences in turn promote new capacities for social relationships. A "developmental issues" perspective (Breger, 1974; Erikson, 1950/1963; Sander, 1975; Sroufe, 1979) is useful for expanding this observation into a more general framework.

Although they have certain similarities, a developmental issues framework is distinctive from classic stage theories in important ways. First, the series of issues that may be outlined are not tasks to be passed or failed; rather, each issue is negotiated in the continuing process of development. Children evolve patterns of adaptation with respect to any given issue, but regardless of how well the issue is engaged, one has no choice but to move on to the negotiation of subsequent issues. There is no concept of developmental arrest, nor is a premium placed on age of accomplishment. Moreover, while issues come to the fore in various developmental periods, an issue is not permanently put behind but rather is negotiated further in subsequent phases of life.

There is, of course, an important way in which a developmental issues position is like a stage theory; it is proposed that adaptation with regard to each issue frames in part the person's negotiation of subsequent issues. However, it is also assumed that negotiating a subsequent issue provides an opportunity for reworking all previous issues.

Table 43.2 outlines a proposed series of issues to illustrate this approach. Adaptation builds on the history of functioning in each previous period, while also providing opportunities for transforming previously established adaptations. For example, consider the second issue. This is labeled "Guided Self-Regulation," because toddlers may achieve varying degrees and styles of self-regulation, but they can do so only within guidance and scaffolding provided by caregivers. Adequate regulation—that is, a balance between free expression of desires and containment of impulses and an ability to remain organized in the face of moderate frustration—requires clear, firm support and containment, as well as encouragement, on the part of parents. When parents are unavailable for support, provoke or ridicule the child when he or she becomes frustrated, and/or harshly punish the child for expressions of emotions or impulsive behaviors, various forms of dysregulation are observed. This guided self-regulation process in general proceeds more smoothly when it has been preceded by an effective attachment relationship (or establishment of trust in Erik Erikson's scheme). As research has clearly shown, infants with a secure attachment relationship are more compliant with parental directions (Londerville & Main, 1981; Matas, Arend, & Sroufe, 1978) and even more "committed" to compliance (Kochanska, 1997) and to maintaining a coordinated relationship (Waters, Kondo-Ikemura, & Richters, 1990). Thus, effective attachment, and the experience with dyadic affect regulation and positive expectations regarding caregivers that is part of it, provides the foundation for beginning autonomy and self-control. Those with secure histories have already learned to count on parental availability and know that parents are dependable and therefore will follow through on what they say. Reciprocally, when parents are firm and supportive with toddlers, the child's trust in them is deepened. Some parents, of course, find this developmental period difficult given the child's strong impulses and labile feelings. Even parents who provided a secure base in infancy may be unable to meet the challenges posed by toddlers. So while early attachment provides a foundation for negotiating Phase 2, it does not by itself determine the outcome.

Forecasting the quality of adaptation in Phase 3 is even more complex. The well-adapted preschool child can flexibly adjust behavior to fit requirements of a particular context (run and shout on the playground, sit quietly and be attentive during story time), can direct his or her own activities, can follow rules without constant adult presence, and can effectively engage peers and sustain interactions despite challenges that inevitably arise. These capacities draw on attachment experiences that color the child's attitudes and expectations about self, other, and relationships, and an early pattern of basic affect regulation. But they also draw on the history of more autonomous regulation during Phase 2 and the supports that are currently available. From infancy, some children bring forward a capacity for engaging the object world with curiosity and positive affect. From the toddler period, if it goes well, they bring forward the capacity to stay organized in the face of frustration and a belief that they can cope with challenges. If emotional support remains available and if opportunities are provided, they now manifest a capacity for self-regulation and are attractive play partners, well liked by teachers and children. On the other hand, children who are lacking in feelings of self-worth, who are easily frustrated and dysregulated, who lack empathy or the skills for positive engagement, or are chronically angry, inhibited, or withdrawn, are at a notable disadvantage for engaging the world of preschool. The cumulative nature of development—the way it builds upon itself—helps to account for the strong intercorrelations among competence indices in the preschool period, including sociometric status, self-confidence, dependence–independence, empathy, ego-resilience, self-control, and rule-abiding behavior (e.g., Sroufe, 1983, 2005a). All of these, and other currently in vogue constructs such as "executive function," build on the same preceding core experiences (Bernier, Whipple, & Carlson, 2010).

As was true in Phase 2, strong support in the preschool period can help those with less adequate

**TABLE 43.2. Salient Issues of Development**

Infancy period

Major issue: Formation of an effective attachment relationship
Subsidiary issues
    Beginning reciprocity
    Dyadic affect regulation
    Attachment/exploration balance

Toddler period

Major issue: Guided self-regulation
Subsidiary issues
    Increased autonomy
    Increased awareness of self and others
    Awareness of standards for behavior
    Self-conscious emotions

Preschool period

Major issue: Self-regulation
Subsidiary issues
    Self-reliance with support (agency)
    Self-management
    Expanding social world
    Internalization of rules and values

School years

Major issue: Competence
Subsidiary issues
    Personal effectance
    Self-integration
    Competence with peers
    Place in group
    Functioning in group
    Loyal friendships
    Competence in school

Adolescence

Major issue: Individuation
Subsidiary issues
    Autonomy with connectedness
    Identity
    Peer network competence
    Place in network
    Functioning in network
    Intimate relationships
    Coordinating school, work, and social life

Transition to adulthood

Major issue: Emancipation
Subsidiary issues
    Launching a life course
    Financial responsibility
    Adult social competence
    Coordinating partnerships and friendships
    Coordinating colleagues, partners, and friends
    Stable partnerships
    Coordinating work, training, career, and life

beginnings move toward increased self-regulation capacities and more positive expectations regarding relationships. Our research has shown that those with histories of insecure attachment are better adjusted during the preschool period if social support for parents has increased in the years since infancy (Sroufe et al., 2005a). We also found that supportive preschool teachers can have a positive impact (Sroufe, 1983). Others have shown that social skill may be increased through play with more competent peers (Hartup, 1999). Again, both developmental history and current support play a role in adaptation. New issues are faced within the framework of prior adaptations, yet transformation remains possible, for better or worse.

The process continues in middle childhood. Having expanded the capacity for self-regulation, having had positive experiences in an expanding social world, and having rapidly acquired the skills needed in social interaction, some children are now well prepared for the more complicated world of middle childhood, with its greater academic and social challenges. For many, self-confidence becomes real-world competence, and interactive skill merges into durable, loyal friendships that can be maintained even given the need to function in the larger group. The basic sense of connection from infancy, the impulse control and autonomy from the toddler period, and the self-management capacities from the preschool period are all called upon. Reciprocally, positive social experiences in middle childhood or developing some special talent can enhance self-esteem now and help children become more able social partners.

Adolescence can be the most challenging developmental period of all in modern society. Social demands are extraordinarily complex, with same- and mixed-gender peer groups, same- and mixed-gender friendships, and beginning intimate relationships. Cognitive and physical changes can be both helpful and daunting. For example, the individual now confronts the future in a new way. Though challenging for all, the issues faced here are certainly easier for some. Whereas many teens develop psychiatric problems, many actually flower. There are no guarantees, of course. However, for some, the foundation for successful negotiation of the issues of adolescence has been laid down every step of the way. The capacity to be vulnerable and to commit in relationships has roots in the trust established in infancy. Autonomy with connectedness already was established once during the toddler phase. Self-regulation (and effective use of social support) has been practiced since the preschool years. And a sense of competence and mastery was firmly established during the years of middle childhood, along with first experiences of close, durable relationships with agemates.

This developmental perspective certainly highlights many features of experiential support beyond the quality of early attachments. At the same time, infant attachment experiences certainly are not trivialized by this description. Development is a cumulative process, which each phase building on all that has gone before, just like the developing embryo or the developing brain (Stiles, 2008). Therefore, the infant–caregiver attachment relationship, coming as it does at the beginning, is of notable importance. It represents an inner core of an emerging self that, while certainly open to modification, remains an important feature of the developmental landscape.

## Goals for the Future

Fifty years ago it was generally accepted in psychology that early experience had little predictive power, that individual characteristics were unstable, and that constructs such as personality might not even be useful. Today we know that early life does leave a lasting legacy, that individual development and behavior are coherent when assessed at an appropriate level of complexity, and that constructs such as personality and attachment not only have validity but are crucial for the field. We also can put aside debates about whether early experience or later experience, or parenting or peer experiences, are more important. We know they are all important, and we know they work together to shape development. Likewise, important progress has been made toward an integrated view of experience and neurophysiology. It is clear that the developing brain is experience-dependent (Stiles, 2008). There is also support for the idea that early experience retains potential for influence even following developmental change, and that representations are the carriers and preservers of early experience. These are monumental achievements, and attachment research has played a vital role in all of this.

What might be important goals for this field going forward? I suggest just four areas that seem of great importance to me. A central theme in all of them is that work in each area would promote our understanding of both attachment and devel-

opment. At the same time, it is important to retain some focus on the core of attachment theory, namely, Bowlby's questions regarding how parent–child interactions influence the nature of the attachment relationships that are formed and how it is that attachment experiences are the foundation for individual differences in personality.

Regarding Bowlby's first question we need more detailed studies regarding exactly what kinds of experience promote later effective secure-base behavior. Ainsworth's Sensitivity Scales, soon to be published in the revision of the classic book (Ainsworth et al., 1978), provide a wealth of ideas about the kind of attunement and responsiveness that are important, but this topic requires a great deal of further exploration. There also are very few data regarding experiences that lead to resistant versus avoidant attachment. A modicum of data suggest that avoidance results from rejection precisely when the infant signals a tender need (e.g., Ainsworth et al., 1978; Isabella, 1993), but the origins of these two patterns—if indeed they are coherent and distinctive—is not really established. Some argue that a security dimension captures what there is in valid individual differences. But if there are distinctive patterns, and if they prove to have distinctive outcomes, this is of great theoretical and practical significance. There are some data supporting different outcomes for avoidant and resistant histories (Sroufe et al., 2005a), but the case is not nearly as strong as it would need to be to conclude that these are distinctive patterns.

A very important developmental question arises from findings concerning the discordance between infant attachment classifications with two parents. In general, studies report significant but moderate concordance between the two classifications (Fox, Kimmerly, & Schafer, 1991; Main & Weston, 1981). Some of the lack of concordance may be due to methodological issues (e.g., including cases in which both parents are not actually attachment figures), but this cannot be the total explanation. Main and Weston (1881), for example, provides information that specific interactive history with the particular parent predicts security and also that considering the two attachments bolsters outcome predictions. Therefore, we can conclude that at least in a substantial number of cases, an infant may be secure with one parent and anxious with another. According to Bowlby's theory, the infant would have two separate working models of attachment. The intriguing question then becomes, how do these disparate models become integrated into a singular state of mind regarding attachment, as is suggested to be the case in all of the adult attachment literature (Hesse, 1999, Chapter 26, this volume)? Main's data suggest the possibility that infant attachment status with the more primary figure might hold sway, but other factors have to be involved as well. To date I know of no studies of this truly critical question.

In general, we need to know much more about how attachment experiences combine with other developmental influences, be they child vulnerabilities (however they may arise), other aspects of parenting, or other features of the environment. We know, for example, that insecure infant attachment is a risk factor for various kinds of later problems, but we currently understand little about why one child with a particular attachment history develops one problem, whereas other children with the same early attachment develop different kinds of problems or no psychiatric problems at all. Such an understanding is critical for the field of developmental psychopathology and embodies the hope for a new approach to psychiatric classification. This example also points us to the more general problem of continuity and change, a core issue for all developmental study. We know by now that continuity depends on supports for pathways being followed and that change is lawful, that is, that it can be predicted to some extent. Over periods of time, representations change or behavior changes, and some intervening variable accounts for some of this change. But at this point our knowledge is rather crude, usually based on broadband predictors (e.g., changes in life stress or parental depression). Thus, we have associations between some measure and some indicator of change, but we still know very little about the process of change. We do not even know, for example, whether attachment representations change gradually or quickly, or much about how they change. Do certain kinds of experiences lead to more rapid change and others to gradual change? Is gradual change sustained better? Do changes in representations of partners lead to changes in representations of parents? There are myriad questions about attachment and the process of development.

Finally, it is important to increase research on attachment and the *mind* exponentially. There are many articles and chapters on attachment and the *brain*, and that is a topic for this volume also (see Bretherton & Munholland, Chapter 4, and Coan, Chapter 12, this volume). But little has been written about attachment and the developing mind. With the exception of the connection between unresolved status on the AAI and early trauma

and disorganization, we are not even very far along in understanding the origins and course of adult states of mind regarding attachment. Beyond this, we know little about processes linking attachment experiences and distortions of the mind, including various defensive postures. We know that cognitive skills are rarely impaired in those having histories of insecure attachment, but there is more to the mind than this. There are vast differences in the individual process of finding meaning, and in the meanings individuals make of particular experiences; for example, how it comes to be that the same experience is threatening to some and benign or amusing to others. Perhaps Kahneman's (2011) distinction between fast and slow mental systems is a starting point. The "fast" system, which is intuitive, unreflective, and uncritical (the source of many biases and distortions in thinking and perception), may be more colored by an individual's particular history, especially by trauma and distortions in attachment. Whether this is truly so, the process through which it develops to be this way, and the particular role of attachment in this process, all wait to be discovered.

Attachment theory has proven to be quite robust and generative. Its contributions are apparent in diverse fields of study. Whether it will continue to grow in utility in the future may well hinge on keeping it wed to a developmental perspective, where it was in the beginning.

## References

Ainsworth, M. D. S., Blehar, M., Waters, E., & Wall, S. (1978). *Patterns of attachment.* Hillsdale, NJ: Erlbaum.

Bernier, A., Whipple, N., & Carlson, S. (2010). From external regulation to self-regulation: Early parenting precursors of young children's executive functioning. *Child Development, 81,* 326–339.

Block, J., & Block, J. H. (1980). The role of ego-control and ego-resiliency in the organization of behavior. In W. A. Collins (Ed.), *Minnesota Symposia on Child Psychology: Vol. 13. Development of cognition, affect, and social relations* (pp. 39–101). Hillsdale, NJ: Erlbaum.

Bowlby, J. (1973). *Attachment and loss: Vol. 2. Separation.* New York: Basic Books.

Bowlby, J. (1982). *Attachment and loss: Vol. 1. Attachment.* New York: Basic Books. (Original work published 1969)

Breger, L. (1974). *From instinct to identity.* Englewood Cliffs: Prentice-Hall.

Carlson, E. A. (1998). A prospective longitudinal study of attachment disorganization/disorientation. *Child Development, 69*(4), 1107–1128.

Carlson, E. A., Egeland, B., & Sroufe, L. A. (2009). A

prospective investigation of the development of borderline personality symptoms. *Development and Psychopathology, 21,* 1311–1334.

Carlson, E. A., Jacobvitz, D., & Sroufe, L. A. (1995). A developmental investigation of inattentiveness and hyperactivity. *Child Development, 66,* 37–54.

Carlson, E. A., Sroufe, L. A., & Egeland, B. (2004). The construction of experience: A longitudinal study of representation and behavior. *Child Development, 75*(1), 66–83.

de Wolff, M. S., & Van Ijzendoorn, M. H. (1997). Sensitivity and attachment: A meta-analysis on parental antecedents of infant attachment. *Child Development, 68,* 571–591.

Dozier, M., Stovall-McClough, K., & Albus, K. (2008). Attachment and psychopathology in adulthood. In J. Cassidy & P. R. Shaver (Eds.), *Handbook of attachment* (2nd ed., pp.718–744). New York: Guilford Press.

Elicker, J., Englund, M., & Sroufe, L. A. (1992). Predicting peer competence and peer relationships in childhood from early parent–child relationships. In R. Parke & G. Ladd (Eds.), *Family–peer relationships: Modes of linkage* (pp. 77–106). Hillsdale, NJ: Erlbaum.

Englund, M., Luckner, A., Whaley, G., & Egeland, B. (2004). Children's achievement in early elementary school: Longitudinal effects of parental involvement, expectations, and quality of assistance. *Journal of Educational Psychology, 96,* 723–730.

Erikson, E. (1963). *Childhood and society.* New York: Norton. (Original work published 1950)

Fox, N., Kimmerly, N., & Schafer, W. (1991). Attachment to mother/attachment to father: A meta-analysis. *Child Development, 62,* 210–225.

Groh, A., Fearon, R. P., Bakermans-Kranenberg, M., Van IJzendoorn, M., Steele, R., & Roisman, G. (2014). The significance of attachment security for children's social competence with peers: A meta-analytic study. *Attachment and Human Development, 16*(2), 103–136.

Harris, J. (1998). *The nurture assumption: Why children turn out the way they do.* New York: Free Press.

Hartup, W. (1999). Peer experience and its developmental significance. In M. Bennett (Ed.), *Developmental psychology: Achievements and prospects* (pp. 106–125). Philadelphia: Psychology Press.

Hesse, E. (1999). The Adult Attachment Interview: Historical and current perspectives. In J. Cassidy & P. R. Shaver (Eds.), *Handbook of attachment: Theory, research, and clinical applications* (pp. 395–433). New York: Guilford Press.

Hinde, R. (1979). *Towards understanding relationships.* London: Academic Press.

Isabella, R. (1993). Origins of attachment: Maternal interactive behavior across the first year. *Child Development, 64,* 605–621.

Jacobvitz, D., Hazen, N., & Riggs, S. (1997, March). *Disorganized mental processes in mothers, frightened/frightening caregiving, and disorganized/disoriented behavior in infancy.* Paper presented at the meeting of the Society for Research in Child Development, Washington, DC.

Kagan, J. (1984). *The nature of the child.* New York: Basic Books.

Kagan, J., & Moss, H. (1962). *Birth to maturity.* New York: Wiley.

Kahneman, D. (2011). *Thinking, fast and slow.* New York: Farrar, Straus & Giroux.

Kochanska, G. (1997). Multiple pathways to conscience formation for children with different temperaments: From toddlerhood to age 5. *Developmental Psychology, 33,* 228–248.

Londerville, S., & Main, M. (1981). Security of attachment, compliance, and maternal training methods in the second year of life. *Developmental Psychology, 17,* 289–299.

Macfie, J., Swan, S., Fitzpatrick, K., Watkins, C., & Rivas, E. (2014). Mothers with borderline personality and their young children: Adult attachment interviews, mother–child interactions, and the children's narrative representations. *Development and Psychopathology, 26,* 539–551.

Main, M., Hesse, E., & Kaplan, N. (2005). Predictability of attachment behavior and representational processes at 1, 6, and 19 years of age. In K. E. Grossmann, K. Grossmann, & E. Waters (Eds.), *The power of longitudinal attachment research: From infancy and childhood to adulthood* (pp. 245–304). New York: Guilford Press.

Main, M., & Weston, D. (1981). The quality of the toddler's relationship to mother and father: Related to conflict behavior and to readiness to form new relationships. *Child Development, 52,* 932–940.

Masten, A. S. (2001). Ordinary magic: Resilience processes in development. *American Psychologist, 56*(3), 227–238.

Masters, J., & Wellman, H. (1974). Human infant attachment: A procedural critique. *Psychological Bulletin, 81,* 218–237.

Matas, L., Arend, R., & Sroufe, L. A. (1978). Continuity of adaptation in the second year: The relationship between quality of attachment and later competence. *Child Development, 49,* 547–556.

Mikulincer, M., & Shaver, P. (2007). *Attachment in adulthood: Structure, dynamics, and change.* New York: Guilford Press.

Mischel, W. (1968). *Personality and assessment.* New York: Wiley.

Moffitt, T. (1993). Adolescence-limited and life-course-persistent antisocial behavior: A developmental taxonomy. *Psychological Review, 100,* 674–701.

NICHD Early Child Care Research Network. (1997). The effects of infant child care on infant–mother attachment security: Results of the NICHD study of early child care. *Child Development, 68,* 860–879.

Pederson, D., Gleason, K., Moran, G., & Bento, S. (1998). Maternal attachment representations, maternal sensitivity, and the infant–mother attachment relationship. *Developmental Psychology, 34,* 925–933.

Pianta, R., Egeland, B., & Sroufe, L. A. (1990). Maternal stress in childrens' development: Predictions of school outcomes and identification of protective factors. In J. E. Rolf, A. Masten, D. Cicchetti, K. Neuchterlen, & S. Weintraub (Eds.), *Risk and protective factors in the development of psychopathology* (pp. 215–235). New York: Cambridge University Press.

Posada, G., Jacobs, A., Carbonell, O. A., Alzate, G., Bustamante, M., & Arenas, A. (1999). Maternal care and attachment security in ordinary and emergency contexts. *Developmental Psychopathology, 35*, 1379–1388.

Raby, K. L., Steele, R., Carlson, E., & Sroufe, L. A. (2015). Continuities and changes in infant attachment patterns across two generations. *Attachment and Human Development, 17*(4), 414–428.

Salvatore, J., Kuo, S., Steele, R., Simpson, J., & Collins, W. A. (2011). Recovering from conflict in romantic relationships: A developmental perspective. *Psychological Science, 22*, 376–383.

Sander, L. (1975). Infant and caretaking environment. In E. J. Anthony (Ed.), *Explorations in child psychiatry* (pp. 129–165). New York: Plenum Press.

Schuengel, C., Bakermans-Kranenburg, M., Van Ijzendoorn, M. H., & Blom, M. (1999). Unresolved loss and infant disorganization: Links to frightening maternal behavior. In J. Solomon & C. George (Eds.), *Attachment disorganization* (pp. 71–94). New York: Guilford Press.

Shulman, S., Elicker, J., & Sroufe, L. A. (1994). Stages of friendship growth in preadolescence as related to attachment history. *Journal of Social and Personal Relationships, 11*, 341–361.

Simpson, J., & Overall, N. (2014). Partner buffering of attachment insecurity. *Current Directions in Psychological Science, 23*, 54–59.

Simpson, J., & Rholes, S. (2012). Adult attachment orientations, stress, and romantic relationships. In P. Devine & A. Plant (Eds.), *Advances in experimental social psychology* (Vol. 45, pp. 279–328). Burlington, VT: Academic Press.

Sroufe, L. A. (1979). The coherence of individual development. *American Psychologist, 34*(10), 834–841.

Sroufe, L. A. (1983). Infant–caregiver attachment and patterns of adaptation in preschool. In M. Perlmutter (Ed.), *Minnesota Ssymposia in Child Psychology: Vol. 16. The roots of maladaptation and competence* (pp. 129–135). Hillsdale, NJ: Erlbaum.

Sroufe, L. A. (1986). Appraisal: Bowlby's contribution to psychoanalytic theory and developmental psychology; attachment: separation: loss. *Journal of Child Psychology and Psychiatry, 27*, 841–849.

Sroufe, L. A. (1989). Relationships, self, and individual adaptation. In A. J. Sameroff & R. N. Emde (Eds.), *Relationship disturbances in early childhood: A developmental approach* (pp. 70–94). New York: Basic Books.

Sroufe, L. A. (1997). Psychopathology as an outcome of development. *Development and Psychopathology, 9*, 251–268.

Sroufe, L. A., Egeland, B., & Carlson, E. (1999). One social world: The integrated development of parent–child and peer relationships. In W. A. Collins & B. Laursen (Eds.), *Minnesota Symposia on Child Psychology: Relationships as developmental context* (pp. 241–262). Hillsdale, NJ: Erlbaum.

Sroufe, L. A., Egeland, B., Carlson, E., & Collins, W. A. (2005a). *The development of the person: The Minnesota Study of Risk and Adaptation from Birth to Adulthood.* New York: Guilford Press.

Sroufe, L. A., Egeland, B., Carlson, E., & Collins, W. A. (2005b). The place of early attachment experiences in developmental context. In K. E. Grossmann, K. Grossmann, & E. Waters (Eds.), *The power of longitudinal attachment research: From infancy and childhood to adulthood* (pp. 48–70). New York: Guilford Press.

Sroufe, L. A., Egeland, B., & Kreutzer, T. (1990). The fate of early experience following developmental change: Longitudinal approaches to individual adaptation in childhood. *Child Development, 61*, 1363–1373.

Sroufe, L. A., Fox, N., & Pancake, V. (1983). Attachment and dependency in developmental perspective. *Child Development, 54*(6), 1615–1627.

Sroufe, L. A., & Rutter, M. (1984). The domain of developmental psychopathology. *Child Development, 55*, 17–29.

Stiles, J. (2008). *Fundamentals of brain development.* Cambridge, MA: Harvard University Press.

Troy, M., & Sroufe, L. A. (1987). Victimization among preschoolers: The role of attachment relationship history. *Journal of the American Academy of Child and Adolescent Psychiatry, 26*(2), 166–172.

Waddington, C. (1957). *The strategy of the genes.* London: Allen & Unwin.

Waters, E. (1978). The stability of individual differences in infant-mother attachment. *Child Development, 49*, 483–494.

Waters, E., Kondo-Ikemura, K., & Richters, J. (1990). Learning to love: Milestones and mechanisms in attachment, identity, and identification. In M. Gunnar & L. A. Sroufe (Eds.), *Minnesota Symposia in Child Psychology: Vol. 23. Self-processes in development* (pp. 217–255). Hillsdale, NJ: Erlbaum.

# Author Index

# Subject Index

Page numbers followed by *f* indicate figure; *n*, note; and *t*, table

CPSIA information can be obtained
at www.ICGtesting.com
Printed in the USA
BVHW011342090819
555367BV00005B/14/P

9 781462 525294